Clinical Autonomic Disorders

Evaluation and Management, Second Edition

Clinical Autonomic Disorders

Evaluation and Management, Second Edition

Editor **Phillip A. Low, M.D.**
Professor of Neurology, Mayo Medical School
Chairman, Division of Clinical Neurophysiology, and
Consultant in Neurology, Mayo Clinic, Rochester, Minnesota

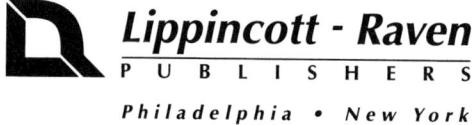

Lippincott - Raven
PUBLISHERS
Philadelphia • New York

Acquisitions Editor: Mark Placito
Developmental Editor: Mattie Bialer
Manufacturing Manager: Dennis Teston
Production Manager: Lawrence Bernstein
Production Editor: Janice G. Lochansky
Cover Designer: Patty Gast
Indexer: Gloria Hamilton
Compositor: Compset, Inc.
Printer: Maple Press

©1997, by Mayo Foundation, Rochester, Minnesota. All rights reserved. This book is protected by copyright. No part of it may be reproduced, stored in a retrieval system, or transmitted, in any form or by any means   electronic, mechanical, photocopy, recording, or otherwise   without the prior written consent of the publisher, except for brief quotations embodied in critical articles and reviews. For information write **Lippincott-Raven Publishers, 227 East Washington Square, Philadelphia, PA 19106-3780.**

Materials appearing in this book prepared by individuals as part of their official duties as U.S. Government employees are not covered by the above-mentioned copyright.

Printed in the United States of America

9 8 7 6 5 4 3 2 1

Library of Congress Cataloging-in-Publication Data

Clinical autonomic disorders : evaluation and management / Phillip A.
   Low, editor. — 2nd ed.
      p.   cm.
      Includes bibliographical references and index.
      ISBN 0-316-53281-9
      1. Autonomic nervous system—Diseases—Treatment.   2. Autonomic
nervous system—Diseases—Diagnosis.   I. Low, Phillip A.
      [DNLM: 1. Autonomic Nervous System Diseases—diagnosis.
2. Autonomic Nervous System Diseases—therapy.   3. Autonomic Nervous
System—physiopathology.   WL 600 C641 1997]
RC407.C56   1997
616.8'8—dc21
DNLM/DLC
for Library of Congress   97-11278

Care has been taken to confirm the accuracy of the information presented and to describe generally accepted practices. However, the authors, editors, and publisher are not responsible for errors or omissions or for any consequences from application of the information in this book and make no warranty, express or implied, with respect to the contents of the publication.

The authors, editors, and publisher have exerted every effort to ensure that drug selection and dosage set forth in this text are in accordance with current recommendations and practice at the time of publication. However, in view of ongoing research, changes in government regulations, and the constant flow of information relating to drug therapy and drug reactions, the reader is urged to check the package insert for each drug for any change in indications and dosage and for added warnings and precautions. This is particularly important when the recommended agent is a new or infrequently employed drug.

Some drugs and medical devices presented in this publication have Food and Drug Administration (FDA) clearance for limited use in restricted research settings. It is the responsibility of the health care provider to ascertain the FDA status of each drug or device planned for use in their clinical practice.

*To my wife, Maureen, whose continuing support and encouragement
has provided sustained impetus to my work on the autonomic nervous system.
Her dedication to the family has given me extra hours in the evenings and
on weekends to write this book.
And to my four wonderful children, Yvette, Rachele, Tori, and Phillip Andrew.
Since the last edition, we have been blessed with two grandchildren, Kate and Michael.*

Contents

Contributing Authors	xi
Preface to the First Edition	xv
Preface	xvii

I: The Scientific Basis

1. Clinical Autonomic Disorders: Classification and Clinical Evaluation 3
   Phillip A. Low, Eduardo Benarroch, and Guillermo A. Suarez

2. The Central Autonomic Network 17
   Eduardo E. Benarroch

3. Spinal Cord and Peripheral Nervous System 25
   Yadollah Harati and Hazem Machkhas

4. The Central Nervous System and Cardiovascular Control in
   Health and Disease 47
   William T. Talman

5. Autonomic Regulation of Circulation 61
   Michael J. Joyner and John T. Shepherd

6. Maintenance of Postural Normotension in Humans 73
   Wouter Wieling and Johannes J. van Lieshout

7. Autonomic Regulation of Temperature and Sweating 83
   Tokuo Ogawa and Phillip A. Low

8. Normal and Abnormal Sweat Gland Function 97
   Kenzo Sato

9. Innervation of the Skin 109
   William R. Kennedy and Gwen Wendelschafer-Crabb

10. Autonomic Regulation of Urinary Bladder 117
    William E. Bradley and Claire C. Yang

11. Autonomic Regulation of Sexual Function 129
    John D. Stewart

12. Autonomic Regulation of Gastrointestinal Motility 135
    Michael Camilleri

13. Autonomic Regulation of Immune Function 147
    Barry G. W. Arnason

14. The Effect of Aging on the Autonomic Nervous System 161
    Phillip A. Low

II: Evaluation of Autonomic Function

15. Laboratory Evaluation of Autonomic Function 179
    Phillip A. Low

16. Laboratory Evaluation of Complex Regional Pain Syndrome 209
    Catherine L. Willner and Phillip A. Low

17. Skin Potentials: Normal and Abnormal 221
    Ronald Schondorf

18. Microneurogaphy and Autonomic Dysfunction 233
    B. Gunnar Wallin and Mikael Elam

19. Thermoregulatory Sweat Test 245
    Robert D. Fealey

20. Evaluation of Pupillary and Lacrimal Function 259
    Shelley Ann Cross

21. Causes and Evaluation of Male Sexual Dysfunction 269
    John D. Stewart

22. Electrophysiologic Evaluation of Sexual Dysfunction 277
    Clare J. Fowler

23. Standardization of Autonomic Function 287
    Phillip A. Low and Michael A. Pfeifer

24. Noninvasive Evaluation of Heart Rate Variability: The Time Domain 297
    Roy Freeman

25. Analysis of Blood Pressure and Heart Rate Variability: Theoretical
    Considerations 309
    John M. Karemaker

26. Time-Frequency Analysis of Cardiovascular Function and Its Clinical
    Applications 323
    Vera Novak, Peter Novak, and Phillip A. Low

27. Transcranial Doppler Evaluation in Disorders of Reduced Orthostatic
    Tolerance 349
    Peter Novak, Vera Novak, Phillip A. Low, and George W. Petty

28. The Neuropathology of Autonomic Neuropathies 369
    Phillip A. Low and Peter J. Dyck

29. Development of an Autonomic Laboratory 383
    Phillip A. Low and Irvin R. Zimmerman

30. Pitfalls in Autonomic Testing 391
    Phillip A. Low

31. Experimental Models of Autonomic Neuropathy 403
    Roger R. Tuck and Stephen Brimijoin

III: Clinical Disorders of Autonomic Function

32. Central Disorders of Autonomic Function 421
    Eduardo E. Benarroch

33. Conditions of Reduced Gravity 429
    Victor A. Convertino

34. Autonomic Disorders of the Pupil, Ciliary Body, and Lacrimal Apparatus 441
    Shelley Ann Cross

35. Autonomic Disorders Associated with Spinal Cord Injury 455
    Yadollah Harati

36. Autonomic Neuropathies 463
    Phillip A. Low and James G. McLeod

37. Diabetic Autonomic Neuropathy 487
    Jannik Hilsted and Phillip A. Low

38. Immune Mechanisms in Diabetic Autonomic and Related Neuropathies 509
    Steven L. Rabinowe

39. Familial Dysautonomia 525
    Felicia B. Axelrod

40. Reflex Sympathetic Dystrophy 537
    Peter R. Wilson

41. Paraneoplastic Autonomic Dysfunction 545
    Ramesh K. Khurana

42. Multiple System Atrophy and Pure Autonomic Failure 555
    Phillip A. Low and Sir Roger G. Bannister

43. Other Extrapyramidal Disorders 577
    Michael J. Aminoff

44. Neurochemical and Pharmacologic Abnormalities in Chronic Autonomic Failure Syndromes 585
    Ronald J. Polinsky

45. Gastrointestinal Dysfunction: Approach to Management 597
    Charlene M. Prather and Michael Camilleri

46. The Diagnosis and Treatment of Urinary Bladder Dysfunction 613
    Claire C. Yang and William E. Bradley

47. Sleep Apnea and Autonomic Failure 633
    Sudhansu Chokroverty

48. Fainting: Approach to Management 649
    Win-kuang Shen and Bernard J. Gersh

49. Postural Tachycardia Syndrome 681
    *Phillip A. Low, Vera Novak, Peter Novak, Paola Sandroni,
    Ronald Schondorf, and Tonette L. Opfer-Gehrking*

50. Distal Small-Fiber Neuropathy 699
    Michael J. Giuliani, John D. Stewart, and Phillip A. Low

51. Mechanisms of Normal and Abnormal Facial Flushing and Sweating 715
    Peter D. Drummond and James W. Lance

52. Autonomic Failure and AIDS 727
Roy Freeman

53. Postprandial Hypotension 737
Robert D. Hoeldtke

54. Hyperthermia and Hypothermia 747
Timothy J. Ingall

55. Management of Orthostatic Hypotension 763
Robert D. Fealey and David Robertson

56. Syndromes of Autonomic Overactivity 777
Jan Fagius

57. Management of the Autonomic Storm 791
Allan H. Ropper

58. Management of Male Sexual Dysfunction 803
John D. Stewart

59. Acral Sympathetic Dysfunction and Hyperhidrosis 809
Ramesh K. Khurana

Subject Index 819

Contributing Authors

Michael J. Aminoff, M.D., F.R.C.P. *Professor of Neurology, Department of Neurology, University of California, 505 Parnassus Avenue, Room 794-M, San Francisco, California 94143*

Barry G. W. Arnason, M.D. *Professor, Department of Neurology, University of Chicago, 5841 South Maryland-MC 2030, Chicago, Illinois 60637*

Felicia B. Axelrod, M.D. *Carl Seaman Family Professor for Dysautonomia Treatment and Research, Departments of Pediatrics and Neurology, New York University Medical Center, 530 First Avenue, New York, New York 10016*

Sir Roger G. Bannister, F.R.C.P., M.Sc., D.M. *Autonomic Department, The National Hospital for Neurology and Neurosurgery, Queen Square, London, WC1*

Eduardo E. Benarroch, M.D. *Associate Professor of Neurology, Department of Neurology, Mayo Clinic, 200 First Street SW, Rochester, Minneosta 55905*

William E. Bradley, M.D. *Clinical Professor, Departments of Urology and Neurology, University of Washington, Seattle, Washington 98195*

W. Stephen Brimijoin, Ph.D. *Professor and Chair of Pharmacology, Department of Pharmacology, Mayo Clinic, 200 First Street SW, Rochester, Minnesota 55905*

Michael Camilleri, M.D. *Professor of Medicine, Department of Internal Medicine, Division of Gastroenterology, Mayo Clinic and Mayo Foundation, 200 First Street SW, Rochester, Minnesota 55905*

Sudhansu Chokroverty, M.D., F.R.C.P., F.A.C.P. *Professor, Department of Neurology, New York Medical College, Valhalla, New York 10595; Professor, Department of Neurology, Robert Wood Johnson Medical School, New Brunswick, New Jersey; Associate Chairman of Neurology, Chairman of Neurophysiology, Director of Sleep Center, Saint Vincents Hospital and Medical Center, 153 West 11th Street, Cronin 466, New York, New York 10011*

Victor A. Convertino, Ph.D. *Senior Research Physiologist, Physiology Research Branch, Armstrong Laboratory, 2507 Kennedy Circle, Brooks AFB, Texas 78235*

Shelley Ann Cross, M.D. *Assistant Professor of Neurology and Consultant in Neurology, Department of Neurology, Mayo Clinic, 200 First Street, SW, Rochester, Minnesota 55905*

Peter D. Drummond, Ph.D. *Senior Lecturer, Psychology Section, Murdoch University, Perth, Western Australia*

Peter J. Dyck, M.D. *Professor, Department of Neurology, Mayo Clinic, 200 First Street SW, Rochester, Minnesota 55905*

Mikael Elam, M.D., Ph.D. *Department of Clinical Neurophysiology, Sahlgren University Hospital, S-41345 Gokberg, Sweden*

Jan Fagius, M.D., Ph.D. *Associate Professor, Department of Neurology, University Hospital, S-751 Uppsala, Sweden*

Robert D. Fealey, M.D. *Assistant Professor of Neurology, Mayo Medical School; Consultant in Neurology, Mayo Clinic and Mayo Foundation, 200 First Street SW, Rochester, Minnesota 55905*

Clare J. Fowler, M.D. *Consultant in Uro-Neurology, The National Hospital for Neurology and Neurosurgery, Queen Square, London WC1N 3BG, England*

Roy Freeman, M.D. *Director, Autonomic and Peripheral Nerve Laboratory, Department of Neurology, Beth Israel Deaconess Medical Center, Harvard Medical School, Boston, Massachusetts 02215.*

Bernard J. Gersh, M.D. *Chief, Division of Cardiology, Georgetown Medical Center, 3800 Reservoir Road NW, Washington D.C. 20007*

Michael J. Giuliani, M.D. *Associate Professor, Department of Neurology, University of Pittsburgh-Presbyterian University Hospital, 200 Lothrop Street, Pittsburgh, Pennsylvania 15213*

Yadollah Harati, M.D., F.A.C.P. *Professor, Department of Neurology, Baylor College of Medicine, One Baylor Plaza, Houston, Texas 77030*

Jannik Hilsted, M.D. *Department of Internal Medicine, Hvidovre Hospital, DK-2650 Hvidovre, Denmark*

Robert D. Hoeldtke, M.D., Ph.D. *Professor, Department of Medicine/Endocrinology, West Virginia University, Robert C. Byrd Health Sciences Center North, Medical Drive, Morgantown, West Virginia 26506*

Timothy J. Ingall, M.B., B.S., Ph.D. *Assistant Professor, Department of Neurology, Mayo Clinic Scottsdale, 13400 East Shea Boulevard, Scottsdale, Arizona 85259*

Michael J. Joyner, M.D. *Associate Professor, Department of Anesthesiology, Mayo Clinic, 200 First Street SW, Rochester, Minnesota 55905*

John M. Karemaker, Ph.D. *Associate Professor, Department of Physiology, Academic Medical Center, University of Amsterdam, 1100 DD Amsterdam, The Netherlands*

William R. Kennedy, M.D., M.S., B.S. *Professor, Department of Neurology, University of Minnesota, 420 Delaware Street, Minneapolis, Minnesota 55455*

Ramesh K. Khurana, M.D., F.A.A.N. *Clinical Associate Professor, Department of Neurology, Univeristy of Maryland School of Medicine, 22 S. Greene Street, Baltimore, Maryland 21201; Assistant Professor, Department of Neurology, The Johns Hopkins University School of Medicine, 601 N. Carolina Street, Suite 5070, Baltimore, Maryland 21287*

James Lance, M.D. *Institute of Neurological Sciences, Prince of Wales Hospital, New South Wales, Australia*

Phillip A. Low, M.D. *Professor, Department of Neurology, Mayo Clinic, 200 First Street SW, Rochester, Minnesota 55905*

Hazem Machkhas, M.D. *Department of Neurology, Baylor College of Medicine, Houston, Texas 77030*

James G. McLeod, M.B., B.S., D.Phil. *Professor, Department of Medicine, University of Sydney, Sydney, NSW 2006 Australia*

Peter Novak, M.D., Ph.D. *Autonomic Disorders Center, Mayo Clinic, 200 First Street SW, Rochester, Minnesota 55905*

Vera Novak, M.D., Ph.D. *Autonomic Disorders Center, Mayo Clinic, 200 First Street SW, Rochester, Minnesota 55905*

Tokuo Ogawa, M.D. *Professor Emeritus, Department of Physiology, Aichi Medical University, Nagakute, Aichi 480-11 Japan*

Tonette L. Opfer-Gehrking *Department of Neurology, Mayo Clinic, Rochester, Minnesota 55905*

George W. Petty, M.D., B.S. *Associate Professor, Department of Neurology, Mayo Medical School, 200 First Street SW, Rochester, Minnesota 55905; Consultant in Neurology, Mayo Clinic, 200 First Street SW, Rochester, Minnesota 55905*

Michael A. Pfeifer, M.D. *Professor and Section Head of Endocrinology and Metabolism, Section of Endocrinology and Metabolism; and Director of Diabetes and Obesity Center, East Carolina University School of Medicine, Brody 2N-72, Greenville, North Carolina 27858*

Ronald J. Polinsky, M.D. *Therapeutic Area Head (CNS), Novartis Pharmaceuticals Corporation, 59 Route 10, East Hanover, New Jersey 07936*

Charlene M. Prather, M.D. *Associate Professor of Medicine, Division of Gastroenterology, Mayo Foundation, 200 First Street SW, Rochester, Minnesota 55905*

Steven L. Rabinowe, M.D. *Chairman, Soble Department of Medicine, Sinai Hospital, Detroit, Michigan 48235*

David Robertson, M.D. *Professor of Medicine, Pharmacology and Neurology; Director of Clinical Research Center, Autonomic Dysfunction Center, Vanderbilt University, 11161 21st Avenue South, Nashville, Tennessee 37232-2195*

Allan H. Ropper, M.D. *Professor, Department of Neurology, Tufts University School of Medicine, St. Elizabeth's Medical Center, 736 Cambridge Street, Boston, Massachusetts 02135*

Paola Sandroni, M.D., Ph.D. *Peripheral Nerve Fellow, Department of Neurology, Mayo Clinic, Rochester, Minnesota 55905*

Kenzo Sato, M.D., Ph.D. *Professor, Department of Dermatology, University of Iowa College of Medicine, 200 Hawkins Drive, Iowa City, Iowa 52242*

Ronald Schondorf, M.D., Ph.D *Assistant Professor, Department of Neurology, McGill University, Sir Mortimer B. Davis Jewish General Hospital, 3755 Chemin de la Cote St. Catherine, Montreal Quebec, Canada H3T 1E2*

Win K. Shen, M.D. *Associate Professor of Medicine and Consultant in Cardiovascular Diseases, Department of Internal Medicine, Mayo Graduate School of Medicine, Mayo Clinic, 200 First Street, Rochester, Minnesota 55905*

John T. Shepherd, M.D., D.Sc., F.R.C.P. *Professor of Physiology and Biophysics, Department of Physiology and Biophysics, Mayo Clinic and Foundation, 200 First Street SW, Rochester, Minnesota 55905*

John D. Stewart, M.B.B.S., F.R.C.P. (C) *Professor of Neurology and Neurosurgery, Department of Neurology and Neurosurgery, McGill University and Montreal Neurological Hospital, 3801 University Street, Montreal Quebec H3A 2B4, Canada*

Guillermo A Suarez, M.D. *Assistant Professor, Department of Neurology, Mayo Clinic, 200 First Street SW, Rochester, Minnesota 55905*

William T. Talman, M.D. *Professor of Neurology and Neuroscience, Department of Neurology, University of Iowa College of Medicine, 200 Hawkins Drive, Iowa City, Iowa 52242*

Roger R. Tuck, M.B., B.S., Ph.D., B.Sc., F.R.A.C.P. *Visiting Neurologist, Department of Neurology, The Canberra Hospital, 161 Strickland Crescent, Deakin, ACT 2600, Australia*

Johannes J. Van Lieshout *Department of Internal Medicine P4, Academic Medical Centre, Meibergareef 9, 1105 AZ Amsterdam, The Netherlands*

B. Gunnar Wallin, M.D. *Professor, Department of Clinical Neurophysiology, Sahlgren University Hospital, S-41345 Goteberg, Sweden*

Gwen Wendelschafer-Crabb *Department of Neurology, University of Minnesota, 420 Delaware Street, Minneapolis, Minnesota 55455*

Wouter Wieling, M.D. *Department of Internal Medicine F4, Academic Medical Centre, Meibergdreef 9 1105 AZ Amsterdam, The Netherlands*

Catherine L. Willner, M.D. *Department of Neurology, Mayo Clinic, 200 First Street SW, Rochester, Minnesota 55905*

Peter R. Wilson, M.B., B.S., Ph.D. *Associate Professor, Department of Anesthesiology, Mayo Clinic, 200 First Street SW, Rochester, Minnesota 55905*

Claire C. Yang, M.D. *Associate Professor, Department ot Urology, University of Washington School of Medicine, Seattle, Washington 98195*

Irvin R. Zimmerman M.S.E.E. *Department of Neurology, Mayo Clinic, 200 First Street SW, Rochester, Minnesota 55905*

Preface to the First Edition

There are a number of excellent books on specific aspects of autonomic function, the majority covering the areas of expertise of the editor. *Clinical Autonomic Disorders* is an attempt, in a single volume, to comprehensively cover all key human autonomic disorders and to incorporate the recent advances of noninvasive laboratory evaluation of autonomic function and management of human autonomic disorders.

We have witnessed, in the past decade and a half, rapid developments in laboratory evaluation, insights into pathophysiologic mechanisms, and advances in the treatment of clinical autonomic disorders. Several disparate areas have developed from this growth. One area is the noninvasive evaluation of autonomic function, which has developed in a wide variety of disciplines, including an extension of the electromyography, electroencephalography, sleep disorder, psychology, peripheral nerve research, and cardiovascular laboratories. A second area is the quantitation of autonomic function. A third is the management, including treatment trials, of autonomic failure. A fourth is the study of basic mechanisms of autonomic dysfunction in experimental animals and in humans.

This rapid growth has left major gaps among these areas. This book attempts to integrate some of these apparently disparate areas and to provide both a human and clinical perspective. One set of aims of *Clinical Autonomic Disorders* is to critically evaluate current noninvasive tests of autonomic function, integrate the simple tests with their basic underlying mechanisms, define the values and limitations of such tests, and to bring together, in a single volume, the large number of autonomic tests that are available. Apart from a critical evaluation of laboratory tests, a special attempt is made to integrate the bedside evaluation with the laboratory.

In keeping with our clinical orientation, basic mechanisms are emphasized, but always with a human perspective. Many of the mechanisms of autonomic function based on animal experiments have been uncritically applied to humans, and these have often been found to be incorrect. The authors have been carefully chosen so that all contributors are not only leaders in their respective fields but are also mainly clinicians.

There are some areas of considerable controversy. In such situations, I have attempted to provide a balance. Reflex sympathetic dystrophy is such an area. I have included one expert who is highly critical (some would say a nihilist) of current concepts and questions all of the standard dogma. This chapter is balanced by a more practical chapter that incorporates standard and recent ideas on the management of sympathetically maintained pain.

Another area of focus is on management of autonomic failure and dysfunction, a requirement that spans the bedside and the laboratory and integrates that information with the cutting edge of management options.

A major cause of autonomic failure and dysfunction is the autonomic neuropathies. In my opinion, no current text does this subject justice, especially on the evaluation aspects. My interest in the neuropathies is the focus of this volume, with detailed coverage on the evaluation and management of the autonomic neuropathies.

The development of autonomic evaluation and management has occurred coincidentally in North America and Europe and in several other countries. A North American emphasis was deliberately chosen. Medications cited follow generic proprietary names used in North America. Drugs that are experimental or are not available in the United States are clearly stated as such.

This book is aimed primarily at the practicing neurologist and the clinical neurophysiologist (i.e., EMG, EEG, evoked potential, autonomic, and sleep laboratories and clinical psychologists). It should also appeal to diverse internists, including the diabetologist, cardiologist, and general practitioner, as well as medical students and laboratory personnel.

The organization of this book is designed so that the enormous amount of information is assimilable. The underlying scientific basis is provided in the early chapters, followed by the evaluation, and finally, the management of autonomic disorders. In the beginning of each chapter the key points are summarized.

This book is the culmination of many years of work on the autonomic nervous system in Sydney, Australia, and at the Mayo Clinic, Rochester, Minnesota. Jim McLeod provided me with encouragement and ideas in my early days in Sydney. It is my privilege to have included him as coauthor of the chapter on the autonomic neuropathies. Peter Dyck has been an important mentor at Mayo and more than anyone else is responsible for my joining the staff of Mayo. I also wish to acknowledge the support and friendship of Jack Whisnant, who, as Chairman of Neurology, had the wisdom to support my founding of the Mayo Autonomic Laboratory in 1982, when it was still an idea. Since then the exponential growth of the laboratory has seen the number of tests performed increase to more than 2800 in 1991.

The continuing interactions with outstanding young men and women have generated many of the ideas and experiments that have taken place in my autonomic and neurophysiology laboratories. These people include Roger Tuck, Timothy Day, Douglas Zochodne, Philip McManis, Megumi Takeuchi, Jeffrey Cohen, Eduardo Benarroch, Paola Sandroni, Catherine Willner, Mikihiro Kihara, Ron Schondorf, and Guillermo Suarez. The research assistance of Toni Opfer-Gehrking has been outstanding, as has been that of Jim Schmelzer, Kim Nickander, Paula Zollman, and Nora Torres. I also wish to acknowledge the support of Carolene Neumann and Carol Proper. Finally, this book would have floundered without the outstanding secretarial support, including literature research, of Anita Payne.

P. A. L.

Preface

The first edition has been very well received. Readers have responded positively to the comprehensive nature of the textbook on autonomic disorders, clinical disorders, autonomic neuropathies, clinical laboratory evaluation, and to the emphasis on management. We have continued to emphasize these themes. The numeric summary on the first page of each chapter has been well received. I also received constructive criticisms and suggestions on the content and organization of the book, which I have attempted to incorporate in the new edition. We have organized the book more systematically, beginning with a chapter on the classification of autonomic disorders and the clinical evaluation of the patient. The chapter on multiple system atrophy and pure autonomic failure was criticized as being under-referenced and lacking detail. This chapter has been extensively revised and its bibliography greatly expanded.

Considerable research advances have necessitated the addition of new chapters and the updating of older ones. New chapters include those on the continuous recordings of cerebral blood flow velocity using transcranial doppler, the time-frequency analysis of cardiovascular function and their clinical applications, the autonomic function under condition of reduced gravity, and spinal cord disorders. Chapters that were less-well received have been eliminated.

The Editor continues to be stimulated by an expanding team of bright and stimulating young minds that have rotated through the Autonomic Disorders Research Center. The number continues to grow. Since the last edition, these have included Drs. Vera Novak, Peter Novak, Paola Sandroni, Mikihiro Kihara, Jiro Fujimura, Arthur Smit, Hideyuki Sasaki, Jong-Chyou Denq, Michael Giuliani, Chia-Lun Wu, Yoshiyuki Mitsui, Victor Gordon, Amnon Mosek, Judith Spies, and Michel Melanson. They have all contributed in various ways to the new edition.

Drs. Eduardo Benarroch, Michael Joyner, Stephen Brimijoin, and Rose Dotson, as close collaborators and Principal Investigators of the Autonomic Disorders Program Project, provide continuing insights into autonomic pathophysiology. Drs. Terrence Lagerlund, George Petty, Vera Novak, and Peter Novak, as co-investigators of my research program on Postural Tachycardia Syndrome (POTS) have contributed greatly to our work on orthostatic intolerance. Tonette Opfer-Gehrking, as program coordinator, continues to provide the glue that holds much of my research program together. I would also like to acknowledge Sue Paxton, Mariana Suarez, Irv Zimmerman, Matt Graham, and Wayne Meeker for their contributions that form, in different ways, the infrastructure that is needed to carry on the autonomic studies that provide the scientific basis of the book.

I would like to acknowledge my colleagues in the Mayo Autonomic Laboratory (Drs. Robert Fealey, Eduardo Benarroch, Guillermo Suarez, and Rose Dotson) and the able allied health personnel for providing the effective interfacing between practice and research.

Finally, I continue to depend on Anita Zeller (nee Payne) who drives approximately 130 miles each day to work with me. This book and my many other academic activities would not be the same without her hard work and dedication.

P. A. L.

SECTION I
The Scientific Basis

CHAPTER 1

Clinical Autonomic Disorders: Classification and Clinical Evaluation

Phillip A. Low, Guillermo A. Suarez, and Eduardo E. Benarroch

---

1. We have classified clinical autonomic disorders into those without and with central nervous system involvement, the autonomic neuropathies, disorders of reduced orthostatic tolerance, paroxysmal autonomic disorders, and medication-related problems.
2. The clinical evaluation is separate from, but complementary to, the laboratory investigation of autonomic function.
3. Specific aims include the *recognition* of the presence and *distribution* of autonomic dysfunction, certain *patterns* of autonomic failure that can be related to specific syndromes, potentially *treatable* disorders, and conditions that warrant *further evaluation*. They also include investigation of those *diverse areas* that defy laboratory measurement, evaluation of autonomic dysfunction as a function of *time*, and determination of the *effect* of autonomic dysfunction on the system and the patient.
4. To achieve these aims, a directed and comprehensive history and examination, followed by routine and specialized laboratory tests, should be incorporated into an approach to the management of the patient with suspected autonomic dysfunction.

INTRODUCTION

The clinical approach to any autonomic disorder begins with a detailed history, examination, and laboratory evaluation followed by a synthesis of the clinical and laboratory information into a plan of management. The autonomic nervous system is extremely diffuse with its pathways permeating all organ systems. Thus, manifestations of dysfunction are protean, and the autonomic expert has a crucial clinical role. The history and examination are essential in order to ascertain whether dysautonomia is present, what systems are involved, and whether further laboratory evaluation is warranted.

For the purpose of this chapter, the clinical evaluation of autonomic function refers to the office, bedside, or prelaboratory evaluation of autonomic failure. The chapter begins with a classification of clinical autonomic disorders, followed by a description of the specific aims of clinical appraisal; an accounting of the guiding principles underlying a clinical autonomic evaluation; a history, examination, and routine tests; and, finally, a plan of management (see Table 1).

The autonomic nervous system is involved with virtually all diseases. All structural pathophysiologic processes involving the brain (neoplastic, infectious, inherited, degenerative, etc.) can cause autonomic syndromes. Many of the acute neurologic conditions such as delirium, coma and the loss of consciousness of epilepsy and stroke are important autonomic crises. Such a classification would be of little practical value, since these conditions are well covered in other classifications. The classification we have developed is practical but abitrary, embracing disorders that clinicians have come to recognize as being uniquely autonomic. We have developed a classification that attempts to organize these disorders by anatomic system and level. We have organized the disorders without central nervous system or peripheral nervous system involvement [pure autonomic failure (PAF) is uniquely defined], within the brain and within the spinal cord, and disorders primarily involving peripheral nerve. Whenever possible, we have adopted an approximately rostral–caudal organization. Finally, we describe three categories that do not neatly fit within this

---

P. A. Low, G. A. Suarez, and E. E. Benarroch: Department of Neurology, Mayo Clinic, Rochester, Minnesota 55905.

TABLE 1. *Classification of clinical autonomic disorders*

1. Autonomic disorders *without* central nervous system or peripheral nervous system involvement
    Pure autonomic failure (PAF; Chapter 42)
2. Autonomic disorders with brain involvement
    I. Associated with multisystem degeneration
        A. Multisystem degeneration: autonomic failure clinically important
            i. Multiple-system atrophy (Chapter 42)
        B. Multisystem degeneration: autonomic failure clinically unimportant
            i. Parkinson's disease (Chapter 43)
            ii. Other extrapyramidal disorders (Chapter 43)
                Inherited olivopontocerebellar atrophy
                Progressive supranuclear palsy
                Corticobasal degeneration
                Machado–Joseph disease
    II. Unassociated with multisystem degeneration
        A. Disorders mainly due to cerebral cortex involvement
            i. Frontal cortex causing urinary/bowel incontinence
            ii. Partial complex seizures
            iii. Insula and adnexae causing cardiac arrhythmias
        B. Disorders of the limbic and paralimbic circuits
            i. Shapiro's syndrome (agenesis of corpus callosum, hyperhidrosis, hypothermia)
            ii. Autonomic seizures
        C. Disorders of the hypothalamus
            i. Wernicke–Korsakoff syndrome
            ii. Diencephalic syndrome
            iii. Neuroleptic malignant syndrome
            iv. Serotonin syndrome
            v. Fatal familial insomnia
            vi. Antidiuretic hormone syndromes (diabetes insipidus and inappropriate ADH)
            vii. Disturbances of temperature regulation (hyperthermia and hypothermia)
            viii. Disturbances of sexual function
            ix. Disturbances of appetite
            x. Disturbances of blood pressure/heart rate and gastric function
            xi. Horner's syndrome
        D. Disorders of the brainstem and cerebellum
            i. Posterior fossa tumors
            ii. Syringobulbia and Arnold–Chiari malformation
            iii. Disorders of blood pressure control (hypertension and hypotension)
            iv. Cardiac arrhythmias
            v. Central sleep apnea
            vi. Syncope and presyncope
            vii. Baroreflex failure
            viii. Horner's syndrome
3. Autonomic disorders with spinal cord involvement
    i. Traumatic tetraplegia
    ii. Syringomyelia
    iii. Subacute combined degeneration
    iv. Multiple sclerosis
    v. Amyotrophic lateral sclerosis
    vi. Tetanus
    vii. Stiff-man syndrome
    viii. Spinal cord tumors
4. Autonomic neuropathies (Chapter 36)
    I. The Acute autonomic neuropathies
        i. Acute panautonomic neuropathy (pandysautonomia)
        ii. Acute paraneoplastic autonomic neuropathy
        iii. Acute cholinergic neuropathy
        iv. Guillain–Barré syndrome
        v. Botulism
        vi. Porphyria
        vii. Drug-induced acute autonomic neuropathies
        viii. Toxic acute autonomic neuropathies
    II. The Chronic peripheral autonomic neuropathies
        A. Distal small fiber neuropathy
        B. Pure cholinergic neuropathies
        C. Pure adrenergic neuropathy
        D. Combined sympathetic and parasympathetic failure
            (Autonomic dysfunction clinically *important*)
            i. Amyloid (Chapter 36)
            ii. Diabetic autonomic neuropathy (Chapter 37)
            iii. Chronic autonomic including panautonomic neuropathy
            iv. Chronic paraneoplastic autonomic including panautonomic neuropathy
            v. Sensory neuronopathy with autonomic failure
            vi. Familial dysautonomia (Riley–Day syndrome; Chapter 39)
        E. Combined sympathetic and parasympathetic failure
            (Autonomic dysfunction usually clinically *unimportant*)
            i. Hereditary neuropathies
            ii. Connective tissue diseases
            iii. Infectious
            iv. Immune mediated
            v. Metabolic: uremia
            vi. Nutritional deficiencies
            vii. Dysautonomia of old age (Chapter 14)
5. Disorders of reduced orthostatic tolerance (Chapters 48,49)
    i. Vasovagal syncope
    ii. Prolonged bed rest
    iii. Dysautonomia associated with mitral valve prolapse
    iv. Postural orthostatic tachycardia syndrome (POTS)
    v. Prolonged weightlessness
    vi. Postexercise syncope
6. Paroxysmal or intermittent acral dysautonomia
    i. Paroxysmal hyperhidrosis (Chapter 59)
    ii. Raynaud's syndrome (Chapter 59)
    ii. Erythromelalgia (Chapter 36)
7. Drugs affecting autonomic regulation
    A. *Anticholinergics:* tricyclic antidepressant (e.g., amitriptyline); antihistamine (e.g., bendadryl); muscarine antagonists (e.g., atropine)
    B. *Vasoconstrictors:* α-receptor agonists (e.g., phenylpropanolamine and midodrine); ephedrine, methylphenidate, amphetamines; ergot derivatives
    C. *Vasodilators:* α-antagonists, clonidine, ganglion blocking agents (e.g., antihypertensives and calcium channel blockers)
    D. *Diuretics*
    E. β-*Antagonists* (e.g., propranolol)

category, but are sufficiently characteristic to warrant their own category. These are the disorders of reduced orthostatic tolerance, the paroxysmal disorders and, finally, medication-related autonomic dysfunction.

Injury to many parts of the cerebral cortex can cause dysautonomia. Where several areas are involved, we have attempted to avoid repetition and instead to classify the disorder at the site that is most relevant. When the cerebral cortex is involved, its areas are interconnected to other areas, in particular the hypothalamus. The two syndromes listed, of incontinence and partial complex seizures, appear to be uniquely cerebral. The frontal lobe is important in continence. Connections with the hypothalamus and limbic system are important in this regulation of bladder and bowel function (Chapters 2 and 33). Partial complex seizures can have a high autonomic content, especially when there is involvement of the amygdaloid or hippocampal regions. Seizures involving other limbic paralimbic structures can also have a prominent autonomic content. These are the cingulate, opercular, anterior frontopolar, and orbitofrontal regions (Chapter 33). The insula and adnexae are arrhythmogenic and may be a mechanism of sudden death in strokes (Chapters 4 and 33). Shapiro's syndrome consists of episodic hyperhidrosis and hypothermia in patients with agenesis of the corpus callosum (Chapter 33).

Structural lesions of the hypothalamus commonly cause dysautonomia (Chapter 33). The Wernicke-Korsakoff syndrome is associated with lesions in several areas, including the mammillary body, cerebellar vermis and peripheral nerve, in addition to the hypothalamic lesion. It is listed here since the hypothermia is likely due to the hypothalamic lesion (Chapter 33). The diencephalic syndrome consists of episodic dysautonomia with pupillary dilatation, flushing, diaphoresis, hypertension, tachycardia, and hyperventilation. There are numerous causes of the syndrome, including acute hydrocephalus, and the neuroleptic malignant syndrome (Chapter 33). The site of the lesion is tentatively localized to the hypothalamus, since one case was associated with necrosis of the anterior and lateral hypothalamic lesions (6), although its pathophysiology and site of the lesion are unproven. The serotonin syndrome consisting of mental and behavioral changes, and motor and autonomic hyperactivity, follows the use of potent serotomimetic agents (Chapter 33). Fatal familial insomnia is a prion disease characterized by intractable insomnia, dysautonomia, and motor dysfunction. The neuropathology is localized to the hypothalamus (anteroventral and dorsomedial nuclei; Chapter 33). Two syndromes of antidiuretic hormone (ADH) secretion can develop in lesions of the hypothalamus. With destructive lesions of the supraoptic and paraventricular vasopressin neurons, diabetes insipidus ensues, resulting in hypovolemia. This mechanism might in important in nondestructive lesions in some patients with orthostatic intolerance, who seem to have episodic impairment of ADH secretion/function. In some of the autonomic syndromes, such as Guillain–Barré syndrome (GBS), the inverse problem of inappropriate ADH secretion can occur. Problems of thermoregulation, due to excessive effects of increased ambient temperature, often in patients with reduced thermoregulatory defenses, can result in heat stress syndromes, including heat exhaustion and heat stroke (Chapter 55). The converse problem of hypothermia can be due to an excessive low ambient temperature or a hypothalamic lesion (Chapters 7, 33, and 55). Disturbances of sexual development, appetite, and electrolyte balance are common with hypothalamic lesions.

The brainstem regulates blood pressure (BP), vasomotor, cardiovagal, sleep, and respiratory functions. Lesions of the brainstem include tumors, structural malformations, infarcts, and inflammatory disorders. Manifestations include cardiac arrhythmias, sleep apnea, orthostatic hypotension, hypertension, syncope, baroreflex failure, and Horner's syndrome (Chapters 33 and 48).

Disorders of the spinal cord result in a disruption of key descending autonomic pathways, ascending sensory and autonomic inputs, and the loss of function of preganglionic sympathetic and parasympathetic neurons. The disease processes include trauma, malformations, vitamin deficiency (B_{12}), demyelinating disease, amyotrophic lateral sclerosis, tetanus, and the stiff-man syndrome.

AIMS OF A CLINICAL EVALUATION

The aims of a clinical evaluation are different from but complementary to those of the laboratory. It is important to have a clear appreciation of the specific aims of the clinical evaluation, which are to

1. Recognize the *presence* and *distribution* of autonomic dysfunction.
2. Recognize *patterns* of autonomic failure that can be related to specific syndromes.
3. Recognize the potentially *treatable* disorders.
4. Recognize the disorders that warrant *further evaluation*.
5. Probe the *diverse areas* involved with dysautonomia and their numerous manifestations that defy laboratory measurement.
6. Evaluate autonomic dysfunction as a function of *time*.
7. Evaluate the *effect* of autonomic dysfunction on the system and the patient.

Recognize the Presence and Distribution of Autonomic Dysfunction

A detailed autonomic system review (see below) is of critical importance, and time invested in obtaining a history will pay handsome dividends. This part of the evaluation will determine which systems are involved. The severity and distribution of autonomic dysfunction should be resolved. One focus should be the diverse systems involved with dysautonomia and their various manifestations, especially those that defy laboratory quantitation (specific aim 5). Another focus should be intermittent autonomic dysfunction, including paroxysmal hyperhidrosis, certain orthostatic presyncopal symptoms, and sympathetically mediated pain, that occurs only at particular times or under specific circumstances (specific aim 6). By listening, probing and, if necessary, prompting, the autonomic historian should end up with a catalogue of autonomic symptoms by autonomic systems.

Recognize Patterns of Autonomic Failure That Can Be Related to Specific Syndromes

In neurologic diagnosis, a catalogue of symptoms is obtained, followed by a deduction of involvement by system and by level and, finally, an understanding of the process is reached. In certain disorders, such as the peripheral neuropathies, pattern recognition is more important than the classic approach (10). The mind-set of the peripheral neurologist is geared to seeking certain core features in the history (and examination) that are of diagnostic importance. For example, the recognition of mononeuropathy multiplex, sensory neuronopathy or acute demyelinating polyradiculoneuropathy patterns is an important step in diagnostic processing. Similarly, pattern recognition is very important in the autonomic neuropathies. For example, the core features of amyloid polyneuropathy (5) are diffuse autonomic failure, a selective loss of pain and temperature, weight loss, and the demonstration of amyloid in subcutaneous fat, rectal tissue, or sural nerve. Similarly, the diagnostic core of diabetic autonomic neuropathy is hyperglycemia and diffuse autonomic failure involving cardiovagal, postganglionic sympathetic sudomotor and adrenergic systems (9). Chronic idiopathic anhidrosis is characterized by heat or exertional dizziness, dyspnea, fatigue, palpitations, and flushing unassociated with orthostatic hypotension and relieved by cooling (11).

Recognize the Potentially Treatable Disorders

The autonomic interviewer has the important charge of recognizing the potentially treatable disorders. Symptoms do not require extensive evaluation when a cause is apparent or the disorder is benign. For example, autonomic testing is not warranted in a patient with orthostatic hypotension on a ganglion-blocking agent. Older patients are quite susceptible to orthostatic hypotension and can become symptomatic when their blood volume is reduced by diuretic therapy or when they receive tricyclic antidepressant therapy. In a tertiary referral center, only one in four patients with orthostatic hypotension had a progressive autonomic disorder, and 38% had hypotension without evidence of autonomic failure (15). A careful history is extremely important because medication adjustment or management of volume status can lead to resolution of orthostatic hypotension. Similarly, patients with chronic heat intolerance and an inability to sweat, who do not have orthostatic hypotension or other symptoms of autonomic failure, likely have chronic idiopathic anhidrosis (11). An autonomic reflex screen (Chapter 15) and thermoregulatory sweat test (TST) (Chapter 19) would document the severity and distribution of anhidrosis and the status of cardiovagal and adrenergic systems. Extensive investigations and imaging studies would be unnecessary.

Treatable disorders include dysautonomia caused by poisons and drugs (Chapter 36). Botulism, mushroom poisoning, and overdoses of prescription (e.g., hypotensive agents) or street drugs (cocaine, amphetamines, crack, or phencyclidine) may result in an autonomic storm (Chapter 57). Also treatable is the autonomic dysfunction observed in thallium or arsenic neuropathy and in drug-induced acute intermittent porphyria or, rarely, the autonomic failure resulting from Vacor poisoning (Chapter 36). Treatable autonomic disorders requiring urgent intervention include the cholinergic crisis in myasthenia gravis, acute autonomic neuropathies, GBS, the acute cholinergic neuropathies, acute panautonomic neuropathy, tetanus, and acute intermittent porphyria.

The management of BP and heart rate (HR) variability in the autonomic neuropathies (mainly GBS, but similar problems may occur in acute panautonomic neuropathy and acute intermittent porphyria), the autonomic instabilities involved with strokes, subarachnoid hemorrhage, and acute brain trauma, and the autonomic hyperreflexia of the tetraplegic, are all extremely important and may be lifesaving (Chapters 56, 57).

A related situation is the recognition of sympathetically mediated pain in causalgia, reflex sympathetic dystrophy (Chapter 40), and certain neuropathies. These patients may be helped, at least temporarily, by sympathetic block or section or by sympatholytic drugs.

Recognize the Disorders That Need Further Evaluation

The autonomic interviewer must separate disorders that are treatable (specific aim 3), serious or emergent. The diagnosis of serious neurologic disease obviously is of high priority. Patients with amyloid neuropathy, PAF, or multiple-system atrophy with autonomic failure (MSA: Shy–Drager syndrome) have serious progressive disorders that require confirmation. Rapidly progressive disorders such as GBS, acute panautonomic neuropathy, and acute sympathetic or parasympathetic storms need urgent confirmation and management because of their rapid development, changing autonomic status, and the need for life-support systems.

Probe the Diverse Areas Involved with Dysautonomia and Their Numerous Manifestations That Defy Laboratory Measurement

Much time, expense, and effort would be required if one chose to quantitate the entire gamut of autonomic symptoms and, usually, this is not warranted. Thus, autonomic clinicians have a particular charge. Their skills must be such that they are able to recognize the various symptoms (specific aim 1), establish core symptoms that might need further evaluation for diagnostic or management purposes, and qualitatively assess all other symptoms. The particular pattern of symptoms may be diagnostic or highly suggestive of certain disorders. For example, patients with postural tachycardia syndrome (POTS—Chapter 16) have little or no orthostatic hypotension, but exhibit marked orthostatic tachycardia on prolonged standing. Associated with these findings are central nervous system symptoms of dizziness and anxiety verging on a panic state and accompanied by tremulousness and palpitations. This gestalt is quite different from the usual symptoms of orthostatic hypotension.

Evaluate Autonomic Dysfunction as a Function of Time

An adequate history may provide a semiquantitative estimation of paroxysmal or fluctuating symptoms that complement the laboratory evaluation. For example, orthostatic hypotension may vary significantly throughout the day, in response to medications (e.g., insulin or Sinemet levodopa/carbidopa) or meals. Often, patients will experience troublesome orthostatism in the early morning or postprandially. Informed autonomic experts can combine evaluation with management to the benefit of patients. An example is that patients are taught to have their supine and standing BP taken in the early morning and are rechecked after sleeping with the head of the bed elevated. Postprandial BP can also be checked with different dietary modifications. This sort of information can be very useful in planning the timing of adrenergic agonist ingestion.

Evaluate the Effect of Autonomic Dysfunction on the System and the Patient

It is important to define not only the presence of autonomic failure or dysfunction, but to supplement that information with an evaluation of its effect on the autonomic organ or system under consideration and on the entire patient. The latter information is important because compensatory mechanisms are often so effective that autonomic failure has minimal effects on the patient. For example, a patient with orthostatic hypotension of several months' duration often does not have cerebral ischemic symptoms because the autoregulated range of cerebral blood flow is shifted to a lower BP (19). A patient who is well compensated does not need to be treated, at least under normal conditions.

GUIDING PRINCIPLES OF CLINICAL AUTONOMIC EVALUATION

There are a number of cardinal rules regarding neurologic history taking and examination. These will not be covered here (4,13). Instead, reference will be made to certain guiding principles that are relevant to the autonomic evaluation.

First, it is important to recognize the strengths and shortcomings of the bedside or office evaluation compared with those of the laboratory. The aims are different, but complementary. Second, it is important to develop the skills necessary to take a proper autonomic history and perform an adequate autonomic examination. Third, the bedside evaluation should not ape a laboratory quantitation. Parameters are measured more accurately in the laboratory. Time is better spent doing things that cannot be done in the laboratory. For example, to have a patient do a Valsalva maneuver or digitally evaluate the HR response to deep breathing is time wasted. The result is a third-rate Valsalva ratio and HR range. Instead, specific aims exist that are best achieved at the bedside. Finally, the particular role of the office or bedside is to coordinate the management of autonomic dysfunction. The role of the clinician is crucial in identifying any problem that needs further evaluation, ascertaining the meaning of autonomic test results, and using these results intelligently to develop a strategy of management.

History

It is helpful, initially, to list the cardinal symptoms. Ask the patient to list, in descending order of concern, their major complaints and their duration: "If I had a magic wand and could wave away your symptoms, what would you like to get rid of most?" The characteristics, onset and evolution, aggravating and relieving factors, and possible relationship to meals and time of day can then be evaluated. Finally, a full system review should be undertaken, with particular reference to autonomic symptoms.

In addition to obtaining a neurologic history, there is a need to specifically evaluate orthostatic dizziness, vasomotor, sudomotor, pupillomotor, bladder, bowel and sexual function (Appendix 1). Orthostatic hypotension is manifest as dizziness, syncope, or near syncope on standing. It is important to obtain an estimate of the severity and its effect on the patient's activities encountered in daily living. An orthostatic intolerance grade has been defined that grades patients by the severity of symptoms, standing time, and interference with ability to perform activities of daily living (Table 2). The standing time to first symptom and to

TABLE 2. *The grading of orthostatic intolerance*

Orthostatic grade by symptoms[a]
Grade 0   Normal orthostatic tolerance.

Grade I
  1. Orthostatic symptoms are infrequent, or only under conditions of increased orthostatic stress.[b]
  2. Able to stand >15 min on most occasions.
  3. Typically has unrestricted activities of daily living.

Grade II
  1. Orthostatic symptoms are frequent, developing at least once a week. Orthostatic symptoms commonly develop with orthostatic stress.
  2. Able to stand >5 min on most occasions.
  3. Some limitation in activities of daily living is typical.

Grade III
  1. Orthostatic symptoms develop on most occasions and are regularly unmasked by orthostatic stresses.
  2. Able to stand >1 min on most occasions.
  3. Marked limitation in activities of daily living is typical.

Grade IV
  1. Orthostatic symptoms are consistently present.
  2. Able to stand <1 min on most occasions.
  3. Seriously incapacitated, being bed or wheelchair bound because of orthostatic intolerance.
  4. Syncope/presyncope are common if the patient attempts to stand.

[a]Symptoms may vary with time and state of hydration and circumstances.
[b]Orthostatic stresses include prolonged standing, a meal, exertion, or heat stress.

TABLE 3. *Symptoms of orthostatic intolerance*

Symptoms	%
Lightheadedness (dizziness)	88
Weakness or tiredness	72
Cognitive (thinking/concentrating)	47
Blurred vision	47
Tremulousness	38
Vertigo	37
Pallor	31
Anxiety	29
Tachycardia or palpitations	26
Clammy feeling	19
Nausea	18

TABLE 4. *Aggravating factors*

Factors	%
Prolonged standing	58
Physical exertion or exercise	53
Environmental warming	32
Postprandial	24
Menstrual cycle	6

though lightheadedness is common, ~50% of patients over the age of 60 have problems of cognitive impairment on standing that clears on sitting or lying down (12). Cognitive problems are typically more obvious to companions than to patients, although not infrequently patients will use phrases like "I feel goofy" (at least in Minnesota). Some patients complain of a retrocollic heaviness or headache on continued standing (16). Patients may feel faint only under certain conditions. Many patients complain of weakness, especially in the legs on standing. Some patients develop ataxia when their BP falls. Aggravating symptoms need to be sought. Apart from continued standing, other orthostatic stressors include exercise, environmental warming, or food ingestion (Table 4). Standing time is most commonly <1 min before the onset of symptoms (Table 5). Indeed, an increase in standing time by 1–2 min results in a dramatic increase in activities of daily living. Although it is well known that patients are often worse on first awakening in the morning, the most common time of day when orthostatic intolerance is worse is no particular time of day (Table 6). It should be emphasized that, although our patients were highly symptomatic, ~75% having frequent symptoms, the majority of patients do not have syncope (Table 7), suggesting that these patients either have sufficient warning to avert syncope or have sufficient compensatory mechanisms to avoid syncope.

Some younger subjects may develop POTS (Chapter 50) characterized by dizziness, palpitations, weakness, tremulousness, anxiety, and nausea after prolonged standing. These patients have significant symptoms of sympathetic activation and β-receptor supersensitivity.

Vasomotor changes initially are perceived as a feeling of coldness ("Doctor, I just can't keep my feet warm"). This symptom often antedates somatic manifestations of a peripheral neuropathy. Later, there are additional skin color and trophic changes. Normal skin wrinkles following several minutes of immersion in water. Adrenergic failure re-

TABLE 5. *Standing time*

Time (min)	%
<1	50
2–5	25
>15	18
6–15	7

presyncope should be sought. More subtle symptoms also should be sought. Since few studies have been primarily focused on symptoms, we undertook a prospective study of patients with orthostatic intolerance who were referred to the Mayo Autonomic Laboratory. We evaluated 90 patients with symptomatic orthostatic intolerance, 60 patients with symptoms but without laboratory confirmation of orthostatic intolerance, and 5 patients with asymptomatic orthostatic intolerance. The data on patients with symptomatic orthostatic intolerance are summarized in Tables 3-7. Al-

TABLE 6. *Relationship of symptoms to the time of day*

Time of day	%
No particular time	50
On awakening	34
Afternoon	10
Evening or night	6

TABLE 7. *Frequency of syncope*

Frequency	%
Never	58
Present but <1 per month	28
>1 per month	14

sults in an absence of wrinkling (2). Generalized sudomotor failure is sought by asking whether patients sweat on a hot day and, if so, their sweat distribution. Patients should be asked whether their clothes get moist. A common response is that they do not know or that their level of activity has declined because of ill-health. Patients should then be asked whether they sweat with a fever. Another clue obtained from observant patients is whether they sweat following a hot bath. The normal response is sweating that persists for several minutes after drying. Patients should be questioned about heat intolerance (they feel hot, flushed, dizzy, dyspneic, and weak but do not sweat). Acral changes are best sought by direct questioning (ask patients whether their socks are moist, like they used to be, and then check them). Patients' socks should feel moist when they are removed in the office.

Secretomotor function should also be determined (ask about dry eyes and mouth).

Gastroparesis may be manifest as anorexia, early satiety, persistent sense of bloating or fullness, frequent nausea, or the vomiting up of undigested food. An important clue to significant gastroparesis is weight loss. The symptoms may be difficult to interpret. For example, a patient may be referred with the combination of weight loss, anorexia, and early satiety. The main differential of these symptoms would be between psychogenic mechanisms or autonomic failure. A trial of metoclopramide (Reglan) might result in resolution of these symptoms, indicating that the patient probably has gastroparesis.

Diarrhea may alternate with obstinate constipation. The diarrhea is often nocturnal, explosive, and quite intermittent. The stools may contain much undigested fats and fiber.

Bladder problems are typically caused by parasympathetic failure. The initial presentation is that of infrequent micturition followed by a delay in initiation with incomplete emptying. In addition, a relatively frequent passage of small quantities of urine may occur due to retention with overflow.

Sexual dysfunction is usually due to erectile failure. Patients initially experience partial failure (infrequent and/or poorly sustained erections) followed later by total failure. Patients should be asked about nocturnal erections and circumstances surrounding erections. Ask whether the erections are firm enough for penetration. A poor man's assessment of erectile function is the postage stamp test. The patient is asked to encircle his penile shaft with a strip of postage stamps. The next morning, the strip should be separated along the perforations if nocturnal erections have occurred. Less commonly, the patient experiences sympathetic failure manifest as an inability to ejaculate. Occasionally, retrograde ejaculation into the bladder occurs. In this case, the urine looks milky.

Patients should be questioned about pupillomotor symptoms: "Have you recently had trouble with your eyes?" They may complain of blurring of vision or glare in bright sunlight. These symptoms usually are related to difficulties with accommodation. Another symptom is poor night vision caused by reduced dark-adapted pupil diameter with sympathetic failure.

A systematized validated *autonomic symptom profile* has been developed that consists of 169 items directed at seven domains of autonomic symptoms with weighted scores. The categories are orthostatic intolerance, sexual failure, bladder disorder, diarrhea, gastroparesis, secretomotor disorder, constipation, and vasomotor and pupillomotor impairment. The profile is constructed such that the presence and severity of each symptom is followed by systematic analysis of aggravating factors. The final result is a score of severity and a report summarizing the patient's autonomic symptomatology. The profile has been validated against patients with different severities of autonomic failure by using the composite autonomic scoring scale (8). It has a sensitivity and specificity of 76% and 87%, respectively, in detecting autonomic failure.

The Autonomic Examination

In addition to a full neurologic examination, it is necessary to pay particular attention to several autonomic indices.

General Evaluation

It is necessary to look for evidence of hypothalamic involvement (dwarfism, sexual immaturity, hypothermia, pallor).

Blood Pressure, Heart Rate, and Temperature

BP and HR should be checked supine and after standing for 1 min. The orthostatic reduction in BP at 5 or 10 min is not usually appreciably greater in older patients. However, if POTS is suspected, then BP and HR, after at least 10 min of standing, are needed because the fall in BP may be delayed and more subtle BP/HR changes may not be obvious in brief recordings. If orthostatic hypotension is suspected but not detected and autonomic laboratory testing is not planned, then it might be worthwhile to have the patient do 12 squats before repeating BP recordings. The presence of orthostatic hypotension without reflex tachycardia is good evidence of generalized sympathetic adrenergic (with cardiovagal) failure. If reflex tachycardia is present, then orthostatic hypotension secondary to hypovolemia cannot be excluded.

Patients with hypothalamic disorders or those with a cold injury may be hypothermic. In such cases, it would be necessary to record core temperature with a low reading thermometer.

Skin Integument and Mucous Membrane

Acral vasomotor changes should be checked. Acrocyanosis, pallor, mottling, or redness should be noted. If sympathetically maintained pain is suspected, the extremities should be compared for temperature, color, sweating, swelling, and trophic changes. The skin should also be palpated for allodynia (pain resulting from nonpainful stimulus) and hyperalgesia (where painful stimulus appears more painful). The response to stroking and deep pressure should be determined. Repetitive touch or pressure testing may need to be evaluated.

Sweating

Sudomotor changes are recognized as dryness and a lack of resistance to a gentle stroke with the examiner's finger pads. More elaborate tests include the use of a roller-shaped resistance meter (20) or the running of a moderately heavy spoon over the skin (20), but they probably are no better than an experienced examiner and certainly are inferior to autonomic laboratory testing.

Dystrophic Changes

Trophic changes are manifest as alopecia or hypertrichosis. Nail changes include thickening, discoloration, and distortion. Lipodystrophy, wasting, and atrophic skin changes may also occur.

Evidence of Charcot's Joints

Neuropathic joints exhibit marked disorganization. They are misshapen, crepitus is present, and the joint has an excessive range of movement. Pain is usually present in Charcot's joints, but is less than would be expected given the amount of disorganization and range of movement.

Pupils and Conjunctiva

The pupillary shape, size, and responses to light and accommodation should be noted. If the pupils are unreactive to direct light, the response to a sustained light stimulus (1 min) should be observed to demonstrate the presence of a tonic pupil. Similarly, the redilatation following constriction may be delayed or slow.

Investigations

Patients suspected of having a neuropathic disorder should have routine tests for that neuropathy (Chapter 37). In addition, the following tests should be performed on patients with orthostatic hypotension:

1. Morning and evening cortisol levels (for evidence of adrenal insufficiency).
2. Plasma catecholamine concentrations (norepinephrine, epinephrine, and dopamine, supine and standing). Supine plasma norepinephrine levels can be measured because of a spillover from postganglionic sympathetic fibers and the level is reduced when widespread postganglionic sympathetic adrenergic failure is present. In preganglionic failure, supine plasma norepinephrine levels are normal, but no increase occurs after patients have been standing for 5–10 min. In most instances, estimation of plasma norepinephrine is the most useful test. Rarely, the combination of catecholamines is needed to diagnose an enzymatic defect in the catecholamine biosynthetic pathway. An example would be a dopamine–β-hydroxylase deficiency in which unrecordable levels of norepinephrine and epinephrine and excessive plasma and cerebrospinal fluid concentrations of dopamine exist (1,17).
3. Tissue biopsy to determine amyloid content (rectal, subcutaneous fat or sural nerve). Properly stained amyloid deposits should be demonstrated. Subcutaneous fat biopsy is the least invasive test and peripheral nerve is the most reliable test.
4. Other tests to be considered are red cell and plasma volume in POTS, leukocyte α-galactosidase in Fabry's disease, and vasoactive intestinal peptide in patients with flushing.
5. Patients with pupillary abnormalities may require pupillography combined with pharmacologic studies (Chapters 21 and 35). Dryness of the eyes would need to be confirmed with the Schirmer's test for tear production and the Rose–Bengal test for conjunctival staining. Patients suspected of having Sjögren's syndrome, with keratoconjunctivitis sicca and xerostomia, should be evaluated using the collagen vascular disease battery (Chapter 37). A minor salivary gland biopsy sample from lip subcutaneous tissue provides definitive evidence of Sjögren's disease when perivascular round cell infiltration is observed.

6. Less frequently, specialized tests that focus on certain organ systems also need to be performed. These include cystometrography–electromyography, gut motility studies, and penile tumescence studies. Patients suspected of having autonomic failure or dysfunction should be evaluated, in addition, in an autonomic laboratory (Chapter 17).

APPROACH TO THE MANAGEMENT OF PATIENTS WITH SUSPECTED AUTONOMIC FAILURE

The clinical and laboratory evaluations of autonomic failure are complementary and, therefore, will be integrated in this section of the discussion.

Step 1: Is Significant Autonomic Dysfunction Present?
The first step is to determine whether significant autonomic dysfunction is present. Based on the history and examination, it should be possible to determine whether this is so. Significance is based on the system involved, its severity, and the effect it has on the activities involved in daily living.

Step 2: What Is the Involvement by System and Level?
It is important to define, clinically, whether dysautonomia involves the sympathetic or parasympathetic nervous system. It is also important to specify the level of involvement. Although the autonomic neuraxis is extensive, it should be possible to determine whether the lesion is central, preganglionic, postganglionic, or involves the neuroeffector. It is also important to specify which organ system is involved.

Step 3: What Is the Pattern of Autonomic Dysfunction?
Specific combinations of symptoms are characteristic of certain autonomic disorders (7):

1. Distal sympathetic neuropathy
2. Pure cholinergic neuropathy
3. Pure adrenergic neuropathy
4. Generalized autonomic failure
5. Paroxysmal or intermittent dysautonomia
6. Sympathetically maintained pain
7. Selective system failure
8. The autonomic storm
9. The acute autonomic neuropathies

Distal sympathetic neuropathy is quite common and is one component of a distal neuropathy. Symptoms consist of distal sudomotor and vasomotor alterations. Overactivity is an early symptom, and patients complain of difficulty in keeping their feet warm. Patients may have excessive perspiration to the point of maceration of the skin in the toe clefts.

Distal sympathetic overactivity may occur in the painful neuropathies. It may be important in causing the pain, or it may merely be a manifestation of painfulness. In the former, sympathetic overactivity may be causing or maintaining the pain (sympathetically maintained pain). Sympathetic blockade, section, or the administration of sympatholytic agents results in pain relief. It is important, however, to realize that overaction does not necessarily indicate that the pain is due to increased sympathetic activity. It may be a symptom in that a distal painful source may result in the augmentation of somatosympathetic reflexes resulting in sympathetic overactivity. In this case, sympathetic blockade would result in a normalization of the dysautonomia, but no amelioration of the pain. This separation is therapeutically important, since the focus of therapy in the former is on the sympathetic outflow while in the latter is on the painful source itself (neuroma, trigger point, etc.). One useful clue that points to the latter is the appearance of an early sudomotor response on quantitative sudomotor axon reflex test (QSART) that is due to augmented somatosympathetic reflexes (Chapter 37).

Distal sympathetic failure results in anhidrosis and an increase in skin blood flow. There may be dependent rubor and acrocyanosis. There may also be subcutaneous edema, possibly due to sympathetic denervation. Sympathetic innervation and denervation of pre- and postcapillary sphincters may cause an imbalance with a resulting alteration in the Starling forces in the microcirculation and tissue edema.

Episodic rubor, with accentuation of pain, may occur via nonsympathetic sensory mechanisms. One syndrome characterized by intermittent redness associated with a severe burning pain is thought to be due to activation of the polymodal C nociceptor and its axon reflex, resulting in a neurogenic flare response in addition to the pain (3). This syndrome has been termed the ABC or angry backfiring C nociceptor syndrome (14).

Pure cholinergic neuropathy is another distinct syndrome. It is less common than the generalized syndrome of adrenergic, cholinergic, and cardiovagal failure. Patients with cholinergic failure do not have orthostatic hypotension. Abnormalities are confined to the cholinergic system and include anhidrosis, atonic bladder, Adie's pupil, alacrima, constipation, cardiovagal failure, and impotence. Disorders causing this syndrome include chronic idiopathic anhidrosis, acute cholinergic neuropathy, Lambert–Eaton Myasthenic Syndrome (LEMS), and botulism (see Chapter 31).

Pure adrenergic neuropathy is usually a laboratory diagnosis. Orthostatic hypotension dominates the symptoms. On laboratory testing, patients exhibit sympathetic adrenergic failure with normal sudomotor tests (TST and QSART). Pure autonomic failure or multiple-system atrophy may be confined to the adrenergic system in ~5% of cases.

Generalized autonomic failure is the most common autonomic syndrome. Patients with this syndrome exhibit cholinergic and adrenergic failure with manifestations as described above. The most common causes of generalized autonomic failure are PAF, MSA, diabetic autonomic neuropathy, GBS, Sjögren's syndrome, and amyloid neuropathy. Less common causes include acute idiopathic and paraneoplastic panautonomic neuropathy.

Paroxysmal or intermittent dysautonomia is less well recognized, but is probably relatively common. Some episodes of dysautonomia occur as part of a clear-cut nonautonomic syndrome and cause no confusion. Examples include partial complex seizure, subarachnoid hemorrhage, and cerebral ischemia. In these syndromes, the primary processes (seizure and ischemia) are readily recognizable and the autonomic discharge may be epileptic, due to pressure or ischemia.

A second category are those patients with episodic dysautonomia in whom the autonomic symptoms predominate. Shapiro's syndrome consists of recurrent idiopathic spontaneous hypothermia with agenesis of the corpus callosum. Associated with this are polydipsia, polyuria, hyponatremia, and autonomic paroxysms characterized by hypertension, tachycardia, and diaphoresis. Some of the symptoms can be related to the sudden norepinephrine increase that has been reported to be due to an increased release and reduced clearance of this amine (18). These patients respond well to clonidine administration.

Episodic hyperhidrosis may occur in the absence of the other components of Shapiro's syndrome. These episodes of hyperhidrosis are sometimes associated with vasomotor changes and respond well to clonidine administration. Essential hyperhidrosis is also often associated with episodic accentuation, usually due to emotional mechanisms.

Episodic autonomic failure may occur reflexly. Well-described syndromes include vasovagal, glossopharyngeal, carotid sinus, cough, and micturition syncope. Some syndromes are due to the abrupt, presumably reflexly mediated, cessation of sympathetic outflow (21). Some cases are triggered by supersensitive receptors such as are found in the carotid sinus (carotid sinus syncope) and trigeminal system (oculocardiac syncope).

Selective system or organ failure is relatively common. Examples include Adie's pupil and Horner's syndrome, megacolon or megaesophagus. An autonomic evaluation is required in order to clarify whether the disorder is truly restricted, since a considerable spectrum of autonomic involvement is associated with the primary disorder.

The autonomic storm is described in Chapter 58 and is comprised of dysautonomic manifestations that occur in a setting which renders diagnosis straightforward.

The acute autonomic neuropathies include acute panautonomic, acute paraneoplastic, panautonomic, acute cholinergic neuropathies, and GBS and botulism. The acute tempo is characteristic. The individual disorders are detailed in Chapter 37.

Step 4: What Is the Cause of the Dysautonomia?
The cause of dysautonomia often logically follows steps 1–3. Many of the acute autonomic neuropathies are quite characteristic. Sometimes the pattern narrows the choice down to a very manageable differential diagnosis. For example, the pattern may be suggestive of an acute panautonomic neuropathy. The laboratory task would then be to determine whether the neuropathy was due to a paraneoplastic or idiopathic cause. Some disorders, such as amyloid or Fabry's disease, may require an additional specific test or tissue diagnosis. The individual disorders are detailed in Chapter 37.

Step 5: Management of Autonomic Failure
This is detailed in the appropriate chapters. The procedures followed in the management of autonomic disorders are similar to those employed for general medical principles.

INDICATIONS FOR LABORATORY EVALUATION

These are detailed in the following chapters, so they are listed, without further comment, here:

1. Diagnosis of generalized autonomic failure
2. Diagnosis of benign autonomic disorders that may mimic life-threatening disorders
3. Diagnosis of distal small fiber neuropathy
4. Evaluation of orthostatic intolerance
5. Evaluation of the course of the autonomic disorder
6. Evaluation of the response to therapy
7. Evaluation of autonomic involvement in the peripheral neuropathies
8. Detection of sympathetic dysfunction in sympathetically maintained pain
9. Research questions

REFERENCES

1. Biaggioni I, et al. Dopamine–beta-hydroxylase deficiency in humans. *Neurology* 1990;40:370–373.
2. Bull C, Henry JA. Finger wrinkling as a test of autonomic function. *BMJ* 1977;1:551–552.
3. Cline MA, et al. Chronic hyperalgesia and skin warming caused by sensitized C nociceptors. *Brain* 1989;112:621–647.
4. DeJong RN. Case taking and the neurologic examination. In:Joynt RJ, ed. *Clinical neurology.* Philadelphia:Lippincott, 1988.
5. Dyck PJ, Lambert EH. Dissociated sensation in amylidosis:compound action potential, quantitative histologic and teased-fiber, and electron microscopic studies of sural nerve biopsies. *Arch Neurol* 1969;20:490–507.
6. Horn E, et al. Hypothalamic pathology in the neuroleptic malignant syndrome. *Am J Psychiatry* 1988;145:617–620.
7. Low PA. Autonomic neuropathy. *Semin Neurol* 1987;7:49–57.
8. Low PA. Composite autonomic scoring scale for laboratory quantification of generalized autonomic failure. *Mayo Clin Proc* 1993;68:748–752.
9. Low PA, Fealey RD. Sudomotor neuropathy. In:Dyck PJ, et al., eds. *Diabetic neuropathy.* Philadelphia:WB Saunders, 1987:140–145.
10. Low PA, Stevens JC. Peripheral neuropathies including autonomic neuropathies. In:Spittell JA, ed. *Clinical medicine.* Hagerstown, MD:Harper and Row, 1985.

11. Low PA, et al. Chronic idiopathic anhidrosis. *Ann Neurol* 1985;18:344–348.
12. Low PA, et al. Prospective evaluation of clinical characteristics of orthostatic hypotension. *Mayo Clin Proc* 1995;70:617–622.
13. Mayo Clinic and Foundation Clinical. *Examinations in neurology.* Chicago:Mosby Year Book, 1991.
14. Ochoa J. The newly recognized painful ABC syndrome:thermographic aspects. *Thermology* 1986;2:65–107.
15. Robertson D, et al. The head and neck discomfort of autonomic failure:an unrecognized etiology of headache. *Clin Auton Res* 1994;4:99–103.
16. Robertson D, Robertson RM. Causes of chronic orthostatic hypotension. *Arch Intern Med* 1994;154:1620–1624.
17. Robertson D, et al. Isolated failure of autonomic noradrenergic neurotransmission:evidence for impaired beta-hydroxylation of dopamine. *N Engl J Med* 1986;314:1494–1497.
18. Sanfield JA, et al. Altered norepinephrine metabolism in Shapiro's syndrome. *Arch Neurol* 1989;46:53–57.
19. Thomas DJ, Bannister R. Preservation of autoregulation of cerebral blood flow in autonomic failure. *J Neurol Sci* 1980;44:205–212.
20. Tsementzis SA, Hitchcock ER. The spoon test:a simple bedside test for assessing sudomotor autonomic failure. *J Neurol Neurosurg Psychiatry* 1985;48:378–380.
21. Wallin BG, et al. Syncope induced by glossopharyngeal neuralgia:sympathetic outflow to muscle. *Neurology* 1984;34:522–524.

APPENDIX: Autonomic Symptoms

Major Complaints: _____
(and duration)

_____

Underline if symptoms are negative/normal, **circle** if positive/abnormal:

Orthostatic
   Lightheadedness/
   Dizziness

☐   0 = never or insignificant
      1 = mild or infrequent
      2 = frequent
      3 = consistent
      4 = consistent with frequent syncope

Precipitating or aggravating Factors: early morning   postprandial   menstrual cycle
                                                                    prolonged standing   exertion/walking

Associated Symptoms: palpitations   nausea   vertigo   headache
                                 blurred vision   weakness   tremulousness   unsteadiness
                                 anxiety   pallor   clammy skin

Vasomotor Symptoms   discoloration (red, white, purplish); coldness
_____

Sweating: reduced in feet, excessive in feet/hands/head
             heat intolerance

Other Symptoms _____

Secretomotor Symptoms   dry mouth; dry eyes; excessive salivation/secretion; gustatory sweating

Postprandial
   Symptoms

☐   0 = never or insignificant
      1 = mild or infrequent
      2 = frequent
      3 = consistent
      anorexia; early satiety; persistent fullness (bloating); vomiting or frequent
      nausea; weight loss: _____ pounds

Abdominal Pain/Cramping _____
_____

Autonomic Diarrhea _____
_____

Obstinate Constipation _____
_____

Bladder Involvement   incontinence; incomplete emptying _____
_____

Sexual Problems   loss of libido; erectile failure; ejaculatory failure
Onset & Severity _____
Sleep Problems   snoring; apnea; stridor _____

Pupils   glare; blurred vision _____
Other Symptoms _____
_____
_____

Family History _____

Medications and Dose _____

_____

Alcohol Intake _____

Autonomic Examination

	BP	HR
Supine:	_____	_____
Standing:	_____	_____
Squats:	_____	_____

Sudomotor _____
Vasomotor _____

Pupils _____
Other _____

Comments _____

_____

_____

CHAPTER 2

The Central Autonomic Network

Eduardo E. Benarroch

---

1. The central autonomic network (CAN), includes the insular, anterior cingulate and ventromedial prefrontal cortices, central nucleus of the amygdala, paraventricular and other nuclei of the hypothalamus, periaqueductal gray matter, parabrachial nucleus, nucleus of the solitary tract, ventrolateral medulla, ventromedial medulla, and medullary lateral tegmental field.
2. The insula is the primary viscerosensory cortex, and the anterior cingulate and ventromedial prefrontal are visceral *premotor* cortices. The central nucleus of the amygdala is involved in emotional and conditioned responses. The hypothalamus integrates autonomic and endocrine responses critical for homeostasis. The periaqueductal gray integrates responses to stress, including pain modulation. The nucleus of the solitary tract is the first relay station for a variety of medullary reflexes controlling cardiovascular and respiratory function. The ventrolateral medulla is directly involved in tonic and reflex control of preganglionic and respiratory motoneurons.
3. The central autonomic areas receive and integrate visceral, humoral, and environmental information. Their main effectors are the preganglionic autonomic neurons, controlled by several hypothalamic and brainstem pathways. Other effectors include neuroendocrine, respiratory, and sphincter motoneurons.
4. The CAN is neurochemically complex. L-glutamate is the main excitatory and γ-aminobutyric acid the main inhibitory neurotransmitters, whereas acetylcholine, monoamines, neuropeptides, purines, and nitric oxide exert a modulatory action. Neuropeptides may act both as endogenous neurotransmitters and as circulating signas, via the circumventricular organs, that are areas lacking a blood–brain barrier.
5. The CAN is involved in tonic, reflex, and adaptive control of autonomic function and its activity is state dependent (i.e., it varies during the sleep–wake cycle or during adaptive behaviors). The function of the CAN is not limited to visceral control; rather, it coordinates autonomic with endocrine, behavioral, and antinociceptive responses to a variety of environmental stimuli.

FUNCTIONAL AND NEUROCHEMICAL ANATOMY

Components of the Central Autonomic Network

The central neural control of autonomic function involves multiple areas distributed throughout the neuraxis (40). These areas are reciprocally interconnected and constitute a functional unit referred to as the *central autonomic network* (CAN) (6,31) (Fig. 1).

The cortical components of this network include the insular cortex, which is the primary viscerosensory cortex, and the anterior cingulate gyrus and ventromedial prefrontal cortex, which are premotor autonomic regions (1,12,36).

The central nucleus of the amygdala and the bed nucleus of the stria terminalis form a unit referred to as the *extended amygdala* that integrates autonomic responses to emotion (29).

The hypothalamus, which integrates autonomic with endocrine responses to maintain homeostasis (32,37,43), includes three functionally distinct longitudinal zones: periventricular, medial, and lateral (43). The periventricular zone is involved in neuroendocrine control and generation

---

E. E. Benarroch: Department of Neurology, Mayo Clinic, Rochester, Minnesota 55905.

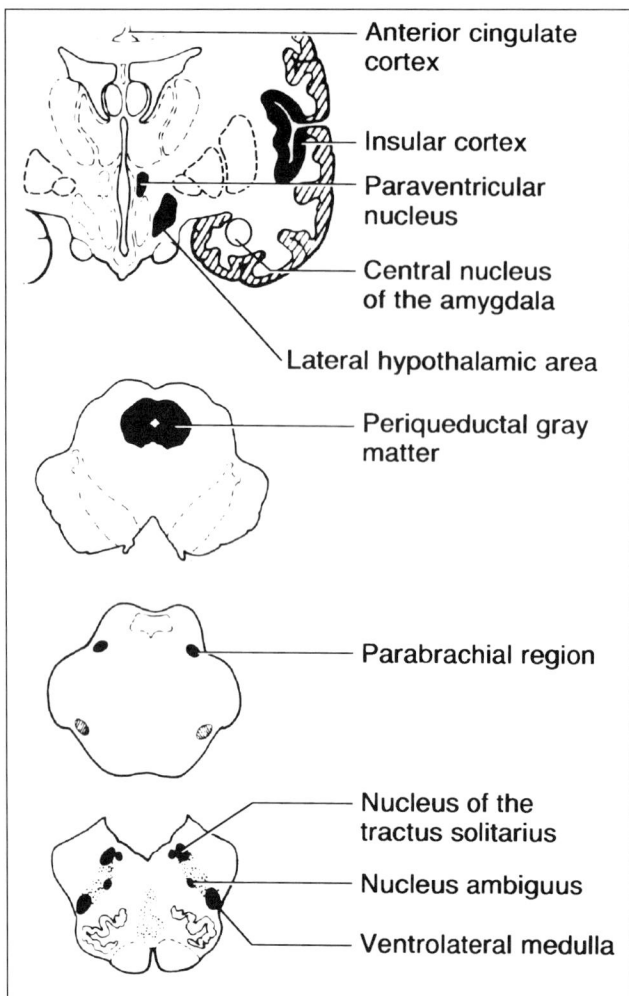

FIG. 1. Components of the central autonomic network.

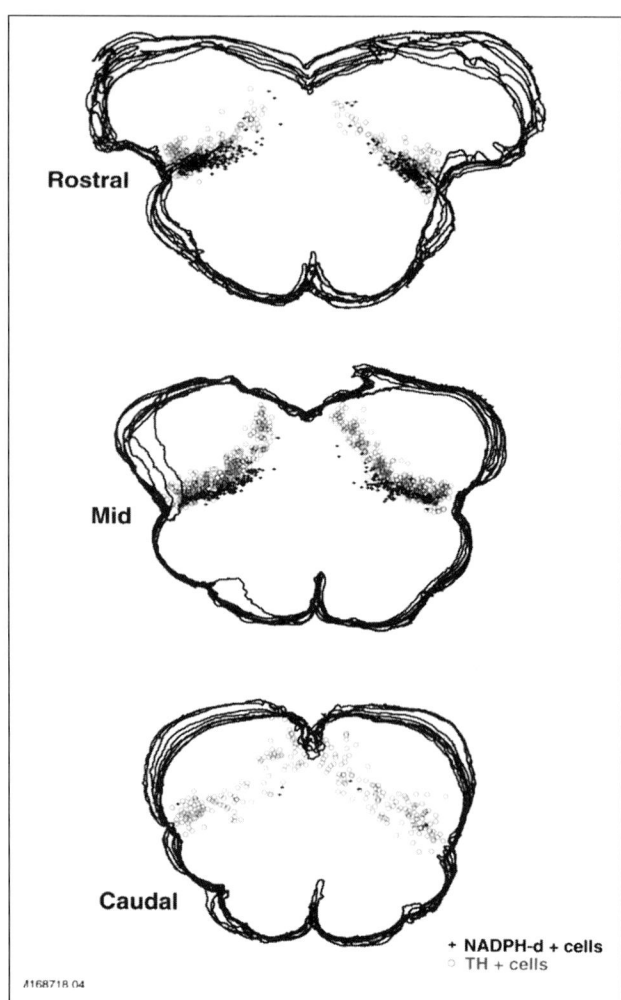

FIG. 2. Composite of sections of human medulla stained for tyrosine hydroxylase (TH) (*open circles*) and nicotinamide–adenine dinucleotide phosphate diaphorase (NADPH) d. The intermediate ventrolateral medulla. TH neurons of the ventrolateral medulla correspond to the A1 (caudal) and C1 rostral groups.

of biological rhythms. It includes the suprachiasmatic nucleus, which is the circadian pacemaker, and the paraventricular (parvicellular division) and other nuclei controlling anterior pituitary function (43). The medial zone includes several discrete nuclei that initiate integrated autonomic and behavioral responses related to homeostasis and reproduction, including the medial preoptic region, critically involved in thermoregulation. The lateral hypothalamic area is involved in behavioral arousal and motivated behavior. All three functional subdivisions contain neuronal groups that project to autonomic centers of the brainstem and spinal cord (25,43).

The periaqueductal gray matter (PAG) of the midbrain integrates autonomic with antinociceptive and behavioral responses to challenging stimuli (5,34). The parabrachial nucleus of the pons participates in relay of visceral and somatosensory information and control of cardiovascular and respiratory function (31). The nucleus of the solitary tract (NTS) is the first relay station for cardiovascular, respiratory, and gastrointestinal afferents (14,31,39); it is a critical component of a variety of medullary reflexes controlling these functions and relays viscerosensory information to all the other areas of the CAN. The intermediate reticular formation of the medulla, particularly the ventrolateral medulla (VLM), contains the interneuronal networks and premotor neurons that directly control the preganglionic sympathetic and respiratory motoneurons (19). Neurons of the ventromedial medulla contribute to innervation of spinal autonomic nuclei. All of these regions have been identified in anatomically and neurochemically in human brain (Fig. 2).

Inputs to the Central Autonomic Network

The central autonomic regions receive and integrate multiple visceral, humoral, and environmental information. Visceral information is conveyed both by medullary and spinal afferents. Afferents for baroreceptors, chemoreceptors, and pulmonary and gastrointestinal receptors project via the vagus and glossopharyngeal nerves to the NTS (41). The NTS is the first relay station both for these general visceral afferents and for taste afferents relayed primarily via the facial nerve (31), and is subdivided into a rostral (taste), intermediate (general visceral), and caudal (commissural) regions (31,42). The intermediate NTS has a viscerotopic organization and is involved in cardiovascular, respiratory, and gastrointestinal reflexes. The commissural NTS receives convergent viscerosensory information and projects to rostral levels of the CAN. The NTS relays viscensory information both directly or via projections to the parabrachial nucleus or VLM. General visceral and taste information is relayed via the parvicellular region of the ventroposteromedial nucleus of the thalamus to the insular cortex (12). The insular cortex is the primary viscerosensory area and contains a viscerotopic map for taste and general visceral afferents (12). Spinal afferents from dorsal root ganglion neurons innervating cardiac, respiratory, and gastrointestinal receptors are carried via the sympathetic nerves and project to the thoracolumbar spinal dorsal horn. Dorsal horn neurons receive convergent visceral and somatic information and project via the spinothalamic, spinoreticular, and spinomesencephalic pathways to relay visceral pain and initiate viscerosympathetic and somatosympathetic responses.

Humoral signals are in part relayed via the circumventricular organs, which are regions that lack a blood–brain barrier. They include the subfornical organ and the vascular organ of the lamina terminalis in the anterior wall of the third ventricle, and the area postrema in the walls of the fourth ventricle. Circulating signals, including angiotensin II and cytokines, act via receptors in these circumventricular organs to affect central autonomic circuits (18).

Other important humoral information is provided by circulating steroids, which act via receptors distributed throughout the CAN, and by changes in composition of the blood or cerebrospinal fluid detected by chemoreceptive neurons in the hypothalamus and medulla.

Information from the external environment and integrated in unimodal and multimodal cortical sensory association areas is relayed to the CAN via paralimbic areas of the cerebral cortex, including the insular, anterior cingulate and ventromedial prefrontal cortex (13).

Outputs of the Central Autonomic Network

The main effectors of the CAN are the preganglionic autonomic neurons. The sympathetic preganglionic neurons (SPNs) are located in the T1–L2 segments of the intermediolateral cell column and form functionally separate units that receive selective supraspinal and primary afferent inputs and innervate selective subpopulations of sympathetic ganglion neurons. These include muscle vasomotor, skin vasomotor, sudomotor, and visceromotor neurons (11). The SPNs receive multiple parallel supraspinal input from the hypothalamus and brain stem.

Preganglionic parasympathetic neurons are located both in the brain stem and sacral spinal cord. The dorsal nucleus of the vagus innervates the gastrointestinal tract, except for the proximal esophagus, innervated by the nucleus ambiguus, and the distal colon and rectum, innervated by the sacral parasympathetic nucleus. Cardiac vagal motoneurons are located in the nucleus ambiguus and dorsal motor nucleus of the vagus (33). The sacral parasympathetic output originates in the sacral parasympathetic nucleus, located in the intermediolateral cell column at S2–S4 segments of the spinal cord, is carried in the pelvic nerves, and facilitates evacuation of the bladder or bowel and penile erection (26).

Other effector mechanisms of the CAN include neuroendocrine, respiratory, and sphincter motoneurons (17). The CAN controls hormonal systems both via connections of the hypothalamus with the pituitary gland and through the autonomic innervation of peripheral endocrine organs, including the adrenal medulla, juxtaglomerular apparatus, pancreas, and gut (15,38).

Neurochemistry

The areas of the CAN are reciprocally interconnected via neurochemically complex pathways. L-glutamate is the main excitatory transmitter, and γ-aminobutyric acid (GABA) the main inhibitory transmitter, that mediate rapid point-to-point information within the CAN. Acetylcholine, monoamines, neuropeptides, and purines exert a modulatory action. The catecholaminergic innervation originates in norepinephrine- and epinephrine-synthesizing neurons of the lateral tegmentum of the pons and medulla. These include the A1–A3 and A5 groups of norepinephrine-synthesizing neurons and the C1–C3 groups of epinephrine-synthesizing neurons. These groups are well defined in human brain (4,7,20–21) (Fig. 2). The CAN contains essentially all of the neuropeptide families so far described in the brain. Important examples are substance P, neuropeptide Y, corticotropin-releasing hormone (CRH), and opioids. Some peptides, such as angiotensin II, vasopressin, and cytokines may act both as endogenous neurotransmitters and as circulating signals, via the circumventricular organs.

Nitric oxide (NO), purines (e.g., adenosine) and eicosanoids may be important local modulators. Neurons synthesizing NO are identified by their reactivity to NADPH-diaphorase (Fig. 2) and include most preganglionic and some brainstem and hypothalamic neurons. NO acts as rapid diffusible intercellular messenger. Circulating steroids or locally produced neurosteroids may exert important influence on central autonomic control via both genomic and nongenomic mechanisms (24).

FUNCTIONAL ASPECTS

The CAN is involved in tonic, reflex, and adaptive control of autonomic function, and integrates autonomic with hormonal, immunomodulatory, and pain-controlling responses to internal or external environmental challenges.

Ventrolateral Medulla and Tonic Control of Sympathetic Outflow

Sympathetic preganglionic neurons have low level of activity at rest and are continuously modulated by the interactions of a variety of excitatory and inhibitory postsynaptic influences affecting their membrane ionic currents (11). Supraspinal inputs originate from the paraventricular and other hypothalamic nuclei, the A5 region, the C1 area of the rostral VLM, the ventromedial medulla, and the caudal raphe (31). Segmental inputs to SPNs arise from primary somatic and visceral afferents.

The rostral VLM, including the C1 group of epinephrine-synthesizing neurons, provides tonic excitation of SPNs. These inputs are mediated by L-glutamate, which may coexist with epinephrine, neuropeptide Y, substance P, and other neuropeptides in neurons of the rostral VLM. Tonic activity of neurons of the rostral VLM may reflect intrinsic pacemaker activity, inputs from an *oscillatory* propriobulbar network, inputs from the central respiratory generator, and synchronizing inhibitory influences from the baroreceptors (14,19,41). These neurons are topographically organized according to their target organs and control sympathetic outflows to the heart, blood vessels, and adrenal medulla. Neurons of the rostral VLM mediate a variety of reflexes controlling sympathetic function, including those initiated from baroreceptors, cardiac receptors, and chemoreceptors (14,19,41). Some of these neurons may act as *oxygen sensors* and mediate sympathoexcitatory responses to hypoxia and ischemia (43). These neurons receive direct input from the amygdala, hypothalamus, and PAG and thus mediate sympathetic responses to emotional states (5,23,34,38).

Neurons of the ventromedial medulla contribute glutamatergic innervation to SPNs and may play a supplementary role in maintaining basal arterial pressure. These neurons may contain serotonin, GABA, substance P, opioid, and other neuropeptides (22). Whereas glutamate produces fast excitation of SPNs, catecholamines, serotonin, and neuropeptides have a modulatory effect (19).

Nucleus of the Solitary Tract and Medullary Reflexes

The central control of autonomic function involves a variety of medullary reflexes. The NTS is a critical relay station for cardiovascular, respiratory, and gastrointestinal afferents (31). The intermediate NTS has a viscerotopic organization and is involved in baroreceptor, cardiac, chemoreceptor, and respiratory reflexes that control sympathetic, cardiac vagal, and respiratory activity, as well as gastrointestinal vagovagal reflexes controlling gastrointestinal motility and secretion (3,14,31).

The baroreflex is the most important mechanism of moment-to-moment control of arterial pressure. The baroreflex circuit has been extensively investigated (3,14,39) and provides a good model for other medullary cardiorespiratory reflexes (Fig. 3). The arterial baroreceptors are mechanoreceptors located in the carotid sinus and aortic arch and innervated by branches of the IXth or Xth nerve, respectively. They are stimulated by an increase in arterial pressure and initiate a reflex activation of cardiac vagal inputs (producing bradycardia), inhibition of sympathetic outflow (resulting in vasodilatation) and inhibition of release of vasopressin. The first central station for these afferents is the NTS. Baroreceptive NTS neurons directly activate cardiovagal neurons of the nucleus ambiguus and dorsal vagal nucleus, and inhibit sympathoexcitatory neurons of the rostral VLM, via a GABAergic interneuron in the caudal VLM (3,8,14,40). The baroreflex produces tonic inhibition of vasopressin producing magnocellular neurons of the supraoptic and paraventricular nuclei of the hypothalamus. In humans, bilateral lesions involving the NTS produce either acute hypertension or chronic lability of arterial pressure (35).

Cardiorespiratory Interactions in the Reticular Formation

Tonic and reflex activity of medullary neurons is strongly modulated by respiration. The respiratory rhythm is dominant within the central cardiorespiratory network and involves interaction of a pontine respiratory group in the parabrachial–Kölliker Fuse region, a dorsal respiratory group in the NTS, and a ventral respiratory group in the ambigual–retroambigual regions of the VLM (17). Respiratory, sympathetic, and cardiovagal neurons interact at the level of the NTS and VLM. For example, tonic and baroreflex-induced activity of cardiovagal neurons of the nucleus ambiguus are inhibited during inspiration (33). These interactions likely involve interneuronal networks in the intermediate medullary reticular formation. These networks also coordinate *patterned* reflex responses involving respiratory and autonomic neurons, including vomiting. Sympathoexcitatory neurons of the rostral VLM are intimately related to chemosensitive regions in the ventral medullary surface; these areas contain neurons that primarily respond to changes in PCO_2 and pH of the cerebrospinal fluid (17).

Circadian Rhythms, Sleep, and Autonomic Function

Circadian rhythms, thermoregulation, and the sleep–wake cycle profoundly affect autonomic function and have important implications in human disease. Circadian oscil-

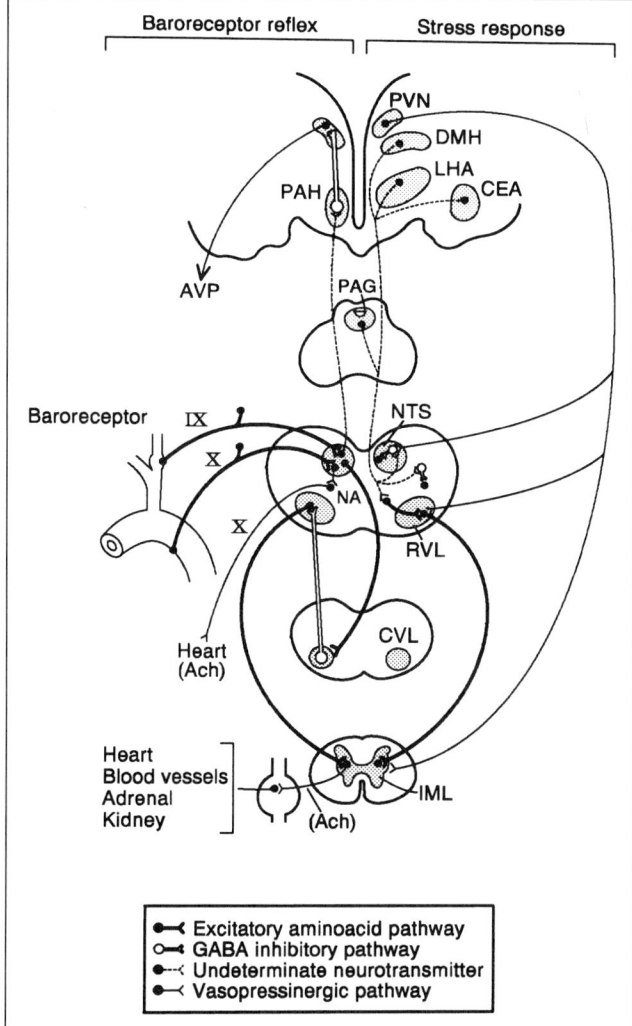

FIG. 3. Central circuits for baroreflex and cardiovascular stress response. Baroreceptor inputs from the carotid sinus and the aortic arch are carried by the glossopharyngeal (IX) and vagus (X) nerves, respectively, and relay in the nucleus of the tractus solitarius (NTS). Baroreceptor activation of NTS neurons result in (1) sympathoinhibition via a relay in the caudal ventrolateral medulla (CVL) that sends a GABAergic input to vasomotor neurons of the rostral ventrolateral medulla (RVL); (2) activation of cardiovagal neurons of the nucleus ambiguus (NA); and (3) inhibition of release of vasopressin (AVP) from the supraoptic and paraventricular nucleus (PVN) via a GABAergic projection from the preoptic–anterior hypothalamic region (PAH) to magnocellular vasopressinergic neurons. The stress response involves a circuit that includes the central nucleus of the amygdala (CEA), lateral hypothalamic area (LHA), dorsomedial nucleus of the hypothalamus (DMH), PVN, and periaqueductal gray matter (PAG). Stimulation of these regions results in sympathoexcitation and inhibition of the baroreflex; this involves direct activation of neurons of the RVL and inhibition of barosensitive neurons of the NTS and NA mediated by local GABAergic interneurons. Preganglionic cardiovagal neurons of the NA and sympathetic neurons of the intermediolateral cell column (IML) are the final effectors of these responses and use acetylcholine (ACh) as their neurotransmitter.

lations depend on the suprachiasmatic nucleus, in part via its projections to the paraventricular nucleus (9). Changes related to thermoregulation, including sleep onset, are integrated by the thermosensitive neurons of the medial preoptic region. Autonomic function varies during the sleep–wake cycle, and this reflects possible interactions between autonomic and sleep-modulating networks at the level of the brain stem and hypothalamus. During non-REM (rapid eye movement) sleep, activation of the parasympathetic and inhibition of the sympathetic outflows produces a tonic decrease in arterial pressure and heart rate, in association with a downward resetting of the thermostat and decrease in body temperature and metabolism. By contrast, REM sleep is characterized by marked phasic fluctuations of sympathetic and parasympathetic activity and by impairment of homeostatic baroreflex responses and thermoregulation.

Integrated Responses to Emotion and Stress

The CAN coordinates the adaptive autonomic, endocrine, and behavioral responses to emotional and stressful stimuli. The patterns of responses vary with the type of stress (23). Acute, transient challenges trigger a short-term response referred to as the *defense reaction*. It includes sympathetic activation, with increase in heart rate, cardiac output, and arterial pressure; redistribution of blood flow to the limbs, secondary to muscle vasodilatation and skin and visceral vasoconstriction; and inhibition of baroreflex responses (15,28,38,41). An integral component of the defense response is the activation of central pain-controlling mechanisms (5). Chronic stress states elicit a *vigilance* reaction, characterized by activation of the hypothalamus–pituitary–adrenocortical system.

The areas involved in processing and initiation of emotional and stress responses include the ventromedial frontal and insular cortices (1,16), the amygdala (10), the paraventricular and other nuclei of the hypothalamus (30,44), and the PAG (5,15,28) (Fig. 3). These regions are intimately interconnected and project to the NTS, vagal nuclei, and ventrolateral and ventromedial reticular formation, which control the sympathetic, parasympathetic, pain-modulating, and motor responses to emotional and stressful stimuli.

The anterior cingulate and orbitofrontal regions of the frontal lobe, together with the amygdala, ventral striatum, and PAG, constitute a functional unit, referred to as the *rostral* limbic system (16). This is involved both in the assessment of emotional content of sensory stimuli and in executive functions related to affective behavior, including regulation of autonomic, endocrine, and motor outputs (2,16). In humans, lesions of the ventromedial prefrontal cortex impair sympathetic skin responses to emotional stimuli (13).

The amygdala is critically involved in emotional and conditioned responses to aversive stimuli. It interprets the emotional or affective significance of incoming sensory information and generates the appropriate autonomic and behavioral responses (29). The amygdala consists of multiple nuclear groups that are subdivided into a basolateral and a centromedial groups (2). The basolateral amygdala has reciprocal connections with the cerebral cortex, and receives highly processed sensory information. The central nucleus of the amygdala, together with the bed nucleus of the stria terminalis, constitute the *extended amygdala*, which projects to several nuclei of the hypothalamus and brainstem that initiate the autonomic, endocrine, and motor components of emotional responses (2,15,29).

The paraventricular nucleus (PVN) of the hypothalamus is an integrative center that plays a critical role in coordination of neuroendocrine and autonomic responses to stress (30,43). It receives humoral, viscerosensory, and external information, contains different subpopulations of *effector* neurons controlling endocrine and autonomic outflows, has access to a variety of external and internal information, and shows a high degree of plasticity of neurotransmitter expression (30,44). The effector neurons of the PVN include (a) magnicellular neurons producing and releasing arginine vasopressin (AVP) and oxytocin to the general circulation, (b) parvicellular neurons producing CRH and other hormones regulating the anterior pituitary, and (c) *mediocellular* neurons that project to autonomic and other regions of the brainstem and spinal cord (14,30).

Activity of magnicellular AVP-secreting neurons is tonically inhibited by the baroreceptor and cardiopulmonary receptor reflexes. On the other hand, AVP secretion increases in response of unloading of baropulmonary or cardiopulmonary receptors (e.g., during hypovolemia), or chemoreceptor stimulation. The pathway involves a relay on the A1 noradrenergic group of the caudal VLM. Norepinephrine, released from A1 projections, activates magnicellular AVP neurons, via α_1 receptor mechanisms (14).

The PVN plays a critical role in stimulation of the pituitary–corticoadrenal axis during stress; it is the sole source of CRH for stimulation of adrenocorticotropin hormone (ACTH)-secreting cells in at the anterior pituitary (44). The full ACTH-releasing potency of the PVN involves not only CRH, but also AVP, angiotensin, and cholecystokinin. As mentioned previously, these neuropeptides can be expressed in CRH neurons, and their expression suppressed by circulating steroids and upregulated following adrenalectomy (44).

The PVN is the *master controller* of autonomic function as it innervates all autonomic relay centers, including the rostral VLM, NTS, parabrachial nucleus, and preganglionic vagal and sympathetic neurons (26,38,44). Neurons in specific regions of the autonomic PVN are organized into functionally specialized units that innervate specific subsets of preganglionic neurons. The paraventriculospinal tract is neurochemically very complex, and contains AVP, oxytocin, enkephalin, and other neuropeptides (27,43).

The PAG is critically involved in integration of autonomic, somatic, and antinociceptive responses to stress, including the defense reaction. The PAG has a high degree of anatomical and functional organization, and is subdivided into longitudinal columns, or modules, with specific inputs and outputs. The lateral PAG is involved in sympathoexcitation, threat or flight responses, and opioid-independent antinociception.

The cardiovascular and pain-suppressing effects of PAG are mediated via its projections to the rostral VLM. In both the PAG and the rostral ventrolateral medulla, there is a topographic organization of neurons in pools controlling specific vascular beds (5). The ventrolateral PAG is involved in sympathoinhibition, motor quiescence, and opioid-dependent analgesia. The effects of the ventrolateral PAG are mediated via its projections to the medullary raphe nuclei (5,34).

REFERENCES

1. Allen GV, et al. Organization of visceral and limbic connections in the insular cortex of the rat. *J Comp Neurol* 1991;311:1–16.
2. Amaral DG, et al. Anatomical organization of the primate amygdaoid complex. In: Aggleton JP, ed. *The amygdala: neurobiological aspects of emotion.* Wiley-Liss, 1992:1–66.
3. Andresen MC, Kunze DL. Nucleus tractus solitarius: gateway to neural circulatory control [Review]. *Annu Rev Physiol* 1994;56:93–116.
4. Arango V, et al. Catecholaminergic neurons in the ventrolateral medulla and nucleus of the solitary tract in the human. *J Comp Neurol* 1988;273:224–240.
5. Bandler R, Shipley MT. Columnar organization in the midbrain periaqueductal gray: modules for emotional expression? *Trends Neurosci* 1994;17:379–389.
6. Benarroch EE. The central autonomic network: functional organization dysfunction and perspective [Review]. *Mayo Clin Proc* 1993;68:988–1001.
7. Benarroch EE, et al. Localization and possible interactions of catecholamine- and NADPH-diaphorase neurons in human medullary autonomic regions. *Brain Res* 1995;684:215–220.
8. Blessing WW, et al. Inhibitory vasomotor neurons in the caudal ventrolateral region of the medulla oblongata. *Prog Brain Res* 1989;81:83–97.
9. Blessing WW, Willoughby JO. Central neural pathways mediating baroreceptor-initiated secretion of vasopressin. In: Hainsworth R, McWilliam PN, Mary DASG, eds. *Cardiogenic reflexes.* Oxford: Oxford University Press, 1987:301–317.
10. Briggs CA. Potentiation of nicotinic transmission in the rat superior cervical sympathetic ganglion: effects of cyclic GMP and nitric oxide generators. *Brain Res* 1991;573:139–146.
11. Cabot JB. Sympathetic preganglionic neurons: cytoarchitecture ultrastructure and biophysical properties. In: Loewy AD, Spyer KM, eds. *Central regulation of autonomic functions.* New York: Oxford University Press, 1990:44–67.
12. Cechetto DF, Saper CB. Role of the cerebral cortex in autonomic function. In: Loewy AD, Spyer KM, eds. *Central regulation of autonomic functions.* Oxford: Oxford University Press, 1990:208–223.
13. Damasio AR, et al. Individuals with sociopathic behavior caused by frontal damage fail to respond autonomically to social stimuli. *Behav Brain Res* 1990;41:81–94.
14. Dampney RA. Functional organization of central pathways regulating the cardiovascular system [Review]. *Physiol Rev* 1994;74:323–364.
15. Davis M. The role of the amygdala in fear-potentiated startle: implications for animal models of anxiety [Review]. *Trends Pharmacol Sci* 1992;13:35–41.

16. Devinsky O, et al. Contributions of anterior cingulate cortex to behaviour [Review]. *Brain* 1995;118:279–306.
17. Feldman JL, Ellenberger HH. Central coordination of respiratory and cardiovascular control in mammals. *Annu Rev Physiol* 1988;50:593–606.
18. Ferguson AV, et al. Circumventricular organs and cardiovascular homeostasis. In: Kunos G, Ciriello J, eds. *Central neural mechanisms in cardiovascular regulation;* vol 2. Basel: Birkhauser, 1992:80–101.
19. Guyenet PG. Role of the ventral medulla oblongata in blood pressure regulation. In: Loewy AD, Spyer KM, eds. *Central regulation of autonomic functions.* New York: Oxford University Press, 1990:145–167.
20. Halliday GM, McLachlan EM. A comparative analysis of neurons containing catecholamine-synthesizing enzymes and neuropeptide Y in the ventrolateral medulla of rats guinea-pigs and cats. *Neuroscience* 1991;43:531–550.
21. Halliday GM, et al. The distribution of neuropeptide Y-like immunoreactive neurons in the human medulla oblongata. *Neuroscience* 1988;26:179–191.
22. Helke CJ, et al. Chemical neuroanatomy of the parapyramidal region of the ventral medulla in the rat. *Prog Brain Res* 1989;81:17–28.
23. Henry JP. Biological basis of the stress response. *News Physiol Sci* 1993;8:69–74.
24. Herbert J. Peptides in the limbic system: neurochemical codes for coordinated adaptive responses to behavioural and physiological demand [Review]. *Prog Neurobiol* 1993;41:723–791.
25. Holstege G. Subcortical limbic projections to brainstem and spinal cord. In: Paxinos G, ed. *The human nervous system.* New York: Academic Press, 1990:261–283.
26. Holstege G, Griffiths D. Organization of micturition. In: Paxinos G, ed. *The human nervous system.* New York: Academic Press, 1990:297–305.
27. Jennings G, et al. Treatment of orthostatic hypotension with dihydroergotamine. *BMJ* 1979;2:307.
28. Jordan D, et al. Hypothalamic inhibition of neurones in the nucleus tractus solitarius of the cat is GABA mediated. *J Physiol* 1988;399:389–404.
29. Ledoux JE. Emotion and the amygdala. In: Aggleton JP, ed. *The amygdala: neurobiological aspects of emotion.* New York: Wiley–Liss, 1992:339–351.
30. Liposits Z. Ultrastructure of hypothalamic paraventricular neurons [Review]. *Crit Rev Neurobiol* 1993;7:89–162.
31. Loewy AD. Central autonomic pathways. In: Loewy AD, Spyer KM, eds. *Central regulation of autonomic functions.* New York: Oxford University Press, 1990:88–103.
32. Loewy AD. Forebrain nuclei involved in autonomic control [Review]. *Prog Brain Res* 1991;87:253–268.
33. Loewy AD, Spyer KM. Vagal preganglionic neurons. In: Loewy AD, Spyer KM, eds. *Central regulation of autonomic functions.* New York: Oxford University Press, 1990:68–87.
34. Lovick TA. Integrated activity of cardiovascular and pain regulatory systems: role in adaptive behavioural responses. *Prog Neurobiol* 1993;40:631–644.
35. Magnus O, et al. Cerebral mechanisms and neurogenic hypertension in man with special reference to baroreceptor control. In: De Jong W, Provoost AP, Shapiro AP, eds. *Hypertension and brain mechanisms;* vol 47. Amsterdam: Elsevier, 1977:199–218.
36. Neafsey EJ. Prefrontal cortical control of the autonomic nervous system: anatomical and physiological observations [Review]. *Prog Brain Res* 1990;85:147–165 (Discussion 165–166).
37. Saper C. Hypothalamus. In: Paxinos G, ed. *The human nervous system.* New York: Academic Press, 1990:389–413.
38. Smith OA, DeVito JL. Central neural integration for the control of autonomic responses associated with emotion [Review]. *Annu Rev Neurosci* 1984;7:43–65.
39. Spyer KM. Annual review prize lecture: central nervous mechanisms contributing to cardiovascular control. *J Physiol* 1994;474:1–19.
40. Spyer KM. The central nervous organization of reflex circulatory control. In: Loewy AD, Spyer KM, eds. *Central regulation of autonomic functions.* New York: Oxford University Press, 1990:168–187.
41. Spyer KM. Neural mechanisms involved in cardiovascular control during affective behaviour. *Trends Neurosci* 1989;12:506–513.
42. Sun M-K, Reis DJ. Hypoxia-activated Ca^{2+} currents in pacemaker neurones of rat rostral ventrolateral medulla *in vitro*. *J Physiol* 1994;476:101–116.
43. Swanson LW. The hypothalamus. In: Bjorklund A, Hokfelt T, Swanson LW, eds. *Handbook of chemical neuroanatomy;* vol 5. Amsterdam: Elsevier, 1987:1–124.
44. Swanson LW. Biochemical switching in hypothalamic circuits mediating responses to stress [Review]. *Prog Brain Res* 1991;87:181–200.

CHAPTER 3

Spinal Cord and Peripheral Nervous System

Yadollah Harati and Hazem Machkhas

1. There is no anatomically identifiable descending autonomic pathway or tract in the spinal cord. Most evidence suggests that the descending autonomic fibers are diffusely disbursed in the spinal cord, all projecting to the intermediolateral and intermediomedial neurons.
2. Many neuropeptides have been localized to the spinal and peripheral autonomic nervous system. Of these, vasoactive intestinal polypeptide, neuropeptide Y, substance P, and the enkephalins are of particular importance.
3. Nitric oxide, an ubiquitous free radical, is now recognized as a major neuronal messenger. Nitrergic autonomic transmission has now been demonstrated at several sites.
4. The ratio of preganglionic to postganglionic neurons is much smaller in the parasympathetic system than in the sympathetic system, and this explains the very specific, controlled, and localized function of the parasympathetic nervous system.
5. The higher the incidence of arm vasomotor or sudomotor disturbances associated with injuries to the lower trunk of the brachial plexus is explained anatomically by the higher density of postganglionic sympathetic fibers in the medial cord of the brachial plexus and median and ulnar nerves.

INTRODUCTION

This chapter discusses the anatomy of the spinal and peripheral components of the autonomic nervous system (ANS). The discussion is limited largely to the anatomic consideration of the ANS in humans, with minimal reference to animal studies. This chapter considers only the general anatomy of the peripheral sympathetic and parasympathetic systems. For specific and more detailed descriptions of the autonomic innervation of different body systems, readers are referred to subsequent chapters or to the standard textbooks of anatomy (76,113).

SPINAL CORD

Descending Autonomic Fibers

Most research suggests that the majority of fibers originating from brainstem "visceral" centers are small-diameter fibers that predominantly travel via the lateral funiculus of the spinal cord, although this is by no means certain. A smaller number of these fibers may descend in the anterior funiculus. However, attempts to identify a group of degenerating fibers in the spinal cord following lesions of the hypothalamus or brainstem have generally been unsuccessful, suggesting that the descending autonomic fibers may be diffusely disbursed in the spinal cord. In addition, although there is no direct anatomic evidence that the reticulospinal and corticospinal tracts contain autonomic fibers, disturbed vasomotor and sudomotor functions following the interruption of reticulospinal pathways or the stimulation of the prefrontal cortex suggest that some fibers in these tracts may be autonomic. Regardless of their pathways, all descending autonomic fibers project to neurons of the intermediolateral (IML) or intermediomedial (IMM) columns of the spinal lateral gray column (Fig. 1).

Intermediolateral and Intermediomedial Cell Columns

The small neurons of the IML and IMM cell columns at the thoracic and upper lumbar regions of the spinal cord

Y. Harati and H. Machkhas: Department of Neurology, Baylor College of Medicine, Houston, Texas 77030.

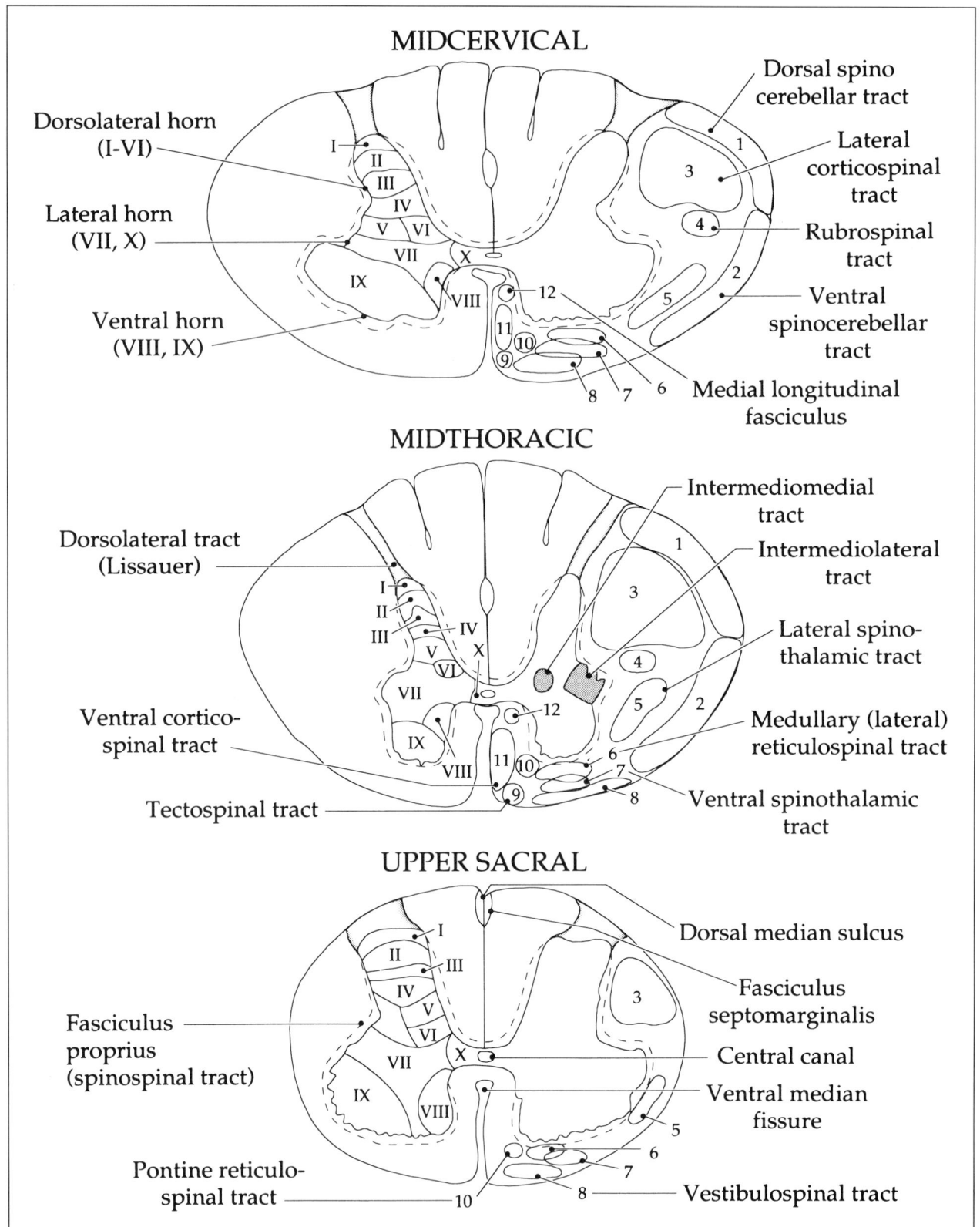

FIG. 1. The approximate relative position of the nerve fiber tracts of the human spinal cord at the midcervical, midthoracic, and upper sacral levels (right half). The pattern of Rexed lamination of the gray matter is shown in the left half.

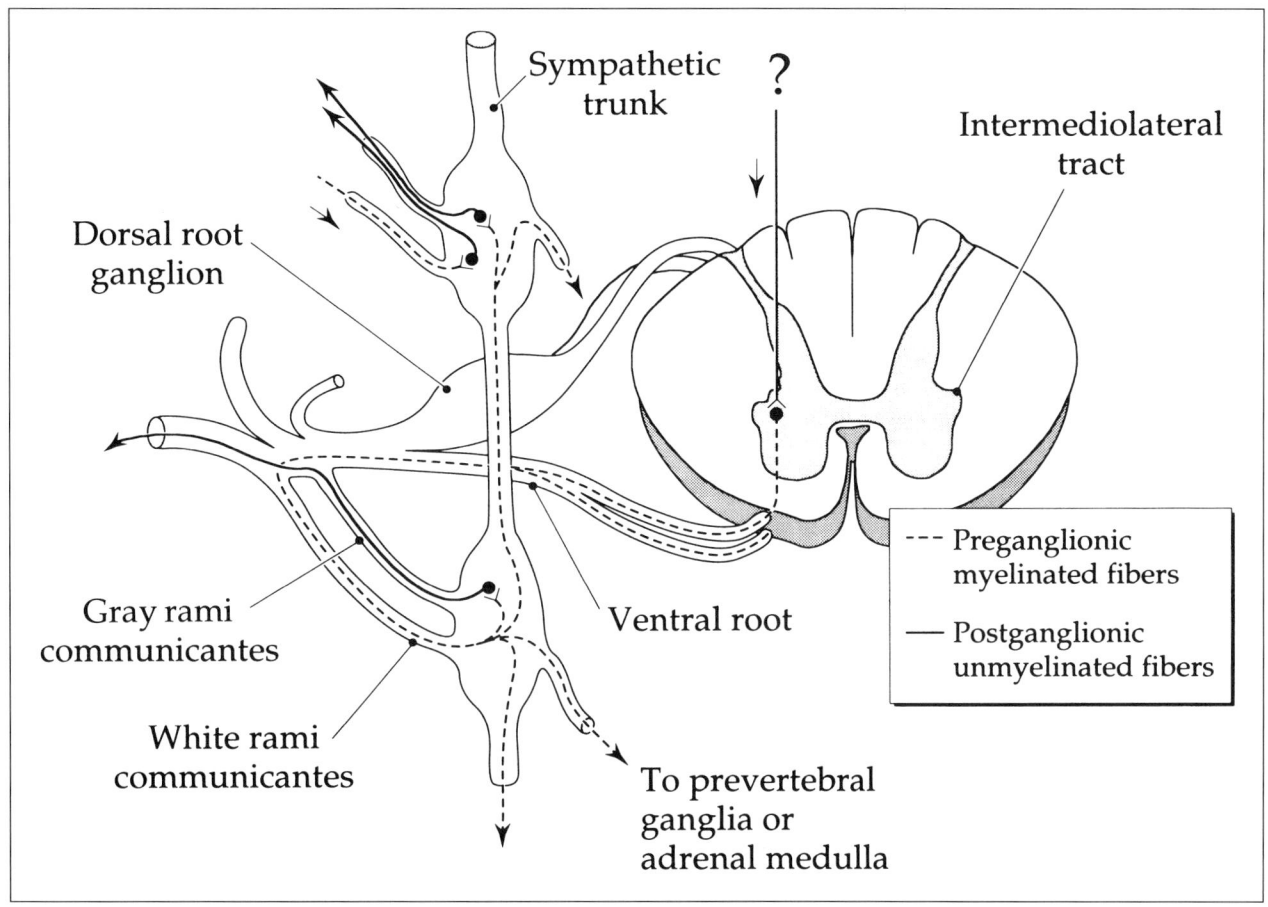

FIG. 2. The efferent sympathetic fibers and their relationship to the sympathetic ganglia.

develop in the embryonic cord from intermediate-zone neuroblasts in the dorsal part of the ventrolateral lamina. Neurons migrating laterally from the central canal form the triangularly shaped IML cell column, and those remaining closer to the canal create the IMM cell column. There is remarkable variability in the number of neurons in the IML, such that the number may vary by as much as fivefold in serial or even in the same sections (49). The IML and IMM cell columns lie within lamina VII of the laminar architecture of the spinal cord[1]. The neurons in these columns form the primary efferent sympathetic autonomic neurons, or preganglionic neurons. Their axons, which precede the autonomic ganglia (hence preganglionic fibers), project onto a postganglionic neuron (secondary efferent neuron) with its cell body in one of the paravertebral sympathetic trunk ganglia or in related ganglia (Fig. 2). The adrenal medulla is unique in that it receives only preganglionic fibers. The preganglionic nerve fibers are finely myelinated with a diameter of 2–5 μm and reach the ganglionic neuron via the ventral spinal root and the white rami communicantes. Because of their myelination, they are almost white when seen *en masse*, contributing to the whitish appearance of the white rami and ventral roots. The preganglionic nerve fibers may course through several ganglia before eventually synapsing in one or several of the 22 pairs of ganglia of the paravertebral sympathetic chain (Fig. 3). The sympathetic pathways originating in different segments of the spinal cord are not necessarily distributed to the same part of the body as the spinal nerve fibers from the same segments. Instead, the sympathetic fibers from T1 generally pass up the sympathetic chain into the head, fibers from T2 into the neck, fibers from T3–6 into the thorax, fibers from T7–11 into the abdomen, and fibers from T12 and L1–2 into the legs. There is, however, significant overlap in the distribution. A stricter regional pattern of distribution is seen in postganglionic fibers, where respective ganglia project to specific parts of the body. The entire sympathetic nervous system originates from the thoracic and upper lumbar spinal cord (thoracolumbar outflow), and the parasympathetic nerves originate from cranial nerves III,

---

[1] The Rexed laminar cytoarchitecture, as described in the cat, may also be applied to the human spinal cord. For observed differences in the cat and human spinal laminar cytoarchitecture, see Shoenen and Faull (97).

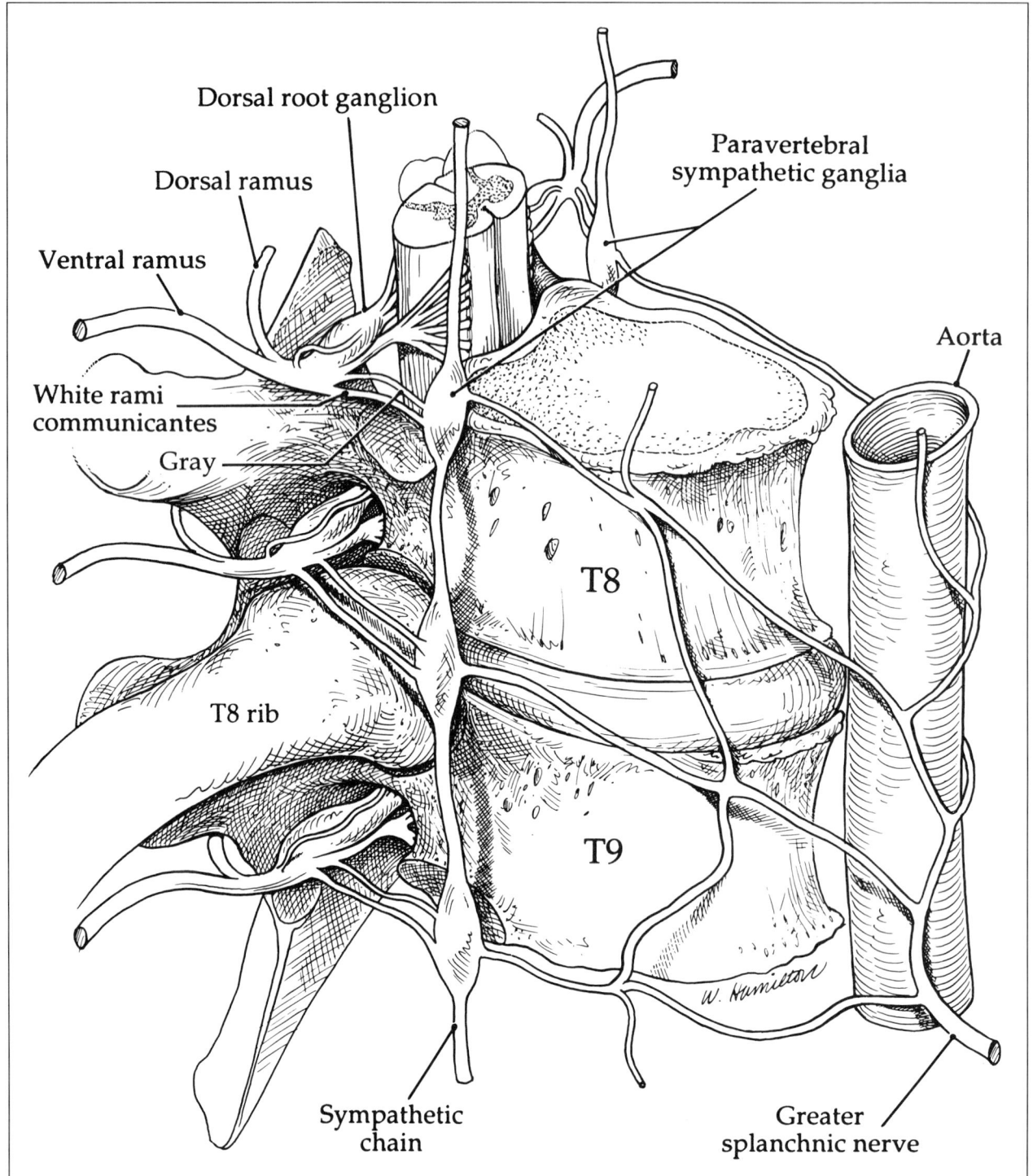

FIG. 3. The thoracic paravertebral sympathetic chain ganglia and their relationship to adjacent structures.

VII, IX, and X, as well as from the second, third, and fourth sacral spinal IML cell columns (craniosacral outflow). The parasympathetic relay ganglia are located near the structures innervated, where they are mostly found in the walls of hollow organs or in the substance of solid viscera (Fig. 4).

The neurons of the human IML (and probably IMM) cell columns have large and often eccentric nuclei, and have an oval, polygonal, spindle, or club shape. They have a mean diameter of 12- to 13-μm (range, 8–23 μm). They exhibit the staining characteristics of motor neurons, with coarse

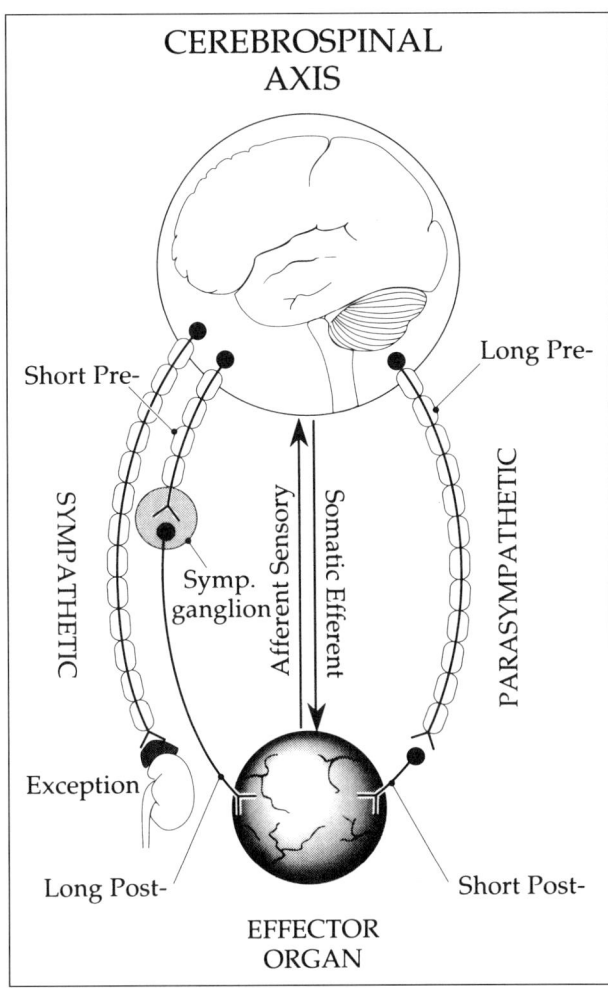

FIG. 4. The major anatomic differences between the sympathetic and parasympathetic systems.

and irregular Nissl substance. The mean cell count at the T6, T7, and T8 spinal cord segments has been shown to be 5,002, 5,004, and 4,654, respectively, with no significant sex differences. Each preganglionic neuron is estimated to project to as many as 20 postganglionic sites on different ganglia. Accordingly, as many as 100,000 postganglionic neurons are controlled by any given spinal segment. Both IML neurons and their preganglionic axons diminish in number with age, and the rate of age-related attrition is ~8% per decade (58).

The main neurotransmitter released by the preganglionic neurons of the IML and IMM cell columns is acetylcholine (ACh). These neurons contain high levels of muscarinic cholinergic receptor binding, acetylcholinesterase (AChE), and high concentrations of several neuropeptides. ACh is stored in agranular vesicles, 30–60 nm in diameter, and is released by exocytosis into the junctional cleft of the autonomic ganglion. Like the ACh released from motor nerve endings, it is hydrolyzed by AChE, and the resultant choline is actively taken up by the nerve terminal. Unlike norepinephrine (NE), the re-uptake of ACh itself into the nerve terminal does not occur. A small fraction of ACh that may diffuse away from the junctional cleft is hydrolyzed by cholinesterase in the effector tissue or in the circulation. Release of ACh triggers excitatory junction potentials (14) that possess a longer latency and time course (100–200 msec) than those of skeletal muscle end-plate potentials. Histochemical and immunohistochemical localization of AChE and choline acetyltransferase, as well as autoradiographic methods that can visualize muscarinic receptors, have aided in the understanding of the distribution of cholinergic autonomic neurons and nerve terminals.

Neuropeptides

The nerve fibers and neurons of the IML and IMM cell columns are also the site of activity for several of the currently known 60 neuropeptides that act as neuromodulators or cotransmitters. A neuromodulator is defined as any substance that modifies the process of neurotransmission. It may be a circulating neurohormonal substance, a locally produced agent such as histamine or bradykinin, or a substance released from the same or neighboring neurons. A neuromodulator may presynaptically increase or decrease the release, or postsynaptically alter the time course or extent of action, of the principal transmitter. A cotransmitter, on the other hand, may act by means of its own receptors to produce synergistic actions with those of the principal neurotransmitter. The presence of neuropeptides in the IML and IMM cell columns suggests that they play a role in the supraspinal or segmental modulation of autonomic reflexes (8).

Some of the neuropeptides that have been localized, among other substances, to the human lateral gray columns include the neuropeptides discussed in the following sections (Fig. 5).

Substance P

Substance P, consisting of an 11-amino-acid residue, is the best-known member of the family of structurally related peptides known as *tachykinins* and is found in appreciable quantities in the intestine, where it may be a chemical mediator in the myenteric reflex. The peptide and its receptors are also widely distributed in the body and are involved in numerous physiologic activities, such as vasodilation, smooth muscle contraction, regulation of respiratory activity (11), stimulation of salivary secretion (53), activation of cells of the immune system (40,56,77,80) and, most importantly, as a neurotransmitter or neuromodulator in the transmission of painful stimuli from the periphery. It is a major neurotransmitter in the brain, where it plays an important memory-promoting role (45), and spinal cord. No substance P-positive preganglionic neurons are found at any level of the spinal cord, but im-

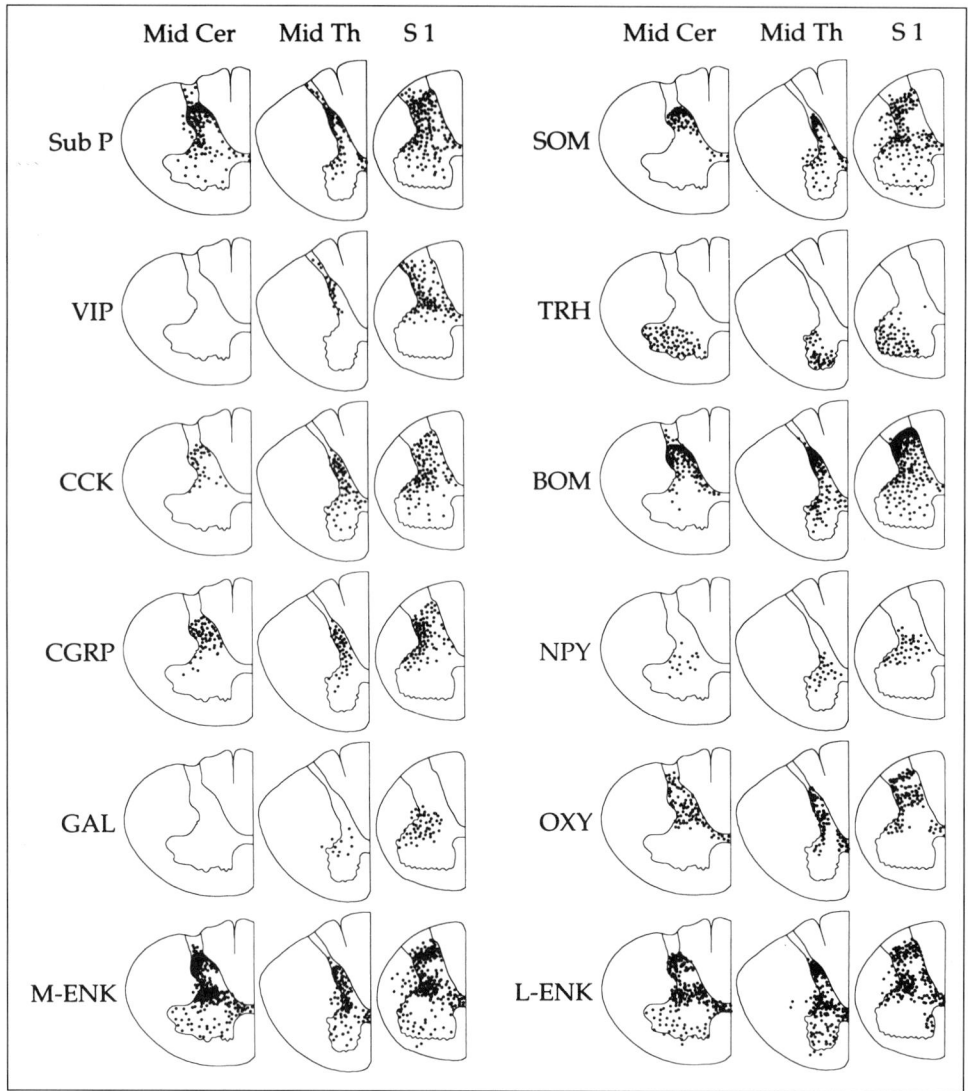

FIG. 5. The concentration of different neuropeptides in the spinal cord at the midcervical, midthoracic, and upper sacral levels. (*Cer* = cervical; *TH* = thoracic; *Sub P* = substance P; *VIP* = vasoactive intestinal peptide; *CCK* = cholecystokinin; *CGRP* = calcitonin gene-related peptide; *GAL* = galanin; *M-ENK* = met-enkephalin; *SOM* = somatostatin; *TRH* = thyrotropin-releasing hormone; *BOM* = bombesin; *NPY* = neuropeptide Y; *OXY* = oxytocin; *L-ENK* = leu-enkephalin.)

munoreactivity exists in several known projections to these columns. Most substance P immunoreactivity in the human spinal cord is observed in the superficial dorsal horn (laminae I–III), lateral lamina V, central gray, intermediate gray, and tract of Lissauer (17). The strongest intensity is in lamina I at the lumbar level. Schoenen (98) found a dense distribution of substance P fibers to the IML cell column and the sacral parasympathetic nuclei. Immunoreactive fibers for substance P (and some other peptides) are not visible in the IML cell columns until relatively late in fetal life (weeks 20–24) (64). About 20% of the spinal and trigeminal ganglion cells, in particular the small neurons giving off nociceptive small unmyelinated (class C) or myelinated (A delta) fibers, contain substance P. With the discovery of potent substance P antagonists (66,101), it has become possible to investigate the physiologic properties of this peptide, including its distribution, synthesis, and metabolism, plus its differential effect from other tachykinins and its roles in disease states and in therapy. While the full spectrum of substance P's direct role in human preganglionic neuron function is not yet fully understood, there is evidence that substance P-mediated central inputs into preganglionic neurons play an important role in blood pressure regulation (82).

Substance P is not the only tachykinin present in mammalian tissue. Recently, two novel tachykinins, neurokinin A (also called neurokinin α, substance K, or neuromedin L) and neurokinin B (also called neurokinin β or neuromedin K), have been isolated from the porcine spinal cord. In human spinal cord, substance K may coexist with substance P in some primary sensory neurons. The function of substance K remains to be determined, although a central role on the expression of male sexual behavior has been demonstrated in rats (24). Its receptor was the first neural polypeptide receptor to be cloned (71).

Somatostatin

Somatostatin is a 14-amino-acid polypeptide with an extremely short half-life. It is primarily secreted in the hypothalamus, where it suppresses anterior pituitary growth hormone secretion, and in the delta cells of the islets of Langerhans, where it depresses secretion of insulin and glucagon. In mammals, somatostatin exists in two forms: somatostatin 14 and an NH_2 terminally extended form, somatostatin 28.

Cell bodies immunoreactive for somatostatin are demonstrated in the IML column and lamina II beginning in fetal week 20 in humans and are present in all the subsequent ages studied (64). It also has a broad distribution within the central nervous system (CNS). In the brain, somatostatin modulates the release of various neurotransmitters and hormones (43). There is also evidence of a role for somatostatin as a CNS neurotransmitter with effects on locomotion and cognitive functions (87). The distribution of somatostatin in the human spinal cord generally resembles that of lower vertebrates and is very similar to that observed in primates. Many somatostatin-positive terminals are observed in the sacral parasympathetic IML nucleus, but only a few of these structures are present in the sympathetic nuclei (32,99). Sacral spine preganglionic parasympathetic neurons also contain somatostatin. The role of somatostatin in the parasympathetic outflow is unclear. There is evidence to suggest that somatostatin exerts a vasodepressive effect through presynaptic inhibition of sympathetic outflow to the blood vessels (88).

Vasoactive Intestinal Polypeptide

Vasoactive intestinal polypeptide (VIP), a "gastrointestinal" 28-amino-acid residue polypeptide that is also a neurotransmitter or neuromodulator with excitatory and inhibitory functions, is almost entirely localized to the sacral cord, in particular the superficial dorsal horn, the intermediate zone, the gray matter adjacent to the central canal, and the small dorsal root ganglion cells. Some VIP-positive fibers cross the midline through the dorsal and ventral commissures, and the ventrally coursing fibers arborize within the region of the sacral parasympathetic nuclei (17,32). Besides the spinal cord, VIP is widely distributed in the bipolar neurons of the cerebral cortex, the median eminence of the hypothalamus, intramural ganglion cells of the intestinal wall, and sympathetic ganglia. Because VIP exists in a variety of functionally different somatic and autonomic neurons, no single function can be attributed to this potent peptide (18). The prominent concentration of VIP in lumbosacral segments, however, suggests that it is probably a major neurotransmitter in the pelvic visceral pathways. VIP, nitric oxide (NO), and ACh are colocalized in the penile nerves, and their synergistic interaction is important for penile vasodilation and erection (34). There have also been claims that VIP is a cotransmitter with ACh in parasympathetic nerves supplying the salivary glands in cats (59). There is evidence that ACh elicits secretion mainly by directly stimulating the secretory cells in the gland, but VIP causes vasodilation mainly by relaxing smooth muscle cells around blood vessels (51). In the adrenal cortex, VIP is thought to act as an agonist that either potentiates the steroidogenic response to adrenocorticotropic hormone or exerts a direct steroidogenic action (27). As will be discussed later, VIP has also been identified in many branches of human vagus nerve.

Thyrotropin-Releasing Hormone

Thyrotropin-releasing hormone (TRH) is a hypothalamic tripeptide that regulates the release of thyrotropin (thyroid-stimulating hormone) and prolactin by the anterior pituitary. It is widespread throughout the CNS of mammals. Although the highest concentrations of TRH in the human spinal cord are at the lamina IX level, which contains motor neurons, a low to moderate density of TRH fiber networks has been described in the thoracic IML cell column (10,32,52,63,114). The presence of TRH terminals in the IML cell column of humans, however, has not been observed by others (17), and the innervation of the sacral parasympathetic cell column has been shown to be relatively sparse (32). At least in rats, TRH in the IML cell column can coexist with either serotonin or substance P, or both, in fibers and terminals apposed to preganglionic sympathetic neurons (5). The exact role of TRH in the ANS is not very clear. There is evidence that caudal raphe nuclei regulate vagal activity to the viscera through projections containing TRH and serotonin (103). It is also well established that intravenous administration of TRH increases heart rate and blood pressure, and also acts to induce catecholamine secretion from the adrenal medulla (54). However, the exact sympathetic pathways that mediate this response are not well established.

Cholecystokinin

Cholecystokinins (CCKs), hormones related to gastrin, are synthesized in the duodenum and cause secretion of pancreatic juice and the ejection of bile. Of several types of CCKs with different amino acid residues, only CCK 58 and CCK 8 have been found in nerve tissues, with CCK 8 being the most abundant. These two CCKs are broadly distributed in the human CNS, especially in the cerebral cortex, hippocampus, amygdala, and substantia nigra (20). There is a dense network of CCK-immunoreactive small to medium-sized fibers in the superficial dorsal horn of the spinal cord and in the IML cell column, but a lesser density in the ventral horn. Unlike substance P and bombesin, CCK immunoreactivity is mainly concentrated in the thoracic and lumbar spinal levels (17,98). The exact role of CCK in the ANS is unclear. There is evidence to suggest a neuromodulatory effect on the release of other neurotransmitters (20).

Bombesin

Bombesin, a 14-amino-acid peptide, was originally isolated from some European amphibians (*Bombina bombina*) (3). It is similar to substance P in that it depolarizes dorsal horn neurons. The spinal distribution of bombesin has been demonstrated for humans and is very similar to that of substance P, but has a greater intensity (17). Bombesinlike neuropeptides (e.g., gastrin-releasing peptides and neuromedins) have been demonstrated in nonhuman mammals, with the highest distribution in the dorsal horn and dorsal root ganglion cells (35). Bombesin is thought to act primarily as a neuromodulator that stimulates sympathetic release of epinephrine and decreases appetite by releasing CCK (13).

Calcitonin Gene-Related Peptide

Calcitonin gene-related peptide (CGRP), a 37-amino-acid peptide produced by alternate processing of the primary transcript of the calcitonin gene, is one of the first novel bioactive peptides to be discovered by the technique of molecular genetics (91). CGRP is widely distributed in the CNS and peripheral nervous system (39), and is colocalized with other peptides, including substance P, CCK, somatostatin, and VIP, and with NO. It plays a key role in the transfer of nociceptive messages from primary afferent fibers to spinothalamic neurons (12,95). CGRP in humans exists in two forms: CGRP I (or α) and CGRP II (or β). They differ by only one amino acid residue, and both are potent vasodilators (81). CGRP concentrations are greatest in the dorsal part of the spinal cord, with smaller concentrations in the ventral spinal cord, pituitary gland, and hypothalamus and very low concentrations in the cerebral cortex (106). There are few CGRP-containing fibers in the thoracic IML cell column, but they are more numerous in the sacral parasympathetic region (32). Although the exact role of CGRP in autonomic function is not known, its depletion in the dorsal and lateral gray columns of the spinal cord, along with substance P and substance K, has been reported in the context of multiple-system atrophy (2). There is also mounting evidence of a major role for CGRP, in close conjunction with NO, in modulating nonadrenergic and noncholinergic vasodilation (42).

Neuropeptide Y

Neuropeptide Y (NPY), a polypeptide containing 36 amino acid residues, belongs to the pancreatic polypeptide family. It is present in many parts of the brain, where it is the most abundant peptide, and in the ANS (83). At the human thoracic and sacral spine levels, large heavily varicosed fibers have been demonstrated that are closely associated with nonimmunoreactive preganglionic neurons (32). Much of the NPY in the ANS, however, is located in noradrenergic neurons, where it functions as a cotransmitter of NE and ATP. There is evidence that it is stored separately from NE in large nondense vesicles at the nerve endings (29). NPY is primarily localized in sympathetic neurons innervating the blood vessels, the heart, and the vas deferens (7). The predominant role of NPY is in creating and maintaining long-lasting peripheral vasoconstriction in situations of high sympathetic activity, such as stress (118). This is achieved through direct effect of NPY on smooth muscle as a cotransmitter, and also secondary to the neuromodulatory action of prejunctional reduction of the release of NE and ATP, and postjunctional potentiating effect on NE-induced vasoconstriction (15,62). There is mounting evidence in support of a role of NPY in essential hypertension (16,26,68).

Galanin

Galanin is a peculiar 29/30-amino-acid neuropeptide that was first described in 1983 (104) and that does not belong to any known peptide family. It is abundant throughout the nervous system, with high concentrations in the hypothalamus, locus coeruleus, and the hippocampus (6). Galanin has few immunoreactive fibers in the thoracic IML cell column and a moderate number of fibers in the sacral parasympathetic region (32). It is also known to coexist with epinephrine and NE in the sympathetic nerves innervating the pancreas. This coexistence, along with the fact that epinephrine mediates the stress-induced inhibition of insulin secretion, suggest a possible role for galanin in the response to stress (25). Other actions of galanin include impairment of cognitive skills (19) and stimulation of feeding (55). In the spinal cord, galanin acts as an antinociceptive substance, whose gene expression is upregulated by lesions of peripheral branches of primary sensory neurons, and that may play an important role in the control of nervous impulses that underlie pain states that occur after peripheral nerve injury (112).

Oxytocin

Oxytocin is a 9-amino-acid peptide synthesized in hypothalamic cells that project either to the neurohypophysis or to sites within the CNS. Its primary functions are stimulation of uterine contraction and lactation in females. Its role in the CNS appears to be that of a neuroregulator that induces maternal and reproductive behaviors, and influences the formation of social bonds (41). Although oxytocin-positive fibers are found in laminae I, III, IV, and X, there are conflicting reports of its presence in the IML cell columns (47,57,98,102). At least a few descending fibers terminate in the IML cell columns, the central gray area, and the marginal zone of the dorsal horns (47). Oxytocin (and vasopressin)-containing fibers, which connect the brain paraventricular nuclei and the spinal autonomic centers, may participate in the regulation of processes in the periphery in which these peptides are also involved, such as control of blood pressure and lactation.

Enkephalins

The enkephalins are a group of peptides ("naturally occurring opiates"), two of which—methionine enkephalin and leucine enkephalin—have been extensively studied in different parts of the nervous system. These two enkephalins act as endogenous ligands for opiate receptors and can induce analgesia if infused into appropriate areas of the brainstem. At the spinal cord level, immunoreactive fibers for enkephalins are most numerous in the lateral region of lamina II and are thinner than those containing substance P (17,99). Both thoracic and sacral autonomic cell groups also contain a dense innervation of enkephalin-positive, thicker fibers. Most of these fibers arise from the dorsolateral white matter. There is also a small to moderate number of fibers in other laminae. Occasional small and predominantly bipolar immunoreactive perikarya are seen at the dorsal horn level, especially lamina II (17,32). The general distribution of enkephalin immunoreactivity, however, is consistent at all levels of the spinal cord in comparatively similar quantities. The immunoreactive fibers appear between 20 and 24 weeks of gestation (64) and by week 32 are well visualized (98).

Of different opiate receptors (μ, δ, κ, and σ), only the μ- and δ-receptors have some effect on autonomic function. Their agonists have little effect on the resting autonomic outflow, but appear to modulate certain evoked autonomic reflexes, such as pain-evoked changes in cardiovascular activity, volume-evoked micturition reflex, and gastrointestinal motility (115).

Nitric Oxide

NO is an ubiquitous free radical that has long been suspected to have important biological activity. This was first confirmed when NO was identified as the molecule responsible for endothelium-derived relaxing factor activity (31). Subsequently, an explosion of interest and knowledge has identified NO to be a major neuronal messenger (109) with a wide distribution in a variety of CNS neurons. The localization of NO was greatly facilitated when it was discovered that NO synthase [the enzyme that generates NO from L-arginine (70)] immunoreactivity and NADPH-diaphorase staining are very intimately colocalized in the CNS (21) and, subsequently, NO synthase was identified as the enzyme responsible for this strong neuronal NADPH-diaphorase histochemical reaction (44,110).

In human CNS, NO synthase is found in the cortex (96), subcortical white matter (67), striatum (93), hypothalamus (94), and brainstem (9,50). It is also widely present in the spinal cord, where NO synthase immunoreactivity was found in laminae I and II, in the ventral horn, and in the dorsal root ganglia, as well as in the IML cell column at the thoracic levels (100,105). In the latter location, NADPH-diaphorase-reactive sympathetic preganglionic neurons form interconnected clusters (Fig. 6). The abundance of NADPH-diaphorase-reactive neurons in the human IML suggests a role for NO release from preganglionic terminals in the regulation of sympathetic outflow to various target organs (100). This is supported by the identification of abundant NO-containing fibers in the sympathetic ganglia in rats (4). Postganglionic NO-mediated neuroeffector transmission has also been demonstrated in human bladder

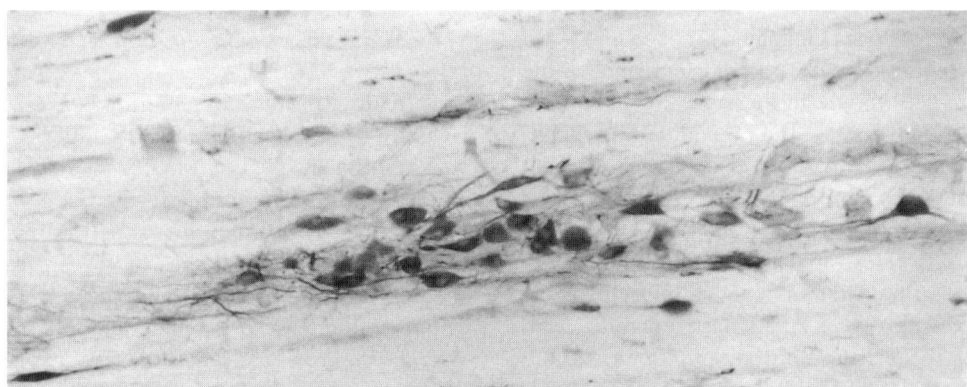

FIG. 6. Sagittal section from T1 segment of human spinal cord demonstrates NADPH Diaphorase positive intreconnected clusters of sympathetic preganglionic neurons (Reproduced with permission from Ref. 100.)

and respiratory tract, as well as in a variety of organs in animals (85). There is now mounting evidence for an important role for NO in neuronal toxicity, particularly in several neurodegenerative disorders with autonomic failure (22, 100). The elucidation of the various functions of NO as a neurotransmitter promises to yield exciting new information, but is compounded by the fact that NO synthase frequently coexists with other neurotransmitters, including glutamate, γ-aminobutyric acid, serotonin, acetylcholine, catecholamines, and a variety of neuropeptides (108).

SYMPATHETIC RELAY GANGLIA

A ganglion (meaning "knot" in Greek) is a group of nerve cell bodies located outside the CNS. The sympathetic ganglia include collections of cells on the sympathetic trunks (paravertebral ganglia), prevertebral ganglia in the autonomic plexuses, and the intermediate ganglia. Sympathetic ganglia are extremely complex, both anatomically and pharmacologically. Each ganglion is invested by a fairly dense fibrous connective tissue capsule that is continuous with the epineurium of the pre- and postganglionic nerve trunks. Their neurons are multipolar (20–60 μm in diameter) and receive cholinergic synapses from a variable number of preganglionic fibers. Conversely, each preganglionic fiber synapses with several neurons. Preganglionic axons lose their myelin sheath before they reach the cell bodies. Besides relatively large neurons with ovoid or spherical nuclei, delicate neurofibrils, and abundant rough endoplasmic reticulum, each sympathetic ganglion contains a smaller percentage of a second smaller cell type that is intensely fluorescent, resembles the cells of the adrenal medulla and, like those, gives a positive chromaffin reaction [small intensely fluorescent (SIF) cells]. SIF cells are known to exist singly or in richly vascularized, compact clusters of varying sizes (65). Although they are known to contain many peptides, the exact role of SIF cells in the overall functioning of the sympathetic nervous system is still not completely understood. Claims that they may represent interneurons situated between pre- and postganglionic elements have not been fully substantiated. Similarly, their role as endocrinelike, dopamine-containing cells, at least in humans, is not clear. Such a role was recently supported by morphologic evidence of the existence of an SIF-cell nodule in the superior mesenteric ganglia of six fetuses (116). The SIF-cell nodule was encapsulated by dense connective tissue and contained afferent blood vessels and nerves.

Embryologically, ganglion cells are derived from the neural crest that proliferates rapidly to form a bilateral series of oval-shaped primordial spinal ganglia, which migrate laterally and ventrally. A small part separates from the ventral regions of each primordial spinal ganglia and migrates toward the sides of the aorta to form the sympathochromaffin cells of the sympathetic trunk ganglia. Some of the cells of the thoracic and upper lumbar regions migrate still farther and eventually form subsidiary prevertebral sympathetic ganglia, such as the celiac, superior mesenteric, and renal, or contribute to the cells of the medulla of the adrenal glands.

There are usually 10–12 thoracic ganglia, 4 lumbar, and 4–5 sacral (Fig. 7). The cervical sympathetic ganglia are fused to form three interconnected ganglia: the superior, middle, and cervicothoracic (stellate). A true inferior cervical ganglion exists in 20% of humans.

Cervical Sympathetic Ganglia

The Superior Cervical Ganglion

The superior cervical ganglion is the largest of the cervical sympathetic ganglia, ~2.5–3.0 cm long, and contains >1 million large neurons (78). The preganglionic fibers for this ganglion emerge in the white rami communicantes of the uppermost thoracic spinal nerves and ascend to it in the cervical sympathetic trunk. An unknown number of preganglionic fibers pass without interruption through this ganglion and relay at a higher level in the internal carotid ganglia. The superior cervical ganglion sends gray rami communicantes (postganglionic fibers) to the upper four cervical spinal nerves, as well as branches to the inferior and superior vagal ganglia and hypoglossal nerve, inferior glossopharyngeal ganglion, carotid body, superior jugular bulb, and associated jugular glomus, and some branches to the posterior cranial fossa meninges. The right and left cardiac branches take a different course in the neck and thorax, but both contribute to the formation of the cardiac plexus on the ascending aorta and the aortic arch. The superior cervical ganglion also sends branches to the common, internal, and external carotid arteries, forming a delicate plexus that extends to some of the divisions of the external carotid artery (e.g., facial artery and middle meningeal artery) and reaches to the salivary gland, otic ganglion, and facial ganglion. The fibers of the facial sweat glands leave the branches of the external carotid artery to join the trigeminal nerve branches before reaching the sweat glands.

The Middle Cervical Ganglion

The middle cervical ganglion is a small ganglion that is usually formed from the fusion of the fifth and sixth cervical ganglia. It exists normally in ~60% of individuals, is ~0.7–0.8 cm long and is located at about the level of the sixth cervical vertebra, just superior to the inferior thyroid artery. Its visceral branches supply the thyroid and parathyroid glands, esophagus, and trachea. At least the nerve fibers to the thyroid gland contain NPY, which may stimulate hormone secretion (90). The cardiac branch arising from this ganglion is the largest sympathetic cardiac nerve contributing to the cardiac plexus. This ganglion contributes postganglionic gray rami communicantes to the fifth and sixth cervical nerves and sometimes also to the

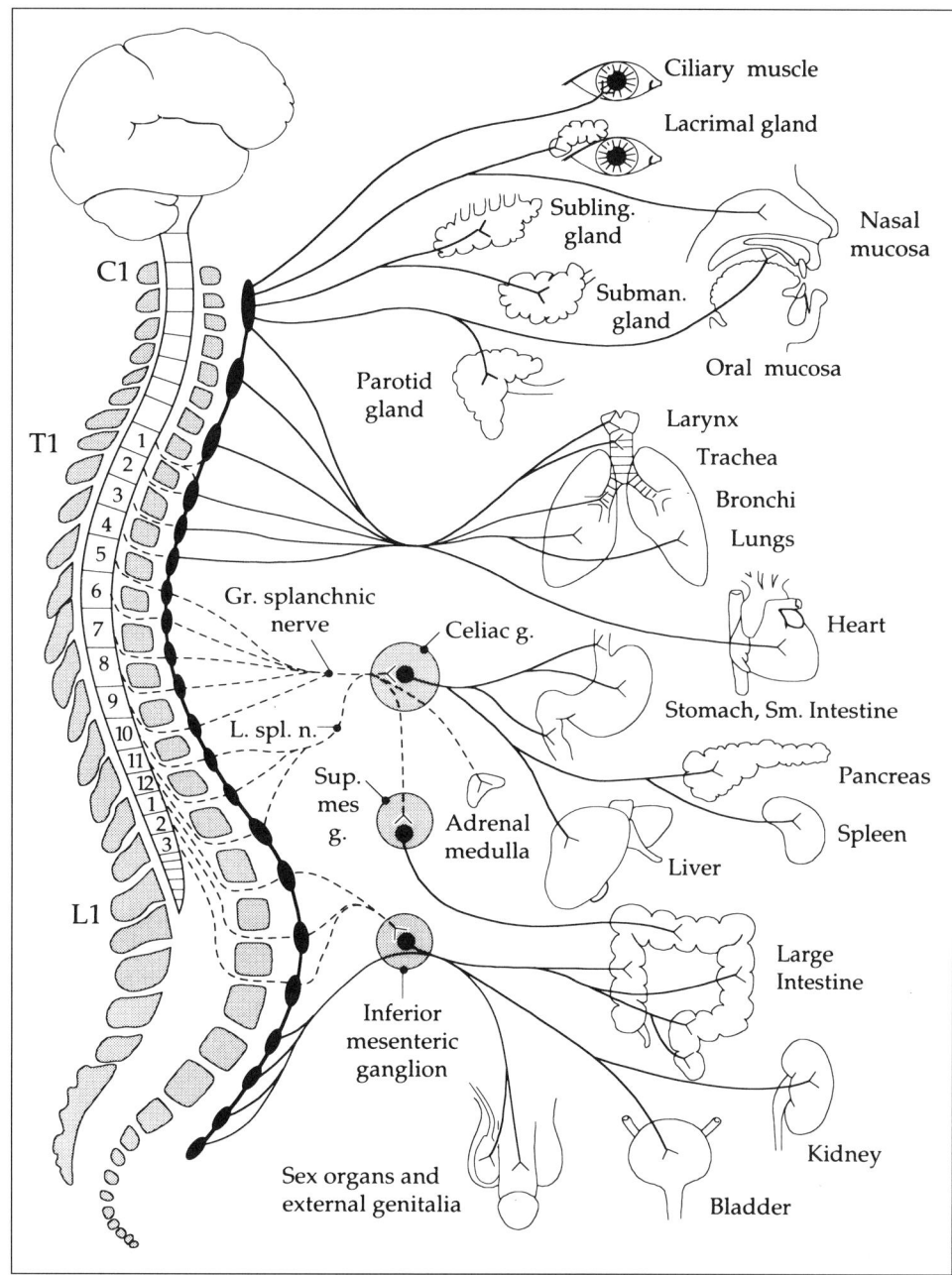

FIG. 7. Sympathetic innervation of different organs (*dotted lines*), preganglionic myelinated fibers (*solid lines*), and postganglionic unmyelinated fibers. (*L. spl. n.* = lesser splanchnic nerve; *Sup. mes. g.* = superior mesenteric ganglion; *g* = ganglion.)

fourth and seventh. There are fine connections between this ganglion, the phrenic nerve, the recurrent laryngeal nerves, and possibly the vagus nerve.

The Cervicothoracic Ganglion

The cervicothoracic (stellate) ganglion is an irregularly fusiform ganglion that is formed by the fusion of the lower two cervical and first and sometimes the second thoracic ganglia. It is 2.8 cm long and is anterior to the seventh cervical transverse process and the neck of the first rib. It is posterior to the origin of the vertebral artery, the first part of the subclavian artery, and the apex of the lung. The cervicothoracic ganglion sends gray rami communicantes to the seventh and eighth cervical and first thoracic spinal nerves, a cardiac branch to the cardiac plexus, and branches to the nearby vessels, phrenic nerve, and sometimes the vagus nerve. The branches to the vertebral arteries extend to the basilar artery and as far as the posterior cerebral arteries, where they meet a plexus from the internal carotid. The resulting vertebral plexus is considered the main intracranial extension of the sympathetic system. The preganglionic fibers for the upper limbs originate from the IML cell columns of the T2–T6 segments and ascend by means of the sympathetic trunk to synapse in the cervicothoracic ganglion. From there, postganglionic fibers enter the lower trunk of the brachial plexus, pass mainly into the medial cord, and then extend into the median and ulnar nerves and, to a lesser extent, into other branches of the plexus. An injury to the lower trunk of the brachial plexus, therefore, is more likely to cause vasomotor or sudomotor disturbances than is a lesion of the upper plexus. The second and third thoracic ventral roots contain most of the vasoconstrictor fibers for the upper limb, and interruption of the sympathetic trunk below the third thoracic ganglion results in near-complete sympathetic denervation of the upper limb. In Telford's operation for sympathectomy, besides cutting the sympathetic trunk below the third thoracic ganglion, the rami communicantes connected with the second and third thoracic ganglia are also severed. Generally, in sympathectomies, the ganglia are removed or preganglionic fibers are cut, rather than the postganglionic fibers, because the latter may regenerate (113).

Thoracic Paravertebral Ganglia

The thoracic paravertebral ganglia are longitudinally connected ganglia found at the side of and near the vertebrae (see Fig. 3). Eleven pairs of thoracic ganglia can be identified in >70% of individuals, the first of which is usually fused with the inferior cervical ganglion, forming the stellate ganglion. The thoracic ganglia are relatively small, each containing ~90,000–100,000 neurons. Fine branches from the upper fifth or sixth thoracic ganglia contribute to the thoracic aortic, pulmonary, cardiac, and esophageal plexuses, and the large branches of the lower sixth or seventh ganglia supply the aorta and also form the greater, lesser, and least splanchnic nerves. The noradrenergic neurons giving rise to cardiac branches also contain NPY, which may excite the cardiac muscle directly as well as inhibit the vagal postganglionic neurons within the heart. The greater splanchnic nerve consists mainly of myelinated preganglionic efferent and visceral afferent fibers, and ends mainly in the celiac ganglion but also in the aortorenal ganglion and the adrenal gland. The lesser splanchnic nerve ends in the aortorenal ganglion, and the least splanchnic (renal) nerve terminates in the renal plexus. Of the different splanchnic nerves, only the greater splanchnic nerve is present in all individuals; the lesser is found in 94% and the least in 56% (48).

Lumbar Sympathetic Ganglia

The lumbar ganglia are extraordinarily variable in number, but there are usually four. They are located retroperitoneally and anterior to the spinal column, and along the medial margin of the psoas major muscle, contributing extensively to the rich sympathetic innervation of the abdominal and pelvic cavities. On average, each ganglion contains 60,000–85,000 nerve cell bodies. Of these neurons, ~75% are noradrenergic, about half also contain NPY (60), and a very small percentage also contain somatostatin (46). The remaining 25% of neurons represent cholinergic sympathetic neurons, and some also contain VIP and CGRP.

Virtually all sympathetic plexuses in the abdomen receive branches from the lumbar ganglia via the four lumbar splanchnic nerves. Vascular branches to the iliac arteries and proximal femoral arteries originate from all lumbar ganglia and pass to the aortic and renal plexuses. Many NE- and NPY-containing postganglionic fibers of the lumbar ganglia travel in the femoral and obturator nerves and their branches, and provide vasoconstrictor nerve fibers to their corresponding arteries. Beyond the proximal thigh, the sympathetic nerve supply to the lower limb is largely uncertain. Sympathetic denervation of lower-limb vessels, however, is usually achieved by removing the upper three lumbar ganglia and severing all preganglionic fibers to the limb.

Pelvic Sympathetic Trunk

There are four or five small, interconnected pelvic sympathetic ganglia. The right and left sympathetic chains meet and fuse at the coccygeal level. They contribute extensively to the inferior hypogastric (pelvic) plexus. No white rami communicantes are present at the sacral trunk ganglia level, but each ganglion supplies one or more gray rami communicantes containing postganglionic sympathetic fibers to the sacral and coccygeal spinal nerves. The pelvic plexuses are located on each side of the rectum and lower part of the bladder, and supply branches to the pelvic viscera and genitalia. These branches contain postganglionic fibers but also afferent sensory fibers. The details of the functional anatomy of the pelvic plexuses in humans are still incomplete and are best described in relation to the organs they innervate.

Plexuses of the Autonomic Nervous System

A detailed description of the many autonomic plexuses located in the thoracic, abdominal, and pelvic cavities is beyond the scope of this chapter. It is sufficient to mention that the cardiac, pulmonary, celiac, and hypogastric plexuses, which are aggregates of nerves and ganglia, are somewhat continuous and interconnected by their extensions, which pass along most branches of the large vessels. Many of these extensions are named after the blood vessels (e.g., the superior mesenteric plexus and the hypogastric plexus).

PARASYMPATHETIC NERVOUS SYSTEM

The peripheral part of the parasympathetic nervous system (craniosacral outflow) consists of the autonomic fibers that arise from cranial nerves III, VII, IX, and X, as well as those from the IML horns of the spinal cord at the origin of the second, third, and fourth sacral nerves (Fig. 8). The parasympathetic preganglionic neurons give rise to relatively long myelinated preganglionic fibers that synapse with postganglionic neurons in the many small ganglia located near or within the wall of individual innervated organs. In contrast to the sympathetic fibers, the postganglionic parasympathetic fibers are therefore short (1 mm to several centimeters). The ratio of preganglionic to postganglionic neurons, in contrast to the sympathetic system, is usually much smaller: 1:15–1:20. The disparity between the sympathetic and parasympathetic systems in the ratio of preganglionic to postganglionic neurons correlates with the wide range of sympathetic autonomic effects and the massive sympathetic outflow possible during strenuous physical activity and stressful situations. Such massive sympathetic discharges may evoke simultaneous diverse

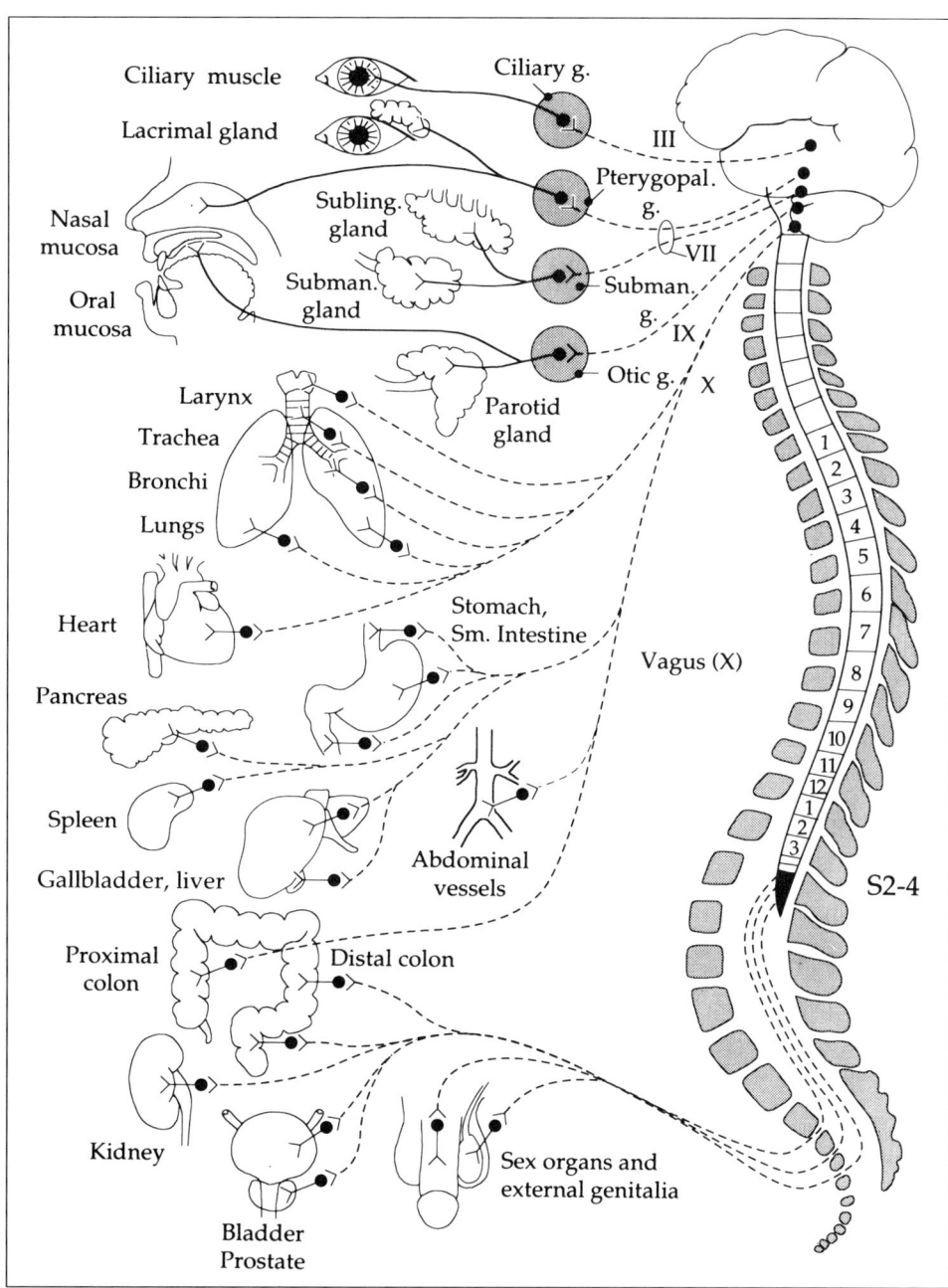

FIG. 8. Parasympathetic innervation of different organs (craniosacral outflow). (Dotted lines denote preganglionic long myelinated nerve fibers, and solid lines, postganglionic short unmyelinated fibers.)

responses, including increases in arterial pressure, blood flow to active muscles, muscle glycolysis, cellular metabolic rate, blood glucose concentration, muscle strength, and mental activity, as well as contraction of sphincters and decreased gastrointestinal peristalsis. A disorder that predominantly affects the sympathetic nervous system may therefore render the body incapable of dealing appropriately with strenuous physical or emotional stimulation. In contrast, the smaller disproportion between the number of preganglionic and postganglionic neurons in the parasympathetic system promotes a more localized disruption and favors the very specific controlled function of the parasympathetic system.

Oculomotor Parasympathetic Fibers

The parasympathetic preganglionic fibers for the eye originate in the Edinger–Westphal oculomotor nucleus. They travel in the inferior division of the oculomotor nerve, pass through the superior orbital fissure, and exit in the motor root of the ciliary ganglion, where they synapse. The ciliary ganglion, which is <2 mm long, lies in fat-filled connective tissue in the posterior orbit, just anterior to the superior orbital fissure, and contains ~3,000 multipolar, cholinergic neurons (79). The postganglionic fibers of the ciliary ganglion cells (the short ciliary nerves) reach the globe near the optic nerve and travel between the choroid and sclera to supply the smooth muscle fibers of the iris sphincter (sphincter pupillae), the ciliary muscle, and the blood vessels. The nerve fibers in the choroid contain VIP and may contribute to the VIP innervation of the ciliary muscles and the choroidal blood vessels (69). There is also evidence for an important role of neurally derived NO in the control of choroidal blood flow (117). Both iris sphincter and ciliary muscle fibers have ACh receptors. Focusing of the eye lens is controlled almost entirely by the parasympathetic innervation of the ciliary muscles. Excitation of parasympathetic fibers caused by approaching objects provokes contraction of the ciliary muscles, which, in turn, relaxes the lens ligaments, thus allowing the lens to become more convex and thereby increasing its refractory powers. This allows the eye to keep the object constantly in focus.

The ratio of postganglionic fibers innervating the iris sphincter to fibers innervating the ciliary muscles is ~30:1. This ratio is an important anatomic basis for light–near dissociation (see Chapter 34).

Facial Parasympathetic Fibers

The facial parasympathetic fibers originate in the superior salivatory nucleus near the motor nucleus and travel via the nervous intermedius of Wrisberg, often called "the sensory root" of the facial nerve. These preganglionic fibers are destined for the submandibular ganglion, which has postganglionic connections to the submandibular and sublingual glands, and for the pterygopalatine ganglion (sphenopalatine ganglion), which has postganglionic connections to the glands of the palatal and nasal mucosa as well as the lacrimal glands. The sensory root also contains many parasympathetic efferent fibers that, when stimulated, cause vasodilation of vessels in the areas supplied by the facial nerve.

The pterygopalatine ganglion is small (3 mm long) and contains ~56,500 closely packed, ovoid neurons with dense dendritic connections (78). Most of these neurons stain strongly for AChE and contain VIP and its gene-related peptide: peptide histidine methionine (PHM) (61). The ACh- and VIP-containing postganglionic fibers originating from this ganglion provide vasodilatory and secretory input to a number of arteries, veins, and glands of the face, nasal and oral mucosa, tongue, eyes, and cerebral arteries. Because the vasodilatory responses are largely unaffected by atropine, this may suggest an important role for VIP and PHM coreleased with ACh (59). The postganglionic neurons of the submandibular ganglion are also strongly AChE positive, and at least some contain VIP and PHM (61,107). VIP and PHM may modify the content of human salivary proteins, such as amylase (52).

Glossopharyngeal Parasympathetic Fibers

The glossopharyngeal nerve (cranial nerve IX) is closely related anatomically and physiologically to the vagus nerve (Fig. 9). Its autonomic pathways also have several features in common with the facial nerve. It has 3–5 slender fila, or rootlets, as it emerges from the medulla in a groove between the olive and the inferior cerebellar peduncle above the rootlets of the vagus nerve. The glossopharyngeal and vagus nerves share common nuclei of origin, but the glossopharyngeal nerve also carries parasympathetic secretomotor fibers from the inferior salivatory nuclei. The glossopharyngeal nerve is a mixed nerve containing motor fibers that extend to the stylopharyngeus muscle, parasympathetic secretomotor fibers that travel to the parotid gland, and sensory fibers that go to the pharynx, tonsils, and posterior tongue. The nerve leaves the skull through the central part of the jugular foramen. It has two ganglia: superior and inferior. The smaller superior ganglion is situated at the jugular foramen and has no branches; the larger inferior ganglion lies in the lower border of the petrous bone and has many branches, including the tympanic, carotid, pharyngeal, muscular, tonsillar, and lingual branches. The unipolar cells of these ganglia convey gustatory and tactile sensation from the posterior third of the tongue and general sensation from the posterior tongue, fauces, tonsils, nasopharynx, inferior surface of the soft palate, uvula, eustachian tube, and tympanic cavity. The sensory branch also innervates a small cutaneous area in front of the tragus, together with a small area of the adja-

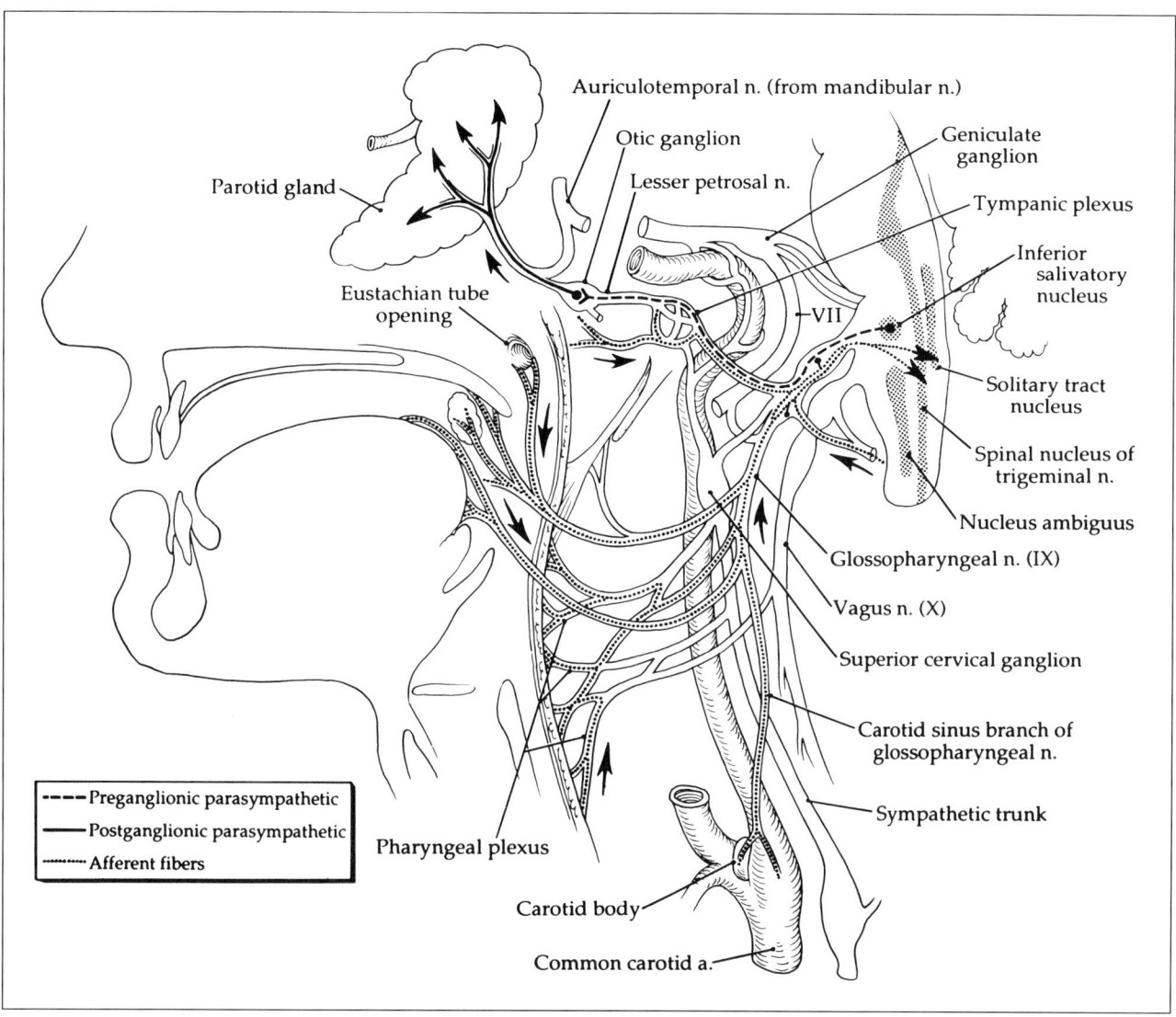

FIG. 9. The course and distribution of the major branches of the glossopharyngeal nerve and its relationship to the vagus nerve. (*n* = nerve.)

cent anterior wall of the outer auditory meatus. In the upper neck, the glossopharyngeal nerve lies in front of the vagus nerve and passes between the internal carotid artery and internal jugular vein, before passing superficially to the internal carotid artery behind the styloid process. It then travels across the lateral surface of the stylopharyngeus muscle, which plays a role in elevating the pharynx, and between the constrictors of the pharynx. The motor branches to the stylopharyngeus muscle are believed to originate in the nucleus ambiguus.

Of the branches of the glossopharyngeal nerve, two are of particular importance in the ANS: the branch to the carotid sinus and body, and the branch to the otic ganglion. The carotid sinus nerve, which arises just below the jugular foramen and descends on the internal carotid artery, contains the primary afferent fibers of the chemoreceptors in the carotid body (carotid glomus) and of the baroreceptors lying in the carotid sinus wall. These fibers project to the neurons at the middle third of the nucleus tractus solitarius and show a graded increase in impulse traffic as the partial pressure of oxygen is lowered or the partial pressure of carbon dioxide is raised in the blood flow to the carotid body. The carotid bodies are also innervated by a plexus of other glossopharyngeal nerve branches, vagal and sympathetic (from the superior cervical ganglion) components. Each carotid body contains islands of two types of cells: type I (glomus cells) and type II (probably glial cells), surrounded by fenestrated sinusoidal capillaries. Unmyelinated endings of glossopharyngeal nerve fibers are found at intervals between type I and II cells. Although there is no consensus, these nerve endings are believed to be involved in chemoreception and in sensing oxygen tension.

These functions are believed to be primarily mediated by NO (37) and substance P (84).

The carotid sinus, a small dilation in the internal carotid artery just below the common carotid bifurcation into the external and internal carotid branches, receives intertwined and extensively branched myelinated nerve-fiber endings of the carotid sinus nerve, which innervate baroreceptors. The impulses generated by these receptors in response to the absolute level of, and changes in, arterial pressure reach the tractus solitarius in the medullary area via the carotid sinus nerve branch of the glossopharyngeal nerve.

The glossopharyngeal nerve branch to the otic ganglion serves as the anatomic connection between the intracranial pathways of this nerve and those of the facial nerve. It contains preganglionic parasympathetic secretomotor fibers for the parotid glands, originating in the inferior salivatory nucleus. The fibers reach the otic ganglion via the tympanic plexus and the lesser petrosal nerve. Additional preganglionic fibers to the otic ganglion may travel via the chorda tympani nerve, indicating some preganglionic input from the facial nerve. Postganglionic fibers leave the ganglion via the auriculotemporal nerve, which conveys them to the parotid gland. Some otic ganglion neurons may project directly to the vasculature of the jaw and the cerebral circulation or weakly innervate the sweat glands around the lips. The neurons of the otic ganglion and their axons stain positively for AChE, but contain few VIP-staining axons (107).

Vagus Nerve

The vagus nerve accounts for 75% of all parasympathetic nervous system activity (Fig. 10 and Table 1). It carries fibers that contain special and general visceral efferents and afferents, and provides both excitatory and inhibitory inputs to its final effectors. It has four nuclei in the medulla: the dorsal nucleus, nucleus ambiguus, nucleus solitarius, and spinal trigeminal nucleus. At least some of the neurons in these nuclei contain substance P (38). The 8–10 vagus nerve rootlets emerge from the medulla, below the glossopharyngeal nerve, at a sulcus immediately dorsal to the prominence of the inferior olive, and unite to form the nerve trunk. The trunk leaves the skull through the jugular foramen within the same dural sleeve as the glossopharyngeal and accessory nerves. Immediately outside the skull, it expands into the superior and inferior ganglia of the vagus nerve. Both ganglia are exclusively sensory, containing somatic, special visceral, and general visceral afferent neurons. All efferent fibers originating in the medulla pass uninterrupted through both ganglia. The superior (jugular) ganglion is ~4 mm in diameter and communicates with the nearby cranial roots of the accessory nerve, the inferior glossopharyngeal ganglion, the facial nerve, and the superior cervical sympathetic ganglion. Despite these connections with other cranial nerves, there is little functional evidence for the direct vagal control of any cranial structure. The second branch of the vagus nerve, the auricular branch, is in fact a somatic afferent nerve, which, after joining a ramus from the inferior ganglion of the glossopharyngeal nerve, supplies cutaneous sensory fibers to the concha of the external ear (posterior wall and floor of the external acoustic meatus and the outer surface of the tympanic membrane). Irritation of the external auditory canal and the tympanic membrane by cerumen or syringing may, therefore, cause abnormal reflexes, resulting in coughing, vomiting, or even cardiac inhibition. The inferior vagal ganglion (nodose ganglion), which is ~25 mm long and contains ~30,000 neurons, communicates with the superior sympathetic ganglion, the hypoglossal nerve, and a loop between the first and second cervical spinal nerves. It also connects with the cranial part of the accessory nerve. The pharyngeal branch, which consists chiefly of filaments from the cranial accessory nerve, is the main motor nerve of the pharynx and emerges from the upper part of the inferior vagal ganglion. Most of this ganglion's neurons are concerned with visceral sensation in the heart, lung, larynx, and gastrointestinal tract. The ganglion also gives off other branches, including those to the carotid sinus branch of the glossopharyngeal nerve and to the superior laryngeal nerve, which divides into internal (sensory) and external (motor) nerves.

Below their inferior ganglion, both vagal nerves communicate with branches of the cervical sympathetic trunks, forming a mixed parasympathetic–sympathetic network. In the neck region, the right vagus nerve gives rise to the right recurrent laryngeal nerve, which curves backward below and behind the subclavian artery and, after coursing near the medial surface of the thyroid, enters the larynx. It car-

TABLE 1. *Primary branches of the vagus nerve*

Immediately extracranial
Meningeal
Auricular
Neck
Pharyngeal
Carotid body
Superior laryngeal
Right recurrent laryngeal nerve
Cardiac
Thorax
Cardiac
Left recurrent laryngeal nerve
Pulmonary
Esophageal
Abdomen
Gastric
Celiac
Hepatic
Renal

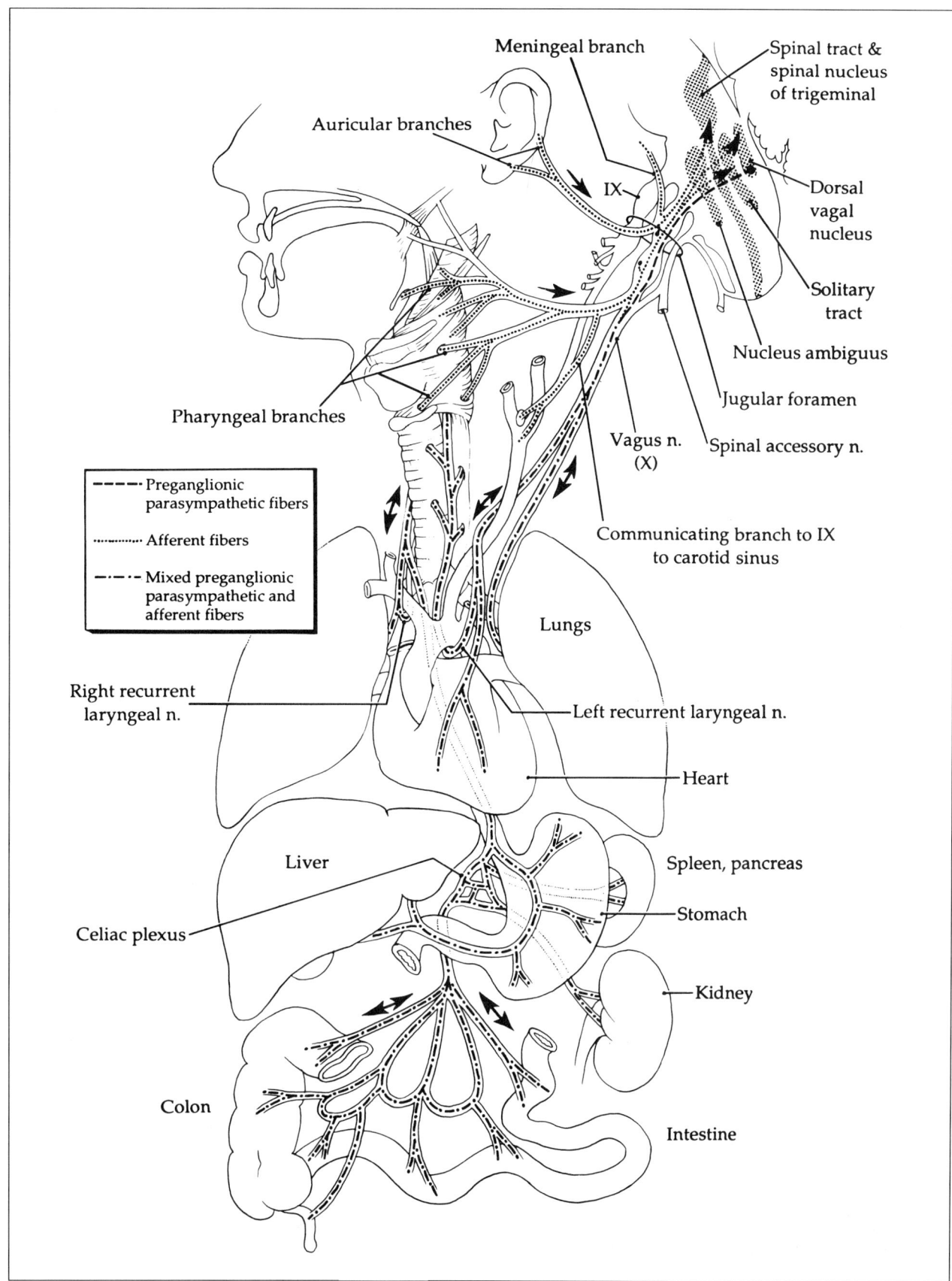

FIG. 10. The course and distribution of the major branches of the vagus nerve.

ries afferent fibers from laryngeal stretch receptors and supplies all laryngeal muscles except the cricothyroid. The left recurrent laryngeal nerve arises from the vagus nerve on the left of the aortic arch and, like the right nerve, contributes motor, sensory, glandular, and vascular fibers to the upper trachea and esophagus, and also supplies fibers to the laryngeal muscles. Both nerves also contribute fibers to the deep cardiac plexus.

The major vagal preganglionic nerve fibers to the heart travel via the branches arising from the thoracic vagal nerves, recurrent laryngeal nerves, and superior cervical rami. They richly anastomose with the cardiac sympathetic nerves, forming the ventral and dorsal cardiopulmonary plexuses. The right and left coronary cardiac nerves and the left lateral cardiac nerve emerge from these plexuses. There is substantial anatomic variation among individuals in the number and distribution of these cardiac nerves. The parasympathetic nerve fibers reach the intrinsic subpericardial ganglia, each containing from 5 to >150 neurons. The sinus node contains more of the right vagal and sympathetic fibers, and the atrioventricular node contains more left vagal and sympathetic fibers. The vagal innervation of the cardiac ventricles is largely concentrated in the conducting tissue and is less dense than that in the atria. Of the atrial ganglia cells, most are AChE positive and some also contain somatostatin (23,28). The combined effect of ACh and somatostatin is thought to be responsible for some of the effects of vagal stimulation on the human heart. VIP and enkephalinlike immunoreactivity have also been described in the axons of the atrial myocardium (86). (For further discussion on the innervation of the heart, see Chapter 4.)

The vagal preganglionic fibers to the airways and lungs travel via the posterior and anterior pulmonary branches of the vagus nerve, which, along with nerve fibers from the second to sixth thoracic sympathetic trunk, form the posterior and anterior pulmonary plexuses. Many small parasympathetic ganglia are found in the submucosal, subchondrial, and extrachondrial regions of the trachea and bronchi and near branches of the nearby blood vessels. Many of the neurons of these ganglia contain AChE and a few also contain VIP (51,74). The short postganglionic fibers that are closely associated with the submucosal secretory cells and the smooth muscles controlling the airway diameter contain VIP, which is known to relax the airway smooth muscles (73) and to act as a potent vasodilator of the pulmonary arteries (36,60).

A detailed microscopic study of the relationship of the vagus nerve to the intrinsic neurons of the alimentary tract is not available. The major vagal input to the gastrointestinal tract occurs primarily in the esophagus and stomach, but may extend to the proximal small intestine and parts of the colon (89). The esophageal branches arise above and below the pulmonary branches and form the esophageal plexuses. The striated muscles of the upper part of the esophagus are controlled by vagal motor nerves, whereas the smooth muscles of the lower part are under autonomic control. The vagal postganglionic neurons that contain VIP (1) are responsible for the relaxation of the lower esophageal sphincter.

The left vagus nerve supplies the anterior and superior parts of the stomach and the right vagal nerve supplies the posterior and inferior surfaces. A detailed description of the anatomy and physiology of the enteric nervous system and its relationship to vagal nerves may be found in the text by Furness and Costa (30). It is sufficient to mention that the vagus nerve influences both gastric motility and secretion, and that both ACh and peptide-containing neurons (in particular gastrin-releasing peptides) mediate these functions.

The distention of the gallbladder following vagotomy suggests the existence of a tonic input from the vagus nerve, mediated by intrinsic cholinergic or VIP-containing neurons or their interaction with the excitatory effects of CCK released from the duodenum (92). The branches of the vagus nerve to the gallbladder arise from hepatic branches, which in turn form the hepatic plexuses. There is probably little or no vagal input to the liver (72).

Branches of the right vagus nerve innervate the pancreatic islets. Conflicting studies suggest that stimulation of this nerve may elicit increased insulin and glucagon secretions (74). Some of the postganglionic ACh- and VIP-containing nerve endings within the pancreas provide the predominant autonomic secretomotor innervation to the pancreatic exocrine and endocrine cells [for detailed information, see Walsh (111)].

CONCLUSION

This chapter provides an overview of some aspects of the complex spinal and peripheral ANS. This system is distributed throughout the body and controls a wide range of visceral functions, in part through the interplay of its sympathetic and parasympathetic components. It is, however, not completely independent of the somatic elements of the CNS, being intimately responsive to changes in somatic activities. Additionally, the transmitters and peptides released by the unmyelinated primary sensory neurons can modify peripheral autonomic function, indicating a close relationship between the sensory neurons and the peripheral autonomic nerves. The exact roles of many of the neuropeptides identified in the ganglia and nerve endings of the human ANS are gradually being identified, further expanding our understanding of its complexity. Although the sympathetic and parasympathetic divisions of the ANS often perform as physiologic antagonists, their complementary actions are also required in many functions. Therefore, a full understanding of the peripheral ANS is not possible without an appreciation of the central autonomic and somatic nervous structures.

ACKNOWLEDGMENT

This work was made possible by the generous support of Claude and Andrea Walker and their parents from Taylor, Louisiana.

REFERENCES

1. Aggestrup S, et al. Regulatory peptides in the lower esophageal sphincter of man. *Regul Pept* 1985;10:167–178.
2. Anand P, et al. Marked depletion of dorsal spinal cord substance P and calcitonin gene-related peptide with intact skin flare responses in multiple system atrophy. *J Neurol Neurosurg Psychiatry* 1988;51:192–196.
3. Anastasi A, et al. Isolation and structure of bombesin and alytesin, two analogous active peptides from the skin of the European frog bombina and alytes. *Experientia* 1971;27: 166–167.
4. Anderson CR, et al. The distribution of nitric oxide synthase containing autonomic preganglionic terminals in the rat. *Brain Res* 1993;614:78–85.
5. Appel NM, et al. Thyrotropin releasing hormone in spinal cord: coexistence with serotonin and with substance P in fibers and terminals apposing identified preganglionic sympathetic neurons. *Brain Res* 1987;415:137–143.
6. Bedecs K, et al. Galanin: 10 years with a neuroendocrine peptide. *Int J Biochem Cell Biol* 1995;27:337–349.
7. Benarroch EE. Neuropeptides in the sympathetic system: presence, plasticity, modulation, and implications. *Ann Neurol* 1994;36:6–13.
8. Benarroch EE, et al. Segmental analysis of neuropeptide concentrations in normal human spinal cord. *Neurology* 1990;40:137–144.
9. Benarroch EE, et al. Localization and possible interactions of catecholamine and NADPH-diaphorase neurons in human medullary autonomic regions. *Brain Res* 1995;684:215–220.
10. Bennett GW, et al. Regional distribution of immunoreactive-thyrotrophin-releasing hormone and substance P, and indoleamines in human spinal cord. *J Neurochem* 1986;46:1718–1724.
11. Bonham AC. Neurotransmitters in the CNS control of breathing. *Respir Physiol* 1995;101:219–230.
12. Bourgoin S, et al. Opioidergic control of the spinal release of neuropeptides: possible significance for the analgesic effect of opioids. *Fundam Clin Pharmacol* 1994;8:307–321.
13. Bray GA. The nutrient balance hypothesis: peptides, sympathetic activity, and food intake. *Ann NY Adac Sci* 1993;676:223–241.
14. Burnstock G. Autonomic neuromuscular junctions: current developments and future directions. *J Anat* 1986;146:1–30.
15. Burnstock G, Milner P. Structural and chemical organization of the autonomic nervous system with special reference to non-adrenergic, non-cholinergic transmission. In: Bannister R, Mathias CJ, eds. *Autonomic failure: a textbook of clinical disorders of the autonomic nervous system.* 3rd ed. Oxford: Oxford Medicine, 1992:107–125.
16. Chalmers J, et al. Neuropeptide Y in the sympathetic control of blood pressure in hypertensive subjects. *Clin Exp Hypertens* 1989;11(Suppl 1):59–66.
17. Chung K, et al. Immunohistochemical localization of seven different peptides in the human spinal cord. *J Comp Neurol* 1989;280: 158–170.
18. Costa M, et al. Colocalization of VIP with other neuropeptides and neurotransmitters in the autonomic nervous system. *Ann NY Acad Sci* 1988;27:103–109.
19. Crawley JN. Functional interactions of galanin and acetylcholine: relevance to memory and Alzheimer's disease. *Behav Brain Res* 1993;57:133–141.
20. Crawley JN, Corwin RL. Biologic actions of cholecystokinin. *Peptides* 1994;15:731–755.
21. Dawson TM, et al. Nitric oxide synthase and neuronal NADPH-diaphorase are identical in brain and peripheral tissues. *Proc Natl Acad Sci USA* 1991;88:7797–7801.
22. Dawson VL, Dawson TM. Physiological and toxicological actions of nitric oxide in the central nervous system. *Adv Pharmacol* 1995;34:323–342.
23. Day S, et al. Somatostatin in the human heart and comparison with guinea-pig and rat heart. *Br Heart J* 1985;53:153–157.
24. Dornan WA, et al. Site specific effects of intracerebral injections of three neurokinins (neurokinin A, neurokinin K, and neurokinin gamma) on the expression of male rat sexual behavior. *Physiol Behav* 1993;54:249–258.
25. Drews G, et al. Non-additivity of adrenaline and galanin effects on Rb-86 efflux and membrane potential in mouse β-cells suggests sharing of common targets. *Biochem Biophys Acta* 1993;1175: 214–218.
26. Edvinsson L, et al. Increased plasma levels of neuropeptide Y-like immunoreactivity and catecholamines in severe hypertension remain after treatment to normotension in man. *Regul Pept* 1991;32: 279–287.
27. Edward AV, Jones CT. Autonomic control of adrenal function. *J Anat* 1993;183:291–307.
28. Franco-Cereceda A, et al. Somatostatin: an inhibitory parasympathetic transmitter in the human heart? *Eur J Pharmacol* 1986;132: 101–102.
29. Fried G, et al. Evidence for differential localization of noradrenaline and neuropeptide Y (NPY) in neuronal storage vesicles isolated from rat vas deferens. *J Neurosci* 1985;5:450–458.
30. Furness JB, Costa M. *The enteric nervous system.* Edinburgh: Churchill-Livingstone, 1987.
31. Garthwaite J. Glutamate, nitric oxide and cell–cell signaling in the nervous system. *Trends Neurosci* 1991;14:60–67.
32. Gibson SJ, et al. A comparison of the distributions of eight peptides in spinal cord from normal controls and cases of motor neuron disease with special reference to Onuf's nucleus. *Brain Res* 1988; 474:255–278.
33. Gilbert RFT, et al. The effects of monamine neurotoxins on peptides in the rat spinal cord. *Neuroscience* 1982;7:69–87.
34. Giuliano FA, et al. Neural control of penile erection. *Urol Clin North Am* 1995;22:747–766.
35. Go VL, Yaksh TL. Quantification of bombesin-like peptides in mammalian spinal cord. *Ann NY Acad Sci* 1988;547:70–75.
36. Greenberg B, et al. Vasoactive intestinal peptide causes non-endothelial dependent relaxation in human and bovine pulmonary arteries. *Blood Vessels* 1987;24:45–50.
37. Grimes PA, et al. Nitric oxide synthase occurs in neurons and nerve fibers of the carotid body. *Adv Exp Med Biol* 1994;360:221–224.
38. Halliday GM, et al. Distribution of substance P-like immunoreactive neurons in the human medulla oblongata: colocalization with monoamine-synthesizing neuron. *Synapse* 1988;2:353–370.
39. Harmann PA, et al. Calcitonin gene-related peptide (CGRP) in the human spinal cord a light and electron microscopic analysis. *J Comp Neurol* 1988;269:371–380.
40. Hartung H, et al. Substance P: binding properties and studies on cellular responses in guinea pig macrophages. *J Immunol* 1986;136: 3856–3863.
41. Higuchi T. Oxytocin: a neurohormone, neuroregulator, paracrine substance. *Jpn J Physiol* 1995;45:1–21.
42. Holzer P, et al. Sensory nerves, nitric oxide, and NANC vasodilation. *Arch Int Pharmacodyn Ther* 1995;329:67–79.
43. Hoyer D, et al. Molecular pharmacology of somatostatin receptors. *Naunyn Schmiedebergs Arch Pharmacol* 1994;350: 441–453.
44. Huang PL, et al. Targeted disruption of the neuronal nitric oxide synthase gene. *Cell* 1993;75:1273–1286.
45. Huston JP, Hasenohrl RU. The role of neuropeptides in learning: focus on the neurokinin substance P. *Behav Brain Res* 1995;66:117–127.
46. Järvi R, et al. Somatostatin-like immunoreactivity in human sympathetic ganglia. *Cell Tissue Res* 1987;249:1–5.
47. Jenkins JS, et al. Vasopressin, oxytocin and neurophysins in the human brain and spinal cord. *Brain Res* 1984;291:111–117.
48. Jit I, Mukerjee RN. Observations on the anatomy of the human thoracic sympathetic chain and its branches, with an anatomical assessment of operations for hypertension. *J Anat Soc India* 1960;9: 55–82.
49. Kennedy PGE, Duchen LW. A quantitative study of intermediolateral column cells in motor neuron disease and the Shy–Drager syndrome. *J Neurol Neurosurg Psychiatry* 1985;48:1103–1106.

50. Kowall NW, Mueller MP. Morphology and distribution of nicotinamide adenine dinucleotide phosphate (reduced form) diaphorase reactive neurons in human brainstem. *Neurosci* 1988;26:645–654.
51. Laitinen A, et al. VIP-like immunoreactive nerves in human respiratory tract: light and electron microscopic study. *Histochemistry* 82:313–320, 1985.
52. Lechan RM, et al. Distribution of immunoreactive human growth hormone–like material and thyrotropin-releasing hormone in the rat central nervous system: evidence for their coexistence in the same neurons. *Endocrinology* 1983;112:877–884.
53. Leeman SE, Hammerschlag R. Stimulation of salivary secretion by a factor extracted from hypothalamic tissue. *Endocrinology* 1967; 81:803–810.
54. Lehnert H, et al. Extrapituitary effects of corticotropin-releasing hormone and thyrotropin-releasing hormone. *Neuropsychobiology* 1993;28:54–61.
55. Leibowitz SF. Neurochemical–neuroendocrine systems in the brain controlling macronutrient intake and metabolism. *Trends Neurosci* 1992;15:491–497.
56. Lotz M, et al. Substance P activation of rheumatoid synoviocytes: neural pathway in pathogenesis of arthritis. *Science* 1987;235: 893–895.
57. Loupe F, et al. Localization of oxytocin binding sites in the human brainstem and upper spinal cord: an autoradiographic study. *Brain Res* 1989;500:223–230.
58. Low PA, et al. Splanchnic preganglionic neurons in man. I. Morphometry of preganglionic cytons. *Acta Neuropathol* 1977;40: 55–61.
59. Lundberg JM. Evidence for coexistence of vasoactive intestinal polypeptide (VIP) and acetylcholine in neurons of cat exocrine glands: morphological, biochemical and functional studies. *Acta Physiol Scand* 1981;112(Suppl 496):1–57.
60. Lundberg JM, et al. Coexistence of multiple peptides and classic transmitters in airway neurons: functional and pathophysiologic aspects. *Am Rev Respir Dis* 1987;136:(6pt2)S16–S22.
61. Lundberg JM, et al. Coexistence of peptide HI (PHI) and VIP in nerves regulating blood flow and bronchial smooth muscle tone in various mammals including man. *Peptides* 1984;5:593–606.
62. Lundberg JM, et al. Neuropeptide Y (NPY)-like immunoreactivity in peripheral noradrenergic neurons and effects of NPY on sympathetic function. *Acta Physiol Scand* 1982;116:477–480
63. Manaker S, et al. Autoradiographic localization of thyrotropin releasing hormone (TRH) receptors in human spinal cord. *Neurology* 1985;35:328–332.
64. Marti E, et al. Ontogeny of peptide- and amine-containing neurons in motor, sensory, and autonomic regions of rat and human spinal cord, dorsal root ganglia, and rat skin. *J Comp Neurol* 1987;266:322.
65. Matthews MR. Small, intensely fluorescent cells and the paraneuron concept. *J Electron Microsc Tech* 1989;12:408–416.
66. McLean S, et al. Activity and distribution of binding sites in brain of a nonpeptide substance P (NK$_1$) receptor antagonist. *Science* 1991; 251:437–439.
67. Meyer G, et al. Morphology of neurons in the white matter of the adult human neocortex. *Exp Brain Res* 1992;88:204–212.
68. Michel MC, Rascher W. Neuropeptide Y: a possible role in hypertension? *J Hypertens* 1995;13:385–395.
69. Miller AS, et al. Vasoactive intestinal polypeptide immunoreactive nerve fibres in the human eye. *Aust J Ophthalmol* 1983;2:185–193.
70. Moncada S, et al. Nitric oxide: physiology, pathophysiology and pharmacology. *Pharmacol Rev* 1991;43:109–142.
71. Nakanishi S. Mammalian tachykinin receptors. *Annu Rev Neurosci* 1991;14:123–136.
72. Nobin A, et al. Organization of the sympathetic innervation in liver tissue from monkey and man. *Cell Tissue Res* 1978;195:371–380.
73. Palmer JBD, et al. VIP and PHM and their role in noradrenergic inhibitory responses in isolated human airways. *J Appl Physiol* 1986;61:1322–1328.
74. Palmer JP, et al. Evaluation of the control of glucagon secretion by the parasympathetic nervous system in man. *Metab Clin Exp* 1979; 28:549–552.
75. Partanen M, et al. Catecholamine- and acetylcholinesterase-containing nerves in human lower respiratory tract. *Histochemistry* 1982; 76:175–188.
76. Paxinos G. *The human nervous system.* San Diego: Academic, 1990.
77. Payan DG, et al. Substance P recognition by a subset of human T lymphocytes. *J Clin Invest* 1984;74:1532–1539.
78. Pearson J, Pytel B. Quantitative studies of sympathetic ganglia and spinal cord intermediolateral gray columns in familial dysautonomia. *J Neurol Sci* 1978;39:37–59.
79. Perez GM, Keyser RB. Cell body counts in human ciliary ganglia. *Invest Ophthalmol Vis Sci* 1987;27:1428–1431.
80. Perianin A, et al. Substance P primes human neutrophil activation: a mechanism for neurological regulation of inflammation. *Biochem Biophys Res Commun* 1989;161:520–524.
81. Petermann JB, et al. Identification in the human central nervous system, pituitary, and thyroid of a novel calcitonin gene-related peptide and partial amino acid sequence in the spinal cord. *J Biol Chem* 1987;262:542–545.
82. Pilowsky PM, et al. Substance P and serotonergic inputs to sympathetic preganglionic neurons. *Clin Exp Hypertens* 1995;17:335–344.
83. Potter EK. Neuropeptide Y as an autonomic neurotransmitter. *Pharmacol Ther* 1988;37:251–273.
84. Prabhakar NR, et al. Analysis of carotid chemoreceptor responses to substance P analogue in anesthetized cats. *J Auton Nerv Syst* 1995; 52:43–50.
85. Rand MJ, Li CG. Nitric oxide in the autonomic and enteric nervous systems. In: Vincent SR, ed. *Nitric oxide in the nervous system.* San Diego: Academic, 1995:227–279.
86. Rechardt L, et al. Peptidergic innervation of human atrial myocardium: an electron microscopical and immunocytochemical study. *J Auton Nerv Syst* 1986;17:21–32.
87. Reisine T, Bell GI. Molecular properties of somatostatin receptors. *Neuroscience* 1995;67:777–790.
88. Rioux F, et al. Somatostatin: interaction with the sympathetic nervous system in guinea pigs. *Neuropeptides* 1981; 1:319–327.
89. Roman C, Gonella J. Extrinsic control of digestive tract motility. In: Johnson LR, ed. *Physiology of the gastrointestinal tract.* 2nd ed. New York: Raven, 1990:507–553.
90. Romco HE, et al. Origins of the sympathetic projections to rat thyroid and parathyroid glands. *J Auton Nerv Syst* 1986;17:63–70.
91. Rosenfield MG, et al. Production of a novel neuropeptide encoded by the calcitonin gene via tissue-specific RNA processing. *Nature* 1983;304:129–135.
92. Ryan JP. Motility of the gallbladder. In: Johnson LR, ed. *Physiology of the digestive tract.* 2nd ed. New York: Raven, 1987:695–721.
93. Sajin B, et al. Compartmentalization of NADPH-diaphorase staining in the developing human striatum. *Neurosci Lett* 1992;140: 117–120.
94. Sangruchi T, Kowall NW. NADPH-diaphorase histochemistry of the human hypothalamus. *Neuroscience* 1991;40:713–724.
95. Satoh M. Transmission and modulation of nociceptive information in the spinal dorsal horn. *Nippon Yakurigaku Zasshi* 1993;101: 289–298.
96. Scherer-Singler U, et al. Demonstration of a unique population of neurons with NADPH-diaphorase histochemistry. *J Neurosci Methods* 1983;9:229–234.
97. Schoenen J, Faull RLM. Spinal cord: cytoarchitectural, dendroarchitectural, and myeloarchitectural organization. In: Paxinos, G, ed. *The human nervous system.* San Diego: Academic, 1990.
98. Schoenen J, et al. Substance P, enkephalins, somatostatin, cholecystokinin, oxytocin, and vasopressin in human spinal cord. *Neurology* 1985;35:881–890.
99. Schroder HD. Somatostatin in the caudal spinal cord: an immunohistochemical study of the spinal centers involved in the innervation of pelvic organs. *J Comp Neurol* 1984;223:400–414.
100. Smithson IL, Benarroch EE. Organization of NADPH-diaphorase-reactive neurons and catecholaminergic fibers in human intermediolateral cell column. *Brain Res* 1996;723:218–222.
101. Snider RM, et al. A potent nonpeptide antagonist of the substance P (NK$_1$) receptor. *Science* 1991;251:435–436.
102. Sofroniew MV. Projections from vasopressin, oxytocin, and neurophysin neurons to neural targets in the rat and human. *J Histochem Cytochem* 1980;28:475–478.

103. Tache Y, et al. Caudal raphe–dorsal vagal complex peptidergic projections: role in gastric vagal control. *Peptides* 1995;16:431–435.
104. Tatemoto K, et al. Galanin: a novel biologically active peptide from porcine intestine. *FEBS Lett* 1983;164:124–128.
105. Terenghi G, et al. Immunohistochemistry of nitric oxide synthase demonstrates immunoreactive neurons in spinal cord and dorsal root ganglia of man and rat. *J Neurol Sci* 1993;118:34–37.
106. Tschopp FA, et al. Calcitonin gene-related peptide and its binding sites in the human central nervous system and pituitary. *Proc Natl Acad Sci USA* 1985;82:248–252.
107. Uddman R, et al. Neuronal VIP in salivary glands: distribution and release. *Acta Physiol Scand* 1980;110:31–38.
108. Vincent SR. Localization of nitric oxide neurons in the central nervous system. In: Vincent SR, ed. *Nitric oxide in the nervous system.* San Diego: Academic, 1995:83–102.
109. Vincent SR. Nitric oxide: a radical neurotransmitter in the central nervous system. *Prog Neurobiol* 1994;42:129–160.
110. Vincent SR, Hope BT. Neurons that say NO. *Trends Neurosci* 1992;15:109–113.
111. Walsh JH. Gastrointestinal hormones. In: Johnson LR, ed. *Physiology of the gastrointestinal tract.* 2nd ed. New York: Raven, 1987: 181–284.
112. Weisenfeld-Hallin Z, Bartfai T, Hokfelt T. Galanin in sensory neurons in the spinal cord. *Front Neuroendocrinol* 1992;13:319–343.
113. William PL, et al. *Gray's anatomy.* 37th British ed. Edinburgh: Churchill-Livingstone, 1989.
114. Winokur A, et al. TRH and TRH receptors in the spinal cord. *Ann NY Acad Sci* 1989;553:314–324.
115. Yaksh TL. Opioid receptor systems and the endorphins: a review of their spinal organization. *J Neurosurg* 1987;67:157–176.
116. Yuan W, Wang Y. A new structure of small intensely fluorescent cells in superior mesenteric ganglions of human fetus. *Chin Med J* 1995;108:52–54.
117. Zagvazdin YS, et al. Neural nitric oxide mediates Edinger–Westphal nucleus evoked increase in choroidal blood flow in the pigeon. *Invest Ophthalmol Vis Sci* 1996;37:666–672.
118. Zukowska-Grojec Z. Neuropeptide Y: a novel sympathetic stress hormone and more. *Ann NY Acad Sci* 1995;771:219–233.

CHAPTER 4

The Central Nervous System and Cardiovascular Control in Health and Disease

William T. Talman

---

1. Central nervous system (CNS) lesions may cause electrocardiographic (ECG) changes and cardiac arrhythmias. The arrhythmias, although potentially fatal, may be treatable.
2. Parasympathetic–sympathetic balance is important in maintenance of normal cardiac rhythm. Parasympathetic influence tends to lessen and adrenergic stimulation to increase the tendency for ventricular arrhythmias.
3. Asymmetric sympathetic activity, particularly that favoring left-sided sympathetic pathways to the heart, is especially arrhythmogenic.
4. Cardiac arrhythmias and ischemic ECG changes resulting from central lesions are most common in hemorrhagic strokes and subarachnoid hemorrhage, where they may appear as frequently as 70% of the time.
5. ECG changes secondary to CNS lesions are typically difficult to distinguish from those of primary heart disease; recognition is important because their presence is associated with a worsened prognosis.
6. Sympathetic activation and catecholamine release may cause the changes; these precipitating factors may occur with stressful stimuli and do not depend on either central or cardiac lesions.
7. Stimulation of either the left stellate ganglion or the left cardiac nerve may cause ST depression and T-wave peaking; ST elevation and deep T-wave inversion may follow right-sided stimulation.
8. Toxic effects of catecholamines on cardiac myocytes or increased cardiac contractility and oxygen demand due to actions at calcium channels may explain ECG changes after central lesions.
9. CNS lesions may also alter regulation of arterial pressure. Effects may be mediated through the autonomic nervous system, the neuroendocrine system, and renal mechanisms effecting fluid and electrolyte balance.
10. Centrally mediated arterial hypertension is most commonly associated with lesions directly or indirectly affecting the medulla oblongata or, less commonly, with lesions affecting the hypothalamus.
11. Chronic dysfunction such as normal pressure hydrocephalus may also contribute to hypertension in humans.
12. In contrast, discrete lesions of the ventral medulla oblongata or the spinal cord may result in hypotension.
13. Circumscribed central lesions rarely cause orthostatic hypotension, which is nonetheless a common feature of diffuse neurodegenerative disorders of the autonomic nervous system.

INTRODUCTION

The central nervous system (CNS) plays an important role in modulating autonomic and neurohumoral influences on cardiovascular function in health and disease. This chapter reviews clinically relevant cardiovascular disturbances that are associated with lesions of the CNS and summarizes the current state of knowledge regarding central anatomy and physiology of central cardiovascular control.

CARDIOVASCULAR DISTURBANCES CAUSED BY CENTRAL LESIONS

Cardiac Arrhythmias

Cardiac arrhythmias are the most immediately life-threatening of the potential cardiovascular disturbances as-

---

W. T. Talman: Chief of the Neurology Service, Veterans Affairs Medical Center; and Department of Neurology, University of Iowa College of Medicine, Iowa City, Iowa 52240.

sociated with CNS disease. They have long been recognized as a complication of CNS disease (37,169), and the need for aggressive management has been emphasized for decades (144). Arrhythmias may be of supraventricular or ventricular origin and may occur with a variety of central disorders, including subarachnoid hemorrhage, head injury, cerebral ischemia, multiple sclerosis, and cerebral tumors (33,48,52,55,59,64,80,82,106,126,145,170,202). Transient arrhythmias may even occur as a result of neurosurgical manipulation of brain (80). The arrhythmias may occur in the context of concomitant intrinsic heart disease (154), but many patients who have died from such arrhythmias have had no demonstrable cardiac disease at postmortem examination. Experimental studies have clearly shown that potentially fatal arrhythmias can occur without heart disease. Even in the presence of ischemic cardiac disease, the influence of the CNS may be decisive. For example, the threshold for ventricular fibrillation during coronary artery occlusion decreases if the hypothalamus is stimulated during the period of occlusion (165). In contrast, ventricular fibrillation threshold may increase if cortical hypothalamic pathways have been interrupted (177). Far less dramatic central events may likewise lead to serious cardiac arrhythmias. For example, stress created by conditioning to aversive stimuli can affect the threshold for arrhythmias both in the normal heart and in the heart compromised by disease or toxins (165).

Clearly, cardiac arrhythmias would further compromise the prognosis of patients with already serious intracranial disease. In one population of patients, those with subarachnoid hemorrhage, arrhythmias may be particularly devastating and contribute to the high incidence (4%–5%) of sudden death seen in that condition (145), but the complication is by no means restricted to subarachnoid hemorrhage. Both in animal subjects and in patients, an increased incidence of arrhythmias has been documented with other central vascular lesions as well. In cats, ischemia in the distribution of the left middle cerebral artery led to major arrhythmias in 60% of the animals and sudden death in 45% (202). Between 5% and 8% of patients studied died suddenly after intracerebral hemorrhages (73,81). This potential for clinically significant cardiac arrhythmias in patients with cerebral lesions, and particularly in patients with subarachnoid hemorrhages, has led some to suggest that treatment of arrhythmias in these patients should be just as aggressive as it is in patients who have sustained an acute myocardial infarction (145). Although optimal therapy is not known, some have reported that muscarinic blockade with atropine for supraventricular bradyarrhythmias and β-blockade for tachyarrhythmias may be effective (145). One study suggests that augmenting muscarinic receptor activation may also be an effective means of decreasing potentially fatal ventricular arrhythmias associated with cardiac ischemia and sympathetic activation (38). Of course, under some circumstances, viz. arrhythmogenic seizures, the best therapy for arrhythmias is direct treatment of the underlying central condition (118).

The efficacy of each of these therapies supports a neurogenic basis for arrhythmias promoted by central events. Much additional direct and indirect evidence confirms that the arrhythmias occur coincident with disturbances in autonomic activity.

A balance in that activity seems critical to normal cardiac function. In intact, normally innervated hearts, sympathetic–parasympathetic interactions regulate myocardial electrical stability (152). Cardiac sympathetic stimulation speeds sinoatrial depolarization, which, in turn, increases the frequency of sinus node firing and leads to sinus tachyarrhythmias (107,168,204). In general, adrenergic stimulation also increases the ventricle's propensity to develop arrhythmias. Vagal stimulation, on the other hand, slows or abolishes depolarization of the sinus node, decreases sinoatrial firing rate (204), and increases electrical stability (182). These vagally mediated changes decrease the incidence of ventricular fibrillation in experimental animals (182) and ventricular tachycardia in humans (152). The balance between sympathetic–parasympathetic influences on cardiac excitability may be altered in pathologic conditions. For example, during cardiac ischemia, an imbalance may result from differing effects of ischemia on the sympathetic and vagal innervation of the ventricles (13,174,198), supersensitivity to catecholamines due to interruption of sympathetic innervation on normal myocardial cells distal to an infarct (8,92), or changes in coronary vasomotor tone (206). Resultant alterations in autonomic activity may predispose one to cardiac arrhythmias (92,198) and sudden death (206). Similarly imbalanced autonomic influences on the heart can be effected by stimulation of autonomic afferents. Vagal afferent stimulation may initiate depressor reflexes with hypotension and bradycardia while stimulation of sympathetic afferents may initiate sympathoexcitatory responses associated with increased heart rate and blood pressure (174).

Central mechanisms underlying arrhythmogenesis may change as the lesion evolves. For example, after acute experimental subarachnoid hemorrhage, the pathophysiologic basis for immediate neurogenic cardiac arrhythmias is more directly related to suddenly increased intracranial pressure than to actual presence and location of blood in the subarachnoid space (53). Such early arrhythmias result from combined vagal and sympathetic effects whereas more delayed arrhythmias may depend less on direct neural influences than on levels of circulating or intracardiac catecholamines (53,55,140). The neural and neurohumoral influences on rhythm may result from direct actions on cardiac conduction or through neurogenic myocardial injury (see below).

Experimental studies reveal that asymmetric augmentation of cardiac sympathetics resulting from selective stimulation of one cardiac nerve is particularly deleterious because it reduces ventricular fibrillation threshold (7,26,69). Such asymmetric activation may also result from central disturbances (124,165). Asymmetry favoring the left cardiac sympathetic nerve is more highly associated with arrhythmias than is that favoring the right side. In contrast, direct electrical stimulation of the left (but not the right) cardiac sympathetic nerve, stellate ganglion, or middle cervical ganglion produces ventricular and supraventricular arrhythmias (7,26,69). For arrhythmias to develop, activity of the left sympathetics apparently only needs to be relatively increased with respect to activity of the right side. Cooling or removal of the right stellate ganglion alone may lead to similar arrhythmias (173). It seems likely that the increased incidence of arrhythmias with stimulation of the left stellate ganglion is related to resultant decreased ventricular refractory period (79). In support of this mechanism, stimulation of the left stellate ganglion affects the refractory period more than does stimulation on the right (79). The decreased refractory period may mediate the increased incidence of ventricular fibrillation of perfused or ischemic cardiac muscle during asymmetric alteration in cardiac sympathetic activity (76,173,199). Interestingly, some have shown that blockade of the left stellate ganglion with 1% lidocaine may even block centrally induced arrhythmias (94).

It seems likely that altered cardiac autonomic activity similarly accounts for cardiac arrhythmias associated with naturally occurring central disorders such as subarachnoid hemorrhage, other cerebrovascular accidents (145), and epilepsy (17,196). The sudden infant death syndrome (31,102) and sudden death in adults (141) may also have an underlying, though undefined, central disturbance. Other conditions in which central influences on the autonomic nervous system may play a role include digitalis-induced arrhythmias (58,137) and the idiopathic long QT syndrome (172). Prolongation of the QT interval, a common electrocardiographic (ECG) result of autonomic stimulation or localized central lesions (141,186) is itself associated with an increased incidence of potentially fatal ventricular arrhythmias (172). There is some indication that sudden death in patients with the prolonged QT syndrome may be caused by imbalances in left versus right sympathetic innervation to the heart (124,172) and treatment with β-adrenergic antagonists may improve survival even among patients without CNS lesions (193). The specific relationship between the syndrome and a central disorder has not been determined.

Though potential central influences on cardiac rhythm may be profound, they may be enhanced further by coexistent peripheral nerve disease. For example, in the Guillain–Barré syndrome, there is an increased incidence of arrhythmias and sudden death secondary to increased sympathetic activity (63,116,180). An increased incidence of sudden death also has been described in patients with diabetic autonomic neuropathy (120).

There is now substantial evidence that peripheral catecholamines, released as a result of central lesions, may generate cardiac arrhythmias. Intravenous infusion of norepinephrine or epinephrine can cause arrhythmias and conduction disturbances that are identical to those associated with central lesions (113). Combined treatment with atropine and propronalol can block fatal arrhythmias in animals exposed to severe cerebral ischemia (203), and interruption of sympathetic nerves may eliminate central neurogenic arrhythmias (64). β-Blockade alone was reported to eliminate centrally induced arrhythmias in one study (203), but it was ineffective in another (64). Still others have reduced the incidence of arrhythmia by selectively interrupting the vagus nerves (178).

The inference from therapeutic results that central disturbances can lead to increased activation of cardiac sympathetics has been supported by direct measurements of sympathetic activity. In one study, electrical stimulation of the hypothalamus increased sympathetic nerve activity (153) and was associated with almost immediate frequency-dependent increases in activity in the inferior cardiac nerve (148,149). These findings strongly support sympathetic involvement in arrhythmogenesis, but the role of vagal parasympathetic activity has not been proven. Vagus nerve activity does not increase with hypothalamic stimulation that would be arrhythmogenic (153), and ventricular arrhythmias associated with diencephalic or hypothalamic stimulation have been shown to be sympathetically, not vagally, mediated (85,128,197).

Central stimulation outside the diencephalon can also elicit cardiac arrhythmias. For example, stimulation of amygdala, hippocampus, anterior cingulate gyrus, temporal pole, subiculum, and parabrachial nucleus has been reported to be arrhythmogenic (5,27,39,156). The arrhythmias in these instances did not depend on spread of current or seizures (86) although seizures themselves may be arrhythmogenic (17,39,42,130,195,196) and represent one cause of sudden death (118).

The evidence cited in the preceding paragraphs has dealt primarily with studies using central stimulation to support the possibility that CNS lesions produce cardiac arrhythmias. However, it is worth noting that most of the clinical situations in which central processes are associated with arrhythmias involve irritative lesions. For example, arrhythmias are frequently associated with intracranial hemorrhages (particularly subarachnoid) and lesions such as trauma, surgery, and tumors that may also be epileptogenic. It does not follow that all arrhythmogenic lesions are irritative. Some may lead to arrhythmias by altering the symmetry of sympathetic activity. For example, arrhythmias have been reported in patients with multiple sclerosis (170), and sympathetic imbalance that might contribute to arrhythmias has been reported in Alzheimer's disease (3). It appears that development of arrhythmias with a central process depends not only on the nature of the lesion but also on the location of the disturbance in the brain and the age of the affected individual (67,68). Lesions affecting the limbic system have the highest correlation with appearance of a long QT interval that may lead to cardiac arrhythmias (104). Furthermore, changes in sympathetic nerve activity, plasma catecholamine levels, and ECG changes, all of which tend to predispose one to arrhythmias, seem more likely to occur following lesions in the right than in the left hemisphere (67). However, whether there is indeed "dominance" of one hemisphere in autonomic control is yet to be proven.

There is now considerable thought that the syndrome of sudden death may represent a cardiac manifestation of a central disturbance that is not associated with a gross CNS lesions (121). It certainly appears that the syndrome may occur as a result of a cardiac electrical event that is independent of coronary occlusion (122,135,142) but may be triggered by the autonomic nervous system. As noted the ventricular fibrillation threshold may be significantly lowered by stimulation of cardiac sympathetic nerves (121,173,199). Studies have suggested that the sympathetic activation leads to an influx of calcium into cardiac myocytes and that it is the intracellular calcium that predisposes one to arrhythmias (12). Blocking that buildup of intracellular calcium with an intracellular calcium chelator has effectively diminished the arrhythmogenesis of sympathetic stimulation.

Detrimental sympathetic activation mediated by the CNS clearly does not depend on the presence of central lesions but can result from naturally occurring events in the CNS (25,49,51,100,119,121,139,177). As noted previously, stress itself can lead to arrhythmias. The effects of stress on the heart appear to be multifactorial. They include genetic and developmental factors as well as factors relating to the nature of stress and the situation under which stress occurs (45,50,171). The individual faced with inescapable, unavoidable stress seems particularly prone to sudden death (25,51,194,201). In one case seen recently at the University of Iowa, a young woman had repeated pseudoseizures that were repeatedly documented by telemetric electroencephalographic monitoring. When told that her spells were pseudoseizures and did not require treatment with the antiepileptic medications that had been initiated previously, she became extremely anxious. From then on, with frequent typical pseudoseizures, she had transient cardiac asystole that corrected to a normal sinus rhythm without intervention within 30–45 sec. With addition of oral muscarinic antagonists, but no other change in her medical regimen, the patient has remained symptom free for $1\frac{1}{2}$ years.

An extreme example of stress-related sudden death also occurred with the Northridge, California, earthquake in 1994. On the day of the temblor, the incidence of sudden death increased fivefold over that of control periods (112). Because the number of sudden deaths occurring in the days after the earthquake actually fell, the incidence during the week of the quake did not exceed that of comparable periods. Thus, sudden death under stressful conditions may occur in individuals predisposed to the fatal outcome. Perhaps 40% of occurrences of sudden death without such signal stresses may in fact be related to less notable stresses affecting those at risk (112,136). Although stress clearly seems to predispose one to sudden death, the precise mechanism through which it does so is not known. Potentially sympathetic activation during stress may favor left cardiac sympathetic nerves, or the overwhelming central activation may lead to sudden death through intense release of catecholamines. Cannon, in his classic work, seems to have spoken to the latter possibility when he suggested that activation of the "sympathoadrenal" axis caused death related to a voodoo spell (25).

Myocardial Injury

As mentioned previously, CNS lesions may cause overt rhythm disturbances and/or ECG changes that suggest a predisposition for those rhythm disturbances. In addition, central lesions may lead to ECG changes suggesting myocardial ischemia or injury without any change in cardiac rhythm (1,2,23,202) (Fig. 1). Failure to recognize the relationship between these changes and underlying disease may lead to errant diagnoses and treatment and may worsen prognosis (181). Though it is critical to recognize the potential for centrally mediated ECG changes, accurate assessment is often difficult because the ECG abnormalities may closely resemble those that occur in patients with ischemic cardiac disease. In addition, coronary vascular disease may be significantly increased in patients with ischemic cerebrovascular disease that may cause ECG changes (157,160). Therefore, it is prudent to provide care in an appropriately monitored setting until a myocardial infarction has been excluded even when a CNS event may be the cause of ECG changes.

ECG changes that do occur secondary to CNS disease may take a variety of forms, but the most common abnormalities are prolongation of the QT interval, depression of ST segments, flattening or inversion of T waves, and U waves (22,33,41,48,56,62,77,82,83,89,126,132). In addition, one may identify elevation and peaking or notching of the T waves, elevation of ST segments, increased amplitude of the P wave, increases in QRS voltage, and the appearance of Q waves (41,48,62,77,82,83). Clearly, ECG changes secondary to CNS disease may directly resemble those due to primary cardiac ischemia. Adding to diagnostic difficulties, ECG changes associated with CNS disease and ischemic cardiac disease may evolve similarly. With central lesions, the ECG usually reverts to normal within 2 weeks, but U waves and QT prolongation may persist (22,56,77) (Fig. 2).

Unfortunately, no single feature or combination of features in the ECG indicates unequivocally that the changes

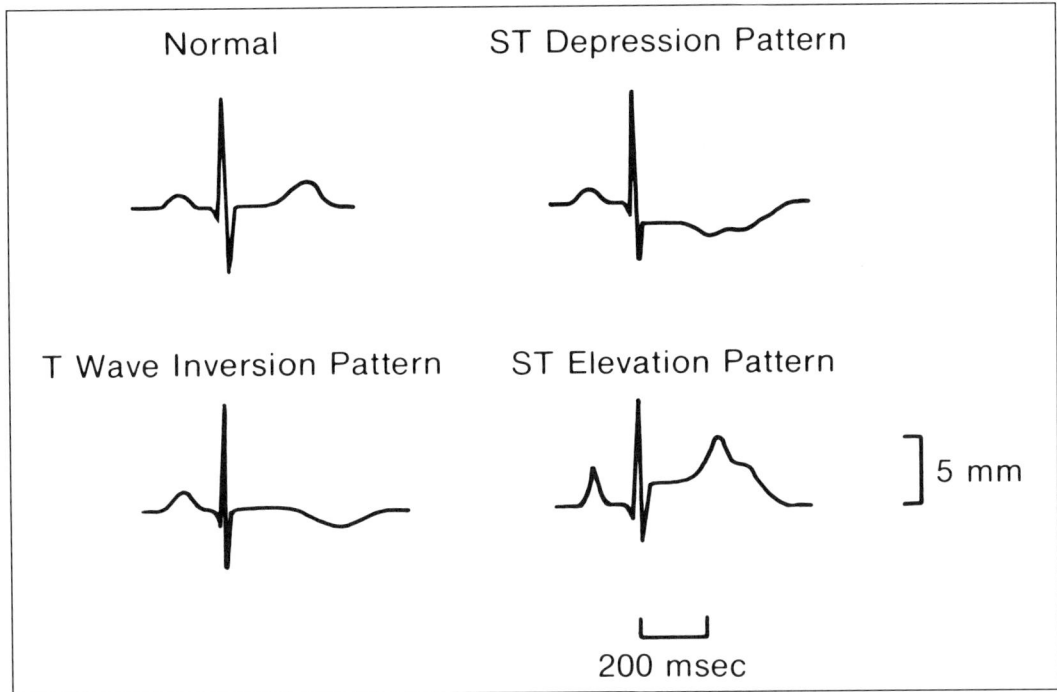

FIG. 1. Schematic representation of common electrocardiographic changes seen with central lesions. The normal pattern, as seen with a cardiac rate of 70 beats/min, is shown at the top left. The QT interval is prolonged in each of the representative abnormal patterns. Other abnormalities include U waves **(top right and bottom right)**, ST depression and T-wave inversion **(top right)**, T-wave inversion without ST changes **(bottom left)**, and peaked P and T waves accompanying ST elevation **(bottom right)**. From Talman (186), with permission.

are due to myocardial ischemia or a central lesion. If the changes are related to CNS disease, they do not have any localizing value or diagnostic value with respect to the underlying central event. It would appear that they may accompany virtually any central event, but certain lesions are associated with the highest incidence of the changes. The incidence may be as high as 70% in patients with intracerebral hemorrhages, 40% in patients with nonhemorrhagic strokes, and 70% in patients with subarachnoid hemorrhage (22,33,56,74,77,109,117,126). Similar changes have also been reported in patients with brain tumors, spinal cord lesions, meningitis, multiple sclerosis, and hydrocephalus (74,80,82,83,89,132). Even manipulation of the basal forebrain during neurosurgical procedures has resulted in similar ECG changes (57).

Particularly in patients with apparent occlusive cerebrovascular disease, the physician must be careful not to conclude that a cardiac event with infarction and possible embolization to the brain has occurred because of the ECG changes. Such changes have been seen in patients who have been thoroughly analyzed and found not to have a myocardial infarction, even though cardiac enzymes may have been elevated during the time of the ECG changes (89,91,127). In fact, the cardiac enzyme changes do reflect myocardial necrosis but not that related to coronary occlusive disease, as will be discussed below. In the face of such profound ECG changes with enzymes that suggest the presence of myocardial necrosis, it is not at all surprising that the ECG changes, even in the absence of coronary disease, are associated with a significantly increased mortality (41,48,83). With such changes, 80% of patients in one study died after subarachnoid hemorrhage, whereas only 33% of patients without changes died (83).

There is much speculation about potential pathophysiologic mechanisms for the ECG changes. Virtually identical changes can be elicited experimentally through peripheral stimulation of cardiac sympathetics or through intravenous infusion of high concentrations of norepinephrine (103, 108,205). Considerable evidence suggests that release of catecholamines upon cardiac myocytes leads to the ECG changes of ischemia (167,185). Such ECG changes have been correlated with postmortem evidence of micronecrotic changes representing contraction band necrosis in the myocardium (29,30,62,105,109,147,163,179). As would be expected since the ECG changes themselves are associated with increased morbidity and mortality in patients with central lesions, similarly increased morbidity and mortality are seen in patients with central lesions and elevations of plasma catecholamines (10,72). To some extent, the myocardial changes may be reversible (75) and thus

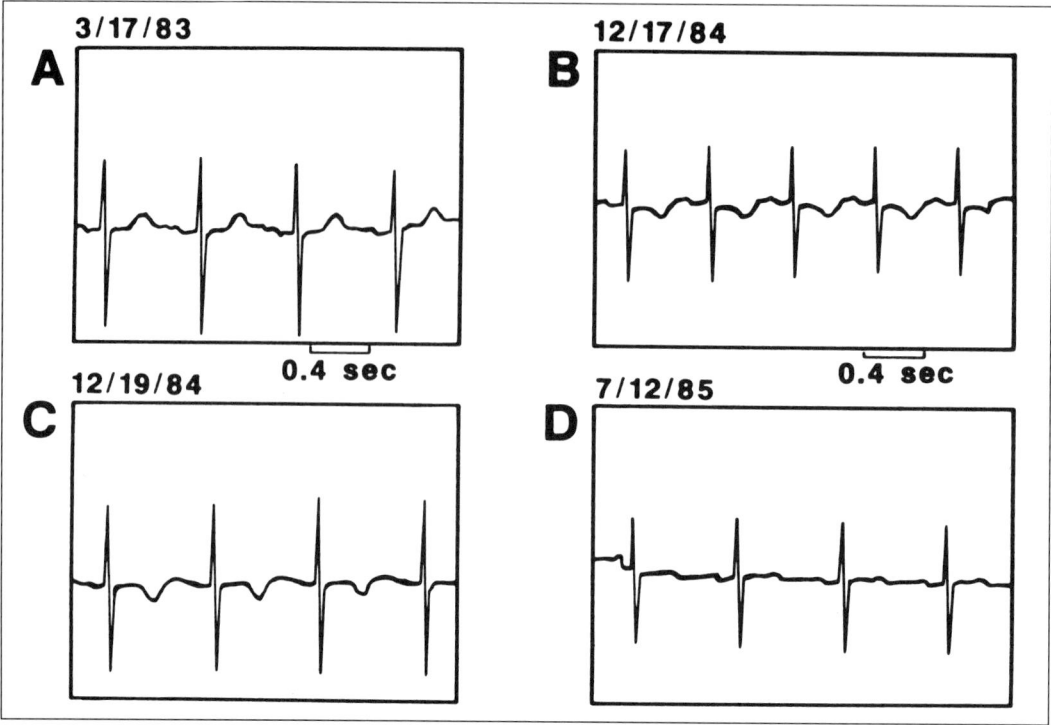

FIG. 2. Evolution of electrocardiographic abnormalities seen in a 66-year-old man who came to the Veterans Affairs Medical Center (Iowa City, IA, U.S.A.) on December 17, 1984, because of encephalopathy that resulted from head trauma and secondary subarachnoid hemorrhage. His previously normal electrocardiographic pattern **(A)** was replaced by ST depression and T-wave inversion on admission **(B)**. Over the ensuing 7 months, the pattern evolved toward normal **(C,D)**. There were never enzymatic changes of myocardial damage; postmortem examination of his heart after his death due to septicemia revealed patent coronary arteries and neither acute nor chronic myocardial injury. From Talman (187), with permission.

may not be found in some patients who have manifested typical ECG changes.

It seems certain that the ECG changes do not result from alterations in electrolytes as was once suggested (22,48,83). The changes can clearly occur without any accompanying electrolyte or metabolic disturbance (56,80,89).

The evidence just cited has led to an hypothesis that ECG and morphologic changes occurring in the presence of brain lesions are neurogenically mediated. Some have questioned this hypothesis (154), which is nonetheless supported by well-controlled experimental studies where sympathetic tone has been increased, with or without an increase in vagal tone, in otherwise completely normal experimental animals (22,70,90,93,103,108,125,129,131,140,205). Furthermore, when sympathetic activity is increased by either electrical (131) or mechanical (70) stimulation of the hypothalamus or orbital frontal cortex (71), typical signs of myocardial damage appear on the ECG. A clinical correlate of this experimental model has been seen in patients with tumors of the basal forebrain and parasellar structures (80) and in patients who have sustained rupture of an aneurysm into the hypothalamus (47). Both of these lesions could, at least in part, produce ECG changes through mechanical stimulation of extensive connections that pass between the basal forebrain and hypothalamus to the brainstem. Again, experimental evidence supports this potential pathophysiologic mechanism as it is known that mechanical stimulation can produce physiologic responses that resemble those following local excitation of central structures (87,190).

It may be that hypothalamic stimulation, stimulation of projections into the ventrolateral medulla, or direct stimulation of ventrolateral medulla may produce ischemic ECG changes by direct actions on coronary vasomotor control (18,19,65,98,99). Although experimental studies that have activated some of these centers have relied on chemical or electrical excitation, similar excitation could be produced by an endogenous epileptogenic or irritant focus. However, the complexity of the pathogenic mechanisms for the ECG changes has increased with the recognition that such epileptogenic foci may actually be associated with an increased incidence of true atherosclerotic coronary vascular disease (6,66). These evaluations have further emphasized the need for both careful cardiologic and neurologic evaluation of patients with such changes in their ECG.

Studies of the effects on the heart and the ECG when stimuli are delivered to the peripheral sympathetic nervous system have also provided support for the neurogenic mediation of ECG changes. With stimulation of the stellate ganglia (103,205) or the cardiac nerves (108), typical ECG changes may develop. The type of ECG change may depend on whether the stimulus is delivered to cardiac sympathetics on the left or the right side of the body (108,205). When the stimulus is delivered to the right stellate ganglion or right cardiac nerve, ST elevation and deep T-wave inversion occurs (108,205). In contrast, stimulation to the left stellate ganglion elicits ST depression, elevation and peaking of the T waves, and an increase in the QT interval (205). Stimulation of the left ventrolateral cardiac nerve also increases the amplitude of the T wave (108). Although it is known that a majority of projections from the hypothalamus to the intermediolateral column of the spinal cord terminate ipsilaterally (164), it is not known whether such disparate ECG changes are determined by the side of the lesion in the CNS.

Evidence strongly supports a role for sympathetic activation in the ECG changes of central lesions, but the pathophysiologic mechanisms at the cellular level are less clear. Certainly the changes could result from sympathetically mediated increases in both myocardial oxygen demand (61,175) and coronary vasoconstriction (18,19,143). However, there is also substantial evidence suggesting that catecholamines themselves may be toxic to the myocardium, even when their release upon cardiac myocytes is not associated with a neural effect on myocardial blood flow and metabolism. Such toxicity can be seen with the intravenous administration of norepinephrine in high concentrations (167,185). Such high concentrations of catecholamine as well as the myocardial toxicity may be seen in patients with subarachnoid hemorrhages, and the outcome in those patients has been shown to be inversely related to the plasma level of epinephrine and norepinephrine at the time of the patient's admission (10). If catecholamine levels can be decreased, the incidence of myocardial toxicity can be reduced. For example, in experimental animals subjected to subarachnoid hemorrhage, the incidence of myocardial necrosis is markedly reduced if the catecholamine response to the hemorrhage is attenuated by pretreatment of the animal with reserpine (78,129). The relationship between myocardial damage and plasma catecholamines is further supported by evidence that concentrations of catecholamines are increased not only in plasma (55) but also in cardiac tissue itself (140). Very probably the catecholamines in cardiac tissue are released by intrinsic cardiac sympathetic nerves, as it is known that the microscopic foci of myocardial damage predominantly lie immediately adjacent to intracardiac nerve terminals (62).

Once again, however, we may be at least one step away from the actual cellular mechanism of myocardial toxicity. There is one interesting hypothesis that may prove to explain the toxicity. Intense stimulation with catecholamines is thought to lead to opening of receptor-activated calcium channels that in turn promote excessive myocardial contraction. These events, by increasing metabolic demand without adequate increases in coronary blood flow, would ultimately lead to release of radicals and resultant myocardial necrosis (163).

Although the role of the sympathetic nervous system in production of myocardial damage with central lesions is supported by both clinical and experimental evidence, the role of the parasympathetic nervous system in the development of such damage is not clear, and efforts to define that role have led to conflicting results. For example, myocardial damage following experimental head trauma has developed despite vagal blockade (78), but myocardial damage that results from stimulation of the vagus nerves has been prevented by systemic administration of muscarinic antagonists (125). In that negative ionotropic and chronotropic influences that impair sympathetic input to the heart become more pronounced with greater prevailing levels of tonic sympathetic activity (114,115), it may be that vagal influences on myocardial damage depend on prevailing levels of sympathetic activity. Clearly, well-defined experimental studies will be needed to clarify the role of the vagus and of interactions between vagal and sympathetic influences on the heart in the genesis of myocardial damage.

HYPERTENSION AND HYPOTENSION

Central influences on arterial pressure are mediated through the autonomic nervous system, the neuroendocrine system, and renal mechanisms of electrolyte balance. Each may be variably influenced by stimulation or lesions of different sites in the CNS. Thus, different CNS lesions may not only lead to different responses of arterial pressure, but mechanisms underlying the same response may differ. Some central processes may lead to hypertension while others cause hypotension.

Bilateral lesions in the nucleus tractus solitarii cause acute neurogenic hypertension (43). Chemical disturbances in the region may be as effective as gross structural lesions in producing hypertension (189,192). Hypertension resulting from lesions in the nucleus tractus solitarii results not only from a marked increase in vasomotor tone and total peripheral resistance (44) but also from neurohumoral changes such as increased plasma levels of vasopressin (184). Although large bilateral lesions in this nucleus often lead to pulmonary edema and death in experimental animals, smaller lesions may be compatible with survival and may lead to lability of arterial pressure for the remainder of the animal's life (20,138,188) (Fig. 3). Chronic lability of arterial pressure may also be seen in humans after ischemic, degenerative, or destructive lesions of the nucleus tractus solitarii (11,101,123,134).

Another form of neurogenic hypertension, the *Cushing response*, has been recognized in humans for years (34). The response consists of a triad of physiologic changes in-

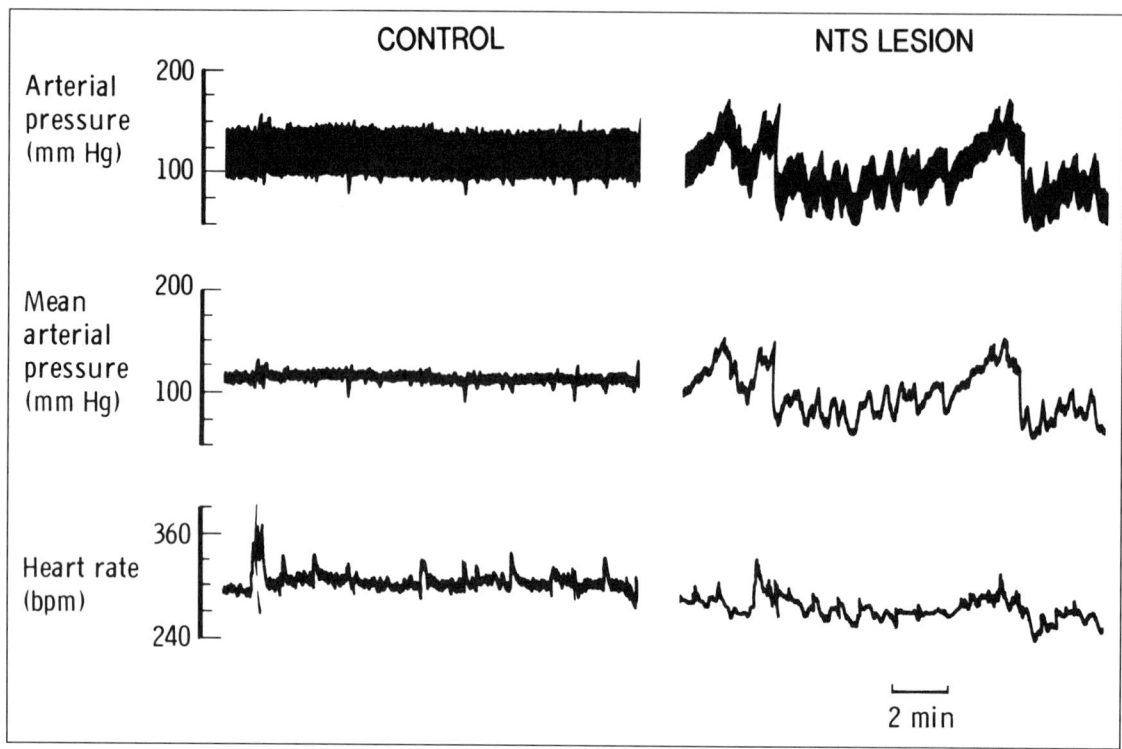

FIG. 3. Chronic lability of arterial pressure following a small midline lesion in the nucleus tractus solitarii of a rat. The labile pattern in an awake freely moving operated rat **(right)** is compared with the normal pattern in an awake unoperated control animal. Similar lability follows interruption of baroreceptor afferent fibers before they have entered the brain stem. In addition to lability, animals with nucleus tractus solitarius lesions show exaggerated arterial pressure responses to any environmental stimulus or behavior response (111,191).

cluding hypertension, bradycardia, and apnea. Cushing suggested that these responses result from distortion of the medulla and that the graded increase in arterial pressure that accompanied increases in intracranial pressure served to maintain cerebral arterial pulse pressure and thus cerebral blood flow (34). Although the response may accompany increased intracranial pressure and herniation, a similar triad may develop during ischemia or distortion of the dorsal medullary reticular formation along the floor of the fourth ventricle (87). Thus, the Cushing response is not an absolute indicator of herniation. Its diagnostic value is further limited in that it infrequently accompanies herniation (150), the response can consist of an increase in arterial pressure alone, or it may appear in its fully developed form as a result of a spinal lesion without herniation at all (87).

Hypertension has also been described as a result of tumors in the posterior fossa (54,155). This form of hypertension may present a complex diagnostic enigma because it may be clinically and biochemically indistinguishable from that of pheochromocytoma (54,155). It is likely that the hypertension resulting from posterior fossa lesions results from local distortion of the brain stem (155). Clearly, such distortion can lead to an increase in sympathetic activity and in levels of circulating catecholamines. Although the nucleus that mediates the hypertension produced by such lesions is not known, there are a number of nuclei in addition to the nucleus tractus solitarii in the medulla that could be responsible. In experimental animals, fulminant hypertension has also been produced by lesions in the caudal portion of the ventral medulla (15). A group of noradrenergic neurons, the A1 cell group (35), is located in the caudal ventrolateral medulla and from that site projects to vasopressinergic neurons in the hypothalamus (16,166). Lesions that affect the A1 group also interrupt these projections and consequently lead to release of vasopressin in concentrations that are sufficient to produce pressor responses (14). The caudal ventrolateral medulla also sends inhibitory projections to neurons of the rostral ventrolateral medulla, a site that influences tonic levels of arterial pressure through maintenance of tonic sympathetic nerve activity (24,36,161). Hypertension following lesions of the caudal region is also related to removal of that inhibitory input and consequent increased vasomotor tone.

Hypertension also may result from lesions that directly affect the hypothalamus in humans (146), but the humoral or neural mechanisms for that hypertension have not been determined. In experimental animals, on the other hand, hypothalamic lesions have led to hypertension that is dependent on release of adrenal medullary catecholamines. With central lesions lying rostral to the hypothalamus, hypertension is distinctly unusual unless the lesion results in epilepsy that does lead to increases of arterial pressure (42,130,195). Thus, lesions at many different levels of the CNS may produce hypertension. It is unclear, however, whether the CNS plays any role in the pathogenesis of essential hypertension. Some investigators have suggested such a role because they observed that distortion of the brain stem by ectatic branches of the basilar artery may be associated with hypertension in humans (4,95,96). Hypertension has also been produced by placement of a pulsatile balloon adjacent to the brain stem in experimental animals (97).

A significant association with hypertension has also been found with normal pressure hydrocephalus in humans (60). Similarly, hypertension correlates with increased ventricular size in experimental animals (9,158,159). Although both normal pressure hydrocephalus in humans and the animal model share hydrocephalus as a common feature, the precise site of origin of hypertension is unknown.

Focal structural lesions of the CNS have not been identified in patients with essential hypertension. Potentially, the relevant central process may be chemical or metabolic rather than structural. Numerous central disturbances involving both neurotransmitters and biosynthetic enzymes have been identified in genetic models of hypertension (84,110,133,151,162,200). Evidence even suggests that the tendency to hypertension can be transmitted to an animal by transplantation of brain tissue from an animal genetically predisposed to hypertension (40). These observations, as well as evidence that modification of certain putative central neurotransmitter mechanisms may lead to hypertension, suggest that identification of central neurochemical disturbances and the molecular basis for these disturbances may open important avenues of investigation into the role played by the CNS in hypertensive disease (46).

Hypotension may also follow central lesions. One such lesion that has been described in humans and in experimental animals involves the rostral ventrolateral medulla or fiber tracts projecting from that area to the intermediolateral cell column in the spinal cord. Profound hypotension has been described with such lesions and, under certain circumstances, without support of blood pressure, these lesions have led to death (150,161). The level to which blood pressure falls after such lesions is similar to that produced by transection of the rostral spinal cord. Evidence has shown that life support during the period of hypotension may enable the organism to recover sufficiently so that, even without support of blood pressure, arterial pressure returns fully to baseline levels despite a permanent destructive lesion in the medulla (28). Although the mechanism by which such physiologic recovery occurs has not been fully elucidated, there is some evidence to suggest that other central sites may assume an increased role in blood pressure homeostasis with the loss of the rostral ventrolateral medulla (32). With spinal cord transections in which blood pressure similarly falls, there is evidence in patients to suggest that, even with permanently absent autonomic control, those patients can maintain their arterial pressure through neuroendocrine mechanisms (183). However, even while resting blood pressure in the supine position may be normal, blood pressure may fall precipitously when such patients assume an upright posture.

Aside from the situation in cord transection, it is unclear whether other solitary lesions of the CNS lead to orthostatic hypotension. This condition may develop in experimental animals that have been subjected to lesions of the vestibular nuclei or to the fastigial nucleus of the cerebellum (45). Central lesions have been identified in patients with orthostatic hypotension (88), but the lesions were not confined to a single nuclear area. Typically, when orthostatic hypotension has been seen in humans with central lesions, the lesions have represented diffuse central processes that are often of a degenerative nature and involve both peripheral and central structures (176).

There is a common misperception that interruption of the baroreceptor reflex may lead to orthostatic hypotension; in fact, though, the role of lesions of peripheral or central baroreflex mechanisms in the development of orthostatic hypotension is suspect. Central interruption of the baroreflex arc does not lead to orthostatic hypotension (45). It is possible that some of the posturally related decreases in arterial pressure accompanying central lesions may be the result of direct compression of brain stem structures that are involved in blood pressure control. Just such hypotensive spells have been described with distortion of the nucleus tractus solitarii (190). Blood pressure may also be indirectly affected by such central lesions that may produce marked effects on eating and drinking behavior as well as loss of fluid through repeated vomiting and excess diuresis. Thus, when faced with a patient manifesting orthostatic hypotension and a single central lesion, the clinician would be wise to investigate abnormalities of fluid balance, drug intolerance, or general inanition before attributing orthostatic hypotension to the central event.

CONCLUSION

The CNS, through its modulation of autonomic activity, plays an important role in maintaining homeostasis in the cardiovascular system and in integrating cardiovascular responses with behaviors. Central disturbances then can lead to profound alterations in cardiac or vascular control manifested by cardiac arrhythmias, myocardial necrosis, hypertension, and lability of arterial pressure. Clearly, some of these disturbances can themselves further compromise the prognosis of patients with primary central lesions. Rapid recognition and appropriate treatment of the cardiovascular complications as well as the underlying condition is critical for effective management of many such patients.

ACKNOWLEDGMENTS

This work was supported in part by a Merit Review and Clinical Investigator Award from the Department of Veterans Affairs, National Institutes of Health HL32205 and HL14388, and an American Heart Association Grant in Aid.

REFERENCES

1. Abildskov JA, Vincent GM. The autonomic nervous system in relation to electrocardiographic wave form and cardiac rhythm. In: Randall WC, ed. *Neural regulation of the heart*. New York: Oxford University Press, 1977:409–424.
2. Abildskov JA, et al. The electrocardiogram and the central nervous system. *Prog Cardiovasc Dis* 1970;13:210–216.
3. Aharon-Peretz J, et al. Increased sympathetic and decreased parasympathetic cardiac innervation in patients with Alzheimer's disease. *Arch Neurol* 1992;49:919–922.
4. Akimura T, et al. Essential hypertension and neurovascular compression at the ventrolateral medulla oblongata: MR evaluation. *Am J Neuroradiol* 1995;16:401–405.
5. Anand BK, Dua S. Circulatory and respiratory changes induced by electrical stimulation of limbic system (visceral brain). *J Neurophysiol* 1956;19:393–400.
6. Annegers JF, et al. Heart disease mortality and morbidity in patients with epilepsy. *Epilepsia* 1984;25:699–704.
7. Armour JA, et al. Arrhythmias induced by local cardiac nerve stimulation. *Am J Physiol* 1972;223:1068–1075.
8. Barber MJ, et al. Transmural myocardial infarction in the dog produces sympathectomy in noninfarcted myocardium. *Circulation* 1983;67:787–796.
9. Bendel P, Eilam R. Quantitation of ventricular size in normal and spontaneously hypertensive rats by magnetic resonance imaging. *Brain Res* 1992;574:224–228.
10. Benedict CR, Loach AB. Sympathetic nervous system activity in patients with subarachnoid hemorrhage. *Stroke* 1978;9:237–244.
11. Biaggioni I, et al. Baroreflex failure in a patient with central nervous system lesions involving the nucleus tractus solitarii. *Hypertension* 1994;23:491–495.
12. Billman GE, et al. Elevated myocardial calcium and its role in sudden cardiac death. *FASEB J* 1991;5:2586–2592.
13. Bishop VS, et al. Cardiac mechanoreceptors. In: Shepherd JT, Abboud FM, eds. *Handbook of physiology*, sect 2: The cardiovascular system, vol 3: Peripheral circulatory and organ blood flow. Bethesda, MD: American Physiological Society, 1983:497–555.
14. Blessing WW, et al. Destruction of noradrenergic neurons in rabbit brain stem elevates plasma vasopressin, causing hypertension. *Science* 1982;217:661–663.
15. Blessing WW, et al. Hypertension, bradycardia, and pulmonary edema in the conscious rabbit after brain stem lesions coinciding with the A1 group of catecholamine neurons. *Circ Res* 1981;49:949–958.
16. Blessing WW, et al. Hypothalamic projections of medullary catecholamine neurons in the rabbit: demonstration by formaldehyde–glutaraldehyde-induced catecholamine fluorescence and HRP retrograde transport. *Brain Res Bull* 1982;9:279–286.
17. Blumhardt LD, et al. Electrocardiographic accompaniments of temporal lobe epileptic seizures. *Lancet* 1986;1:1051–1056.
18. Bonham AC, et al. Electrical stimulation in perifornical lateral hypothalamus decreases coronary blood flow in cats. *Am J Physiol* 1987;252:H474–H484.
19. Bonham AC, et al. Neurogenic regulation of coronary blood flow: evidence for a central nervous system pathway. *Circ Res* 1987;61(Suppl 2):II-42–II-46.
20. Buchholz RA, et al. Comparison of 1-hour and 24-hour blood pressure recordings in central or peripheral baroreceptor-denervated rats. *Hypertension* 1986;8:1154–1163.
21. Burch GE, et al. A new electrocardiographic pattern observed in cerebrovascular accidents. *Circulation* 1954;9:719–723.
22. Burch GE, et al. Acute myocardial lesions following experimentally induced intracranial hemorrhage in mice: a histological and histochemical study. *Arch Pathol* 1967;84:517–521.
23. Byer E, et al. Electrocardiogram with large, upright T-waves and long Q-T intervals. *Am Heart J* 1947;33:796–906.
24. Calaresu FR, Yardley CP. Medullary basal sympathetic tone. *Annu Rev Physiol* 1988;50:511–524.
25. Cannon WB. "Voodoo" death. *Am Anthropol* 1942;44:169–181.
26. Cardinal R, et al. Mapping of ventricular tachycardia induced by thoracic neural stimulation in dogs. *Can J Physiol Pharmacol* 1986;64:411–418.
27. Chamberlin NL, Saper CB. Topographic organization of cardiovascular responses to electrical and glutamate microstimulation of the parabrachial nucleus in the rat. *J Comp Neurol* 1992;326:245–262.
28. Cochrane KL, Nathan MA. Normotension in conscious rats after placement of bilateral electrolytic lesions in the rostral ventrolateral medulla. *J Auton Nerv Syst* 1989;26:199–211.
29. Connor RCR. Fuchsinophilic degeneration of myocardium in patients with intracranial lesions. *Br Heart J* 1970;32:81–84.
30. Connor RCR. Myocardial damage secondary to brain lesions. *Am Heart J* 1969;78:145–148.
31. Coryllos E. Vagal dysfunction and sudden infant death syndrome. *NY State J Med* 1982;82:731–735.
32. Cox BF, Brody MJ. Evidence for two functionally distinct vasomotor subregions of rostral ventral medulla. *Clin Exp Hypertens [A]* 1988;10(Suppl 1):11–18.
33. Cropp GJ, Manning GW. Electrocardiographic changes simulating myocardial ischemia and infarction associated with spontaneous intracranial hemorrhage. *Circulation* 1960;22:25–38.
34. Cushing H. Some experimental and clinical observations concerning states of increased intracranial tension. *Am J Med Sci* 1902;124:375–400.
35. Dahlström A, Fuxe K. Evidence for the existence of monoamine-containing neurons in the central nervous system. I. Demonstration of monoamines in the cell bodies of brain stem neurons. *Acta Physiol Scand* 1964;62:5–55.
36. Dampney RAL. The subretrofacial nucleus: its pivotal role in cardiovascular regulation. *NIPS* 1990;5:63–67.
37. Danilewsky B. Experimentelle Beitrage zur Physiologie des Gehirns. *Pflugers Arch* 1875;11:128–138.
38. De Ferrari GM, et al. Prevention of life-threatening arrhythmias by pharmacologic stimulation of the muscarinic receptors with oxotremorine. *Am Heart J* 1992;124:883–890.
39. Delgado JMR, et al. Cardiovascular phenomena during seizure activity. *J Nerv Ment Dis* 1960;130:477–487.
40. Deschepper CF, et al. Hypertension induced by brain grafts from fetal spontaneously hypertensive rats. *Hypertension* 1994;23(Part 1):765–773.
41. Dimant J, Grob D. Electrocardiographic changes and myocardial damage in patients with acute cerebrovascular accidents. *Stroke* 1977;8:448–455.
42. Doba N, et al. Changes in regional blood flow and cardiodynamics associated with electrically and chemically induced epilepsy in cat. *Brain Res* 1975;90:115–132.
43. Doba N, Reis DJ. Acute fulminating neurogenic hypertension produced by brainstem lesions in the rat. *Circ Res* 1973;32:584–593.
44. Doba N, Reis DJ. Role of central and peripheral adrenergic mechanisms in neurogenic hypertension produced by brain stem lesions in rat. *Circ Res* 1974;34:293–301.
45. Doba N, Reis DJ. Role of the cerebellum and the vestibular apparatus in regulation of orthostatic reflexes in the cat. *Circ Res* 1974;34:9–18.
46. Dominiczak AF, Lindpaintner K. Genetics of hypertension: a current appraisal. *NIPS* 1994;9:246–251.
47. Doshi R, Neil-Dwyer G. A clinicopathological study of patients following a subarachnoid hemorrhage. *J Neurosurg* 1980;52:295–301.
48. Eisalo A, et al. Electrocardiographic abnormalities and some laboratory findings in patients with subarachnoid hemorrhage. *Br Heart J* 1972;34:217–226.
49. Ekman P, et al. Autonomic nervous system activity distinguishes among emotions. *Science* 1983;221:1209–1210.

50. Ely DL. Hypertension, social rank, and aortic atherosclerosis in CBA/J mice. *Physiol Behav* 1981;26:655–661.
51. Engel GL. Psychologic factors in instantaneous cardiac death. *N Engl J Med* 1976;294:664–665.
52. Estanol BV, Marin OSM. Cardiac arrhythmias and sudden death in subarachnoid hemorrhage. *Stroke* 1975;6:382–386.
53. Estanol BV, et al. Cardiac arrhythmias in experimental subarachnoid hemorrhage. *Stroke* 1975;8:440–447.
54. Evans CH, et al. Astrocytoma mimicking the features of pheochromocytoma. *N Engl J Med* 1972;286:1397–1399.
55. Feibel JJ, et al. Myocardial damage and cardiac arrhythmias in cerebral infarction and subarachnoid hemorrhage: correlation with increased systemic catecholamine output. *Trans Am Neurol Assoc* 1976;101:242–244.
56. Fentz V, Gormsen J. Electrocardiographic patterns in patients with cerebrovascular accidents. *Circulation* 1962;25:22–28.
57. Finkelstein D, Nigaglioni A. Electrocardiographic alterations after neurosurgical procedures. *Am Heart J* 1961;66:772–784.
58. Gillis RA, Quest JA. The role of the nervous system in the cardiovascular effects of digitalis. *Pharmacol Rev* 1979;31:19–97.
59. Goldstein DS. The electrocardiogram in stroke: relationship to pathophysiological type and comparison with prior tracings. *Stroke* 1979;10:253–258.
60. Graff-Radford NR, Godersky JC. Idiopathic normal pressure hydrocephalus and systemic hypertension. *Neurology* 1987;37:868–871.
61. Granata L, et al. Coronary inflow and oxygen usage following cardiac sympathetic nerve stimulation in unanesthetized dogs. *Circ Res* 1965;16:114–120.
62. Greenhoot JH, Reichenbach DD. Cardiac injury and subarachnoid hemorrhage: a clinical, pathological, and physiological correlation. *J Neurosurg* 1969;30:521–531.
63. Greenland P, Griggs RC. Arrhythmic complications in the Guillain–Barré syndrome. *Arch Intern Med* 1980;140:1053–1055.
64. Grossman MA. Cardiac arrhythmias in acute central nervous system disease. *Arch Intern Med* 1976;136:203–207.
65. Gutterman DD, et al. Role of medullary lateral reticular formation in baroreflex coronary vasoconstriction. *Brain Res* 1991;557:202–209.
66. Guttstein WH, et al. Neural factors contribute to atherogenesis. *Science* 1978;199:449–451.
67. Hachinski VC, et al. Asymmetry of sympathetic consequences of experimental stroke. *Arch Neurol* 1992;49:697–702.
68. Hachinski VC, et al. Effect of age on autonomic and cardiac responses in a rat stroke model. *Arch Neurol* 1992;49:690–696.
69. Hageman GR, et al. Cardiac dysrhythmias induced by autonomic nerve stimulation. *Am J Cardiol* 1973;32:823–830.
70. Hall R, et al. Myocardial changes after hypothalamic stimulation in the intact, conscious dog. *Circulation* 1972;46(Suppl 2):II-1180 (abst).
71. Hall RE, et al. Orbital cortical influences on cardiovascular dynamics and myocardial structure in conscious monkeys. *J Neurosurg* 1977;46:638–647.
72. Hamill RW, et al. Catecholamines predict outcome in traumatic brain injury. *Ann Neurol* 1987;21:438–443.
73. Hamman L. Sudden death. *Bull Johns Hopkins Hosp* 1934;55:387–415.
74. Hammer WJ, et al. Observations on the electrocardiographic changes associated with subarachnoid hemorrhage with special reference to their genesis. *Am J Med* 1975;59:427–433.
75. Hammermeister KE, Reichenbach DD. QRS changes, pulmonary edema, and myocardial necrosis associated with subarachnoid hemorrhage. *Am Heart J* 1969;78:94–100.
76. Han JK, et al. Adrenergic effects on ventricular vulnerability. *Circ Res* 1964;14:516–524.
77. Harrison MT, Gibb BH. Electrocardiographic changes associated with cerebrovascular accident. *Lancet* 1964;2:429–430.
78. Hawkins WC, Clower BR. Myocardial damage after head trauma and simulated intracranial hemorrhage in mice: the role of the autonomic nervous system. *Cardiovasc Res* 1971;5:524–529.
79. Haws CW, Burgess MJ. Effects of bilateral and unilateral stellate stimulation on canine ventricular refractory periods at sites of overlapping innervation. *Circ Res* 1978;42:195–198.
80. Hayashi S, et al. Studies of electrocardiographic patterns in cases with neurosurgical lesions. *Jpn Heart J* 1961;2:92–111.
81. Helpern M, Rabson SM. Sudden and unexpected death: general considerations and statistics. *NY State J Med* 1945;45:1197–1201.
82. Hersch C. Electrocardiographic changes in head injuries. *Circulation* 1961;23:853–860.
83. Hersch C. Electrocardiographic changes in subarachnoid haemorrhage, meningitis, and intracranial space-occupying lesions. *Br Heart J* 1964;26:785–793.
84. Hershowitz M, et al. The muscarinic cholinergic receptors in the posterior hypothalamus of hypertensive and normotensive rats. *Eur J Pharmacol* 1983;86:229–236.
85. Hockman CH, et al. ECG changes resulting from cerebral stimulation. II. A spectrum of ventricular arrhythmias of sympathetic origin. *Am Heart J* 1966;71:695–700.
86. Hoff EC, Green HD. Cardiovascular reactions induced by electrical stimulation of the cerebral cortex. *Am J Physiol* 1936;117:411–422.
87. Hoff JT, Reis DJ. Localization of regions mediating the Cushing response in CNS of cat. *Arch Neurol* 1970;23:228–240.
88. Hsu CY, et al. Orthostatic hypotension with brain stem tumors. *Neurology* 1984;34:1137–1143.
89. Hugenholtz PG. Electrocardiographic abnormalities in cerebral disorders: report of six cases and review of the literature. *Am Heart J* 1962;63:451–461.
90. Hunt D, Gore L. Myocardial lesions following experimental intracranial hemorrhage: prevention with propranolol. *Am Heart J* 1972;83:232–236.
91. Hunt D, et al. Electrocardiographic and serum enzyme changes in subarachnoid hemorrhage. *Am Heart J* 1969;77:479–488.
92. Inoue H, Zipes DP. Results of sympathetic denervation in the canine heart: supersensitivity that may be arrhythmogenic. *Circulation* 1987;75:877–887.
93. Jacobson SA, Danufsky P. Marked electrocardiographic changes produced by experimental head trauma. *J Neuropathol Exp Neurol* 1954;13:462–466.
94. James TN, Spence CA. Distribution of cholinesterase within the sinus node and AV node of the human heart. *Anat Rec* 1966;155:151–162.
95. Jannetta PJ, Gendell HM. Neurovascular compression associated with essential hypertension. *Neurosurgery* 1978;2:165.
96. Jannetta PJ, et al. Neurogenic hypertension: etiology and surgical treatment. I. Observations in 53 patients. *Ann Surg* 1985;201:391–398.
97. Jannetta PJ, et al. Neurogenic hypertension: etiology and surgical treatment. II. Observations in an experimental nonhuman primate model. *Ann Surg* 1985;202:253–261.
98. Jones LF, Brody MJ. Characterization of coronary vasoconstriction produced by rostral ventrolateral medulla stimulation in rats. *Am J Physiol (Heart Circ Physiol)* 1992;262:H437–H442.
99. Jones LF, et al. Patterns of hemodynamic responses associated with central activation of coronary vasoconstriction. *Am J Physiol Regul Integr Comp Physiol* 1992;262:R276–R283.
100. Jonsson A, Hansson L. Prolonged exposure to a stressful stimulus (noise) as a cause of raised blood pressure in man. *Lancet* 1977;1:86–87.
101. Kemp E. Arterial hypertension in poliomyelitis. *Acta Med Scand* 1957;157:109–118.
102. Kinney HC, et al. Decreased muscarinic receptor binding in the arcuate nucleus in sudden infant death syndrome. *Science* 1995;269:1446–1450.
103. Klouda MA, Borynjolfsson G. Cardiotoxic effects of electrical stimulation of the stellate ganglia. *Ann NY Acad Sci* 1969;156:271–280.
104. Koepp M, et al. Electrocardiographic changes in patients with brain tumors. *Arch Neurol* 1995;52:152–155.
105. Koskelo P, et al. Subendocardial haemorrhage and ECG changes in intracranial bleeding. *BMJ* 1964;1:1479–1480.
106. Koudstaal PJ, et al. Holter monitoring in patients with transient and focal ischemic attacks of the brain. *Stroke* 1986;17:192–195.
107. Kralios FA, Miller CK. Sympathetic neural effects on regional atrial recovery properties and cardiac rhythm. *Am J Physiol* 1981;240:H590–H596.
108. Kralios FA, et al. Local ventricular repolarization changes due to sympathetic nerve-branch stimulation. *Am J Physiol* 1975;228:1621–1626.

109. Kreus KE, et al. Electrocardiographic changes in cerebrovascular accidents. *Acta Med Scand* 1969;185:327–334.
110. Krukoff TL, et al. Gene expression of brain nitric oxide synthase and soluble guanylyl cyclase in hypothalamus and medulla of two-kidney, one clip hypertensive rats. *Hypertension* 1995;26:171–176.
111. LeDoux JE, et al. Hierarchic organization of blood pressure responses during the expression of natural behaviors in rat: mediation by sympathetic nerves. *Exp Neurol* 1982;78:121–133.
112. Leor J, Poole WK, Kloner RA. Sudden cardiac death triggered by an earthquake. *N Engl J Med* 1996;334:413–419.
113. Lepeschkin E, et al. Effect of epinephrine and norepinephrine on the electrocardiogram of 100 normal subjects. *Am J Cardiol* 1960;5:594–603.
114. Levy MN. Cardiac sympathetic–parasympathetic interactions. *Fed Proc* 1984;43:2598–2602.
115. Levy MN. Sympathetic–parasympathetic interactions in the heart. *Circ Res* 1971;29:437–445.
116. Lichtenfield P. Autonomic dysfunction in the Guillain–Barré syndrome. *Am J Med* 1971;50:772–780.
117. Lichtlen P, Schaub F. EKG-Veranderungen bei zerebralen Insult. *Cardiologia* 1962;40:159–168.
118. Liedholm LJ, Gudjonsson O. Cardiac arrest due to partial epileptic seizures. *Neurology* 1992;42:824–829.
119. Light KC, et al. Psychological stress induces sodium and fluid retention in men at high risk for hypertension. *Science* 1983;220:429–431.
120. Lloyd-Mostyn RH, Watkins PJ. Defective innervation of heart in diabetic autonomic neuropathy. *BMJ* 1975;3:15–17.
121. Lown B. Sudden cardiac death: the major challenge confronting contemporary cardiology. *Am J Cardiol* 1979;43:313–328.
122. Lown B, et al. Basis for recurring ventricular fibrillation in the absence of coronary heart disease and its management. *N Engl J Med* 1976;294:623–629.
123. Magnus O, et al. Cerebral mechanisms and neurogenic hypertension in man, with special reference to baroreceptor control. *Prog Brain Res* 1977;47:199–218.
124. Malliani A, et al. Neural mechanisms in life-threatening arrhythmias. *Am Heart J* 1980;100:705–715.
125. Manning GW, et al. Vagal stimulation and the production of myocardial damage. *Can Med Assoc J* 1937;37:314–318.
126. Marion DW, et al. Subarachnoid hemorrhage and the heart. *Neurosurgery* 1986;18:101–106.
127. Marriott HJ. *Practical electrocardiography.* 6th ed. Baltimore: Williams and Wilkins, 1977.
128. Mauck HP Jr, et al. ECG changes resulting from cerebral stimulation. I. Anomalous atrioventricular excitation elicited by electrical stimulation of the mesencephalic reticular formation. *Am Heart J* 1964;68:98–101.
129. McNair JL, et al. Effect of reserpine pretreatment on myocardial damage associated with stimulated intracranial hemorrhage in mice. *Eur J Pharmacol* 1970;9:1–6.
130. Meldrum BS, Horton RW. Physiology of status epilepticus in primates. *Arch Neurol* 1973;28:1–9.
131. Melville KI, et al. Cardiac ischemic changes and arrhythmias induced by hypothalamic stimulation. *Am J Cardiol* 1963;12:781–791.
132. Millar K, Abildskov JA. Notched T waves in young persons with central nervous system lesions. *Circulation* 1968;37:597–603.
133. Mohring J, et al. Decreased vasopressin content in brain stem of rats with spontaneous hypertension. *Naunyn Schmiedebergs Arch Pharmacol* 1980;315:83–84.
134. Montgomery BM. The basilar artery hypertensive syndrome. *Arch Intern Med* 1961;108:559–569.
135. Moss AJ. Prediction and prevention of sudden cardiac death. *Annu Rev Med* 1980;31:1–14.
136. Muller JE, Verrier RL. Triggering of sudden-death lessons from an earthquake. *N Engl J Med* 1996;334:460–461.
137. Natelson BH. Stress, predisposition and the onset of serious disease: implications about psychosomatic etiology. *Neurosci Biobehav Rev* 1991;7:511–527.
138. Nathan MA, Reis DJ. Chronic labile hypertension produced by lesions of the nucleus tractus solitarii in the cat. *Circ Res* 1977;40:72–81.
139. Obrist PA, et al. Sympathetic influences on cardiac rate and contractility during acute stress in humans. *Psychophysiology* 1974;11:405–427.
140. Offerhaus I, Van Gool J. Electrocardiographic changes and tissue catecholamines in experimental subarachnoid hemorrhage. *Cardiovasc Res* 1969;3:433–440.
141. Oppenheimer SM, et al. Cerebrogenic cardiac arrhythmias: cerebral electrocardiographic influences and their role in sudden death. *Arch Neurol* 1990;47:513–519.
142. Oppenheimer SM, et al. Insular cortex stimulation produces lethal cardiac arrhythmias: a mechanism of sudden death. *Brain Res* 1991;550:115–121.
143. Pace JB. Autonomic control of the coronary circulation. In: Randall WC, ed. *Neural regulation of the heart.* New York: Oxford University Press, 1977:313–344.
144. Parizel G. Life-threatening arrhythmias in subarachnoid hemorrhage. *Angiology* 1973;24:17–21.
145. Parizel G. On the mechanism of sudden death with subarachnoid hemorrhage. *J Neurol* 1979;220:71–76.
146. Penfield W. Diencephalic autonomic epilepsy. *Arch Neurol Psych* 1929;22:358–374.
147. Pfister CW, de Pando B. Cerebral hemorrhage simulating acute myocardial infarction. *Dis Chest* 1962;42:206–207.
148. Pitts RF, Bronk DW. Excitability cycle of the hypothalamus–sympathetic neurone system. *Am J Physiol* 1941;135:992–996.
149. Pitts RF, et al. An analysis of hypothalamic cardiovascular control. *Am J Physiol* 1941;134:359–383.
150. Plum F, Posner JB. *The diagnosis of stupor and coma.* 3rd ed. Philadelphia: FA Davis, 1980.
151. Plunkett LM, Saavedra JM. Increased angiotensin II binding affinity in the nucleus tractus solitarius of spontaneously hypertensive rats. *Proc Natl Acad Sci USA* 1985;82:7721–7724.
152. Prystowsky EN, et al. Effect of autonomic blockade on ventricular refractoriness and atrioventricular nodal conduction in humans: evidence supporting a direct cholinergic action on ventricular muscle refractoriness. *Circ Res* 1981;49:511–518.
153. Ranson SW, et al. Autonomic responses to electrical stimulation of hypothalamus, preoptic region and septum. *Arch Neurol Psych* 1935;33:467–477.
154. Reichek N. Heart and head, 1985 [Editorial]. *Ann Neurol* 1985;18:13–20.
155. Reis DJ, Doba N. Hypertension as a localizing sign of mass lesions of brain stem. *N Engl J Med* 1972;287:1355.
156. Reis DJ, Oliphant MC. Bradycardia and tachycardia following electrical stimulation of the amygdaloid region in monkey. *J Neurophysiol* 1964;27:893–912.
157. Rem JA, et al. Value of cardiac monitoring and echocardiography in TIA and stroke patients. *Stroke* 1985;16:950–956.
158. Ritter S, Dinh TT. Progressive postnatal dilation of brain ventricles in spontaneously hypertensive rats. *Brain Res* 1986;370:327–332.
159. Ritter S, et al. Cerebroventricular dilation in spontaneously hypertensive rats (SHRs) is not attenuated by reduction of blood pressure. Brain Res 1988;450:354–359.
160. Rokey R, et al. Coronary artery disease in patients with cerebrovascular disease: a prospective study. *Ann Neurol* 1984;16:50–53.
161. Ross CA, et al. Tonic vasomotor control by the rostral ventrolateral medulla: effect of electrical or chemical stimulation of the area containing C1 adrenaline neurons on arterial pressure, heart rate and plasma catecholamines and vasopressin. *J Neurosci* 1984;4:474–494.
162. Saavedra JM, et al. Changes in central catecholaminergic neurons in the spontaneously (genetic) hypertensive rat. *Circ Res* 1978;42:529–534.
163. Samuels MA. Neurogenic heart disease: a unifying hypothesis. *Am J Cardiol* 1987;60:15J–19J.
164. Saper CB, et al. Direct hypothalamo-autonomic connections. *Brain Res* 1976;117:305–312.
165. Satinsky J, et al. Ventricular fibrillation induced by hypothalamic stimulation during coronary occlusion. *Circulation* 1971;44(Suppl 2):II-60(abst).
166. Sawchenko PE, Swanson LW. Central noradrenergic pathways for the integration of hypothalamic neuroendocrine and autonomic responses. *Science* 1981;214:685–687.

167. Schenk EA, Moss AJ. Cardiovascular effects of sustained norepinephrine infusions II. Morphology. *Circ Res* 1966;18:605–615.
168. Scher AM, et al. Sympathetic and parasympathetic control of heart rate in the dog, baboon and man. *Fed Proc* 1972;31:1219–1225.
169. Schiff M. Untersuchungen uber die motorischen Functionen des Gross-Hirns. *Naunyn Schmiedebergs Arch Pharmacol* 1875;3:171–179.
170. Schroth WS, et al. Multiple sclerosis as a cause of atrial fibrillation and electrocardiographic changes. *Arch Neurol* 1992;49:422–424.
171. Schwartz PJ. Cardiac sympathetic innervation and the sudden infant death syndrome: a possible pathogenetic link. *Am J Med* 1976;60:167–172.
172. Schwartz PJ, et al. The long Q-T syndrome. *Am Heart J* 1975;89:378–390.
173. Schwartz PJ, et al. Effects of unilateral stellate ganglion blockade on the arrhythmias associated with coronary occlusion. *Am Heart J* 1976;92:589–599.
174. Shepherd JT. Cardiac mechanoreceptors. In: Fozzard HA, et al., eds. *The heart and cardiovascular system.* New York: Raven, 1986:1535–1558.
175. Shipley RE, Gregg DE. The cardiac response to stimulation of the stellate ganglia and cardiac nerves. *Am J Physiol* 1945;143:396–401.
176. Shy GM, Drager GA. A neurological syndrome associated with orthostatic hypotension: a clinical–pathological study. *Arch Neurol* 1960;2:511–527.
177. Skinner JE. Regulation of cardiac vulnerability by the cerebral defense system. *J Am Coll Cardiol* 1985;5:88B–94B.
178. Smith M, Ray CT. Cardiac arrhythmias, increased intracranial pressure and the autonomic nervous system. *Chest* 1972;61:125–133.
179. Smith RP, Tomlinson BE. Subendocardial haemorrhages associated with intracranial lesions. *J Pathol Bacteriol* 1954;68:327–334.
180. Smith SA, Smith SE. Heart rate variations in the Guillain–Barré syndrome. *BMJ* 1980;281:1009–1010.
181. Srivastava SC, Robson AO. Electrocardiographic abnormalities associated with subarachnoid hemorrhage. *Lancet* 1964;2:431–434.
182. Stull JT, Mayer SE. Biochemical mechanisms of adrenergic and cholinergic regulation of myocardial contractility. In: Berne RM, Sperelakis N, eds. *Handbook of physiology,* sect 2: The cardiovascular system, vol 1: The heart. Bethesda, MD: American Physiological Society, 1979:741–774.
183. Sved AF, McDowell FH, Blessing WW. Release of antidiuretic hormone in quadriplegic subjects in response to head-up tilt. *Neurology* 1985;35:78–82.
184. Sved AF, et al. Vasopressin contributes to hypertension caused by nucleus tractus solitarius lesions. *Hypertension* 1985;7:262–267.
185. Szakacs JE, Mehlman B. Pathologic changes induced by *l*-norepinephrine: quantitative aspects. *Am J Cardiol* 1960;5:619–627.
186. Talman WT. Cardiovascular regulation and lesions of the central nervous system. *Ann Neurol* 1985;18:1–12.
187. Talman WT. The central nervous system and cardiovascular regulation. In: Weintraub MI, Fass AE, eds. *Heart and brain: interactions of cardiac and neurologic disease.* Costa Mesa, CA: PMA, 1991:1–28.
188. Talman WT, et al. Chronic lability of arterial pressure in the rat does not evolve into hypertension. *Clin Sci* 1980; 59(Suppl):405s–407s.
189. Talman WT, et al. Acute hypertension after the local injection of kainic acid into the nucleus tractus solitarii of rats. *Circ Res* 1981;48:292–298.
190. Talman WT, Reis DJ. Baroreflex actions of substance P microinjected into the nucleus tractus solitarii in rat: a consequence of local distortion. *Brain Res* 1981;220:402–407.
191. Talman WT, et al. Chronic lability of arterial pressure produced by destruction of A2 catecholaminergic neurons in rat brainstem. *Circ Res* 1980;46:842–853.
192. Talman WT, et al. Antagonism of the baroreceptor reflex by glutamate diethyl ester, an antagonist to L-glutamate. *Brain Res* 1981;217:186–191.
193. Towbin JA. New revelations about the long-QT syndrome. *N Engl J Med* 1995;333:384–385.
194. Trichopoulos D, et al. Psychological stress and fatal heart attack: the Athens (1981) earthquake natural experiment. *Lancet* 1983;1:441–443.
195. Van Buren JM. Some autonomic concomitants of ictal automatism: a study of temporal lobe attacks. *Brain* 1958;81:505–528.
196. Van Buren JM, Ajmone-Marsan C. A correlation of autonomic and EEG components in temporal lobe epilepsy. *Arch Neurol* 1960;3:683–703.
197. Verrier RL, et al. Effect of posterior hypothalamic stimulation on ventricular fibrillation threshold. *Am J Physiol* 1975; 228:923–927.
198. Verrier RL, Lown B. Behavioral stress and cardiac arrhythmias. *Annu Rev Physiol* 1984;46:155–176.
199. Verrier RL, et al. Ventricular vulnerability during sympathetic stimulation: role of heart rate and blood pressure. *Cardiovasc Res* 1974;8:602–610.
200. Versteeg DHG, et al. Catecholamine content of individual brain regions of spontaneously hypertensive rats (SH rats). *Brain Res* 1976;112:429–434.
201. Voridis EM, et al. Holter monitoring during 1981 Athens earthquakes. *Lancet* 1983;1:1281–1282.
202. Weidler DJ. Myocardial damage and cardiac arrhythmias after intracranial hemorrhage: a critical review. *Stroke* 1974;5:759–764.
203. Weidler DJ, et al. Cardiac arrhythmias secondary to acute cerebral ischemia: prevention by autonomic blockade. *Circulation* 1976;53–54(Suppl 2):II-102(abst).
204. West TC, et al. Drug alteration of transmembrane potentials in atrial pacemaker cells. *J Pharmacol Exp Ther* 1956;117: 245–252.
205. Yanowitz F, et al. Functional distribution of right and left stellate innervation to the ventricles: production of neurogenic electrocardiographic changes by unilateral alteration of sympathetic tone. *Circ Res* 1966;18:416–428.
206. Zipes DP, et al. Sudden cardiac death: neural–cardiac interactions. *Circulation* 1987;76(Suppl 1):I-202–I-207.

CHAPTER 5

Autonomic Regulation of Circulation

Michael J. Joyner and John T. Shepherd

1. The upright posture and muscular exercise are two common activities that pose challenges to circulatory homeostasis in humans. These activities allow the expanding complexity and the integrative nature of autonomic circulatory control to be explored.
2. With standing, there is a shift of blood volume from the thorax to the legs, such that venous return and cardiac output are reduced. Vasoconstriction elicited by the combined actions of the venoarteriolar, cardiopulmonary, and arterial baroreflexes increases systemic vascular resistance. Arterial baroreflexes also increase heart rate. Together these actions maintain mean arterial pressure at the supine value.
3. At the onset of exercise, there is a rapid central command related to the motor signals sent by higher brain centers that stimulates the brainstem cardiovascular centers. This feed-forward signal is responsible for the immediate cardiovascular changes observed at the beginning of exercise. A central command signal may also play a role in the upward resetting of the arterial baroreflexes observed with exercise.
4. With exercise, the increased contractile activity of the skeletal muscles causes metabolites to be released. These metabolites can (a) cause local vasodilation, (b) act to inhibit sympathetic neurotransmission, and (c) activate a powerful vasoconstricting muscle chemoreflex. The balance between the potentially competing effects of the metabolites can differ with static and rhythmic exercise.
5. During both standing and exercise, the autonomic nervous system plays the dominant role in integrating the various local and reflex mechanisms to regulate arterial blood pressure and meet the needs of the entire organism.
6. In recent years, a number of vasoactive substances (such as nitric oxide) produced by the vascular endothelium have been shown to have marked effects on arterial pressure. Newer evidence indicates that there can be both acute and chronic interactions between the endothelium and autonomic nerves. These interactions will be the focus of much future research related to the reflex control of the circulation.

INTRODUCTION

The overall behavior of the cardiovascular system is governed by complex interactions between local and neurohumoral mechanisms that act in combination to control cardiac output, systemic vascular resistance, and local organ blood flow to regulate mean arterial pressure (50,53). Figure 1 illustrates the complexity of this system. However, blood pressure does not always remain within a narrow range. It varies throughout the day, and the target pressure that the system seeks to maintain appears to shift in concert with either increased or decreased physical or emotional stress (36) (Fig. 2).

M. J. Joyner: Department of Anesthesiology, Mayo Clinic, Rochester, Minnesota 55905.
J. T. Shepherd: Department of Physiology and Biophysics, Mayo Clinic and Foundation, Rochester, Minnesota 55905.

Rather than cataloging the components that contribute to the circulatory system, this chapter considers the complexity and integrative nature of circulatory regulation in terms of how the arterial blood pressure is regulated during two common human activities—upright posture and muscular exercise. The responses to these activities will then be used to highlight how various local and neurohumoral mechanisms interact. These maneuvers also highlight the central role that skeletal muscle, which can account for >40% of lean body mass, plays in the regulation of arterial pressure by virtue of the total size of its vascular bed.

UPRIGHT POSTURE

Assumption of the upright posture shifts blood volume from the thorax to the abdomen and lower extremities (Fig. 3), thereby reducing venous return and cardiac filling

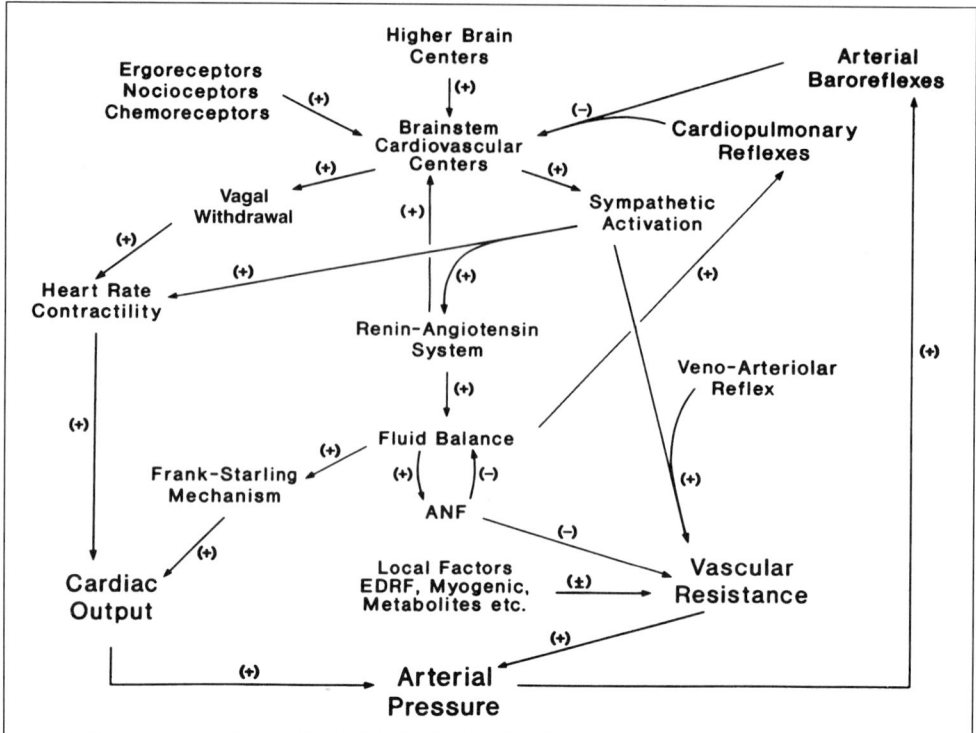

FIG. 1. The expanding complexity of some of the major local and systemic mechanisms that participate in the autonomic control of circulation. ANF, atrial natriuretic factor; EDRF, endothelium-derived relaxing factor.

pressure (42,54). These factors lead to reduced cardiac output that, if unopposed, reduces arterial blood pressure and could ultimately precipitate syncope. In a recumbent position, ~25%–30% of the circulating blood volume is in the thorax. Upon standing, this volume is estimated to fall by 26%–30%, resulting in a shift of 6–8 ml/kg of blood to the lower part of the body (54). The fluid shift begins immediately, and up to 50% of the total change can be achieved within seconds of standing. This rapid reduction in central blood volume also causes a fall in stroke volume of ~40% brought about by the decrease in cardiac filling pressure. There is a simultaneous reflex increase in heart rate, caused primarily by withdrawal of vagal activity to the sinus node. The changes in heart rate compensate (in part) for the reduction in stroke volume and, as a result, cardiac output declines by only 20%. The augmented sympathetic outflow also increases the systemic vascular resistance and, as a consequence, the mean arterial blood pressure is maintained at or near the supine level, although the pulse pressure is reduced (42,54). A complex series of mechanisms are important in this maintenance of mean arterial pressure.

Venoarteriolar Axon Reflexes

With standing, venous distention in the dependent legs, sufficient to increase venous transmural pressure to ≥25 mm Hg, stimulates a local axon reflex that constricts arterial inflow to the skin, muscle, and adipose tissue (23,24). In a series of studies conducted in normal subjects, paraplegic and quadriplegic patients, and patients undergoing spinal anesthesia [to eliminate central nervous system (CNS) and spinal reflexes], Henriksen and colleagues (23,24) demonstrated that this venoarteriolar axon reflex can elicit up to 40% of the total increase in limb vascular resistance with standing, and thus may be an important adjunct to the postural reflexes mediated by the CNS. The receptor sites appear to dwell in small veins and the effector sites are located in the arterioles supplying the dependent tissues.

Cardiopulmonary Reflexes

The peripheral vasoconstriction provided by the venoarteriolar reflexes is reinforced by the cardiopulmonary reflexes. A number of sensors are located in the thoracic cavity and, depending on their location, they can modulate the autonomic outflow to cause the systemic vessels to constrict or dilate and the heart rate to increase or decrease (27,30,51,52,60). Mechanoreceptors subserved by unmyelinated vagal afferents exist in all four cardiac chambers. They exert a tonic inhibitory influence on the brainstem cardiovascular centers, which is augmented by increasing stretch (i.e., increased blood volume). The reductions in central blood volume and pressure that occur with standing unload these receptors, thus evoking a reflex increase in sympathetic outflow that is vital in defending arterial blood pressure by constricting both systemic resistance

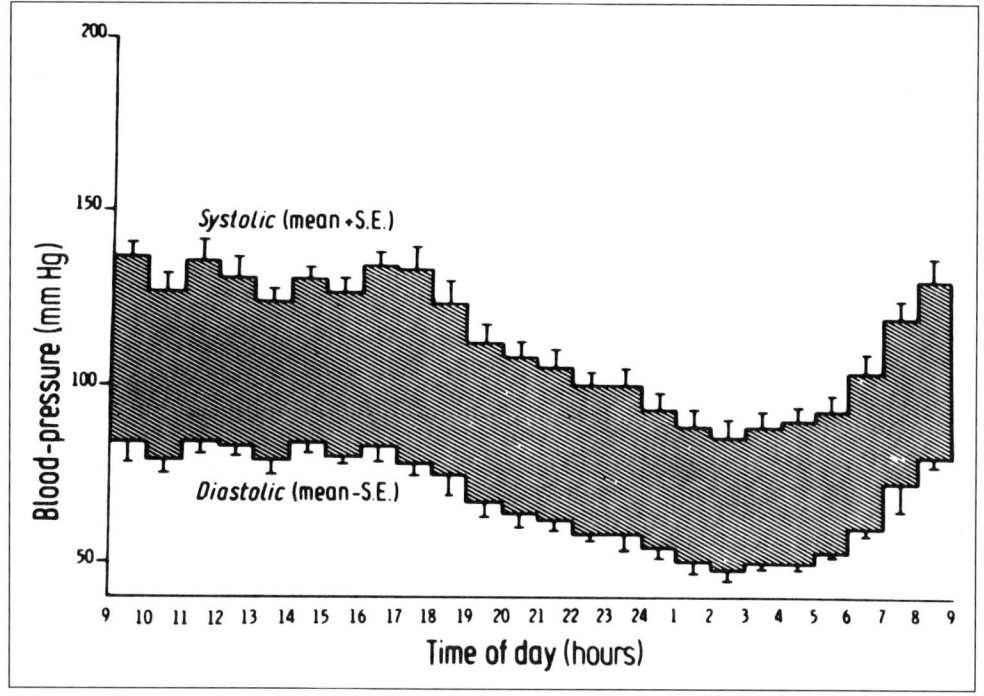

FIG. 2. The 24-hr averages of systolic and diastolic arterial pressure in normotensive subjects, demonstrating the daily variation in arterial blood pressure. From Millar-Craig et al. (36), with permission.

vessels and splanchnic capacitance vessels. The constriction of the splanchnic capacitance vessels serves to maintain the cardiac filling pressure (10,52). The lungs also have receptors that, when activated by stretch, inhibit the vasomotor center. These could also contribute to an increase in the sympathetic outflow when the thoracic volume is reduced upon standing (51).

In humans, lower body suction has been used to study the cardiovascular responses to venous pooling (Fig. 4). During mild levels of suction, there is a reduction in central blood volume and peripheral vasoconstriction and no change in heart rate. These responses have been attributed to "selective" unloading of the cardiopulmonary receptors. The concept is that since arterial pressure does not change, and because there is no rise in heart rate, then "arterial baroreceptors" are not stimulated during mild venous pooling and the vasoconstriction results from unloading of cardiopulmonary receptors. In some heart transplant patients, the vasoconstrictor responses to mild venous pooling are attenuated, suggesting a key role for ventricular receptors in causing this response (40). Evidence in normals, however, indicates that even very low levels of venous pooling are associated with changes in the mechanical deformation of the aortic mechanoreceptors that are reflected in the usual measure of arterial pressure, suggesting that aortic receptors might also contribute to the vasoconstriction (58). Taken together, these observations highlight the difficulty of studying the contribution of the cardiopulmonary receptors in regulating vascular tone in conscious humans.

Atrial or ventricular mechanoreceptors, or both, with vagal afferents may also inhibit the release of antidiuretic hormone from the posterior pituitary (6,52,59). The reduction of cardiac volume with standing should also operate locally to suppress the release of atrial natriuretic factor, or factors, that normally promote diuresis and vasodilation (20). Together these actions preserve or increase the circulating plasma volume and thereby attempt to maintain (in the long term) the cardiac filling pressure and compensate for the reduced central blood volume. The increased sympathetic outflow, acting on β-receptors in the juxtaglomerular cells, increases the renin output. The resultant increase in the level of circulating angiotensin II then acts directly on the resistance vessels to cause vasoconstriction and also on the sympathetic nerve terminals to increase the norepinephrine output. It may also produce an increase in the sympathetic outflow by stimulating the brainstem cardiovascular centers.

During space flight (when zero gravity is reached) or during immersion in water, the opposite events occur as blood is displaced to the thoracic cavity (42,54).

Pulmonary Stretch Receptors

Pulmonary vagal afferents sensitive to increases in lung volume promote two differing effects on the peripheral sympathetic outflow (51). First, when stimulated by lung inflation, they can inhibit sympathetic outflow to limb vessels, so that most of the sympathetic outflow to skeletal

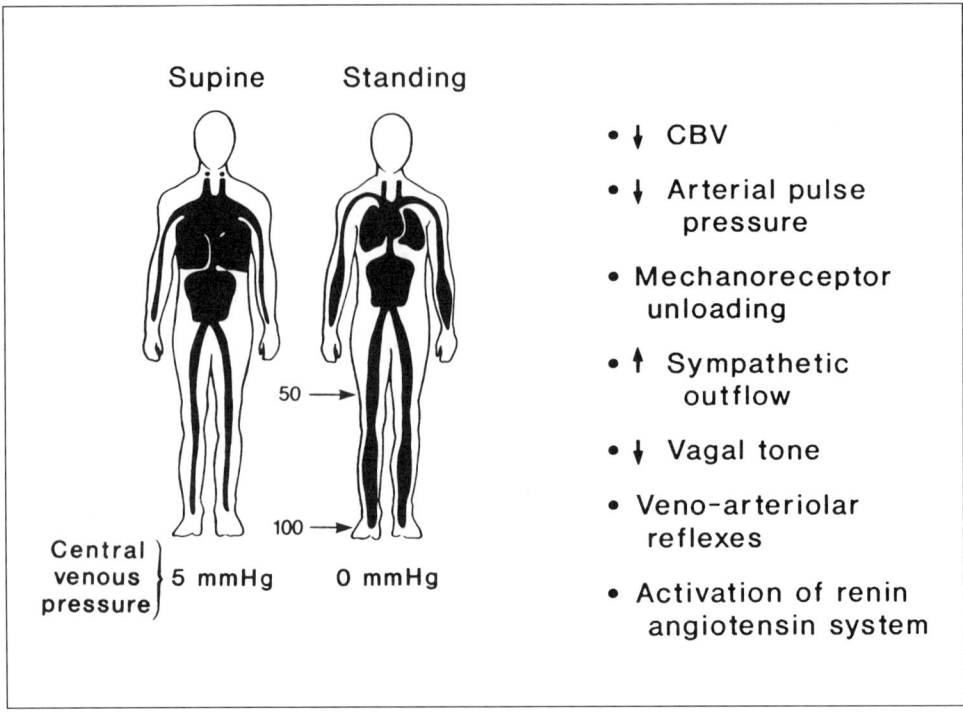

FIG. 3. The shift in blood volume and some of the consequential physiologic responses that occur. CBV, circulating blood volume. Adapted from Rowell (42) and Smith (54).

muscles takes place at the end of expiration or early during inspiration. This occurs without a change in the overall sympathetic outflow (19,47). There are also periodic changes in arterial pressure, which occur in synchrony with inspiration and expiration, that can affect the activity of arterial baroreceptors (19). Of more importance to the maintenance of upright posture are the deep breaths that cause venoconstriction. This venoconstriction, combined with the thoracic pumping action of the negative intrathoracic pressure with breathing, helps maintain venous return (12). In many subjects, vasovagal syncope is preceded by deep and prolonged sighing, presumably in an attempt to augment cardiac filling and oppose the impending decrease in arterial pressure.

Arterial Baroreflexes

Mechanically sensitive afferents from the aorta (vagus nerve) and carotid sinus (glossopharyngeal nerve) are stimulated when stretched by increases in arterial blood pressure (31). Individual nerve fibers that respond preferentially to the level of systolic, diastolic, or pulse pressure have been identified (1,4,13,14,31). The increased afferent activity that accompanies an increase in blood pressure inhibits sympathetic outflow and slows heart rate, with the reverse happening when pressure falls. Therefore, these receptor systems can cause rapid changes in heart rate, cardiac contractility, and venous capacitance. In experimental animals, the carotid sinus baroreceptors can be surgically

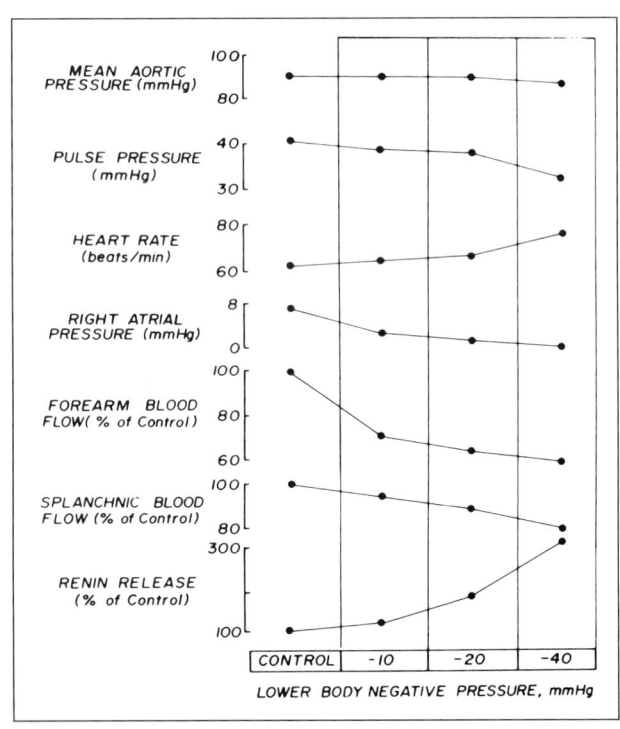

FIG. 4. Circulatory effects of graded venous pooling with lower-body negative pressure (suction) in humans. The changes associated with negative pressures of up to −20 mmHg stem predominantly from the unloading of cardiopulmonary receptors. Both arterial and cardiopulmonary reflexes contribute at higher levels of suction. From Shepherd and Vanhoutte (53), with permission.

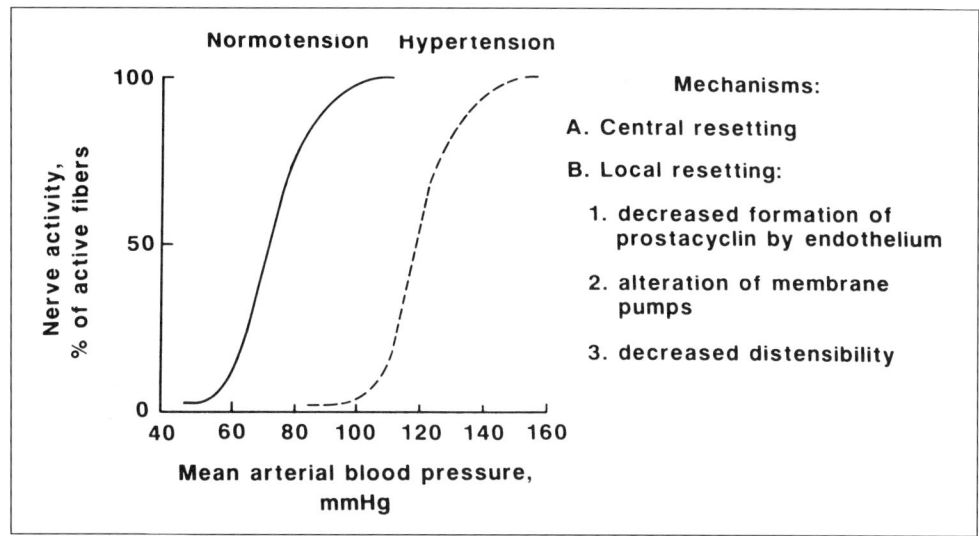

FIG. 5. Proposed mechanisms of arterial baroreflex resetting in the context of hypertension. Besides central resetting, local factors that alter the compliance of the receptors may also play a role. Similar mechanisms are thought to operate in the resetting observed for other situations. From Shepherd (50), with permission.

isolated and their functions studied (35,63,64). In humans, infusions of vasoactive drugs, or the use of neck collars that apply positive or negative pressure to the neck and thus alter the transmural pressure at the carotid sinus, are used to study the arterial baroreflexes. Drug infusions yield information only about heart rate, as they directly alter vascular resistance. The interpretation of neck pressure or suction studies can be confused by the activation of other receptors, because any reflex changes in pressure caused by the carotid receptors are buffered by the aortic and possibly cardiopulmonary receptors (31).

Arterial baroreflexes are usually characterized as a negative-feedback system that attempts to lower arterial pressure when it is high and raise arterial pressure when low. This concept is illustrated by a hypothetical stimulus–response curve obtained in an isolated carotid sinus preparation (Fig. 5). When the carotid sinus pressure is held at a variety of levels and the reflex changes in arterial pressure, heart rate, or efferent sympathetic traffic are measured, a sigmoidal curve is obtained. Such curves have led to a number of important concepts concerning baroreceptor function, including the concept of a so-called set or operating point that normally lies midway on the linear portion of the stimulus–response curve.

The set-point is thought to represent the target pressure that the arterial baroreflexes attempt to defend. The location of the set-point on the steep linear portion of the stimulus–response curve allows for equally effective buffering of either increases or decreases in the arterial pressure. Baroreflex resetting is a key feature of the arterial baroreflex system that reflects a changing of the set-point of the system with time, without a change in the shape of the curve. The resetting can occur rapidly, on the order of seconds to minutes, or it can be long term (see Fig. 5). Either CNS alterations or local factors operating at the receptor level are thought to be responsible for the resetting (13,14,57). During exercise, there is a rapid upward resetting that is likely to be centrally mediated (8,18). Substances produced in the vascular endothelium lining the site of the receptors can also cause resetting (14). In both the experimental and clinical setting of human hypertension, the arterial pressure defended by the reflexes is increased and the operating point is shifted, thereby reinforcing the hypertensive state (31,50). In experimental settings, a rise in arterial pressure usually evokes a fall in heart rate in the "negative feedback" manner just described. However, heart rate and arterial pressure normally rise or fall together in response to common physical and mental stressors.

When a person assumes the upright posture, the carotid receptors are shifted above the heart and the distending pressure they sense is reduced, both in absolute terms and relative to the aortic receptors. The aortic receptors appear to respond preferentially to static changes in pressure (4). They also appear to maintain a sustained increase in sympathetic outflow in response to prolonged small reductions in pressure (44,46). The carotid receptors are thought to respond more vigorously to rapid changes in arterial pressure and to reset quickly (4). In this way, the carotid reflexes operate best by buffering the immediate changes in arterial pressure that occur upon standing, with the aortic receptors playing an important role as the upright posture is continued. The interaction between the aortic and carotid receptors may be a particularly "human" problem associated with the upright posture. In most animals, the receptors are anatomically similar with respect to their orientation to the heart. This factor and the previously discussed limitations of drug infusions and neck collars make it difficult to conduct studies of the differential effects of the carotid and aortic reflexes in humans.

Interaction of Cardiopulmonary and Arterial Reflexes

Although the carotid and cardiopulmonary reflexes are usually studied in isolation, during standing they are both unloaded simultaneously. It appears that unloading of the cardiopulmonary receptors with low levels of venous pooling increases the responsiveness of the carotid reflexes to augment both heart rate and vascular resistance (9,20,42). In this way, the reflexes operate synergistically and reinforce each other to maintain arterial pressure with standing.

EXERCISE

The key difference between rest and exercise is volitional activation of the skeletal muscles. This produces a large increase in the use of adenosine triphosphate by the contractile machinery, and this is accompanied by circulatory (and respiratory) events that augment oxygen delivery to the active muscles. CNS signals related to the increased motor commands to the spinal cord appear to stimulate the brainstem cardiovascular centers directly (21,29,48), and the metabolic products of contraction appear to promote vasodilation and modulate sympathetic neurotransmission locally in the vascular beds perfusing the active muscles (49). Certain metabolites can also stimulate blood pressure, raising sensory nerves in the contracting muscles (2,28,32,39,43,61). The interaction of these events and the reflex responses to them mediate many of the complex physiologic responses to exercise (Fig. 6) (39,42).

Types of Exercise

Two types of exercise are normally considered. Static (or isometric) exercise consists of held contractions, with little or no external muscle shortening. Common examples are the sustained holding of a suitcase or stabilization of a heavy object. Rhythmic (or dynamic) exercise involves repetitive contractions, such as running or cycling. In both types of exercise, the mass of the active muscles involved

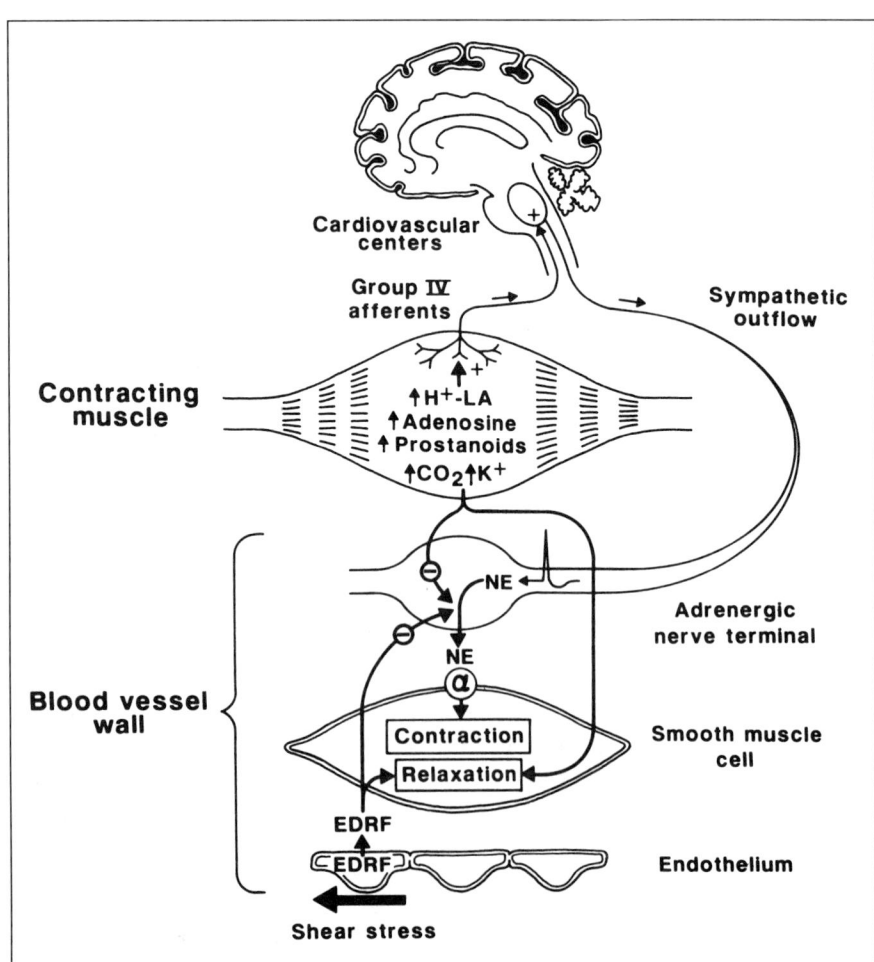

FIG. 6. Local and reflex circulatory effects of factors released by contracting muscles. These factors can (a) directly dilate skeletal muscle resistance vessels, (b) modulate sympathetic neurotransmission, and (c) activate sympathoexcitatory chemosensitive afferents. The increase in blood flow they elicit may also act locally to release endothelium-derived relaxing factor (EDRF), which could contribute to the hyperemia and also inhibit sympathetic neurotransmission. LA, lactate; NE, norepinephrine.

can be as small as a finger or forearm, and range up to the simultaneous use of both arms and legs. The division between static and dynamic exercise is somewhat artificial, however, and represents the ends of a continuum; most human activity is a mixture of both (5). However, the key difference between the two forms of exercise is that the held contractions of static exercise compress the skeletal muscle vessels and reduce or, if the force is sufficient, stop blood flow to the active muscles. During rhythmic exercise involving a small mass of active muscles, the regular relaxations between contractions allow up to a hundredfold (300 ml/100 ml/min) increases in muscle blood flow, resulting from the actions of the local vasodilating factor, or factors, released from the contracting muscles (3,42). These differing effects on muscle blood flow are responsible for the different cardiovascular responses (Fig. 7).

In the case of static exercise, there is a progressive increase in arterial pressure as the various cardiovascular control systems attempt to perfuse the active muscles in the face of the mechanical obstruction to flow (2,39). In contrast, during rhythmic exercise of a large muscle mass (10 kg), maximum metabolic vasodilation in the active muscle could theoretically overwhelm the pumping capacity of the heart in normal subjects (~20–25 L/min), so that blood pressure would fall if the sympathetic nervous system did not restrain flow to the active muscles and cause reflex constriction of the renal and splanchnic vessels (15,41). In fact, marked hypotension during supine or even head-down cycling is observed in patients who suffer from orthostatic hypotension (33). Normally the increases in muscle blood flow and cardiac output are also matched by augmented venous return as the skeletal-muscle pump returns blood from the limbs to the heart (7,15,42,49). The net results of these interactions during upright, large-muscle-mass rhythmic exercise are increases in cardiac output of up to 20–25 L/min (30–40 L/min in elite endurance athletes), along with marked increases in systolic pressure, reductions in diastolic pressure, and only modest increases in mean arterial pressure (15,42). Heart rate can increase to ~200 beats/min and stroke volume will return and then slightly surpass the resting supine value as the muscle pumps the direct blood volume centrally (Fig. 8) (7,15).

Central Command

The first excitatory signal to reach the brainstem cardiovascular centers during both static and rhythmic exercise has been termed *central command*. This refers to a signal received by the brainstem cardiovascular centers that is proportional to the motor commands that initiate and sustain the voluntary muscle contractions (21,29,39,48,62). It is an old idea that was first enunciated in the early 1900s and has been used since to describe the instantaneous changes in the circulation and respiration upon the onset of voluntary exercise (29). Studies in cats have furnished di-

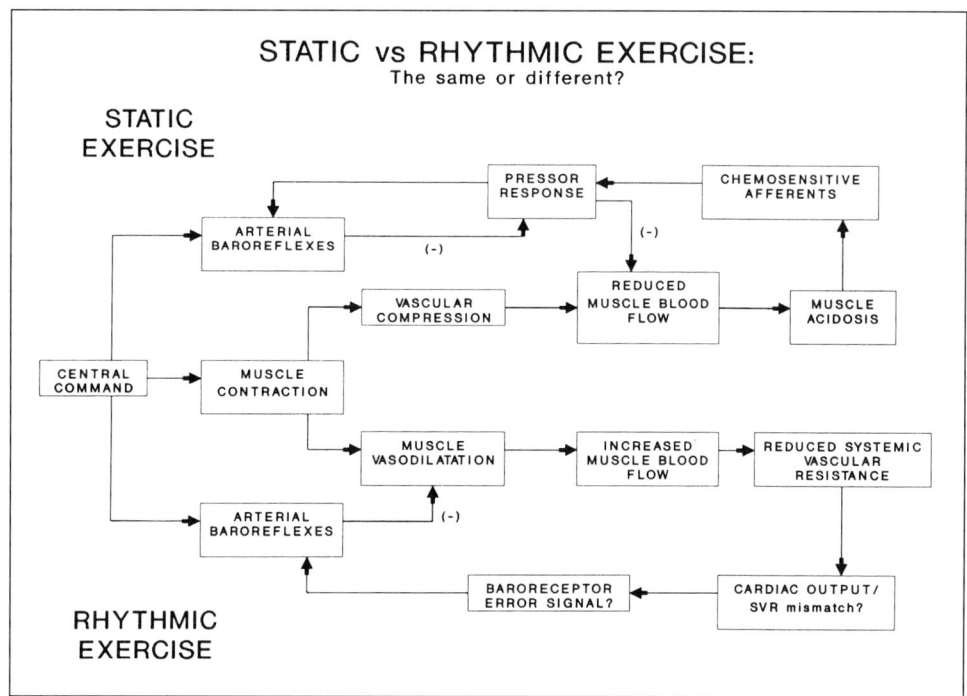

FIG. 7. The similarities and differences between static and rhythmic exercise. The essential difference is that static exercise compresses muscle vessels and rhythmic exercise causes their dilation. SVR, systemic vascular resistance. From Joyner and Shepherd (26), with permission.

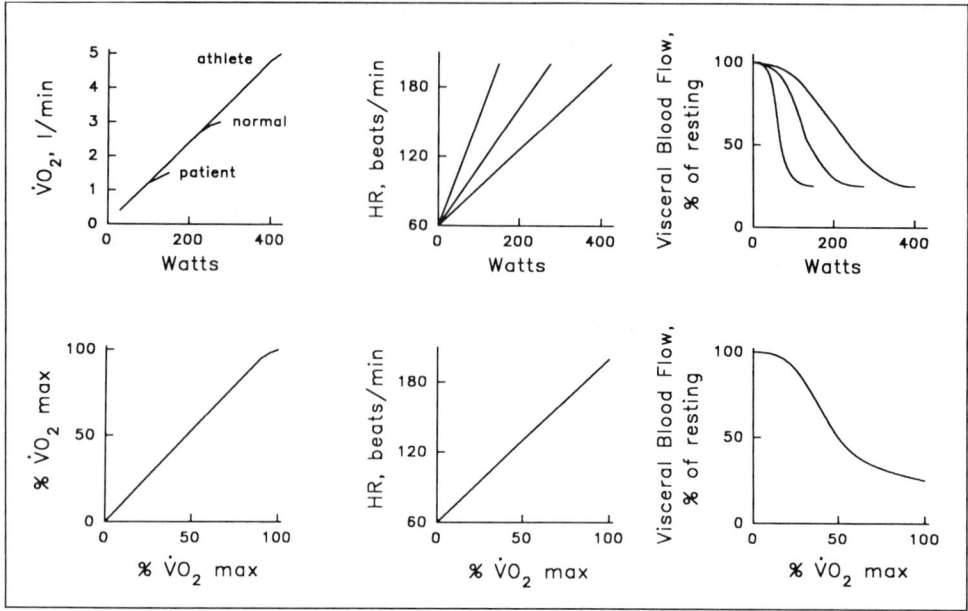

FIG. 8. Cardiovascular adjustments to incremental rhythmic leg exercise in patients with limited peak cardiac outputs (5–10 L/min), normal subjects (peak cardiac output, 20–25 L/min), and champion athletes (peak cardiac outputs, 30–40 L/min). The differences in cardiac output primarily result from the differences in stroke volume. At a given percentage of maximum oxygen uptake ($\dot{V}O_2$max), visceral blood flow is reduced equally in all three groups, demonstrating that the reflex mechanisms responsible for the vasoconstriction respond to the relative intensity of the exercise and not the absolute level. In humans, current concepts favor that a mixture of mechanisms, including the arterial baroreflexes, muscle chemoreflexes, and central command, is responsible for the increase in vasoconstrictor outflow to the periphery. Central command is also considered the prime regulator of heart rate (HR). Data from Clausen (15) and Rowell (42).

rect neurophysiologic evidence for the existence of central command, and it remains a key concept in our understanding of autonomic control during exercise (21). In the current schemes, central command is a feed-forward signal originating from higher brain centers that is responsible for the immediate increases in heart rate, blood pressure, and respiration seen at the onset of exercise. In humans, central command has been best studied during small-muscle-mass (handgrip) static and rhythmic exercise, in which it can clearly increase heart rate and cardiac output through vagal withdrawal and cause vasoconstriction in vascular beds other than skeletal muscle (32,62).

There is also some evidence that, at the onset of exercise, central command can mediate a cholinergic vasodilation in the forearm (but not leg) muscles (17,45). There can also be marked neurally mediated "active" forearm vasodilation when some subjects are exposed to mental or emotional stress. Recent evidence indicates that the vasodilating substance nitric oxide (NO) participates in this dilation. It is not yet clear whether the NO is released directly from autonomic (nitroxidergic) nerves or as a result of sympathetic–cholinergic stimulation of the vascular endothelium. The potential role of vasodilating autonomic nerves in the reflex control of the circulation remains poorly understood (16).

Arterial Baroreflexes

At the onset of either static or rhythmic exercise involving a small or large mass of active muscles, the carotid (and presumably aortic) receptors are reset to a higher operating (set) point, so that the target mean arterial pressure that these reflexes defend is increased (8,18). In animal studies, baroreflex control of heart rate has also exhibited a parallel shift (35,63,64). This also appears to be true in humans, except during fairly heavy dynamic exercise, when arterial pressure regulation is reset but baroreflex control of the heart rate may be slightly diminished (8). The mechanism of receptor resetting is unclear, but its speed (almost instantaneous) suggests that CNS signals may play a key role. Baroreflex resetting is thought to play a permissive role in allowing blood pressure to increase with exercise.

The reduction in vascular resistance associated with heavy rhythmic exercise of a large muscle mass could, if unopposed, threaten arterial pressure. Various lines of evidence favor the view that sympathetic nerves to the resistance vessels that perfuse active muscles act to restrain the metabolic vasodilation in the active muscles.

In summary, the resetting of the arterial baroreflexes allows the arterial pressure to increase with exercise. The causes of the resetting are unclear, but its speed suggests a

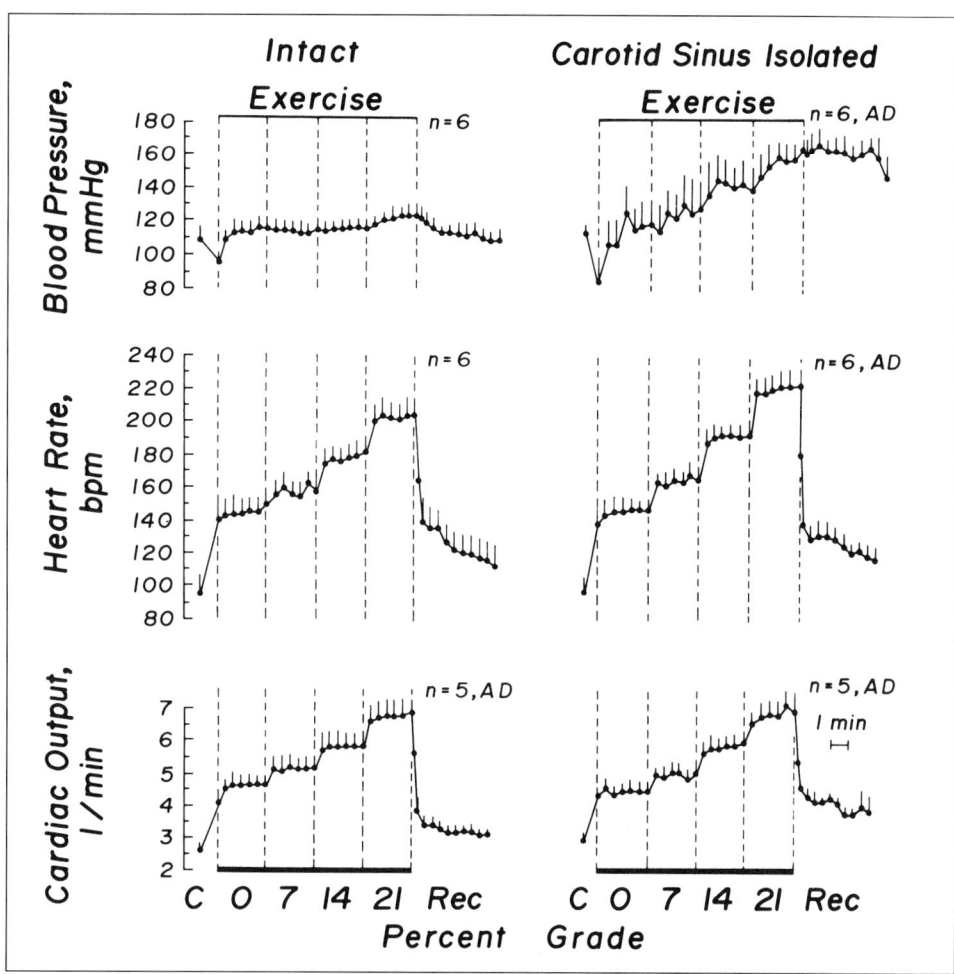

FIG. 9. Hemodynamic responses to graded exercise in dogs with aortic denervation (AD). With the carotid sinus intact **(left)**, there is little change in the mean arterial pressure (MAP), but cardiac output and heart rate rise with each level of exercise. The pressure in a surgically isolated carotid sinus **(right)** is held constant at a low level. This demonstrates the key role of the arterial receptors in regulating arterial blood pressure, but not heart rate or cardiac output, during exercise. In dogs, the arterial baroreflexes may act to limit the increase in arterial pressure; in humans, they may play a more critical role in maintaining adequate arterial blood pressure. From Walgenbach and Donald (63) and Walgenbach and Shepherd (64), with permission.

CNS mechanism. The role of the arterial baroreflexes in regulating cardiac output and heart rate during exercise appears to be less prominent than that of vascular resistance (22,55). This is demonstrated by the observation that cardiac output and heart rate respond normally but mean arterial pressure is increased (compared with control) in dogs, following isolation of the carotid sinuses with low-pressure perfusion during exercise (Fig. 9) (63,64). In humans, the participation of arterial baroreflexes in the sympathetic restraint of muscle vasodilation during large-muscle-mass exercise is likely, but poorly understood (26,56).

Ergoreceptors

Small, unmyelinated, chemosensitive afferents located in the skeletal muscles are also important in the autonomic responses to exercise (2,28,39). Their activation leads to an increase in blood pressure and augmented sympathetic outflow to skeletal muscles (28,32,39). The chemosensitive afferents are stimulated by metabolites and other factors released from the contracting muscles. However, based on studies in anesthetized animals and conscious humans, it appears that skeletal-muscle acidosis plays a decisive role in stimulating these afferents *in vivo* (28,61). This is best demonstrated in patients with McArdle's disease, whose congenital lack of myophosphorylase prevents the development of muscle lactic acidosis during ischemic exercise. These patients do not exhibit the increases in muscle sympathetic nerve activity normally associated with such exercise (41). Their condition also confirms the concept that the ergoreceptors and not central command are the key regulators of sympathetic outflow to muscle during small-muscle-mass exercise (32,62). Based on these observations, the chemosensitive (ergoreceptor) afferents are thought to subserve a so-called muscle chemoreflex, whereby a mismatch between muscle blood flow and metabolism in contracting muscles causes an increase in muscle acidosis (2,43). This muscle acidosis stimulates the afferents to evoke reflex increases in arterial pressure to improve blood flow to the contracting muscles and reduce the mismatch between flow and metabolism.

Ergoreceptor-mediated sympathetic activation is particularly important in static exercise, when muscle blood flow is mechanically obstructed. In dogs, the muscle chemoreflex also restores or improves blood flow to underperfused, rhythmically contracting muscles (43). In humans, however, the increases in sympathetic outflow to resistance vessels elicited by the muscle chemoreflex may limit its ability to augment muscle blood flow (25,65).

Future Directions

The vascular endothelium produces many vasoactive substances, including prostanoids and NO. Some of these substances cause vasodilation, whereas others cause constriction. These substances appear to play important roles in regulating both local organ blood flow and whole body arterial pressure. It has become clear that there are significant interactions between autonomic nerves and the vascular endothelium (11). For example, endothelial factors produced in the carotid sinus can contribute to resetting of carotid baroreceptors by modulating the mechanoreceptors that sense distension in that region (34). It also appears that there are long-term trophic interactions between autonomic (sympathetic) nerves and the vascular endothelium that play a role in regulating the balance of contracting and relaxing factors released by the endothelium (38). NO may also be directly released from autonomic nerves in regions like the cerebral and penile circulation and perhaps skeletal muscle (16). There are also autonomic nerves located in the coronary circulation and skeletal muscle that release acetylcholine that may reach the vascular endothelium where it stimulates muscarinic receptors that evoke NO release. Finally, substances released by the vascular endothelium can also modulate the release and actions of various vasoactive substances from autonomic nerves (37). Taken together, these observations indicate that a fuller understanding of the complex interactions between the vascular endothelium and autonomic nervous system will constitute one of the next major advances in our understanding of cardiovascular reflexes.

CONCLUSION

The basic "architecture" of the autonomic nervous system and the various reflexes subserved by its component parts have been known for many years, although a variety of details continue to emerge and be refined. The ability of the cardiovascular system to meet the demands of the upright posture and exercise demonstrate the dominant role that the autonomic nervous system plays in regulating arterial pressure so that the various local and organ level adaptations and mechanisms are modulated in concert for the benefit of the entire organism. The concept that the vascular endothelium might be an important "target tissue" for the autonomic nervous system and vice versa is the current focus of much research.

ACKNOWLEDGMENTS

The authors thank Mrs. Janet Beckman, Mrs. Kathleen Street, and Mr. Robert Lorenz for their help in preparing both the manuscript and the figures.

REFERENCES

1. Abboud FM, Thames MD. Interaction of cardiovascular reflexes in circulatory control. In: Shepherd JT, Abboud FM, eds. *Handbook of physiology,* sect 2: The cardiovascular system, vol 3: Peripheral circulation and organ blood flow, part 2. Bethesda, MD: American Physiological Society, 1983:675–753.
2. Alam M, Smirk FH. Observations in man upon a blood pressure raising reflex arising from the voluntary muscles. *J Physiol (Lond)* 1937; 89:372–383.
3. Andersen P, Saltin B. Maximal perfusion of skeletal muscle in man. *J Physiol (Lond)* 1985;366:233–249.
4. Angell-James JE, Daly M de B. Comparison of the reflex vasomotor responses to separate and combined stimulation of the carotid sinus and aortic arch baroreceptors by pulsatile and non-pulsatile pressures in the dog. *J Physiol (Lond)* 1970;209:257–293.
5. Asmussen E. Similarities and dissimilarities between static and dynamic exercise. *Circ Res* 1981;48(Suppl 1):I-3–I-10.
6. Banner NR, et al. Altered cardiovascular and neurohumoral responses to head-up tilt after heart–lung transplantation. *Circulation* 1990; 82:863–871.
7. Bevegård S. Studies on the regulation of the circulation in man. *Acta Physiol Scand* 1962;57(Suppl 200):1–36.
8. Bevegård BS, Shepherd JT. Circulatory effects of stimulating the carotid arterial stretch receptors in man at rest and during exercise. *J Clin Invest* 1966;45:132–142.
9. Bevegård S, et al. Blood pressure and heart rate regulating capacity of the carotid sinus during changes in blood volume distribution in man. *Acta Physiol Scand* 1977;99:300–312.
10. Bishop VS, et al. Cardiac mechanoreceptors. In: Sheperd JT, Abboud FM, eds. *Handbook of Physiology,* sect 2: The cardiovascular system, vol 3: Peripheral circulation and organ blood Flow, part 2. Bethesda, MD: American Physiological Society, 1983: 497–555.
11. Broten TP, et al. Role of endothelium-derived relaxing factor in parasympathetic coronary vasodilation. *Am J Physiol* 1992;262:H1579–H1584.
12. Browse NL, Hardwich PJ. The deep breath–venoconstriction reflex. *Clin Sci* 1969;37:125–135.
13. Chapleau MW, Abboud FM. Determinants of sensitization of carotid baroreceptors by pulsatile pressure in dogs. *Circ Res* 1989;65:566–577.
14. Chapleau MW, et al. Peripheral and central mechanisms of baroreflex resetting. *Clin Exp Pharmacol Physiol* 1989;15(Suppl):31–43.
15. Clausen JP. Effect of physical training on cardiovascular adjustments to exercise in man. *Physiol Rev* 1977;57:779–815.
16. Dietz NM, et al. Nitric oxide contributes to the rise in forearm blood flow during mental stress in humans. *J Physiol (Lond)* 1994;480: 361–368.
17. Duprez DA, et al. Vascular responses in forearm and calf to contralateral static exercises. *J Appl Physiol* 1989;66:669–674.

18. Ebert TJ. Baroreflex responsiveness is maintained during isometric exercise in humans. *J Appl Physiol* 1986;61:797–803.
19. Eckberg DL, et al. Respiratory modulation of muscle sympathetic and vagal cardiac outflow in man. *J Physiol (Lond)* 1985;365:181–196.
20. Edwards BS, et al. Atrial stretch, not pressure, is the principal determinant controlling the acute release of atrial natriuretic factor. *Circ Res* 1988;62:191–195.
21. Eldridge FL, et al. Stimulation by central command of locomotion, respiration and circulation during exercise. *Respir Physiol* 1985;59:313–337.
22. Hales JRS, Ludbrook J. Baroreflex participation in redistribution of cardiac output at onset of exercise. *J Appl Physiol* 1988;64:627–634.
23. Henriksen O, Sejrsen P. Local reflex in microcirculation in human skeletal muscle. *Acta Physiol Scand* 1977;99:19–26.
24. Henriksen O, Skagen K. Local and central sympathetic vasoconstrictor reflexes in human limbs during orthostatic stress. In: : Christensen NJ, Henriksen O, Lassen NA, eds. *The sympathoadrenal system* (Alfred Benzon Symposium 23). Copenhagen: Munksgaard, 1988:83–94.
25. Joyner MJ. Does the pressor response to ischemic exercise improve blood flow to contracting muscles in humans? *J Appl Physiol* 1991;71:1496–1501.
26. Joyner MJ, Shepherd JT. Arterial baroreflexes and exercise. In: Kircheim HR, Person D, eds. *Baroreceptor reflexes, integrative functions, and clinical aspects.* Berlin: Springer-Verlag, 1991:237–255.
27. Joyner MJ, et al. Sustained increases in sympathetic outflow during prolonged lower body negative pressure in humans. *J Appl Physiol* 1990;68:1004–1009.
28. Kaufman MP, Rybicki KJ. Discharge properties of group III and IV muscle afferents: their responses to mechanical and metabolic stimuli. *Circ Res* 1987;61(Suppl I):I-60–I-65.
29. Krogh A, Linhard J. The regulation of respiration and circulation during the initial stages of muscular work. *J Physiol (Lond)* 1913;47:112–136.
30. Mancia G, Donald DE. Demonstration that the atria, ventricles, and lungs each are responsible for a tonic inhibition of the vasomotor center in the dog. *Circ Res* 1975;36:310–318.
31. Mancia G, Mark AL. Arterial baroreflexes in humans. In: Shepherd JT, Abboud FM, eds. *Handbook of physiology,* sect 2: The cardiovascular system, vol 3: Peripheral circulation and organ blood flow, part 2. Bethesda, MD: American Physiological Society, 1983:755–793.
32. Mark AL, et al. Microneurographic studies of the mechanisms of sympathetic nerve responses to static exercise in humans. *Circ Res* 1985;57:461–469.
33. Marshall RJ, et al. Blood pressure during supine exercise in idiopathic orthostatic hypotension. *Circulation* 1961;24: 76–81.
34. Matsuda T, et al. Modulation of baroreceptor activity by nitric oxide and S-nitrosocysteine. *Circ Res* 1995;76:426–433.
35. Melcher A, Donald DE. Maintained ability of carotid baroreflex to regulate arterial pressure during exercise. *Am J Physiol* 1981;241:H838–H849.
36. Millar-Craig MW, et al. Circadian variation of blood-pressure. *Lancet* 1978;1:795–797.
37. Miller VM, Vanhoutte PM. Role of the endothelium in modulating vascular adrenergic receptor actions. *Prog Clin Biol Res* 1989;286:33–39.
38. Milner P, et al. Interactions between sensory perivascular nerves and the endothelium in brain microvessels. *Int J Microcirc Clin Exp* 1995;15:1–9.
39. Mitchell JH, Schmidt RF. Cardiovascular reflex control by afferent fibers from skeletal muscle receptors. In: Shepherd JT, Abboud FM, eds. *Handbook of physiology,* sect 2: The cardiovascular system, vol 3: Peripheral circulation and organ blood flow, part 2. Bethesda, MD: American Physiological Society, 1983:623–658.
40. Mohanty, PK, et al. Impairment of cardiopulmonary baroreflex after cardiac transplantation in humans. *Circulation* 1987;75:914–921.
41. Pryor SL, et al. Impairment of sympathetic activation during static exercise in patients with muscle phosphorylase deficiency (McArdle's disease). *J Clin Invest* 1990;85:1444–1449.
42. Rowell LB. *Human circulation: regulation during physical stress.* New York: Oxford University Press, 1986.
43. Rowell LB, Sheriff DD. Are muscle "chemoreflexes" functionally important? *NIPS* 1988;3:250–253.
44. Sanders JS, et al. Arterial baroreflex control of sympathetic nerve activity during elevation of blood pressure in normal man: dominance of aortic baroreflexes. *Circulation* 1988;77: 279–288.
45. Sanders JS, et al. Evidence for cholinergically mediated vasodilations at the beginning of isometric exercise in humans. *Circulation* 1989;79:815–824.
46. Sanders JS, et al. Importance of aortic baroreflex in regulation of sympathetic responses during hypotension: evidence from direct sympathetic nerve recordings in humans. *Circulation* 1989;79:83–92.
47. Seals DR, et al. Influence of lung volume on sympathetic nerve discharge in normal humans. *Circ Res* 1990;67: 130–141.
48. Secher NH. Heart rate at the onset of static exercise in man with partial neuromuscular blockade. *J Physiol (Lond)* 1985;368:481–490.
49. Shepherd JT. Circulation to skeletal muscle. In: Shepherd JT, Abboud FM, eds. *Handbook of physiology,* sect 2: The cardiovascular system, vol 3: Peripheral circulation and organ blood flow, part 1. Bethesda, MD: American Physiological Society, 1983:319–370.
50. Shepherd JT. Increased systemic vascular resistance and primary hypertension: the expanding complexity. *J Hypertens* 1990;8(Suppl 7):S15–S27
51. Shepherd JT. The lungs as receptor sites for cardiovascular regulation. *Circulation* 1981;63:1–10.
52. Shepherd JT, Mancia G. Reflex control of the human cardiovascular system. *Rev Physiol Biochem Pharmacol* 1986;105:1–99.
53. Shepherd JT, Vanhoutte PM. *The human cardiovascular system: facts and concepts.* New York: Raven, 1979.
54. Smith JJ. *Circulatory response to the upright posture.* Boca Raton, FL: CRC, 1990:187.
55. Sprangers RLH, et al. Initial blood pressure fall on stand up and exercise explained by changes in total peripheral resistance. *J Appl Physiol* 1991;70:523–530.
56. Strange S, et al. Cardiovascular responses to carotid sinus baroreceptor stimulation during moderate to severe exercise in man. *Acta Physiol Scand* 1990;138:145–153.
57. Tan W, et al. A central mechanism of acute baroreflex resetting in the conscious dog. *Circ Res* 1989;65:63–70.
58. Taylor JA, et al. "Non-hypotensive" hypovolaemia reduces ascending aortic dimensions in humans. *J Physiol* 1995;483:289–298.
59. Thames MD, et al. Neural control of renin secretion in anesthetized dogs: interaction of cardiopulmonary and carotid baroreceptors. *Circ Res* 1978;42:237–245.
60. Thoren P. Role of cardiac vagal C-fibers in cardiovascular control. *Rev Physiol Biochem Pharmacol* 1979;86:1–94.
61. Victor RG, et al. Sympathetic nerve discharge is coupled to muscle cell pH during exercise in humans. *J Clin Invest* 1988;82:1301–1305.
62. Victor RG, et al. Effects of partial neuromuscular blockade on sympathetic nerve responses to static exercise in humans. *Circ Res* 1989;65:468–476.
63. Walgenbach SC, Donald DE. Inhibition by carotid baroreflex of exercise-induced increases in arterial pressure. *Circ Res* 1983;52:253–262.
64. Walgenbach SC, Shepherd JT. Role of arterial and cardiopulmonary mechanoreceptors in the regulation of arterial pressure during rest and exercise in conscious dogs. *Mayo Clin Proc* 1984;59:467–475.
65. Williams CA, et al. Sympathetic control of the forearm blood flow in man during brief isometric contractions. *Eur J Appl Physiol* 1985;54:156–162.

CHAPTER 6

Maintenance of Postural Normotension in Humans

Wouter Wieling and Johannes J. van Lieshout

1. Active or passive changes in posture evoke different initial (first 30 sec) cardiovascular effects. Circulatory readjustment is usually completed within 1 min.
2. The orthostatic response can be classified into three stages: the initial response (first 30 sec), the early phase of circulatory stabilization (1–2 min upright), and prolonged orthostatic stress (at least 5 min upright).
3. The initial and early-phase circulatory adjustments are governed by the neural system. Integrity of sympathetic outflow to the peripheral resistance and splanchnic capacitance vessels, rather than cardiac effector mechanisms, is essential.
4. Under normal circumstances, activation of the sympathetic nervous system and the renin–angiotensin–aldosterone system is involved in the maintenance of blood pressure during prolonged orthostasis. The vasopressin level only increases markedly during hypotensive orthostatic stress.
5. Arterial (and especially carotid) baroreceptor control of peripheral resistance and splanchnic capacitance vessels is the single most important component in the maintenance of postural normotension in humans. The skeletal muscle pump of the lower body can compensate in part for the neural system.
6. The dynamics of the underlying cardiovascular control mechanisms should be taken into account when investigating orthostatic circulatory control.

INTRODUCTION

Once humans assumed the upright posture, this increased their vulnerability to the effects of gravity on the circulation. The brain, the organ most susceptible to hypoxia, is in the most disadvantageous location (1,3,10,23). The crucial problem posed by the upright posture is the vertical displacement of blood below the heart (Fig. 1) resulting in a decline in venous return. Because the heart cannot pump out what it does not receive, ventricular stroke volume declines and arterial pressure tends to fall. A series of cardiovascular-regulatory mechanisms or reflexes (11) is activated to offset this assault on the circulation. Its purpose is directed at maintaining the level of arterial pressure and cerebral perfusion irrespective of the effect of gravity. To achieve this, stroke volume, cardiac output, and peripheral vascular resistance are modulated, with arterial pressure as the controlled variable. The *latency* (reflex time), *time constant* (a measure of the time from the onset of counterregulation to full power), and *gain* (power to counteract the disturbance) differ for the various components of this compensatory system (7,11,46).

The cardiovascular control system includes the following major subsets of the pressure-buffering components (in chronologic order): the *neurocardiovascular* or *neural* system, the *humorocardiovascular* or *humoral* system, the *capillary-fluid-shift* system, and the *renal-body-fluid control* system. This order does not parallel the ranking of these controls with respect to their gain. The renal-blood-fluid system acts as a slow, long-term blood pressure integral controller. The humoral and, especially, the neural control systems serve as fast, fine-tuning feedback mechanisms that serve to match the needs of the body more closely (7,11). The main sensory receptors involved in or-

---

W. Wieling and J. J. van Lieshout: Department of Medicine, University of Amsterdam Academic Medical Centre, Amsterdam, The Netherlands.

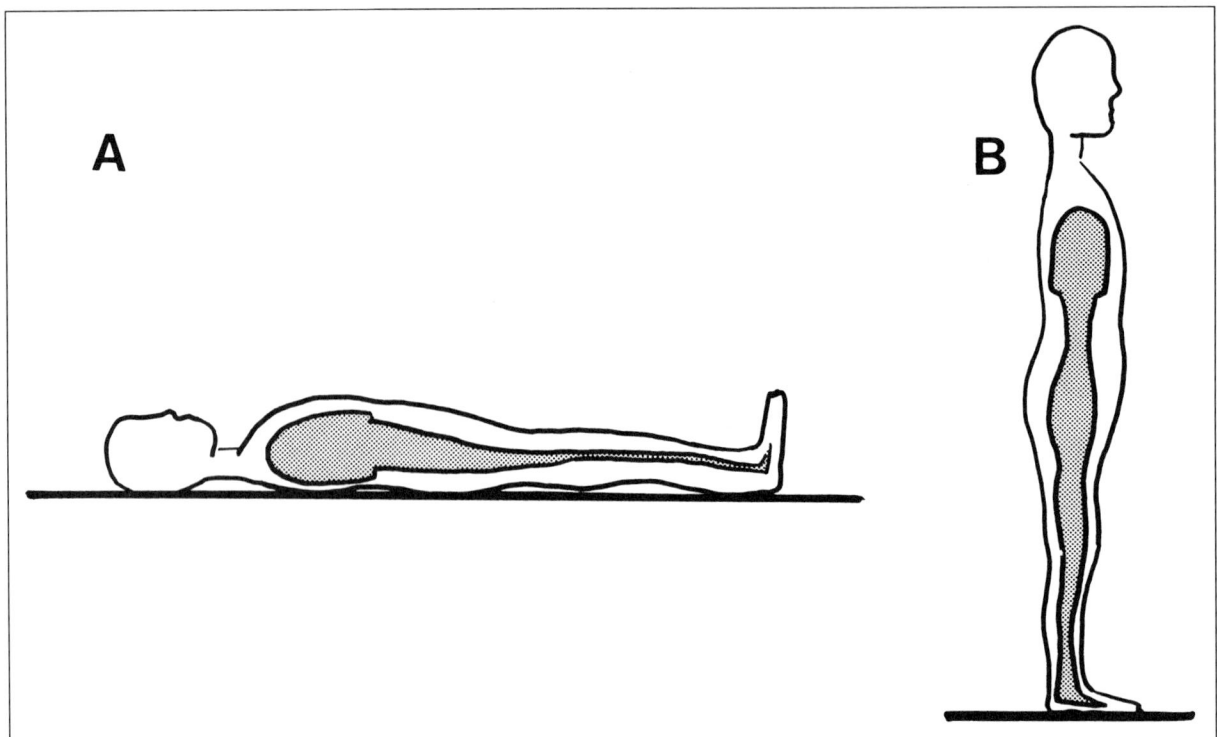

FIG. 1. Influence of gravity on intravascular fluid shifts. Modified from Rowell (23).

thostatic reflex adjustments are the arterial baroreceptors located in the aortic arch, and carotid sinuses and receptors located in the heart and lungs (Fig. 2). The arterial baroreceptors are stretch receptors, which react to changes in arterial pressure. The cardiopulmonary receptors may be considered to function as rapidly acting volume receptors ideally suited to detect changes in the filling of the central venous circulation. The arterial and cardiopulmonary reflex mechanisms are discussed in detail in the previous chapter; the present chapter focuses on their role in orthostatic reflex adjustments. The first section of this chapter deals with gravity's influence on cardiovascular hemodynamics during orthostatic stress. The second part is concerned with the compensatory adjustment of the human body. As part of this discussion, the circulatory responses to postural changes are described for healthy subjects, aged 20–45 years. Factors important for maintenance of postural normotension are identified (Table 1).

INFLUENCE OF GRAVITY ON CARDIOVASCULAR HEMODYNAMICS IN HUMANS

When humans stand up from the supine position, it is estimated that 300–800 ml of blood is transferred from the chest to the distensible venous capacitance system below the diaphragm (Fig. 1) (23,29,30). Up to 50% of this total shift occurs within 5–10 sec. Venous pooling is the term commonly used to describe this process. Assumption of the upright position causes not only a fluid shift within the vascular tree, but also largely influences intravascular pressures; the intravascular pressure decreases above and increases below the venous *hydrostatic indifference point* (HIP), which is the point in the vascular tree where pressure is independent of posture. In humans, the venous HIP is at the diaphragmatic level (3,10). The large increase in capillary transmural pressure below the HIP produces continued net filtration into the tissue spaces. Estimations based on changes in hematocrit or plasma protein concentration indicate that the transcapillary fluid shift equilibrates—10 min after the change in posture, resulting in a net fall in plasma volume of ~10% (12,20,38).

TABLE 1. *Factors involved in the maintenance of postural normotension in humans*

1. Adequacy of circulating blood volume
2. Sympathetic outflow to the peripheral resistance and splanchnic capacitance vessels
3. Carotid and aortic baroreceptor reflexes
4. Cardiopulmonary reflexes
5. Venoarterial reflexes
6. Myogenic response
7. Renin-angiotensin and vasopressin systems
8. Skeletal muscle pump of the lower body

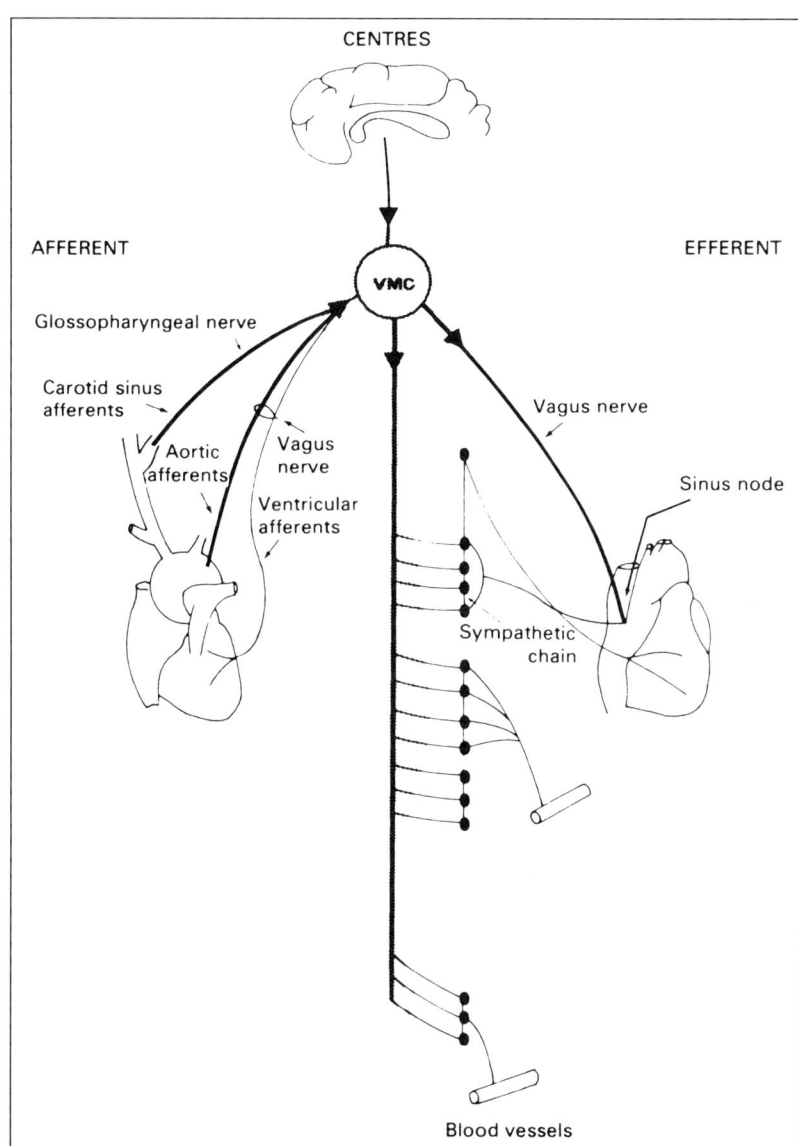

FIG. 2. Schematic drawing of the afferent and efferent pathways of the baroreceptor reflex arc. Nerve fibers from the lungs (not shown) and the heart join the vagus nerve as cardiopulmonary afferents toward the vasomotor centers (VMC) in the brainstem. From van Lieshout et al. (41), with permission of the Biochemical Society and Portland Press.

Mechanical factors play an important role in promoting venous return in the upright posture. First, the static increase in skeletal muscle tone involved in active standing opposes pooling of blood in limb veins even in the absence of movement of the subject (30,46). Second, activation of the muscle pump of the legs during tiptoeing or walking, in the presence of competent venous valves, pumps blood back to the heart. The leg-muscle pump can be considered as a "second heart" (23). Third, the respiratory pump may also contribute; with inspiration, intrathoracic pressure decreases and the intraabdominal pressure increases, thereby promoting venous return (23,28). A sighing respiration often precedes an actual faint; it has been suggested that this helps to prevent syncope by enhancing the abdominothoracic pump and by inducing venoconstriction. However, continuous deep breathing and the consequent hypocapnia cause vasodilation in skeletal muscle and vasoconstriction in the brain and can promote the development of a fainting response.

The importance of mechanical factors in opposing gravitational pooling of venous blood has been clearly demonstrated in patients with autonomic disturbances (5,40,45). Abdominal contraction and leg crossing have been shown to be beneficial to combat the orthostatic hypotension in these patients (Figs. 3 and 4). These maneuvers, which involve tensing of large skeletal muscle groups, translocate venous blood pooled below the diaphragm back to the chest and thereby partially restore the cardiac filling pressure, stroke volume and, thereby, cardiac output (Fig. 4) (36,42).

The instantaneous and fast venous pooling of blood below the diaphragm on assumption of the upright posture results in a rapid diminution of the volume of blood directly available to the cardiac ventricles, which is of paramount

76 / THE SCIENTIFIC BASIS

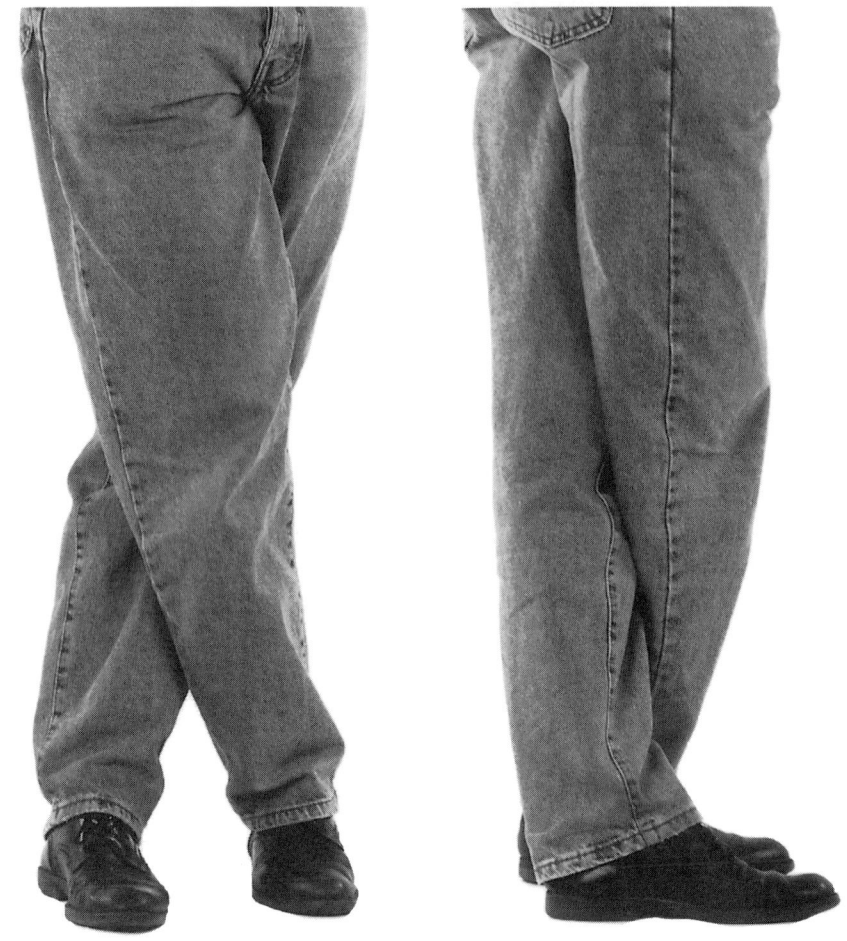

FIG. 3. Legs in the crossed position from the front and from aside (cocktail-party posture). From Wieling (42), with permission of Academic Press.

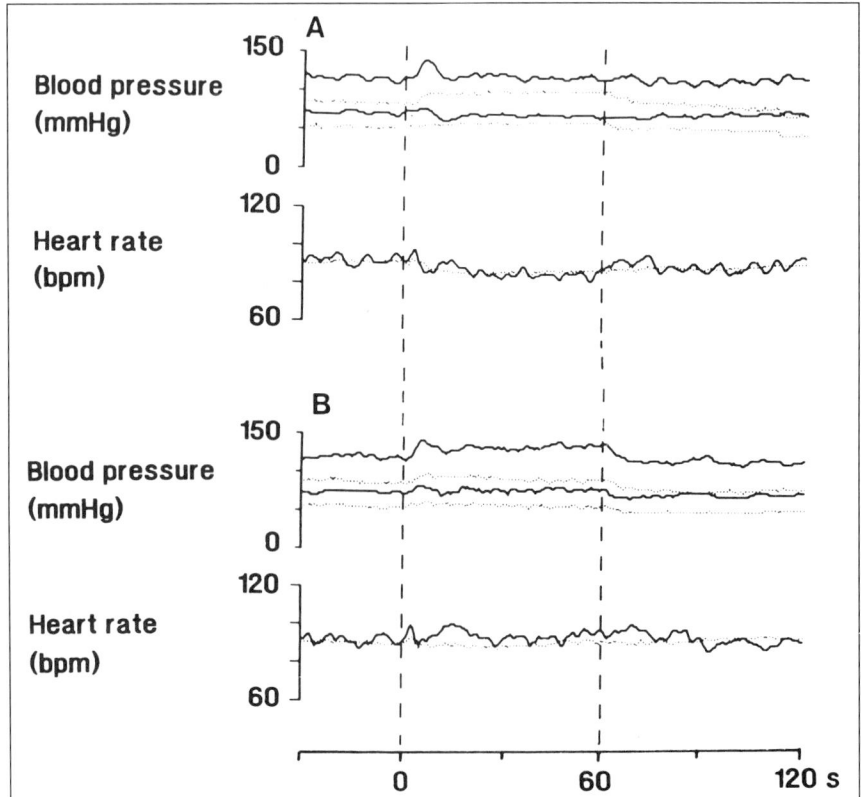

FIG. 4. Circulatory responses to abdominal contraction **(A)** and leg crossing **(B)** in healthy subjects (n = 6; *continuous lines*) and patients with orthostatic hypotension (n = 7; *dotted lines*). Modified from Wieling (42), with permission of Academic Press.

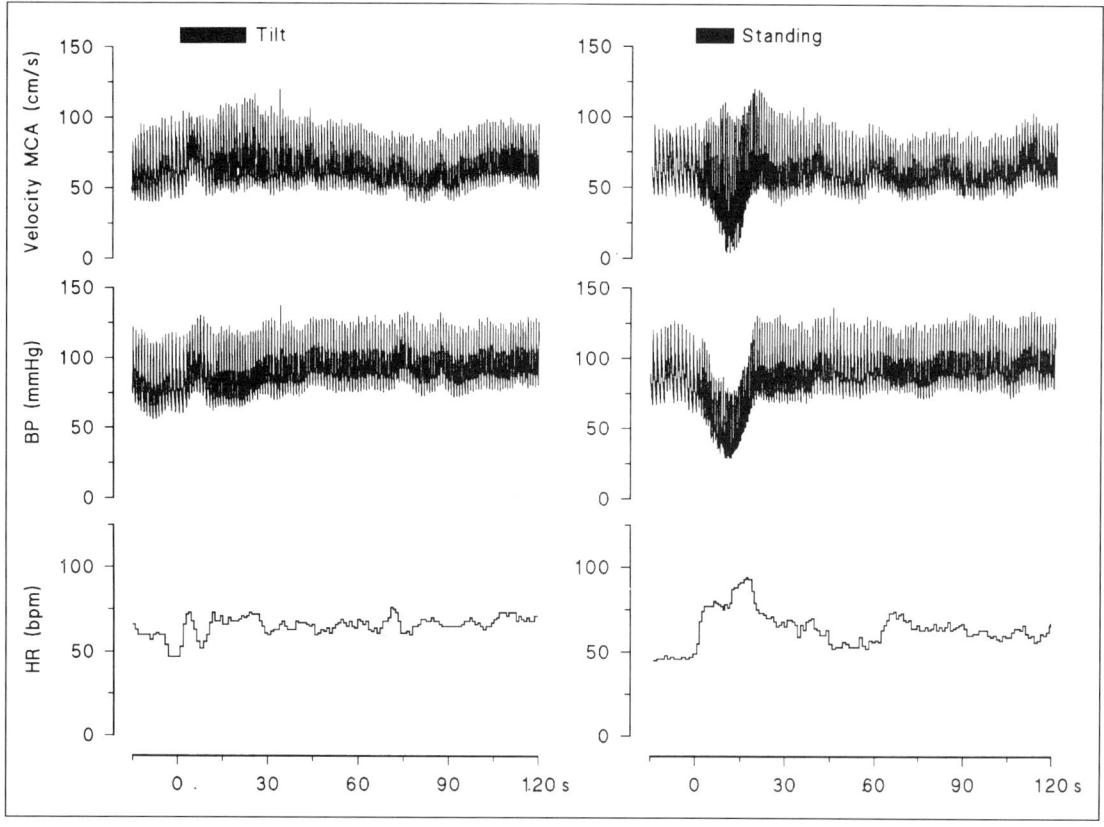

FIG. 5. Changes in arterial pressure, heart rate, and flow velocity in the middle cerebral artery (MCA) in a healthy 25-year-old man evoked by a passive 70° head-up tilt **(left)** and standing **(right)**. Note the dip in arterial pressure and MCA velocity upon active change of posture.

importance for the beat-to-beat adjustment of arterial pressure. Unless compensatory adjustments are promptly instituted, arterial pressure falls and the subject faints. The next section discusses neurohumoral reflex adjustments, which oppose the gravitational forces imposed on the cardiovascular system once a person has assumed the upright posture.

ADJUSTMENTS OF THE BODY TO ORTHOSTATIC STRESS

Speed is the hallmark of the circulatory adjustment to orthostatic stress. In healthy subjects, circulatory stabilization is usually reached within 1 min. In the ensuing minutes, blood pressure and heart rate change only minimally. The initial circulatory responses brought about by an active change of posture (stand up) differ from those elicited by passive change (tilt up) (Fig. 5) (4,8,15,33,47).

We have found it useful to classify the orthostatic response according to the *initial response* (the first 30 sec), the *early phase of stabilization* (1–2 min upright), and *prolonged orthostasis* (at least 5 min upright), as well as according to the active (standing up) or passive (head-up tilt) nature of orthostasis (43,44). The circulatory adjustment to postural change in the initial phase and the early phase of stabilization is governed exclusively by the neural system (23,46).

Initial Circulatory Response to Head-Up Tilt

Despite a fall in venous return on head-up tilting, a reduction in stroke volume does not take place until after ~6 beats of normal stroke output, because of the amount of blood initially available in the lungs and heart. Stroke volume then gradually diminishes until it reaches a new stable level (Figs. 1 and 7) (30,33). The orthostatic drop in arterial and cardiac filling pressures is perceived by the carotid sinus and aortic arch baroreceptors and by cardiopulmonary receptors (Fig. 2), and produces an increase in heart rate and vasoconstriction (6,10,30,46). Central modulation of vasomotor outflow is reinforced by the venoarteriolar axon reflex. The latter, which is a local axon reflex initiated by the elevated hydrostatic pressure below the HIP, constricts arterial inflow to the skin, muscle, and adipose tissue. This reflex is reported to elicit up to 40% of the total increase in limb vascular resistance with standing and thus may be an important adjunct to the cardiovascular reflexes mediated by the central nervous system (14). A myogenic response of the smooth muscle of the resistance ves-

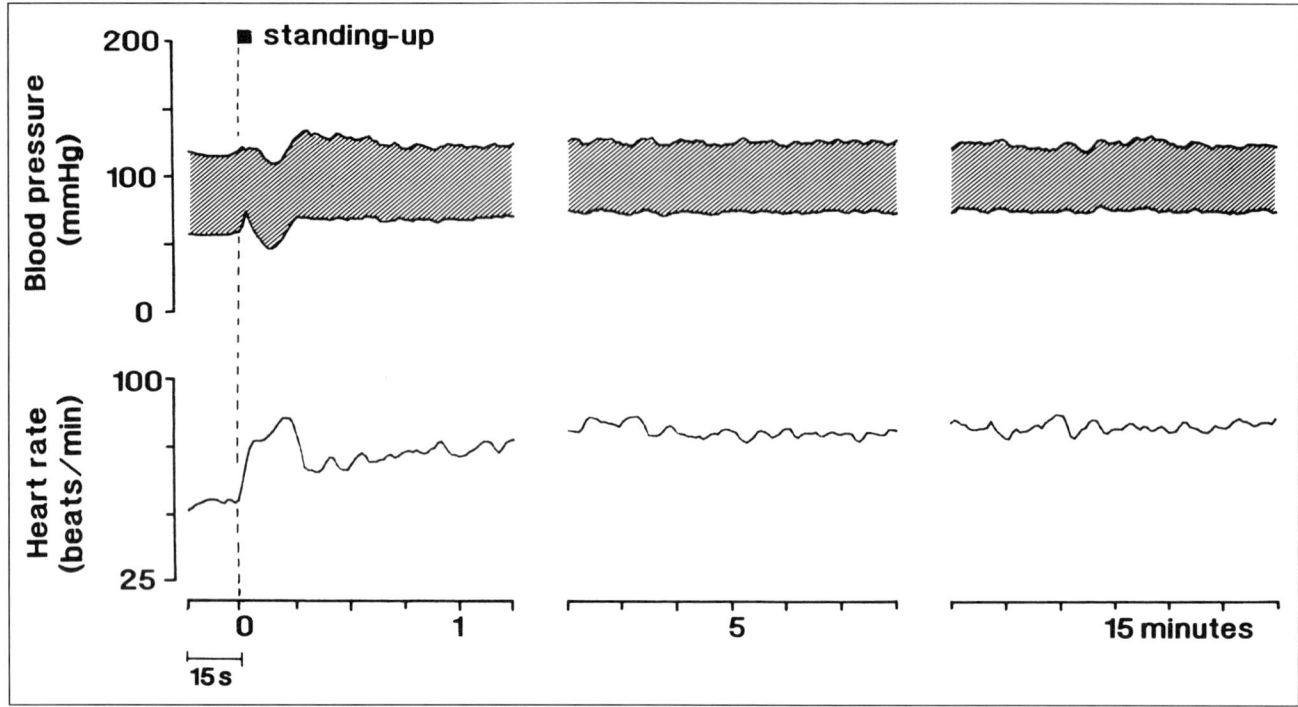

FIG. 6. Initial and early steady-state responses and circulatory adjustment to prolonged standing (averaged over ten male subjects with a mean age of 28 years; range, 22–40 years). Adapted from Wieling and Wesseling (46), with permission of W. B. Saunders.

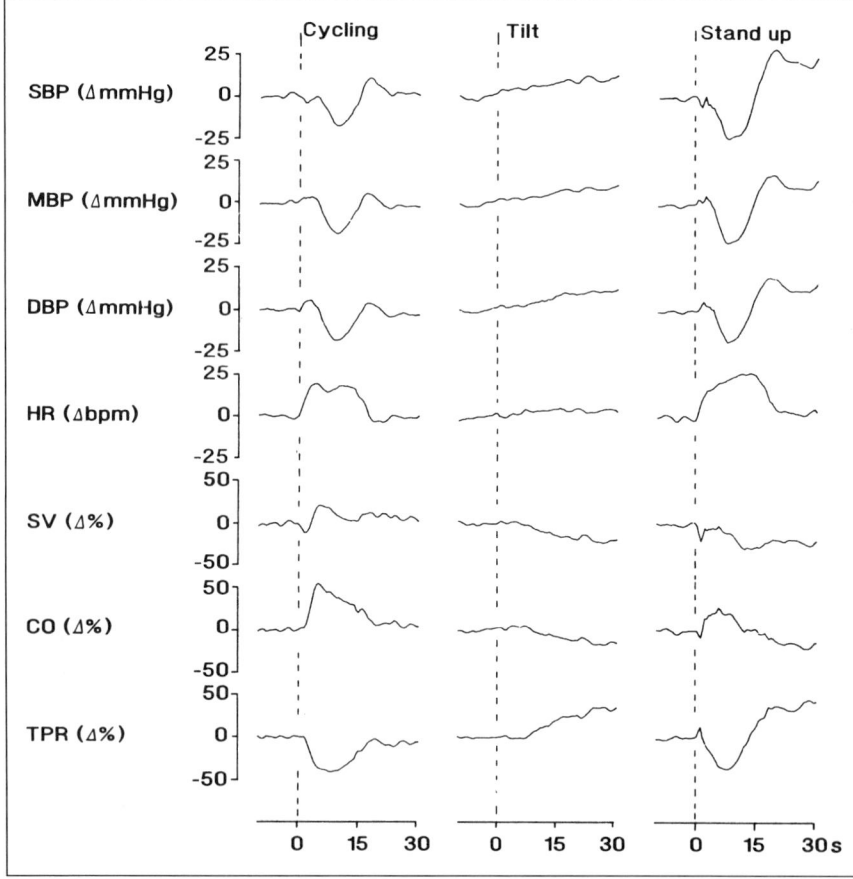

FIG. 7. The beat-to-beat hemodynamic changes during cycling, head-up tilt, and standing in eight subjects (expressed as absolute or percentage changes from control). Note the abrupt transient fall in blood pressure and total peripheral resistance, and rise in cardiac output on cycling and standing, which contrasts with the gradual changes in tilt. SBP, systolic blood pressure; MBP, mean blood pressure; DBP, diastolic blood pressure; HR, heart rate; SV, stroke volume; CO, cardiac output; TPR, total peripheral resistance. Adapted from Sprangers et al. (33), with permission of the American Physiological Society.

sels in the dependent parts to the increased transmural pressure probably also contributes (10).

The gradual increase in diastolic pressure at heart level on tilt can be related to the rise in peripheral vascular resistance (10,33), while the change in systolic pressure is only small (see Fig. 5). Neural adjustments result in an increase in mean arterial pressure of 5–10 mmHg at heart level in the upright posture. The aortic receptors, which are located just above heart level, thus sense an increased, instead of a decreased, mean arterial pressure, and only pulse pressure is perceived as reduced for these receptors. The mean pressure sensed by the carotid receptors, in contrast, drops and remains below the recumbent level, since they are located ~20–25 cm above the heart in upright adults. The hydrostatic effect lowers the effective pressure at the level of the carotid baroreceptors by ~15 mmHg (10,46). Thus, the carotid baroreceptors are likely to be most important in the maintenance of arterial blood pressure and in defending the constancy of perfusion pressure of the brain during orthostasis. Accordingly, in humans who have undergone bilateral carotid denervation, orthostatic blood pressure control is impaired (9,46). Cardiopulmonary receptors act in concert with arterial baroreceptors to effect the necessary adjustments in sympathetic outflow, but are not essential for the cardiovascular adjustments to orthostatic stress [for a review, see Wieling and Wesseling (46)].

When the change of posture is not to fully upright, the gravitational stress is a function of the sine of the angle of tilt and not of the angle itself. Thus, a 30° head-up tilt represents 50% of the full gravity factor and a 70° tilt corresponds to 94% of the full gravity factor (3,10,32). With tilt times between 2 and 5 s, the speed of the maneuver has little or no influence on the orthostatic response to upright tilting (32). Peripheral vascular, rather than cardiac effector, mechanisms are essential to the adjustment of arterial pressure to the upright posture. Autonomic blockade of the heart does not affect orthostatic tolerance in normal subjects; arterial pressure is maintained by greater peripheral vasoconstriction (23,46).

The contribution of venoconstriction in retarding orthostatic volume displacement as a result of elevated hydrostatic pressure below the HIP is another issue. Reflex venoconstriction in the lower limbs appears of little importance. Muscle veins in human limbs have little smooth muscle and little or no sympathetic innervation. The cutaneous veins are richly innervated, but venoconstriction of these vessels is not a consistent response to the upright posture; if it occurs, it is only transient (27). The capacity of cutaneous veins to contain blood seems primarily determined by thermoregulatory and psychological stimuli. Heat markedly increases venous capacity and thus reduces orthostatic tolerance. Cold has the opposite effect.

In humans, intact innervation of the splanchnic bed is of paramount importance for orthostatic tolerance. The upright posture is accompanied by constriction of splanchnic resistance vessels increasing systemic vascular resistance. Constriction of splanchnic resistance vessels is also thought to cause a passive expulsion of blood out of the large venous reservoir of the splanchnic bed by elastic recoil of venous vessels (13,23). Active capacitance responses in the highly distensible splanchnic circulation containing a large volume of blood are of potentially great importance in mobilizing additional venous blood to maintain cardiac filling pressures (13,19,23,27). The rich innervation and the great sensitivity and rapidity of reflex responses of these vessels to very low frequencies of sympathetic discharge appear indicative of their importance in responding to postural changes (13).

Initial Circulatory Response to Standing Up

An active change in posture evokes a characteristic initial circulatory response that differs distinctly from the response to a passive tilt (Figs. 5 and 7). Comparable events are observed at the onset to other forms of whole body exercise (Fig. 8) (4,33,42). Two main effects are thought to be involved. First, the effort of standing compresses the venous vessels in the contracting muscles of the legs and increases intraabdominal pressure (3,35). This causes an immediate translocation of blood toward the heart and increases right atrial pressure (Fig. 8) and thereby the cardiac output (Fig. 7) (33,35). Second, active standing induces a drop in total peripheral resistance, which is not found upon head-up tilt. The increase in cardiac output is not sufficient to make up for this drop in total peripheral resistance, and the result is a transient fall in systemic blood pressure (Fig. 7). The pronounced release in vasoconstrictor tone has been previously attributed to the steep rise in right atrial pressure activating cardiopulmonary afferents and thereby causing reflex vasodilatation (33). However, a recent study suggests that nonautonomically mediated, instantaneous increase in flow in the exercising muscles is the main factor involved in the vasodilatation, since it also occurs in patients with autonomic failure (47).

The abrupt increase in heart rate upon standing, which peaks at ~3 sec after the onset of standing up (Figs. 5 and 7), results from abrupt inhibition of cardiac vagal tone, as this response is absent after parasympathetic blockade. This is a general exercise reflex that operates as soon as voluntary (static) muscle contractions are performed. A more gradual secondary increase in heart rate starts ~5 sec after standing up, and rises to a secondary peak at ~12 sec (Fig. 7). This increase is elicited by the dual effects of further reflex inhibition of cardiac vagal tone and an increase in sympathetic tone. These effects can be attributed to diminished activation of the arterial baroreceptors by the temporary fall in blood pressure. Arterial pressure recovers after ~7 sec because of decreased stimulation of the arterial baroreceptors and cardiopulmonary receptors. The mag-

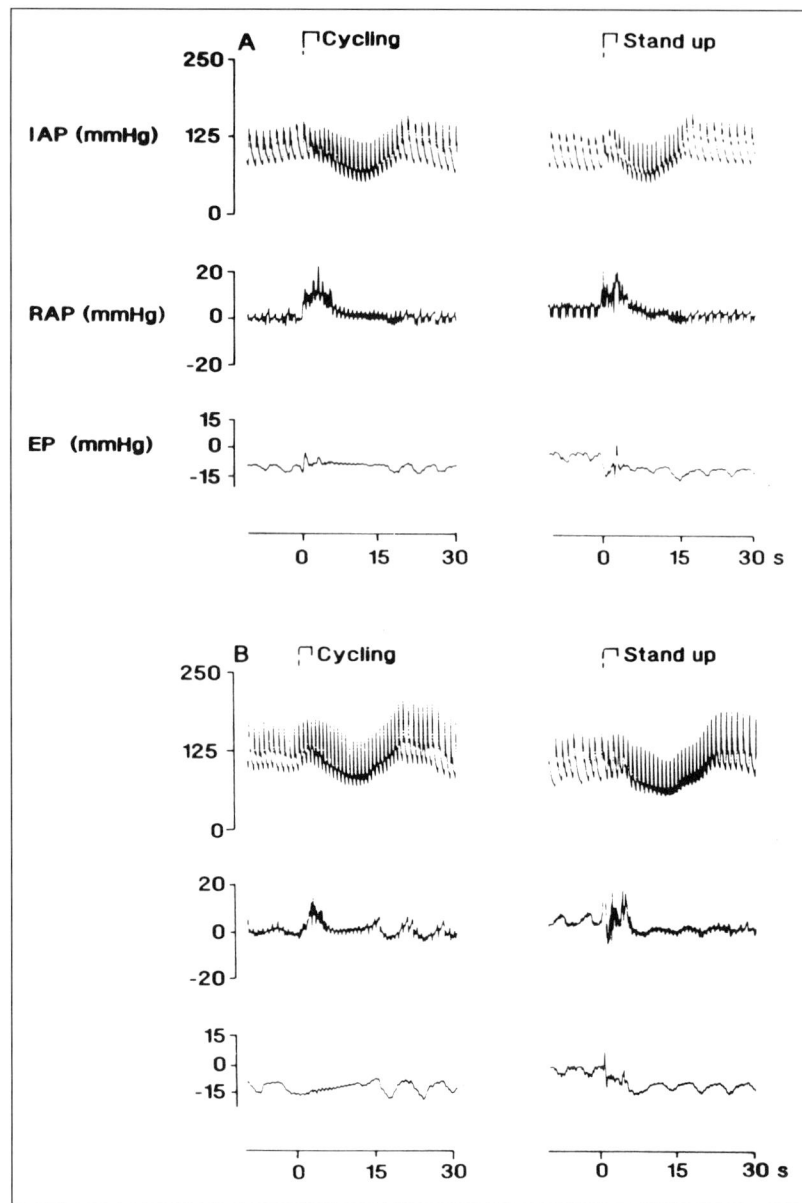

FIG. 8. Intraarterial pressure (IAP), right atrial pressure (RAP), and esophageal pressure (EP) transients induced by cycling and standing (*open squares*) in two subjects **(A and B)**. The duration of each maneuver is indicated at the *top* of each tracing. The fall in blood pressure in all four maneuvers is preceded by a 10- to 15-mmHg rise in the RAP. Because EP does not change, except briefly at the onset of the maneuvers, the change in RAP is an index for the mechanical stimulation of the cardiopulmonary receptors. Adapted from Sprangers et al. (33), with permission of the American Physiological Society.

nitude of the initial blood pressure fall and overshoot and rise in initial heart rate on active standing is increased by lengthening the period of preceding rest (4,36).

Blood pressure and heart rate recovery is complete ~30 sec after the onset of standing up, such that the early phase of stabilization has been attained.

Early Phase of Stabilization (After 1–2 min Upright) and Prolonged Orthostasis (at Least 5 min Upright)

The normal blood pressure response after 1–2 min standing consists of an increase in diastolic pressure by ~10 mmHg, with little or no change in systolic pressure at heart level. The heart rate increase amounts to ~10 beats/min (Fig. 6). The responses of heart rate and blood pressure in the early phase of stabilization are commonly used in the clinical evaluation of neural circulatory control (43). Few further changes in heart rate and blood pressure are observed during continued orthostatic stress (Fig. 6).

The main features (in comparison to the supine circulation) are, approximately, intrathoracic blood volume reduced by ~30%, stroke volume reduced by 30%–40%, heart rate increased by 15%–30%, cardiac output decreased by ~20%, arteriovenous oxygen difference increased by 20%, mean arterial pressure raised by 0–10%, diastolic pressure increased by ~10%, and systolic pressure usually unchanged (10,30). The circulatory adjustments during prolonged standing and head-up tilt are reported to be similar (1,31), but detailed data are lacking.

The neural control system continues to play the central role in the maintenance of arterial pressure during prolonged standing. It has been suggested that sustained unloading of the cardiopulmonary receptors underlies the steady-state sympathetic outflow during prolonged orthostatic stress (17). However, activation of these receptors does not appear to be necessary for orthostatic blood pressure adjustment; patients with heart–lung transplants do not suffer orthostatic hypotension (16).

The activity of various humoral mechanisms is altered by postural changes. The contribution of the humoral system to circulatory orthostatic adjustments depends on the effective circulating blood volume, which is the component of blood volume that the volume-regulatory system responds to by initiating renal retention of water and sodium (26). When the effective blood volume is adequate, the humoral system is minimally involved in the early steady-state circulatory adjustment. It becomes more important during prolonged orthostasis, particularly in combating imminent arterial hypotension in the volume-depleted state (30,34). Under normal circumstances, the sympathetic nervous system and the renin–angiotensin–aldosterone system (RAAS) are activated in response to standing (18,22,48). Plasma catecholamine levels rise within minutes. Renin release and the subsequent formation of angiotensin occur more slowly (19,22,45). The plasma vasopressin level does not normally change much in response to standing, but increases markedly during severe orthostatic stress and vasovagal syncope (30,41). If salt intake is normal, blood pressure is maintained during passive head-up tilt when renin release is pharmacologically inhibited by propranolol (21) or angiotensin formation is prevented by an angiotensin-converting enzyme inhibitor (24). Under these circumstances, the sympathetic nervous system and vasopressin act in concert to maintain arterial pressure (2). However, blood pressure falls when a sodium-depleted state is also induced (24). Thus, the RAAS and vasopressin can compensate for each other (25). During severe orthostatic stress, both activation of the RAAS and vasopressin release are necessary for maintaining arterial pressure (2,24). Under these circumstances, vasopressin may rise sharply to levels that promote reabsorption of water by the kidney tubules and have profound vasoconstrictor effects (2,30). Notwithstanding the important role of the humoral systems during severe orthostatic stress, they cannot supplant the functions of the neural system.

REFERENCES

1. Amberson WR. Physiological adjustments to the standing posture. *Bull School Med Univ Md* 1943;27:127–145.
2. Bennett T, Gardiner SM. Involvement of vasopressin in cardiovascular regulation. *Cardiovasc Res* 1985;19:57–68.
3. Blomqvist CG, Stone HL. Cardiovascular adjustments to gravitational stress. In: Shepherd JT, Abboud FM, eds. *Handbook of Physiology*, sect 2: The cardiovascular system. Bethesda, MD: American Physiological Society, 1983:1025–1063.
4. Borst C, et al. Mechanisms of initial heart rate response to postural change. *Am J Physiol* 1982;12:H676–H681.
5. Bouvette CM, et al. The role of physical countermaneuvers in the management of orthostatic hypotension: efficacy and biofeedback augmentation. *Mayo Clin Proc* 1996;71:847–853.
6. Burke D, et al. Postural effects on muscle nerve sympathetic activity in man. *J Physiol (Lond)* 1977;272:399–414.
7. Cowley AW. Long-term control of arterial pressure. *Physiol Rev* 1992;72:231–278.
8. Dambrink JHA, et al. Circulatory adaptation to orthostatic stress in healthy 10–14 year-old children investigated in a general practice. *Clin Sci* 1991;81:51–58.
9. Eckberg DL, Sleight P. *Human baroreflexes in health and disease.* Oxford: Oxford University Press, 1992.
10. Gauer OH, Thron HL. Postural changes in the circulation. In: Hamilton WF, Dow P, eds. *Handbook of Physiology*, sect 2: Circulation. Washington, DC: American Physiological Society 1965:2409–2437.
11. Guyton AC. Control theory and its application to arterial pressure regulation: proportional control, integral control, gain, and damping mechanisms. In: Guyton AC, ed. *Circulatory physiology. III. Arterial pressure and hypertension.* Philadelphia: WB Saunders, 1980: 30–54.
12. Hagan RD, et al. Plasma volume changes with movement to supine and standing positions. *J Appl Physiol* 1978; 45:414–418.
13. Hainsworth R. The importance of vascular capacitance in cardiovascular control. *News Physiol Sci* 1990;5:250–254.
14. Hendriksen O, Skagen K. Local and central sympathetic vasoconstrictor reflexes in human limbs during orthostatic stress. In: Christensen NJ, Hendriksen O, Lassen NA, eds. *The sympathoadrenal system: physiology and pathophysiology* (Alfred Benzon Symposium 23). Copenhagen: Munksgaard, 1986:83–94.
15. Imholz BPM, et al. Orthostatic circulatory control in the elderly evaluated by non-invasive continuous blood pressure measurement. *Clin Sci* 1990;79:73–79.
16. Jacobsen TN, et al. Relative contributions of cardiopulmonary and sinoaortic baroreflexes in causing sympathetic activation in human skeletal muscle circulation during orthostatic stress. *Circ Res* 1993; 73:367–378.
17. Joyner MJ, et al. Sustained increases in sympathetic outflow during prolonged lower body negative pressure in humans. *J Appl Physiol* 1990;68:1004–1009.
18. Kala R, et al. Effect of short-term upright posture on plasma angiotensin II in man. *Scand J Clin Invest* 1974;33:87–94.
19. Low PA, et al. The splanchnic autonomic outflow in Shy–Drager syndrome and idiopathic orthostatic hypotension. *Ann Neurol* 1978;4: 511–514.
20. Lundevall J, Bjerkhoel P. Failure of hemoconcentration during standing to reveal plasma volume decline induced in the erect posture. *J Appl Physiol* 1994;77:2155–2162.
21. Morganti A, et al. Role of the sympathetic nervous system in mediating the renin response to head-up tilt. *Am J Cardiol* 1979;43:600–604.
22. Oparil S, et al. Role of renin in acute postural homeostasis. *Circulation* 1970;41:89–95.
23. Rowell LB. Human cardiovascular control. Oxford: Oxford University Press, 1993:1–162.
24. Sancho JR, et al. The role of the renin–angiotensin–aldosterone system in cardiovascular homeostasis in normal human subjects. *Circulation* 1976;53:400–405.
25. Schadt JC, Ludbrook J. Hemodynamic and neurohumoral responses to acute hypovolemia in conscious mammals. *Am J Physiol* 1991;260: H305–H318.
26. Schrier RW. Pathogenesis of sodium and water retention in high-output and low-output cardiac failure, nephrotic syndrome, cirrhosis, and pregnancy. *N Engl J Med* 1988;319:1065–1072 and 1127–1134.
27. Shepherd JT. Role of venoconstriction for circulatory adjustment to orthostatic stress. In: Christensen NJ, Hendriksen O, Lassen NA, eds. *The sympathoadrenal system: physiology and pathophysiology* (Alfred Benzon Symposium 23). Copenhagen: Munksgaard, 1986:103–115.
28. Shepherd JT, Vanhoutte PM. *Veins and their control.* Philadelphia: WB Saunders, 1975:171–180.
29. Sjöstrand T. Volume and distribution of blood and their significance in regulating the circulation. *Physiol Rev* 1953;33:202–225.
30. Smith JJ, Ebert J. General response to orthostatic stress. In: Smith JJ, ed. *Circulatory response to the upright posture.* Boca Raton, FL: CRC, 1990:1–46.

31. Smith JJ, et al. Cardiovascular response of young men to diverse stresses. *Aerospace Med* 1974;45:583–590.
32. Sprangers RLH, et al. Initial cardiovascular response to change in posture: influence of angle and speed of tilt. *Clin Physiol* 1991;11:211–220.
33. Sprangers RLH, et al. The initial blood pressure fall upon stand up and onset of exercise explained by changes in total peripheral resistance. *J Appl Physiol* 1991;70:523–530.
34. Streeten DHP. *Orthostatic disorders of the circulation: mechanisms, manifestations, and treatment.* New York: Plenum, 1987.
35. Tanaka H. Cardiac output and blood pressure during active and passive standing. *Clin Physiol* 1996;16:157–170.
36. Ten Harkel ADJ, et al. Effects of leg muscle pumping and tensing on orthostatic arterial pressure: a study in normal subjects and in patients with autonomic failure. *Clin Sci* 1994;87:553–558.
37. Ten Harkel ADJ, et al. The assessment of cardiovascular reflex tests: influence of posture and period of preceding rest. *J Appl Physiol* 1990;68:147–153.
38. Thompson WO, et al. The effect of posture upon the composition and volume of the blood in man. *J Clin Invest* 1928;5:573–609.
39. Van Lieshout JJ, et al. Combatting orthostatic dizziness dizziness in autonomic failure by physical maneuvers. *Lancet* 1992;339:897–898.
40. Van Lieshout JJ, et al. Orthostatic hypotension caused by sympathectomies performed for hyperhidrosis. *Neth J Med* 1990;36:53–57.
41. Van Lieshout JJ, et al. The vasovagal response. *Clin Sci* 1991;81:575–586.
42. Wieling W. External support and physical maneuvers. In: Robertson D, Low PA, Polinsky (eds). *Primer on the autonomic nervous system.* San Diego; Academic Press 1996:319–324.
43. Wieling W. Non-invasive continuous recording of heart rate and blood pressure in the evaluation of neurocardiovascular control. In: Bannister R, Mathias CJ, eds. *Autonomic failure: a textbook of clinical disorders of the autonomic nervous system.* 3rd ed. Oxford: Oxford University Press, 1992:291–311.
44. Wieling W, et al. Classification of orthostatic disorders based on the short-term circulatory response upon standing. *Clin Sci* 1991;99:241–248.
45. Wieling W, et al. Physical manoeuvers that reduce postural hypotension in autonomic failure. *Clin Auton Res* 1993;3:57–65.
46. Wieling W, Wesseling KH. Importance of reflexes in the circulatory adjustments to postural change. In: Hainsworth R, ed. *Cardiovascular reflex control in health and disease.* London: WB Saunders, 1993:35–65.
47. Wieling W, et al. Circulatory response evoked by a 3 s bout of dynamic leg exercise in humans. *J Physiol (Lond)* 1996;494:601–611.
48. Zanchetti AS. Neural regulation of renin release. Circulation 1977;56:691–698.

CHAPTER 7

Autonomic Regulation of Temperature and Sweating

Tokuo Ogawa and Phillip A. Low

1. The main thermoreceptor input derives from the preoptic and anterior hypothalamic (POAH) areas. Other inputs are from the midbrain, medulla, spinal cord, skin, and possibly abdominal viscera.
2. The two types of thermosensitive neurons in the POAH are warm-sensitive and cold-sensitive, with the former predominating. The activities of those neurons are modified by thermal inputs from other receptors that converge on the POAH.
3. The POAH thus serves to integrate thermal information and establish a set-point. The posterior hypothalamus plays a minor integrative role, if any.
4. In addition to thermal inputs, the POAH also receives inputs from structures of the central nervous system (CNS), and POAH activity is influenced by various CNS activities, such as mental activity, sleep, exercise, and biological clock. On the other hand, POAH activity influences other CNS activities, such as feeding activity.
5. Thermoregulatory responses are affected by humoral conditions, such as plasma osmolarity, volume, hypercapnia and hypocapnia, and pH changes. Progesterone depresses the activity of warm-sensitive neurons in the POAH and is responsible for postovulatory hyperthermia in women.
6. Norepinephrine, serotonin, and acetylcholine are believed to be neurotransmitters in the POAH. Arginine vasopressin, thyrotropin-releasing hormone, adrenocorticotropin hormone, and α-melanocyte-stimulating hormone are endogenous thermolytic substances. Bombesin inhibits both thermosensitive and nonthermosensitive neurons in the POAH, resulting in poikilothermia. Other neuropeptides that have been reported to modulate thermoregulation include neurotensin, vasoactive intestinal peptide, cholecystokinin octapeptide, and somatostatin.
7. Thermoregulatory effector mechanisms in humans include behavioral and autonomic ones, the latter consisting of shivering and nonshivering thermogenesis (NST) for heat production and cutaneous vasomotor response and sweating for heat dissipation. Heat exchange between the body and the environment occurs through radiation, conduction and convection, and evaporation. The rate of heat loss is regulated by adjusting cutaneous blood flow and sweating.
8. The shivering center is located in the dorsomedial posterior hypothalamus and receives thermal inputs from the POAH. Shivering occurs secondary to increased inputs from cold receptors to the POAH. Spinal neurons are reached via tectospinal and rubrospinal tracts. It is a major thermogenetic response to cooling in humans, except in neonates, in whom NST is important.
9. Skin vasculature, comprising capillaries and arteriovenous anastomoses, are influenced by ambient temperature directly and by neural influences. Norepinephrine is the major neurotransmitter, but nonadrenergic, noncholinergic mechanisms appear to be also present.
10. Emotional or mental sweating affects the palms and soles, and thermal sweating occurs over the general body surface. The latter is directly controlled by the POAH center.

T. Ogawa: Department of Physiology, Aichi Medical University, Nagakute, 480-11 Japan.
P. A. Low: Department of Neurology, Mayo Clinic, Rochester, Minnesota 55095.

INTRODUCTION

The human thermoregulatory system is outlined in Fig. 1. The major central mechanism is located in the hypothalamus, where thermal information from central and peripheral thermoreceptors is integrated and from which efferent thermoregulatory discharges arise. Of all the effector mechanisms, sweating is especially unique in humans, and its regulation is discussed in a separate section of this chapter.

THERMORECEPTORS AND THERMAL AFFERENTS

The most important thermal information originates from thermosensitive neurons in the preoptic and anterior hypothalamic (POAH) areas, where the integration of thermal inputs is believed to take place. Other thermal information comes from the midbrain, medulla, spinal cord, skin and, possibly, abdominal viscera (Fig. 2).

Preoptic Area–Anterior Hypothalamus

There are two types of thermosensitive neurons: the warm-sensitive ones, which account for 20%–40% of neuronal population, and the cold-sensitive ones, which constitute 5%–10%. Some of these neurons receive thermal information from the remote thermoreceptors. Warm-sensitive neurons increase their activity when peripheral temperature increases, and the activity of cold-sensitive neurons is augmented by peripheral temperature decrease.

Brainstem

Warm-sensitive and cold-sensitive neurons are present in the medullary reticular formation. Some respond to changes in skin temperature, while others receive inputs from the spinal cord, the midbrain, and the POAH, and send output to the POAH (45). Thermosensitive neurons have been identified in the midbrain reticular formation and the raphe nucleus; the population of cold-sensitive neurons exceeds that of warm-sensitive ones in the former and vice versa in the latter (41,77). They may be primary thermosensitive neurons and may also relay thermal signals from the periphery to the hypothalamus. Nonthermal afferents that modulate thermal information may also exist in the brain stem.

Spinal Cord

Selective warming and cooling of the spinal cord elicit thermoregulatory responses, demonstrating the presence of spinal thermosensitive structures, but the localization re-

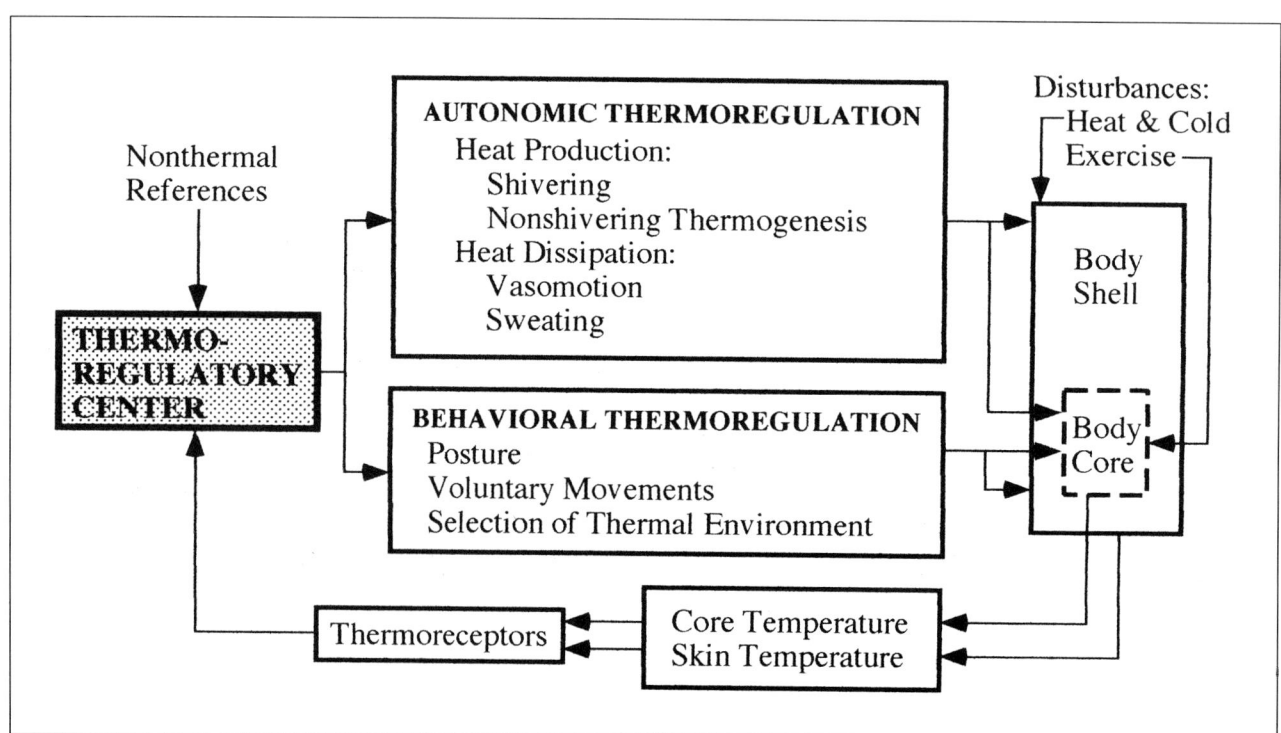

FIG. 1. The human thermoregulatory system.

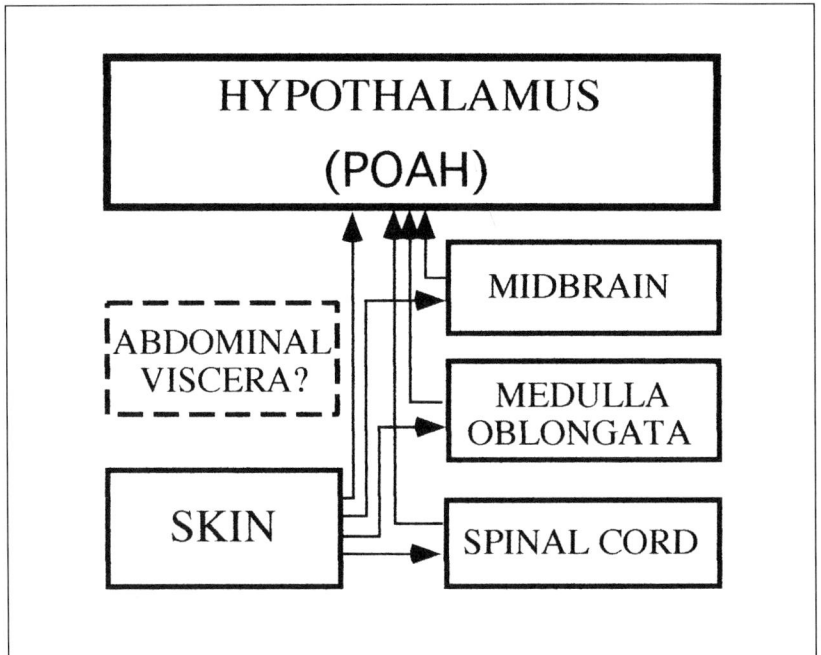

FIG. 2. Sites of thermoreceptors and thermal afferents.

mains unclear (48,111). The afferents are located in the spinothalamic tract (112).

Skin

Skin temperature is sensed mainly by specific cold and warm thermoreceptors. However, nociceptors and other nonspecific receptors may be involved in the sensation of extreme cold or heat. Cold receptors are free nerve endings with terminals that protrude into the basal epidermal cells (40). Warm receptors are also assumed to be free endings, but located somewhat deeper in the dermis.

Primary afferents from cutaneous cold receptors consist of A-δ and C fibers, and primary afferents from warm receptors are made up of C fibers. They enter the spinal cord via the dorsal root and, a few segments higher, connect to second-order neurons in the dorsal horn. However, primary thermal afferents from the face enter the brainstem via the trigeminal nerve and descend to the nucleus tractus spinalis nervi trigemini and to the dorsal horn of the cervical cord. Cutaneous thermal information ascends mainly in the contralateral spinothalamic tract and reaches the hypothalamus and the cerebral cortex via the midbrain (raphe nucleus) and the thalamus. Cutaneous thermoreceptors respond with constant-discharge frequency to a constant local temperature (static response), but respond to a rapid change in temperature with a transient, excessive change in discharge frequency (dynamic response). The degree and rate of the temperature change are matched by the dynamic response of the thermoreceptors. The response is also influenced by the temperature to which the thermoreceptors have adapted (60).

Abdominal Viscera

It has long been known that selective intra-abdominal heating or cooling induces thermoregulatory responses. Afferent thermal impulses have been recorded from the splanchnic nerve (37,101), but thermoreceptors have not been identified in the abdominal viscera.

CENTRAL INTEGRATION

Role of the Anterior Hypothalamus

Thermosensitive neurons in the POAH not only detect brain temperature but also integrate thermal information received from different regions of the body. Many thermoregulatory phenomena are readily explained by the assumption that body temperature is regulated to match a set-point. Diurnal fluctuation of body temperature, its variability during the menstrual cycle, and fever are attributed to shifts in this set-point. Various hypotheses have been proposed concerning the nature, or determinant, of the set-point. Body temperature might be determined by a dynamic balance between the activities of warm-sensitive and cold-sensitive neurons (Fig. 3). The activities of warm-sensitive neurons decrease and those of cold-sensitive ones increase during a fever or in response to the administration of a pyrogen (13,24,126). Similar changes are induced by the administration of progesterone, which is considered to be responsible for a higher body temperature during the luteal phase (78).

Thermal inputs from cutaneous thermoreceptors contribute little to thermal equilibrium, and the relative impor-

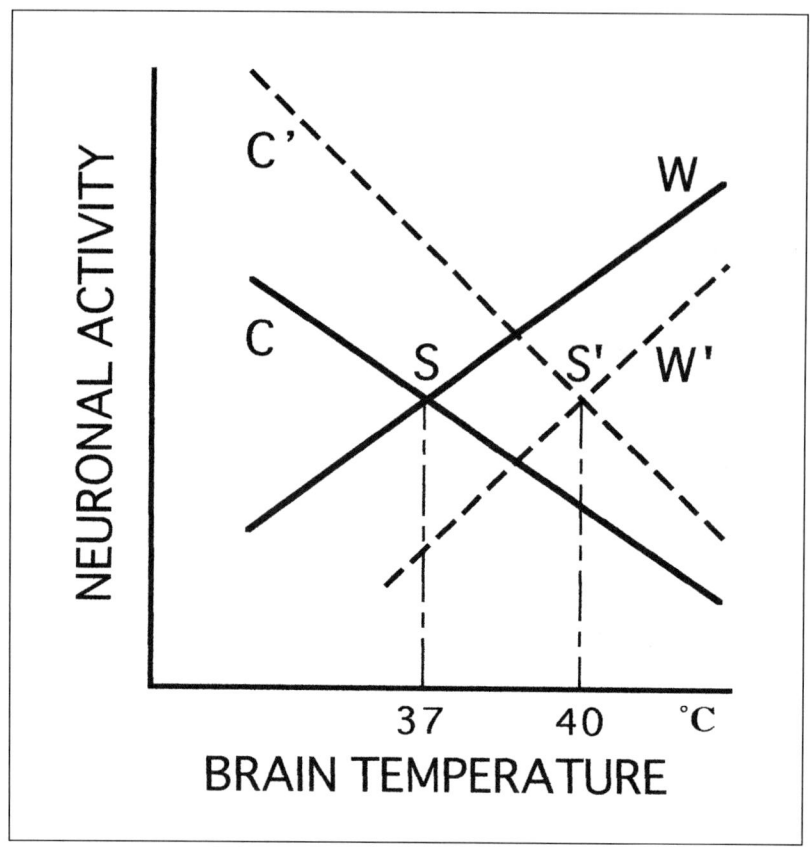

FIG. 3. Thermal characteristics of warm-sensitive (W) and cold-sensitive (C) neurons that possibly determine the set-point (S). Their changes to W' and C', respectively, cause a shift of S to S' during fever.

tance of skin to brain temperature has been determined to range between 0.14 and 0.33 (12). However, the alteration in skin temperature following a rapid change in the thermal environment is largely responsible for rapid, transient thermoregulatory responses, which take place before any appreciable change in brain temperature (68).

Role of the Posterior Hypothalamus

The posterior hypothalamus was once considered the site of final integration of thermal information. However, evidence suggests a more minor role for this structure; it is now regarded as the site of integration for thermogenesis or shivering, or merely a part of the efferent pathways for the shivering reflex (33,64). Only few thermosensitive neurons have been detected in the posterior hypothalamus, and some respond to thermal stimulation of the POAH and the spinal cord.

Modulation by Other Central Regulatory Mechanisms

The central thermoregulatory mechanism is not mediated only by the integration of thermal inputs. Thermoregulatory responses occur through the interaction and intervention of various regulatory mechanisms. Abundant neuronal connections have been identified between the POAH and other hypothalamic and brain areas (16). Afferent neurons from the mediobasal hypothalamus, medial forebrain bundle, sulcal prefrontal cortex, hippocampal formation, amygdala, midbrain reticular formation, and raphe nucleus have been found to project to the POAH.

Hypothalamic thermoregulatory processing can be modified by higher brain activities, as evidenced by the changes in thermoregulatory responses during sleep, mental stress, and emotional excitement (see also the section *Nonthermal Factors That Affect Central Sudomotor Drive*).

The elevation in body temperature seen during exercise is considered a regulated process and not the result of impaired thermal balance due to heat production exceeding dissipation. Core temperature during exercise is linearly related to metabolic rate, but not necessarily to the rate of heat production (82). Individual differences in the degree of body temperature increase are minimized when body temperature is related to the relative value of oxygen consumption to his or her maximum (% $\dot{V}O_2$ max) (106). However, this is a controversial mechanism. The involvement of nonthermal factors has also been suggested, and these include mental excitement accompanying work performance or central motor command.

It is well known that body temperature affects feeding behavior. A rise in POAH temperature facilitates the activity of glucoreceptive neurons in the ventromedial hypothalamus (VMH), which is the satiety center, and inhibits glucose-sensitive neurons in the lateral hypothalamus, the feeding center (79). POAH neurons not only send axons to the VMH and lateral hypothalamus, but receive projections from those areas. The VMH may be involved in diet-induced thermogenesis, as stimulation of the VMH has been shown to increase nonshivering thermogenesis (NST) (97).

Thermoregulatory responses are affected considerably by changes in body-fluid balance, such as osmolarity, volume, distribution, electrolyte concentrations, and pH. Most commonly encountered is the dehydration that arises after profuse sweating. Heat-dissipating responses are reduced during dehydration. Body temperature is linearly related to plasma osmolarity (34,81). Dehydration elicits mainly a central effect, by hyperosmolarity (5,27) (Fig. 4A). Many warm-sensitive neurons in the POAH are inhibited by an increase in local osmolarity (76) and also receive projections from the hepatoportal osmoreceptors (58). Hypovolemia and hypervolemia, without changes in osmolarity, have also been shown to cause a rise and fall in body temperature, respectively (26).

Hypercapnia usually causes cutaneous vasodilation and augmentation of sweating, accompanied by a drop in core temperature. Conversely, hypocapnia brought about by sustained hyperventilation causes cutaneous vasoconstriction and reduced sweat production, accompanied by a rise in core temperature. The mechanism of the CO_2 effect may not be a simple one because of the variety of effects that carbon dioxide has on many functions, such as cardiovascular function, ventilatory activity, and cellular metabolism (43). Relatively mild hypercapnia may cause an increase in heat production due to the facilitative effect of carbon dioxide on cellular metabolism.

Neurotransmitters and Neuromodulators

Various intracerebral substances, including monoamines, acetylcholine, prostaglandins, and peptides, have been studied to determine their role as neurotransmitters or neuromodulators. Norepinephrine, serotonin, and acetylcholine are believed to act as neurotransmitters in the thermoregulatory processing that takes place in the POAH region, but there are major differences among animal species. Hypothetical neuronal circuit models have been proposed for monkeys (72) and sheep (4), but they may apply only to those particular animals. The role of dopamine is disputed.

Prostaglandin E plays a crucial role in fever as the putative final mediator (70). However, it is unlikely that it participates in the normal thermoregulatory process (22).

A number of hypothalamic neuropeptides have been identified, and many are reported to be important in the central thermoregulatory mechanism. Arginine vasopressin is thought to be an endogenous thermolytic substance that prevents excessive hyperthermia during fever (53). Adrenocorticotropin hormone and α-melanocyte-stimulating hormone may also be endogenous thermolytic peptides (17).

Thyrotropin-releasing hormone (TRH) also exerts different effects on the thermoregulatory responses of different species. In humans, TRH is considered to be thermolytic, because the intravenous administration of TRH causes cutaneous vasodilation and augmentation of sweating, with a resulting drop in core temperature (116) (Fig. 4B,C). Interestingly, TRH fails to augment sweating in patients with Parkinson's disease (Watanabe and Kihara, unpublished data), suggesting the involvement of dopamine in the thermolytic effect of TRH. TRH induces hyperthermia in rats; intravenously administered TRH in rats is transported to the brain, where it is rapidly concentrated in the hypothalamus (74).

Bombesin appears to repress the central thermoregulatory mechanism, resulting in a poikilothermic condition (119). It inhibits both thermosensitive and nonthermosensitive neurons in the POAH (42). Modulation of thermoregulatory activities by other neuropeptides has also been reported. These include neurotensin (42), vasoactive intestinal peptide (VIP) (18), cholecystokinin octapeptide (54), and somatostatin (11).

Endogenous opioids, such as β-endorphin and met-enkephalin, exhibit diverse thermoregulatory effects for different species, environments, and doses, and with or without restraint; they may participate in changes of body temperature provoked by stress (17).

EFFECTOR MECHANISMS

Thermoregulatory responses can be divided into two groups: autonomic and behavioral (Fig. 1). The behavioral group is phylogenetically older and plays a major role in natural living of many animals; the autonomic response has been defined only in birds and mammals.

Autonomic thermoregulatory systems possess no specific effectors except for sweat glands, but make use of various organs with other functions, such as those in the circulatory, respiratory, metabolic, and motor systems. Autonomic thermoregulatory responses in humans consist of shivering and NST, which promote heat production, and cutaneous vasomotor response and sweating, which produce heat dissipation. Heat exchange between the human body surface and its environment occurs through radiation, conduction, convection (nonevaporative, or dry, heat loss or gain), and evaporation (evaporative, or wet, heat loss). The rate of dry heat loss is regulated by adjusting the cutaneous blood flow and that of wet heat loss is controlled by sweating.

Shivering

Shivering arises when there is an increased input to the central thermoregulatory mechanism derived from the cold

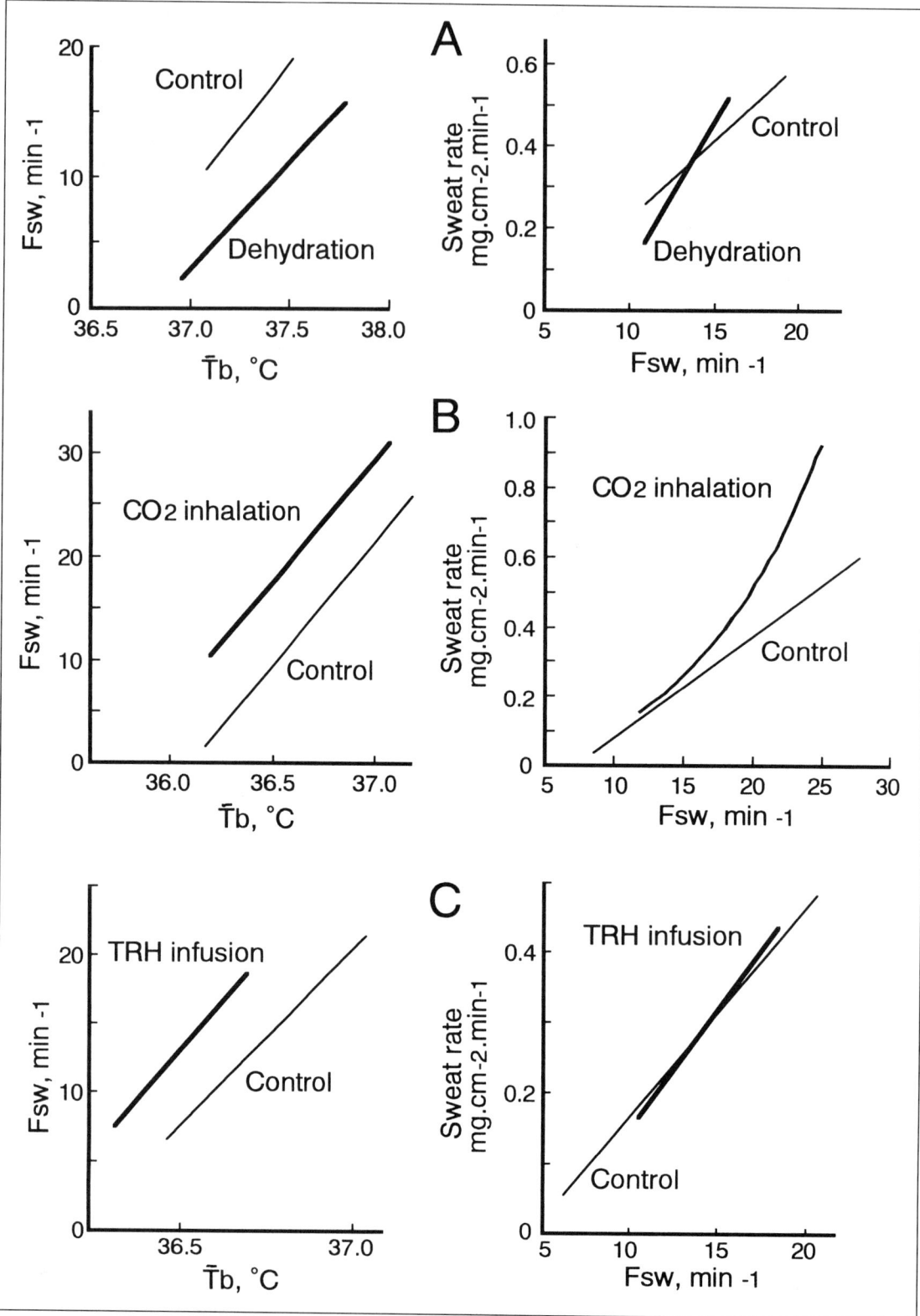

FIG. 4. Changes in characteristics of the frequency of sweat expulsions (Fsw) during thermal dehydration **(A)**, 6% CO_2 inhalation **(B)**, and thyrotropin-releasing hormone (TRH) infusion **(C)**. Plots of Fsw against mean body temperature (Tb) are shown in the *left column*, and plots of local sweat rate against Fsw in the *right column*. From Ogawa and Sugenoya (94), with permission.

receptors. It is functionally an autonomic (involuntary) phenomenon, but the somatic nervous system and skeletal muscles are involved. To some extent, therefore, shivering can be inhibited consciously and voluntarily by muscle contractions. Because flexor and extensor muscles contract synchronously, minimal external work is performed by shivering muscles and most of the liberated chemical energy is converted to heat. Shivering is a major thermogenetic response to cooling in humans, except in neonates, for whom NST is important to thermoregulation.

The center for shivering control is assumed to be in the posterior hypothalamus (113). The efferent pathway travels through the midbrain tegmentum, the pons, and the lateral part of the medullary reticular formation, and reaches spinal motor neurons via the tectospinal and rubrospinal tracts (9). However, the rhythm of shivering is not dictated by the efferent discharge, but is generated at the spinal level and involves a negative-feedback circuit that operates through Renshaw cells (114).

Nonshivering Thermogenesis

NST is heat production that does not involve muscle contraction. It can be classified into obligatory NST, which includes basal metabolic heat production and diet-induced thermogenesis, and thermoregulatory NST, which is caused by cold stimulation. Thermoregulatory NST is observed predominantly in cold-acclimated animals and neonates. It is induced by a weaker cold stimulus than that required for shivering and produces a shift of the threshold temperature for shivering to a lower level. Brown adipose tissue is the most important site of the thermoregulatory NST. This tissue is markedly developed in rodents and hibernating mammals and is hypertrophied by cold acclimatization. In humans, it functions effectively for thermoregulation only in neonates and is replaced by white adipose tissue as they grow.

The regulatory center for NST is located in the POAH. Brown adipose tissue is innervated by adrenergic sympathetic nerve fibers and is known to be stimulated through a β-adrenergic receptor mechanism. However, brown adipose tissue also possesses α_1-receptors, and these increase in number with cold acclimatization (99). Furthermore, thyroid hormone is required for thermogenesis at brown adipose tissue (36).

Vasomotor Response

Skin temperature is directly influenced by ambient temperature. It is regulated through changes in skin blood flow effected by constriction and dilation of the cutaneous vasculature. Abundant arteriovenous anastomoses, present in the hands and feet and especially at the finger and toe tips, are responsible for a remarkable change in skin blood flow at the extremities.

In a cool environment, arteriovenous anastomoses close and superficial cutaneous veins constrict, so that the blood flow slows down and much of the blood is directed to deep veins, the venae comitantes, a pair of which accompany each limb artery. A countercurrent heat-exchange system operates between the veins and artery: arterial blood is cooled as it travels toward the periphery, and venous blood is warmed as it returns to the core. Accordingly, the skin temperature of the extremities is lowered by much more than that of the trunk, and finger and toe temperatures can approach ambient temperature. In a warm environment, arteriovenous anastomoses open and superficial veins dilate, enabling blood to pass through them rapidly. In this situation, the countercurrent heat-exchange system hardly works, so the skin temperature of the distal limbs rises. Finger blood flow begins to increase at a lower ambient temperature than does toe blood flow.

Cutaneous vasculature is innervated primarily by adrenergic vasoconstrictor nerve fibers. Neuropeptide Y, a potent vasoactive substance, coexists with norepinephrine in these neurons and may take a part in cutaneous vasoconstriction (98). As the ambient temperature rises, their activity decreases, resulting in "passive" vasodilation. Another massive increase in blood flow is closely associated with sweating activity. This "active" vasodilation occurs because of increased activity in a vasodilator mechanism. Although specific vasodilator nerve fibers have been demonstrated in animals, their presence in humans is debated. It has been proposed that bradykinin, produced locally by the action of kallikrein, which is released from activated sweat glands, could be responsible for local vasodilation (29). However, this hypothesis has been strongly disputed (103), mainly because the vasodilation persists after atropinization, which blocks sweating. Alternatively, cholinergic sudomotor nerve terminals have been observed to contain vasoactive peptides, which are assumed to be released as cotransmitters with acetylcholine, and these could affect active vasodilation (see the section *Classification and Innervation of Sweat Glands*). Vasodilator mechanisms have been observed in human fingers. β-Adrenoreceptors are present in the finger and have been reported to accelerate arteriovenous shunt flow when stimulated by circulating catecholamines (20). A cholinergic vasodilator mechanism has been reported in human fingers that seems to be confined to capillary flow (19). Naloxone increases blood flow in the human hand, suggesting the presence of endogenous opioid control and a possible role of opioid antagonists (3).

When the fingers, hands, or feet are exposed to severe cold, the local blood vessels constrict, but dilate after several minutes. Thereafter, vasoconstriction and dilation occur alternately and are referred to as *cold-induced vasodilation*, *hunting reaction*, or *Lewis' reaction* (63). This phenomenon can be attributed to episodic opening of the arteriovenous anastomoses and is caused by a direct local effect, as it persists in sympathectomized or denervated hands. The vasodilative response is facilitated, and its threshold temperature is raised, in a cooler environment (125) and in cold-acclimated people (65).

In general, skin blood flow increases locally as the result of direct heating, but the mechanism for this is not clear. Local heating of the hand to 37°–41°C, however, may produce a decrease in finger blood flow due to the constriction of the arteriovenous anastomoses (75). Heat-induced vasoconstriction may be effective in reducing heat gain through the hand when the ambient temperature is higher than the body temperature.

Cardiac output increases markedly in a hot environment, compared with that in the cold, resulting in a greatly increased cutaneous blood flow, while visceral blood flow is rather decreased (104).

Evaporative Heat Loss

Evaporation in the absence of sweating is called *insensible water loss*. It consists of evaporation through the airway and the skin, and is not controlled by thermoregulatory mechanisms in humans. However, panting is a major autonomic means of heat dissipation in some animals.

Sweating is by far the most important heat-dissipating response to heat in humans. Evaporation, mostly of sweat, is the only means of heat dissipation, which can take place when ambient temperature exceeds skin temperature. The regulation of sweating activity is discussed in a separate section in this chapter.

Efferent Autonomic Pathways

The sympathetic efferent pathways, including the vasomotor and sudomotor ones, are assumed to follow similar but different courses within the CNS.

In animals, the descending pathways from the hypothalamus to the lower brainstem are considerably diverse (35,38). It has been demonstrated in rats that efferent signals from the POAH project dominantly to the ipsilateral salivary glands for thermally induced salivary secretion (52). The pathways from the brain stem to the intermediolateral nucleus of the spinal cord originate at the solitary nucleus, the ventrolateral reticular formation, and the raphe nucleus (1,66). A tract has been identified that arises in the hypothalamus, especially the ventrolateral nucleus, and leads directly to the intermediolateral nucleus (96, 107). However, the relationship between each autonomic function and its pathway has not been elucidated. The efferent pathways mainly travel ipsilaterally, though some cross to the contralateral side at the pontine and bulbar levels and at the spinal segmental levels (80). Therefore, sweating activity in patients with unilateral brain stem lesions, such as Wallenberg's syndrome, is reduced, but not lost, on the ipsilateral side. In rats, the efferent vasomotor pathway partly crosses within and below the POAH, but the innervation is stronger ipsilaterally (50), whereas the pathway for shivering shows crossing somewhere below the POAH and the innervation is equal on both sides (51).

Monoaminergic fibers that are derived from the ventrolateral medulla and raphe nucleus and descend to the intermediolateral nucleus of the spinal cord (21,23) are assumed to have an inhibitory effect on the cardiovascular system. There may also be sweat-inhibitory efferents derived from the medulla, as have been demonstrated in studies of the sweating response of the cat foot pad (124,129).

According to Foerster (25), descending vasoconstrictor and sudomotor pathways travel in the lateral funiculus, ventral to the lateral corticospinal tract, and are arranged in order according to the body areas they innervate: fibers innervating the upper limbs and the trunk are located medial to those innervating the lower limbs. However, this arrangement has been the subject of some dispute. There have been claims that the distribution of the vasomotor and sudomotor pathways is not identical (49), and that the main vasopressor pathway descends in the periphery of the lateral funiculus and is arranged in order in cats, monkeys (55), and dogs (6). However, an extensive experimental study in patients who had undergone anterolateral cordotomy has revealed that vasomotor and sudomotor pathways lie essentially within the same area, though they do not exactly overlie each other. These pathways are located within the medial part of the equatorial plane, extending from the base of the posterior and lateral horns across the medial half of the lateral funiculus (80). The inhibitory pathways are located in the ventral and dorsal parts of the lateral funiculus (21,44).

Preganglionic neurons are located in the intermediolateral nucleus of spinal segments T1 to L3 (occasionally, also, C8 or L4, or both). Preganglionic fibers exit the cord in the anterior root, enter the sympathetic chain via the white ramus, and synapse with postganglionic neurons in paravertebral ganglia at the corresponding and several adjacent levels, cranially and caudally. In the human paravertebral ganglia, there are abundant enkephalin-containing preganglionic fibers innervating selectively postganglionic sudomotor neurons (47). Postganglionic fibers join the spinal nerve via the gray ramus and extend to cutaneous effectors. Those fibers innervating cutaneous blood vessels, pilomotor muscles, and sweat glands follow a similar course, though their activities are, in general, not coincidental. The area of skin covered by the preganglionic fibers from each segment (the sympathetic dermatome) is wider than the sensory dermatome, and its outline is rather irregular and asymmetrical (100). Furthermore, the distribution of vasomotor innervation may not correspond to that of sudomotor innervation, especially in the lower body (83).

Exceptionally, facial sweat glands appear to be dually innervated. In addition to the sympathetic fibers that accompany the external carotid artery and its branches, it is likely that the sympathetic fibers join the branches of the trigeminal nerve distal to the gasserian ganglion (110).

REGULATION OF SWEATING

Classification and Innervation of Sweat Glands

Sweat glands are conventionally classified as either apocrine or eccrine glands, based on their secretory processes. However, there are no distinct differences between them: eccrine secretion can be observed in apocrine glands, and apocrine-like secretion is also seen in the superficial cells of eccrine glands. In humans, they can be characterized morphologically as well as ontogenically, although sweat glands of mixed types have been identified in the axillary, perianal, and nasal ala skins (46,109). The apocrine gland opens into the lumen of a hair follicle, whereas the eccrine gland opens directly onto the skin. Thus, the terms *epitrichial* and *atrichial* have been proposed to replace *apocrine* and *eccrine*, respectively (10). The apocrine glands are restricted to a few hairy areas, such as the axilla, areola of the nipple, and perineum. These glands have a poor secretory capacity and are of little physiologic significance. They become functional during preadolescence. On the other hand, eccrine glands are distributed throughout nearly the whole body surface and have a high secretory capacity. Their activation is believed to commence after fetal week 28 and is completed by $2\frac{1}{2}$ years of age (62).

Eccrine glands are innervated by sympathetic postganglionic nerve fibers, which are cholinergic. Phylogenetically, they are believed to have developed from apocrine-type adrenoceptive glands, and retain α- and β-receptor mechanisms (see Chapter 8). Several neuropeptides in the nerve terminals surrounding the eccrine gland, including VIP, calcitonin gene-related peptide, atrial natriuretic peptide, and galanin, have been identified as possible cotransmitters (67,120,122).

Human apocrine glands appear to be innervated by adrenergic fibers, which may participate only in the contraction of the myoepithelium. The production of apocrine sweat may be stimulated by humoral epinephrine. Apocrine secretion is not blocked by sympathectomy. Apocrine glands do not respond to thermal stimuli and secrete scanty sweat in response to severe mental stress.

Distribution and Density of Sweat Glands

Human skin has 2.5–5.0 million sweat glands, but not all are functional. Because the development of sweat glands is completed early in life and the final number of functional glands depends on the thermal environment during this period (62), people born in the tropics have a greater number of functional sweat glands than do people from colder climates. The number of functional sweat glands may increase in some individuals in association with acclimatization to heat, but the probability of this differs with ethnic group (57).

Sweat glands are, in general, more densely distributed on bare body areas, especially on the palms, soles, and forehead. However, individual sweat glands on the palms and soles are smaller, whereas those on the back of the trunk are much larger and have a superior secretory capacity. The rate of sweating is relatively high for the head and ventral and dorsal aspects of the trunk, and is generally low for the extremities, but there is considerable individual variation (62).

Thermal and Mental Sweating

The major role of human sweating is thermoregulation. This thermal sweating occurs over the general body surface when temperatures exceed thermoneutral values or is seen during exercise, but does not affect the palms and soles. The palms and soles in wakeful human subjects sweat even in the absence of thermal sweating, and mental excitement increases the rate with a short latency. This is called *mental sweating*, and its central mechanism may involve the cerebral neocortex, limbic system, and hypothalamus. Differences in sudomotor as well as vasoconstrictor components of skin sympathetic nerve activity between nerves innervating glabrous and hairy skin have been demonstrated microneurographically at different ambient temperatures (95). An excessive response to emotional stress may precipitate palmar hyperhidrosis, accompanied often by a plantar hyperhidrosis. It occurs most commonly in young, nervous females. Annoyance with this excessive sweating may aggravate hyperhidrosis, thus causing continuous problems. Furthermore, repeated stimulation can cause palmar sweat glands to increase their secretory capacity (see the section *Peripheral Factors That Affect Sweat Gland Activity*).

Various mental stresses also affect general body surface sweating. In the presence of thermal sweating, these stresses cause phasic responses in the generalized sweating. The pattern of response varies with different kinds of mental stress and among individuals, and does not always resemble the response pattern of palmar and plantar sweating: sweating on the general body surface may be augmented or depressed during mental stress, while palmar sweating is always augmented (86). Conversely, palmar sweating is influenced by thermal conditions and does not occur when it is cold. There appears to be some interaction between the central mechanisms of thermal and mental sweating (92).

Sweating from the axilla often occurs even when there is no thermal sweating elsewhere. It is characterized by a much lower threshold temperature and is less responsiveness to thermal load. The feature of the sweating response in the axilla is, however, identical to that on the general body surface, but not to that on the palm (118). Forehead sweating resembles axillary activity in some individuals.

Many normal persons exhibit sweating on the face, especially on and around the nose and lips, when they taste spicy or acidic food. This type of gustatory sweating is assumed to be a local reflex, but its regulatory pathway is not clear. Gustatory sweating is often also observed following injuries or inflammation of the parotid gland or its vicinity (auriculotemporal syndrome, or Frey's syndrome), injuries involving the submandibular area (chorda tympani syndrome), and after cervical or thoracic sympathectomy. Such instances of gustatory sweating are attributed either to misdirection of the regenerated fibers (32) or to cross-excitation of sudomotor nerve fibers by adjacent parasympathetic nerve fibers supplying the salivary gland, especially (31) (for details, see Chapter 51).

Central Sudomotor Drive–Sweat Expulsion

In spontaneous sweating, sweat is discharged in a pulsatile fashion with an irregular rhythm, the rate ranging from several to >20 expulsions/min. These sweat expulsions arise synchronously over the general body surface, and their rate is highly related to both the ambient temperature (89) and body temperature (115). Therefore, they are considered to reflect a centrally derived sudomotor drive. Sweat expulsions are also observed for palmar and plantar sweating, and are synchronous over the palms and soles. They are considered to reflect the central drive for mental sweating. Expulsions on the palm and sole are largely synchronized with those for the general body surface in some individuals, but are only partly synchronized in others (92). The microneurographic recording of skin sympathetic activity reveals burst discharges that coincide with sweat expulsions (117). Changes in regional sweating rates, due to modifications of sudomotor drive in the efferent pathways or in the periphery, do not affect either the rate or the synchronism of sweat expulsions (89). Thus, by analyzing characteristics of sweat expulsions, response of the higher central mechanism and more peripheral mechanisms involving efferent pathway and effector can be estimated separately (92). A few examples of results of the analysis are shown in Fig. 4.

Recruitment and Distribution of Thermal Sweating

Thermal sweating, even in response to a local stimulus, occurs uniformly over the general body surface. Thermal sweating is initiated nearly simultaneously over the whole body in the upright standing or sitting positions, whereas it occurs first on the lower body and extends over the upper body in the supine posture. Furthermore, when an individual lies on one side, the onset of sweating is considerably delayed over the lower side of the body and its rate is remarkably reduced. This phenomenon is known as *hemihidrosis*. Such variability in the recruitment patterns of sweating is attributed to a reflex induced by skin pressure (121).

Semihidrosis is primarily a reflex suppression of sweating over one side of the body, brought about by pressure applied to a certain skin area on the ipsilateral side. Pressure on the lateral chest and scapular area is especially effective, causing unilateral suppression of sweating over the upper body surface. The extent of the sweat-suppressed area depends on the area where pressure is applied. If the site of pressure application is moved caudally on the lateral chest, the sweat-suppressed area shifts caudally, which suggests that this reflex pathway involves spinal segments (93). Pressure over one side of the iliac crest, trochanter, and sole causes hemihidrosis over the lower body. Sweating from the corresponding area on the contralateral side is, in general, augmented. It may likely result from reciprocal innervation. When pressure is applied bilaterally, sweating on both sides of body is inhibited, e.g., sweating over the whole upper body is reduced in an individual lying supine.

Nonthermal Factors That Affect Central Sudomotor Drive

As already noted, mental activity induces phasic changes in the generalized sweating activity. Occasionally, a transient increase in thermal sweating in response to a strong emotional stimulus may be accompanied by a transient rise in tympanic temperature, which is assumed to be elicited secondarily by a rise in brain temperature (T. Ogawa et al., unpublished data).

Sweating increases during exercise. The onset of and subsequent increases in sweating precede the rise in body temperature, but the possible involvement of thermal or neural information from the acting muscles has been ruled out. Instead, nonthermal factors have been assumed to be involved in the control of increased sweating activity, especially in the initial period of exercise. These factors may consist of the mental excitement that accompanies the commencement of exercise or the irradiation of the central motor command.

Heat-dissipating activities including thermal sweating and cutaneous vasodilation are enhanced during sleep, especially in its initial phase. The phenomena are attributed to a downward shift of the set-point temperature (91,105). The shift is superimposed by the declining phase of circadian rhythm of body temperature in nocturnal sleep. In general, the deeper the non-REM (rapid eye movement) sleep, the higher the sweat rate. Sweating is usually suppressed during REM sleep, but may show an abrupt increase in association with emotional dream (91). Palmar sweating is completely absent throughout sleep.

Dehydration results in a diminished rate of sweating, accompanied by an elevated core temperature. As already discussed, this effect has been attributed largely to an increase in plasma osmolarity (27). Similarly, the increased rate of sweating that occurs with rehydration is effected largely by a reduction in osmolarity (15). In patients with renal failure, sweating activity is enhanced after hemodialysis, which reduces plasma osmolarity despite a minimal change in volume. Hypercapnia and hypocapnia cause an increase and decrease in the rate of sweating, respectively, and the mechanism involved in these changes has been discussed. These conditions appear to affect not only the central thermoregulatory mechanism, but also peripheral effector mechanisms (Fig. 4B) (92). The peripheral effect of carbon dioxide may be exerted either directly on sweat gland activity or indirectly by its vasodilative property, or both may operate.

Peripheral Factors That Affect Sweat Gland Activity

Skin temperature is important in thermoregulation, not only as an input to the central regulatory mechanism, but also as a local effect on the secretory activity of sweat glands. Local warming facilitates local sweating activity, the temperature quotient (Q_{10}) effect being around 2–3 (73,87). It is thought that the amount of transmitter released at the neuroglandular junction is increased (69), and that the responsiveness of secretory cells to this transmitter is enhanced (85).

Ample blood flow to the sweat gland is a prerequisite for sustained activity. Sweating in an area where blood flow is occluded soon ceases because of fatigue at the neuroglandular junction and dulling of the secretory mechanism caused by anoxia. Active cutaneous vasodilation accompanies sweating, the mechanism of which has been discussed. Vasoactive peptides that are thought to be cotransmitters released at the sudomotor nerve terminals include VIP (128), atrial natriuretic peptide (127), and calcitonin gene-related peptide (61). These peptides have been shown to augment sweating when administered locally, even though they have no sudorific effect *per se*.

In the event of profuse sweating or sweating in a hot and humid environment, the rate of sweat drippage increases, but then starts to decline within an hour and continues to decrease until sweat drippage stops. This phenomenon, known as *hidromeiosis*, is considered to be a local effect caused by the constant wetting of the epidermis. Osmosis of water causes swelling of the horny layer and, especially, the keratin ring in the intraepidermal duct, resulting in narrowing or occlusion of the orifices of the sweat ducts (56,108). Drying will restore sweating in the local area. The greater the rate of sweat drippage at the peak of sweating, the faster the sweat rate declines. Meanwhile, only the rate of sweat drippage declines; the rate of evaporation is unchanged (14,94).

Sweat glands can be conditioned by repeatedly immersing a local area in warm water for several days. This causes an increase in the secretory capacity of the local sweat glands. Increased sweating capacity in association with heat acclimation is attributed partly to such adaptation of the sweat glands (30). Dry heat, such as radiant heat, is less effective than moist heat in producing this change. The occurrence of hidromeiosis is delayed and the rate of sweating decline is slowed after training with repeated hot baths (88).

Effects of Gender and Age on Sweating

Functional glands in the neonate have only a weak sweat-secretory capacity, and the threshold body temperature for thermal sweating is high (28). Sweating capacity increases rapidly after birth and continues to increase with age during infancy and childhood. Less secretory capacity of sweat glands in children than adults is counterbalanced by higher density of sweat glands in children because of their smaller body surface area. Many investigators have reported that the rate of sweating during exercise is lower in children than adults (2,7). The maximum rate of sweating in children seems inferior to that in adults.

Gender differences in sweating activity become obvious after puberty. The threshold temperature for generalized sweating is higher and its sensitivity to body temperature is lower in females. This is mainly due to differences in thermal balance mechanisms. However, the secretory capacity of sweat glands is also lower in females (71). Many studies have demonstrated that in women the threshold body temperature for sweating is higher in the luteal phase than in the follicular phase of the menstrual cycle (8,39,59).

A tendency has been noted that the sweating response to a heat load is delayed and the threshold body temperature for thermal sweating rises with advancing age. Because of wide individual variation, however, many studies have failed to obtain statistically significant differences in sweating activity among different age groups (84). Reports of age-related changes in the magnitude of the sweating response have met with controversy (84,130). At least in very old men (>70 years) and women (>80 years), however, a distinct reduction in sweat gland function is noted, especially in the extremities. The ability to augment sweating capacity in association with heat acclimatization may be limited in elderly men (123), although physically fit men appear to be minimally affected (102). The effect of sweat gland conditioning is generally diminished in the aged, especially in men, and this may at least partly account for the reduced improvement in sweating capacity in elderly men (90).

REFERENCES

1. Amendt K, et al. Bulbospinal projections to the intermediolateral cell column: a neuroanatomical study. *J Auton Nerv Syst* 1979;1: 103–117.
2. Araki K, et al. Age difference in sweating during muscular exercise. *Jpn J Phys Fitness Sports Med* 1979;28: 239–248.
3. Archer AG, et al. Naloxone increases blood flow in the human hand. *J Physiol* 1985;363:315–321.
4. Bacon M, Bligh J. Interaction between the effects of spinal heating and cooling and of injections into a lateral cerebral ventricle of noradrenaline, 5-hydroxytryptamine and carbachol on thermoregulation in sheep. *J Physiol* 1976;254:213–227.

5. Baker MA, Doris PA. Effect of dehydration on hypothalamic control of evaporation in the cat. *J Physiol* 1982;322:457–468.
6. Barman SM, Wurster RD. Visceromotor organization within descending spinal sympathetic pathways in the dog. *Circ Res* 1975;37:209–214.
7. Bar-Or O. Climate and the exercising child: a review. *Int J Sports Med* 1980;1:53–65.
8. Bittel J, Henane R. Comparison of thermal exchanges in men and women under neutral and hot conditions. *J Physiol* 1975;250:475–489.
9. Birzis L, Hemingway A. Descending brain stem connections controlling shivering in cat. *J Neurophysiol* 1956;19:37–43.
10. Bligh J. A thesis concerning the processes of secretion and discharge of sweat. *Environ Res* 1967;1:28–45.
11. Brown M, et al. Somatostatin-28, somatostatin-14 and somatostatin analogs: effects on thermoregulation. *Brain Res* 1981; 214:127–135.
12. Cabanac M. Temperature regulation. *Annu Rev Physiol* 1975;37:415–439.
13. Cabanac M, et al. Effect of temperature and pyrogens on single unit activity in the rabbit's brain stem. *J Appl Physiol* 1968;24:645–652.
14. Candas V, et al. Sweating and sweat decline of resting men in hot humid environments. *Eur J Appl Physiol* 1983;50: 223–234.
15. Candas V, et al. Hydration during exercise: effect on thermal and cardiovascular adjustments. *Eur J Appl Physiol* 1986;55:113–122.
16. Chiba T, Murata Y. Afferent and efferent connections of the medial preoptic area in the rat: a WGA–HRP study. *Brain Res Bull* 1985; 14:261–272.
17. Clark WG, Lipton JM. Brain and pituitary peptides in thermoregulation. *Pharmacol Ther* 1983;22:249–297.
18. Clark WG, et al. Hyperthermic responses to vasoactive intestinal peptide (VIP) injected into the third cerebral ventricle of cats. *Neuropharmacology* 1978;17:883–885.
19. Coffman JD, Cohen RA. Cholinergic vasodilator mechanisms in human fingers. *Am J Physiol* 1987;252:H594–H597.
20. Cohen RA, Coffman JD. β-Adrenergic vasodilator mechanism in the finger. *Circ Res* 1981;49:1196–1201.
21. Coote JH, Maclead VH. The influence of bulbospinal monoaminergic pathways on sympathetic nerve activity. *J Physiol* 1974;241:453–475.
22. Cranston WI, et al. Is brain prostaglandin synthesis involved in responses to cold? *J Physiol* 1975;249:425–434.
23. Dahlstrom A, Fuxe K. Evidence for the existence of monoamine neurons in the central nervous system. *Acta Physiol Scand* 1965;64 (Suppl 247):1–85.
24. Eisenmann JS. Pyrogen-induced changes in the thermosensitivity of septal and preoptic neurons. *Am J Physiol* 1969;216:330–334.
25. Foerster O. *Handbuch der Neurologie*. Berlin: Springer-Verlag, 1936.
26. Fortney SM, et al. Effect of blood volume on sweating rate and body fluids in exercising humans. *J Appl Physiol* 1981;51:1594–1600.
27. Fortney SM, et al. Effect of hyperosmolarity on control of blood flow and sweating. *J Appl Physiol* 1984;57:1688–1695.
28. Foster KG, et al. The response of the sweat glands of the new-born baby to thermal stimuli and to intradermal acetylcholine. *J Physiol* 1969;203:13–29.
29. Fox RH, Hilton SM. Bradykinin formation in human skin as a factor in heat vasodilation. *J Physiol* 1958;142:219–232.
30. Fox RH, et al. The nature of the increase in sweating capacity produced by heat acclimatization. *J Physiol* 1964;171:368–376.
31. Gardner WJ. Cross talk: the paradoxical transmission of a nerve impulse. *Arch Neurol* 1966;14:149–156.
32. Gardner WJ, McCubbin JW. Auriculotemporal syndrome: gustatory sweating due to misdirection of regenerated nerve fibers. *JAMA* 1956;160:272–277.
33. Gilbert TM, Blatteis CM. Hypothalamic thermoregulatory pathways in the rat. *J Appl Physiol* 1977;43:770–777.
34. Greenleaf JE, Castle BL. Exercise temperature regulation during hypohydration and hyperhydration. *J Appl Physiol* 1971;30:847–853.
35. Grofova I, et al. Mesencephalic and diencephalic afferents to the superior colliculus and periaqueductal gray substance demonstrated by retrograde axonal transport of horseradish peroxidase in the cat. *Brain Res* 1971;146:205–220.
36. Gunn TR, Gluckman PD. The endocrine control of the onset of thermogenesis at birth. *Baillieres Clin Endocrinol Metab* 1989;3:869–886.
37. Gupta BN, et al. Cold-sensitive afferents from the abdomen. *Pflügers Arch* 1979;380:203–204.
38. Hancock MB. Cells of origin of hypothalamospinal projections in the rat. *Neurosci Lett* 1976;3:179–184.
39. Hassemer V, Brück K. Influence of menstrual cycle on shivering, skin blood flow, and sweating responses measured at night. *J Appl Physiol* 1985;59:1902–1912.
40. Hensel H, Andres KH, During MV. Structure and function of cold receptors. *Pflügers Arch* 1974;352:1–10.
41. Hori T, Harada Y. Responses of midbrain raphe neurons to local temperature. *Pflügers Arch* 1976;364:205–207.
42. Hori T, et al. Responses of preoptic thermosensitive neurons to poikilothermia-inducing peptides: bombesin and neurotensin. *Pflügers Arch* 1986;407:558–560.
43. Houdas Y, et al. Quantitative influence of CO_2 inhalation on thermal sweating in man. *Aerospace Med* 1973;44:265–268.
44. Illert M, Gabriel M. Descending pathways in the cervical cord of cats affecting blood pressure and sympathetic activity. *Pflügers Arch* 1972;335:109–124.
45. Inoue S, Murakami N. Unit responses in the medulla oblongata of rabbit to changes in local and cutaneous temperature. *J Physiol* 1976;259:339–356.
46. Ito T. Morphological connections of the human apocrine and eccrine sweat gland: occurrence of the so-called "mixed sweat glands"—a review. *Okajimas Folia Anat Jpn* 1988;65:315–336.
47. Järvi R, Pelto-Huikko M. Localization of neuropeptide Y in human sympathetic ganglia: correlation with met-enkephalin, tyrosine hydroxylase and acetylcholinesterase. *Histochem J* 1990;22:87–94.
48. Jessen C, Simon-Oppermann C. Production of temperature signals in the peripherally denervated spinal cord of the dog. *Experientia* 1976;32:484–485.
49. Johnson DA, et al. Autonomic pathways in the spinal cord. *J Neurosurg* 1952;9:599–605.
50. Kanosue K, et al. Hypothalamic network for thermoregulatory vasomotor control. *Am J Physiol* 1994;267: R283–R288.
51. Kanosue K, et al. Hypothalamic network for thermoregulatory network. *Am J Physiol* 1994;267:R275–R282.
52. Kanosue K, et al. Modes of action of local hypothalamic and skin thermal stimulation on salivary secretion in rats. *J Physiol* 1990; 424:459–471
53. Kasting NW. Vasopressin: a homeostatic effector in the febrile process. *Neurosci Biobehav Rev* 1982;6:215–222.
54. Katsuura G, Itoh S. Effect of cholecystokinin octapeptide on body temperature in the rat. *Jpn J Physiol* 1981;31:849–858.
55. Kerr FWL, Alexander S. Descending autonomic pathways in the spinal cord. *Arch Neurol* 1964;10:249–261.
56. Kerslake DM. *The stress of hot environments*. London: Cambridge University Press, 1972.
57. Knip AS. Acclimatization and maximum number of functioning sweat glands in Hindu and Dutch females and males. *Ann Human Biol* 1975;2:261–277.
58. Koga H, et al. Convergence of hepatoportal osmic and cardiovascular signals on preoptic thermosensitive neurons. *Brain Res Bull* 1987;20:581–596.
59. Kolka MA, Stephenson LA. Control of sweating during the human menstrual cycle. *Eur J Appl Physiol* 1989;58:890–895.
60. Konietzny H, Hensel H. The dynamic response of warm units in human skin nerves. *Pflügers Arch* 1977;370:111–114.
61. Kumazawa K, et al. Modulatory effects of calcitonin gene-related peptide and substance P on human cholinergic sweat secretion. *Clin Auton Res* 1994;4:319–322.
62. Kuno Y. *Human perspiration*. Springfield, IL: Charles C Thomas, 1956.
63. Lewis T. Observations upon reactions of vessels of human skin to cold. *Heart* 1930;15:177–208.
64. Lipton JM, et al. Effects of brainstem lesions on temperature regulation in hot and cold environments. *Am J Physiol* 1974;226:1356–1365.
65. Livingstone SD. Changes in cold-induced vasodilatation during Arctic exercises. *J Appl Physiol* 1976;40:455–457.

66. Loewy AD, Burton H. Nuclei of the solitary tract: efferent projections to the lower brain stem and spinal cord of the cat. *J Comp Neurol* 1978;181:421–450.
67. Lundberg JM, et al. Vasoactive intestinal polypeptide in cholinergic neurons of exocrine glands: functional significance of coexisting transmitters for vasodilation and secretion. *Proc Soc Natl Acad Sci USA* 1980;77:1651–1655.
68. McCaffrey TV, et al. Role of skin temperature in the control of sweating. *J Appl Physiol* 1979;47:591–597.
69. McIntyre BA, et al. Mechanism of enhancement of eccrine sweating by localized heating. *J Appl Physiol* 1968;25:255–260.
70. Milton AS. Prostaglandins in fever and the mode of action of antipyretic drugs. In: Milton AS, ed. *Pyretics and antipyretics*. Berlin: Springer-Verlag, 1982: 257–303 (*Handbook of experimental pharmacology;* vol 60).
71. Morimoto T, et al. Sex differences in physiological reactions to thermal stress. *J Appl Physiol* 1967;22:526–532.
72. Myers RD. Hypothalamic mechanism of pyrogen action in the cat and monkey. In: Wolstenholme GEW, Bligh J, eds. *Pyrogen and fever.* London: Churchill, 1971:131–153.
73. Nadel ER, et al. Importance of skin temperature in the regulation of sweating. *J Appl Physiol* 1971;31:80–87.
74. Nagai Y, et al. Blood level and brain distribution of thyrotropin releasing hormone (TRH) determined by radioimmunoassay after intravenous administration in rats. *J Pharmacobiodyn* 1980;3:500–506.
75. Nagasaka T, et al. Heat-induced vasoconstriction in the finger: a mechanism for reducing heat gain through the hand heated locally. *Pflügers Arch* 1986;407:71–75.
76. Nakashima T, et al. Osmosensitivity of preoptic thermosensitive neurons in hypothalamic tissue slice *in vitro*. *Pflügers Arch* 1985; 405:112–117.
77. Nakayama T, Hardy JD. Unit responses in the rabbit's brain stem to changes in brain and cutaneous temperature. *J Appl Physiol* 1969; 27:848–857.
78. Nakayama T, et al. Action of progesterone on preoptic thermosensitive neurons. *Nature* 1975;258:80.
79. Nakayama T, et al. Effects of preoptic thermal stimulation on the ventromedial hypothalamic neurons in rats. *Neurosci Lett* 1981;26: 177–181.
80. Nathan PW, Smith MC. The location of descending fibres to sympathetic preganglionic vasomotor and sudomotor neurons in man. *J Neurol Neurosurg Psychiatry* 1987;50:1253–1262.
81. Nielsen B. Effects of changes in plasma volume and osmolarity on thermoregulation during exercise. *Acta Physiol Scand* 1974;90: 725–730.
82. Nielsen B. Regulation of body temperature and heat dissipation at different levels of energy and heat production in man. *Acta Physiol Scand* 1966;68:215–227.
83. Normell LA. Distribution of impaired cutaneous vasomotor and sudomotor function in paraplegic man. *Scand J Clin Lab Invest* 1974; 33(Suppl 318):25–41.
84. Ogawa T. Influence of aging on sweating activity. In: Kligman AM, Takase Y, eds. *Cutaneous aging.* Tokyo: University of Tokyo Press, 1989:111–125.
85. Ogawa T. Local effect of skin temperature on threshold concentration of sudorific agents. *J Appl Physiol* 1970;28:18–22.
86. Ogawa T. Thermal influence on palmar sweating and mental influence on generalized sweating in man. *Jpn J Physiol* 1975;25: 525–536.
87. Ogawa T, Asayama M. Quantitative analysis of the local effect of skin temperature on sweating. *Jpn J Physiol* 1986;36:417–422.
88. Ogawa T, et al. Effects of sweat gland training by repeated local heating. *Jpn J Physiol* 1982;32:971–981.
89. Ogawa T, Bullard RW. Characteristics of subthreshold sudomotor neural impulses. *J Appl Physiol* 1972;33:300–305.
90. Ogawa T, Ohnishi N. Trainability of sweat glands in the aged. In: Yousef MK, ed. *Milestones in environmental physiology.* The Hague: Academic, 1989:63–71.
91. Ogawa T, et al. Sweating during night sleep. *Jpn J Physiol* 1967; 17:135–148.
92. Ogawa T, Sugenoya J. Pulsatile sweating and sympathetic sudomotor activity. *Jpn J Physiol* 1993;43:275–289.
93. Ogawa T, et al. Dermatomal inhibition of sweating by skin pressure. In: Szelényi Z, Székely M, eds. *Contribution to thermal physiology.* Budapest: Akadémiai Kiadó, 1981:413–415 (*Advances in physiological sciences;* vol 32).
94. Ogawa T, et al. Temperature regulation in hot–humid environments, with special reference to the significance of hidromeiosis. *J Therm Biol* 1984;9:121–125.
95. Okamoto T, et al. Different thermal dependency of cutaneous sympathetic outflow to glabrous and hairy skin in humans. *Eur J Appl Physiol* 1994;68:460–464.
96. Ono T, et al. Paraventricular nucleus connections to spinal cord and pituitary. *Neurosci Lett* 1978;10:141–146.
97. Perkins MN, et al. Activation of brown adipose tissue thermogenesis by the ventromedial hypothalamus. *Nature* 1981;289:401–402.
98. Pernow J, et al. Vasoconstrictor effects *in vivo* and plasma disappearance rate of neuropeptide Y in man. *Life Sci* 1987;40:47–54.
99. Raasmaja A, et al. Increased alpha-adrenergic receptor density in brown adipose tissue of cold-acclimated rats and hamsters. *Eur J Pharmacol* 1985;106:489–498.
100. Richter CP, Woodruff BG. Lumbar sympathetic dermatomes in man determined by the electrical skin resistance method. *J Neurophysiol* 1945;8:323–338.
101. Riedel W. Warm receptors in the dorsal abdominal wall of the rabbit. *Pflügers Arch* 1976;361:205–206.
102. Robinson S, et al. Acclimatization of older men to work in the heat. *J Appl Physiol* 1965;20:583–586.
103. Rowell LB. Active neurogenic vasodilatation in man. In: Vanhoutte PM, Leusen I, eds. *Vasodilatation.* New York: Raven, 1981: 1–17.
104. Rowell LB. Human cardiovascular adjustments to exercise and thermal stress. *Physiol Rev* 1974;54:75–159.
105. Sagot JC, et al. Sweating responses and body temperature during nocturnal sleep in humans. *Am J Physiol* 1987;252:R462–R470.
106. Saltin B, Hermansen L. Esophageal, rectal and muscle temperature during exercise. *J Appl Physiol* 1966;21:1757–1762.
107. Saper CB, et al. Direct hypothalamo-autonomic connections. *Brain Res* 1976;117:305–312.
108. Sarkany I, et al. Occlusion of the sweat pore by hydration. *Br J Dermatol* 1965;77:101–104.
109. Sato K, et al. Morphology and development of an apoeccrine sweat gland in human axillae. *Am J Physiol* 1987;251:R160–R180.
110. Schliak H, et al. Untersuchungen zur Frage der Schweissdrüseninnervation im Bereich des Gesichts. *Acta Anat (Basel)* 1972;81: 421–438.
111. Simon E. Temperature regulation: the spinal cord as a site of extrahypothalamic thermoregulatory functions. *Rev Physiol Biochem Pharmacol* 1974;71:1–76.
112. Simon E, Iriki M. Sensory transmission of spinal heat and cold sensitivity in ascending spinal neurons. *Pflügers Arch* 1971;328:103–120.
113. Stuart DG, et al. Effects of septal and hypothalamic lesions on shivering. *Exp Neurol* 1962;5:335–347.
114. Stuart D, et al. The rhythm of shivering. I. General sensory contributions. *Am J Phys Med* 1966;45:61–74.
115. Sugenoya J, Ogawa T. Characteristics of central sudomotor mechanism estimated by frequency of sweat expulsions. *Jpn J Physiol* 1985;32:783–794.
116. Sugenoya J, et al. Effects of thyrotropin releasing hormone on human sudomotor and cutaneous vasomotor activities. *Eur J Appl Physiol* 1988;57:632–638.
117. Sugenoya J, et al. Identification of sudomotor activities in cutaneous sympathetic nerves by using sweat expulsion as effector response. *Eur J Appl Physiol* 1990;61:302–308.
118. Sugenoya J, et al. Occurrence of mental and thermal sweating on the human axilla. *Jpn J Physiol* 1982;32:717–726.
119. Tache Y, et al. Bombesin-induced poikilothermy in rats. *Brain Res* 1980;188:525–530.
120. Tainio H, et al. The distribution of substance P-, CGRP-, galanin-, and ANP-like immunoreactive nerves in human sweat glands. *Histochem J* 1987;19:375–380.
121. Takagi K, Sakurai T. A sweat reflex due to pressure on the body surface. *Jpn J Physiol* 1950;1:22–28.

122. Vaalasti A, et al. Vasoactive intestinal polypeptide (VIP)-like immunoreactivity in the nerves of human axillary sweat glands. *J Invest Dermatol* 1985;85:246–248.
123. Wagner JA, et al. Heat tolerance and acclimatization to work in the heat in relation to age. *J Appl Physiol* 1972;33:616–622.
124. Wang GH, Brown VW. Suprasegmental inhibition of an autonomic reflex. *J Neurophysiol* 1956;19:564–572.
125. Werner J. Influences of local and global temperature stimuli on the Lewis reaction. *Pflügers Arch* 1977;367:291–294.
126. Wit A, Wang SC. Temperature-sensitive neurons in preoptic/anterior hypothalamic region: actions of pyrogen and acetyl salicylate. *Am J Physiol* 1968;215:1160–1169.
127. Yamashita Y, et al. Effects of atrial natriuretic peptide on human sweating activity [in Japanese]. *Auton Nerv Syst* 1989;26:523–530.
128. Yamashita Y, et al. Local effect of vasoactive intestinal polypeptide on human sweat-gland function. *Jpn J Physiol* 1987;37:929–936.
129. Yokota T, et al. Analysis of inhibitory influence of bulbar reticular formation upon sudomotor activity. *Jpn J Physiol* 1963;13:145–154.
130. Yousef MK, et al. Thermoregulatory responses of the elderly population. *Sangyo Ika Daigaku Zasshi* 1986;8:219–227.

CHAPTER 8

Normal and Abnormal Sweat Gland Function

Kenzo Sato

1. Humans and apes are unique in their ability to regulate body temperature by evaporative heat loss through eccrine sweating.
2. Disorders of eccrine sweating include sweat retention, hyperhidrosis, and hypohidrosis.
3. Hypohidrosis caused by chronic neuropathy may be associated with glandular atrophy. In contrast, sweat glands from hyperhidrotic areas usually are hypertrophic and display higher ionic channel activity.
4. The eccrine sweat gland has two components: the secretory coil, which secretes an isotonic fluid, and the duct, which reabsorbs sodium chloride, producing hypotonic sweat.
5. The primary neurotransmitter is acetylcholine (ACh), but catecholamine, vasoactive intestinal polypeptide, atrial natriuretic peptide, calcitonin gene-related peptide, galanin, and possibly adenosine 5'-triphosphate (ATP) are present in periglandular nerves.
6. ACh-mediated sweating is mediated by intracellular Ca^{2+} increase.
7. Isoproterenol (β-adrenergic) sweating represents <20% of the maximal muscarinic sweat response and is mediated by cyclic adenosine 3',5'-monophosphate accumulation.
8. Currently the best model of sweat secretion following ACh release and receptor binding is the following sequence: an influx of extracellular Ca^{2+} by activation of receptor-coupled Ca^{2+} channels, causing a net efflux of potassium chloride and water; this produces cellular shrinkage with activation of cotransporters that return Na^+, K^+, and $2Cl^-$ intracellularly; this creates an isotonic solution that in turn stimulates (Na, K)-ATPase activity in the sweat duct, resulting in a hypotonic sweat solution.

INTRODUCTION

The eccrine sweat gland (or eccrine sweating) has been a favorite research target by investigators from at least five different scientific disciplines: (a) sports medicine and thermoregulatory physiology, (b) dermatology, (c) neurology, (d) membrane physiology, and (e) psychoneurophysiology.

Sports physiologists' interest in sweating and thermoregulation continues as athletic competitions intensify in all age groups and at both professional and amateur levels. Since thermoregulatory sweating is also associated with loss of fluids and electrolytes, which can lead to dehydration in endurance athletic competitions, the search for optimal methods of replacing lost water and electrolytes is an increasingly popular area of investigation by sport physiologists.

The eccrine sweat gland is one of the major cutaneous appendages. As primary-care physicians for various skin disorders, dermatologists are the physicians who treat such disorders of eccrine sweating as sweat retention, hyperhidrosis, hypohidrosis, bromidrosis, and dyshidrosis. Furthermore, the possible role of the eccrine sweat gland as a modifier of various cutaneous disorders has been the subject of intense interest for many dermatologists. As the most salient cutaneous effector organ of sympathetic nervous system, clinical study of abnormal sweating has helped neurologists diagnose neurologic disorders associated with autonomic neuropathy.

Because of its easy accessibility via a simple skin biopsy, the human eccrine sweat gland has the potential to be a model system for studying the mechanisms of membrane transport and signal transduction during exocrine secretion. Cystic fibrosis is a genetic disease of the cyclic adenosine 3',5'-monophosphate (cAMP)-dependent chloride channel (widely known as the cystic fibrosis transport regulator or CFTR) affecting many exocrine secretory ep-

---

K. Sato: Marshall Dermatology Research Laboratory, University of Iowa College of Medicine, Iowa City, Iowa 52242.

ithelia, including the eccrine sweat gland. The elevated sweat electrolyte concentration and elevated skin potential (due to a greater negative sweat ductal potential) are still used as inexpensive screening diagnostic tests for cystic fibrosis. Because the >400 mutations of CFTR that are known to date cause a wide spectrum of clinical phenotypes, the human sweat gland has the potential to serve as a unique research model for further understanding the correlation between genotypes and phenotypes in cystic fibrosis.

The galvanic skin response, also termed the sympathetic skin response or skin conductance response, can be registered on the skin of palms or soles. Not only is this measurement exploited by lie detector tests, but it is also used to study the function of the sympathetic nervous system innervating the palms and soles. Although the galvanic skin response (or the sympathetic skin response) is presumably caused by the sudomotor activity on the palms and soles induced by various somatosensory triggers, its mechanism is still poorly understood (13,76). If galvanic skin response is a measure of sudomotor activity, why is it not applicable to the sudomotor function of other parts of the body? The answer is not available at present. It is humbling to acknowledge that we do not even know whether the sweat glands of the palms and soles function in the same way as do those in the general hairy skin surface. Our concept of the palmoplantar sweat glands is limited to the fact that they are emotionally triggered as opposed to the sweat glands on the hairy skin, which are triggered by thermoregulatory stimuli.

Since so little is known about the function of the sweat gland in general and since the interests of sweat gland investigators are so diverse, as just indicated, this chapter is not intended to be a comprehensive review of all sweat-gland-related subjects. Rather, I have reviewed a few subjects that will hopefully fill the gap between the clinical aspects and basic science of the eccrine sweat gland.

ECCRINE SWEAT GLANDS AND THERMOREGULATION

Humans are unique in that they are capable of regulating their body temperature when in a hot environment or during physical activity by the evaporative heat loss associated almost exclusively with eccrine sweating. Apes have a limited capacity to thermoregulate in the heat partly by the evaporative cooling of eccrine sweating and perhaps partly by secretion of trichial (apocrinelike) glands (Fig. 1), as is the case with some domestic animals (16). The evaporative cooling of the eccrine glands for apes enables them to maintain their physical well-being and activity without resorting to a variety of thermoregulatory behaviors employed by other mammals, such as panting, moving to a cool place, physical inactivity, and splashing water onto the body surface.

The eccrine sweat gland, one of the largest cutaneous appendages (35 µg per gland × 3 million glands = 100 g

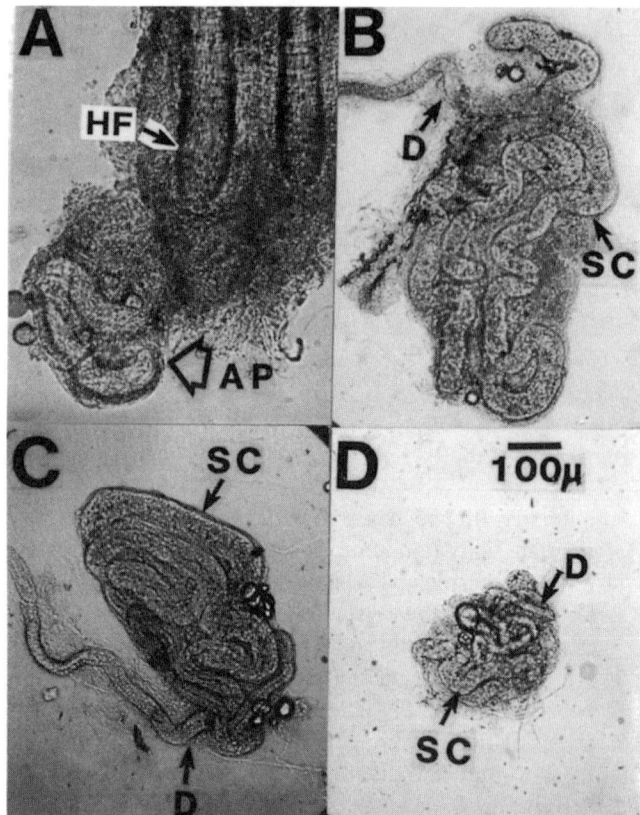

FIG. 1. Isolated eccrine (atrichial) and trichial (hair-associated, or apocrinelike) glands in patas and rhesus monkeys. The role of trichial glands in patas monkey **(A)** is not well known. Patas monkeys are known to have well-developed eccrine sweat glands **(B)** [see Sato et al. (36)] that are comparable in size to those of the rhesus palm **(C)** and human eccrine gland (51). Note that the eccrine gland in the rhesus hairy skin is extremely small **(D)** and less functionally active (17). *SC*, secretory coil; *D*, duct; *AP*, apocrinelike gland; *HF*, hair follicle.

in total) in humans and the most active transporting epithelium, serves a vital function for human survival (38,41, 62,63). Sweating is designed to meet adequately the thermoregulatory demand of the body during vigorous exercise or in the heat. For example, evaporation of 1 g (or ml) of sweat water from the skin surface removes ~0.58 kcal of heat. The maximal sweating rate per gland in an average person is ~10 nl (i.e., 10^{-9}) per minute per gland or 0.6 µl (mg) per hour per gland (48) so that the 1.8 L of sweat secreted per hour (3 million sweat glands × 0.6 µl) can in theory remove as much as 1,044 kcal of heat. Running on a treadmill at 7 miles/hr on a slope of 5° for 1 hr (comparable to running half the distance of a marathon course) consumes about the same amount of energy, most of which is converted into heat, contributing to the elevation of body temperature during running.

Inability to achieve thermal equilibrium by evaporative heat loss leads to hyperthermia, heat exhaustion, or heat stroke. During two heat waves in the early 1980s, ~2,000 elderly and infants succumbed to heat stroke in the midwestern United States. During the heat wave in Chicago in July 1995, nearly 500 people succumbed to heat-related illnesses (22,23). Even without a heat wave, at least 240 deaths are attributed to heat-related illnesses each year in the United States. The question of why some elderly and frail individuals succumbed while others survived in comparable environmental conditions remains unanswered. It is also noteworthy that patients with acute heat stroke typically show dry skin (absence of sweating) in the presence of severe hyperthermia. The pathogenesis of this anomalous anhidrosis in heat stroke has never been fully understood.

HYPERHIDROSIS AND HYPOHIDROSIS

As a dermatologist, I have had the opportunity to see patients with complaints of hyperhidrosis or hypohidrosis. Excessive sweating occurs on the palms and soles or axillae, but can occur in other parts of the body, e.g., arms, face, chest, back, and groin. Occasionally, excessive localized sweating is associated with generalized hypohidrosis or anhidrosis, but it is only the excessive sweating that the patient is aware of. Counseling these patients is not easy, because little is known about the pathogenesis of hyperhidrosis and hypohidrosis and there are no established diagnostic methods or paradigms for clinicians to follow.

If such acute conditions as poisoning, ingestion of drugs, infectious diseases, and heat stroke (and/or tropical anhidrotic asthenia) (27) can be excluded, then decreased sweating (and associated heat intolerance) is usually due to either decreased sweat secretion or to interference with the delivery of secreted sweat to the skin surface, i.e., sweat retention or poral occlusion. When faced with a patient's claims such as the inability to sweat in heat, heat intolerance, or dry skin, the first and foremost considerations in our diagnostic approach are to confirm anhidrosis and localize its distribution and extent. Thermoregulatory sweat testing is instrumental in studying these patients. Testing is done by exposing a patient to a hot and humid

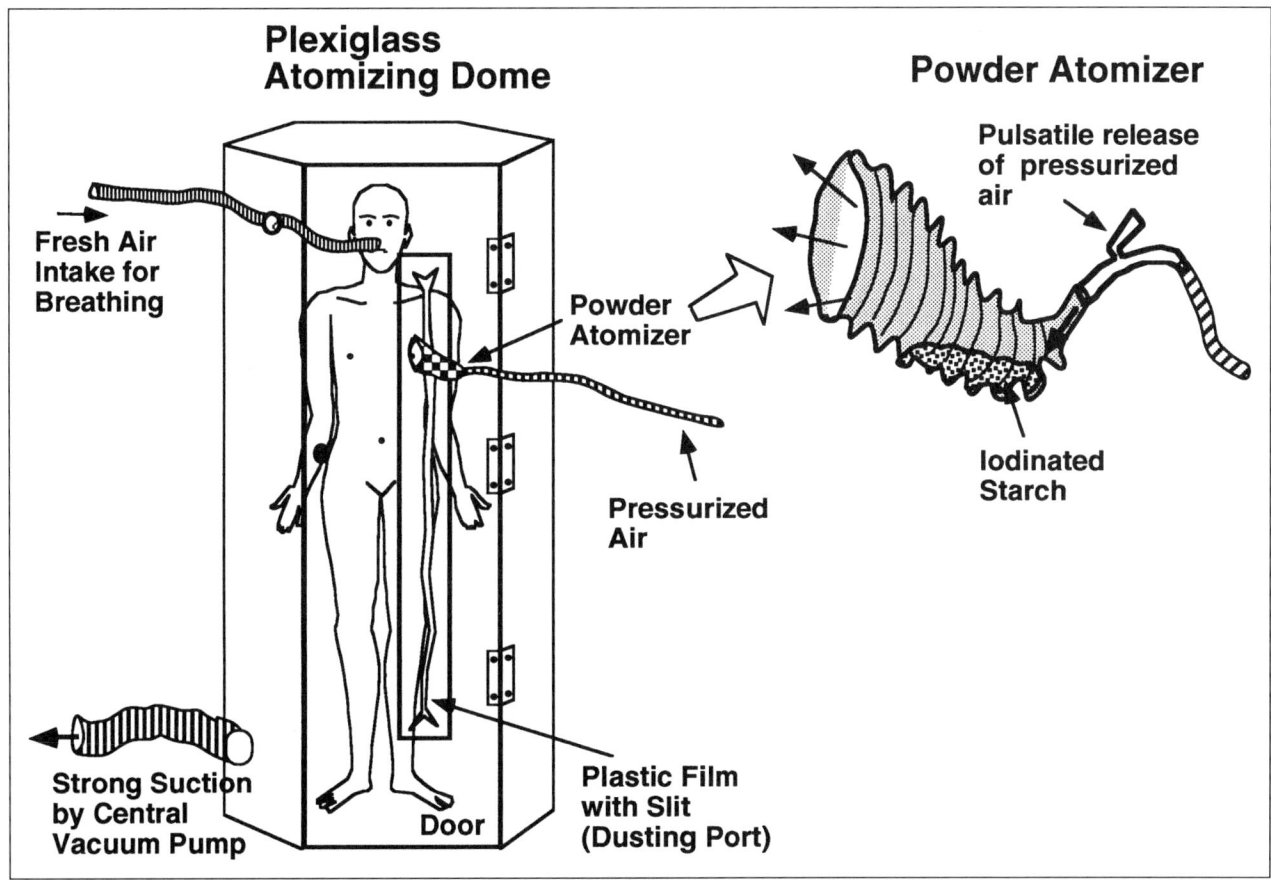

FIG. 2. An improved method for visualizing the regional distribution of thermoregulatory sweating in the clinical setting. After exposing a patient in a sauna until the core temperature is raised by 1°C, the patient is placed in an atomizing dome for dusting the entire body with an indicator powder. We conveniently use iodinated soluble starch (67) for dusting. Strong suction of air from the dome while dusting keeps the examination room free of pollution with the powder. The patient closes the eyes while inside the dusting dome and inhales air from the hose. The starch in the atomizer is stirred by repeated brief releases of pressurized air. The patient turns around while dusting.

environment such as sauna, at 45°–50°C with 60%–70% relative humidity, until core temperature is elevated at least by 1°C. This is followed by visualizing sweating by either dusting an indicator powder (Fig. 2) over the skin or taking sweat pore imprints from various body sites by using iodine-impregnated papers or by other appropriate methods (53).

Having confirmed the presence of anhidrosis, the next critical challenge is to study the pathogenesis of anhidrosis and to differentiate between poral occlusion and lack of sweat secretion. Unfortunately, however, there is no known practical method available for differentiating between these two conditions. We can only discuss some potentially useful approaches and some research oriented methods. First, people with atopic diathesis (a history of asthma or hay fever, dry skin, repeated skin infection, recurrent eczematous problems) are susceptible to poral occlusion. Anhidrosis in these patients can be insidious or acute in onset, but is rarely uniform. Some atopic patients may complain of intense pruritus on exposure to heat. Patients with sweat retention syndrome (including those with atopic diathesis) usually show generalized hypohidrosis with irregular areas of active sweating in intertriginous areas such as the groins, regions near the axillae, and skin folds around the neck, with the areas of sweating showing no relationship to innervation patterns. If the pore imprints from anhidrotic areas show a few profusely active pores, the anhidrosis may be more likely due to poral occlusion because anhidrosis/hypohidrosis caused by chronic neuropathy may be rather uniform. Repeated Scotch-tape stripping may restore sweating in the presence of very superficial poral occlusion, but this is not always the case. Punch biopsy for routine histopathology slides is not always helpful because poral occlusion can rarely be identified and glandular atrophy is very difficult to recognize. One area of future promise is that hypohidrosis caused by chronic neuropathy may be associated with glandular atrophy (Fig. 3). We have already reported that glandular size correlates with *in vivo* sweating in physiologic settings, i.e., people with a history of hypohidrosis (or poor sweaters) tend to have glandular atrophy or smaller sweat glands, whereas heavy sweaters by history have hypertrophic glands associated with a greater thermoregulatory and pharmacologic sweating rate$_{max}$ (51). Thus, glandular isolation and inspection may help differentiate anhidrosis caused by pore occlusion from that caused by chronic neuropathy. This preliminary observation must be extended to a large number of patients for further verification. In contrast, sweat glands isolated from a hyperhidrotic area usually show marked glandular hypertrophy and higher ionic channel activity (10,64), suggesting that the sweat gland may enlarge or shrink in response to repeated stimulation with neurotransmitters or local growth factors. Little is known about such candidate regulatory molecules of sweat gland growth and function. The putative periglandular neurotransmitters include acetylcholine (ACh), norepinephrine (NE), vasoactive intestinal

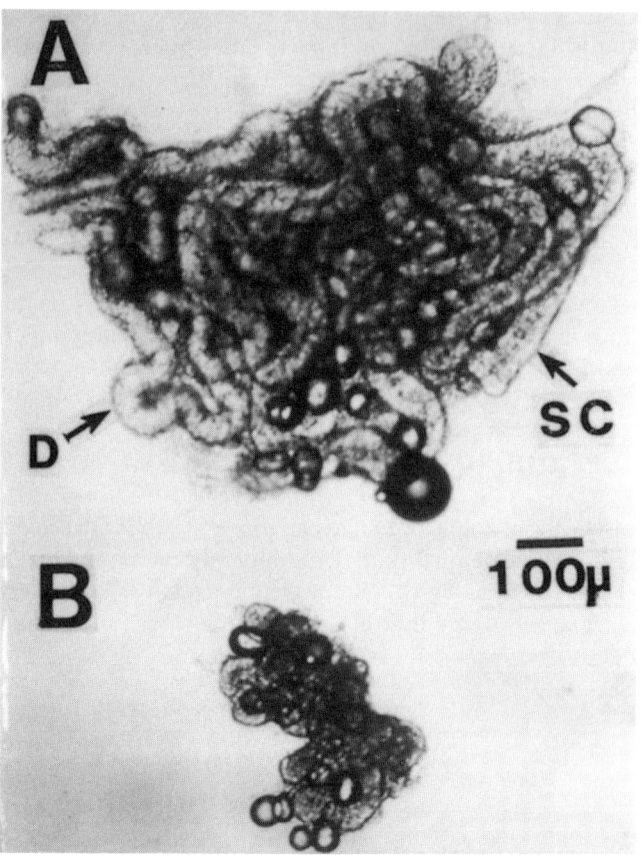

FIG. 3. Glandular atrophy in the anhidrotic area of the trunk **(B)** in a patient with Ross' syndrome (segmental neuropathy with anhidrosis, Adie's tonic pupil, areflexia). Note that the sweat gland isolated from an adjacent normally sweating area is of normal gland size **(A)**. *SC*, secretory coil; *D*, duct.

peptide (VIP), ATP, neurotensins, substance P, and calcitonin gene-related peptides (CGRP) (62). Candidate regulatory peptides of sweat gland origin include epidermal growth factor, kallikrein, interleukins, prostaglandins, and prolactin (15,21,52,62,63,65,68). The development of new investigative model systems holds the key for further understanding of the regulation of glandular function.

ANATOMY OF ECCRINE AND APOECCRINE SWEAT GLANDS

There are three histologically and functionally distinguishable types of sweat glands: eccrine, apocrine, and apoeccrine glands (44,60); however, it is the eccrine sweat gland that is primarily involved in thermoregulation (Fig. 4). The eccrine sweat gland consists of two components (Fig. 5): the secretory coil, which secretes a nearly isotonic primary fluid, and the duct, which reabsorbs NaCl in excess of water, producing hypotonic sweat onto the skin surface. The size of a sweat gland varies as much as fivefold

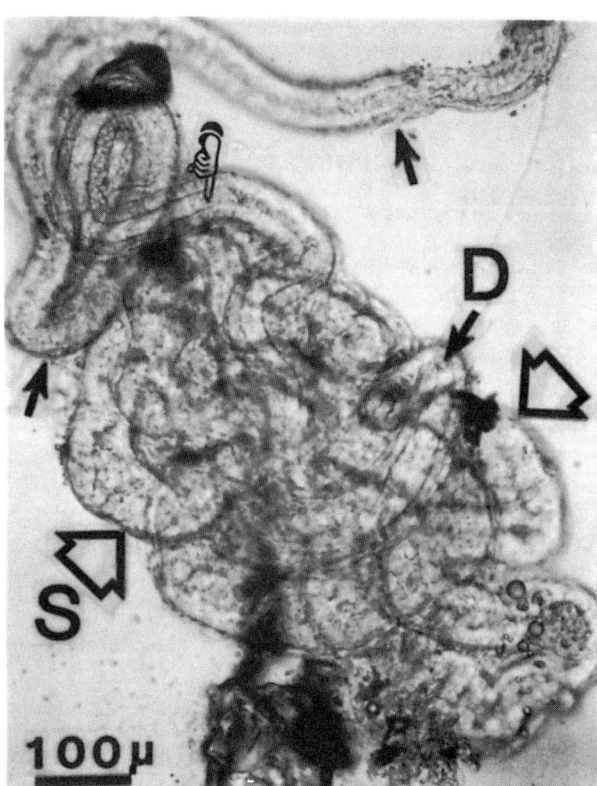

FIG. 4. A human eccrine sweat gland isolated from the upper arm of an adult male. *D* and the *small arrows* indicate the duct, showing the partially dilated luminal cuticular border (*fingertip sign*). *Large open arrows* indicate the secretory coil where the luminal space is not clearly recognized.

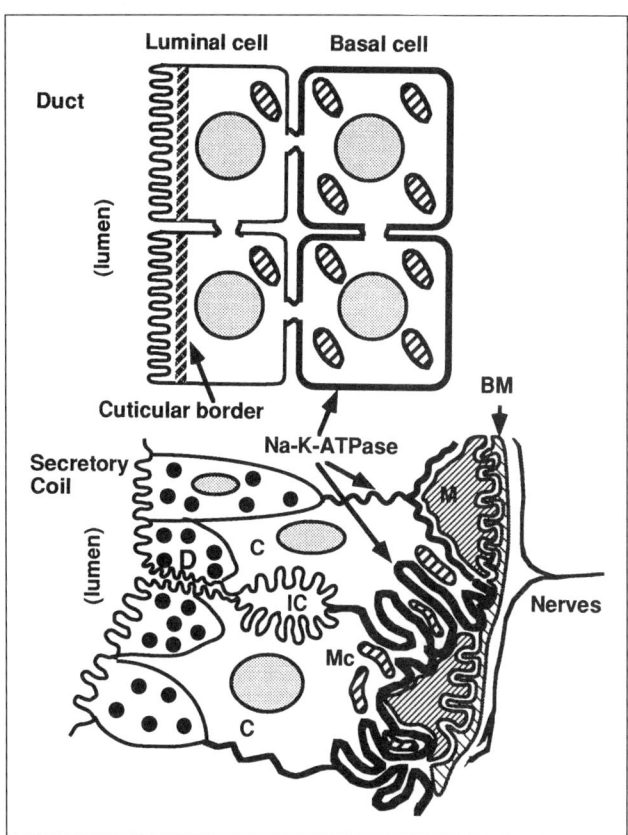

FIG. 5. The sweat duct and the secretory coil. The duct is made up of two cell layers. The luminal duct cell is characterized by luminal membrane villi, a cuticular border, a small number of mitochondria, and the less active (Na, K)-ATPase. In contrast, the basal duct cell is characterized by a large number of mitochondria and strong (Na, K)-ATPase activity in the entire cell membrane. Three types of cell are illustrated in the secretory coil. An intercellular canaliculus (IC) opens into the lumen. Mitochondria (Mc) are more numerous in the basal side of the clear cell (C) above or between the myoepithelial cell (M). Dark cells (D) line the luminal side of the coil. Localization of (Na, K)-ATPase is indicated by a *thick line* on the basal labyrinth. The basement membrane (BM) is present only in the secretory coil, not in the duct.

among different individuals, and size is strongly correlated with individual (and perhaps also regional) differences in the rate of sweating (maximal sweat rate ranges from 2 to 20 nl/min/gland) (48).

The secretory coil is composed of three distinct cell types: clear, dark (mucoid), and myoepithelial cells (7). The fine morphologic appearance of the clear cell is characterized by the presence of intricate basal infoldings and intercellular canaliculi (Fig. 5). The basal infoldings stain densely with ouabain-sensitive (Na, K)-dependent paranitrophenyl phosphatase (7) [which reflects the catalytic activity of (Na, K)-ATPase] and bind labeled ouabain (32). In contrast, the intercellular canaliculi, which are actually pouch openings into the lumen (and thus correspond to the luminal membrane) are free of paranitrophenyl phosphatase activity (34). Mitochondria are more numerous near the basal side of the clear cells, especially in the basal labyrinth (Fig. 6B). However, they are absent or very scarce near the intercellular canaliculi (Fig. 6A), suggesting that energy-requiring membrane transport is more active in the basal side of the cell. These morphologic characteristics support the notion that the basolateral membrane, but not the luminal membrane or the membrane forming the intercellular canaliculi, is site of the Na$^+$ pump. The dark cells are easily discernible because of the presence of many electron-dense dark cell granules in their cytoplasm. Although the function of the dark cell is unknown, periodic acid–Schiff-positive sweat glycoproteins have been traced to the dark cell granules (75).

Myoepithelial cells are located at the periphery of the secretory tubule and are filled with dense myofilaments (Fig. 6). They are spindle shaped and contract in response to cholinergic, but not adrenergic, stimulation (75). The cytoplasm is filled with dense myofilaments that react to anti-actin antibodies. Although the myofilaments also react to antikeratin monoclonal antibodies, and this suggests an epidermal origin of the myoepithelium (5), their significance remains unknown. The long-held hypothesis that the myoepithelium is instrumental in pumping out preformed sweat has been disputed (45). Rather, the myoepithelium

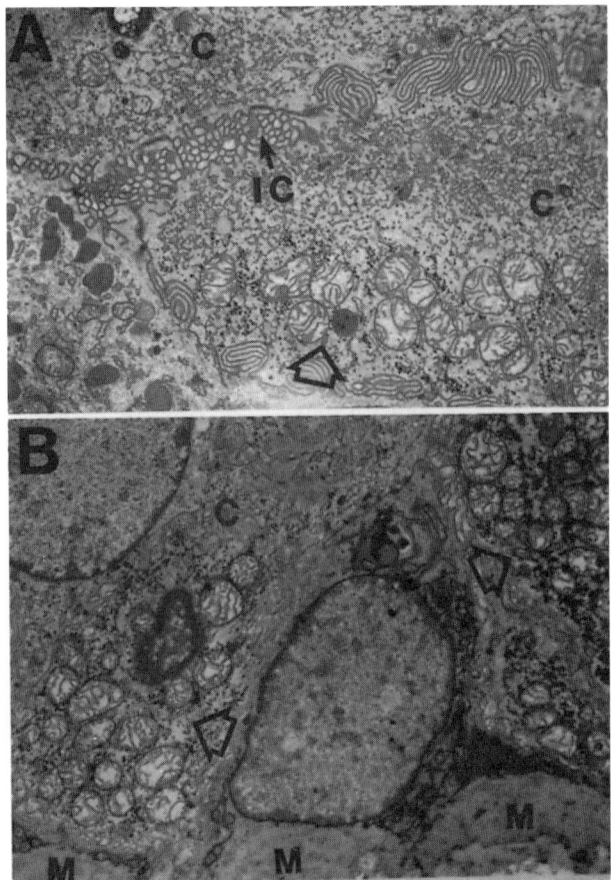

FIG. 6. Localization of mitochondria in the human eccrine clear cell. **A:** Note the absence of mitochondria (*large arrow*) near the intercellular canaliculus (*IC*). *C*, clear cell. **B:** The abundance of mitochondria (*arrows*) near the basal membrane infoldings are shown. *M*, myoepithelium.

may provide mechanical support for the secretory coil wall to resist the increase in luminal hydrostatic pressure (45).

The duct is composed of two layers of cells: the basal and luminal ductal cells. The basal (or peripheral) cells are morphologically and functionally distinct from the luminal cells. The basal ductal cells are replete with mitochondria, and the entire cell membrane is rich in ouabain-sensitive (Na, K)-dependent paranitrophenyl phosphatase activity, the catalytic subunit of (Na, K)-ATPase (Fig. 5) (34), suggesting that the entire basal cell membrane is involved in Na+ pumping for ductal Na+ absorption. In contrast, the luminal ductal cells have fewer mitochondria, much less ouabain-sensitive paranitrophenyl phosphatase activity, and a dense layer of tonofilaments near the luminal membrane (which is often referred to as the *cuticular border* because it resembles the cuticle at the light-microscopic level). The cuticular border thus provides a structural resilience to the otherwise very friable tubular wall. The entire structural organization of the duct is well designed for the most efficient Na+ absorptive function; the luminal membrane serves as the absorptive surface by housing both Na+ and Cl− channels, and the basal ductal cells serve Na+ pumping by providing maximally expanded Na+ pump sites and efficient energy metabolism.

CENTRAL AND PERIPHERAL CONTROL OF SWEATING

Sweat Center and Temperature Set-Point

Evidence abounds that the preoptic hypothalamic area is essential in the regulation of body temperature (2,18). In experimental animals, local heating of the preoptic hypothalamic tissue activates generalized sweating, vasodilatation, and polypnea, whereas local cooling of the preoptic area causes generalized vasoconstriction and shivering (1,14). Thus, elevation of hypothalamic temperature caused by an increase in body temperature provides the strongest stimulus for thermoregulatory sweating responses. Sweating does not commence, however, until the core temperature reaches a certain level [temperature set-point (T_{se})], and only above T_{se} does the sweating rate increase linearly with the increase in core temperature. In pathologic conditions such as diencephalic epilepsy or the syndrome of episodic hyperhidrosis, hypothermia, and agenesis of the corpus callosum (Hines–Bannick syndrome and Shapiro's syndrome, respectively), an episodic decrease in the T_{se} is thought to trigger episodic profuse sweating (19). In addition to the core temperature, Nadel et al. (24,25) observed that the local skin temperature modifies the effect of the core temperature on the sweating rate (Fig. 7). For example, if local cooling decreases the skin temperature from 30°C to 26°C, sweating in the cooled skin area does not start until the core temperature is in-

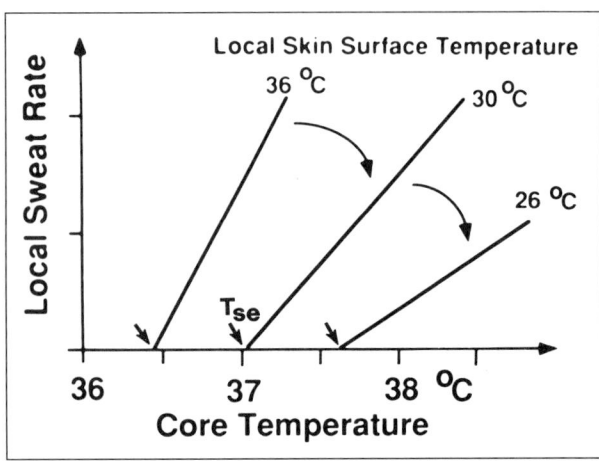

FIG. 7. The relationship between the local skin temperature, the local sweating rate, and the temperature set-point (T_{se}). The underlying assumption is that the T_{se} reflects the degree of central drive (i.e., nerve impulses), but the local temperature effect is complex and could be due to a variety of factors regulating the glandular function.

creased to 37.7°C, and the efficacy of the increase in core temperature is also lowered. On a degree-to-degree basis, however, an increase in core temperature is ~9 times more efficient than an increase in the mean skin temperature in stimulating the sweat center and thus the sweating rate (24,25). The mechanism by which the local temperature modifies the effect of the core temperature is unknown, but it may be due to a combination of factors such as the effect of periglandular temperature on the amount of neurotransmitter released, on the glandular metabolism, on the affinity of receptors to agonists, on membrane transport, or a combination of these factors. To rule out the first possibility—that the effect of local temperature on sweating is simply due to the increased periglandular release of ACh—we directly studied the effect of bath temperature on the sweating rate in the presence of 5 μM methacholine (MCh) by using single-cannulated human eccrine sweat glands *in vitro* (unpublished results) (Fig. 8). Although the sweating rate increased linearly with the increase in bath temperature, the minimal temperature at which sweating was induced varied significantly in different subjects. Furthermore, it was noted that the higher the maximal sweat rate was of a given gland, the lower was the minimal bath temperature at which sweating was initiated. Because sweat glands with a high sweat rate are likely derived from well-acclimatized individuals (51), the minimal bath temperature needed to support sweat secretion may be an additional characteristic of functional glandular activity.

Studies have also indicated that the T_{se} can vary by altering the homeostasis of the body. For example, infusion of hypertonic NaCl (15–20 mM) into the brain of experimental animals increases the body temperature by ~1°C (11). During exercise, elevating the plasma Na+ concentration ([Na]) in humans slows the onset of sweating and raises the plateau level of the core temperature, whereas increasing plasma Ca^{2+} ([Ca]) has an opposite effect (26). Isotonic hypovolemia also reduces the sensitivity of the sweating response, increases the threshold core temperature for the onset of the sweating response, and increases the threshold core temperature for the onset of cutaneous vasodilatation (8). It is tempting to speculate that the paradoxical anhidrosis that is seen frequently in heat-stroke victims is mediated in part by the altered function of the sweat center, which stems from the deranged plasma homeostasis following prolonged sweating.

Periglandular Neurotransmitters

The nerves surrounding the sweat glands are sympathetic, postganglionic fibers, and ACh is the principal terminal neurotransmitter. In addition, catecholamine (71,72), VIP (20,74), atrial natriuretic peptide, CGRP, and galanin (69) have been localized to the periglandular nerves. Adenosine ATP coexists with NE or ACh, and may function as a sympathetic coneurotransmitter (3). Although ATP has not been reported to occur in the sweat gland, we presume that ATP is also presumed to exist in the periglandular nerves. The significance of these peptides or neurotransmitters in sweat gland function is not fully understood. Because immunoreactivity for atrial natriuretic peptide, CGRP, and galanin is also found in the cutaneous sensory nerves, the function of these peptides may not be specifically directed to the sweat gland. In contrast, VIP is not only a stimulant of sweat secretion in a cAMP-mediated fashion, but is a synergistic amplifier of the isoproterenol (ISO)-stimulated cAMP accumulation in the isolated eccrine sweat gland (50). Interestingly, such amplified intracellular cAMP accumulation is further synergistically augmented by ACh, which by itself has no effect on the cAMP level. Although the role of the synergistically amplified cAMP level is not clear, cAMP might be involved in the regulation of intracellular [Ca] (47). The function of periglandular ATP is also unknown; however, extracellular ATP at 1 mM elevates the intracellular [Ca] and stimulates K+ efflux, as does ACh (unpublished data).

PHARMACOLOGIC RESPONSIVENESS OF THE ECCRINE SWEAT GLAND

Human eccrine sweat glands respond best to the intradermal injection of ACh. In contrast, the sweating response to intradermally injected NE and ISO in humans takes 1–2 min and is only transient. The ISO-induced sweat rate is usually <20% of the maximal cholinergic sweat rate (48, 55). α-Adrenergic stimulation (e.g., phenylephrine) also induces sweat secretion, but to a much lesser extent than does β stimulation.

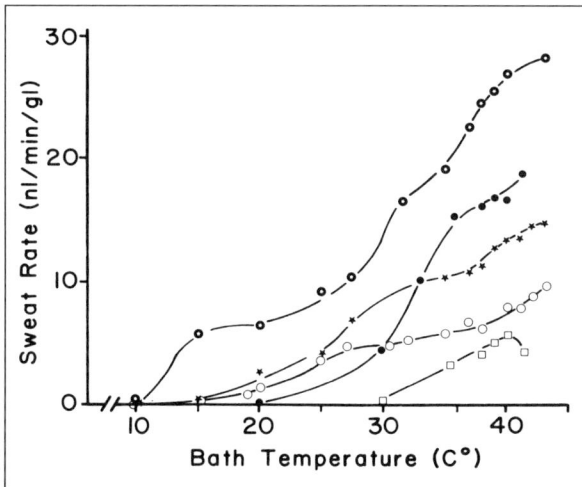

FIG. 8. The effect of bath temperature on the sweat rate in isolated human eccrine sweat glands. Each gland was isolated from the back of a different subject. The bath consisted of Kreb's bicarbonate Ringer's solution containing 5 μM methacholine, and the temperature was increased in steps. *Each line* represents a different sweat gland.

Prostaglandins E1 and E2 stimulate sweat secretion *in vitro*, but their *in vivo* physiologic role in eccrine sweating remains unknown. Histamine, serotonin, and substance P fail to induce sweat secretion *in vitro*. VIP is a strong stimulant of sweat secretion although the sweating response is transient (50). It remains to be studied whether ATP is involved as a regulator of other receptor functions or glandular metabolism. Determining pharmacologic responsiveness of the human eccrine sweat gland had been only of academic interest until it was discovered that patients with cystic fibrosis lack β-adrenergic sweating (48). Furthermore, the maximal cholinergic sweat rate provides an indirect measure of the physiologic sweat gland activity, in that the higher the maximal sweat rate is, the larger is the glandular size and the higher is the pharmacologic sensitivity (51).

STIMULUS–SECRETION COUPLING IN ECCRINE SWEAT SECRETION

In the classic concept of stimulus–secretion coupling, Ca^{2+} is viewed as the major link in the chain of events that is initiated at the cell membrane by the actions of ACh and other agonists that trigger the release of the secretory product (6). A similar link has been postulated in the eccrine sweat gland, with Ca^{2+} serving as an intracellular mediator of cholinergic stimulation (57). Some of the supporting evidence includes the following: cholinergic sweating is absolutely dependent on extracellular [Ca]; a calcium ionophore (A23187), which transports Ca^{2+} across the cell membrane, induces sweat secretion as profusely as does ACh; a blocker of Ca^{2+} transport, such as D600 or verapamil, abolishes sweat secretion; and the strontium ion, which substitutes for Ca^{2+} but diffuses into the cell and bypasses agonist–receptor interaction, induces profuse spontaneous sweat secretion. More recently, the increase in intracellular [Ca] after cholinergic, but not β-adrenergic, stimulation has been directly demonstrated by using fluorescent probes such as quin 2 (56) and fura 2 (12,59) (Fig. 9). In contrast, sweat secretion, which is induced by the β-adrenergic agonist ISO, may be due in large part to accumulated cAMP because cAMP accumulates in the sweat gland during stimulation with ISO but not with ACh. External Ca^{2+} is not required for the ISO-induced cAMP response. Furthermore, sweat secretion can be induced by theophylline (a phosphodiesterase inhibitor that enhances endogenous cAMP) or by dibutyryl cAMP (58). ISO-induced sweating is relatively insensitive to the removal of Ca^{2+} from the external medium; however, the resting intracellular [Ca] may still be necessary for β-adrenergic sweating because prolonged chelation of Ca^{2+} with ethyleneglycol tetraacetic acid (EGTA) in a Ca^{2+}-free medium may eventually abolish β-adrenergic sweating. Intracellular [Ca] is not raised by ISO or other cAMP-elevating agents. Although the role of cAMP as an intracellular mediator of β-adrenergic stimulation has been firmly established, this

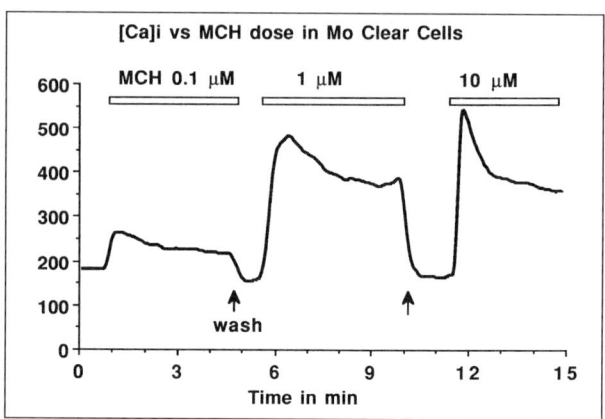

FIG. 9. An increase in the cytoplasmic calcium concentration ($[Ca]_i$) due to methacholine (MCh) stimulation in a dissociated rhesus eccrine clear cell. The Ca^{2+}-sensitive fluorescent probe, fura 2, was used. The excitation wavelengths were 340 and 380 nm, and the emission wavelength was 500 nm. Varying doses of MCh in Ringer's solution were perfused in a microflow chamber mounted in a thermostated fluorescent microscope with a filter wheel.

traditional thesis is still disputed. For example, in the salivary gland, the ISO-activated K^+ and Cl^- currents are inhibited by Ca^{2+} chelation and not mimicked by cAMP and other cAMP-elevating agents such as forskolin. Cook et al. (4) thus postulated that Ca^{2+}, rather than cAMP, is the intracellular mediator of β-adrenergic stimulation, although, as indicated earlier, the effect of complete Ca^{2+} chelation may not be physiologic, and thus the data should be interpreted with caution.

Cyclic guanosine 3',5'-monophosphate (cGMP) was once viewed as the intracellular mediator of cholinergic stimulation in some tissues. In the sweat gland, cGMP does not appear to be directly involved as a mediator of cholinergic sweating because the tissue cGMP level reaches a peak at 2 min and returns to the baseline level within 5 min after MCh stimulation, whereas the sweating response starts within seconds of stimulation and persists for hours (47).

STIMULATION OF MEMBRANE TRANSPORT DURING SWEAT SECRETION

Although the movement of ions in the clear cells during cholinergic sweat secretion was once assumed to conform to Ussing's leak-pump model (73), this model has been replaced by the Na-K-Cl cotransporter model (9,28), with minor modifications (Fig. 10). Some of the observations in the sweat secretory coil that led us to adopt the Na-K-Cl cotransport model (cell B in Fig. 10) include (62) (a) (Na, K)-ATPase (and thus the Na^+ pump) exists in the basolateral membrane (34), (b) the luminal electrical potential in the secretory coil decreases from -1 mV at rest to -6 mV during MCh stimulation, (c) K^+ channels and K^+ conduc-

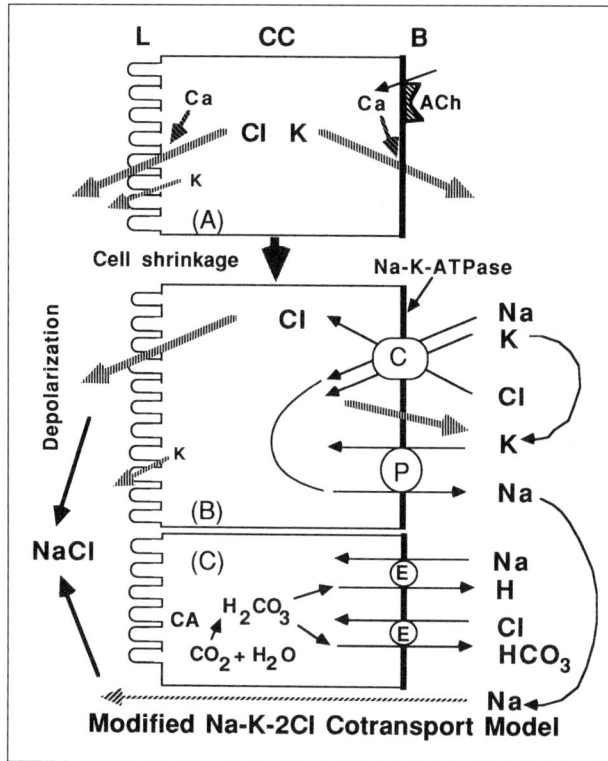

FIG. 10. Modified Na-K-2Cl cotransport model for ionic mechanism of cholinergic eccrine sweat secretion. The initial events are summarized in cell A. Cell B is similar to the original cotransport model, except a small K+ conductance is located across the luminal (apical) membrane. L, luminal or apical membrane; CC, clear cell; B, basolateral membrane; ACh, acetylcholine; Ca, calcium ion; C, Na-K-2Cl cotransporter; P, (Na, K)-ATPase-dependent Na+ pump; IP_3 and IP_4, inositol triphosphate and inositol tetrakisphosphate, respectively; *shaded thick arrows*, conductive downhill flux of ions through ionic channels; CA, carbonic anhydrase; E, exchanger; Na+ movement across the cell junction is indicated with a *shaded arrow* at the bottom of the figure.

tance are present in the basolateral membrane, (d) Cl− channels exist (presumably in the luminal membrane) and are activated because the luminal membrane depolarizes during cholinergic stimulation, (e) sweat secretion is inhibited by the "loop diuretics" such as furosemide an bumetanide, and (f) sweat secretion is dependent on the presence of Cl− and Na+ in the bath (33,35,49).

According to this model, the sequence of events during sweat secretion are as follows. ACh is released from periglandular cholinergic nerve endings in response to nerve impulses and binds to cholinergic receptors that are presumably located in the basolateral membrane of the clear cell. Activation of cholinergic receptors stimulates an influx of extracellular Ca^{2+} into the cytoplasm (see Fig. 8-10) presumably by activating the receptor-coupled Ca^{2+} channels. Because the ACh-induced increase in cytosolic [Ca], potassium chloride (KCl) efflux (33,35,70), cell shrinkage, and sweat secretion *in vitro* are drastically in-

hibited in a Ca^{2+}-free medium, the role of stored endogenous Ca^{2+} may be negligible (56,67) (unpublished observations) and the clear cell relies on external Ca^{2+} for its continuous supply. The increased cytosolic [Ca] subsequently stimulates Cl− channels in the luminal membrane and K+ channels in the basolateral membrane (cell A in Fig. 10), causing a net KCl efflux from the cell (66,70) and thus cell shrinkage (70) (Fig. 11), because water follows the solutes to maintain isosmolarity. Because the cell cytoplasm contains osmotically active organic electrolytes, such as amino acids (which do not leave the cell so readily) in addition to K+ and Cl−, cytoplasmic K+ and Cl− preferentially leave the cell through their respective ion channels, causing a significant decrease in cytoplasmic K+ [K] and Cl− [Cl] concentrations. The decrease in [K] and [Cl] provides a favorable chemical potential gradient (i.e., the driving force) for Na-K-2Cl cotransporters located in the basolateral membrane. Consequently, Na+, K+, and 2Cl− are carried into the cell in an electrically neutral fashion. Because Na+ channels are absent in the clear cell membrane, Na-K-2Cl cotransporters are the only means by which Na+ enters the cells. In fact, when Na-K-2Cl cotransporters are inhibited by bumetanide, the cytoplasmic [Na] does not increase (33). The increase in cytoplasmic [Na] is well known to stimulate Na+ pumps to extrude cytoplasmic Na+ in exchange for extracellular K+, but because the Na-K-2Cl cotransporters are continuously operating, the [Na] remains higher than the prestimulation level (70). One of the interesting features of the Na-K-2Cl cotransport model is that, in the steady state (i.e., during the sustained sweat secretion; see cell B in Fig. 10), K+ and Na+ recycle across the basolateral membrane without a net loss and the only ion that does not recycle is Cl−. Thus, the Cl− that enters into the cell via the Na-K-2Cl cotransporters moves into the lumen through the Ca^{2+}-dependent Cl− channels at the apical membrane. The movement of Cl− across the apical (luminal) membrane, which is down the electrochemical gradient, depolarizes the apical membrane and generates the negative luminal potential (with respect to the bath) (61). The negative luminal potential then attracts Na+ into the lumen across the Na+-conductive intercellular junction (i.e., paracellular pathway) (40). Thus, the Cl−, which enters the lumen across the cell, and the Na+, which diffuses into the lumen by the favorable electrical gradient generated by the Cl− movement, join in the lumen to form NaCl in the isotonic primary fluid. Although the cotransport model may be the major ionic mechanism for sweat secretion, further modifications of the model are needed. For example, we have observed that ISO stimulation is associated with intracellular alkalinization (37). This observation has led us to believe that parallel Na+–H+ and Cl−–HCO_3^- exchangers are also involved in the ionic mechanism of sweat secretion (see cell C in Fig. 10). Furthermore, the presence of such parallel exchangers is further supported by the partial decrease of MCh-induced KCl efflux in the absence of HCO_3 in the perfusate.

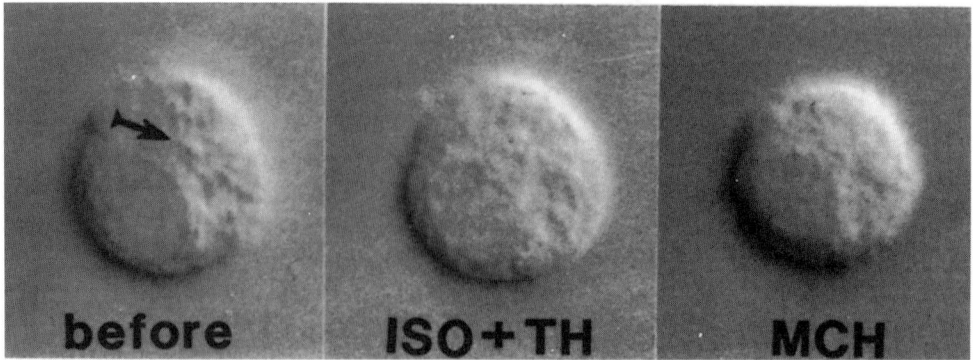

FIG. 11. Methacholine (MCH)-induced cell shrinkage of a rhesus eccrine clear cell. Note that the isoproterenol (ISO; 50 μM) plus theophylline (TH; 1 mM) combination failed to induce cell shrinkage in the same cell. The *arrow* indicates a lipofuscin granule that is present in most clear cells, but rarely in dark cells. Differential interference contrast was used.

REABSORPTION OF SODIUM CHLORIDE BY THE DUCT

The principal function of the sweat duct is to reabsorb Na^+, Cl^-, and HCO_3 from the plasmalike primary fluid in order to conserve these vital electrolytes. The duct consists of the proximal segment, which coils intimately with the secretory coil, and the distal duct, which is relatively straight or slightly helical as it ascends to reach the acrosyringium (i.e., the intraepidermal eccrine sweat duct unit). The major driving force for ductal Na^+ absorption is the ouabain-sensitive (Na, K)-ATPase/Na pump, which is involved in the uphill transport of Na^+ and perhaps also Cl^- (e.g., if Cl^- is reabsorbed from 30 mM in the lumen to 130 mM in the peritubular fluid and the lumen potential is -20 mV, the electrochemical gradient for Cl^- is equivalent to 18 mV uphill; however, if the luminal [Cl] is 50 mM, the net gradient is 6 mV downhill). The proximal duct contains ~10 times greater (Na, K)-ATPase activity than does the distal duct in the monkey-palm sweat gland (43), suggesting that the proximal duct may be more active in reabsorbing NaCl. The duct is made up of two layers of cells. The basal (or peripheral) ductal cells may be involved primarily in ductal NaCl absorption because these cells are rich in (Na, K)-ATPase activity (34), mitochondria, and membrane villi. The fact that the entire cell membrane of the basal cell is equipped with (Na, K)-ATPase (and thus Na^+ pumps) appears to be an elaborate mechanism designed to maximize the Na^+-pumping sites. The luminal cell may be involved by allowing Na^+ and Cl^- ions to enter passively into its cytoplasm and transferring them to the basal cells. However, such a functional partition of the two layers of cells requires the cells to behave like a syncytium through intimate intercellular communication (e.g., through gap junctions). The presence of gap junctions between ductal cells has not yet been observed; recent electrophysiologic studies, however, indicate that ductal cells are indeed electrically coupled (46).

The ionic mechanism of ductal NaCl absorption has been modeled after Ussing's leak-pump model, which was originally developed for the frog skin and the urinary bladder (Fig. 12). The minimum components of the model include the presence of Na^+–K^+ exchange pumps and K^+ conductance at the basolateral membrane and the presence of amiloride-sensitive Na^+ channels across the luminal membrane. Cl^- channels may reside in both the luminal and basolateral membranes. The presence of amiloride-sensitive Na^+ channels at the luminal membrane is suggested because 10^{-5} M amiloride inhibits ductal NaCl absorption (29,39), depolarizes the luminal potential (a luminal negative potential of <20 mV changes to +10–20 mV after amiloride exposure), and increases the luminal membrane resistance (31). The duct is also highly permeable to Cl^- ions because the reduction of luminal Cl^- by replacement with impermeant anions increases the ductal resistance and hyperpolarizes the luminal potential (29,39). Ductal NaCl absorption proceeds as follows: Na^+ passively enters the cell from the ductal lumen through amiloride-sensitive Na channels at the luminal membrane and is pumped out across the basal membrane in exchange for K^+ (Fig. 8-12). Cellular K^+ leaks out passively through K^+ channels at the basolateral membrane, thereby generating the membrane potential. K^+ then recycles back into the cell when it is pumped in, in exchange for cellular Na^+ brought in by the Na^+ pump.

In addition to NaCl absorption, the sweat duct may also absorb HCO_3 either directly or by means of secretion (54). The mechanism of H^+ secretion could consist of either Na^+–H^+ exchange or an H^+ pump (31) (see Fig. 9). The overall pharmacologic regulation of ductal absorptive function is still poorly understood, except that aldosterone is known to increase ductal Na^+ absorption (42).

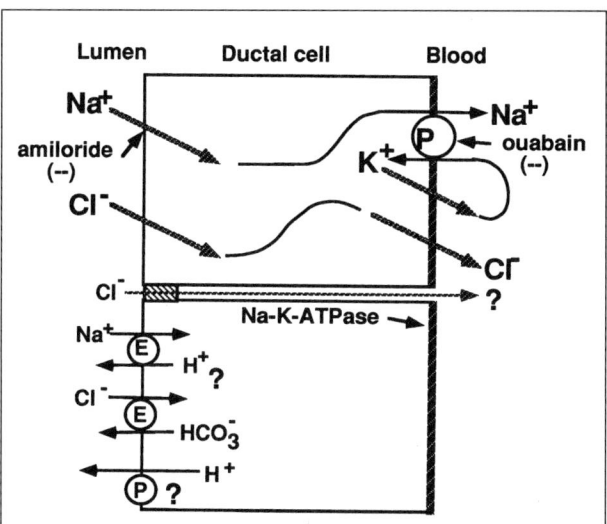

FIG. 12. The ionic mechanism of ductal NaCl absorption according to the modified Ussing's leak-pump model. Because the two cell layers are most likely coupled and behave like a syncytium, the two layers are reduced to a single layer. The **top part** is basically the same as Ussing's model. Possible mechanisms of HCO_3 absorption have been depicted in the **bottom part**. P, Na+ pump; E, exchanger.

ACKNOWLEDGMENTS

This chapter has been supported in part by National Institutes of Health grants DK 27857 and AR 25339. Neal Kane helped in preparation of the manuscript.

REFERENCES

1. Benzinger TH. Heat regulation: homeostasis of central temperature in man. *Physiol Rev* 1969;49:671–759.
2. Boulant JA. Hypothalamic mechanisms in thermoregulation. *Fed Proc* 1981;40:2843–2850.
3. Burnstock G. Physiological and regulatory functions of adenosine. In: Baer HP, Drummond GI, eds. *Physiological and regulatory functions of adenosine and adenine nucleotides.* New York: Raven, 1979: 3–32.
4. Cook DI, et al. Ca^{2+} not cyclic AMP mediates the fluid secretory response to isoproterenol in the rat mandibular gland: whole-cell patch clamp studies. *Pflugers Arch* 1988;413:67–76.
5. Dairkee SH, et al. Monoclonal antibody that defines human myoepithelium. *Proc Natl Acad Sci USA* 1985;82:7409–7413.
6. Douglas WW, Rubin RP. The mechanism of catecholamine release from the adrenal medulla and the role of calcium in stimulus–secretion coupling. *J Physiol (Lond)* 1963;167:288–310.
7. Ellis RA. Eccrine sweat glands. In: Jadassohn J, ed. *Handbuch der Haut und Geschlechtskrankheiten;* vol 1: *Nomale und Pathologische Anatomie der Haut.* Berlin: Springer-Verlag, 1967:224–266.
8. Fortney SM, et al. Effect of blood volume on sweating rate and body fluids in exercising humans. *J Appl Physiol* 1981;51:1594–1600.
9. Geck P, et al. Electrically silent cotransport of Na+,K+ and Cl− in Ehrlich cells. *Biochem Biophys Acta* 1980;600:432–437.
10. Gitter D, Sato K. Localized hyperhidrosis over pretibial myxedema associated with glandular hypertrophy. *J Am Acad Dermatol* 1990;23: 252–254.
11. Greenleaf JE. Hyperthermia and exercise. In: Robertshaw D, ed. *International review of physiology: environmental physiology III;* vol 20. Baltimore: University Park Press, 1979:157–208.
12. Grynkiewicz GM, et al. A new generation of Ca^{2+} indicators with greatly improved fluorescence properties. *J Biol Chem* 1985;260: 3440–3450.
13. Gutrecht JA. Sympathetic skin response. *J Clin Neurophysiol* 1994; 11:519–524.
14. Hammel HT. Regulation of internal body temperature. *Annu Rev Physiol* 1968;30:641–710.
15. Hibino T, et al. Human eccrine sweat contains tissue kallikrein and kininase II. *J Invest Dermatol* 1994;102:214–220.
16. Jenkinson DM. Sweat gland function in domestic animals. In: Botelho S, Brooke F, Sherry W, eds. *The exocrine gland.* Philadelphia: University of Pennsylvania, 1968:201–214.
17. Johnson GS, Elizondo RS. Eccrine sweat gland in *Macaca mulatta*: physiology, histochemistry, and distribution. *J Appl Physiol* 1974;37: 814–820.
18. Johnson RF, Spalding JMK. *Disorders of the autonomic nervous system.* Philadelphia: FA Davis, 1974:5 (*Contemporary neurology*).
19. LeWitt PA, et al. Episodic hyperhidrosis, hypothermia, and agenesis of corpus callosum. *Neurology* 1983;33:1122–1129.
20. Lundberg JM, et al. Vasoactive intestinal polypeptide in cholinergic neurons of exocrine glands: functional significance of coexisting transmitters for vasodilatation and secretion. *Proc Natl Acad Sci USA* 1980;77:1651–1655.
21. Mangal P, et al. Secretion of epidermal growth factor (EGF) in human control subjects and patients with cystic fibrosis. *Clin Res* 1988; 36:671A(abst).
22. Morbidity and Mortality Weekly Report CDC. Heat-related illnesses and deaths—United States, 1994–1995. *JAMA* 1995;274:209– 210.
23. Morbidity and Mortality Weekly Report CDC. Heat-related mortality in Chicago, July, 1995. *JAMA* 1995;274:602.
24. Nadel ER, et al. Importance of skin temperature in the regulation of sweating. *J Appl Physiol* 1971;31:80–87.
25. Nadel ER, et al. Peripheral modifications to the central drive for sweating. *J Appl Physiol* 1971;31:828–833.
26. Nielsen B. Effect of changes in plasma Na and Ca ion concentration on body temperature during exercise. *Acta Physiol Scand* 1974;91: 123–129.
27. O'Brien JP. A study of miliaria rubra, tropical anhidrosis and anhidrotic asthenia. *Br J Dermatol* 1947;59:125–158.
28. O'Grady SM, et al. Characteristics and functions of Na-K-Cl cotransport in epithelial tissues. *Am J Physiol* 1987;253: C177–C192.
29. Quinton PM. Effect of some ion transport inhibitors on secretion and reabsorption in intact and perfused single human sweat glands. *Pflugers Arch* 1981;391:309–313.
30. Quinton PM, Bijman J. Higher bioelectric potentials due to decreased chloride absorption in the sweat glands of patients with cystic fibrosis. *N Engl J Med* 1983;308:1185–1189.
31. Quinton PM, Reddy MM. Cl-conductance and acid secretion in the human sweat duct. *Ann NY Acad Sci* 1989;574:438–446.
32. Quinton PM, Tormey JM. Localization of Na-K-ATPase sites in the secretory and reabsorptive epithelia of perfused eccrine sweat glands: a question to the role of the enzyme in secretion. *Membr Biol* 1976; 29:383–399.
33. Saga K, Sato K. Electron probe X-ray microanalysis of cellular ions in the eccrine secretory coil cells during methacholine stimulation. *J Membr Biol* 1988;107:13–24.
34. Saga K, Sato K. Ultrastructural localization of ouabain-sensitive, K-dependent *p*-nitrophenyl phosphatase activity in monkey eccrine sweat gland. *J Histochem Cytochem* 1988;36:1023–1030.
35. Saga K, et al. K+ efflux from the monkey eccrine secretory cell during the transient of stimulation with agonists. *J Physiol (Lond)* 1988;405: 205–217.
36. Sato F, et al. Functional and morphological changes in the eccrine sweat gland with heat acclimation in the patas monkey. *J Appl Physiol* 1990;69:232–236.
37. Sato F, et al. Interleukin-1α (IL-1α) in human sweat regulates cytoplasmic pH and $[Ca]_i$ and its gene is expressed in the human sweat gland. *Clin Res* 1991;39(2) 520A(abst).
38. Sato K. Inhibition of respiration in the eccrine sweat gland by ethacrynic acid. *Pflugers Arch* 1973;431:233–242.
39. Sato K. Mechanism of eccrine sweat secretion. In: Quinton PM, Martinez JR, Hopfer U, eds. *Fluid and electrolyte abnormalities in exocrine glands in cystic fibrosis.* San Francisco: San Francisco Press, 1982:35–52.

40. Sato K. The physiology and pharmacology of the eccrine sweat gland. In: Goldsmith L, ed. *Biochemistry and physiology of the skin.* London: Oxford University Press, 1983:596–641.
41. Sato K. The physiology, pharmacology and biochemistry of the eccrine sweat gland. *Rev Physiol Biochem Pharmacol* 1977;79:51–181.
42. Sato K, Dobson RL. The effect of intracutaneous d-aldosterone and hydrocortisone on the human eccrine sweat gland function. *J Invest Dermatol* 1970;54:450–459.
43. Sato K, et al. Enzymatic basis for the active transport of sodium in the eccrine sweat gland. II. Localization and characterization of Na-K-ATPase. *J Invest Dermatol* 1971;57:10–16.
44. Sato K, et al. Morphology and development of an apoeccrine sweat gland in human axillae. *Am J Physiol* 1987;252:R160–R180.
45. Sato K, Nishiyama A. Mechanical properties and functions of the myoepithelium in the eccrine sweat gland. *Am J Physiol* 1979;237:C177–C184.
46. Sato K, et al. Membrane transport and intracellular events in control and cystic fibrosis eccrine sweat glands. In: Mastella G, Quinton PM, eds. *Cellular and molecular basis of cystic fibrosis.* San Francisco: San Francisco Press, 1988:171–185.
47. Sato K, Sato F. Cyclic GMP accumulation during cholinergic stimulation of eccrine sweat glands. *Am J Physiol* 1984;247:C234–C239.
48. Sato K, Sato F. Defective β-adrenergic response of cyclic fibrosis sweat glands *in vivo* and *in vitro*. *J Clin Invest* 1984;73:1763–1771.
49. Sato K, Sato F. Effect of periglandular ionic composition and transport inhibitors on rhesus monkey eccrine sweat gland function *in vitro*. *J Physiol (Lond)* 1987;393:195–212.
50. Sato K, Sato F. Effect of VIP on sweat secretion and cAMP accumulation in isolated simian eccrine glands. *Am J Physiol* 1987;253:R935–R941.
51. Sato K, Sato F. Individual variations in structure and function of human eccrine sweat gland. *Am J Physiol* 1983;245:R203–R208.
52. Sato K, Sato F. Interleukin-1α in human sweat is functionally active and derived from the eccrine sweat gland. *Am J Physiol* 1994;266:R950–R959.
53. Sato K, Sato F. Methods for studying eccrine sweat gland function *in vivo* and *in vitro*. *Methods Enzymol* 1990;192;583–599.
54. Sato K, Sato F. Na+, K+, H+, Cl− concentrations in cystic fibrosis eccrine sweat *in vivo* and *in vitro*. *J Lab Clin Med* 1990;115:504–511.
55. Sato K, Sato F. Pharmacological responsiveness of isolated single eccrine sweat glands. *Am J Physiol* 1981;240:R44–R51.
56. Sato K, Sato F. Relationship between quin 2-determined cytosolic [Ca^{+2}] and sweat secretion. *Am J Physiol* 1988;254:C310–C317.
57. Sato K, Sato F. Role of calcium in cholinergic and adrenergic mechanisms of eccrine sweat secretion. *Am J Physiol* 1981;241:C113–C120.
58. Sato K, Sato F. Role of cyclic AMP in beta adrenergic mechanisms of sweat secretion. *Pflugers Arch* 1981;390:49–53.
59. Sato K, Sato F. Stimulation-induced changes in cytosolic calcium in a single dissociated eccrine secretory cell by use of fluorescent dye fura 2. *Clin Res* 1989;37:354A(abst).
60. Sato K, Sato F. Sweat secretion by human axillary apoeccrine sweat gland *in vitro*. *Am J Physiol* 1987;252:R181–R187.
61. Sato K, Sato F. Transepithelial p.d. during Sr^{2+}-induced spontaneous sweat secretion. *Am J Physiol* 1982;242:C360–C365.
62. Sato K, et al. Biology of the eccrine sweat gland. I. Normal sweat gland function. *J Am Acad Dermatol* 1989;20:537–565.
63. Sato K, et al. Biology of the eccrine sweat gland. II. Hyperhidrosis and hypohydrosis. *J Am Acad Dermatol* 1989;20:713–729.
64. Sato K, et al. Functional characteristics of sweat glands isolated from a patient with circumscribed idiopathic hyperhidrosis. *J Invest Dermatol* 1996;106:862(abst).
65. Sato K, et al. Normal and abnormal eccrine sweat gland function. In: Soter NA, Baden HP, eds. *Pathophysiology of dermatologic diseases.* New York: McGraw-Hill, 1990:211–234.
66. Sato KT, et al. Movement of cellular ions during stimulation with isoproterenol in simian eccrine clear cells. *Am J Physiol* 261:R87–R93, 1991.
67. Sato KT, et al. One step iodine starch method for direct visualization of sweating. *Am J Med Sci* 1988;295:528–531.
68. Soos G, Sato F, Sato K. Prolactin and prolactin receptor and their gene expression in the human eccrine sweat gland. *J Dermatol Sci* 1993;6:153(abs).
69. Tainino H, et al. The distribution of substance P-, CGRP-, galanin- and ANP-like immunoreactive nerves in human sweat glands. *Histochem J* 1987;19:375–380.
70. Takemura T, et al. Intracellular ion concentrations and cell volume decrease during cholinergic stimulation of eccrine secretory coil cells. *J Membr Biol* 1991;119:211–219.
71. Uno H. Sympathetic innervation of the sweat glands and piloerector muscle of macaques and human beings. *J Invest Dermatol* 1977;69:112–130.
72. Uno H, Montagna W. Catecholamine-containing nerve terminals of the eccrine sweat glands of macaques. *Cell Tissue Res* 1975;158:1–13.
73. Ussing HH. Transport of electrolytes and water across the epithelia. *Harvey Lect* 1965;59:1–30.
74. Vaalassti A, et al. Vasoactive intestinal polypeptide (VIP)-like immunoreactivity in the nerves of human axillary sweat glands. *J Invest Dermatol* 1985;85:246–248.
75. Yanagawa S, et al. Origin of periodic acid–Schiff-reactive glycoprotein in human eccrine sweat. *J Appl Physiol* 1986; 60:1615–1622.
76. Zimmermann KP, et al. Poststroke autonomic nervous system function: palmar sympathetic skin responses thirty or more days after cerebrovascular accident. *Arch Phys Med Rehabil* 1995;76:250–256.

CHAPTER 9

Innervation of the Skin

William R. Kennedy and Gwen Wendelschafer-Crabb

---

1. Cutaneous nerves can be visualized by immunohistochemically localizing protein gene product 9.5, which reacts with myelinated as well as fine unmyelinated fibers. Neuropeptides and other structures in skin, such as basement membrane or vasculature, can be localized simultaneously.
2. Three-dimensional orientation of nerve to various structures can be ascertained by visualizing very thick immunostained sections with a laser-scanning confocal microscope.
3. Sensory nerves in the epidermis as well as autonomic nerves to sweat glands, arteries, and arrectores pilorum muscles can be identified and evaluated at their terminals.
4. The epidermis contains many very fine nerve fibers that arise from a subepidermal neural plexus. They can be quantified by counting, length determination, and branch analysis.
5. Sweat glands are richly innervated by sympathetic sudomotor nerves, that arise from an adjacent nerve bundle and encircle the secreting tubule with tightly spaced fibers. They can be quantified by determination of their volume per volume of sweat gland.
6. Other nerves associated with the subepidermal neural plexus, hair follicles, arrectores pilorum muscles, and arteries are clearly visualized but more difficult to quantify routinely because of their frequency within sections or problems with imaging.
7. Divergence from normal in the number of nerves, length of nerve, number of branch points, or volume of nerve frequently occurs in neuropathic conditions.
8. The skin biopsy procedure is inexpensive, minimally invasive, results in minimal scarring, has low potential for infection, and does not result in a detectable sensory deficit.
9. Skin biopsy will be increasingly important for diagnosis and has potential for follow-up evaluation of therapeutic endeavors to halt or reverse the progress of polyneuropathy.

INTRODUCTION

This chapter is written from the prospective of using skin biopsies for diagnosis of disorders of the autonomic and peripheral nervous systems and for evaluating response to clinical trials. These ambitious endeavors require knowledge of the normal innervation of skin and the relationship to other structures in skin. The cutaneous innervation includes different types of autonomic motor and somatic sensory nerves that can be identified at their terminals by the end structure that they innervate. Autonomic motor axons innervate sweat glands, blood vessels, and arrectores pilorum muscles. Somatic sensory nerves terminate in the epidermis, on hair follicles, and in a variety of encapsulated receptors. Study of the cutaneous nerves of normal subjects and patients with peripheral nerve disease provides the potential for making correlations with the clinical findings, electrophysiologic tests, and the results of quantitative measurements of touch, thermal sensitivity, sweating, and localized vasomotor reactions performed near the biopsy site.

METHODS

Cutaneous nerves can be clearly visualized by staining 2- to 4-mm punch-biopsy specimens by using immunohistochemical techniques (14,15). Skin samples are held overnight at 4°C in Zamboni's fixative (33) and then stored in 20% sucrose-phosphate-buffered saline until sectioned. Then, 100-μm sections are cut with a freezing microtome

---

W. R. Kennedy and G. Wendelschafer-Crabb: Department of Neurology, University of Minnesota, Minneapolis, Minnesota 55455.

(Leica SM 2000R) and prepared for immunohistochemical staining. Nonimmune sera is used for negative controls. A number of antibodies and lectins for nerve, epidermal cells, basement membrane, endothelial cells, and other structures can be used depending upon the purpose of the particular study. Antibodies are visualized with cyanine 3.18 or cyanine 5.18 fluorophores conjugated to appropriate goat or donkey secondary antibodies (Jackson Immunoresearch, West Grove, PA, U.S.A.). Some sections are treated with 50 µg/ml *Ulex europaeus* agglutinin (UEA I) labeled with fluorescein isothiocyanate (Vector, Burlingame, CA, U.S.A.) to stain blood vessels, sweat gland tubules, and hair follicles (9).

Specimens are initially examined with a Nikon Microphot SA epifluorescence microscope (Melville, NY, U.S.A.) to select areas for further examination in a MRC-1000 Confocal Imaging System equipped with a krypton/argon ion laser (Bio-Rad Life Science, Hercules, CA, U.S.A.). The association of two or three antigens in the same tissue is assessed by double or triple staining with primary antibodies from different species by using appropriate filters for the specific visualization of fluorescein, cyanine 3.18, and cyanine 5.18 (3). Typically, a series of images of optical sections (called a z series) is acquired at 2- to 4-µm intervals throughout the depth of the specimen. Each image can be viewed individually, or the entire series can be projected into a single in-focus image. The visibility of lightly stained fibers in the projections is increased by enhancing the contrast of individual images with computer processing. Quantitation of sudomotor or epidermal nerves is performed from the confocal images by using Images Volumes® from Minnesota Dolametrics, St. Paul, MN or Neurolucida® from MicroBrightField, Colchester, Vermont software systems.

OVERVIEW OF CUTANEOUS STRUCTURES

Figure 1 is a low-magnification confocal image that illustrates many of the structures in nonglabrous skin that are immunostained for nerve and collagen type IV (Col IV), which is found in the basement membrane of follicular structures, the dermatoepidermal basement membrane, and blood vessels. The epidermis occupies the top 100–200 µm of the figure. It consists of four basic layers, including basal cell layer, spinous layer, granular layer, and cornified layer. The epidermis is separated from the papillary dermis by the dermatoepidermal basement membrane (Fig. 2), which contains Col IV as its major component plus several important glycoproteins such as laminin, heparan-sulfate proteoglycan, entactin, and fibronectin. Dermal papillae project from the most superficial layer of the papillary dermis into the epidermis. Each contains one, occasionally two, capillary loops. Most of the nerves that are destined to penetrate the basement membrane and enter the epidermis pass near the capillaries in the dermal papillae.

Hair follicles are partially covered by a network of capillaries, from the bulb region deep in the dermis to nearly the surface of the skin. Sebaceous glands adjacent to the superior segment of the hair follicle also have a surface capillary network. Arrectores pilorum muscles insert onto the hair follicle at the bulge region, just below the position of the sebaceous glands.

Sweat glands are located slightly deeper in the dermis. If associated with a hair follicle, they are found below the sebaceous gland and insertion of the arrector pili muscle. Sweat gland secretory tubules and their convolutions can be visualized with antibody to cytokeratins 8, 18, and 19, or by staining their basement membrane with antibody to Col IV. The heavy yellow and green sudomotor nerves in Fig. A almost obscure the underlying sweat tubule.

GENERAL FEATURES OF CUTANEOUS INNERVATION

The most consistent staining method to visualize human cutaneous nerve fibers is immunohistochemical staining for protein gene product (PGP) 9.5 (5,30). The large dermal nerve trunks in nonglabrous skin contain a variety of unmyelinated autonomic motor nerves plus unmyelinated and myelinated somatic sensory nerves. The nerve trunks branch deep in the dermis to innervate small arteries and arterioles, sweat glands, and the bulb of hair follicles (Fig. 1). Higher in the dermis, nerve branches innervate the arrectores pilorum muscles, hair follicles, and the sweat glands associated with hair follicles. The nerves that innervate the superficial dermis and epidermis can be recognized in middermis by their tree-shaped configuration, each branch innervating a segment of skin. As the branches approach and enter the papillary dermis, they form a nearly horizontal subepidermal plexus before giving off thin branches or single nerve fibers that end near capillary loops, around Merkel's cells, and in different levels of the epidermis.

Epidermis and Papillary Dermis

Although detailed descriptions of the epidermal innervation are available from silver (26) and methylene blue (1) staining methods, more consistent staining of greater numbers of nerves has been obtained with immunoreaction to PGP (PGP-IR)(14,32). Epidermal nerves are extensions of unmyelinated nerves in the subepidermal plexus. We have not observed any nerves that lose the myelinated sheath deep in the dermis to continue as unmyelinated axons toward the surface and enter the epidermis. Epidermal nerves are not invested in a Schwann cell sheath. (8,14,23). The Schwann cell covering terminates where the nerve penetrates the basement membrane (4).

Laser scanning confocal microscopy images of 100-µm-thick sections of nonglabrous skin immunoreacted for PGP

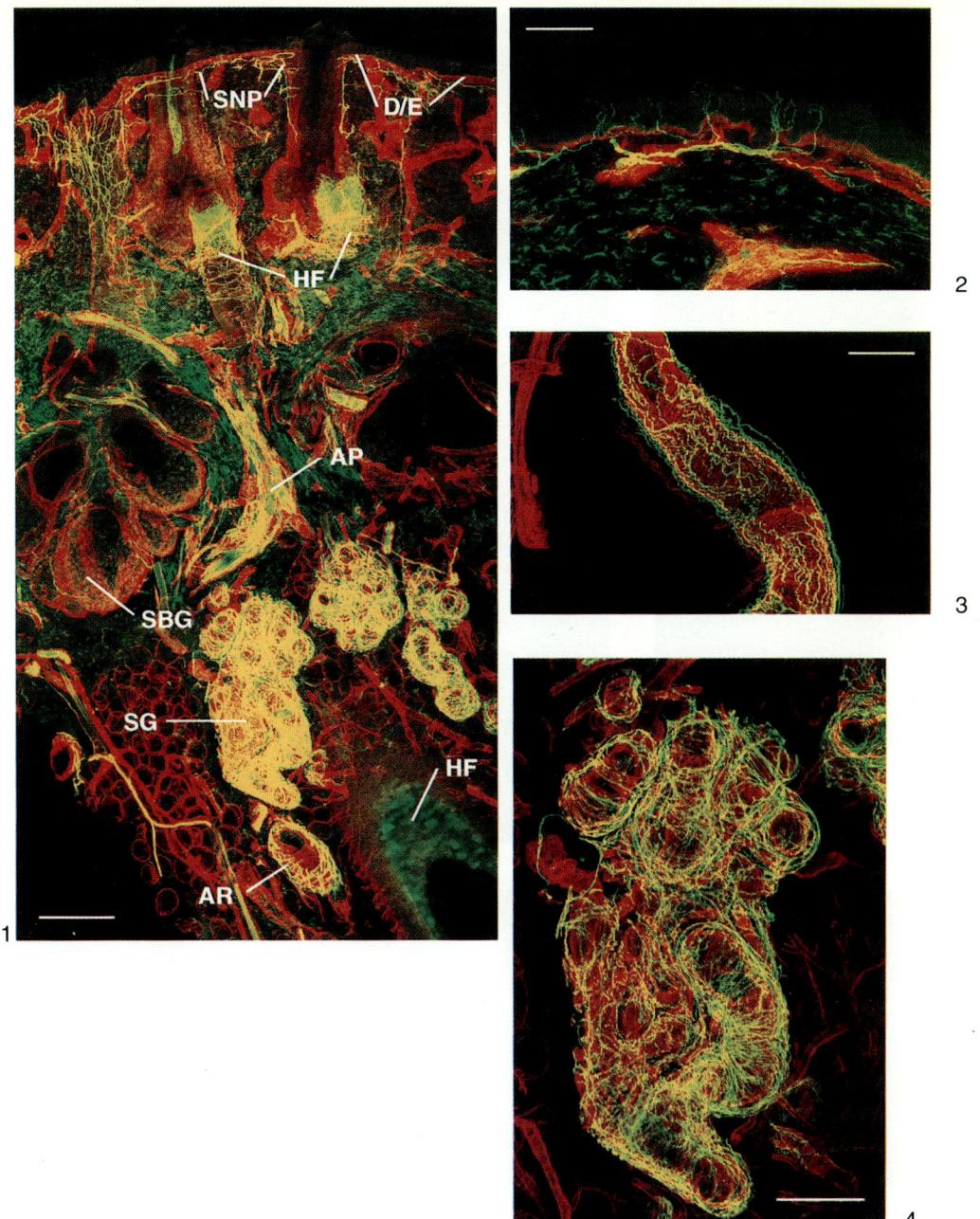

COLOR FIG. 1. (1) Low-magnification laser scanning confocal micrograph of human skin from face. This section of skin was immunostained for basement membrane (type IV collagen—*red*) and nerve (protein gene product 9.5—*green* and *yellow*) to provide an overview of the structures present in human skin. Epidermis, the top layer of skin, is delineated from the papillary dermis by the dermatoepidermal basement membrane (D/E). Papillary dermis contains a plexus of capillaries with loops extending into the dermal papilla. An extensive subepidermal neural plexus (SNP) is visible. Hair follicles (HF) extend from the surface of the skin to the deepest part of the dermis. These are associated with sebaceous glands (SBG) and arrectores pilorum muscles (AP). Sweat glands (SG) are present below the sebaceous glands. A small segment of an artery (AR) is visible at the base of the section. Scale bar = 200 μm. **(2)** Epidermis from human calf contains many fine nerve fibers (immunoreactive protein gene product 9.5, protein—*green* and *yellow*), presumably sensory, that differ in branching patterns. These arise from the subepidermal plexus, which underlies the dermatoepidermal basement membrane (type IV collagen—*red*). Scale bar = 100 μm. **(3)** An arteriole, outlined with immunostaining for type IV collagen (*red*), is distinguished by its characteristic pattern of sympathetic innervation (protein gene product, 9.5—*green* and *yellow*). Scale bar = 100 μm. **(4)** This sweat gland, seen at lower magnification in Fig. 1, is so heavily innervated by autonomic sudomotor nerves that the structure of the secreting tubule can be recognized by the pattern of the nerves enwrapping them. The tubule and capillaries are immunostained for type IV collagen (*red*). Scale bar = 100 μm.

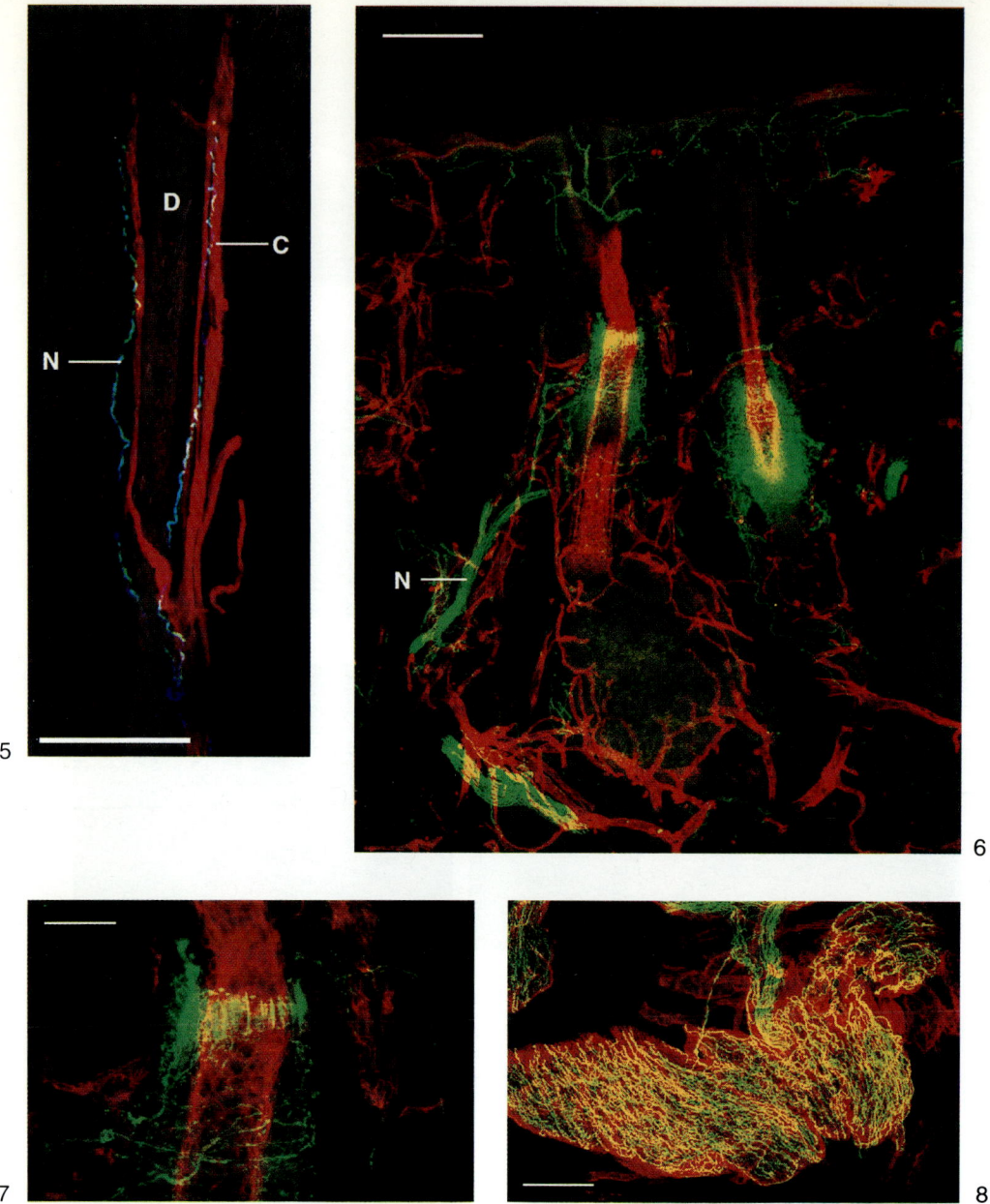

COLOR FIG. 1 cont. (5) The sweat duct (D) is sparsely innervated. One or two nerves (N) associated with capillaries (C) accompany the duct to the surface. This duct is delineated with antibody to type IV collagen, capillaries are stained with fluorescein-labeled *Ulex europaeus* agglutinin type I, and nerves are immunostained for protein gene product 9.5. Scale bar = 100 μm. **(6)** Facial hair follicles are surrounded by an interwoven capillary network (*Ulex europaeus* agglutinin—*red*). All follicles have a band of heavy innervation above the bulge region; in some follicles, this is accompanied by myelinated lanceolate endings (protein gene product 9.5—*green* and *yellow*) (see Fig. 7). These nerves are derived from nerve bundles (N) that ascend from the deep dermis to branch in the bulge region. Nerves to hair follicles are somatic sensory. Scale bar = 200 μm. **(7)** Lanceolate endings (higher magnification of Fig. 6) are endings of myelinated nerves that are arranged in a ringlike structure around the follicle. Finer reticular nerve endings are visible below the lanceolate endings. Scale bar = 40 μm. **(8)** Arrectores pilorum muscles are often present in thick sections of skin. They extend between the papillary dermis and a hair follicle (type IV collagen—*red*). Each muscle is heavily innervated by a wavy, parallel array of autonomic nerve fibers (protein gene product 9.5—*yellow* and *green*). Scale bar = 100 μm.

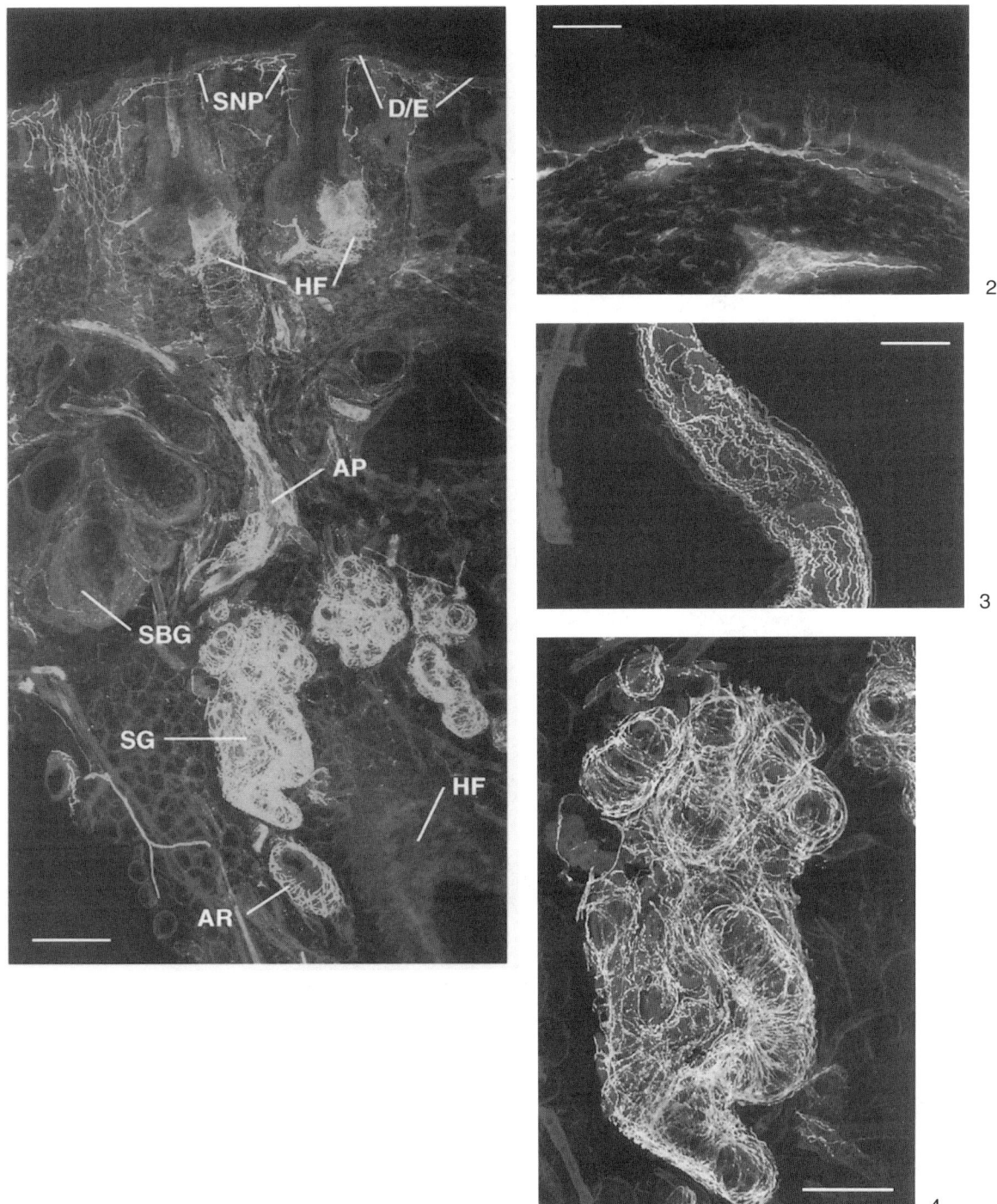

FIGS. 1–4. (1) Low-magnification laser scanning confocal micrograph of human skin from face. This section of skin was immunostained for basement membrane (type IV collagen—red) and nerve (protein gene product 9.5—green and yellow) to provide an overview of the structures present in human skin. Epidermis, the top layer of skin, is delineated from the papillary dermis by the dermatoepidermal basement membrane (D/E). Papillary dermis contains a plexus of capillaries with loops extending into the dermal papilla. An extensive subepidermal neural plexus (SNP) is visible. Hair follicles (HF) extend from the surface of the skin to the deepest part of the dermis. These are associated with sebaceous glands (SBG) and arrectores pilorum muscles (AP). Sweat glands (SG) are present below the sebaceous glands. A small segment of an artery (AR) is visible at the base of the section. Scale bar = 200 μm. (2) Epidermis from human calf contains many fine nerve fibers (immunoreactive protein gene product 9.5, protein—green and yellow), presumably sensory, that differ in branching patterns. These arise from the subepidermal plexus, which underlies the dermatoepidermal basement membrane (type IV collagen—red). Scale bar = 100 μm. (3) An arteriole, outlined with immunostaining for type IV collagen (red), is distinguished by its characteristic pattern of sympathetic innervation (protein gene product, 9.5—green and yellow). Scale bar = 100 μm. (4) This sweat gland, seen at lower magnification in Fig. 1, is so heavily innervated by autonomic sudomotor nerves that the structure of the secreting tubule can be recognized by the pattern of the nerves enwrapping them. The tubule and capillaries are immunostained for type IV collagen (red). Scale bar = 100 μm. See color fig. 1.

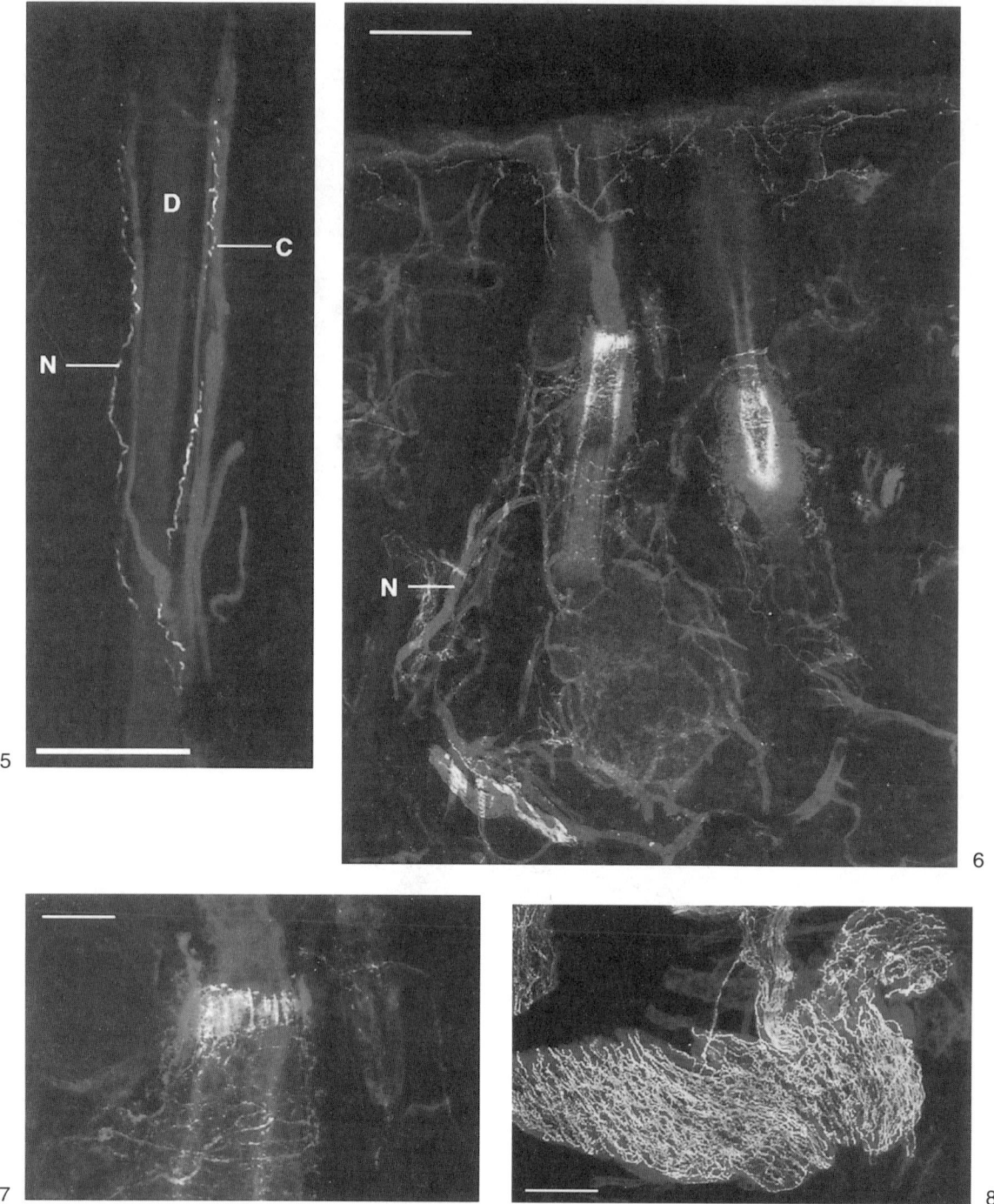

FIGS. 5–8. (5) The sweat duct (D) is sparsely innervated. One or two nerves (N) associated with capillaries (C) accompany the duct to the surface. This duct is delineated with antibody to type IV collagen, capillaries are stained with fluorescein-labeled *Ulex europaeus* agglutinin type I, and nerves are immunostained for protein gene product 9.5. Scale bar = 100 μm. **(6)** Facial hair follicles are surrounded by an interwoven capillary network (*Ulex europaeus* agglutinin—*red*). All follicles have a band of heavy innervation above the bulge region; in some follicles, this is accompanied by myelinated lanceolate endings (protein gene product 9.5—*green* and *yellow*) (see Fig. 7). These nerves are derived from nerve bundles (N) that ascend from the deep dermis to branch in the bulge region. Nerves to hair follicles are somatic sensory. Scale bar = 200 μm. **(7)** Lanceolate endings (higher magnification of Fig. 6) are endings of myelinated nerves that are arranged in a ringlike structure around the follicle. Finer reticular nerve endings are visible below the lanceolate endings. Scale bar = 40 μm. **(8)** Arrectores pilorum muscles are often present in thick sections of skin. They extend between the papillary dermis and a hair follicle (type IV collagen—*red*). Each muscle is heavily innervated by a wavy, parallel array of autonomic nerve fibers (protein gene product 9.5—*yellow* and *green*). Scale bar = 100 μm. *See color Fig. 1.*

9.5 provide a three-dimensional view of epidermis that reveals several morphologic types of epidermal nerves differing in length and branching pattern. Some of these differences were recognized nearly 90 years ago by Botezat (2) and more recently by Novotny and Gommert–Novotny (26) with silver staining methods. We tentatively described five variations (17). The fiber types differ in their length, branching patterns, and surface projections or territories. The types are simple, nearly vertical fibers with short terminal branches near the surface; short fibers that branch immediately after entering epidermis; nerves with multiple branches below or just above the basement membrane that penetrate epidermis for variable distances; single vertical branches with one or two branches in stratum spinosum; and short single branches ending in the basal cell layer. Some of the fiber types can be distinguished in Fig. 2. The functional significance of the varying morphology is unknown.

Calcitonin gene-related peptide (CGRP)-IR and the less frequent substance P (SP)-IR nerves usually have clawlike endings near the capillary loop in the papillary dermis. Neither are commonly observed in the epidermis of human nonglabrous skin (5,11–13). In 100-μm-thick sections of calf and thigh double stained for CGRP-IR and Col IV-IR, we have observed occasional small branches of CGRP nerves penetrating the basement membrane for a few micrometers. We have found very few SP-ir nerves penetrating deep into epidermis of nonglabrous calf skin.

Merkel cells are oval cells that are situated between basal keratinocytes and basement membrane and usually located at the tips of the rete pegs. Their occurrence in nonglabrous skin, as determined by antibodies directed against cytokeratin 8, is sparse in adult human skin, varying from <10 to ~40/mm^2 in the proximal and distal limb areas that are commonly biopsied (19). Merkel cells form neurite complexes (7) with endings of myelinated nerve fibers. The neurite complexes have commonly been considered to be mechanosensory, but Mills and Diamond (24) have reported that destruction of Merkel cells in rat touch domes did not result in loss of mechanosensory sensitivity. They concluded that mechanosensory transduction must reside in the associated nerve endings.

Langerhans' cells are plentiful in epidermis, mainly in the stratum spinosum. Hosoi et al. (10) reported that CGRP-IR nerves are intrinsically associated with Langerhans' cells in human epidermis (biopsy site not stated) and that CGRP is often found at the surface of some Langerhans' cells. Furthermore, in functional assays, CGRP inhibited Langerhans' cell antigen presentation. The findings suggested an modulatory interaction between nerve and immunologic function. However, Hilliges et al. (8) observed, by electron microscopy, membrane–membrane apposition between keratinocytes and epidermal nerves without any specialized structures, but no contacts with other epidermal cells.

Blood Vessels

Arterioles, venules, and capillaries are easily located by staining with UEA I, a lectin that reacts with fucose moieties of the endothelium of blood vessels and follicular structures of the skin, or by staining with antibodies to Col IV in the basement membrane of these vascular structures. Large arteries and veins enter the biopsy specimen in the lower reticular dermis or hypodermis. Nerves localized with PGP 9.5 antibody are woven along the length of arterioles in a characteristic wavy innervation pattern (Fig. 3). Innervation is more sparse on the smaller arterioles in the upper reticular dermis as they approach the surface. Vasomotor axons are also immunoreactive to vasoactive intestinal polypeptide (VIP) and neuropeptide Y (NPY). It is unusual to observe nerve associated with an arteriole at the level of the subepidermal plexus. The association of CGRP-IR and SP-IR nerves with terminal capillary loops was remarked upon above. Veins and venules rarely have even a single axon. Arterioles that enter sweat glands are ~30 μm in diameter and heavily innervated by unmyelinated sympathetic vasomotor axons. These arterioles give off capillaries that are intertwined with the sweat tubule merging into venous capillaries that join veins that exit the sweat capsule.

Sweat Glands

The sympathetic innervation of the sweat gland is derived from 1 or 2 nerve bundles that give rise to multiple unmyelinated sudomotor axons (14). These divide into a complex array of unmyelinated axons in association with the sweat gland tubule. The most common pattern of sweat gland innervation is a circular wrapping of sudomotor axons around the secretory tubule at loosely defined intervals, either singly or in compact bundles of 2 or 5 axons (Fig. 4). Encircling axons occasionally branch, but short, abruptly ending branches are unusual. Sweat ducts from the gland to the surface of the skin are innervated by 1–2 axons and accompanied by 1 or 2 capillaries with periodic interconnections (Fig. 5). The interrelationships between sudomotor nerves (and their neuropeptide content), sweat tubules, and vascularity can be assessed by triple staining for UEA I, PGP 9.5, and a selected neuropeptide. VIP-IR and synaptophysin are always present in the PGP 9.5-IR sudomotor nerves. CGRP-IR is usually present to a lesser extent, but SP-IR axons are sparse.

Hair Follicles

Somatic sensory nerves supply a variety of innervation to hair follicles (Figs. 6 and 7). Myelinated nerves are not frequent in the dermis of nonglabrous skin, even in thick sections. When present, they can sometimes be traced to the lanceolate endings of the hair follicle (Fig. 7). The heaviest innervation of hair is found near the bulge region, where unmyelinated nerves, several immunoreactive for SP, run in circular and longitudinal directions. The nerve plexus of the hair follicle extends to become continuous with the epidermal innervation (Fig. 1, top left).

Arrectores Pilorum Muscles

Arrectores pilorum smooth muscles are commonly encountered in biopsies of hairy skin. From zero to five arrectores pilorum muscles are usually contained in a 3-mm biopsy specimen. The muscles originate near the papillary dermis and project down to insert on the bulge region of a hair follicle. They appear to be wrapped around a sebaceous gland as though providing support to the gland. When immunostained by PGP 9.5-IR, the nerves are in good contrast (Fig. 8) and can be easily quantified. The nerves are also immunoreactive for CGRP and synaptophysin and stain for acetylcholine esterase. In biopsy specimens that are sectioned perpendicular to the surface of the skin, it is possible to observe branching of nerve fibers within the muscle to form an approximately parallel wavy network.

CLINICAL UTILITY OF SKIN BIOPSY

There are potential advantages of using skin biopsies for diagnosis of neuropathy and for therapeutic trials, as compared with nerve biopsy. The information available from the two procedures is not identical, however, and both have a place in clinical usage. Nonglabrous skin is better suited for biopsy, but small biopsies can be made of glabrous skin without complications. The usual punch biopsy is 2–4 mm in diameter; 2- and 3-mm biopsies do not require sutures. The skin biopsy procedure is inexpensive and minimally invasive, results in minimal scarring, has low potential for infection, and does not result in a detectable sensory deficit. The biopsy specimen contains a selection of nerves that are of known autonomic and somatic sensory function, some of which can be quantified. Two or more skin sites can be sampled to determine the extent of proximal–distal involvement in polyneuropathy and to reduce sampling error. Sampling sites can be selected according to the patient's symptoms and results of the neurologic examination and quantitative sensory and clinical neurophysiologic testing. Epidermal nerves, presumed to be somatic sensory nerves, appear to be the most important cutaneous nerves in nonglabrous skin in relation to patient symptoms. Although not of autonomic origin, like autonomic nerves, they are small and unmyelinated, and they are often abnormal in neuropathies that have prominent autonomic features (personal observation). The innocuous nature of the skin biopsy procedure increases the probability that patients will permit a posttherapy biopsy at the completion of a therapeutic trial. Some disadvantages are the absence of somatic motor axons and deficiency of myelinated nerves. Although, autonomic motor nerves to blood vessels, arrectores pilorum muscles, and sweat glands are plentiful in skin, and the nerves of the latter two can be quantified, only sweat glands are reliably present in sufficient numbers in a 3-mm punch biopsy specimen to warrant study.

METHODS FOR QUANTIFICATION OF CUTANEOUS NERVES

Methods to quantify cutaneous nerves have improved in parallel with advances in immunohistochemistry, imaging, and computer technology. Earlier methods consisted of counting short nerve segments (22) and subjective double-blinded grading of immunohistochemically stained dermal nerves from thin (10–20 μm) sections (13,20). Computer analysis of enhanced images from the epifluorescent microscope in immunohistochemically stained skin biopsy specimens increased the reliability and accuracy of quantitation (21,27,29). Recent use of thicker sections added the advantage of increasing the sample of nerves available for study. Thick sections provide a three-dimensional perspective of skin innervation that makes it possible to distinguish nerves in the epidermis from those in the subepidermal plexus and to count the number of epidermal nerve fibers (23), measure nerve length (28), or do both, plus count the number of branch points (16). Laser scanning confocal microscope images of immunohistochemically stained 100-μm-thick sections have provided the most sharply focused images yet available (14), thereby increasing the accuracy of computer volume or surface rendering for quantification of sudomotor (18) or epidermal nerves (16,17).

ABNORMALITIES OF CUTANEOUS NERVES

Diabetic neuropathy is the condition most studied by analysis of skin biopsy specimens. The usual criterion for abnormality has been a reduction in the number of nerve fibers, either detected directly by nerve counts or grid intersections or indirectly by reduced immunofluorescence. Early in the course of diabetes mellitus, however, there appears to be increased innervation of epidermis–subepidermal plexus and sweat glands (27). Several studies have shown a later decrease of nerve fibers in the epidermis–subepidermal plexus and sweat glands that is in general proportional to the duration of diabetes and in parallel with the decreased function found by clinical, electrophysiologic, or quantitative sensory testing methods (16,20,22, 27). Kennedy et al. (16) found a reduced number of epidermal nerve fibers and reduced total epidermal nerve length in diabetic neuropathy; branching of epidermal nerves was also measured, but not found to be increased. They also measured a reduced nerve volume in sweat glands (18). Lastly, nerve counts by McCarthy et al. (23) revealed decreased epidermal nerves in skin from the lower extremities of HIV-positive and HIV-negative patients with sensory neuropathy. Altered cutaneous innervation has also been reported in leprosy (13), Raynaud's phenomena and systemic sclerosis (12), nodular prurigo (25), and psoriasis (11).

Although the number and length of cutaneous nerves appear to be the most obvious deficiencies to evaluate, other features of cutaneous innervation may be found to be important. Other potential criteria of abnormality are altered immunoreactivity, like the absence of SP-IR nerves in lepromatous neuropathy (13) or the reduced number of NPY-IR fibers in diabetic neuropathy (31); selective loss of some of the described morphologic types of epidermal nerve fibers (16); or changes in branching pattern that would be expected to accompany collateral reinnervation after selective denervation (6).

CONCLUSION

Correlation of the severity of abnormalities found in skin biopsies with those from clinical and neurophysiologic and quantitative sensory testing indicates a usefulness for skin biopsy in evaluation of peripheral nerve disease. The techniques for staining, imaging, and quantifying cutaneous nerves are continually improving. Although the importance of skin biopsy in clinical medicine is not yet firmly established, the innocuous nature of the procedure and availability of quantitative information from selected body sites indicate that skin biopsy will be increasingly important for diagnosis and has potential for follow-up evaluation of therapeutic endeavors to halt or reverse the progress of polyneuropathy.

ACKNOWLEDGMENTS

Support for this work was provided by National Institutes of Health NS 31397 and Toray Industries, Tokyo. We are grateful to Ruth Anway and Timothy Johnson for technical assistance.

REFERENCES

1. Arthur RP, Shelley WB. The innervation of human epidermis. *J Invest Dermatol* 1959;32:397–411.
2. Botezat E. Die Nerven der Epidermis. *Anat Anz* 1908;33:45–53.
3. Brelje TC, et al. Multicolor laser scanning confocal immunofluorescence microscopy: practical application and limitations. *Methods Cell Biol* 1993;38:97–181.
4. Cauna N. The free penicillate nerve endings of the human hairy skin. *J Anat* 1973;115:277–288.
5. Dalsgaard CJ, et al. Cutaneous innervation in man visualized with protein gene product 9.5 (PGP 9.5) antibodies. *Histochemistry* 1989;92:385–390.
6. Diamond J, et al. Endogenous NGF and nerve impulses regulate the collateral sprouting of sensory axons in the skin of the adult rat. *J Neurosci* 1992;12:1454–1466.
7. Hashimoto K. The ultrastructure of the skin of human embryos. *J Anat* 1972;111:99–120.
8. Hilliges M, et al. Ultrastructural evidence for nerve fibers within all vital layers of the human epidermis. *J Invest Dermatol* 1995;104:134–137.
9. Holthofer H, et al. *Ulex europaeus* I lectin as a marker for vascular endothelium in human tissues. *Lab Invest* 1982; 47:60–66.
10. Hosoi J, et al. Regulation of Langerhans cell function by nerves containing calcitonin gene-related peptide. *Nature* 1993;363:159–163.
11. Johansson O, et al. Altered cutaneous innervation in psoriatic skin as revealed by PGP 9.5 immunohistochemistry. *Arch Dermatol Res* 1991;283:519–523.
12. Karanth SS, et al. An immunocytochemical study of cutaneous innervation and the distribution of neuropeptides and protein gene product 9.5 in man and commonly employed laboratory animals. *Am J Anat* 1991;191:369–383.
13. Karanth SS, et al. Changes in nerves and neuropeptides in skin from 100 leprosy patients investigated by cytochemistry. *J Pathol* 1989;157:15–26.
14. Kennedy WR, Wendelschafer-Crabb G. The innervation of human epidermis. *J Neurosci* 1993;115:184–190.
15. Kennedy WR, et al. Innervation and vasculature of human sweat glands: an immunohistochemistry–laser scanning confocal fluorescence microscopy study. *J Neurosci* 1994; 14(II Pt 2):6825–6833.
16. Kennedy WR, et al. Quantitation of epidermal nerves in diabetic neuropathy. *Neurology* 1996;47:1042–1048.
17. Kennedy WR, et al. Classification of epidermal nerves. *Neurology* 1996;46(Suppl):A287(abst).
18. Kennedy WR, et al. Quantitative study of nerves in sweat glands in normal and diabetic subjects. *Ann Neurol* 1993;34:269–270.
19. Lacour JP, et al. Anatomical mapping of Merkel cells in human adult epidermis. *Br J Dermatol* 1991;125:535–542.
20. Levy DM, et al. Depletion of cutaneous nerves and neuropeptides in diabetes mellitus: an immunocytochemical study. *Diabetologia* 1989; 32:427–433.
21. Levy DM, et al. Immunohistochemical measurements of nerves and neuropeptides in diabetic skin: relationship to tests of neurological function. *Diabetologia* 1992;35:889–897.
22. Lindberger M, et al. Nerve fibre studies in skin biopsies in peripheral neuropathies. *J Neurol Sci* 1989;93:289–296.
23. McCarthy BG, et al. Cutaneous innervation in sensory neuropathies. *Neurology* 1995;45:1848–1855.
24. Mills LR, Diamond J. Merkel cells are not the mechanosensory transducers in the touch dome of the rat. *J Neurocytol* 1994;24:117–134.
25. Molina FA, et al. Increased sensory neuropeptides in nodular prurigo: a quantitative immunohistochemical analysis. *Br J Dermatol* 1992;127:344–351.
26. Novotny GEK, Gomert-Novotny E. Intraepidermal nerves in human digital skin. *Cell Tissue Res* 1988;254:111–117.
27. Properzi G, et al. Early increase precedes a depletion of VIP and PGP 9.5 in the skin of insulin dependent diabetics: correlation between quantitative immunohistochemistry and clinical assessment of peripheral neuropathy. *J Pathol* 1993;169:269–277.
28. Stocks EA, et al. Steriological estimation of epidermal nerve fibers in normal human skin. *Soc Neurosci Abstr* 1994;20:701.
29. Terenghi G, et al. Image analysis quantification of peptide-immunoreactive nerves in the skin of patients with Raynaud's phenomenon and systemic sclerosis. *J Pathol* 1991;164:245–257.
30. Thompson RJ, Day INM. Protein gene product 9.5: a new neuronal and neuroendocrine marker. In: Marangos PJ, Campbell R, Cohen M, eds. *Neuronal and glial proteins: structure, function and clinical application.* CA: Academic, 1988:209–228 (Neurobiological research; vol 2).
31. Wallengren J, et al. Innervation of the skin of the forearm in diabetic patients: relation to nerve function. *Acta Derm Venereol (Stockh)* 1995;75:37.
32. Wang L, et al. Protein gene product 9.5-immunoreactive nerve fibres and cells in human skin. *Cell Tissue Res* 1990;261:25–33.
33. Zamboni L, de Martino C. Buffered picric acid formaldehyde: a new rapid fixative for electron microscopy. *J Cell Biol* 1967;35:148A (abst).

CHAPTER 10

Autonomic Regulation of Urinary Bladder

William E. Bradley and Claire C. Yang

---

1. Most observations of urinary bladder physiology, pharmacology, and innervation have been made in experimental animals, and there is a paucity of human data. Whether it is appropriate to freely infer human function from animal findings must be the subject of future research.
2. Newer diagnostic methods, such as evoked-potential testing of bladder neural pathways and ambulatory cystometric monitoring, in conjunction with magnetic resonance imaging studies of the central nervous system (CNS), have begun to develop information on human bladder function. It is anticipated that initial studies may be disappointing and that persistence is necessary.
3. The principal location of areas in the CNS concerned with bladder innervation include the frontal cortex, the rostral lateral portion of the pontine tegmentum, and portions of the gray matter of the conus medullaris. The bulk of information on these areas has been gained from animal experimentation, and it will be necessary to apply the new methodologies of diagnosis to define them in humans.
4. The crucial event in the initiation of normal voiding is a coordinated detrusor reflex contraction, with a resultant smooth, sustained rise in intravesical pressure and concurrent relaxation of the external urinary sphincter.
5. The mechanism that coordinates detrusor muscle contraction to evoke dilation of the proximal urethra and total evacuation of intravesical content is undefined.
6. There are four reflex pathways that are crucial to the innervation and neural control of the urinary bladder. Relays between the frontal cortex and the pontine detrusor nucleus constitute the first reflex pathway or loop and represent the mechanism underlying volitional control of bladder function. The second loop, or reflex pathway, consists of long-routed sensory axons extending from the urinary detrusor and ascending in the spinal cord to synapse in the pontine detrusor nucleus. From this nucleus, axons descend in the spinal cord to innervate the smooth muscle cells of the urinary bladder. The third reflex pathway, or loop, consists of afferent sensory axons originating from the bladder and passing into the conus medullaris to synapse on motor neurons in the pudendal nuclei. The fourth reflex pathway is composed of the supraspinal and segmental innervation of the striated muscle cells of the external urinary sphincter. Further work employing newer diagnostic methods is necessary to define those pathways derived from animal experimentation.

INTRODUCTION

During the past decade, considerable experimental data have accumulated concerning urinary bladder function. The bulk of these studies have been conducted in experimental animals. The early investigators of urinary bladder function were concerned about the accuracy of the analogy between human and animal voiding, and considered the fastidious behavior of domestic cats similar to that of humans (5) (Ruch, personal communication, 1965). More recently, animal research has shifted from cats to laboratory rats. Whether bladder function in rats, with undocumented voiding behavior, is analogous to that in humans awaits further study. Certainly the human urinary bladder, deriving innervation from a five-lumbar and five-sacral segment spinal cord, is neurologically distinct from any animal species currently used for investigation. Moreover, the location of the urinary bladder in the bony pelvis of the biped human is anatomically different from that in the quadruped animal.

W. E. Bradley and C. C. Yang: Departments of Urology and Neurology, University of Washington, Seattle, Washington 98108.

In this chapter on human anatomy, physiology, and pharmacology of the urinary bladder, the authors would prefer to cite only human data. However, the paucity of human studies on normal bladder function and the necessary limitations of the study techniques compel use of animal data. Further, there are areas of interest, such as the brainstem and spinal innervation of the bladder, that are not accessible to observation in human studies. Human data are also frequently altered by the presence of pathologic conditions that obscure physiologic conclusions.

New methods have appeared to facilitate greater understanding of the physiology of voiding in humans. These include ultrasound studies of bladder emptying (84) as well as electrophysiologic techniques for documenting bladder innervation (12). Other new methods include ambulatory monitoring of bladder function (7) and transcranial magnetic stimulation of the cerebral cortex to define brain innervation of the external urinary sphincter (33). When the results of these methods are combined with the clinical neurologic examination, insight into normal and abnormal function of the human urinary bladder is increased (78,91). The following reviews offer further information on the anatomy, physiology, and pharmacology of urinary bladder function in both experimental animals and humans (11,28, 35,56,90,108).

Early studies of urinary bladder function included those by Mosso and Pellacani (71) and by Denny-Brown and Robertson (29). Denny-Brown and Robertson, using bladder-filling techniques described in part by Mosso and Pellacani, observed reflex contractions during bladder distention in humans. These contractions, which registered as increases in intravesical pressure, were recorded in response to the retrograde infusion of water through a urethral catheter. This technique, along with the contributions of other investigators, and termed *cystometry* (34), represented a significant advance in the clinical evaluation of bladder function. Cystometry defined the contribution of the smooth muscle component of the bladder, the urinary detrusor, in voiding. The method confirmed the findings of Barrington (5) in cats that detrusor reflex contraction to bladder filling represented the initial step in a series of complex reflex events that constitute the voiding of intravesical contents. However, to assess the role of urethral contraction and relaxation in providing a conduit for the expulsion of urine and prevention of urinary leakage required the development of later methods (1,9).

Use of these methods and other forms of assessment in patients with neurologic diseases suggested a hierarchy of nervous system influences on urinary bladder function (11,28,35,56,90,108). The areas of the central nervous system (CNS) specifically defined in bladder innervation included the cerebral cortex in humans (3) and cats (8,57), the pons in cats (5), and the conus medullaris in humans (11). Similar findings between cat and human investigations encouraged and facilitated the application of evoked-potential studies to identify the pathways of these nuclei in humans (44,47).

Finally, there are beginnings of attempts by urologists to incorporate the skills of the neurologist and the results of the clinical neurologic examination in the interpretation of testing results. Perhaps the latter development is of greater significance than improvements in technology.

CEREBROCORTICAL INNERVATION OF THE URINARY BLADDER

The role of the cerebral cortex in the control of urinary bladder function has been investigated in both experimental animals and in humans. Experiments in cats have used stimulation and ablation (11). Electrical stimulation of the sensorimotor cortex of cats resulted in bladder contraction, whereas stimulation of areas of the limbic system resulted in relaxation (38). Ablation of the sensorimotor cortex of cats had previously resulted in lowered-threshold detrusor reflex contractions (57).

Electrical stimulation of the cerebral cortex and its effect on urinary bladder function in humans has not been investigated. However, the effects of neurologic lesions of the frontal lobes on detrusor function have been documented. Patients with lesions of the anteroinferior portion of the prefrontal area exhibit an unsuppressible or uncontrollable detrusor reflex contraction on bladder filling, known as *detrusor hyperreflexia* (6).

Evoked-potential studies of the cerebral cortex in humans have included electrical stimulation of the pelvic urethral nerve (47) and the dorsal nerve of the penis (44). Stimulation of the pelvic nerve in the urethra was performed using a concentric-ring electrode mounted on an indwelling catheter (94,95). Stimulation of the dorsal nerve of the penis, a terminal sensory division of the pudendal nerve, was accomplished by transcutaneous electrical stimulation. Diphasic responses to stimulation were recorded in the central vertex (pelvic nerve) and 2 cm posterior to the central vertex (dorsal nerve of the penis). The latency of the pudendal cortical evoked response was ~42 msec, and the latency of the pelvic nerve responses was approximately two-thirds longer. Earlier studies in cats that assessed responses recorded in the exposed cerebral cortex evoked by electrical stimulation of the pelvic detrusor nerves and pudendal urethral nerves identified a specific area in the sensorimotor cortex responsible for both responses. This area was similar for both nerves and was in the posteromedial aspect of the sensorimotor cortex (8).

The initial reports of scalp recorded responses evoked by stimulation of the vesicourethral junction provide for development of clinical studies to assess this pathway.

Electroencephalographic (EEG) responses to bladder filling in humans have been reported (10,51), suggesting the participation of the cerebral cortex in detrusor function. Polysomnographic studies of sleep and bladder function have been reported for enuretics (79). Unfortunately, brain activity in these studies was recorded from a single parietal EEG electrode. This form of evaluation merits further trial in patients with problems associated with the cerebral control of voiding.

The recording of downstream influences by responses evoked in the external urinary sphincter by transcranial magnetic stimulation of the motor cortex (33) may be useful for identifying the cerebral innervation of the urethra. The method requires stimulation of the motor neurons located on the medial aspect of the sensorimotor cortex in the interhemispheric cleft. This is difficult to perform in some patients and does not define the laterality of innervation.

Finally, the initial attempts to correlate magnetic resonance imaging (MRI) and computed tomographic findings in patients with acute cerebrovascular occlusion and bladder function studies confirm the prior predictions of the influence of the cerebral cortex upon the urinary bladder.

BASAL GANGLIA AND BLADDER FUNCTION

The basal ganglia have been a subject of interest in the study of bladder innervation since the original observation that patients with Parkinson's disease exhibited abnormal cystometric findings, the most striking of which was detrusor hyperreflexia (73). The precise manner in which lesions of the basal ganglia in humans cause bladder dysfunction or affect normal function is unknown. However, electrical stimulation of different areas in the basal ganglia in cats suppresses spontaneous detrusor reflex contractions (60,61). Subsequent electrophysiologic studies have suggested that detrusor reflex suppression is relayed in part through the pons (85).

THE LIMBIC SYSTEM AND URINARY BLADDER FUNCTION

The influence of the limbic system on urinary bladder function in humans is unknown. Electrical stimulation of different areas of the limbic system in cats has evoked both contraction and relaxation of the urinary bladder (38).

THE THALAMUS AND URINARY BLADDER INNERVATION

The thalamic nuclei are most probably involved in the relay of both pelvic detrusor and pudendal afferent impulses to the cerebral cortex. However, no information is available either for experimental animals or for humans that confirms this conclusion.

CEREBELLAR CONTROL OF BLADDER FUNCTION

There have been clinical reports of urinary bladder symptoms in patients with cerebellar disease (32). A range of cystometric findings in such patients includes detrusor hyperreflexia and detrusor areflexia (58). Understanding the role of the cerebellum in regulating the detrusor reflex and its interaction with the external urinary sphincter in humans has been impeded by the dearth of clinical studies. Correlating neurologic examination findings with MRI and bladder function test findings in patients with cerebellar disease could help define the respective influence of the cerebellar hemispheres and the midline structures. The development of evoked-potential studies for measuring the integrity of afferent pathways to the cerebellum would also help.

Studies in cats using electrical stimulation of the pelvic detrusor nerves and pudendal urethral nerves have confirmed the presence of direct afferent pathways to the anterior vermis (16,17). These pathways have been characterized by tracer studies of spinocerebellar axons obtained from the sacrococcygeal region of cats that project to the anterior vermis (111). Electrical stimulation of the fastigial nucleus of decerebrated cats suppresses spontaneous detrusor reflex contractions, whereas ablation of the anterior vermis and fastigial nuclei accentuates detrusor reflex contractions (16,17). These experiments have demonstrated direct pathways that extend from the anterior vermis and the fastigial nuclei to the pontine nuclei for detrusor contraction. In later experiments conducted in dogs (77), detrusor reflex hyperactivity and coordinated relaxation of the external urethral sphincter were observed following decerebration and cerebellectomy. This finding is surprising in view of the repeated observations that cerebellectomy in decerebrate dogs evokes profound spasticity of the extremities (32). Cerebellectomy would be expected to cause spasticity of the external urethral sphincter and an incoordinate or dyssynergic response to bladder contraction.

The actual effect of a clinical cerebellar deficit on bladder function therefore remains unknown. Intensive human and animal research could give insight into the role of the cerebellum in the control of voiding.

INNERVATION OF THE URINARY BLADDER BY THE PONTINE NUCLEI

The pontine nuclei innervating the urinary bladder in cats have been a subject of research for ~80 years. Whether detrusor reflex contractions in the urinary bladder of humans in response to bladder filling are organized in the dorsolateral tegmentum of the pons in a manner analogous to that found in experimental animals is unknown. There have been only preliminary reports of bladder dysfunction in patients with pontine lesions (54), and no neuropathologic studies of patients with pontine lesions and bladder dysfunction are available.

The rostral and lateral pontine area in the nucleus locus coeruleus is the crucial site for the appearance of detrusor reflex contraction evoked by bladder distention in cats and rats (5,62,96,97,104). In rats, the nuclei for detrusor contraction consist of a complex near the locus coeruleus, but the location of the pontine nucleus for detrusor contraction has not been identified in primates.

There are bilateral descending projections from homologous pontine nuclei to the intermediolateral cell column of the sacral spinal cord (62,96,97,104). These pathways have been established in animals by tracer studies and by recordings of responses evoked in detrusor motor axons by microelectrode stimulation of the pontine nuclei (80). Extracellular microelectrode recordings in the rostral lateral pons and caudal mesencephalon of cats have documented unit responses that were evoked by bladder filling and detrusor reflex contractions (13).

The pharmacologic characteristics of these spinal descending pathways have been investigated in cats. Hydroxydopamine, a catecholamine toxin, was injected bilaterally into the nucleus locus coeruleus of cats (112) and produced reduced catecholamine levels in the injected tissue and detrusor areflexia. The subsequent intrathecal injection of phenylephrine, an α-adrenergic agonist, in the same animals restored detrusor reflex responses. The investigators concluded that the nucleus locus coeruleus in cats is the site of origin of descending adrenergic transmitter pathways to detrusor motor neurons in the sacral spinal cord.

The afferent pathways from the bladder to the pontine nuclei have been defined in cats by electrophysiologic investigations (20,28a), which have indicated that the bulk of bladder afferents are long-routed from their point of entry in the sacral spinal cord to the pontine nuclei. These afferents evoke responses in the pontine nuclei, which descend to elicit efferent impulses in the detrusor motor axons. Electrical stimulation of detrusor afferent axons in cats has confirmed the presence of a long-latency, long-duration evoked response abolished by spinal cord transection. Activation of axons in this spinobulbospinal pathway by bladder distention is crucial to the appearance of a detrusor reflex contraction.

The rostral routing of pathways from the dorsolateral pontine tegmentum has not been studied in conjunction with urinary bladder function. Several pathways from both the nucleus locus coeruleus and proximal areas have been identified by tracer studies (37,52,93). One pathway consisted of axons that contain the immunoreactive peptide substance P and were traced to the mediofrontal cortex. Other noradrenergic-containing axons were found to be extensively distributed to all areas of the cerebral cortex. Cholinergic axons from the dorsolateral pontine tegmentum were traced to the thalamic nuclei, particularly the nonspecific group, as well as to the nucleus dorsomedialis (52).

Future investigation of bladder function in patients with pontine lesions anatomically defined by neurologic examination, MRI and, where available, by postmortem study would help define the function of these nuclei in humans. Evoked-response studies of the spinobulbospinal pathways in animals that might lead to the development of a comparable clinical technique would be particularly helpful.

The proximity of detrusor motor nuclei in the pontine tegmentum to other areas of the reticular formation for the innervation of the external urethral sphincter has been described in cats (56,63). Stimulation of these sphincter-innervating areas evokes electromyographic responses in the external urethral sphincter. Similarly, rises in intravesical pressure elicited by stimulation of the pontine detrusor nuclei have been evoked in an area immediately medial and distinct from that innervating the external urethral sphincter. Animal experiments that define the external urinary sphincter response to decerebration at the intercollicular level would help delineate brainstem function in bladder sphincter coordination. Stimulation of nuclei close to the midline of the medulla in cats evoked monosynaptic excitatory postsynaptic potentials of pudendal motor neurons innervating the external urinary sphincter (63).

ASCENDING AND DESCENDING SPINAL TRACTS FROM THE PELVIC AND PUDENDAL NUCLEI IN THE CONUS MEDULLARIS

The principal afferent and efferent reticulospinal pathways from detrusor motor neurons in the conus medullaris have been identified in patient studies (75,76,92). These tracts were found in the posterior superficial portion of the lateral columns. The spinal pathways for innervation of the external urinary sphincter have not been identified in humans, but they can be assumed to resemble the organization of skeletal muscle, with ascending pathways in the posterior columns and descending tracts in the corticospinal and reticulospinal pathways.

The correlation of clinical findings and the results of bladder function have been utilized in patients with cervical myelopathy. The results are similar to those of previous studies, including the conclusion that ascending pathways are located in the dorsal columns (92).

THE PELVIC AND PUDENDAL NUCLEI OF THE CONUS MEDULLARIS

The anatomy and physiology of the pelvic and pudendal nuclei in the conus medullaris have been explored in humans and experimental animals (18,70,103,107). Methods applied to animals have included both electrophysiologic techniques and tracer studies using horseradish peroxidase (69,70,103) and radioactive proline (74). Methods employed in humans have included neural blocks (88), electrodiagnostic techniques (2,22), histologic examination of postmortem material (100), and the correlation of laboratory findings with the results of neurologic examination (102). By comparing and contrasting data in humans and experimental animals, a concept of the organization of somatic and visceral nuclei is emerging.

The principal nuclei innervating the urinary bladder of cats consist of motor neurons located in the gray matter of the intermediolateral cell column of the sacral spinal cord and motor neurons in the ventral gray matter of the sacral spinal cord in the region of Onuf's nucleus (66,83). The rostral caudal or longitudinal distribution of detrusor nuclei in cats and primates has been found to range from L7 to S2 (82,89).

Horseradish-peroxidase tracer studies of the pelvic nerve in cats have revealed the existence of both segmental and ascending pathways in the sacral spinal cord (70,71, 103). After penetrating Lissauer's tract, a lateral collateral axonal pathway travels to the parasympathetic preganglionic neurons in the intermediolateral cell column. A medial collateral axonal pathway travels to the region of the dorsal commissure. Previous electrophysiologic studies (20,28a) suggested that the bulk of the afferent axons, crucial to the development of the detrusor reflex by activation of the spinobulbospinal pathway, are found in the medial collateral pathway.

The detrusor nucleus in the sacral spinal cord of cats extends 10 mm in the rostral caudal direction, with the bulk of the motor neurons at S2. This would correspond to the S4 segment in humans. The cells of the detrusor nucleus in cats are spindle shaped and located in the gray matter, corresponding to Rexed's laminae V through VII.

The afferent connections to the detrusor nuclei have been demonstrated electrophysiologically in cats (18). Short-latency responses in the detrusor motor nerves were evoked by stimulation of the pudendal urethral nerves.

In humans, sacral nerve blocks have revealed that the detrusor nucleus has a rostral caudal extension going from the S3 to S4 segments that depends on the presence of pre- or postfixation (88). The precise intramedullary location of detrusor motor neurons and their histologic characteristics in the sacral spinal cord have not been described. Sung (100) used as a marker the abnormal intracellular lipid collections in the autonomic neurons found in patients with Fabry's disease, and concluded that Onuf's nucleus in the ventral gray matter of the sacral spinal cord of humans was the site of autonomic neurons innervating the pelvic viscera. This has not correlated with the consistent results of animal studies, however. Perhaps this finding should be accepted as further evidence of the unusual nature of the neurons making up Onuf's nucleus.

The pudendal nuclei in animals and humans have been identified in the location described by Onuf (66,81,83, 103).

Animal studies have included the injection of horseradish peroxidase into the external urinary sphincter (103). The inputs and outputs from the nuclei have been traced by evoked-potential studies (18). In cats, the pudendal nuclei have been found in the ventrolateral gray matter of the S2 segment (103). The longitudinal distribution of the nucleus extends from the caudal portion of the L7 segment to the S2 segment, with maximal density of motor neurons at the S1 segment. In this study, a unimodal dimensional pattern of neurons was observed, which the authors believed to be consistent with an exclusive α motor neuron innervation of the external urinary sphincter. The absence of γ motor neurons was associated with the paucity of muscle spindles in the external sphincter (41,67).

Evoked-potential studies in cats have identified pelvic detrusor afferent axons that synapse on pudendal urethral motor neurons, as well as ipsilateral pudendal urethral afferent axons that synapse on contralateral pudendal urethral motor neurons (18). The stimulation of pelvic detrusor afferents on identified pudendal motor neurons caused the exclusive development of inhibitory postsynaptic potentials (11).

The rostral innervation of the pudendal nuclei has been documented by the stimulation of neurons in the medulla (63) as well as by the tracing of axons from the cerebral cortex (74). This latter study consisted of autoradiographic studies of corticospinal tract neurons extending from the tail portion of area 4 of primates to Onuf's nucleus. The studies indicated bilateral innervation of the pudendal nuclei from ipsilateral cortical neurons.

In humans, evoked-potential studies constitute the principal technique for defining the pathways of the pudendal nucleus. These have included transcutaneous stimulation of the dorsal nerve of the penis, which is the terminal sensory portion of the pudendal nerve. This evokes a contractile response in the bulbocavernosus muscle (30) and the anal sphincter (2). The latencies of responses in these muscles were measured by electromyography, either by a concentric-needle electrode or by a surface electrode placed near the muscle.

The conduction velocity of the dorsal nerve of the penis can be measured (14,53) and excludes the possibility of pudendal neuropathy as a factor in errors in latency measurements of pudendal evoked responses. Stimulation of pudendal nerve afferents in the urethra by indwelling catheters with concentric rings has been employed to evoke responses in the anal sphincter (2,12,22). The latency of evoked responses in the pudendal innervation of the anal sphincter has also been measured by stimulation of the urinary detrusor (2). An important finding in these studies has been the suppression of the pudendal evoked response by increasing bladder distention (12). The cerebrocortical pathway to pudendal motor neurons innervating the external urinary sphincter has also been defined by transcranial magnetic stimulation (9). The effect of cortical lesions on the tone of the anal sphincter has not been delineated in clinical reports.

THORACOLUMBAR SPINAL INNERVATION OF THE URINARY DETRUSOR AND URETHRA

A considerable body of evidence (35,108) indicates that the thoracolumbar spinal cord of cats sends axons to the detrusor muscle and urethra (68). This innervation, which is similar to that in humans and is derived from sympathetic motor neurons extending from T12 to L2, is believed to furnish a number of responses to bladder filling. These responses include depression of transmission through the pelvic ganglia (105), relaxation of the detrusor muscle through activation of β-adrenergic receptors, and increased tonus in the smooth muscle of the urethra through stimulation of α-adrenergic receptors. There is, however, less-compelling evidence that the sympathetic nervous system plays more than a minor role in the function of the human urinary bladder. The observations by Learmonth (59) and Wein et al. (108) indicate that surgical ablation of the sympathetic innervation of the bladder in humans does not have a measurable effect on detrusor reflex function. Hence, bladder function in humans depends on the anatomic and functional integrity of the parasympathetic and somatic innervation of the urinary bladder.

REFLEX PATHWAYS OF MICTURITION

For clinical considerations, the CNS innervation of the urinary bladder is visualized as composed of four interacting loops or reflex arcs (11).

The axonal pathways of the first loop consist of a reflex arc that extends from the pontine nucleus to the dorsomedial aspect of the frontal lobe. Lesions of the frontal lobes and of the basal ganglia result in detrusor hyperreflexia or inability to suppress the detrusor reflex on command during the cystometric examination (Fig. 1). Loop I lesions in humans release the pontine nucleus from volitional control. The axonal pathways of loop I have been defined by tracer studies in animals (37,52,93). Similar studies in humans will require evoked-potential studies, MRI, and correlation with the neurologic examination findings and results of bladder function tests.

The spinobulbospinal pathway that goes from the urinary bladder to the pontine nucleus and returns to detrusor motor axons constitutes loop II, or the second crucial reflex (see Fig. 1). This pathway has been well defined in experimental animals by using electrophysiologic and tracer methods (11). Ruch (personal communication, 1965) suggested that this routing of bladder sensory afferents provided for gain or amplification of the time course of the detrusor reflex contraction. The evidence for interruption of this pathway in humans is the presence of detrusor hyperreflexia. There is no currently known method that can define abbreviation of detrusor reflex contraction.

A third important pathway, consisting of pelvic detrusor afferents to the pudendal nucleus, has been defined in experimental animals (59) and in humans (12) (Fig. 2). In cats, bladder distention affects detrusor reflex activity by invoking inhibition of pudendal motor neuron impulses (18,21). In humans, the suppression of an evoked urethroanal sphincter response by bladder distention represents a similar effect (12).

The fourth important reflex circuit consists of the supraspinal and segmental innervation of the external urinary sphincter (Fig. 3). The afferent pathway of the supra-

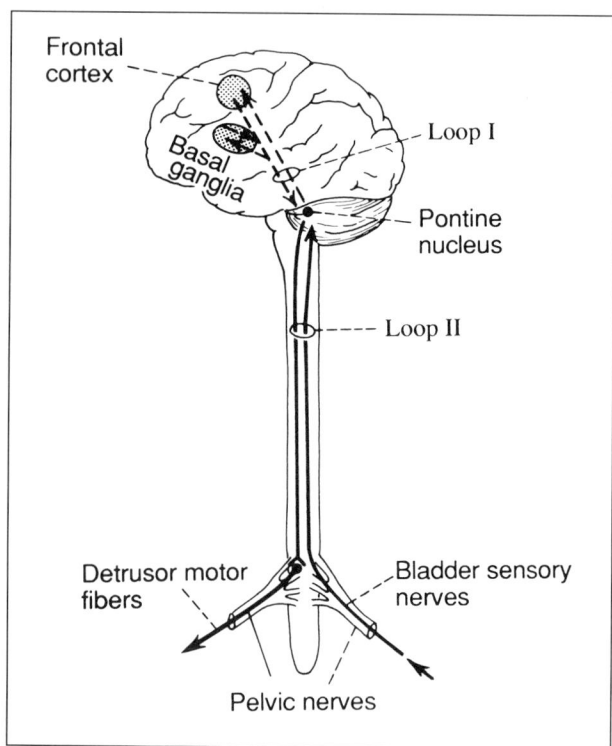

FIG. 1. Loops, or reflex pathways, I and II are the cerebral and spinal neural networks, respectively, for innervation of the smooth muscle of the urinary detrusor. Loop I consists of the cerebral pathways innervating the pontine detrusor nucleus. These include the frontomedial portion of the cerebral cortex as well as the basal ganglia and other subcortical nuclei. Loop II consists of long-routed sensory axons that extend from the urinary detrusor to the pontine detrusor nucleus. Descending axons from the pons synapse in the intermediolateral cell column of the sacral spinal cord. Motor axons transit from the detrusor nuclei in the sacral spinal cord to synapse in the pelvic ganglia, and course as postganglionic motor axons to innervate smooth muscle cells in the bladder.

spinal portion of this loop can be tested by measuring the latency of the cortical evoked response during stimulation of the dorsal nerve of the penis (44). The integrity of the descending limb can be evaluated by transcranial magnetic stimulation of the motor cortex (33). The segmental portion of this reflex can be identified by stimulation of the pudendal afferent innervation of the urethra (12) or of the dorsal nerve of the penis and measuring the latency of the response evoked in the anal sphincter (2).

PERIPHERAL INNERVATION OF THE URINARY BLADDER

In animals and humans, the neuroanatomic innervation of the urinary detrusor consists of axons in the hypogastric nerves originating in the thoracolumbar spinal cord and of axons in the pelvic nerve. The pelvic nerves formed from the S2 to S4 ventral roots in humans combine with the hy-

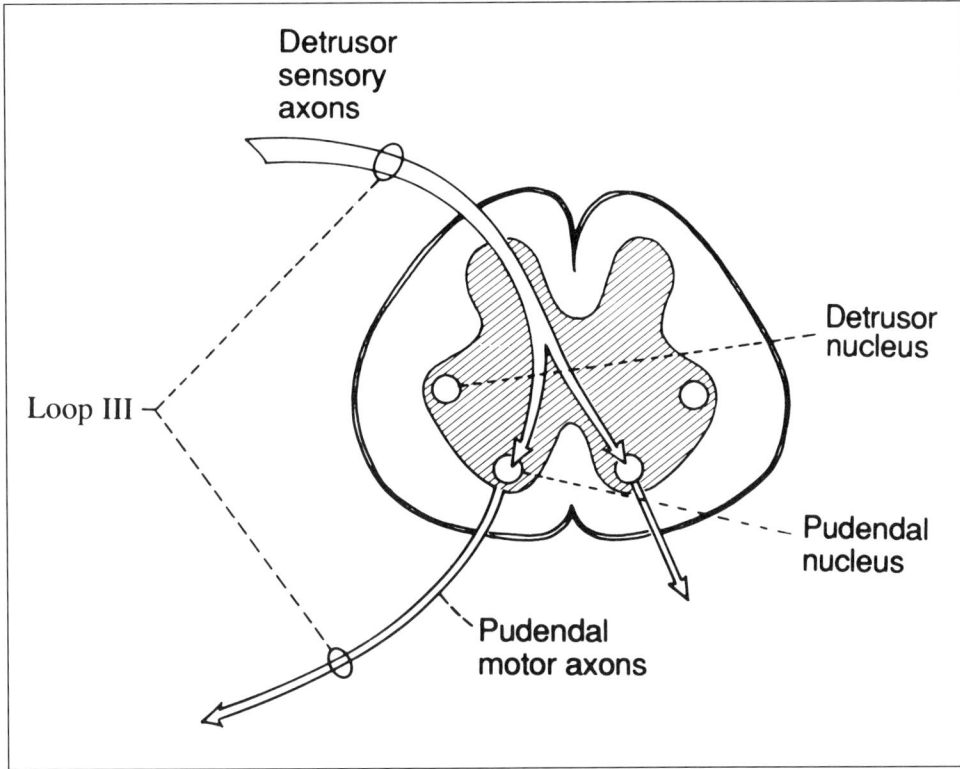

FIG. 2. Loop, or reflex pathway, III comprises bladder afferents that convey sensory impulses to motor neurons in the pudendal nuclei in the sacral spinal cord. The sensory input from the urinary bladder evoked by increasing distention suppresses tonic motor impulses in the pudendal motor axons innervating the external urinary sphincter.

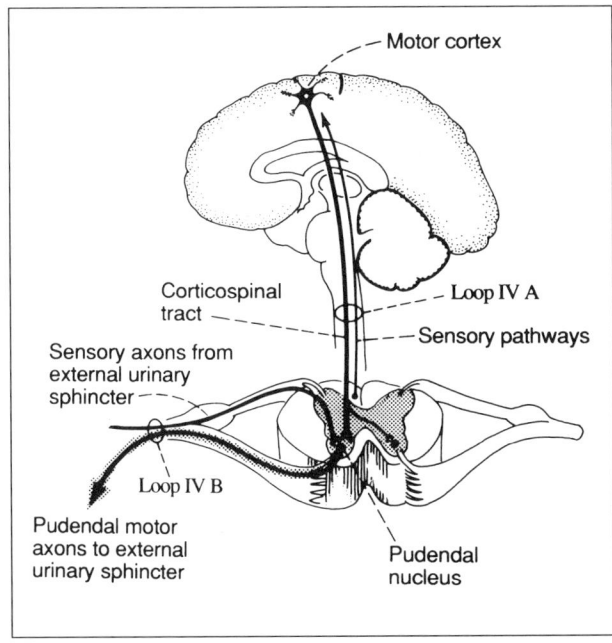

FIG. 3. Loops, or reflex pathways, IV A and IV B represent the supraspinal and segmental innervation, respectively, of the external urinary sphincter.

pogastric nerves to form the pelvic plexus and, more distally, the vesical plexus (35). Axons from the vesical plexus innervate the bladder and urethra. The pudendal axons originate from the sacral plexus and innervate the external urinary sphincter and penis, or clitoris. The preganglionic axonal input from the vesical and prostatic plexuses innervates ganglia as the axons follow a tortuous course in the smooth muscle bundles of the urinary detrusor (19,31,86). The preganglionic input terminates at axodendritic and occasional axosomatic synapses on neurons in the ganglia. Most sympathetic axons synapse in the hypogastric plexus, whereas the preganglionic parasympathetic axons synapse in ganglia located in the pelvic plexus and intramural ganglia. There are two types of neurons in the ganglia—cholinergic and adrenergic (45)—but the population of cholinergic neurons is greater than that of adrenergic neurons. The ganglia are situated principally in the area of the trigone and bladder neck.

The axons that innervate the urinary detrusor are rarely myelinated. Motor axons have been identified in the dorsal roots and afferent axons have been found in the ventral roots of cats (24). Whether this arrangement exists in humans, and to what extent, is unknown. In addition to preganglionic input, neurons in the isolated pelvic ganglion of rats receive afferent sensory input that synapses on postganglionic neurons (87). There does not appear to be an underlying anatomic mechanism for the coordination of detrusor muscle contraction (106), although there is physiologic evidence of this in cats (25). The coordination of detrusor muscle contraction during voiding is an important concept that warrants investigation in humans.

Intraganglionic events have been analyzed electrophysiologically in the isolated pelvic ganglion of rats (86) and in cat vesical ganglia (42). Responses in postganglionic axons as well as intracellular neural responses have been recorded following stimulation of preganglionic axons. Pelvic nerve ganglionic transmission is cholinergic, and shows blockade of synaptic transmission following the administration of anticholinergic agents (42). Postganglionic responses are facilitated after repetitive stimulation of preganglionic input. Stimulation of the hypogastric nerve depresses pelvic ganglion transmission (19,98). This depression is attributed to activation of intraganglionic adrenoreceptors (46,105).

As the postganglionic axons continue in the smooth muscle of the urinary detrusor, free nerve endings appear. Based on the results of dorsal rhizotomy and the resultant degeneration experiments done in cats, these are believed to be sensory nerve endings (106). There is no morphologic distinction between the sensory ending and the conducting axon (43,64,65). There are also occasional pacinian corpuscles. Pacinian corpuscles are innervated by noradrenergic fibers in cats (55). In humans, acetylcholinesterase-positive nerve endings in the submucosa of the urinary detrusor and urethra have been tentatively identified as sensory endings (39). These endings are more abundant in the region of the trigone.

The motor innervation of the smooth muscle cells of the urinary detrusor is accomplished by postganglionic axons originating from the pelvic ganglia. The neuromuscular unit is less specialized than that in striated muscle. Swellings or varicosities appear in the terminal axons. The vesicles in the varicosities contain neurotransmitters. The vesicles in the axonal varicosities of the human urinary detrusor muscle contain acetylcholine, and an adrenergic agent (15,40,99), and the neural impulses in the postganglionic axon that occur during reflex responses evoke the release of the neurotransmitter by exocytosis from a synapse *en passage.* The neurotransmitter diffuses into a domain of the smooth muscle cells (35). Dependent on the level of excitability of an individual smooth muscle cell, there is cell depolarization and contraction (26). The principal neurotransmitter that evokes contraction in the urinary detrusor of humans is acetylcholine (15,99). Potassium channel openers have been described in the guinea-pig urinary bladder and may modulate excitability (48).

The urinary bladder consists of a rostral portion, the urinary detrusor, and the trigone, which is near the posterior bladder neck. The bladder neck and urethra serve as a conduit for the expulsion of intravesical contents through the external urinary meatus.

The human urinary detrusor is arranged in three layers (109,110): an outer layer of connective tissue, a middle layer of smooth muscle arranged in a collagen framework (101), and an inner layer consisting of a submucosal stroma on which rests a mucosal layer of transitional epithelium. There is a rich blood supply (50).

The trigone is a distinct area in the posterior bladder base. It is defined by the ureteral entry zones and the bladder neck, and consists of dense collagen and a deep portion that is a continuation of the detrusor muscle. The trigone transmits contraction of the urinary detrusor to facilitate opening of the proximal urethra and provides traction on the ureter to prevent vesicoureteral reflux during voiding.

The urinary detrusor muscle bundles form arcades or loops as they descend toward the bladder base. These loops consist of a trigonal loop and a detrusor loop at the bladder base, with their concavities facing in opposite directions (109,110). Upon detrusor muscle contraction of the rostral detrusor bundles, there is separation of the arcades or loops and passage of intravesical urine into the proximal urethra.

Studies of the collagen architecture of the human urinary detrusor muscle utilizing scanning electron microscopy have confirmed an extensive distribution of fibers through the mucosal layer and smooth muscle fascicles. There was evidence of separation and investment of individual smooth muscle fascicles such that fascicles could perform individual contraction (50,72).

The urethra in the male consists of a preprostatic, prostatic, and membranous portion, as well as the penile urethra (39). The urethra is composed of layers of smooth muscle in a collagen framework similar to that of the urinary detrusor. In the region of the membranous urethra of humans, there is striated muscle, which is divided into an intramural portion and an extramural portion. The intramural aspect has been designated the *external urethral sphincter* and, histochemically, is of the slow-twitch fiber type. The extramural portion is referred to as the *periurethral striated muscle,* and is derived from the proximal fibers of the levator ani; histochemically it is made up of both slow- and fast-twitch fibers (41). Muscle spindles are rarely seen in the human external urinary sphincter, similar to observations made in cats (67).

The female urethra extends from the bladder neck to the external urinary meatus. It descends from a site posterior to the pubic symphysis and travels in the anterior wall of the vagina for a distance of ~4 cm. The female urethra is composed of smooth muscle bundles in a dense collagen framework (4,27,49). The organization and concentration of collagen and smooth muscle have been defined in cats by stereomorphometry. The striated muscle sphincter is less well developed than that in males and is deficient posteriorly. The urethral sensory and motor innervation consists of pelvic and hypogastric nerves proximally and the pudendal nerve distally (23). In animal investigations, the pudendal innervation has occasionally been found to extend to the region of the bladder neck.

In summary, many questions remain about normal human urinary bladder function. As methods improve to resolve these questions, there will continue to be differing interpretations based on the investigators' backgrounds and training. Hopefully the training of clinical urologists in the neurosciences will facilitate greater insight into the process of micturition.

REFERENCES

1. Andersen JT, Bradley WE. Urethral pressure profilometry. *J Urol* 1977;118:423–427.
2. Andersen JT, et al. Electrophysiological techniques for the study of urethral and vesical innervation. *Scand J Urol Nephrol* 1976;10:189–194.
3. Andrew J, Nathan PW. Lesions of the anterior frontal lobes and disturbances of micturition and defecation. *Brain* 1964;87:233–262.
4. Augsberger HR, et al. Morphology and stereology of the female canine urethra correlated with the urethral pressure profile. *Acta Anat (Basel)* 1993;148:197–205.
5. Barrington FJF. The relation of the hind brain to micturition. *Brain* 1921;44:23–53.
6. Bates P, et al. The standardization of terminology of lower urinary tract function. *J Urol* 1979;121:551–554.
7. Bhatia NN, et al. Urodynamics: continuous monitoring. *J Urol* 1982;128:963–968.
8. Bradley WE. Cerebro-cortical innervation of the urinary bladder. *Tohoku J Exp Med* 1980;131:7–13.
9. Bradley WE. Cystometry and sphincter electromyography. *Mayo Clin Proc* 1976;51:329–335.
10. Bradley WE. Electroencephalography and bladder innervation. *J Urol* 1977;118:412–414.
11. Bradley WE. Physiology of the urinary bladder. In: Walsh PC, et al., eds. *Campbell's urology*. 5th ed. Philadelphia: WB Saunders, 1986:129–185.
12. Bradley WE. Urethral electromyelography. *J Urol* 1972;108:563–564.
13. Bradley WE, Conway CJ. Bladder representation in the pontine–mesencephalic reticular formation. *Exp Neurol* 1966;16:237–249.
14. Bradley WE, et al. Measurement of the conduction velocity of the dorsal nerve of the penis. *J Urol* 1984;131:1127–1129.
15. Bradley WE, Sundin T. The physiology and pharmacology of urinary tract dysfunction. *Clin Neuropharmacol* 1982;5:131–158.
16. Bradley WE, Teague CT. Cerebellar influence on the micturition reflex. *Exp Neurol* 1969;23:399–411.
17. Bradley WE, Teague CT. Cerebellar regulation of the micturition reflex. *J Urol* 1969;101:396–399.
18. Bradley WE, Teague CT. Electrophysiology of pelvic and pudendal nerves in the cat. *Exp Neurol* 1972;35:378–393.
19. Bradley WE, Teague CT. Innervation of the vesical detrusor muscle by the ganglia of the pelvic plexus. *Invest Urol* 1968;6:251–266.
20. Bradley WE, Teague CT. Spinal cord organization of micturition reflex afferents. *Exp Neurol* 1968;22:504–516.
21. Bradley WE, Teague CT. Synaptic events in pudendal motoneurons of the cat. *Exp Neurol* 1977;56:237–240.
22. Bradley WE, et al. Detrusor and urethral electromyelography. *J Urol* 1975;114:891–894.
23. Bradley W, et al. Sensory innervation of the mammalian urethra. *Invest Urol* 1973;10:287–289.
24. Coggeshall RE. Law of separation of function of the spinal roots. *Physiol Rev* 1980;60:716–755.
25. Conway CJ, Bradley WE. Measurement of spread of excitation in the urinary detrusor muscle during reflex induction. *J Urol* 1969;101:533–538.
26. Creed KE, et al. Electrical and mechanical activity recorded from rabbit urinary bladder in response to nerve stimulation. *J Physiol (Lond)* 1983;338:149–164.
27. Cullen C, et al. Histology of the canine urethra, I. Morphometry of the female urethra. *Anat Rec* 1981;199:177–186.
28. De Groat WC. Nervous control of the urinary bladder of the cat. *Brain Res* 1975;87:201–211.
28a. De Groat WC, Ryall RW. Reflexes to sacral parasympathetic neurones concerned with micturition in the cat. *J Physiol (Lond)* 1969;200:87–108.
29. Denny-Brown D, Robertson EC. On the physiology of micturition. *Brain* 1933;56:149–190.
30. Dick H, et al. Pudendal sexual reflexes. *Urology* 1974;3:376–379.
31. Dixon JS, et al. Intramural ganglia of the human urinary bladder. *Br J Urol* 1983;55:195–198.
32. Dow RS, Moruzzi G. *The physiology and pathology of the cerebellum*. Minneapolis: University of Minnesota Press, 1958.
33. Eardley I, et al. A new technique for assessing the efferent innervation of the human striated urethral sphincter. *J Urol* 1990;144:948–951.
34. Ek A, Bradley WE. History of cystometry. *Urology* 1983;22:335–350.
35. Fletcher TF, Bradley WE. Neuroanatomy of the bladder–urethra. *J Urol* 1978;119:153–160.
36. Fowler CJ. Investigation of the neurogenic bladder. *J Neurol Neurosurg Psychiatry* 1996;60:6–13.
37. Gatter KC, Powell TPS. The projection of the locus coeruleus upon the neocortex in the macaque monkey. *Neuroscience* 1977;2:441–445.
38. Gjone R, Setekleiv J. Excitatory and inhibitory bladder responses to stimulation of the cerebral cortex in the cat. *Acta Physiol Scand* 1963;59:337–348.
39. Gosling JA, et al. *Functional anatomy of the urinary tract: an integrated text and colour atlas*. Baltimore: University Park Press, 1982.
40. Gosling JA, et al. The autonomic innervation of the human male and female bladder neck and proximal urethra. *J Urol* 1977;118:302–305.
41. Gosling JA, et al. A comparative study of the human external sphincter and periurethral levator ani muscles. *Br J Urol* 1981;53:35–41.
42. Griffith WH III, et al. An intracellular investigation of cat vesical pelvic ganglia. *J Neurophysiol* 1980;43:343–354.
43. Habler HJ, et al. Receptive properties of myelinated primary afferents innervating the inflamed urinary bladder of the cat. *J Neurophysiol* 1993;69:395–405.
44. Haldeman S, et al. Pudendal evoked responses. *Arch Neurol* 1982;39:280–283.
45. Hamberger B, Norberg K-A. Adrenergic synaptic terminals and nerve cells in bladder ganglia of the cat. *Int J Neuropharmacol* 1965;4:41–45.
46. Hanani M, Mandley N. Intracellular recording from intraneural neurons in the guinea pig urinary bladder. *J Neurophysiol* 1995;74:2358–2365.
47. Hansen MV, et al. Cerebral evoked potentials after stimulation of the posterior urethra in man. *Electroencephalogr Clin Neurophysiol* 1990;77:52–58.
48. Hashitani H, et al. Effects of Y-26763, a novel K-channel opener, in electrical responses of smooth muscles in the guinea pig bladder. *J Urol* 1996;155:1454–1458.
49. Hickey DS, et al. Arrangement of collagen fibrils and muscle fibres in the female urethra and their implications for the control of micturition. *Br J Urol* 1982;54:556–561.
50. Hoseler FE, Monson FC. Microvasculature of the rabbit urinary bladder. *Anat Rec* 1995;243:438–448.
51. Inoue M, et al. Rhythmic slow wave observed on nocturnal sleep encephalogram in children with idiopathic nocturnal enuresis. *Sleep* 1987;10:570–579.
52. Jones BE, Webster HH. Neurotoxic lesions of the dorsolateral pontomesencephalic tegmentum–cholinergic cell area in the cat. *Brain Res* 1988;451:13–32.
53. Kaneko S, Bradley WE. Penile electrodiagnosis: value of bulbocavernosus reflex latency versus nerve conduction velocity of the dor-

sal nerve of the penis in diagnosis of diabetic impotence. *J Urol* 1987;137:933–935.
54. Khurana RK. Autonomic dysfunction in pontomedullary stroke. *Ann Neurol* 1982;12:86.
55. Kunamoto K, et al. Noradrenergic fibers in the pacinian corpuscle of the cat urinary bladder. *Acta Anat (Basel)* 1993; 146:46–52.
56. Kuru M. Nervous control of micturition. *Physiol Rev* 1965;45:425–494.
57. Langworthy OR, Kolb LC. The encephalic control of tone in the musculature of the urinary bladder. *Brain* 1933;56:371–382.
58. Leach GE, et al. Urodynamic manifestations of cerebellar ataxia. *J Urol* 1982;128:348–350.
59. Learmonth JA. A contribution to the neurophysiology of the urinary bladder in man. *Brain* 1931;54:147–176.
60. Lewin RJ, et al. Extrapyramidal inhibition of the urinary bladder. *Brain Res* 1967;4:301–307.
61. Lewin RJ, Porter RW. Inhibition of spontaneous bladder activity by stimulation of the globus pallidus. *Neurology* 1965;15:1049–1052.
62. Loewy AD, et al. Descending projections from the pontine micturition center. *Brain Res* 1978;172:533–538.
63. Mackel R. Segmental and descending control of the external urethral and anal sphincters in the cat. *J Physiol (Lond)* 1979;294:105–122.
64. Maggi CA, Melli A. The role of neuropeptides in the regulation of the micturition reflex. *J Auton Pharmacol* 1986;6:133–162.
65. Maggi CA, et al. Cystometric evidence that capsacian-sensitive nerves modulate the afferent branch of micturition reflex in humans. *J Urol* 1989;142:150–154.
66. Mannen T, et al. Preservation of a certain motoneurone group of the sacral cord in amyotrophic lateral sclerosis: its clinical significance. *J Neurol Neurosurg Psychiatry* 1977;40:464–469.
67. Martin WD, et al. Innervation of feline perineal musculature. *Anat Rec* 1974;180:15–30.
68. Morgan C, et al. The spinal distribution of sympathetic preganglionic and visceral primary afferent neurons that send axons into the hypogastric nerves of the cat. *J Comp Neurol* 1986;243:23–40.
69. Morgan C, et al. Location of bladder preganglionic neurons within the parasympathetic nucleus of the cat. *Neurosci Lett* 1979;14:189–194.
70. Morgan C, et al. The distribution of visceral primary afferents from the pelvic nerve to Lissauer's tract and the spinal gray matter and its relationship to the sacral parasympathetic nucleus. *J Comp Neurol* 1981;201:415–440.
71. Mosso A, Pellacani P. Sur les fonctions de la vessie. *Arch Ital Biol* 1882;1:97–128.
72. Murakomo M, et al. Three-dimensional arrangement of collagen and elastin fibers in the human urinary bladder: a scanning EM study. *J Urol* 1995;154:251–256.
73. Murnaghan GF. Neurogenic disorders of the bladder in Parkinsonism. *Br J Urol* 1961;33:403–409.
74. Nakagawa S. Onuf's nucleus of the sacral cord in a South American monkey (*Saimiri*): its location and bilateral cortical input from area 4. *Brain Res* 1980;191:337–344.
75. Nathan PW, Smith MC. The centrifugal pathway for micturition in the spinal cord. *J Neurol Neurosurg Psychiatry* 1958;21:177–189.
76. Nathan PW, Smith MC. The centripetal pathway from the bladder and urethra within the spinal cord. *J Neurol Neurosurg Psychiatry* 1951;14:262–280.
77. Nishizawa O, et al. Effect of cerebellectomy on reflex micturition in the decerebrate dog as determined by urodynamic evaluation. *Urol Int* 1989;44:152–156.
78. Nitte VW, et al. Role of urodynamics in the evaluation of voiding function in men after cerebrovascular accident. *J Urol* 1996;155:263–266.
79. Norgaard JP, et al. Sleep cystometries in children with nocturnal enuresis. *J Urol* 1989;141:1156–1159.
80. Noto H, et al. Excitatory and inhibitory influences on bladder activity elicited by electrical stimulation in the pontine micturition center in the rat. *Brain Res* 1989;492:99–115.
81. Oliver J, et al. Spinal cord distribution of the somatic innervation of the external urethral sphincter of the cat. *J Neurol Sci* 1970;10:11–23.
82. Oliver JE, et al. Spinal cord representation of the micturition reflex. *J Comp Neurol* 1969;137:329–346.
83. Onuf (Onufrowicz) B. On the arrangement and function of the groups of the sacral region of the spinal cord in man. *Arch Neurol Psychopathol* 1900;3:387–411.
84. Perkash I, Friedland GW. Real-time gray-scale transrectal linear array ultrasonography in urodynamic evaluation. *Semin Urol* 1985;3:49–59.
85. Porter RW. A pallidal response to detrusor contraction. *Brain Res* 1967;4:381–383.
86. Purinton PT, et al. Innervation of the pelvic viscera in the rat: evoked potentials in nerves to bladder and penis (clitoris). *Invest Urol* 1976;14:28–32.
87. Purinton T, et al. Sensory perikarya in autonomic ganglia. *Nature* 1971;231:63–64.
88. Rockswold GL, et al. Effect of sacral nerve blocks on the function of the urinary bladder in humans. *J Neurosurg* 1974;40:83–89.
89. Rockswold GL, et al. Innervation of the urinary bladder in higher primates. *J Comp Neurol* 1980;193:509–520.
90. Rockswold GL, Chou SN. Urological problems associated with central nervous system disease. In: Youmans JR, ed. *Neurological surgery*. 3rd ed. Philadelphia: WB Saunders, 1990,814–832.
91. Sakakibara R, et al. Micturitional disturbance after acute hemispheric stroke: analysis of the lesion site by CT and MRI. *J Neurol Sci* 1996;137:47–56.
92. Sakakibara K, et al. The location of the paths subserving micturition: studies in patients with cervical myelopathy. *J Auton Nerv Syst* 1995;55:165–168.
93. Sakanaka M, et al. Evidence for the existence of a substance P–containing pathway from the nucleus laterodorsalis tegmenti (Castaldi) to the medial frontal cortex of the rat. *Brain Res* 1983;259:123–126.
94. Sarica Y, et al. Cerebral responses elicited by stimulation of the vesico-urethral junction in diabetics. *Electroencephalogr Clin Neurophysiol* 1996;100:55–61.
95. Sarica Y, et al. Cerebral responses evoked by stimulation of the vesico-urethral function in man. *Electroencephalogr Clin Neurophysiol* 1986;65:130–136.
96. Satoh K, et al. Descending projection of the nucleus tegmentalis laterodorsalis to the spinal cord. *Neurosci Lett* 1978;8:9–15.
97. Satoh K, et al. Localization of the micturition center at dorso-lateral pontine tegmentum of the rat. *Neurosci Lett* 1978;8:27–33.
98. Saum WR, de Groat WC. Parasympathetic ganglia: activation of an adrenergic inhibitory mechanism by cholinomimetic agents. *Science* 1972;175:659–661.
99. Sibley GNA. A comparison of spontaneous and nerve-mediated activity in bladder muscle from man, pig and rabbit. *J Physiol (Lond)* 1984;354:431–443.
100. Sung JH. Autonomic neurons affected by lipid storage in the spinal cord in Fabry's disease: distribution of autonomic neurons in the sacral cord. *J Neuropathol Exp Neurol* 1979;38:87–98.
101. Swaiman KF, Bradley WE. Quantitation of collagen in the wall of the human urinary bladder. *J Appl Physiol* 1967;22:122–124.
102. Taylor MC, et al. The conus demyelination syndrome in multiple sclerosis. *Acta Neurol Scand* 1984;69:80–89.
103. Thor KB, et al. Organization of afferent and efferent pathways in the pudendal nerve of the female cat. *J Comp Neurol* 1989;288:263–279.
104. Tohyama M, et al. Organization and projections of the neurons in the dorsal tegmental area of the rat. *J Hirnforsch* 1978;19:165–176.
105. Tsurusaki M, et al. Alpha$_2$-adrenoceptors mediate the inhibition of cholinergic transmission in parasympathetic ganglia of the rabbit urinary bladder. *Synapse* 1990;5:233–240.
106. Uemura E, et al. Distribution of sacral afferent axons in cat urinary bladder. *Am J Anat* 1973;136:305–313.
107. Vereecken RL, et al. Electrophysiological exploration of the sacral conus. *J Neurol* 1982;227:135–144.
108. Wein AJ, Levin RM, Barrett DM. Voiding function: relevant anatomy, physiology, and pharmacology. In: Gillenwater JY, et al.,

eds. *Adult and pediatric urology.* Chicago: Year Book Medical, 1987:800–862.
109. Woodburne RT. Structure and function of the urinary bladder. *J Urol* 1960;84:79–85.
110. Woodburne RT. The sphincter mechanism of the urinary bladder and the urethra. *Anat Rec* 1961;141:11–20.
111. Xu Q, Grant G. The projection of spinocerebellar neurons from the sacrococcygeal region of the spinal cord in the cat. *Arch Ital Biol* 1990;128:209–228.
112. Yoshimura N, et al. Mediation of micturition reflex by central norepinephrine from the locus coeruleus in the cat. *J Urol* 1990;143:840–843.

CHAPTER 11

Autonomic Regulation of Sexual Function

John D. Stewart

1. The sympathetic, parasympathetic, and somatic nervous systems act in a coordinated manner to control the physiologic responses that occur during sexual intercourse.
2. These responses include erectile tissue engorgement and detumescence, glandular secretion, and contraction and relaxation of smooth and striated muscle.
3. The central nervous system areas involved are mainly in the hypothalamus. Sympathetic fibers arise from the lower thoracic and upper lumbar spinal cord; parasympathetic and somatic fibers arise from the sacral cord.
4. Lesions in either the central or peripheral nervous systems, or both, can produce sexual dysfunction.

INTRODUCTION

The complete sexual act can be divided into four phases—excitement, plateau, orgasm, and resolution—collectively designated as the sexual response cycle (21). These phases are mediated through the combined and integrated activities of the somatic and autonomic nervous systems that innervate the organs and structures in the reproductive tract. For a variety of reasons, the physiologic features of the male sexual responses have been better characterized than their counterparts in females. Despite the obvious anatomic differences between males and females, however, many of the physiologic sexual responses are similar: erectile tissue engorgement and detumescence, glandular secretion, and contraction of smooth and striated muscles.

This chapter describes the neurologic control of these physiologic responses as a background for understanding sexual dysfunction resulting from disorders of the autonomic nervous system.

ANATOMY

Male Sexual Organs

These principally comprise the penis, testes, epididymis, vas deferens, seminal vesicles, and prostate gland. The erectile tissue of the penis consists of three longitudinal bundles: the corpora (Fig. 1). The paired corpora cavernosa principally subserve erectile function. The single corpus spongiosum surrounds the urethra and expands distally to form the glans penis; it is mainly involved with urination and ejaculation. The corpora cavernosa consist of many blood-filled spaces called lacunae (or sinusoids). The walls of the lacunae are the trabeculae, which consist of bundles of smooth muscle and fibroelastic tissue. The outermost circumferential layer of trabecular tissue is denser and is termed the tunica albuginea. The corpus spongiosum is similar in structure, but the trabeculae are finer and the surrounding tunica is thinner. Each of the three corpora is surrounded by fascia.

The arteries of the penis comprise a cavernosal artery within each corpus cavernosum, a pair of smaller arteries within the corpus spongiosum, and two dorsal arteries (Fig. 1). These are branches of the internal pudendal artery, which in turn arises from the internal iliac artery. Within the corpora cavernosa are numerous helicine arteries that branch off from the cavernosal arteries and open directly into the lacunar spaces.

The venous drainage system of the corpora consists of small veins that lie among the lacunae and that coalesce to form larger emissary veins. These pierce the tunica albuginea to drain into the deep dorsal vein of the penis.

Two muscles of the perineum important to sexual function are the bulbocavernosus (bulbospongiosus) and ischiocavernosus muscles. The bulbocavernosus muscle surrounds the expanded proximal end of the corpus spongiosum (which contains the urethra) and has an important role in ejaculation. The ischiocavernosus muscle attaches anteri-

---

J. D. Stewart: Department of Neurology, McGill University, Montreal, Quebec, H3A 2B4, Canada.

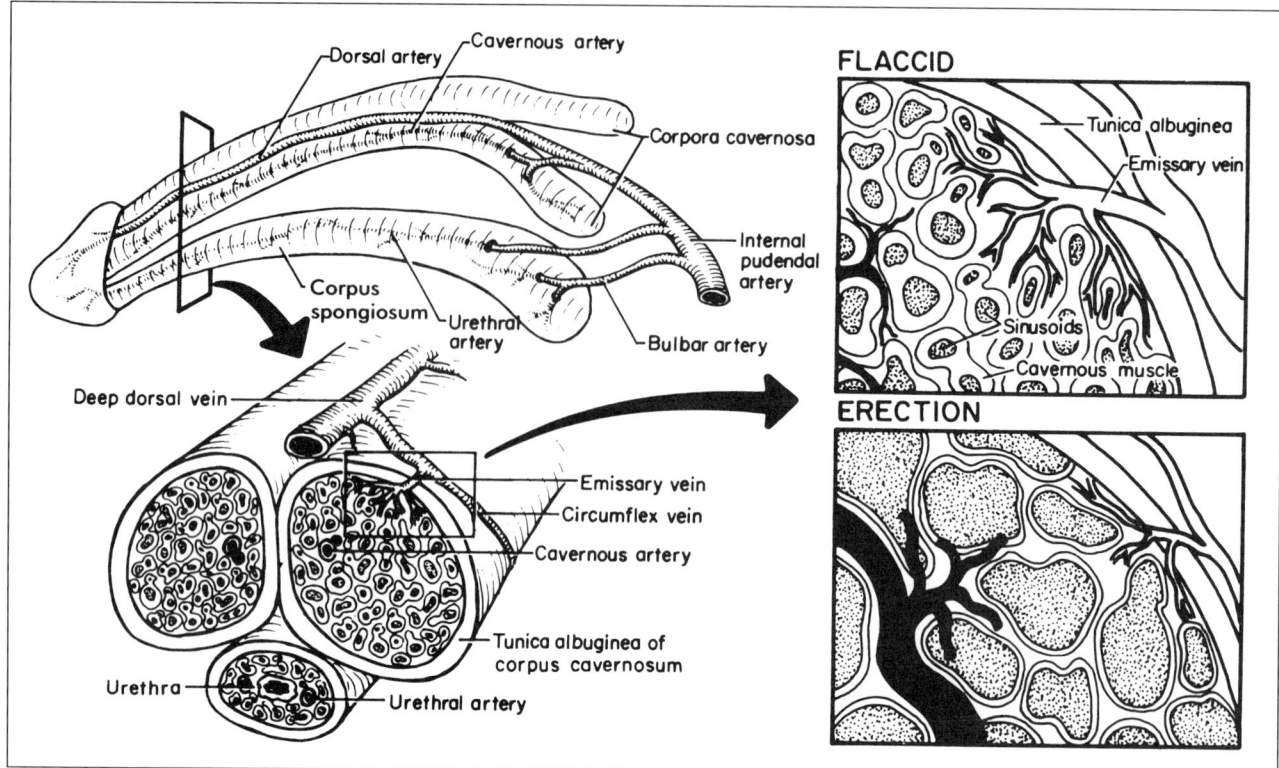

FIG. 1. The anatomy of the penis. Note that during erection the expansion of the lacunae (sinusoids) with blood compresses the veins against the tunica albuginea, partially occluding them and thereby reducing venous outflow. From de Groat and Steers (6); modified and adapted from Lue and Tanagho (20a), with permission.

orly over the base of the penis and may help to impair venous return from the corpora cavernosa during erection.

The testes have the dual role of being an endocrine gland for producing testosterone and are also the site for spermatozoa formation. The epididymis lies above the testis and is the repository for maturing spermatozoa. The vas deferens connects the epididymis with the posterior urethra. The seminal vesicles are paired glands that lie behind the prostate gland and beneath the bladder. Their secretions form the bulk of seminal fluid, which is important for the survival of spermatozoa outside the male genital tract. Prostatic secretions constitute a smaller amount of the seminal fluid.

Female Sexual Organs

The external organs include the mons pubis, the labia, the clitoris, the bulb of the vestibule, and the greater vestibular (Bartholin's) glands. The clitoris is an erectile structure, homologous to the penis, consisting of two corpora cavernosa and a glans. Deep to the labia lie the two other structures containing erectile tissue: the paired bulbs of the vestibule. These elongated masses lie on either side of the vaginal orifice and connect together anteriorly with the clitoris. Each bulb is covered by the thin bulbocavernosus (bulbospongiosus) muscle. The clitoris and bulbs of the vestibule have the same internal structure as the penile corpora cavernosa. The greater vestibular glands lie posteriorly, and their ducts open near the vaginal orifice.

The internal organs comprise the vagina, uterus, fallopian tubes, and ovaries. The vagina is a fibromuscular tube, and the muscular part is nonstriated. It is lined with stratified epithelium that contains no glands, but can produce some secretions. The bulbospongiosus muscles surround the orifice of the vagina. These muscles arise posteriorly from the perineal body, with fibers passing forward on each side of the vagina, covering the bulbs of the vestibule, and attaching anteriorly to the corpora cavernosa of the clitoris. These muscles rhythmically contract during orgasm, and contraction of the anterior fibers as well as of the smaller ischiocavernosus muscle probably contributes to erection of the clitoris by compressing the deep dorsal vein.

INNERVATION OF THE SEXUAL ORGANS

Three sets of nerves innervate the sexual organs (Fig. 2): (a) thoracolumbar sympathetic nerves, (b) sacral parasympathetic nerves, and (c) pudendal somatic nerves.

toris, and bulbs of the vestibule; and (c) smooth muscle in the seminal vesicles, prostate, vagina, and uterus.

Parasympathetic Nerves

The cell bodies of the parasympathetic nerves lie in the sacral spinal cord. Preganglionic fibers leave through the S2–4 ventral roots, travel in the cauda equina, and then enter the pelvis through the foramina of the sacral nerve roots. They then form the pelvic nerves (nervi erigentes) that join the pelvic (inferior hypogastric) plexus (Fig. 2). This plexus is a mix of sympathetic and parasympathetic pre- and postganglionic fibers and ganglia. The postganglionic parasympathetic fibers innervate (a) erectile tissue in the penis/clitoris; (b) smooth muscle and glandular tissue in the urethra, seminal vesicles, prostate gland, vagina, and uterus; and (c) blood vessels and possibly secretory epithelium in various pelvic structures involved in sexual function.

Somatic Nerves

The cell bodies for the motor fibers of the pudendal nerves are located in the medial part of the ventral horn of the sacral spinal cord, called Onuf's nucleus. Motor and sensory fibers lie in the S2–4 dorsal and ventral roots and spinal nerves (the same as contain the parasympathetic fibers to the genitalia) within the cauda equina. They pass through the foramina of the sacral nerve roots to join the sacral plexus. The pudendal nerves themselves arise from this plexus and pass forward into the perineum. The first branch is the inferior rectal (hemorrhoidal) nerve that innervates the external anal sphincter. The next, the perineal nerve, supplies the muscles of the perineum, including the bulbocavernosus and ischiocavernosus muscles, the external urethral sphincter, and the skin of the perineum and scrotum or labia. The final branch of the pudendal nerve is the (sensory) dorsal nerve of the penis or clitoris.

CENTRAL NERVOUS SYSTEM

Animal studies have shown that hypothalamic and limbic areas and pathways are involved in sexual arousal. In particular, the hypothalamic medial preoptic area is thought to be an important integrating area (5,11,14). Electrical stimulation of this region produces erections, and conversely sexual behavior is suppressed by lesions there. Stimulation of other hypothalamic areas also causes erection, as well as other copulatory reactions, and sometimes ejaculation. Descending pathways travel in the medial forebrain bundle in the tegmentum of the midbrain, the ventrolateral pons, and medulla, and then down the lateral column of the spinal cord. They terminate in the lower thoracic, lumbar, and sacral areas of the spinal cord.

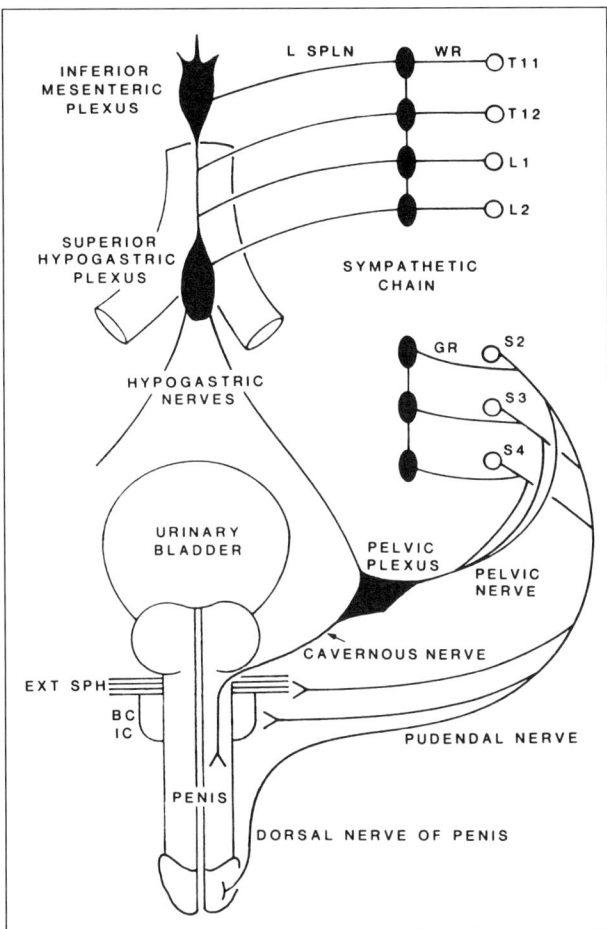

FIG. 2. Schematic drawing to show the sympathetic, parasympathetic, and somatic efferent nerve pathways to the male genitalia. WR, white rami; LSPLN, lumbar splanchnic nerves; GR, gray rami; EXT SPH, external sphincter of the urinary bladder; BC and IC, bulbocavernosus and ischiocavernosus muscles. From de Groat and Steers (5), with permission.

Sympathetic Nerves

The preganglionic fibers arise from the intermediolateral column of the lower thoracic and upper lumbar spinal cord and leave the cord in the T11–L2 ventral roots to enter the sympathetic chain. Thereafter, sympathetic fibers take a variety of routes (Fig. 2). Some fibers synapse with postganglionic fibers within the chain; others pass through uninterruptedly to reach the inferior mesenteric and superior hypogastric plexuses, synapsing there with postganglionic sympathetic fibers. These then travel to pelvic organs via the hypogastric nerves, pelvic plexus, and cavernous nerves. Other sympathetic nerve fibers travel with parasympathetic nerves to the pelvic plexus. A third group joins the mainly somatic nerve fibers in the pudendal nerves.

The sympathetic nerves innervate (a) blood vessels in the reproductive organs; (b) erectile tissue of the penis, cli-

The neurotransmitters involved in the central sexual reflex pathways include the monoaminergic transmitters, 5-hydroxytriptymine, dopamine, and noradrenaline, and neuropeptides such as oxytocin, opioid peptides, and γ-aminobutyric acid (4,11).

HORMONAL REGULATION

The hormonal control of sexual function involves complex interactions among the hypothalamus, pituitary gland, and the sexual and reproductive organs.

In males, the two gonadotropins of importance are leutinizing hormone (LH) and follicle-stimulating hormone (FSH). The major action of LH is to control the synthesis of testosterone within the testis, and FSH stimulates spermatogenesis. The release of these two gonadotropins from the pituitary gland is controlled by the hypothalamus. The anterior pituitary also secretes the hormone prolactin. This has no identified physiologic function in the normal male, but men with prolactin-secreting pituitary tumors often suffer from erectile impotence. Potency is restored by reducing the prolactin level to normal with the dopamine agonist bromocriptine or by surgical removal of the tumor. Testosterone is involved in causing and maintaining libido rather than in the physiologic control of erections or ejaculation. Hypogonadal men (e.g., after orchidectomy for carcinoma of the prostate) can therefore have successful sexual intercourse, though libido is lower than normal (19,26).

In females, LH and FSH stimulate the ovaries to produce estrogen and progesterone, which are responsible for the maturation of the sexual organs at menarche and the control of the menstrual cycle. The hormonal factors involved in the maintenance of libido are poorly understood.

PHYSIOLOGY OF THE SEXUAL RESPONSE CYCLE

Males

Penile Erection

Erections can occur from local stimulation of the genitalia (reflexogenic or spinal erections), psychogenic stimuli (psychogenic or supraspinal erections), or both. In reflexogenic erections, cutaneous sensory receptors are activated and the signals transmitted to the spinal cord via the pudendal nerves. Ascending pathways carry some signals to the brain while local spinal pathways, involving interneurons, activate the parasympathetic nerves to produce an erection. Psychogenic erections are initiated by a variety of stimuli such as auditory, visual, olfactory, or imaginative. The higher centers and descending pathways stimulate activity in the parasympathetic pelvic efferents to produce an erection. Reflexogenic and psychogenic mechanisms act synergistically in most situations of sexual arousal.

An erection occurs because of blood pooling within the cavernous tissue. The sequence of events is as follows (18): The cavernosal and helicine arteries dilate, increasing the blood flow into the cavernous tissue. The smooth muscle in the trabecular walls of the lacunar spaces of the cavernosae relaxes to accommodate the increased blood flow. This relaxation of the arteries and the trabecular walls occurs from both a reduction of tonic smooth muscle contraction and active relaxation. The expansion of the cavernosae forces their outermost parts against the rigid surrounding tunica albuginea. This compresses the emissary veins, cutting down on the venous outflow from the lacunar spaces (Fig. 1). Venous occlusion thus occurs passively. In addition, contraction of the ischiocavernosus muscle (and the bulbocavernosus muscle in females) may constrict the proximal parts of the corpora cavernosa to contribute to venous occlusion.

Detumescence results from contraction of the smooth muscle of both the helicine arteries and the trabeculae. The arterial constriction reduces the blood flow to the lacunar spaces. Contraction of the trabeculae promotes emptying of the lacunae, and by pulling the outermost lacunar walls away from the tunica albuginea, the draining veins are opened.

Emission, Ejaculation, and Orgasm

Emission occurs by the contractions of smooth muscle in the epididymis, vas deferens, seminal vesicles, and prostate gland. This deposits spermatozoa and seminal fluid into the proximal urethra. Contraction of the sphincters of the bladder neck prevents reflux of semen into the bladder (retrograde ejaculation). These events seem to be principally mediated by the sympathetic nerves.

Ejaculation consists of the semen being rapidly transmitted down the urethra and released in spurts. This is accomplished by rhythmic contractions of the bulbocavernosus, ischiocavernosus, and periurethral striated muscles. Neural control is principally mediated by the somatic nerve fibers in the pudendal nerve.

Orgasm comprises the pleasurable sensations associated with emission and ejaculation: the buildup and then expulsion of semen. These sensations are principally signalled through the pudendal somatic sensory afferents.

Neural and Neurotransmitter Control of Erection and Detumescence

The tone of the smooth muscle in the penile arteries and the trabeculae of the cavernosal tissue is controlled by complex interactions of proerectile and antierectile neural mechanisms.

Adrenergic Nerves: These release norepinephrine that acts on α-receptors to cause contraction of the smooth muscle in the erectile tissue arteries (i.e., vasoconstriction) and the walls of the trabeculae. Tonic activity in these nerves thus helps to maintain flaccidity. Other substances such as adenosine triphosphate and neuropeptides are cotransmitters in those neurons (3).

Cholinergic Nerves: These nerves play an important part in mediating erections. One major action of acetylcholine is to act prejunctionally to inhibit the antierectile activity of adrenergic nerves (11,15,25). A second action is to react with muscarinic receptors on endothelial cells to release nitric oxide (NO), which relaxes vascular and trabecular smooth muscle cells (see below) (6–8,10,20,27).

Nonadrenergic, Noncholinergic Nerves: The genitalia are richly innervated by neurons displaying immunoreactivity for vasoactive intestinal polypeptide (VIP). This neurotransmitter is a powerful relaxer of vascular and trabecular smooth muscle (1,13,22,23). It is uncertain as to how much of this action is direct or is mediated through the release of NO from the endothelium (12,17,22). In addition to cholinergic and VIPergic nerves, there are also neurons that synthesize and release NO (nitrergic nerves) (2,24,28). Many postganglionic parasympathetic nerves supplying pelvic vascular and erectile tissues are both cholinergic and VIPergic; some may in addition be partly nitrergic (11). Colocalization of VIP and NO in some neurons has also been shown (16). The temporal pattern of release and the relative roles of these proerectile neurotransmitters is not known with certainty (11).

Endothelial Factors: Signals from cholinergic and VIPergic nerves stimulates NO release from the endothelium; nitrergic nerves release NO from their endings. Local physical effects on the endothelium such as increased blood flow further stimulate NO release (25). It is thought that neurally released NO is more important than endothelial NO under physiologic conditions (11). In addition to NO, there may be other endothelium-derived relaxing factors. There are also vasoconstrictor peptides produced by vascular endothelial cells, e.g., the very potent constrictor endothelin (27,29). These may play a role in the maintenance of penile flaccidity (9).

Summary: Proerectile neuropharmacologic mechanisms include the following: Relaxation of the penile arteries and cavernosal trabeculae is mediated by the parasympathetic nerves releasing acetylcholine that in turn activates NO release. This is augmented by VIP and NO release from the same as well as from other nerves. This is accompanied by inactivation of sympathetic noradrenergically mediated tonic vasocostriction and cavernosal trabeculae contraction. Blood flow into the lacunae increases, the cavernosae expand, and venous occlusion occurs passively. Detumescence occurs from a reversal of the above neural signals, with constriction of the arteries and contraction of the trabeculae. The reduced volume of the cavernosal tissue passively opens the venules draining the lacunar spaces.

Females

The physiologic events occurring in the female sexual response cycle is similar to that in the male (20–22). The equivalent of erection is engorgement of the clitoris and the bulbs of the vestibule, presumably brought about by the same neurovascular mechanisms as penile erection. The bulbocavernosus and ischiocavernosus muscles may help to impair venous drainage from the clitoris. Vasocongestion occurs also in other pelvic structures: the labia, vagina, and uterus. Vaginal lubrication increases, although the mechanisms are unclear. Some may come from the cervix, some from Bartholin's glands; it is also thought that the vaginal epithelium can "sweat" during sexual arousal (21). Orgasm is accompanied by the rhythmic contraction of the vagina and the muscles of the pelvic floor.

REFERENCES

1. Benson GS. Penile erection: in search of a neurotransmitter. *World J Urol* 1983;1:209–212.
2. Bredt DS, Snyder SH. Nitric oxide: a novel neuronal messenger. *Neuron* 1992;8:3–11.
3. Burnstock G. The changing face of autonomic neurotransmission. *Acta Physiol Scand* 1986;126:67–91.
4. Crowley WR, Zelman FP. The neurochemical control of mating behaviour. In: Adler N, ed. *Neuroendocrinology of reproduction: physiology and behaviour.* New York: Plenum, 1981:451–484.
5. De Groat WC, Steers WD. The neuroanatomy and neurophysiology of penile erection. In: Tanagho E, Lue T, McClure T, eds. *Contemporary management of impotence and fertility.* Baltimore: Williams and Wilkins, 1988:3–27.
6. De Groat WC, Steers WD. Autonomic regulation of the urinary bladder and sexual organs. In: Loewy AD, Spyer KM, eds. *Central regulation of autonomic functions.* New York: Oxford University Press, 1990:310–333.
7. De Tejada IS, et al. Cholinergic neurotransmission in human corpus cavernosum. I. Responses of isolated tissue. *Am J Physiol* 1988;254:H459–H467.
8. De Tejada IS, et al. Impaired neurogenic endothelium-mediated relaxation of penile smooth muscle from diabetic men with impotence. *N Engl J Med* 1989;320:1025–1030.
9. De Tejada IS, et al. Role of endothelin in the local control of penile smooth muscle tone. *J Vasc Med Biol* 1989;1:112.
10. Furchgott RF, Zawadzki JV. The obligatory role of endothelial cells in the relaxation of arterial smooth muscle by acetylcholine. *Nature* 1980;288:373–376.
11. Giuliano FA, et al. Neural control of penile erection. *Urol Clin North Am* 1995;22:747–766.
12. Grider JR, et al. Stimulation of nitric oxide from muscle cells by VIP: prejunctional enhancement of VIP release. *Am J Physiol* 1992;262:G774–G778.
13. Gu J, et al. Decrease of vasoactive intestinal polypeptide (VIP) in the penises from impotent men. *Lancet* 1984;2:315–317.
14. Hart BL, Leedy MG. Neurological basis of male sexual behavior. In: Adler N, Pfaff D, Goy RW, eds. *A handbook of behavioral neurobiology.* New York: Plenum, 1985:7:373–422.
15. Hedlund H, et al. Pre- and post-junctional adreno- and muscarinic receptor functions in the isolated human corpus spongiosum urethrae. *J Auton Pharmacol* 1984;4:241249.

16. Junemann KP, et al. Nitric oxide synthase in coexistence with vasoactive intestinal polypeptide in nerve terminals of human corpus cavernosum. *Int J Impotence Res* 1994;6:A3(abst).
17. Kimura K, et al. The relaxation of human corpus cavernosum caused by nitric oxide [in Japanese]. *Nippon Hinyokika Gakkai Zasshi* 1993;84:1660–1664.
18. Krane RJ, et al. Impotence. *N Engl J Med* 1989;321:1648–1659.
19. Kwam M, et al. The nature of androgen action on male sexuality: a combined laboratory–self-report study on hypogonadal men. *J Clin Endocrinol Metab* 1983;57:557–562.
20. Levin RJ. The physiology of sexual function in women. *Clin Obstet Gynecol* 1980;7:213–252.

20a. Lue TF, Tanagho EA. Functional anatomy and mechanism of penile erection. In: Tanagho E, Lue T, McClure T, eds. *Contemporary management of impotence and infertility.* Baltimore: Williams and Wilkins, 1988:39–50.

21. Masters WH, Johnson VE. *Human sexual responses.* Boston: Little Brown, 1966.
22. Ottesen B, Fahrenkrug J. Vasoactive intestinal polypeptide and other preprovasoactive intestinal polypeptide-derived peptides in the female and male genital tract: localization, biosynthesis, and functional and clinical significance. *Am J Obstet Gynecol* 1995;172:1615–1631.
23. Polak JM, et al. Vipergic nerves in the penis. *Lancet* 1981;2:217–219.
24. Rajfer J, et al. Nitric oxide as a mediator of relaxation of the corpus cavernosum on response to nonadrenergic, noncholinergic neurotransmission. *N Engl J Med* 1992;326:90–94.
25. Rubanyi GM, et al. Flow-induced release of endothelium-derived relaxing factor. *Am J Physiol* 1986;250:H1145–H1149.
26. Skakkebach NE, et al. Androgen replacement with oral testosterone undecanoate in hypogonadal men: a double blind controlled study. *Clin Endocrinol* 1981;14:49–61.
27. Vane JR, et al. Regulatory functions of the vascular endothelium. *N Engl J Med* 1990;323:27–36.
28. Vincent SR. Nitric oxide: a radical neurotransmitter in the central nervous system. *Prog Neurobiol* 1994;42:129–160.
29. Yanagisawa M, et al. A novel potent vasoconstrictor peptide produced by vascular endothelial cells. *Nature* 1988;332:411–415.

CHAPTER 12

Autonomic Regulation of Gastrointestinal Motility

Michael Camilleri

1. The autonomic regulation of gastrointestinal motor function consists of extrinsic control by the parasympathetic and sympathetic nervous systems and intrinsic control by the enteric plexuses.
2. The enteric nervous system constitutes a semi-autonomous system with specific "programs" for motor responses, such as peristaltic reflexes and regional rate of contraction by the pacemaker systems.
3. There is autonomic regulation of function by levels of innervation. The enteric nervous system mediates peristalsis, the prevertebral ganglia mediate entero-enteric reflexes, the brainstem mediates enterogastric reflexes, and higher centers mediate satiety.
4. Sympathetic innervation has an important inhibitory influence on gut smooth muscle. When lacking, uncoordinated or excessive contractility results in conditions such as achalasia, Hirschsprung's disease, or chronic idiopathic intestinal pseudo-obstruction.
5. The autonomic nervous system provides the main pathways for afferent function in the gut. The predominant afferents are C fibers that ascend through a three-neuron chain to the higher centers and reflex centers in the brain. Descending modulation of afferent pathways and reflex loops modulates motor and sensory functions of the gastrointestinal tract.

INTRODUCTION

The gastrointestinal tract constitutes one of the largest organs whose motor, transport, secretory, storage, and excretory functions are controlled by the autonomic nervous system. At every level, the gut is composed of four layers: mucosa, submucosa, muscularis, and serosa. The innermost layer, or mucosa, is primarily concerned with the processes of digestion and absorption; the surface epithelium and lamina propria of the mucosa are separated from the submucosa by the specialized, circumferentially oriented smooth muscle, called the muscularis mucosae. The latter probably functions to bring surface absorptive or digestive cells into intimate contact with luminal content; it may also play a role in mixing of intraluminal contents. The submucosa is composed of connective, lymphatic, and vascular tissue. The muscularis propria (or externa) is composed of two muscle layers: an inner, thicker layer in which the long axis of cells is oriented in a circular direction; and an outer layer that is thinner and has longitudinally oriented smooth muscle cells. In the esophagus and small intestine, the longitudinal layer covers the whole circumference of the viscus; in the colon, it is separated into three bands or taeniae coli. The stomach also has a third oblique orientation of smooth muscle fibers. Each smooth muscle is 40–100 μm long and 2–8 μm in diameter, and the spindle-shaped cells are tightly packed with little connective tissue and with special contacts to allow for electrical coupling among the cells (*electrical syncytium*). Thus, gap junctions between the smooth muscle cells permit sheets of muscle to be controlled by the innervation of a few cells at the nerve–muscle interface. The outermost serosal layer is composed of a thin sheet of mesothelial cells and connective tissue.

The gastrointestinal tract also contains neural tissue and other cells that contain hormones, transmitters, and autocoids (18). Nerve cell bodies and plexuses are found in various plexuses (6). The classically recognized plexuses

M. Camilleri: Department of Internal Medicine, Division of Gastroenterology, Mayo Clinic and Mayo Foundation, Rochester, Minnesota 55905.

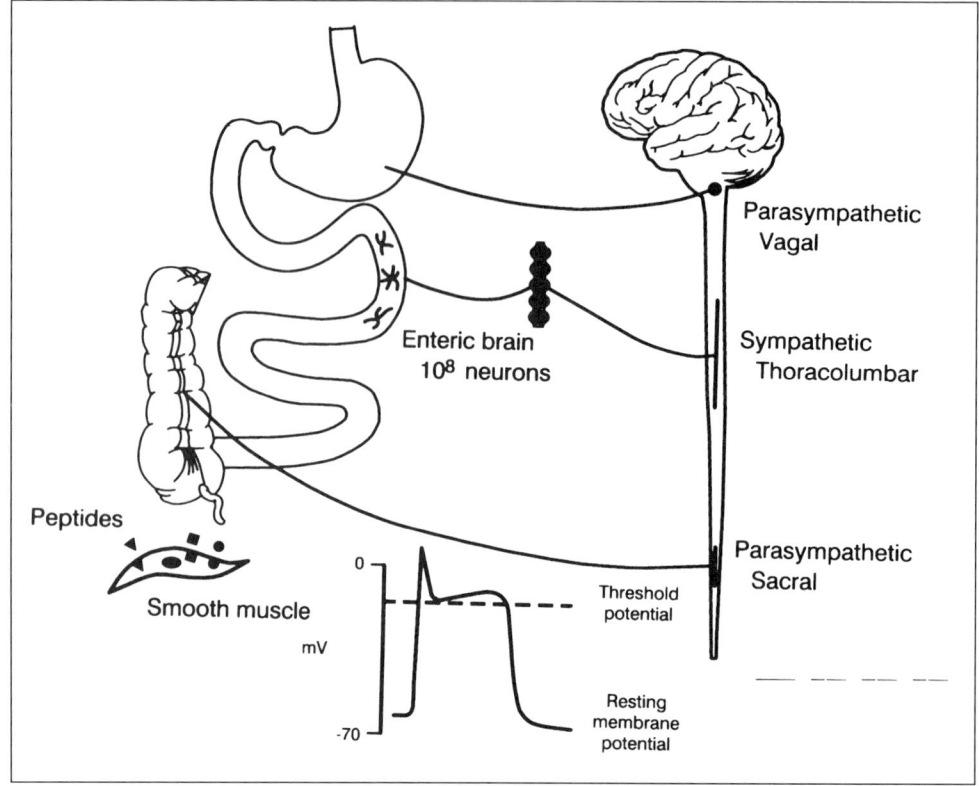

FIG. 1. Control of gut motility: extrinsic autonomic neural control, enteric nervous system, and smooth muscle function. From Camilleri and Phillips (3), with permission.

(Fig. 1) are the myenteric (Auerbach's) plexus found between the two muscular layers of the muscularis externa, and the submucosal (Meissner's) plexus. However, other plexuses of nerve-fiber bundles occur in the muscle layers in the mucosa, beneath the serosa, and around arteries. These intrinsic nerves communicate with structures outside the gut via extrinsic nerves. The latter convey afferent and efferent information to and from the central nervous system and prevertebral ganglia via the sympathetic and parasympathetic nerves. Thus, the intrinsic or enteric nervous system constitutes an important third arm (11) of the autonomic nervous system.

In this chapter, the autonomic factors controlling gastrointestinal motility (Fig. 1) are discussed, with particular emphasis on the recently recognized organization and function of the enteric nervous system. Understanding the hard-wiring of the autonomic regulation of gastrointestinal motility provides the basis for the approach to the diagnosis and management of motility disorders of the gut, which is discussed further in Chapter 45.

EXTRINSIC NEURAL CONTROL

The digestive tract can function fairly normally in the absence of extrinsic nerves because of the functional autonomy arising from intrinsic reflexes that are mediated by nerve ganglia within the wall of the intestine. Thus, extrinsic nerves mainly "modulate" the intrinsic reflexes and integrate activity in different regions of the alimentary canal (18). Nevertheless, the modulatory effects of extrinsic nerves on gastrointestinal motility are demonstrable either from anatomic, electrical, or pharmacologic observations; from studies of stimulation in experimental animals; or by the significant alterations in motor function of the gut in various neurologic disorders (2). Summaries of the wiring and functions of extrinsic neural pathways (15) to the digestive tract are presented in Fig. 2 and in Table 1. Table 2 summarizes the levels of neural control of gastrointestinal motor and sensory functions. There is limited information about the supraspinal control of gut motility, although it is clear that brainstem centers are involved in enterogastric and gastrocolic reflexes. A bulbar inhibitory center projects to the spinal inhibitory center and probably to the paravertebral ganglia that mediate responses such as intestinointestinal inhibitory reflexes. Direct projections from the brainstem on the sacral segments of the spinal cord also indicate significant supraspinal control of the distal digestive tract. Central areas that potentially influence gut motility are located in various cortical and hypothalamic areas, the lower part of the amygdala, and the fastigial nucleus in the cerebellum. Higher centers mediate behavioral responses

TABLE 1. *Wiring and functions of extrinsic neural control*

Region	Parasympathetic Wiring	Parasympathetic Function	Sympathetic Wiring	Sympathetic Function	Central mechanism
Esophagus Cervical	Vagus nerve; recurrent laryngeal branch	Peristalsis in response to burst of spike activity	Superior cervical ganglion	Stimulation of upper esophageal sphincter tone	*Motor:* nucleus ambiguus, cortico-bulbar pathways
	Glossopharyngeal and vagus nerve	Sensation			*Sensory:* nucleus of tractus solitarus
Thoracic	Vagus nerve	Peristalsis by successive firing of vagal fibers	Celiac ganglion T6–9 spinal cord	Stimulation of lower esophageal sphincter tone	*Motor:* dorsal motor nucleus of vagus, corticobulbar pathways *Swallowing:* afferent modulation of central program
	Vagus nerve to nodose ganglia	Sensation			
Stomach	Vagus nerve	Peristalsis (cholinergic), inhibitory (nonadrenergic), e.g., receptive relaxation	Celiac ganglion T6-9 spinal cord	Inhibition and relaxation (e.g., antrofundal reflex)	*Motor and sensory:* Dorsal motor nucleus of vagus, thoracic spinal cord; nucleus ambiguus
	Vagus nerve	Stretch and chemosensation	Spinal root ganglia T7-11	Mechanosensation (e.g., gastrogastric or enterogastric distention or nutrient reflexes)	
Small and large intestines	Vagus nerve	Small bowel and proximal colon peristalsis and sensation	Celiac ganglion to duodenum; superior and inferior mesenteric ganglia via splanchnic nerves to small bowel and via lumbar colonic nerves to colon; T9-10 spinal cord	Motor inhibition; distention reflexes	Nucleus of tractus solitarus (*sensory*), dorsal motor nucleus of vagus (*sensory and motor*); thoracic spinal cord; spinal cord base of dorsal horn (*motor parasympathetic*); parasympathetic nucleus (*sensory*)
	Sacral S2-4	Distal colon peristalsis and sensation			
Ileocecal sphincter	Vagus nerve	Sphincter contraction	Splanchnic and lumbar colonic nerves	Sphincter contraction (α effect); possibly also inhibitory β-effect	T9-10 spinal cord; ? vagal nucleus (*motor*)
Internal anal sphincter	S2-4	Sphincter relaxation	Lumbar splanchnic nerves; inferior mesenteric ganglia via hypogastric nerves	Sphincter contraction (α effect); possibly inhibitory β effect; ? participates in rectoanal inhibitory reflex; mediation of vesico-anal reflex	T9-10 spinal cord; spinal cord base of dorsal horn (*parasympathetic*)
External anal sphincter	S2-4 via pudendal nerves	Voluntary control; sensation			Lateral part of ventral horn of spinal cord (*motor and sensory*)

T, thoracic; S, sacral.

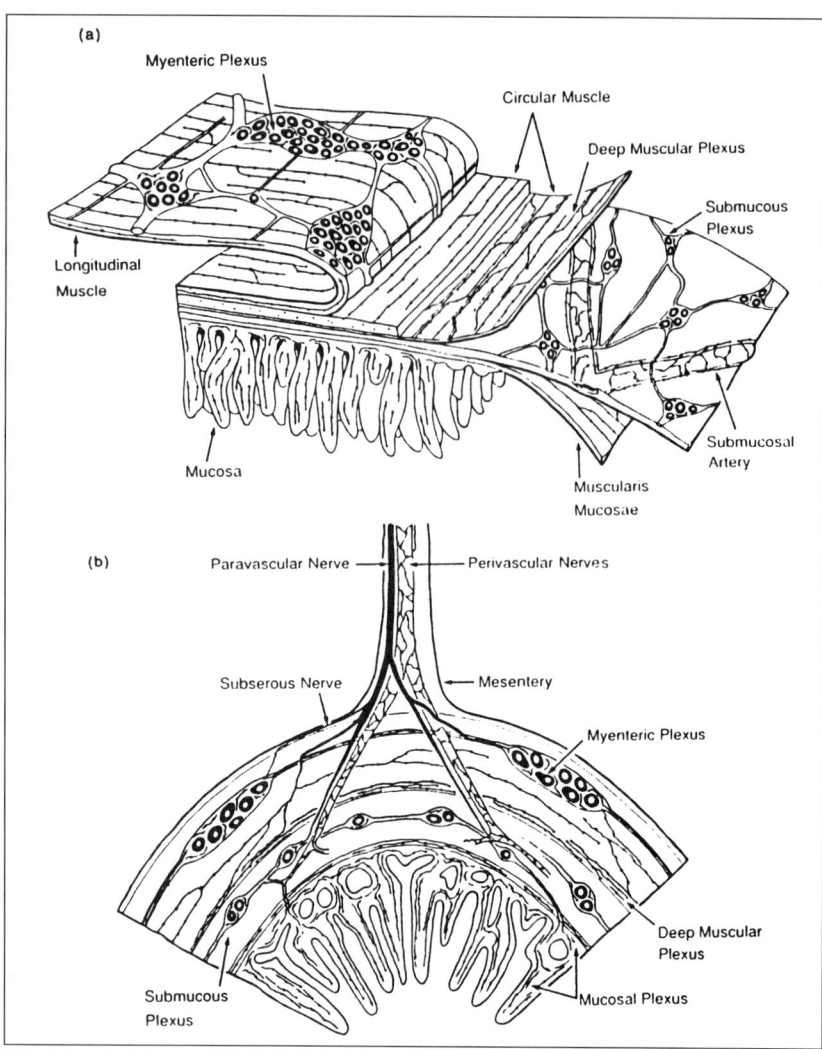

FIG. 2. Diagrammatic representation of the enteric plexuses in whole mounts of intestine **(A)** and in transverse section **(B)**. From Furness et al. (6), as modified from Furness and Costa (7), with permission.

(such as satiety) that, in turn, alter gut motility (e.g., by intake of food). In general, the extrinsic neural control of the gut results in stimulation, mediated through the vagus nerve, and inhibition via sympathetic routes, such as the lumbar colonic nerves.

It is important to realize that at the level of the diaphragm, almost half of the vagal nerve fibers are afferents (1). Autonomic afferents reach various central nervous structures, and neurons of nucleus tractus solitarius (e.g., gustatory and probably pain mechanosensation) and dorsal motor nucleus of vagus (e.g., glucoreceptors) may exhibit a specific response to a given type of stimulus. A greater understanding of the modulation by these afferent projections on the efferent discharges arising from central structures would provide important insights into the extrinsic neural control of the gut.

THE ROLE OF PREVERTEBRAL SYMPATHETIC GANGLIA

Prevertebral (celiac, superior mesenteric, and inferior mesenteric) ganglia function as relay stations between the central nervous system and the periphery (10,11). The different prevertebral ganglia are interconnected with one another bidirectionally, and principal ganglion cells of each ganglion receive spinal preganglionic input. They are also involved in multiplication of centrifugal impulses, integration of impulse flow from central and peripheral sources, and participation in peripheral reflex activity (10). Thus,

TABLE 2. *Levels of neural control of gut motility*

Function	Level of control
Peristalsis	Enteric nervous system
Migrating motor complex	
Enteroenteric sympathetic reflexes	Prevertebral ganglia
Enterogastric, gastrocolic reflex	Brainstem
Satiety	Higher centers

prevertebral ganglia mediate at least two types of intestinal inhibitory reflexes: first, spinal reflexes that are mediated through the spinal cord, dorsal root ganglia, and preganglionic autonomic neurons; and, second, peripheral reflexes (16) involving neural afferent projections to the prevertebral ganglia and efferent projections of noradrenergic neurons. The latter reflexes involve peptidergic fibers and may be involved in the *crosstalk* that occurs between different regions (10) of the digestive tract, including peristalsis and the responses to intestinal distention (enteroenteric reflexes).

THE ENTERIC NERVOUS SYSTEM

The enteric nervous system is a network of nerve cells and nerve fibers embedded in the wall throughout the gastrointestinal tract (6). It consists of two major ganglionated plexuses—the myenteric and submucous plexuses—and plexuses of nerve-fiber bundles in the muscle layers, mucosa, subserosa, and around arteries (Fig. 2). The myenteric plexus contains a large number of closely spaced ganglia interlinked by nerve-fiber bundles and extending from the pharyngoesophageal junction to the internal anal sphincter. Each ganglion contains a variable number of nerve cell bodies (up to 100), and the human gut contains a total of $\sim 10^8$ nerve cell bodies in the enteric plexuses. This number is roughly equivalent to the number of neurons in the spinal cord.

The submucous plexus is confined to the small and large intestines, and its ganglia are either large or small and form overlapping, but interlinked, plexuses. The larger ganglia lie closer to the inner surface of the circular muscle; the smaller ganglia are juxtamucosal and appear to be involved in the control of water and electrolyte secretion.

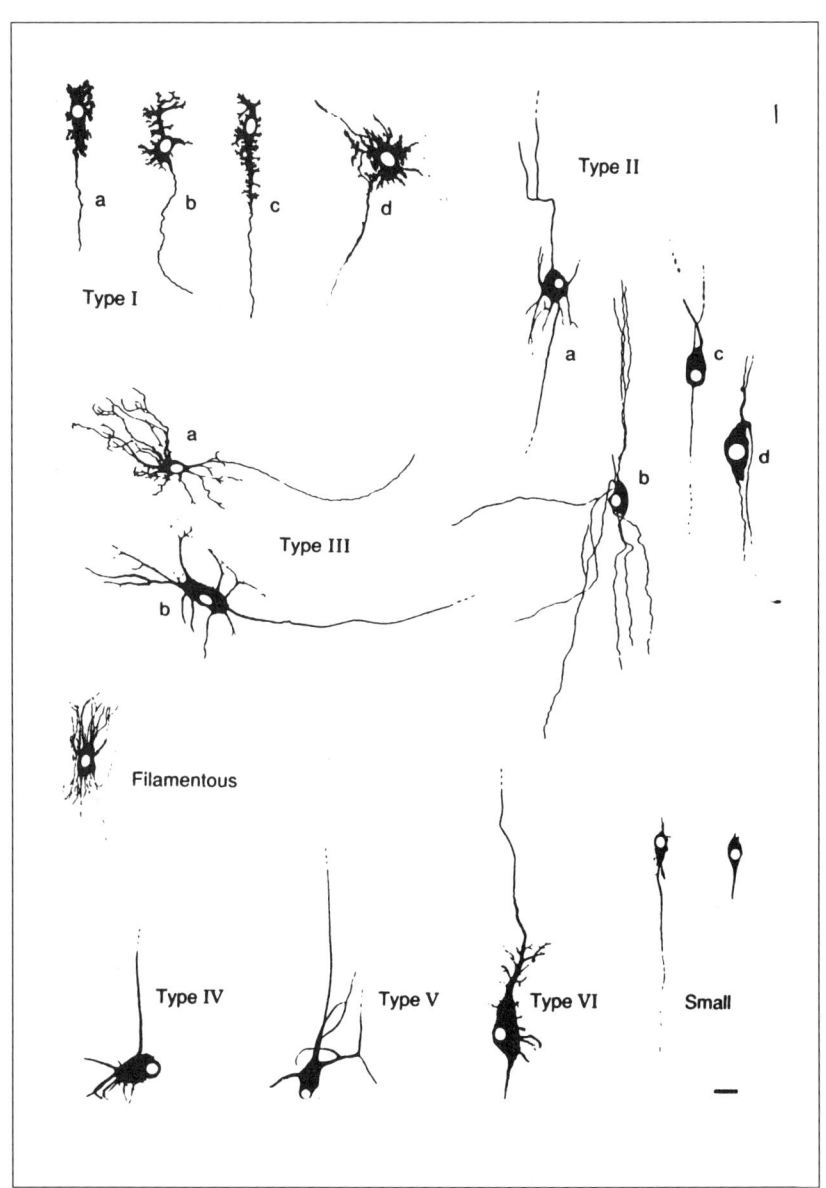

FIG. 3. Morphology of neurons in myenteric plexuses. These drawings are taken from whole-mount preparations of the small intestine (Dogiel types I and II, and Stach types IV, V, and VI) or large intestine (Dogiel type III). From Furness et al. (6), with permission.

Other nerve plexuses are developed to a variable extent in different animal species. A *longitudinal muscle plexus* consists of fine nerve-fiber bundles throughout the thickness of the longitudinal muscle, oriented parallel to the muscle fibers. The *deep muscular plexus of Cajal* is a dense layer of nerve bundles found near the inner surface of the circular muscle. There is increasing evidence that the interstitial cells of Cajal function as the pacemakers of the gut. Finally, a *mucosal plexus* is located throughout the lamina propria with fibers close to epithelial cells, connective tissue components, muscularis mucosae, blood vessels, and immunocompetent cells. The mucosal plexus itself has subglandular, periglandular, and villous components.

The neurons of the enteric plexuses in animal species have been extensively studied, and correlations of shape (Fig. 3), biophysical characteristics, and synaptic inputs have been established morphologically, electrophysiologically, and histochemically (6). Thus, among neurons of the myenteric plexus, Dogiel type I (monoaxonal neurons with broad dendrites often joining the cell soma via one narrow neck), filamentous, and small neurons are of the S type electrophysiologically, exhibiting fast excitatory postsynaptic potentials of ≥10 mV amplitude. In contrast, Dogiel type II (multiaxonal) neurons are of the AH type electrophysiologically, exhibiting long-lasting hyperpolarizations that last several seconds. In the submucous plexus of the guinea-pig small intestine, characterization of transmitter content has demonstrated clear functional specificity of neurons. Thus, neurons containing vasoactive intestinal polypeptide are noncholinergic and secretomotor, whereas neurons containing both choline acetyltransferase (ChAT), which results in synthesis of acetylcholine, and neuropeptide Y are cholinergic secretomotor neurons; ChAT and substance P are sensory neurons; and neurons containing ChAT only are interneurons. Further characterization of human enteric plexuses and their neurons in health and disease is necessary to enhance our understanding of the mechanisms that lead to gastrointestinal motor dysfunction.

OVERALL FUNCTIONS OF THE ENTERIC NERVOUS SYSTEM

Like the central nervous system, the enteric nervous system is an independent integrative system (the "little brain") consisting of sensory neurons, motor neurons, and interneurons (19,20). Sensory neurons are specialized for detecting thermal, chemical (e.g., glucose, lipid, pH, and osmolality), and mechanical (e.g., stretch) stimuli and transform the information into action potential codes. Interneurons are synaptically connected into networks that process sensory information and control the activity of motor neurons. Thus, they "decipher" the action potential codes from sensory and other interneuronal circuits and respond to these inputs by relaying the message to other interneurons that are organized in program circuits. The latter determine the stereotyped responses that are relayed to

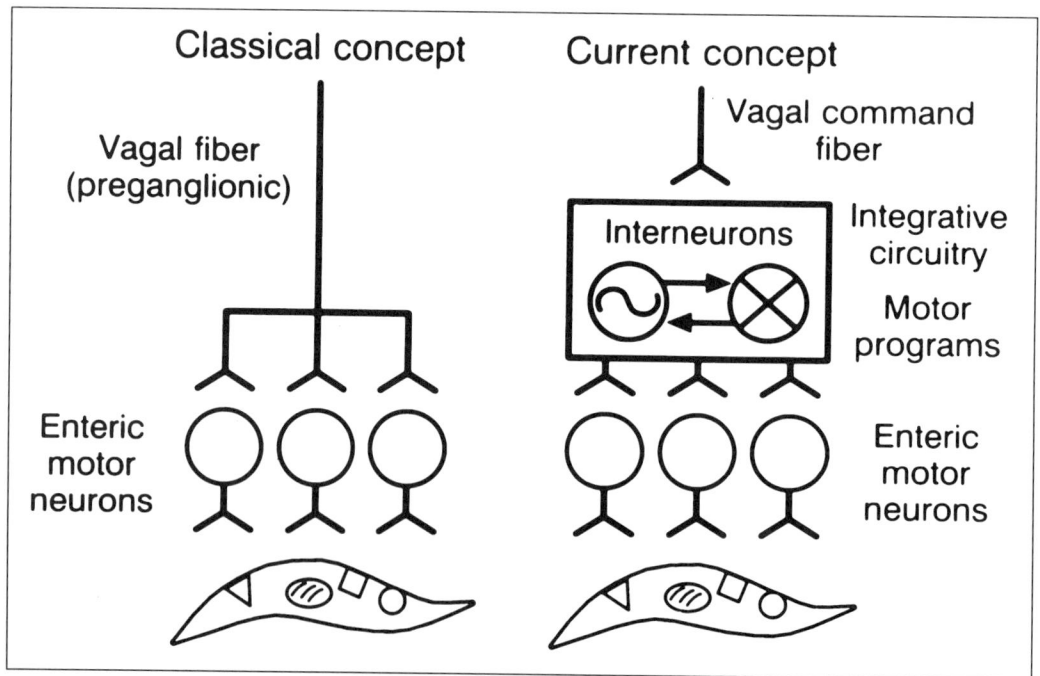

FIG. 4. Classic and current concepts of interaction between extrinsic and enteric plexuses. According to the classic concept, preganglionic cholinergic fibers synapse with a small number of enteric neurons; according to the novel concept, vagal command fibers synapse with preprogrammed circuits with "hard-wired" functions. Modified from Wood and Wingate (20), with permission 1987.

the effector systems (e.g., smooth muscle contraction and epithelial cell secretion) through the motor neurons.

Thus, the current concept (Fig. 4) is that local integrative circuits of the enteric nervous system are organized for functional operations that may be independent of preganglionic parasympathetic output (19). This concept differs from the classic concept of vagal innervation where preganglionic fibers were thought to synapse directly with the enteric ganglion cells that directly innervate the effector (e.g., motor or secretory) cells. Such a concept is untenable because there are an estimated 100 million neurons in the enteric nervous system, or 10,000 postganglionic neurons for each preganglionic vagal fiber. In contrast, the current concept suggests that ganglion cells are organized in *hardwired* programs of the "little brain" or enteric nervous system and receive modulating commands from the "big brain" or central nervous system via the efferent vagal fibers. It is believed that stereotyped programs of the semiautonomous enteric nervous system are selected on the basis of the sensory inputs from the periphery, or "commands" by the central nervous system.

SPECIFIC FUNCTIONS OF THE ENTERIC NERVOUS SYSTEM

The enteric nervous system is intricately involved in specific gastrointestinal motor functions. It provides a pacemaker system, controls contractile activity and reflex programs such as the peristaltic reflex, and transfers or transforms information leading to integrated responses.

Gastrointestinal muscle fibers are coupled to form electrical syncytia in which electrical currents spread from cell to cell. Electrical pacemakers intrinsic to the musculature evoke action potentials that propagate between muscle fibers, thereby triggering an excitatory response within the muscle fibers, resulting in an organized contraction. These action potentials are initiated simultaneously around the circumference of the bowel by the synchronous pacemaker potentials. Propagation in the long axis of the viscus occurs more slowly.

Control of the contractile activity of the gut depends on the effects of excitatory or inhibitory motor neurons. In sphincteric muscle, inhibitory neurons are normally off and are switched on when the sphincter needs to be opened as part of the coordinated events in a region, such as the lower esophageal, the antroduodenal, or the anorectal regions. In nonsphincteric muscle, activation of inhibitory neurons determines the length of a contracting segment by controlling the distance of spread of myogenic excitation within the syncytium. Failure of such inhibitory control may result in motor dysfunction, as in the contracted segment of Hirschsprung's disease, achalasia of the lower esophageal sphincter; conversely, excessive inhibitory activity may result in paralytic ileus (20).

The enteric nervous system also controls the peristaltic reflex, which is a stereotyped sequence of muscular contractions and relaxations, respectively above and below an

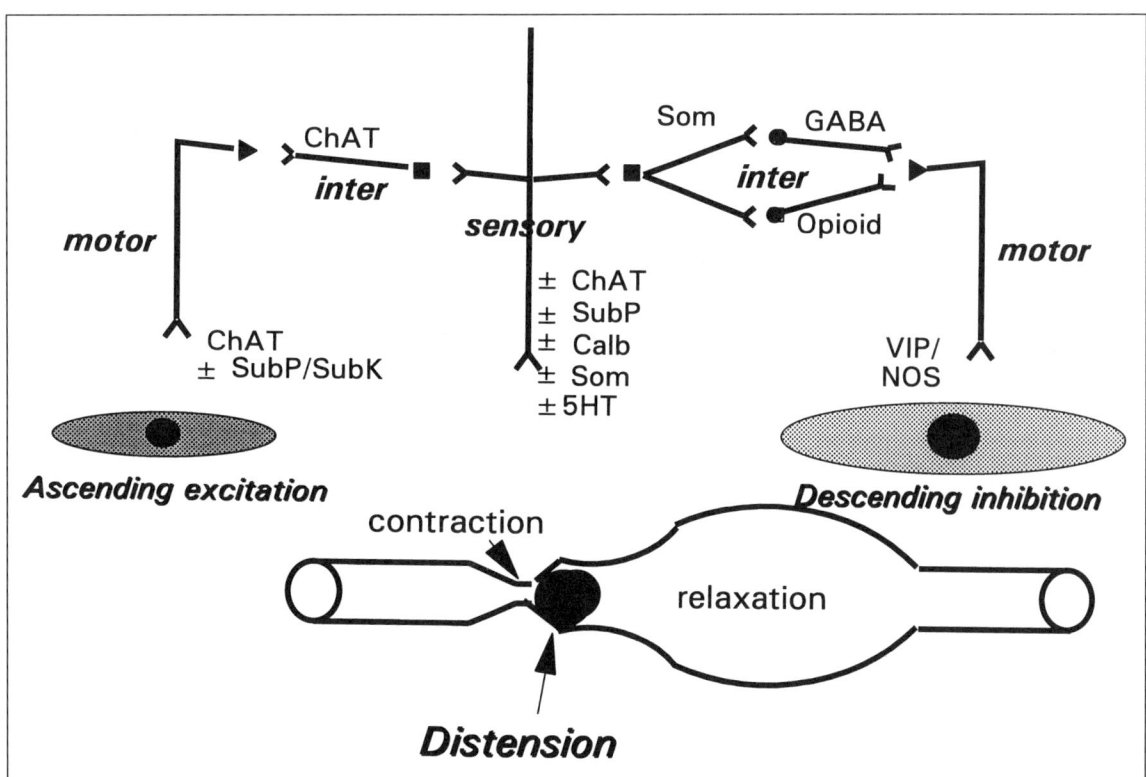

FIG. 5. Schematic of transmitters involved in the peristaltic reflex.

area where intramural stretch receptors are activated (19). Orad to the stimulus, contraction of the circular muscle occurs; caudad to the distention, the circular muscle is inhibited and the longitudinal muscle shortens. A fundamental neural circuit expressed repeatedly along the intestine mediates this reflex to accomplish aborad propulsion of intraluminal contents. The operation of synaptic or transmembrane channels that are opened by stimuli of a certain intensity serves to link these repetitive circuits and determine the distance of propulsion. Enteric neurons often contain more than one transmitter or peptide, and the nature of the incoming electrical stimulus may determine which transmitter is released and, hence, which response to elicit in the effector organ. The main excitatory transmitters are acetylcholine and tachykinins, and the main inhibitory transmitters involved in the descending limb of the peristaltic reflex are vasoactive intestinal polypeptide, nitric oxide, and interneurons containing somatostatin, opioids, and γ-aminobutyric acid (Fig. 5).

Enteric neural circuits also serve to transfer and transform information by propagation of action potentials along nerve fibers and by chemical transmission at synapses. This function serves to integrate sensory input and presynaptic modulation (parasympathetic and sympathetic) and to set up the appropriate effector response.

INTEGRATION BETWEEN ENTERIC AND EXTRINSIC AUTONOMIC NERVOUS SYSTEMS FOR MOTOR FUNCTION

The integration between the enteric and extrinsic autonomic nervous systems occurs through the excitatory vagal pathway (cholinergic fibers that stimulate programs involving myenteric cholinergic neurons) and sympathetic pathways. Vagal preganglionic fibers affect gut motility by influencing "command neurons" in the myenteric plexus, stimulating programmed patterns of neural activity that is *hard-wired* in intrinsic enteric neuronal circuits (19). The sympathetic postganglionic fibers inactivate neural circuits that generate motor activity while permitting continuous activity of inhibitory intrinsic motor neurons. Vagal fibers also activate nonadrenergic inhibitory motoneurons. Loss of this adrenergic or vagal nonadrenergic modulation may result in excessive or uncoordinated motor responses in the gut, as occurs in various disease processes where the extrinsic neural control is impaired (2).

VISCERAL AFFERENT FUNCTIONS

Sensory information that is coded by sensory neurons in the form of action potentials is processed by networks in the central nervous system, prevertebral ganglia, and the enteric nervous system. Afferent fibers predominate over efferent fibers by a ratio of 30:1 in the vagus nerve (9); the cell bodies are located in the nodose ganglion, and the synapses in the brain stem lead to vagovagal reflexes. Vagal afferents appear to be primarily concerned with visceral reflexes and behavior mediated by the central nervous system and project to the nucleus of the solitary tract, the area postrema in the fourth ventricle, and the dorsal motor nucleus of the vagus. Visceral afferents also traverse along sympathetic fibers to either the cell bodies in the dorsal root ganglion with synapses occurring in the spinal cord, mainly in laminae I and V, or to cell bodies in enteric ganglia and synapses in the prevertebral ganglia. Concurrence of somatic and visceral nociceptive inputs to the same relay neurons and pathways in the central nervous system results in visceral referred pain.

Sensory pathways serve several homeostatic functions, such as control of peristalsis, alterations in mucosal blood flow, and secretion via local axon reflexes (13) or reflex loops centered in the prevertebral ganglia (17), spinal, or supraspinal levels (12). These extrinsic reflexes are involved in the process of luminal "sampling," and homeostatic responses to enteric events such as intestinointestinal reflexes or viscerointestinal reflexes that may be involved in postoperative ileus or the phenomenon of *meteorism* in patients with ureteric colic. The anatomy, physiology, and transmitters involved in reflex control at prevertebral ganglia have been reviewed in detail by Szurszewski and Miller (17). Afferent activation in the digestive tract will also lead to conscious perception of stimuli arising from the alimentary tract. Thus, when the afferent input changes its character or the viscus is inflamed or injured, the signal is relayed beyond homeostatic or reflex centers to the higher senses. Perception of visceral stimulus occurs through a network of fibers and centers that show a general organization based on three order neurons similar to that of somatic sensation.

In general, visceral afferents tend to respond to distention either at mucosal or deeper levels, as well as to chemical, osmotic, and thermal stimulation (14). Receptors that convey these types of sensory stimuli have been characterized functionally but not structurally in the gastrointestinal tract except for the pacinian corpuscles present in the mesentery (12). Previously, noxious stimuli were believed

TABLE 3. *Mechanisms of hyperalgesia*

Peripheral sensitization due to inflammation or chemical injury activating nociceptive and "silent" afferents
Stimulation of nerve endings, e.g.,
    High-threshold, pain-encoding or nociceptive fibers
    Low-threshold fibers that encode pain with repetitive or large areas of stimulation
Change in afferent function or receptive field size by sensitization of dorsal horn neuron
Affective-motivational modulation increasing cortical perception, imparting autonomic and emotional components to pain

---

Reprinted with permission from Camilleri et al. (2a).

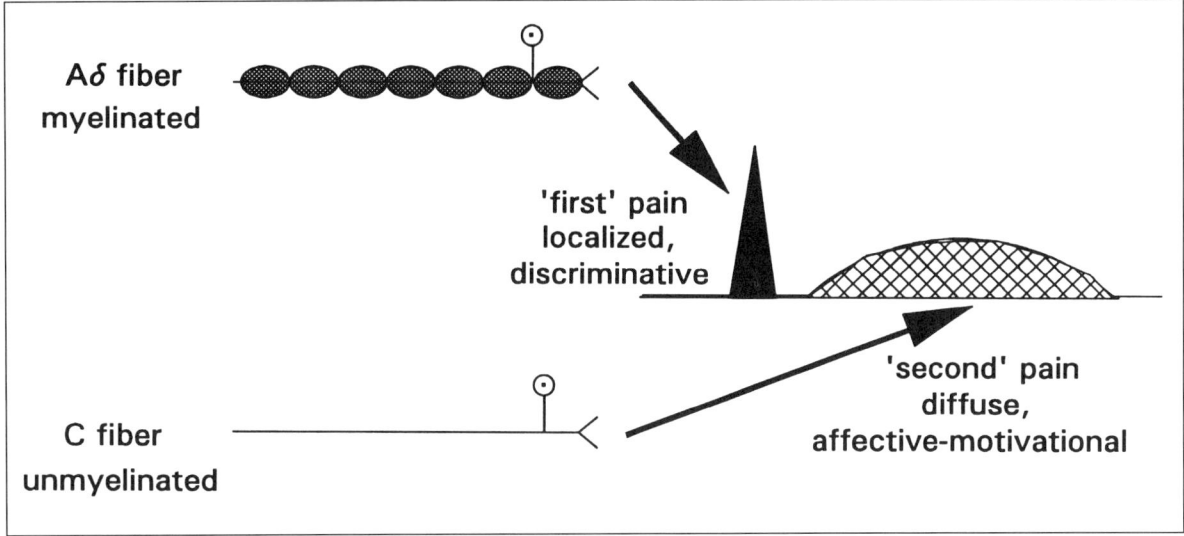

FIG. 6. Types of afferent fibers and characteristics of pain mediated by those fibers. From Camilleri et al. (4), with permission.

to be relayed exclusively by sympathetic pathways. The vagus nerve is predominantly an afferent nerve at the level of the diaphragm (9); it is believed that vagal and sacral parasympathetic fibers also mediate visceral perception. Visceral sensitivity is controlled either in the peripheral receptors, the spinal cord by altering signal processing in the dorsal horn or second-order neurons, or in the higher centers above the brainstem where conscious perception occurs. Visceral sensation has two major characteristics: sensory discriminative function and affective–motivational

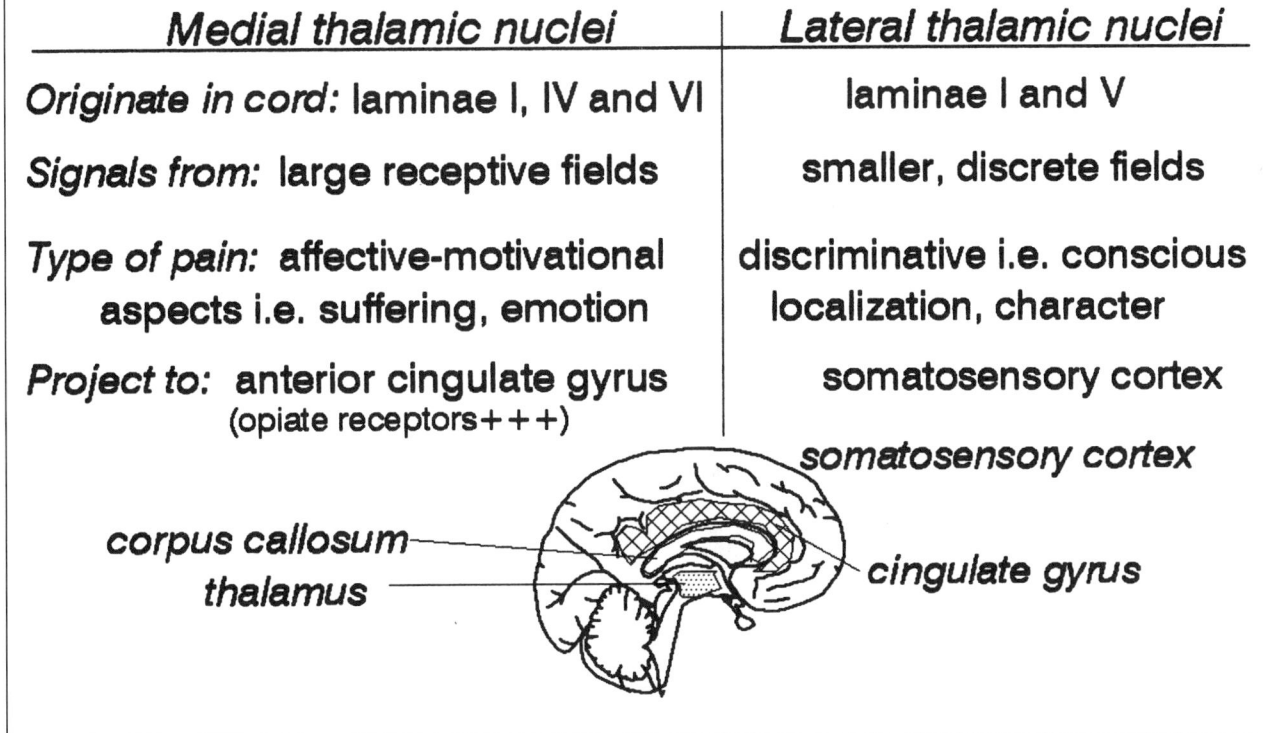

FIG. 7. Central projection of nociceptive spinothalamic tract neurons. Note that the type of pain sensed depends on the location of thalamic nuclei and projection of the third-order neuron to somatosensory cortex or cingulate gyrus. From Camilleri et al. (4), with permission.

perception that imparts the characteristic emotional and autonomic components to visceral pain.

There are two predominant diameters of primary sensory afferents (Table 3) (5). Myelinated A-δ fibers range from 0.4 to 3.0 μm in diameter, whereas unmyelinated C fibers are 2.0–12.0 μm in diameter. A-δ, small myelinated fibers are responsible for the sensation of "first" pain in the soma (Fig. 6). This is well localized, discriminative, and lasting as long as the stimulus C or unmyelinated fibers are responsible for the longer lasting "second" pain and convey afferent impulses from polymodal sensory receptors or afferent signals involving recruitment of multiple nonnoxious sensory afferent stimuli (5). Second pain tends to be more diffuse, lasting beyond the duration of the stimulus, and is associated with affective–motivational aspects of pain.

The dorsal horn neurons are the site of convergence of visceral and somatic signals. This convergence on the same neurons in lamina V of the dorsal horn is responsible for "convergence–projection" or "referred pain" of a visceral stimulus.

Visceral afferents project centrally via two ascending pathways (5): the spinothalamic and spinoreticular tracts. The spinothalamic tract contains fibers arising from wide-dynamic-range (50%) and nociceptive-specific (30%) neurons. Spinothalamic tract neurons project to the medial or lateral thalamic nuclei (Fig. 7), which are respectively associated with affective–motivational and discriminative types of pain. Fibers directed to the medial thalamus also project to the reticular formation and mediate arousal and possibly autonomic responses. The third-order neurons arising in the medial thalamic nucleus project diffusely to the frontal, parietal, and limbic regions of the cortex, including the anterior cingulate gyrus which is rich in opiate receptors (Fig. 7). This series of central projections constitutes the more medially located, phylogenetically older nervous system and is involved in homeostasis, integrative function, and the affective–motivational aspects of visual pain. The third-order neuron arising from the lateral thalamic nuclei is relayed to the somatosensory cortex.

The second major ascending pathway is the spinoreticular tract, which projects to the medial thalamus (Fig. 8) via the reticular formation in the pons and medulla (e.g., nucleus gigantocellularis and the nucleus paragigantocellularis) or in the mesencephalon (e.g., the periaqueductal grey). Central projections from the reticular formation to the hypothalamus result in some of the autonomic as well as the emotional responses to painful stimulation. More-

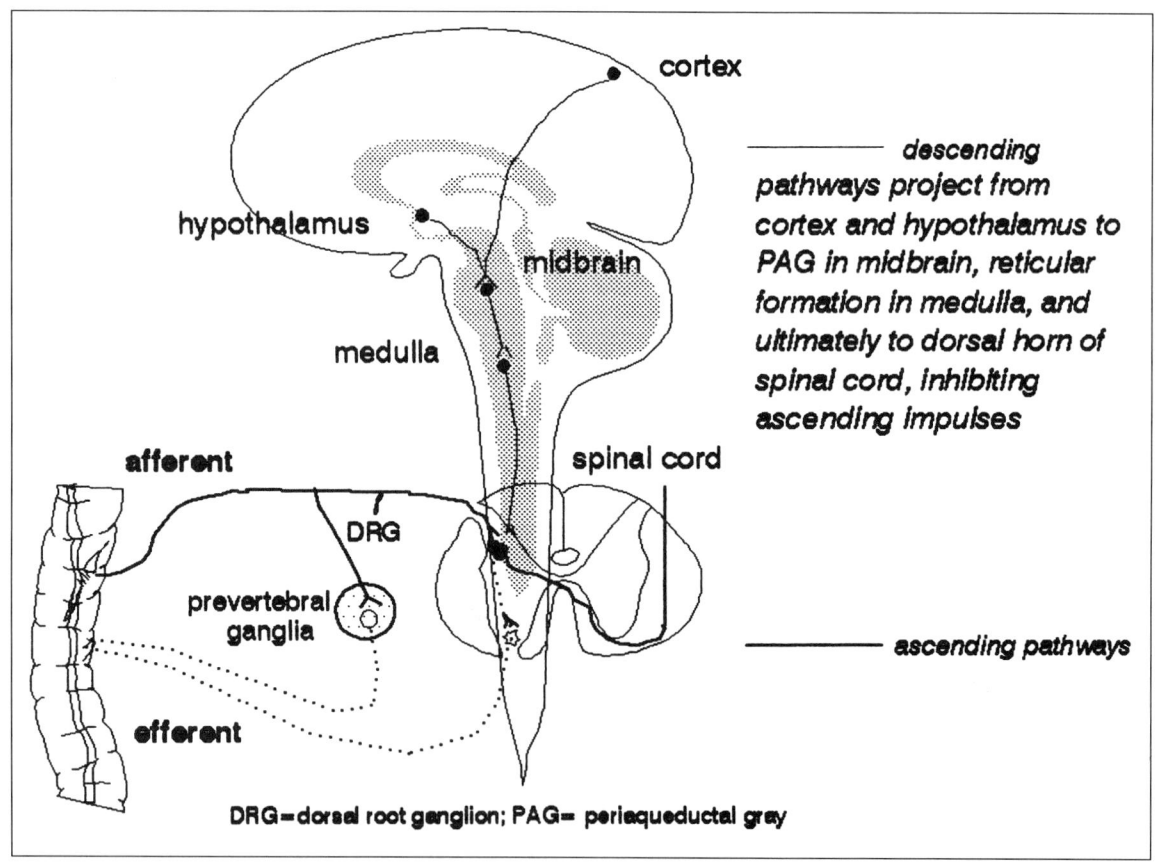

FIG. 8. Schema showing descending modulation of sensory pathways. From Camilleri et al. (4), with permission.

over, from these reticular neurons arise the descending pathways that modulate the function of dorsal horn neurons and, hence, the spinal control of afferent input.

SUPRASPINAL MODULATION OF PAIN

Supraspinal modulation originates in the frontal cortex and hypothalamus, and traverses to the brainstem to reach the dorsal horn neurons in the spinal cord (Fig. 8). The main transmitters include norepinephrine, serotonin, and opioids, and descending pathways inhibit nociceptive-specific dorsal horn neurons. Supraspinal modulation constitutes a powerful negative-feedback system that explains analgesia produced by hypnosis or by counterirritation.

RELEVANCE OF VISCERAL AFFERENT SENSITIVITY TO CLINICAL SYNDROMES

In virtually all functional gastrointestinal syndromes from the level of the esophagus to the anal sphincter, investigators have consistently demonstrated a subpopulation of patients who have increased visceral perception that is attributed to afferent sensitivity. Thus, in clinical syndromes such as noncardiac chest pain, nonulcer dyspepsia, irritable bowel syndrome and, possibly, proctalgia fugax, there is evidence of excessive visceral afferent function.

CONCLUSION

The extrinsic autonomic nervous system and enteric nervous system are intricately involved in the regulation of gastrointestinal motility. Stereotyped programs, hard-wired within the enteric nervous system, are set off by central modulation or by sensory input at the periphery. Understanding these controls of gut motility provides a framework for greater comprehension of the mechanisms that result in gut dysmotility. The autonomic nervous system is also intimately involved in the sensory connections between the gut and the central nervous system. Further progress in these areas may lead to insights into the derangement of gut functions occurring in neurologic disorders that affect gut function, or in common diseases such as irritable bowel syndrome and functional dyspepsia, which constitute almost 50% of the referral population in gastroenterology clinics in the Western world.

REFERENCES

1. Andrews PLR, et al. Vagal afferent discharge from mechanoreceptors in different regions of the ferret stomach. *J Physiol (Lond)* 1980;298:513–524.
2. Camilleri M. Disorders of gastrointestinal motility in neurologic diseases. *Mayo Clin Proc* 1990;65:825–846.
3. Camilleri M, Phillips SF. *Gastroenterol Clin North Am* 1989;18:405–424.
4. Camilleri M, et al. Gastrointestinal sensation: mechanisms and relation to functional gastrointestinal disorders. *Gastroenterol Clin North Am* 1996;25:247–258.
5. Cross SA. Pathophysiology of pain. *Mayo Clin Proc* 1994;69:375–383.
6. Furness JB, et al. The normal structure of gastrointestinal innervation. *J Gastroenterol Hepatol* 1990;1:1–9.
7. Furness JB, Costa M. *The enteric nervous system.* London: Churchill-Livingstone, 1987.
8. Gershon MD, Erde SM. The nervous system of the gut. *Gastroenterology* 1981;80:1571–1594.
9. Grundy D. Speculations on the structure/function relationship for vagal and splanchnic afferent endings supplying the gastrointestinal tract. *J Auton Nerv Syst* 1988;22:175–180.
10. Kreulen DL, Szurszewski JH. Reflex pathways in the abdominal prevertebral ganglia: evidence for a colo-colonic inhibitory reflex. *J Physiol (Lond)* 1979;295:21–32.
11. Langley JN, Anderson HK. On the innervation of the pelvic and adjoining viscera. I. The lower portion of the intestine. *J Physiol (Lond)* 1895;18:67–105.
12. Mayer EA, Gebhart GF. Basic and clinical aspects of visceral hyperalgesia. *Gastroenterology* 1994;107:271–293.
13. Maggi CA, Meli A. The sensory–efferent function of capsaicin-sensitive sensory neurons. *Gen Pharmacol* 1988;19:1–43.
14. Mei N. Sensory structures in the viscera. In: Autrum H, et al., eds. *Progress in sensory physiology;* vol 4. Berlin: Springer-Verlag, 1983:1–42.
15. Roman C, Gonella J. Extrinsic control of digestive tract motility. In: Johnson LR, ed. *Physiology of the gastrointestinal tract.* 2nd ed. New York: Raven, 1987:507–553.
16. Szurszewski JH, Krier J. Sympathetic regulation of gastrointestinal motility. In: Dyck PJ, et al., eds. *Peripheral neuropathy.* 2nd ed. Philadelphia: WB Saunders, 1984:265–284.
17. Szurszewski JH, Miller S. Physiology of prevertebral ganglia. In: Johnson LR, ed. *Physiology of the gastrointestinal tract.* 3rd ed. New York: Raven, 1994:795–877.
18. Weisbrodt NW. Motility of the small intestine. In: *Johnson LR, ed. Physiology of the gastrointestinal tract.* 2nd ed. New York: Raven, 1987:631–663.
19. Wood JD. Enteric neurophysiology. *Am J Physiol* 1984;247:G585–G598.
20. Wood JD, Wingate DL. Gastrointestinal neurophysiology: unit 20. In: *The UTP slide lecture series.* Timonium, MD: Milner Fenwick, 1987.

CHAPTER 13

Autonomic Regulation of Immune Function

Barry G. W. Arnason

1. The sympathetic nervous system (SNS) modulates immune function.
2. SNS axons innervate the spleen and lymphoid tissues, and nerve endings contact T cells, monocytes and, to a lesser extent, B cells.
3. Lymphocytes and macrophages have β_2-adrenergic receptors. The rank order of density of receptors is B cells > C8 + T suppressor cells, macrophages > CD8 + cytotoxic T cells > CD4 + T cells with few receptors. The neurotransmitters are norepinephrine and epinephrine.
4. Immunocytes respond to adrenergic agonists by a rise in intracellular cyclic AMP.
5. Other receptors on immunocytes include vasoactive intestinal peptide (T cells), muscarinic acetylcholine, substance P, somatostatin, enkephalins, and endorphins.
6. β-Agonists inhibit many immune responses. β-Antagonists upregulate adrenergic receptors on the cell surface.
7. Chemical postganglionic adrenergic ablation with 6-hydroxydopamine results in a functional postganglionic axotomy. Immune alterations include a marked increase of T-cell-independent antibody response, augmentation of T-cell proliferative responses, increased severity of autoimmune myasthenia gravis and experimental allergic encephalomyelitis, altered kinetics of natural killer cells, a reduction in the ratio of CD8+ : CD4+ cells, and an upregulation of β_2-adrenergic receptors on splenic lymphocytes.
8. Most patients with progressive multiple sclerosis (MS) have impaired sympathetic function. The patients with impaired SNS have upregulated β-adrenergic receptors. β-Adrenergic receptors are upregulated during MS attacks.
9. Most progressive MS patients with impaired parasympathetic function have upregulated muscarinic acetylcholine receptors.
10. Not only does the SNS modulate immune function, the latter also affects the SNS. Mediators include interleukin 1, interleukin 2, interferon γ, and tumor necrosis factor α.

INTRODUCTION

Interactions between the sympathetic nervous system (SNS) and the immune system are discussed in this chapter. Some readers may be unfamiliar with immune mechanisms. Accordingly, a brief discussion of some of the general principles of immune regulation and of the cell types responsible for immune responses is provided as an introduction to the discussion that follows. This capsule overview must be recognized as selective and simplified, but since the modulatory role of the SNS on immune responses is not uniform, some orientation is required.

THE IMMUNE SYSTEM

The immune system can be divided into two arms—humoral and cellular. Humoral responses are mediated by antibodies released by B cells, cellular responses by T cells, and by monocyte-derived macrophages. T-cell progenitors proliferate within the thymus, mature there, and then migrate to peripheral lymphoid organs such as the lymph nodes and spleen. Two-thirds of mature T cells bear a surface marker protein named CD4 (antigen cluster designation 4) and one-third a surface marker protein named CD8. The two proteins are mutually exclusive on mature T cells. B cells, in contrast to T cells, mature in the bone marrow as do monocytes that are destined to become macrophages. Since both the thymus and the bone marrow receive a SNS innervation (see later) a modulatory role for the SNS in im-

---

B. G. W. Arnason: Department of Neurology, University of Chicago, Chicago, Illinois 60637.

munocyte maturation can be envisaged. Evidence that this is the case has recently been advanced [reviewed by Madden and Felten (82)]. 6-Hydroxydopamine (6OHDA) treatment destroys sympathetic nerves (see later). Thymic denervation with 6OHDA is followed by enhanced thymocyte proliferation, indicating an inhibitory role for the SNS in thymocyte maturation (75).

Immune responses can be divided into two phases—inductive and effector. The inductive phase is generated primarily within the lymphoid organs and the effector phase outside them, extracellularly in the case of antibody-mediated responses and on the surfaces of target cells in the case of T-cell-mediated and/or macrophage-mediated responses.

B-cell responses can be subdivided into two broad groupings—T-cell independent and T-cell dependent. T-cell-independent responses involve the production of immunoglobulin (Ig) M class antibody directed chiefly against carbohydrate and lipid antigens such as those found on bacteria. T-cell-dependent responses involve a switch by B cells from an initial synthesis of IgM antibody to subsequent synthesis of IgG and other classes of immunoglobulins. This switch is triggered by signal molecules provided by a distinct subpopulation of T cells, known as Th2 (T helper type 2) cells, which carry the CD4 (antigen cluster designation 4) surface marker protein. The major signaling molecules released by T cells are proteins called cytokines. The three major cytokines released by Th2 cells that act on B cells are known as interleukins (ILs) 4, 5, and 10. IgG responses, like IgM responses, may be directed against carbohydrates and lipids but are also directed against proteins. Antigenic sites on proteins are known as epitopes, and the folded conformation (i.e., three-dimensional shape) of the protein determines the epitopes.

B cells carry surface IgM. IgM molecules have constant and variable domains. The variable domains are responsible for antigen recognition, and a large repertoire of B-cell clones exists each with its own distinct variable domain. Only a minuscule proportion of this repertoire binds any given epitope. Once the appropriate epitope binds to the surface IgM of B cells of any given clone, the cells of that clone pass through numerous mitotic cycles in order to expand the population. Only after clonal expansion has been achieved is immunoglobulin with the requisite antigen-binding variable domains released into the circulation. Once antibody enters the circulation it binds to free-floating antigens (e.g., bacteria) or to cell surface-bound antigens wherever they are found.

T-cell responses are quite different. T cells recognize only short peptide sequences. The critical feature for recognition is amino acid sequence rather than the conformation; i.e., the epitopes recognized by T cells are in general distinct from those recognized by B cells. T cells recognize antigen by means of T-cell receptors for antigen. T-cell receptors have variable and constant domains; the variable domains are responsible for antigen binding. The repertoire of T-cell receptors for antigen is vast and, like B cells, the clonal expansion of T cells bearing the receptor for any given antigenic peptide occurs during the inductive phase of the immune response. For a T-cell response to be initiated, antigenic epitopes must be presented to them by so-called antigen-presenting cells (APCs). Macrophages are one of the principal APC types. Viruses and bacteria that reside intracellularly, once they have infected the APCs, are degraded and their proteins digested into small peptides that are embedded into a cleft found in the proteins of the major histocompatibility complex (MHC). The peptide–MHC complex is then transposed to and inserted into the cell membrane, so that the captured peptide is sited on the external surface of the cell and becomes accessible to T cells. For autoimmune responses, self proteins must be pinocytosed by APCs and degraded into small peptide fragments that are then processed as just described. T cells employ their antigen receptors to recognize cleaved peptides presented by MHC molecules on the surface of APCs.

There are class I and class II MHC alleles. Nonameric (i.e., nine-amino-acid containing) peptides are presented by class I MHC alleles to that population of T cells that bear the CD8 marker. MHC class I alleles are constitutively expressed on the surfaces of most cells within the body, with the brain a notable exception. In the brain, MHC class I alleles are constitutively expressed only on microglia. Astrocytes, oligodendroglia and, to a lesser extent neurons, can be induced to express MHC class I alleles by interferon (IFN)-γ as will be discussed further.

T cells bearing CD8 markers have two assigned functions—cytotoxicity and suppression. Two CD8 subpopulations can be distinguished by means of monoclonal antibodies that bind to a cell surface protein named CD28. CD8-positive cytotoxic T cells express CD28, whereas CD8-positive suppressor cells do not. Once clonal expansion has been achieved, newly activated T cells move from the lymphoid organs into the circulation and then into the tissues in search of targets. Cytotoxicity requires target cells to present antigen to effector cells in the context of surface-bound MHC class I alleles. Cytotoxicity is mediated by perforin, a cytokine released by CD8-positive cytotoxic T cells that have contacted antigenic peptide-bearing MHC class I alleles on target cells. Perforin binds to target cell membranes and polymerizes within them to form a pore that functions as an ion channel. Once channels have formed, the target cell condenses, its DNA fragments, and the cell disintegrates. In contrast, CD8-positive suppressor cells release inhibitory cytokines, including interleukin 10 and transforming growth factor (TGF) β_1 plus others that remain uncharacterized. TGF-β_1 inhibits several functions of immune cells (to be discussed), including IL-2-induced T- and B-cell proliferation, generation of cytotoxic T cells, cytokine production by monocytes and macrophages, IL-1 receptor expression on T cells, mitogen-induced T-cell proliferation, IFN-γ-induced MHC class II expression, and production of oxygen intermediates by macrophages. In contrast, TGF-$β_1$ stimulates other cell types such as fibroblasts.

Class II MHC alleles present larger peptides (12–16 amino acids) than those presented by class I MHC alleles, and this presentation is restricted to CD4 cells. Again epitopes are presented in a cleft on the external surface of MHC class II molecules. CD4 cells have been assigned two effector functions—help for B cells by Th2 cells (discussed previously), and delayed-type hypersensitivity (DTH). The T cells that mediate DTH responses are known as Th1 cells. MHC class II alleles are restricted in their tissue distribution. They are constitutively expressed on immunocytes but rarely on other cell types. They are not expressed in the brain except on some microglial cells. They can, however, be induced on astrocytes by IFN-γ, but not on oligodendrocytes or neurons.

The effector arm of a DTH response involves interaction within the target tissue between CD4-positive Th1 cells and antigen-presenting macrophages. Having been offered antigen, CD4-positive Th1 cells release lymphotoxin, a protein that directly damages target cells. They also release IFN-γ, which activates macrophages. Activated macrophages release proteases, lipases, eicosanoids (i.e., prostaglandins), free radicals, and cytokines. Among the cytokines released by macrophages are IL-1, which stimulates T cells, and tumor necrosis factor α (TNF) α, which has different effects on different tissues. TNF-α is toxic to oligodendrocytes but stimulates astrogliosis. Activated macrophages also perform important cytotoxic, phagocytic, and scavenger functions. Thus, in a DTH response, macrophages function as (a) APCs to CD4-positive T cells, (b) providers of stimulatory signals to T cells by means of IL-1, and (c) participants in destruction of cells that abut the site of the response. Cells destined to be destroyed in a DTH response need not themselves present antigen directly to the T cells; they may simply abut the APCs, i.e., they can be innocent bystanders.

The T-cell system may seem cumbersome but has its advantages. If cytotoxic T cells, whose function is to attack cells that present antigens on their surfaces (e.g., virally infected cells), were to respond to free-floating antigen, the short-range responses for which they are designed would be dissipated far from appropriate targets, such as virally infected cells. The system permits the killing of infected cells while sparing others. Similar considerations apply to the short-range tissue damage that occurs in DTH responses.

B- and T-cell responses require a proliferative phase once antigen has been recognized. Proliferation expands the limited number of clones contained within the repertoire that are programmed to respond to any given antigen. Once expanded, the B cells and T cells are poised to become effectors. For B cells, this involves antibody release; for T cells, this involves migration from the lymphoid organs into the circulation and then out of the circulation into the tissues in a search for appropriate targets. Circulating activated T cells must cross endothelial cells to enter target organs. Attachment to the endothelium is achieved by means of adhesion molecules reciprocally expressed on activated T cells and on the endothelium. The expression of adhesion molecules on both cell types is augmented by released cytokines such as IFN-γ, a product of activated T cells, and by IL-1 and TNF-α released by activated macrophages. Thus, a possible direct effect of the SNS on cell trafficking either by a direct action on endothelial cells, on immunocytes, or on both becomes a consideration as does the possibility that adhesion molecule expression may be influenced by SNS-mediated effects on release of IFN-γ, IL-1, and TNF-α.

THE SYMPATHETIC NERVOUS SYSTEM AND IMMUNE RESPONSES

The lymphoid organs receive SNS innervation. This innervation is not confined to blood vessels. SNS noradrenergic axons can be traced into the periarteriolar lymphatic sheath and surrounding white pulp of the spleen, the cortex but not the germinal centers of lymph nodes, the cortex and corticomedullary region of the thymus, and into gut-associated lymphoid tissues including the appendix and Peyer's patches [reviewed by Bellinger et al. (14), Felten et al. (46), and Madden and Felten (82)]. Nerve endings contact T cells, monocytes and, to a lesser extent, B cells. In rodents, splenic SNS innervation develops postnatally as the immune system is maturing. SNS innervation of the thymus also develops postnatally in rodents. Splenic SNS innervation is maintained until senescence and then declines (14,45). The thymus remains innervated even after it involutes (14). Neuropeptide Y (NPY) is associated with noradrenergic axons in rat thymus and spleen (14,82).

Interactions between the SNS and the immune system are dynamic. Splenic norepinephrine content falls as an immune response is rising and rises as the response begins to decline (39). The magnitude of the early decline correlates directly with the magnitude of the response that will occur (40). No such early decline or subsequent rise is seen in other organs, such as the heart, over the course of an immune response, establishing regional specificity. Similarly, in actively induced experimental allergic encephalomyelitis (EAE), splenic norepinephrine content falls early in disease and rebounds with overshoot at the time of peak disease (81). The rebound provides an immunosuppressive environment and contributes to recovery (78,79,134). Products of activated immune system cells act on SNS nerve endings to lessen SNS-mediated restraint early in an immune response, with the obverse occurring as a herald of the waning of an immune response.

Innervation of the lymphoid organs during postnatal development is also influenced by lymphoid cells. Athymic nude mice lack T cells. Such mice have higher numbers of sympathetic fibers in the spleen than do normal mice, and splenic norepinephrine levels are increased in them (16). SNS innervation of the kidney is normal in athymic mice, again indicating a regional specificity of the effect. Thymus transplantation or thymocyte injection into newborn nude mice restores splenic norepinephrine levels to their normal values. MRL/lpr mice develop systemic lupus erythematosus with massive splenomegaly secondary to an increase in T-cell number. The norepinephrine content of the spleen is reduced below normal levels in such mice, and the number of noradrenergic fibers detectable within the spleen is subnormal (22). These findings indicate that T-cell products exert an inhibitory influence on sympathetic nerve fiber development.

Immune system cells carry neurotransmitter receptors. Lymphocytes and macrophages have β_2-adrenergic receptors, the number varying from one cell type to another (2,52,137). B cells carry the most receptors, followed in descending order by CD8-positive T suppressor cells and macrophages, then by CD8-positive cytotoxic T cells, and lastly by CD4-positive T cells which have few receptors (69,76,84). The receptors respond to norepinephrine, which is released by SNS nerves within the lymphoid organs, and even more so to epinephrine, release of which is controlled by splanchnic nerve input to the adrenal medulla. Whether they also respond to NPY is not known. NPY is known to facilitate the actions of norepinephrine in promoting vasoconstriction and salivation (48).

Immunocytes respond to adrenergic agonists with a brisk elevation of intracellular cyclic adenosine 3',5'-monophosphate (cAMP) (19,49). The hierarchy of the response is not determined solely by β-adrenergic receptor number. The greatest response is observed in CD8-positive suppressor T cells; B cells respond less vigorously even though they carry more receptors (69,84). The cAMP response to β-adrenergic agonists depends primarily on the number of receptors coupled to adenylate cyclase as measured by the number of receptors that are in an agonist-dependent high-affinity state. It is believed that suppressor T cells respond best because they express more functional high-affinity β-adrenergic receptors than do other leukocyte subsets. Under some circumstances, IL-1 and TNF-α, both of which are released by activated macrophages, can uncouple β-adrenergic receptors (50).

Immunocytes carry receptors for other transmitters. The hierarchy varies, depending on the receptor [reviewed by Payan et al. (103)]. Vasoactive intestinal peptide (VIP) receptors are confined to T cells (38); muscarinic acetylcholine receptors are found on all types of immunocytes. VIP inhibits T-cell proliferation, whereas muscarinic acetylcholine agonists stimulate T-cell proliferation (7,98,107). VIP is also implicated in T-cell homing to the Peyer's patches. Lymphocytes also carry receptors for substance P, somatostatin, enkephalins, and endorphins. Substance P degranulates mast cells and basophils, decreases intracellular cAMP, augments T-cell proliferation, enhances macrophage phagocytosis, and induces IL-1 and TNF secretion (57,100,101). Selective denervation of substance P nerve fibers to lymph nodes with capsaicin reduces the severity of adjuvant-induced arthritis in rats and of antibody responses to sheep red blood cells, while ablation of substance P fibers to the joints reduces the severity of arthritis in the denervated joints (14,59) [reviewed by Madden and Felten (82)]. Somatostatin inhibits proliferation of both the B and T cells (102); α-endorphin also inhibits immune responses. Individual axon terminals may release more than one neurotransmitter, and neurotransmitters released by one axon may influence the release from others. Thus, an array of responses and a fine tuning of their kinetics under the influence of neurotransmitters seem likely. The situation is potentially complex, and a consideration of such matters lies beyond the scope of this chapter. Further discussion will be restricted to the roles of β-adrenergic (i.e., sympathetic) and muscarinic acetylcholine (i.e., parasympathetic) receptors in the immune system with the caveat that these are but two players in an orchestra.

Effects of Adrenergic Agonists and Antagonists on Immune Responses

β-Adrenergic agonist drugs inhibit many immune responses [reviewed by Chelmicka-Schorr and Arnason (28)]. They reduce T-cell proliferative responses triggered by mitogenic lectins or by IL-2 (13,36,66), a cytokine released by activated Th1-type T cells that induces both proliferation of the cells that produce it (autocrine stimulation) and of other activated T cells in the vicinity (i.e., paracrine stimulation). Activated T cells respond to released IL-2 because they generate IL-2 receptors. β-Adrenergic agonists cause IL-2 production by activated T cells to be downregulated (70). The expression of IL-2 receptors is reduced as well, especially on CD8-positive T suppressor cells (36,44,138). B-cell proliferation (inductive phase) in response to lectins is inhibited by β-adrenergic agonists. Antibody secretion (effector phase) is also reduced (42,133). The β-adrenergic agonist isoproterenol protects against EAE whether given during the inductive or effector phases of the immune response. Maximal protection is achieved when it is given during both phases (33). β-Adrenergic agonists also protect against recurrences of EAE (135). Finally, β-adrenergic agonists inhibit cytotoxic T-cell and natural killer (NK) cell responses (58,60,74) (to be discussed). Not all effects of β-adrenergic agonists are inhibitory. Epinephrine increases circulating IL-6 levels (41).

Resting immunocytes are in the G_0 stage of the cell cycle. An immune response requires that they enter G_1 as the first step in cell activation. An increase in intracellular cAMP is critical for the transition from G_0 to G_1. For transition out of G_1 into the subsequent S phase of the cell cycle, lowering of intracellular cAMP level is essential. Since adrenergic agonists elevate the intracellular cAMP content, they can trigger cell movement from G_0 into G_1. Several groups of investigators have reported an increased generation of cytotoxic lymphocytes and of immunoglobulin-secreting B cells when β-adrenergic agonists are added early to *in vitro* assays (26,68,72,83,85,110,111,125). It seems likely that, under this circumstance, β-adrenergic agonists drive resting cells from G_0 to G_1. β-Agonists are rapidly degraded in culture and, accordingly, are unlikely to still be available by the time the cell is ready to move into the S phase of the cell cycle. For this reason, the net result of early exposure to β-agonists can be an augmented response. In contrast, the addition of β-adrenergic agonists to responses already under way is overwhelmingly inhibitory, as already discussed, and is anticipated because the rise in the intracellular cAMP content that β-adrenergic agonists occasion blocks proliferation. Isoproterenol increases the rate of inactivation of the delayed rectifier K^+ current in T cells (117). This action may be a major contributor to the antiproliferative effect of β-adrenergic agonists on T-cell proliferation.

The density of adrenergic receptors on the cell surface diminishes after exposure to a β-adrenergic agonist (1) and, in the obverse of the above, the number of adrenergic receptors expressed on the surface of immunocytes rises following exposure to β-adrenergic antagonists. This situation resembles denervation hypersensitivity, in which the number of β-adrenergic receptors rises. Exposure to β-adrenergic antagonists enhances immune responses. Propranolol augments antibody production to T-cell-independent antigens (89), increases lectin-driven T-cell proliferation (28,96), elevates IL-2 receptor expression on lymphocytes (86), and worsens the severity of EAE, a DTH-type Th1-type T-cell-mediated autoimmune disease (24,28). Not all of the effects that SNS neurons exert on cells of the immune system are mediated by neurotransmitters. Freshly isolated newborn rodent sympathetic ganglia contain a high molecular weight peptide, not yet characterized, that profoundly inhibits lymphocyte proliferation (30).

Sympathetic Ablation

One way to explore the interactions between the SNS and the immune system is to determine the consequences of SNS ablation on immune responses in experimental animals. Ablation can be achieved surgically or by treatment with 6OHDA (127). This drug is picked up by SNS nerve endings, oxidizes within them, and in this way destroys SNS axon terminals. In rodents, there is a critical period in neonatal life when SNS endings must make contact with target organs. During this period, nerve cells die if they fail to receive neurotrophic signals provided by nerve growth factor (NGF), which is released from cells destined to become targets of sympathetic innervation. 6OHDA treatment of newborn rodents destroys nerve endings. Absent nerve endings, contact with target tissues is precluded, cytons die, and a permanent sympathectomy ensues. Splenic norepinephrine levels are reduced by 95%–99% following 6OHDA treatment of newborn rodents. Sympathectomized mice are smaller than their littermates. They also exhibit bilateral ptosis and enlarged spleens but otherwise appear healthy.

In adult rodents treated with 6OHDA, SNS endings are again destroyed, so that a functional axotomy is achieved. The cytons do not die, however, and nerve endings regrow over subsequent weeks so that function is gradually restored. 6OHDA treatment in adults produces less complete denervation than that achieved in newborns. Splenic norepinephrine levels are reduced by 85%–90% in axotomized animals. NPY levels are also markedly reduced in the spleens of 6OHDA-treated animals (14).

Damage following 6OHDA treatment of newborns cannot be presumed to be confined to the SNS. The drug can also damage central nervous system (CNS) catecholaminergic neurons because it readily crosses the still imperfectly developed blood–brain barrier. Note, however, that direct injection of 6OHDA intraventricularly depletes central norepinephrine but lessens rather than augments the severity of EAE (78) and that intraperitoneal administration of 6OHDA to newborn rats is not followed by a significant decrease in CNS norepinephrine levels. The CNS is spared in adults treated with 6OHDA, but the resulting compromise in SNS function achieved is less complete and also transient. It is therefore desirable, when feasible, to employ both treatments and to compare the results obtained in sympathectomized and axotomized animals both with each other and with controls.

The following abnormalities in immune function have been observed after SNS ablation:

1. A marked increase in T-cell-independent antibody responses (93). T-cell-independent B-cell responses do not require conventional T-cell help but are known to be under the influence of suppressor T cells. The finding of an increased response most probably indicates augmented B-cell function following SNS ablation, although a failure of T suppressor cell influence perhaps contributes. The increase in response is of the order of three- to fivefold in sympathectomized mice and of two- to threefold in axotomized mice, depending on the antigen.

2. A modest increase at best (17,136) [no increase in some studies, including our own (3,93)] in Th2-cell-dependent antibody responses in both sympathectomized and axotomized animals. In one study, phosphorylcholine was used as the antigen (93). This agent is a T-cell-independent antigen, but when coupled to keyhole limpet hemocyanin it becomes dependent on Th2-cell help. While T-cell-independent responses to phosphorylcholine were increased threefold in sympathectomized mice, Th2-cell-dependent

responses to the same antigen were completely normal. The results suggest limited direct influence of the SNS on CD4-positive Th2 cells, a finding in keeping with the paucity of β_2-adrenergic receptors on CD4-positive T cells.

3. Augmentation of the T-cell proliferative responses *in vitro* following stimulation with mitogenic lectins such as concanavalin A (92). The increase is of the order of twofold, and cell cycling time is accelerated as well. The basis for this effect is not known, but one possibility is a failure of the antiproliferative action of CD8-positive suppressor T cells as a consequence of sympathetic ablation. B-cell proliferation in response to mitogenic lectins is also increased in SNS-ablated animals (89).

4. Augmentation in the severity of experimental autoimmune myasthenia gravis (EAMG) in Lewis rats, as shown by a greater decline in the acetylcholine receptor content at the myoneural junction than is observed in controls (3). EAMG is induced by immunizing rats or mice with neuromuscular junction-type nicotinic acetylcholine receptor. EAMG is antibody mediated, but the B-cell response is totally dependent on Th2-cell help. At the onset of disease, there is a brisk influx of macrophages into the region of the myoneural junction, and it is thought that this contributes to lesion formation. Antiacetylcholine receptor antibody titers are no different in SNS-ablated animals with EAMG than in similarly immunized controls, a finding in keeping with data already cited that T-cell-dependent antibody responses are at best minimally affected by SNS ablation. Accordingly, the greater severity of disease is more appropriately ascribed to augmented macrophage function, or less probably to a failure of CD8-positive suppressor T-cell function, or the two may operate together.

Macrophage function rises following SNS ablation. Peritoneal exudate macrophages from sympathectomized animals release 2–3 times as much TNF-α as control macrophages following *in vitro* stimulation with bacterial lipopolysaccharide (31,32). It is also known that isoproterenol, a β-adrenergic agonist, decreases IL-1 and TNF-α release from macrophages (32,56,63) and decreases their phagocytic capacity; it is also recognized that norepinephrine decreases the IFN-γ-induced tumoricidal activity of macrophages. Arguing by analogy, sympathetic ablation might be anticipated to cause the obverse of these effects in the form of increased phagocytosis and cytocidal activity.

EAMG can be adoptively transferred by administration of antiacetylcholine receptor antibody. The disease occurs within 24 hrs and is accompanied by a brisk macrophage influx into the region of the myoneural junction. Adoptively transferred EAMG is less severe in recipients treated with the β-adrenergic drug terbutaline than in saline-injected controls given the same dose of antibody even though the extent of macrophage influx into the region of the myoneural junction is unaltered (35). The data are consistent with the postulate that increased macrophage function accounts for the increased severity of disease in SNS-ablated rats.

5. An increase in the clinical severity of EAE in Lewis rats (29). The onset of disease is not accelerated, and the histologic picture does not differ appreciably from that observed in controls, a finding that discounts any major inhibiting effect of SNS ablation on cell movement out of the lymph nodes or into target tissues. EAE is a disease of DTH. CD4-positive Th1-type effector T cells, once they have entered the CNS, release lymphotoxin, which has a noxious effect on oligodendrocytes. They also release IFN-γ, which activates macrophages, at all times abundant in EAE lesions. Macrophages in turn release IL-1 and TNF-α, both of which may contribute to lesion formation. There is once again reason to believe that CD8-positive suppressor T cells may exert an inhibiting influence on lesion formation in EAE and that macrophages may also exert a suppressive influence in late stages of the disease rather than the noxious one that they exert at disease onset. The augmenting effect of SNS ablation on EAE could depend on a directly induced increase in DTH effector cell function despite the fact, as already pointed out, that CD4-positive T cells have very few β_2-adrenergic receptors. Onset of disease is not accelerated in SNS-ablated rats, as might be expected if DTH effector cell induction were augmented after SNS ablation. Conversely, when lymph node cells from actively immunized sympathectomized donors are given to normal recipients, the adoptively transferred EAE is more severe than when the same number of cells from similarly immunized control rats is given to normal recipients. The data indicate either a direct increase in the generation of DTH effector cells in sympathectomized rats or failure of suppression.

Augmented macrophage function may also partially explain the results observed. As already noted, EAE can be adoptively transferred with lymph node cells from actively immunized rats. Adoptively transferred EAE is more severe in SNS-ablated hosts than in controls given the same dose of cells obtained from actively immunized normal donors (34). Adoptively transferred disease occurs within a few days of cell inoculation, and the difference between groups is perhaps best ascribed to an augmented activity of macrophages in sympathectomized hosts. Adjuvant-induced arthritis, another T-cell-mediated autoimmune disease and a model for rheumatoid arthritis, is also more severe in SNS-ablated rats, including rats in which only the lymph nodes draining the site of antigen injection are denervated, than in controls (14,82).

6. The β_2-adrenergic agonist terbutaline suppresses experimental allergic neuritis (EAN) in Lewis rats (77). Demyelination is decreased as is wallerian degeneration in peripheral nerves. Electrophysiologic parameters are improved. The drug is effective even if given after symptom onset. EAN is a DTH-mediated disease and provides a model for the Guillain–Barré syndrome of humans. The beneficial effect of terbutaline in EAN may depend on the

inhibiting effect of β-adrenergic agonists on macrophage function as already discussed.

7. Protection of MRL/lpr/lpr mice from early death as a consequence of systemic lupus erythematosus (105). An autoimmune disease spontaneously develops in MRL/lpr/lpr mice that is characterized by immune complex-mediated glomerulonephritis, splenomegaly, massive lymph node enlargement, arthritis, the production of a variety of autoantibodies, and premature demise. The sparing effect of SNS ablation is not understood but may relate to better clearance of immune complexes by macrophages whose function, as already discussed, is augmented in sympathectomized mice. Treatment of MRL/lpr/lpr mice with isoproterenol, a β-adrenergic agonist, leads to increased anti-DNA antibody production and a worsening of glomerulonephritis (37). As mentioned earlier, splenic norepinephrine content is reduced in MRL/lpr/lpr mice compared to controls. The reduction precedes the onset of splenomegaly.

8. Altered kinetics of NK cells (106). NK cells comprise a distinct population of lymphocytes. They are larger than T cells, do not mature in the thymus, contain characteristic intracellular granules, function as killer cells, are not MHC restricted, and are believed to have a role in the immune surveillance of tumor cells. In mice, the number of NK cells in the spleen is low at birth, rises over the next 4–6 weeks, and then declines. NK cell function, as measured by the ability of NK cells (74) to kill target cells that have been selected for their sensitivity to NK cell-mediated killing, rises as NK cell number rises and falls as NK cell number declines. In sympathectomized mice, the number of NK cells in the spleen, and their function as measured *in vitro*, rise sooner but also decline earlier than in controls. The basis for this change is unknown. It may indicate that the SNS modulates NK cell trafficking into and out of the spleen, for which there is considerable evidence.

9. A shift in cell representation within the spleen in sympathectomized mice such that the proportion of CD8-positive cells is reduced relative to that of CD4-positive cells (91). There is also a decrease in the B-cell number even while B-cell responses to T-cell-independent antigens are, as already mentioned, increased. The data imply a role for the SNS in cell trafficking into the spleen, possibly a role in the survival of B cells and CD8-positive T cells, and even a role in cell maturation within the thymus or bone marrow, or both, in early life. In mice axotomized as adults, the number of B cells in the spleen is also decreased, but the number of CD8-positive T cells is unaltered. This discordance for CD8-positive T cells between sympathectomized and axotomized mice perhaps hints that SNS innervation in early life is important for the maturation of CD8-positive T cells.

10. An upregulation of $β_2$-adrenergic receptor number on splenic lymphocytes of axotomized mice (90). This finding suggests denervation hypersensitivity of lymphoid cells as a consequence of SNS ablation. In sympathectomized mice, the overall β-adrenergic receptor density on unfractionated splenic lymphoid cells is unchanged, a point of contrast with axotomized mice. This finding should be interpreted cautiously. The numbers of B cells and CD8-positive T cells are both considerably reduced relative to CD4-positive cells after sympathectomy and, because both B and CD8-positive T cells have many more β-adrenergic receptors than do CD4-positive T cells, a decline in CD8-positive T-cell and B-cell representation could offset an increase in the number of receptors per cell. To settle this issue, the number of receptors on the T-cell subsets of sympathectomized mice must be determined.

Taken in aggregate, the findings outlined suggest the augmentation of a wide array of immune responses as a consequence of SNS denervation. Arguing by extension, the data would imply that increased SNS function, as might be expected under stressful situations, should be associated with a decline in immune function. Evidence of this is furnished by the considerable body of data (already reviewed) indicating that SNS agonist drugs inhibit many immune responses.

SYMPATHETIC NERVOUS SYSTEM–IMMUNE INTERACTIONS IN HUMAN DISEASE

Considerations of the sort just discussed may have a bearing on human disease. Patients with orthostatic hypotension caused by failed SNS function have been reported to have upregulated β-adrenergic receptors on their peripheral blood lymphocytes [see not only Bannister et al. (11) and Hui and Connolly (64), but also Zoukos et al. (140)]. Whether their immune responsiveness is abnormal has not been studied to our knowledge. $β_2$-Adrenergic receptor density on lymphocytes has been found to be elevated in essential hypertension [reviewed by Brodde et al. (23)]. A transient increase in blood lymphocyte $β_2$-adrenergic receptor representation has been described after vigorous exercise (23). This is accompanied by an increase in circulating catecholamine level and depends on a flushing into the circulation of specific $β_2$-receptor-rich lymphocyte subsets such as CD8-positive cytotoxic/suppressor cells and NK cells (95,132). Indomethacin treatment increases β-adrenergic receptors on lymphocytes for unknown reasons (51). It has also been reported that β-adrenergic responsiveness of peripheral blood mononuclear cells is blunted in the context of endogenous depression (53).

Multiple sclerosis (MS) is characterized by attacks and remissions with progressive disability as one attack follows another. Patients who begin with exacerbating-remitting MS may, after a time, suffer a relentlessly progressive disease. Other cases are progressive from the outset. What causes the disease to switch from one mode to the other is not known. Patients with progressive MS are almost invariably spastic, indicating damage to the descending tracts. Most such patients exhibit impaired SNS function as exemplified by the impaired sympathetic skin responses in the lower extremities (10,71,128). It is also known that nonspecific CD8-positive suppressor T-cell function is persistently subnormal in patients with progressive MS, a finding that bespeaks an increase in overall immune responsiveness (8,9).

My colleagues and I reasoned that, if SNS function were defective in progressive MS, then the immune cells of such patients might exhibit denervation hypersensitivity and upregulated β-adrenergic receptors. Accordingly, we undertook to measure β-adrenergic receptors on peripheral blood cells obtained from MS patients and to compare them with such findings in age-matched controls. A two- to threefold increase in $β_2$-adrenergic receptors on CD8-positive, CD28-negative T cells (suppressors) was found in progressive MS patients but not in stable ones (69–71). The data indicate an acquired abnormality.

Although denervation hypersensitivity may contribute to the upregulation of $β_2$-adrenergic receptors on CD8-positive suppressor cells in MS, the major cause would appear to be immune system activation. When T cells are activated with nonspecific mitogenic lectins such as concanavalin A, the number of β-adrenergic receptors on T cells increases, indicating that activation of the immune system alone, for whatever reason, upregulates β-adrenergic receptor density. The recent finding that β-adrenergic receptors are increased on circulating T cells during MS attacks [see not only Zoukos et al. (138,139), but also Karaszewski et al. (69–71)], even in mildly affected patients with presumably normal SNS function, is consistent with this view. Also consistent are observations that, in rats with EAE, an increase in splenocyte β-adrenergic receptor density can be detected prior to disease onset. Receptor density falls with recovery and increases again with relapses (79,81) (E. Chelmicka-Schorr, personal communication). The finding of increased numbers of β-adrenergic receptors on lymphocytes from patients with rheumatoid arthritis, a disease in which SNS function is normal, also argues for activation of the immune system as the major cause for upregulation of β-adrenergic receptors on lymphocytes (139). Note in addition that β-adrenergic receptors on lymphocytes are increased following exposure to IL-1, IL-2, and glucocorticoid, all three of which are released during an immune response (70,139).

The response to β-adrenergic agonists as measured by a rise in the intracellular cAMP content is significantly greater for the CD8-positive cells from patients with progressive MS than for the CD8-positive T cells from controls, indicating that the receptors are functional (69). Treatment of patients with progressive MS by using the β-adrenergic agonist terbutaline reduces the β-adrenergic receptor density to normal or near-normal levels [E. Chelmicka-Schorr, A. Reder, and B. G. W. Arnason, unpublished observations; see also Aarons et al. (1) and Van den Berg et al. (131)]. Terbutaline preferentially reduces $β_2$-adrenergic receptor number on CD8-positive cytotoxic/suppressor cells, less so on CD4-positive cells, and not at all on B cells (84). It remains to be seen whether β-adrenergic agonists can favorably affect the course of the disease.

Relatively little is known regarding the role of parasympathetic nerves as modulators of the immune response. In one study of mice, in which parasympathetic nerves in the neck were severed, a decrease in immune responses in local lymph nodes was noted (5). Attempts to directly demonstrate parasympathetic cholinergic innervation of the organs of the immune system have failed (82). Nonetheless, immune cells do carry muscarinic acetylcholine receptors and possibly also nicotinic acetylcholine receptors (88,107). There is firm evidence that muscarinic cholinergic agonists augment immune responses (87,107,122) and even trigger a modest T-cell proliferative response *in vitro*. Less compelling evidence has been brought forward to indicate an upregulation of nicotinic acetylcholine receptors on T cells (they are reported to be absent on B cells and macrophages) in the draining lymph nodes during the late stages of adjuvant-induced arthritis (88).

Given that SNS function is compromised in progressive MS, my colleagues and I reasoned that parasympathetic function might also be compromised, and there is evidence for this. It has been reported that the normal RR beat variation, a vagally mediated response, is reduced in progressive MS (112,120). If parasympathetic function is compromised in progressive MS, then the acetylcholine receptors might be upregulated. We measured muscarinic acetylcholine receptors on lymphocytes from patients with progressive MS and found them to be upregulated twofold on CD4-positive T cells, a highly significant alteration (7). No such increase was observed in patients with stable MS. There was also an increase in receptors on CD8-positive T cells from patients with progressive MS, but the difference from controls did not reach statistical significance. Lymphocytes have both M_1- and M_2-type muscarinic acetylcholine receptors, but the increase appeared to be selective for M_2-type receptors. M_1 receptors act via the phosphatidylinositol route, whereas M_2 receptors couple to cyclic guanosine 3',5'-monophosphate. $β_2$-Adrenergic receptor levels are higher on CD8-positive T cells than on CD4-positive T cells. The reverse holds for muscarinic acetylcholine receptors (43). In progressive MS, cholinergic receptors are selectively increased on CD4-positive T cells, while adrenergic receptors are selectively increased on CD8-positive, CD28-negative suppressor T cells. The data hint at some sort of reciprocal interaction. We have studied the effect of the muscarinic antagonist scopolamine on EAE. It has a modest ameliorating effect on the disease (6) and potentiates the protective effect of the β-adrenergic agonist isoproterenol (unpublished observations).

Effects of Cytokines on the Sympathetic Nervous System

If the nervous system "talks" to the immune system via the SNS and possibly via parasympathetic nerves, it seems likely that the immune system "talks back." That such "back talk" occurs has been established for the CNS.

During an immune response, activated macrophages release IL-1β to the circulation. The IL-1β passes into the brain in the medial hypothalamic region, which lacks a blood–brain barrier, and activates hypothalamic neurons in the organum vasculosum lateral terminalis. One consequence of this activation is fever. SNS nerves to blood vessels have a major role in the generation of the febrile response (108). During fever, cutaneous vessels constrict while visceral ones dilate. The IL-1β-driven relay from the hypothalamus to the SNS must, therefore, exhibit regional specificity. A second consequence of IL-1-induced activation of hypothalamic neurons is anorexia, which may lessen the availability of nutrients essential to the growth of invading microorganisms. A role for corticotropin-releasing factor (CRF) in anorexia has been proposed (109), as has a role for TNF-α (see later). A third consequence is activation of the hypothalamic–pituitary–adrenal axis. Here a crucial role for CRF is established. IL-1β, whether generated during the course of an immune response or given either intraperitoneally or intracerebroventricularly, causes an increased production (and turnover) of CRF by neurons of the paraventricular nucleus (15). The relay from the organum vasculosum lateral terminalis to the paraventricular nucleus involves prostaglandin. A role for norepinephrine is also possible since norepinephrine levels fall in the hypothalamus during immune responses.

As is well known, CRF stimulates adrenocorticotropic hormone (ACTH) release from the pituitary. ACTH in turn causes cortisol to be released from the adrenal cortex. Cortisol inhibits immune responses, with selectivity for Th1-type T-cell responses and sparing of Th2-type T-cell responses. Cortisol also inhibits macrophages, the source of the IL-1β that initiates the negative feedback loop just described.

CRF is also known to be involved in regulation of sympathetic outflow. Central CRF projections activate descending pathways to the sympathetic nerves (130). One consequence of this activation is a three- to fivefold increase in the firing rate of splenic SNS nerves and an increased release of norepinephrine in selected target organs such as the spleen (4,61,65,123,126). Recall that splenic norepinephrine levels rise at the peak of an immune response as a herald of its impending decline. The rise is ascribable to IL-1β-driven, centrally mediated activation of SNS nerves to immune system organs. IL-1 and CRF antagonists, given intracerebrally, block the splenic norepinephrine rise as does chlorisondamine, a selective blocker of transmission at SNS ganglia (82,123). Intracerebroventricular administration of CRF drastically decreases splenic NK cell activity. Blood NK cell activity is much less affected, pointing to an influence within the spleen that is lacking in the blood. The splenic NK cell effect is blocked by chlorisondamine (82,123).

From the preceding, it is evident that centrally acting IL-1β activates two distinct negative feedback loops. The two loops act jointly, perhaps synergistically, to inhibit immune responses (25,61,65,108,109). Activation of either loop causes splenic macrophage IL-1β secretion and splenic NK function to fall (25,61,123). Activation of both loops causes a still greater fall. Interestingly, secretion of the inhibitory cytokine TGF-β$_1$ is not affected by activation of either loop, indicating cytokine specificity in addition to regional specificity. Lewis rats exhibit a defective CRF response to IL-1β and, accordingly, a diminished glucocorticoid surge in response to immune challenge (121). The deficient glucocorticoid response is thought to explain the propensity of Lewis rats to develop autoimmune diseases. Whether the hypothalamic–SNS feedback loop is also compromised in Lewis rats and whether this, too, contributes to propensity to develop autoimmunity is not known.

TNF-α is released by activated macrophages, circulates, binds to hypothalamic neurons, and inhibits appetite. For this reason, TNF-α is sometimes called cachectin. Both TNF-α and IL-1β elicit slow-wave sleep when injected into the lateral ventricles (114). Augmentation of γ-aminobutyric acid-gated Cl$^-$ conductance has been proposed as an explanation for the somnogenic effect of IL-1 (94). Both TNF-α and IL-1β can be detected within hypothalamic neurons (20,21) and are possibly synthesized within hypothalamic neurons.

The effects of cytokines on the CNS are not restricted to the hypothalamus. IL-2 or IL-1β inhibit long-term potentiation in hippocampal slices (73,124), an action that might adversely affect memory. Both IL-2 and IL-1β also modulate neuronal discharge frequency in the hypothalamus (18,62). Cytokine effects are not restricted to neurons. For example, TNF-α inhibits K$^+$ current expression in cultured oligodendrocytes and causes process retraction (118).

The effects of cytokines on the SNS are mediated not only via the central feedback loop just discussed but also by a direct local action of cytokines on SNS axons. IL-1β is known to increase norepinephrine turnover in the spleen but not the heart (4,97). The decrease in the norepinephrine content of the spleen observed at the onset of an immune response probably depends on a local effect of IL-1β. The rebound in the norepinephrine content of the spleen, observed as the immune response begins to decline, surely depends on the central effects of IL-1β.

Most of the evidence in support of the view that the immune system influences the neuronal activity of SNS fibers within immune organs, and that regulation varies with the state of activation of immune system cells, has come from *in vitro* work. SNS neurons can be maintained in tissue culture in the presence or absence of nonneuronal supporting cells. TNF-α inhibits the repetitive stimulation-induced release of norepinephrine from supporting cell-depleted superior cervical ganglion neuronal cultures and increases Ca^{2+} current density as well (115,116). On the other hand, when supporting cells are present, TNF-α increases norepinephrine release in response to nicotinic agonist treatment, and nicotinic acetylcholine receptors are upregulated (115). Conditioned medium from supporting cell-containing neuronal cultures pulsed with TNF-α increases norepinephrine release from supporting cell-depleted neuronal cultures. The findings indicate that a directly inhibitory effect of TNF-α on SNS neurons is overridden in mixed cultures by the stimulatory effect of a TNF-α-induced soluble factor secreted by non-neural supporting cells (119). Supporting cells are always present *in vivo*, and their possible role as "intermediates" in cytokine-mediated effects on SNS neurons must at all times be borne in mind.

Tyrosine hydroxylase (TH) is the rate-limiting enzyme in catecholamine biosynthesis. The expression of TH mRNA is decreased when spleen cells are added to superior cervical ganglion cultures (12). If the spleen cells are stimulated with the mitogenic lectin concanavalin A and then added to the ganglion cultures, TH mRNA expression is further reduced. NPY mRNA expression is also decreased in SNS cultures exposed to concanavalin A-stimulated splenocytes (12). The "factor" released by spleen cells that inhibits TH and NPY mRNA appears to act directly on neurons rather than through nonneuronal supporting cells. Nonetheless, supporting cells do influence neurotransmitter synthesis. Norepinephrine and NPY levels are lower in SNS neurons cocultured with nonneuronal supporting cells than in neurons cultured alone.

SNS neurons synthesize and release substance P *in vitro*, provided nonneuronal supporting cells are present. Coculture of superior cervical ganglion neurons with spleen cells substantially increases expression of PPT-A mRNA (the precursor of substance P) and of substance P itself, a point of contrast with the effect of spleen cells on TH mRNA and norepinephrine. Conditioned medium from concanavalin A-stimulated lymphocytes also increases PPT-A mRNA expression, pointing to the presence of a soluble mediator (12,66). IL-1β duplicates the effect of conditioned medium. The macrophage is the major accepted source of IL-1β, but it transpires that superior cervical ganglion neurons in tissue culture synthesize and secrete IL-1β (47) so that "endogenous" IL-1β released by neurons may explain spontaneous substance P induction in culture. Substance P production is presumed to be a response to injury since substance P levels are low in sympathetic ganglia *in situ* (47) and presynaptic electrical activity suppresses substance P synthesis *in vitro* as does depolarization with 40 mM KCl or 2–30 μg/ml veratrine. Substance P is localized *in vivo* to neuronal perikarya and intraganglionic processes and is not detected in nerve terminals, so it probably subserves some intraganglionic role. Exogenously applied IL-1β markedly increases neuronal substance P levels *in vitro*; the IL-1β effect is blocked by an IL-1β antagonist and by dexamethosone (47,48,67). Importantly, the effect of IL-1β is not seen in pure cultures of SNS neurons. These findings indicate that IL-1β acts on supporting cells that then secrete a substance P inducer (47,48,54). IL-1β has long been known to induce NGF production by Schwann cells. IL-1β also induces supporting cells, presumably Schwann cells, to produce leukemia inhibitory factor (LIF), a pleiotropic cytokine, and LIF turns out to be the substance P inducer (113). Substance P production is blocked by inhibitors of LIF. Dexamethosone blocks the IL-1β effect but not that of LIF (48), pointing to an inhibitory action of dexamethosone on supporting cells rather than on neurons. Thus, IL-1β released by neurons (or by macrophages) causes supporting cells to release LIF, which in turn induces substance P production by neurons. Cultured SNS neurons can be driven toward an adrenergic or a cholinergic phenotype depending on culture conditions. LIF also increases cholineacetyltransferase levels in SNS neurons.

Cytokines released by T cells can also affect SNS neurons. IL-2, released by activated Th1-type T cells, enhances chick and rat SNS neurite outgrowth (55). IFN-γ, another product of activated T cells, lowers substance P levels in SNS neurons, providing a possible counterbalance to IL-1β (54). A neuronal protein that shares both epitopes and biologic activities with IFN-γ has been characterized (80,99). The neuronal protein is capable of inducing both MHC class I and MHC class II molecule expression, and both it and IFN-γ, when injected intracerebroventricularly, alter behavior (104). SNS neurons require NGF for survival. IFN-γ salvages NGF-deprived SNS neurons at least for a time (27). When IL-6, another cytokine produced by many cell types, including lymphocytes, is added to cultured PC-12 cells, differentiation to a neuronal phenotype is induced (129). The PC-12 tumor is a rat pheochromocytoma.

A clear picture of the roles of cytokines, be they neuron derived or immunocyte derived, on SNS function has yet to emerge. Understanding of the roles of neurotransmitters and other neuron-derived products on immunocyte function is also imperfect. Nonetheless, it is evident that there is considerable interaction between the sympathetic and immune systems, and that there is overlap in the signaling systems that they use. The hypotension, lassitude, fatigue, myalgia, and headache that characterize systemic viral illnesses may depend considerably on actions of circulating cytokines on SNS nerves throughout the body.

ACKNOWLEDGMENTS

Original work reported herein was supported by grant PO 1 NS24575, from the National Institutes of Health, and by grants from the National Multiple Sclerosis Society, the Brain Research Foundation, and the Butz Foundation.

REFERENCES

1. Aarons RD, et al. Decreased beta adrenergic receptor density on human lymphocytes after chronic treatment with agonists. *J Pharmacol Exp Ther* 1982;224:1.
2. Abrass CK, et al. Characterization of the β-adrenergic receptor of the rat peritoneal macrophage. *J Immunol* 1985;135:1338.
3. Agius MA, et al. Sympathectomy enhances the severity of experimental autoimmune myasthenia gravis (EAMG). *J Neuroimmunol* 1987;16:11.
4. Akiyoshi M, et al. Interleukin-1 increases norepinephrine turnover in the spleen and lung in rats. *Biochem Biophys Res Commun* 1990;173:1266.
5. Alito AE, et al. Autonomic nervous system regulation of murine immune responses as assessed by local surgical sympathetic and para-

sympathetic denervation. *Acta Physiol Pharmacol Latinoam* 1987;37:305.
6. Anlar B, et al. Effect of cholinergic agonists and antagonists on experimental allergic encephalomyelitis. *J Neuroimmunol* 1991;(Suppl 1):58.
7. Anlar B, et al. Increased muscarinic cholinergic receptor density on CD4+ lymphocytes in progressive multiple sclerosis. *J Neuroimmunol* 1992;36:171.
8. Antel JP, et al. Activated suppressor cell dysfunction in progressive multiple sclerosis. *J Immunol* 1986;137:137.
9. Arnason BGW, Antel JA. Suppressor cell function in multiple sclerosis. *Ann Immunol* 1970;129:159.
10. Arnason BGW, et al. Blood lymphocyte β-adrenergic receptors in multiple sclerosis. *Ann NY Acad Sci* 1988;540:585.
11. Bannister R, et al. Beta-receptor numbers and thermodynamics in denervation supersensitivity. *J Physiol (Lond)* 1981;319:369.
12. Barbany G, et al. Lymphocyte-mediated regulation of neurotransmitter gene expression in rat sympathetic ganglia. *J Neuroimmunol* 1991;32:97.
13. Beckner SK, Farrar WL. Potentiation of lymphokine-activated killer cell differentiation and lymphocyte proliferation by stimulation of protein kinase C or inhibition of adenylate cyclase. *J Immunol* 1988;140:208.
14. Bellinger DL, et al. Innervation of lymphoid organs and implications in development, aging, and autoimmunity. *Int J Immunopharmacol* 1992;14:329.
15. Berkenbosch F, et al. Neuroendocrine, sympathetic and metabolic responses induced by interleukin-1. *Neuroendocrinology* 1989;50:570.
16. Besedovsky HO, et al. T lymphocytes affect the development of sympathetic innervation of mouse spleen. *Brain Behav Immun* 1987;1:185.
17. Besedovsky HO, et al. Immunoregulation mediated by the sympathetic nervous system. *Cell Immunol* 1979;48:346.
18. Bindoni M, et al. Interleukin 2 modifies the bioelectric activity of some neurosecretory nuclei in the rat hypothalamus. *Brain Res* 1988;462:10.
19. Bourne HR, et al. Modulation of inflammation and immunity by cyclic AMP. *Science* 1974;184:19.
20. Breder CD, et al. Interleukin-1 immunoreactive innervation of the human hypothalamus. *Science* 1988;240:321.
21. Breder CD, Saper CB. Tumor necrosis factor immunoreactive innervation in the mouse brain. *Soc Neurosci* 1988;14:1280.
22. Breneman SM, et al. Splenic norepinephrine is decreased in MRL-lpr/lpr mice. *Brain Behav Immun* 1993;7:135.
23. Brodde O-E, et al. Dynamic exercise-induced increase in lymphocyte beta-2-adrenoreceptors: abnormality in essential hypertension and its correction by antihypertensives. *Clin Pharmacol Ther* 1987;41:371.
24. Brosnan CF, et al. Prazosin, an α_1-adrenergic receptor antagonist, suppresses experimental autoimmune encephalomyelitis in the Lewis rat. *Proc Natl Acad Sci USA* 1985;82:5915.
25. Brown R, et al. Suppression of splenic macrophage interleukin-1 secretion following intracerebroventricular injection of interleukin-1β: evidence for pituitary–adrenal and sympathetic control. *Cell Immunol* 1991;132:84.
26. Campbell KS, et al. Further characterization of the beta-2 adrenoceptor mediated enhancement of the murine primary antibody response *in vitro*. *Fed Proc* 1985;44:1488.
27. Chang JY, et al. Interferon suppresses sympathetic neuronal cell death caused by nerve growth factor deprivation. *J Neurochem* 1990;55:436.
28. Chelmicka-Schorr E, Arnason BGW. Nervous system–immune system interactions. In: Waksman BH, ed. *Proceedings of the Association for Research in Nervous and Mental Diseases: immunologic mechanisms in neurologic and psychiatric disease*. New York: Raven, 1990:67.
29. Chelmicka-Schorr E, et al. Chemical sympathectomy augments the severity of experimental allergic encephalomyelitis. *J Neuroimmunol* 1988;17:347.
30. Chelmicka-Schorr E, et al. Sympathetic nervous system and PC12 pheochromocytoma-derived factors suppress stimulation of lymphocytes. *Brain Behav Immun* 1988;4:23.
31. Chelmicka-Schorr E, et al. Sympathetic nervous system and macrophage function. *Ann NY Acad Sci* 1992;650:40.
32. Chelmicka-Schorr E, et al. Sympathetic nervous system modulates macrophage function. *Int J Neuropharmacol* 1992;14:841.
33. Chelmicka-Schorr E, et al. The β-adrenergic agonist isoproterenol suppresses experimental allergic encephalomyelitis in Lewis rats. *J Neuroimmunol* 1989;25:203.
34. Chelmicka-Schorr E, et al. Sympathectomy augments adoptively transferred experimental allergic encephalomyelitis. *J Neuroimmunol* 1992;37:99.
35. Chelmicka-Schorr E, et al. The β_2-adrenergic agonist terbutaline suppresses acute passive transfer experimental autoimmune myasthenia gravis (EAMG). *Int J Immunopharmacol* 1993;15:19.
36. Chouaib S, et al. Prostaglandin E_2 acts at two distinct pathways of T lymphocyte activation: inhibition of interleukin 2 production and down-regulation of transferrin receptor expression. *J Immunol* 1985;135:1172.
37. Colburn K, et al. β-Adrenergic receptor stimulation increases anti-DNA antibody production in MRL/lpr mice. *J Rheumatol* 1990;17:138.
38. Danek A, et al. Specific binding sites for vasoactive intestinal polypeptide on nonadherent peripheral blood lymphocytes. *J Immunol* 1983;131:1173.
39. Del Rey A, et al. Immunoregulation mediated by the sympathetic nervous system. *Cell Immunol* 1981;63:329.
40. Del Rey A, et al. Sympathetic immunoregulation: difference between high- and low-responder animals. *Am J Physiol* 1982;242:R30.
41. DeRijk RH, et al. Induction of plasma interleukin-6 by circulating adrenaline in the rat. *Psychoneuroendocrinology* 1994;19:155.
42. Diamantstein T, Ulmer A. The antagonistic action of cyclic GMP and cyclic AMP on proliferation by B and T lymphocytes. *Immunology* 1975;28:113.
43. Eva C, et al. [^{3}H]N-Methylscopolamine binding to muscarinic receptors in human peripheral blood lymphocytes: characterization, localization on T-lymphocyte subsets and age-dependent changes. *Neuropharmacology* 1989;28:719.
44. Feldman RD, et al. β-Adrenergic receptor-mediated suppression of interleukin 2 receptors in human lymphocytes. *J Immunol* 1987;139:3355.
45. Felten SY, et al. Decreased sympathetic innervation of spleen in aged Fischer 344 rats. *Neurobiol Aging* 1987;8:159.
46. Felten DL, et al. Noradrenergic sympathetic neural interactions with the immune system: structure and function. *Immunol Rev* 1987;100:225.
47. Freidin M, et al. Cultured sympathetic neurons synthesize and release the cytokine interleukin 1β. *Proc Natl Acad Sci USA* 1992;89:10440.
48. Freidin M, Kessler JA. Cytokine regulation of substance P expression in sympathetic neurons. *Proc Natl Acad Sci USA* 1991;88:3200.
49. Garovoy MR, et al. Antibody dependent lymphocyte mediated cytotoxicity mechanism and modulation by cyclic nucleotides. *Cell Immunol* 1975;20:197.
50. Gulick T, et al. Interleukin 1 and tumor necrosis factor inhibit cardiac myocyte β-adrenergic responsiveness. *Proc Natl Acad Sci USA* 1989;86:6753.
51. Güllner HG, et al. Indomethacin increases leucocyte β-adrenoreceptors in man. *Clin Sci* 1980;59:397.
52. Hadden JW, et al. Lymphocyte blast transformation. I. Demonstration of adrenergic receptors in human peripheral lymphocytes. *Cell Immunol* 1970;1:583.
53. Halper JP, et al. Blunted β-adrenergic responsivity of peripheral blood mononuclear cells in endogenous depression. *Arch Gen Psychiatry* 1988;45:241.
54. Hart RP, et al. Substance P gene expression is regulated by interleukin-1 in cultured sympathetic ganglia. *J Neurosci Res* 1991;29:282.
55. Haugen PK, Letourneau PC. Interleukin-2 enhances chick and rat sympathetic, but not sensory, neurite outgrowth. *J Neurosci Res* 1990;25:443.
56. Koff WC, Dunegan MA. Modulation of macrophage-mediated tumoricidal activity by neuropeptides and neurohormones. *J Immunol* 1985;135:350.
57. Hartung H-P, et al. Substance P: binding properties and studies on cellular responses in guinea pig macrophages. *J Immunol* 1986;136:3856.

58. Hellstrand K, et al. Evidence for a β-adrenoceptor-mediated regulation of human natural killer cells. *J Immunol* 1985;134:4095.
59. Helme RD, et al. The effect of substance P on the regional lymph node antibody response to antigenic stimulation in capsaicin-pretreated rats. *J Immunol* 1987; 139:3470.
60. Henney CS. On the mechanism of T-cell mediated cytolysis. *Transplant Rev* 1973;17:37.
61. Hori T, et al. Immune cytokines and regulation of body temperature, food intake, and cellular immunity. *Brain Res Bull* 1991;27:309.
62. Hori T, et al. Effects of interleukin-1 and arachidonate on the preoptic and anterior hypothalamic neurons. *Brain Res Bull* 1988;20:75.
63. Hu X, et al. The effect of norepinephrine on endotoxin-mediated macrophage activation. *J Neuroimmunol* 1991;31:35.
64. Hui KKP, Connolly ME. Increased numbers of beta receptors in orthostatic hypotension due to autonomic dysfunction. *N Engl J Med* 1981;304:1473.
65. Ichijo T, et al. Central interleukin-1 beta enhances splenic sympathetic nerve activity in rats. *Brain Res Bull* 1994;34:547.
66. Johnson DL, et al. Effects of β-adrenergic agents on the murine lymphocyte response to mitogen stimulation. *J Immunopharmacology* 1981;3:205.
67. Jonakait GM, et al. Interleukin-1 specifically increases substance P in injured sympathetic ganglia. *Ann NY Acad Sci* 1990;594:222.
68. Kamat R, Henney CS. Studies on T cell clonal expansion. II. The *in vitro* differentiation of pre-killer and memory T cells. *J Immunol* 1976;116:1490.
69. Karaszewski JW, et al. Increased high affinity beta-adrenergic receptor densities and cyclic AMP responses of CD8 cells in multiple sclerosis. *J Neuroimmunol* 1993;43:1.
70. Karaszewski JW, et al. Increased lymphocyte beta-adrenergic receptor density in progressive multiple sclerosis is specific for the CD8+, CD28− suppressor cell. *Ann Neurol* 1991;30:42.
71. Karaszewski JW, et al. Sympathetic skin responses are decreased and lymphocyte beta-adrenergic receptors are increased in progressive multiple sclerosis. *Ann Neurol* 1990;27:366.
72. Kasahara K, et al. Suppression of the primary immune response by chemical sympathectomy. *Res Commun Chem Pathol Pharmacol* 1977;16:687.
73. Katsuki K, et al. Interleukin-1 β inhibits long-term potentiation in the CA3 region of mouse hippocampal slices. *Eur J Pharmacol* 1990;181:323.
74. Katz P, et al. Mechanisms of human cell-mediated cytotoxicity. I. Modulation of natural killer cell activity by cyclic nucleotides. *J Immunol* 1982;129:287.
75. Kendall MD, Al-Shawaf AA. Innervation of the rat thymus gland. *Brain Behav Immun* 1991;5:9.
76. Khan MM, et al. Beta-adrenergic receptors on human suppressor, helper, and cytolytic lymphocytes. *Biochem Pharmacol* 1986;35:1137.
77. Kim DH, et al. The $β_2$-adrenergic agonist terbutaline suppresses experimental allergic neuritis in Lewis rats. *J Neuroimmunol* 1994;51:177.
78. Leonard JP, et al. Hypothalamic noradrenergic pathways exert an influence on neuroendocrine and clinical status in experimental autoimmune encephalomyelitis. *Brain Behav Immun* 1991,5:328.
79. Leonard JP, et al. Splenic noradrenergic and adrenocortical responses during the preclinical and clinical stages of adoptively transferred experimental autoimmune encephalomyelitis (EAE). *J Neuroimmunol* 1990;26:183.
80. Lungdahl Å, et al. Interferon-gamma-like immunoreactivity in certain neurons of the central and peripheral nervous system. *J Neurosci Res* 1989;24:451.
81. MacKenzie FJ, et al. Changes in lymphocyte β-adrenergic receptor density and noradrenaline content of the spleen are early indicators of immune reactivity in acute experimental allergic encephalomyelitis in the Lewis rat. *J Neuroimmunol* 1989; 23:93.
82. Madden KS, Felten DL. Experimental basis for neural–immune interactions. *Physiol Rev* 1995;75:77.
83. Madden KS, et al. Sympathetic denervation augments lymphocyte proliferation *in vivo*. *FASEB J* 1988;2:A1262 (abst).
84. Maisel AS, et al. A new method for isolation of human lymphocyte subsets reveals differential regulation of β-adrenergic receptors by terbutaline treatment. *Clin Pharmacol Ther* 1989;46:429.
85. Makino A, Reed CE. Epinephrine inhibition of hemolytic plaque forming cells (PPC) following *in vitro* immunization. *Fed Proc* 1970;29:431.
86. Malec P, Nowak A. Propranolol enhances *in vitro* interleukin 2 receptor expression on human lymphocytes. *Immunol Lett* 1988;17:319.
87. Maśliński W. Cholinergic receptors of lymphocytes. *Brain Behav Immun* 1989;3:1.
88. Maslinski W, et al. Nicotinic receptors of rat lymphocytes during adjuvant polyarthritis. *J Neurosci Res* 1992;31:336.
89. Miles K. *The sympathetic nervous system and the immune response in mice* [PhD dissertation]. Chicago: University of Chicago, 1984.
90. Miles K, et al. β-Adrenergic receptors on splenic lymphocytes from axotomized mice. *Int J Immunopharmacol* 1984;6:171.
91. Miles K, et al. Sympathetic ablation alters lymphocyte membrane properties. *J Immunol* 1985;135:797s.
92. Miles K, et al. Sympathetic nervous system and immune response in mice. *Neurology* 1984;34 (Suppl 1):259.
93. Miles K, et al. The sympathetic nervous system modulates antibody response to thymus-independent antigens. *J Neuroimmunol* 1981;1:101.
94. Miller LG, et al. Interleukin-1 augments γ-aminobutyric acid$_A$ receptor function in brain. *Mol Pharmacol* 1991;39:105.
95. Murray DR, et al. Sympathetic and immune interactions during dynamic exercise: mediation via a beta 2-adrenergic-dependent mechanism. *Circulation* 1992;86:203.
96. Nakazawa H, et al. *In vivo* and *in vitro* effects of chronic propranolol administration on the immune response in mice. *J Allergy Clin Immunol* 1976;61:200.
97. Niijima A, et al. Interleukin 1-β on efferent activity of the splenic and adrenal branch of the splanchnic nerve. *Neurosci Res Suppl* 1989;9:S34.
98. O'Dorisio MS, et al. Vasoactive intestinal polypeptide modulation of lymphocyte adenylate cyclase. *J Immunol* 1981;127:2551.
99. Olsson T, et al. Neuronal interferon-γ immunoreactive molecule: bioactivities and purification. *Eur J Immunol* 1994; 24:308.
100. Payan DG, et al. Specific stimulation of human T lymphocytes by substance P. *J Immunol* 1983;131:1613.
101. Payan DG, Goetzl EJ. Modulation of lymphocyte function by sensory neuropeptides. *J Immunol* 1985;135:783s.
102. Payan DG, et al. Inhibition by somatostatin of the proliferation of T-lymphocytes and Molt-4 lymphoblasts. *Cell Immunology* 1984;84:433.
103. Payan DG, et al. Neuropeptide modulation of leukocyte function. *Ann NY Acad Sci* 1987;496:182.
104. Peng Z-C, et al. Interferon-γ and a factor derived from trypanosomes cause behavioural changes in the rat. *Behav Brain Res* 1994;31:538.
105. Renold FK, et al. 6-Hydroxydopamine (6OHDA) neonatal sympathectomy prolongs survival of MRL/lpr mice. *Arthritis Rheum* 1988;31:S38.
106. Reder AT, et al. The effect of chemical sympathectomy on natural killer cells in mice. *Brain Behav Immun* 1989;3:110.
107. Richman DP, Arnason BGW. Nicotinic acetylcholine receptor: functionally distinct receptor present on human lymphocytes. *Proc Natl Acad Sci USA* 1979;76:4632.
108. Saigusa T. Participation of interleukin-1 and tumor necrosis factor in the responses of the sympathetic nervous system during lipopolysaccharide-induced fever. *Pflugers Arch* 1989;416:225.
109. Saito M, et al. Possible role of the sympathetic nervous system in responses to interleukin-1. *Brain Res Bull* 1991; 27:305.
110. Sanders VM, Munson AE. Beta-adrenoceptor mediation of the enhancing effect of norepinephrine on the murine primary antibody response *in vitro*. *J Pharmacol Exp Ther* 1984;230:183.
111. Sanders VM, Munson AE. Kinetics of the enhancing effect produced by norepinephrine and terbutaline on the murine primary antibody response *in vitro*. *J Pharmacol Exp Ther* 1984;231:527.
112. Senaratne MPJ, et al. Evidence for cardiovascular autonomic nerve dysfunction in multiple sclerosis. *J Neurol Neurosurg Psychiatry* 1984;47:947.
113. Shadiack AM, et al. Interleukin-1 induces substance P in sympathetic ganglia through the induction of leukemia inhibitory factor (LIF). *J Neurosci* 1993;13:2601.

114. Shoham S, et al. Recombinant tumor necrosis factor and interleukin 1 enhance slow-wave sleep. *Am J Physiol* 1987;253:R142.
115. Soliven B, Albert J. Tumor necrosis factor modulates Ca^{2+} currents in cultured sympathetic neurons. *J Neurosci* 1992;12:2665.
116. Soliven B, Albert J. Tumor necrosis factor modulates the inactivation of catecholamine secretion in cultured sympathetic neurons. *J Neurochem* 1992;58:1073.
117. Soliven B, Nelson DJ. Beta-adrenergic modulation of K^+ current in human T lymphocytes. *J Membr Biol* 1990;117:263.
118. Soliven B, et al. Tumor necrosis factor produces process retraction and potassium current inhibition in oligodendrocytes. *Soc Neurosci* 1989;15:352.
119. Soliven B, Wang N. Tumor necrosis factor-α regulates nicotinic responses in mixed cultures of sympathetic neurons and nonneuronal cells. *J Neurochem* 1995;64:883.
120. Sterman AB, et al. Disseminated abnormalities of cardiovascular autonomic functions in multiple sclerosis. *Neurology* 1985;35:1665.
121. Sternberg EM, et al. Inflammatory mediator-induced hypothalamic–pituitary–adrenal axis activation is defective in streptococcal cell wall arthritis-susceptible Lewis rats. *Proc Natl Acad Sci USA* 1989; 86:2374.
122. Strom TB, et al. Cholinergic augmentation of lymphocyte-mediated cytotoxicity: a study of the cholinergic receptor of cytotoxic T lymphocytes. *Proc Natl Acad Sci USA* 1974;71:1330.
123. Sundar SK, et al. Brain IL-1-induced immunosuppression occurs through activation of both pituitary–adrenal axis and sympathetic nervous system by corticotropin-releasing factor. *J Neurosci* 1990; 10:3701.
124. Tancredi V, et al. Interleukin-2 suppresses established long-term potentiation and inhibits its induction in the rat hippocampus. *Brain Res* 1990;525:149.
125. Teh H-S, Paetkau V. Regulation of immune responses. II. The cellular basis of cyclic AMP effects on humoral immunity. *Cell Immunol* 1976;24:220.
126. Terao A, et al. Tissue-specific increase in norepinephrine turnover by central interleukin-1, but not by interleukin-6, in rats. *Am J Physiol* 1994;266:R400.
127. Thoenen H, Tranzer JP. The pharmacology of 6-hydroxydopamine. *Annu Rev Pharmacol* 1973;13:169.
128. Thomaides TN, et al. Physiological assessment of aspects of autonomic function in patients with secondary progressive multiple sclerosis. *J Neurol* 1993;240:139.
129. Satoh T, et al. Induction of neuronal differentiation in PC12 cells by B-cell stimulatory factor 2/interleukin 6. *Mol Cell Biol* 1988;8:3546.
130. Tucker DC, Saper CB. Specificity of spinal projections from hypothalamic and brainstem areas which innervate sympathetic preganglionic neurons. *Brain Res* 1985;360:159.
131. Van den Berg W, et al. Clinical implications of drug-induced desensitization of the beta receptor after continuous oral use of terbutaline. *J Allergy Clin Immunol* 1982;69:410.
132. Van Titts LJH, et al. Catecholamines increase lymphocyte $β_2$-adrenergic receptors via a $β_2$-adrenergic, spleen-dependent process. *Am J Physiol* 1990;258(Endocrinol Metab 21):E191.
133. Vischer TL. The differential effect of cyclic AMP on lymphocyte stimulation by T- or B-cell mitogens. *Immunology* 1976;30:735.
134. Wesselmann U, et al. Altered splenic catecholamine concentrations during experimental allergic encephalomyelitis. *Pharmacol Biochem Behav* 1987;26:851.
135. Wiegmann K, et al. β-Adrenergic agonists suppress chronic/relapsing experimental allergic encephalomyelitis (CREAE) in Lewis rats. *J Neuroimmunol* 1995;56:201.
136. Williams JM, et al. Sympathetic innervation of murine thymus and spleen: evidence for a functional link between the nervous and immune systems. *Brain Res Bull* 1981;6:83.
137. Williams LT, et al. Identification of β-adrenergic receptors in human lymphocytes by (-)[^{3}H]alprenolol binding. *J Clin Invest* 1976;57:149.
138. Zoukos Y, et al. Increased expression of high affinity IL-2 receptors and β-adrenoreceptors in peripheral blood mononuclear cells is associated with clinical and MRI activity in multiple sclerosis. *Brain* 1994;117:307.
139. Zoukos Y, et al. β-Adrenergic receptor density and function of peripheral blood mononuclear cells are increased in multiple sclerosis: a regulatory role for cortisol and interleukin-1. *Ann Neurol* 1992; 31:657.
140. Zoukos Y, et al. β-Adrenoceptor expression on circulating mononuclear cells of idiopathic Parkinson's disease and autonomic failure patients before and after reduction of central sympathetic outflow by clonidine. *Neurology* 1993;43:1181.

CHAPTER 14

The Effect of Aging on the Autonomic Nervous System

Phillip A. Low

---

1. The underlying mechanisms of aging are complex and uncertain. The role of oxidative stress causing excessive mitochondrial DNA mutations and that of apoptosis may be very important.
2. The effects of aging on the autonomic nervous system are heterogeneous, varying by autonomic system and level.
3. Cardiovagal function is impaired.
4. Orthostatic hypotension occurs. The mechanisms are likely multifactorial and include reduced baroreflex responsiveness and impaired neuroeffector function. These deficits are only partly compensated for by an increase in muscle sympathetic activity and an increase in plasma norepinephrine.
5. Sudomotor function is affected. An increase in thermoreceptor threshold and a reduction in capacity result in altered thermoregulation. The impairment is greater in the lower extremities than in the trunk, suggesting a length-dependent process.
6. The effect of age on the autonomic nervous system does, however, appear to be greatly modulated by genetic, dietary, cultural, fitness, and other factors, resulting in considerable, and often marked, individual, and group differences.

MECHANISMS OF AGING

The effects of aging on the autonomic nervous system are complex and heterogeneous by tissue, system, and level of the autonomic neuraxis. The mechanism(s) of aging are controversial, and have included (a) a stochastic process, (b) developmental mechanisms, (c) programmed aging, and (d) free-radical mechanisms (82). Stochastic processes have been discussed in mathematical terms (139), or mechanisms such as the accumulation of multiple somatic mutations, "error catastrophe," and protein glycosylation (82). Developmental mechanisms include those immune and neuroendocrine mechanisms of aging (82,139). The last two theories are supported by significant observational and experimental evidence. One involves aging as programmed cell death (apoptosis), and the other invokes free-radical induced mitochondrial DNA (mtDNA) mutations as the primary mechanism.

Oxidative stress has been suggested to be a major pathogenetic mechanism of aging, and the mitochondrion is a selective focus of it action (174). mtDNA is unusually susceptible to oxidative damage with aging (133) and undergoes excessive mutations (144). These dysfunctional mitochondria have increased free-radical leakage (144). There is the vicious cycle of oxidative damage to inner membrane proteins (of mitochondria) leading to a defective electron transport chain, with increased superoxide and hydrogen peroxide production, which in turn further damages membrane proteins, and the cycle repeats (144). An accumulation of these somatic mutations during the life of an individual causes an energy deficit leading to normal aging. There is a close relationship between the burden of mtDNA mutations and the severity of impairment in mitochondrial energy metabolism (66,92,94). A wide variety of mtDNA mutations have been identified in organs with a great dependence on oxidative metabolism, such as the brain, heart, skeletal muscle, kidney, and endocrine system (165). In neural tissue, there is considerable heterogeneity of response. For instance, mitochondria of human basal ganglia are particularly susceptible to oxidative mutation (22,152).

There is an exponential increase in mutations with increasing age (66,92,94,176). More than 10 different types of deletions have been identified in the mtDNA of various tissues of elderly people (171). Some of these deletions were found only in a certain tissues, but others appeared to

---

P. A. Low: Department of Neurology, Mayo Clinic, Rochester, Minnesota 55905.

be widespread in distribution. The 4,977-base-pair deletion is the most prevalent and abundant one among these deletions (171). Evidence in support of the importance of oxidative stress in the genesis of mtDNA mutations includes a reduced susceptibility in mitochondria with increase superoxide dismutase (90).

A related but different mechanism of aging is that of apoptosis. Apoptosis, or programmed cell death, is a normal physiologic cell death process of eliminating unwanted cells during embryonic and adult development. Apoptosis involves many death and survival genes that are regulated by extracellular factors, including free-radical mechanisms. There are multiple inducers and inhibitors of apoptosis that interact with target cell-specific surface receptors and transduce the signal by second messengers to program cell death. The regulation of apoptosis is elusive, but defective regulation leads to etiology of various ailments, including aging. The number of apoptotic neurons increases with aging, and aging is suggested to accelerate the process (11,17,181).

There are numerous modulators of apoptosis. These include the bcl-2 proto-oncogene, which protects various cell types from apoptotic cell death and is expressed in the developing and adult nervous system. Examples of its action include its ability to reduce the dependence of sensory neurons on nerve growth factor (40), and its inhibition of apoptotic death of motor neurons after axotomy of the sciatic nerve in mice. Another molecule of importance with apoptosis is Fas CD95. Its role during aging has been determined in young, and old CD2-fas-transgenic mice. Fas expression and ligand-induced apoptosis were decreased on T cells from old mice compared with young mice. These results suggest that T-cell senescence with age is associated with defective apoptosis, and that the CD2-fas transgene allows maintenance of Fas apoptosis function and T-cell function in aged mice comparable to that of young mice (182).

While there is general agreement that the autonomic nervous system is affected by aging, there appears to be a lack of appreciation of its heterogeneous effects by autonomic system and level. There is good agreement on the major observations. Problems arise when generalizations and extrapolations are made from these observations. For example, it is well accepted that plasma supine norepinephrine (NE) increases with aging (184). Some investigators have extrapolated these findings to suggest that sympathetic function, in general, is increased (126), without separately considering age-related alterations on effector function, baroreflexity, and preganglionic neurons. The net effect may be very different from a single index of a single level of function. The autonomic neuraxis is also heterogeneously involved within a system. For instance, sympathetic sudomotor function may be affected in the lower but not in the upper extremity and one nerve may be affected more than another. There may also be marked differences between the sympathetic and parasympathetic systems and their innervation of different organ systems. Burnstock (14) has summarized some of the complexities of the autonomic infrastructure that occur with aging. Neuroeffector transmission is complex. There is a multiplicity of transmitters, cotransmission, neuromodulation, and "chemical coding" of individual autonomic neurons, as well as complex projections and central connections. Changes in expression of autonomic nerves and cotransmitters occur with aging. It is suggested that when one undertakes neuropathologic analysis, compensatory increases in innervation should be considered as well as loss or damage to nerves. For instance certain populations of nitric oxide-positive cells increases with aging (6).

There is, sometimes, marked variability among individuals that can be related in significant degrees to genetic, cultural, conditioning, and dietary factors. The presence of concomitant disease and the effects of medication may also significantly affect autonomic function. For example, an increase in blood pressure (BP) with aging occurs in Western societies but not in more "primitive" societies (87). The rest of this chapter focuses on autonomic functions that are of particular interest to the clinician evaluating patients with autonomic failure. The regulation of cardiovagal function, postural normotension, baroreflexes, and indices of peripheral sympathetic and pupillary functions are reviewed and followed by a synthesis. Genitourinary function is covered elsewhere (Chapters 10, 11, and 58).

CARDIOVAGAL HEART RATE TESTS

Resting and Maximal Heart Rate Variability

It has long been known that resting heart rate (HR) decreases with increasing age (64). HR is under combined sympathetic and parasympathetic control, although para-

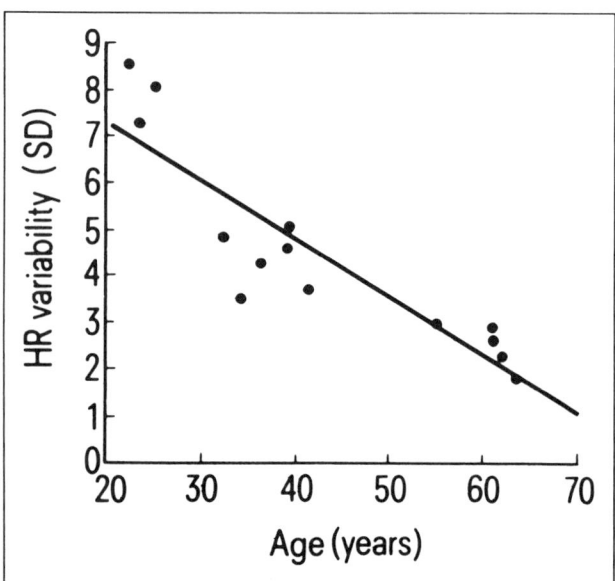

FIG. 1. The beat-to-beat heart rate variation at rest expressed as the standard deviation of mean heart rate sampled over 30 beats for each subject. From Waddington et al. (163), with permission.

TABLE 1. Summary of some published studies on heart rate responses to deep breathing

Year	Authors	No. of subjects	Age range	Duration of test	Cycles/min	Position	Effect of age and comments
1973	Wheeler and Watkins (172)	25	20–50	1 min	6	Supine	SA blocked by atropine; age effect present
1976	Hellman and Stacy (53)	24	21–65	2 min	6	Sitting	Slope = −0.35
1978	Bennett et al. (7)	31	18–60	? 1 min	12 and 6	Supine	Uncertain
1979	Sundkvist et al. (154)	25	<50	1 min	5	Supine	Not evaluated
1979	Hilsted and Jensen (59)	10	20–40	1 min	5	Supine	No effect but narrow range
1980	Watkins and Mackay (168)	54	20–49	1 min	6	Supine	Not evaluated
1981	Dyrberg et al. (31)	28	30–48	1 min	6	Supine	Uncertain
1982	Pfeifer et al. (126)	22	47±3	6 min	5	Supine	Not evaluated
1982	Smith (149)	174	16–89	1 min	5	?	Decline with age
1982	Wieling et al. (173)	133	10–65	1 min	6	Supine	10–29; 20 beats/min 30–49; 15 beats/min 50–65; 12 beats/min
1983	Persson and Solders (125)	75	21–70	1 min	6	Supine	Progressive red with age
1983	Pfeifer et al. (127)	103	19–82	5 min	5	Supine	R-R = −0.0007 × age + 0.072
1985	Oikawa et al. (122)	162	4–77	2 min	6	Supine	Log-linear red with age
1985	Ewing et al. (37)	71	16–65	?	6	Sitting	Decrease with age
1985	Kaijser and Sachs (76)	52	20–80	10 cycles	6	? Sitting	Decrease > age 60
1985	Masaoka et al. (108)	143	20–80	1 min 1 repeat	6	Supine	HRV = 41.1−0.46 × age
1986	Low et al. (100)	35	10–30 31–40 41–50 51–60 61–70	1 min	6	Supine	>25 beats/min >18 beats/min >15 beats/min >12 beats/min >10 beats/min
1986	Solders (151)	128	40–74	1 min	6	Supine	Added 53 patients
1986	O'Brien et al. (116)	310	18–85	10 sec	1		Decrease with age
1986	Gautschy et al. (46)	120	22–92	1 min	6	Sitting	Decrease with age
1986	Vita et al. (161)	70	25–71	≥1 min	6	Sitting	Reduced with age
1986	Bergstrom et al. (8)	56	16–59	1 min	6	Supine	Decrease with age
1986	Clark and Mapstone (20)	85	31–92	1 min	6	Sitting	Decrease with age
1990	Low et al. (101)	122	10–83	1.3 min	8	Supine	Decrease with age
1990	Ingall et al. (68)	72	5–85	1 min	6	Semisitting	Decrease with age
1992	Ziegler et al. (183)	120	15–67	various	6	Supine	Decrease with age
1996	Braune et al. (10)	137	18–85	1 min	6	? Supine	Decrease with age
1996	Low et al.	357	10–83	1 min	6	Supine	Decrease with age

HRV, heart rate variability; SA, sinoatrial node.

sympathetic influences predominate in human subjects under resting conditions. Intrinsic HR (HR following combined sympathetic–parasympathetic blockade), which is a reflection of sinoatrial node function, is reduced with aging and can be predicted by this equation: intrinsic HR = 120 − 0.6 × age (26,74). Cardiac electrophysiologic studies have demonstrated a progressive decline in sinoatrial conduction and sinus node recovery time with age (26).

HR variability declines with age (46,161,163). Resting variation, expressed as the standard deviation of mean HR, regresses linearly with age (Fig. 1). Following parasympathetic blockade by atropine, older subjects respond with a smaller HR increment, indicating that the reduction in HR variability is likely due to a lower vagal tone in elderly subjects (25,112).

HEART RATE RESPONSE TO DEEP BREATHING

All studies involving large numbers of normal subjects have revealed a progressive reduction in forced sinus arrhythmia, quantitated as the mean range of the HR response to deep breathing, with increasing age (8,10, 20,37,46,53,68,101,103,108,122,125,126,149,161,168,173) (Table 1). All large studies have either demonstrated a linear relationship to age, with slopes of 0.34–0.41 (53,68,

TABLE 2. *Summary of published studies on heart rate responses to Valsalva maneuver*

Year	Authors	No. of subjects	Age range	Duration of blowing	mm Hg	No. of reports	Position	Effect of age and comments
1996	Levin (93)	200	? 10–69	10	40	1	Semisupine	Less in elderly
1973	Ewing et al. (38)	37	24–63	15	40	2	?	No controls
1978	Bennett et al. (7)	19	18–56	15	40	2	Supine	No conclusion
1981	Dyrberg et al. (31)	28	30–48	15	40	?	Supine	No conclusion
1983	Persson and Solders (125)	75	21–70	20	40	?	Supine	Weak regression with age found
1985	Kaijser and Sachs (76)	46	21–80	20	40	2	? Sitting	New and published data combined
1985	Ewing et al. (37)	135	16–69	15	40	?	Sitting	No regression with age
1986	Vita et al. (161)	70	25–71	10	40	2	Sitting	No regression with age
1986	O'Brien et al. (116)	310	18–85	15	40	2	Supine	Regression with age found
1986	Clark and Mapstone (20)	85	31–92	15	40	2	Sitting	Regression with age found
1986	Gautschy et al. (46)	120	22–92	15	40	2	Sitting	Regression with age found
1990	Ingall et al. (68)	76	7–85	10	40	2	Semisitting	Regression with age found
1986	Low et al. (101)	35	11–69	10	40	2	Supine	Regression with age found
1990	Low et al. (103)	155	10–83	15	40	3	Supine	Regression with age found
1992	Ziegler et al. (183)	120	15–67	15	40		Supine	Impairment with age
1996	Braune et al. (10)	137	18–85	15	50% of max. EP	?	? Supine	No regression with age

EP, expiratory pressure.

108), or have expressed their data in logarithmic format. Kaijser and Sachs (76) reported a reduction in the HR response with age, but only in subjects >60 years of age.

The Mayo Autonomic Laboratory normative database of 557 normal subjects includes 376 subjects who were evaluated for HR response to deep breathing. Ages ranged from 10 to 83 years and no significant differences were found between the sexes (103). However, a significant regression with age was found (Fig. 15-8): $y = 37.5448 * \log_{10} 0.9832x$ ($p < 0.001$), where y = HR range in beats/min and x = age in years.

The Valsalva Ratio

The effect of age on the Valsalva ratio is controversial. Some workers have reported a lack of variability with age (37,161), whereas others have observed a difference (20, 46,101,103,116,125) (Table 2). Reported slopes have been similar. Ingall et al. (68) reported a slope of 0.01 per year, which is very similar to ours (103).

Valsalva ratio, studied in 425 subjects aged 10–83 years, showed a gender difference. Hence, the data for males and females are described separately (Figs. 15-7 and 15-10): for males (n = 205), $y = 2.15982 - 0.00755x$ ($p < 0.001$); and, for females (n = 220), $y = 2.00273 - 0.00868x - 0.00021x^2$, where y = Valsalva ratio and x = age in years.

The less consistent effect of age on Valsalva ratio than on respiratory sinus arrhythmia likely relates to the smaller change and greater complexity of the maneuver. Whereas respiratory sinus arrhythmia is a relatively pure test of cardiovagal function, many factors, including blood volume, antecedent period of rest (157), cardiac sympathetic and peripheral sympathetic functions (Chapters 6 and 19), and NE response, affect the Valsalva maneuver. Age may affect different components of the Valsalva maneuver in different directions.

Heart Rate Response to Standing

Initially promoted as an age-independent test of parasympathetic function (36), the HR response to standing, dubbed the 30:15 ratio (Chapter 24), is clearly age related (46,116,161,173) (Fig. 2). The response is usually determined by using the ratio of the maximum HR (typically around beat 30) to the minimum HR (about beat 15). The underlying BP alterations and composite mechanisms are described in the section on *Orthostatic hypotension of old age*.

Heart Rate Response to Coughing

Coughing results in cardioacceleration, peaking at ~3 sec, followed by a return to normal rates (169). Like sev-

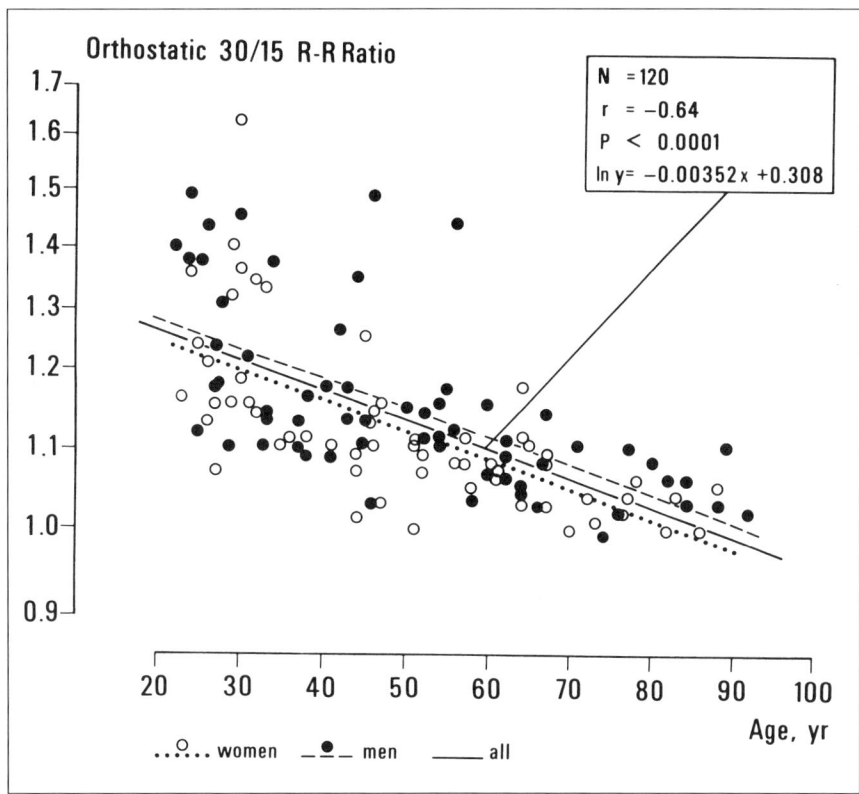

FIG. 2. The orthostatic 30:15 ratio as a function of increasing age, studied in 120 normal subjects. From Gautschy et al. (46), with permission.

eral other vagal reflexes, there is progressive impairment with increasing age (16,169,170).

Heart Rate Response to Facial Cold Stimulus

The exposure of the face to a sudden cold stimulus, such as by immersion in cold water (facial immersion test) or exposure to a cold wind (cold-face test), results in reflex bradycardia and peripheral vasoconstriction (39,51). The bradycardiac response is reported to be increased (91) or reduced (4,76) in older subjects. There was no gender difference.

Frequency Analysis

Total power spectral density with patients supine becomes progressively lower with increasing age, usually in a log-linear fashion (178). The high-frequency component, usually between 0.2 and 0.3 Hz, and widely accepted as representing parasympathetic activity, is also reduced with age in a log-linear fashion (143,183). The normal response with tilt-up is a reduction in the power due to parasympathetic power and an increase in low-frequency power. With aging Mayer waves (~0.1 Hz by autoregressive methodology) become progressively reduced (72,178). A full description of methodology, interpretations, and applications is discussed elsewhere (Chapters 26, 27).

Baroreflexes

When systemic pulse pressure, or mean arterial pressure, is reduced, baroreceptors in the carotid sinus and aortic arch are activated (81). Baroreceptor afferents synapse at the nucleus of tractus solitarius, and activation results in an increase in HR, vasoconstriction of the splanchnic and systemic vasculature, and restoration of BP. This topic is detailed in Chapter 6. In addition to arterial baroreceptors, there are also low-pressure or cardiopulmonary baroreceptors that respond to a reduction in central venous pressure (185). The central pathways and efferents are the same as for arterial baroreceptors.

Acute baroreceptor denervation results in reduced buffering of BP so that BP fluctuates widely (23,69,84). This lability tends to dissipate, however, over days or weeks. Baroreflexes may be depressed in old age (29,49,131,145). The components of this impairment have been dissected (77). Baroreceptors are embedded in the media–adventitial junction (1). Since they detect deformation, atherosclerotic stiffening of the carotid sinus results in reduced sensitivity. Afferent fibers in the carotid sinus and aortic arch undergo axonal degeneration with increasing age (1,58). Baroreflex efferents are also impaired because of reduced vagal modulation of HR and decreased responsiveness of the sinoatrial node. The effect of aging on baroreflex regulation of muscle sympathetic activity to the lower limbs has been compared with its influence on parasympathetic outflow to the sinus node (32). Aging had a significant effect on baroreflex control of cardiac interval, whereas the response of posture on baroreflex gain for MSNA was either not significantly affected by aging (32) or only mildly impaired (70).

Aging does result in several alterations of cardiac sympathetic function. Adrenergic input to the heart is impaired (134). HR and cardiac output with exercise are reduced in healthy old subjects compared with their young counterparts. This difference dissipates with β-adrenergic blockade (21), indicating a diminished role for adrenergic influences in the hearts of older subjects. The HR increment with atropine, considered an index of vagal efferent activity, is reduced (25,112). The HR increase with isoproterenol is also diminished (63,177).

Central nervous system alterations, such as the loss of dopamine and NE in human hypothalamus, have been documented (2). A dynamic central autonomic dysfunction involving defective modulation of catecholaminergic receptors in response to physiologic stress has been postulated (134).

In the peripheral nervous system, there is evidence of impaired ganglionic transmission in aged experimental animals (134). Degenerative changes such as inclusion bodies, myelin disorganization, lipofuscin accumulation (52), and the disappearance of catecholaminergic histofluorescence in aged human ganglia, have been described (57). There is reduced neurotransmitter release at specific neuroeffector junctions, including the heart and certain blood vessels, and many tissues exhibit reduced effector responsiveness (134).

Exercise Capacity and Aging

Exercise capacity in both males and females is reduced with aging (42,110,142). There is a reduced HR increment and left ventricular contractile response with exercise, resulting in a reduction in cardiac output, oxygen consumption, and exercise capacity. The HR increment during exercise is attenuated with aging, due to both less withdrawal of cardiac vagal tone and diminished β-adrenergic responsiveness (153). The latter also appears to contribute to an attenuation in the left ventricular contractile response to exercise despite greater β-adrenergic stimulation. There are some gender-specific differences in cardiovascular indices (35,42).

Much has been attributed to the increased muscle sympathetic nerve activity and arterial plasma NE spillover rates at supine rest (70,114,167,179,184) (Fig. 3). The increase in supine NE is inconsistent and is not seen in some studies (83,115), and the muscle sympathetic response to tilt-up is attenuated (70). The larger increment in NE with standing in older subjects should be viewed in the context of a reduced response with more prolonged or strenuous exercise (83). Considering the greater orthostatic fall in BP

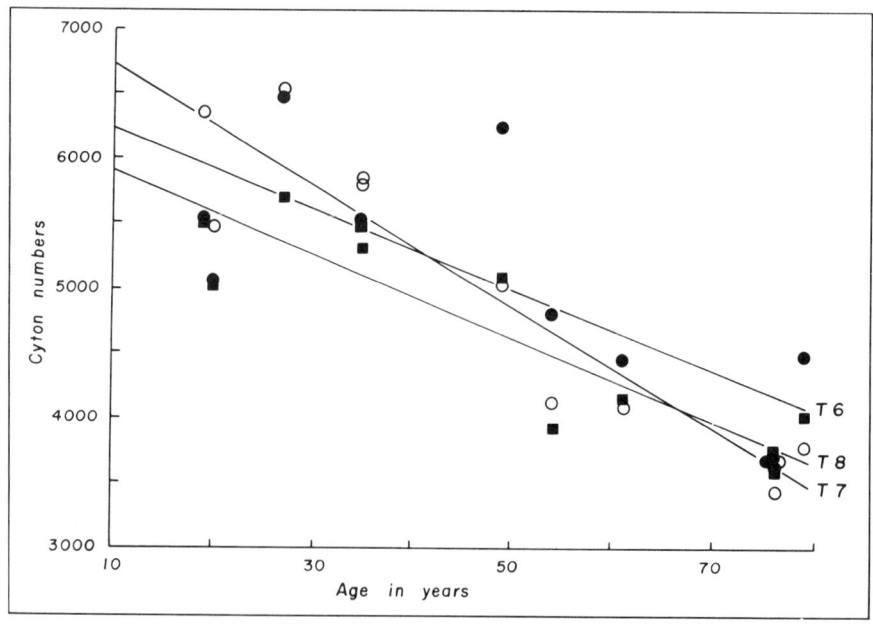

FIG. 3. Progressive reduction of preganglionic sympathetic neuron numbers in the intermediolateral column. T6, *open circles*; T7, *closed circles*; and T8, *open squares*.

in the elderly, the increase in NE is not disproportionate. Overall, with aging, sympathetic tone is normal or increased at rest and, during brief dynamic exercise, and performance is unimpaired with moderate-intensity exercise performance, but is clearly impaired with more intense or protracted exercise. Of particular interest is the observation in older people that aerobic exercise training lowers HR at rest and increases muscle sympathetic activity. The sympathetic neural response and plasma catecholamine responses to stress are also augmented in trained individuals (115). At least in men, there is an improvement in left ventricular performance during peak exercise (142).

ORTHOSTATIC HYPOTENSION OF OLD AGE

Orthostatic hypotension (reduction of systolic BP by >30 mmHg or mean BP by >15 mmHg) has been reported to be relatively common in patients >70 years of age (15,73,96,137,148), although it is typically mild or asymptomatic (24,135,137). The cardiovascular alterations in elderly subjects (aged 60–69 years) have been analyzed in detail (148). They have, compared with younger subjects, in the upright posture, lesser increments in HR and diastolic pressure, but no significant differences from younger age groups in the response of thoracic blood volume, cardiac output, or total vascular resistance. Beginning at about age 75, however, there is an increasing incidence of orthostatic hypotension, which averages ~14%–20% at age 75 and older. We evaluated the effect of 80° upright tilt in 271 normal controls aged 10–83. The normative data are listed in Table 3. The fall in systolic BP by age and gender for the 99th percentile at 1 min of upright tilt was 23.6, 26.5, 29.4, and 32.4 for both males and females of ages 20, 40, 60, and 80 years, respectively. After 5 min of upright tilt, there was a significant difference by gender but not by age. The values for males were 28.5 mmHg for all ages and 32.0 for females. In conclusion, the results show a significant age effect, with a modest gender effect, manifested in the greater reduction in systolic BP at 5 min.

In many older subjects, the BP changes may not be present under normal conditions, but may develop under conditions of orthostatic stress. Significant orthostatic hypotension may develop postprandially (95). Other stresses could include bed rest for more than a few days (deconditioning of vascular reflexes), volume depletion (absolute or relative) resulting from diuretic or hypotensive drug therapy or drugs with hypotensive side effects (111), and intercurrent illness with pyrexia or diarrhea. These patients may develop orthostatic light-headedness or fatigue and do occasionally faint.

The basis of the orthostatic hypotension or reduced orthostatic tolerance in old age is likely to be multifactorial because several components of the cardiovascular system are affected by aging (28,103). First, there is 5%–8% attrition of preganglionic neurons per decade, beginning in early adulthood (100); this becomes symptomatic when ~50% of neurons are lost (97). Excellent concordance was found in preganglionic neuron counts with preganglionic myelinated fiber counts in ventral spinal root and rami communicantes of the same level at autopsy (99,100). Second, aging is associated with baroreflex impairment, involving the receptor, afferent and efferent fibers, and the sinoatrial node (see below). Third, α_2- and possibly α_1-adrenoceptors exhibit reduced potency with aging (28,33,67). Fourth, β-adrenoceptor-mediated cardioacceleration and inotropic response are reduced in older people (13,142,160). This impairment is thought to be due to reduced adenylate cyclase activity rather than a change in receptor density (78,89). Fifth, older patients are often on diuretics that significantly reduce blood volume. Even recommended doses of diuretics may result in severe orthostatic hypotension in older patients (15,175). Sixth, supine BP increases with age, and the BP fall on standing is significantly dependent on supine BP. In a study of 75 healthy controls and in 500 patients with diabetes mellitus, Gert van Dijk et al. (47) reported that the most important determinant for the reduction in systolic BP was supine BP. Using stepwise regression analysis, they found that supine BP accounted for 24% of the variance. Seventh, the tendency toward orthostatic hypotension in the elderly is also due to the structural and functional changes in the circulation itself, and to an impaired skeletal muscle pump (148). Increasing age is associated with a decline in total muscle mass (9,48). There is an ~40% reduction in muscle area between the second and seventh decades of life (138).

The maintenance of orthostatic normotension may be different in the elderly. Arginine vasopressin has been found to participate in BP maintenance especially when other pressor systems are endogenously or pharmacologically impaired. The elderly, like subjects with autonomic failure, have a greater reliance on vasopressin, as indicated

TABLE 3. *Orthostatic reduction in systolic blood pressure; 99th percentile*

Time (min)	Gender	mmHg			
		20 Years	40 Years	60 Years	80 Years
1	Male	23.6	26.5	29.4	32.4
1	Female	23.6	26.5	29.4	32.4
5	Male	28.5	28.5	28.5	28.5
5	Female	32.0	32.0	32.0	32.0

by the greater fall in BP following the use of vasopressin antagonists (27).

The mechanism underlying postprandial orthostatic hypotension is uncertain. Since it occurs after an oral but not an intravenous glucose load, the suggestion has been made that it may be due to the gut release of a vasodilator peptide (60). Somatostatin, which blocks the release of some gut peptides, may prevent postprandial orthostatic hypotension (61). A somatostatin analogue, octreotide, can be used to treat postprandial orthostatic hypotension. The drug has been used to treat orthostatic hypotension in general and the prevention and treatment postprandial orthostatic hypotension in particular (61,62,130). It also has an effect on gut motility, increasing the intensity of contractions and the duration of migrating complex in the small intestine (50). It delays small bowel transit time in healthy subjects (162). One disadvantage is that it has to be administered by injection.

Sudomotor Function

The aged tolerate thermoregulatory stress less well than do the young (3,105). The effects of age on the sudomotor neuraxis (thermoreceptor, afferent pathway, central processing, central sympathetic pathways, preganglionic and postganglionic fibers, and the eccrine sweat gland) are complex.

The full complement of eccrine glands develops in the embryonic state (88), and no new glands develop after birth. Their distribution reveals area differences with the greatest density on the palms and soles. They vary in density from $400/cm^2$ on the palm to $\sim 80/cm^2$ on the thigh and upper arm. The total numbers are ~ 2–5 million (54, 88). The density of sweat glands has been reported to decline with increasing age (120,129), especially beyond the age of 60 years (117); the changes are more marked on lower extremities than on the trunk; there are no gender differences. The density of *active* sweat glands has been reported to be reduced (75,106,147) or unchanged (54) with age.

Morphologic changes that occur with advanced age include degeneration of unmyelinated axons supplying the gland, a reduced density of microvessels, periglandular fibrosis, and the accumulation of pigmented granules in clear and dark cells, especially in exposed areas (109).

Part of the explanation for the liability of older subjects to heat stroke likely relates to their higher thermoreceptor threshold (43,54,55,146,164). However, there is considerable individual variation, and physical fitness and acclimation may negate age-related differences (120). There are significant regional and gender differences in age effects. For example, the threshold is more increased in the extremities than in the trunk in men but not in women (43). There has also been considerable variability among reports (180).

Several studies have focused on sweating capacity. The sweat rate, as the result of heat stress, has been reported to be reduced, and the temperature rise greater—factors that are suggestive of impaired thermoregulation in older subjects (54,55,132). However, a number of other variables are at least as important as aging. Physical fitness greatly affects sweat capacity and may be more important than aging *per se* (120). Older subjects are often on medications with anticholinergic properties. They are frequently prescribed diuretics that, by reducing blood volume, may significantly affect the sweat response. Finally, these patients often are afflicted with neurologic diseases, such as cerebral infarction, which may reduce sweat capacity. Many of the studies of aging have, in fact, used hospitalized patients with these confounding problems. An example of this is an often-cited study by Foster et al. (43), who studied 28 men and 18 women age 70 and over and compared their responses with younger subjects. They studied chemically evoked (acetylcholine or methacholine) and thermoregulatory sweating. From a knowledge of the sweat volume and number of sweat droplets, they derived the secretion rate per sweat gland. The major findings were that sweat threshold was increased and sweat output was reduced in the elderly. The reduction was due to a decrease in output per gland rather than a reduction in gland density. They also noted that the reduction was greatest at the periphery and least on the chest. One flaw in this study was that all subjects were patients with disease, including a disproportionate number with cerebrovascular disease.

We have studied a group of 357 normal individuals who were physically active and did not have illnesses or take medications that may have affected the sweat response. Studies were performed at four sites: the forearm and three lower extremity locations. The forearm site was supplied by the ulnar nerve. The lower extremity sites were the upper lateral leg, lower medial leg, and proximal foot and their innervation was peroneal, saphenous, and sural nerves, respectively. The axon reflex-mediated sweat response to iontophoresed acetylcholine declined with age in the distal lower-extremity sites (proximal foot and distal leg) (Table 4). There was no change with age in the forearm and proximal leg. In both sexes, the slope was steeper in the lower compared with the upper extremity, which is suggestive of a length-dependent mechanism of autonomic failure.

The thermoregulatory sweat test may be abnormal in elderly women (>65 years) (27,51): there is considerable variability. The distribution of the thermoregulatory sweat response, determined semiquantitatively as percent anterior surface anhidrosis, has been studied in 35 normal subjects (19 men and 16 women) aged 20–75 years (41). No significant regression was found for either gender with age although the mean age was a relatively young 52 years.

TABLE 4. *Regression of QSART (left side) sweat volumes with age for males and females for standard sites in human subjects: based on a normative database of 357 normal subjects evenly distributed by age and gender*

Variable	Intercept		Gender		Age		Gender* age	
	$b0$	p	$b1$	p	$b2$	p	$b3$	p
Forearm	4.5291	0.0001	−1.6188	0.0001	−0.0072	0.5752	0.0020	0.7989
Proximal leg	4.0209	0.0001	−1.0076	0.0026	−0.0163	0.1410	0.0011	0.8724
Distal leg	5.5929	0.0001	−1.5921	0.0001	−0.0437	0.0002	0.0075	0.3049
Proximal foot	4.5174	0.0001	−1.5171	0.0001	0.0310	0.0066	0.0101	0.1548

QSART, quantitative sudomotor axon reflex test; b, slope of regression line.

Heat acclimatization results in a lowered sweat threshold and increased gain (sweat rate/°C rise in temperature). This process may be more limited in older subjects (164) although this view is not universally accepted (136). Secretory activity per sweat gland increases with acclimation (44,121), and this may be impaired in the elderly (120). The process has been ascribed to increased aldosterone production or elevated ductal sensitivity to this hormone (80).

SYMPATHETIC FUNCTION

Preganglionic Sympathetic Neurons

There is a progressive reduction in preganglionic sympathetic neurons of the intermediolateral column in humans, beginning in adult life (Fig. 3). Morphometric analyses, at the neuronal level (100), were completed in 12 human thoracic spinal cords (T6, T7, and T8) obtained fresh at autopsy from subjects who died of conditions unrelated to the autonomic nervous system. Each morphometric analysis was performed on celloidin-embedded and cresyl violet-stained material. The intermediolateral counts correlated well with the preganglionic axonal counts at both the same ventral spinal root (98) and the rami communicantes (99). The counts were slightly, but not significantly, higher in males and they did not differ by level. There was an attrition of ~5%–8% per decade (99,100).

Lipofuscin pigment accumulates progressively in human autonomic ganglia with aging (128). The distribution and tinctorial characteristics of lipofuscin appear to be different for old and young cells (113). The distribution is diffuse in neurons of young mice; in aged animals, its distribution is multifocal, being perinuclear, near the axon hillock and principal dendrites (113). Young neurons are Sudan black and periodic acid–Schiff positive and give a green-yellow fluorescence at a wave length of 3,650 A, while old cells are more easily stained with Nile blue and ferric ferricyanide and give an orange-yellow fluorescence. Other alterations include a random arrangement of rough endoplasmic reticulum and swollen mitochondria and Golgi apparatus (141). Their NE content is histochemically reduced (57).

Postganglionic Neurons

There is a small attrition in human postganglionic neurons at the superior cervical ganglion with age (155). In rats, age-related changes are well described for the superior cervical and celiac–superior mesenteric ganglia (5). There is a progressive reduction in density in older animals. Changes occur earlier in the splanchnic system than in the superior mesenteric system. Kennedy et al. (79) reported that the postganglionic sudomotor axon of 60-week-old rats regenerated more slowly and less completely than in younger rats. This impaired regenerative capacity may be due to reduced transport of structural proteins in older animals (85). The superior cervical ganglion has been reported to be even more susceptible to aging than other ganglia (45). Changes in the human postganglionic sympathetic sudomotor axon has been described under sudomotor function, above.

In human sural nerve, it is not possible to separate sympathetic fibers from somatic C fibers reliably. The proportion of unmyelinated fibers that are sympathetic in function is very small in rat peripheral nerve (18). It appears to be similarly small in humans, based on measurements of dopamine–β-hydroxylase (12). It is known that unmyelinated fibers are affected by age (119). Changes consist of the development of denervated bands of Bugner (158), collagen pockets, miniature profiles (119), a shift in unmyelinated fiber diameter histogram to a smaller diameter peak (119), and a reduction in fiber density (30,118). Denervated bands are presumed to be Schwann's cell processes that previously encased unmyelinated fibers that have since been lost (Chapter 28). Similarly, the collagen of collagen pockets is thought to have replaced unmyelinated fibers. The smaller diameter peak (Chapter 28) is due to the large number of miniature regenerated fibers (71,119). The diameter distribution shift from a distribution to a bimodal pattern could be a more sensitive index of unmyelinated fiber pathology than unmyelinated of fiber density (118).

Norepinephrine

Supine plasma free NE is a useful, though insensitive, index of postganglionic sympathetic function. It is found in

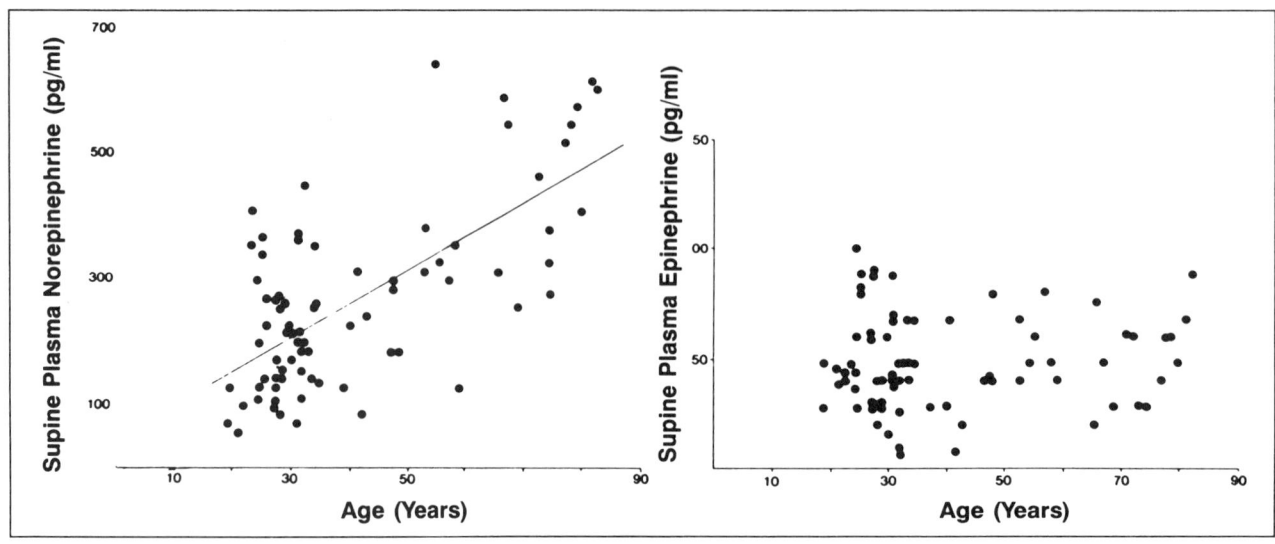

FIG. 4. The effect of aging on plasma norepinephrine and epinephrine concentrations in human subjects. From Pfeifer et al. (126), with permission.

the circulation because of spillover of NE from postganglionic sympathetic terminals. Supine plasma NE increases with age (124,134,184), whereas epinephrine does not. In a typical study, Pfeifer et al. (126) studied 77 subjects, ranging in age from 19 to 82 years, and found a linear relationship between age and plasma NE ($r = 0.68$, $p < 0.01$), but no relationship between age and epinephrine (Fig. 4). The mechanism of increase is controversial. The increase could be due to increased release or reduced clearance. Release has been suggested to be increased based on the microneurographic finding of increased sympathetic traffic in muscle nerves of older subjects (167) and in individuals with normal clearance (140). However, reduced clearance with normal release has also been reported (34). The methodology of the studies has been criticized (19). Specifically, the site of sampling of venous NE may be unsatisfactory and, ideally, should be either the pulmonary artery or the tissue of interest (19).

TABLE 5. *Percentage change in blood flow (or peripheral resistance) with increasing age for female and male control subjects*

Stimulus	Gender	Intercept	Regression coefficient (b)	Significance of b
Inspiratory Gasp				
Finger	F	55.99	−0.38	NS
	M	53.17	−0.05	NS
Toe	F	45.96	−0.01	NS
	M	63.00	−0.34	NS
Cold pressor text				
Finger	F	71.76	−0.44	$p<0.025$
	M	50.22	−0.47	NS
Toe	F	44.10	−0.16	NS
	M	59.50	−0.55	$p<0.01$
Valsalva maneuver				
Finger	F	69.23	−0.51	$p<0.025$
	M	52.10	−0.11	NS
Toe	F	61.03	−0.23	NS
	M	69.58	−0.45	NS
Peripheral resistance				
Finger	F	327.27	−2.47	NS
	M	215.28	0.07	NS

NS, not significant.

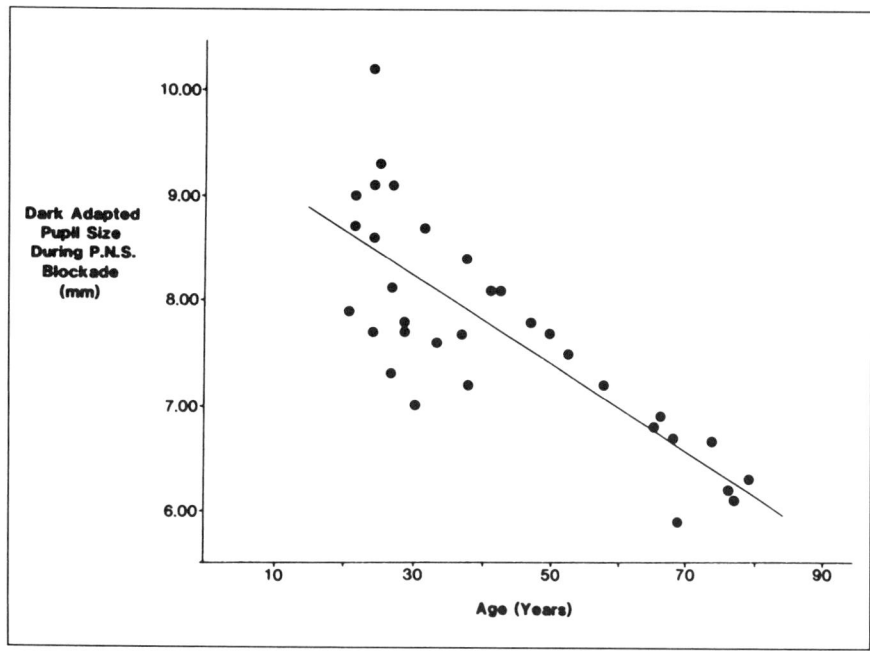

FIG. 5. The relationship between age and dark-adapted pupil size during parasympathetic nervous system (PNS) blockade in normal men. Dark-adapted pupil size decreases with age (pupil size = $-0.04 \times$ age + 9.6; $r = -0.81$; n = 34; $p < 0.001$). From Pfeifer et al. (126), with permission.

Skin Vasomotor Reflexes

The maintenance of postural normotension depends on the integrity of sympathetic innervation of the muscle resistance and venous capacitance beds. Reflex vasoconstriction of skin, muscle, and certain venous beds occurs in concert and is affected by neuropathy (101). Because of the relative ease and noninvasiveness of studying skin blood flow, skin vasomotor reflexes have been studied as indices of sympathetic vasoconstrictor status. The reliability and reproducibility of the tests have been questioned. Skin vasomotor reflexes at the level of the fingerpad, measured using laser Doppler flowmetry, in response to standing and the Valsalva maneuver have been reported to correlate well with the results of the conventional autonomic function test. The responses were reported to be reduced in older subjects (70–89 years) (123). Our experience, recording from both the upper and lower extremities, was less favorable.

We measured the reduction in skin blood flow of fingerpads and toepads in response to inspiratory gasp, Valsalva maneuver, tilt, and contralateral cold stimulus (102). The pads were chosen because of their distal location and because their sympathetic innervation is purely vasoconstrictor. Blood flow was measured using laser Doppler flowmeters. Ages ranged from 10 to 69 years in 34 females and 29 males. All tests yielded a negative slope with increasing age. The slope infrequently reached statistical significance, however (Table 5). Two factors may explain this lack of significance. First, there was considerable variability in the responses that could be related to moment-to-moment alterations in skin sympathetic activity and blood flow. Second, some aged individuals exhibited large responses (102).

Venoarteriolar Reflex

During limb dependency, when venous pressure is increased by 25 mmHg, reflex arteriolar vasoconstriction reduces blood flow by 50% (56). The receptors for this venoarteriolar reflex are located in small veins, and the neural pathway appears to involve a sympathetic C-fiber local axon reflex. The vasoconstrictor response (percent vasoconstriction) was not different between males and females (males = $57.7 \pm 13.8\%$, n = 22; females = $56.8 \pm 17.6\%$, n = 23; $p > 0.05$) and did not significantly regress with increasing age (110). The lack of an observable age effect should be interpreted cautiously. There is marked variability in skin sympathetic activity from moment to moment, depending on skin temperature and, especially, emotional factors (166). A small change with age in tests such as skin vasomotor and venoarteriolar reflexes could be buried within the resting variability of sympathetic activity.

Autonomic Control of the Pupil

Resting dark-adapted pupil diameter decreases with increasing age (150,156) and likely reflects autonomic impairment. The miosis of the aged has been interpreted to be due to sympathetic impairment (86) and not to mechanical alterations (65). However, since the pupil is dually innervated by sympathetic pupillodilator fibers and parasympathetic pupilloconstrictor fibers, the nature of the autonomic lesion requires pharmacologic dissection. There has recently been a resurgence of interest in using pupillometry to evaluate autonomic function noninvasively. The rates of pupillodilatation and constriction have been used as indices of sympathetic function because sympathetic denervation causes the pupil to dilate more slowly in darkness and to constrict more slowly in light (104). Studies suggest that pupillometric recordings should be supplemented with pharmacologic blockade of the interfering system. For example, following parasympathetic blockade, dark-adapted pupillary size is a good index of sympathetic activity (127). Control of iris function progressively declines with increasing age (Fig. 5).

Pupil cycle time has been resurrected as a test of parasympathetic function (107), but Thompson (159), who popularized the test, has urged caution in its interpretation because it is also affected by lesions of the optic nerve, sympathetic pathways, and myoneural junction; narrow-angle glaucoma; and the level of retinal illumination; and is less accurate when pupil movements are weak (159).

SYNTHESIS

In conclusion, aging is a complicated, multifactorial process that clearly affects the autonomic nervous system. Its impact on the autonomic neuraxis is at multiple levels and heterogeneous. Future research should be focused on basic mechanisms at a fundamental level, and the insights gained from these studies should be applied to defined systems at specific levels.

REFERENCES

1. Abraham A. The structure of baroreceptors in pathological conditions in man. In: Kezdi P, ed. *Baroreceptors and hypertension.* Oxford: Pergamon, 1967:273.
2. Adolfsson R, et al. Post-mortem distribution of dopamine and homovanillic acid in human brain, variations related to age, and a review of the literature [Review]. *J Neural Transm* 1979;45:81–105.
3. Al-Khawashki MI, et al. *Heat stroke and temperature regulation.* Sydney: Academic, 1983.
4. Arnold RW, et al. Sensitivity to vasovagal maneuvers in normal children and adults. *Mayo Clin Proc* 1991;66:797–804.
5. Baker DM, Santer RM. Morphometric studies on pre- and paravertebral sympathetic neurons in the rat: changes with age. *Mech Ageing Dev* 1988;42:139–145.
6. Belai A, et al. Effect of age on NADPH–diaphorase-containing myenteric neurones of rat ileum and proximal colon. *Cell Tissue Res* 1995;279:379–383.
7. Bennett T, et al. Assessment of methods for estimating autonomic nervous control of the heart in patients with diabetes mellitus. *Diabetes* 1978;27:1167–1174.
8. Bergstrom B, et al. Autonomic nerve function tests: reference values in healthy subjects. *Clin Physiol* 1986;6:523–528.
9. Booth FW, et al. Effect of aging on human skeletal muscle and motor function [Review]. *Med Sci Sports Exerc* 1994;26:556–560.
10. Braune S, et al. Cardiovascular parameters: sensitivity to detect autonomic dysfunction and influence of age and sex in normal subjects. *Clin Auton Res* 1996;6:3–16.
11. Bright J, et al. Apoptosis: programmed cell death in health and disease [Review]. *Biosci Rep* 1994;14:67–81.
12. Brimijoin S, Dyck PJ. Axonal transport of dopamine–beta-hydroxylase and acetylcholinesterase in human peripheral neuropathy. *Exp Neurol* 1979;66:467–478.
13. Buhler FR, et al. Plasma catecholamines and cardiac, renal and peripheral vascular adrenoceptor-mediated responses in different age groups of normal and hypertensive subjects. *Clin Exp Hypertens* 1980;2:409–426.
14. Burnstock G. Changes in expression of autonomic nerves in aging and disease. *J Auton Nerv Syst* 1990;30(Suppl):S25–S34.
15. Caird FI, et al. The cardiovascular system. In: Brocklehurst JC, ed. *Textbook of geriatric medicine and gerontology.* Edinburgh: Churchill Livingstone, 1985:230.
16. Cardone C, et al. Cough test to assess cardiovascular autonomic reflexes in diabetes. *Diabetes Care* 1990;13:719–724.
17. Carson DA, Ribeiro JM. Apoptosis and disease [Review]. *Lancet* 1993;341:1251–1254.
18. Chad D, et al. Sympathetic postganglionic unmyelinated axons in the rat peripheral nervous system. *Neurology* 1983;33:841–847.
19. Christensen NJ. Sympathetic nervous activity and age. *Eur J Clin Invest* 1982;12:91–92.
20. Clark CV, Mapstone R. Age-adjusted normal tolerance limits for cardiovascular autonomic function assessment in the elderly. *Age Ageing* 1986;15:221–229.
21. Conway J. Effect of age on the response to propranolol. *Int Z Klin Pharmakol Ther Toxikol* 1970;4:148–150.
22. Corral-Debrinski M, et al. Mitochondrial DNA deletions in human brain: regional variability and increase with advanced age. *Nature Genet* 1992;2:324–329.
23. Cowley AW Jr, et al. Role of baroreceptor reflex in daily control of arterial blood pressure and other variables in dogs. *Circ Res* 1973;32:564–576.
24. Dambrink JH, Wieling W. Circulatory response to postural change in healthy male subjects in relation to age. *Clin Sci* 1987;72:335–341.
25. Dauchot P, Gravenstein JS. Effects of atropine on the electrocardiogram in different age groups. *Clin Pharmacol Ther* 1971;12:274–280.
26. De Marneffe M, et al. Variations of normal sinus node function in relation to age: role of autonomic influence. *Eur Heart J* 1986;7:662–672.
27. De Paula RB, et al. Contribution of vasopressin to orthostatic blood pressure maintenance in essential hypertension. *Am J Hypertens* 1993;6:794–798.
28. Docherty JR. Aging and the cardiovascular system [Review]. *J Auton Pharmacol* 1986;6:77–84.
29. Duke PC, et al. The effects of age on baroreceptor reflex function in man. *Can Anaesth Soc J* 1976;23:111–124.
30. Dyck PJ, Lambert EH. Dissociated sensation in amylidosis: compound action potential, quantitative histologic and teased-fiber, and electron microscopic studies of sural nerve biopsies. *Arch Neurol* 1969;20:490–507.
31. Dyrberg T, et al. Prevalence of diabetic autonomic neuropathy measured by simple bedside tests. *Diabetologia* 1981;20:190–194.
32. Ebert TJ, et al. Effects of aging on baroreflex regulation of sympathetic activity in humans. *Am J Physiol* 1992;263:H798–H803.
33. Elliott HL, et al. Effect of age on the responsiveness of vascular alpha-adrenoceptors in man. *J Cardiovasc Pharmacol* 1982;4:388–392.
34. Esler M, et al. Age-dependence of noradrenaline kinetics in normal subjects. *Clin Sci* 1981;60:217–219.
35. Evans SL, et al. Physiological determinants of 10-km performance in highly trained female runners of different ages. *J Appl Physiol* 1995;78:1931–1941.
36. Ewing DJ, et al. Immediate heart rate response to standing: simple test of autonomic neuropathy in diabetes. *BMJ* 1978;1:145–147.

37. Ewing DJ, et al. The value of cardiovascular autonomic function tests: 10 years experience in diabetes. *Diabetes Care* 1985;8:491–498.
38. Ewing DJ, et al. Vascular reflexes in diabetic autonomic neuropathy. *Lancet* 1973;2:1354–1356.
39. Fagius J, Sundlof G. The diving response in man: effects on sympathetic activity in muscle and skin nerve fascicles. *J Physiol* (Lond) 1986; 377:429–443.
40. Farlie PG, et al. bcl-2 transgene expression can protect neurons against developmental and induced cell death. *Proc Natl Acad Sci USA* 1995;92:4397–4401.
41. Fealey RD, et al. Thermoregulatory sweating abnormalities in diabetes mellitus. *Mayo Clin Proc* 1989;64:617–628.
42. Fleg JL, et al. Impact of age on the cardiovascular response to dynamic upright exercise in healthy men and women. *J Appl Physiol* 1995;78:890–900.
43. Foster KG, et al. Sweat responses in the aged. *Age Ageing* 1976; 5:91–101.
44. Fox RH, et al. The nature of the increase in sweating capacity produced by heat acclimatization. *J Physiol* 1964;171:368–376.
45. Gabella G. The structure of smooth muscles of the eye and the intestine. In: Bulbring E, Shuba MF, eds. *Physiology of smooth muscle.* New York: Raven, 1976:265–277.
46. Gautschy B, et al. Autonomic function tests as related to age and gender in normal man. *Klin Wochenschr* 1986;64:499–505.
47. Gert van Dijk J, et al. Effects of supine blood pressure on interpretation of standing up test in 500 patients with diabetes mellitus. *J Auton Nerv Syst* 1994;47:23–31.
48. Graves JE, et al. Exercise, age, and skeletal muscle function [Review]. *South Med J* 1994;87:S17–S22.
49. Gribbin B, et al. Effect of age and high blood pressure on baroreflex sensitivity in man. *Circ Res* 1971;29:424–431.
50. Haruma K, et al. Effect of octreotide on gastrointestinal pressure profiles in health and in functional and organic gastrointestinal disorders. *Gut* 1994;35:1064–1069.
51. Heistad DD, et al. Vasoconstrictor response to simulated diving in man. *J Appl Physiol* 1968;25:542–549.
52. Helen P. Fine-structural and degenerative features in adult and aged human sympathetic ganglion cells. *Mech Ageing Dev* 1983;23:161–175.
53. Hellman JB, Stacy RW. Variation of respiratory sinus arrhythmia with age. *J Appl Physiol* 1976;41:734–738.
54. Hellon RF, Lind AR. Observations on activity of sweat glands with special reference to influence of ageing. *J Physiol* 1956;133:132–144.
55. Hellon RF, et al. Physiological reactions of men of 2 age groups to hot environment. *J Physiol* 1956;133:118–131.
56. Henriksen O. Local sympathetic reflex mechanism in regulation of blood flow in human subcutaneous adipose tissue. *Acta Physiol Scand Suppl* 1977;450:1–48.
57. Hervonen A, et al. Effects of ageing on the histochemically demonstrable catecholamines and acetylcholinesterase of human sympathetic ganglia. *J Neurocytol* 1978;7:11–23.
58. Hilgenberg F. Neurohistologic studies of the carotid sinus baroreceptors in hypertension. In: Kezdi P, ed. *Baroreceptors and hypertension.* Oxford: Pergamon, 1967:293.
59. Hilsted J, Jensen SB. A simple test for autonomic neuropathy in juvenile diabetics. *Acta Med Scand* 1979;205:385–387.
60. Hoeldtke RD, Israel BC. Treatment of orthostatic hypotension with octreotide. *J Clin Endocrinol Metab* 1989;68:1051–1059.
61. Hoeldtke RD, et al. Prevention of postprandial hypotension with somatostatin. *Ann Intern Med* 1985;103:889–890.
62. Hoeldtke RD, et al. Hemodynamic effects of octreotide in patients with autonomic neuropathy. *Circulation* 1991;84:168–176.
63. Hoffmann VH, et al. Dependence on age of the effects of catecholamines in man. I. Effect of noradrenaline, adrenaline and isoprenaline on blood pressure and heart rate [in German]. *Z Gesamte Inn Med* 1975;30:89–95.
64. Howell TH. The pulse rate in old age. *J Gerontol* 1948;3:272–275.
65. Hreidarsson AB. Pupil motility in long-term diabetes. *Diabetologia* 1979;17:145–150.
66. Hsieh RH, et al. Age-dependent respiratory function decline and DNA deletions in human muscle mitochondria. *Biochem Mol Biol Int* 1994;32:1009–1022.
67. Hyland L, Docherty JR. An investigation of age-related changes in pre- and postjunctional alpha-adrenoceptors in human saphenous vein. *Eur J Pharmacol* 1985;114:361–364.
68. Ingall TJ, et al. The effect of ageing on autonomic nervous system function. *Aust NZ J Med* 1990;20:570–577.
69. Ito CS, Scher AM. Hypertension following arterial baroreceptor denervation in the unanesthetized dog. *Circ Res* 1981;48:576–591.
70. Iwase S, et al. Age-related changes of sympathetic outflow to muscles in humans. *J Gerontol* 1991;46:M1–M5.
71. Jacobs JM, Love S. Qualitative and quantitative morphology of human sural nerve at different ages. *Brain* 1985;108:897–924.
72. Jarisch WR, et al. Age-related disappearance of Mayer-like heart rate waves. *Experientia* 1987;43:1207–1209.
73. Johnson RH, et al. Effect of posture on blood pressure in elderly patients. *Lancet* 1965;1:731–733.
74. Jose AD, Collison D. The normal range and determinants of the intrinsic heart rate in man. *Cardiovasc Res* 1970;4:160–167.
75. Juniper K Jr, Dykman RA. Skin resistance, sweat-gland counts, salivary flow, and gastric secretion: age, race, and sex differences, and intercorrelations. *Psychophysiology* 1967;4:216–222.
76. Kaijser L, Sachs C. Autonomic cardiovascular responses in old age. *Clin Physiol* 1985;5:347–357.
77. Karemaker JM, et al. Aging and the baroreflex. In: Amery A, Staessen J, eds. *Handbook of hypertension.* Amsterdam: Elsevier Science, 1989.
78. Kelly J, O'Malley K. Adrenoceptor function and ageing [Review]. *Clin Sci* 1984;66:509–515.
79. Kennedy WR, et al. Reinnervation of sweat glands in the mouse: axonal regeneration versus collateral sprouting. *Muscle Nerve* 1988; 11:603–609.
80. Kirby CR, Convertino VA. Plasma aldosterone and sweat sodium concentrations after exercise and heat acclimation. *J Appl Physiol* 1986;61:967–970.
81. Kirchheim HR. Systemic arterial baroreceptor reflexes [Review]. *Physiol Rev* 1976;56:100–177.
82. Knight JA. The process and theories of aging [Review]. *Ann Clin Lab Sci* 1995;25:1–12.
83. Kohrt WM, et al. Effects of age, adiposity, and fitness level on plasma catecholamine responses to standing and exercise. *J Appl Physiol* 1993;75:1828–1835.
84. Koike H, et al. Influence of cardiopulmonary vagal afferent activity on carotid chemoreceptor and baroreceptor reflexes in the dog. *Circ Res* 1975;37:422–429.
85. Komiya Y. Slowing with age of the rate of slow axonal flow in bifurcating axons of rat dorsal root ganglion cells. *Brain Res* 1980; 183:477–480.
86. Korczyn AD, et al. Sympathetic pupillary tone in old age. *Arch Ophthalmol* 1976;94:1905–1906.
87. Kotchen JM, et al. Blood pressure trends with aging [Review]. *Hypertension* 1982;4(Suppl 3):128–134.
88. Kuno Y. *Human perspiration.* Springfield, IL: Charles C Thomas, 1956.
89. Kusiak JW, Pitha J. Decreased response with age of the cardiac catecholamine sensitive adenylate cyclase system. *Life Sci* 1983;33: 1679–1686.
90. Larsen PL. Aging and resistance to oxidative damage in *Caenorhabditis elegans. Proc Natl Acad Sci USA* 1993;90:8905–8909.
91. LeBlanc J, et al. Effects of age, sex, and physical fitness on responses to local cooling. *J Appl Physiol* 1978;44:813–817.
92. Lee HC, et al. Differential accumulations of 4,977 bp deletion in mitochondrial DNA of various tissues in human ageing. *Biochim Biophys Acta* 1994;1226:37–43.
93. Levin AB. A simple test of cardiac function based upon the heart rate changes induced by the Valsalva maneuver. *Am J Cardiol* 1966; 18:90–99.
94. Lezza AM, et al. Correlation between mitochondrial DNA 4977-bp deletion and respiratory chain enzyme activities in aging human skeletal muscles. *Biochem Biophys Res Commun* 1994;205:772–779.
95. Lipsitz LA, et al. Postprandial reduction in blood pressure in the elderly. *N Engl J Med* 1983;309:81–83.
96. Low PA. Autonomic neuropathy. *Semin Neurol* 1987;7:49–57.

97. Low PA. Quantitation of autonomic responses. In: Dyck PJ, et al., eds. *Peripheral neuropathy.* Philadelphia: WB Saunders, 1984: 1139–1165.
98. Low PA, Dyck PJ. Splanchnic preganglionic neurons in man. II. Morphometry of myelinated fibers of T7 ventral spinal root. *Acta Neuropathol (Berl)* 1977;40:219–225.
99. Low PA, Dyck PJ. Splanchnic preganglionic neurons in man. III. Morphometry of myelinated fibers of rami communicantes. *J Neuropathol Exp Neurol* 1978;37:734–740.
100. Low PA, et al. Splanchnic preganglionic neurons in man. I. Morphometry of preganglionic cytons. *Acta Neuropathol (Berl)* 1977; 40:55–61.
101. Low PA, et al. Comparison of distal sympathetic with vagal function in diabetic neuropathy. *Muscle Nerve* 1986;9:592–596.
102. Low PA, et al. Evaluation of skin vasomotor reflexes by using laser Doppler velocimetry. *Mayo Clin Proc* 1983;58:583–592.
103. Low PA, et al. The effect of aging on cardiac autonomic and postganglionic sudomotor function. *Muscle Nerve* 1990;13:152–157.
104. Lowenstein O, Loewenfeld IE. Mutual role of sympathetic and of parasympathetic in shaping of the pupillary reflex to light. *Arch Neurol Psychiatry* 1950;64:341–377.
105. Lybarger JA, Kilbourne EM. *Homeostatic function and aging.* New York: Raven, 1985.
106. MacKinnon PC. Variations with age in the number of active palmar digital sweat glands. *J Neurol Neurosurg Psychiatry* 1954;17:124–126.
107. Martyn CN, Ewing DJ. Pupil cycle time: a simple way of measuring an autonomic reflex. *J Neurol Neurosurg Psychiatry* 1986;49:771–774.
108. Masaoka S, et al. Heart rate variability in diabetes: relationship to age and duration of the disease. *Diabetes Care* 1985;8:64–68.
109. Montagna W. *Advances in biology of skin.* Oxford: Pergamon, 1965.
110. Moy S, et al. The venoarteriolar reflex in diabetic and other neuropathies. *Neurology* 1989;39:1490–1492.
111. Muller OF, et al. The hypotensive effect of imipramine hydrochloride in patients with cardiovascular disease. *Clin Pharmacol Ther* 1960;2:300–307.
112. Nalefski LA, Brown CFG. Action of atropine on the cardiovascular system in normal persons. *Arch Intern Med* 1950;86:898–907.
113. Nandy K. Properties of neuronal lipofuscin pigment in mice. *Acta Neuropathol (Berl)* 1971;19:25–32.
114. Ng AV, et al. Age and gender influence muscle sympathetic nerve activity at rest in healthy humans. *Hypertension* 1993;21:498–503.
115. Ng AV, et al. Endurance exercise training is associated with elevated basal sympathetic nerve activity in healthy older humans. *J Appl Physiol* 1994;77:1366–1374.
116. O'Brien IA, et al. Heart rate variability in healthy subjects: effect of age and the derivation of normal ranges for tests of autonomic function. *Br Heart J* 1986;55:348–354.
117. Oberste-Lehn H, Montagna W, eds. *Advances in biology of skin.* Oxford: Pergamon, 1965:17–34.
118. Ochoa J. Recognition of unmyelinated fiber disease: morphologic criteria. *Muscle Nerve* 1978;1:375–387.
119. Ochoa J, Mair WGP. The normal sural nerve in man. II. Changes in the axons and Schwann cells due to ageing. *Acta Neuropathol (Berl)* 1969;13:217–239.
120. Ogawa T. Influence of aging on sweating activity. In: Kligman AM, Takase Y, eds. *Cutaneous aging.* Tokyo: University of Tokyo, 1988: 111–125.
121. Ogawa T, et al. Effects of sweat gland training by repeated local heating. *Jpn J Physiol* 1982;32:971–981.
122. Oikawa N, et al. Quantitative evaluation of diabetic autonomic neuropathy by using heart rate variations: determination of the normal range for the diagnosis of autonomic neuropathy. *Tohoku J Exp Med* 1985;145:233–241.
123. Oimomi M, et al. Autonomic nervous function determined by changes of periflux blood flow in the aged. *Arch Gerontol Geriatr* 1986;5:159–163.
124. Pedersen EB, Christensen NJ. Catecholamines in plasma and urine in patients with essential hypertension determined by double-isotope derivative techniques. *Acta Med Scand* 1981;198:373–377.
125. Persson A, Solders G. R-R variations: a test of autonomic dysfunction. *Acta Neurol Scand* 1983;67:285–293.
126. Pfeifer MA, et al. Differential changes of autonomic nervous system function with age in man. *Am J Med* 1983;75:249–258.
127. Pfeifer MA, et al. Quantitative evaluation of sympathetic and parasympathetic control of iris function. *Diabetes Care* 1982;5:518–528.
128. Pick J, et al. The fine structure of sympathetic neurons in man. *J Comp Neurol* 1964;122:19–67.
129. Pinkus H. Anatomy of skin 1954. *Dermatologica* 1956;112:44–62.
130. Raimbach SJ, et al. Prevention of glucose-induced hypotension by the somatostatin analogue octreotide (SMS 201-995) in chronic autonomic failure: haemodynamic and hormonal changes. *Clin Sci* 1989;77:623–628.
131. Randall O, et al. Determinants of baroreflex sensitivity in man. *J Lab Clin Med* 1978;91:514–519.
132. Rees J, Shuster S. Pubertal induction of sweat gland activity. *Clin Sci* 1981;60:689–692.
133. Richter C, et al. Normal oxidative damage to mitochondrial and nuclear DNA is extensive. *Proc Natl Acad Sci USA* 1988;85:6465–6467.
134. Roberts J, Turner H. Age-related changes in autonomic function of catecholamines. *Rev Biol Res Aging* 1987;3:257–298.
135. Robinson BJ, et al. Do elderly patients with an excessive fall in blood pressure on standing have evidence of autonomic failure? *Clin Sci* 1983;64:587–591.
136. Robinson S, et al. Acclimatization of older men at work in heat. *J Appl Physiol* 1965;20:583–586.
137. Rodstein M, Zeman FD. Postural blood pressure changes in the elderly. *J Chronic Dis* 1957;6:581–588.
138. Rogers MA, Evans WJ. Changes in skeletal muscle with aging: effects of exercise training [Review]. *Exerc Sport Sci Rev* 1993; 21:65–102.
139. Rosenberg B, Juckett DA. Quantitative evidence that the genetic basis of human mortality operates at the translation level: a preliminary assessment. *Mech Ageing Dev* 1992;64:149–160.
140. Rubin PC, et al. Noradrenaline release and clearance in relation to age and blood pressure in man. *Eur J Clin Invest* 1982;12:121–125.
141. Santer RM, et al. Glyoxylic acid fluorescence and ultrastructural studies of neurones in the coeliac–superior mesenteric ganglion of the aged rat. *Cell Tissue Res* 1970;211: 475–485.
142. Seals DR, et al. Exercise and aging: autonomic control of the circulation [Review]. *Med Sci Sports Exerc* 1994;26:568–576.
143. Sega S, et al. A comparison of cardiovascular reflex tests and spectral analysis of heart rate variability in healthy subjects. *Clin Auton Res* 1993;3:175–182.
144. Shigenaga MK, et al. Oxidative damage and mitochondrial decay in aging. *Proc Natl Acad Sci USA* 1994;91:10,771–10,778.
145. Shimada K, et al. Age-related changes of baroreflex function, plasma norepinephrine, and blood pressure. *Hypertension* 1985;7: 113–117.
146. Shoenfeld Y, et al. Age and sex difference in response to short exposure to extreme dry heat. *J Appl Physiol* 1978;44:1–4.
147. Silver AF, et al. Aging. In: Montagna W, ed. *Advances in biology of skin.* Oxford: Pergamon, 1965:129–150.
148. Smith JJ, et al. Hemodynamic response to the upright posture [Review]. *J Clin Pharmacol* 1994;34:375–386.
149. Smith SA. Reduced sinus arrhythmia in diabetic autonomic neuropathy: diagnostic value of an age-related normal range. *BMJ* 1982;285:1599–1601.
150. Smith SE, et al. Pupillary signs in diabetic autonomic neuropathy. *BMJ* 1978;2:924–927.
151. Solders G. *Autonomic dysfunction in polyneuropathy* [MD thesis]. Stockholm: Karolinska Institute, 1986.
152. Soong NW, et al. Mosaicism for a specific somatic mitochondrial DNA mutation in adult human brain. *Nature Genet* 1992;2: 318–323.
153. Stratton JR, et al. Beta-adrenergic effects on left ventricular filling: influence of aging and exercise training. *J Appl Physiol* 1994;77: 2522–2529.
154. Sundkvist G, et al. Respiratory influence on heart rate in diabetes mellitus. *BMJ* 1979;1:924–925.
155. Takahashi K. A clinicopathologic study on the peripheral nervous system of the aged: sciatic nerve and autonomic nervous system. *Geriatrics* 1966;21:123–133.

156. Tan ET, et al. Parasympathetic denervation of the iris in alcoholics with vagal neuropathy. *J Neurol Neurosurg Psychiatry* 1984;47:61–64.
157. Ten Harkel ADJ, et al. Assessment of cardiovascular reflexes: influence of posture and period of preceding rest. *J Appl Physiol* 1990;68:147–153.
158. Thomas PK, Ocha J. Microscopic anatomy of peripheral nerve fibers. In: Dyck PJ, et al., eds. *Peripheral neuropathy*. Philadelphia: WB Saunders, 1984:39–96.
159. Thompson HS. The pupil cycle time. *J Clin Neuro Ophthalmol* 1987;7:38–39.
160. Vestal RE, et al. Reduced beta-adrenoceptor sensitivity in the elderly. *Clin Pharmacol Ther* 1979;26:181–186.
161. Vita G, et al. Cardiovascular reflex tests: assessment of age-adjusted normal range. *J Neurol Sci* 1986;75:263–274.
162. Von der Ohe MR, et al. Differential regional effects of octreotide on human gastrointestinal motor function. *Gut* 1995;36:743–748.
163. Waddington JL, et al. Resting heart rate variability in man declines with age. *Experientia* 1979;35:1197–1198.
164. Wagner JA, et al. Heat tolerance and acclimatization to work in the heat in relation to age. *J Appl Physiol* 1972;33:616–622.
165. Wallace DC. 1994 William Allan Award Address: mitochondrial DNA variation in human evolution, degenerative disease, and aging. *Am J Hum Genet* 1995;57:201–223.
166. Wallin BG, Fagius J. Peripheral sympathetic neural activity in conscious humans. *Annu Rev Physiol* 1988;50:565–576.
167. Wallin BG, et al. Plasma noradrenaline correlates to sympathetic muscle nerve activity in normotensive man. *Acta Physiol Scand* 1981;111:69–73.
168. Watkins PJ, Mackay JD. Cardiac denervation in diabetic neuropathy. *Ann Intern Med* 1980;92:304–307.
169. Wei JY, Harris WS. Heart rate response to cough. *J Appl Physiol* 1982;53:1039–1043.
170. Wei JY, et al. Post-cough heart rate response: influence of age, sex and basal blood pressure. *Am J Physiol* 1983;245:R18–R24.
171. Wei YH. Mitochondrial DNA alterations as ageing-associated molecular events [Review]. *Mutat Res* 1992;275:145–155.
172. Wheeler T, Watkins PJ. Cardiac denervation in diabetes. *BMJ* 1973;4:584–586.
173. Wieling W, et al. Reflex control of heart rate in normal subjects in relation to age: a data base for cardiac vagal neuropathy. *Diabetologia* 1982;22:163–166.
174. Wilson PD, Franks LM. The effect of age on mitochondrial ultrastructure and enzymes. *Adv Exp Med Biol* 1975;53:171–183.
175. Wollner L, Spalding JMK. The autonomic nervous system. In: Brocklehurst JC, ed. *Textbook of geriatric medicine and gerontology*. Edinburgh: Churchill Livingstone, 1985:449.
176. Yang JH, et al. A specific 4977-bp deletion of mitochondrial DNA in human ageing skin. *Arch Dermatol Res* 1994;286:386–390.
177. Yin FC, et al. Age-associated decrease in ventricular response to haemodynamic stress during beta-adrenergic blockade. *Br Heart J* 1978;40:1349–1355.
178. Yo Y, et al. Effects of age and hypertension on autonomic nervous regulation during passive head-up tilt. *Hypertension* 1994;23:182–186.
179. Young JB, et al. Enhanced plasma norepinephrine response to upright posture and oral glucose administration in elderly human subjects. *Metabolism* 1980;29:532–539.
180. Youssef MK. *Man in stressful environments: thermal and work physiology*. Springfield: Charles C Thomas, 1987.
181. Zhang L, et al. Identification of neuronal programmed cell death *in situ* in the striatum of normal adult rat brain and its relationship to neuronal death during aging. *Brain Res* 1995; 677:177–179.
182. Zhou T, et al. Prevention of age-related T cell apoptosis defect in CD2-fas-transgenic mice. *J Exp Med* 1995; 182:129–137.
183. Ziegler D, et al. Assessment of cardiovascular autonomic function: age-related normal ranges and reproducibility of spectral analysis, vector analysis, and standard tests of heart rate variation and blood pressure responses. *Diabetic Med* 1992;9:166–175.
184. Ziegler MG, et al. Plasma noradrenaline increases with age. *Nature* 1976;261:333–335.
185. Zoller RP, et al. The role of low pressure baroreceptors in reflex vasoconstrictor responses in man. *J Clin Invest* 1972;51:2967–2972.

SECTION II
Evaluation of Autonomic Function

CHAPTER 15

Laboratory Evaluation of Autonomic Function

Phillip A. Low

---

1. Laboratory evaluation is strongly indicated when generalized autonomic failure is suspected and to recognize benign autonomic disorders that mimic life-threatening disorders, detect distal small fiber neuropathy, diagnose partial autonomic failure, diagnose autonomic neuropathy, and evaluate sympathetically maintained pain (SMP) or the presence of orthostatic intolerance.
2. Evaluation is desirable in monitoring the course of autonomic failure and the response to therapy, characterizing the peripheral neuropathies, studying patients with syncope, amyotrophic lateral sclerosis, extrapyramidal and cerebellar degenerations, and in addressing research questions.
3. The aims are to detect the presence of autonomic failure, quantitate the severity, apportion the type (sudomotor, adrenergic, or cardiovagal) and distribution of deficits, and determine the site of the autonomic lesion.
4. We routinely study quantitative sudomotor axon reflex test (QSART) distribution, orthostatic blood pressure (BP) and heart rate (HR) response to tilt, HR response to deep breathing, the Valsalva ratio, beat-to-beat BP to Valsalva maneuver, tilt and deep breathing, and the thermoregulatory sweat test.
5. The QSART uses an axon reflex pathway and tests the integrity of the postganglionic sympathetic sudomotor axon. The distribution of abnormalities is particularly useful in monitoring a neuropathy.
6. The photoplethysmographic BP recording (Finapres) is a noninvasive method of measuring beat-to-beat BP. It generates an arterial waveform that is indistinguishable from that of a peripheral arterial waveform.
7. Tests to detect SMP are based on the premise that altered sympathetic vasomotor and sudomotor tone occurs in the majority, if not all, of these patients. The finding of altered sympathetic tone is a useful index although the ultimate diagnosis of SMP remains a clinical charge.
8. Cardiovagal and sudomotor tests are sensitive and reproducible. Similar tests of adrenergic function are less sensitive and specific. Orthostatic BP, norepinephrine measurements, or sustained handgrip are insensitive. The evaluation of phases of the Valsalva maneuver provides additional sensitivity.
9. The evaluation of baroreflex indices using BP–HR correlations, and the use of impedance cardiography to obtain additional cardiovascular indices, are useful in selected patients.
10. Tests such as the skin vasomotor reflexes, venoarteriolar reflex, and the neurogenic flare response do not appear to have sufficient sensitivity or specificity to warrant their inclusion as routine tests of autonomic function.

INTRODUCTION

The autonomic laboratory evaluation is an extension of the clinical evaluation. Since the last edition of this book, there has been considerable activity in clinical autonomic testing on several fronts. There is now a better understanding of the indications for laboratory evaluation, greater availability of autonomic function tests, a better understanding of the strengths and weaknesses of the tests, and a more critical evaluation of available tests. The American Academy of Neurology has published a position paper on autonomic function tests (2). The academy has also championed the implementation of autonomic tests. By the time this edition appears, three CPT codes of autonomic tests will be available. The tests to be described in large part reflect the philosophy of the Mayo Autonomic Laboratories, which has gained wide acceptance. There is a heavy emphasis on

P. A. Low: Department of Neurology, Mayo Clinic, Rochester, Minnesota 55905.

noninvasive tests and quantitative methodology. The aims of autonomic testing are followed by a description of the indications for laboratory quantitation, routine tests of autonomic function, and then more specialized tests for special problems. Finally, less useful tests of autonomic function are briefly described.

INDICATIONS FOR LABORATORY EVALUATION OF AUTONOMIC FAILURE

The most common referrals to the Mayo Autonomic Laboratory are suspected generalized autonomic failure (autonomic neuropathies, multiple-system atrophy, pure and autonomic failure), distal small fiber neuropathy, orthostatic intolerance [postural orthostatic tachycardia syndrome (POTS) and syncope], and peripheral neuropathies. The suggested indications for the laboratory evaluation of autonomic failure are described below.

Diagnosis of Generalized Autonomic Failure

Perhaps the main reason for referring patients for autonomic evaluation is the suspicion of generalized autonomic failure (93,95). The most common causes are diabetic autonomic neuropathy, amyloid neuropathy, Sjogren's syndrome, the panautonomic neuropathies (idiopathic and paraneoplastic) (93,161), pure autonomic failure, and multiple-system atrophy. Laboratory confirmation is important. The diagnosis of the disorder has a serious prognostic impact in disorders such as multiple-system atrophy or pure autonomic failure. In diabetes and amyloidosis, the development of generalized autonomic failure significantly worsens the prognosis.

It should be possible to delineate the severity and distribution by autonomic system (cardiovagal, adrenergic, or sudomotor), autonomic failure (detailed in the section on *Aims*), and level (preganglionic versus postganglionic). It is possible to quantitate the deficits and provide a three-dimensional profile of the autonomic involvement.

Diagnosis of Benign Autonomic Disorders That May Mimic Life-Threatening Disorders

Certain autonomic disorders such as the benign syncopes and chronic idiopathic anhidrosis mimic the more malignant generalized autonomic disorders. For instance, the benign syncopes such as neurocardiogenic (vasovagal) and micturition syncope often need to be studied to rule out generalized autonomic failure. Chronic idiopathic anhidrosis cannot be diagnosed without the demonstration of normal adrenergic and cardiovagal function. Patients with POTS may have the disorder *sui generis* or as a result of an autonomic neuropathy. An autonomic screen is necessary to clarify this differential diagnosis.

Diagnosis of Distal Small Fiber Neuropathy

Distal small fiber neuropathy is common, often distressing, and very difficult to diagnose. Routine nerve conduction studies and electromyography are usually normal, since the brunt of the disorder is on unmyelinated fibers. Peripheral autonomic surface potentials will detect a small minority of cases (44). The quantitative sudomotor axon reflex test (QSART) or the thermoregulatory sweat test (TST) are abnormal in ~80% of cases (149).

Detection of Mild or Limited Autonomic Neuropathy

The advent of autonomic testing has provided a pathophysiologic explanation for symptoms in many syndromes or symptoms that previously defied explanation. A number of disorders, such as orthostatic intolerance, pseudo-obstruction syndrome, heat intolerance, and syncope may have an underlying restricted autonomic neuropathy. The detection of autonomic failure may provide improved understanding of pathophysiology and may impact on treatment. For instance, patients with syncope who have peripheral adrenergic failure may worsen with β-blockers and improve with volume expansion or a vasoconstrictor.

Evaluation of Orthostatic Intolerance

Orthostatic intolerance is common, is typically mild, and warrants no evaluation. A subset of patients with syncope or highly symptomatic orthostatic intolerance may be severely incapacitated. Two such entities are POTS and certain varieties of neurocardiogenic syncope (Chapter 48). The role of autonomic testing is to evaluate the presence and severity of orthostatic intolerance (Chapter 49) and to determine whether there is underlying autonomic failure.

Evaluation of the Course of the Autonomic Disorder

These twin attributes of quantitation and noninvasiveness render autonomic laboratory evaluation ideally suited to monitor the alterations of autonomic function over time. The patient's autonomic deficits may change in type, distribution, or in severity. These quantities have hitherto not been readily quantifiable.

Evaluation of the Response to Therapy

The autonomic deficits may lessen in response to treatment. With therapy being evaluated for the neuropathies—e.g., antioxidants, aldose reductase inhibitors, tight glucose control, gangliosides, fish oil etc. for diabetic neuropathy, 3,4-diaminopyridine for the Lambert–Eaton myasthenic syndrome, and immunotherapy for the immune-mediated neuropathies—quantitative methods are needed to evaluate the response to therapy.

Evaluation of Autonomic Involvement in the Peripheral Neuropathies

In the peripheral neuropathies, there is a typical pattern of autonomic involvement, with a length-dependent distribution of sympathetic deficits (maximal distally). However, some neuropathies have an early impairment of cardiovagal function (e.g., diabetes and Chaga's neuropathy), and the distribution of the sudomotor deficit may be multifocal (e.g., leprosy). The combination of routine tests—QSART, cardiovagal tests, beat-to-beat blood pressure (BP_{BB}) responses to tilt, beat-to-beat Valsalva maneuver (VM_{BB}), and the TST—described in detail below enables such an analysis.

Detection of Sympathetic Dysfunction in Sympathetically Maintained Pain

Patients with unilateral limb pain in whom the suspicion of complex abnormal regional pain syndrome I, also known as sympathetically maintained pain (SMP) and reflex sympathetic dystrophy (RSD) or causalgia, will have sympathetic overreaction. Although the pathophysiology of complex abnormal regional pain syndrome is unresolved as to whether sympathetic dysfunction is primary or incidental, sympathetic asymmetry, especially sudomotor asymmetry, is a reliable feature that helps in its recognition (26,98).

Research Questions

The autonomic laboratory can be used to evaluate changes in autonomic function in response to therapy in clinical treatment trials and neuroepidemiologic studies. The techniques can also be used to gain basic information in human subjects.

AIMS OF LABORATORY EVALUATION OF AUTONOMIC FUNCTION

These aims are

1. To detect the presence of autonomic failure.
2. To quantitate the severity and apportion the type of deficits (sudomotor, adrenergic, or cardiovagal).
3. To determine the distribution of autonomic failure.
4. To determine the site of the autonomic lesion.
5. To detect the presence of altered sympathetic manifestations.

The strategy by which the aims are achieved is detailed in the section *Evaluation of Autonomic Function*.

The Autonomic Reflex Laboratory

All studies of autonomic function are performed in the autonomic reflex laboratory with the subject supine and rested. The room temperature is maintained at 23°C, with the exception of the RSD screen, which is done at 20°C, and ideally the room is humidity controlled. Tests of autonomic function are broadly grouped into three categories. The first is the autonomic reflex screen comprising QSART recordings from the forearm and three lower-extremity sites, heart rate response to deep breathing (HR_{DB}), Valsalva ratio (VR), and BP_{BB} to VM, and tilt-up. The second is the sympathetic dysfunction screen comprising a side-by-side comparison study of the affected and contralateral extremity by using telethermography, resting sweat output (RSO), and QSART measurements bilaterally and simultaneously. Additional indices can be measured using bioelectric impedance analysis or the "contour" method of determining stroke volume (see below). The third category are specialized studies such as prolonged tilt, infusions of phenylephrine or isoproterenol, or research protocols. Research studies are often recorded using impedance cardiography, transcranial Doppler, electroencephalography, and microneurography.

ROUTINE TESTS OF AUTONOMIC FUNCTION

A number of tests have been in relatively common use long enough to be considered routine. Not all routine tests have been well validated (see Chapter 23). These tests are considered to be sufficiently useful that a complete autonomic laboratory should probably have them available:

1. QSART distribution
2. HR_{DB}
3. VR
4. HR response to standing
5. BP_{BB} to the VM
6. BP_{BB} and HR response to tilt
7. Salivation test
8. Tests to detect SMP or RSD
    a. Telethermography or infrared thermometry
    b. RSO
    c. QSART
9. TST (Chapter 19)
10. Sustained handgrip
11. Plasma catecholamines
12. Frequency analysis (Chapters 25 and 26)

Not all these tests are done in the Mayo Autonomic Reflex Laboratory. The tests that are routinely done in the Mayo Autonomic Reflex Laboratory are listed in Table 1. The tests should follow a specific sequence.

Patient Preparation: No food, coffee, or nicotine are permitted for 3 hrs before the study. Anticholinergics (including antidepressant, antihistamine, and over-the-counter

TABLE 1. *Routine tests of autonomic function*

Autonomic reflex screen
1. QSART distribution
2. Heart rate response to deep breathing
3. Valsalva ratio
4. Beat-to-beat blood pressure and heart rate responses to the Valsalva maneuver
5. Beat-to-beat blood pressure responses to tilt

Reflex sympathetic dystrophy screen
1. Thermographic skin temperature distribution
2. Side-by-side comparative resting sweat output study
3. Side-by-side comparative QSART study

QSART, quantitative sudomotor axon reflex test.

cough and cold medication), 9-α-fludrocortisone (Florinef), diuretics, sympathomimetic (α- and β-agonists), and parasympathomimetic agents are forbidden for 48 hr. Short-acting α- and β-antagonists are discontinued for 24 hrs, and long-acting ones for 48 hrs, at the discretion of the referring physician. Analgesics, including opioids, are avoided the day of the test. Compressive clothing, including Jobst stockings and corsets, are not worn the morning of the test.

QUANTITATIVE SUDOMOTOR AXON REFLEX TEST

Physiologic Basis

The principle of the test can be surmised from Fig. 1. The neural pathway consists of an axon *reflex* mediated by the postganglionic sympathetic sudomotor axon. The axon terminal is activated by acetylcholine. The impulse travels antidromically, reaches a branch point, and then travels orthodromically to release acetylcholine from nerve terminals. Acetylcholine traverses the neuroglandular junction and binds to M_3 muscarinic receptors on eccrine sweat glands (156) to evoke the sweat response. Acetylcholinesterase in subcutaneous tissue cleaves acetylcholine to acetate and choline, resulting in its inactivation and cessation of the sweat response.

Physiologic Setup

The physiologic setup to measure the QSART is presented in Fig. 2 (93,95). Nitrogen gas of low humidity is piped through to the sudorometer, then to a multicompartmental sweat capsule attached to skin, and returns to the sudorometer. The stimulus is acetylcholine applied by iontophoresis by using a constant current generator. An alternative stimulus is carbachol, which is not broken down by acetylcholinesterase and hence has a longer action (88). The resultant axon reflex-mediated sweat response is recorded from a second population of sweat glands by a sudorometer and a multicompartmental sweat cell. Output from the sudorometer is displayed and analyzed on a computer console (Chapter 29).

Multicompartmental Sweat Cell

A key component of the QSART is the multicompartmental sweat cell (Chapter 29 and Fig. 3). Compartment C is the stimulus compartment and can be loaded with acetylcholine via cannulae E and connected to the anode of a constant current generator via post F. Compartment A is separated from C by compartment B and two narrow

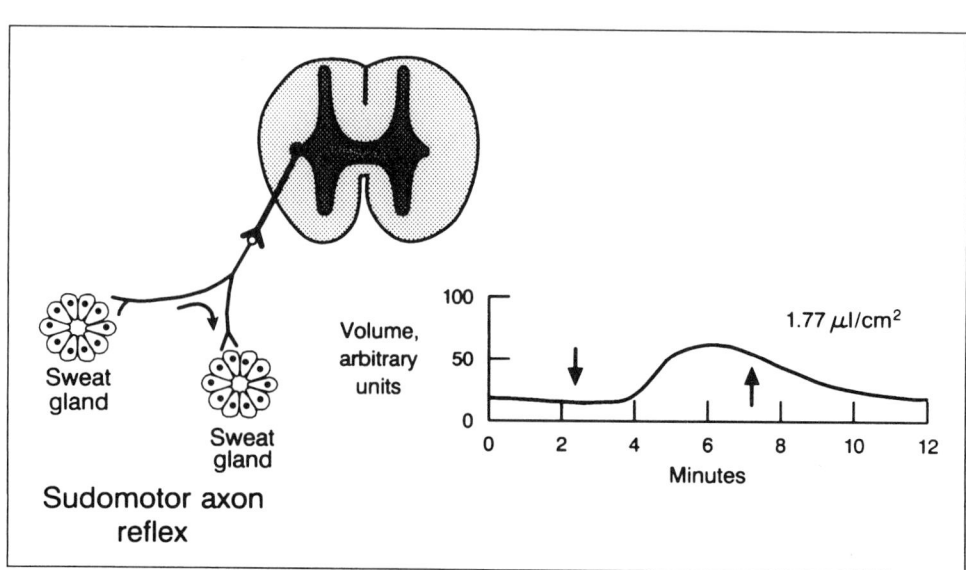

FIG. 1. Left: The neural substrate for the axon reflex sweat response (see the text). **Right:** A representative axon reflex sweat response. From Low et al. (96), with permission.

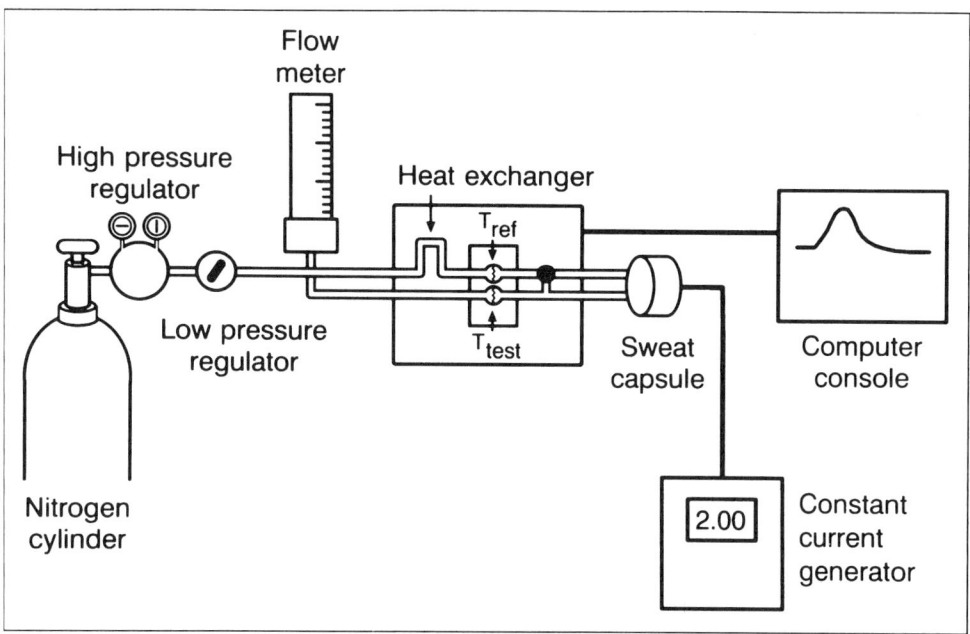

FIG. 2. The sudorometer and attachments. See the text for details.

ridges, which blocks diffusion but not the axon *reflex*. The sweat output in A is evaporated by N_2 gas, and the gas flow of altered thermal mass returns to the sudorometer. Post G permits the attachment of the sudorometer to the limb by straps.

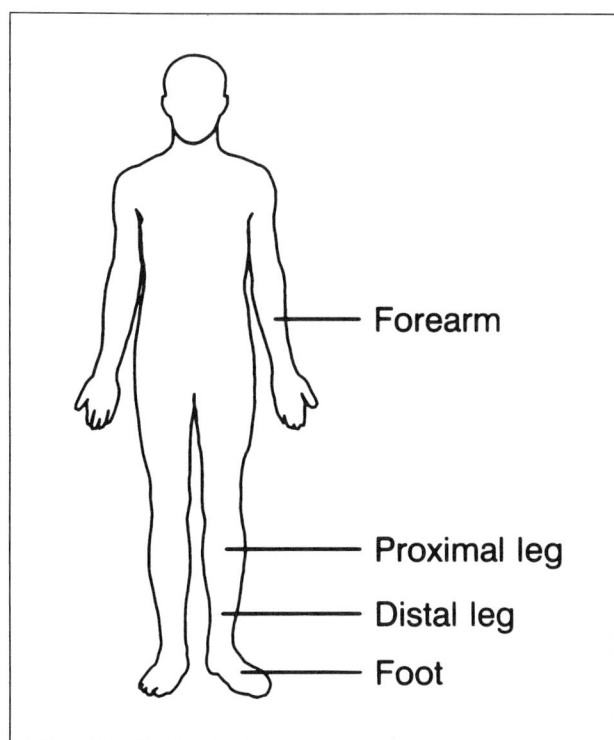

FIG. 3. Quantitative sudomotor axon reflex test recording sites.

Sealed cells are also available. Compartments A and C are sealed so that gas flowing through these compartments provides a "capsule" baseline that differs slightly from the patient baseline, since the latter has the additional component of skin surface with its moisture content. We also have is a larger cell to record insensible perspiration from a wider area of skin.

Constant-Current Generator

The stimulus is a constant current of 2 mA applied for 5 min, and the sweat response is recorded during the stimulus and subsequently for 5 min. The solution consists of 10% acetylcholine loaded into the outer compartment (C).

Reproducibility

The tests are sensitive and reproducible in controls (100) and in patients with diabetic neuropathy (97). Tests repeated on 2 different days have a high coefficient of regression. Tests repeated daily at the identical site may evoke local skin alterations, possibly to the sweat duct after about repetition 3 or 4, but this "tolerance" is highly variable. The coefficient of variation is ≤20% (96,100).

Recording Sites

The recordings are symmetric so that, in normal individuals, the left side is not significantly different from the right (see the section *Normative Data*). We routinely record from the left but will study the right side when clinically warranted, e.g., following left sural nerve biopsy or with unilateral symptoms. Standard recording sites (Fig. 3) are the medial forearm (75% of the distance from the ulnar epicondyle to the pisiform bone), the proximal leg (lateral aspect, 5 cm distal to the fibular head), the distal leg (medial aspect, 5 cm proximal to the medial malleolus), and the proximal foot (on a flat surface over the extensor digitorum brevis muscle). The innervations of the forearm, proximal leg, distal leg, and proximal foot are by ulnar, peroneal, saphenous, and sural (mainly) nerves, respectively.

Abnormal QSART

There are several recognized abnormal QSART patterns (Fig. 4). The response may be (1) normal, (2) reduced, (3) absent, (4) excessive, or (5) persistent. Short latencies are common with patterns 4 and 5. Pattern 5, consisting of persistent sweat response when the stimulus ceases, is often seen in patients with hyperalgesia, such as painful diabetic and other neuropathies, in mild neuropathies, and in florid RSD. QSART recordings have been done in many neuropathies, including diabetic neuropathy (97), multiple-system atrophy, progressive autonomic failure (29), Sjogren's syndrome (97), Lambert–Eaton myasthenic syndrome (110), atopic dermatitis (58), aging (101), idiopathic autonomic neuropathy (150) and distal small fiber neuropathy (149), and Parkinson's disease and related extrapyramidal and cerebellar disorders (137).

Interpretation

A normal test result indicates integrity of the postganglionic sympathetic sudomotor axon. An absent response indicates a lesion of the axon, providing iontophoresis is successful and eccrine sweat glands are present. Since the axonal segment mediating the axon is likely to be short, the test likely evaluates relatively distal function (96). A reduced or absent sweat response indicates postganglionic sympathetic sudomotor failure. In peripheral neuropathies, the distribution of sweat responses is particularly important. In distal small fiber neuropathy, the most distal site or two alone may be reduced or absent. As the disease progresses, sudomotor failure advances to more proximal sites. In preganglionic or central disorders, the QSART is unimpaired. With increasing duration of the preganglionic lesion, however, the QSART may become impaired, suggestive of a transsynaptic defect. Used in conjunction with

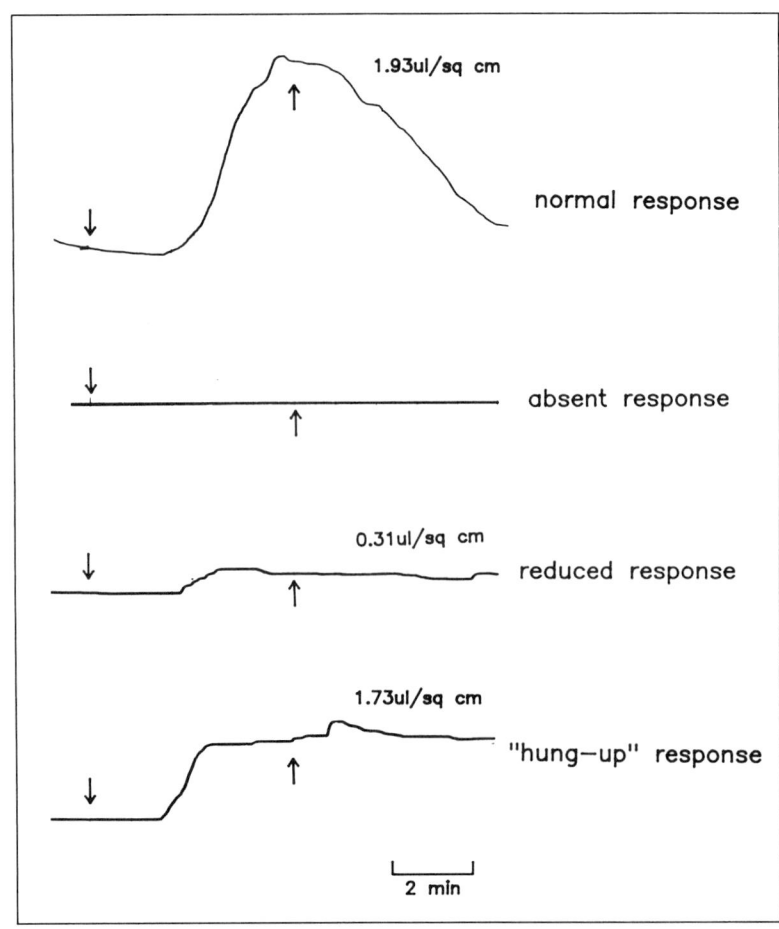

FIG. 4. Patterns of quantitative sudomotor axon reflex test responses.

TABLE 2. *Site of sympathetic lesion*

QSART	TST	Site of the lesion
Abnormal	Abnormal	Postganglionic
Normal	Abnormal	Preganglionic

QSART, quantitative sudomotor axon reflex test; TST, thermoregulatory sweat test.

the TST, the QSART can differentiate a preganglionic from postganglionic lesion (Table 2). The presence of resting sweat activity (RSA) indicates sweat gland activity at a skin temperature that is normally subthreshold at room temperature. Since there is little circulating acetylcholine, the mechanism is likely that of spontaneously active sympathetic sudomotor axons. Circumstantial evidence in support of this mechanism is the association of symptoms suggestive of overactivity of other small fibers. Patients with RSA often have a painful neuropathy with burning dysesthesiae, vasomotor changes, such as cyanosis or pallor, as well as excessive sweating. The presence of persistent sweat activity (PSA) likely has a similar significance and often occurs with RSA. Since it is unlikely that continuous activity occurs at the level of the sweat gland, the mechanism of PSA is likely to be due to repetitive firing of the sympathetic sudomotor axon. It is known that the damaged axon may fire spontaneously and on stimulation and may have more persistent activity than normal axons. The most common clinical situations associated with PSA are mild or painful neuropathies. The latency is sometimes markedly reduced in the context of painful neuropathies with RSA and PSA. In the QSART, transmission time along the axon takes milliseconds (axonal conduction velocity is ~1 m/sec) and transmission delay at the neuroglandular junction is also measured in milliseconds. Latency from receptor occupancy to sweat secretion takes seconds. Hence, the major mechanism of the long latency of 0.5–2.0 min is the time needed to iontophorese acetylcholine. The mechanism of the very short latency (sometimes 10–30 sec) is unknown. One possibility is that the small response is induced by electrical stimulation alone since the damaged axon with RSA and PSA may have a reduced threshold and may respond to painful stimulation as has been observed clinically. The response is likely an augmented somatosympathetic reflex.

Comparison of Tests of Sudomotor Function

Tests of sudomotor function differ in the mode of stimulation and of recording the evoked response. Some of these tests are summarized in Table 3. Several tests in vogue are summarized in Table 4. The clinical tests that are currently in vogue are the QSART, the skin potential test, the TST, and the Silastic imprint test. These are compared in Tables 4 and 5. The different tests evaluate different aspects of sudomotor function. The Silastic imprint method is a good and quantitative one that differs from QSART recordings in several essential respects. The two methods are complementary: the Silastic method provides a sweat output histogram and a count of the number of activated glands, whereas the QSART recording provides a dynamic quantitation of sweat output. The principles of the two methods are quite different. The Silastic method depends on the function of directly stimulated sweat gland (the denervated gland losing its sudomotor response), whereas the QSART depends on the integrity of the axon reflex rather than sweat gland function. Perhaps because of the longer pathway tested in the QSART (sympathetic C → branch point → sympathetic C), this test detects sudomotor failure before the Silastic method. The second major advantage is its dynamic sudorometry so that one is able, for instance, to determine whether there is PSA or to study somatosympathetic reflexes. The sweat-spot test (133) provides a simple

TABLE 3. *Methods to measure sweat output in human subjects*

Tests	Principles	References
Minor's method	Iodine–alcohol–castor oil application, sweat droplets turn violet-black	List and Peet (92)
Sweat imprint method	Soft impression mold showing sweat imprint	Kennedy et al. (82)
Guttmann method	Indicator powder; moisture turns powder purple	Guttmann (60)
Tannic acid method	Sweat droplet seen as a brown dot	Silverman and Powell (141)
Starch-paper iodine paint	Hard copy of Minor's method	Randall (129)
Starch–iodine paper	Iodine impregnated starch paper	MacMillan and Spalding (105)
Bromophenol blue-soaked filter paper	Sweating turns bromophenol blue from light tan to dark blue	Herrmann et al. (69)
Skin resistance or potential recordings	Sweating causes reduction in skin resistance or generates skin potential alteration	Richter (131); Shahani et al. (139)
Prism method	Sweat droplets seen through prism	Netsky (118)
Conductivity change	Humidity increase changes conductivity of silk fiber coated with a salt	Darrow (32)
QSART	Humidity change or thermal mass change	Low et al. (100)
Sweat spot	Iodine–starch paint on skin	Ryder et al. (133)

QSART, quantitative sudomotor axon reflex test.

TABLE 4. Some currently used tests of sudomotor function

Test	Stimulus	Afferent limb	Efferent limb	Normal response
Skin potential recording	Electric shock; deep breath	Type-II and type-III mechanoreceptor pathways	Sympathetic efferent	Skin potential response
Silastic imprint method	Iontophoresis of pilocarpine	No neural pathway; direct stimulation of muscarinic receptors		Silastic imprint of droplets
QSART	Iontophoresis of acetylcholine	Sympathetic (antidromic)	Sympathetic (orthodromic)	Sudorometric sweat response
TST	Whole body warming	Somatic and sympathetic sweat glands	Hypothalamus to eccrine sweating	Indicator powder turns purple with onset of sweating

QSART, quantitative sudomotor axon reflex test; TST, thermoregulatory sweat test.

semiquantitative evaluation of sudomotor function. The stimulus is intradermal acetylcholine, and the response is viewed on the skin, which has been painted with starch iodine. In a group of 50 normal subjects, no effect of gender or age was found. In most of the more accurate tests, a large difference by gender and a significant effect of age are seen (see the section *Normative Data*).

Requirements for Heart Rate Recordings

For HR recordings, the patient lies supine on the tilt table for 20 min before the commencement of tilt-up. The optimal placement of electrodes is at sites where movement artifacts are minimal during the autonomic maneuvers. In our experience, the simplest and best electrode sites are the interscapular area just medial to the tips of the scapula. An alternative placement is at the supraclavicular areas. The reference electrode site is not critical. We use the left midaxillary line at nipple level. The RR interval is converted to HR that is displayed continuously on our computer console. For details, see Chapter 29.

Heart Rate Response to Deep Breathing

HR_{DB} is affected by a number of confounding variables (see Chapter 15) (123), which are summarized in Table 6. It is unaffected by the time of day, gender of the subject, and the amount of preceding rest in relaxed subjects. The effects of age are detailed in Chapter 14. The rate of breathing has a profound influence on the RR variation. The variation is maximal at a breathing rate of 5–6 breaths/min (8,123,174). The procedure that we follow is as follows (97): The subject breathes maximally at a rate of 6 breaths/min (inspiratory and expiratory cycles of 5 sec

TABLE 5. Comparison of QSART, silastic imprint, and skin potential recordings

Parameter	QSART	Silastic Imprint	Skin potential
Principle	Sympathetic axon reflex	Direct sweat gland muscarinic response	Somatosympathetic response
Stimulus	Acetylcholine	Pilocarpine	Various
Neural pathway			
Afferent	Sympathetic C	Nil	Groups II and III
Efferent	Sympathetic C	Nil	Sympathetic B and C
Effector	Sweat gland	Sweat gland	Sweat gland secretion
Response characteristics			
Latency	Long (1–2 min)	? Brief	Brief (sec)
Turn on	Rapid	Rapid	Rapid
Turn off	Relatively fast (2–3 min)	Extremely slow (>2 hr)	Fast (sec)
Neuropathy detection	Sensitive	Sensitive	Sensitive
Advantages	Sensitive, reproducible, accurate, quantitative	Sensitive, reproducible, accurate, quantitative	Standard EMG equipment
Disadvantages	Time-consuming, special equipment, rare problem with thick skin	Time-consuming, special equipment, rare problem with thick skin	Variable (habituation), less accurate, many factors may affect the response
Dynamic recording	Yes	No	Yes
Sweat histogram	No	Yes	No

QSART, quantitative sudomotor axon reflex test; TST, thermoregulatory sweat test; EMG, electromyography.

TABLE 6. *Some factors that affect the heart rate responses to deep breathing*

1. Age
2. Rate of breathing
3. Analytical methods
4. Hypocapnia
5. Influence of sympathetic activity
6. Position of the subject
7. Salicylates and other medications
8. Depth of breathing
9. Obesity

each). The subject is taught to establish inspiratory and expiratory rhythms so that breathing is smooth and maximal. The subject is instructed to follow an oscillating bar for a period of 10 sec. Alternatively, the subject can is asked to "breathe innnn" and "breathe outtt" by the technician. Another approach is to have the subject follow a sine wave visually or auditorily. Eight cycles are recorded and repeated after a rest period. Following 5 min of rest, the procedure is repeated. The five largest consecutive responses are read from the computer by using a cursor, averaged, and the HR range (maximum − minimum) derived. The analytical method significantly affects the derived results. The three main methods of evaluating HR_{DB} are E:I ratio, HR range, and mean circular resultant. The three methods are compared in Table 7. For our recordings of eight cycles, the preferred analytical method is the HR method. Hyperventilation can result in a progressive reduction in HR range, presumably due to hypocapnia. Sympathetic activation will attenuate the E:I ratio markedly but has only a minimal effect on HR range. The confounding variables of HR_{DB} are discussed in Chapters 23 and 24. The position of the subject, the salicylates, and the depth of breathing have modest effects on HR_{DB}. There is some variation among laboratories on the number of responses to average, whether to include the first response, and which responses to include. Bennett et al. (14) consider the first response, which is often larger, preferable to an averaged value. With continued hyperventilation, there is hypocarbia (18,70) with inhibition of sinus arrhythmia. Weight gain of 10% has been reported to reduce, and weight loss increase,

parasympathetic function (71). There is also some variability among individual responses, and some responses are marred by artifact or ectopic beats. Based on these considerations, we have standardized our testing by routinely recording eight cycles and determining the mean of the five consecutive largest responses. We find this approach preferable to the mean of all or the last few responses. We reject the first response if it is more than double the subsequent responses. Control values should be established for the particular laboratory. This approach is better than the adoption of some generic control range. The control values currently used in the Mayo Autonomic Reflex Laboratory are described in the section *Normative Data*.

Valsalva Ratio

For VR, the subject, rested and recumbent, is asked to maintain a column of mercury at 40 mm Hg (not exceeding 50 mm), for 15 sec via a bugle with an air leak (to ensure an open glottis). The responses should be repeated until two responses of similar BP_{BB} and HR are obtained. We will perform up to four maneuvers. The factors that affect the VR are listed in Table 8. The VR is derived from the maximum HR generated by the VM divided by the lowest HR occurring within 30 sec of peak HR (97,102). The choice of 40 mm Hg is made because a pressure of 40 mm Hg seems to yield reproducible results whereas the VR at <20 mm is inadequate and at >60 mm results in less reproducibility (85). Our studies also suggest 40 mm Hg as a practical optimal pressure (13). It is important that BP_{BB} recordings be also recorded during the maneuver, since the HR responses are baroreflex responses to changes in BP. The increase in HR occurs in response to the fall in BP, and the baroreflex response to the overshoot is responsible for the transient bradycardia. In dysautonomic patients, there typically is a loss of both the BP overshoot and the reflex bradycardia. Our criterion for an adequate VM is the generation of two reproducible BP curves. It should be noted that identical expiratory pressures may result in very different BP curves. If the BP excursions are minimal, then a reduced VR is not meaningful. If a fall in BP (early phase II) is not generated (as might occur in patients with a "flat top" response), then the VR may also be spuriously low. Additionally, a normal VR may occur in patients with impaired cardiovagal function if sympathetically mediated

TABLE 7. *Methods of evaluating heart rate response to deep breathing: effect of various parameters on results*

Parameter	HR (max–min)	E : I ratio	MCR
Artifact	Marked	Marked	Nil
Shifting HR	Marked	Marked	Minimal
Mean HR	Nil	Marked	Mild
Regularity of respiratory cycling	Negligible	Marked	Marked
Time to reach stable value	30 sec	30 sec	3 min

HR, heart rate; E : I, expiration–inspiration; MCR, mean circular resultant.

TABLE 8. *Some factors that affect the Valsalva ratio*

Age
Gender
Position of the subject
Expiratory pressure
Duration of effort
Inspiratory volume
Volume status
Medications

HR alterations are sufficiently large to result in an increase and reduction in HR (102,162).

Response to Standing

A detailed evaluation of the phases and mechanisms of the response to standing has been reported (20,47,143). The cardiovascular responses to standing has been analyzed in detail by Smith et al. (143), who divided the response into two phases: an immediate phase (0–30 sec) and the stable period (30 sec to 20 min). The immediate response in healthy young adults is characterized by a sharp decrease in BP and total systemic resistance at 5–10 sec, followed by a rapid rebound and overshoot. A corresponding HR increment follows in 3–5 sec and then tapers. Over the first 30 sec, there is a steady parallel decline in thoracic blood volume and stroke volume; there is also an initial surge in cardiac output followed by a steady decrease. During the stabilized response (30 sec to 20 min), the hemodynamic variables are relatively steady, showing average increases in HR of ~15%–30%, in diastolic pressure of 10%–15%, and in total vascular resistance of 20%–40%. During minutes 5–20, there are also decreases in thoracic blood volume averaging ~25%–30%, in cardiac output of 15%–30%, and in pulse pressure of ~5%–10%. It is evident that, in normal human subjects, assumption of the upright posture results in profound hemodynamic changes, most of them occurring during the first 30 sec. The initial HR responses to standing consist of a tachycardia at 3 sec and then 12 sec, followed by a bradycardia at 20 sec. The initial cardioacceleration is an exercise reflex, while the subsequent tachycardia and bradycardia are baroreflex mediated. The 30:15 ratio (RR interval at beat 30)/(RR interval at beat 15) has been recommended as an index of cardiovagal function and is described in detail in Chapter 23. The test is inferior to HR_{DB} because of its more complex physiology and because the confounding variables are less well clarified.

Comparison of Different Tests of Cardiovagal Function

There has been much enthusiasm in evaluating the sensitivity of various tests of cardiovagal function. Ziegler et al. (176) evaluated cardiovagal function in 261 patients with diabetes of different severity by using spectral analysis, vector analysis, and standard tests of HR variation, and concluded that the most frequently abnormal indices were the coefficient of variation, midfrequency spectral power at rest, mean circular resultant, and the maximum/minimum 30:15 ratio and VR. Much of this emphasis on sensitivity is misplaced. Tests of cardiovagal function are almost all sensitive, with little to choose among them. HR_{DB} is probably preferable to most others. Both afferent and efferent pathways are vagal, most patients are able to cooperate with the procedure, and the confounding variables are well studied. Other procedures such as the VM, standing up, and squatting have complex physiology involving sympathetic and central mechanisms as well.

Photoplethysmographic Blood Pressure Recordings

The Finapres technique, a noninvasive method of measuring BP_{BB}, generates an arterial waveform that is indistinguishable from that of a peripheral arterial waveform. The principle of the technique is based on servoplethysmometry using the volume clamp technique of Penaz (122) and further developed by Wesseling et al. (171,172). An infrared sensor records finger volume (plethysmograph) and is mounted inside a finger cuff. The blood volume seen by the plethysmograph is clamped to a set-point value by cuff pressure by means of an electropneumatic wide-band servosystem. This computerized servo or feedback system continuously counterbalances intraarterial pressure to keep the pressure difference across the arterial wall, the transmural pressure, at zero (172). At zero transmural pressure, cuff pressure equals intramural arterial pressure. The Finapres recorded pressures have been calibrated against intraarterial pressures and accurately reflect intrabrachial (78,159,160) or radial BP (120). The calibration appears to hold during autonomic maneuvers. Close correlation is present during the VM (78,120,160), coughing (159), and tilt (79). It has been reported that the Finapres may underread the systolic BP during exercise when arteriovenous shunts open up (119).

The Finapres recordings just described are reliable under optimal conditions. Our recordings are done from the middle digit of the index finger, unless otherwise stated. Criteria that we use are agreement (within 15%) with manual recordings of systolic and diastolic BP and with morphology. An adequate recording should have sharp contours and show a dicrotic notch. It should be recognized that there are a number of confounding variables in the noninvasive recording of BP_{BB} from digital arteries:

1. Warmth of the hand. It is extremely important that the hand and, in particular, the fingers be warm. A cold hand results in spuriously high Finapres recordings. It is our impression that an excessively vasodilated hand results in a spuriously low reading.
2. Position of the hand. We have the hand held in a relaxed semiopen position "as if holding a can of pop."
3. The shoulder girdle needs to be relaxed. Many patients respond to tilt-up by tightening their thoracic outlet. In some patients, this maneuver will reduce the arterial wave amplitude.
4. The arm must not be excessively extended or abducted, both maneuvers that can reduce BP. In our opinion, it is preferable to have the hand 1–3 inches *below* the apex beat to avoid this confounding effect.
5. Patients with excessive acral vasoconstriction in response to tilt-up may have a spuriously *high* Finapres recording. Presumably, the mechanism is the same for both cold and vasoconstricted fingers (119). Patients

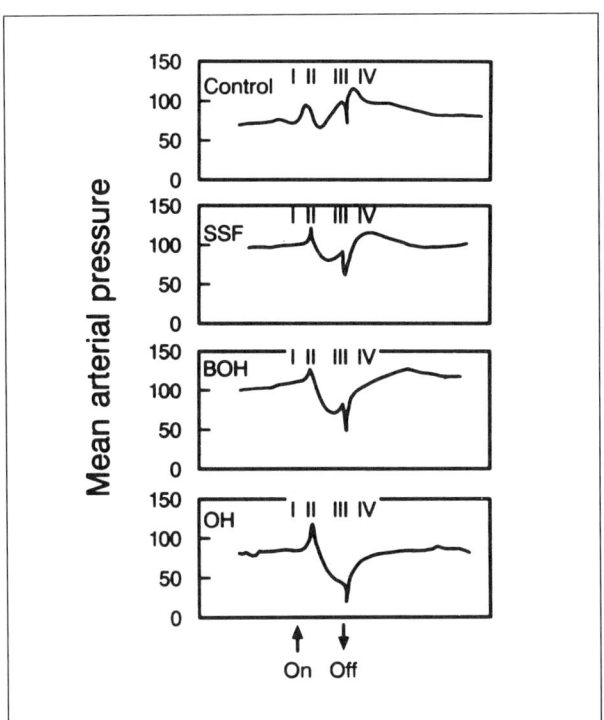

FIG. 5. Representative mean blood pressure responses in a control subject and in patients with sympathetic sudomotor failure (SSF), borderline orthostatic hypotension (BOH), and frank orthostatic hypotension (OH). From Sandroni et al. (136), with permission.

with orthostatic intolerance and a hyperadrenergic state can have good agreement between manual sphygmomanometric recordings of brachial artery with Finapres with the patient supine but significant divergence with a higher reading on Finapres on tilt-up (Chapter 30).

Beat-to-Beat Blood Pressure Response to the Valsalva Maneuver

BP_{BB} responses to the VM, tilt, and deep breathing are recorded using Finapres simultaneously with the HR recordings. The Mayo laboratory computer console displays the systolic, mean, and diastolic BP at a resolution of 100 H_2. The dynamic alterations during tilt and the VM are particularly important in detecting adrenergic failure. There are four main phases in the VM (Fig. 5). In phase I, there is a transient rise in BP due to increased intrathoracic and intraabdominal pressure causing mechanical compression of the aorta (31,81). In early phase II (phase II_e), the reduced preload (venous return) (23) and reduced stroke volume (21) lead to a fall in cardiac output in spite of tachycardia (31) caused by a withdrawal of cardiovagal influence (23). Total peripheral resistance increases (35,85) as a result of efferent sympathetic discharge to muscle (35) and an increase in plasma epinephrine concentration (132) and, within 4 sec after the increase in sympathetic discharge, the fall in BP is arrested (35). This is late phase II (II_L). In normal subjects, phase II_L is so efficient that, by the beginning of phase III, mean arterial pressure is at the resting mean arterial pressure level or above. Phase III, like phase I, is mechanical, lasting 1–2 sec, during which BP falls. The major mechanism is the sudden fall in intrathoracic pressure. Additional factors may be an increase in left ventricular afterload (22) and sudden expansion of intrathoracic vessels (40). There is a further burst of sympathetic activity during this phase (165). In phase IV, venous return (173) and cardiac output (21) have returned to normal while the arteriolar bed remains vasoconstricted, hence the overshoot of BP above baseline values. In the clinical autonomic laboratory setting, with studies done on the patients lying supine, phase IV may be more dependent on cardiac adrenergic tone than on systemic peripheral resistance (136). Intravenous 10 mg phentolamine resulted in the expected elimination of late phase II, but *augmented* rather than blocked phase IV. In contrast, 10 mg intravenous propranolol completely blocked phase IV (Fig. 6).

Valsalva-type maneuvers, which are performed during activities of daily living, include straining at stool, abdominal compression, and micturition. These maneuvers, in patients with generalized autonomic failure, can result in a progressive fall in BP (syncope may occur) without an ensuing overshoot. Indeed, the hypotension may persist for over a minute beyond the maneuver. In Fig. 5, examples of sudomotor sympathetic failure, borderline orthostatic hypotension (BOH), and OH show a progressive increase in abnormalities in phases II and IV. The use of the VM phases to evaluate adrenergic function has been validated in two ways. First, we undertook pharmacologic dissection of the maneuver (136). Late phase II is primarily under peripheral α adrenergic control, being selectively blocked by phentolamine, while phase IV is completely blocked by propranolol, indicating β-adrenoreceptor dependence. Next, we evaluated the maneuver in a control and three age- and sex-matched patient groups with graded adrenergic failure (136). One group had generalized autonomic failure with an orthostatic fall in systolic BP during tilt of >30 mm Hg. A second group had a lesser orthostatic fall in BP (<30>10 mmHg), and a third group had well-documented peripheral autonomic failure (absent QSART responses) but did not have OH. In contrast to controls, all the patient groups, including group 3, exhibited a significant reduction in II_I. An excessive BP fall in phase II and an absent phase IV overshoot were observed in the group with florid OH. Intermediate changes were seen in the borderline OH group. The BP_{BB} changes during the VM, when coupled with BP responses to tilt, provide a significantly improved evaluation of adrenergic failure when compared with bedside BP recordings. Patients with peripheral adrenergic failure, as in neuropathic patients with involvement of autonomic C fibers, will have absent late phase II and have some increase in early phase II. Patients with more severe autonomic failure, involving more widespread limb and splanchnic adrenergic, and cardiovagal impairment, will have a large early phase II and absent late phase II, with a

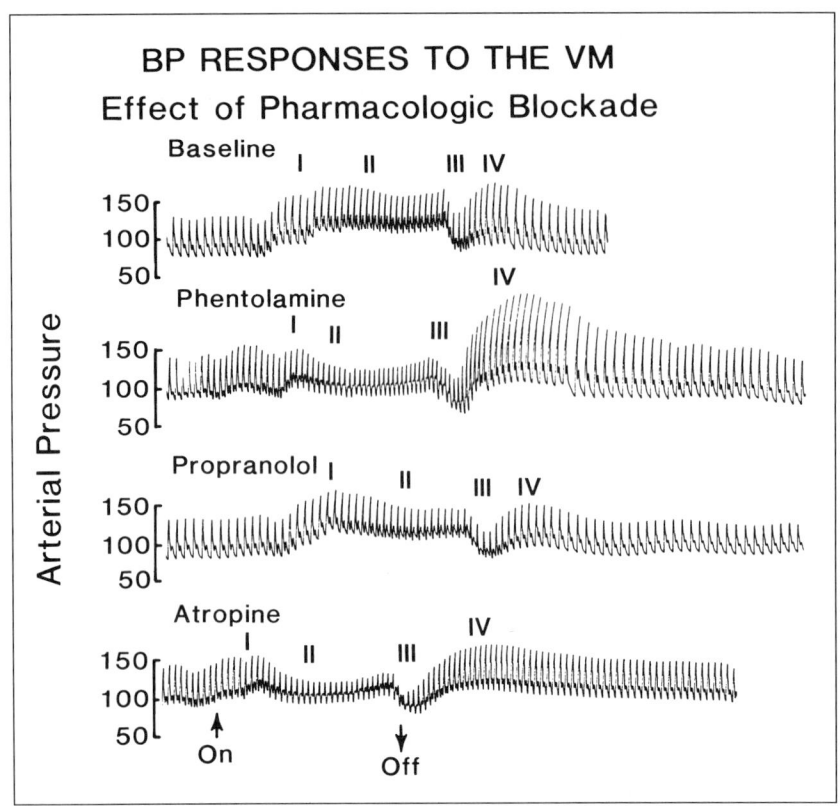

FIG. 6. Blood pressure response to pharmacologic agents. Phentolamine augments and propanolol blocks phase IV.

preserved phase IV. When phase IV is absent, cardiac adrenergic innervation has failed. One caveat is that phase IV can be small or, less often, absent in normal individuals, if phase II is modest or absent. Based on our laboratory experience, we have summarized the gradations of alterations of the VMs in different types and degrees of autonomic failure (Table 9).

Beat-to-Beat Blood Pressure Response to Tilt-Up

Orthostatic BP recordings to tilt are recorded using BP_{BB} and with a sphygmomanometer cuff with the patient supine and following tilt to 80°. We currently use an automated tilt table. The current emphasis is a slow tilt (>10–20 sec). A rapid tilt, achieved within 4 sec, as was recommended in the previous edition, is no longer considered necessary. The rate of tilt does not apparently affect the responses (147). Cuff recordings are obtained at 1 and 5 min after tilt-up. It is important to perform the upright tilt procedure at a standard time after the patients lie down since the orthostatic reduction in BP is greater following 20 min of preceding rest than 1 min, increasing from a mean systolic/diastolic decrement of 8/9 to 17/19 mmHg (154); we routinely perform tilting at the end of the study. BP_{BB} recordings of systolic, mean, and diastolic BP, acquired by Finapres, are continuously displayed on the computer console, as is the HR, derived from electrocardiographic (ECG) leads and an ECG monitor. It is also important to ensure that the arm is at heart level since arm position influences BP measure-

TABLE 9. *Components of Valsalva maneuver in types of autonomic failure*

Condition	Phase I	Phase II$_e$	Phase II$_l$	Phase III	Phase IV	VR
Normal	Present Effort	Present	Present	Present	Large amplitude Long duration	Normal
Vagal lesion	Normal	Reduced	Normal	Normal	Normal	Reduced
Mild lesion sympathetic	Normal	Mild increase	Reduced or absent	Normal	Present Normal	—
Moderate fail sympathetic	Normal	Increased	Absent	Normal	Variable, could be reduced	Reduced or normal
Sympath fail with OH	Normal	Marked increase	Absent	Normal	Absent	Usually reduced

VR, Valsalva ratio; OH, orthostatic hypotension.

ments (167). Several methods have been used to maintain proper arm position. The Finapres-containing digit can be held at a fixed position, at heart level, at the anterior axillary line (154). A second method is to perform the supine recordings with the patient's arm at heart level and then, following upright tilt, to extend the arm to rest it on an armrest, again at heart level. We prefer the third method where the arm is abducted onto an armrest and remains at heart level, at all angles of tilt. If the pulse contour becomes smaller with abduction to heart level, it is preferable and permissible to lower the arm to 2 inches below heart level.

During upright tilt, normal individuals undergo a transient reduction in systolic, mean, and diastolic BP followed by recovery within 1 min (79). The decrement is modest (<10 mm Hg, mean BP). Patients with adrenergic failure have a marked and progressive reduction in BP and pulse pressure (Fig. 7). The HR response is typically attenuated, but in patients whose cardiac adrenergic innervation is spared, HR response is intact and may be increased. Indices of mild adrenergic impairment have been incorporated into an orthostatic intolerance grade to tilt-up (Table 10). Criteria include excessive oscillations in BP, an excessive reduction ($\geq$50%) in pulse pressure, a transient (first minute) reduction in systolic BP >30 mmHg, an excessive increment in HR ($\geq$30 beats/min), and a failure of total systemic resistance to increment. Premonitory signs of syncope are a progressive reduction in BP (especially diastolic BP), total peripheral resistance, and pulse pressure, and loss of BP (and HR) variability. Some of these indices are expected abnormalities in a failure of arteriolar vasoconstriction (total pulmonary resistance and diastolic BP). Some are signs of increased vascular capacitance (reduction in pulse pressure, and excessive HR increment). The increased oscillations are indicative of intact compensatory mechanisms (but are abnormal since they indicate a system under stress), whereas the gradual loss of variability indicates the failure of compensation.

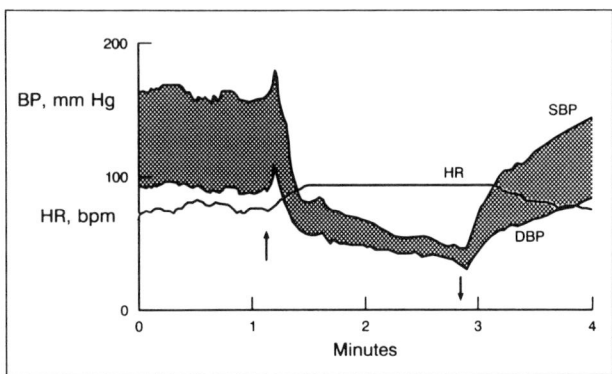

FIG. 7. Blood pressure and heart rate response to tilt in a patient with adrenergic failure. There is a progressive reduction in systolic blood pressure (SBP), diastolic blood pressure (DBP), and pulse pressure during upright tilt. *Arrows* indicate tilt-up followed by tilt-down.

TABLE 10. *Orthostatic intolerance grade to tilt-up*

Grade 0: Normal
Grade 1: Any of the following changes: excessive BP oscillations PP reduction ($\geq$50%) HR increment ($\geq$30 beats/min)
Grade 2: Transient OH with recovery
Grade 3: Sustained asymptomatic OH SBP >30 mmHg DBP >15 mmHg MBP >20 mmHg
Grade 4: Sustained symptomatic OH

BP, blood pressure; PP, pulse pressure; HR, heart rate; OH, orthostatic hypotension; SBP, systolic blood pressure; DBP, diastolic blood pressure; MBP, mean blood pressure.

Composite Autonomic Scoring Scale

The autonomic reflex screen has been used to develop a 10-point composite autonomic scoring scale (CASS) of autonomic function. The scheme allots four points for adrenergic and three points each for sudomotor and cardiovagal failure. Each score is normalized for the confounding effects of age and gender. The details of the scoring scale are presented in Table 11. Patients with a score of $\leq$3 on the CASS have only mild autonomic failure, those with scores of 7–10 have severe failure, and those with scores between these two ranges have moderate autonomic failure. The sensitivity and specificity of the method were assessed by evaluating the CASS in four groups of patients with known degrees of autonomic failure: 18 with multisystem atrophy, 20 with autonomic neuropathy, 20 with Parkinson's disease, and 20 with peripheral neuropathy but no autonomic symptoms. The composite scores (means $\pm$ SD) for these four groups, respectively, were 8.5 $\pm$ 1.3, 8.6 $\pm$ 1.2, 1.5 $\pm$ 1.1, and 1.7 $\pm$ 1.3. Patients with symptomatic autonomic failure had scores of $\geq$5, those without symptomatic autonomic failure had scores of $\leq$4, and no overlap existed in these groups.

Normative Data

Extensive normative data are available in the Mayo Autonomic Reflex Laboratory. We recently reviewed our normative data on 557 normal subjects. Distribution by age and gender is shown in Table 12. Our normative database by test is

QSART	357 subjects
QSART (left vs right sides)	39
Deep breathing	376
RSO	43
VR	425
Orthostatic BP/HR	270

TABLE 11. *Composite autonomic scoring scale*

Sudomotor subscore
If at least three QSART sites are studied, the following scoring criteria should be utilized:
0. Normal
1. Any of the following alterations:
    a. Single QSART site abnormal or
    b. Length-dependent pattern (distal sweat volume $<\frac{1}{3}$ of forearm or proximal leg values) or
    c. Persistent sweat activity at foot (TST anhidrosis present but <25%)
2. Any of the following alterations:
    a. Single QSART site <50% of lower limit
    b. Two or more QSART sites reduced (TST anhidrosis 25%–50%)
3. Two or more QSART sites <50% of lower limit (TST % anhidrosis >50%)

If only two QSART sites are utilized, the following scoring scale should be utilized:
0. Normal
1. a. Single QSART site abnormal or
   b. Length-dependent pattern (distal sweat volume $<\frac{1}{3}$ of proximal value) or
   c. Persistent sweat activity at foot
2. a. Single QSART site <50% of lower limit
   b. Two QSART sites reduced
3. a. Two or more QSART sites <50% of lower limit
   b One site absent and other site reduced

Cardiovagal subscore
1 = HR_{DB} mildly reduced but above <50% of minimum
2 = HR_{DB} reduced to <50% of minimum
3 = Both HR_{DB} and Valsalva ratio reduced to <50% of minimum

Adrenergic subscore
The adrenergic subscore is based on alterations in beat-to-beat blood pressure (BP) on the Valsalva maneuver and tiltup (Finapres and manual). A score of 1 is given for the following changes in Valsalva maneuver:
 a. Phase II_e reduction <40> 20 mmHg MBP (<50 years; 30–40, if >50 years) or
 b. II_l does not return to baseline or
 c. Pulse pressure reduction to ≤50% of baseline

If the Valsalva maneuver is *normal*, a score of 1 can be assigned if the following changes occur on *tiltup*:
 a. Excessive oscillations in MBP (>20 mmHg occupying at least 50% of the duration of tiltup)
 b. Fall in pulse pressure >50%
 c. Transient fall in SBP >20 mmHg with recovery (within 1 min)
 d. SBP reduction ≥20 mmHg beyond 1 min
 e. DBP reduction ≥10 mmHg beyond 1 min
 f. Overshoot ≥20 mmHg following tiltback

A score of 2 is assigned if phase II_e of Valsalva maneuver is >40 mmHg MBP. If a score of 1 is determined from the Valsalva maneuver, it can be increased to 2 if the following changes on tiltup occur:
 a. Transient fall in SBP >30 mmHg with recovery within 2 min
 b. SBP reduction ≥20 mmHg beyond 1 min
 c. DBP reduction ≥10 mmHg beyond 1 min

A score of 3 is assigned if the following changes occur in the Valsalva maneuver:
 a. Phase II_e reduction >40 mmHg + absent II_l and IV;

One additional point is assigned if a reduction in manual SBP ≥30 mmHg occurs beyond 2 min and is sustained for at least 2 min

QSART, quantitative sudomotor axon reflex test; TST, thermoregulatory sweat test; HR, heart rate; MBP, mean blood pressure; SBP, systolic blood pressure; DBP, diastolic blood pressure.

TABLE 12. *Demography: age and gender*

Gender	Age (years)							Total
	≤20	21–30	31–40	41–50	51–60	61–70	≥70	
Male	22	54	49	46	46	39	14	270
Female	24	57	56	58	45	28	19	287
Total	46	111	105	104	91	67	33	557

TABLE 13. *Regression of QSART (left side) sweat volumes with age for males and females for standard sites in human subjects: based on a normative database of 357 normal subjects evenly distributed by age and gender*

Variable	Intercept		Gender		Age		Gender/age*	
	b0	p	b1	p	b2	p	b3	p
Forearm	4.5291	0.0001	−1.6188	0.0001	−0.0072	0.5752	0.0020	0.7989
Proximal leg	4.0209	0.0001	−1.0076	0.0026	−0.0163	0.1410	0.0011	0.8724
Distal leg	5.5929	0.0001	−1.5921	0.0001	−0.0437	0.0002	0.0075	0.3049
Proximal foot	4.5174	0.0001	−1.5171	0.0001	0.0310	0.0066	0.0101	0.1548

QSART, quantitative sudomotor axon reflex test.

TABLE 14. *Male QSART responses: mean, 5th, and 95th percentile values*

Sites	20 Years			40 Years			60 Years		
Forearm	2.67	0.76	5.06	2.67	0.76	5.06	2.67	0.76	5.06
Proximal leg	2.67	1.27	4.54	2.32	0.93	4.19	1.97	0.58	3.84
Distal leg	3.28	1.37	5.27	2.55	0.98	4.55	1.83	0.59	3.82
Proximal foot	2.58	0.87	4.48	2.17	0.78	4.07	1.75	0.68	3.65

QSART, quantitative sudomotor axon reflex test.

TABLE 15. *Female QSART responses: mean, 5th, and 95th percentile values*

Sites	20 Years			40 Years			60 Years		
Forearm	1.15	0.20	2.78	1.15	0.20	2.78	1.15	0.20	2.78
Proximal leg	1.48	0.36	3.17	1.48	0.36	3.17	1.48	0.36	3.17
Distal leg	1.83	0.61	2.85	1.26	0.39	2.28	0.68	0.18	1.70
Proximal foot	1.27	0.23	3.07	1.05	0.18	2.85	0.84	0.12	2.64

QSART, quantitative sudomotor axon reflex test.

QSART

Normative data were available on 357 subjects. A consistent gender difference was found with females having approximately one-half the sweat volumes of males. A series of equations are provided in Table 13 that describe the normative data by age and gender. The mean, 5th percentile, and 95th percentile values are given for patients aged 20, 40, and ≥60 years in Table 14 for males and in Table 15 for females.

Resting Sweat Output

RSO data were recorded from 43 subjects. The actual numbers used for each site are listed in Table 16. There were no significant effects of age or gender, and there were no significant differences by side. The mean values followed by the 5th–95th percentile values are listed in the table.

Heart Rate Response to Deep Breathing

Normative data were evaluated in 376 subjects who were evaluated for HR response to deep breathing. Breakdown by gender was approximately equal. Distribution by gender was approximately equal. There were 91, 81, 67, 60, 48, and 29 subjects aged ≤29, 30–39, 40–49, 50–59, 60–69, and ≥70 years, respectively. Ages ranged from 10 to 83 years, and no significant differences were found between the sexes. However, a significant regression with age was found (Fig. 8): $y = 37.5448 * \log_{10} 0.9832x$ ($p < 0.001$), where y = HR range in beats/min and x = age in years. The values for 2.5 percentile, mean, and 97.5 percentile for ages 20, 40, 60, and 80 are listed in Table 17. The values up to the age of 60 years are robust. Beyond age

TABLE 16. *Control values for resting sweat output*

Sites	n	Percentile values		
		Mean	5th	95th
Hypothenar	41	0.53	0.49	0.20–0.87
Forearm	41	0.08	0.10	0.06–0.12
Distal leg	42	0.12	0.12	0.09–0.72
Proximal foot	43	0.16	0.16	0.12–0.58

TABLE 17. *Heart rate response to deep breathing: 2.5, 5, 95, and 97.5 percentile values*

Parameter	20 Years	40 Years	60 Years	80 Years
2.5; 5.0	13; 14	9; 10	7; 7	7; 7
95; 97.5	41; 43	33; 36	27; 29	27; 29

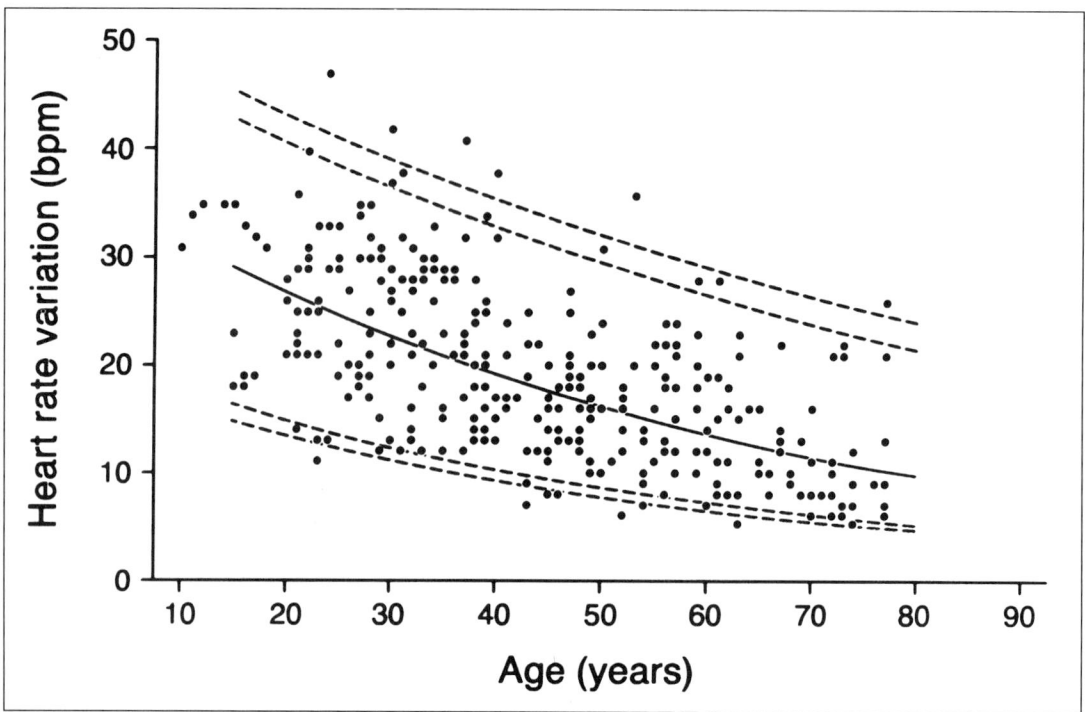

FIG. 8. Heart rate response to deep breathing: there is a significant effect of age.

60, the points are too few and a curve was not fitted. The values at 60 years were used for this and subsequent tables.

The Valsalva Ratio

The effect of age on the VR is controversial. Some workers have reported a lack of variability with age (30,154), while others have observed a difference (16,37, 91,92,105,119) (Table 18). Reported slopes have been similar. Ingall (Ch. 14 (48)) reported a slope of 0.01 per year, which is very similar to ours (91). VR, studied in 425 subjects aged 10–83 years, showed a gender difference. Hence, the data for males and females are described separately (Figs. 9 and 10). Distribution by gender was even (205 males and 220 females). There were 110, 85, 80, 67, 53, and 30 subjects aged ≤29, 30–39, 40–49, 50–59, 60–69, and ≥70 years, respectively. For males (n = 205), $y = 2.15982 - 0.00755x$ ($p < 0.001$). For females (n = 220), $y = 2.00273 - 0.00868x - 0.00021x^2$, where y = VR and x = age in years. The less consistent effect of age on VR than on respiratory sinus arrhythmia likely relates to the smaller change and greater complexity of the maneuver. Whereas respiratory sinus arrhythmia is a relatively pure test of cardiovagal function, many factors, including blood volume, antecedent period of rest (146), cardiac sympathetic and peripheral sympathetic functions (Chapters 4 and 18), and norepinephrine response, affect the VM. Age may affect different components of the VM in different directions. The values for 2.5 percentile, mean, and 97.5 percentile for ages 20, 40, 60, and 80 are listed in Table 18.

Orthostatic Blood Pressure

A total of 270 subjects (129 males and 141 females) were studied. Distribution by gender was even. There were 54, 64, 52, 49, 32, and 19 subjects aged ≤29, 30–39, 40–49, 50–59, 60–69, and ≥70 years, respectively. BP and HR were recorded beat to beat for 5 min. Normative data for HR increment and BP decrement to tilt-up are shown in Tables 19 and 20. Orthostatic BP decrement increased by age but was not different by gender.

TABLE 18. *Valsalva ratio: 2.5, 5, 95, 97.5 percentile values*

Parameter	20 Years		40 Years		60 Years		80 Years	
	Males	Females	Males	Females	Males	Females	Males	Females
2.5; 5.0	1.50; 1.59	1.41; 1.46	1.36; 1.44	1.47; 1.51	1.21; 1.29	1.36; 1.39	1.21; 1.29	1.36; 1.39
95; 97.5	2.87; 2.97	2.73; 2.97	2.52; 2.60	2.64; 2.88	2.18; 2.23	2.41; 2.65	2.18; 2.23	2.41; 2.65

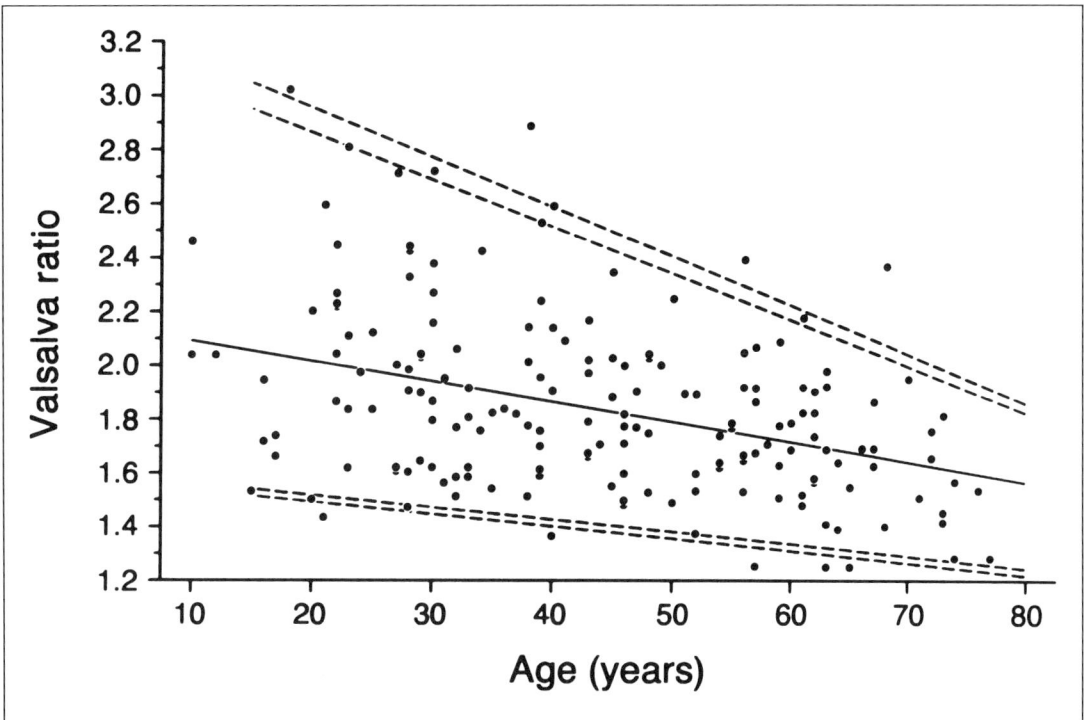

FIG. 9. Valsalva ratio: effect of age in males.

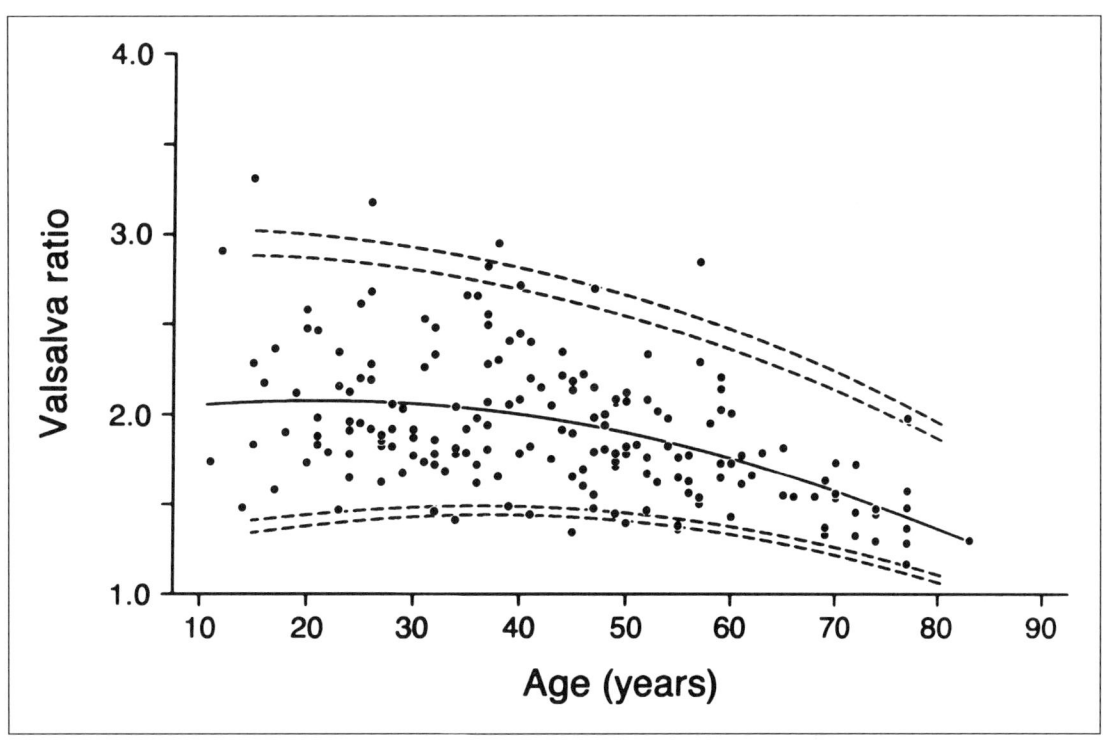

FIG. 10. Valsalva ratio: effect of age in females.

TABLE 19. *Heart rate increment after 1 min of tiltup: 95 and 97.5 percentile values for males and females*

Percentile	20 Years		40 Years		60 Years		80 Years	
	Male	Female	Male	Female	Male	Female	Male	Female
95	34	31	30	27	26	23	21	19
97.5	40	34	36	30	32	26	27	22

Salivation Test

Five gauze pads are deposited within a container and weighed. The subject's sublingual gutter is wiped with a different gauze pad that is discarded. The subject then chews on a preweighed gauze pad each minute for 5 min. At the end of the 5 min, the pads, which have been deposited in the original container, are weighed together with the container, and the original weight is subtracted. Salivation <7.5 mL/5 min is reduced for adults.

Tests to Detect Sympathetically Maintained Pain, (Complex Abnormal Regional Pain Syndrome, and Reflex Sympathetic Dystrophy)

The rationale for our battery of tests on patients with SMP is that altered sympathetic effect is a useful index although the ultimate diagnosis of SMP remains a clinical charge. The increased sympathetic effect may be sudomotor (altered RSO), vasomotor (altered temperature), or reflex sudomotor (altered QSART indices). All studies in patients with suspected sympathetic dysfunction are done on homologous sites in upper or lower extremities and consist of (a) measurements of RSO, (b) measurements of resting skin temperature, and (c) QSART recordings.

Patient Preparation: Patients should be indoors for at least 30 min. In addition, they should have at least 10 min of additional equilibration within the autonomic reflex laboratory before the recordings.

For upper-extremity studies, males and females are asked to undress to the waist and are provided with a sleeveless gown. Women should remove their brassiere. For lower-extremity studies, men and women are asked to undress to their underwear. Women should remove their stockings.

Measurement of Resting Sweat Output

First, large capsules (5.31 cm^2) are strapped on.
Next, recordings are done bilaterally and simultaneously at identical sites. For both the upper and lower extremities, four sites are studied. The hypothenar eminence and the medial forearm are used when the upper extremity is affected, and recordings are made over the extensor digitorum brevis muscle and the distal medial leg bilaterally when the lower extremity is affected.

RSO is then recorded over 5 min in the four sites simultaneously. The RSO over the last of the 5 min is read by the computer. The choice of 5 min is a compromise between the attainment of equilibrium and practicality. By 3–4 min, near steady-state conditions are achieved. Our control values are listed in Table 16.

Measurement of Resting Skin Temperature

Using infrared thermometry, the skin temperature pattern can be compared for evidence of vasomotor asymmetry. This asymmetry is used as an index of differences in skin blood flow. We have used two methods of obtaining this information. The first is simpler and less expensive. Skin temperature is determined by infrared thermometry. For the upper extremity, the ventral aspect of the forearm is divided horizontally into medial and lateral thirds and vertically into upper, middle, and lower thirds, resulting in six areas. The thenar, middle, and hypothenar areas of the palm are studied as are the distal pads of each of the fingers. For the lower extremity, the thigh and anterior leg are each divided into six areas. The skin over the extensor digitorum brevis is studied, as are the pads on each toe. Each area of skin temperature is compared with the identical contralateral areas and charted (Fig. 11).

Measurement of Resting Skin Temperature by Telethermography

For telethermographic recordings, we currently use the following frames, all of which include both sides:

Upper extremity
1. Anterior aspect of upper arm
2. Radial aspect of forearms
3. Palmar aspect of forearms
4. Dorsal aspect of forearms
5. Palmar aspect of hands and fingers
6. Dorsal aspect of hands and fingers

A second identical set of recordings are obtained, beginning 20 mins after commencing the first set of recordings.

TABLE 20. *Blood pressure decrement after 1 min of tiltup: 95 and 97.5 percentile values*

Percentile	20 Years	40 Years	60 Years	80 Years
95	17	20	23	26
97.5	21	24	26	29

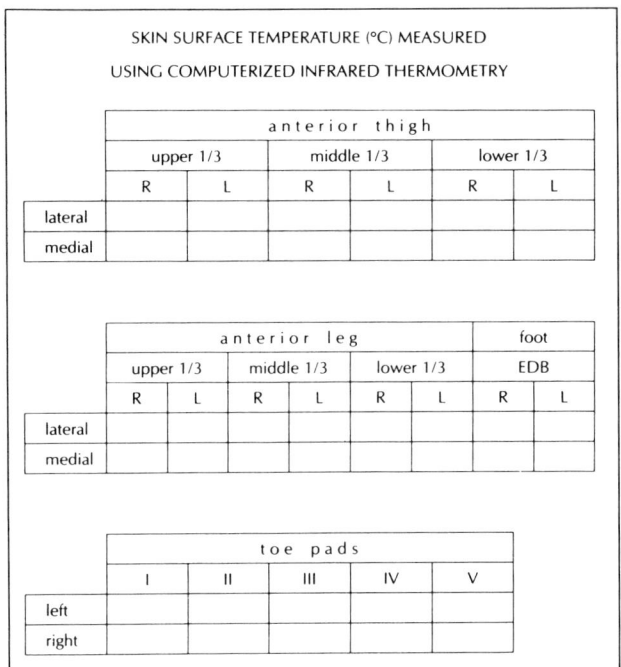

FIG. 11. The areas compared in the telethermographic evaluation of patients with limb pain.

Lower extremity
1. Anterior thighs
2. Anterior legs
3. Dorsa of feet
4. Plantar aspect of feet
5. Posterior thighs
6. Posterior legs

A second identical set of recordings are obtained, beginning 20 min after commencing the first set of recordings.

The particular frames chosen for RSD is less critical than those suggested for radiculopathy studies. We do not do the additional frames, because thermography lacks the sensitivity and specificity to detect radiculopathy (62,146).

QSART Recordings

QSART recordings are done over the medial forearm for upper-extremity studies. For lower-extremity studies, recordings are made over the extensor digitorum brevis muscle and the medial distal leg. All recordings are done simultaneously and bilaterally.

Interpretation

Criteria and laboratory grading of abnormality are described in detail elsewhere (26) and summarized in Table 21. The QSART, skin temperatures, and RSO may be increased or reduced, resulting in an asymmetric pattern of response. For sudomotor tests (QSART and RSO), a grading scheme from 0 (normal) to 3, in increasing abnormality, evaluates the magnitude of side-to-side differences and the diffuseness of the asymmetry. It also recognizes an absolute deficit. A difference between sides of ≥50% in RSO is considered significant. A difference of 25%–50% is scored only if the changes are diffuse. Such differences are more relevant when sweat volumes are large.

For temperature differences, a difference ≥1°C is abnormal, especially if it is found in several different sites. A smaller difference (0.5°–1°C) is considered significant only if multiple sites are involved and is given a grade of only 1. The abnormal site is usually colder but not invariably, since the findings depend on the stage of autonomic dysfunction.

TABLE 21. *Laboratory-based reflex sympathetic dystrophy grading scale*

QSART index
1. a. Unilateral reduction or increase in sweat volume by 25%–50% on the affected side when compared with the contralateral side; or
    b. Ultrashort latency, ipsilateral, contralateral or both
    c. Persistent sweat activity, ipsilateral, contralateral, or both
2. Single QSART site with an increase or decrement by at least 50% on the affected side
3. a. Two or more QSART sites with an increase or decrement by at least 50% on the affected side
    b. Bilateral increase or reduction by >50%

Vasomotor index
1. a. Skin temperature asymmetry (increase or reduction) on affected side by ≥0.5°C diffusely
    b. or by 1° over pads, cooler on affected side
2. a. Skin temperature asymmetry (increase or reduction) on affected side by ≥1.0°C limited distribution, or skin temperature asymmetry ≥1.0°C diffuse but atypical distribution
3. Skin temperature asymmetry (increase or reduction) ≥1.0°C diffuse, maximal distally

Resting sweat index
1. a. Unilateral reduction or increase ≥25% and <50%
    Abnormal morphology
2. b. Unilateral reduction or increase by ≥50% involving a single site
3. c. Two sites with an increase or reduction of ≥50%

QSART, quantitative sudomotor axon reflex test.

A major advantage of telethermography over thermometry is the more reliable detection of diffuse versus focal temperature changes. Thermography has the advantage of demonstrating patterns of abnormality. It is useful in distinguishing the diffuse pattern, maximal distally, of SMP, from, for instance, local pathology, as in arthritis or local injury.

Synthesis of Clinical with Laboratory Evaluation

We have recently reviewed our data on laboratory evaluation of RSD and briefly described our prospective clinical and laboratory evaluation of RSD (98). We concluded that the best current clinical approach to the diagnosis of RSD is to combine clinical and laboratory criteria. Of the clinical criteria, particular emphasis is placed on

1. Severity of pain
2. Distribution of pain (diffuse)
3. Allodynia

Patients with RSD will have pain of moderate or greater severity; have diffuse distribution of pain, maximal distally; and have allodynia to light stroking, pressure, and joint movement. The criteria are summarized in Table 22. These clinical criteria are combined with laboratory evaluation, which focuses on QSART asymmetry and RSO to a greater extent than skin vasomotor alterations.

This approach results in the following modification of our current scale:

I. *Definite RSD:* Allodynia to touch, pressure, and joint movement + side-to-side asymmetry of the QSART (grade 3) or RSO (grade 3 asymmetry)
II. *Probable RSD:* Clinical RSD probability scoring scale (probable) + any of the following on the laboratory RSD scale:-
   a. QSART3 or RSO3
   b. QSART2 + RSO2 or VM2
III. *Possible RSD:* Chronic limb pain + QSART1 or RSO1 or VM1

Sustained Handgrip

Sustained muscle contraction causes a rise in systolic and diastolic BP and HR. The stimulus derives from exercising muscle and central command (19,37,46,48,55,164). Efferents travel to muscle and heart, resulting in increased cardiac output, BP, HR, and muscle vasoconstriction. There is an effort-dependent and time-dependent increase in muscle sympathetic activity (135). The BP rise is mediated by an increase in cardiac output and peripheral resistance. The importance of central command versus muscle afferents has been controversial (57). Hultman and Sjoholm (76) compared BP and HR responses to voluntary and nonvoluntary (electrically stimulated) static exercise in human subjects and found identical results, suggesting that the pressor response is reflex in nature (23). The early HR increase is due to vagal withdrawal (19) while the late components are due to sympathetic activation. The increase in BP in healthy humans is mainly from the increase in cardiac output (91) and is unrelated to position or muscle mass (134). Skin blood flow increases during isometric handgrip (153). This autonomic maneuver has been adapted as a clinical test of sympathetic autonomic function (45). These authors recommend 30% maximal contraction for up to 5 min (45). BP is measured using a sphygmomanometer cuff. A normal response has been suggested to be an increment in the diastolic BP by ≥ 16 mmHg, and 11–15 mmHg is borderline (45). Many patients are unable to sustain their effort for 5 min. An effort at 30% of normal for 3 min is probably adequate. The test is of limited sensitivity and specificity. Confounding variables are not well known (Chapter 23).

Plasma Catecholamines

Plasma norepinephrine (NE) results from a spillover of NE from sympathetic postganglionic nerve terminals, and the supine value is a index of net sympathetic activity (126,166,177), being affected by the rate of NE secretion and clearance (43,125). It has been used as an index to separate postganglionic from preganglionic failure. In a disorder where the lesion is preganglionic, resting supine NE is normal, but the response to standing would be reduced or absent due to failure of activation. In a postganglionic lesion, the supine values would be reduced if the lesion is very widespread. The test should be done with the patient supine and standing. Standing NE is a more sensitive index of adrenergic function than are supine values. Attempts at improving the sensitivity have included using indices of NE biosynthesis by measuring urinary and plasma metabolites as well as NE such as vanillylmandelic acid and plasma dihydroxyphenylglycol (27,73).

TABLE 22. *Clinical reflex sympathetic dystrophy probability scoring system*

Parameter	Definite	Probable	Possible	Not-RSD
1a. Allodynia (touch)				
1b. Allodynia (pressure)	3/3	2/3	1/3	0/3
1c. Allodynia (movement)				
2a. Vasomotor (history)				
2b. Vasomotor (exam)				
2c. Swelling (history)	4/4	$\geq$2/4	$\leq$1/4	0/4
2d. Swelling (exam)				

TABLE 23. Neural pathways of some autonomic reflexes

Test	Stimulus	Afferent	Main central structures	Efferent	Normal response
Deep breathing	Six deep breaths/min	Vagus	NTS	Vagus	Inspiratory increase, expiratory decrease in HR
Facial immersion	Ice water	Cranial nerve V	Medullary centers	Vagus; sympathetic	Bradycardia; vasoconstriction
Valsalva maneuver	Expiratory pressure 40 mm for 10–15 sec	Cranial nerves IX and X	NTS	Vagus; sympathetic	HR increase; then fall; vasoconstriction; four BP phases
Lower-body negative pressure	Vacuum to legs and abdomen	As above	As above	As above	HR increase; then fall; vasoconstriction; PP reduction
Neck suction	Negative pressure to neck	As above	As above	As above	As above
Carotid massage	Firm massage of carotid bulb	Cranial nerve IX	As above	As above	As above
Coughing	Three deep coughs	As above	As above	As above	HR increase
Response to standing	Standing up quickly	Baroreceptor and muscle	Mainly NTS	Vagus; sympathetic	Increase, then fall in HR; vasoconstriction
Squat	Stand, squat, then stand	As above	As above	As above	As above, but greater vagal and orthostatic stress
Pupil cycle time	Light to edge of pupil	Optic nerve	Edinger–Westphal nucleus	Cranial nerve III	Cycles of dilation–constriction
Inspiratory gasp	Single gasp	Spinal nerve	Spinal cord	Sympathetic adrenergic	Vasoconstriction
IV phenylephrine	Cranial nerves IX and X	NTS	—	Sympathetic cardiovagal	BP rise; HR fall
Nitroglycerin	Sublingual nitroglycerine	Cranial nerves IX and X	NTS	Sympathetic cardiovagal	BP fall; HR rise
Contralateral cold stimulus	Hand immersion in ice-cold water	Pain and cortex; temperature	Sympathetic hypothalamus fibers	Adrenergic	Vasoconstriction; BP rise
Reflex heating	Heat to trunk	Spinothalamic	Thalamus; hypothalamus	Sympathetic efferents	Skin vasodilation
Venoarteriolar reflex	Limb dependent <40 cm	Sympathetic axon reflex	Postganglionic sympathetic	Sympathetic axon reflex	Skin vasoconstriction
Mental arithmetic	Serial 7s for ~2 min	Nil	Cortex	Sympathetic efferents	Skin vasoconstriction; BP rise
Startle	Sudden loud noise	Auditory	Auditory cortex; hypothalamus	Sympathetic efferents	HR increase; BP rise; pupillodilatation
Sustained handgrip	30% of maximum grip for up to 5 min	Muscle afferent; central command	Cortex; hypothalamus	Sympathetic efferents; vagus	Rise in BP and HR
Reflex heating	Heating of trunk	Spinothalamic track	Hypothalamus	Sympathetic efferents	Reflex vasodilatation of hand
Exercise	Muscle contraction and intent	Muscle afferent; central command	Cortex	Sympathetic efferents	Rise in BP and HR
24-hr HR monitor	Variable	Variable	NTS	Vagus	Sleep-associated changes

HR, heart rate; BP, blood pressure; PP, pulse pressure; NTS, nucleus of tractus solitarius; IV, intravenous.

ADDITIONAL TESTS OF AUTONOMIC FUNCTION

There are many tests of autonomic function (10,94). The neural pathways of some routine and nonroutine tests of autonomic function are shown in Table 23. The following two sections describe some less commonly used or more complicated tests to be followed by a few less valuable tests.

MIBG–SPECT Study

The quantitative uptake of the radiopharmaceutical iodine-123–metaiodobenzylguanidine (MIBG), an NE analogue, can be measured by single-photon-emission computed tomography (SPECT), which is an index of the functional integrity of presynaptic sympathetic terminals in the heart. Since ischemia *per se* may reduce MIBG uptake, the influence of perfusion defects are evaluated by technetium flow studies. Studies in the rat heart demonstrate that MIBG uptake is mainly dependent on uptake-1 and uptake-2 activity (33) and a linear relationship between MIBG and NE content (68). In a single human autopsy study, the severity of nerve fiber loss correlated with the reduction in MIBG uptake (151). Dynamic studies demonstrated at least biexponential clearance patterns of MIBG from the heart. These ratios, calculated from dynamic and static studies, are helpful in elucidating the uptake at nonvesicular sites, which reflects the severity of sympathetic nervous system abnormalities in the heart.

Normative data on small groups of patients are available. For instance, Tsuchimochi et al. (158) evaluated age and gender differences in normal myocardial adrenergic neuronal function in 29 subjects (18 men and 11 women; age range, 21–79 years; mean age, 42 ± 17 years) with no cardiac disorders. Early (15 min) and late (3–4 hr) planar images, and SPECT images at 3–4 hrs after MIBG injection (111 MBq), were evaluated. There were no significant differences in the global heart values based on age or gender, but there was a significant inverse correlation between the inferior-to-anterior wall count ratio and age, affecting especially inferior wall uptake. Studies have been done on patients with autonomic failure, mainly in diabetic subjects. There is a progressive increase in impairment of MIBG uptake from patients without cardiovagal impairment to those with severe autonomic failure (28,89,106,111,138). Groups with sympathetic failure, on tilt studies or on reduced RR interval of low-frequency power, tended to have more impaired MIBG uptake (111). A correlation between global or regional myocardial [^{123}I]MIBG uptake, however, and duration of diabetes, hemoglobin A_{1c}, body mass index, or QT interval length was not observed (138). Patients with long QT interval had more abnormal MIBG uptake (115,170) but a linear correlation was not found (170). Claus et al. (28) studied 25 diabetic patients and 19 healthy subjects. MIBG scans in all normal subjects showed homogeneous uptake of activity. In 12 of 25 patients, the results of at least two HR variation tests were abnormal, whereas the results of 17 of 25 MIBG–SPECT studies were abnormal. No significant correlation was found between MIBG–SPECT results and spectral analysis of HR variation. Schnell et al. (138) evaluated 20 diabetic patients with and 22 diabetic patients without cardiovagal neuropathy, and nine control subjects. MIBG study findings were normal in only six diabetic patients without (27%) and one diabetic patient with (5%) cardiovagal neuropathy.

Severe impairment is usually found in patients with orthostatic hypotension. Abnormalities have been reported in pure autonomic failure, multiple-system atrophy, amyloid neuropathy, and myotonic dystrophy (61,70,104,117).

Skin Vasomotor Reflexes

Skin blood flow is measured by a laser Doppler flowmeter or by plethysmography, and the vasoconstrictor response to an autonomic maneuver is determined. Studies are usually done on the toepads or fingerpads because the sympathetic innervation to these sites is purely vasoconstrictor, and vasoconstriction can be induced by such maneuvers as inspiratory gasp (34), response to standing (for the finger), contralateral cold stimulus, or VM (99). The pathways of these reflexes are complex. For instance, the response to standing is mediated by the venoarteriolar reflex, by low- and high-pressure baroreceptors and, to a lesser extent, by increases in epinephrine, NE, and renin. The test can be used to detect the presence of sympathetic denervation in the peripheral neuropathies, as in diabetic or amyloid neuropathy (99,130,140). A shortcoming of the test is the marked sensitivity of skin sympathetic fibers to emotional and temperature changes so that there is much ambient fluctuation (99). More optimistic reports are also available (3,49). Faes et al. (49) evaluated reflex cooling and, using their paradigm, found the test to be reproducible. Changes in skin temperature ($p < 0.001$) and skin blood flow ($p < 0.005$) in response to cooling were significantly greater in the control group than in the group with spinal analgesia. Repeated skin temperature measurements on 42 occasions (test–retest period of 4 weeks) in eight healthy subjects and 34 diabetic patients indicated a reliability coefficient of 80%. Abbot et al. (3) studied fingertip skin blood flow as measured by laser Doppler flowmetry (as laser Doppler flux) under environmental conditions promoting vasodilation in Scottish patients with diabetes mellitus and Indian patients with leprosy and reported that the test separated normal from neuropathic patients satisfactorily.

Orthostatic Stress Tests

Some patients with adrenergic failure do not sustain an orthostatic drop in BP on routine upright tilt, but they may do so after a meal or a warm bath. To elicit orthostatism in these patients, orthostatic stress tests can be undertaken. Four stresses that we have employed are sublingual trinitroglycerin, postexercise tilt, lower-body negative pressure, and prolonged tilt. The principle of all three stress tests is the same. The subject is subjected to a vasodilatory stimulus. In the trinitroglycerin stress test (77,102), 0.6 g trinitroglycerin is administered sublingually to the subject, who remains supine. The tilt is repeated 5 min later. An alternative approach is to repeat the study after the subject has done 12 squats. Especially with young subjects, extension of the period of upright tilt to 20 min (5) or the application of lower-body negative pressure (148) may induce presyncope or orthostatism that is not found during 5 min of tilt.

Blood Pressure and Heart Rate Response to Prolonged Tilt

For patients with the "benign" disorders of reduced orthostatic tolerance (Chapters 48,49), POTS, or recurrent vasodepressor syncope, a prolonged tilt for up to 60 min is recommended. The extended time is needed to examine whether orthostatic tachycardia and excessive oscillations in HR and BP develop. Vasodepressor and vasovagal presyncope is sought. There is the sudden reduction in HR and BP associated with presyncopal symptoms. Fitzpatrick et al. (52) studied patients by using prolonged tilt up for to 60 min and suggested a tilt duration of 40 min. Patients who develop vasodepressor syncope will do so within 40 min.

Other Cardiovascular Heart Rate Tests

There are numerous potential tests of cardiovagal function. These include resting HR variation and HR response to coughing and to facial immersion. Coughing results in inspiration, an expiratory effort against a closed glottis followed by an explosive expiration as the glottis suddenly opens (175). The HR response consists of a cardioacceleration that is maximal at ~2–3 sec after the last cough and a return to resting values in ~12–14 sec (168,169). The mechanism is thought to be cholinergic due initially to muscular contraction followed by baroreflex response to a fall in BP (25). The diving response has also been adapted as a test of cardiovagal function (50,83). The application of cold stimulus to both first divisions of the trigeminal nerve results in reflex bradycardia. An alternative approach to evaluating cardiovagal function is 24-hr monitoring (15). In patients with cardiac arrhythmia, pupillary responses of parasympathetic function are useful (4,108).

Heart Rate Response to Drinking

The HR response to drinking a glass of fluid is mediated by cardiac adrenergic activity. One method is to drink 120 ml of a cola at 4°C within 40 sec. The normal response is an increases in HR by 10–20 beats/min (54,127,152). This HR increment is blocked by propranolol (54) and sympathetic denervation (152) and is associated with an increase in NE (127) but not prevented by atropine (54). The stimulus is thought to be mechanical stimulation and distension of the esophagus and stomach (54,116).

Heart Rate Response to Squatting

Squatting has been standardized as a simple noninvasive test of parasympathetic and sympathetic function. Subjects stand for 3 min, squat for 1 min, and then stand again (in inspiration). Marfella et al. (107) reported that atropine abolished the increase in heart period on squatting, and propranolol did the converse on standing. Their study, which included 558 control subjects 20–74 years of age and 558 diabetics, derived vagal and sympathetic ratios, i.e., the bradycardia and tachycardia relative to baseline. They provided similar information in another smaller study. The bradycardic response is likely an accentuated 30:15 ratio. The orthostatic response following squatting is a standing test with greater orthostatic stress. The test has been used by a number of workers, typically involving a series of squats. Whether the squat test as described has sufficient sensitivity and specificity awaits further studies. The physiology of the response is rather complex. These workers have made a good beginning.

Determination of Baroreflex Sensitivity

The baroreflex is one of the most important regulators of moment-to-moment BP control. Baroreflex sensitivity (the change in heart period resulting from a change in BP) can be quantitated in human subjects. Baroreflex sensitivity can be determined under dynamic (59,103,145) and steady-state conditions (86,87,102) by using pharmacologic approaches or carotid sinus stimulation (41,64). In both methods, the BP is changed by a direct-acting α-agonist, usually phenylephrine, and the heart period response to mean BP is determined. In the dynamic method, analysis involves plotting each heart interval against the preceding systolic BP value. A simple linear regression is fitted, and the slope of the regression of systolic BP on heart period is a measure of reflex sensitivity. There is an unknown delay (reflex latency) after the pressure change before the change in heart period occurs. The practical way in which this latency is handled is to calculate two regression slopes by (a) relating systolic BP to its corresponding heart period and (b) relating systolic BP to the subsequent pulse interval. The slope with the highest correlation coefficient is accepted. A new computer-assisted method of analyzing baroreflex sensitivity, using the same raw data, has been developed, termed time-related analysis (144). The results are essentially identical to the "Oxford" method but do provide a direct estimation of reflex latency. The steady-state method relates the change in heart period to change in mean BP. By a suitable range of phenylephrine doses, e.g., 25–300 mg, on the pressor end and by obtaining a dose–response relationship on the hypotensive end (tilt, lower-body negative pressure, or trinitroglycerin or nitroprusside), in normal subjects a sigmoid relationship obtains (86,87). Typical doses of nitroprusside are 50–200 mg, resulting in a 10- to 20-mm Hg fall in mean BP. The curve is computer fitted by probit transformation followed by linear regression analysis or directly by using a program to fit sigmoid curves. The indices of mean gain and heart period range are obtained (86,87,102). Baroreflex gain can also be estimated by relating the heart period to the systolic BP value of the preceding beat (157). These workers regressed heart period and systolic BP beginning with the end of forced expiration and proceeding to the 5th second of the overshoot. The individual values obtained during phase IV of the VM correlate well ($r = 0.9$) with those after phenylephrine injection (157), with the former generating greater slopes.

An alternative method that obviates the use of pharmacologic agents uses instead a neck suction device, which generates a regulated negative pressure to the carotid sinus. This method enables the quantitative assessment of the carotid sinus to sinoatrial node baroreflex (41). The neck suction-derived baroslopes yielded results that were qualitatively and quantitatively similar to those of the standard phenylephrine method (39).

Determination of Denervation Supersensitivity

The denervated end-organ is supersensitive to its neurotransmitter (24). This principle is the basis of several tests of autonomic function, including the pupillary response to dilute pilocarpine (Chapter 21) and the excessive pressor response to directly acting α-agonists. The BP and HR response to intravenous phenylephrine should include low doses (25 mg) to detect denervation supersensitivity. At this dose, normal individuals lack a pressor response. Patients with postganglionic adrenergic denervation have an upregulation of α-receptors and respond with a large BP increment (102,113,142).

Blood Pressure and Heart Rate Response to Intravenous Tyramine

Tyramine is an indirect-acting α-agonist that releases NE presynaptically. It is often given is doses of 10, 20, and 40 mg/kg (36) and often used in conjunction with phenylephrine to provide a full analysis. If a patient had a postganglionic lesion, the pressor response to tyramine would be reduced (because there are fewer functional postganglionic terminals) and there may be a supersensitive response to phenylephrine (because of denervation supersensitivity) (see also Chapter 44).

Isoproterenol Infusion Test

The number of subjects who develop presyncope and syncope during upright tilt is increased by intravenous isoproterenol (6). In many of these individuals, brief head-up tilt was normal (6). The inotropic stimulation and decreased ventricular volume provoked by the combined use of isoproterenol and tilt have been thought to activate unmyelinated ventricular mechanoreceptor afferents intensely and hence a vagally mediated cardioinhibitory reflex (155). We use two infusions of isoproterenol at doses of 0.01 and 0.02 mg/kg/min. A minimum recovery period of 10 min between infusions is required. A HR increase of >50 beats/min or subjective sensation of anxiety, dizziness, or palpitations indicates that the infusion should be promptly terminated. The α-adrenergic antagonist phentolamine and the β-adrenergic antagonist propranolol should be available in order to counteract rapidly any untoward side effects of adrenergic stimulation. In our hands, such intervention has never been required.

Impedance Cardiography

Physiologic and hemodynamic indices can be measured noninvasively by impedance cardiography. The instrument will measure and display a total of 12 cardiodynamic parameters: cardiac output/cardiac index, HR, stroke volume/stroke index, peak flow/peak flow index, ejection fraction, end-diastolic volume/end-diastolic index, contractility index, thoracic fluid index, acceleration index, ventricular ejection time, ejection ratio ("preload index"), and systolic time ratio. Thoracic bioimpedance has been found to correlate strongly with indicator or thermal dilution determinations of cardiac output measured with indwelling catheters (9,16) and with cardiac output measured with the indirect Fick rebreathing technique (42). With accurate electrode placement, the day-to-day reproducibility of the parameters measured shows a coefficient of variation of ~5% and a strong linear correlation (slope 1.04, $r = 0.94$) between days (S. Textor, unpublished observations). Although there is debate as to whether the bioimpedance technique accurately measures the absolute values of cardiac output, it is clear that this technique accurately measures relative changes in cardiac output over a wide range of conditions (16,17).

Norepinephrine Response to Edrophonium

Intravenous edrophonium injection, using the same dose (10 mg) as used in the tensilon test for myasthenia gravis, results in the preganglionic release of acetylcholine and postganglionic release of NE. It has been proposed as a test of preganglionic function, assuming the postganglionic adrenergic neurons are intact (56,109). The NE increment occurs within 2–8 min of injection. In one study (56), four parkinsonian patients and one patient with multiple-system atrophy had a normal NE increment while six of seven patients with pure autonomic failure did not. Adequate dose–response studies and the sensitivity and specificity of the method remain to be established.

Neuroendocrine Tests

Pancreatic polypeptide as measured by radioimmunoassay (84) is reduced in vagal failure and is blocked by anticholinergic medication and by vagotomy. Its release is stimulated by food ingestion and insulin hypoglycemia. The values are not gender related but increase with age (see also Chapter 14).

Evaluation of Splanchnic–Mesenteric Bed

Superior Mesenteric Flow

The splanchnic–mesenteric bed is one of the least accessible vascular beds to evaluate, in spite of its great importance as a venous baroreflex-sensitive capacitance bed. It can be evaluated indirectly by the handling of an indicator dye such as indocyanine green, which is cleared by the liver (74). A more dynamic evaluation of splanchnic flow is that of measuring superior mesenteric artery flow by duplex scanning. Ultrasonic imaging combined with a pulsed Doppler unit (duplex scanning) enables the noninvasive assessment of blood flow of the superior mesenteric artery (80,128). Doppler frequency spectra are used to determine peak systolic, late systolic, and end-diastolic velocity and to compute the mean velocity. In contrast to other flows such as common carotid (80), celiac, or femoral arteries (112), which remain unchanged in response to a standard meal, there is a threefold increase in superior mesenteric artery flow velocity, with end-diastolic velocity showing proportionally the greatest increase. At rest, blood flow through the mesenteric artery is 6.3 ± 2.6 ml/sec and 9.5 ± 2.1 ml/sec in the carotid artery. After the test meal, mesenteric artery blood flow increases and reaches maximal hyperemia after 45 min. The mean ($\pm$SEM) of the superior mesenteric blood flow, based on 70 subjects, was reported to be 517 ± 19 ml/min. There was neither significant difference in flow between sexes, nor correlation between flow and age ($r = 0.042$). The means of the coefficients of variability were 6.8% over the short term and 8.2% in long-term studies (128). Interstudy reproducibility of repeated superior mesenteric arterial flow volume measurements is reported to be good ($r = 0.98$) (163). The accuracy of measurement has been compared to an arterial model. The areas under the time–frequency curves result in a consistent overestimate when compared with the arterial model, measured by planimetry. A correction factor of 1.47 between flow velocities calculated after planimetry and real flow was established. Correction for this factor resulted in a flow velocity of 19.5 ± 4.7 cm/sec and a blood flow rate of 377 ± 166 ml/min in the volunteers.

NONROUTINE OR LESS USEFUL TESTS OF AUTONOMIC FUNCTION

Venoarteriolar Reflex

During limb dependency, when venous pressure is increased by 25 mmHg, reflex arteriolar vasoconstriction reduces blood flow by 50% (65). This venoarteriolar reflex has its receptors in small veins, and its neural pathway appears to be a sympathetic C-fiber local axon reflex (65,66). Henrikson et al. (67) suggested that the function of the reflex is to increase total peripheral resistance, compensating by up to 45% the orthostatic decrease in cardiac output. It may also lessen the orthostatic increase in tissue fluid by adjusting the precapillary-to-postcapillary resistance ratio. The reflex has been reported to be a sensitive test of peripheral adrenergic function (130). We have not found a satisfactory degree of sensitivity or subspecificity (114).

Neurogenic Flare Test

Neurogenic inflammation or the axon flare response refers to an the development of an area of redness several centimeters in diameter developing ~15–30 sec after a painful stimulus and lasting several min. The neural pathway is an axon reflex traveling antidromically and then orthodromically along a polymodal C nociceptor (75). There is clear involvement of substance P, histamine, vasoactive intestinal peptide and somatostatin, but other peptides and prostaglandins have also been implicated (53,90). One synthesis of the data is as follows. A painful stimulus results in the release of substance P (and maybe vasoactive intestinal peptide and somatostatin), causing mast cell degranulation and histamine release to produce the wheal. With passage of the impulse along the efferent limb, there is neurotransmitter release and a flare results. Retreatment with capsaicin blocked the flare but not the wheal, suggesting that it blocks the effector side of the reflex perhaps by depleting nerve terminals of vasodilator peptides (7). The flare response has been used as a test of unmyelinated C-fiber function in the neuropathies. With axonal degeneration of these C-fiber terminals, the reflex becomes attenuated or lost. The hyperemia has been detected by with a laser Doppler probe and the flare and QSART responses simultaneously recorded with a sudorometer and laser probe (121). The test offers the potential of simultaneously evaluating polymodal C-fiber and sympathetic function. The sensitivity and specificity are probably too low to recommend this technique as a clinical test (12).

Mental Stress

Mental stress, as with mental arithmetic (serial sevens from 100 or 1,000), results in an increase in BP and HR. The rise in BP is used as an index of sympathetic adrenergic function. The mental stress results in a centrally mediated sympathetic discharge. The pressor response is due to an increase by ~50% in cardiac output with no change or a reduction in peripheral sympathetic nerve activity and a fall in total peripheral resistance of 30% (51,72).

Cold-Face Test

The diving response has also been adapted as a test of cardiovagal function (83). The application of cold stimulus to both first divisions of the trigeminal nerve resulted in reflex bradycardia. The test can be coupled with recording of skin blood flow by laser Doppler (11) or plethysmographic techniques (63).

Safety of Autonomic Function Tests

The noninvasive autonomic tests have an extremely high value–safety ratio. There are a small number of potential risks.

The VM increases intrathoracic pressure. It also increases intraocular and intracranial pressure. There is a small theoretical potential risk of intraocular hemorrhage and of lens dislocation. Upright tilt may induce syncope, and prolonged tilt may induce cardiac arrhythmias in those so predisposed. In published reports of ~100 studies, totaling ~4,000 cases, no complications with sequelae were reported. The larger studies are especially illustrative. The DCCT study evaluated cardiovascular tests of autonomic function in 1,441 patients in 29 centers over a mean duration of $6\frac{1}{2}$ years without complications (1). The Rochester Diabetic Neuropathy Study (38), involving 380 patients who are studied yearly, is now into year 8 with no complications. Over this time, 1,400 tests (QSART, cardiovascular HR tests, and adrenergic tests) were performed. The Mayo Autonomic Reflex Laboratory has now completed ~20,000 cardiovascular HR tests without complications.

Iontophoresis, like other tests that involve the administration of a current source, requires precautions for electrical safety. There is a small and largely controllable risk of local skin injury. In >40,000 iontophoretic tests performed at the Mayo Clinic in Rochester, Minnesota, iontophoresis had resulted in local skin injuries in only two cases, and these injuries were relatively minor. No injuries have been encountered in the last 3,000 tests since minor modifications in the test have been undertaken.

No symptomatic arrhythmias have been encountered on tilt, and no intraocular complications have been encountered. Patients can develop extrasystoles and, during prolonged tilt, rare cases of sinoatrial arrest can occur. Piha and Voipio-Pulkki (124) analyzed the ECG tracings of 925 consecutive subjects. The ECG was taken during a battery of cardiovascular autonomic reflex tests that included the VM, deep-breathing test, and orthostatic and isometric handgrip. The frequency of ventricular extrasystoles increased during or after the tests, compared with the resting phase, in 11% of healthy subjects, in 11% of diabetic subjects, and in 23% of subjects with a previous myocardial infarction ($p = 0.001$ versus healthy subjects). In patients with previous myocardial infarction, the most dysrhythmogenic individual tests were orthostatic and isometric handgrip. In nine subjects, other cardiac rhythm disturbances were detected (including nonsustained ventricular tachycardia, conduction block, and atrial fibrillation). In all cases, the dysrhythmias were asymptomatic and resolved without medical intervention.

The TST has been performed since at least 1940. The largest systematically analyzed data are from the Mayo Thermoregulatory Sweat Laboratory. Since 1982, a total of 4,661 sweat tests were undertaken. Complications were minimal, comprising chemical dermatitis in 0.13%, skin irritation in 0.6%, claustrophobia requiring premature cessation of the test in 2%, infrared burns (first degree) in 0.1%, and epistaxis in one technician on one occasion due to irritation by alizarin.

Approach to the Laboratory Evaluation of Autonomic Function

Step 1 is to detect the presence and severity of autonomic failure.

Step 2 is to determine the type of autonomic involvement: sudomotor, cardiovagal, or adrenergic.

Step 3 is to determine the distribution of postganglionic sudomotor deficit by using QSART measurements at four sites. If a more detailed distribution of sympathetic denervation is sought, the TST can be done to define the pattern of anhidrosis (Chapter 19).

Step 4 is an attempt to determine the site of the abnormality. One way to localize the site of the lesion is by combining results of the TST and the QSART (Table 4).

Step 5 is to seek evidence of generalized autonomic failure. The presence of orthostatic hypotension indicates widespread sympathetic failure, providing relative or absolute hypovolemia can be excluded. In patients with neuropathy, HR abnormalities to deep breathing and VM indicate impairment of cardiac autonomic function usually indicating generalized autonomic failure since cardiac autonomic failure usually lags behind distal failure (vagal failure occurs early in diabetic neuropathy). Other indices of generalized autonomic failure are widespread abnormalities of the QSART, total or subtotal anhidrosis, and evidence of adrenergic failure (Table 12).

REFERENCES

1. The effect of intensive treatment of diabetes on the development and progression of long-term complications in insulin-dependent diabetes mellitus: the Diabetes Control and Complications Trial Research Group. *N Engl J Med* 1993;329:977–986.
2. Clinical autonomic testing report of the Therapeutics and Technology Assessment Subcommittee of the American Academy of Neurology. *Neurology* 1996;46:873–880.
3. Abbot NC, et al. Vasomotor reflexes in the fingertip skin of patients with type 1 diabetes mellitus and leprosy. *Clin Auton Res* 1993;3:189–193.
4. Adler FH. *Physiology of the eye: clinical applications*. St Louis: CV Mosby, 1950.

5. Allen SC, et al. A study of orthostatic insufficiency by the tiltboard method. *Am J Physiol* 1945;143:11–20.
6. Almquist A, et al. Provocation of bradycardia and hypotension by isoproterenol and upright posture in patients with unexplained syncope [see Comments]. *N Engl J Med* 1989;320:346–351.
7. Anand P, et al. Topical capsaicin pretreatment inhibits axon reflex vasodilatation caused by somatostatin and vasoactive intestinal polypeptide in human skin. *Br J Pharmacol* 1983;78:665–669.
8. Angelone A, Coulter NA. Respiratory sinus arrhythmia: a frequency dependent phenomenon. *J Appl Physiol* 1964;19:479–482.
9. Appel PL, et al. Comparison of measurements of cardiac output by bioimpedance and thermodilution in severely ill surgical patients. *Crit Care Med* 1986;14:933–935.
10. Appenzeller O. *The autonomic nervous system.* Amsterdam: Elsevier Biomedical, 1976.
11. Arnold RW, et al. Sensitivity to vasovagal maneuvers in normal children and adults. *Mayo Clin Proc* 1991;66:797–804.
12. Benarroch EE, Low PA. The acetylcholine-induced flare response in evaluation of small fiber dysfunction. *Ann Neurol* 1991;29:590–595.
13. Benarroch EE, et al. Analysis of Valsalva maneuver in normal subjects. *Ann Neurol* 1989;26:186A(abst).
14. Bennett T, et al. Assessment of methods for estimating autonomic nervous control of the heart in patients with diabetes mellitus. *Diabetes* 1978;27:1167–1174.
15. Bennett T, et al. Twenty-four hour monitoring of heart rate and activity in patients with diabetes mellitus: a comparison with clinic investigations. *BMJ* 1976;1:1250–1251.
16. Bernstein DP. Continuous noninvasive real-time monitoring of stroke volume and cardiac output by thoracic electrical bioimpedance. *Crit Care Med* 1986;14:898–901.
17. Boer P, et al. Measurement of cardiac output by impedance cardiography under various conditions. *Am J Physiol* 1979;237:H491–H496.
18. Borgdorff P. Respiratory fluctuations in pupil size. *Am J Physiol* 1975;228:1094–1102.
19. Borst C, et al. Cardiac acceleration elicited by voluntary muscle contractions of minimal duration. *J Appl Physiol* 1972;32:70–77.
20. Borst C, et al. Mechanisms of initial heart rate response to postural change. *Am J Physiol* 1982;243:H676–H681.
21. Brooker JZ, et al. Alterations in left ventricular volumes induced by Valsalva manoeuvre. *Br Heart J* 1974;36: 713–718.
22. Buda AJ, et al. Effect of intrathoracic pressure on left ventricular performance. *N Engl J Med* 1979;301:453–459.
23. Candel S, Ehrlich DE. Venous blood flow during the Valsalva experiment including some clinical applications. *Am J Med* 1953;15:307–315.
24. Cannon WB, Rosenblueth A. *The supersensitivity of denervated structures: a law of denervation.* New York: Macmillan, 1949.
25. Cardone C, et al. Autonomic mechanisms in the heart rate response to coughing. *Clin Sci* 1987;72:55–60.
26. Chelimsky TC, et al. Value of autonomic testing in reflex sympathetic dystrophy. *Mayo Clin Proc* 1995;70:1029–1040.
27. Christensen NJ, et al. Plasma dihydroxyphenylglycol (DHPG) as an index of diabetic autonomic neuropathy. *Clin Physiol* 1988;8:577–580.
28. Claus D, et al. Investigation of parasympathetic and sympathetic cardiac innervation in diabetic neuropathy: heart rate variation versus meta-iodo-benzylguanidine measured by single photon emission computed tomography. *Clin Auton Res* 1994;4:117–123.
29. Cohen J, et al. Somatic and autonomic function in progressive autonomic failure and multiple system atrophy. *Ann Neurol* 1987;22:692–699.
30. Coote JH, et al. The reflex nature of the pressor response to muscular exercise. *J Physiol (Lond)* 1971;215: 789–804.
31. Corbett JL. *Some aspects of the autonomic nervous system in normal and abnormal man* [PhD thesis]. Oxford: University of Oxford, 1969.
32. Darrow CW. Sensory, secretory and electrical changes in the skin following bodily excitation. *J Exp Psychol* 1927;10:197–226.
33. Degrado TR, et al. Uptake mechanisms of meta-[^{123}I]iodobenzylguanidine in isolated rat heart. *Nucl Med Biol* 1995;22:1–12.
34. Delius W, Kellerova E. Reactions of arterial and venous vessels in the human forearm and hand to deep breath or mental strain. *Clin Sci* 1971;40:271–282.
35. Delius W, et al. Manoeuvres affecting sympathetic outflow in human muscle nerves. *Acta Physiol Scand* 1972;84:82–94.
36. Demanet JC. Usefulness of noradrenaline and tyramine infusion tests in the diagnosis of orthostatic hypotension. *Cardiology* 1976; 61(Suppl 1):213–224.
37. Donald KW, et al. Cardiovascular responses to sustained (static) contractions. *Circ Res* 1967;20:15.
38. Dyck PJ, et al. The Rochester Diabetic Neuropathy Study: reassessment of tests and criteria for diagnosis and staged severity. *Neurology* 1992;42:1164–1170.
39. Ebert TJ, et al. Repetitive ramped neck suction: a quantitative test of human baroreceptor function. *Am J Physiol* 1984;247:H1013–H1017.
40. Eckberg D. Parasympathetic cardiovascular control in human disease: critical review of methods and results. *Am J Physiol* 1980;239: H581–H593.
41. Eckberg DL, et al. A simplified neck suction device for activation of carotid baroreceptors. *J Lab Clin Med* 1975;85:167–173.
42. Edmunds AT, et al. Cardiac output measured by transthoracic impedance cardiography at rest, during exercise and at various lung volumes. *Clin Sci* 1982;63:107–113.
43. Esler M, et al. Determination of norepinephrine apparent appearance and release in human plasma. *Life Sci* 1979;25:1461–1470.
44. Evans BA, et al. The peripheral autonomic surface potential in suspected small fiber peripheral neuropathy. *Muscle Nerve* 1988;11: 982(abst).
45. Ewing DJ, et al. Cardiovascular responses to sustained handgrip in normal subjects and in patients with diabetes mellitus: a test of autonomic function. *Clin Sci Mol Med* 1974;46:295–306.
46. Ewing DJ, et al. Correlation of cardiovascular and neuroendocrine tests of autonomic function in diabetes. *Metabolism* 1986;35:349–353.
47. Ewing DJ, et al. Immediate heart rate response to standing: simple test of autonomic neuropathy in diabetes. *BMJ* 1978;1:145–147.
48. Ewing DJ, et al. The value of cardiovascular autonomic function tests: 10 years experience in diabetes. *Diabetes Care* 1985;8:491–498.
49. Faes TJ, et al. The validity and reproducibility of the skin vasomotor test: studies in normal subjects, after spinal anaesthesia, and in diabetes mellitus. *Clin Auton Res* 1993;3:319–324.
50. Fagius J, Sundlof G. The diving response in man: effects on sympathetic activity in muscle and skin nerve fascicles. *J Physiol (Lond)* 1986;377:429–443.
51. Fencl U, et al. Changes of blood flow in forearm muscle and skin during an acute emotional stress (mental arithmetic). *Clin Sci* 1959; 18:491–498.
52. Fitzpatrick AP, et al. Methodology of head-up tilt testing in patients with unexplained syncope. *J Am Coll Cardiol* 1991;17:125–130.
53. Gamse R, et al. Several mediators appear to interact in neurogenic inflammation. *Acta Physiol Hung* 1987;69:343–354.
54. Gayheart PA, et al. An alpha-adrenergic coronary constriction during esophageal distention in the dog. *J Cardiovasc Pharmacol* 1991; 17:747–753.
55. Gelsema AJ. *Somatic reflex input in cardiovascular control* [PhD thesis]. Amsterdam: University of Amsterdam, 1985.
56. Gemmill JD, et al. Noradrenaline response to edrophonium in primary autonomic failure: distinction between central and peripheral damage. *Lancet* 1988;1:1018–1021.
57. Goodwin GM, et al. Cardiovascular and respiratory responses to changes in central command during isometric exercise at constant muscle tension. *J Physiol (Lond)* 1972;226: 173–190.
58. Greene RM, et al. Sweating patterns in atopic dermatitis patients. *Arch Dermatol Res* 1989;281:373–376.
59. Gribbin B, et al. Effect of age and high blood pressure on baroreflex sensitivity in man. *Circ Res* 1971;29:424–431.
60. Guttmann L. The management of the quinizarin sweat test (QST). *Postgrad Med J* 1947;23:353–366.
61. Hakusui S, et al. A radiological analysis of heart sympathetic functions with meta-[^{123}I]iodobenzylguanidine in neurological patients with autonomic failure. *J Auton Nerv Syst* 1994;49:81–84.
62. Harper CM Jr, et al. Utility of thermography in the diagnosis of lumbosacral radiculopathy. *Neurology* 1991;41:1010–1014.

63. Heath ME, Downey JA. The cold face test (diving reflex) in clinical autonomic assessment: methodological considerations and repeatability of responses. *Clin Sci* 1990;78:139–147.
64. Heidorn GH, McNamara AP. Effect of carotid sinus stimulation on the electrocardiograms of clinically normal individuals. *Circulation* 1956;14:1104–1113.
65. Henriksen O. Local sympathetic reflex mechanism in regulation of blood flow in human subcutaneous adipose tissue. *Acta Physiol Scand Suppl* 1977;450:1–48.
66. Henriksen O, et al. Autoregulation of blood flow in human cutaneous tissue. *Acta Physiol Scand* 1973;89:538–543.
67. Henriksen O, et al. Contribution of local blood flow regulation mechanisms to the maintenance of arterial pressure in upright position during epidural blockade. *Acta Physiol Scand* 1983;118: 271–280.
68. Herman LM, et al. Meta-iodobenzylguanidine uptake in the hypertensive–diabetic rat heart: a marker for myocardial dysfunction? *Can J Physiol Pharmacol* 1994;72:1162–1167.
69. Herrmann F, et al. Studies on sweating. IV. A new quantitative method of assaying sweat-delivery to circumscribed areas of the skin surface. *J Invest Dermatol* 1951;17:241–249.
70. Hirayama M, et al. A scintigraphical qualitative analysis of peripheral vascular sympathetic function with meta-[123I]iodobenzylguanidine in neurological patients with autonomic failure. *J Auton Nerv Syst* 1995;53:230–234.
71. Hirsch J, et al. Nutritionally-induced changes in parasympathetic function. *Brain Res Bull* 1991;27:541–542.
72. Hjemdahl P, et al. Differentiated sympathetic activation during mental stress evoked by the Stroop test. *Acta Physiol Scand Suppl* 1984;527:25–29.
73. Hoeldtke RD, et al. Assessment of norepinephrine secretion and production. *J Lab Clin Med* 1983;101:772–782.
74. Hoeldtke RD, et al. Hemodynamic effects of octreotide in patients with autonomic neuropathy. *Circulation* 1991;84:168–176.
75. Hokfelt T, et al. Experimental immunohistochemical studies on the localization and distribution of substance P in cat primary sensory neurons. *Brain Res* 1975;100:235–252.
76. Hultman E, Sjoholm H. Blood pressure and heart rate response to voluntary and nonvoluntary static exercise in man. *Acta Physiol Scand* 1982;115:499–501.
77. Hume L, et al. Provocation of postural hypotension by nitroglycerin in diabetic autonomic neuropathy. *Diabetes Care* 1980;3:27–30.
78. Imholz BP, et al. Continuous non-invasive blood pressure monitoring: reliability of Finapres device during the Valsalva manoeuvre. *Cardiovasc Res* 1988;22:390–397.
79. Imholz BPM, et al. Orthostatic circulatory control in the elderly evaluated by noninvasive continuous blood pressure measurement. *Clin Sci* 1990;79:73–79.
80. Jager K, et al. Measurement of mesenteric blood flow by duplex scanning. *J Vasc Surg* 1986;3:462–469.
81. Johnson RH, Spalding JMK. *Disorders of the autonomic nervous system.* Philadelphia: FA Davis, 1974.
82. Kennedy WR, et al. Quantitation of the sweating deficit in diabetes mellitus. *Ann Neurol* 1984;15:482–488.
83. Khurana RK, et al. Cold face test in the assessment of trigeminal–brainstem–vagal function in humans. *Ann Neurol* 1980;7:144–149.
84. Koch MB, et al. Can plasma human pancreatic polypeptide be used to detect diseases of the exocrine pancreas? *Mayo Clin Proc* 1985;60:259–265.
85. Korner PI, et al. Reflex and mechanical circulatory effects of graded Valsalva maneuvers in normal man. *J Appl Physiol* 1976;40:434–440.
86. Korner PI, et al. Central nervous system control of baroreceptor reflexes in the rabbit. *Circ Res* 1972;31:637–652.
87. Korner PI, et al. "Steady-state" properties of the baroreceptor–heart rate reflex in essential hypertension in man. *Clin Exp Pharmacol Physiol* 1974;1:65–76.
88. Lang E, et al. Stimulation of sudomotor axon reflex mechanism by carbachol in healthy subjects and patients suffering from diabetic polyneuropathy. *Acta Neurol Scand* 1995;91:251–254.
89. Langer A, et al. Metaiodobenzylguanidine imaging in diabetes mellitus: assessment of cardiac sympathetic denervation and its relation to autonomic dysfunction and silent myocardial ischemia. *J Am Coll Cardiol* 1995;25:610–618.
90. Lembeck F. Mediators of vasodilatation in the skin. *Br J Dermatol* 1983;109(Suppl 25):1–9.
91. Lind AR. The circulatory effects of sustained voluntary muscle contraction. *Clin Sci* 1964;27:229–244.
92. List CF, Peet MM. Sweat secretion in man. I. Sweating responses in normal persons. *Arch Neurol Psychiatry* 1938;39:1228–1237.
93. Low PA. Autonomic neuropathy. *Semin Neurol* 1987;7:49–57.
94. Low PA. Quantitation of autonomic responses. In: Dyck PJ, et al., eds. *Peripheral neuropathy.* Philadelphia: WB Saunders, 1984: 1139–1165.
95. Low PA. Sudomotor function and dysfunction. In: Asbury AK, McKhann GM, McDonald WI, eds. *Diseases of the nervous system.* Philadelphia: WB Saunders, 1986:596–605.
96. Low PA, Opfer-Gehrking TL, Kihara M. *In vivo* studies on receptor pharmacology of the human eccrine sweat gland. *Clin Auton Res* 1992;2:29–34.
97. Low PA, et al. Comparison of distal sympathetic with vagal function in diabetic neuropathy. *Muscle Nerve* 1986;9:592–596.
98. Low PA, et al. Clinical characteristics of patients with reflex sympathetic dystrophy (sympathetically maintained pain) in the USA. In: Janig W, Stanton-Hicks M, eds. *Progress in pain research management.* Seattle: IASP, 1996:49–66.
99. Low PA, et al. Evaluation of skin vasomotor reflexes by using laser Doppler velocimetry. *Mayo Clin Proc* 1983;58:583–592.
100. Low PA, et al. Quantitative sudomotor axon reflex test in normal and neuropathic subjects. *Ann Neurol* 1983;14:573–580.
101. Low PA, et al. The effect of aging on cardiac autonomic and postganglionic sudomotor function. *Muscle Nerve* 1990;13:152–157.
102. Low PA, et al. The sympathetic nervous system in diabetic neuropathy: a clinical and pathological study. *Brain* 1975;98:341–356.
103. Ludbrook J, et al. The variable-pressure neck-chamber method for studying the carotid baroreflex in man. *Clin Sci Mol Med* 1977; 53:165–171.
104. Machida K, et al. Abnormal sympathetic innervation of the heart in a patient with myotonic dystrophy detected with I-123 MIBG cardiac SPECT. *Clin Nucl Med* 1994;19:968–972.
105. Macmillan AL, Spalding JM. Human sweating response to electrophoresed acetylcholine: a test of postganglionic sympathetic function. *J Neurol Neurosurg Psychiatry* 1969;32:155–160.
106. Mantysaari M, et al. Noninvasive detection of cardiac sympathetic nervous dysfunction in diabetic patients using [123I]metaiodobenzylguanidine. *Diabetes* 1992;41:1069–1075.
107. Marfella R, et al. The squatting test: a useful tool to assess both parasympathetic and sympathetic involvement of the cardiovascular autonomic neuropathy in diabetes. *Diabetes* 1994;43:607–612.
108. Martyn CN, Ewing DJ. Pupil cycle time: a simple way of measuring an autonomic reflex. *J Neurol Neurosurg Psychiatry* 1986;49:771–774.
109. Matthews DM, et al. Noradrenaline response to edrophonium (Tensilon) and its relation to other autonomic tests in diabetic subjects. *Diabetes Res* 1987;6:175–180.
110. McEvoy KM, et al. 3,4-Diaminopyridine in the treatment of Lambert–Eaton myasthenic syndrome. *N Engl J Med* 1989;321:1567–1571.
111. Miyanaga H, et al. Clinical usefulness of 123I-metaiodobenzylguanidine myocardial scintigraphy in diabetic patients with cardiac sympathetic nerve dysfunction. *Jpn Circ J* 1995;59:599–607.
112. Moneta GL, et al. Duplex ultrasound measurement of postprandial intestinal blood flow: effect of meal composition. *Gastroenterology* 1988;95:1294–1301.
113. Moorhouse JA, et al. Vascular responses in diabetic peripheral neuropathy. *BMJ* 1966;1:883–888.
114. Moy S, et al. The venoarteriolar reflex in diabetic and other neuropathies. *Neurology* 1989;39:1490–1492.
115. Muller KD, et al. 123I-metaiodobenzylguanidine scintigraphy in the detection of irregular regional sympathetic innervation in long QT syndrome. *Eur Heart J* 1993;14:316–325.
116. Nakai M. Cardiovascular responses to gastric hypo-osmolar stimulation in anesthetized dogs. *Jpn J Physiol* 1993;43:335–346.

117. Nakata T, et al. Cardiac sympathetic denervation in transthyretin-related familial amyloidotic polyneuropathy: detection with iodine-123–MIBG. *J Nucl Med* 1995;36:1040–1042.
118. Netsky MG. Studies on secretion in man. I. Innervation of the sweat glands of the upper extremity: newer methods of studying sweating. *Arch Neurol Psychiatry* 1948;60:279–287.
119. Nijboer JA, et al. The difference in blood pressure between upper arm and finger during physical exercise. *Clin Physiol* 1988;8:501–510.
120. Parati G, et al. Comparison of finger and intra-arterial blood pressure monitoring at rest and during laboratory testing. *Hypertension* 1989;13:647–655.
121. Parkhouse N, LeQuesne PM. Quantitative objective assessment of peripheral nociceptive C fibre function. *J Neurol Neurosurg Psychiatry* 1988;51:28–34.
122. Penaz J. Photoelectric measurement of blood pressure, volume and flow in the finger. In: Albert R, Vogt WS, Helbig W, eds. *Digest of the International Conference on Medicine and Biological Engineering*. Dresden: Conference Committee on the 10th International Conference on Medicine and Biological Engineering, 1973:104.
123. Pfeifer MA, et al. Quantitative evaluation of cardiac parasympathetic activity in normal and diabetic man. *Diabetes* 1982;31: 339–345.
124. Piha SJ, Voipio-Pulkki LM. Cardiac dysrhythmias during cardiovascular autonomic reflex tests. *Clin Auton Res* 1993;3:183–187.
125. Polinsky RJ, et al. Decreased sympathetic neuronal uptake in idiopathic orthostatic hypotension. *Ann Neurol* 1985;18:48–53.
126. Polinsky RJ, et al. Pharmacologic distinction of different orthostatic hypotension syndromes. *Neurology* 1981;31:1–7.
127. Puddey IB, et al. Fluid temperature and volume dependence of the dissociated plasma epinephrine and norepinephrine response to drinking. *J Clin Endocrinol Metab* 1986;62:438–440.
128. Qamar MI, et al. Transcutaneous Doppler ultrasound measurement of superior mesenteric artery blood flow in man. *Gut* 1986;27:100–105.
129. Randall WC. Quantitation and regional distribution of sweat glands in man. *J Clin Invest* 1946;25:761–767.
130. Rayman G, et al. Blood flow in the skin of the foot related to posture in diabetes mellitus. *BMJ* 1986;292:87–90.
131. Richter CP. Instructions for using the cutaneous resistance recorder, or "dermometer" on peripheral nerve injuries, sympathectomies, and paravertebral blocks. *J Neurosurg* 1946;3:181–191.
132. Robertson D, et al. Comparative assessment of stimuli that release neuronal and adrenomedullary catecholamines in man. *Circulation* 1979;59:637–643.
133. Ryder RE, et al. Acetylcholine sweatspot test for autonomic denervation. *Lancet* 1988;1:1303–1305.
134. Sadomoto T, et al. Cardiovascular reflexes during isometric exercise: role of muscle mass and gravitational stress. *Aviat Space Environ Med* 1987;58:211–217.
135. Saito M, et al. Responses in muscle sympathetic nerve activity to sustained hand-grips of different tensions in humans. *Eur J Appl Physiol* 1986;55:493–498.
136. Sandroni P, et al. Pharmacological dissection of components of the Valsalva maneuver in adrenergic failure. *J Appl Physiol* 1991;71:1563–1567.
137. Sandroni P, et al. Autonomic involvement in extrapyramidal and cerebellar disorders. *Clin Auton Res* 1991;1:147–155.
138. Schnell O, et al. Scintigraphic evidence for cardiac sympathetic dysinnervation in long-term IDDM patients with and without ECG-based autonomic neuropathy. *Diabetologia* 1995;38:1345–1352.
139. Shahani BT, et al. Sympathetic skin response: a method of assessing unmyelinated axon dysfunction in peripheral neuropathies. *J Neurol Neurosurg Psychiatry* 1984;47:536–542.
140. Shore AC, et al. Posturally induced vasoconstriction in diabetes mellitus. *Arch Dis Child* 1994;70:22–26.
141. Silverman JJ, Powell VE. Simple technique for outlining sweat pattern. *War Med* 1945;7:178–180.
142. Smith AA, Dancis J. Exaggerated response to infused norepinephrine in familial dysautonomia. *N Engl J Med* 1964;270:704–707.
143. Smith JJ, et al. Hemodynamic response to the upright posture [Review]. *J Clin Pharmacol* 1994;34:375–386.
144. Smith SA, et al. Estimation of sinoaortic baroreceptor heart rate reflex sensitivity and latency in man: a new microcomputer assisted method of analysis. *Cardiovasc Res* 1986;20: 877–882.
145. Smyth HS, et al. Reflex regulation of arterial pressure during sleep in man: a quantitative method of assessing baroreflex sensitivity. *Circ Res* 1969;24:109–121.
146. So YT, et al. The role of thermography in the evaluation of lumbosacral radiculopathy. *Neurology* 1989;39:1154–1158.
147. Sprangers RL, et al. Initial circulatory responses to changes in posture: influence of the angle and speed of tilt. *Clin Physiol* 1991;11:211–220.
148. Stevens PM, Lamb LE. Effects of lower body negative pressure on the cardiovascular system. *Am J Cardiol* 1965;16:506–515.
149. Stewart JD, et al. Small-fiber peripheral neuropathy: diagnostic value of sweat tests and autonomic cardiovascular reflexes. *Ann Neurol* 1989;26:145A(abst).
150. Suarez GA, et al. Idiopathic autonomic neuropathy: clinical, neurophysiologic, and follow-up studies on 27 patients. *Neurology* 1994;44:1675–1682.
151. Takano H, et al. Atrophic nerve fibers in regions of reduced MIBG uptake in doxorubicin cardiomyopathy. *J Nucl Med* 1995;36:2060–2061.
152. Takeshima R, Dohi S. Circulatory responses to baroreflexes, Valsalva maneuver, coughing, swallowing, and nasal stimulation during acute cardiac sympathectomy by epidural blockade in awake humans. *Anesthesiology* 1985;63:500–508.
153. Taylor WF, et al. Cutaneous vascular responses to isometric handgrip exercise. *J Appl Physiol* 1989;66:1586–1592.
154. Ten Harkel ADJ, et al. Assessment of cardiovascular reflexes: influence of posture and period of preceding rest. *J Appl Physiol* 1990;68:147–153.
155. Thoren P. Role of cardiac vagal C-fibers in cardiovascular control [Review]. *Rev Physiol Biochem Pharmacol* 1979;86:1–94.
156. Torres NE, et al. Characterization of muscarinic receptor subtype of rat eccrine sweat gland by autoradiography. *Brain Res* 1991;550:129–132.
157. Trimarco B, et al. Valsalva maneuver in the assessment of baroreflex responsiveness in borderline hypertensives. *Cardiology* 1983;70:6–14.
158. Tsuchimochi S, et al. Age and gender differences in normal myocardial adrenergic neuronal function evaluated by iodine-123–MIBG imaging. *J Nucl Med* 1995;36:969–974.
159. Van Lieshout EJ, et al. Cardiovascular response to coughing: its value in the assessment of autonomic nervous control. *Clin Sci* 1989;77:305–310.
160. Van Lieshout EJ, et al. Monitoring of finger blood pressure. *J Neurol Neurosurg Psychiatry* 1987;50:503–504.
161. Van Lieshout JJ, et al. Acute dysautonomia associated with Hodgkin's disease. *J Neurol Neurosurg Psychiatry* 1986;49: 830–832 [erratum in *J Neurol Neurosurg Psychiatry* 1986;49:1461].
162. Van Lieshout JJ, et al. Pitfalls in the assessment of cardiovascular reflexes in patients with sympathetic failure but intact vagal control. *Clin Sci* 1989;76:523–528.
163. Van Oostayen JA, et al. Activity of Crohn disease assessed by measurement of superior mesenteric artery flow with Doppler US. *Radiology* 1994;193:551–554.
164. Vissing SF, Victor RG. Central motor command activates sympathetic outflow to the skin during static exercise. *Acta Physiol Scand* 1989;136(Suppl 584):44.
165. Wallin BG, Eckberg DL. Sympathetic transients caused by abrupt alterations of carotid baroreceptor activity in humans. *Am J Physiol* 1982;242:H185–H190.
166. Wallin BG, et al. Plasma noradrenaline correlates to sympathetic muscle nerve activity in normotensive man. *Acta Physiol Scand* 1981;111:69–73.
167. Webster J, et al. Influence of arm position on measurement of blood pressure. *BMJ* 1984;288:1574–1575.
168. Wei JY, Harris WS. Heart rate response to cough. *J Appl Physiol* 1982;53:1039–1043.
169. Wei JY, et al. Post-cough heart rate response: influence of age, sex and basal blood pressure. *Am J Physiol* 1983;245:R18–R24.
170. Wei K, et al. Association between QT dispersion and autonomic dysfunction in patients with diabetes mellitus. *J Am Coll Cardiol* 1995;26:859–863.

171. Wesseling KH, et al. Effects of peripheral vasoconstriction on the measurement of blood pressure in a finger. *Cardiovasc Res* 1985; 19:139–145.
172. Wesseling KH, et al. On the indirect registration of finger blood pressure after Penaz. *Funkt Biol Med* 1982;1:245–250.
173. Wexler L, et al. Velocity of blood flow in normal human venae cavae. *Circ Res* 1968;23:349–359.
174. Wheeler T, Watkins PJ. Cardiac denervation in diabetes. *BMJ* 1973;4:584–586.
175. Widdicombe JG. Mechanism of cough and its regulation [Review]. *Eur J Respir Dis* 1980;110(Suppl):11–20.
176. Ziegler D, et al. Prevalence of cardiovascular autonomic dysfunction assessed by spectral analysis, vector analysis, and standard tests of heart rate variation and blood pressure responses at various stages of diabetic neuropathy. *Diabetic Med* 1992;9:806–814.
177. Ziegler MQ, et al. The sympathetic nervous system defect in primary orthostatic hypotension. *N Engl J Med* 1977; 296:293–297.

CHAPTER 16

Laboratory Evaluation of Complex Regional Pain Syndrome

Catherine Willner and Phillip A. Low

1. This chapter briefly reviews pathophysiology, clinical features, laboratory evaluations, diagnostic considerations, and treatment modalities for the complex regional pain syndromes, also called reflex sympathetic dystrophy and causalgia.
2. The roles of the autonomic and somatic nervous systems, and of the vasomotor and local tissue control factors, in these clinical pain problems are complex and incompletely understood.
3. Animal models of various types of nerve injuries are beginning to provide further insight about these complex pain syndromes.
4. There are diagnostic pitfalls and disagreements about the characteristics and appropriate interventions in evaluating and caring for patients with these syndromes.
5. A distinction is still made between the syndromes on the basis of definable neural injury, but there are clearly border zones, where visceral or deeper tissue nerves may be injured but poorly detected.
6. Diagnostic criteria for these syndromes are evolving, but it is argued that they should include pain types, clinical symptoms, signs, and objective laboratory studies as well as operantly defined responses to treatments or interventions.
7. Sympathetically maintained pain is part of a group of characteristics that may or may not be present in a patient who meets other criteria for diagnosis of complex regional pain syndromes, and diagnostic sympatholytic procedures can result in more than sympathetic blockade, making the operant definition questionable.
8. Treatment options will be better defined when pathophysiological mechanisms are better understood. Well-controlled, blinded, and pain-categorized studies are few. Invasive and other treatments are briefly reviewed.
9. When pain is the predominant feature, control or relief, by a variety of means with normalization of the use of an affected limb is an optimal goal, but attempts should still be made to determine and document the efficacy of treatments used because some incur significant expense and potential risk to patients.
10. Physicians working with these complex problems are encouraged to participate in efforts aimed at better definition of diagnostic evaluations and studies of treatment modalities.

INTRODUCTION

The physiologic responses of the autonomic nervous system, and the sympathetic nervous system in particular, in relation to nociception and potential threat to the integrity of an organism are complex but fairly well understood and accepted. The responses observed to onset of acutely painful or threatening stimuli include an increase in sympathetic activity, measurable as tachycardia, hypertension, shift of blood flow to muscles for escape or defense (sometimes resulting in peripheral cutaneous vasospasm), and other accompaniments such as sweating, piloerection, and mydriasis (see Chapter 1). As is commonly discussed, these same generalized physiologic parameters are often not present in patients presenting with complaints of chronic

---

C. Willner and P. A. Low: Department of Neurology, Mayo Clinic, Rochester, Minnesota 55905.

pain, though alterations in functions usually considered to be modified by the autonomic system, such as limb temperature, perfusion, and sweating, are seen in many different circumstances long after there should have been somatic healing and resolution of a nociceptive response. The development of several specific models of neuropathic injury in animals has begun to unravel this physiology, but extensive discussion is beyond the scope of this chapter, which is directed at evaluation and treatment of people with chronic pain syndromes (6,34,50,63). Extensive studies of both the behaviors that appear to accompany neuropathic pain and a variety of parameters related to the peripheral microenvironment, neuropeptides, blood flow, and central nervous system alterations have been performed using several models of injury (1,6,13,21,62,64,78,79,95). For all the usual reasons related to translation of animal behavior to a subjective human experience such as pain, the insights provided to date are far from satisfying, but they provide some capability to delineate specific mechanisms, and they often show wide variability in physiologic changes, underscoring the complexity of the systems involved in pain and, where humans are concerned, suffering.

This chapter discusses the evaluation of patients who have significant pain, especially in a body region or limb, that is associated with physiologic signs that suggest abnormal functions usually to some degree regulated or controlled by the autonomic nervous system. These features are not confined to a single clinical diagnostic category. Critical discussion of the potential roles of the autonomic nervous system must include the recognition of the complex interrelationships of the somatic, visceral, and autonomic nervous systems, including plasticity of responses in the central nervous system, local tissue inflammatory, neuropeptide, and metabolic alterations, vasoregulation, and hormonal influences, as well as social, emotional, cultural, cognitive, and psychogenic issues. The complexities of the relationship of the microenvironment, perfusion, and the autonomic nervous system are only beginning to be explored in humans (37,57,80,81,88,91). Stipulations reminding us of the complexity of human physiology and experience are relevant to the discussion of any chronic or significant pain problem that persists beyond the anticipated time required to heal an injury (76). Dissatisfaction with the terminologies used to describe, define, and diagnose various pain syndromes is widely apparent and frustrates all physicians, caregivers, and patients because of the implications and assumptions imposed as we attempt to improve the functioning of patients with chronic refractory or recurrent pain complaints. This frustration, and the limitations of our understanding, should not justify classifying all chronic pain as "central" or somatiform, though criticisms are worthy of further review and debate (90).

The field of pain medicine continues to evolve rapidly, and because it includes multiple traditional medical disciplines, there is naturally a struggle to define acceptable terminology and practice. Though almost anyone asked has an opinion, there is usually great disagreement about the various pain syndromes with autonomic features. There is, however, at least some agreement that the naming of specific pain diagnoses should, for now, be more generalized and not assume identification of a specific pathology or mechanism (75,85). There is, however, reason to attempt to hypothesize potential mechanisms involved in maintaining specific types of pain in any clinical situation as an approach to identifying appropriate therapeutic options (24, 79). The approaches to patients who have pain complaints will, without doubt, change as better understanding of potential mechanisms involved in all chronic pain syndromes evolves. This bias toward a pathophysiologic focus is an idealistic goal but one worth aiming toward because of the cost to society and individuals of the extensive interventions often made available to patients with chronic pain. Potential alteration of the autonomic nervous system has been hypothesized to be involved in a variety of pain syndromes as different as chronic headaches and chronic pelvic pain of visceral origin and has lead to use of invasive procedures for sympatholysis that are not without risk and expense (9,14,16,27,30,33,43,44,46,48,49,67). The controversies involved are widely discussed in the literature (10,19,90). A partial list of potential mechanisms whereby the sympathetic nervous system might play a role in chronic pains is presented in Table 1, and the potential mechanisms are discussed extensively in several reviews (11,48,57, 65,74,79,82).

The focus of this chapter remains the evaluation and management of the syndromes previously termed causalgia and reflex sympathetic dystrophy. It is relevant to reemphasize that, if a list of clinical features were generated that included all the variations in physical change possible in response to injury or disuse because of pain or swelling, this list could come close to approximating the broader definitions that have been offered. The current taxonomy of the International Association for the Study of Pain (IASP) has designated these disorders to be included in the category of complex regional pain syndromes (CRPS), classifying type I as what used to be referred to as reflex sympa-

TABLE 1. *Potential pain mechanisms involving the sympathetic nervous system*

Adrenergic receptor modification (peripheral or central)
Denervation supersensitivity (circulating catecholamines)
Microcirculatory alterations (sympathetic "shunting")
Wide-dynamic-range neuron modification/upregulation
Cotransmittor alterations
Chronic inflammatory mediator modification
Upregulation or alternation of central sympathetic activity
    (loss of descending inhibition, or primary myelinated
    afferent inhibition, reorganization of central reflexes after
    partial deafferentation)

TABLE 2. *International Association for the Study of Pain Taxonomy*

Reflex sympathetic dystrophy

Definition	Continuous pain in a portion of an extremity after trauma that may include fracture but does not involve a major nerve; associated with sympathetic hyperactivity.
Site	Usually the distal extremity adjacent to a traumatized area.
System	Peripheral nervous system; possibly the central nervous system.
Main features	The pain follows trauma (usually mild), not associated with significant nerve injury; the pain is described as burning, continuous, exacerbated by movement, cutaneous stimulation, or stress. Onset usually weeks after injury.

Causalgia

Definition	Burning pain, allodynia, and hyperpathia, usually in the hand or foot, after partial injury of a nerve or one of its major branches.
Site	In the region of the limb innervated by the damaged nerve.
Main features	Onset usually immediately after partial nerve injury or may be delayed for months. Causalgia of the radial nerve is very rare. The nerves most commonly involved are the median, sciatic, tibial, and ulnar. Spontaneous pain, described as constant, burning; exacerbated by light touch, stress, temperature change, movement of involved limb, visual and auditory stimuli (e.g., a sudden sound or bright light), or emotional disturbances.

Complex Regional Pain Syndrome, Type I (Reflex Sympathetic Dystrophy) (I-4)

Definition	CRPS Type I is a syndrome that usually develops after an initiating noxious event, is not limited to the distribution of a single peripheral nerve, and is apparently disproportionate to the inciting event. It is associated at some point with evidence of edema, changes in skin blood flow, abnormal sudomotor activity in the region of the pain, or allodynia or hyperalgesia.
Site	Usually the distal aspect of an affected extremity or with a distal to proximal gradient.
System	Peripheral nervous system; possibly the central nervous system.
Main features	Pain often follows trauma, which is usually mild and is not associated with significant nerve injury. It may follow a fracture, a soft tissue lesion, or immobilization related to visceral disease, e.g., angina or stroke. The onset of symptoms usually occurs within one month of the inciting event. The pain is frequently described as burning and continuous and exacerbated by movement, continuous stimulation, or stress. The intensity of pain fluctuates over time, and allodynia or hyperalgesia may be found which are not limited to the territory of a single peripheral nerve. Abnormalities of blood flow occur including changes in skin temperature and color. Edema is usually present and may be soft or firm. Increased or decreased sweating may appear. The symptoms and signs may spread proximally or involve other extremities. Impairment of motor function is frequently seen.
Associated symptoms and signs	Atrophy of the skin, nails, and other soft tissues, alterations in hair growth, and loss of joint mobility may develop. Impairment of motor function can include weakness, tremor, and, in rare instances, dystonia. Symptoms and signs fluctuate at times. Sympathetically maintained pain may be present and may be demonstrated with pharmacological blocking or provocation techniques. Affective symptoms or disorders occur secondary to the pain and disability. Guarding of the affected part is usually observed.
Laboratory findings	Noncontact skin temperature measurement indicates a side-to-side asymmetry of greater than 1°C. Due to the unstable nature of the temperature changes in this disorder, measurements at different times are recommended. Measurements of skin blood flow may show an increase or a reduction. Testing of sudomotor function, both at rest and evoked, indicates side-to-side asymmetry. The bone uptake phase of a three-phase bone scan may reveal a characteristic pattern of subcutaneous blood pool changes. Radiographic examination may demonstrate patchy bone demineralization.
Usual course	Variable.
Relief	In cases with sympathetically maintained pain, sympatholytic interventions may provide temporary or permanent pain relief.
Complications	Phlebitis, inappropriate drug use, and suicide.
Social and physical impairment	Inability to perform activities of daily living and occupational and recreational activities.
Pathology	Unknown.
Diagnostic criteria	1. The presence of an initiating noxious event, or a cause of immobilization. 2. Continuing pain, allodynia, or hyperalgesia with which the pain is disproportionate to any inciting event. 3. Evidence at some time of edema, changes in skin blood flow, or abnormal sudomotor activity in the region of the pain. 4. This diagnosis is excluded by the existence of conditions that would otherwise account for the degree of pain and dysfunction. Note: Criteria 2–4 must be satisfied.
Differential diagnosis	CRPS Type II (causalgia) unrecognized local pathology (e.g., fracture, strain, sprain), traumatic vasospasm, cellulitis, Raynaud's disease, thromboangiitis obliterans, thrombosis.

From IASP (44,45), with permission.

TABLE 3. *Proposed definition of reflex sympathetic dystrophy and causalgia (abbreviated)*

Definition
A syndrome of continuous diffuse limb pain, often burning in nature and usually consequent to injury or noxious stimulus and disuse, presenting with variable sensory, motor, autonomic, and trophic changes; causalgia represents a specific presentation of reflex sympathetic dystrophy associated with peripheral nerve injury.

Clinical features
The symptoms and changes spread independently of both the source and site of the precipitating event, presenting with a glove-and-stocking anatomic distribution. Clinical findings include disturbances of

Autonomic deregulation: alterations in blood flow, hyper/hypohidrosis, edema.
Sensory abnormalities: hypo/hyperesthesias, allodynia to cold, and mechanical stimulation.
Motor dysfunction: weakness, tremor, joint stiffness.
Trophic changes: skin, hair, nails.
Psychological reactive disturbances: anxiety, depression, hopelessness (as with other chronic pain patients).

These features manifest diffusely but not necessarily uniformly in the entire distal extremity. They occur at a variable time after the onset of the syndrome, spreading proximally and occasionally to the opposite side as the syndrome progresses. Dominating symptoms are spontaneous pain, swelling, and weakness.

Diagnostic tests
Autonomic: bilateral symmetrical, multidigital temperature measures by surface thermistors or thermography show consistent discrepancies (cooler or warmer) on the affected side.
Sensory: lowered thresholds to pinprick, light touch, and cold.
Motor: reduced measures of strength as well as active and passive range of motion.
Block response: sympathetic block usually abolishes diffuse burning pain and allodynia, also raises skin temperature to 35°–36°C, and abolishes the vasoconstrictor response to cold stimulation.
Bone scan: three-phase scanning shows distinctive diffuse patterns of altered flow, pooling, and delayed periarticular uptake or decreased flow.

Nonspecific confirmatory tests can be used to further quantify changes and follow progress. These include radiographic densitometry testing of osteopenia and water displacement plethysmography for measures of swelling, plus tests of sudomotor function, such as skin conductivity or potentials, or quantitative sweat testing.

Adapted from Abram et al. (2), with permission.

---

thetic dystrophy and type II as what previously was called causalgia (identified nerve injury). Both the previous and the current classifications of CRPS Type I (because of length) are delineated in Table 2 (45) and discussed widely (2,10,66,68,71,80). Emphasis remains that these are diagnoses of exclusion, which require that a treating physician identify reversible pathology, including large or small vessel occlusion, nonhealing fracture, infections, and inflammatory or connective tissue diseases. Identification of any of these processes essentially excludes the diagnosis of a CRPS. However, it must be remembered that the autonomic nervous system may still play a role in the maintenance of pain under these circumstances. Treatment must be focused first, however, on any primary underlying process.

This chapter is divided into two primary sections: diagnostic considerations and treatment modalities. It is hoped that the reader will appreciate the presentation of these topics as a common ground for continued research to improve the care rendered to all patients with chronic pain.

DIAGNOSTIC CONSIDERATIONS

The IASP criteria for CRPS are clinical, descriptive, and intended not to imply mechanism or causality. It is argued by some that no specific tests are useful for diagnosis. However, for purposes of attempting better delineation of the pathophysiology, it is still relevant to classify the symptoms, signs, and laboratory changes more specifically as outlined in Table 3, which is an older proposed definition of RSD. These clinical features are likely a natural part of healing of many injuries, but the course and evolution of such changes as they become more chronic are not well documented and epidemiologic studies are lacking. The original descriptions of clinical stages and degrees of severity are important to acknowledge but may relate more to failure to remobilize an extremity than to a specific pathophysiology (77). The development of significant pain and vasomotor changes in a limb usually seeming more severe than warranted by the initial insult heralds consideration of the diagnosis of CRPS type I. With nerve or radicular involvement documented, the classification is CRPS type II.

Clinical Presentations

The development of diffuse and usually spontaneous pain, often described as burning, throbbing, or intensely aching, is characteristic. It often differs from the pain of an original injury or surgical healing. The symptoms are often exacerbated by a dependent position or movement of the extremity. The responses to external changes in temperature, emotions, and spontaneous variability should be reviewed with the patient. The severity of the pain(s) should be rated especially as this relates to responses to treatments. Use of a visual analogue scale or other measurements of pain severity can be helpful. Examination findings include several features: hyperpathia (i.e., an exaggerated response to painful stimuli), allodynia (i.e., the perception of usually nonpainful stimuli as painful), summation (persistent or increasing pain after repeated stimuli), and subjectively abnormal sensory perceptions are often present. Although the

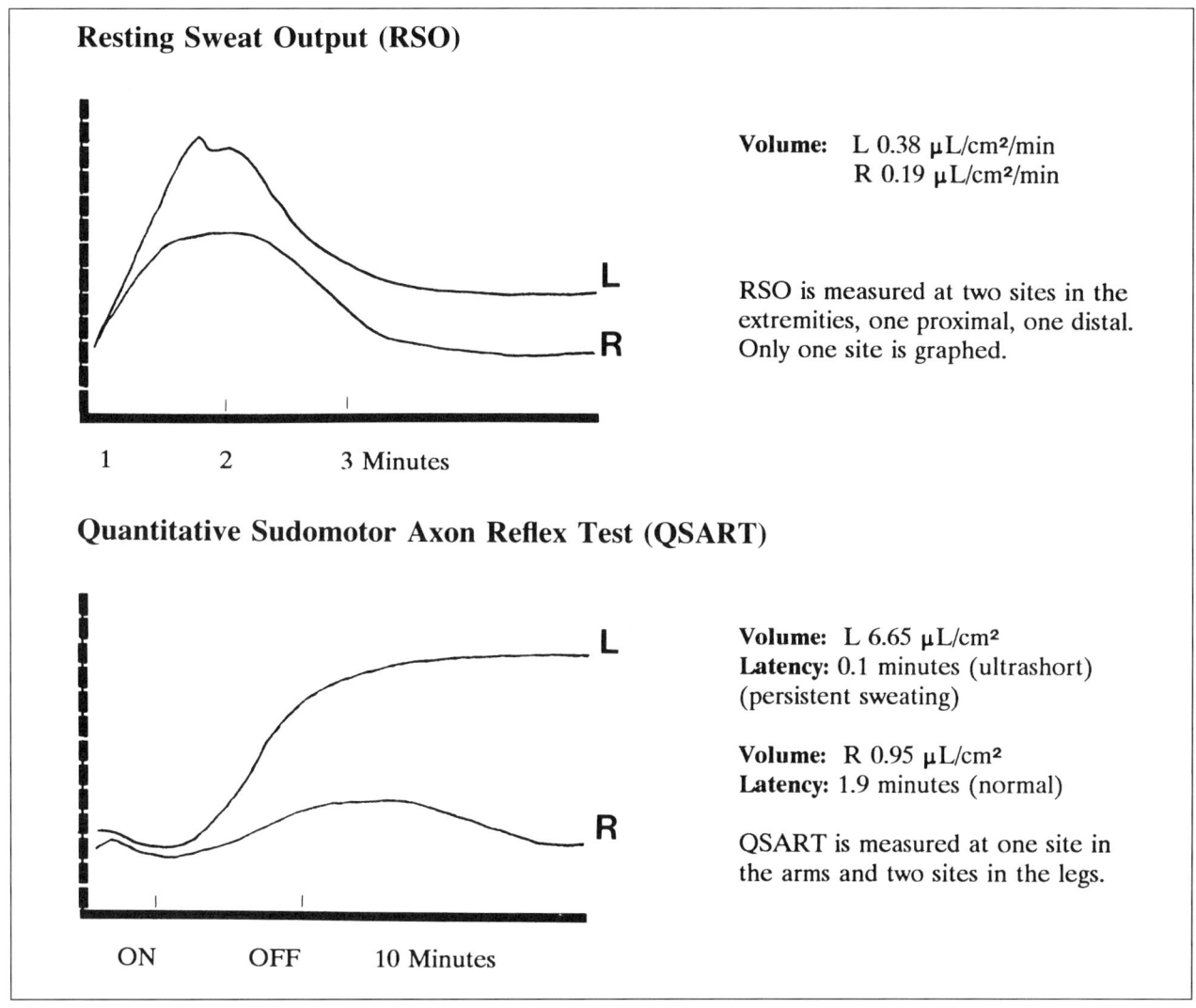

FIG. 1. Example of part of the laboratory studies performed on a 30-year-old woman with a 5-month history of left leg pain. The left leg was 5°C cooler diffusely, more prominent distally. Pain was burning and diffuse; there was allodynia to touch and to cold greater than hot, though temperature discrimination was poor.

sensory examinations of these patients are difficult and tedious to perform, they should be undertaken and meticulously documented. Given the degree of swelling that is often present, it is tempting to attribute these changes to difference in skin thickness, to edema, or to altered perfusion, but this is probably an oversimplification. An accurate and detailed sensory examination is also a prerequisite for documentation of peripheral nerve injury to classify the condition appropriately.

The features that most obviously indict the autonomic nervous system in these disorders are vasomotor instability and sudomotor instability. Changes in the patterns of temperature control, blood flow, and sweating may at various times resemble sympathetic hyperactivity or hypoactivity in individual patients. There may also be confounding features suggesting a mixed picture of autonomic function. Attempts to define a course or natural progression for these features often yield unpredictable results. More importantly, whether these changes are primary or secondary to the processes causing the pain remains uncertain.

Motor symptoms, including posturing, tremulousness, or even dystonia, remain controversial, and motor examination is often completely compromised by limb protection and posture. Reflexes can be hyperactive simply on this basis, so if absent in a specific pattern, they may point to identification of a peripheral nerve or root injury. The reduction in spontaneous movement could be due to a variety of factors, including simply pain or edema, but other explanations cannot be completely excluded. Opinions about the causes of these findings range from central or segmental motor disturbances to purely psychogenic syndromes. An interesting hypothesis about neglect has recently been pre-

TABLE 4. *Kozin's criteria for reflex sympathetic dystrophy*

Definite reflex sympathetic dystrophy
Pain and tenderness in the distal extremity
Signs and/or symptoms of vasomotor instability
Swelling in the extremity—often with periarticular prominence
(Dystrophic skin changes usually present)

Probably reflex sympathetic dystrophy
Pain and tenderness
 and
Vasomotor instability
 or
Swelling
No pain, but mild to moderate tenderness may be present
(Dystrophic skin changes occasionally present)

Doubtful reflex sympathetic dystrophy
Unexplained pain and tenderness in an extremity

Compiled from Kozin et al. (53–55).

TABLE 5. *Putative diagnostic criteria for reflex sympathetic dystrophy[a]*

Clinical symptoms and signs
Burning pain
Hyperpathia/allodynia
Temperature/color changes
Edema
Hair/nail growth changes

Laboratory results
Thermometry/thermography
Bone x-ray studies
Three-phase bone scan
Quantitative sweat test
Response to sympathetic blockade

Interpretation
>6 Probable RSD
3–5 Possible RSD
<3 Unlikely RSD

RSD, reflex sympathetic dystrophy.
[a]As proposed by Wilson (94), modified from Gibbons et al. (28a).

sented (26). Until these features are better delineated (perhaps in animal models of causalgia), it remains pertinent to document the changes present and characterize changes in response to treatments that have been reported (96).

Laboratory Studies

Supplementary to clinical examination findings, the documentation of asymmetry of skin temperature, as measured by infrared thermometry or thermography, can define patterns of cutaneous blood flow. Responses to thermal challenge can also be measured. In our laboratory, the patient is unclothed in the area of interest (symmetrically), the patient's surface temperature is allowed to equilibrate to room temperature, and two separate temperature measurements are recorded. Patients are asked to remain indoors for at least 30 min before coming to the laboratory and to refrain from using substances such as nicotine, caffeine, and certain medications that have vasoactive effects. Use of transcutaneous electrical nerve stimulation, central nervous system stimulators, compressive garments, or splints is prohibited on the day of the test when possible. A temperature asymmetry of at least 1°C is considered significant. However, caution about overinterpretation of thermographic results is warranted because, for example, it has been demonstrated that patients can control this variable through methods such as biofeedback (84). We have also seen clear cases where proximal constrictive garments have been used to produce swelling in factitious disorders. The pattern of changes on thermography usually documents the site and pattern of constriction, and careful physical examination will usually confirm this suspicion.

The degree of swelling can also be measured, either by circumferential comparison or by water displacement. Any skin discoloration, and any variable and observed environmental influence or internal precipitants (i.e., pain changes), are recorded in the patient record.

Alterations in sudomotor function are quantified by both the resting sweat output and the quantitative sudomotor axon reflex test (QSART) (61). Examples of these recordings are presented in Fig. 1. The interpretation of these variables—resting skin temperature, resting sweat output, and QSART (response to acetylcholine iontophoresis)—is based on asymmetry of results between limbs and on the proximal-to-distal changes observed in one limb. The presence of ultrashort latencies on the QSART studies is frequently seen in patients with pain and is considered important to document. Retrospective blinded analysis of these data relative to a simpler clinical diagnosis of reflex sympathetic dystrophy (in older terminology but using published criteria) has suggested correlation of both resting and stimulated sudomotor changes with prediction of a clinical diagnosis and possibly responsiveness to sympatholytic procedures (16). Correlation of skin temperature changes tended to predict response to sympathetic blockade (warmer symptomatic limb, but this also usually correlated with shorter duration of symptoms). Interpretation of these data is limited because they represent retrospective analysis and the numbers undergoing sympatholytic treatment were small enough to make conclusions less than reassuring. That no true placebo or sham procedures were performed is only one primary reason for this concern about interpretation related to treatment (see below).

Other studies that are often considered include electrophysiologic testing. Unfortunately, just as the motor exam is poorly tolerated, electrophysiologic studies including electromyography and somatosensory evoked potentials are also often poorly tolerated and technically limited by patients' difficulties in cooperating. Study findings that are abnormal obviously assist in classifying CRPS into type I or II if this is not already obvious clinically.

Findings on plain radiographic studies can include patchy periarticular osteoporosis or more diffuse demineralization (39). In the lower extremities, these changes may correlate better with disuse and non-weight-bearing. Metabolic bone diseases need to be considered in the differential diagnoses related to these radiographic findings (42). Radionuclide scintigraphy documenting early blood flow and pooling as well as delayed uptake is referred to as the three-phase bone scan. The clinical criteria for diagnosis and interpretation of findings are traditionally those of Kozin et al., outlined in Table 4 (53–55). The traditional interpretation defined positive results as reduced early blood flow (first phase), asymmetry of pooling (second phase), and an increase in the periarticular uptake in the late, or third, phase. Findings in a retrospective study assessing factors that affect sensitivity and specificity in 63 patients who had undergone imaging as part of the diagnostic evaluation for unexplained upper-extremity pain, using the criteria of Kozin et al., suggested a substantial increase in sensitivity for patients who had had symptoms for <6 months (64% versus 50% in patients with symptoms for >6 months), with specificity not affected (94% versus 96%, respectively) (93). This same group of investigators also looked at the predictive value of the three-phase bone scan in a retrospective review of 119 patients and found that the results of early phases (blood flow and pooling) really only improved the sensitivity of lower-extremity studies, whereas use of only the later uptake images was adequate for upper-extremity pain diagnosis (18). These and the other earlier statistics regarding sensitivity and specificity are difficult to interpret because of the relatively small numbers of patients who met the clinical criteria for the diagnosis. Larger studies with higher prevalence of pain and the older clinical diagnosis of reflex sympathetic dystrophy have suggested higher sensitivity indices (93). Recent reviews of the predictive value, though, have reemphasized the wide variability in the literature and suggested that these changes not be included in the clinical diagnosis criteria so far as the upper extremities are concerned (59). Bone scans can, however, identify other explanations for pain such as stress or occult fractures, infections, or inflammatory processes that require different interventions than simply analgesia. Some variations of presentation in the pediatric population have been described (32).

For purposes of consistent data interpretation, though still utilizing "older" terminology, we favor specific identification of the pain types and severities, autonomic symptoms, exam findings, and ancillary lab data as outlined in Table 5. This approach permits the most accurate method for assessing interventions and outcome-based studies. Acceptance of the newer terminology of CRPS simply serves to reinforce how much is left to learn about chronic pain associated with apparent autonomic accompaniments.

TREATMENT MODALITIES

The variety of modalities used in the treatment of pain syndromes with autonomic features serves as a reminder about two important points. First, there are likely multiple mechanisms underlying similar symptomatic complaints and clinical findings and, second, we are not yet skilled enough to ascertain specific pathophysiology to target treatment with universal efficacy. Historically, the more recent literature addressing the regional pain syndromes has yielded attempts to discriminate pains that are sympathetically maintained from those that are not. This has, in a simplistic fashion, been done on the basis of circular reasoning by operant definition. If a patient had an even partial response to some type of intervention purported to be sympatholytic, then the pain could be called sympathetically maintained. A variety of research-supported mechanisms hypothetically explain how the sympathetic nervous system might maintain or alter pain perception and experience (see Table 1), but the system itself is complex and not different from the somatic nervous system to any great degree in that both peripheral and central as well as dynamic factors need to be considered. Unfortunately, the types of treatments argued to produce sympatholysis are really not always purely affecting the sympathetic nervous system. The wide differences in opinions about these issues are argued heatedly in the pain literature. Some of the obvious concerns are addressed as each topic is visited. The major criticism is often simply that patients with chronic pain syndromes are perhaps even more likely to be placebo responders than the general population. This remains to be proven but is not a minor point when considering the efficacy of invasive procedures. The same caveats emphasized in this chapter in the first edition remain important. Ideally, if patients could be separated according to specific symptom complexes that were completely control matched, then treatments would be easier to judge. Efforts are further along in this regard, but only in relation to pain types such as allodynia in response to specific treatment modalities. To control for all of the variables related to the somatic, autonomic, and psychosocial axes while studying anatomic and physiologic parameters is a formidable task, but obviously this significantly impacts interpretation of treatment outcomes. The same criticisms related to existing data apply: (a) diagnostic criteria are not uniform, (b) series are often small and uncontrolled, (c) measures of outcome are vaguely defined (i.e., pain reduction is not clarified as to pain type), and (d) follow-up studies are constricted or absent. The point was made previously that the presence or absence of nerve injury (hence the designation of type I versus type II in the categories of CRPS) likely affects long-term prognosis (47). And the issue of visceral, vascular, or articular nerve injury remains an issue and is not easily ascertained with usual electrophysiologic studies. In our clinical studies, it seems reasonable to hypothesize that patients with reduced QSART responses in a colder affected limb likely are exhibiting loss of small fiber function (and possibly upregulation or denervation hypersensitivity to circulating catecholamines). Studies looking at catecholamines and cotransmitters like neuropeptide Y and other parameters of the microenvironment at painful sites will hopefully provide a better understanding of alterations in the peripheral tissue, nociceptors, and altered receptor function. As mentioned in opening paragraphs, the neural injury models of Bennett and Xie (6) among others, demonstrate the wide variability of these substrates in relationship to behavioral responses purported to represent neuropathic pain symptoms, but they are yielding data about treatment outcomes, including sympatholysis and various medications available for use in humans.

The opinions about appropriateness of available treatments are slowly shifting but still ultimately depend on a patient's point of entry into the medical system, recognition of the potential diagnosis and, often, personal bias that is sometimes simply related to the physician's specific discipline. A sentiment that is verbalized frequently (though not specifically tested in a controlled fashion) in circles of physicians caring for patients with chronic pain syndromes involving the limbs and meeting the criteria of CRPS is that any modality which reduces subjective pain enough to remobilize the limb to normalize its use is the most successful approach. The sooner this is done after the onset of symptoms, the better.

Discussion of specific therapeutic modalities is separated into categories somewhat along the lines of medical disciplines. It must be emphasized that well-controlled trials proving efficacy are rare, though the literature is replete with anecdotal and case presentation data. Extensive reviews are available (60,82,83,94). The order of presentation and the extent of discussion are not intended to imply any ranking of treatment selection, though it is likely now generally agreed that physical therapy to remobilize a painful limb is paramount to recovery when it occurs. Medications are discussed last because decisions about which ones might be useful are sometimes derived from other interventions such as invasive blocks or infusions.

Physical Modalities

The mainstays of physical therapy techniques are the reduction of swelling and the normalization of temperature and limb use patterns. Techniques include methods to attempt pain reduction but also programs for desensitization, which, in practice, often initially worsen the subjective experience of pain. Specific modalities used include such approaches as use of passive and active range of motion, massage, ultrasound, transcutaneous electrical nerve stimulation, cutaneous desensitization with brisk rubs, light touch, and contrast baths (i.e., alternating exposure to cold and heat at specific temperatures). Additionally, thermal and myofascial biofeedback, relaxation and stress management techniques, and a variety of other therapies have been reported to be useful (5,38,92). Extensive reviews of these therapies are available, though they tend to engender many of the same criticisms directed toward other interventions, cited above.

Invasive Procedures

These techniques are generally performed by physicians specifically trained in their use. Procedures available include a number of different approaches: myofascial injections (trigger points), nerve blocks, intravenous procedures, acupuncture, ablative surgical techniques, and implantable stimulatory or infusion pump devices. For specific technical discussions regarding procedures, the reader is referred elsewhere (1,3,17,70,75).

Sympathetic Blocks

The original concept of interfering with the autonomic nervous system to attempt to control causalgic pain probably stems from the surgical denervation of periarterial neural plexuses (68). The instillation of a local anesthetic agent at the site of sympathetic ganglia remains a frequently used technique, though there are numerous theoretical reasons why use of these procedures has been called into question. Documentation of efferent sympathetic blockade by recording a rise in temperature of the limb and reduction of hyperhidrosis, when present, helps to confirm a technically successful block; however, the interpretation of these results is not without controversy (7). Because of the complexity of the anatomy at the most frequently blocked sites (the stellate ganglion for upper extremities and the L2–4 paravertebral chain for the lower extremities), the possible contribution of somatic overflow block is often not documented nor even considered. At the stellate site, development of Horner's syndrome is often considered evidence of successful blockade, but this can occur without change in the temperature or autonomic function of the limb. The meaning of pain relief in this setting is of uncertain significance so far as pathologic mechanisms are concerned. In one study (29), morphine injected at the site of the usual stellate block reportedly did not result in any symptomatic improvement. Documentation of a change in the subjective perception of pain or sensory complaints, duration of the changes, and the relationship to evolution of the results of the block can sometimes provide useful guidance for future therapies. For example, if a block achieves very brief pain relief, but the technical results of the block last for hours, it is difficult to argue that this pain is "sympathetically maintained." If one is to assess the usefulness of these or any procedures applied to the care of these patients, it is of paramount importance to document any changes in all of the features of the syndrome described by the patients. This is a time-consuming task and often only possible in the strictest of research settings, and choices about methodologies to document sympatholysis vary (8).

Successful sympathetic blockade may reduce only certain features of a patient's pain, but this finding can be useful in unmasking other underlying abnormalities that may be contributing to (or inciting) the autonomic features. The physiologic effect of efferent sympathetic blockade is a combination of vasodilatation, reduction in norepinephrine release with potential change in blood flow, tissue perfusion, and alteration of the microenvironment that can affect multiple somatic and neuroreceptor functions, all of which might alter pain in an extremity (20,65,82). Sympatholysis has been reported to alter some of the signs attributed to neuropathic pain in rat neural injury models (51).

Regional Intravenous Blockades

This technique, which is often referred to as the Bier block, involves placement of a tourniquet to isolate the systemic blood flow physiologically in the distal extremity and then introduction of pharmacologically active medications into the venous circulation at that site (35). Guanethidine, the use of which was reported in early studies, is no longer available (36), but a wide variety of substances have been tried, including steroids, local anesthetics, reserpine, bretylium, and droperidol (7,22,23,35,50). Of importance, studies using droperidol failed to show efficacy, but using a small sample, which was randomized and cross-controlled, the investigators reported patients who claimed pain relief when saline and heparin (placebo) alone were instilled (50). This is noteworthy because the prolonged application of the tourniquet itself is not comfortable. One can question whether there is some relative large fiber block from compression, or whether there is simply reduction of pain following release from the discomfort of the procedure. The possible role of heparin as part of the placebo in relation to this report is uncertain.

Intravenous Infusions

Systemic sympatholytic procedures have been recently advocated, including the use of intravenous phentolamine, a short-acting α-blocker (3,70). The arguments waged for use of this approach are related to ease of administration and relative safety, but compromised by the difficulty in blocking all side effects for the purposes of placebo control and certainly limited on the basis of the of the substance's expense, which, at this writing, still exceeds the usual cost of a sympathetic block. In certain pain clinic settings, this approach has been expanded to include sequential administration of a number of pharmacologically active medications, including lidocaine and narcotics in addition to phentolamine, which in usual protocols also calls for use of β-blockers to prevent some of the inevitable side effects of isolated α-blockade. These techniques are widely discussed elsewhere and, though theoretically intriguing, they remain to be thoroughly tested specifically as related to the prediction of long-term response to treatments they purportedly mimic (25,89). Even on just theoretical grounds, it can be argued that systemic administration of a medication may imply that more is occurring than just peripheral sympathetic blockade, which obviously must impact interpretations about the meaning of response to these interventions. Whether response to systemic intravenous sympathetic blockers correlates to response to oral sympatholytics remains to be documented in a large controlled study.

Somatic (or Mixed) Blocks

Because peripheral nerves vary in the number of sympathetic and nociceptive (as well as motor and sensory) fibers they carry, discussion of specific peripheral nerve blocks is beyond the scope of this chapter. However, a few useful guiding principles are worth mentioning. Because nerve fibers differ in their sensitivity to local anesthetics (both in degree and duration of effective block), these procedures can sometimes be helpful in diagnosing the pain source. If a proximal (epidural or spinal) block is used, the level of the block and type of anesthetic used can result in different effects on the somatic and sympathetic systems (58,86). Thus, to reach diagnostic conclusions from the use of these blocks, it is crucial to carry out preblock and postblock evaluations of motor, cutaneous, and autonomic functions over time as they relate the patient's symptoms and signs. This is also a tedious process.

In general, smaller (C) fibers, including somatic nociceptive and autonomic fibers, are blocked first, and the effect lasts longer than that of larger myelinated somatic fibers (87). Motor function may also return before somatic cutaneous function. It can be helpful to determine whether the pain is affected only when all fibers are blocked or whether it returns when cutaneous sensation in response to pinprick or temperature is restored. The reverse order of fiber sensitivity is described for compressive blocks (which relates to the preceding discussion about Bier blocks). These diagnostic approaches were used in an attempt to define the role of mechanoreceptors in the production of allodynia (12,87). Many research questions are being explored in this regard. Obviously, use of these techniques requires time-consuming methods to establish their relative efficacy. Establishing the appropriate role of these invasive techniques requires better controlled scientific studies. In the clinical setting at this time, it is easy to argue that if a few sympathetic block procedures assist the patient to recover that they are appropriate and beneficial. This argument falls short when one attempts to justify the continued use (for example, we have seen patients who have received over a hundred such procedures with nonsustained benefits). Similar caution applies to the use of indwelling catheters for administration epidurally (or rarely intrathecally in the acute setting) of narcotics, anesthetics, or other pharmacologically active substances. Repeated use of invasive procedures of any type is potentially harmful to both the tissues and the nerves, so the benefits must be weighed against these risks. It is our opinion that blocks without remobilization are contraindicated and that their usefulness is limited.

Surgeries and Implantable Devices

In addition to placement of temporary epidural catheters, implantation of tunneled ports for intrathecal administration of medications is sometimes advocated, primarily for narcotics. Implantable spinal cord stimulators are also sometimes suggested and, as techniques for percutaneous introduction have become more widely known, use of these expensive devices has become more popular. Their long-term efficacy is reported as high in some hands, but good long-term multicenter studies are lacking. These procedures are debated in the pain and neurosurgical literature and are not discussed further here (4,33). Having waxed and waned in popularity over the years, surgical sympathectomy is only rarely indicated, and many patients seem to report complications such as pain at the margin of the sympathectomy or, in the leg, pain of lumbar plexopathy, perhaps related to the surgical approaches (9,40,56,63). Caution in interpretation of case reports is warranted especially as new techniques for percutaneous sympatholysis become more widely available (75).

Medications

The variety of pharmacologic approaches used in the setting of the diagnostic criteria of CRPS also emphasizes the relative lack of complete understanding of these disorders. In general, polypharmacy is the rule, simple analgesics usually afford minimal benefits, and other analgesic adjuvants help sometimes but not consistently. These substances range from α-blocking and vasoactive substances like phenoxybenzamine and calcium channel blockers to purported anti-inflammatory medications like steroids (and nonsteroidal anti-inflammatory drugs) to adjuvants normally belonging to classes of neurotransmitter modulators like the antidepressants or membrane-active medications like the oral anesthetics and anticonvulsants. Obviously, there is overlap in activity. The ready acceptance and use of this widely varying pharmacopoeia simply emphasize our frustration with specific successful treatments. Often the goal is symptom management more than true analgesia. Extensive discussion of each of these is beyond the scope of this chapter. All of the usual criticisms about controlled studies apply. There are trials reportedly ongoing with use of the newer (wider spectrum than selective serotonin reuptake inhibitors) neurotransmitter modulators like Zoloft (Effexor) and tramadol (Ultram) (which has μ-agonist activity somewhat like desipramine), and planned studies are anticipated with medications in the anticonvulsant classes, including Neurontin and Lamictal. These agents have been suggested to be useful in reducing presumed pain behaviors in animal models of neuropathic pain (1) (G. Bennett, personal communication). In an early review (41), symptoms were reportedly worsened with use of barbiturates.

The studies reporting efficacy of steroids, especially the early studies using the criteria of Kozin et al., were not placebo controlled and other forms of intervention were not disclosed, but there was some evidence for accelerated return of function and pain reduction (53,54,82). Calcitonin treatment has been advocated in small studies suggesting that when administered subcutaneously (100 units of salmon calcitonin daily for 3 weeks), and in comparison to physical therapy alone, the treatment was beneficial (30,31,72). Phenoxybenzamine has been reported to be effective in reducing pain and edema when the drug is administered in doses ranging from 40 to 120 mg/day over 4–6 weeks. Unfortunately, little information about the actual criteria for diagnosis and the pain features was delineated (28). Use of calcium channel blockers has also been studied, although no results of well-controlled trials with careful standards of diagnosis have been published. The findings in one series of 13 patients treated with nifedipine (with a dosage that was increased gradually from 10 to 30 mg t.i.d.) suggested that about half of the patients experienced symptom improvement ranging from reduction of burning pain and dysesthesias to improvement in cold intolerance (69). Whether these changes correlated with actual objective changes in tissue perfusion was not specified.

Case reports previously listed, including the use of phenytoin, nitroglycerin, dimethylsulfoxide, and various opiates and antidepressants, have been expanded to include the use of electroconvulsive therapy (ECT) (15,43,52,82).

CONCLUSION

This chapter has focused briefly on the diagnosis and treatment of a complex group of disorders. There are obvious gaps in this discussion, including the conspicuous absence of comments regarding the psychological profiles of these patients, absence of opinion about the concept of pain symptom spread, and no mention of possible genetic or hereditary predisposition to the development of chronic pain with autonomic changes. Interested readers should review the basic science literature as it pertains to nociception, neurogenic function in chronic inflammation, and the current chronic pain models. The potential roles of the autonomic nervous system in production, maintenance, or alteration of pain perception are only beginning to be understood at the cellular level. Even more intriguing is that many of the features considered part of the traditional descriptions of CRPS can occur in patients without complaints of pain. It is hoped that better controlled trials, which are under way, of clinical interventions will offer insight into the appropriate utilization of health care resources for patients with such difficult and chronic syndromes as those discussed.

REFERENCES

1. Abram SE, Yaksh TL. Systemic lidocaine blocks nerve injury induced hyperalgesia and nociceptor driven spinal sensitization in the rat. *Anesthesiology* 1994;80:383–391.
2. Abram SE, et al. Proposed definition of reflex sympathetic dystrophy. In: Stanton-Hicks M, et al., eds. *Reflex sympathetic dystrophy.* Boston: Kluwer, 1989:207–210.
3. Arner S. Intravenous phentolamine test: diagnostic and prognostic use in RSD. *Pain* 1991;46:17–22.
4. Barolat G, Schwartzman R, Woo R. Epidural spinal cord stimulation in the management of reflex sympathetic dystrophy. *Stereotact Funct Neorosurg* 1989;53:29–39.
5. Barowsky EI, Zweig JB, Moskowitz J. Thermal biofeedback in the treatment of symptoms associated with reflex sympathetic dystrophy. *J Child Neurol* 1987;2:229–232.
6. Bennett GJ, Xie Y. A peripheral mononeuropathy in rat that produces disorders of pain like those seen in man. *Pain* 1988;33:87–107.
7. Benson HT, Chomka CM, Brunner EA. Treatment of reflex sympathetic dystrophy with regional intravenous reserpine. *Anesth Analg* 1980;59:500–502.
8. Benson HT, et al. Sign of complete sympathetic blockade: sweat test or sympathogalvanic response? *Anesth Analg* 1985;64:415–419.
9. Bergan JJ, Conn J, Jr. Sympathectomy for pain relief. *Med Clinic North Am* 1968;52:145–159.
10. Bonica JJ. Causalgia and other reflex sympathetic dystrophies. New York: Raven, 1979 (Bonica JJ, ed; *Advances in pain research and therapy;* vol 3).
11. Campbell JN, Meyer RA, Raja SN. Is nociceptor activation by alpha-1 adrenoreceptors the culprit in sympathetically maintained pain? *Am Pain Soc* 1992;1:3–11.
12. Campbell JN, et al. Myelinated afferents signal the hyperalgesia associated with nerve injury. *Pain* 1988;32:89–94.
13. Chaball D, Russell LC, Burchiel KJ. The effect of intravenous lidocaine, tocainide and mexiletine on spontaneously active fibers originating in rat sciatic neuromas. *Pain* 1988;38:333–338.
14. Chalkley JE, Lander C, Rowlingson JC. Probable reflex sympathetic dystrophy of the penis. *Pain* 1986;25:223–225.
15. Chaturvedi SK. Phenytoin in reflex sympathetic dystrophy. *Pain* 1989;36:379–380.
16. Chelimsky TC, et al. Value of autonomic testing in RSD. *Mayo Clin Proc* 1995;70:1029–1040.
17. Cousin MJ, Bridenbaugh PO, eds. *Neural blockade in clinical anesthesia and management of pain.* 2nd ed. Philadelphia: Lippincott, 1988:7–14.
18. Davidoff G, et al. Predictive value of the three-phase technetium bone scan in diagnosis of the reflex sympathetic dystrophy syndrome. *Arch Phys Med Rehabil* 1989;70:135–137.
19. Dellemijn PLI, et al. The interpretation of pain relief and sensory changes following sympathetic blockade. *Brain* 1994;117:1475–1487.
20. Devor M. Nerve pathophysiology and mechanisms of pain in causalgia. *JANS* 1983;7:371–384.
21. Devor M, Janig W, Michaelis M. Modulation of activity in dorsal root ganglion neurons by sympathetic activation in nerve injured rats. *J Neurophysiol* 1994;71:38–47.
22. Duncan KH, et al. Treatment of upper extremity reflex sympathetic dystrophy with joint stiffness using sympatholytic Bier blocks and manipulation. *Orthopedics* 1988;11:883–886.
23. Ford AU, Forrest WH, Eltherington L. The treatment of reflex sympathetic dystrophy with intravenous regional bretylium. *Anesthesiology* 1988;68:137–140.
24. Galer BS. Neuropathic pain of peripheral origin: advances in pharmacologic treatment. *Neorology* 1995;45(Suppl 9):S17–S25.
25. Galer BS. Peak pain relief is delayed and duration of relief is extended following intravenous phentolamine infusion: preliminary report. *Reg Anaesth* 1995;20:444–447.
26. Galer BS, Butler S, Jensen MP. Case reports and hypothesis: a neglect-like syndrome may be responsible for the motor disturbance in reflex sympathetic dystrophy (CRPS-I). *J Pain Symptom Manage* 1995;10:385–391.
27. Gellman H, et al. Reflex sympathetic dystrophy in cervical cord injury patients. *Clin Orthop* 1988;233:126–131.
28. Ghostine SY, et al. Phenoxybenzamine in the treatment of causalgia: report of 40 cases. *J Neorosurg* 1984;60:1263–1268.
28a. Gibbons, et al. Interscalene blocks for chronic upper extremity pain. *Reg Anaesth* 1988;13:50.
29. Glynn C, Casale R. Morphine injected around the stellate ganglion does not modulate the sympathetic nervous system nor does it provide pain relief. *Pain* 1993;53:33–37.
30. Gobelet C, Waldburger M, Meier JL. The effect of adding calcitonin to physical treatment on reflex sympathetic dystrophy. *Pain* 1992;48:171–175.
31. Gobelet C, et al. Calcitonin and reflex sympathetic dystrophy syndrome. *Clin Rheumatol* 1986;5:382–388.
32. Goldsmith DP, et al. Nuclear imaging and clinical features of childhood neurovascular dystrophy: comparison with adults. *Arthritis Rheum* 1989;32:480–485.
33. Goodman RR, Brisman R. Treatment of lower extremity reflex sympathetic dystrophy with continuous intrathecal morphine infusion. *Appl Neurophysiol* 1987;50:425–426.
34. Goris R, Dongen LM, Winters HA. Are toxic oxygen radicals involved in the pathogenesis of reflex sympathetic dystrophy? *Free Radic Res Commun* 1987;3:13–18.
35. Hannington-Kiff JG. Antisympathetic drugs in limbs. In: Wall PD, Melzack R, eds. *Testbook of Pain.* Edinburgh: Churchill Livingstone, 1984:566–573.
36. Hannington-Kiff JG. Intravenous regional sympathetic block with guanethidine. *Lancet* 1974;1:1019–1020.
37. Hardin RN, et al. Norepinephrine and epinephrine levels in affected versus unaffected limbs in sympathetically maintained pain. *Clin J Pain* 1994;10:324–330.
38. Headley B. Historical perspective of causalgia: management of sympathetically maintained pain. *Phys Ther* 1987;67:1370–1374.
39. Herrmann LG, Reineke HG, Caldwell JA. Post-traumatic painful osteoporosis: a clinical and roentgenological entity. *Am J Roentgenol Radium Ther* 1942;47:353–361.
40. Herz DA, et al. Second thoracic sympathetic ganglionectomy in sympathetically maintained pain. *J Pain Symptom Manage* 1993;8:483–491.
41. Horton P, Berster JC. Reflex sympathetic dystrophy syndrome and barbiturates: a study of 25 cases treated with barbiturates compared with 124 cases treated without barbiturates. *Clin Rheumatol* 1984;3:493–499.
42. Huaux JR, et al. Reflex sympathetic dystrophy syndrome: an unusual mode of presentation of osteomalacia. *Arthritis Rheum* 1986;29:918–925.
43. Hyland WT. Treating reflex sympathetic dystrophy with transdermal nitroglycerin. *Plast Reconstr Surg* 1989;83:195.
44. IASP. Classification of chronic pain, prepared by the Subcommittee on Taxonomy: descriptions of chronic pain syndromes and definition of pain terms. *Pain* 1986;(Suppl 3).
45. IASP. Classification of chronic pain. In: Merskey H, Bogduk N, eds. *Description of complex regional pain syndromes and definition of pain terms.* 2nd ed. Seattle: IASP, 1994.
46. Jaeger B, Singer E, Kroening R. Reflex sympathetic dystrophy of the face. *Arch Neurol* 1986;43:693–695.
47. Jaeger B, Singer E, Whitenack SH. Nerve injury complications: management of neurogenic pain syndromes. *Hand Clin* 1986;2:217–234.
48. Janig W, Kollman W. The involvement of the sympathetic nervous system in pain: possible neuronal mechanisms. *Arzneimittel forschung* 1984;34:1066–1073.
49. Katz MM, Hungerfor DS. Reflex sympathetic dystrophy affecting the knee. *J Bone Joint Surg [Br]* 1987;69:797–803.
50. Kettler RE, Abram SE. Intravenous regional droperidol in the management of reflex sympathetic dystrophy: a double-blind, placebo controlled, crossover study. *Anesthesiology* 1988;69:933–936.
51. Kim SH, et al. Effects of sympathectomy on a rat model of peripheral neuropathy. *Pain* 1993;55:85–92.

52. King JH, Nuss S. *Pain* 1993;55:393–396.
53. Kozin F, et al. The reflex sympathetic dystrophy syndrome. I. Clinical and histological studies: evidence for bilaterality, response to corticosteroids and articular involvement. *Am J Med* 1976;60:321–331.
54. Kozin F, et al. The reflex sympathetic dystrophy syndrome (RSDS). II. Roentgenographic and scintigraphic evidence of bilaterality and of periarticular accentuation. *Am J Med* 1976;60:332–338.
55. Kozin F, et al. The reflex sympathetic dystrophy syndrome (RSDS). III. Scintigraphic studies, further evidence for the therapeutic efficacy of systemic corticosteroids, and proposed diagnostic criteria. *Am J Med* 1981;70:23–30.
56. Krames RC, Robers WJ, Gillette RG. Post-sympathectomy neuralgia: hypothesis on peripheral and central neuronal mechanisms. *Pain* 1996;64:1–9.
57. Kurvers HA, et al. Reflex sympathetic dystrophy: result of autonomic denervation? *Clin Sci* 1994;87:663–669.
58. Ladd AL, et al. Reflex sympathetic imbalance: a response to epidural blockade. *Am J Sports Med* 1989;17:660–668.
59. Lee GW, Weeks PM. The role of bone scintigraphy in diagnosing reflex sympathetic dystrophy. *J Hand Surg [Am]* 1995;20:458–463.
60. Loh L, Nathan PW. Painful peripheral states and sympathetic blocks. *J Neurol Neurosurg Psychiatry* 1978;41:664–671.
61. Low PA, et al. Quantitative sudomotor axon reflex test in normal and neuropathic subjects. *Ann Neurol* 1983;14:573–580.
62. Munglani R, et al. Changes in neuronal markers in a mononeuropathic rat model: relationship between neuropeptide Y, pre-emptive drug treatment and long term mechanical hyperalgesia. *Pain* 1995;63:21–32.
63. Munn JS, Baker WH. Recurrent sympathetic dystrophy: successful treatment by contralateral sympathectomy. *Surgery* 1987;102:102–105.
64. Na HS, Leem JW, Chung JM. Abnormalities of mechanoreceptors in a rat model of neuropathic pain: possible involvement in mediating mechanical allodynia. *J Neurophysiol* 1993;70:522–528.
65. Nathan PW. Pain and the sympathetic nervous system. *JANS* 1983;7:363–370.
66. Perl ER. Causalgia and reflex sympathetic dystrophy revisited. In: Boivie J, Hannson P, Lindblom U, eds. *Touch, temperature, and pain in health and disease*. Seattle: IASB, 1994:231–248. *Progress in pain research and management*; vol 3.
67. Poehling GG, Pollock FE, Koman LA. Reflex sympathetic dystrophy of the knee after sensory nerve injury: arthroscopy. *J Arthroscop Related Surg* 1988;4:31–35.
68. Procacci P, Maresca N. Reflex sympathetic dystrophies and algodystrophies: historical and pathogenic considerations. *Pain* 1987;31:137–146.
69. Prough DS, et al. Efficacy of oral nifedipine in the treatment of reflex sympathetic dystrophy. *Anesthesiolog* 1985;62:796–799.
70. Raja SN, et al. Systemic alpha-adrenergic blockade with phentolamine: a diagnostic test for sympathetically maintained pain. *Anesthesiol* 1991;74:691–698.
71. Richards RL. Causalgia: a centennial review. *Arch Neurol* 1967;16:339–350.
72. Rico H, Merono E, Bomex-Castresana F. Scintigraphic evaluation of reflex sympathetic dystrophy: comparative study of the course of the disease under two therapeutic regimens. *Clin Rheumatol* 1987;67:233–237.
73. Robbrecht W, et al. Painful muscle spasms complicating algodystrophy: central or peripheral disease. *J Neurol Neurosurg Psychiatry* 1988;51:563–567.
74. Roberts WJ. A hypothesis on the physiological basis for causalgia and related pains. *Pain* 1986;24:297–311.
75. Rocco AF. Radiofrequency lumbar sympatholysis: the evolution of a technique for managing sympathetically maintained pain. *Reg Anaesth* 1995;20:3–12.
76. Rowbotham MC. Chronic pain: from theory to practical management. *Neurology* 1995;45(Suppl 9):S5–S10.
77. Rowlingson JC. The sympathetic dystrophies. In: Stem JM, Wakefield CA, eds. *Pain management*. Boston: Little, Brown, 1983:117–129.
78. Sato J, Perl ER. Adrenergic excitation of cutaneous pain receptors induced by peripheral nerve injury. *Science* 1991;25:1608–1610.
79. Scadding JW. Development of ongoing activity, mechanosensitivity and adrenaline sensitivity in severed peripheral nerve axons. *Exp Neurol* 1981;73:345–364.
80. Schott GD. Mechanisms of causalgia and related clinical conditions: the role of the central and of the sympathetic nervous system. *Brain* 1986;109:717–738.
81. Schwartzman RJ. Reflex sympathetic dystrophy and causalgia. *Neuro Clin* 1992;10:953–973.
82. Schwartzman RJ, McLellan TL. Reflex sympathetic dystrophy: a review. *Arch Neurol* 1987;44:551–561.
83. Shelton RM, Lewis CW. Reflex sympathetic dystrophy: a review. *J Am Acad Dermatol* 1987;22:513–520.
84. Sherman RA, Barja RH, Bruno GM. Thermographic correlates of chronic pain: analysis of 125 patients incorporating evaluations by a blind panel. *Arch Phys Med Rehabil* 1987;68:273–279.
85. Stanton-Hicks M, et al. Reflex sympathetic dystrophy: changing concepts and taxonomy. *Pain* 1995;63:127–133.
86. Strong WE, et al. Does the sympathetic block outlast sensory block? A thermographic evaluation. *Pain* 1991;46:173–176.
87. Torebjork HE, Hallin RG. Perceptual changes accompanying controlled referential blocking of A and C fibre response in intact human skin nerves. *Exp Brain Res* 1973;16:321–332.
88. Torebjork HE, et al. Noradrenaline-evoked pain in neuralgia. *Pain* 1995;63:11–20.
89. Verdugo RJ, Campero M, Ochoa JL. Phentolamine sympathetic block in painful polyneuropathies. II. Further questioning of the concept of 'sympathetically maintained pain.' *Neurology* 1994;44:101–1014.
90. Verdugo RJ, Ochoa JL. Use and misuse of conventional electrodiagnosis, quantitative sensory testing, thermography and nerve block in the evaluation of painful neuropathic syndromes. *Muscle Nerve* 1993;16:1056–1062.
91. Wall PD. Noradrenaline-evoked pain in neuralgia [Editorial]. *Pain* 1995;63:1–2.
92. Watson HK, Carlson L. Treatment of reflex sympathetic dystrophy of the hand with an active "stress loading" program. *J Hand Surg [Am]* 1987;12:779–785.
93. Werner R, et al. Factors affecting the sensitivity and specificity of the three-phase technetium bone scan in the diagnosis of reflex sympathetic dystrophy in the upper extremity. *J Hand Surg [Am]* 1989;14:520–523.
94. Wilson PR. Sympathetically maintained pain: diagnosis, measurement and efficacy of treatment. In: Stanton-Hicks M, ed. *Pain and the sympathetic nervous system*. Boston: Kluwer, 1990.
95. Woolf CJ, Shortland P, Coggeshall RE. Peripheral nerve injury triggers central sprouting of myelinated afferents. *Nature* 1992;355:75–78.
96. Yokota T, Furukawa T, Tsujkagoshi H. Motor paresis improved by sympathetic block: a motor form of reflex sympathetic dystrophy? *Arch Neurol* 1989;46:683–687.

CHAPTER 17

Skin Potentials: Normal and Abnormal

Ronald Schondorf

1. Evoked electrodermal activity (EDA) refers to the electrical activity that originates from sweat glands and the adjacent epidermal and dermal tissues and is recorded with macroelectrodes applied to the skin surface. Measurement of spontaneously occurring evoked EDA has been proposed as an easily obtainable index of sudomotor function.
2. The central organization of sympathetic sudomotor activity directed to palmar and plantar skin differs significantly from the activity directed to thermoregulatory nonpalmar/nonplantar skin sites. Despite this difference in organization, many investigators have used the spontaneous or evoked palmar and plantar EDA as an index of sympathetic sudomotor activity.
3. Evoked EDA, the sympathetic skin response, has been found to be abnormal in several types of axonal neuropathies.
4. Despite these abnormalities, the correlation of an abnormal sympathetic skin response with more generalized abnormalities of sympathetic sudomotor dysfunction, autonomic dysfunction, or small fiber sensory neuropathy is surprisingly poor.
5. The utility of the sympathetic skin response as a test of central autonomic dysfunction requires further clarification.

INTRODUCTION

The autonomic nervous system is affected in many diseases of the peripheral and central nervous systems. The objective evaluation of the presence or absence of autonomic dysfunction requires a specialized laboratory and equipment as well as personnel skilled in the performance and interpretation of standardized tests of autonomic function (4,56) (Chapters 15, 16, 25–27). There has been increased interest, however, in defining simple and sensitive tests of autonomic function that can be performed at the bedside (29) or with standard clinical electrophysiologic techniques and equipment found in any well-equipped electromyography laboratory. Measurement of spontaneously occurring or evoked electrodermal activity (EDA) has been proposed as an easily obtainable index of sudomotor function (43,82). The terms sympathetic skin response (SSR) or peripheral autonomic surface potential (PASP) have been used by these and other investigators who have used this technique in the assessment of peripheral neuropathy. This chapter focuses on the properties of the generator of EDA and the central organization of neural circuits involved in the genesis or modulation of EDA. The utility of EDA as a test of autonomic function has been recently reviewed (1,33) and is critically evaluated.

THE GENERATOR OF ELECTRODERMAL ACTIVITY

EDA refers to the electrical activity that originates from sweat glands and adjacent epidermal and dermal tissues and is recorded with macroelectrodes applied to the skin surface. This phenomenon was first noted by Tarchanoff (90) at the end of the 19th century. Recording EDA in this manner has also been termed endosomatic in contrast to the exosomatic recordings of concomitant fluctuations in skin conductance or resistance (10,18,19,56). Resting skin potential is consistently negative (-25 to -40 mV) relative to the body interior (17,20). At a normal ambient temperature, the palmar or plantar skin is ordinarily 10–25 mV more negative than other skin regions (17), and spontaneous fluctuations in skin potential may be recorded from these skin sites. The presence of spontaneous or evoked EDA depends on the integrity of the cutaneous innervation at the site of recording (Fig. 1) and is abolished by section

R. Schondorf: Department of Neurology, McGill University, Sir M. B. Davis Jewish General Hospital, Montreal, Quebec, Canada H3T 1E2.

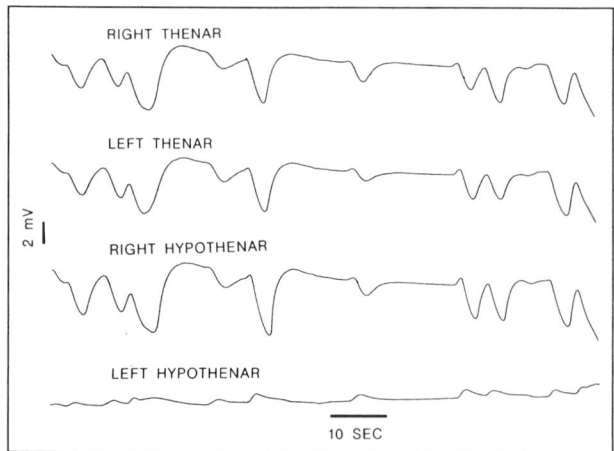

FIG. 1. Spontaneous electrodermal activity (EDA) recorded from both thenar and hypothenar eminences in a patient with a left ulnar neuropathy. The large amplitude synchronous evoked EDA is significantly attenuated in the cutaneous territory innervated by the left ulnar nerve.

of the corresponding peripheral nerve, sympathectomy, or iontophoresis with atropine (48,49,55,70,71,87). Conversely, electrical stimulation of the distal end of cut peripheral cutaneous nerve or postganglionic sympathetic efferent fibers evokes a wave of EDA in glabrous skin (55,85,87). Microneurographic recordings from cutaneous nerves have demonstrated synchronous activity in nerve fascicles that occurs before fluctuations in EDA or skin resistance (51,97). The effect of this spontaneous activity on skin resistance may be mimicked by selective electrical stimulation of these fascicles via the microneurographic electrode (46,47).

Electrical stimulation of the distal end of cut peripheral nerve afferents or of the sympathetic trunk gives rise to a transient negative potential and a longer-duration positive potential from the glabrous skin of animals (55,70,85). The afterpositivity recorded with macroelectrodes appears only after higher frequencies of stimulation (85). If continuous repetitive stimulation is employed, the intraluminal negativity begins to decay within 30 sec and becomes positive by the end of minute 3. In contrast, the macroelectrode recordings show surface positivity early in minute 1 of electrical stimulation. The source of the initial negativity of the EDA is the sweat gland itself. Negative potentials of similar latency have been recorded with microelectrodes placed in the lumen of individual sweat glands during peripheral nerve stimulation or intraarterial injection of methacholine (85,88); positive intraluminal potentials are never seen.

The source of the surface positivity of EDA is less clear. The waveform of the EDA is significantly distorted by AC amplification, both in terms of amplitude of the evoked response and the artifactual introduction of a positive afterpotential (45,110). In addition, if differential amplification is used and recordings are made from two active skin sites, the negative potential arriving at the indifferent electrode (G2) may be reflected as a late positivity (under G1). A late positivity is obtained, however, even if very long time constants or DC amplifiers are used and the inactive electrode referred to a skin site inactivated by a local anesthetic or skin drilling (84,110).

The morphologic characteristics of the diphasic potential may be modified under certain conditions. A diphasic EDA recorded from the finger pulp converts to a monophasic negativity following occlusion of the local circulation for 10–15 min (88,107). Pressure on one side of the chest changes the ipsilateral diphasic EDA to a monophasic negativity whereas the contralateral EDA remains diphasic (108). Cholinergic blockade abolishes both the positive and negative components of skin potentials, but a negative EDA recovers before the positive component of the EDA (17). A diphasic EDA is more likely to be obtained from the palm following strong arousal stimuli (110). Lloyd suggested that the afterpositivity reflects a secretory potential secondary to sweat duct filling and reabsorption, as it was prolonged and more prominent following repetitive nerve stimulation that would tend to maximize sweat output (55). Richter (73), however, recorded only slow positive potentials from the skin of a patient with congenital absence of sweat glands, whereas other normal subjects consistently demonstrated biphasic EDA. Moreover, positive potentials are not recorded from individual sweat glands (85).

There is evidence that an epidermal component may contribute to the level and polarity of EDA. Edelberg and colleagues (20,24) noted that the size of exosomatic or endosomatic recordings of EDA was immediately influenced by the type of ionic medium in contact with skin, a maneuver not likely to affect immediately the relatively protected sweat glands deep within the skin but likely to modify an epidermal contribution to EDA. Moreover, the maximal conductance that is predicted by multiplying known values for individual sweat gland conductance by the sweat gland density gives a value only half that of the actually measured value (22), suggesting that other components in the skin may contribute to generation of the EDA. Positive potentials are recorded from microelectrodes applied to the epidermal surface of the skin, and these persist post mortem after negative sweat gland potentials are no longer recordable (85).

Edelberg (17) proposed a two-effector model in which the epidermis and sweat gland are each represented by an individual generator and resistance that are connected in parallel. The transcutaneous potential of the epidermal component, although still negative with respect to the body interior, is 15- to 25-mV positive relative to the sweat gland (17). Under resting conditions, the resistance of the epidermal component is high, and therefore EDA largely reflects sweat gland activity. As sweating progresses, the epidermis becomes more hydrated and the epidermal resistance is decreased, thereby allowing the relatively positive epidermal potential to become more evident. A surface positivity may then be recorded.

Those conditions that limit maximal sweat gland activity (such as tourniquet ischemia, skin pressure, or recovery from cholinergic blockade) will limit skin hydration and eliminate surface positivity. Surface positivity has been noted to occur in conjunction with increased skin absorption of ambient moisture but not during active expulsion of sweat (23). The interaction of the two components, sweat gland and epidermal, makes the absolute amplitude of the evoked EDA difficult to interpret (36). The lack of tight correlation between skin conductance and sudorometric measurements of sweat gland activity is also explained by the complex interaction of independent components of skin conductance (21).

The data just reviewed suggest that the level of EDA reflects the complex interaction between surface potentials originating from the sweat gland and epidermis. The epidermal potential likely depends on the degree of hydration of the epidermis that, in turn, relies on sweat gland activity. Despite the complex nature of the EDA, the synchrony of EDA activity at homologous skin sites does suggest that EDA can be used as an index of the presence of sympathetic sudomotor activity although it cannot quantitate the absolute level of that activity. It may not follow conclusively, however, that absence of EDA is solely due to abnormalities in function or sympathetic denervation, because diseases that may modify epidermal conductivity (e.g., trophic changes of skin, and callus) may theoretically modify or attenuate EDA.

CENTRAL MODULATION OF ELECTRODERMAL ACTIVITY

Spontaneous Evoked Electrodermal Activity

At normal ambient temperatures, synchronized spontaneous EDA is recorded from the volar surface of the hands and feet. Examples of this tightly synchronized activity are presented in Figs. 1 and 2. In these and all subsequent records of EDA, the indifferent electrode is placed on an inactive skin-drilled site (84). Arousal stimuli such as loud noises, light flash, inspiratory gasp, and mental arithmetic all increase the frequency and amplitude of the spontaneous EDA.

At normal ambient temperature, EDA is generally not recorded from other skin sites; once ambient temperature is increased, however, an orderly recruitment of synchronous EDA may be observed in nonpalmar and nonplantar skin (Fig. 3) (foot to thigh to hand to forearm) (74,80). An example of this tightly synchronized spontaneous EDA recorded at 40°C from the anterior aspects of both thighs and the dorsa of both feet is presented in Fig. 3. As a general rule, tightly synchronous activity of skin sites at some distance from each other suggests that spontaneous EDA arises from a centrally generated rhythmic input to structures in the skin (9,100).

The rhythmicity from nonpalmar and nonplantar skin sites differs significantly from that recorded simultaneously from palmar and plantar skin, indicating the existence of two main types of sudomotor activity that we term emotive (palmar and plantar) and thermoregulatory (nonpalmar and nonplantar). Similar observations have been obtained by using sudorometric techniques (67,68) (Chapter 7) and in microneurographic recordings made simultaneously from fascicles of cutaneous sympathetic postganglionic axons in the median nerve and lateral cutaneous nerve of the forearm (7). At normal ambient temperatures, no activity has been recorded from the lateral cutaneous nerve although activity synchronous with the palmar EDA was recorded from the median nerve. In contrast, increasing the ambient temperature heightens sympathetic activity in the lateral cutaneous nerve of the forearm. The microneurographic data confirm the notion that regional differences in spontaneous EDA reflect differences in the central organization of sudomotor input to palmar and plantar and nonpalmar and nonplantar skin.

The differentiation of sudomotor activity into emotive and thermoregulatory types is not absolute, however. As

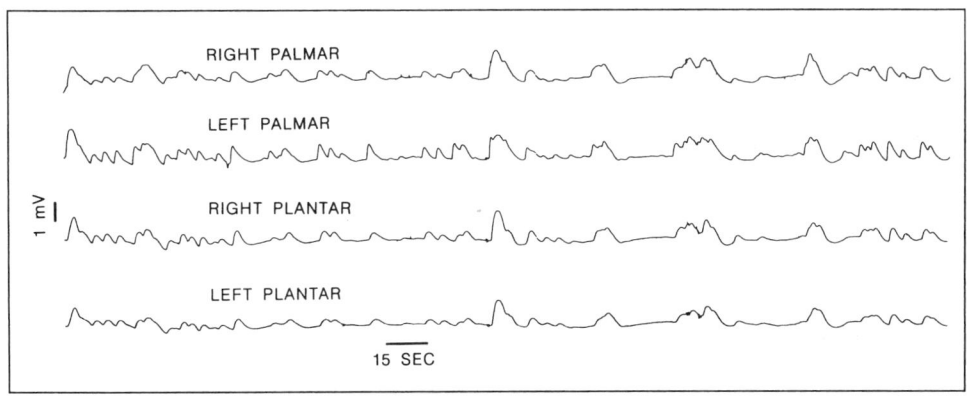

FIG. 2. A sample of tightly synchronized spontaneous electrodermal activity recorded from homologous sites from both palms and soles.

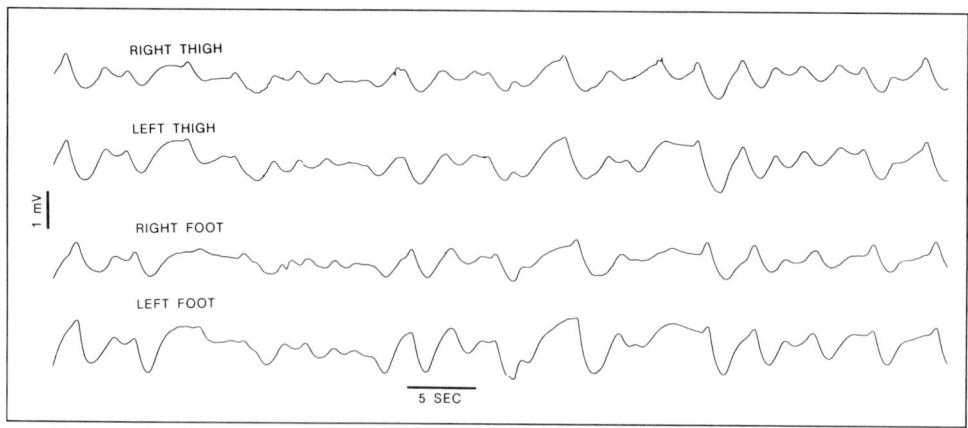

FIG. 3. A sample of tightly synchronized spontaneous electrodermal activity recorded from homologous sites from the anterior aspect of both thighs and the dorsa of both feet at an ambient temperature of 40°C. At normal ambient temperature, no activity was recorded from any site.

shown in Fig. 4, EDA recorded from the dorsa of the feet at an ambient temperature of 40°C is increased when the subject is asked to perform difficult mathematical calculations rapidly, a maneuver that reliably increases the palmar and plantar EDA (8,13).

There are few data regarding the central organization of thermoregulatory sudomotor activity. Most data have been obtained in EDA recordings from the footpads of cats, which possess no sweat glands that participate in thermoregulatory activity (9,12,45,98–100). Indeed, Wang and Chun (101) described *decreased* EDA in cats at high ambient temperatures. Studies of spontaneous EDA in humans have devoted little attention to the site of recording, although again most observations have been made from palmar and plantar sites (87).

In a series of studies summarized in a review and a monograph, Wang (98–100) studied the effects of chronic ablations of selected portions of the central nervous system (CNS) on spontaneous EDA in cats. The presence of spontaneous synchronized EDA depends on supraspinal inputs to sympathetic sudomotor neurons, as this EDA is present only in the forepaws of cats with low thoracic cord lesions; only low-level desynchronized EDA exists in all four limbs of cats with a high transection of the spinal cord.

Removal of the orbitofrontal cortex was observed to enhance spontaneous EDA (63), but synchronized EDA remained even when the entire neocortex and rhinencephalon were removed. Removal of the striatum resulted in desynchronization of EDA that persisted when transections were extended to involve structures rostral to the superior colliculus, although more caudal lesions were associated with progressively less EDA. Transection of the brainstem just caudal to the inferior colliculus completely abolished spontaneous EDA. The presence of EDA in chronic spinal cats and its absence in cats with transection caudal to the inferior colliculus suggest the existence of

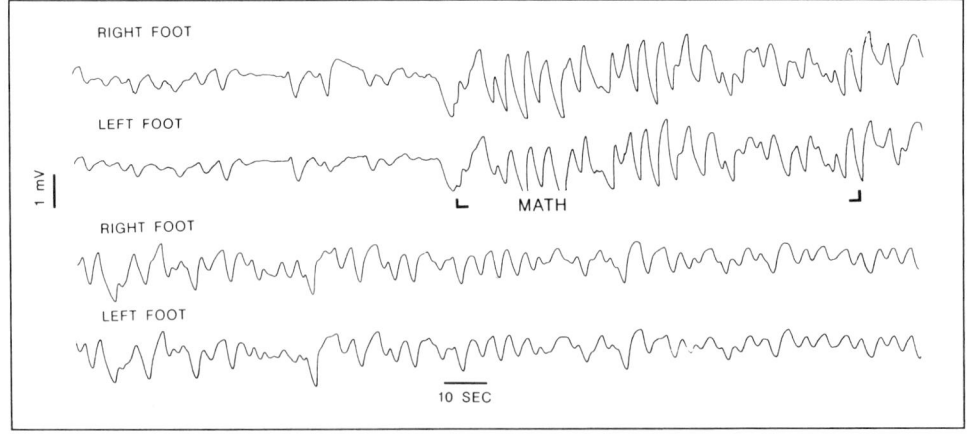

FIG. 4. Spontaneous electrodermal activity (EDA) recorded from the dorsa of both feet at an ambient temperature of 40°C. Between the marks, the subject was asked to perform a complex multiplication. Note the synchronous increase in evoked EDA during the calculation.

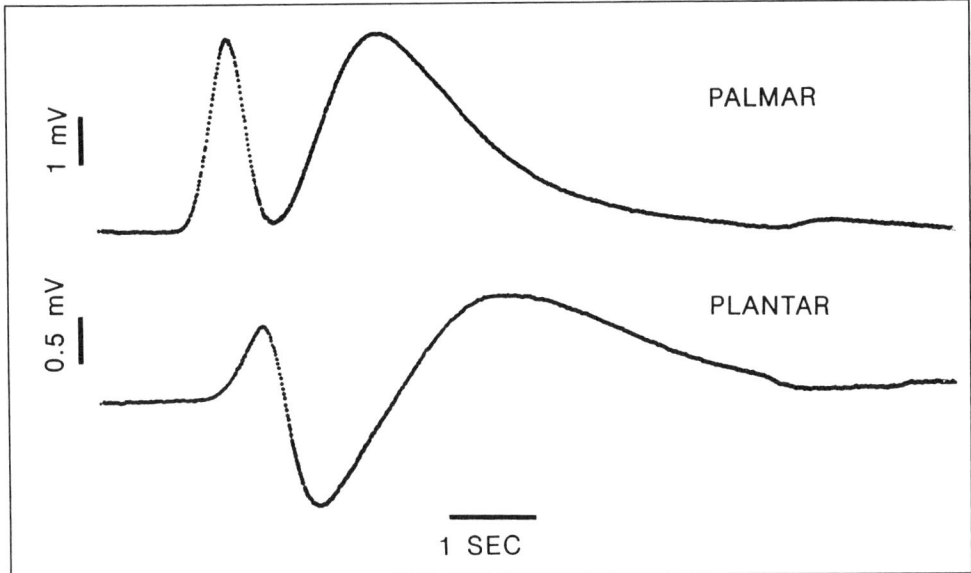

FIG. 5. Averages of four sympathetic skin responses (negativity *upward*) recorded from the palm and sole evoked by electrical stimulation of the sural nerve with surface electrodes. An early negativity is followed by a positive potential and subsequent late long-duration negativity.

tonic inhibitory inputs that project from the brainstem to spinal circuits that are involved in the genesis of EDA. Within the acutely isolated spinal cord itself, inhibition of spontaneous EDA can be observed following noxious cutaneous input originating from dermatomes adjacent to the site of recording, but stimulation of remote cutaneous sites consistently increases EDA (38).

Evoked Evoked Electrodermal Activity

Electrophysiologic Properties of the Sympathetic Skin Response

Electrical stimulation of peripheral nerve afferents evokes a wave of EDA that is generally biphasic, consisting of an initial negativity followed by a positive potential. A late negativity may be observed in ~30% of normal subjects (80). All three components of the SSR are shown in Fig. 5. In some cases, the initial potential may be positive (Fig. 6) and the morphologic appearance of the potential may even change during the period of recording (4). Table 1 summarizes the reported peak-to-peak amplitudes and latencies to onset of the SSR recorded from plantar and palmar skin cited in different studies. The average latency to onset of the evoked palmar response is 1.44 sec, and the average latency to onset of the plantar response is 1.97 sec. The difference in latencies largely results from the increased efferent peripheral conduction time in the legs (30). As shown in Table 1, the amplitude of the SSR is significantly attenuated at a low-pass filter setting of >0.5 Hz. The SSR also normally diminishes with age. Among normal subjects >60 years of age, 50% may have an absent plantar SSR (15). This may be due in a part to the diminution of sweat gland density that occurs with aging (31).

All investigators have noted that the SSR tends to habituate with repetitive stimuli (25,35,43,83) and, in general, stimuli should be delivered at irregular intervals of >30 sec to assure reproducibility of the SSR. Habituation and variability of the evoked reflex response are both observed

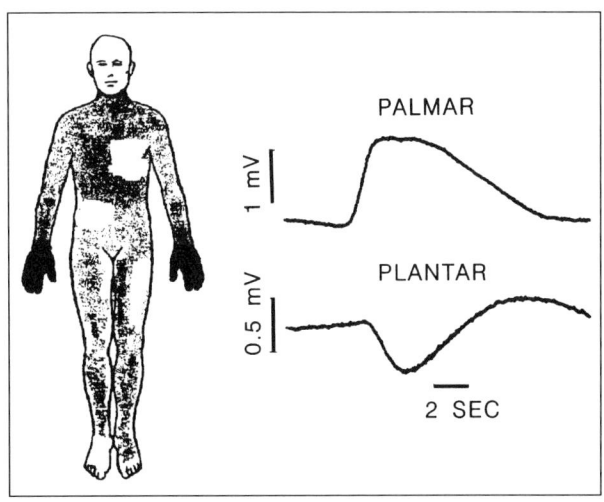

FIG. 6. Comparison of the thermoregulatory sweat test (TST) and sympathetic skin response in a diabetic subject with burning pain localized to the thoracic anhidrotic areas. The presence of the sympathetic skin response (SSR) is in marked contrast to the sudomotor abnormalities demonstrated with the TST. Sweat gland counts taken from the dorsum of the anhidrotic foot were also markedly decreased.

TABLE 1. *Electrophysiological properties of the sympathetic skin response.*

Study	Bandpass (Hz)	Palmer response		Plantar response	
		Latency (sec)	Amplitude (mV)	Latency (sec)	Amplitude (mV)
Baba et al. [3]	2–4,000	1.34 + 0.11	1.79 + 0.83	...	...
Elie and Guiheneue [25]	0.1–100	1.49 + 0.07	2.9 + 1.7	2.7 + 0.12	1.4 + 0.8
Knezevic and Bajada [43]	2–5,000	1.52 + 0.13	0.48 + 0.10	2.07 + 0.16	0.10 + 0.04
Linden and Berlit [53]	1–2,000	1.23 + 0.34	2.13 + 1.62	1.9 + 0.36	1.03 + 0.71
Opsomer et al. [69]	1–1,000	1.38 + 0.07	0.42 + 0.16	1.94 + 0.08	0.14 + 0.05
Schondorf and Gendron [80]	0.1–3,000	1.48 + 0.24	2.54 + 1.27	2.04 + 0.31	2.17 + 1.62
Shahani et al. [83]	0.5–2,000	1.39 + 0.07	0.81 + 0.32	1.88 + 0.11	0.64 + 0.28
Soliven et al. [86]	1.6–3,200	1.31 + 0.18	0.79 + 0.35	1.93 + 0.17	0.39 + 0.23
Tzeng et al. [92]	2–5,000	1.24 + 0.16	0.91 + 0.37	1.83 + 0.18	0.51 + 0.21
Valls-Sole et al. [95]	2–1,000	1.53 + 0.24	0.47 + 0.18	2.10 + 0.25	0.16 + 0.09
Van den Bergh and Kelly [96]	?	1.4 + 0.1	0.18 + 0.09	1.8 + 0.1	0.08 + 0.05
Yokota et al. [112]	0.53–1,000	1.34 + 0.1	5.53 + 3.24	1.84 + 0.28	1.64 + 1.08

when recording microneurographically from cutaneous sympathetic postganglionic axons in the median nerve (78). To correct for the variability of the SSR, many investigators average four consecutive SSRs whereas others measure the amplitude of the largest SSR. Baba et al. (3) have suggested that the changing morphologic appearance of the SSR may cancel the phases and attenuate the response amplitude. In our experience with observing the morphologic characteristics of single SSRs and averaging four consecutive SSRs, phase cancellation has not proved to be a significant problem (80). Ideally, while recording, the indifferent electrode should be placed on an inactivated skin-drilled site (79,80,84); however, a reasonable approximation of an inactivated site at normal ambient temperature can often be obtained by placing the indifferent electrode on an adjacent thermoregulatory skin site or on a nail bed.

Additional insight into the central organization of the SSR has been obtained by magnetic stimulation. In normal subjects, transcranial magnetic stimulation of the motor strip delivered via a flat probe positioned over C3 and C4 elicited palmar and plantar SSRs similar both in latency and in amplitude to those evoked by median nerve stimulation (76). These responses were also present in one patient with a predominantly sensory neuropathy although, in this case, no SSR was evoked by median nerve stimulation (77). Magnetic stimulation of the neck with the center of the coil placed between the seventh cervical and first thoracic spinous processes evoked two positive palmar potentials at latencies of 400 and 600 msec and a negative potential ~325 msec later (94). The positive potentials did not habituate with repetitive stimulation, were blocked by iontophoresis of atropine into the skin under the recording site, and were enhanced by iontophoresis of pilocarpine. They were therefore assumed to represent the activation of efferent sudomotor fibers. The later negative potential was thought to represent the SSR evoked by stimulation of cervicothoracic dorsal roots. The latency between onset of the positive and negative potentials (325 msec) would then represent an approximation of the central reflex time of the SSR. These intriguing results, although clearly requiring further confirmation, suggest that the delay of the afferent limb of the SSR is negligible compared with the time required for central processing and efferent conduction.

Central Organization of the Sympathetic Skin Response

In cats the SSR is maximally evoked by stimulation of myelinated group II afferents (40). The excitatory wave is followed by 20–30 sec of inhibition, as assessed by standard conditioning and testing paradigms. Electrical stimulation or ablation of selected CNS sites has yielded additional insight into the central organization of circuits involved in the genesis or modulation of the SSR. EDA is evoked by electrical stimulation of orbitofrontal, pericruciate, and parietal cortex, posterior hypothalamus, dorsal thalamus, and ventrolateral brainstem reticular formation (12,32,37,45,81,98–100). The EDA evoked by stimulation of the frontal cortex does not involve a hypothalamic relay and is probably mediated by a double descending system: one involving corticoreticulospinal pathways and a direct corticospinal one (81). Inhibition of the SSR is obtained by stimulation of the orbitofrontal cortex, caudate nucleus, anterior lobe of the cerebellum and, most strikingly, the ventromedial brainstem reticular formation (100,106). Removal of the forebrain markedly enhances the SSR (87,103). The amygdala does not appear to participate in the genesis of the SSR (91). Section of the neuraxis caudal to the inferior colliculus abolishes the SSR, an effect reversed by block of tonic activity within the ventromedial reticular formation (102). The isolated spinal cord can mediate SSR, albeit at a level lower than with the neuraxis intact.

The neuroantomic substrate underlying the SSR in humans remains largely unknown. A recent study (44) evaluated SSR in 49 patients with early or late (6–12 months) hemispheric brain infarction in the territory of the internal carotid artery and in nine patients with lateral medullary syndrome. In all cases of cortical infarction, palmar SSR amplitudes were decreased bilaterally relative to control values. Patients with brainstem infarction had similar decreases although ipsilateral SSR amplitude tended to be lower than the contralateral SSR. Another study (53) evaluated 29 patients after cerebrovascular infarction: left middle cerebral artery (12), right middle cerebral artery (9), pontine ischemia (6), and medullary ischemia (2). Most had a bilateral decrease in SSR amplitude, with some having a side-to-side differentiation in amplitude or latency. The bilateral diminution of the SSR in most cases does underscore the central complexity the neural substrate mediating the SSR in humans.

CLINICAL UTILITY OF ELECTRODERMAL ACTIVITY AND THE SYMPATHETIC SKIN RESPONSE

Despite the complexity of the SSR, this reflex has been used as an easily obtainable index of autonomic function and has been suggested as being useful in the early recognition of dysautonomia. In the past 3 years, numerous publications have described SSR abnormalities in a variety of neuropathies, disorders of the central nervous system, reflex sympathetic dystrophy, and essential hyperhidrosis. In this section, we review the data and evaluate the clinical utility and limitations of the SSR and suggest further investigations that may shed additional light on the role of SSR as a clinical electrophysiologic tool.

What Constitutes an Abnormal Sympathetic Skin Response?

There is as yet no clear consensus as to what constitutes an abnormal SSR. Most investigators have used the parameters of SSR amplitude and latency and some have also used response to different stimuli to define an abnormal SSR. Owing to its extreme variability, most investigators have considered the SSR to be abnormal only when it is absent although, as noted previously, plantar SSR may normally be absent in many normal elderly individuals. Yokota et al. (112) have suggested two other criteria of amplitude abnormality: an absence of SSR in one of four limbs only or a reduction of SSR amplitude by 50% between ipsilateral and contralateral limbs. This clearly necessitates simultaneous recording of the SSR from both palmar and plantar sites (four channels) and, in the author's opinion, is the preferred method of evaluating the SSR.

An absent SSR is not necessarily indicative of abnormal sympathetic sudomotor function. SSR evoked by median nerve stimulation was not obtained following ischemic conduction block of the arm in normal control subjects although SSR was still evoked by cough or deep inspiration (93). This dependence on the integrity of peripheral nerve afferents constitutes one of the major limitations of the SSR as a clinical test of sudomotor function. As will be seen, SSR evoked by peripheral nerve stimulation is absent in at least 50% of patients with obvious diabetic neuropathy. However, SSR evoked by deep inspiration was absent in only three of 68 diabetic patients, 19 of whom had symptomatic autonomic neuropathy (50). These very important observations underscore the requirement for multiple types of stimulation (peripheral nerve stimulation, acoustic stimulation, and inspiratory gasp) before one may conclude that emotive sympathetic sudomotor function is impaired.

The significance of an abnormal SSR latency remains unclear. Although in some studies the latency to onset of the SSR was occasionally prolonged in patients with neuropathies, there is significant overlap between much of the normal and neuropathic population (79,92,95). In one study of patients with multiple sclerosis, abnormally delayed palmar or plantar SSRs were noted in 85% of patients, whereas SSR amplitude was normal (26). Two other studies of patients with multiple sclerosis have noted SSR amplitude abnormalities only (34,112). One can therefore only speculate whether an abnormal SSR latency reflects abnormal central reflex processing.

Sympathetic Skin Response and Peripheral Neuropathy

Shahani et al. (83) measured the SSR in 33 patients with axonal, demyelinating, and mixed neuropathies of a variety of causes. The SSR was absent in most of the patients with axonal neuropathies. Similar results were obtained by Van den Bergh and Kelly (96). In three patients with absent SSR, sural nerve biopsy showed a decreased number of myelinated and unmyelinated axons (83). Surprisingly, in this study, SSR was absent in only one of four patients with clinically evident dysautonomia. This observation led to the suggestion that SSR was a better index of dysfunction of unmyelinated axons than of dysautonomia. In a subsequent study of 53 patients with neuropathy, however, SSR was absent in 19 of 22 patients with clinically evident dysautonomia, whereas only four of 31 subjects without dysautonomia had absent SSR (82).

Despite the suggestion of Shahani et al. (83), an abnormal SSR correlates poorly with the clinical impression of small fiber sensory neuropathy. Abnormal SSRs were obtained in only six of 63 patients referred with symptoms suggestive of mild small fiber peripheral neuropathy but without clinically significant dysautonomia (27). In a study of one family with familial amyloid polyneuropathy, SSRs were absent in four members who had symptomatic neuropathy and SSRs were of low amplitude in some asymptomatic carriers. In two of the four symptomatic patients, however, the SSR was present within the normal range despite the presence of a symptomatic small fiber neuropathy (62).

The SSR is absent in a variety of axonal and demyelinating neuropathies of defined etiology. SSRs were found to be absent in four of 21 (11) and five of 36 (105) patients with chronic renal failure. In these patients, the SSR was absent only if significant abnormalities of nerve conduction were observed (105). In three studies of patients with alcoholic neuropathy (61,65,95), ~60% had an absent plantar SSR, but only 13% had an absent palmar SSR. The likelihood of obtaining SSR abnormalities correlated with the presence of peripheral neuropathy and impaired nutritional status (61,65). Navarro et al. (64) reported a single case of absent SSR and absent sweat gland response to iontophoresed pilocarpine in one patient with Sjogren's syndrome who showed no evidence of more widespread neuropathy or autonomic dysfunction. The SSR was absent from at least one limb in nine of 24 patients with Guillain–Barré syndrome (89) and in three of nine patients with acute sensory ataxic neuropathy (2).

The SSR has been most commonly studied in patients with diabetic neuropathy. Soliven et al. (86) studied 47 diabetic patients who manifested clinical symptoms and signs of peripheral neuropathy; 37 of them had symptoms of autonomic involvement. The symptoms included orthostatic hypotension (13 patients), gastroparesis (20 patients), bladder dysfunction (four patients), and impotence in 24 of the 30 men. The plantar SSR was lacking in 31 of 47 patients, 90% of whom had signs of autonomic involvement. However, only 28 (76%) of the patients with autonomic involvement had an absent SSR.

Niakan and Harati (66) studied 72 diabetics with neuropathy. The SSR was absent in only the lower extremities in 33 patients and was lacking in both the upper and lower extremities in 27. Thus, 80% of patients had an abnormal SSR. This population also exhibited significant autonomic dysfunction. Of the patients, 15% had orthostatic hypotension on physical examination; 15% of the patients had a history of postural dizziness, 24% had gustatory sweating, and 7% had gastrointestinal abnormalities; and 44 (80%) of 54 men were impotent. Almost all patients had trophic skin changes.

Maselli et al. (59) studied 39 diabetics, 33 of whom had autonomic involvement: 11 had orthostatic hypotension, 18 had gastroparesis, nine had recurrent diarrhea and 22 of the 28 men were impotent. In this severely affected population, the presence or absence of the SSR correlated with the presence or absence of the quantitative sudomotor axon reflex test (QSART) (57), which serves as an index of postganglionic sympathetic sudomotor function.

Watahiki et al. (106) studied 67 diabetics, 21 of whom showed clinical signs of dysautonomia. The palmar SSR was absent in only six patients; the SSR was present in 36 others but was decreased in amplitude. The plantar SSR was not assessed. Jha and Nag (39) studied 34 diabetics, 15 of whom showed symptomatic orthostatic intolerance. The SSR was not recordable in eight of 19 asymptomatic diabetics and was not obtained in 10 of 15 diabetics with symptomatic autonomic dysfunction.

The presence of clinically apparent autonomic dysfunction occurs only late in the course of diabetic neuropathy and is associated with poor prognosis (28). The data just reviewed show that SSR is abnormal in advanced diabetic neuropathy, although it is not possible to ascertain from these studies the utility of the SSR in the evaluation of early sympathetic sudomotor dysfunction in the context of diabetes. One might argue that, considering the obvious symptomatology in these subjects, it is surprising that SSR was not absent in virtually all cases studied.

The question arises as to whether the SSR is a good index of more generalized sympathetic sudomotor dysfunction. The data reported by Maselli et al. (59) just cited show a good correlation between gross abnormalities revealed by QSART and an absent SSR. Martyn and Reid (58), however, were able to elicit the SSR from two of four diabetic patients with clear loss of sweating in the lower extremities and compensatory hyperhidrosis over the upper trunk and face. Navarro et al. (65) compared the sweat response to iontophoresed pilocarpine and the SSR in 30 patients with alcoholic neuropathy. The pilocarpine response in the foot was abnormal in 18 patients and the plantar SSR was absent in 16. In only 10 patients were the results of both tests abnormal. Baser et al. (6) compared the SSR and sweat response with intradermal methacholine in nine patients with progressive autonomic failure or multiple-system atrophy. The SSR was present in five of nine patients despite evidence of a significantly attenuated sweat response to methacholine. Schondorf and Gendron (79) compared the SSR, the thermoregulatory sweat test (TST) (see Chapter 19), and the sweat gland response to iontophoresed pilocarpine (41,42) in 20 patients with neuropathy (17 diabetic, two Guillain–Barré, and one chronic inflammatory demyelinating polyradiculopathy. Only two patients had symptoms of autonomic dysfunction. In 16 patients in whom TST and SSR were measured, the TST result was abnormal in three who had a normal SSR, and the SSR was abnormal in five who had a normal TST result. An example of such a discrepancy is shown in Fig. 6. The response to pilocarpine was assessed in 17 patients and was abnormal in three patients with a normal SSR but was normal in six cases with an abnormal SSR. In marked contrast to the SSR, there was close concordance of the TST result and the sweat gland response to pilocarpine. Some have inferred preganglionic sympathetic sudomotor dysfunction based on absence of a plantar SSR following peripheral nerve stimulation or deep inspiration and presence of normal acetylcholine sweat response from the dorsum of the foot (109). Since emotive or thermoregulatory sudomotor pathways may be selectively impaired, such conclusions may not be warranted.

The data just reviewed show that although the SSR is abnormal in the context of neuropathy, it is of little use in determining the presence or absence of more widespread sudomotor dysfunction. There are several likely reasons for this discrepancy. The respective central organization of pathways controlling thermoregulatory and emotive EDA differs considerably, the absent SSR may be due to sensory nerve afferent dysfunction, the absent SSR may reflect trophic skin changes that occur with some long-standing neuropathies, and the SSR amplitude itself is not linearly related to sweat gland number and depends to a large degree on background sympathetic activity (46,47).

Sympathetic Skin Response and Central Nervous System Disease

The usefulness of SSR in evaluating CNS disease has received scant attention. Some patients with amyotrophic lateral sclerosis have absent SSRs (5,14,60). SSR was found to be abnormal in 13 of 17 patients with multiple-system atrophy or progressive autonomic failure (72), although this same group of investigators later found that SSR was present in five of nine such patients (6). SSRs were abnormal in most patients with Shy–Drager syndrome, sporadic olivopontocerebellar atrophy, and striatonigral degeneration but were normal in patients with familial forms of cerebellar degeneration (111). SSR does not seem to be impaired in patients with Alzheimer's disease (104). Some studies have noted abnormal SSR amplitude (34,54,112) in 17 of 29 and in 21 of 28 patients with clinically definite multiple sclerosis, whereas one study noted abnormally prolonged SSR latencies in 60 of 70 patients (26). The authors of the latter study advanced the interesting notion that the SSR may be used as an additional electrophysiologic tool in establishing the laboratory diagnosis of multiple sclerosis. Since these patients were severely affected, no inferences can be made regarding the utility of the SSR in establishing the diagnosis of equivocal cases of multiple sclerosis. This concept requires further study.

The SSR has also been used to study reflex sympathetic dystrophy (RSD) and essential hyperhidrosis. In one study, SSR amplitude was absent or diminished in seven of 12 affected limbs (16), whereas it was abnormal in 15 of 24 patients with chronic RSD (75). Whether the SSR is useful as a diagnostic test of RSD or as a means of establishing prognosis in this condition is unclear. Abnormalities of the morphology of the SSR in palmar hyperhidrosis have been noted in two studies. In one study (49), palmar SSR amplitudes were either increased or reduced in amplitude but followed by several successive waves after the initial reduced response. Another group of investigators (52) noted an absent palmar SSR in 20% of patients. The variable morphology of the SSR is most likely due to the high level of background sympathetic activity and the nonlinear response characteristics of the SSR (46,47). Clearly, an attenuated amplitude in these patients cannot reflect reduced peripheral sympathetic sudomotor function. These data once again underscore the lack of relationship between SSR amplitude and the sweat response.

CONCLUSIONS

The SSR is in patients with a variety of axonal neuropathies. The limitations of the technique have been discussed. The SSR does not appear to be a reliable index of thermoregulatory sudomotor dysfunction, nor does it appear particularly sensitive in the early detection of small fiber sensory neuropathy. There is little data regarding the utility of the SSR in detecting early autonomic failure in diseases of the peripheral or central system, but it appears unlikely that this test will have sufficient power or sensitivity. A more rigorous approach must be adopted by those who use the SSR. Age-related normative data must be derived for each laboratory. It is suggested that palmar and plantar responses to electrical stimulation of peripheral nerve afferents, acoustic stimuli, and inspiratory gasp be recorded simultaneously from all four limbs and that the synchronous spontaneous EDA be evaluated as well. Simultaneous assessment of palmar and plantar sweat gland density and magnetic stimulation of central reflex pathways may also help to elucidate the significance of an absent SSR.

REFERENCES

1. Arunodaya GR, Taly AB. Sympathetic skin response: a decade later. *J Neurol Sci* 1995;129:81–89.
2. Arunodaya GR, Taly AB, Swamy HS. Sympathetic skin response in acute sensory ataxic neuropathy. *J Neurol Sci* 1995;130:35–38.
3. Baba M, et al. Sympathetic skin response in healthy man. *Electromyogr Clin Neurophysiol* 1988;28:277–283.
4. Bannister R, Mathias C. Testing autonomic reflexes. In: Bannister R, ed. *Autonomic failure: a textbook of clinical disorders of the autonomic nervous system.* 2nd ed. Oxford: Oxford University Press, 1988:289–307.
5. Barron SA, et al. Sympathetic cholinergic dysfunction in amyotrophic lateral sclerosis. *Acta Neurol Scand* 1987;75: 62–63.
6. Baser SM, et al. Sudomotor function in autonomic failure. *Neurology* 1991;41:1564–1566.
7. Bini G, et al. Regional similarities and differences in thermoregulatory vaso- and sudomotor tone. *J Physiol (Lond)* 1980;306:553–565.
8. Bini G, et al. Thermo-regulatory and rhythm generating mechanisms governing the sudomotor and vasoconstrictor outflow in human cutaneous nerves. *J Physiol (Lond)* 1980;306:537—552.
9. Bloch V. Le controle central de l'activite electrodermale. *J Physiol (Paris)* 1965;57(Suppl 13):1–132.
10. Christie MJ. Electrodermal activity in the 1980's: a review. *J R Soc Med* 1981;74:616–622.
11. D'Alpa F, et al. Sympathetic skin response in chronic renal failure. *Acta Neurol (Napoli)* 1988;10:280–285.
12. Davison MA, Koss MC. Brainstem loci for activation of electrodermal response in the cat. *Am J Physiol* 1975;229:930–934.
13. Delius W, et al. Manoeuvres affecting sympathetic outflow in human skin nerves. *Acta Physiol Scand* 1972;84:177–186.
14. Dettmers C, et al. Sympathetic skin response abnormalities in amyotrophic lateral sclerosis. *Muscle Nerve* 1993;16:930–934.

15. Drory VE, Korczyn AD. Sympathetic skin response: age effect. *Neurology* 1993;43:1818–1820.
16. Drory VE, Korczyn AD. The sympathetic skin response in reflex sympathetic dystrophy. *J Neurol Sci* 1995;128:92–95.
17. Edelberg R. Biopotentials from the skin surface: the hydration effect. *Ann NY Acad Sci* 1968;148:252–262.
18. Edelberg R. Electrical properties of the skin. In: Brown CC, ed. *Methods in psychophysiology.* Baltimore: Williams and Wilkins, 1967:1–53.
19. Edelberg R. Electrical properties of skin. In: Elden HR, ed. *Biophysical properties of the skin;* vol 1. New York: John Wiley and Sons, 1971:513–550.
20. Edelberg R. Electrophysiologic characteristics and interpretation of skin potentials. *USAF School Aerospace Med* 1963:1–9.
21. Edelberg R. Independence of galvanic skin response amplitude and sweat production. *J Invest Dermatol* 1964;42:443–448.
22. Edelberg R. Relation of electrical properties of skin to structure and physiologic state. *J Invest Dermatol* 1977;69:324–327.
23. Edelberg R. Response of cutaneous water barrier to ideational stimulation: a GSR component. *J Comp Physiol Psychol* 1966;61:28–33.
24. Edelberg R, et al. Some membrane properties of the effector in the galvanic skin response. *J Appl Physiol* 1960;15:691–696.
25. Elie B, Guiheneuc P. Sympathetic skin response: normal results in different experimental conditions. *Electroencephalogr Clin Neurophysiol* 1990;76:258–267.
26. Elie B, Louboutin JP. Sympathetic skin response (SSR) is abnormal in multiple sclerosis. *Muscle Nerve* 1995;18:185–189.
27. Evans BA, et al. The peripheral autonomic surface potential in suspected small fiber peripheral neuropathy. *Muscle Nerve* 1988;11:982.
28. Ewing DJ, et al. The natural history of diabetic autonomic neuropathy. *Q J Med* 1980;49:95–108.
29. Ewing DJ, et al. The value of cardiovascular autonomic function tests: 10 years experience in diabetes. *Diabetes Care* 1985;8:491–498.
30. Fagius J, Wallin BG. Sympathetic reflex latencies and conduction velocities in normal man. *J Neurol Sci* 1980;47:433–448.
31. Ferrer T, et al. Sympathetic sudomotor function and aging. *Muscle Nerve* 1995;18:395–401.
32. Girardot MN, Koss MS. A physiological and pharmacological analysis of the electrodermal response in the rat. *Eur J Pharmacol* 1984;98:185–191.
33. Gutrecht JA. Sympathetic skin response. *J Clin Neurophysiol* 1994;11:519–524.
34. Gutrecht JA, et al. Sympathetic skin response in multiple sclerosis. *J Neurol Sci* 1993;118:88–91.
35. Hoeldtke RD, et al. Autonomic surface potential analysis: assessment of reproducibility and sensitivity. *Muscle Nerve* 1992;15:926–931.
36. Holmquest D, Edelberg R. Problems in the analysis of the endosomatic galvanic skin response. *Psychophysiology* 1964;1:48–54.
37. Isamat F. Galvanic skin responses from stimulation of limbic cortex. *J Neurophysiol* 1961;24:176–181.
38. Ito K, et al. Excitatory and inhibitory electrodermal reflexes evoked by cutaneous stimulation in acute spinal cats. *Jpn J Physiol* 1978;28:737–747.
39. Jha S, Nag D. Sympathetic skin response and autonomic dysfunction in diabetes. *Indian J Physiol Pharmacol* 1995;39:149–153.
40. Karl H, et al. Electrodermal reflexes induced by activity in somatic afferent fibers. *Brain Res* 1975;87:145–150.
41. Kennedy WR, Navarro X. Sympathetic sudomotor function in diabetic neuropathy. *Arch Neurol* 46:1182–1186.
42. Kennedy WR, et al. Quantitation of the sweating deficiency in diabetes mellitus. *Ann Neurol* 1984;15:482–488.
43. Knezevic W, Bajada S. Peripheral autonomic surface potential. *J Neurol Sci* 1985;67:239–251.
44. Korpelainen JT, et al. Suppressed sympathetic skin response in brain infarction. *Stroke* 1993;24:1389–1392.
45. Koss MC, Davison MA. Characteristics of the electrodermal response. *Naunyn Schmiedebergs Arch Pharmacol* 1976;295:153–158.
46. Kunimoto M, et al. Neuro-effector characteristics of sweat glands in the human hand activated by irregular stimuli. *Acta Physiol Scand* 1992;146:261–269.
47. Kunimoto M, et al. Non-linearity of skin resistance response to intraneural electrical stimulation of sudomotor nerves. *Acta Physiol Scand* 1992;146:385–392.
48. Lader MH, Montagu JD. The psycho-galvanic reflex: a pharmacological study of the peripheral mechanism. *J Neurol Neurosurg Psychiatry* 1962;25:126–133.
49. Lefaucher JP, et al. Abolition of sympathetic skin responses following endoscopic thoracic sympathectomy. *Muscle Nerve* 1996;19:581–586.
50. Levy DM, et al. Quantitative measures of sympathetic skin response in diabetes: relation to sudomotor and neurological function. *J Neurol Neurosurg Psychiatry* 1992;10:902–908.
51. Lidberg L, Wallin BG. Sympathetic skin nerve discharges in relation to amplitude of skin resistance responses. *Psychophysiology* 1981;18:268–270.
52. Lin TK, et al. Abnormal sympathetic skin response in patients with palmar hyperhidrosis. *Muscle Nerve* 1995;18:917–919.
53. Linden D, Berlit P. Sympathetic skin responses (SSRs) in monofocal brain lesions: topographical aspects of central sympathetic pathways. *Acta Neurol Scand* 1995;91:372–376.
54. Linden D, Diehl RR, Berlit P. Subclinical autonomic disturbances in multiple sclerosis. *J Neurol* 1995;242:374–378.
55. Lloyd D. Action potential and secretory potential of sweat glands. *Proc Natl Acad Sci USA* 1961;47:351–362.
56. Low PA. Quantitation of Autonomic Responses. In: Dyck PJ, et al., eds. *Peripheral neuropathy;* vol 1. Philadelphia: WB Saunders, 1984:1139–1478.
57. Low PA, et al. Quantitative sudomotor axon reflex test in normal and neuropathic subjects. *Ann Neurol* 1983;14:573–580.
58. Martyn CN, Reid W. Sympathetic skin response [Letter]. *J Neurol Neurosurg Psychiatry* 1985;48:489–490.
59. Maselli RA, et al. Comparison of sympathetic skin response with quantitative sudomotor axon reflex test in diabetic neuropathy. *Muscle Nerve* 1989;12:420–423.
60. Masur H, et al. Sympathetic skin response in patients with amyotrophic lateral sclerosis. *Funct Neurol* 1995;10:131–135.
61. Miralles R, et al. Autonomic neuropathy in chronic alcoholism: evaluation of cardiovascular, pupillary and sympathetic skin responses. *Eur Neurol* 1995;35:287–292.
62. Montagna P, et al. Sympathetic skin response in familial amyloid polyneuropathy. *Muscle Nerve* 1988;11:183–184.
63. Murray M, Wang GH. Sweating in chronic rostrocortical and caudocortical cats. *Arch Ital Biol* 1967;105:393–398.
64. Navarro X, et al. The value of the absence of the sympathetic skin response in Sjogren's syndrome. *Muscle Nerve* 1990;13:460.
65. Navarro X, et al. Comparison of sympathetic sudomotor and skin responses in alcoholic neuropathy. *Muscle Nerve* 1993;16:404–407.
66. Niakan E, Harati Y. Sympathetic skin response in diabetic peripheral neuropathy. *Muscle Nerve* 1988;11:261–264.
67. Ogawa T. Thermal influence on palmar sweating and metal influence on generalized sweating in man. *Jpn J Physiol* 1975;25:525–536.
68. Ogawa T, et al. Comparison of sudomotor neural activities between palmar and non-palmar sweating. In: *Proceedings of the 28th International Congress of Neurovegetative Research, Japan,* Nov 1977:236–238.
69. Opsomer RJ, et al. Sympathetic skin responses from the limbs and the genitalia: normative study and contribution to the evaluation of neurologic disorders. *Electroencephalogr Clin Neurophysiol* 1996;101:25–31.
70. Patton HD. Secretory innervation of the cat's footpad. *J Neurophysiol* 1948;11:217–227.
71. Pavesi G, et al. Sympathetic skin response (SSR) in the foot after sural nerve biopsy. *Muscle Nerve* 1995;18:1326–1328.
72. Ravits JM, et al. A comparative study of electrophysiologic tests of autonomic function in patients with primary autonomic failure. *Muscle Nerve* 1986;9:657.
73. Richter CP. A study of the electrical skin resistance and the psychogalvanic reflex in a case of unilateral sweating. *Brain* 1927;50:216–235.
74. Rickles WH Jr, Day JL. Electrodermal activity in non-palmer skin sites. *Psychophysiology* 1968;4:421–435.

75. Rommel O, et al. Sympathetic skin response in patients with reflex sympathetic dystrophy. *Clin Auton Res* 1995;5:205–210.
76. Rossini PM, et al. Sudomotor skin responses following nerve and brain stimulation. *Electroencephalogr Clin Neurophysiol* 1993;89:442–446.
77. Rossini PM, et al. Sudomotor skin responses to brain stimulation do not depend on nerve sensory fiber functionality. *Electroencephalogr Clin Neurophysiol* 1993;89:447–451.
78. Satchell P, Seers CP. Evoked skin sympathetic nerve responses in man. *J Neurol Neurosurg Psychiatry* 1987;50:1015–1021.
79. Schondorf R, Gendron D. Evaluation of sudomotor function in patients with peripheral neuropathy. *Neurology* 1990;40:386.
80. Schondorf R, Gendron D. Properties of electrodermal activity recorded from non palmar/plantar skin sites. *Neurology* 1990;40:128.
81. Sequeira H, et al. Fronto-parietal control of electrodermal activity in the cat. *J Auton Nerv Syst* 1995;53:103–114.
82. Shahani BT, et al. RR interval variation and the sympathetic skin response in the assessment of autonomic function in peripheral neuropathy. *Arch Neurol* 1990;47:659–664.
83. Shahani BT, et al. Sympathetic skin response: a method of assessing unmyelinated axon dysfunction in peripheral neuropathies. *J Neurol Neurosurg Psychiatry* 1984;47:536–542.
84. Shakel B. Skin drilling: a method of diminishing galvanic skin-potentials. *Am J Psychol* 1959;72:114–121.
85. Shaver BA, et al. Origin of the galvanic skin response. *Proc Soc Exp Biol Med* 1962;110:559–564.
86. Soliven B, et al. Sympathetic skin response in diabetic neuropathy. *Muscle Nerve* 1987;10:711–716.
87. Sourek K. *The nervous control of skin potentials in man*. Prague: Rozpravy Ceskoslovenske Akademie Ved, Roenik 75: Sesit 1 1965;1–97.
88. Takagi K, Nakayama T. Peripheral effector mechanism of galvanic skin reflex. *Jpn J Physiol* 1959;9:1–7.
89. Taly AB, et al. Sympathetic skin response in Guillain–Barre syndrome. *Clin Auton Res* 1995;5:215–219.
90. Tarchanoff J. Uber die galvanischen Erscheinungen an der Haut des Menschen bei Reizung der Sinnesorgane und bie verschiedenen Formen der psychischen Tatigkeit. *Pflugers Arch* 1890;46:46–55.
91. Tranel D, Damasio H. Intact electrodermal skin conductance responses after bilateral amygdala damage. *Neuropsychologia* 1989;27:4:381–390.
92. Tzeng SS, et al. The latencies of sympathetic skin responses. *Eur Neurol* 1993;33:65–68.
93. Uncini A, et al. The sympathetic skin response: normal values elucidation of afferent components and application limits. *J Neurol Sci* 1988;87:299–306.
94. Uozumi T, et al. Sudomotor potential evoked by magnetic stimulation of the neck. *Neurology* 1993;43:1397–1400.
95. Valls-Sole J, et al. Abnormal sympathetic skin response in alcoholic subjects. *J Neurol Sci* 1991;102:233–237.
96. Van den Bergh P, Kelly JJ. The evoked electrodermal response in peripheral neuropathies. *Muscle Nerve* 1986;9:656–657.
97. Wallin BG. Sympathetic nerve activity underlying electrodermal and cardiovascular reactions in man. *Psychophysiology* 1981;18:470–476.
98. Wang GH. The galvanic skin reflex: a review of old and recent works from a physiologic point of view. Part 1. *Am J Phys Med* 1957;36:295–320.
99. Wang GH. The galvanic skin reflex: a review of old and recent works from a physiologic point of view. Part 2. *Am J Phys Med* 1958;37:35–57.
100. Wang GH. *The neural control of sweating*. Madison, WI: University of Wisconsin Press, 1964:3–128.
101. Wang GH, Chun WS. Sweating under different ambient temperatures in normal, striatal and thalamic cats. *Arch Ital Biol* 1967;105:379–391.
102. Wang GH, et al. Brainstem reticular system and galvanic skin reflex in acute decerebrate cats. *J Neurophysiol* 1956;19:350–355.
103. Wang GH, et al. Effects of transection of central neuraxis on galvanic skin reflex in anesthetized cats. *J Neurophysiol* 1956;19:340–349.
104. Wang SJ, et al. Cardiovascular autonomic functions in Alzheimer's disease. *Age Ageing* 1994;23:400–404.
105. Wang SJ, et al. Sympathetic skin response and R-R interval variation in chronic uremic patients. *Muscle Nerve* 1994;17:411–418.
106. Watahiki Y, et al. Sympathetic skin response in diabetic neuropathy. *Electromyogr Clin Neurophysiol* 1989;29:155–159.
107. Yokota T. Studies on the galvanic skin reflex (I). *J Physiol Soc Jpn* 1957;19:98.
108. Yokota T. Studies on the galvanic skin reflex (III). *J Physiol Soc Jpn* 1957;19:724–725.
109. Yokota T, et al. Dysautonomia with acute sensory motor neuropathy: a new classification of acute autonomic neuropathy. *Arch Neurol* 1994;51:1022–1031.
110. Yokota T, et al. Studies on the diphasic wave form of the galvanic skin reflex. *Electroencephalogr Clin Neurophysiol* 1959;11:687–696.
111. Yokota T, et al. Sympathetic skin response in patients with cerebellar degeneration. *Arch Neurol* 1993;50:422–427.
112. Yokota T, et al. Sympathetic skin response in patients with multiple sclerosis compared with patients with spinal cord transection and normal controls. *Brain* 1991;114:1381–1394.

CHAPTER 18

Microneurography and Autonomic Dysfunction

B. Gunnar Wallin and Mikael Elam

1. Techniques that monitor sympathetic effector function are easy to perform but difficult to interpret because neuroeffector mechanisms are complex and incompletely known, respond slowly to neural drive, and are influenced by microenvironmental, hormonal, mechanical, and chemical stimuli.
2. These difficulties are circumvented in direct intraneural recordings of sympathetic impulse traffic (microneurography).
3. Although only two sympathetic subdivisions can be studied (i.e., those to skin and muscle), microneurography has provided important new information on (1) the functional organization of the sympathetic nervous system, (2) specific sympathetic reflex mechanisms, (3) hormonal–sympathetic interaction, (4) the correlation between sympathetic nerve activity and release of transmitter, (5) sympathetic neuroeffector transmission, and (6) sympathetic drug effects.
4. This chapter summarizes both the normal characteristics of sympathetic nerve activity to muscle and skin and the studies that have expanded the knowledge of sympathetic pathophysiologic mechanisms.
5. Selected references will only include recent studies, whereas discussion of older references can be found in previous reviews [53,60].

METHODS

Intraneural recordings are made with tungsten microelectrodes that have an uninsulated tip of a few micrometers in diameter. The electrodes are inserted manually through intact skin into an underlying nerve. A low-impedance reference electrode is placed subcutaneously a short distance away. Mostly multiunit activity is obtained, but activity from single units has been recorded both in skin nerves and in muscle nerves. Recordings are commonly obtained from the peroneal, tibial, or median nerves, but small cutaneous nerve branches in arms, legs, and the face have also been used. All nerve fascicles in the proximal aspects of extremities are composed of a mixture of muscle and skin nerve fibers; distally, fascicles contain fibers connected only to a defined skin area or to a muscle. Therefore, mixed nerves are impaled as far distally as possible to obtain recordings from pure muscle or skin nerve fascicles. Action potentials can be recorded only when the electrode tip has penetrated the perineural sheath enveloping a nerve fascicle. This rules out the possibility of *crosstalk* between fascicles. During the search for a suitable recording site, subjects may experience minor discomfort, but they feel nothing during the actual recording. Transient paresthesia in the recorded extremity persists for a few days following the experiment in ~10% of the subjects. A description of the technique has been given by Vallbo et al. (53). For quantitative analysis of multiunit neurograms, bursts of impulses are detected either visually or by computer programs. When comparing different segments of a record obtained with unchanged electrode site, the strength of activity during a given time period is usually expressed as the number of bursts multiplied by their mean voltage area or amplitude. Since burst areas and amplitudes cannot be compared between different electrode sites, only the number of bursts are used for interindividual (intersite) comparisons.

The recording electrodes can also be used for evoking action potentials by intraneural electrical stimulation. Stimulation-induced cutaneous sympathetic effector responses can be detected by monitoring blood flow or sweat activity. Local anesthetic blocks of the nerve proximal or

B. G. Wallin and M. Elam: Department of Clinical Neurophysiology, University of Goteberg, Sahlgren Hospital, Sweden.

distal to the stimulation site may differentiate between effector responses caused by reflexes or by orthodromic impulses in directly stimulated sympathetic efferents. Proximal anesthetic blocks are advantageous during intraneural stimulation of sympathetic fibers, as afferent nociceptor C fibers are coactivated, making stimulation very painful in unanesthetized subjects.

NORMAL SYMPATHETIC ACTIVITY

Functional Organization of Sympathetic Outflow

The sympathetic impulses in both skin and muscle fascicles are clustered into synchronized bursts that are separated by more or less complete neural inactivity. A similar bursting pattern has been described repeatedly in recordings from various sympathetic nerves in experimental animals. The *average* firing rate in single sympathetic neurons is low at rest, but the clustering of impulses into bursts leads to *instantaneous firing frequencies* (i.e., rates calculated from the interval between two successive spikes) that occasionally exceed 50 Hz at average frequencies of <1 Hz (27). Bursts in multifiber recordings presumably stem from the simultaneous activation of many fibers and brief high-frequency firing in individual fibers. Increases of activity probably depend more on recruitment of additional fibers than on multiple firing in the same fiber.

Resting sympathetic outflow depends on an excitatory supraspinal drive, as activity is virtually absent below a complete spinal transection. The central neuronal network responsible for this excitatory drive probably also discharges in bursts, as transient or permanent arterial baroreceptor deafferentation abolishes the cardiac rhythmicity of (MSA), but the impulses still continue to occur in bursts. The bursting pattern has functional implications, in that both sympathetic transmitter release and neuroeffector transmission may be more efficient with irregular than with regular nerve traffic.

At one time, sympathetic reactions were thought to occur in parallel in different nerves. This view of a diffusely acting system led to adoption of the term "sympathetic tone" to describe the strength of a presumed global level of sympathetic activity. However, this concept has not proved tenable because no common sympathetic tone exists. Direct nerve recordings obtained in both experimental animals and humans have revealed clear-cut differences in the nerve traffic between different sympathetic subdivisions, thus indicating that sympathetic outflows to various regions are controlled separately. For example, Fig. 1 shows

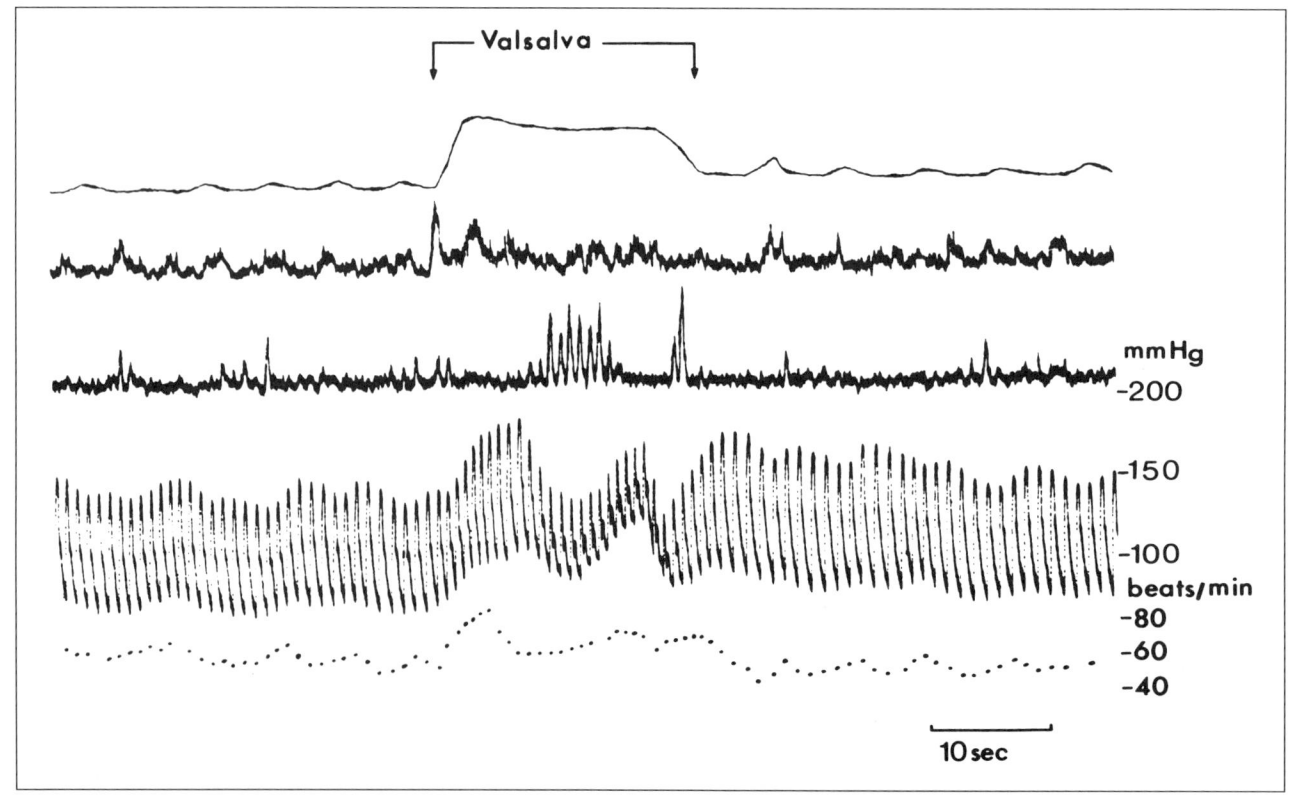

FIG. 1. The effect of the Valsalva maneuver on skin sympathetic activity (SSA) and muscle sympathetic activity (MSA) recorded simultaneously from the left (SSA) and right (MSA) peroneal nerves. *First trace:* Respiratory movements, inspiration upward. *Second trace:* SSA, integrated nerve signal. *Third trace:* MSA, integrated nerve signal. *Fourth trace:* Blood pressure. *Fifth trace:* Heart rate. From Wallin et al. (58), with permission.

that the character of skin sympathetic activity (SSA) and MSA is different at rest and that responses to the Valsalva maneuver also differ. Although MSA is similar in different extremity nerves under resting conditions, this is not always so. With some maneuvers, MSA outflow to arm muscle and outflow to leg muscle do not change in parallel, and differences among SSAs recorded from different arm and leg nerves have also been reported. Taken together, these results suggest that there are several populations of spinal sympathetic neurons, each subjected to its own supraspinal drive, which may or may not resemble that of other populations. Thus, the sympathetic system can be regarded as consisting of a number of subdivisions (each controlled by its own reflex mechanisms) that can be activated in varying combinations and to different degrees, depending on the functional demands.

Muscle Sympathetic Nerve Activity

Sympathetic outflow to muscle is dominated by vasoconstrictor impulses destined to muscle blood vessels, and an increase in MSA is associated with intramuscular vasoconstriction. MSA bursts show cardiac rhythmicity, and their duration correlates with that of the corresponding cardiac interval. The cardiac rhythmicity is due to inhibitory reflex influence from arterial baroreceptors (see below), and there is a reflex latency from the R wave in the electrocardiogram to the peak of the related sympathetic burst. In a given individual the mean latency is reproducible regardless of heart rate, but between individuals it varies between 1.1 and 1.5 sec. The latency is longer in tall than in short subjects and correlates with the length of the extremity recorded from, that is, with the length of the postganglionic fibers involved. This indicates that a large part of the latency can be attributed to peripheral conduction time. The conduction velocity in the sympathetic fibers of muscle nerves, as calculated from such latencies, is 0.7 m/sec in the median and 1.1 m/sec in the peroneal nerve. When comparing reflex latencies between individual neural discharges, strong bursts have shorter latencies than do weak bursts (57). This may indicate that increased central excitability is associated with shortening of central synaptic delays or recruitment of faster conducting nerve fibers.

In a given subject, the variations in MSA are small except during specific MSA-stimulating maneuvers (to be discussed). Resting activity is also remarkably constant in recordings repeated >10 years apart (12). This property makes it possible to monitor long-term changes in MSA, in both the context of disease and therapeutic interventions. In contrast, the number of MSA bursts per minute at rest varies markedly among individuals. Some subjects exhibit only sporadic bursts separated by long intervals; other subjects show long sequences of repeated bursts with only minor interposed silent periods. The burst incidence increases with age, body mass index (41), and waist-to-thigh ratio (36), and males have higher levels of activity than do females (32). Genetic factors may be important for the interindividual differences of activity, since homozygotic twins had much fewer differences in level of activity than did age-matched pairs of subjects who were unrelated (59). Peripheral sympathetic outflow depends on an excitatory supraspinal drive, but whether the interindividual differences in MSA are due to differences in central excitatory drive or peripheral inhibitory influence is unclear. However, alterations in central drive are probably responsible for the MSA decrease seen during deepening stages of non–rapid eye movement (non-REM) sleep as well as the marked transient increases in MSA during REM sleep.

Reflex Regulation of Muscle Sympathetic Activity

The main control of MSA is exerted by *arterial baroreceptors*, and their regulating influence is responsible for both the cardiac rhythmicity of MSA and the inverse relationship between variations in arterial blood pressure and the occurrence of sympathetic bursts. The effects evoked from carotid and aortic arterial baroreceptors differ, however. Dynamic stimulation of the carotid baroreceptors is effective in influencing MSA, but static stimuli have minor effects. In contrast, static stimulation of aortic baroreceptors elicits maintained MSA changes. These findings suggest that the static MSA changes evoked by posture (which mainly alter carotid but not aortic arterial baroreceptor firing) are elicited only to a minor extent from arterial baroreceptors.

The relationship of MSA to the respiratory cycle, with bursts occurring most frequently during late expiration and early inspiration, is probably a consequence of a primary central respiratory rhythm, but a respiratory rhythmicity of MSA may also be secondary to respiration-induced changes in blood pressure (26,46).

Alterations in central blood volume influence MSA by means of *cardiopulmonary volume (low-pressure) receptors*. The MSA increases during lower-body negative pressure and during the classic tilt-table test stem in part from the unloading of these receptors. The Valsalva maneuver, which is associated with a marked increase in MSA, probably also unloads both arterial and cardiopulmonary baroreceptors. Systemic *chemoreceptor* stimulation, trigged by hypoxia and hypercapnia, increases MSA. This probably contributes to the MSA increase seen during voluntary apnea.

Isometric handgrip contraction leads to an increase of MSA in nerves to noncontracting muscles that is attenuated after endurance training of the forearm muscles (50). The MSA increase is due mainly to reflex effects from *intramuscular chemosensitive receptors* in the activated muscles, whereas central command is of less importance and contributes mainly at high voluntary efforts (54). A comparison of finger extension and handgrip to exhaustion suggests that MSA responses increase with increasing mass of the contracting muscle (45). The location of the exercising muscle also appears to be important. A possible explanation is that muscles differ in metaboreceptor sensitivity. Alternatively, contraction of larger muscle groups may be associated with greater shifts in blood pressure and central blood volume, leading to baroreceptor-mediated inhibition of MSA that may counteract the metaboreflex-induced MSA increase. This mechanism has been suggested to explain the slower rise in MSA during isometric leg exercise (38). Two recent studies have compared peroneal MSA in nerves to exercising and nonexercising muscles during weak unilateral toe extension: one study found similar MSA increases to both legs (19) whereas the other found lower MSA to the exercising limb (56).

The popular sympathoexcitatory cold pressor test elicits a successive rise in MSA, presumably mediated by *cutaneous cold or pain receptors*, or both. Face immersion in cold water also increases MSA. Although evoked in part by cutaneous receptors, this diving reflex is more complex and differs functionally from the cold pressor test. *Pain* induced by electrical stimulation of skin nerves has little or no effect on MSA, whereas pain induced by mechanical pressure of a hard object against a fingernail or toenail or against the supraorbital or maxillary bone causes prompt and marked increases in nerve traffic (35). Mechanical stimulation of *receptors in the pharynx and larynx* in paralyzed patients under general anesthesia causes pronounced increases in MSA. Bladder filling increases MSA, possibly through the activation of *stretch receptors in the bladder wall*.

In contrast to these cardiovascular and physical stress stimuli, an arousal stimulus or short-lasting *mental stress* does not increase MSA. During mental stress of longer duration, differences in task difficulty and the subject's reactions are of importance. In one study, MSA in the peroneal nerve in the leg increased after the first minute of 4 min of mental arithmetics, but there was no change in the radial nerve in the arm. When stress was induced by delayed auditory feedback, MSA in the tibial nerve increased already during the first minute of stress (28). Thus, sympathetic outflows may differ not only between different stressors and organs but also between different anatomic locations of the same type of effector organ.

Relationship of Muscle Sympathetic Activity to Transmitter Release

Intraneurally recorded MSA and norepinephrine (NE) concentrations in, and spillover to, forearm venous plasma have been positively correlated at rest in normotensive and hypertensive subjects, in patients with cardiac failure, and in patients with liver cirrhosis and ascites. Several factors may contribute to the correlation: (a) muscles are responsible for ~20% of the total NE spillover, (b) NE spillover to forearm venous plasma derives mainly from muscle, and (c) at rest the strength of MSA correlates to noradrenaline spillover in the heart and the kidney (60). On a group basis, several maneuvers associated with MSA increases are also followed by increases in plasma NE levels, but individual increases in MSA and NE concentration often show a poor correlation. Furthermore, the increase in MSA seen during systemic hypoxia is not associated with an increase in plasma NE concentration. That there may be a lack of correlation between levels of MSA and plasma NE in some situations is not surprising: the plasma concentration depends both on spillover and on clearance of NE, it is affected by changes of blood flow, and it depends on the site of blood sampling and the timing between maneuvers and sampling.

Skin Sympathetic Nerve Activity

Sympathetic activity in skin nerve fascicles consists of vasoconstrictor impulses to skin capillaries and arteriovenous shunts, mixed with sudomotor impulses to sweat glands and possibly also piloerector and vasodilator impulses. The conduction velocity in vasoconstrictor fibers is ~0.8 m/sec, whereas sudomotor fibers conduct at ~1.3 m/sec. Since the different types of impulses can be recorded in the same electrode site and cannot be distinguished from each other in the neurogram, meaningful quantification of the different components of SSA is difficult to achieve. At rest at normal room temperature, spontaneous SSA consists of irregular bursts of impulses that vary in strength and duration but show no clear relationship to the cardiac rhythm or spontaneous blood pressure variations. Simultaneous recordings of SSA from two nerves have shown similar discharge patterns to the hands and feet, but comparisons of nerve traffic to hairy and glabrous skin showed less coordination. During non-REM sleep, both decreased SSA (52) and unchanged SSA (34) have been reported, illustrating the difficulties in quantitating the mixture of vasomotor and sudomotor traffic comprising SSA. Clear increases in SSA are seen during REM sleep and in association with K complexes in non-REM stage 2.

Reflex Regulation of Skin Sympathetic Activity

The skin is a thermoregulatory organ, and therefore SSA varies tonically with ambient and body temperature. At a comfortable ambient temperature, a relaxed subject exhibits little spontaneous SSA. In the median nerve, body cooling selectively activates vasoconstrictor fibers whereas body heating inhibits vasoconstrictor fibers (which results in passive vasodilation) and activates sudomotor and, presumably, also (active) vasodilator fibers. At very high ambient temperatures, however, there is evidence suggesting that vasoconstrictor traffic increases again, which may be a reflex protecting against overheating.

Any stimulus that causes arousal evokes a short-lasting generalized reflex discharge in SSA, which contains both vasoconstrictor and sudomotor impulses. Maneuvers or situations that evoke mental stress lead to a more long-lasting increase in SSA, which occasionally may persist long after the end of the stimulus. An inspiratory gasp is also followed by a strong reflex burst of SSA. The vasoconstrictor component of SSA in nerves to hands and feet shows no baroreceptor sensitivity, in that it exhibits no cardiac rhythmicity and no relationship to blood pressure variations. However, bursts of sudomotor activity display cardiac rhythmicity, which may be due to excitatory influence from cardiopulmonary (low pressure) receptors. This is suggested by (a) the absence of relationship between SSA and arterial blood pressure variations and (b) the finding that sudomotor discharges are inhibited by blood volume displacement from the chest to the lower body (6). Presumably, this reflex counteracts excessive volume loss in warm environments.

Thermoregulatory and other cutaneous reflex effects interact. In warm subjects, arousal, a deep breath, mental stress, or painful stimuli coactivate vasoconstrictor and sudomotor fibers, which constitutes the basis for *cold sweat*. In cold subjects, the same stimuli evoke cutaneous vasodilation. The transition from vasoconstriction to vasodilation occurs at a skin temperature around 28°C in the hand and 33°C in the foot. Thus, when studying skin blood flow, careful temperature control is necessary and, to avoid ambiguous results, subjects should probably be either warm or cold rather than thermoneutral.

Skin Sympathetic Neuroeffector Transfer

The relationship between sympathetic nerve traffic and effector responses is complex and only partially understood. As mentioned previously, transmitter release and vascular responses may vary depending on the pattern of stimulation. Neuroeffector transfer at sweat glands is also complex. When sudomotor fibers in the median nerve were stimulated electrically, a given stimulus evoked different skin resistance responses depending on the degree of previous sudomotor nerve traffic (Fig. 2). These findings prove that measurements of skin resistance variations cannot reliably quantitate sympathetic sudomotor nerve activity.

HORMONAL INFLUENCES ON SYMPATHETIC NERVE ACTIVITY

Among hormonal factors, the effects of altered plasma insulin levels and glucose metabolism are most extensively studied. Intravenous infusion of insulin or 2-deoxy-D-glucose increases both MSA and the sudomotor component of SSA, whereas the vasoconstrictor component of SSA is inhibited (1). In part, the effects may be due to central nervous system glucopenia. However, insulin also has a direct sympathoexcitatory effect, since MSA increases markedly during a euglycemic hyperinsulinemic clamp. The MSA increase is abolished by pretreatment with dexamethasone

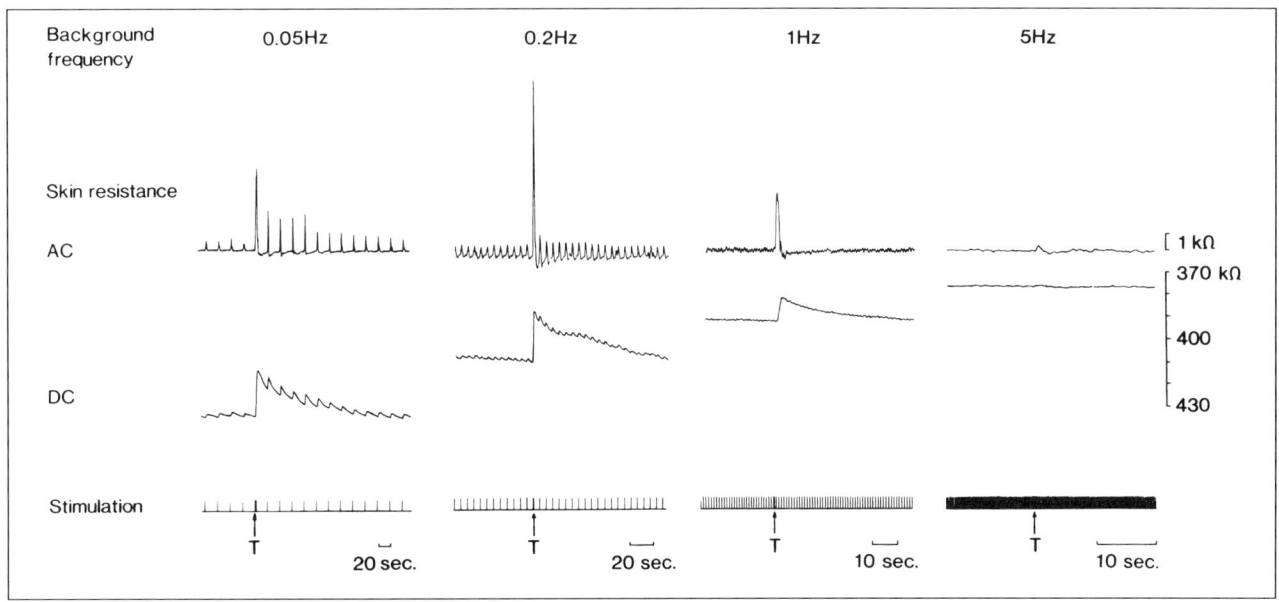

FIG. 2. Effects of intraneural stimulation of a skin fascicle in the median nerve upon skin resistance recorded within the innervation zone in the index finger. At each background frequency, a train (T) of six impulses at 20 Hz was added. In this subject, the maximum change in skin resistance (AC) evoked by the train occurred at a background frequency of 0.2 Hz. Note the potentiation (at 0.05 and 0.2 Hz) of skin resistance changes in response to the first few background stimuli after the train. Spontaneous sympathetic activity was abolished by regional local anesthesia of the axillary plexus. From Kirnö et al. (25), with permission.

(43), interpreted as indicating a centrally mediated effect of insulin. Interestingly, the insulin-induced increase in MSA during a euglycemic clamp is not associated with increased arterial pressure, possibly because the sympathoexcitation is limited to muscle vasoconstrictor fibers. In agreement with this notion, total body NE spillover is not significantly increased (17). This underlines the lack of a simple relationship between MSA and blood pressure levels, which is important when considering the pathophysiology of hypertension (cf. below).

A centrally mediated MSA increase has been demonstrated after subcutaneous injection of thyrotropin-releasing hormone. Hypothyreotic patients have augmented resting MSA. MSA has been shown to correlate negatively with serum levels of free triiodothyronine and thyroxine, and positively with thyroid-stimulating hormone, suggesting an inverse relationship between thyroid function and sympathetic nerve activity (29).

Blood pressure reductions induced by atrial natriuretic factor are associated with a less pronounced reflex increase in MSA than are similar pressure reductions induced by sodium nitroprusside, suggesting that atrial natriuretic factor has a relative sympathoinhibitory effect. This was recently suggested to be due to modulation of ganglionic neurotransmission (13).

The MSA increase following oral (15,22) or intravenous (37) alcohol administration has been suggested to be mediated via secretion of corticotropin-releasing hormone, since the alcohol-induced sympathoexcitation was abolished by dexamethasone (37).

SYMPATHETIC ACTIVITY IN PATHOLOGIC CONDITIONS

Many nervous lesions may produce pathologic sympathetic activity that can be detected in microneurographic recordings. These abnormalities may be qualitative or quantitative in nature. Quantitative abnormalities arise if the number of sympathetic impulses reaching the effector is reduced (or increased), resulting in weakened (or exaggerated) but qualitatively normal reflex responses. A qualitative abnormality implies that reflex effects are evoked by a stimulus that normally is ineffective, or that the manifestation of a reflex effect is reversed, for example, if a normally inhibitory response is altered into an excitatory one.

In principle, it would be possible to use intraneural recordings of sympathetic nerve activity for diagnostic purposes in patients with qualitative abnormalities. Unfortunately, such abnormalities are rare. To diagnose quantitative abnormalities is difficult for two main reasons. First, there are large interindividual differences among normal subjects, both in terms of the strength of MSA and SSA at rest and in their responsiveness to various stimuli. This makes it difficult to define meaningful normal values. Second, if a dysfunction is due to a reduction in the number of functioning postganglionic sympathetic fibers, it may be impossible to find a recording site with an acceptable signal-to-noise ratio for sympathetic activity. However, because occasionally it is also not possible to find a sympathetic recording site in normal subjects, microneurographic failure in a single trial has little diagnostic significance. The consequence of these limitations is that microneurography is useful for controlled studies that compare groups of subjects but not as a diagnostic tool in individual patients.

Peripheral Neuropathies

Sympathetic failure as part of a *generalized polyneuropathy* is common. Large-diameter fiber involvement in polyneuropathy is usually characterized by reduced nerve conduction velocity in both somatomotor and sensory axons, but these results are not applicable to unmyelinated fibers. In a study of patients with polyneuropathy of varying causes, MSA and SSA were normal (when detected). The conduction velocity in postganglionic fibers was normal also in patients who had marked slowing in myelinated fibers and clinical symptoms of autonomic failure. However, inability to detect sympathetic activity in microneurographic recordings was significantly more frequent, especially in patients with diabetic polyneuropathy. These findings suggest that impulses in postganglionic sympathetic (and perhaps also sensory unmyelinated) fibers are propagated with a normal velocity as long as the fibers conduct, and that the successive loss of functioning fibers leads to disappearance of detectable activity. Clinical symptoms of sympathetic failure probably appear when too few fibers remain to achieve adequate control of effector organ function.

Some patients with *acute inflammatory polyneuropathy* (the Guillain–Barré syndrome) develop hypertension and tachycardia, symptoms that indicate sympathetic overactivity rather than failure. In such patients, MSA was abnormally increased during the acute phase of the disease, as concluded from findings of much lower levels of activity at repeated recordings after recovery. A probable explanation for this is that the neuropathy affected sympathoinhibitory afferent fibers from arterial or cardiopulmonary baroreceptors, or both, resulting in reduced inhibition of sympathetic outflow.

Paroxysms of hypertension were reported in a patient with a history of *neck and mediastinal irradiation*. Microneurography revealed loss of cardiac rhythmicity in MSA but preserved responses to lower-body negative pressure. Probably, therefore, the neuropathy had selectively affected arterial baroreceptor fibers.

Syncope

Episodes of blood pressure reduction and syncope may sometimes represent physiologic reflex reactions but can also be due to peripheral neural lesions. *Vasovagal syncope* belongs to the first category and is generally caused by emotional reactions but may also be elicited by peripheral reflexes as a protective reaction in unfavorable homeostatic situations. Such syncope is associated with sudden withdrawal of MSA, but whether active vasodilation also contributes is uncertain. Animal research has indicated that the withdrawal of vasoconstrictor activity may be a reflex effect caused by strong activation of cardiac ventricular receptors, but, because syncope with MSA withdrawal has also been demonstrated in a patient without innervated ventricular receptors (after heart transplantation), alternative mechanisms must exist. In a patient with *carotid sinus hypersensitivity*, carotid massage was found to cause inhibition of MSA together with asystole and blood pressure reduction (49).

In contrast to vasovagal syncope, *fainting during attacks of glossopharyngeal neuralgia* is probably caused by a nerve lesion. The neuralgic attacks are evoked from the back of the mouth and throat by mechanical stimuli (eating, coughing, etc.). Some patients with this disorder faint in conjunction with the pain attack. In this type of syncope, there is also a sudden withdrawal of MSA, which contributes to vasodilation and blood pressure reduction. Because pain fibers from the throat and baroreceptor fibers from the carotid sinus both run in the glossopharyngeal nerve, it has been suggested that there is a pathologic synapse (a so-called ephapse) somewhere along this pathway where the pain impulses are misdirected to the baroreceptor fibers. Presumably, there is profound sympathetic inhibition when this barrage of impulses reaches the vasomotor centers in the brainstem.

The findings described in this section illustrate that the diversity of sympathetic aberrations in peripheral nerve lesions depends on the character of the reflex and the locus of the neuropathy. Lesions anywhere in an excitatory reflex arc can be expected to reduce the strength of sympathetic activity (and the effector response), but the effects of lesions in an inhibitory reflex arc may vary. If the damage is in the afferent limb, the effects should be the opposite of those arising from damage to the efferent limb; if both limbs are affected, the disturbance may vary, depending on which lesion dominates.

Central Dysautonomia

In patients with traumatic *spinal cord transection*, MSA and SSA were almost completely absent below the level of transection, indicating that spinal sympathetic activity depends on an excitatory supraspinal drive. The baroreceptor-induced cardiac rhythmicity of MSA was lost, and reflex discharges in MSA and SSA were more difficult to evoke below the lesion and not stronger than normal; nevertheless, marked blood pressure increases often occurred. Thus, the episodes of high blood pressure evoked by skin stimuli below the lesion in patients with spinal cord injury cannot be explained by supersensitivity of the decentralized preganglionic sympathetic neurons. A qualitative abnormality was noted, however, in that skin pinches, electrical skin stimuli, and pressure over the bladder provoked simultaneous SSA and MSA increases. As MSA is normally unaffected by such stimuli, it means that the stimulus caused vasoconstriction in a larger than normal vascular bed, and this, together with the lack of functioning baroreflexes, may contribute to the blood pressure increases seen in spinal cord-injured patients.

Only a few recordings of probable sympathetic nerve activity have been performed in patients with degenerative central dysautonomias. In one patient with the *Shy–Drager syndrome*, resting MSA was weak but increased markedly in strength after the oral administration of L-threo-3,4-dihydroxyphenylserine. This suggests that, at least in some Shy–Drager patients, loss of sympathetic function may stem from a biochemical defect rather than from an anatomic loss of sympathetic neurons.

Compared with a group of age-matched controls, resting MSA was found to be increased and the MSA response to 30° head-up tilt decreased in patients with *amyotrophic lateral sclerosis* (48). The underlying reason is unclear, and no difference was found between the groups with regard to blood pressure or heart rate.

Hypertension

Studies comparing resting MSA in patients with essential hypertension and normotensive controls have reached varying results, partly due to too small materials and to confounders such as age and body weight. Recent studies using age- and weight-matched study groups have indicated an augmented MSA in patients with *borderline hypertension* (14,20). In contrast, no significant increase in MSA was found in established *essential hypertension* (18). Patients with *accelerated hypertension* have been shown to have higher MSA than subjects with benign hypertension (30). Increased MSA has also been reported in association with *renovascular hypertension* (31) and hypertension in *chronic renal failure* (4).

Established and/or borderline hypertensive patients have shown elevated MSA responses during the cold pressor test, lower-body negative pressure, apnea during hypoxia and during mental stress, but not in response to the isometric handgrip test. A recent study in normotensive offspring of hypertensive patients demonstrated an MSA increase during mental stress that was not found in offspring of normotensive parents. However, no significant difference in resting MSA was found (33).

Sleep Apnea

Hypertension is common in patients with sleep apnea, a syndrome associated with augmented MSA in the awake state and accentuated sympathoexcitation during apneic episodes in sleep (2,21,51,61). This sympathoexcitation is

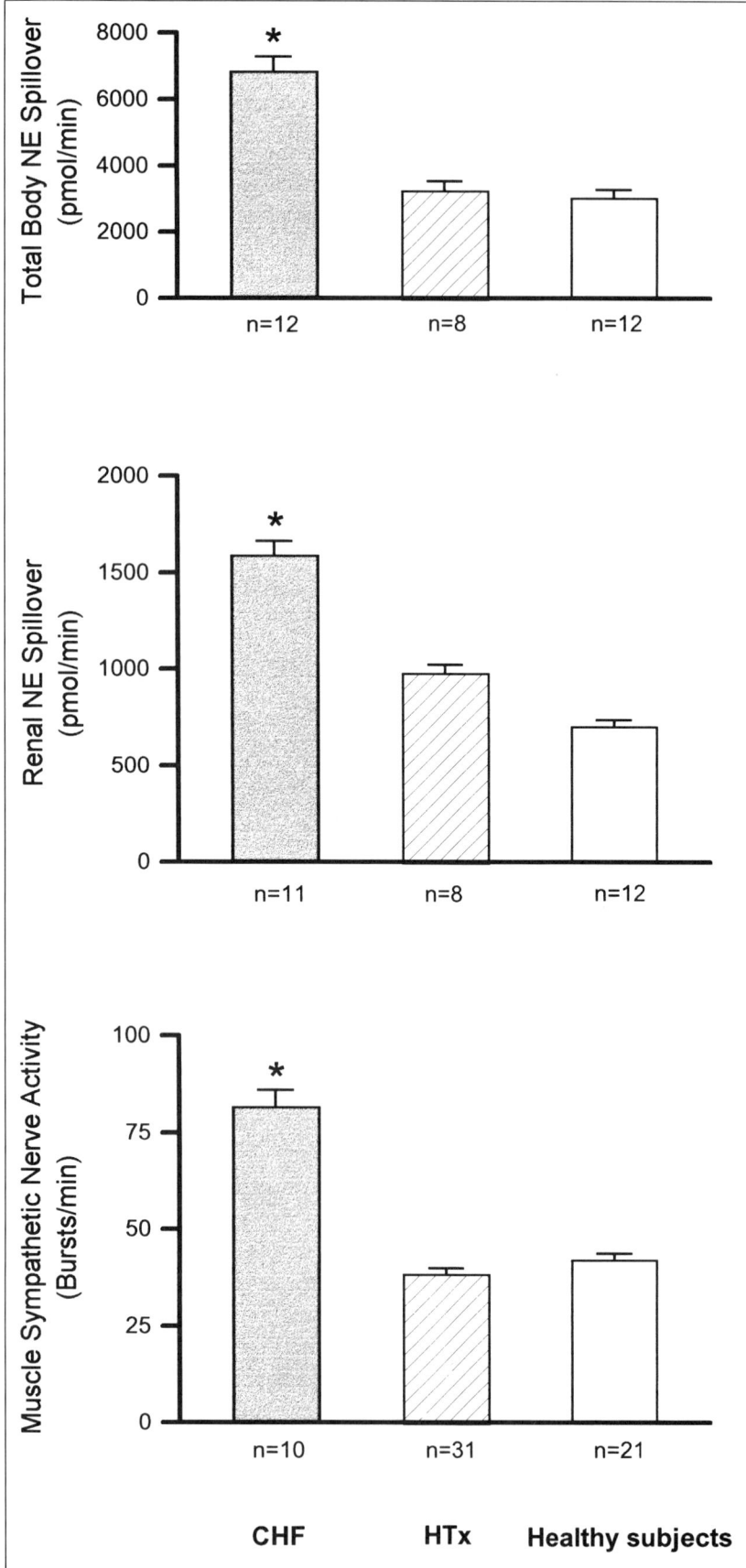

FIG. 3. MSA □, total body □, and renal □ norepinephrine spillovers are markedly increased in patients with severe congestive heart failure. One year after cardiac transplantation, these indices of sympathetic activity do not differ from age- and weight-matched healthy controls.

reduced by therapy with continuous positive airway pressure (51). The sustained MSA increase in these patients may depend on a reduced baroreflex sensitivity (3), which in turn may represent an adaptive response to the repetitive nocturnal blood pressure surges.

Heart Failure

Several studies have shown increased MSA and plasma concentrations of NE in patients with moderate to severe chronic heart failure. One study has shown significantly increased MSA also in mild heart failure of New York Heart Association class I–II (16). A recent study combining nerve recording with measurements of NE kinetics showed that an increased cardiac NE spillover precedes changes in MSA and total body spillover (39).

The mechanisms underlying sympathoexcitation in heart failure are not clear, but impaired baroreflexes may contribute. The administration of digitalis glycosides does not affect resting MSA in healthy subjects (44) but reduces MSA in heart-failure patients, an effect thought to be mediated partly by arterial and/or low-pressure reflexes.

After cardiac transplantation, an early study found that MSA remained markedly augmented (42), but in several subsequent studies MSA and NE spillover were normalized (11,23,40) (Fig. 3) The reduction in MSA occurs within 1 month postoperatively.

Pain

Acute pain gives rise to an immediate increase in SSA, and a recent study has shown that also MSA increases in response to several nociceptive stimuli (see above). An augmented sympathetic outflow is often suggested to contribute to various types of chronic pain syndromes. Clinical signs of skin sympathetic disturbances in affected patients (asymmetrical vasomotor or sudomotor function) is often taken as evidence for a neural disturbance. However, the few published accounts of intraneural recordings in patients with this type of pain syndrome revealed no abnormality in sympathetic outflow to the affected area (10), but intracutaneous administration of NE elicited the characteristic pain sensations. A possible explanation is that sympathetically maintained pain is due to alterations in neuroeffector mechanisms rather than in neural activity.

The notion that chronic fibromyalgic pain may be caused by a tension-induced increase in MSA, resulting in muscle ischemia, is based partly on the beneficial effect of regional sympathetic blocks in this syndrome. However, a recent study showed no difference in resting MSA between patients with chronic fibromyalgia and age-matched healthy controls, nor did the responses to isometric handgrip and mental stress differ. Given the sympathetic modulation of sensory afferent transmission, a beneficial effect from chemical sympathectomy does not necessarily indicate primary sympathetic involvement in the generation of a pain syndrome.

Peridural and intradural local anesthetic blocks are important for the diagnosis and treatment of chronic pain states, especially neuropathic pain, but it has been questioned whether such procedures are effective in achieving a sympathetic block. In microneurographic studies, however, peridural anesthesia with the spinal level of sensory blockade at T9 or higher completely eliminated MSA and SSA in the peroneal nerve. This finding indicates that peridural and intradural anesthesia can be used as pharmacologic tools to evaluate the influence of sympathetic activity on effector organ function. It was also demonstrated that intrathecal opiate administration did not affect sympathetic nerve activity whereas epidurally administered clonidine had a sympathoinhibitory effect (24). Presumably, this inhibition was mediated by a systemic/central rather than a regional/spinal mechanism, and equal sympathoinhibition was produced by intramuscular injection of clonidine.

General Anesthetic Procedures

MSA is reduced during induction of anesthesia with propofol, thiopental sodium, and metohexital sodium and during maintenance of anesthesia with isoflurane. In contrast, nitrous oxide and desflurane (8) increase MSA, whereas etomidate and sevoflurane (9) have no effects. Interestingly, both clonidine (5) and the opioid analgesic alfentanil (62) have been shown to reduce the desflurane-induced blood pressure increase without diminishing its sympathoexcitatory effect.

Laryngoscopy and intubation lead to a massive increase of both MSA and SSA. The baroreflex sensitivity of MSA is reduced during propofol anesthesia (47), although reflex responses to a hypertensive stimulus have been shown to remain (7). Surgical procedures may increase the strength of MSA dramatically, with associated increases in blood pressure, effects that are reduced or eliminated by additional doses of anesthetic drugs.

CONCLUSION

Microneurography was developed in a laboratory of clinical neurophysiology, and initially physiological and neurological applications were most common. More recently, the technique has spread to several clinical disciplines and the development has been especially fruitful in cardiology, hypertension, endocrinology, and anesthesiology. No diagnostic use of the technique has been reported, but it can be applied to quite complicated clinical settings (e.g., surgery and intensive care). With proper training and precautions, the method is safe and has the attraction that it may differentiate neural from effector disturbances in clinical autonomic disorders.

ACKNOWLEDGMENT

This work was supported by Swedish Medical Research Council grant 3546.

REFERENCES

1. Berne C, Fagius J. Metabolic regulation of sympathetic nervous system activity: lessons from intraneural recordings. *Int J Obes* 1993; 17(Suppl 3):S2–S6.
2. Carlson JT, et al. Augmented resting sympathetic activity in awake patients with obstructive sleep apnea. *Chest* 1993;103:1763–1768.
3. Carlson JT, et al. Depressed baroreflex sensitivity in patients with obstructive sleep apnea. *Am J Respir Crit Care Med* 1996;154:1490–1496.
4. Converse RL Jr, et al. Sympathetic overactivity in patients with chronic renal failure. *N Engl J Med* 1992;327:1912–1918.
5. Devcic A, et al. The effects of clonidine on desflurane-mediated sympathoexcitation in humans. *Anesth Analg* 1995;80:773–779.
6. Dodt C, et al. Central blood volume influences sympathetic sudomotor nerve traffic in warm humans. *Acta Physiol Scand* 1995;155:41–51.
7. Ebert TJ, Muzi M. Propofol and autonomic reflex function in humans. *Anesth Analg* 1994;78:369–375.
8. Ebert TJ, Muzi M. Sympathetic hyperactivity during desflurane anesthesia in healthy volunteers: a comparison with isoflurane. *Anesthesiology* 1993;79:444–453.
9. Ebert TJ, et al. Neurocirculatory responses to sevoflurane in humans: a comparison to desflurane. *Anesthesiology* 1995;83:88–95.
10. Elam M. Is sympathetic nerve activity abnormal in reflex sympathetic dystrophy? *Funct Neurol* 1993;8(Suppl 6):71–78.
11. Elam M, et al. Is sympathetic neural hyperactivity in chronic heart failure affected by heart transplantation? *Eur Heart J* 1993;14:521–525.
12. Fagius A, Wallin BG. Long-term variability and reproducibility of resting human muscle nerve sympathetic activity at rest, as reassessed after a decade. *Clin Auton Res* 1993;3:201–205.
13. Floras JS. Inhibitory effect of atrial natriuretic factor on sympathetic ganglionic neurotransmission in humans. *Am J Physiol* 1995;269 (*Regul Integr Comp Physiol* 38):R406–R412.
14. Floras JS, Hara K. Sympathoneural and haemodynamic characteristics of young subjects with mild essential hypertension. *J Hypertens* 1993;11:647–655.
15. Grassi GM, et al. Effects of alcohol intake on blood pressure and sympathetic nerve activity in normotensive humans: a preliminary report. *J Hypertens* 1989;7(Suppl 6):S20–S21.
16. Grassi G, et al. Sympathetic activation and loss of reflex sympathetic control in mild congestive heart failure. *Circulation* 1995;92:3206–3211.
17. Gudbjörnsdottir S, et al. The effect of metformin and insulin on sympathetic nerve activity, norepinephrine spillover and blood pressure in obese, insulin resistant, normoglycemic, hypertensive men. *Blood Pressure* 1994;3:394–403.
18. Gudbjörnsdottir S, et al. Sympathetic nerve activity and insulin in obese normotensive and hypertensive men. *Hypertension* 1996;27: 276–280.
19. Hansen J, et al. Muscle metaboreflex triggers parallel sympathetic activation in exercising and resting human skeletal muscle. *Am J Physiol* 1994;266(*Heart Circ Physiol* 35):H2508–H2514.
20. Hara K, Floras JS. Influence of naloxone on muscle sympathetic nerve activity, systemic and calf haemodynamics and ambulatory blood pressure after exercise in mild essential hypertension. *J Hypertens* 1994;13:447–461.
21. Hedner J, et al. Is high and fluctuating muscle nerve sympathetic activity in the sleep apnoea syndrome of pathogenetic importance for the development of hypertension? *J Hypertens* 1988;6(Suppl 4): S529–S531.
22. Iwase S, et al. Effect of oral ethanol intake on muscle sympathetic nerve activity and cardiovascular functions in humans. *J Auton Nerv Syst* 1995;54:206–214.
23. Kaye DM, et al. Cyclosporine therapy after cardiac transplantation causes hypertension and renal vasoconstriction without sympathetic activation. *Circulation* 1993;88:1101–1109.
24. Kirnö K, et al. Epidural clonidine depresses sympathetic nerve activity in humans by a supraspinal mechanism. *Anesthesiology* 1993; 78:1021–1027.
25. Kirnö K, et al. Can galvanic skin response be used as a quantitative estimate of sympathetic nerve activity in regional anesthesia? *Anesth Analg* 1991;73:138–142.
26. Macefield V, Wallin BG. Modulation of muscle sympathetic activity during spontaneous and artificial ventilation and apnoea in humans. *J Auton Nerv Syst* 1995;53:137–147.
27. Macefield VG, et al. The discharge behaviour of single vasoconstrictor motoneurones in human muscle nerves. *J Physiol (Lond)* 1994; 481:799–809.
28. Matsukawa T, et al. Increased muscle sympathetic nerve activity during delayed auditory feedback in humans. *Jpn J Physiol* 1995;45: 905–911.
29. Matsukawa T, et al. Altered muscle sympathetic nerve activity in hyperthyroidism and hypothyroidism. *J Auton Nerv Syst* 1993;42:171–176.
30. Matsukawa T, et al. Elevated sympathetic nerve activity in patients with accelerated essential hypertension. *J Clin Invest* 1993;92: 25–28.
31. Miyajima E, et al. Muscle sympathetic nerve activity in renovascular hypertension and primary aldosteronism. *Hypertension* 1991;17: 1057–1062.
32. Ng AV, et al. Age and gender influence muscle sympathetic nerve activity at rest in healthy humans. *Hypertension* 1993;21:498–503.
33. Noll G, et al. Increased activation of sympathetic nervous system and endothelin by mental stress in normotensive offspring of hypertensive parents. *Circulation* 1996;93:866–869.
34. Noll G, et al. Skin sympathetic nerve activity and effector function during sleep in humans. *Acta Physiol Scand* 1994;151:319–329.
35. Nordin M, Fagius J. Effect of noxious stimulation on sympathetic vasoconstrictor outflow to human muscles. *J Physiol (Lond)* 1995; 489:885–894.
36. Parker Jones P, et al. Gender differences in muscle sympathetic nerve activity: effect of body fat distribution. *Am J Physiol* 1996;270(*Endocrinol Metab* 33):E363–E366.
37. Randin D, et al. Suppression of alcohol-induced hypertension by dexamethasone. *N Engl J Med* 1995;332:1733–1737.
38. Ray CA, Mark AL. Augmentation of muscle sympathetic nerve activity during fatiguing isometric leg exercise. *J Appl Physiol* 1993;75: 228–232.
39. Rundqvist B, et al. Increased cardiac adrenergic drive precedes generalized sympathetic activation in human heart failure. *Circulation* 1997;95:169–175.
40. Rundqvist B, et al. Normalization of total body and regional sympathetic hyperactivity in heart failure after cardiac transplantation. *J Heart Lung Transplant* 1996;15:516–526.
41. Scherrer U, et al. Body fat and sympathetic nerve activity in healthy subjects. *Circulation* 1994;89:2634–2640.
42. Scherrer U, et al. Cyclosporine-induced sympathetic activation and hypertension after heart transplantation. *N Engl J Med* 1990;323: 693–698.
43. Scherrer U, et al. Suppression of insulin-induced sympathetic activation and vasodilation by dexamethasone in humans. *Circulation* 1993;88:388–394.
44. Schobel HP, et al. Differential effects of digitalis on chemoreflex responses in humans. *Hypertension* 1994;23:302–307.
45. Seals DR. Influence of activity muscle size on sympathetic nerve discharge during isometric contractions in humans. *J Appl Physiol* 1993;75:1426–1431.
46. Seals DR, et al. Respiratory modulation of muscle sympathetic nerve activity in intact and lung denervated humans. *Circ Res* 1993;72: 440–454.
47. Sellgren J, et al. Sympathetic muscle nerve activity, peripheral blood flows, and baroreceptor reflexes in humans during propofol anesthesia and surgery. *Anesthesiology* 1994;80:534–544.
48. Shindo K, et al. Microneurographic analysis of muscle sympathetic nerve activity in amyotrophic lateral sclerosis. *Clin Auton Res* 1993; 3:131–135.
49. Smith ML, et al. Sympathoinhibition and hypotension in carotid sinus hypersensitivity. *Clin Auton Res* 1992; 2:389–392.

50. Somers VK, et al. Forearm endurance training attenuates sympathetic nerve response to isometric handgrip in normal humans. *J Appl Physiol* 1992;72:1039–1043.
51. Somers VK, et al. Sympathetic neural mechanisms in obstructive sleep apnea. *J Clin Invest* 1995;96:1897–1904.
52. Takeuchi S, et al. Sleep-related changes in human muscle and skin sympathetic nerve activities. *J Auton Nerv Syst* 1994;47:121–129.
53. Vallbo ÅB, et al. Somatosensory, proprioceptive and sympathetic activity in human peripheral nerves. *Physiol Rev* 1979;59:919–957.
54. Victor RG, et al. Central command increases muscle sympathetic nerve activity during intense intermittent isometric exercise in humans. *Circ Res* 1995;76:127–131.
55. Wallin BG. Assessment of sympathetic mechanisms from recordings of postganglionic efferent nerve traffic. In: Hainsworth R, Mark AL, eds. *Cardiovascular reflex control in health and disease.* London: WB Saunders 1994:65–93.
56. Wallin BG, et al. Coherence between the sympathetic drives to relaxed and contracting muscles of different limbs of human subjects. *J Physiol (Lond)* 1992;455:219–233.
57. Wallin BG, et al. Coupling between variations in strength and baroreflex latency of sympathetic discharges in human muscle nerves. *J Physiol (Lond)* 1994;474:331–338.
58. Wallin BG, et al. Regional control of sympathetic outflow in human skin and muscle nerves. In: Umbach W, Koepchen HP, eds. *Central rhythmic and regulation.* Stuttgart: Hippocrates, 1974:190–195.
59. Wallin BG, et al. Possible genetic influence on the strength of human muscle nerve sympathetic activity at rest. *Hypertension* 1993;22:282–284.
60. Wallin BG, et al. Renal noradrenaline spillover correlates with muscle sympathetic activity in humans. *J Physiol (Lond)* 1996;491:881–887.
61. Watanabe T, et al. Enhanced muscle sympathetic nerve activity during sleep apnea in the elderly. *J Auton Nerv Syst* 1992;37:223–226.
62. Yonker-Sell AE, et al. Alfentanil modifies the neurocirculatory responses to desflurane. *Anesth Analg* 1996;82:162–166.

CHAPTER 19

Thermoregulatory Sweat Test

Robert D. Fealey

1. The thermoregulatory sweat test (TST) is useful for assessing the integrity of central and peripheral sympathetic sudomotor pathways.
2. The proper technique for performing the TST involves controlling the ambient air temperature and humidity, as well as the patient's skin temperature, so that a maximal sweat response is produced in a tolerable fashion. Operating conditions to ensure an adequate heat stimulus should be as follows: air temperature 45°–50°C, relative humidity, 35%–40%, and skin temperature 39.0°–39.5°C.
3. One needs to be familiar with the normal variants of the sweat response and have normative data regarding oral and skin temperature changes at which maximal recruitment of sweating has occurred. In our laboratory, we continue the test until the continuously monitored oral temperature reaches 38.0°C or is 1.0°C higher than the initial temperature, whichever of the two is greater. The mean oral temperature rise we have noted in our patients is 1.5°C, a value significantly higher than the 1.0°C cited in the literature.
4. The sweat test report should describe the heating stimulus, the patient's initial and final central (oral or equivalent) temperature rise, the sweat distribution, and some estimate of the percentage of the body surface that does not sweat.
5. The percentage of body surface anhidrosis provides a useful index of the degree of autonomic failure in the characterization of the multiple system atrophy syndromes; the distribution of anhidrosis is helpful in characterizing the anatomic–pathologic pattern of involvement of autonomic peripheral nerves in diabetic, leprosy, idiopathic small fiber, amyloid, and other neuropathies.
6. The TST can be used in conjunction with axon–reflex sweat tests (such as the quantitative sudomotor axon reflex test or QSART) to determine whether a lesion is pre- or postganglionic.
7. In localized hyperhidrotic conditions, the TST can demonstrate whether the excessive sweating is "compensatory" and due to widespread anhidrosis elsewhere.
8. The completeness of surgical sympathectomy is well demonstrated by the TST.
9. Difficulties encountered with the TST include the duration and untidiness of the test, the rare irritant skin reactions to the indicator powder, and the ~5% incidence of incomplete studies due to patient intolerance of the heat stress or enclosed environment. There's also a need for careful documentation of the distribution of anhidrosis via photograph or computerized drawing to enable quantitation of results. Variables confounding interpretation of results include advanced age, prior use of anticholinergic drugs, skin lotions, and hydration status.
10. Positive attributes of the TST include the ability to screen the entire anterior body surface for pre- or postganglionic sympathetic lesions, the relative noninvasiveness and simplicity of the test, and the ability to quantitate the result in terms of percentage of body surface anhidrosis.

INTRODUCTION

The thermoregulatory sweat test (TST) is useful in assessing the integrity of central and peripheral sympathetic sudomotor pathways. The sweat response is mediated by preganglionic centers, including the hypothalamus, bulbospinal pathways, intermediolateral cell columns, and white rami and postganglionic pathways, including the sympathetic chain and postganglionic sudomotor axons to sweat glands (Fig. 1) (33,34).

R. D. Fealey: Department of Neurology, Mayo Clinic, Rochester, Minnesota 55905.

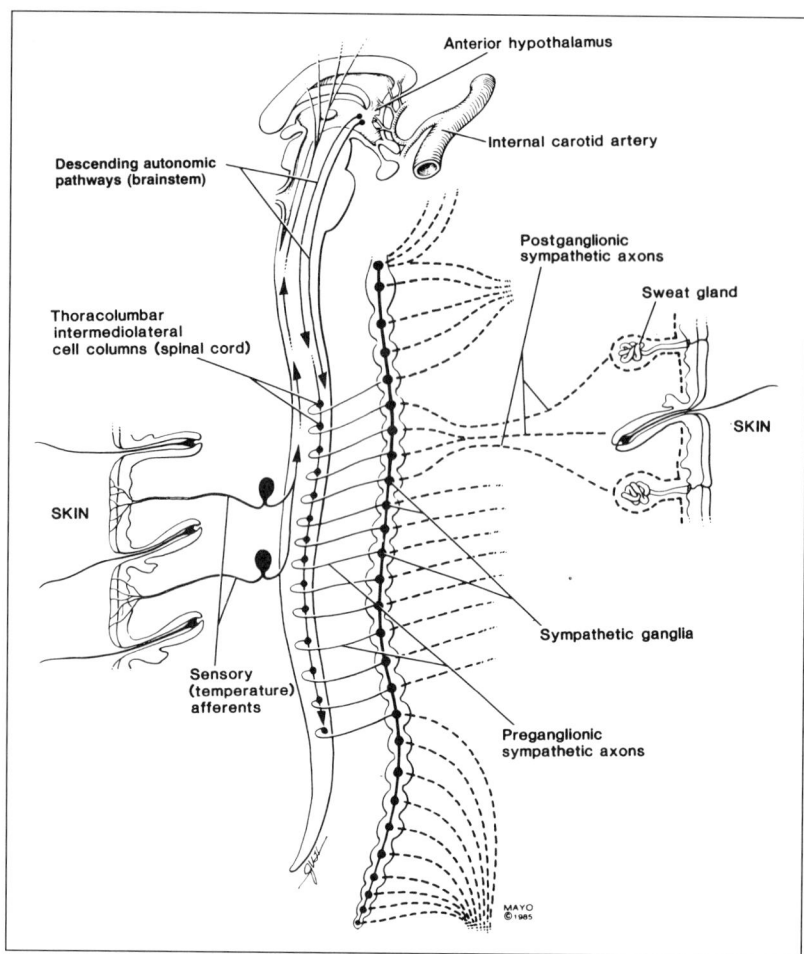

FIG. 1. Thermoregulatory sweating pathways: skin thermal afferents and central blood temperature affect sympathetic sudomotor efferents. From Fealey et al. (17), with permission.

As sweat rate has been shown to be directly proportional to the mean and local skin temperature as well as the central (blood/core) temperature (32,44), a maximal sweat response and recruitment of intact efferent sudomotor units are realized by raising central and mean skin temperature. Central blood temperature is estimated by measuring oral or tympanic membrane temperature (44).

The proper technique for performing the TST includes controlling the ambient air temperature and humidity as well as the patient's skin temperature to produce a reproducible maximal response. To avoid hydromeiosis (reduced sweat rate at high temperatures and levels of skin moisture), some degree of sweat evaporation must also take place (49,51). To avoid injury and confounding somatosympathetic reflex sweating, the skin temperature should not exceed 40.0°C (18).

The TST conducted in the Mayo Clinic Thermoregulatory Laboratory is a modification of Guttmann's quinizarin sweat test (17,24,36). Unclothed subjects lie supine on a movable cart and are enclosed (head included) in the heated environment. Suitable parameters include an ambient (air) temperature of 45°–50°C, relative humidity of 35%–40%, and a skin temperature between 38.5° and 39.5°C. In normals, the skin temperature will be <39.0°C even with an ambient temperature of 45°–50°C. To achieve this temperature, the skin is separately heated by overhead infrared heaters that are carefully regulated by skin temperature feedback control. A specially constructed sweat cabinet provides these parameters, and subjects are heated for ~45–65 min until a maximal sweat response has occurred.

The average response of skin, oral temperature, and sweat rate in 50 healthy controls, aged 20–75 years, is shown in Fig. 2. For our control data, the mean temperature rise during the TST was 1.2°C, with 38.0°C as end-point oral temperature. The mean skin temperature was 39.0°C, and the average time of heating was 45 min.

The mean oral temperature increase for 504 patients tested in 1994 was 1.5°C, using 38.0°C *or* a 1.0°C rise above baseline (whichever yielded the *higher* temperature), as an end point.

Our observations indicate that the often-quoted 1.0°C oral temperature rise as an end point for the TST (4) is inadequate in many cases, especially in those with low initial temperatures (<36.5°C) and in the elderly. At 38.0°C, most subjects will have reached a sweat rate maximum and activated normally innervated skin. This end point is more important rather than some arbitrary amount of time spent in the sweat cabinet. It is not necessary to raise the oral temperature to 38.0°C, however, if generalized sweating occurs at a lower body temperature. For reasons of patient

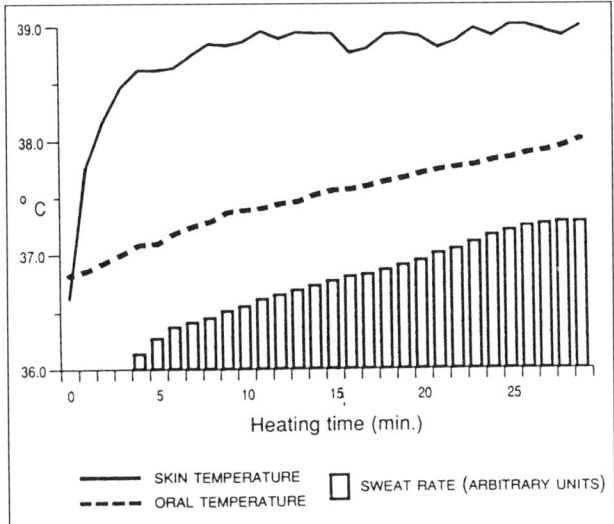

FIG. 2. Composite profile of mean skin temperature, oral (central) temperature, and sweat rate in 35 laboratory control subjects.

mometer held in place between cheek and gum by a sponge. This site's temperatures are identical to sublinqual and are not disturbed by mouth opening, talking, or respiration.

Sweating on the skin surface is best visualized by application of an indicator powder to the area of the body of interest before heating. It is best to powder as much of the exposed body surface as possible so that symmetry and distribution of sweating can be determined. The powder has an indicator substance and changes color when it becomes wet. We have

comfort and safety, we do not raise oral temperature to >38.5°C or extend the heating period beyond 65 min.

Regarding the magnitude of physical stress of the TST, Wilkinson and Johnson (66), using heating criteria just a bit less vigorous than ours, showed only minimal cardiovascular stress during a TST. Nevertheless, oral (or equivalent) and skin temperatures still have to be continuously monitored to avoid burning insensitive skin or causing relative hyperthermia (>38.5°C).

The probe used in our laboratory for the continuous measurement of oral temperature has a thermistor ther-

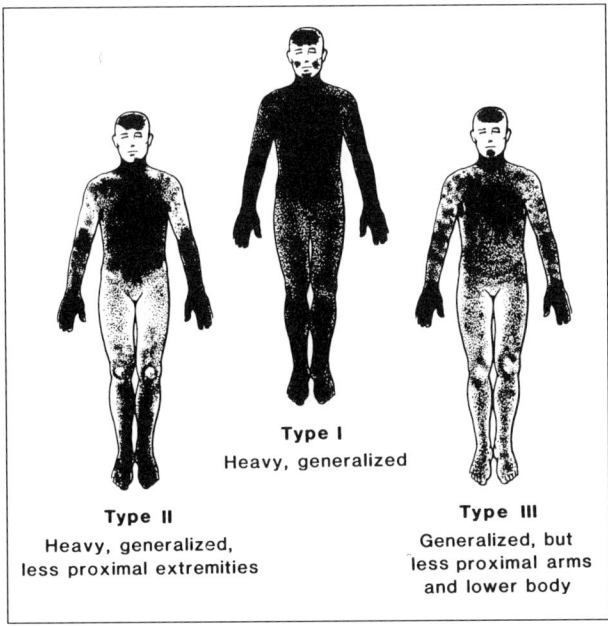

FIG. 3. Normal thermoregulatory sweating patterns (sweating areas in *black*). Modified from Fealey et al. (7), with permission.

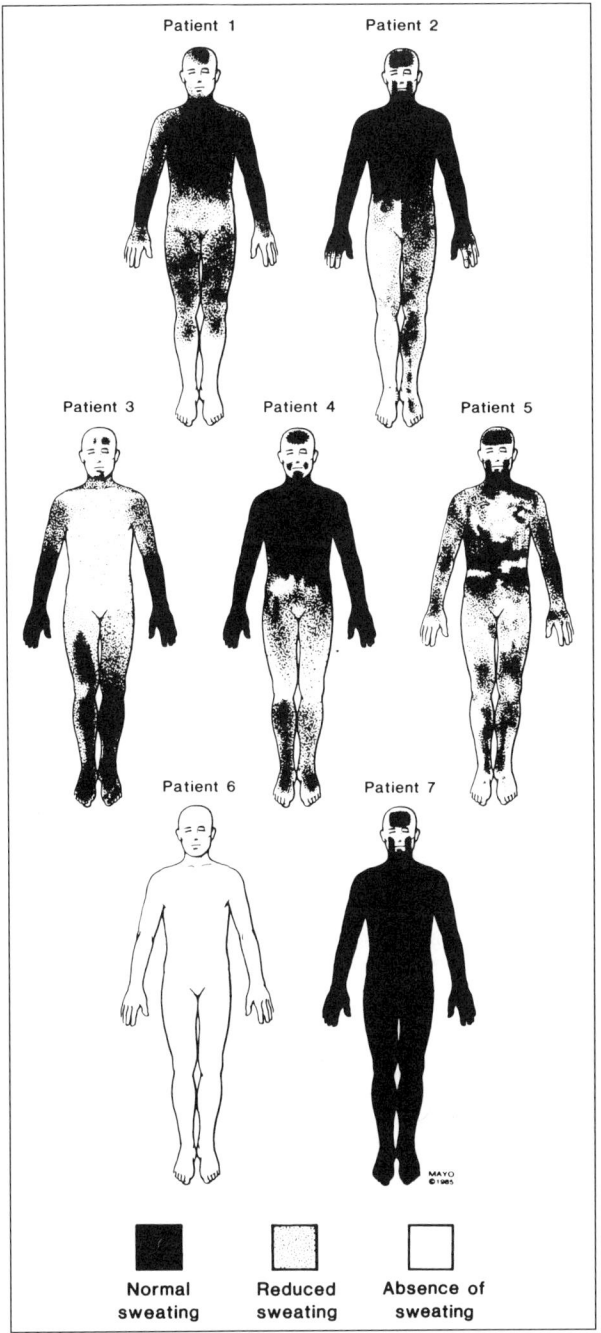

FIG. 4. Sweat distribution patterns: Examples from patients having diabetes mellitus (sweating in *shaded* areas). Modified from Low and Fealey (40), with permission.

used alizarin red (36) mixed with corn starch and sodium carbonate (50, 100, and 50 g, respectively). The powder mixture is light orange when dry and purple when wet (see Fig. 14). Others (57) have used iodinated corn starch (light orange/brown when dry and dark blue when wet). Older techniques, e.g., painting the skin with an iodine solution (45), are still used effectively (28), but the techniques are more time consuming. Quinizarin powder (24) is not recommended because it generally is not available in the United States and is sensitizing. Care should be taken to minimize patient and technician exposure to alizarin, because it can irritate skin and mucous membranes.

Investigators need to be aware of the normal patterns of the sweat response (17,20,31,33,34) and have normative data regarding testing conditions and oral and skin temperature responses accompanying the distributions. The normal variants in sweat distributions seen our TST laboratory are shown in Fig. 3. These results are based on 50 controls (30 female, 20–75 years of age). Areas of "normal" anhidrosis may occur over bony prominences (e.g., patellae and clavicles) and (when tested in the supine position) in the lateral calves and inner thighs. The proximal extremities are frequently lighter sweating than distal but left–right symmetry is always the rule. Males tend to show Type I (heavy, generalized) pattern while females usually show type II (heavy generalized, less proximal extremities) or type III (generalized, but less proximal arms and lower body). The elderly of both sexes tend to exhibit types II and III and the lighter sweating areas have a higher threshold of activation (20).

An age-related loss of sweating has been reported to occur in the higher-threshold sweating areas just noted (20), but this has not been fully confirmed, and some of that study's control subjects had cerebral infarction [recently demonstrated by Korpelainen et al. (30) to have a potential effect on contralateral sweating responses].

We have noted anhidrosis in elderly women (≥70 years of age) (R. D.Fealey, unpublished observations, 1988), who have normal neurologic exam and autonomic inventory results except for their report of dry skin for years. Whether these subjects represent a variant of chronic idiopathic anhidrosis (42) or truly reflect the known loss of preganglionic autonomic neurons (37) with aging is unclear. Others (11) have not noted loss of sweat capacity in healthy, active women with aging.

SWEAT DISTRIBUTION PATTERNS

We have described seven types of thermoregulatory sweat patterns or distributions that are used in reporting test results. Examples shown in Fig. 4 and described next are from patients with diabetes mellitus:

1. *Distal* anhidrosis is characterized by sweat loss greatest in the fingers, the legs below the knees, and the lower anterior abdomen (patient 1).
2. *Segmental* anhidrosis involves large contiguous zones of the body surface bordered by areas of normal sweat-

TABLE 1. *Disorders with potential thermoregulatory sweat test disturbances*

Generalized primary autonomic failure
  Pure autonomic failure or Bradbury–Eggleston syndrome
  Multiple system atrophy with autonomic failure:
    Shy–Drager syndrome
  Idiopathic autonomic neuropathy (62)
  Acute pandysautonomia (panautonomic neuropathy)

Partial primary autonomic failure
  Chronic idiopathic anhidrosis
  Chronic idiopathic intestinal pseudo-obstruction
  Adie's syndrome with segmental autonomic failure
    (Ross' syndrome)
  Postural orthostatic tachycardia syndrome

Anhidrosis due to central nervous system causes
  Tumors: hypothalamic, parasellar, and posterior fossa
  Multiple cerebral infarcts
  Wernicke's encephalopathy
  Tabes dorsalis
  Traumatic, infectious (i.e., AIDS), and inflammatory
    myelopathies
  Parkinson's disease
  Hereditary system degenerations
  Syringomyelia
  Dysautonomia of advanced age
  Multiple sclerosis

Anhidrosis due to peripheral nervous system causes
  Porphyria
  Lambert–Eaton myasthenic syndrome
  Paraneoplastic autonomic dysfunction (autonomic
    neuropathy, enteric neuronopathy, and subacute
    sensory neuropathy)
  Uremic neuropathy
  Connective tissue diseases (e.g., Sjögren's syndrome)
  Tangier and Fabry's diseases
  Vincristine and heavy metal neuropathies
  Leprosy
  B_{12} deficiency
  Chronic Chagas' disease
  Propafenone toxicity (21)

Anhidrosis due to iatrogenic causes
  Psychotropic drugs (phenothiazines, butyrophenones,
    and tricyclic antidepressants)
  Antiparkinsonian drugs [anticholinergics like Cogentin
    (benztropine mesylate) and Artane (trihexyphenidyl)]
  Surgical sympathectomy and skin incisions

Anhidrosis due to skin disorders
  Cholinergic urticaria
  Psoraisis
  Hypohidrotic ectodermal dysplasia
  Scleroderma
  Radiation injury

Disorders with excessive sweating
  Essential hyperhidrosis
  Autonomic hyperreflexia
  Paroxysmal localized hyperhidrosis
  Perilesional hyperhidrosis
  Syringomyelia
  Familial dysautonomia (Riley–Day syndrome, hereditary
    sensory and autonomic neurotherapy type III)

ing (patient 2). These usually respect sympathetic dermatomal borders.

3. *Focal* sweat loss is confined to isolated dermatomes or peripheral nerve territories or small, localized skin areas (patients 4 and 5).
4. *Global* anhidrosis occurs by definition when >80% of the body surface is involved (patient 6).
5. *Regional* anhidrosis (patient 3) refers to large anhidrotic areas (but <80%) that blend gradually into sweating areas and that may or may not be contiguous; anhidrosis of the trunk alone and anhidrosis of the proximal parts of all four extremities would be examples of this pattern.
6. *Mixed* patterns are combinations of any of the above in the same patient (as in patient 5, showing focal and distal patterns of anhidrosis).
7. *Normal* sweat distribution (patient 7) has no areas of anhidrosis or minor areas of sweat loss observed in controls, as previously described above and shown in Fig. 3.

REPORTING RESULTS

Data regarding the patient's age, sex, identification number, clinical problem, and date of the TST are indicated on the report. The temperature and humidity ranges, the time exposed to the heat stress, and the initial and final oral temperatures are indicated.

The body of the report includes a brief anatomic description of the results and states the clinical significance of the findings.

The anatomic figure on the form is shaded in by the technician, depicting the *distribution* or pattern of sweating/anhidrosis. The accuracy of the drawing is verified by the reporter before the patient showers. Alternatively, the areas of anhidrosis are photographed with a video-disc camera and are reviewed by the reporter on a monitor (see Fig. 14 at the end of this chapter for some examples). These images can be digitized and stored for comparison studies and/or incorporated into the report. They provide the detail needed to generate a computerized body image. This digitized image is then used, with a pixel-counting program, to determine the percentage of anterior body surface anhidrosis (TST%) and is suitable for ink-jet printer output for a permanent record (13). Another method of deriving the TST% uses planimetric area readings directly from the drawing. An accurate planimeter with a resolution of 0.005 cm2 is required (16).

THE THERMOREGULATORY SWEAT TEST IN CLINICAL DISORDERS OF THE AUTONOMIC NERVOUS SYSTEM

The TST is helpful in identifying autonomic involvement in many neurologic disorders (Table 1), including primary autonomic failure, secondary autonomic failure due to neuropathy (diabetes, primary systemic amyloid, lepromatous, idiopathic small fiber, and paraneoplastic), myelopathy (syrinx, spinal cord injury, and multiple sclerosis), surgical sympathectomy, and disorders of sweat

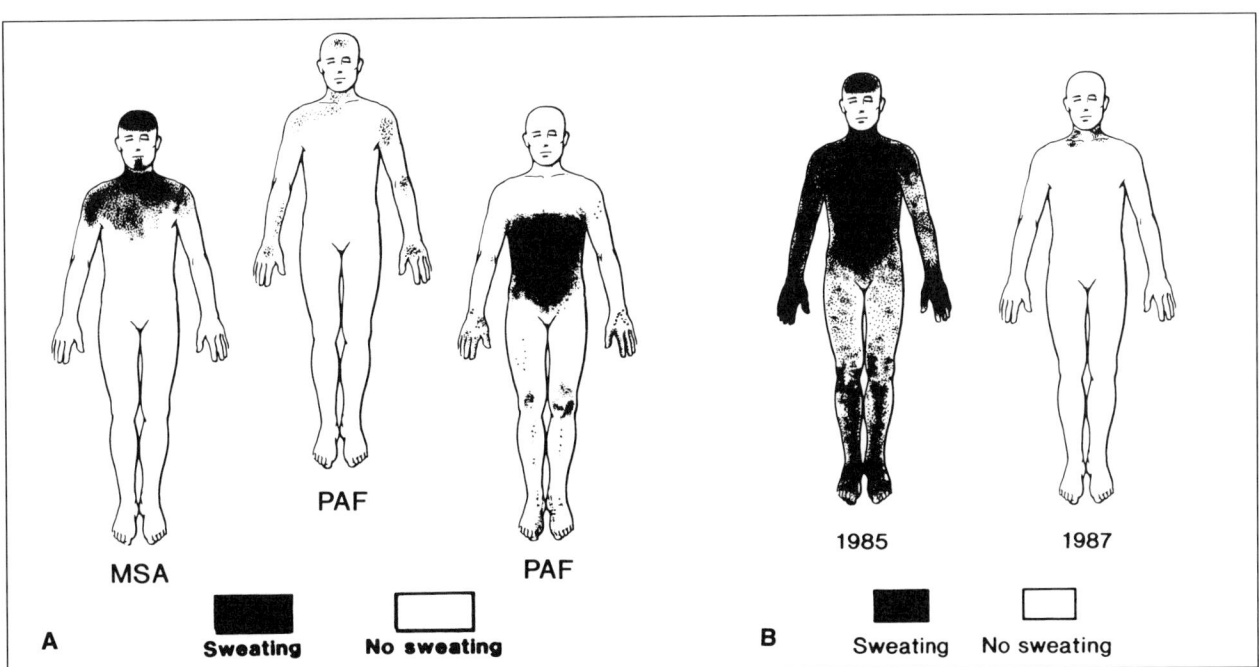

FIG. 5. A: Sweat loss patterns in pure autonomic failure (PAF) and multiple system atrophy (MSA). From Cohen et al. (9), with permission. **B:** Progressive sweat loss in a patient with an L-dopa responsive, extrapyramidal disorder and mild orthostatic hypotension in 1985 and severe MSA unresponsive to L-dopa with disabling autonomic failure by 1987. From Low and Fealey (37), with permission.

glands and skin (10,53). The TST can monitor disease progression or recovery. In addition, skin areas not readily accessible to other techniques are so with the TST, and several patterns are diagnostic.

THE THERMOREGULATORY SWEAT TEST IN SPECIFIC DISEASES

The TST in primary autonomic failure syndromes is characterized by widespread anhidrosis (4,9,16,56). Median values of body surface anhidrosis (TST%) were 91% and 97% for patients with pure autonomic failure and multiple-system atrophy, respectively (9). Typical sweat distributions are shown in Fig. 5. Note how isolated segments of sweating may remain and how global (>80%) anhidrosis is the rule in these syndromes. Sweat loss tends to occur in conjunction with other signs of autonomic failure, although it can occur early. Sweating may be preserved in acral (more peripheral) parts and totally absent elsewhere; rarely are patients fully aware of their sweat loss. Clinical deterioration is accompanied by progressive sweat loss on serial studies (Fig. 5B) and the severity of clinical autonomic failure in the patients with extrapyramidal and cerebellar system disorders regresses significantly with the TST% (55).

Acute pandysautonomia or panautonomic neuropathy (38) typically produces widespread postganglionic sudomotor failure manifest by near complete anhidrosis on the TST. In most cases, scattered "islands" of sweating several centimeters in diameter remain that may become confluent with recovery of sweating. Incomplete recovery of sweating has been the most common observation made in cases followed for up to 6 years.

A subacute course of idiopathic autonomic neuropathy has recently been summarized by Suarez et al. (62). The disorder is likely immune mediated and often is postinfectious, and the spectrum of autonomic involvement ranges from panautonomic to selective adrenergic or cholinergic. TST abnormalities may be global, glove and stocking (distal), or strikingly segmental. Postganglionic anhidrosis is the rule when TST anhidrosis is further tested with acetylcholine iontophoresis via the quantitative sudomotor axon reflex (sweat) test (QSART).

In yet other disorders, isolated sudomotor failure in combination with gastrointestinal dysfunction occurs acutely or chronically, resulting in large areas of anhidrosis (8). More commonly, one sees isolated sudomotor failure as a chronic disorder causing heat intolerance and fatigue, a condition we refer to as *chronic idiopathic anhidrosis* (42).

Chronic Idiopathic Anhidrosis

In 1985, we described eight patients with chronic idiopathic anhidrosis. Individuals were heat intolerant and became hot, flushed, dizzy, dyspneic, and weak but did not sweat when the ambient temperature was high or when they exercised. The TST was markedly abnormal in all patients, frequently showing global anhidrosis or striking regional or segmental defects (Fig. 6). Four patients had preganglionic sudomotor lesions (abnormal TST with normal QSART). No patients had postural hypotension, and all but one had otherwise normal secretomotor function; three patients had pupillary abnormalities, but none had Adie's pupils. One patient with progressive segmental anhidrosis with initially preserved QSART responses in areas of thermoregulatory anhidrosis subsequently lost the response at follow-up 5 years later similarly to the case reported by Faden et al. (15). Long-standing, widespread anhidrosis without generalized autonomic failure is common, and several patients recover remarkably to near normal sweating over the course of 1–5 years.

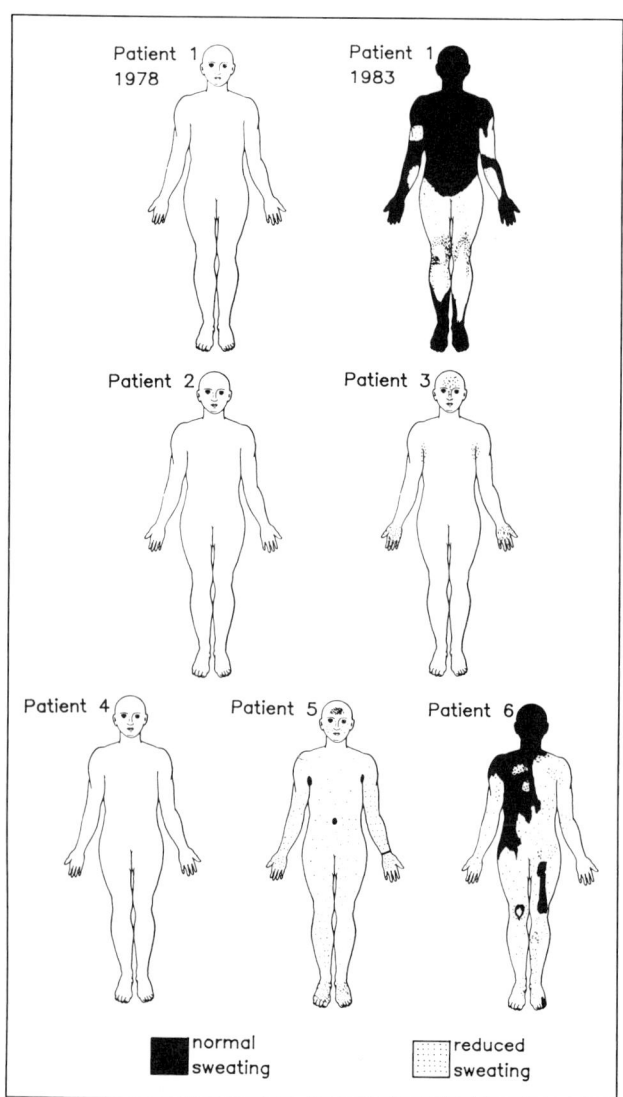

FIG. 6. The spectrum of thermoregulatory sweat test abnormalities seen in chronic idiopathic anhidrosis. From Low et al. (42), with permission.

Ross' Syndrome

Segmental anhidrosis associated with Adie's pupils was reported by Ross in 1958 (54). Since then, others have reported similar cases (12,25,43,50,60). The anhidrosis is most often asymmetric and rarely are other features of generalized autonomic failure present.

THE THERMOREGULATORY SWEAT TEST IN SECONDARY DISORDERS OF THE AUTONOMIC NERVOUS SYSTEM

Central Disorders

These are lesions affecting the intermediolateral cell columns in the spinal cord, the descending autonomic bulbospinal tracts (Fig. 7), and efferent hypothalamic projections (Fig. 8).

Body surface areas exhibiting TST anhidrosis on a central basis as a rule show normal postganglionic sweating when tested with acetylcholine iontophoresis (e.g., the QSART, described in Chapter 14).

With long-standing central or preganglionic lesions, the postganglionic response may be lost due to transsynaptic effects (9), making it difficult to tell the origin of the autonomic lesion producing TST anhidrosis. Faden et al. (15) observed this phenomenon in their report of a patient with chronic idiopathic anhidrosis.

The TST is one of the few methods available to test hypothalamic function directly. Tumors of the anterior and posterior hypothalamus or of the pineal region and disorders with probable hypothalamic abnormality such as anorexia nervosa can be associated with global anhidrosis. Figure 8 depicts global anhidrosis in a patient with an inferiorly extending pineal tumor, which returned to near normal 6 months following surgical resection of the lesion.

Segmental spinal cord lesions may produce a zone of perilesional hyperhidrosis in the last preserved dermatome and noticeable within the first few minutes of heating during the TST (24), and this may represent either a compensatory or irritative phenomenon.

Patients with upper thoracic and cervical cord transections can be safely tested with little threat of autonomic hyperreflexia and spinal reflex sweating as long as the urinary bladder is emptied beforehand (18).

Patients with chronic multiple sclerosis affecting the spinal cord and brainstem frequently show regional, segmental, or global anhidrosis. In the largest study published to date, Noronha and colleagues (46) found TST abnormalities in 25 of 60 patients, the extent of anhidrosis positively correlated with the Kurtzke disability score and pyramidal tract involvement. With the mean 1.2°C oral temperature rise, most patients experienced a temporary aggravation of their symptoms that was reversed within a few hours when their body temperature had returned to normal levels. Interestingly, bladder distention failed to produce spinal re-

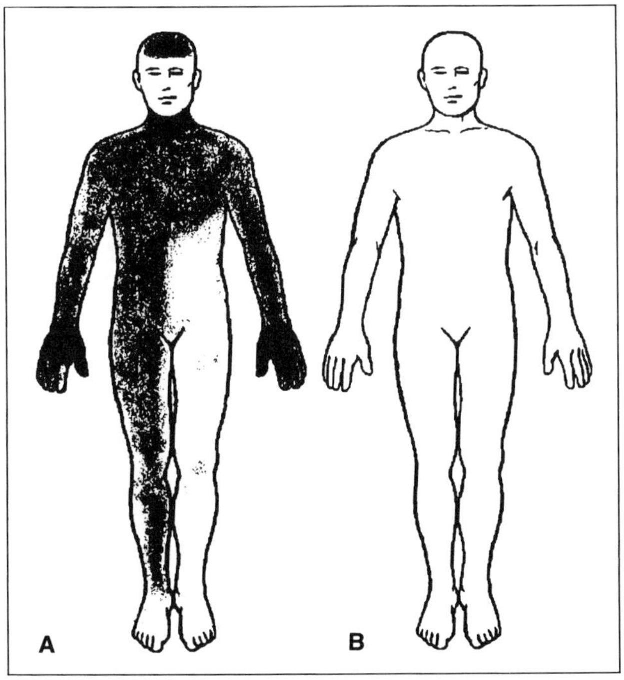

FIG. 7. Incomplete myelopathy at T3 **(A),** and complete cord transection at C6 **(B)** (sweating areas in *black*).

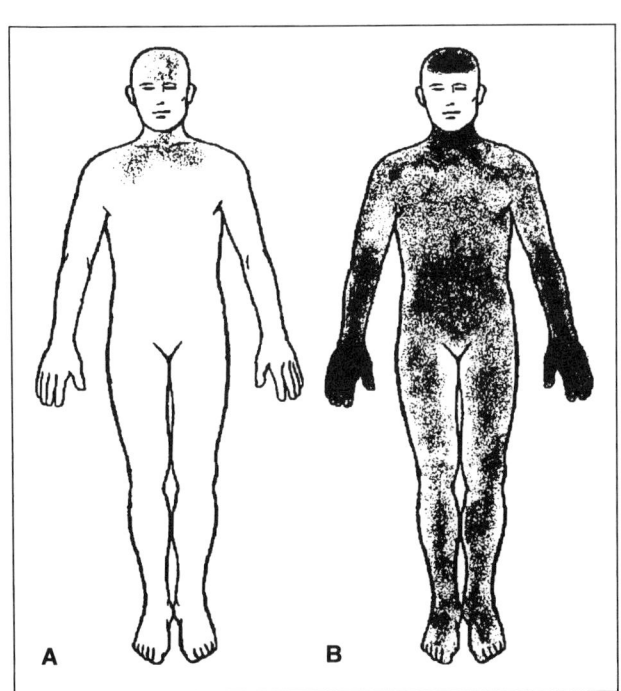

FIG. 8. Anhidrosis produced by hypothalamic compression from pineal tumor **(A),** and postoperative recovery of sweating **(B)** (sweating areas in *black*).

flex sweating even in totally anhidrotic patients, most likely because of the longitudinal distribution of cervical and thoracic cord lesions as well as a less than complete interruption of descending inhibitory pathways.

Traumatic spinal cord injury produces global anhidrosis with complete cervical cord lesions, segmental anhidrosis below the level of the lesion in thoracic cord lesions, variable loss in the legs with lumbar cord lesions, and little or no significant loss with cauda equina lesions (18,52).

Excessive sweating especially of the head occurs in autonomic hyperreflexia (dysreflexia), which occurs with cord lesions above the T5 level and is not thermoregulatory sweating but rather an uninhibited somatosympathetic reflex response from the intact but isolated cord below the lesion. Prior removal of the usual mechanisms (full bladder or rectum) triggering dysreflexia will help prevent this from occurring during the TST. Quadraplegic subjects (as well as other neurologically impaired individuals) tolerate the TST surprisingly well as long as oral and skin temperatures are monitored during the test (18).

Peripheral Disorders

Lesions of the sympathetic chain or white rami produce segmental deficits of sweating. A classic lesion of this sort is the apical lung (Pancoast) tumor. The patient in Fig. 9 noted pain and loss of sweating in the right arm. There was no Horner's pupil. The TST shows anhidrosis of the right T2 (primarily) to T4 sympathetic dermatomes. (Facial sweating is derived from T2 and not T1.) This pattern of anhidrosis also occurs with surgical sympathectomy (T2 ganglionectomy).

Thermoregulatory sweating abnormalities were demonstrated in all six patients with Guillain–Barré syndrome (64), exemplifying probable lesions affecting the sympathetic chains or white rami. Chronic inflammatory demyelinating polyradiculopathy may also cause areas of anhidrosis (26).

Diabetes mellitus produces distinct peripheral neurologic disorders, including length-dependent neuropathy, multifocal mononeuropathy, painful truncal radiculopathy, and autonomic neuropathy (3,5,13,14,17,23,36,40,47,48,63).

The ability to examine the whole anterior body surface in detail and the common involvement of sudomotor nerves in diabetes particularly suits the TST for the evaluation of this disorder.

Peripheral neuropathy may produce distal sweat loss in the lower extremities and, as the neuropathy advances, the fingertips and the lower anterior abdomen become affected (see Fig. 4, patient 1).

Painful truncal radiculopathy has a distinct clinical presentation and a characteristic TST pattern of patchy to complete asymmetric anhidrosis primarily in the anterior distribution of one or several adjacent thoracic dermatomes (see Fig. 4, patients 4 and 5; and Fig. 14).

The degree of sweat loss (TST%) correlates closely with the clinical severity of diabetic autonomic neuropathy

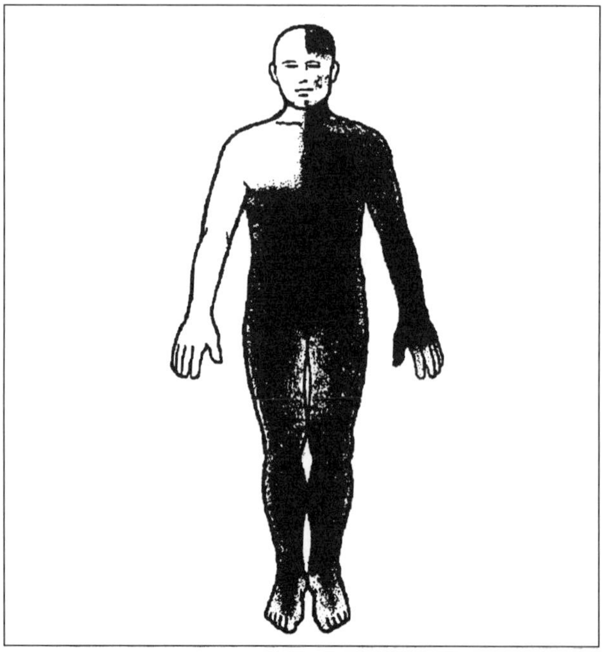

FIG. 9. Right head, upper trunk, and upper extremity sweat loss due to right-sided Pancoast's tumor. Distal anhidrosis due to peripheral neuropathy was also present.

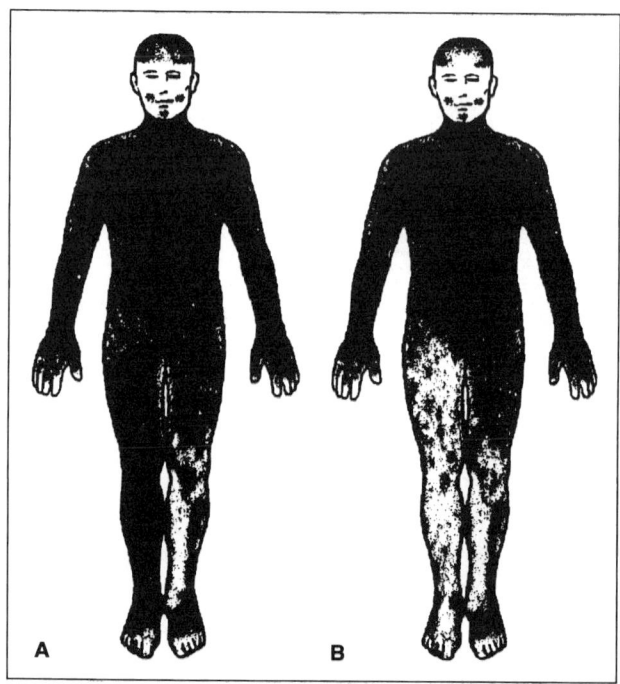

FIG. 10. Thermoregulatory sweat test (TST) monitoring of a diabetic with progressive polyradiculoneuropathy (sweating areas in *black*). **A:** At the initial visit, TST% was 9%. **B:** At 9 months later, TST% was 27%.

(17); this quantitative parameter coupled with digital photography documentation provides a possible means to monitor the course of the disease (Fig. 10).

Deficits ranging from unilateral "autosympathectomy" (Fig. 4, patient 2) to global anhidrosis (Fig. 4, patient 6) can be seen. There are occasional diabetics who have a mild peripheral neuropathy and a perfectly normal TST (Fig. 4, patient 7).

When diabetic anhidrosis shown by TST is further tested with acetylcholine iontophoresis, a postganglionic lesion is usually found. Infrequently, the TST abnormality is preganglionic (normal acetylcholine iontophoretic sweating), compatible with neuropathologic observations (2).

In primary systemic amyloidosis and inherited amyloid neuropathy, sudosympathetic nerves are often involved; hence, there are usually TST abnormalities. Postganglionic anhidrosis is the rule, although preganglionic lesions can occur. Anhidrosis in a "glove and stocking" distribution often with an upper-body (head especially) segmental sweat loss occurs commonly (39).

Neuropathies associated with collagen vascular diseases will commonly produce patchy anhidrosis, greatest in the distal lower extremities. Sjogren's syndrome may be associated with larger areas of absent sweating affecting proximal and distal extremities asymmetrically. Recently, we have seen several cases that seem to have a variant of Sjogren's syndrome, with lymphoplasmacytic infiltrates on lip minor salivary gland biopsy but negative extractable nuclear antigen antibodies. Direct involvement of sweat glands as well as small cutaneous nerves may occur.

Paraneoplastic autonomic neuropathy produces widespread postganglionic and/or preganglionic anhidrosis corresponding to the clinical severity of autonomic failure (59). Cytotoxic T-cell-mediated destruction of enteric and other ganglionic neurons may be causative. About 25% of patients with subacute sensory neuronopathy of Denny-Brown can have a significant degree of autonomic neuropathy and thermoregulatory anhidrosis (29).

Lepromatous nerve involvement has long been known to produce deficits of sweating often in patches affecting the cooler areas of the body (7,55). Such areas are usually anesthetic as well. As expected, patchy to complete (i.e., distally) anhidrosis in acral body parts, scattered circular areas in the distribution of peripheral nerve branches on the trunk and extremities (Figs. 11 and 14) occur. The TST can monitor the response of the skin neuropathic lesions during therapy (digital photographs of the serial TSTs are suggested).

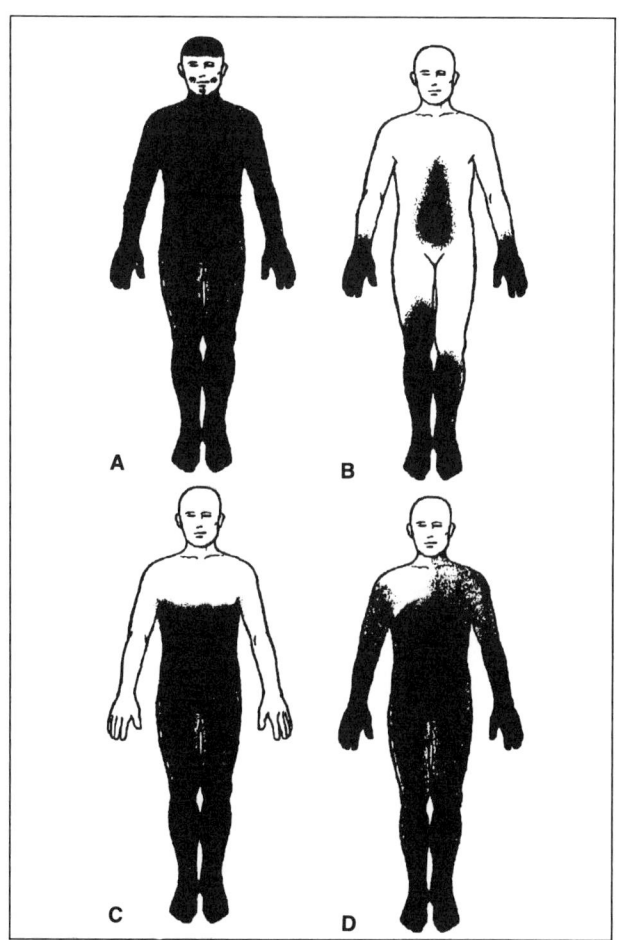

FIG. 12. Essential hyperhidrosis type I **(A)** and type II **(B)**. Effect of sympathectomy on the patient A at 3 months **(C)** and at 3 years **(D)** (sweating areas in *black*).

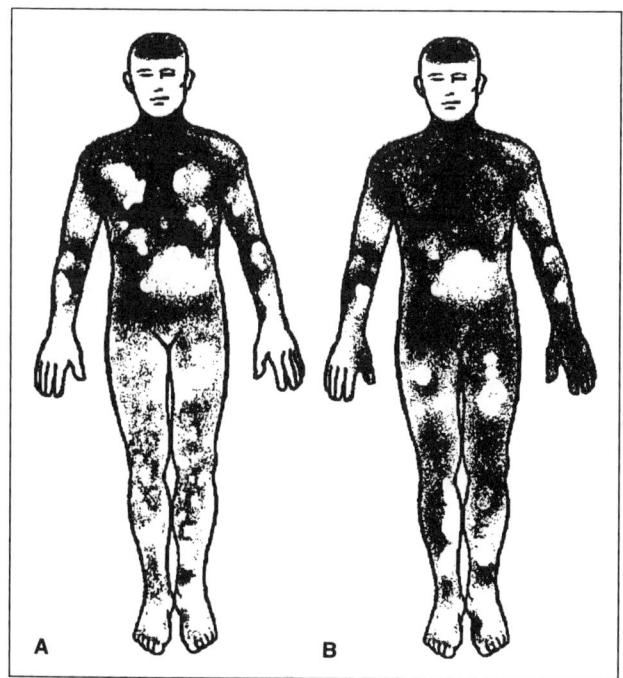

FIG. 11. Multifocal and distal anhidrosis in a patient with leprosy at time of diagnosis **(A)** and 2 years after treatment **(B)**. Note the recovery of sweating in the left hand, upper trunk, and proximal legs (sweating areas in *black*).

Painful "small fiber" neuropathies often are the cause of the "burning feet" syndrome, and often no cause is found (61). The TST has been used to investigate this syndrome and showed convincing distal anhidrosis in 72% of patients diagnosed clinically. The results of electromyography and clinical neurologic exam are often normal in these patients. The deficits are often striking (Fig. 14).

ESSENTIAL HYPERHIDROSIS

Figure 12 shows the two varieties of essential hyperhidrosis encountered in the TST laboratory. The patient in Fig. 12A has excessive sweating of the hands and feet, normal to heavy generalized sweating, and no areas of anhidrosis (type I). The patient in Fig. 12B also has excessive sweating of hands and feet, but exhibits large areas that lack sweating (type II). Type II is less commonly encountered, and both patterns may be seen in related family members.

The TST of the patient in Fig. 12A following bilateral T2 ganglionectomy treatment is shown in Fig. 12C. A transient Horner's syndrome occurred on the left. After 3 years, there was a partial return of sweating (Fig. 12D).

The effects of sympathectomy (22) or pharmacologic blockade (35) on the TST are immediate and do not require axonal degeneration. The extent of surgical denervation and the occurrence of regeneration can be readily monitored via the TST (see Fig. 14).

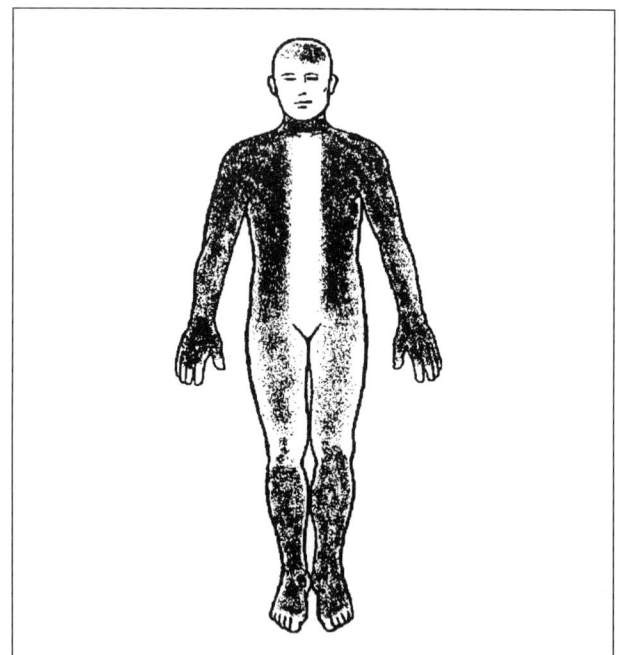

FIG. 13. Anhidrosis due to radiation damage to dermis. The striking rectangular truncal deficit defines the radiation port; the rest of the trunk was shielded behind lead (sweating areas in *black*).

DERMATOLOGIC DISORDERS

Skin disorders associated with focal anhidrosis on TST include psoriasis, scleroderma, exfoliative dermatitis, cholinergic uturcaria (65), and some forms of icthyosis. Hypohidrotic ectodermal dysplasia may show areas of reduced sweating, but quantitative techniques may be necessary (27) to demonstrate an abnormality unequivocally. Radiation damage (Fig. 13) can produce striking rectangular deficits, the sharp margins demonstrating the location of lead shields defining the radiation ports used.

DIFFICULTIES AND PITFALLS IN INTERPRETATION

The interpreter must be aware of the normal patterns of thermoregulatory sweating (see Fig. 3), including areas where anhidrosis may be normal, such as over bony prominences or over the lateral calves.

Patients having just worn pressure wraps (i.e., ace bandages or abdominal binders) may show anhidrosis in the areas that were covered, which usually is easily recognized by the straight edges of the deficit.

Severely dehydrated patients may sweat less overall (19) but generally do not have focal defects. Anticholinergic drugs (including most tricyclic antidepressants) may inhibit thermoregulatory sweating and should be stopped 48 hr before the TST is done.

The application of skin lotions (i.e., moisturizing creams) may produce a discoloration where alizarin covers the skin, making it difficult to discern areas of anhidrosis, and so lotions are prohibited on the day of the TST.

Anhidrosis in elderly patients may present an interpretative challenge because the effect of aging on the autonomic nervous system may be responsible for the regional anhidrosis (most often affecting the lower body half and proximal arms) seen especially in women over age 65 (R. D. Fealey, personal observations, 1988). Foster et al. (20) found evidence of an age-related reduction in sweat gland response to thermal stimulation. While there is evidence for attrition of intermediolateral cell columns of the spinal cord (41), the evidence for failure of sweating with age is somewhat inconclusive (10). Senile atrophy of the skin and differences in sweat gland training between young and old may also be operative. A certain percentage of elderly who report years of being unable to sweat much but who are otherwise healthy may have a variety of chronic idiopathic anhidrosis (42).

Some difficulties encountered with the TST include the untidiness and duration of the test, and the possibility of skin heat injury or skin irritation (due to the indicator powder alizarin). Contact dermatitis occurs rarely, with an observed frequency of 1 : 1,000 subjects, and is readily treated with oral and topical agents. More common but not harmful is the persistence of purple discoloration of small

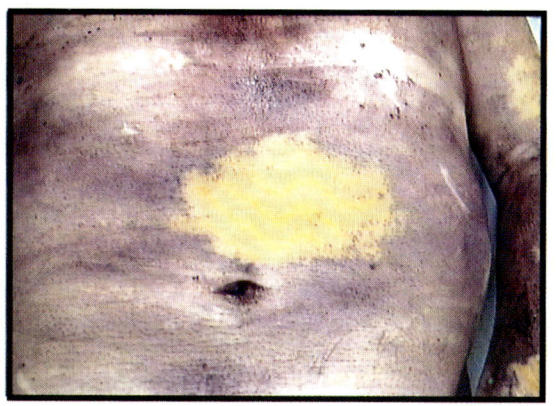
Leprosy neuropathy

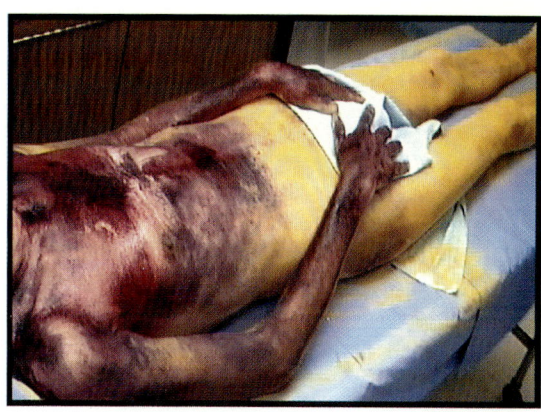
AIDS myelopathy

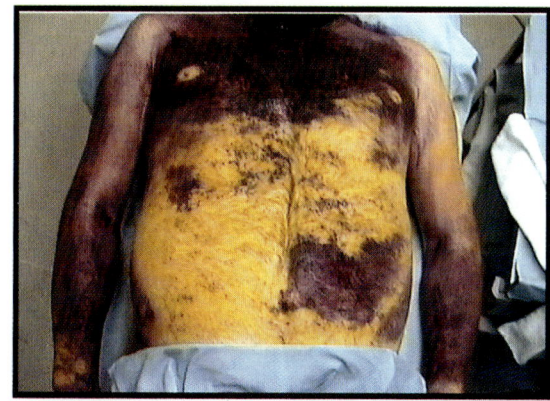
Diabetic neuropathy

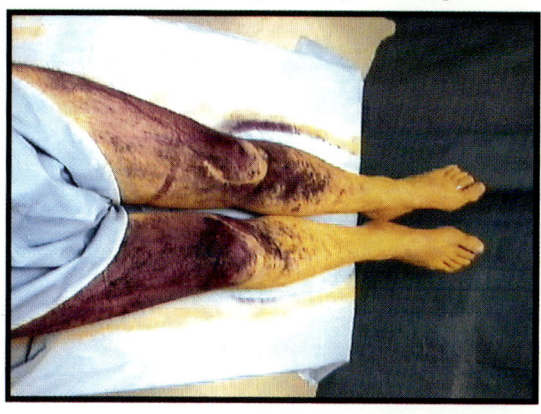
Small fiber neuropathy

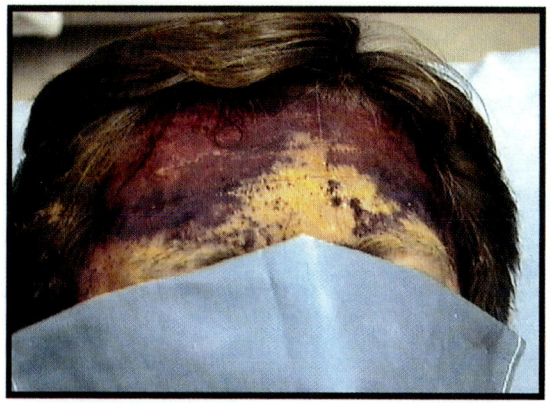
Horner's syndrome

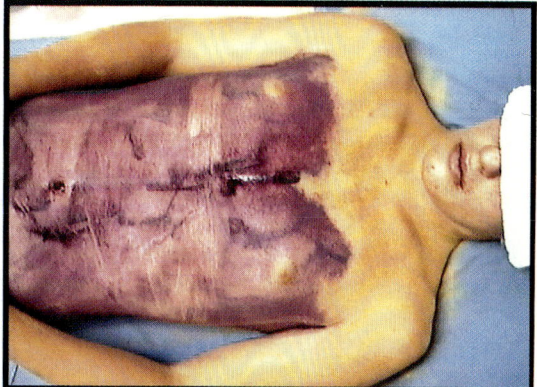
T_2 sympathectomy

COLOR FIG. 2. Thermoregulatory sweat test Digital photo images (from **top left** to **bottom right**): the multifocal lesions of *borderline leprosy*; a patient with orthostatic hypotension, spastic neurogenic bladder and a "sweat level" due to *AIDS-associated myelopathy*; striking *truncal anhidrosis due to diabetic neuropathy*; stocking distribution sweat loss in a patient with *small fiber neuropathy* (burning feet and a normal electromyogram), medial forehead anhidrosis due to an *internal carotid sympathetic plexus* lesion in a patient with chronic cluster headache; and a patient with essential hyperhidrosis 1 month after bilateral *2nd thoracic sympathetic ganglionectomy* (abnormal anhidrotic areas are *orange-yellow* in all photos).

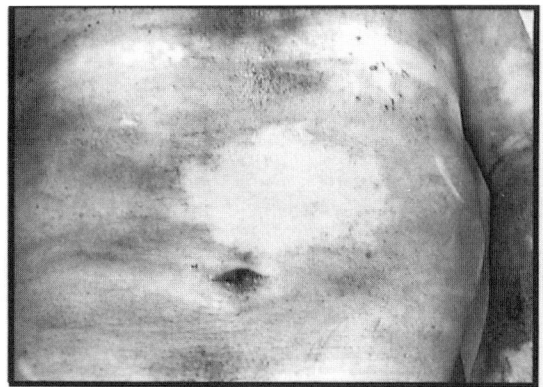
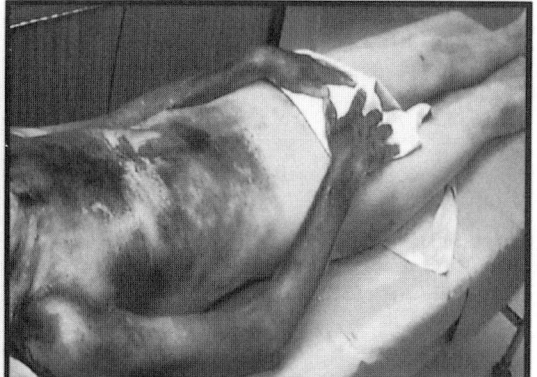
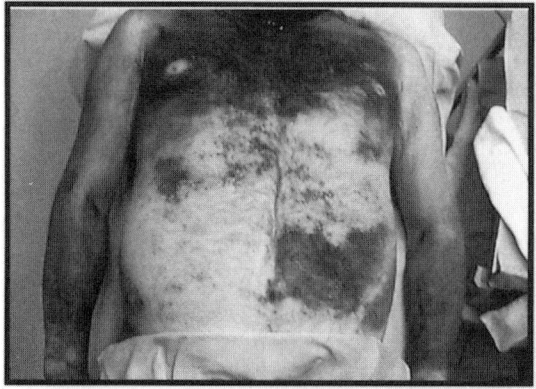
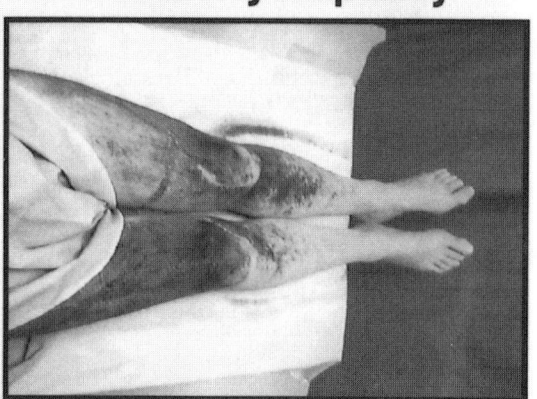
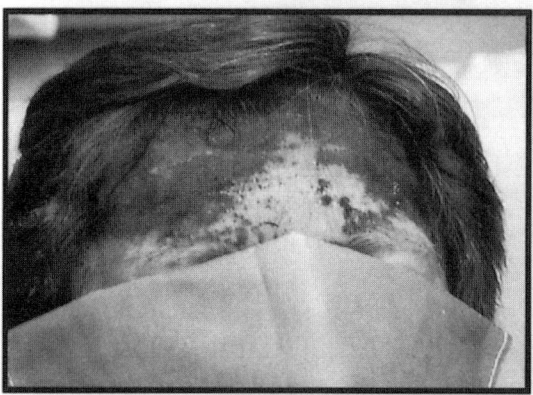
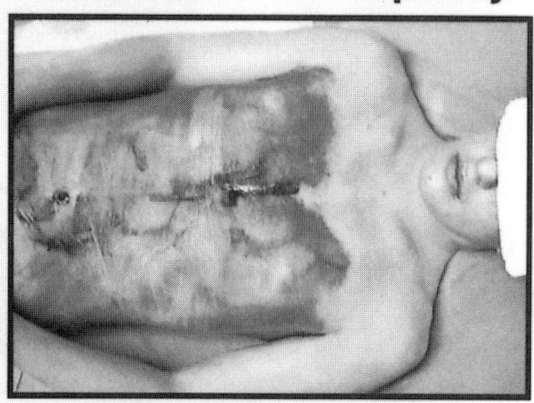

FIG. 14. Thermoregulatory sweat test Digital photo images (from **top left** to **bottom right**): the multifocal lesions of *borderline leprosy;* a patient with orthostatic hypotension, spastic neurogenic bladder and a "sweat level" due to *AIDS-associated myelopathy;* striking *truncal anhidrosis due to diabetic neuropathy;* stocking distribution sweat loss in a patient with *small fiber neuropathy* (burning feet and a normal electromyogram), medial forehead anhidrosis due to an *internal carotid sympathetic plexus* lesion in a patient with chronic cluster headache; and a patient with essential hyperhidrosis 1 month after bilateral *2nd thoracic sympathetic ganglionectomy* (abnormal anhidrotic areas are *orange-yellow* in all photos). *See color figure 2.*

skin areas that takes several days to wash out. Because of repeated exposure, our laboratory technicians wear masks, gloves, and goggles during the application of indicator powder to minimize inhalation, oral ingestion, or eye contact. We have recently installed a ventilated hood to trap airborne indicator dust, further protecting personnel, patients, and equipment.

It is not yet established that the TST can be used for controlled trials to monitor progression of disease or response to treatment because of its inherent qualitative assessment of sweat production. However, by using quantitative measures such as the percentage of body surface anhidrosis derived from digital photographs of the sweat distribution coupled with a measurable and reproducible testing stimulus as described in this chapter, it should be possible to produce data capable of use in trials and complementary to anatomically focused techniques of autonomic testing.

REFERENCES

1. Altomare DF, et al. Acetylcholine sweat test: an effective way to select patients for lumbar sympathectomy. *Lancet* 1994;344:976–978.
2. Appenzeller O, Richardson EP. The sympathetic chain in patients with diabetic and alcoholic polyneuropathy. *Neurology* 1966;16:1205–1207.
3. Asbury AK. Focal and multifocal neuropathies of diabetes. *Diabetic Neuropathy* Philadelphia: WB Saunders, 1978:56–65.
4. Bannister R, Ardill L, Fentem P. Defective autonomic control of blood vessels in idiopathic orthostatic hypotension. *Brain* 1967;90:725–746.
5. Barany FR, Cooper EH. Pilomotor and sudomotor innervation in diabetes. *Clin Sci* 1956;15:533–1540.
6. Bonnin M, Skinner SL, Whelan RF. Holmes–Adies' syndrome with progressive autonomic degeneration. *Aust NZ J Med* 1961;10:304–307.
7. Boyle A, Ramu G. Assessment of cutaneous autonomic nerve functions in leprosy. *Lepr India* 1982;54:518–524.
8. Camilleri M, Fealey RD. Idiopathic autonomic denervation in eight patients presenting with functional gastrointestinal disease: a causal association? *Dig Dis Sci* 1990;35:609–616.
9. Cohen J, et al. Somatic and autonomic function in progressive autonomic failure and multiple system atrophy. *Ann Neurol* 1987;22:692–699.
10. Collins KJ. Autonomic control of sweat glands and disorders of sweating. In: Bannister R, ed. *Autonomic failure: a textbook of clinical disorders of the autonomic nervous system.* 2nd ed. Oxford: Oxford University Press, 1988:748–765.
11. Drinkwater BL, et al. Sweating sensitivity and capacity of women in relation to age. *J Appl Physiol* 1982;53:671–676.
12. Drummond PD, Edis RH. Loss of facial sweating and flushing in Holmes–Adie syndrome. *Neurology* 1990;40:847–849.
13. Dyck PJ, et al. Ten steps in characterizing and diagnosing patients with peripheral neuropathy. *Neurology* 1996;47:10–17.
14. Dyck PJ, Karnes J, O'Brien PC. Diagnosis, staging and classification of diabetic neuropathy and associations with other complications. In: Dyck PJ, et al., eds. *Diabetic neuropathy.* Philadelphia: WB Saunders, 1987:36–44.
15. Faden AI, Chan P, Mendoza E. Progressive isolated segmental anhidrosis. *Neurology* 1982;39:172–175.
16. Fealey RD. Thermoregulatory sweat test. In: Daube JR, ed. *Clinical neurophysiology.* Philadelphia: FA Davis, 1996:396–402.
17. Fealey RD, Low PA, Thomas JE. Thermoregulatory sweating abnormalities in diabetes mellitus. *Mayo Clin Proc* 1989;64:617–628.
18. Fealey RD, et al. Effect of traumatic spinal cord transection on human upper gastrointestinal motility and gastric emptying. *Gastroenterology* 1984;87:69–75.
19. Fortney SM, et al. Effect of blood volume on sweating rate and body fluids in exercising humans. *J Appl Physiol* 1981;51:1594–1600.
20. Foster KG, et al. Sweat responses in the aged. *Age Ageing* 1976;5:91–101.
21. Galasso PJ, Stanton MS, Vogel H. Propafenone-induced peripheral neuropathy. *Mayo Clin Proc* 1995;70:469–472.
22. Golueke PJ, et al. Dorsal sympathectomy for hyperhidrosis: the posterior paravertebral approach. *Surgery* 1988;103:568–572.
23. Goodman JI. Diabetic anhidrosis. *Am J Med* 1966;41:831–835.
24. Guttmann L. The management of the quinizarin sweat test (Q.S.T.). *Postgrad Med J* 1947;23:353–366.
25. Hedges TR, Gerner EW. Ross' syndrome (tonic pupils plus). *Br J Opthalmol* 1975;59:387–391.
26. Ingall TJ, McLeod JG, Tamura N. Autonomic function and unmyelinated fibers in chronic inflammatory demyelinating polyradiculoneuropathy. *Muscle Nerve* 1990;13:70–76.
27. Kanai M, et al. Acetylcholine-induced activation of the eccrine sweat glands in a case of hypohidrotic congenital ectodermal dysplasia. *J Electron Microsc (Tokyo)* 1989;38:371–381.
28. Khurana RK. Oculocephalic sympathetic dysfunction in posttraumatic headaches. *Headache* 1995;35:614–620.
29. Khurana RK. Paraneoplastic autonomic dysfunction. In: *Primer on the autonomic nervous system.* New York: Academic, 1996:266–269.
30. Korpelainen JT, Sotaniemi KA, Myllyla VV. Asymmetric sweating in stroke: a prospective quantitative study of patients with hemispheral brain infarction. *Neurology* 1993;43:1211–1214.
31. Kuno Y. *Human perspiration.* Springfield, IL: Charles C Thomas, 1956.
32. Libert JP, Candas V, Vogt JJ, Mairiaux P. Central and peripheral inputs in sweating regulation during thermal transients. *J Appl Physiol* 1982;52:1147–1152.
33. List CF, Peet MM. Sweat secretion in man. I. Sweating responses in normal persons. *Arch Neurol Psychiatry* 1938;39:1228–1237.
34. List CF, Peet MM. Sweat secretion in man. II. Sweating responses in normal persons. *Arch Neurol Psychiatry* 1938;40:27–43.
35. Lofstrom JB, Lloyd JW, Cousins MJ. Sympathetic neural blockade of the upper and lower extremity. In: Cousins MJ, Bridenbaugh PO, eds. *Neural blockade in clinical anesthesia and management of pain.* Philadelphia: JB Lippincott, 1980:355–382.
36. Low PA, et al. The sympathetic nervous system in diabetic neuropathy: a clinical and pathological study. *Brain* 1975;98:341–356.
37. Low PA, Okazaki H, Dyck PJ. Splanchnic preganglionic neurons in man. I. Morphometry of preganglionic cytons. *Acta Neuropathol (Berl)* 1977;40:55–61.
37a. Low PA, Fealey RD. Tests of sweating. I: Bannister R, ed. *Autonomic failure.* 3rd ed. Oxford: Oxford University Press, 1991 [in press].
38. Low PA, et al. Acute panautonomic neuropathy. *Ann Neurol* 1983;13:412–417.
39. Low PA, et al. The splanchnic autonomic outflow in amyloid neuropathy and Tangier disease. *Neurology (NY)* 1981;31:461–463.
40. Low PA, Fealey RD. Sudomotor neuropathy. In: Dyck PJ, et al., eds. *Diabetic neuropathy.* Philadelphia: WB Saunders, 1987:140–145.
41. Low PA, Fealey RD. The sympathetic neuron, pathological studies, and clinical evaluation of sympathetic sudomotor function. In: Bannister R, ed. *Autonomic failure: A textbook of clinical disorders of the autonomic neurons system.* 3rd ed. Oxford: Oxford University Press, 1991.
42. Low PA, et al. Chronic idiopathic anhidrosis (CIA). *Ann Neurol* 1985;18:344–348.
43. Lucey DD, Van Allen MW, Thompson HS. Holmes–Adie's syndrome with segmental hypohidrosis. *Neurology* 1967;17:763–769.
44. McCaffrey TV, et al. Role of skin temperature in the control of sweating. *J Appl Physiol* 1979;47:591–597.
45. Minor V. *Dtsch Z Nervhlk* 1928:101.
46. Noronha MJ, Vas CJ, Aziz H. Autonomic dysfunction (sweating responses) in multiple sclerosis. *J Neurol Neurosurg Psychiatry* 1968;31:19–22.
47. Odel HM, Roth GM, Keating FR Jr. Autonomic neuropathy simulating the effects of sympathectomy as a complication of diabetes mellitus. *Diabetes* 1955;4:92–98.
48. Olsson Y, Sourander P. Changes in the sympathetic nervous system in diabetes mellitus. *J Neuro-Visceral Relat* 1968;31:86.
49. Pandolf KB, et al. Heat intolerance as a function of percent of body surface involved with miliaria rubra. *Am J Physiol* 239 *(Regul Integrative Comp Physiol)* 1980;8:R226–R232.

50. Petajan JH, et al. Progressive sudomotor denervation and Adie's syndrome. *Neurology* 1965;15:172–176.
51. Pinnagoda J, et al. Transepidermal water loss with and without sweat gland inactivation. *Contact Dermatitis* 1989;21:16–22.
52. Pollock L, et al. Defects in regulatory mechanisms of autonomic function in injuries to spinal cord. *J Neurophysiol* 1951;14:85–93.
53. Quinton PM. Sweating and its disorders. *Annu Rev Med* 1983;34:429–452.
54. Ross AT. Progressive selective sudomotor denervation. *Neurology* 1958;8:809–817.
55. Sabin TD, Swift TR. Leprosy. In: Dyck PJ, et al., eds. *Peripheral neuropathy;* vol 2. Philadelphia: WB Saunders, 1984:1955–1987.
56. Sandroni P, et al. Autonomic involvement in extra-pyramidal and cerebellar disorders. *Clin Auton Res* 1991;1:147–155.
57. Sato KT, et al. One-step iodine starch method for direct visualization of sweating. *Am J Med Sci* 1988;295:528–531.
58. Schondorf R, Low PA. Idiopathic postural orthostatic tachycardia syndrome: an attenuated form of acute pandysautonomia? *Neurology* 1993;43:132–137.
59. Sodhi N, et al. Autonomic function in intestinal pseudo-obstruction caused by paraneoplastic syndrome. *Dig Dis Sci* 1989;34:1937–1942.
60. Spector RH, Bachman DL. Bilateral Adie's tonic pupil with anhidrosis and hyperthermia. *Arch Neurol* 1984;41:342–343.
61. Stewart JD, Low PA, Fealey RD. Distal small fiber neuropathy: results of tests of sweating and autonomic cardiovascular reflexes. *Muscle Nerve* 1992;15:661–665.
62. Suarez GA, et al. Idiopathic autonomic neuropathy: clinical, neurophysiologic, and follow-up. *Neurology* 1994;44:1675–1682.
63. Thomas PK, Brown MJ. Diabetic polyneuropathy. In: Dyck PJ, et al., eds. *Diabetic neuropathy*. Philadelphia: WB Saunders, 1987:56–65.
64. Tuck RR, McLeod JG. Autonomic dysfunction in Guillain–Barr syndrome. *J Neurol Neurosurg Psychiatry* 1981;44:983–990.
65. Tupker RA, Doeglas HM. Water vapour loss threshold and induction of cholinergic urticaria. *Dermatologica* 1990;181:23–25.
66. Wilkinson R, Johnson RH. Catecholamine concentrations during exposure of resting man to the heat of a standard sweat test. *Clin Exp Pharmacol Physiol* 1988;15:789–793.
67. Yamamoto K, et al. Possible mechanism of anhidrosis in a symptomatic female carrier of Fabry's disease: an assessment by skin sympathetic nerve activity and sympathetic skin response. *Clin Auton Res* 1996;6:107–110.

CHAPTER 20

Evaluation of Pupillary and Lacrimal Function

Shelley Ann Cross

1. The parasympathetic innervation to the eye originates in the Edinger–Westphal nucleus of the third-nerve nuclear complex and travels with the third nerve to the ciliary ganglion, in the orbit. From there, postganglionic fibers supply the pupillary constrictor and the ciliary muscle of accommodation.
2. The parasympathetic innervation to the lacrimal glands originates in the tegmentum of the pons dorsal to the superior salivary nucleus. It travels for part of its course with the nervus intermedius (the sensory root of the seventh nerve), emerges from the temporal bone as the greater superficial petrosal nerve, and then passes to the sphenopalatine ganglion. Postganglionic fibers supply the lacrimal glands and stimulate the production of tears.
3. The sympathetic pathway to the eye begins in the posterolateral hypothalamus. Axons descend in the anterolateral brainstem and the intermediolateral cord to the spinal center of Budge–Waller, between C8 and T2. Presynaptic neurons exit the spinal cord, ascend in the sympathetic chain, and synapse in the superior cervical ganglion. Postganglionic neurons ascend in the sheath of the internal carotid artery to the cavernous sinus and then leave the artery and enter the orbit with the third nerve. They supply the dilator muscle of the pupil and Muller's muscle of the upper lid.
4. Sensory fibers for taste on the anterior two-thirds of the tongue (seventh nerve) travel for part of their course in proximity to the parasympathetic fibers for lacrimation and salivation.
5. Parasympathetic fibers for salivation follow two parallel pathways. Fibers from the superior salivary nucleus pass to the nervus intermedius (a rootlet of the seventh nerve) on their way to the submandibular and sublingual ganglia where they synapse and then supply the submandibular and sublingual salivary glands, respectively. Fibers from the inferior salivary nucleus travel with the ninth nerve. They cross the tympanic cavity lying near fibers for lacrimation, ending in the otic ganglion where postganglionic fibers supply the parotid gland.
6. The pupil is largely under parasympathetic control with modulating sympathetic influences. Both sympathetic and parasympathetic afferents have prenuclear input from the telencephalon, diencephalon, and brainstem.
7. The pupillary light reflex begins with light striking the retina and follows ganglion cell axons in the optic nerve, chiasm, and tracts. Just before reaching the lateral geniculate body, fibers branch off entering the dorsal midbrain and synapsing with interneurons that contact the Edinger–Westphal nucleus. The efferent pathway is that of the parasympathetic outflow traveling with the third nerve to the pupillary constrictor.

INTRODUCTION

This chapter describes the anatomy of autonomic innervation to the iris, ciliary body, and lacrimal glands. It also discusses the normal physiology of these structures as it relates to autonomic function. Chapter 34 enumerates pathologic conditions and their explication by objective measures of autonomic function, including topical agents, pupillography, and various measures of tear production.

ANATOMY

The Iris

The iris forms a diaphragm between the anterior and posterior chambers of the eye. In its center is the pupil, a

---

S. A. Cross: Mayo Clinic, Rochester, Minnesota 55905.

round opening permitting light to enter the eye. Through changes in the size of the pupil, the iris regulates the amount of light entering the eye and controls the depth of focus. The iris is supplied by sympathetic and parasympathetic fibers, with the addition of sensory innervation provided by the ophthalmic division of the fifth cranial nerve. These three types of fibers travel via the short and long ciliary nerves, which pierce the sclera and enter the globe posteriorly near the optic nerve. They form a plexus from which the iris muscles, ciliary muscles, and vessel walls are supplied.

The Ciliary Body

The ciliary body, via the ciliary muscle it contains, regulates the shape and hence the refractive power of the lens of the eye. The ciliary muscle receives mainly parasympathetic with some sympathetic innervation. The circular portion of the muscle, the contraction of which rounds up the lens for focus at near, is largely parasympathetically innervated. Radially oriented muscle fibers, the contraction of which pulls the lens flatter for focus at distance, may be at least partially sympathetically innervated (19).

The Lacrimal Apparatus

Tears are produced by the lacrimal gland, the accessory lacrimal glands, and the goblet cells of the conjunctiva. They drain out of the eye through the lacrimal puncta and canaliculi to the lacrimal sac, which communicates with the nasal cavity. The lacrimal gland is in the upper, outer quadrant of the orbit immediately behind the orbital rim within the lacrimal fossa of the frontal bone. The main lacrimal gland has parasympathetic innervation and functions primarily during reflex tear secretion. The accessory lacrimal glands provide nonreflex basal tear secretion (20).

Parasympathetic Pathway

The parasympathetic innervation to the pupillary constrictor and the ciliary muscle of accommodation originates in visceral nuclei in the dorsal mesencephalon (Figs. 1 and 2). The main nuclei are the Edinger–Westphal nuclei located dorsal and medial to the oculomotor nuclear complex and composed of medial and lateral visceral cell columns. Two other nuclear groups, the anterior median nuclei and the nucleus of Perlia, may also have parasympathetic projections to the ciliary ganglion. The parasympathetic fibers travel with the third nerve. In the subarachnoid space and the cavernous sinus, the fibers generally occupy a medial and superior position. They move slightly medially and inferiorly in the anterior cavernous sinus (16). In diabetic patients with pupillary-sparing oculomotor palsies, the pathologic lesions have been located deep in the third nerve consistent with the concept that the autonomic fibers are superficially located (1). The ciliary ganglion (Fig. 3) contains the cell bodies of postganglionic neurons that innervate the iris sphincter and ciliary body. It is located in the apex of the orbit between the optic nerve and the lateral rectus muscle in close association with the inferior division of the third nerve. Most of the fibers in it are preganglionic parasympathetic axons synapsing to supply the iris sphincter and ciliary body, although there are a few sympathetic postganglionic fibers passing through without synapsing to supply mainly the vessels of the iris, and a few afferent sensory fibers that eventually join the nasocil-

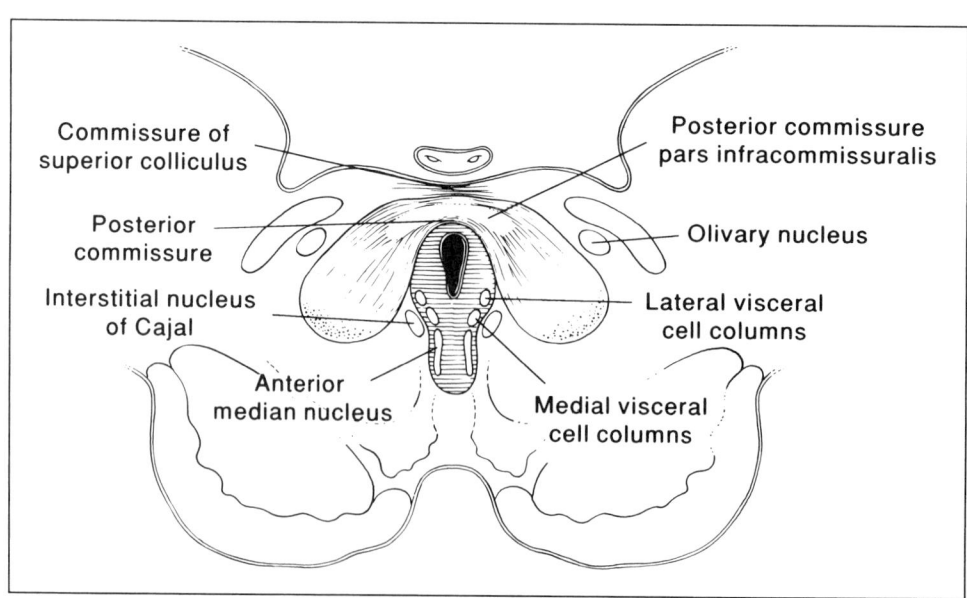

FIG. 1. Parasympathetic ocular motor nuclei in the dorsal mesencephalon.

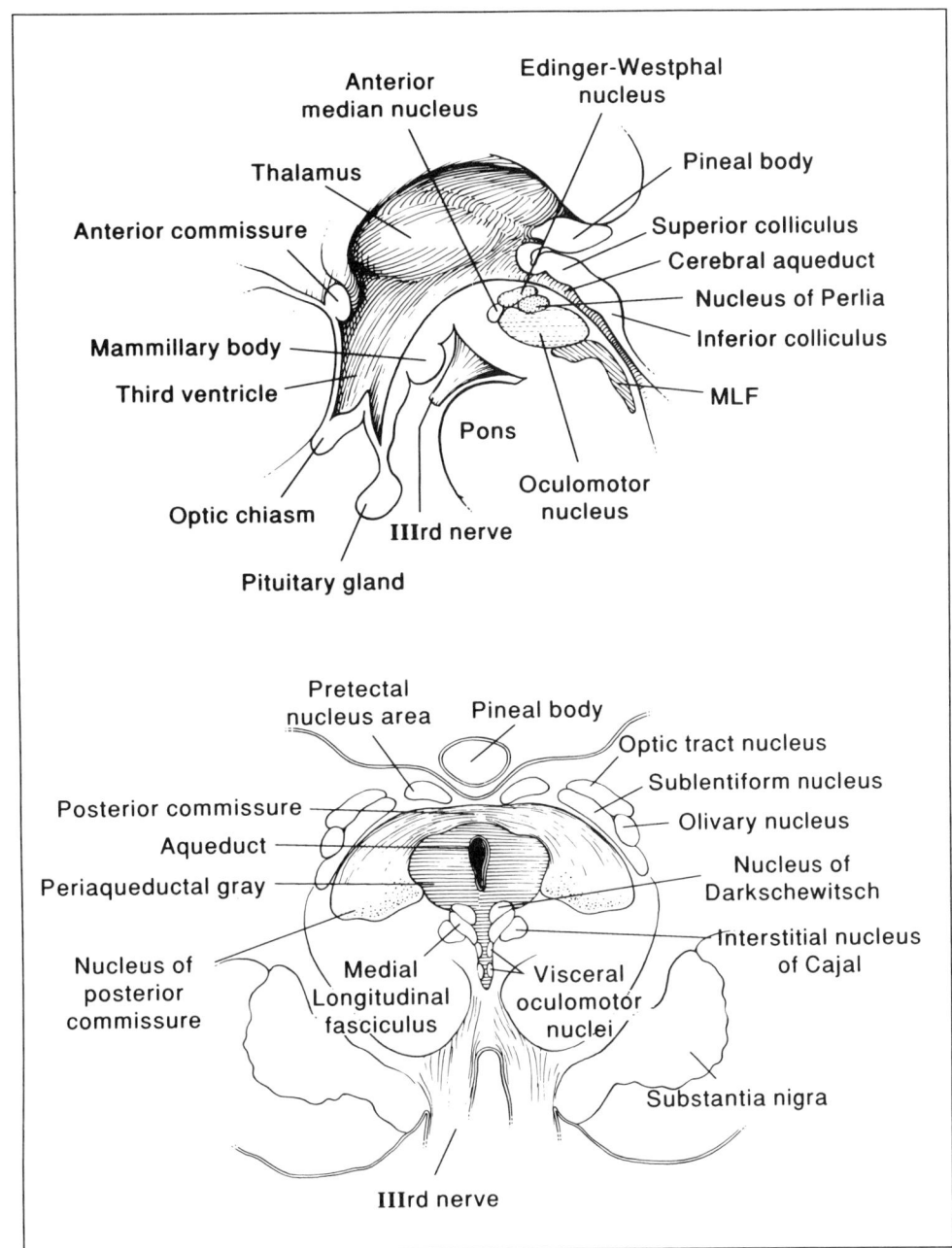

FIG. 2. Major pretectal nuclei in the mesencephalon.

iary branch of the ophthalmic division of the fifth nerve. About 3% of the parasympathetic fibers synapsing in the ganglion give rise to axons that supply the iris sphincter, while ~94% supply the ciliary muscle. Therefore, >90% of the mesencephalic parasympathetic outflow is concerned with accommodation and not with pupillary constriction (21). Controversy exists about whether there is a direct parasympathetic pathway from the dorsal mesencephalon to the ciliary muscle and iris sphincter without a synapse in the ciliary ganglion (6,15).

The first-order parasympathetic neurons responsible for the secretion of tears are in the tegmentum of the pons, dorsal to the superior salivary nucleus (Fig. 4). They traverse the facial nucleus and join the sensory root of the seventh nerve, the nervus intermedius, which emerges from the lateral pons between the seventh and eighth nerves. The nervus intermedius passes to the cerebellopontine angle and joins the rest of the seventh nerve entering the internal auditory meatus. The fibers destined for the lacrimal gland travel through the geniculate ganglion of the seventh nerve and then emerge from the temporal bone in the floor of the middle fossa as the greater superficial petrosal nerve. This nerve passes under the gasserian ganglion in Meckel's cave and enters the vidian canal at the anterior end of the fora-

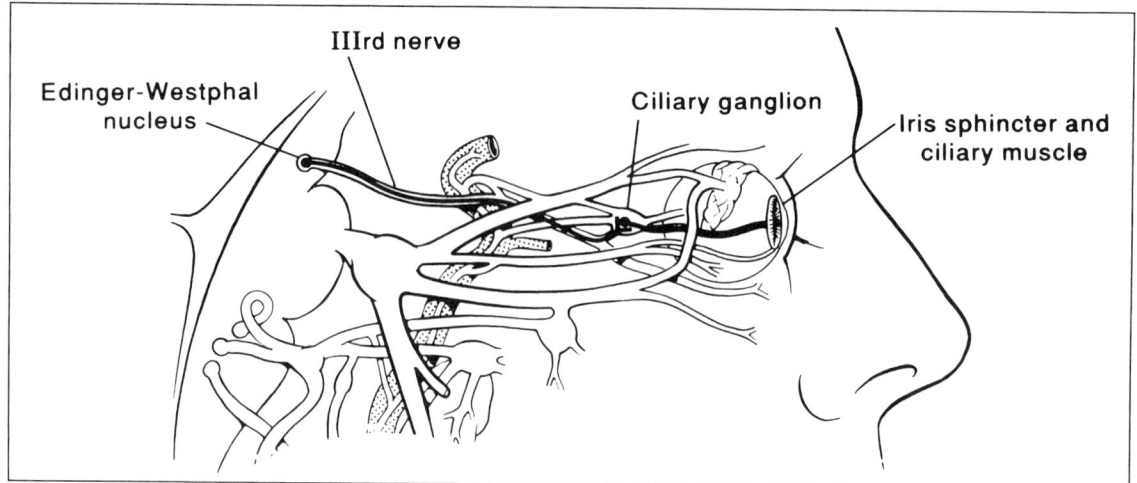

FIG. 3. Parasympathetic outflow to the iris sphincter and ciliary muscle.

men lacerum. At this point, the greater superficial petrosal nerve joins the deep petrosal nerve to form the vidian nerve, which then passes to the sphenopalatine ganglion.

In this ganglion, the preganglionic axons synapse with postganglionic parasympathetic neurons. The sphenopalatine ganglion sends branches to the pharynx, palate, palatine tonsil, the mucus membranes of the nose, and sends orbital branches to the lacrimal gland, the periosteum, and the striated muscles of the orbit. Those going to the lacrimal gland leave the splenopalatine ganglion, enter the

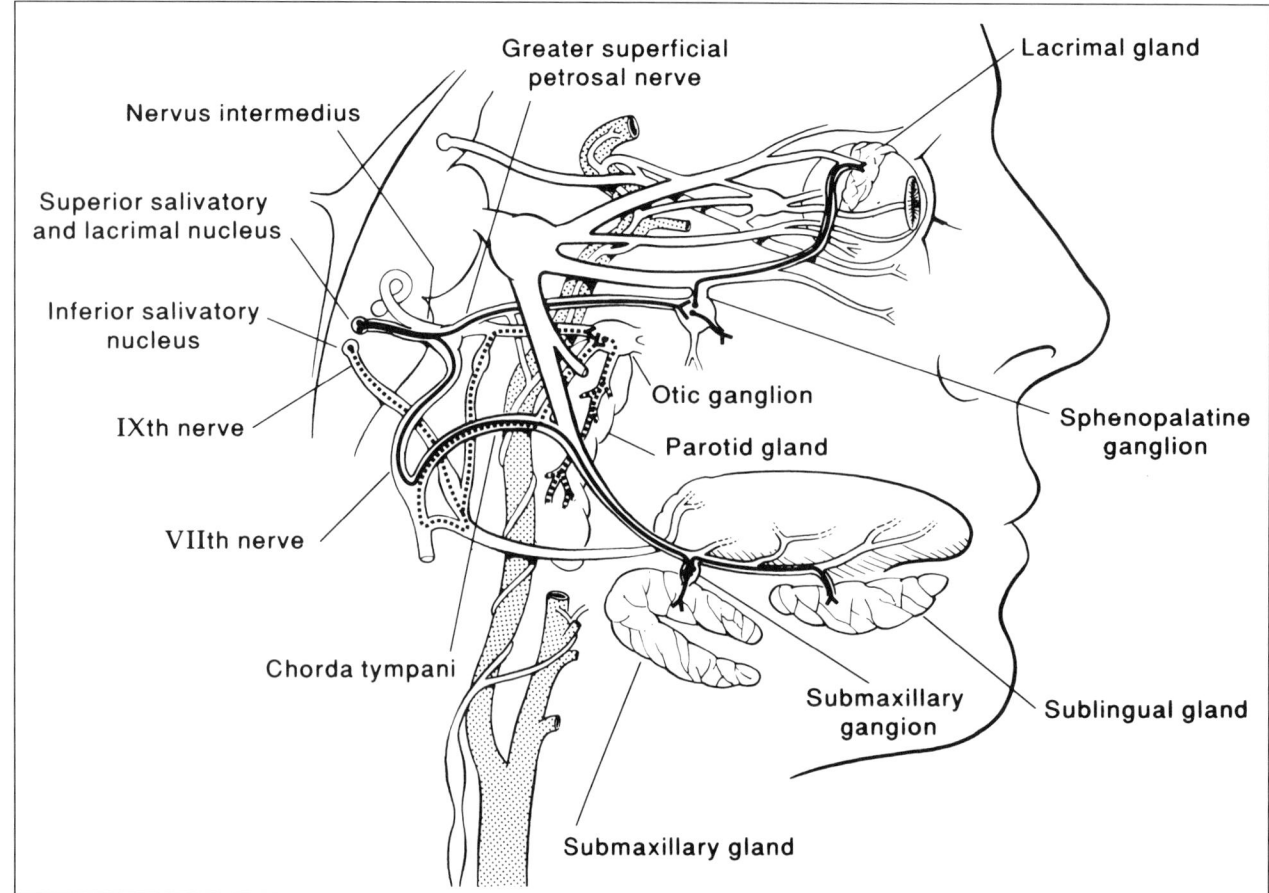

FIG. 4. Parasympathetic outflow for lacrimation and salivation: *solid lines* indicate outflow from the superior salivatory nucleus, and *broken lines* indicate outflow from the inferior salivatory nucleus.

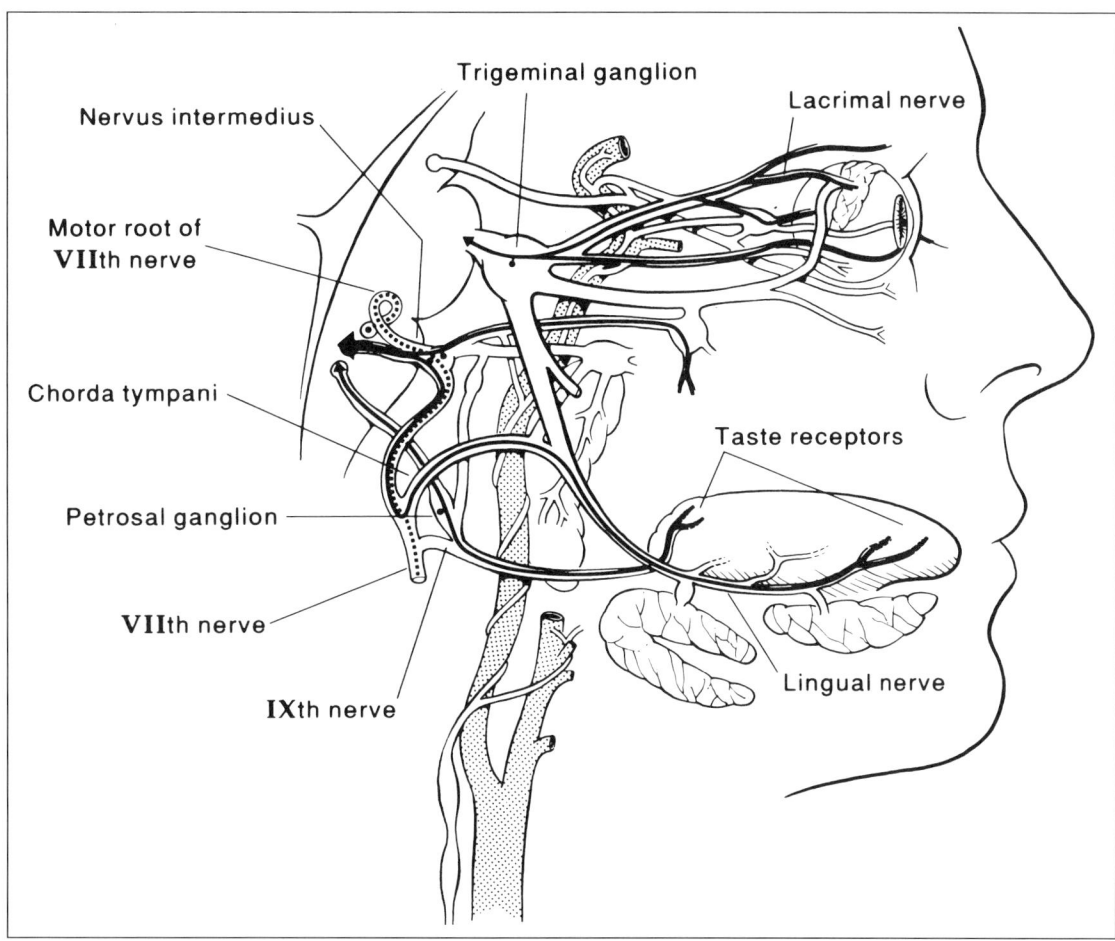

FIG. 5. Sensory afferents for lacrimal and salivary reflexes: *solid lines* indicate afferents traveling via cranial nerves V, VII, and IX, and *broken lines* show motor fibers to the face in cranial nerve VII.

maxillary division of the fifth nerve, and pass through the inferior orbital fissure. They then travel in the lateral wall of the orbit and reach the lacrimal gland through an anastomosis between the zygomaticotemporal branch of this division and the lacrimal nerve (a branch of the ophthalmic division of the fifth nerve). They terminate between the cells and around the ducts in the gland. Sympathetic outflow to the gland is mainly vasomotor and is derived from fibers in the cervical sympathetic chain and the carotid plexus. Some sympathetic fibers travel with the vidian nerve to the deep petrosal nerve and go with the parasympathetic fibers. Others travel with the carotid plexus and the ophthalmic division of the fifth nerve. The sensory pathway for the lacrimal reflex is shown in Fig. 5.

The Sympathetic Pathway

The iris dilator muscle is controlled by the sympathetic nervous system. Fibers originate in the posterolateral regions of the hypothalamus (Fig. 6). Most descend directly without synapse, while other fibers probably do contain synapses in the tegmental region of the pons and mesencephalon. In the spinal cord, the fibers descend in the anterolateral column (12) and synapse with preganglionic neurons of the peripheral sympathetic pathway in the intermediolateral cell column between C8 and T2, the ciliospinal center of Budge–Waller. Most of the fibers destined for the eye leave the spinal cord in the first ventral thoracic root. They travel to the sympathetic paravertebral chain as the white rami communicates and ascend without synapse through the stellate ganglion, mainly in the anterior loop of the ansa subclavia of Vieussens, and ascend further through the inferior and middle cervical ganglia to synapse in the superior cervical ganglion.

This ganglion is located below the base of the skull, between the internal jugular vein and the internal carotid artery. Its cell bodies are adrenergic postganglionic neurons. The ratio of preganglionic to postganglionic fibers is 1:11 to 1:17 (21). There are two main groups of postganglionic efferents; those that supply C1 through C4 (as gray rami) and the ninth, tenth, and twelfth nerves, and those

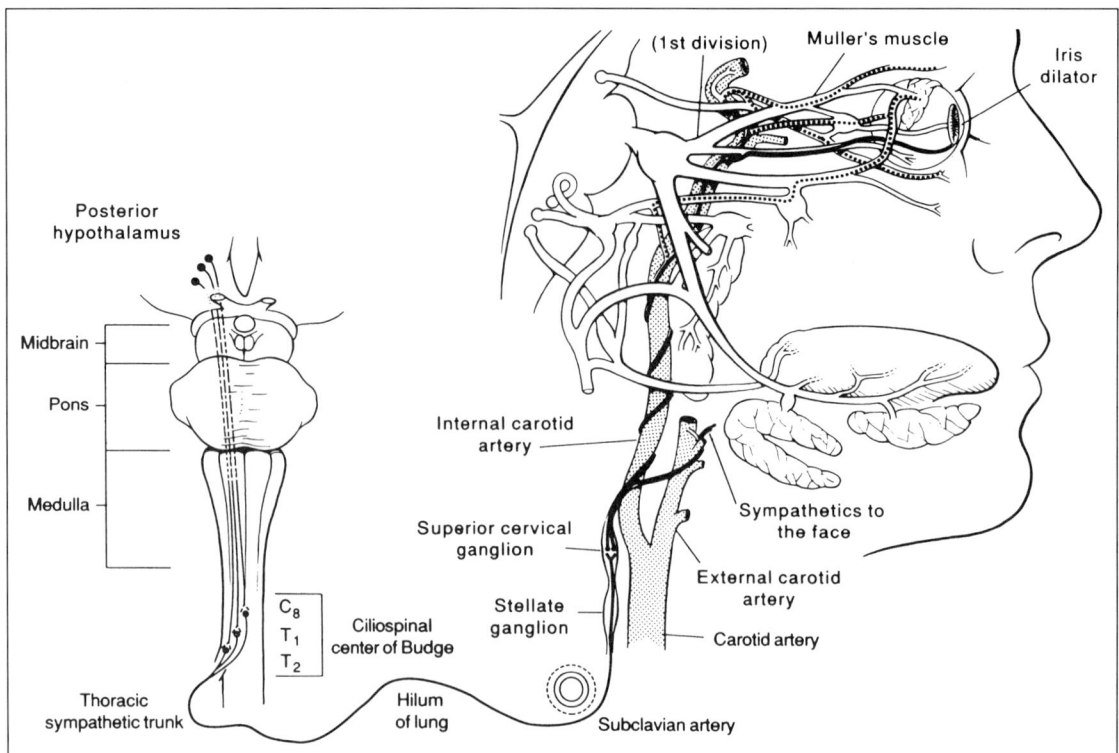

FIG. 6. Sympathetic outflow to the eye: *solid lines* indicate fibers to the dilator of the pupil, and *broken lines* indicate sympathetics to Muller's muscle in the upper lid, a similar muscle in the lower lid, and the vessels of the lacrimal gland.

that supply the pharynx, heart, and sympathetic targets in the head via the external and internal carotid plexus. The proximity of this ganglion to the lower cranial nerves explains its frequent involvement when these nerves are damaged by trauma and infection.

The fibers destined for the eye travel in a plexus surrounding the internal carotid artery while those destined for sweat glands travel with the external carotid (Fig. 6). The fibers around the internal carotid artery enter the skull with this artery via the carotid canal and foramen lacerum and proceed to the cavernous sinus. As the carotid enters the skull, some of the sympathetic fibers join the tympanic branch of the glossopharyngeal nerve to form the tympanic plexus on the promontory of the middle ear and, after passing through this plexus, they rejoin the internal carotid plexus. The carotid canal is in close relation to the gasserian ganglion.

In the cavernous sinus are sympathetic fibers destined for intracranial vessels, as well as fibers destined for the eye. The latter leave the carotid, travel briefly with the sixth nerve and then the third nerve, and finally join the ophthalmic division of the fifth nerve. Some of the branches are distributed to the arteries in the cavernous sinus and orbit, regulating blood flow to these areas. Other fibers leave the carotid plexus to form the deep petrosal nerve, which joins the greater superficial petrosal nerve to form the vidian nerve, which then joins the sphenopalatine ganglion. This carries visceral efferent fibers of the seventh nerve, some of which supply the lacrimal gland. Most of the sympathetic fibers pass through the superior orbital fissure along with cranial nerves III, IV, and VI and the first division of cranial nerve V and then travel with this last nerve, following the nasociliary nerve to the pupil and ciliary body.

Postganglionic fibers of the sympathetic system supply the vessels of the orbit, the intrinsic muscles of the eye, the melanocytes of the uveal tract, the extrinsic ocular muscles, the smooth muscle of Muller and a similar muscle in the lower lid, the lacrimal gland, and possibly the pigment layer of the retina (4). The fibers that innervate the pupillary dilator muscle enter the orbit with the nasociliary nerve, bypass the ciliary ganglion, and reach the eye via the long ciliary nerves. Other sympathetic fibers pass through the ciliary ganglion, but do not synapse there (as it is a parasympathetic ganglion), and comprise vasomotor efferents for the eye. Sympathetic fibers are present, therefore, in both the long and the short ciliary nerves.

Taste

Sensory fibers from the taste buds in the anterior two-thirds of the tongue travel with the lingual branch of the mandibular nerve and then join the chorda tympani, which passes through the middle ear to the facial canal and then along with the facial nerve to the geniculate ganglion

(Fig. 5). From the geniculate ganglion, the gustatory fibers pass centrally as the nervus intermedius. When this nerve enters the pons, the fibers turn caudally to the tractus solitarius and synapse in the rostral end of the nucleus solitarius. Gustatory fibers from the posterior third of the tongue reach the nucleus solitarius via the glossopharyngeal nerves.

Salivation

Preganglionic salivary neurons originate in two sets of nuclei in the brainstem and follow two separate pathways to their respective parasympathetic ganglia (Fig. 5). Neurons in the superior salivary nucleus leave the lower pons with the lacrimal fibers in the nervus intermedius, pass through the geniculate ganglion without synapsing, travel down the seventh nerve, and leave the facial canal with the chorda tympani. They then join the lingual nerve and pass to the submandibular ganglion and sublingual ganglion where they synapse with postganglionic neurons that innervate the submandibular and sublingual salivary glands. Salivary neurons from the inferior salivary nucleus leave the medulla with fibers of the ninth nerve, pass through the jugular foramen along with the tenth and eleventh nerves, pass through the petrous ganglion of the ninth nerve without synapsing, branch at the base of the skull, ascend as the tympanic nerve to the tympanic cavity, and then divide into branches forming the tympanic plexus. They then join the greater superficial petrosal nerve, pass through the anterior surface of the petrous bone to the middle fossa as the lesser superficial petrosal nerve, and leave through the foramen ovale to end in the otic ganglion. Here the preganglionic fibers synapse with neurons that supply the parotid gland. The otic ganglion has a sensory root from fibers of the ninth and seventh nerves via the lesser superficial petrosal nerve, a motor root from fibers to the internal pterygoid muscle, and a sympathetic root from the carotid sympathetic plexus. It gives rise to three communicating nerves: the nerve to the pterygoid canal, a twig to the chorda tympani, and the auriculotemporal nerve, which supplies the postganglionic secretory fibers to the parotid gland. Two motor branches supply the tensor tympani and the tensor veli palatini.

THE PHYSIOLOGY OF THE NORMAL PUPIL

The Balance Between Sympathetic and Parasympathetic Influences

The size of the pupil under different circumstances reflects the balance between sympathetic and parasympathetic control. Parasympathetic innervation is of primary importance, and sympathetic innervation plays a supporting role (18). With age, the pupils become smaller and less reactive. This change has been attributed to loss of sympathetic tone (8), but in actuality both sympathetic and parasympathetic inputs to the iris are diminished (14). When an individual is alert, parasympathetic influences are inhibited and the hypothalamus maintains a level of sympathetic tone. Stimulation of the hypothalamus can provoke mydriasis, widening of the palpebral fissures, and a rise in blood pressure. As the individual becomes tired, the pupils become smaller and oscillatory fatigue waves or fluctuating changes in pupillary size become apparent. In states of fatigue and sleep, sympathetic activity is reduced and the resulting predominance of parasympathetic influence results in miosis. During sleep, the pupils are small, but reactive to light. This represents a release phenomenon, since inhibitory influences from the cortex, hypothalamus, and reticular activating system are diminished (18).

Sensory and Emotional Sympathetic Stimulation

Sensory and emotional stimuli cause the pupils to dilate. Two mechanisms achieve this: the radially arranged fibers of the dilator muscle contract because of sympathetic stimulation, and the circumferentially oriented sphincter muscle relaxes because of inhibition of parasympathetic tone. In anesthetized animals, the active component is abolished, and the pupils dilate by inhibition of the sphincter alone (18). Adrenergic substances, such as norepinephrine and epinephrine, traveling in the bloodstream stimulate the dilator muscle directly and cause a larger pupil. In patients with Horner's syndrome, massive catecholamine release or intravenous epinephrine or norepinephrine will dilate the abnormal more than the normal pupil because of the denervation supersensitivity of the former. When the neck is pinched or some other painful stimulus is given, the pupil will dilate (ciliospinal reflex). Pupillary dilitation to noxious electrical stimulation is an accurate predictor of the level of sensory spinal block during combined epidural–general anesthesia (9).

Supranuclear Inhibition of Parasympathetic Innervation

A number of supranuclear pathways can inhibit constriction of the pupils. When an eye adapted to light is suddenly exposed to darkness, the pupils dilate. If the sympathetic innervation that controls the iris dilator is abolished, the dilation will still occur, although not to the same degree. There must be, therefore, some inhibitory influence on the Edinger–Westphal and anterior median nuclei (11).

Supranuclear Control of Sympathetic Innervation

Cortical and subcortical influences regulate the iris dilator muscle. Stimulation in limbic areas, including the cingulate gyrus, the subcallosal and postorbital regions, the olfactory tubercle, and the piriform cortex can dilate the pupil (5). Stimulation of neocortex, including area 8 of Broadman, sensory motor areas, and the occipital lobe can result in pupillary dilatation as well. This dilatation is abolished by an ipsilateral hypothalamic lesion (13). Stimulation of a wide area in the ventrolateral hypothalamus will cause rapid and maximal pupillary dilatation due to sympathetic excitation. Stimulation of the diencephalon or the cortex in sympathectomized cats and monkeys causes pupillary dilation and abolition of the light reflex, indicating that pupillary dilatation results from parasympathetic inhibition as well as sympathetic stimulation (3,10). Even in the case of a severe cervical spinal cord lesion interrupting descending sympathetic fibers, mydriasis can occur with arousal or painful stimuli, indicating brain stem inhibition of pupillary constriction. There are probably also inhibitory pathways from the spinal cord and the reticular activating system acting on the Edinger–Westphal nucleus directly inhibiting the motor neurons for pupillary constriction (18).

The Pupillary Light Reflex

The pupillary light reflex (Fig. 7), constriction of the pupils in the response to light, begins with retinal photoreceptors that synapse with bipolar cells that in turn synapse with retinal ganglion cells whose axons travel as the optic nerve, chiasm, and tracts. Just before these axons reach the lateral geniculate body, they send collaterals to the mesencephalon via the brachium of the superior colliculus. These fibers synapse in the pretectal region of the mesencephalon in a number of small subnuclei. These pretectal subnuclei send ipsilateral and contralateral fibers to the Edinger– Westphal nucleus. Cutting the brachium to the superior colliculus on each side abolishes light reflexes, and stimulation of the brachium can produce pupillary constriction (7). The Edinger–Westphal nucleus sends parasympathetic efferents as part of the third nerve to the pupillary constrictor. The pupillary light reflex sets the pupils at a size that is optimal for visual acuity. The latent period of pupillary light reaction is relatively long, as would be expected in a function controlled by smooth muscle.

The Direct and Consensual Light Reflexes

When light is shined in either eye, both pupils constrict. The constriction of the eye being stimulated is the direct response, and the constriction in the contralateral eye is the consensual response. These direct and consensual responses are, practically speaking, equal in magnitude, as long as there is no lesion in the parasympathetic or sympathetic pathways.

The Near Response

When fixation is shifted from a far object to a near one, the eyes converge, the lenses undergo the optical change termed accommodation, and both pupils constrict. This triad of activity is called the near response. These three functions are separate, and any one of them can be selectively abolished or elicited without affecting the others. The near response is stimulated by a pathway that begins in the occipital cortex and whose fibers descend to a ventrolateral position in the upper midbrain. This ventrolateral location explains the sparing of the near reflex in the more dorsal and medial lesions of the tectum and posterior commissure. It also explains pupillary light–near dissociation, as ventrolaterally located pathways for pupillary constriction associated with voluntary and involuntary effort to look at near objects can be relatively uninterrupted by more dorsomedial pretectal lesions that impair the pupillary light reflex. A number of places in Broadman's areas 18 and 19, when stimulated, cause pupillary constriction together with convergence and accommodation (2). The final common pathway of the near response arises in various cell groups in the oculomotor and Edinger–Westphal nuclei. The pupillary constriction to light and the near response have a single final pathway via the parasympathetic innervation to the constrictor of the pupil. From the aspect of the clinical examination, the light reflex is more useful than near response because the latter has subjective features. If the near response is poor, it is difficult to be certain that the patient made a good effort. For practical purposes, the near response is important only when it is more prominent than the light response, as, for example, in Argyll Robertson or tonic pupils.

Benign Conditions Affecting Pupillary Size

About 20% of individuals have pupillary inequality with normal reactivity to light and darkness. This benign or simple anisocoria may well be due to asymmetries of supranuclear inhibitory control on visceral nuclei, and it has no clinical significance. It tends to decrease in light. Its main importance is that it be recognized in order to avoid extensive evaluations for a benign condition. When some normal individuals look in extreme lateral gaze, the pupil on that side becomes larger and the opposite one becomes smaller. This is Tourney's phenomenon, which may result from central inhibition of mesencephalic visceral oculomotor nuclei (17). It is quite rare. Hippus is physiologic pupillary unrest. In ordinary illumination, due to varying levels of sympathetic and parasympathetic tone, pupils of a young healthy person are in constant motion. This is similar to, but not identical to, the oscillatory pupillary movements that occur with reduced alertness from variation in reticular activating system input to pupillary control.

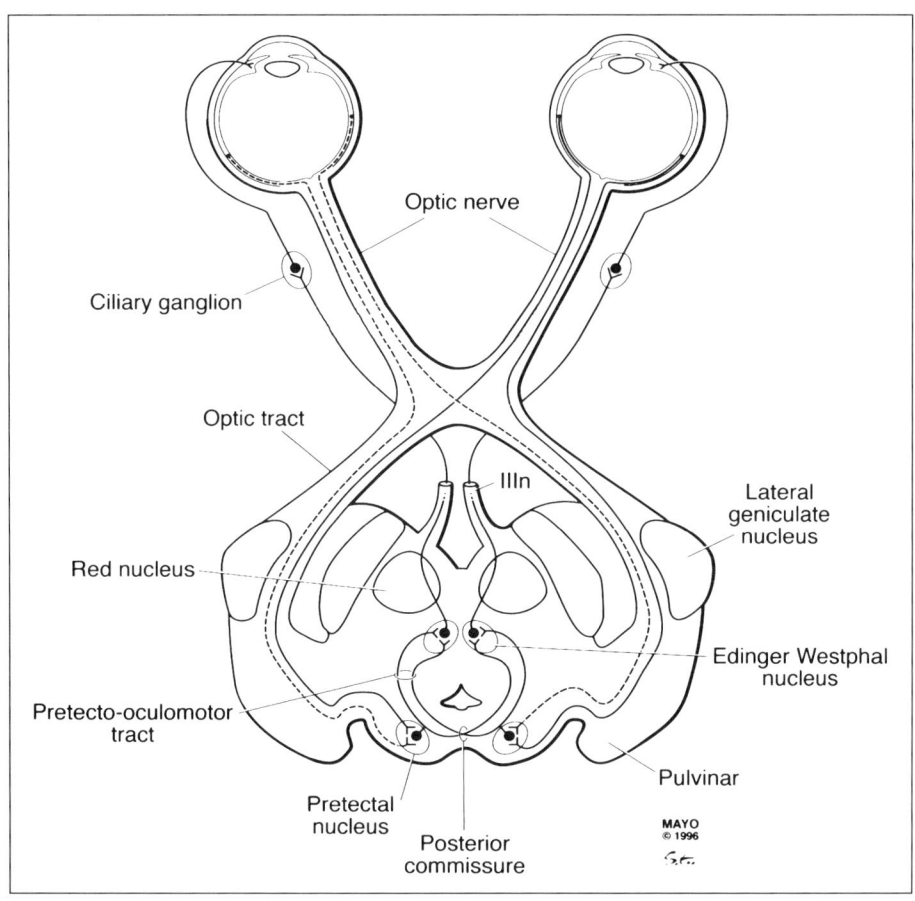

FIG. 7. Pupillary light reflex.

Lacrimation

Nonreflex basal tear production occurs continuously for protection and maintenance of the cornea and sclera. It is under parasympathetic and probably some sympathetic influence. Reflex tears are stimulated by sensory stimuli via afferent impulses from the first division of the cranial nerve V and the retina via strong light exposure. The efferent pathway is parasympathetic. Psychogenic tearing occurs in response to emotions and is controlled by corticolimbic and hypothalamic input. Parasympathomimetic drugs directly induce, and anticholinergic drugs directly inhibit, tear production. Tearing is a component of yawning, coughing, and vomiting.

REFERENCES

1. Asbury AK, et al. Oculomotor palsy in diabetes mellitus: a clinicopathological study. *Brain* 1970;93:555–566.
2. Barris RW. A pupillo-constrictor area in the cerebral cortex of the cat and its relationship to the pretectal area. *J Comp Neurol* 1936;63:353–369.
3. Bonvallet MS, Zbrozyna A. Les commandes reticulaires du systeme autonome et en particulier de l'innervation sympathetique et parasympatique de la pupille. *Arch Ital Biol* 1963;101:174–207.
4. Duke-Elder S. *System of ophthalmology;* vol 2. St Louis: CV Mosby, 1961.
5. Harris AJ, et al. The afferent path of the pupillodilator reflex in the cat. *J Neurophysiol* 1944;7:231–243.
6. Jaeger RJ, Benevento LA. A horseradish peroxidase study of the innervation of the internal structures of the eye: evidence for a direct pathway. *Invest Ophthalmol Vis Sci* 1980;19:575–583.
7. Karplus JP, Kreidl A. Ueber dri Bahn des Pupillarreflexes (die reflectorische Pupillenstarre). *Pflugers Arch Gesamte Physiol Mensch Tiere* 1913;149:115–155.
8. Korczyn AD, et al. Sympathetic pupillary tone in old age. *Arch Ophthalmol* 1976;94:1905–1906.
9. Larson MD, et al. Pupillary assessment of sensory block level during combined epidural/general anesthesia. *Anesthesiology* 1993;79: 42–48.
10. Lowenfeld IE. Mechanisms of reflex dilatation of the pupil: histological review and experimental analysis. *Doc Ophthalmol* 1958;12: 185–448.
11. Lowenstein O, Loewenfeld IE. The pupil. In: Davison H, ed. *The eye;* vol 3. New York: Academic, 1962:231–267.
12. Nathan PW, Smith MC. The location of descending fibers to sympathetic neurons supplying the eye and sudomotor neurons supplying the head and neck. *J Neurol Neurosurg Psychiatry* 1986;49:187–194.
13. Parsons JH. The physiology of pupil reactions. *Trans Ophthalmol Soc UK* 1924;44:1–11.
14. Pfeifer MA, et al. Differential changes of autonomic nervous system function with age in man. *Am J Med* 1983;75:249–258.
15. Slamovits TL, Miller NR, Burde RM. Intracranial oculomotor nerve paresis with anisocoria and pupillary parasympathetic hypersensitivity. *Am J Ophthalmol* 1987;104:401–406.
16. Sunderland S, Hughes ESR. The pupillo-constrictor pathway and the nerves to the ocular muscles in man. *Brain* 1946;69:301–309.

17. Tournay A. Sur l'anisocorie normale dans le regard lateral extreme. *Arch Ophthalmol* 1927;44:574–576.
18. Walshe, Hoyt W. The Pupil: Embryology, anatomy, innervation and reflex movements of the iris. In: Miller, Williams, Wilkins, eds. *Clinical neuro-ophthalmology*. 1984:400–441.
19. Walshe, Hoyt W. Accommodation: Embryology, anatomy, innervation and normal function. In: Miller, Williams, Wilkins, eds. *Clinical neuro-ophthalmology*. 1984:442–457.
20. Walshe, Hoyt W. Anatomy, physiology, and testing of normal lacrimal secretion. In: Miller, Williams, Wilkins, eds. *Clinical neuro-ophthalmology*. 1984:458–468.
21. Warwick R. The ocular parasympathetic nerve supply and its mesencephalic sources. *J Anat* 1954;88:71–93.
22. Wolf GA Jr. The ratio of preganglionic neurons to postganglionic neurons in the visceral nervous system. *J Comp Neurol* 1941;75:235–243.

CHAPTER 21

Causes and Evaluation of Male Sexual Dysfunction

John D. Stewart

1. Male sexual dysfunction can consist of reduced libido, impaired erections, or abnormal ejaculation. Each of these can have a psychogenic or organic origin. Sometimes both are present, with organic sexual dysfunction giving rise to secondary psychogenic factors.
2. The causes of organic sexual dysfunction fall into the following categories: vascular, neurogenic, and endocrine abnormalities; medication side-effects; and toxins.
3. A thorough clinical evaluation (which may include psychiatric evaluation) can establish the cause of dysfunction in many patients.
4. Tests available for further elucidating the cause include blood tests, intracavernosal injections of vasoactive substances, penile blood pressure or circulatory studies, nocturnal penile tumescence studies, arteriography and cavernosography, and neurophysiologic studies.
5. The choice of tests should be dictated by the findings yielded by the clinical evaluation.

INTRODUCTION

The physiology of male sexual function is described in Chapter 11. There are a variety of types of male sexual dysfunction, but the emphasis in this chapter is on erectile dysfunction—the consistent inability to attain and maintain a penile erection sufficient for satisfactory sexual intercourse. The frequency of this problem has probably been seriously underestimated in the past; it is now thought that as many as 20–30 million American men may be affected (23,48). This chapter describes the clinical and laboratory approaches to making an accurate diagnosis as a prelude to the rational choice of treatment. There is also an emphasis on distinguishing organic from psychogenic erectile impotence. As clinically useful as this distinction is, it is important to recognize its limitations (62):

> Literature on the assessment and treatment of erectile dysfunction has narrowly focused on a dichotomized etiologic model, erroneously pitting organic against psychologic elements as mutually exclusive causal agents. A more sophisticated model recognizes that physiologic, affective, and cognitive factors all contribute to normal erectile function, and any or all of them contribute to abnormal erectile function. The cause of most erectile problems is likely to be multifactorial, and assessment should focus on delineating not only etiologic factors, but also factors most likely to affect treatment recommendation and contribute to a good prognosis.

Organic causes include endocrine, vascular, or neurogenic abnormalities, medication side-effects, and toxins; more than one of these organic factors may be present—"mixed" sexual dysfunction. The treatment of male sexual dysfunction is discussed in Chapter 58.

CAUSES

Male sexual dysfunction can be classified into the following categories: diminished libido, erectile impotence, and ejaculatory disorders (Table 1). Each of these categories is further divided into psychogenic or organic causes, or a combination of both.

Diminished Libido

Reduced libido is often psychogenic in origin, resulting from depression, anxiety, or both. The most common organic cause is probably any form of chronic ill health.

J. D. Stewart: Departments of Neurology and Neurosurgery, Montreal Hospital, Montreal, Quebec H3A 2B4 Canada.

Endocrine disorders—such as primary or secondary hypogonadism, excessive endogenous estrogens, Addison's disease, hypothyroidism, and some pituitary adenomas—can all produce diminished libido (70). Other causes include some chronic hepatic diseases and temporal lobe damage (9,28,53). Most medications that cause sexual dysfunction impair erection or ejaculation and not libido. Those that do depress libido include reserpine, propranolol, cimetidine, tricyclic antidepressants, monoamine oxidase inhibitors, fenfluramine, sedatives, and narcotics (3, 29,47). Estrogens given for suppression of prostatic carcinoma can also suppress libido. Excessive prolonged alcohol intake can impair both libido and erection. Testicular atrophy and liver disease may both play a role in reduced libido (17,63), but one study has shown that sexual dysfunction in half of the patients is psychogenic (61). Erectile dysfunction in some alcoholics probably stems from autonomic peripheral neuropathy (14,61).

Erectile Dysfunction

Psychogenic factors, principally depression or anxiety, are important and common causes of erectile dysfunction. Organic erectile impotence can be caused by vascular problems, neurologic abnormalities (or a combination of both), endocrine factors, medications, and toxins (notably alcohol) (Table 1). Combinations of these factors can occur, e.g., the diabetic male with vascular insufficiency and peripheral neuropathy.

Vascular causes include decreased arterial inflow, as is seen in patients with severe arteriosclerosis of the common or internal iliac arteries, and overly rapid venous drainage ("venous leakers").

Disorders of the central and the peripheral nervous systems, or both, give rise to neurogenic erectile impotence. Intracranial causes of sexual dysfunction are rare. Patients with temporal lobe lesions and temporal lobe seizures may have impaired erections as well as reduced libido (9,28, 53). Bilateral lesions made in the region of the ansa lenticularis and hypothalamus for the treatment of hyperkinetic behavior have precipitated erectile failure (19).

Spinal cord injuries that produce paraplegia are the commonest central lesions causing sexual dysfunction (10,15, 16,18,27,50,57,60). Damage above the sacral cord interferes with psychogenic erections but not the spinal reflexes involved in erection and ejaculation, so many of these patients can have sexual activity following genital stimulation. Sacral cord and conus medullaris lesions abolish sexual function because the parasympathetic and somatic pathways are destroyed. Other myelopathies, such as multiple sclerosis, can impair male sexual function to a variable extent, depending on the site and severity of the demyelinating plaques (7,36,59). In the peripheral nervous system, damage to the cauda equina produces an effect similar to that caused by a distal spinal cord (conus medullaris) lesion. Peripheral neuropathies may also cause sexual dysfunction, particularly those that involve small myelinated and unmyelinated fibers. By far the commonest neuropathy to cause sexual dysfunction is diabetic neuropathy: ~40% of male diabetics have erectile dysfunction (22). Peripheral autonomic disorders, such as acute pandysautonomia, also interfere with sexual function (Chapter 37). In disorders such as multiple-system atrophy and pure autonomic failure (Chapter 42), there is degeneration of either or both central and peripheral components of the autonomic nervous system, so that erectile dysfunction is often an early manifestation of autonomic impairment. Pelvic and urologic surgery can also damage the autonomic nerves in the pelvis (5).

The major endocrine cause of erectile failure is hyperprolactinemia secondary to a pituitary adenoma or to medications associated with overproduction of prolactin (α-methyldopa, phenothiazines, or reserpine).

Medications that can cause erectile failure include many of the antihypertensive, anticholinergic, antipsychotic, antidepressant, and antihistamine agents, as well as some diuretics (3,25,29,47). Alcohol-induced erectile failure has

TABLE 1. *Causes of male sexual dysfunction*

Decreased libido
Psychogenic
Organic
   Chronic ill health
   Endocrine: hypogonadism, excessive estrogens, Addison's disease, hypothyroidism, pituitary adenomas, Cushing's syndrome, hepatic disease, temporal lobe damage
   Medications
   Alcohol

Erectile impotence
Psychogenic
Organic
   Vascular: arterial insufficiency, excessive venous leakage
   Neurogenic: myelopathies; conus medullaris, cauda equina and sacral plexus lesions; peripheral neuropathies; peripheral and/or central autonomic disorders
Endocrine
   Hyperprolactinemia, hypothyroidism, hyperthyroidism
   Medications
   Alcohol
   Peyronie's disease

Ejaculatory abnormalities
Psychogenic
Organic
   Neurogenic retrograde ejaculation: postprostatectomy; diabetes mellitus
   Neurogenic anejaculation: myelopathies, diabetes mellitus, retroperitoneal surgery
   Medications

been just discussed. Smoking and the use of street drugs such as marijuana and cocaine are frequently cited as contributing factors in sexual dysfunction, but critical analyses of these factors are lacking (4).

Ejaculatory Disorders

Disturbances of ejaculation include premature, retarded, retrograde ejaculation, and anejaculation (38,69).

Premature ejaculation is a common problem but is not due to neurologic dysfunction. Retrograde ejaculation is the propulsion of semen from the proximal urethra back into the bladder. This occurs because of dysynergia of the muscles of the pelvic floor, the base of the bladder, and the urethral sphincters. Semen is expelled backward up the urethra into the bladder instead of down the urethra, though the sensation of orgasm is usually preserved. One cause is transurethral resection of the prostate, which often results in an open bladder neck so that the semen takes the path of least resistance into the bladder. Retrograde ejaculation is also quite common in diabetic males and is thought to be due to dysfunction of the sympathetic innervation of the internal urethral sphincter. The diagnosis can be confirmed by examining a postcoital urine specimen for the presence of spermatozoa. Because retrograde ejaculation is usually accompanied by the sensation of orgasm, it is only a problem for those men who wish to procreate.

Anejaculation is uncommon and may result from spinal cord injury, transverse myelitis, multiple sclerosis, retroperitoneal lymph node dissection with damage to the sympathetic chain, and diabetes mellitus; it can also be psychogenic (32,69). Anejaculation, with or without failure of orgasm, can result from a variety of medications, including some antihypertensives, thioridazine, some tricyclic antidepressants, and levodopa.

It should be stressed that psychogenic sexual dysfunction and organic sexual dysfunction are not mutually exclusive. Organic dysfunction frequently produces secondary anxiety that can exacerbate the original problem, an important point to be remembered when evaluating and treating men with sexual dysfunction. It is also important to attribute causality of sexual dysfunction with caution. For example, in a diabetic man with erectile impotence, the cause could be assumed to be vascular or neurogenic or both; however, it could be neither of these but psychogenic (64).

CLINICAL EVALUATION

The evaluation of a man with erectile dysfunction begins with the clinical history taking and examination, either of which may rapidly point to an obvious cause, such as spinal cord injury, overt depression, severe peripheral vascular disease, or peripheral neuropathy. Less obvious causes may be implicated by a family history of diabetes mellitus, use of the medications already listed, heavy alcohol intake, claudication in the legs, or other neurologic symptoms. Concomitant impairment of bladder and bowel, with or without somatic neurologic symptoms in the legs, suggests a lesion of the conus medullaris, cauda equina, or sacral plexus. Associated dysautonomic symptoms indicate a generalized dysautonomic disorder. Psychiatric symptoms, particularly depression and anxiety, may not be volunteered by the patient and should be sought carefully. Important clues to a psychogenic versus organic etiology can be gained from detailed questioning about erections. When spontaneous erections occur during sleep or upon wakening but are unsatisfactory at times of attempted intercourse, the cause is likely psychogenic. This is also true if satisfactory erections occur during masturbation or with one partner but fail with another.

On general examination, signs of liver failure and hypogonadism, testicular atrophy, Peyronie's disease, and vascular insufficiency in the legs should all be sought. A careful neurologic examination should be done to seek evidence of myelopathy, cauda equina or sacral plexus damage, or peripheral neuropathy. In particular, this involves a sensory examination of the genital and perianal area, and rectal sphincter evaluation. In patients with peripheral neuropathy, the signs may be very subtle if only the small-diameter fibers are involved.

If at the end of the clinical evaluation there is a high suspicion that the source of the impotence is psychogenic, the next best step, before an extensive laboratory evaluation, is a referral for psychological evaluation.

LABORATORY TESTING

There is now a large battery of tests available for evaluating erectile dysfunction. Many of them are of unknown sensitivity and specificity, and there is little consensus as to what constitutes a reasonable evaluation of the impotent male (6,26). I advocate choosing from the tests described below, depending on the conclusions from the clinical evaluation, and using simple and inexpensive tests first (Table 2). The goal is to confirm or identify the specific cause so that treatment can be tailored to that cause. In practice, however, the treatments available are often effective regardless of the specific cause of the erectile failure.

Blood Tests

Blood tests should include a fasting blood sugar determination to detect undiagnosed diabetes, with a glucose tolerance test or determination of 2-hr postprandial glucose levels for confirmation if the fasting value is abnormal; and liver and thyroid function tests. Prolactin and testosterone levels may also be determined.

TABLE 2. *Laboratory testing for erectile dysfunction*[a]

Blood tests
    Fasting glucose, 2-hr postprandial glucose, glucose tolerance test
    Liver function tests
    Thyroid function tests
    Prolactin
    Testosterone

Diagnostic intracavernosal injection

Penile vascular studies
    Penile–brachial index
    Doppler, ultrasonography
    Cavernosometry
    Cavernosography
    Arteriography

Penile tumescence studies
    Sleep laboratory studies
    Home studies
    Erotic stimulation studies

Imaging studies
    Conventional arteriography
    Cavernosography

Neurophysiologic studies

Psychological profile

[a]This table is a summary of the tests that may be used in establishing the cause of male sexual dysfunction. I advocate selecting those tests that are relevant to the individual patient depending on the history and physical examination.

Intracavernosal Injections

Both the investigation and the management of erectile dysfunction have been fundamentally altered by the introduction of injections of vasoactive agents into the corpora cavernosa of the penis (12,65). The three agents that have been used are papaverine, phentolamine, and prostaglandin E_1 (PGE_1). A number of variables determine the sensitivity and specificity of this type of testing. PGE_1 has been shown to be best in terms of erections achieved and the lowest rate of prolonged erection, the most significant complication (33,41,44,51). The dose chosen for initial testing should be low, with repeated injections at higher doses carried out depending on the response. Erectile responsiveness can be enhanced by self-stimulation, vibratory stimulation, visual erotic stimuli, or by applying a penoscrotal tourniquet (20,30,39,66). From a diagnostic point of view, if a poor response is obtained, the cause is likely to be vascular—either arterial insufficiency or venous leakage. If a good response is obtained from a low-dose injection, the cause is most likely to be psychogenic, neurologic, or endocrine (13,33,42); however, some patients with vasculogenic erectile dysfunction respond to low doses (41). Because both psychogenic and organic impotence respond well to intracorporeal injections, patients and their physicians may opt for this as long-term treatment without pursuing other investigations to define the cause of the erectile dysfunction more precisely.

Penile Vascular Studies

The penile brachial index (PBI) is a simple and useful test for vascular insufficiency (1,35). The penile blood pressure is recorded with a special cuff and a Doppler ultrasound velocity detector. The penile blood pressure is then compared with that in the arm to calculate the PBI. Normal values are ≥ 0.8. A PBI of <0.6 is highly suggestive of vascular insufficiency. Values between 0.6 and 0.8 are ambiguous.

Refinements in Doppler technology have led to the development of systems that can estimate blood flow through the penile arteries and ultrasonographically image the cavernosae (44). These techniques have largely replaced PBI testing. The new Doppler/ultrasonography methods are also being used to evaluate penile responses to intracavernous injections in attempts to define more accurately patients with arterial or venous dysfunction (44).

Cavernosometry, which is a technique specifically aimed at quantifying veno-occlusive dysfunction (44), involves infusing fluids into the corpora cavernosae, with venous outflow resistance being determined by the flow rate required to sustain an erection. An extension of this study is cavernosography, in which contrast is infused into the corpora with the draining veins being visualized radiographically (45,56).

Arteriography can be used to assess the major vessels of the legs and pelvic organs. A patient with vasculogenic impotence may have severe stenosis of the common iliac or internal or external iliac arteries. If this is not found, then more selective arteriography of the branches of the internal iliac artery, including the deep and dorsal penile arteries, may be performed (49).

These last three techniques—cavernosometry, cavernosography, and arteriography—are invasive methods that require experienced operators; they are used in highly selected patients.

Nocturnal Penile Tumescence Studies

The rationale behind tests of nocturnal penile tumescence (NPT) is that normal men have recurrent spontaneous erections several times per night during sleep (24,34,55). These occur during the rapid eye movement (REM) phase of sleep. NPT studies evaluate whether spontaneous erections occur and, by electroencephalographic recording, whether the normal phases of sleep have occurred. Erections can be evaluated either by direct observation or with monitors that record penile diameter or rigidity. There are three outcomes to such studies. If it can be established that in the presence of normal sleep patterns there were no erections, then it is likely that the erectile dysfunction is organic (but see below). If normal sleep patterns and spontaneous erections occurred, then the erectile dysfunction is most likely psychogenic. If the sleep patterns were abnormal, particularly lacking in REM phases, and no erections have occurred, then the latter problem may be secondary to a sleep disorder such as that caused by hypnotic medications, alcohol intake, or both.

One problem with sleep and NPT studies are that they are time-consuming and expensive. Patients may not sleep well in the artificial environment of a laboratory, so tests showing abnormal results may need to be repeated for confirmation.

An important criticism of NPT studies is that they have never been validated in patients shown to have psychogenic or organic impotence with criteria independent of the NPT measurements themselves (67). Indeed it has long been recognized that psychological factors can interfere with nocturnal erections. Further, full erections may not occur during sleep even in normal potent males with normal sleep patterns (54). In addition, earlier recording methods could document increases in penile diameter during sleep but not the quality (particularly rigidity) of the erection; penile diameter may increase without rigidity (52). This problem has been largely overcome by the use of devices that assess rigidity (discussed in the next section). Finally, there is the problem that erections occurring in the awake state are a better reflection of sexual functioning than is NPT (46). Methods for assessing awake erections are discussed later. For all of these reasons, NPT studies are of doubtful sensitivity and specificity.

An alternative to the sleep-laboratory approach is to have the patient apply snap gauges in his own home (21). These gauges have three preset snap-release fasteners that break open at different forces, depending on the increased diameter of the penis during erection. During a normal erection, all three fasteners should be released. Shortcomings include the fact that only one erection is required to break the snap gauge, and therefore the number of spontaneous erections cannot be established; this method also cannot assess the duration and rigidity of erections (52).

Penile Rigidity Studies

Traditional tumescence studies are based on increases in penile circumference. Because considerable expansion can occur without rigidity, a technique has been devised for continuous recording of both penile tumescence and rigidity; both the degree and duration of rigidity can therefore be established (11). The computerized device stores and redisplays the data. Such recordings can be made during sleep or with electroencephalographic recording in a sleep laboratory, or because the instrument is portable, in the patient's home. Some of the important drawbacks to classic NPT studies apply to home monitoring (40). There has also been a problem in establishing normative data and establishing criteria for the several patterns of apparently abnormal recordings (40).

Another method is that of erotic stimulation testing, the usual stimulus being videotapes (37,43,68,71). This may well be a useful, quick, and economical technique to distinguish organic from psychogenic erectile impotence (68).

Neurophysiologic Tests

A variety of tests have been devised, and are described in Chapter 23, that attempt to show whether a patient's sexual dysfunction is neurogenic in origin, particularly a disorder of the peripheral autonomic and somatic neuronal circuits.

Psychological Profile Testing

In an attempt to separate psychogenic from organic impotence, the Minnesota Multiphasic Personality Inventory (MMPI) has been used. One study concluded that this accurately discriminated between these two groups of patients (8), but a later study came to the opposite conclusion (58). The authors of the latter study conclude that the MMPI is only helpful in identifying patients with severe psychopathology, and in assessing the patient's reaction to having a penile implant. A further study evaluated the ability of the MMPI to discriminate between psychogenic and organic causes in impotent diabetic men; NPT, vascular, and endocrine studies were also done in these patients (31). The results showed that the MMPI resulted in a high degree of misclassification. These authors also pointed out that erectile impotence is often not strictly psychogenic or organic but a composite of both. Thus, the MMPI and other psychological profile testing should be used and interpreted with caution in the evaluation of male sexual dysfunction.

Another approach is to use standardized psychological questionnaires specifically designed for the evaluation of sexual dysfunction. However, it is felt that professionally conducted psychosocial interviews with patient and partner are the best way to assess the complexities of sexuality and relationships (2,62). For comprehensive reviews, see references 2 and 62.

CONCLUSIONS

The commonest abnormality of male sexual function is erectile failure. This is categorizable into psychogenic and organic causes, with the latter being further divided into endocrine, vascular, neurologic, or due to medications or toxins. An important caveat is that there are often important components of psychogenic and organic factors in any individual patient, so causality should not be viewed as strictly an "either–or" situation. In many patients, the cause is easily diagnosed by history and examination. When this is not the case, a selected group of blood tests plus the response to intracavernosal injection of a vasoactive substance are relatively simple ways of further elucidating the cause. If there is still doubt about the diagnosis, then further investigations should be judiciously selected from those available, depending on local resources. It is important to realize that no single test enables the physician to determine with absolute certainty the cause and degree of erectile dysfunction, and in particular to quantify the psychogenic and organic contributions to the dysfunction.

REFERENCES

1. Abelson D. Diagnostic value of the penile pulse and blood pressure: a Doppler study of impotence in diabetics. *J Urol* 1975;113:636–639.
2. Ackerman MD, Carey MP. Psychology's role in the assessment of erectile dysfunction: historical precedents, current knowledge, and methods. *J Consult Clin Psychol* 1995;63:862–876.
3. Anonymous. Drugs that cause sexual dysfunction. *Med Lett Drugs Ther* 1980;22:108–110.
4. Anonymous. NIH releases consensus statement on impotence. *Am Fam Physician* 1993;48:147–150.
5. Benet AE, Melman A. The epidemiology of erectile dysfunction. In: Melman A, ed. *The urologic clinics of North America: impotence.* Philadelphia: WB Saunders, 1995;22:699–709.
6. Benson GS. The clinical evaluation of the patient presenting with erectile dysfunction: what is reasonable? *Semin Urol* 1990;8:94–99.
7. Betts CD, et al. Erectile dysfunction in multiple sclerosis: associated neurological and neurophysiological deficits, and treatment of the condition. *Brain* 1994;117:1303–1310.
8. Beutler LE, et al. Psychological screening of impotent men. *J Urol* 1976;116:193–197.
9. Blumer D, Walker AE. Sexual behaviour in temporal lobe epilepsy. *Arch Neurol* 1967;16:7–43.
10. Bors E, Comarr E. Neurological disturbances of sexual function with special reference to 529 patients with spinal cord injury. *Urol Surv* 1960;10:191–222.
11. Bradley WE, et al. New method for continuous measurement of nocturnal penile tumescence and rigidity. *Urology* 1985;26:4–9.
12. Brindley GS. Cavernosal alpha-blockade: a new technique for investigating and treating erectile impotence. *Br J Psychiatry* 1973;143:332–337.
13. Buvat J, et al. Is intracavernous injection of papaverine a reliable screening test for vascular impotence? *J Urol* 1986;135:476–478.
14. Cohen JA, et al. Autonomic neuropathy in alcoholics is not related to hepatic injury. *Can J Neurol Sci* 1990;17:249.
15. Comarr AE, Vigue M. Sexual counselling among male and female patients with spinal cord and/or cauda equina injury. Part I. *Am J Phys Med* 1978;57:107–122.
16. Comarr AE, Vigue M. Sexual counselling among male and female patients with spinal cord and/or cauda equina injury. Part II. *Am J Phys Med* 1978;57:215–227.
17. Cornely CM, et al. Chronic advanced liver disease and impotence: cause and effect? *Hepatology* 1984;4:1227–1230.
18. Courtois FJ, et al. Clinical approach to erectile dysfunction in spinal cord injured men: a review of clinical and experimental data. *Paraplegia* 1995;33:628–635.
19. De Groat WC, Steers WD. Autonomic regulation of the urinary bladder and sexual organs. In: Loewy AD, Spyer KM, eds. *Central regulation of autonomic functions.* New York: Oxford University Press, 1990:310–333.
20. Donatucci CF, Lue TF. The combined intracavernous injection and stimulation test: diagnostic accuracy. *J Urol* 1992;148:61–62.
21. Ek A, et al. Nocturnal penile rigidity measured by the snap-gauge band. *J Urol* 1983;129:964–966.
22. Ewing DJ, et al. The natural history of diabetic autonomic neuropathy. *Q J Med* 1980;193:95–108.
23. Feldman HA, et al. Impotence and its medical and psychosocial correlates: results of the Massachusetts Male Aging Study. *J Urol* 1994;151:54–61.
24. Fischer C, et al. Evaluation of nocturnal penile tumescence in the differential diagnosis of sexual impotence. *Arch Gen Psychiatry* 1979;36:431–437.
25. Gitlin MJ. Psychotropic medications and their effects on sexual function: diagnosis, biology, and treatment approaches. *J Clin Psychiatry* 1995;55:406–413.
26. Haldeman S, et al. Assessment: neurological evaluation of male sexual dysfunction. *Neurology* 1995;45:2287–2292.
27. Hanson RW, Franklin MR. Sexual loss in relation to other functional losses for spinal cord injured males. *Arch Phys Med Rehabil* 1976;57:291–293.
28. Hierons R, Saunders M. Impotence in patients with temporal lobe lesions. *Lancet* 1966;2:761–764.
29. Horowitz JD, Goble AJ. Drugs and impaired male sexual function. *Drugs* 1979;18:206–217.
30. Janssen E, et al. Visual stimulation facilitates penile responses to vibration in men with and without erectile disorder. *J Consult Clin Psychol* 1994;62:1222–1228.
31. Jefferson TW, et al. An evaluation of the Minnesota multiphasic personality inventory as a discriminator of primary organic and primary psychogenic impotence in diabetic males. *Arch Sex Behav* 1989;18:117–126.
32. Jones DR, et al. Ejaculatory dysfunction after retroperitoneal lymphadenectomy. *Eur Urol* 1993;23:169–171.
33. Jüneman KP, Alken P. Pharmacotherapy of ED: a review. *Int J Impotence Res* 1989;1:71–76.
34. Karacan I, et al. Nocturnal erections, differential diagnosis of impotence, and diabetes. *Biol Psychiatry* 1977;12:373–380.
35. Kempczinski RF. Role of the vascular diagnostic laboratory in the evaluation of male impotence. *Am J Surg* 1979;138:278–282.
36. Kirkeby JH, et al. Erectile dysfunction in multiple sclerosis. *Neurology* 1988;38:1366–1371.
37. Kockott G, et al. Psychophysiological aspects of male sexual inadequacy: results of an experimental study. *Arch Sex Behav* 1980;9:477–493.
38. Lakin M. The evaluation and nonsurgical management of impotence. *Semin Nephrol* 1994;14:544–550.
39. Lanigan D, et al. A modified papaverine test and the use of venous constriction in erectile dysfunction. *Int J Impotence Res* 1993;5:119–122.
40. Levine LA, Lenting EL. Use of nocturnal penile tumescence and rigidity in the evaluation of male erectile dysfunction. In: Melman A, ed. *The urologic clinics of North America: impotence.* Philadelphia: WB Saunders, 1995;22:775–788.
41. Lipshultz LI. Injection therapy for erectile dysfunction [Editorial and Comment]. *N Engl J Med* 1996;334:913–914.
42. Lue T. Impotence: a patient's goal-directed approach to treatment. *World J Urol* 1990;8:67–74.
43. Melman A, et al. Evaluation of the first 70 patients in the Center for Male Sexual Dysfunction of Beth Israel Medical Center. *J Urol* 1984;131:53–55.
44. Meuleman EJ, Diemont WL. Investigation of erectile dysfunction: diagnostic testing for vascular factors in erectile dysfunction. In: Melman A, ed. *The urologic clinics of North America: impotence.* Philadelphia: WB Saunders, 1995;22:803–819.
45. Montague DK, ed. *Disorders of male sexual function.* Chicago: Year Book Medical, 1988.
46. Morales A, et al. Diurnal penile tumescence recording in the etiological diagnosis of erectile dysfunction. *J Urol* 1994;152:1111–1114.
47. Moss HB, Procci WR. Sexual dysfunction associated with oral antihypertensive medication: a critical survey of the literature. *Gen Hosp Psychiatry* 1982;4:121–129.
48. NIH Consensus Development Panel on Impotence. Impotence. *JAMA* 1993;270:83–90.

49. Padula G, Reiss H. Radiologic evaluation: arteriography and cavernosography. In: Montague DK, ed. *Disorders of male sexual function.* Chicago: Year Book Medical, 1988:60–74.
50. Phelps G, et al. Sexual experience and plasma testosterone in male veterans after spinal cord injury. *Arch Phys Med Rehabil* 1983; 64:47–52.
51. Porst H. Diagnostic use and side-effects of vaso-active drugs: a report on over 2100 patients with erectile failure. *Int J Impotence Res* 1990; 2:222(abst).
52. Rundell OH, et al. Nocturnal penile tumescence. In: Montague DK, ed. *Disorders of male sexual function.* Chicago: Year Book Medical, 1988:75–85.
53. Saunders M, Rawson M. Sexuality in male epileptics. *J Neurol Sci* 1970;10:577–583.
54. Schiavi RC. Luteinizing hormone and testosterone during nocturnal sleep: relation to nocturnal penile tumescent cycle. *Arch Sex Behav* 1977;6:97–104.
55. Schiavi RC, Fisher C. Assessment of diabetic impotence: measurement of nocturnal erections. *Clin Endocrinol Metab* 1982;11: 769–784.
56. Shabsigh R, et al. Venous leaks: anatomic and physiological observations. *J Urol* 1991;146:1260–1265.
57. Slot O, et al. Erectile and ejaculatory function of males with spinal cord injury. *Int Disabil Stud* 1989;11:75–77.
58. Staples RB, et al. A re-evaluation of MMPI discriminators of biogenic and psychogenic impotence. *J Consult Clin Psychol* 1980;48:543–545.
59. Szasz G, et al. Sexual dysfunctions in multiple sclerosis. *Ann NY Acad Sci* 1984;436:443–452.
60. Talbot HS. The sexual function in paraplegics. *J Urol* 1955;73:91–100.
61. Tan ETH, et al. Erectile impotence in chronic alcoholics. *Alcohol Clin Exp Res* 1984;8:297–301.
62. Tiefer L, Schuetz-Mueller D. Psychological issues in diagnosis and treatment of erectile disorders. *Urol Clin North Am* 1995;22:767–773.
63. Van Thiel DH. Ethanol: its adverse effects upon the hypothalamic–pituitary–gonadal axis. *J Lab Clin Med* 1983;101:21–33.
64. Veves A, et al. Aetiopathogenesis and management of impotence in diabetic males: four years experience from a combined clinic. *Diabetic Med* 1995;12:77–82.
65. Virag R. Intracavernous injection of papaverine for erectile failure. *Lancet* 1982;2:938.
66. Vruggink PA, et al. Enhanced pharmacological testing in patients with erectile dysfunction. *J Androl* 1995;16:163–168.
67. Wasserman MD, et al. Theoretical and technical problems in the measurement of nocturnal penile tumescence for the differential diagnosis of impotence. *Psychosom Med* 1980;42:575–585.
68. Wincze JP, et al. A comparison of nocturnal penile tumescence and penile response to erotic stimulation during waking states in comprehensively diagnosed groups of males experiencing erectile difficulties. *Arch Sex Behav* 1988;17:333–348.
69. Witt MA, Grantmyre JE. Ejaculatory failure. *World J Urol* 1993; 11:89–95.
70. Zonszein J. Diagnosis and management of endocrine disorders of erectile dysfunction. In: Melman A, ed. *The urologic clinics of North America: impotence.* Philadelphia: WB Saunders, 1995;22:789–802.
71. Zukerman M, et al. Nocturnal penile tumescence and penile responses in the waking state in diabetic and nondiabetic sexual dysfunctionals. *Arch Sex Behav* 1985;14:109–130.

CHAPTER 22

Electrophysiologic Evaluation of Sexual Dysfunction

Clare J. Fowler

1. Sexual dysfunction commonly occurs as a consequence of disease of the central or peripheral nervous system.
2. Because very little research into female sexual disorders has been carried out, investigative techniques that have been developed are mostly directed at evaluating male erectile dysfunction (MED).
3. The advent of intracorporeal pharmacotherapy altered both management and investigation of MED. A good response to an intracorporeal injection effectively excludes arterial insufficiency as a possible cause of erectile failure. The differential diagnosis then lies between neurogenic or psychogenic causes, and it is in these circumstances that various neurophysiologic investigations may be used to detect a possible underlying neurologic pathology.
4. Electrophysiologic measurement of the bulbocavernous (BC) reflex was extensively used in the past, but its poor sensitivity and specificity are now widely acknowledged.
5. Cortical evoked potentials can be recorded in response to electrical stimulation of the pudendal nerve, but they are rarely of greater value than a careful neurologic examination to detect spinal cord disease. There is little evidence that the pudendal evoked potential is superior to the tibial response in demonstrating the spinal cord disease that is causing MED.
6. Both the BC reflex and pudendal evoked potential are conveyed in large myelinated fibers and do not test the functionally important autonomic innervation.
7. MED in diabetics is probably multifactorial, and autonomic function tests in diabetics with impotence may fail to reveal an abnormality.
8. Estimations of cutaneous thermal thresholds may be useful to demonstrate a generalized small fiber neuropathy in men with diabetes and MED.
9. MED occurs as one of the early symptoms in multiple system atrophy (MSA), and sphincter electromyography (EMG) is indicated if MSA is suspected. Sphincter EMG can reveal changes of chronic reinnervation indicating that there has been loss of anterior horn cells in Onuf's nucleus: a neuropathologic feature of MSA.
10. Sympathetic skin responses can be recorded from the genital region, and these are often absent in diabetics with MED.
11. The exact nature of the neurophysiologic recordings made from the penis using either needle or surface electrodes—single-potential analysis of cavernosus electrical activity or so-called SPACE—when recorded on a fast time base, remains to be determined. However, these waveforms do appear to reflect the autonomic innervation of the genital region and therefore represent a significant advance in methods available to investigate MED.
12. In summary, no single test as yet distinguishes between psychogenic and neurogenic MED, but tests of penile autonomic innervation using either sympathetic skin responses or by recording *corpus cavernosum EMG* are most relevant.

C. J. Fowler: The National Hospital for Neurology and Neurosurgery, London WCIN 3BG, England.

INTRODUCTION

Sexual function requires complex neural connections between higher cortical centers and the genitalia, which are innervated by sacral somatic and autonomic nerves. Therefore, many different diseases of either the central nervous system or the peripheral nervous system can disrupt sexual function in men and women. These neurologic disorders include cortical lesions, multiple system atrophy (MSA) spinal cord disease, cauda equina lesions, sacral or pudendal nerve injury in the pelvis, and small fiber or autonomic neuropathy.

Primary hyposexuality and secondary impotence have been well described in patients with temporal lobe damage or seizure disorders (5,27,50), but whether they are due to temporal lobe disease or are the result of anticonvulsant therapy is the subject of controversy (53). Erectile failure may be one of the earliest symptoms in MSA (1). Spinal cord disease is highly likely to cause sexual dysfunction (6) in men or women. Cauda equina lesions cause loss of somatic and erotic sensitivity in the genital region in both men and women and erectile failure in men. Damage to the peripheral nerves in the pelvis at the time of surgery or from trauma can also cause erection disorders. There is a high prevalence of impotence in diabetic men, in whom the problem may be multifactorial (36) although autonomic neuropathy can be a significant factor (17).

Little attempt has been made to evaluate scientifically the sexual response of women, although there is no doubt that neurologic disorders do result in significant dysfunction. However, no known effective treatments exist, and although the problems are those of altered psychosexual involvement, passivity and pleasure, medical attention has not focused on these matters. Therefore, the most common symptom of sexual dysfunction requiring investigation is erectile dysfunction in men.

INTRACORPOREAL PHARMACOTHERAPY

The management and investigation of male erectile dysfunction (MED) was fundamentally altered by the introduction of an effective medical means of treating erectile failure, i.e., intracorporeal injection of vasoactive agents. Before this was available, the principal aim when investigating MED was to establish whether the problem was organic: if thought to be psychogenic, psychosexual counseling was recommended. The advent of intracorporeal injections meant that the reliance on psychotherapy diminished and a somewhat simplified management algorithm adopted: a good response to intracorporeal pharmacotherapy effectively excludes a vascular etiology for MED, and the problem can then be reasonably attributed to either a psychological or neurologic cause.

Having found an effective treatment, many patients and their physicians opt for this on a pragmatic basis and no attempt is made to differentiate between the two possible pathogeneses. It is in these circumstances, however, that neurophysiologic methods might be employed. There is little to be gained by neurophysiologic investigations in men with established neurologic disease, but a diagnosis may be pursued in a small number of cases because of the patient's own curiosity, medicolegal reasons, or possibly insurance purposes.

This chapter describes the various tests that have been used to investigate MED, with a brief description of the recording method for each test together with an evaluation of its use.

THE BULBOCAVERNOUS REFLEX

For many years, electrophysiologic measurement of the bulbocavernous (BC) reflex was considered to be valuable in the investigation of erectile failure. This reflex consists of contraction of BC muscles when the glans penis is lightly touched or squeezed. The BC reflex latency was measured electrophysiologically using needle electrodes in the muscle to record the response to electrical stimulus applied to the dorsal nerve of the penis (47). Subsequent studies showed that a reflex contraction of the urethra or anal sphincter, or the pelvic floor, can be recorded in response to electrical stimulation of the dorsal nerve (3,13,55,59). Thought at first to be a polysynaptic flexor response with two components, subsequent studies using a single fiber needle electrode demonstrated such low variability of the latency of the first component that the reflex is now thought to be oligosynaptic (57).

Recording Methods

Various recording methods have been used to record the BC reflex. The stimulus is applied either by ring electrodes to the shaft of the penis (13,52) or by using a hand-held bipolar stimulator (3,32,58). The intensity of stimulation needed is very variable: in some men the response may be obtained at low intensities whereas in others a stimulus intensity approaching uncomfortable strengths may be necessary. Most studies have used concentric needle electrodes to record from the BC (32,34,47) or sphincter muscle (3,4,13,59). Either the minimum latency of a number of consecutive responses is measured or the onset latency of an averaged series.

Value of the Bulbocavernous Reflex in the Investigation of Impotence

Damage to the cauda equina would be expected to produce abnormalities of this sacral segmental S2–S4 reflex. Following an acute cauda equina injury, the presence of a recordable BC reflex has been shown to have some prognostic value for assessing bladder and sexual function (14), but an abnormal response is not inevitable in a patient with a cauda equina lesion (3,4). However, such patients rarely present with impotence as an isolated complaint, and there is usually prominent somatic sensory loss also.

Early studies showed that the BC latency in some men with impotence considered due to peripheral neuropathy was prolonged in comparison to values obtained from control subjects (10,13). However, the response latency was normal in other patients who were also known to have neurogenic impotence. Further studies of the latency of the BC reflex in diabetics have all yielded much the same findings (9,16,20,28,40,43,49,52): the latency may be abnormally prolonged in those men with severe generalized peripheral neuropathy whereas the response can be within control range in other diabetic men with MED in whom the problem is not thought to be vascular insufficiency. Although refinements in the technique have been suggested (45,52), even these have not improved the diagnostic sensitivity of the test to a level where an abnormality can be demonstrated in all patients with established neurogenic impotence.

Not only may the BC reflex be normal in a proportion of patients with definite peripheral neuropathy and neurogenic impotence, but the response may be abnormally prolonged in men with neuropathy and good erection. A study of six men with hereditary motor and sensory neuropathy demonstrated extreme prolongation of the response in four, none of whom were troubled by sexual dysfunction (60).

Although measurement of the BC reflex has done much over the years to increase awareness of neurogenic causes of erectile failure, the test lacks the necessary specificity to be of diagnostic value in individual patients. This is because the neural pathways examined by the electrophysiologic reflex measurement are mainly those that subserve somatic innervation. The BC reflex is conveyed in large myelinated fibers with conduction velocities 10–15 times faster than those of the functionally important autonomic fibers. Although somatic sensation conveyed by the pudendal nerve is important in the complex responses involved in sexual arousal, it is the autonomic innervation that is important in producing and maintaining an erection (7). An abnormal BC reflex may provide evidence of a coexistent large fiber neuropathy, but it does not test the functionally important class of small nerve fibers or autonomic innervation.

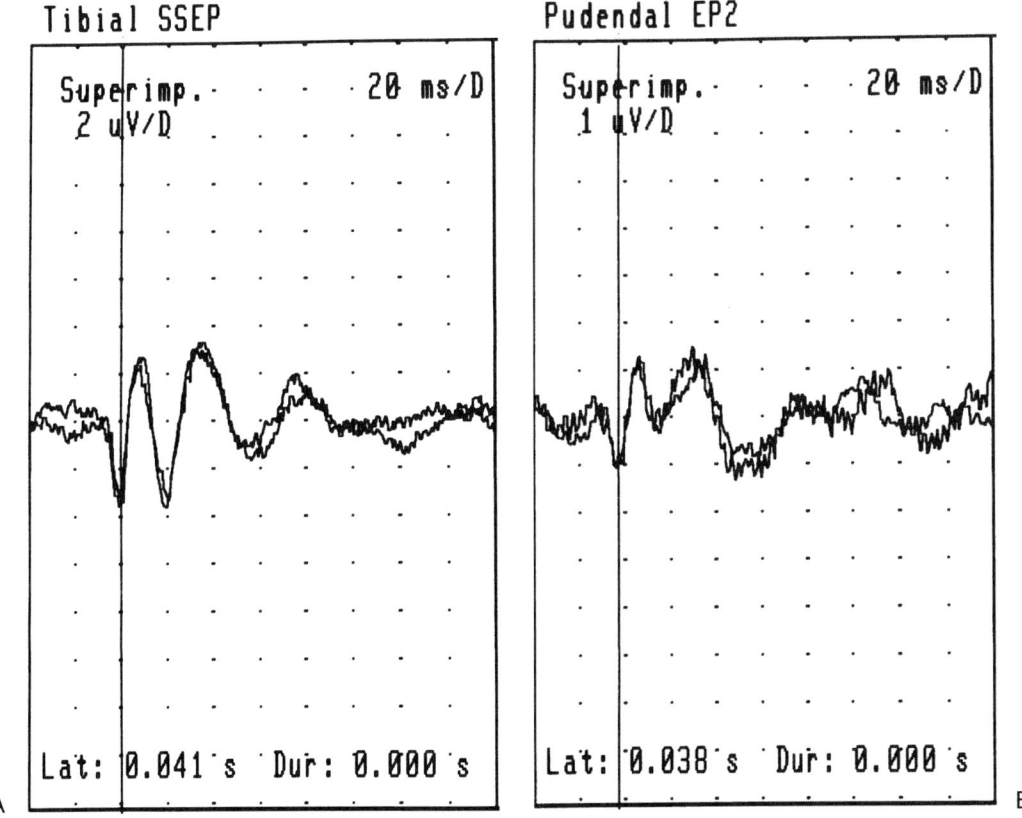

FIG. 1. A: Tibial evoked potential (×2 superimposed). Recordings were made at F_z-C_z 2 cm in response to stimulation of the right tibial nerve averaging 50 epochs. **B:** Pudendal evoked potential recorded from the same individual by using the recording site and conditions as for the tibial. Note the lower gain used for recording the tibial evoked potential.

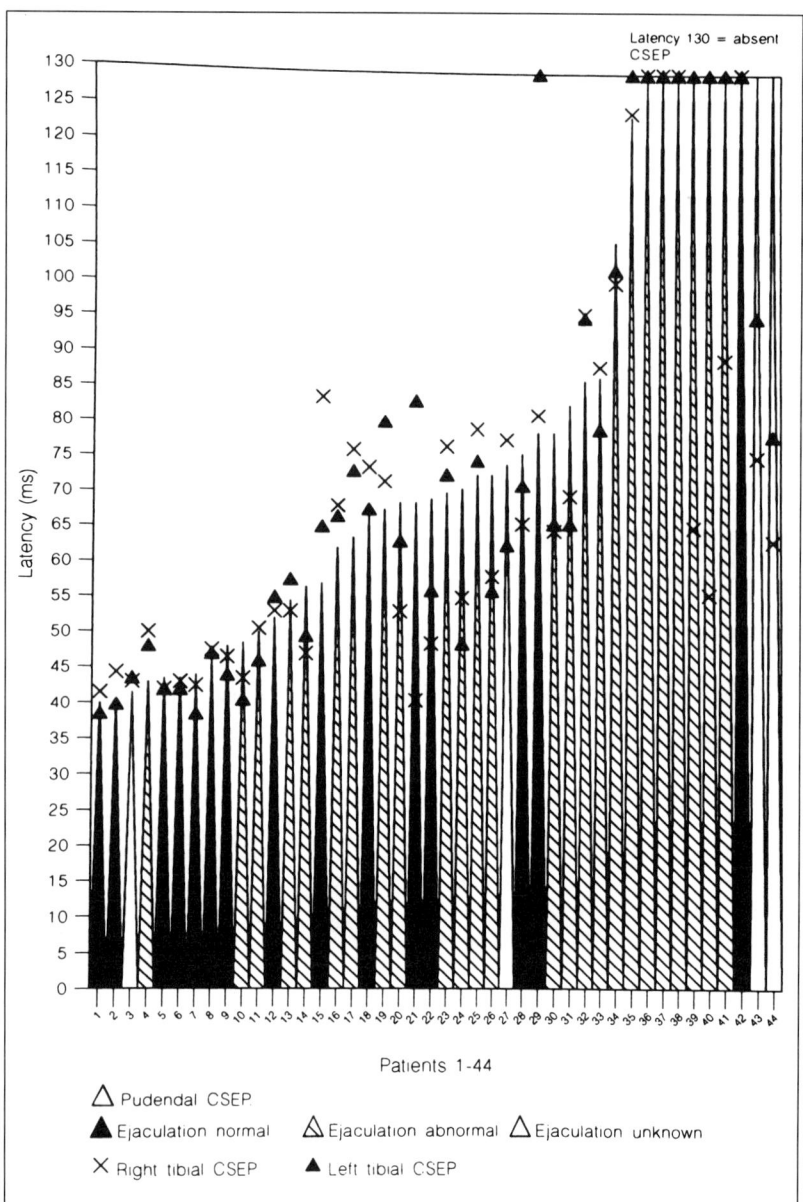

FIG. 2. The latencies of the pudendal and tibial cortical evoked potentials in 44 men with multiple sclerosis and erectile dysfunction. From Betts et al. (2), with permission.

PUDENDAL CORTICAL EVOKED POTENTIALS

Measurement of the cortical response evoked by electrical stimulation of the pudendal nerve was also much used in the investigation of MED. Introduced in the early 1980s (25), it was suggested at first that measurement of the BC reflex and pudendal evoked potential together provided a comprehensive examination of the innervation of the genital region and, for some while, many different research groups employed these electrophysiologic tests (16,23,26, 45,52). However, the limitations of the pudendal evoked potential in terms of which group of fibers they test are similar to those of the BC reflex, and a number of studies have now cast doubt over the value of this test in individual patients.

The pudendal evoked potentials are as easily obtained as the tibial responses and have a similar waveform and even similar latencies despite the much longer conduction distance over which the tibial response is conveyed (Fig. 1). This relative delay of the pudendal response is attributed to slower central conduction in the spinal cord (24). There have been several reports giving control values (16,19, 29,41,56) and a number of studies that have looked at the correlation between subject height and the latency of the P1 response (38,52).

Recording Methods

The methods of stimulation used for the BC reflex can be employed to stimulate for the pudendal evoked potential, but the stimulus intensity needed is lower so that a faster rate of stimulation, i.e., 1.5–4.7 Hz, can be used. The intensity should be $2\frac{1}{2}$ times that of threshold and should never be uncomfortable. If recordings are made from only a single channel, the active electrode should be placed 2 cm posterior to C_z and referred to F_z. Recording electrodes can be placed laterally to either side of the center, but the maximum response is recorded in the midline (25).

Value of the Pudendal Evoked Potential in the Investigation of Male Erectile Dysfunction

Sexual dysfunction as a complication of spinal cord injury is well recognized (6), but erectile failure may also occur as an early symptom of progressive spinal cord disease such as multiple sclerosis (MS). MED due to spinal cord disease is more likely to be confused with psychogenic MED because erections in response to tactile stimulation may still occur, as well as periods of nocturnal penile tumescence (22). The pudendal evoked potential can demonstrate abnormal spinal conduction and has been particularly used in studies of MED in MS. A study of 29 men with MS with MED showed that the pudendal evoked potential was delayed in 26 of them (31), and subsequent studies have confirmed that results of the test are usually abnormal in this group of men, although they may also be abnormal in men with MS who do not have MED (22).

Furthermore, a study that looked at the relative value of the pudendal cortical response and the tibial evoked potential found that the former provided no more information about responsible spinal cord involvement than did the latter (2) (Fig. 2).

A number of studies have now taken a critical look at the value of this measurement in the investigation of MED and have mostly concluded that it added little to the clinical examination in detecting spinal cord disease. In a study of 48 men with MS and MED, the majority had unequivocal bilateral pyramidal signs in their legs, and in only two patients were there no neurologic abnormalities in the lower limb (2). In a general study of the clinical application of the pudendal evoked potential used to investigate MED in 280 men, much the same conclusion was reached, i.e., the clinical examination was as good as the evoked potential in demonstrating neurologic disease (44). It was abnormal in only 7% of 106 men who had what was thought to be nonneurogenic erectile failure. Likewise, in a study that looked at the number of patients with a variety of urogenital complaints including MED, only one of 110 was found with an abnormal evoked pudendal potential and normal neurologic examination findings (8). In summary, therefore, the current view is that although the pudendal evoked potential may be useful if objective evidence of penile sensory dysfunction is required, it does not have a place in routine clinical assessment of MED.

SPHINCTER ELECTROMYOGRAPHY

The indications for performing sphincter electromyography (EMG) in the investigation of MED are limited. Sphincter EMG is of great value, however, in the investigation of MSA, and erectile impotence may be the earliest symptom of that condition (1). The anterior horn cells of the striated sphincter lie within Onuf's nucleus in the sacral spinal cord, and these cells appear to show selective atrophy in MSA resulting in denervation of the striated muscle of both sphincters. Using standard EMG techniques, changes of chronic reinnervation can be readily demonstrated in the motor units of the sphincter in MSA (30,48). Why MED occurs as a heralding symptom in MSA is not know: it may occur 7–8 years before the diagnosis is recognized and often precedes the development of urinary symptoms. The presence of this complaint in patients with MSA is not associated with postural hypotension or other features of autonomic failure.

Sphincter EMG is clearly not feasible as a routine investigation in those with MED alone, but it is worthwhile in men with additional complaints such as atypical parkinsonism, bladder symptoms, postural hypotension, or cerebellar ataxia. Establishing the diagnosis at an early stage may spare patients inappropriate urologic surgery and lead to the institution of effective medical management of incontinence.

AUTONOMIC FUNCTION TESTS IN MALE ERECTILE DYSFUNCTION

The most common cause of peripheral neuropathy with autonomic involvement is diabetes mellitus, and the high incidence of MED in this condition is well known (36). Several different factors are associated with the development of MED in diabetics, including increasing age, alcohol consumption, poor glycemic control, symptoms of intermittent claudication, and retinopathy, as well as symptoms of neuropathy (35). A study of autonomic function tests—heart rate changes with Valsalva maneuver, blood pressure response to sustained handgrip, and postural fall in blood pressure—in diabetic men with MED alone showed that these responses among the group were almost normal (18). A longitudinal study conducted in this same group 5 years later showed that six of 14 men still had MED as their only symptom and that the results of their autonomic function tests have remained normal, whereas the other eight had either developed other symptoms of autonomic neuropathy, died, or had abnormal autonomic function test results (17). From this, it was concluded that MED could occur in the absence of other evidence of autonomic neuropathy in some men, whereas MED appeared to be the earliest symptom of a progressive autonomic dysfunction in others. In a large study of diabetics with MED (39), single-breath beat-to-beat variation was found to be especially valuable in detecting abnormality, but no test of autonomic function was sufficiently sensitive to make it useful as a screening investigation in this context. The 30/15 heart rate variation response to standing was found to yield the highest incidence of abnormality among a battery of laboratory tests applied to a group of 30 men with a number of different underlying causes of MED (33).

OTHER TESTS IN SMALL FIBER NEUROPATHY

An alternative approach used to demonstrate a relevant generalized small fiber neuropathy had been to estimate cutaneous thermal thresholds. Sensation of warming is conveyed by unmyelinated afferents and cooling by small myelinated afferents—the same class of peripheral nerve fibers that comprise the autonomic nervous system. A generalized peripheral neuropathy that involves these fiber types is likely to impair the perception of thermal and pain sensation as well as produce symptoms of autonomic failure. Because the severity of neuropathy in diabetics appears to be length dependent, it has been recommended that perception of thermal sensation on the feet be tested in diabetic men with MED (20). Others have recommended testing thermal sensitivity in the genital region (46), although these nerve fibers are relatively shorter and testing sensation in the feet would theoretically maximize the possibility of demonstrating an abnormality.

SYMPATHETIC SKIN RESPONSES

Although there are limitations with the sympathetic skin response (SSR) recordings (see Chapter 17), this response is of value in assessing directly the autonomic innervation of the genital region. In a study that evaluated a battery of tests in the investigation of MED, SSR testing of the foot—the genital region was not tested—resulted in a high incidence of abnormality (33). Using the standard technique for recording the SSR, Ertekin et al. (15) demonstrated that this could be recorded in the perineum and found that it was present in all healthy control subjects (Fig. 3). In a study of diabetics with MED, the response was demonstrated to be unrecordable from the genital region, whereas it could still be recorded from the hand in a high proportion of men (12). Some, however, still had a genital SSR, so unfortunately the test can not be considered as sufficiently discriminating to be used as a reliable clinical test. In a study that evaluated the value of the SSR recorded from the limbs and genital region in 42 patients with urinary and/or sexual complaint, SSR abnormalities were demonstrated in those patients with polyneuropathy (42). More had SSR abnormality recorded from the lower limbs than from the genital region, but two patients had normal neurophysiologic investigations, i.e., BC reflex and pudendal evoked potentials, in whom the SSRs from the genital region were abnormal.

No difference was demonstrated between a patient group and controls in the SSR recorded from the genital region in

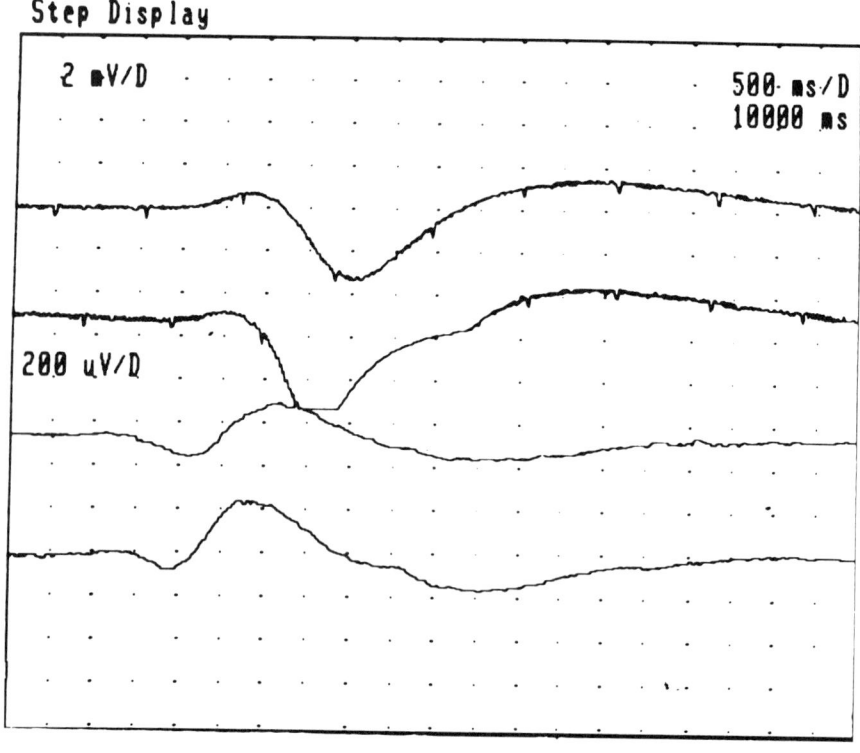

FIG. 3. Sympathetic skin responses recorded simultaneously from the foot (*top two traces*) and the genital region (*bottom two traces*) in response to stimulations of the left median nerve. Note the lower gain and longer latency for the response in the recordings from the foot.

men with chronic alcoholism and MED; it was concluded that the problem in this group was not the result of an autonomic peripheral neuropathy (11). In a study of 18 men (11) with premature ejaculation, genital and hand SSRs were found to be suppressed during pharmacotherapy-induced erection as a generalized bodily reaction. The same did not occur in control subjects, and the phenomenon was explained as indicating that specific and regional suppression of genital sympathetic activity could not be properly adjusted in patients with premature ejaculation.

CORPUS CAVERNOSUM ELECTROMYOGRAPHY

In 1989, a method was described for recording activity using a concentric needle electrode (61) inserted through the skin and tunica albuginea into the corpus cavernosum. Using a bandpass of 2–100 Hz, spike potentials in the flaccid penis were recorded. With visual sexual stimulation and the development of an erection, electrical activity decreased. When this method was used to investigate men who had neurogenic erectile MED caused either by pelvic operations or by trauma, differences were found between the patient and control studies (21). Similar activity can be recorded using either needle or surface recording electrodes, and it has been claimed that the activity is EMG generated by the corpus cavernosum (21,61). Using a faster time base, single-potential analysis of cavernosus electrical activity (SPACE) (51) has been has been described. Although there is little doubt that the activity that these authors are reporting is physiologic, some doubt must exist as to whether it is being generated by the smooth muscle of the penis (62). Smooth muscle EMG is notoriously difficult to record, and the similarity between the published pictures of the corpus cavernosum EMG recordings and the ongoing sympathetic activity that can be recorded from the hands and feet by surface electrodes and similar filter settings needs to be explained (62) (Fig. 4).

Reports of SPACE recordings in a large number of men with MED have now shown low amplitude and infrequent activity in patients with diabetics (37,54).

Although some controversy remains about the nature of these recordings, they certainly represent a significant advance both in terms of providing a direct measure of autonomic innervation of the genital region as well as in raising awareness of the inadequacies of former means of neurophysiologic testing in investigation of MED.

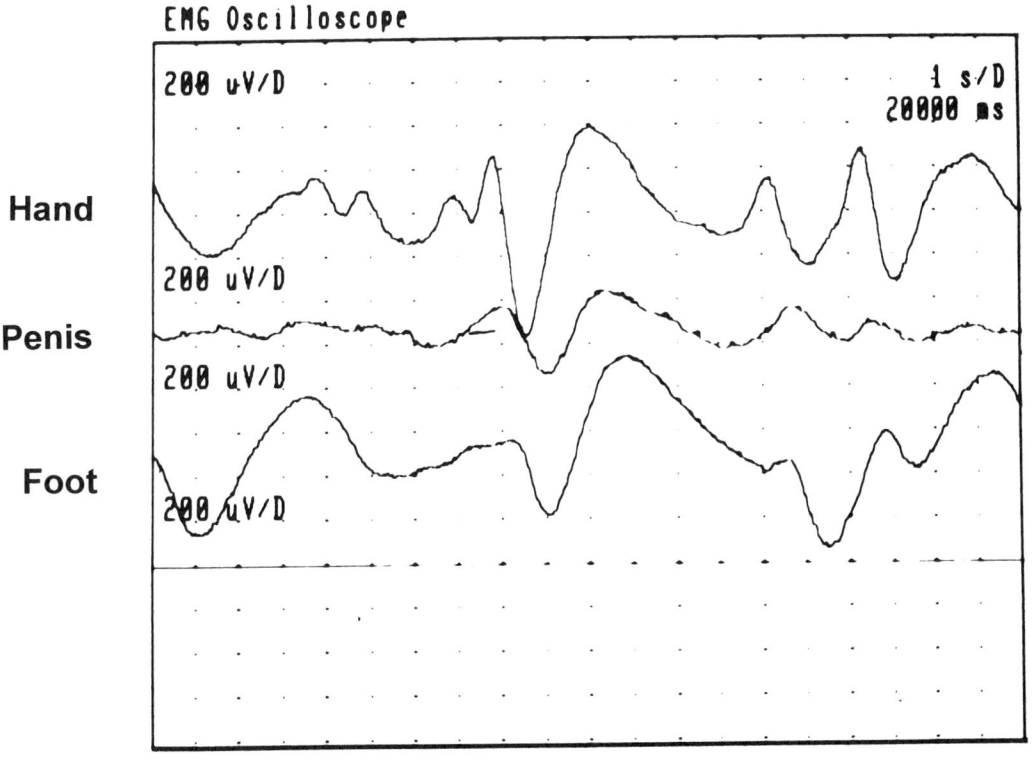

FIG. 4. Recording electrodermal skin responses simultaneously from hand **(top)**, penis **(middle)**, and foot **(bottom)** in response to an alerting noise.

CONCLUSION

With the introduction of various new forms of effective treatment for MED, the need to establish a definite organic basis or neurologic cause has diminished. Neurophysiologic investigations are therefore indicated only in quite special circumstances or as a research technique. It is now generally accepted that tests that examine somatic genital innervation such as the BC reflex and pudendal evoked potentials are of limited use, that tests that evaluate generalized autonomic involvement are poorly sensitive, and that specific tests of penile autonomic innervation by using either SSRs or recording corpus cavernosum EMG are more valuable.

REFERENCES

1. Beck RO, et al. Genitourinary dysfunction in multiple system atrophy: clinical features and treatment in 62 cases. *J Urol* 1994;151:1336–1341.
2. Betts CD, et al. Erectile dysfunction in multiple sclerosis: associated neurological and neurophysiological deficits and treatment of the condition. *Brain* 1994;117:1303–1310.
3. Bilkey WJ, et al. Clinical application of sacral reflex latency. *J Urol* 1983;129:1187–1189.
4. Blaivas JG, et al. The bulbocavernosus reflex in urology: a prospective study of 299 patients. *J Urol* 1981;126: 197–199.
5. Blumer D, Walker AE. Sexual behavior in temporal lobe epilepsy. *Arch Neurol* 1967;16:7–43.
6. Bors EH, Comarr AE. Neurological disturbances of sexual function with special references to 529 patients with spinal cord injury. *Urol Surv* 1960;10:191–222.
7. De Groat WC, Steers WD. Neuroanatomy and neurophysiology of penile erection. In: *Contemporary management of impotence and infertility*. Baltimore: Williams and Wilkins, 1988:3–27.
8. Delodovici ML, Fowler CJ. Clinical value of the pudendal somatosensory evoked potential. *Electroencephalogr Clin Neurophysiol* 1995;96:509–515.
9. Desai KM, et al. Neurophysiological investigation of diabetic impotence: are sacral response studies of value? *Br J Urol* 1988;61:68–73.
10. Dick HC, et al. Pudendal sexual reflexes: electrophysiologic investigations. *Urology* 1974;3:376–379.
11. Ertekin C, et al. Sympathetic skin potentials and bulbocavernosus reflex in patients with chronic alcoholism and impotence. *Eur Neurol* 1990;30:334–337.
12. Ertekin C, et al. Autonomic sympathetic nerve involvement in diabetic impotence. *Neurourol Urodyn* 1989;8:589–598.
13. Ertekin C, Reel F. Bulbocavernosus reflex in normal men and in patients with neurogenic bladder and/or impotence. *J Neurol Sci* 1976;28:1–15.
14. Ertekin C, et al. Bulbocavernosus reflex in patients with conus medullaris and cauda equina lesions. *J Neurol Sci* 1979;41:175–181.
15. Ertekin C, et al. Skin potentials (SP) recorded from the extremities and genital regions in normal and impotent subjects. *Acta Neurol Scand* 1987;76:28–36.
16. Ertekin C, et al. The value of somatosensory evoked potentials and bulbocavernosus reflex in patients with impotence. *Acta Neurol Scand* 1985;71:48–53.
17. Ewing DJ, et al. The natural history of diabetic autonomic neuropathy. *Q J Med* 1980;193:95–108.
18. Ewing DJ, et al. Vascular reflexes in diabetic autonomic neuropathy. *Lancet* 1973;2:1354–1356.
19. Fernandez-Gonzalez F, Suarez T. Pudendal nerve evoked potentials: neurophysiology and clinical applications. In: Morocutti C, Rizzo PA, eds. Amsterdam: Elsevier Science, 1985:97–106.
20. Fowler CJ, et al. The value of testing for unmyelinated fibre, sensory neuropathy in diabetic impotence. *Br J Urol* 1988;61:63–67.
21. Gerstenberg TC, et al. Standardized evaluation of erectile dysfunction in 95 consecutive patients. *J Urol* 1989;141:857–862.
22. Ghezzi A, et al. Erectile impotence in multiple sclerosis: a neurophysiological study. *J Neurol* 1995;242:123–126.
23. Goldstein I. Evoked-response evaluation. In: Barrett DM, Wein AJ, eds. *Controversies in neuro-urology.* New York: Churchill-Livingstone, 1984:117–129.
24. Guerit JM, Opsomer RJ. Bit-mapped imaging of somatosensory evoked potentials after stimulation of the posterior tibial nerves and dorsal nerve of the penis/clitoris. *Electroencephalogr Clin Neurophysiol* 1991;8:228–237.
25. Haldeman S, et al. Evoked responses from the pudendal nerve. *J Urol* 1982;128:974–980.
26. Herman CW, et al. Testing for neurogenic impotence: a challenge. *Urology* 1986;27:318–321.
27. Hierons R, Saunders M. Impotence in patients with temporal lobe lesions. *Lancet* 1966;2:761–764.
28. Kaneko S, Bradley WE. Penile electrodiagnosis: value of bulbocavernosus reflex latency versus nerve conduction velocity of the dorsal nerve of the penis in diagnosis of diabetic impotence. *J Urol* 1987;137:933–935.
29. Kaneko S, et al. Evoked central somatosensory potentials after penile stimulation in man. *Urology* 1983;21:58–59.
30. Kirby RS, et al. Urethro-vesical dysfunction in progressive autonomic failure with multiple system atrophy. *J Neurol Neurosurg Psychiatry* 1986;49:554–562.
31. Kirkeby HJ, et al. Erectile dysfunction in multiple sclerosis. *Neurology* 1988;38:1366–1371.
32. Krane RJ, Siroky MB. Studies on sacral-evoked potentials. *J Urol* 1980;124:872–876.
33. Kunesch E, et al. Neurological risk profile in organic erectile impotence. *J Neurol Neurosurg Psychiatry* 1992;55:275–281.
34. Lavoisier P, et al. Bulbocavernosus reflex: its validity as a diagnostic test of neurogenic impotence. *J Urol* 1989;141:311–314.
35. McCulloch DK, et al. The natural history of impotence in diabetic men. *Diabetologia* 1984;26:437–440.
36. McCulloch DK, et al. The prevalence of diabetic impotence. *Diabetologia* 1980;18:279–283.
37. Merckx LA, et al. Electromyography of cavernous smooth muscle during flaccidity: evaluation of technique and normal values. *Br J Urol* 1993;72:353–358.
38. Nikiforidis G, et al. Reduced variance of latencies in pudendal evoked potentials after normalization for body height. *Neurourol Urodyn* 1995;14:239–252.
39. Nisen HO, et al. Cardiovascular reflexes in the neurological evaluation of impotence. *Br J Urol* 1993;71:199–203.
40. Nogueira MC, et al. Neurophysiological investigations of two hundred men with erectile dysfunction: interest of bulbocavernosus reflex and pudendal evoked responses. *Eur Urol* 1990; 18:37–41.
41. Opsomer RJ, et al. Pudendal cortical somatosensory evoked potentials. *J Urol* 1986;135:1216–1218.
42. Opsomer RJ, et al. Sympathetic skin responses from the limbs and the genitalia: normative study and contribution to the evaluation of neurourological disorders. *Electroencephalogr Clin Neurophysiol* 1996;101:25–31.
43. Parys BT, et al. Bulbocavernosus reflex latency in the investigation of diabetic impotence. *Br J Urol* 1988;61:59–62.
44. Pickard RS, et al. The clinical application of dorsal penile nerve cerebral-evoked response recording in the investigation of impotence. *Br J Urol* 1994;74:231–235.
45. Porst H, et al. Neurophysiological investigations in potent and impotent men. *Br J Urol* 1988;61:445–450.
46. Robinson LQ, et al. Results of investigation of impotence in patients with overt or probable neuropathy. *Br J Urol* 1987;6:583–587.
47. Rushworth G. Diagnostic value of the electromyographic study of reflex activity in man. *Electroencephalogr Clin Neurophysiol* 1967;25:65–73.
48. Sakuta M, et al. Anal muscle electromyograms differ in amyotrophic lateral sclerosis and Shy–Drager syndrome. *Neurology* 1978;28:1289–1293.
49. Sarica Y, Karacan I. Bulbocavernosus reflex to somatic and visceral nerve stimulation in normal subjects and in diabetics with erectile impotence. *J Urol* 1987;138:55–58.

50. Saunders M, Rawson M. Sexuality in male epileptics. *J Neurol Sci* 1970;10:577–583.
51. Stief CG, et al. Single potential analysis of cavernous electrical activity in impotent patients: a possible diagnostic method for autonomic cavernous dysfunction and cavernous smooth muscle degeneration. *J Urol* 1991;146:771–776.
52. Tackmann W, et al. Bulbocavernosus reflex latencies and somatosensory evoked potentials after pudendal nerve stimulation in the diagnosis of impotence. *J Neurol* 1988;235:219–255.
53. Toone BK. Sexual disorders in epilepsy. In: *Recent advances in epilepsy.* Edinburgh: Churchill-Livingstone, 1985.
54. Truss MC, et al. Single potential analysis of cavernous electrical activity: four years' experience in more than 500 patients with erectile dysfunction. *Eur Urol* 1993;24:358–365.
55. Varma JS, et al. Electrophysiological observations on the human pudendo-anal reflex. *J Neurol Neurosurg Psychiatry* 1986;49:1411–1416.
56. Vodusek DB. Pudendal SEP and bulbocavernosus reflex in women. *Electroencephalogr Clin Neurophysiol* 1990;77:134–136.
57. Vodusek DB, Janko M. The bulbocavernosus reflex: a single motor neuron study. *Brain* 1990;113:813–820.
58. Vodusek EDB, et al. Direct and reflex responses in perineal muscles on electrical stimulation. *J Neurol Neurosurg Psychiatry* 1983;46:67–71.
59. Vodusek DB, et al. EMG single fibre EMG and sacral reflexes in assessment of sacral nervous system lesions. *J Neurol Neurosurg Psychiatry* 1982;45:1064–1066.
60. Vodusek DB, Zidar J. Pudendal nerve involvement in patients with hereditary motor and sensory neuropathy. *Acta Neurol Scand* 1987;76:457–460.
61. Wagner G, et al. Electrical activity of corpus cavernosum during flaccidity and erection of the human penis: a new diagnostic method? *J Urol* 1989;142:723–725.
62. Yarnitsky D, et al. Corpus cavernosum electromyogram: spontaneous and evoked electrical activities. *J Urol* 1995;153:653–654.

CHAPTER 23

Standardization of Autonomic Function

Phillip A. Low and Michael A. Pfeifer

1. Certain key aspects of autonomic function can be measured noninvasively with precision, accuracy, and reproducibility in clinical laboratories.
2. Autonomic failure is important to detect and quantitate because autonomic failure adversely affects function, is amenable to improvement, and may adversely affect morbidity and mortality.
3. Good clinical autonomic tests should be sensitive, specific, reproducible, physiologically and clinically relevant, noninvasive, relatively easy to perform and standardize, and affordable; the necessary technology should be available; and confounding variables should be well known.
4. Subjects should be adequately prepared for the test to minimize the effects of confounding variables.
5. A reasonable clinical screen might involve two cardiovascular heart rate (HR) tests (i.e., HR response to deep breathing and the Valsalva ratio), the quantitative sudomotor axon reflex test (QSART) distribution, and tests of adrenergic function (beat-to-beat blood pressure and HR responses to tilt and the Valsalva maneuver).
6. A reasonable clinical research screen might involve HR response to deep breathing, the Valsalva ratio, HR, and blood pressure recording supine and after 1 and 5 min upright or after upright tilt, QSART recordings, and dark-adapted pupil size after parasympathetic blockade. More rigorous patient preparation and baseline and final studies in duplicate are suggested.

INTRODUCTION

The noninvasive evaluation of autonomic function lends itself to detailed and repeated testing, a capability ideally suited to monitor the course of a neuropathy and its response to therapy. The proliferation of tests and laboratories has led to a large variety of test batteries comprising a large number of different tests. When the same tests are done, they are usually done under different conditions, rendering results difficult to compare. There are certain pitfalls (Chapter 30) and a lack of agreement in the optimal tests, the number of tests, the test conditions, and even the normative values. The ready acceptance of "bedside" testing has correctly emphasized the relative simplicity of the test procedure, without a corresponding acknowledgment, however, of the complexity of the test physiology and the many compounding variables. There is a great need for standardization, but adequate standardization is more demanding in tests of autonomic function than in other neurophysiologic tests because the variables include the condition of the subject, the ambient conditions, and the interaction with the tester in addition to the test procedure. This chapter focuses particular attention on standardization in the preparation of the subject, the test, and the interpretation (20,24,45). The following suggestions are based on the experience of the authors and a critical reading of the literature. As this is an evolving field, the recommendations should change with time. Obviously, the needs of a particular patient or clinical trial may mandate specific modifications.

JUSTIFICATION FOR TESTS OF AUTONOMIC FUNCTION IN THE PERIPHERAL NEUROPATHIES

The justification for tests of autonomic function is predicated on the assumption that we can measure aspects of autonomic function that are clinically and physiologically

---

P. A. Low: Department of Neurology, Mayo Clinic, Rochester, Minnesota 55905.

Michael A. Pfeifer: Department of Internal Medicine, Southern Illinois University, Springfield, Illinois 62794-9230.

relevant, with precision, accuracy, and reproducibility, without patient or investigator distress or exhaustion, using tests that are practicable in a clinical laboratory. The argument is enhanced if clinically relevant aspects of autonomic function are amenable to improvement. The criteria for tests of autonomic function are discussed below. Evidence suggests that the function of unmyelinated and small myelinated fibers may improve as the neuropathy improves (21,34). Fagius and colleagues (17,18) found a statistically significant improvement in the heart rate (HR) response to deep breathing (HR_{DB}) in aldose reductase inhibitor–treated patients and suggestive evidence of improvement in skin potentials in the foot. We found an improvement in cholinergic function following treatment of Lambert–Eaton myasthenic syndrome with 3,4-diaminopyridine (34). There is some suggestion that these fiber populations are at least as amenable as somatic fibers to improve (21). There is good clinical evidence that sympathetic fibers have a great propensity to regenerate (8).

Autonomic cardiovascular indices track well with cardiovascular exercise performance. The worse the cardiovascular autonomic neuropathy is, the more abnormal is cardiovascular performance and systemic peripheral resistance responses (40), so autonomic neuropathy may contribute to exercise intolerance. The fatigability of patients with multiple sclerosis has been in part ascribed to autonomic failure (37).

Another reason for undertaking autonomic evaluation relates to the poorer prognosis of patients who have autonomic failure (13,39,41). Ewing and colleagues (13) suggested that autonomic failure, detected in cardiovascular HR tests, associated with the presence of clinical signs of autonomic dysfunction, bears a very poor prognosis: 56% of 73 patients died in 5 years. Sampson and colleagues (41) reported a less ominous prognosis showing a mortality of 25% in 10 years among similar patients (but younger and without renal failure at the beginning of the study). In the same report, an isolated abnormality in cardiovascular HR tests was not associated with an increase in mortality. The lengthening of the QT interval in diabetic patients correlates with abnormal results in clinical autonomic tests and has been suggested to play a possible role in unexpected death (5,6,12). A related problem is the occurrence of painless myocardial infarction in these patients (Chapter 37).

Diabetics with impaired autonomic function may have an increase in blood pressure (BP) instability (requiring pharmacologic treatment) and an increase in intraoperative mortality (11,22). Denervation supersensitivity is present in ~25% of patients with diabetic neuropathy (31). The supersensitivity response may result in dangerously high BP responses to cough and cold medications containing phenylephrine or phenylpropanolamine or in response to local application or infiltration of vasoactive agents, i.e., injections of epinephrine and local anesthetic.

CRITERIA FOR SATISFACTORY TESTS OF AUTONOMIC FUNCTION

Based on experience with clinical trials and the use of tests in a clinical noninvasive laboratory setting, a set of criteria has emerged that candidate tests should able to fulfill:

1. *The test should be sensitive.* Tests such as HR_{DB}, Valsalva ratio, all indices of spectral and vector analyses of HR variation (20,46), thermoregulatory sweat test, and quantitative sudomotor axon reflex test (QSART) are tests of demonstrated sensitivity (25,26, 37) and will detect an abnormality in the great majority of subjects, so normal results provide reassurance that significant autonomic failure is absent. The sensitivity declines with age, though, and concern has been expressed that HR_{DB} and Valsalva ratio may lack sensitivity for patients beyond the age of 65 (10). The use of the maximal HR increment in response to the Valsalva maneuver has been recommended instead (10). Although the effect of age undoubtedly corrodes the sensitivity of autonomic function tests in the elderly, sufficient sensitivity exists for patients ≥60 years of age (Chapter 14). Tests of the venoarteriolar reflex, neurogenic flare response, and skin vasomotor reflexes are of low sensitivity (7,28,35) and thus would not be satisfactory.

2. *The test should be specific.* The test should be specific (low false-positive rate) for detecting autonomic failure. There is typically a trade-off between sensitivity and specificity [type I (α) and type II (β) errors] in the choice of control ranges. For instance, if we rejected all values that fall within the control values based on several hundred controls, then the specificity would be very high, but the sensitivity would likely be unacceptably low. If values that fall outside the 10th and 90th percentiles are taken as abnormal, the sensitivity would be enhanced but specificity reduced. A reasonable compromise is to use the 2.5–97.5 percentile values.

3. *The test should be reproducible.* Tests such as HR_{DB}, Valsalva ratio, and the QSART have coefficients of variation of <20%, whereas skin vasomotor reflexes and the neurogenic flare responses have considerably higher variability. In evaluating tests, it is important to compare a new test against an established test by using an adequate range of abnormalities. The evaluation of a new test might be biased positively by selecting only patients with advanced failure and comparing these against controls.

4. *The system tested should be physiologically and clinically relevant.* In evaluating a generalized neuropathy, such as diabetic autonomic neuropathy, the testing of HR_{DB} has been a particularly valid because of the early and prominent involvement of cardiovagal function. On the other hand, in the evaluation of a length-dependent toxic neuropathy, or a distal small fiber neuropathy (43), the most sensitive test is one, such as the

QSART, that will detect acral deficits. In patients with Adie's pupil, testing of HR_{DB}, although very sensitive, would be the wrong because the wrong system would be tested, whereas the pupillary response to dilute pilocarpine is the correct test even though it is less well validated.

5. *The test should be noninvasive.* Tests that involve the use of needles, such as microneurography or intraarterial or intravenous access, or the infusion of vasoactive agents are considered invasive.
6. *The test should be relatively easy and not excessively time consuming.* Most published tests meet this requirement. Some more recent tests, such as power spectral analysis, require longer periods of data acquisition because the patients need to remain stationary. If only cardiovagal function needs to be evaluated, recording requires only 5–10 min with patients resting supine. Tests of the effect of tilt-up on the electroencephalogram and transcranial Doppler or on superior mesenteric flow are more time consuming and require much postacquisition data reduction and complicated analysis. These tests are therefore of more limited routine utility. The time taken to perform the test should not be excessive. Based on the suggested algorithm, a full evaluation can be achieved in $\sim$1 hr.
7. *The test should be relatively easy to standardize.* Most tests that are easy to do are also easy to standardize, at least superficially. Because these noninvasive tests evaluate effector function, the well-standardized stimulus may be several steps removed from the true stimulus (see also Chapter 30).
8. *The necessary technology should be readily available.* The ready availability of the test instruments is critically important. The long-standing availability of the electrocardiogram (ECG) has ensured the popularity of cardiovascular HR tests. The limited availability to date of the QSART and data acquisition units for photoplethysmographic BP recording (Finapres) has limited their wider use.
9. *Equipment should be affordable.*
10. *Confounding variables should be well known.* Many variables affect tests of autonomic function. We have selected HR_{DB}, VR, and the QSART because the confounding variables for these tests are well known. The influence of these variables can be handled by adequate patient preparation, whereas variables such as age can be matched by an adequate selection of controls.

HOW MANY TESTS?

The number of tests recommended depends on the particular aspects of the autonomic nervous system that require testing. It is customary to evaluate parasympathetic and sympathetic functions separately. Most tests of parasympathetic function are sensitive and reproducible, whereas sympathetic adrenergic failure has been most difficult to quantitate reproducibly. Statistically, it would be preferable to rely on a single test, or a single test in each category, rather than on a battery of tests. For parasympathetic evaluation, HR_{DB} has been suggested to be the best and thus the recommended single test (38). Although there is general agreement with this, others suggest that no single test is sufficiently reliable and recommend instead a battery of five tests to evaluate parasympathetic and sympathetic functions (16). The simple addition of more tests of a single system, e.g., tests of cardiovagal function, is a procedure that has rapidly diminishing returns, generates more confusion when less well-validated tests are added, and leads to patient and clinician exhaustion. A reasonable compromise, incorporated into the recently approved CPT codes for cardiovagal function, is to undertake at least two tests of cardiovagal function.

Another shortcoming in many of the batteries proposed in the literature is the clustering of tests of a single system and autonomic level. For instance, the majority of the proposed batteries lack a test of distal autonomic function. Neuropathic patients have distal motor, sensory, and autonomic symptoms (Chapter 36), so it would be prudent to measure distal sympathetic function in addition to somatic function. The cardiovagal tests require that subjects be in sinus rhythm, so parasympathetic function cannot be evaluated in patients with cardiac arrhythmias, no matter how many cardiovagal tests are run.

For a clinical laboratory, the following suggestions are a reasonable compromise. The most reliable single test of parasympathetic function is HR_{DB} (20). A second test, the VR or the 30:15 ratio, should be added because there are certain pitfalls in the use of respiratory sinus arrhythmia as a test of cardiovagal function (Chapter 30). For clinical testing at the Mayo Autonomic Reflex Laboratory, we use a tilt table, so the 30:15 ratio is less reliable (9). We also routinely determine the Valsalva maneuver by BP_{BB} recordings, so, for us, the Valsalva maneuver is more relevant. If photoplethysmographic BP_{BB} is evaluated, the BP information enhances the validity of the Valsalva ratio, and a quantitative analysis of individual phases of the Valsalva maneuver can be used to provide a sensitive index of adrenergic function (42). The 30:15 ratio is, physiologically, a more complicated test (9) that depends significantly on muscle contraction (which is not controlled) and requires more subject cooperation, and the confounding variables are less well evaluated. It probably has a greater coefficient of variation and thus is less desirable than the other two tests.

SELECTION OF INDIVIDUAL TESTS OF AUTONOMIC FUNCTION

There are numerous tests of autonomic function. Some that are potentially useful as routine clinical tests or have

TABLE 1. *Evaluation of qualities of some tests of autonomic function*

Test	1	2	3	4	5	6	7	References	Comments
RR variation	Yes	Yes	4	Yes	3	4	Yes	20	Single best cardiovagal test
Valsalva ratio	Yes	Yes	3	Yes	3	4	Yes	13	Next best cardiovagal test
30 : 15 ratio	Yes	Yes	3	Yes	3	4	Yes	14	Less well validated than above two
Pupil cycle time	Yes	Yes	3	?Yes	3	3	Yes	33	Needs better validation
Pancreatic polypeptide	Yes	Yes	NA	NA	3,4	2	Yes	23	Infusion of insulin; limited information
CMG with i.v. bethanechol	Yes	No	2	Yes	?	1	No	**Chapter 46**	—
NPT	Yes	Yes	3	Yes	3	2	Yes	**Chapter 21**	Needs sleep-lab facilities
Heart rate spectral analysis	Yes	Yes	3	Yes	?	1	?Yes	**Chapter 26**	Limited experience; cumbersome
QSART	Yes	Yes	3	Yes	3	3	Yes	25,29	Needs specialized equipment
Postural blood pressure	Yes	Yes	2	Yes	2	4	Yes	**Chapter 15**	—
D-A pupil size	Yes	Yes	4	Yes	4	2	Yes	37	PNS blockade needed; rubeosis affects
Handgrip	Yes	Yes	2	Yes	2	2	?Yes	15	Not well validated; uncomfortable
Norepinephrine	Yes	Yes	2	Yes	2	3	Yes	**Chapter 15**	Standing more sensitive than supine; insensitive
TST	Yes	Semi	3	Yes	?	2	Yes	**Chapter 19**	Cumbersome; messy; subject heated up
Skin sympathetic response	Yes	Semi	2	Yes	2	3	?	**Chapter 17**	Limited recording sites; habituation
Sweat imprint	Yes	Yes	2,3	Yes	3	2	Yes	**Chapter 15**	Needs special equipment
Skin VM reflexes	Yes	Semi	2	Yes	2	3	?	28	Marked variability; not recommended
Venoarteriolar reflex	Yes	Yes	2	?	2	3	?	35	Marked variabilty; not recommended
QT interval	Yes	Yes	2	Yes	4	4	Yes	6,12	Affected by ischemia
Spectral analysis	No	Yes	3	Yes	3	3	Yes	46	Needs standardization
Squat test	Yes	Yes	2,3	?Yes	?Yes	2	?	32	—

1 = standardized; 2 = quantitative; 3 = sensitivity; 4 = specificity; 5 = reproducibility; 6 = ease of use; 7 = suitability for longitudinal studies.

CMG, congenital myasthenia gravis; D-A, Dark adapted; NPT, nocturnal penile tumescence; PASP, pulmonary artery systolic pressure; PNS, parasympathetic nervous system; QSART, quantitative sudomotor axon reflex test; TST, thermoregulatory sweat test; VM, Valsalva maneuver.

been suggested as being suitable for clinical trials are listed below and evaluated in Table 1. The list is incomplete. Chapter 15 describes these and other tests in detail.

Tests of parasympathetic function
1. RR variation (HR_{DB})
2. Valsalva ratio
3. HR response to standing
4. HR response to coughing
5. Spectral analysis of the respiratory component of the RR interval
6. HR response to squatting
7. Pupil cycle time
8. Pancreatic polypeptide
9. Cystometrogram with intravenous bethanechol
10. Nocturnal penile tumescence

Tests of sympathetic function
1. QSART
2. BP supine and standing
3. Beat-to-beat BP to the VM
4. Dark-adapted pupil size after parasympathetic blockade
5. Sustained handgrip
6. Plasma norepinephrine
7. Thermoregulatory sweat test
8. Sympathetic skin responses
9. Sweat imprint
10. Skin vasomotor reflexes
11. Venoarteriolar reflex
12. Squatting test
13. Spectral analysis of BP response to tilt-up (Chapter 26)

RECOMMENDATIONS FOR TESTS OF AUTONOMIC FUNCTION

The consensus statement of the San Antonio Conference on Diabetic Neuropathy (2) addressed the issue of tests of autonomic function as part of its overall discussion on diabetic neuropathy. Its comments on noninvasive tests of autonomic function read in part as follows:

These are suitable for routine screening for autonomic dysfunction or for monitoring the progress of autonomic neuropathy. When performed in a carefully controlled manner, the following tests have been validated and shown to be reliable and reproducible, to correlate with each other and with tests of peripheral somatic nerve function, and to have prognostic value:

1. Tests of HR control (mainly parasympathetic). Heart rate response to
   a. Valsalva maneuver
   b. Deep breathing
   c. Standing
2. Tests of blood pressure control (mainly sympathetic). Blood pressure response to
   a. Standing or tilting
   b. Sustained handgrip
3. Tests of sudomotor control, i.e.:
   a. Temperature-induced sweating
   b. Chemically-induced sweating (i.e., acetylcholine or pilocarpine)

The panel recommends that

1. Symptoms possibly reflecting autonomic neuropathy should not, by themselves, be considered markers for its presence.
2. Noninvasive validated measures of autonomic neural reflexes should be used as specific markers of autonomic neuropathy if end-organ failure is carefully ruled out and other important factors, such as concomitant illness, drug use, and age, are taken into account. An abnormality of more than one test on more than one occasion is desirable to establish the presence of autonomic dysfunction.
3. Independent tests of both parasympathetic and sympathetic function should be performed.
4. A battery of quantitative measures of autonomic reflexes should be used to monitor improvement or deterioration of autonomic nerve function, although their utility for monitoring patients over time has not been clearly established.

These recommendations provide an important perspective of autonomic testing *vis-à-vis* other tests of diabetic neuropathy and provide broad guidelines. They lack specificity for individual autonomic laboratories, however, and do not critically evaluate available tests of autonomic function. The following specific recommendations are provided in an attempt to meet the needs of individual clinical laboratories and investigators.

The 1988 consensus panel focused on the use of autonomic tests in clinical trials and did not address the choice of autonomic tests in the clinical autonomic laboratory (2).

Recently, the Therapeutics and Technology Committee of the American Academy of Neurology (3) has published a position paper on the evaluation of autonomic function. In its executive summary, it considered that autonomic function tests are *safe,* defined as acceptability of risk for a given evaluation, by a provider with specified training, at a specified type of facility. The committee has a long history of neurologic test evaluation. A test is graded as *established* when it is accepted as appropriate for the given indication in the specified patient population. The grade *investigational* is used when there is insufficient evidence to determine appropriateness, but further study is considered warranted. The use of the technology should largely be confined to research protocols. The grades in decreasing order are established, promising, investigational, doubtful, and unacceptable. The values of specific tests are summarized below and in Table 2.

Specific Validated Tests

Cardiovascular heart rate tests are *established.* The strong positive recommendation is based on class I and II evidence. The HR_{DB} and the Valsalva ratio are especially well validated.

Sudomotor tests are *established* for the QSART, sweat imprint, skin potential recordings, and the thermoregulatory sweat test. The strong positive recommendation is based on well-designed clinical studies in the case of the QSART and on extensive experience with the thermoregulatory sweat test (class I and II evidence). The sympathetic skin response is established by extensive experience but may, in the future, be superseded.

Adrenergic tests are *established* for standard tilt testing, prolonged tilt testing, and beat-to-beat BP analysis of the VM based on class I and II evidence. They are investigational for BP response to sustained handgrip.

TABLE 2. *Evaluation summary of autonomic function tests*

Test	Application	Rating	Quality of evidence ratings (class)	Strength of evidence ratings
Cardiovagal heart rate	Diagnosing and monitoring the course of autonomic neuropathy	Established	I, II	B
Adrenergic	Diagnosing and monitoring the course of autonomic neuropathy	Established	I, II	B
Sudomotor	Diagnosing autonomic neuropathy	Established	I, II	B
Skin vasomotor	—	Investigational	III	D
Neurogenic flare	—	Investigational	III	D

Less Well-Validated Tests

Certain other tests that appear to have limited sensitivity and specificity include those of skin vasomotor reflexes and of venoarteriolar reflex, and the related (though not strictly autonomic) neurogenic flare test.

SUGGESTED TESTS FOR A CLINICAL AUTONOMIC REFLEX SCREEN

1. HR_{DB}
2. Valsalva ratio
3. BP_{BB} recording of Valsalva maneuver
4. BP_{BB} and HR during at least 5 min of tilt
5. QSART recordings from four standard sites

These comprise the routine battery employed in the Mayo Autonomic Reflex Laboratory. The entire battery can be completed in an adequately prepared subject in ~1 hr by two technicians. The battery has been selected to provide a noninvasive evaluation of cardiovagal function (HR_{DB} and Valsalva ratio), postganglionic sudomotor function (distribution of the QSART value), and adrenergic function (beat-to-beat BP and HR responses to tilt and Valsalva maneuver) and are described in greater detail in Chapter 15. Among the various tests of cardiovagal function, the most reliable are HR_{DB}, Valsalva ratio, and HR response to standing up. There are a number of methods of evaluating HR variation. The recommendation is that at least two tests of cardiovagal function should be used. Power spectral analysis of the respiratory component of HR variation is a sensitive and reproducible method (46) that is useful in specific laboratories. There is a great need for standardization of spectral analysis algorithms. The details of testing are very important. All of the autonomic tests described evaluate effector function. The major controllable variables are the stimulus, the procedure, the subject, and the analysis.

Patient Preparation

Patients should be adequately prepared. Preparation of patients for the clinical laboratory and preparation for clinical trials differ in some details. For routine study, we adopt a practical rather than optimal preparation. Patients are not permitted food, coffee, or nicotine for 3 hrs before the study. Anticholinergics (including antidepressants, antihistamines, and over-the-counter cough and cold medications), 9-α-fludrocortisone (Florinef), diuretics, and sympathomimetic (α- and β-agonists) and parasympathomimetic agents are forbidden for 48 hrs. α-Antagonists and β-antagonists are discontinued for 24 hrs at the discretion of the referring physician. Patients should not wear compressive clothing, including Jobst stockings or corsets, on the morning of the test. They must avoid the use of alcohol for 12–14 hr prior to testing. Diabetics should have no evidence of hypoglycemia or have needed treatment for hypoglycemia within the preceding 12 hrs. Patients who are obviously distraught or in pain should not be tested.

Sequence of Tests

We recommend the following sequence of tests:

1. QSART
2. HR and Finapres response to deep breathing
3. HR and Finapres response to Valsalva maneuver
4. HR and Finapres response to tilt

The QSART is described in greater detail in Chapter 15. A skin thermistor probe is attached to the dorsum of left foot at midfoot level. The foot is warmed and maintained at 31°C with an infrared lamp. Four sites on the left are used and are studied with patients supine. All recordings can be done simultaneously. If only two sudorometers are available, the proximal lateral foot sites can be recorded with subjects lying on their right, and the forearm and distal medial leg can be recorded with subjects lying on their left. This positioning ensures horizontal capsule placement.

ECG electrode placement should be such that movement artifact is minimized. One approach is to attach ECG electrodes at the left and right interscapular sites just medial to the scapular tips, with a ground electrode at the left midaxillary region. This positioning of active electrodes, in contact with the tilt table, prevents electrode movement and reduces artifacts. All HR studies are done with subjects supine. Deep breathing is done with each subject lying on a single pillow. Subjects are trained to alternately inspire and expire deeply with 5 sec each for the inspiratory and expiratory cycles, which should be smooth and forceful without an intervening pause; the maneuvers should not be an inspiratory gasp, followed by a pause and then an expiratory grunt. A total of 8–25 continuous cycles is an adequate sample. Eight cycles are chosen to provide an adequate sample for determinations of HR range. The test should ideally be repeated after a 5-min rest. A total of 25 cycles is used when mean circular resultant is to be determines.

The duration of preceding rest affects the results of BP and HR responses to tilt (44), presumably by the redistribution of intravascular fluid. Such a redistribution could presumably affect the Valsalva maneuver as well. We therefore recommend that the Valsalva maneuver be done third, when ~30 min will have elapsed. The Valsalva maneuver is performed, with patients *supine*, at an expiratory pressure of 40 mmHg for 15–20 sec. The test should be repeated until two reproducible recordings are obtained. In practical terms, this means 2–4 recordings. Reproducible recordings are usually obtained after the second or third recording, and patient distress begins after about the fourth maneuver. The servomechanism on the Finapres device is turned off for the maneuver. Chapter 15 provides details on the analysis of the BP_{BB} evaluation. BP and HR responses to tilt are recorded for 5 min with patients supine. Two sphygmomanometric recordings of BP are also taken. Patients are tilted to 80°. BP and HR are continuously recorded for 5 min, and also recorded with the cuff at 1 and 5 min, followed by a return of patients to the supine position.

Patients with suspected syncopal disorders need more prolonged tilt. In many studies, the number of subjects who experienced syncope during upright tilt was increased by intravenous isoproterenol (4) or by prolonged tilt (up to 60 min) (19). This area of autonomic testing is more specialized and carries a small risk of cardiac arrhythmia. For a more detailed description, see Chapters 15 and 48.

The thermoregulatory sweat test is very important in several clinical situations. We suggest the following indications:

1. When multifocal autonomic failure is suspected as in certain autonomic neuropathies, such as leprosy (Chapter 19).
2. In combination with the QSART, to define the site (preganglionic versus postganglionic) of the lesion (25).
3. To detect the severity and distribution of sudomotor failure in chronic idiopathic anhidrosis (27).
4. To detect certain characteristic patterns of sudomotor failure that aid neurologic evaluation (Chapter 20). For instance, the completeness of sympathectomy and the dermatologic pattern of anhidrosis can be helpful in neurologic diagnosis. The distal pattern of anhidrosis in distal small fiber neuropathy is seen in 72% of patients.
5. In the differential diagnosis of certain neurologic disorders. For instance, Parkinson's disease is usually associated with <40% anhidrosis, whereas multiple-system atrophy and pure autonomic failure are associated with usually >70% anhidrosis (42).
6. To monitor the course of a neuropathy and, possibly, the response of a dysautonomia to treatment.

INTERPRETATION OF TESTS OF AUTONOMIC FUNCTION

Detailed interpretation of tests is covered in Chapter 15. HR_{DB} is interpretable by several different methods (Table 3). The most widely used are the HR range (RR interval), the expiration–inspiration (E/I) ratio, and the mean circular resultant. The number of respiratory cycles studied will vary from 8 to 25, depending on the paradigm followed. The HR range is simply the peak HR minus the trough HR. At Mayo, we routinely obtain 8 inspiration–expiration cycles at 10 sec/cycle. Subjects are instructed to follow an oscillating bar for 10 sec. The five largest consecutive responses are read from the computer by using a cursor, averaged, and the HR range (maximal − minimal) derived. To avoid an excessive biasing of results by the initial response, we include the first response, providing it is not more than twice the range of subsequent responses. If a cycle is marred by artifact, the next cycle is accepted. Recordings that are uneven or marred by artifacts should be repeated. This method is affected by drifting HR but is relatively insensitive to mean HR or tachycardia. Another approach, with the mean circular resultant paradigm, is to use the middle 5 min of a 6-min recording (1).

The E/I ratio ($RR_{max.}/RR_{min.}$) is affected by drifting HR and greatly affected by resting tachycardia, with tachycardia suppressing the E/I ratio. The HR range is therefore better if the patient has resting tachycardia than is E/I ratio.

The mean circular resultant provides a direct measure of the synchronization between HR variation and respiration. This algorithm has the advantage of being virtually unaffected by shifting mean HR, ectopic beats, or resting tachycardia. It does require the use of a specific algorithm, a prolonged period of recording since the value is highly cyclic, and is significantly affected by asynchrony of respiration resulting in lower values.

Power spectral analysis is covered in detail in Chapters 25 and 26. Spectral power likely has all of the qualities for a test of autonomic function. We recommend it cautiously because the current methodology is insufficiently standardized. In particular, measurement of respiration is essential (Chapter 26) and not routinely used in clinical laboratories. After agreement on duration of recording, respiration, details of the conditions of recording, algorithm for bad point removal, filter settings, and methods of analysis, the method will likely be acceptable and could become a first-line technique to evaluate cardiovagal function.

The Valsalva ratio should be read as the peak HR following the onset of the maneuver divided by the minimal HR within 30 sec of the peak HR. QSART responses are described in Chapter 15.

TABLE 3. *Methods of evaluating heart rate (HR) response to deep breathing*

Parameter	$HR_{max.-min.}$	EI ratio	MCR
Artifact	Marked	Marked	Nil
Shifting HR	Marked	Marked	Minimal
Mean HR	Nil	Marked	Mild
Regularity of respiration	Negligible	Marked	Marked
Time to stable value	30 sec	30 sec	3 min

EI, expiratory–inspiratory; MCR, mean circular resultant.

Clearly normal or abnormal results, especially when internally consistent, need not be repeated. For instance, patients who have orthostatic hypotension with beat-to-beat BP responses showing an exaggerated phase II, and absent late phases II and IV, have adrenergic failure. Patients with borderline or mildly abnormal results should be retested for confirmation, or the results should be interpreted with caution, since autonomic tests tend to be indirect tests of autonomic pathways.

SUGGESTED TESTS FOR CLINICAL TRIALS

For clinical trials, confounding variables need to be even more rigorously controlled. We recommend the following tests, although the choice of autonomic function tests is determined by the specific aims of the study. Sometimes only a single test is needed. Under those circumstances, some standardized evaluation of HR variation (deep breathing, spectral analysis, and mean circular resultant) is reasonable. The following comprise a reasonable fuller autonomic battery:

1. HR_{DB}
2. Valsalva ratio
3. HR and BP recording with patients supine and after 1 and 5 min upright or after upright tilt
4. QSART recordings
5. Dark-adapted pupil size after parasympathetic blockade
6. Spectral analysis of HR and BP

PATIENT PREPARATION

Patients should be adequately prepared and the physiologic condition standardized. Eating, caffeine (coffee or tea), smoking, volume depletion, posture, many medications, exercise, and anxiety can affect the autonomic nervous system. Therefore, in an ideal situation, studies for the purposes of clinical trials should be performed under the following conditions:

1. The study is done in the morning after an overnight (8 hr) fast. Patients who are diabetic should have their glucose normalized, with insulin if necessary.
2. Patients should be calm, relaxed, and comfortable, with an empty bladder, and should not be in pain. A total of 20–30 min of supine rest is required in a temperature-controlled quiet laboratory maintained at 23°C.
3. Patients should avoid the use of tobacco products, aspirin, and coffee or tea for 8 hrs and alcohol for 12 hrs before the test. The use of anticholinergic agents (including antidepressant medications, antihistamines, and over- the-counter cough and cold medications), fludrocortisone, and diuretics is discontinued for 48 hrs. The use of vasoactive agents (α- and β-agonists) and α- and β-antagonists is discontinued for 24 hrs.
4. Patients should remove compressive clothing and Jobst stockings.
5. Patients should not have had an acute illness in the preceding 48 hrs.
6. Patients should avoid vigorous unaccustomed exercise in the preceding 24 hrs.
7. The test(s) should be done after patients have been taught and have practiced the procedure.

The tests are done as described above. The cardiovascular HR studies have been well validated. The QSART is well validated, but only limited experience is available outside of the Mayo Autonomic Reflex Laboratory. The photoplethysmographic volume clamp technique (Finapres device) is potentially very important in the evaluation of adrenergic function, but information on its sensitivity, specificity, and reproducibility is lacking. The components of the Valsalva maneuver, e.g., the magnitude of late and early phase II or phase IV, are considerably more sensitive than postural BP recordings (42). We recommend, for the time being, that sphygmomanometric recordings be continued. In clinical trials, it would seem worthwhile to have a small number of centers compare the Finapres recordings of phases of the VM with the standard BP comparisons. At Mayo, we currently do both in clinical trials. The baseline and final sets of recordings are extremely important. It is suggested that the beginning and final sets of recordings be done in *duplicate* and the means used.

TRAINING AND EXPERIENCE

The training of autonomic clinical neurophysiologists is still being defined, as is the training for autonomic technicians. The Mayo Clinical Neurophysiology Technology Program model consists of an intensive 2-year program in electromyography, electroencephalography, sleep laboratory, and autonomic testing, leading to an associate degree. The autonomic component alone includes 20 lectures, a series of tutorials, laboratory demonstrations, and 3 months of laboratory experience. Extrapolating from our experience with the program, it is likely that clinicians will need a thorough grounding in basic neurophysiology, including sudomotor, cardiovascular neurophysiology, extended cardiopulmonary resuscitation training, and instrumentation.

Autonomic clinical neurophysiologists should be experienced in autonomic testing. Tentatively, trained clinical neurophysiologists (electromyography or electroencephalography) may need 6 months of additional training, whereas trainees without such a background will likely need 12 months of training. These people would qualify to take the American Board of Psychiatry and Neurology examination in added qualifications in clinical neurophysiology.

CONCLUSION

Our attempt at generating standardized clinical and research tests of autonomic function is aimed at providing a starting point. We have deliberately attempted to be specific to the degree that other investigators may legitimately disagree. It is our earnest hope that subsequent editions of this book will find autonomic testing so standardized and advanced that this chapter will no longer be needed.

REFERENCES

1. Diabetes Control and Complications Trial (DCCT). Design and methodologic considerations for the feasibility phase: the DCCT Research Group. *Diabetes* 1986;35:530–545.
2. American Diabetes Association American Academy of Neurology. Consensus statement: report and recommendations of the San Antonio Conference on Diabetic Neuropathy [Review]. *Diabetes Care* 1988;11:592–597.
3. Clinical autonomic testing report of the Therapeutics and Technology Assessment Subcommittee of the American Academy of Neurology. *Neurology* 1996;46:873–880.
4. Almquist A, et al. Provocation of bradycardia and hypotension by isoproterenol and upright posture in patients with unexplained syncope [see Comments]. *N Engl J Med* 1989;320:346–351.
5. Bellavere F, et al. Analysis of QT versus RR ECG interval variations in diabetic patients shows a longer QT period in subjects with autonomic neuropathy. *Diabetologia* 1984;27:255(abst).
6. Bellavere F, et al. Prolonged QT period in diabetic autonomic neuropathy: a possible role in sudden cardiac death? *Br Heart J* 1988;59:379–383.
7. Benarroch EE, Low PA. The acetylcholine-induced flare response in evaluation of small fiber dysfunction. *Ann Neurol* 1991;29:590–595.
8. Bloor K. Gustatory sweating and other responses after cervico-thoracic sympathectomy. *Brain* 1969;92:137–146.
9. Borst C, et al. Mechanisms of initial heart rate response to postural change. *Am J Physiol* 1982;243:H676–H681.
10. Braune S, et al. Cardiovascular parameters: sensitivity to detect autonomic dysfunction and influence of age and sex in normal subjects. *Clin Auton Res* 1996;6:3–16.
11. Burgos LG, et al. Increased intraoperative cardiovascular morbidity in diabetics with autonomic neuropathy. *Anesthesiology* 1989;70:591–597.
12. Chambers JB, et al. QT prolongation on the electrocardiogram in diabetic autonomic neuropathy [see Comments]. *Diabetic Med* 1990;7:105–110.
13. Ewing DJ, et al. The natural history of diabetic autonomic neuropathy. *Q J Med* 1980;49:95–108.
14. Ewing DJ, et al. Cardiovascular responses to sustained handgrip in normal subjects and in patients with diabetes mellitus: a test of autonomic function. *Clin Sci Mol Med* 1974;46:295–306.
15. Ewing DJ, et al. Immediate heart rate response to standing: simple test of autonomic neuropathy in diabetes. *BMJ* 1978;1:145–147.
16. Ewing DJ, et al. The value of cardiovascular autonomic function tests: 10 years experience in diabetes. *Diabetes Care* 1985;8:491–498.
17. Fagius J, Jameson S. Effects of aldose reductase inhibitor treatment in diabetic polyneuropathy: a clinical and neurophysiological study. *J Neurol Neurosurg Psychiatry* 1981;44:991–1001.
18. Fagius J, et al. Limited benefit of treatment of diabetic polyneuropathy with an aldose reductase inhibitor: a 24-week controlled trial. *Diabetologia* 1985;28:323–329.
19. Fitzpatrick AP, et al. Methodology of head-up tilt testing in patients with unexplained syncope. *J Am Coll Cardiol* 1991;17:125–130.
20. Genovely H, Pfeifer MA. RR-variation: the autonomic test of choice in diabetes. *Diabetes Metab Rev* 1988;4:255–271.
21. Hreidarsson AB. Pupil size in insulin-dependent diabetes: relationship to duration, metabolic control, and long-term manifestations. *Diabetes* 1982;31:442–448.
22. Knuttgen D, et al. Diabetic autonomic neuropathy: abnormal cardiovascular reactions under general anesthesia. *Klin Wochenschr* 1990;68:1168–1172.
23. Krarup T, et al. Impaired response of pancreatic polypeptide to hypoglycaemia: an early sign of autonomic neuropathy in diabetics. *BMJ* 1979;2:1544–1546.
24. Low PA. Quantitation of autonomic function. In: Dyck PJ, et al., eds. *Peripheral neuropathy*. Philadelphia: WB Saunders, 1993:729–745.
25. Low PA, Fealey RD. Sudomotor neuropathy. In: Dyck PJ, et al., eds. *Diabetic neuropathy*. Philadelphia: WB Saunders, 1987:140–145.
26. Low PA, et al. Comparison of distal sympathetic with vagal function in diabetic neuropathy. *Muscle Nerve* 1986;9:592–596.
27. Low PA, et al. Chronic idiopathic anhidrosis. *Ann Neurol* 1985;18:344–348.
28. Low PA, et al. Evaluation of skin vasomotor reflexes by using laser Doppler velocimetry. *Mayo Clin Proc* 1983;58:583–592.
29. Low PA, et al. The effect of aging on cardiac autonomic and postganglionic sudomotor function. *Muscle Nerve* 1990;13:152–157.
30. Low PA, et al. Quantitative sudomotor axon reflex test in normal and neuropathic subjects. *Ann Neurol* 1983;14:573–580.
31. Low PA, et al. The sympathetic nervous system in diabetic neuropathy: a clinical and pathological study. *Brain* 1975;98:341–356.
32. Marfella R, et al. The squatting test: a useful tool to assess both parasympathetic and sympathetic involvement of the cardiovascular autonomic neuropathy in diabetes. *Diabetes* 1994;43:607–612.
33. Martyn CN, Ewing DJ. Pupil cycle time: a simple way of measuring an autonomic reflex. *J Neurol Neurosurg Psychiatry* 1986;49:771–774.
34. McEvoy KM, et al. 3,4-Diaminopyridine in the treatment of Lambert–Eaton myasthenic syndrome. *N Engl J Med* 1989;321:1567–1571.
35. Moy S, et al. The venoarteriolar reflex in diabetic and other neuropathies. *Neurology* 1989;39:1490–1492.
36. Nordenbo AM, Boesen F, Andersen EB. Cardiovascular autonomic function in multiple sclerosis. *J Auton Nerv Syst* 1989;26:77–84.
37. Pfeifer MA, et al. Autonomic neural dysfunction in recently diagnosed diabetic subjects. *Diabetes Care* 1984;7:447–453.
38. Pfeifer MA, et al. Quantitative evaluation of cardiac parasympathetic activity in normal and diabetic man. *Diabetes* 1982;31:339–345.
39. Rathmann W, et al. Mortality in diabetic patients with cardiovascular autonomic neuropathy. *Diabetic Med* 1993;10:820–824.
40. Roy TM, et al. Autonomic influence on cardiovascular performance in diabetic subjects. *Am J Med* 1989;87:382–388.
41. Sampson MJ, et al. Progression of diabetic autonomic neuropathy over a decade in insulin-dependent diabetics. *Q J Med* 1990;75:635–646.
42. Sandroni P, et al. Autonomic involvement in extrapyramidal and cerebellar disorders. *Clin Auton Res* 1991;1:147–155.
43. Stewart JD, et al. Distal small fiber neuropathy: results of tests of sweating and autonomic cardiovascular reflexes. *Muscle Nerve* 1992;15:661–665.
44. Ten Harkel ADJ, et al. Assessment of cardiovascular reflexes: influence of posture and period of preceding rest. *J Appl Physiol* 1990;68:147–153.
45. Wieling W, van Lieshout JJ. The assessment of cardiovascular reflex activity: standardization is needed. *Diabetologia* 1990;33:182–183.
46. Ziegler D, et al. Assessment of cardiovascular autonomic function: age-related normal ranges and reproducibility of spectral analysis, vector analysis, and standard tests of heart rate variation and blood pressure responses. *Diabetic Med* 1992;9:166–175.

CHAPTER 24

Noninvasive Evaluation of Heart Rate Variability

The Time Domain

Roy Freeman

---

1. Assessment of heart rate variability in health and disease has now attained widespread use in a diverse group of disciplines.
2. Respiration is the most common stimulus used to provoke heart rate variability, and measurement of the respiratory sinus arrhythmia is the basis of several sensitive and specific measures of cardiovagal function.
3. The heart rate (HR) change in response to a Valsalva maneuver is a widely used indirect measure of autonomic function. The Valsalva ratio, the ratio of the shortest RR interval (the tachycardia) during or after phase II of the maneuver to the longest RR interval (the bradycardia) in phase IV of the maneuver, is the most commonly used measure derived from the maneuver.
4. This orthostatic stress of standing evokes a sequence of compensatory cardiovascular responses to maintain cardiovascular homeostasis. The heart rate tachycardia and subsequent bradycardia provoked by standing is the basis of another commonly used test of autonomic function.
5. Other physiologic perturbations to provoke heart rate variability include lying to standing, squatting, passive tilting, coughing, carotid sinus massage and other baroreflex stimuli, mental stress, exercise, apneic facial immersion, cold stimuli, and infusions of vasoactive pharmacologic agents.
6. These tests are influenced by a number of confounding variables that should be considered when establishing a database of normal heart rate variability values and in interpreting test results.

INTRODUCTION

Vagal nerve traffic cannot be measured directly in humans. The assessment of HR variability has thus become the most widely used indirect measure of cardiac vagal nerve function. Reverend Stephen Hales (1677–1761) (49) and Albrecht von Haller (1708–1777) (50) are credited with making the first observations of rhythmic variations in the heart rate. Although well recognized as a physiologic phenomenon in the ensuing centuries, it was only widely appreciated in the 1960s and 1970s that a decrease in heart rate variability accompanied autonomic failure and that this loss of heart rate variability could be used as a measure of autonomic function (98).

The clinical utility of HR variability was first recognized in obstetrics, where it was used as a marker of fetal distress. Hon and Lee (57) first suggested that HR slowing and alterations in interbeat intervals might be a sign of fetal distress requiring rapid delivery. Wheeler and Watkins (112) drew attention to the important role of vagal cardiac innervation in the mediation of HR variability. They documented the reduction or loss of HR_{BB} variability of diabetics with autonomic neuropathy and demonstrated that HR variability was "abolished" by atropine but "unaltered" by sympathetic blockade. These authors hypothesized that the loss of heart rate variability associated with diabetic autonomic neuropathy was due to vagal cardiac denervation.

Careful review of figures in their manuscript reveals that heart rate variability is not completely abolished, but rather only the high-frequency heart rate oscillations are lost (Fig. 1A-C). The low-frequency oscillations are in fact retained

---

R. Freeman: Autonomic and Peripheral Nerve Laboratory, Department of Neurology, Beth Israel Deaconess Medical Center, Harvard Medical School, Boston, Massachusetts 02215.

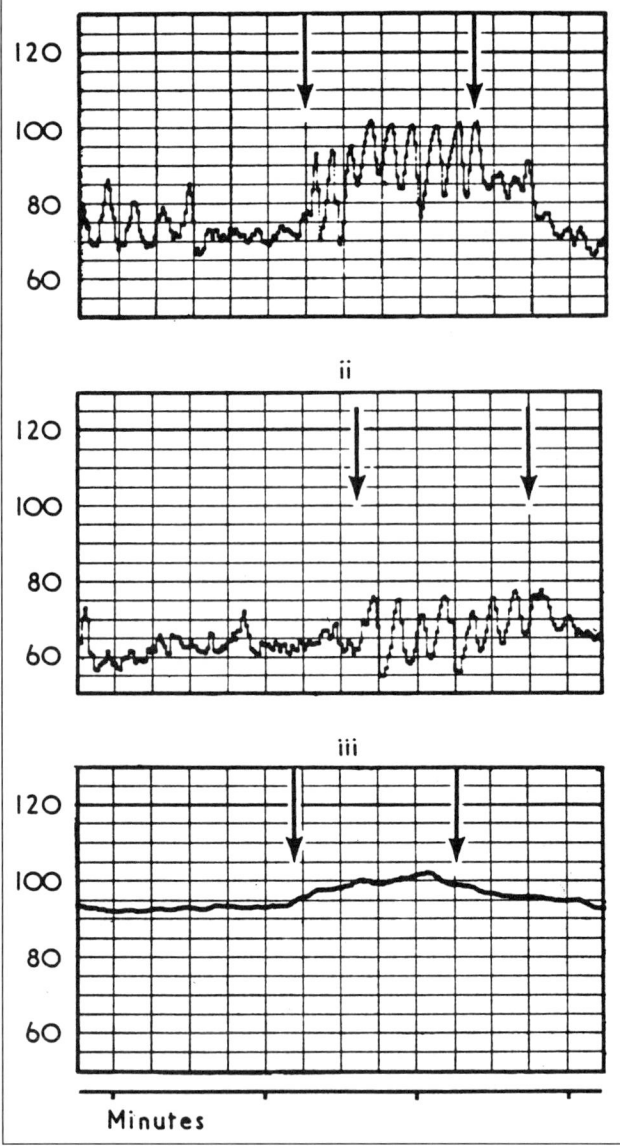

FIG. 1. The effect of intravenous propranolol and atropine on beat-to-beat variation in heart rate in a healthy man aged 30 years **(A)** before drug administration, **(B)** after 10 mg propranolol, and **(C)** after 1.8 mg atropine. *Arrows* mark points between which breaths were taken. From Wheeler and Watkins (112), with permission.

during cholinergic blockade with atropine (Fig. 1C) and are subsequently abolished by sympathetic blockade with propranolol (Fig. 1B). Nevertheless, this important manuscript drew clinical attention to the important role played by the vagus nerve in the mediation of heart rate variability. It is of some interest that in the same year, Sayers (97), using frequency domain techniques, drew attention to the mid- and low-frequency as well as high-frequency oscillations in HR_{BB}. These lower-frequency oscillations, usually determined by analysis of the heart rate power spectrum, have been the subject of an extensive body of research in the ensuing years.

In 1982, Ewing and Clarke (32) advocated a battery of five tests suitable for bedside autonomic function testing. These tests—the average inspiratory–expiratory heart rate difference with six deep breaths, the Valsalva ratio, the 30:15 ratio, the diastolic blood pressure (BP) response to isometric exercise, and the systolic BP fall to standing—they suggested, provided an assessment of both sympathetic and parasympathetic nervous system function. With some modifications, this test battery still forms the core of the cardiovascular autonomic evaluation performed by many autonomic laboratories.

More recently, the time domain measures of HR have gained widespread use in the field of clinical cardiology. Wolf et al. (119) first noted an increased risk of postmyocardial infarction mortality in patients with decreased heart rate variability. It is hypothesized that reduced heart rate variability after myocardial infarction is a reflection of reduced vagal modulation of HR and increased prominence of sympathetic nervous system modulation which results in a predisposition to arrhythmogenesis. A decrease in measures of heart rate variability has been associated with an increase in mortality and of arrhythmic complications in patients who suffered an acute myocardial infarction (13,37,63,74,87).

Assessment of HR variability in health and disease has now attained widespread use in a diverse group of disciplines that include neurology, cardiology, psychology, psychophysiology, obstetrics, anesthesiology, and psychiatry. Respiration is the most common stimulus used to provoke heart rate variability although other physiologic perturbations include a Valsalva maneuver, standing to lying, lying to standing, squatting, passive tilting, coughing, carotid sinus massage and other baroreflex stimuli, mental stress, exercise, apneic facial immersion, cold stimuli, and infusions of vasoactive pharmacologic agents. The increased availability of powerful desktop computers and the resulting ease with which cardiovascular signals can be acquired

TABLE 1. *Time domain statistical measures of heart rate (HR) variability with respiration*

Maximum minus minimum HR difference
Maximum minus minimum RR interval difference
Maximum/minimum HR
Maximum/minimum RR interval
Standard deviation (SD) of RR intervals
SD of the HR
Histogram displays of RR intervals
Coefficient of variation of HR
Coefficient of variation of RR intervals
SDNN index (see text for definition)
SDANN index (see text for definition)
MSSD (mean square successive difference)
rMSSD (root mean square successive difference)
MSD (mean successive difference)
SDSD (SD of the successive differences in RR intervals)
Histogram displays of RR interval differences
Mean circular resultant

and processed digitally have resulted in an array of measures of heart rate variability in the time and frequency domain. This chapter covers the most commonly used time domain tests of heart rate variability.

RESPIRATORY SINUS ARRHYTHMIA

Heart rate variability with deep respiration is the simplest and most widely performed measure of autonomic function. This test provides a sensitive, specific, and reproducible indirect measure of cardiac vagal nerve function.

There are a number of determinants of the heart rate fluctuations with respiratory activity, which include

1. Neural coupling within the central nervous system such that there is overflow from the respiratory center to the medullary vagal efferent neurons resulting in inhibition of vagal efferent activity with inspiration (68).
2. Changes in baroreflex sensitivity with respiratory phase; the baroreflex gain is greatest during late inspiration and early expiration and least during late expiration and early inspiration (26).
3. Arterial baroreceptor-mediated heart rate responses to the blood pressure changes that occur during the respiratory cycle (81).
4. The Hering–Breuer reflex—a stretch reflex from the lungs and thoracic wall provoked by inspiration; inspiration excites stretch receptor afferents in the lung and chest wall (53).
5. The Bainbridge reflex—an increase in central venous volume and the resulting changes in cardiac filling provide a mechanical stimulus to cardiopulmonary structures that produces an increase in HR (2,3).
6. Local intracardiac or sinus node stretch reflexes (60, 65).

Despite these multiple mechanisms that involve several reflex arcs, respiratory sinus arrhythmia has provided a valuable window for determining autonomic nervous system control of cardiovascular function and an important index of autonomic nervous system pathology.

A variety of statistical measures of respiratory-mediated heart rate variability have been used as tests of autonomic function. In the report just described, Wheeler and Watkins (112) first suggested that the difference between the maximum and minimum heart rates with deep respiration might serve as a clinical measure of cardiac vagal autonomic function. This observation was confirmed by Katona and Jih (61), who, in 1975, measured the heart period and respiratory sinus arrhythmia of anesthetized dogs while controlling vagal nerve activity by cooling and rewarming the cervical vagus nerve. They defined *parasympathetic cardiac control* as the decrease in the average heart period caused by the elimination of parasympathetic influences on the heart while leaving sympathetic nervous system influences unaltered. They determined respiratory sinus arrhythmia or the *variation in heart period* as the peak-to-trough change in RR interval over a series of respiratory cycles (Fig. 2). These authors demonstrated a linear relationship between parasympathetic control and the variation in heart period, thus supporting the use of the magnitude of respiratory sinus arrhythmia as a noninvasive measure of parasympathetic cardiac control. This linear relationship was unchanged by modifying vagal tone with alterations in blood pressure or by changes in cardiac sympathetic function induced by β-adrenoreceptor blockade (61). These findings were subsequently replicated in humans with cholinergic pharmacologic blockade using fractionated doses of atropine (40).

In the ensuing years, others workers have advocated a variety of time domain statistical measures. Another sim-

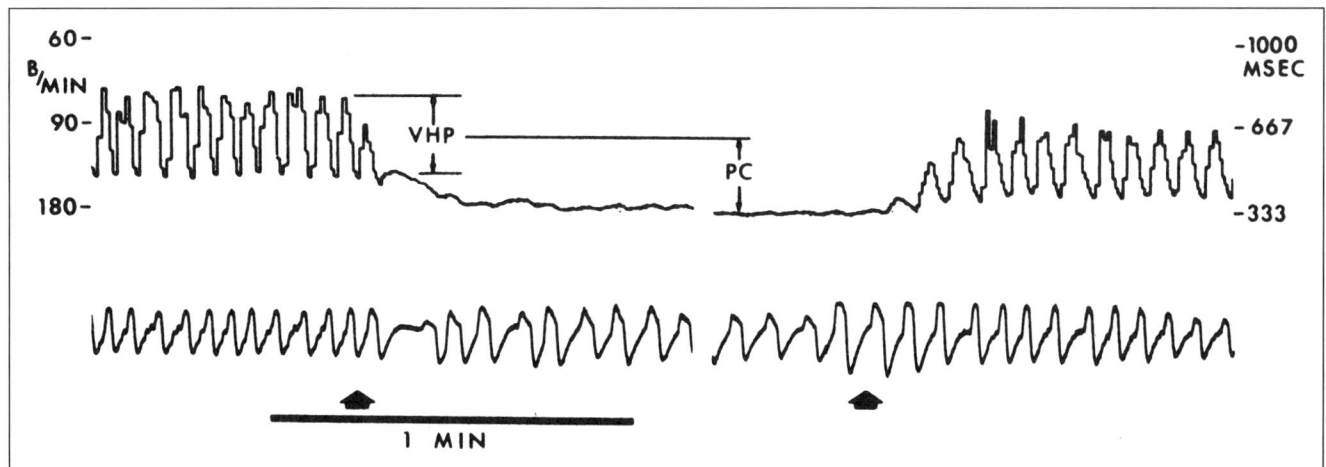

FIG. 2. The effect of bilateral vagal cooling: heart period **(top)** and respiration **(bottom)**. The region between the *arrows* denotes cooling. Respiratory variation of heart period (VHP) is eliminated, and average heart period and parasympathetic cardiac control (PC) are reduced. Rewarming restores original conditions. From Katona and Jih (61), with permission.

ply determined and widely performed measure is the *inspiratory–respiratory ratio* or E:I ratio—the ratio between the shortest RR interval during inspiration to the longest RR interval during expiration (102). The mathematics of the E:I ratio would suggest that this estimation might be more directly influenced by the resting HR (51), but empirically this is not necessarily the case (99).

The laboratory or bedside tests of HR variability with deep breathing are usually performed with patients supine (22,31,99,100,102,115), where vagal tone is greatest; however, some authors have advocated the seated position (34, 80,86). A careful study of a small number of subjects did not show that subject position or the duration of rest preceding the test procedure influenced the measures of heart rate variability with deep respiration. Typically, the test is performed over six respiratory cycles, although some have advocated ten cycles (73), five cycles (22,100), the mean of the five largest responses from eight respiratory cycles (70) or three cycles (84). Bennett et al. (9) suggested that the heart rate response to a single maximal inspiration may provide a more powerful stimulus to HR variability than do repeated deep breaths. This has also been advocated by others (86,94,99), although the heart rate response to a single maximal inspiration may show less reproducibility (28,114).

The tests just described require only a standard electrocardiographic (ECG) recording. The accessibility of sophisticated microcomputer technology has resulted in time domain heart rate variability measures of increasing mathematical complexity. The standard deviation of the mean RR interval is a commonly determined measure of cardiovascular autonomic function. The standard deviation provides a statistical measure of the variability or spread of the RR intervals around the average heart rate. The results of this determination depend on the number of observations (RR intervals) and the mean HR. Unrecognized ectopic beats and other artifacts can significantly effect this measure. The standard deviation may be complemented by the display of the histogram of the RR intervals (18,19, 83,99) and by geometric analytical methods (19,75). To minimize the dependence of the standard deviation on the resting heart rate, the coefficient of variation may be used (the standard deviation divided by the mean RR interval).

The role of vagal modulation of heart rate variability becomes proportionately less as the duration of monitoring increases, such that if the standard deviation of RR intervals is calculated over 24 hrs, <5% of the RR interval variance is due to vagal modulation (12,109). The standard deviation of the RR intervals (the square root of the variance) thus provides a measure of heart rate variability over a range of frequencies—the variance is the mathematical equivalent of the total power of the HR power spectrum. This relationship is described by Parseval's theorem.

The standard deviation (SD) of so-called *normal-to-normal* (NN) RR intervals derived from 24-hr Holter monitoring is a frequently used time domain measure of HR variability in clinical cardiology. The SDNN and two derivations of this measure—the SDNN index and SDANN index—show a significant association with mortality from all causes in myocardial infarction survivors. The SDNN index—the mean of the standard deviation of the RR intervals in the 5-min segments of the 24-hr ECG record—is a time domain measure of heart rate variability that correlates with heart rate variability between 0.0033–0.04 Hz (very low frequency power) and 0.04–0.15 Hz (low-frequency power) of the heart rate power spectrum, whereas the SDANN index is defined as the standard deviation of the average RR intervals in the 5-min segments of the ECG record and correlates with the ultra-low-frequency power (<0.0033 Hz) of the heart rate power spectrum (12,64).

Gundersen and Neubauer (48) proposed that a measure based on successive differences in the RR intervals, i.e., the actual differences between adjacent RR intervals, would be more sensitive than the standard deviation to short-term fluctuations in HR. The mean square successive difference (MSSD) is the average of the square of the differences between successive beats (48), the rMSSD is its square root (11), the mean successive difference (MSD) (31) is the average of the differences between successive beats, and the SDSD is the standard deviation of the successive differences (76). Unlike the standard deviation, these measures depend on the sequence of RR intervals. The measurements are theoretically robust against gradual trends in heart rate over time and are independent of mean HR (51) (although not in all studies) (120). They are, however, sensitive to ectopic beats such as premature ventricular contractions, i.e., a short interval followed by a long compensatory pause (51). A histogram of the RR interval differences may be used to provide a graphic display of the number of such ectopic beats and other artifacts (18). The rMSSD provides a measure of short-term heart rate variability and correlates with energy in the high frequency of the heart period power spectrum (>0.15 Hz).

The SD, MSSD, rMSSD, and MSD when performed in the laboratory are most commonly determined during spontaneous, normal respiration with patients usually supine (22,86,99) and rarely standing (31,120). Heart rate variability determined by this test may be greater when supine (10,31). The duration of measurement is usually longer than the duration of the tests assessing the heart rate response to deep breathing (31,99,120).

Ewing et al. (29,35) drew attention to the large, irregular, episodic changes in heart rate that occur in normal subjects. They quantified these steps using a threshold value of a 50-msec difference from the preceding RR interval (NN50) and demonstrated a reduced number of these steps in diabetic subjects with autonomic neuropathy, some diabetics without autonomic neuropathy, and patients with cardiac transplants. The number of such steps or *RR counts* in normal subjects shows an inverse relationship with age, and the steps show a significant increase during sleep (29,

35). Of diabetic subjects with normal cardiovascular reflexes, 24% had 24-hr RR count results that were less than the lower 95% confidence limit for healthy controls related to age. Based on these results, the authors suggested that this method of heart rate variability analysis is more sensitive than the conventional tests of cardiovascular reflexes (35). This measure and the related pNN50 (the proportion of differences in consecutive normal RR intervals that are >50 msec) correlate with the rMSSD and power in the high frequency of the HR power spectrum (>0.15 Hz) (11,12,64).

The mean circular resultant, a determination based on vector analysis, has been proposed as a method that is resistant to nonrespiratory sources of variability such as ectopic heartbeats and slow trends in HR. In this method, RR intervals are recorded as time events plotted or wrapped on a circle with the periodicity of a single respiratory cycle. The distribution of the points on the circle is determined by vector analysis, giving a result in arbitrary units. Regular distribution of the events on the circle would result in a small vector and denote reduced HR variability. In contrast, clustering of the events on the circle would result in a large vector and suggest normal HR variability. A total of 5 min of carefully controlled respiration is required (44,111). Although this measure has not attained widespread use, it was the sole test of HR variability with respiration in the DCCT study (1).

A number of factors influence respiratory-mediated HR variability. Respiratory sinus arrhythmia is dependent on the both the frequency and the depth of respiration; i.e., the magnitude of change in heart rate at a given respiratory rate depends on the tidal volume and, for a specific tidal volume, the magnitude of HR variability depends on the breathing frequency. Several time and frequency domain studies have suggested that the amplitude of the HR increase is maximal at respiratory rates of 5–10 breaths/min. Smaller changes in HR occur at lower and higher respiratory rates for a given tidal volume (15,23,41,56,72). The maximal HR response in subjects with an autonomic neuropathy occurs at lower respiratory rates (41,72).

The well-established relationship between age and HR variability has been expressed in most studies as a linear decline in the heart rate response to deep breathing with increasing age (70,80,86,89,91,99,117,120). These studies suggest a decline in heart rate variability of 3–5 beats/min per decade in control subjects (regression slope coefficients ranging from ~0.35 to 0.46) The use of a single normative value for all ages will thus reduce the diagnostic discrimination of this test and may result in false-negative test results in younger patients and false-positive results in older patients.

The time of testing may also influence the heart rate response. There is a well-established circadian variation in measures of HR variability characterized by increased heart rate variability observed at night, particularly during sleep, and decreased HR variability in the morning (29,35,43,48,77).

There is also an association between anthropometric indices of body habitus and measures of HR variability (42,54,55,90). Body weight and body mass index are significant predictors of both the E:I ratio and the difference between maximum and minimum heart rates with deep respiration. A 1 SD increase in the body weight or body mass index results in a decrease in the E:I ratio of 0.010–0.014 and a decrease in the maximum minus minimum heart rate difference of 0.49–0.72 beats/min. An increase in these anthropometric indices across the distribution (5–95 percentile) results in a decrease in the E:I ratio of 0.032–0.037 and a decrease in the maximum minus minimum heart rate difference of 1.56–2.39 beats/min (42).

Other factors that influence HR variability include alterations in blood gases (25), physical fitness (21,45,46), food ingestion (93), medications, particularly those with anticholinergic side effects (59,69), and body position in some (10,31) but not all studies (104). There are thus a number of confounding variables to be considered in establishing a database of normal HR variability values and in interpreting test results.

THE HEART RATE RESPONSE TO A VALSALVA MANEUVER

The cardiovascular response to a Valsalva maneuver is the basis of several widely used measures of baroreflex and autonomic function. In a standard Valsalva maneuver, the subject performs a forced expiration against a fixed resistance with a closed glottis. The hemodynamic response to the resulting sudden, transient increase in intrathoracic and intraabdominal pressure in normal subjects may be subdivided in to four phases (Fig. 3). In phase I, there is a transient rise in BP and a fall in HR that is predominantly due to compression of the aorta and propulsion of blood into the peripheral circulation. The hemodynamic changes during this phase are mainly secondary to mechanical factors and are not accompanied by an increase in muscle sympathetic activity (20) or affected by α-adrenergic blockade (66,96). Phase II consists of a fall in BP early in the phase, with a subsequent recovery of BP later in the phase. These BP changes are accompanied by an increase in heart rate. The fall in cardiac output due to impaired venous return to the heart results in compensatory cardioacceleration and an increase in muscle sympathetic activity (20) and peripheral resistance (66). In phase III, a fall in BP and increase in HR occur with cessation of expiration. Phase IV of the maneuver is characterized by an increase in BP above the baseline value (the overshoot) due to the residual vasoconstriction and now normal venous return. In a pharmacologic study of four subjects, the BP overshoot in phase IV was significantly decreased by propranolol, unaffected by atropine, and enhanced by phentolamine (96). These results suggest

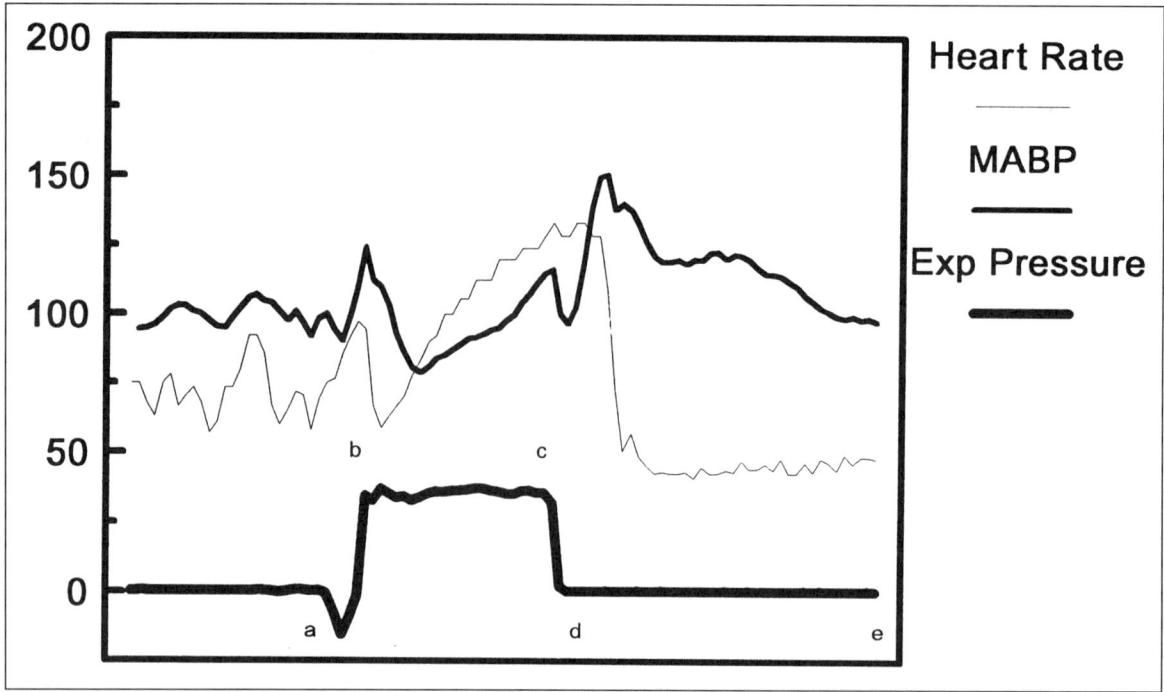

FIG. 3. The normal hemodynamic response to a Valsalva maneuver *a–b*, phase I; *b–c*, phase II; *c–d*, phase III; and *d–e*, phase IV. MABP, mean arterial blood pressure; Exp Pressure, expiratory pressure.

that cardioacceleration plays the central role in the BP overshoot. This BP increase in phase IV is responsible for the baroreflex-mediated bradycardia.

The HR change in response to this maneuver is a widely used indirect, sensitive, specific, and reproducible measure of autonomic function (4,36,71,85,98). The Valsalva ratio—the ratio of the shortest RR interval (the tachycardia) during or after phase II of the maneuver to the longest RR interval (the bradycardia) in phase IV of the maneuver—is the most commonly used measure derived from the maneuver (4,36,67,71). Other statistical measures of the heart rate response to the maneuver include the tachycardia ratio—the ratio of the shortest RR interval during the maneuver to the longest RR interval before the maneuver—which may be more reproducible but more dependent on resting heart rate than is the Valsalva ratio (4).

The availability of accurate, noninvasive, BP_{BB} pressure measurements has significantly enhanced this test of autonomic function (58). Previously, the noninvasive use of this test was limited to measuring the magnitude of the heart rate response to the maneuver to provide an indirect measure of cardiac vagal function. Continuous, noninvasive blood pressure measurements provide a direct assessment of the cardiovascular response to the maneuver and permit the determination of baroreflex and sympathetic nervous system function. The noninvasive BP measurements have enabled investigators to determine the latencies of the HR responses to the Valsalva maneuver (38). In one study, 79% of diabetic subjects had an abnormal tachycardia latency (defined as the latency from the lowest blood pressure of phase III of the Valsalva maneuver to the tachycardia) and 84% of diabetic subjects had an abnormal bradycardia latency (defined as the latency from the blood pressure overshoot to the bradycardia in phase IV).

The maneuver is most frequently performed with an expiratory pressure of 40 mmHg and duration of expiration of 15 sec. Few studies, however, have critically analyzed the effects of expiratory pressure and test duration on the hemodynamic changes that accompany the Valsalva maneuver (24). In one study, the HR and BP responses correlated significantly with the expiratory pressures when measured over a range of 20 to 50 mmHg (7). The reported duration of expiration for the Valsalva maneuver ranges from 10 sec to "as long as the patient is able" (24). At high expiratory pressures (50 mmHg) the Valsalva ratio and phase II HR increase but not the phase IV HR decrease correlated with the duration of expiration (7). These authors proposed that fifteen sec was a practical test duration (7).

The noninvasive measurement of BP has also drawn attention to an important pitfall in the assessment of the HR response to a Valsalva maneuver in patients with isolated sympathetic vasomotor lesions but intact cardiovagal function. Van Lieshout et al. (106) noted high Valsalva ratios in two such patients due to the significant tachycardia that occurred in response to the blood pressure fall in phase II of the maneuver, despite the absence of a postmaneuver bradycardia in phase IV of the maneuver. Thus, a normal or high-normal Valsalva ratio, generally regarded as a sign of preserved sympathetic nervous system–mediated vasoconstriction, may be misinterpreted. This observation emphasizes the importance of interpreting the HR response in conjunction with BP_{BB} measurements. The absence of a postmaneuver bradycardia despite the presence of a normal Valsalva ratio may provide some clue to the presence of this phenomenon. These BP changes may be replicated by α-adrenergic blockade with phentolamine, which also results in a significant increase in the Valsalva ratio (96).

Consistent with this observation is the observed superior correlation between the Valsalva ratio and the HR response in phase II compared with the HR response in phase IV of the maneuver (7). A detailed physiologic study of such patients revealed that they demonstrated large blood pressure falls in phase II and a normal phase IV resulting in a significantly enhanced baroreflex stimulus. The patients had a normal HR increase in phase II, but 75% did not develop the reflex bradycardic response that is characteristic of phase IV (88).

Investigators have suggested that one maneuver (84,86,94) or three maneuvers (32) be performed, selecting the best (70) or average (38) of the three maneuvers. There is also some controversy as to whether the Valsalva ratio should be determined by measuring the shortest RR interval during the maneuver (70) or, since HR continues to increase after the maneuver ceases, the shortest RR interval during and after the maneuver (86).

The hemodynamic response to the Valsalva maneuver may be attenuated by the buffering effect of blood within the thoracic cavity. Thus, the patient position during, and duration of rest preceding, the maneuver significantly affect test results (104). Some investigators advocate the seated position for this test as the cardiovascular effects are likely to be greater (32,115). A decline in the Valsalva ratio with age has been reported in some (70,86,89) although not all (34,108) studies.

THE HEART RATE RESPONSE TO STANDING

The hemodynamic response to standing provides the physiologic basis of a commonly performed measure of autonomic function. Transferring from the supine to upright posture results in the translocation of 300–800 mL of blood from the central intravascular compartment to dependent regions. This orthostatic stress evokes a sequence of compensatory cardiovascular responses to maintain homeostasis.

The HR response to active standing is bimodal. There is an abrupt increase in heart rate that peaks at ~3 sec, followed by a more gradual increase that peaks at ~12 sec after standing (14). The initial increase in HR is mediated by the sudden inhibition of vagal tone while the more gradual increase is due to further vagal inhibition and increased sympathetic nervous system activity. The immediate HR increase is most likely an *exercise reflex* evoked by muscle contraction and is also observed with other voluntary muscle contractions (14). Reduced baroreflex activity due to transient hypotension is responsible for the later increase in HR. Sprangers et al. (101) suggested that this initial fall in blood pressure was due to a reflex release of vasoconstrictor tone. They proposed that the decrease in peripheral resistance was predominantly mediated by cardiopulmonary receptors stimulated by the translocation of blood to the intrathoracic compartment by the muscle contractions accompanying standing (107). More recently, Wieling et al. (116) have argued that the time course of this response is faster than might be expected for a sympathetic nervous system reflex mediated by cardiopulmonary afferent nerve fibers. They have proposed that the fall in peripheral resistance is due to local, nonautonomically mediated, postexercise vasodilation in active muscle groups. In addition, central command (47) and cholinergic mediated vasodilation (95) may play a contributory role in evoking this decrease in peripheral resistance. This transient fall in blood pressure and increase in heart rate is followed by a return of the HR and BP to a new baseline after ~30 sec. An *overshoot* in BP evokes the transient bradycardia (14,118). This response is thus dependent on an intact sympathetic nervous system, parasympathetic nervous system, and baroreflex.

The 30:15 ratio assesses this physiologic response by comparing the ratio of the heart rate increase that occurs at ~15 sec after standing with the relative bradycardia that occurs at ~30 sec after standing. When cardiovagal function is deficient or abolished by atropine, the bradycardia does not occur (30,33). This ratio thus provides a measure of cardiac vagal function (6,30,82).

Ewing et al. (33) proposed that the 30:15 ratio be determined as the ratio between the shortest RR interval at or around the 15th beat and the longest RR interval at or around the 30th beat. While the smallest RR interval occurs at or close to RR interval number 15 and the largest RR interval heart rate occurs close to RR interval number 30, there is variability (SD of up to ±7 RR intervals) and the absolute maximum-to-minimum RR interval ratio is usually considerably higher (117). The sensitivity of this test measuring the heart rate response to standing may be increased by enlarging the window during which the test peak and trough heart rates are calculated (120) or even by measuring the ratio of the absolute maximum-to-minimum heart rate after standing (82,86,117). There is a low correlation between indices of the HR response to postural change and those of HR variability provoked by deep breathing ($r = 0.14$), which suggests that different physiologic mechanisms are involved (117).

The magnitude of the HR response depends on the period of rest that precedes standing (104). Recording of the heart rate for this test is usually initiated at the onset of standing (32,113) to allow for the early heart rate increase, although some studies have reported test results after measuring the HR only once the test subjects are erect (86). There is an inverse relationship between measures of the heart rate response to standing and age (108,117).

Sundkvist et al. (103) dissected the HR response to passive tilting by measuring the acceleration index (the shortest RR interval after standing minus the baseline RR interval, all divided by the baseline RR interval) and the brake index (the longest RR interval after standing minus the shortest RR interval, all divided by the baseline RR interval). They suggested that the acceleration index provides a measure of baroreceptor-mediated vagal withdrawal while the brake index assesses the vagal response to the sympathetic nervous system–mediated increase in peripheral resistance. Others (14,30) have suggested that the RR interval lengthening does not occur after passive tilting.

In patients with isolated sympathetic vasomotor lesions but intact cardiovagal function, absence of the normal bradycardic response that is typically observed 20–30 sec after standing does not imply cardiovagal dysfunction but rather an absence of sympathetic nervous system–mediated vasoconstriction (106). As with the Valsalva maneuver, the heart rate response to standing should also be interpreted in relationship to the BP_{BB} measurements (88,106).

THE HEART RATE RESPONSE TO LYING DOWN

A related test measures the heart rate response to assuming the supine position. After lying down, there is a decrease in the RR interval that is maximal around the third or fourth beat, which is followed by an increase in the RR interval value (greater than the resting value) at approximately the 25th–30th beat. Autonomic blockade studies with atropine and propranolol have suggested that the initial RR interval shortening is mediated by the vagus nerve while the latter lengthening of the RR interval is predominantly mediated by the sympathetic nervous system. The initial tachycardia is most likely a manifestation of the *exercise or muscle–heart reflex* (5,6).

THE HEART RATE RESPONSE TO SQUATTING

Marfella et al. (78,79) have delineated the cardiovascular response to squatting in a group of controls and diabetic subjects. In their test, protocol subjects stood still for 3 min, squatted down for 1 min, and finally stood up during inspiration. Squatting resulted in lengthening of the RR interval that is abolished by atropine, suggesting a vagal-mediated response while the shortening of the RR interval that occurred after standing from a squatting position was attenuated by propranolol. A vagal ratio based on this test (the ratio between the RR interval mean before squatting and the longest RR interval after squatting) was calculated that was outside the 99% confidence interval in 42% of diabetic patients and 1.3% of the control subjects, whereas a sympathetic ratio (the ratio between the baseline RR interval and the shortest RR interval after standing) was outside the 99% confidence interval in 40% of diabetic patients and 0.8% of the control subjects. The test results showed an inverse correlation with age (79).

THE HEART RATE RESPONSE TO COUGHING

Coughing generates a sudden large intrathoracic pressure transient of 25–250 mmHg that results in hypotension and cardioacceleration (92,110). The HR response, which may increase by >30%, has been quantified by several investigators (92,110). A short cough evokes a decrease in RR interval length (maximal 2–3 sec after coughing), with a return to the resting RR interval 18–20 sec later (16). The cough-induced cardioacceleration is predominantly under cholinergic control and related to both the contraction of abdominal and thoracic musculature as well as the cough-induced arterial hypotension (16,17). The cardioacceleration is abolished by atropine but not propranolol, suggesting a cholinergic mechanism. Increasing age is associated with a decline in the amplitude and rapidity of the chronotropic response to cough. The clinical utility of this provocative maneuver has been questioned by others (105).

THE HEART RATE RESPONSE TO APNEIC FACIAL IMMERSION

The diving reflex in mammals is provoked by facial cooling and consists of bradycardia, apnea, decreased cardiac output, and vasoconstriction (39). This complex cardiovascular reflex is thought to prolong survival by decreasing myocardial oxygen consumption and shunting blood to the vital organs. As a clinical test, the diving reflex assesses trigeminal–vagal–cardiac and trigeminal–sympathetic–vascular smooth muscle pathways and does not directly involve the baroreflex or its primary central connections (27). The test can also be performed on uncooperative or unconscious patients (62). Some, however, have suggested that this test does not add significantly to other measures of autonomic function (8). Although trigeminal afferent pathways do not directly interact with the central baroreflex pathways, baroreflex-mediated bradycardia is enhanced by facial immersion. Eckberg et al. (27) have argued that the augmented vagal response represents an interaction that occurs "downstream" from the anatomically discrete central terminations of the trigeminal and baroreceptor afferent fibers.

Khurana et al. (62) demonstrated that in humans the bradycardia induced by simulated diving (apneic facial immersion) could be replicated by the application of cold compresses to the face—the cold face test. The cutaneous receptors of the ophthalmic division of the trigeminal nerve were the most sensitive site for the elicitation of this reflex. The bradycardia induced by the test in control subjects was attenuated in patients with diabetes mellitus, brainstem stroke, multiple sclerosis, and the Shy–Drager syndrome. Based on data derived from a quantitative methodologic study, Heath and Downey (52) proposed that cold compresses at 0°C, applied bilaterally to the whole face for 40–60 sec, produced the maximum bradycardia and peripheral vasoconstriction. The mean, maximum bradycardia in controls was 22.2% [cf. 21.4 (62)]. Venous occlusion plethysmographic measurements revealed decreased blood flow in the finger (72.5%), toe (59%), and calf (44.4%) (52).

REFERENCES

1. The Diabetes Control and Complication Trial Research Group. The effect of intensive diabetes therapy on the development and progression of neuropathy: the Diabetes Control and Complications Trial Research Group. *Ann Intern Med* 1995;122: 561–568.
2. Bainbridge FA. The influence of venous filling upon the rate of the heart. *J Physiol (Lond)* 1915;50:65–84.
3. Bainbridge FA. The relation between respiration and the pulse rate. *J Phsyiol (Lond)* 1920;54:192–202.
4. Baldwa VS, Ewing DJ. Heart rate response to Valsalva manoeuvre: reproducibility in normals, and relation to variation in resting heart rate in diabetics. *Br Heart J* 1977;39:641–644.
5. Bellavere F, Ewing DJ. Autonomic control of the immediate heart rate response to lying down. *Clin Sci* 1982;62:57–64.
6. Bellavere F, et al. Standing to lying heart rate variation: a new simple test in the diagnosis of diabetic autonomic neuropathy. *Diabetic Med* 1987;4:41–43.
7. Benarroch EE, et al. Use of the photoplethysmographic technique to analyze the Valsalva maneuver in normal man. *Muscle Nerve* 1991; 14:1165–1172.
8. Bennett T, et al. Cardiovascular reflex responses to apnoeic face immersion and mental stress in diabetic subjects. *Cardiovasc Res* 1976;10:192–199.
9. Bennett T, et al. Assessment of methods for estimating autonomic nervous control of the heart in patients with diabetes mellitus. *Diabetes* 1978;27:1167–1174.
10. Bennett T, et al. Assessment of vagal control of the heart in diabetes: measures of R-R interval variation under different conditions. *Br Heart J* 1977;39:25–28.
11. Bigger JT Jr, et al. Comparison of time- and frequency domain-based measures of cardiac parasympathetic activity in Holter recordings after myocardial infarction. *Am J Cardiol* 1989;64:536–538.
12. Bigger JT Jr, et al. Correlations among time and frequency domain measures of heart period variability two weeks after acute myocardial infarction. *Am J Cardiol* 1992;69:891–898.
13. Bigger JT Jr, et al. Frequency domain measures of heart period variability and mortality after myocardial infarction. *Circulation* 1992; 85:164–171.
14. Borst C, et al. Mechanisms of initial heart rate response to postural change. *Am J Physiol* 1982;243:H676–H681.
15. Brown TE, et al. Important influence of respiration on human R-R interval power spectra is largely ignored. *J Appl Physiol* 1993;75: 2310–2317.
16. Cardone C, et al. Autonomic mechanisms in the heart rate response to coughing. *Clin Sci* 1987;72:55–60.
17. Cardone C, et al. Cough test to assess cardiovascular autonomic reflexes in diabetes. *Diabetes Care* 1990;13:719–724.
18. Cashman PMM. The use of R-R interval and difference histograms in classifying disorders of sinus rhythm. *J Med Eng Technol* 1977; 1:20–28.
19. Cripps TR, et al. Prognostic value of reduced heart rate variability after myocardial infarction: clinical evaluation of a new analysis method. *Br Heart J* 1991;65:14–19.
20. Delius W, et al. General characteristics of sympathetic activity in human muscle nerves. *Acta Physiol Scand* 1972;84:65–81.
21. De Meersman RE. Heart rate variability and aerobic fitness. *Am Heart J* 1993;125:726–731.
22. Dyrberg T, et al. Prevalence of diabetic autonomic neuropathy measured by simple bedside tests. *Diabetologia* 1981;20:190–194.
23. Eckberg DL. Human sinus arrhythmia as an index of vagal cardiac outflow. *J Appl Physiol* 1983;54:961–966.
24. Eckberg DL. Parasympathetic cardiovascular control in human disease: a critical review of methods and results [Review]. *Am J Physiol* 1980;239:H581–H593.
25. Eckberg DL, et al. Modulation of human sinus node function by systemic hypoxia. *J Appl Physiol* 1982;52:570–577.
26. Eckberg DL, et al. Phase relationship between normal human respiration and baroreflex responsiveness. *J Phsyiol (Lond)* 1980;304: 489–502.
27. Eckberg DL, et al. Trigeminal–baroreceptor reflex interactions modulate human cardiac vagal efferent activity. *J Physiol (Lond)* 1984;347:75–83.
28. Espi F, et al. Testing for heart rate variation in diabetes: single or repeated deep breaths? *Acta Diabetol Lat* 1982; 19:177–181.
29. Ewing DJ, et al. New method for assessing cardiac parasympathetic activity using 24 hour electrocardiograms. *Br Heart J* 1984;52: 396–402.
30. Ewing DJ, et al. Autonomic mechanisms in the initial heart rate response to standing. *J Appl Physiol* 1980;49:809–814.
31. Ewing DJ, et al. Cardiac autonomic neuropathy in diabetes: comparison of measures of R-R interval variation. *Diabetologia* 1981; 21:18–24.
32. Ewing DJ, Clarke BF. Diagnosis and management of diabetic autonomic neuropathy. *BMJ* 1982;285:916–918.
33. Ewing DJ, et al. Immediate heart-rate response to standing: simple test for autonomic neuropathy in diabetes. *BMJ* 1978;1:145–147.
34. Ewing DJ, et al. The value of cardiovascular autonomic function tests: 10 years experience in diabetes. *Diabetes Care* 1985;8:491–498.
35. Ewing DJ, et al. Twenty four hour heart rate variability: effects of posture, sleep, and time of day in healthy controls and comparison with bedside tests of autonomic function in diabetic patients. *Br Heart J* 1991;65:239–244.
36. Ewing DJ, et al. Vascular reflexes in diabetic autonomic neuropathy. *Lancet* 1973;2:1354–1356.
37. Farrell TG, et al. Risk stratification for arrhythmic events in postinfarction patients based on heart rate variability, ambulatory electrocardiographic variables and the signal-averaged electrocardiogram. *J Am Coll Cardiol* 1991;18:687–697.
38. Ferrer MT, et al. Baroreflexes in patients with diabetes mellitus. *Neurology* 1991;41:1462–1466.
39. Finley JP, et al. Autonomic pathways responsible for bradycardia on facial immersion. *J Appl Physiol* 1979;47:1218–1222.
40. Fouad FM, et al. Assessment of parasympathetic control of heart rate by a noninvasive method. *Am J Physiol* 1984;246:H838–H842.
41. Freeman R, et al. Transfer function analysis of respiratory sinus arrhythmia: a measure of autonomic function in diabetic neuropathy. *Muscle Nerve* 1995;12:76–84.
42. Freeman R, et al. The relationship between heart rate variability and measures of body habitus. *Clin Auton Res* 1995;5:261–266.
43. Furlan R, et al. Continuous 24-hour assessment of the neural regulation of systemic arterial pressure and RR variabilities in ambulant subjects. *Circulation* 1990;81:537–547.
44. Genovely H, Pfeifer MA. RR-variation: the autonomic test of choice in diabetes. *Diabetes Metab Rev* 1988;4:255–271.
45. Goldberger AL, et al. Atropine unmasks bed-rest effect: a spectral analysis of cardiac interbeat intervals. *J Appl Physiol* 1986;61: 1843–1848.
46. Goldsmith RL, et al. Comparison of 24-hour parasympathetic activity in endurance-trained and untrained young men [see Comments]. *J Am Coll Cardiol* 1992;20:552–558.
47. Goodwin GM, et al. Cardiovascular and respiratory responses to changes in central command during isometric exercise at constant muscle tension. *J Physiol (Lond)* 1972;226: 173–190.
48. Gundersen HJG, Neubauer B. A long-term diabetic autonomic nervous abnormality. *Diabetologia* 1977;13:137–140.
49. Hales S. *Statical essays*. London: Innys and Manby, 1733.

50. Haller A. *Elementa physiologicae corporis humini.* Lausanne, Sumpithus MM Bousquet et Suliorum 1760.
51. Harry J, Freeman R. Assessing heart rate variability: a computer simulated comparison of methodologies. *Muscle Nerve* 1993;16:267–277.
52. Heath ME, Downey JA. The cold face test (diving reflex) in clinical autonomic assessment: methodological considerations and repeatability of responses. *Clin Sci (Colch)* 1990;78:139–147.
53. Hering E. Uber eine reflectorische Beziehung zwischen und Herz. *Sitzber Akad Wiss Wien* 1871;64:333–353.
54. Hirsch J, et al. Nutritionally-induced changes in parasympathetic function. *Brain Res Bull* 1991;27:541–542.
55. Hirsch J, et al. Heart rate variability as a measure of autonomic function during weight change in humans. *Am J Physiol* 1991;261:R1418–R1423.
56. Hirsch JA, Bishop B. Respiratory sinus arrhythmia in humans: how breathing pattern modulates heart rate. *Am J Physiol* 1981;241:H620–H629.
57. Hon EH, Lee ST. Electronic evaluation of the fetal heart rate patterns preceding fetal death: further observations. *Am J Obstet Gynecol* 1965;87:814–826.
58. Imholz BP, et al. Continuous non-invasive blood pressure monitoring: reliability of Finapres device during the Valsalva manoeuvre. *Cardiovasc Res* 1988;22:390–397.
59. Jakobsen J, et al. Heart rate variation in patients treated with antidepressants: an index of anticholinergic effects? *Psychopharmacology (Berlin)* 1984;84:544–548.
60. James TN. The sinus node as a servomechanism [Review]. *Circ Res* 1973;32:307–313.
61. Katona PG, Jih F. Respiratory sinus arrhythmia: noninvasive measure of parasympathetic cardiac control. *J Appl Physiol* 1975;39:801–805.
62. Khurana RK, et al. Cold face test in the assessment of trigeminal–brainstem–vagal function in humans. *Ann Neurol* 1980;7:144–149.
63. Kleiger RE, et al. Decreased heart rate variability and its association with increased mortality after acute myocardial infarction. *Am J Cardiol* 1987;59:256–262.
64. Kleiger RE, et al. Stability over time of variables measuring heart rate variability in normal subjects. *Am J Cardiol* 1991;68:626–630.
65. Koizumi K, et al. Cardiac and autonomic system reactions to stretch of the atria. *Brain Res* 1975;87:247–261.
66. Korner PI, et al. Reflex and mechanical circulatory effects of graded Valsalva maneuvers in normal man. *J Appl Physiol* 1976;40:434–440.
67. Levin AB. A simple test of cardiac function based upon the heart rate changes induced by a Valsalva maneuver. *Am J Cardiol* 1966;18:90–99.
68. Levy MN, et al. Effects of respiratory center activity on the heart. *Circ Res* 1966;18:67–78.
69. Low PA, Opfer-Gehrking TL. Differential effects of amitriptyline on sudomotor, cardiovagal, and adrenergic function in human subjects. *Muscle Nerve* 1992;15:1340–1344.
70. Low PA, et al. The effect of aging on cardiac autonomic and postganglionic sudomotor function. *Muscle Nerve* 1990;13:152–157.
71. Low PA, et al. The sympathetic nervous system in diabetic neuropathy: a clinical and pathological study. *Brain* 1975;98:341–356.
72. Mackay JD. Respiratory sinus arrhythmia in diabetic neuropathy. *Diabetologia* 1983;24:253–256.
73. Mackay JD, et al. Diabetic autonomic neuropathy: the diagnostic value of heart rate monitoring. *Diabetologia* 1980;18:471–478.
74. Malik M, Camm AJ. Significance of long term components of heart rate variability for the further prognosis after acute myocardial infarction. *Cardiovasc Res* 1990;24:793–803.
75. Malik M, et al. Heart rate variability in relation to prognosis after myocardial infarction: selection of optimal processing techniques. *Eur Heart J* 1989;10:1060–1074.
76. Malpas SC, Maling TJ. Heart-rate variability and cardiac autonomic function in diabetes. *Diabetes* 1990;39:1177–1181.
77. Malpas SC, Purdie GL. Circadian variation of heart rate variability. *Cardiovasc Res* 1990;24:210–213.
78. Marfella R, et al. Detection of early sympathetic cardiovascular neuropathy by squatting test in NIDDM. *Diabetes Care* 1994;17:149–151.
79. Marfella R, et al. The squatting test: a useful tool to assess both parasympathetic and sympathetic involvement of the cardiovascular autonomic neuropathy in diabetes. *Diabetes* 1994;43:607–612.
80. Masaoka S, et al. Heart rate variability in diabetes: relationship to age and duration of the disease. *Diabetes Care* 1985;8:64–68.
81. Melcher A. Respiratory sinus arrhythmia in man: a study in heart rate regulating mechanisms. *Acta Physiol Scand Suppl* 1976;435:1–31.
82. Mitchell EA, et al. Diabetic autonomic neuropathy in children: immediate heart-rate response to standing. *Aust Paediatr J* 1983;19:175–177.
83. Murray A, et al. RR interval variations in young male diabetics. *Br Heart J* 1975;37:882–885.
84. Mustonen J, et al. Testing of autonomic cardiovascular regulation: methodological considerations. *Clin Physiol* 1989;9:249–257.
85. Nathanielsz PW, Ross EJ. Abnormal response to Valsalva maneuver in diabetics: relation to autonomic neuropathy. *Diabetes* 1967;16:462–465.
86. O'Brien IA, et al. Heart rate variability in healthy subjects: effect of age and the derivation of normal ranges for tests of autonomic function. *Br Heart J* 1986;55:348–354.
87. Odemuyiwa O, et al. Comparison of the predictive characteristics of heart rate variability index and left ventricular ejection fraction for all-cause mortality, arrhythmic events and sudden death after acute myocardial infarction. *Am J Cardiol* 1991;68:434–439.
88. Opfer-Gehrking TL, Low PA. Impaired respiratory sinus arrhythmia with paradoxically normal Valsalva ratio indicates combined cardiovagal and peripheral adrenergic failure. *Clin Auton Res* 1993;3:169–173.
89. Persson A, Solders G. R-R variations: a test of autonomic dysfunction. *Acta Neurol Scand* 1983;67:285–293.
90. Peterson HR, et al. Body fat and the activity of the autonomic nervous system. *N Engl J Med* 1988;318:1077–1083.
91. Pfeifer MA, et al. Differential changes of autonomic nervous system function with age in man. *Am J Med* 1983;75:249–258.
92. Rowe JW, et al. Post-cough heart rate response: influence of age, sex, and basal blood pressure. *Am J Physiol* 1983;245:R18–R24.
93. Ryan SM, et al. Spectral analysis of heart rate dynamics in elderly persons with postprandial hypotension. *Am J Cardiol* 1992;69:201–205.
94. Ryder REJ, Hardisty CA. Which battery of autonomic tests? *Diabetologia* 1990;33:177–179.
95. Sanders JS, et al. Evidence for cholinergically mediated vasodilation at the beginning of isometric exercise in humans. *Circulation* 1989;79:815–824.
96. Sandroni P, et al. Pharmacological dissection of components of the Valsalva maneuver in adrenergic failure. *J Appl Physiol* 1991;71:1563–1567.
97. Sayers BM. Analysis of heart rate variability. *Ergonomics* 1973;16:17–32.
98. Sharpey-Schafer EP, Taylor PJ. Absent circulatory reflexes in diabetic neuritis. *Lancet* 1960;1:559–562.
99. Smith SA. Reduced sinus arrhythmia in diabetic autonomic neuropathy: diagnostic value of an age-related normal range. *BMJ* 1982;285:1599–1601.
100. Smith SE, Smith SA. Heart rate variability in healthy subjects measured with a bedside computer-based technique. *Clin Sci* 1981;61:379–383.
101. Sprangers RL, et al. Initial blood pressure fall on stand up and exercise explained by changes in total peripheral resistance. *J Appl Physiol* 1991;70:523–530.
102. Sundkvist G, et al. Respiratory influence on heart rate in diabetes mellitus. *BMJ* 1979;1:924–925.
103. Sundkvist G, et al. Abnormal diastolic blood pressure and heart rate reactions to tilting in diabetes mellitus. *Diabetologia* 1980;19:433–438.
104. Ten Harkel ADJ, et al. Assessment of cardiovascular reflexes: influence of posture and period of preceding rest. *J Appl Physiol* 1990;68:147–153.
105. Van Lieshout EJ, et al. Cardiovascular response to coughing: its value in the assessment of autonomic nervous control. *Clin Sci* 1989;77:305–310.
106. Van Lieshout JJ, et al. Pitfalls in the assessment of cardiovascular reflexes in patients with sympathetic failure but intact vagal control. *Clin Sci* 1989;76:523–528.

107. Vissing SF, et al. Relation between sympathetic outflow and vascular resistance in the calf during perturbations in central venous pressure: evidence for cardiopulmonary afferent regulation of calf vascular resistance in humans. *Circ Res* 1989;65: 1710–1717.
108. Vita G, et al. Cardiovascular reflex tests: assessment of age-adjusted normal range. *J Neurol Sci* 1986;75:263–274.
109. Vybiral T, et al. Effect of passive tilt on sympathetic and parasympathetic components of heart rate variability in normal subjects. *Am J Cardiol* 1989;63:1117–1120.
110. Wei JY, Harris WS. Heart rate response to cough. *J Appl Physiol* 1982;53:1039–1043.
111. Weinberg CR, Pfeifer MA. An improved method for measuring heart-rate variability: assessment of cardiac autonomic function. *Biometrics* 1984;40:855–861.
112. Wheeler T, Watkins PJ. Cardiac denervation in diabetes. *BMJ* 1973;4:584–586.
113. Wieling W. Heart rate variability in healthy subjects: effect of age and derivation of normal ranges for tests of autonomic function [Letter]. *Br Heart J* 1987;57:109–110.
114. Wieling W. Reduced sinus arrhythmia in diabetic autonomic neuropathy [Letter]. *BMJ* 1983;286:1285.
115. Wieling W, van Lieshout JJ. The assessment of cardiovascular reflex activity: standardization is needed. *Diabetologia* 1990;33:182–183.
116. Wieling W, et al. Circulatory response evoked by a 3 s bout of dynamic leg exercise in humans. *J Physiol (Lond)* 1996;494:601–611.
117. Wieling W, et al. Reflex control of heart rate in normal subjects in relation to age: a data base for cardiac vagal neuropathy. *Diabetologia* 1982;22:163–166.
118. Wieling W, et al. Testing for autonomic neuropathy: heart rate changes after orthostatic manoeuvres and static muscle contractions. *Clin Sci* 1983;64:581–586.
119. Wolf M, et al. Sinus arrhythmia in acute myocardial infarction. *Med J Aust* 1978;2:52–53.
120. Ziegler D, et al. Assessment of cardiovascular autonomic function: age related normal ranges and reproducibility of spectral analysis, vector analysis, and standard tests of heart rate variation and blood pressure responses. *Diabetic Med* 1992;9:166–175.

CHAPTER 25

Analysis of Blood Pressure and Heart Rate Variability

Theoretical Considerations

John M. Karemaker

---

1. Blood pressure (BP) and heart rate (HR) variability can be analyzed by frequency analysis techniques, which can detect different rhythms in the signal, such as respiratory-related and slower rhythms (Mayer waves).
2. Discussed are the two techniques most used for analysis of HR and BP variability: fast Fourier transform and autoregressive spectral analysis.
3. In the spectrum of relatively brief registrations (a few minutes), the best established rhythms are the respiratory rhythm and a "10-sec" rhythm observed in the BP and in the HR.
4. In humans, the respiratory variability in BP is mainly mechanically induced, and the accompanying HR variability is under baroreflex control via the vagus nerves.
5. The 10-sec BP variability, which is related to sympathetic activity to the vasculature, can be explained as a synergy between reflex corrections of BP perturbations and the sluggishness of the sympathetic response. HR 10-sec variations are mediated by both sympathetic and vagal activity.
6. Because cardiovascular control behaves as a bounded but poorly predictable system, analysis techniques from chaos theory have been introduced that look into the patterns of variation that were formerly considered as nonrhythmic "background" noise.
7. These newer analyses study aspects as the "1/f" (1 divided by the frequency) character of the power spectra and measures for complexity of the HR signal.
8. Many studies have demonstrated significant changes in either spectral peaks or chaos theory–derived measures under certain conditions.
9. For routine clinical applications, however, the sensitivity and the specificity of the proposed new diagnostic tools have rarely been studied. The best proven application is the detection of abnormalities in cardiac vagal control.
10. It is concluded that analysis of BP and HR variability in the frequency domain has been useful in pathophysiologic research into the nature of cardiovascular regulation. For reliable clinical applications, more research needs to be done.

INTRODUCTION: RHYTHMS IN BLOOD PRESSURE AND HEART RATE

One of the most important aims in the evaluation of blood pressure (BP) and heart rate (HR) registration is the quest

---

J. M. Karemaker: Department of Physiology, University of Amsterdam Academic Medical Center, 1105 AZ Amsterdam, The Netherlands.

for signs of abnormal and normal autonomic control and, in this context, the analysis of BP and HR variability may be valuable. It is well known that BP and HR are not constant but constantly varying. This variability has many components, most of which are commonly observed in daily clinical practice and are more or less taken for granted. We are not amazed that HR rises when a person gets upset, and we do not expect BP to remain constant under such circumstances. Conversely, one would not expect

BP to rise to values over 200/120 mmHg even under severe stress. But how often does this occur in normal daily life? Our knowledge of the normal range of BP and HR has vastly expanded since the advent of ambulatory methods for unobtrusively tracking a patient's BP and HR in normal daily life. With the increased amount of BP data now available, we are currently confronted with the problem of making sense of this seemingly overwhelming amount of information.

Figure 1, which is taken from the thesis by Van Montfrans (57), shows the 1-min averages of BP and HR in a borderline hypertensive patient over a 24-hr. period. Obviously, there is a great deal of variability, but most prominent is the day–night rhythm. The sudden jumps between successive points are generally situationally induced, for instance by changes in posture, activity, or emotion. Even when a normal subject sits quietly in a chair, however, beat-to-beat variability occurs (Fig. 2). One can discern the well-known respiratory variations both in HR and in BP. These variations are most conspicuous in the systolic BP. A different and slower rhythm is seen in the diastolic BP fluctuations. These low-frequency variations in BP constitute the well-known Mayer waves, named after the man who, in 1876, described prominent slowly recurring BP variations (mostly 6–9/min) in experimental animals (33). When studying the effects of asphyxia and hypercarbia, Traube (52) had described BP oscillations with the same frequency in 1865, an observation later amplified by Hering (22) in 1869.

The tradition to name a phenomenon after its discoverer produced chaos in nomenclature, which Schweitzer (48) tried to resolve in 1945 by his proposition to name any BP (or HR) wave coupled to the respiratory cycle after Traube and Hering, and any rhythm slower than the respiratory one after Mayer. Despite the resolution of the problem with the nomenclature, little insight was gained into the origin of the waves. In their 1958 book on reflexogenic areas in the circulation, Heymans and Neil (23) presented an overview of the proposed explanations for the Mayer waves. The underlying mechanism was still not conclusively established, but all opinions on the effector mechanism accepted the sympathetic outflow to the vasculature to be the final common pathway. This was later conclusively demonstrated in experiments by Preiss and Polosa (40) and by Fernandez de Molina and Perl (18) by direct recordings of sympathetic nerve activity in phase with the BP waves. Although low-frequency BP waves had been observed in experimental animals for many decades, Sayers and colleagues (24) were the first, in the 1970s, to apply systematic signal analysis to recordings obtained in humans, and demonstrated prominent low-frequency rhythms occurring in humans as well. Since then, this kind of analysis has blossomed, especially in recent years. This can be ascribed to a number of factors: (a) the popularization of

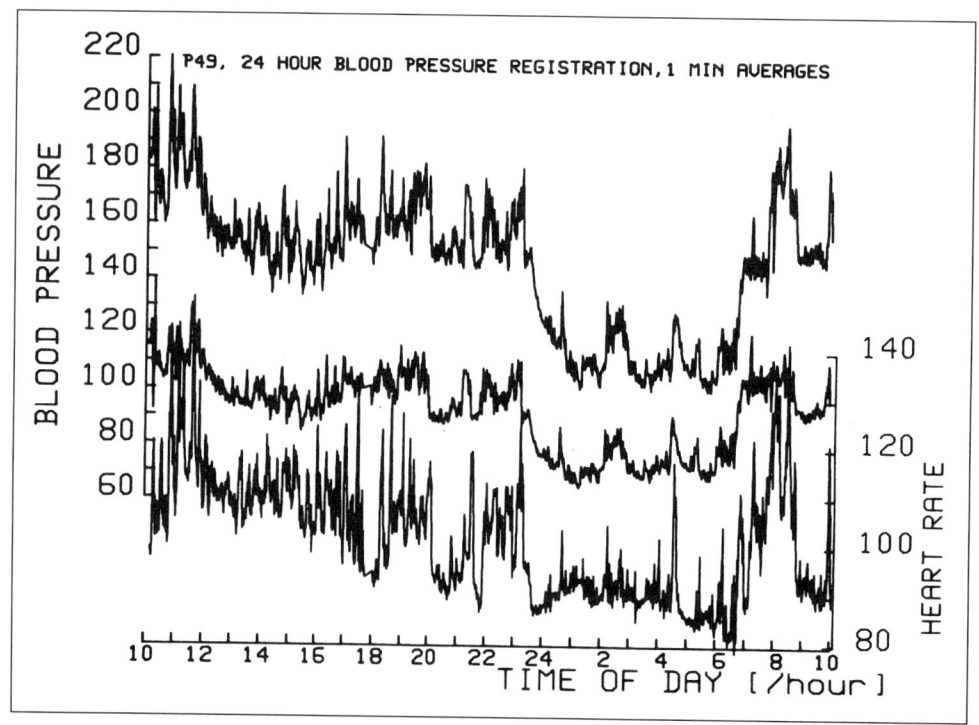

FIG. 1. Example of 24-hr continuous ambulatory blood pressure recording. Values of systolic pressure (*top curve*), diastolic pressure (*middle curve*), and heart rate (*lower curve*) are averaged over 1-min periods. From Van Montfrans (57), with permission.

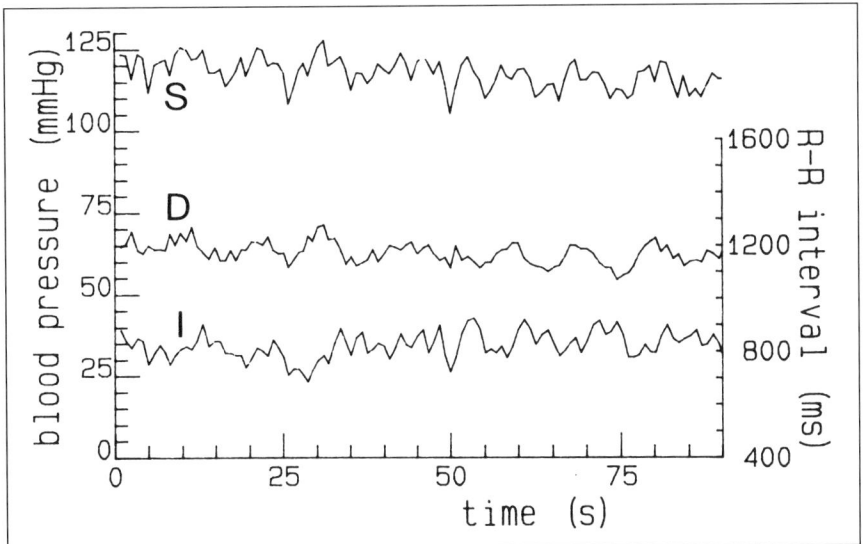

FIG. 2. Beat-to-beat values of blood pressure and heart period in a test subject who is sitting quietly. Note the spontaneous fluctuations in pressure and RR interval. S, systolic pressure; D, diastolic pressure; I, RR interval. From DeBoer (11), with permission.

the fast Fourier transform (FFT) and related computational techniques, which make decomposition of any signal into its constituent frequency components feasible for smaller computer systems; (b) progress in the development of physiologic theories in which the presence or absence of specific frequencies in the spectrum of HR and BP variability has been linked to changes in the balance between sympathetic and parasympathetic outflow; (c) the availability of techniques that accurately and noninvasively measure beat-to-beat HR and BP, a prerequisite for the above-mentioned analysis; and (d) the widespread use of increasingly powerful personal computers.

In more recent years, prompted by the development of mathematics of nonlinear dynamical systems, much attention has been devoted to analysis of cardiovascular variability in terms of *chaos*. In daily use, this term has a different meaning from what mathematicians have come to understand by it: a system that can be well defined by a more or less elaborate set of deterministic or statistical rules that describe its behavior in time. Due to nonlinear interactions, however, the condition of the system can be predicted for only a very brief period because very small, seemingly insignificant variations in the initial conditions can quickly lead to large deviations from an expected

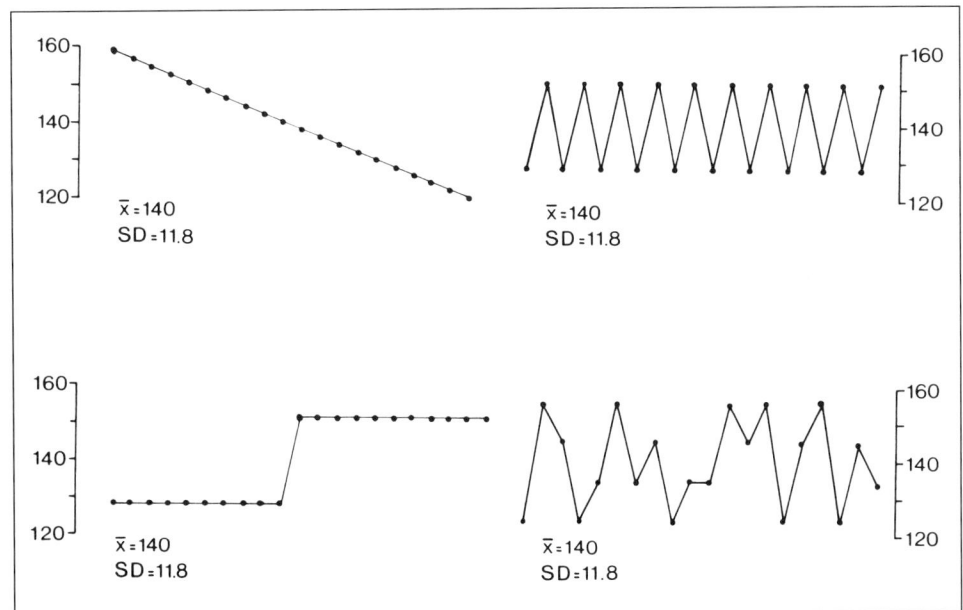

FIG. 3. Four hypothetical signals, all with identical means and standard deviations (SD). From DeBoer et al. (13), with permission.

course. Over time, the system remains within boundaries and many of its parameters can be derived by observation.

In the following sections, the developments in these various fields are analyzed. In the process, both the useful and the doubtful applications of these newer techniques are presented.

ANALYSIS OF VARIABILITY IN THE CONSTITUENT FREQUENCIES

The first question to consider is what is the purpose of resolving a signal in the time domain into (theoretical) sine and cosine components? Fourier's proposition is that most signals that vary around some mean value can be reconstructed as a sum of sines and cosines at different frequencies. Figure 3 shows why such analysis can occasionally make more sense than simple computation of the basic statistical properties of a signal. The figure from DeBoer et al. (13) shows that the information contained in a signal is not fully represented by the mean value and standard deviation. The time sequence in the deviations around the mean tells an equally important story. This is exactly what Fourier analysis can furnish. Specifically, if oscillations of more or less constant frequencies occur, they will show up as peaks in the spectrum. The spectrum can be considered as the distribution of the total variance in the signal over the different constituent (underlying) frequencies (Fig. 4). Therefore, the dimension of the y-axis is variance/hertz and the integral of the whole curve over the frequency axis is the original (total) variance.

A number of different techniques are available for computing the Fourier spectrum from a data set. The following is an overview of the techniques used most often. Although, in principle, the different techniques should yield the same results from the same data set, there may be problems inherent to particular techniques.

Analysis of Heart Rate Variability

HR variability analysis, which is considered first here because it is an essentially discontinuous signal, is defined as the number of heartbeats per unit of time, usually taken as 1 min. To arrive at a value for each heartbeat, a "trick" is used: the duration of each heart period is converted into a beats/min value. Even then, the HR signal only has a value at the conclusion of each heart period, as it is measured in between cardiac activities. Preferably, the onset of the P wave should be used (in the following sections, HR variability will be interpreted as the autonomic influence on the sinus node). For convenience, though, usually the moment of occurrence of the R wave is used because it is easily detected in the standard electrocardiogram (ECG). When the ECG is lacking, the upstroke of the pulse wave can be used instead.

There are essentially three different methods for arriving at a tractable signal for rhythm analysis of HR variability: (a) forming an interpolated, quasi-continuous HR signal, (b) replacing the R waves with unit spikes (delta functions) at their exact moments of occurrence, or (c) replacing the R waves with values equal to the just-completed heart period and placed at regular intervals, the mean heart period of the total period of analysis. Figure 5 depicts these three different HR signals as derived from an ECG recording. [More details on the mathematics of how to formulate power spectra from these different signals are provided by DeBoer and colleagues (11,12)].

Theoretically, the different methods of generating the input data for spectral analysis yield different results. In practice, however, most of these differences are negligible, so the method may be chosen according to what best suits the purposes of the situation.

Techniques for Spectrum Estimation

This section presents an overview of the computational techniques for estimating a spectrum. For more practical or theoretical information, see Bendat and Piersol (5) and Press et al. (41). The description that follows is restricted to those methods that are commonly referred to in most publications on the topic.

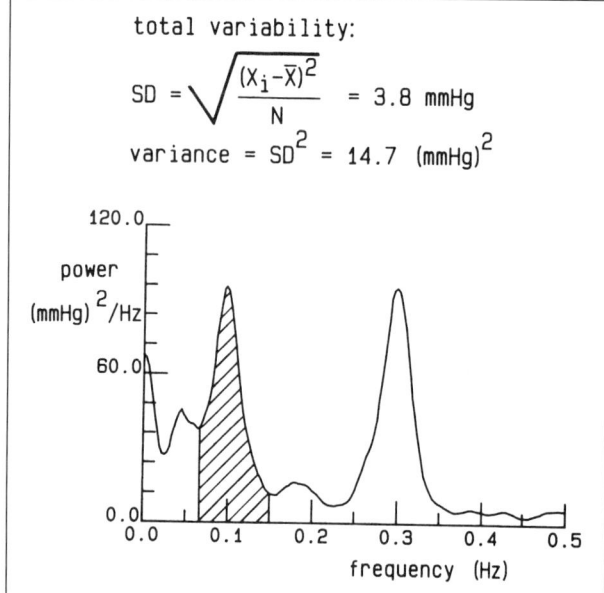

FIG. 4. Power spectrum of systolic blood pressure variability. The total variance is divided by the Fourier transform over the frequency axis. The *total area under the curve* equals the total variance, and the *hatched area* shows the amount of variance that can be ascribed to variability in the 0.1-Hz band, i.e., a rhythm in systolic blood pressure that recurs every 10 sec. Provided by Dr. R. W. DeBoer, published with permission.

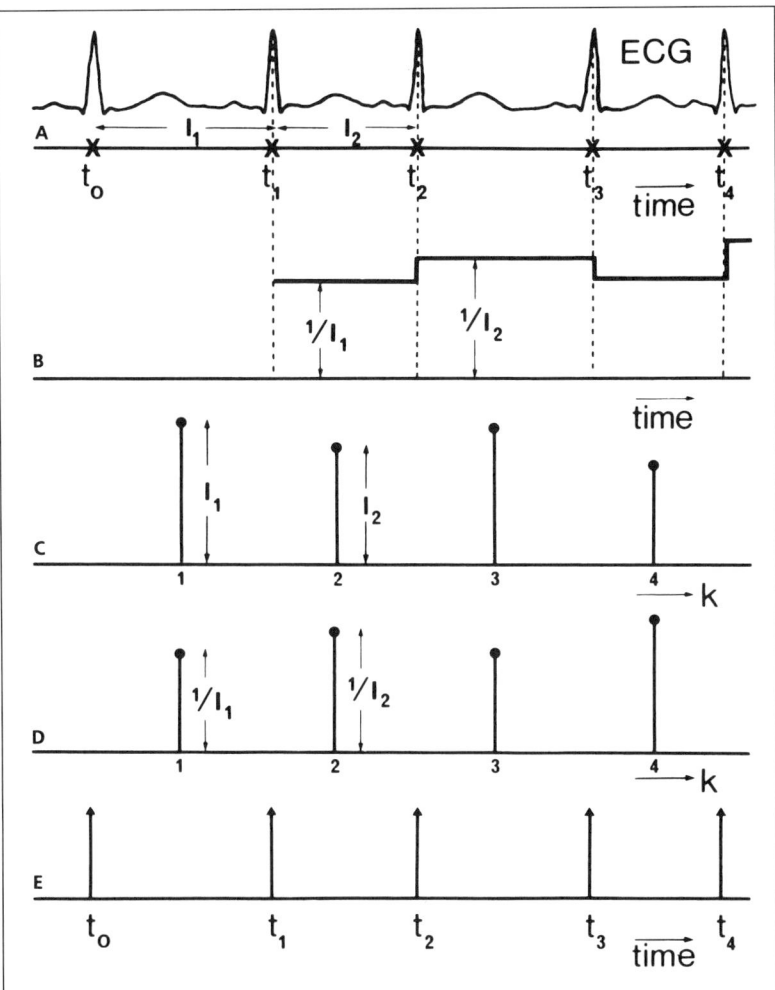

FIG. 5. **A:** Event series representing R waves of the electrocardiogram (ECG). **B:** Heart rate signal derived from A. In real time, the value for heart rate in a particular interval is displayed during the next interval (this time shift may be corrected for off-line). Standard spectral techniques can be applied after regular sampling of this signal. **C:** Interval series derived from A. For spectral analysis, the values are placed at regular intervals equal to the mean heart period. **D:** Series of inverse intervals, treated as in C. **E:** The events of A have been replaced by spikes (delta functions); the spectrum of this signal represents the spectrum of counts. From DeBoer et al. (12), with permission.

Fast Fourier Transform

In most instances, the computationally most efficient method is the FFT, which was designed as a fast implementation of the discrete Fourier transform for equidistantly sampled processes. As indicated previously, HR variability data can basically be considered as being derived from an irregularly sampled process. When the FFT algorithm is applied directly to the HR or RR interval series, as sequentially measured in time, this yields a spectrum that is measured in cycles per beat (instead of cycles per second or hertz). By multiplying the number axis by the average HR, as observed in the measurement period, a spectrum is created that may look like the one depicted in Fig. 6B. This does not really look like a curve that can lead to any conclusions. However, because the estimate for each point of the spectrum is very unreliable [the standard deviation of the estimate is as great as the quantity being estimated (5)], this warrants smoothing the curve by averaging adjacent points, which results in the better-looking curves shown in Fig. 6C-D. This allows better recognition of the spectral regions or bands where variability (i.e., power or squared amplitude in the Fourier transform) is concentrated. A large amount of this power may be present at very low frequencies, as in the example. This is actually misleading: at the lowest possible frequency, i.e., 0 Hz or a steady level, no power can be present, because the variability was analyzed after subtraction of the average value from the signal first. Moreover, to suppress spurious low-frequency variability, a linear or even quadratic trend that might exist in the signal is very often subtracted before the FFT is applied.

Are there, indeed, such low-frequency changes in HR? Yes, but this is very difficult to interpret. To illustrate this point, let the total duration of the recording to be analyzed be 5 min [as recommended in the recently proposed "standards of measurement" (8)]. During this period, the test subject must be in very stable condition to ensure a good spectral estimate. If this subject has an average HR of 60 beats/min in this 5-min period, then there are 300 successive heart periods from which to compute the spectrum. The FFT needs a power-of-two number as the input data

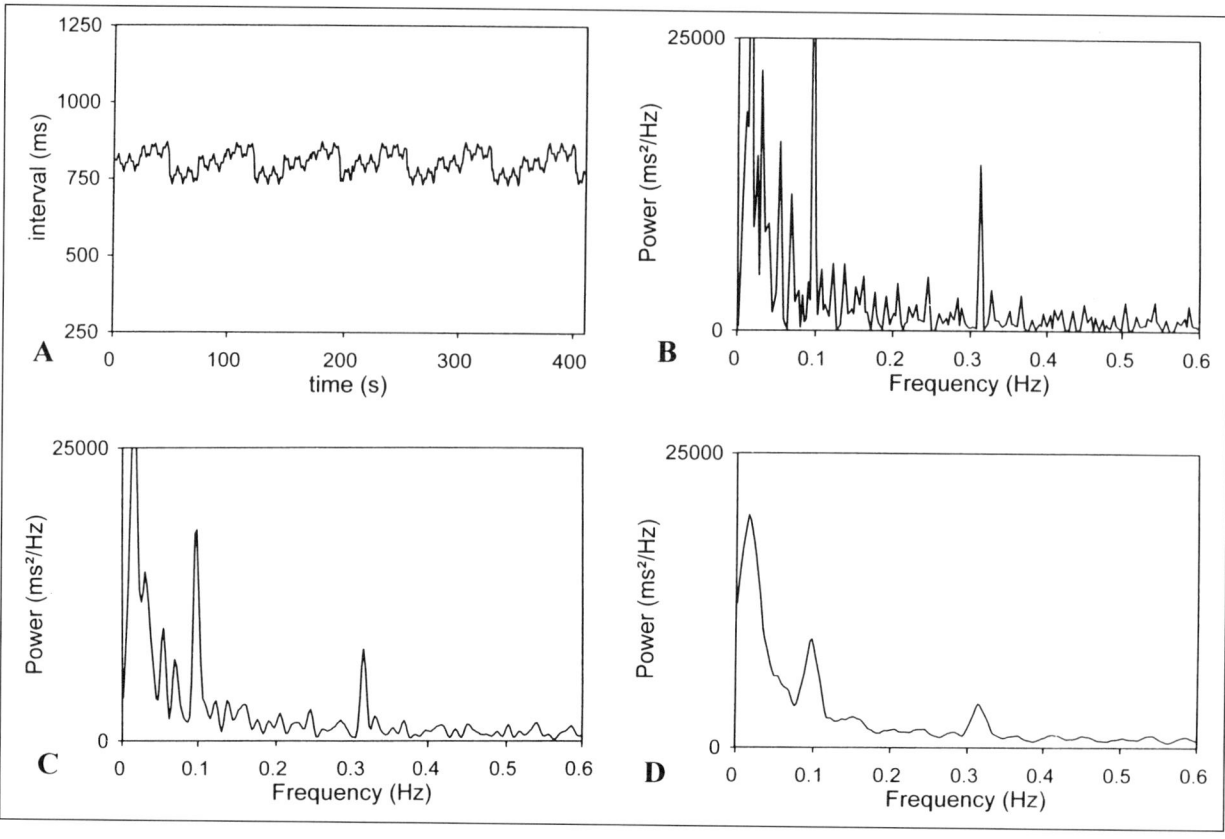

FIG. 6. A: Artificial heart period signal (512 data points) with periodicities of 0.31, 0.1, and 0.013 Hz. Mean heart period is 801 msec, and standard deviation is 36 msec. **B:** Unsmoothed Fourier transform of heart rate variability shown in A. **C:** Fourier transform after smoothing, using a 5-point triangular window to average adjacent points. **D:** As in C, smoothed using a 15-point window.

set; therefore, either 44 data points must be discarded to get 300 − 44 = 256, or 212 "dummy" points need to be added to get 300 − 212 = 512. Because these extra points must not influence the spectrum, it is customary to add a set of leading and trailing zeros to the data set (i.e., the set after subtraction of the average value): this is known as *zero padding*. Either way, in a 5-min set, it is not possible to recognize a lower frequency than that of a sine wave that occurs at least once in the period of measurement, or 1/300 Hz. Because the FFT computes the spectrum in discrete steps of frequency, the resolution over the whole frequency axis is 1/300 Hz in this example. Averaging the adjacent frequency points in the smoothing operation would have further decreased the resolution. From this reasoning, it is clear that it is very difficult to appraise the power in the lowest frequency range. Formally, because the variability value at 0 Hz by definition must be zero, the lowest peak cannot be relied on to represent a genuine peak. It might just be the effect of a high content of low-frequency power that is truncated to zero near the *y*-axis. Moreover, irregularities in the signal, such as ventricular extrasystoles or missed R waves, or one or more deep sighs can sufficiently disturb to the spectral estimation so that the whole picture is seriously distorted, as is shown in Fig. 7.

Autoregressive Spectral Estimation

The previously described method for spectral estimation basically attempts to develop the spectrum from a sum of sinusoids that approximates the original signal. Another way of making a spectral estimate is to try to find a time series that describes each point in the signal as a weighted sum of previous values plus some remnant variation (*noise*). The set of weighing coefficients that performs this task defines a model for the internal structure of the data set. Such a model also defines an estimate for the spectrum of the signal. The advantage of the method is that we may try to describe the signal "parsimoniously" by a small number of coefficients. A very smooth-looking spectrum result shows nothing of the peaked aspect that characterizes the output of the FFT. Figure 8A is an example of such autoregressive spectrum, computed for the same set shown in Fig. 6A. Based on appearance, Fig. 8A is preferable to Fig. 6B. However, this technique also has its disadvantages. Obviously, the chosen number of coefficients defines the number of spectral frequencies that are detected. When the number of coefficients is increased, this may generate numerous spurious peaks (see Fig. 8B), especially on noisy input data sets. Therefore, either rigid information

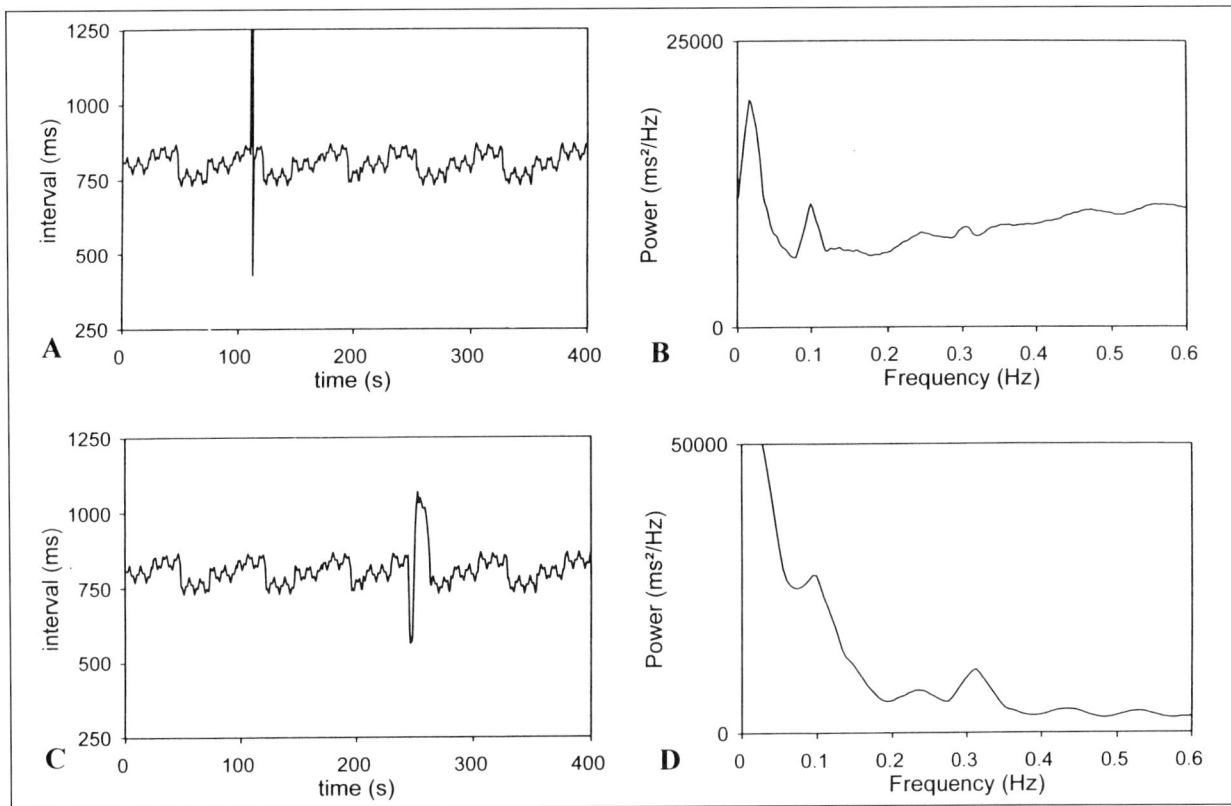

FIG. 7. A: Signal as in 6A, with one trigger error, resulting in one longer and one shorter period. **B:** The spectrum is distorted to such an extent that the respiratory peak at 0.31 Hz almost disappears. **C:** Signal with one (simulated) deep sigh. Now the low-frequency part of the spectrum is seriously distorted (D, note the adapted y-scale).

theory–derived criteria are needed to define the model order [as recommended by Camm et al. (8)] or this method should be combined with the more conservative spectral estimates to choose the model order reliably and thus avoid spurious peaks [as mentioned by Press et al. (41)].

Analysis of Blood Pressure Variability

Only HR variability has been considered so far, because this is the most problematic signal to contend with in frequency analysis techniques. Because the BP signal is continuous, the problem of irregularly sampled signals might not be anticipated. This overly simplistic approach is misleading, however, in that the frequency content of the original BP signal is not important for slow-wave detection. The main frequencies in the analogue BP tracing are the fundamental frequency (i.e., HR) and its harmonics. The slower variations that extend over a number of heart periods are of greater interest.

Therefore, it has become customary to characterize the BP signal by using a set of indices per heartbeat: systolic, diastolic, and (true) mean BP, as observed in a particular heart period. Consequently, the same techniques that were described for HR variability spectral estimation can be applied to the analysis of BP variability. Moreover, the same problems that were mentioned earlier apply.

Cross-Spectral Analysis of Blood Pressure and Heart Period

Spectral analysis techniques can be valuable in detecting evidence of abnormal autonomic control in the varying BP and HR signals. Before describing this technique, however, it is necessary to additionally explain the technique of cross-spectral analysis.

Up to this point, only single signals have been considered, in which periodicities were identified by the FFT or related techniques. In the event of two signals, however, such as systolic BP and HR, which are both varying in time (Fig. 9A), the spectra of both signals look very much alike (see Fig. 9B,C). Therefore, one may wish to examine whether the two signals are changing together in some time-locked fashion. In applied statistics, the linear relationship between two signals is investigated by computing the regression and correlation coefficients. A comparable method is available in spectral analysis. However, because two complete spectra are involved, the answer will, again, be a function of frequency: the cross-spectrum is com-

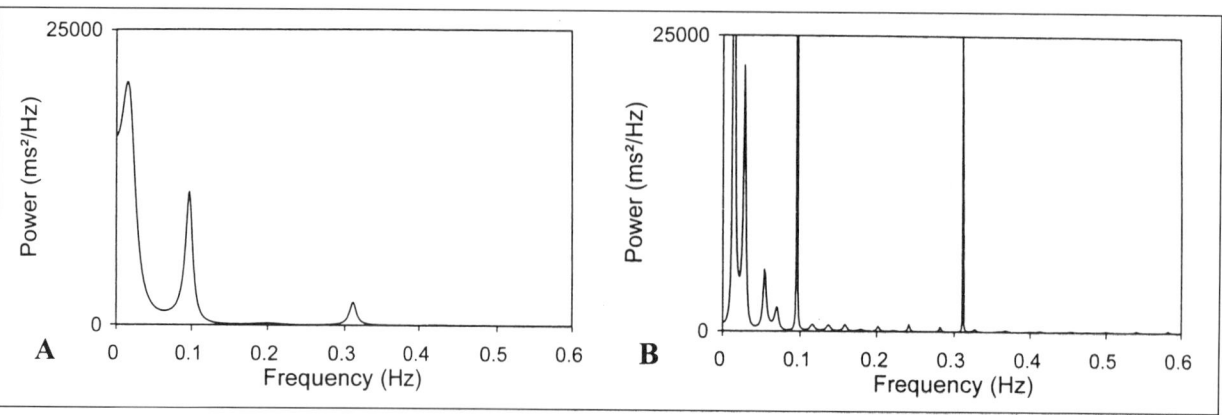

FIG. 8. A: Autoregressive spectrum of the 512 data points used in Fig. 6A. The model has been adapted with 15 poles (cf. Fig. 6D). **B:** As in A, the model has now been adapted with 60 poles (cf. Fig. 6B,C).

puted, which gives the coherence (comparable to the squared correlation in a certain frequency region) and the phase (see Fig. 9D). Coherence ranges between 0 and 1 and phase ranges between −180° and +180°. The term *phase* represents the difference angle between two sinusoids of the same periodicity. When the phase angle in Fig. 9D is negative, the variation in systolic pressure leads the variation in heart period at that same frequency. Because one may shift one sinus curve over a multiple of 360° with respect to the other one, the judgment on "leading" or "lag-

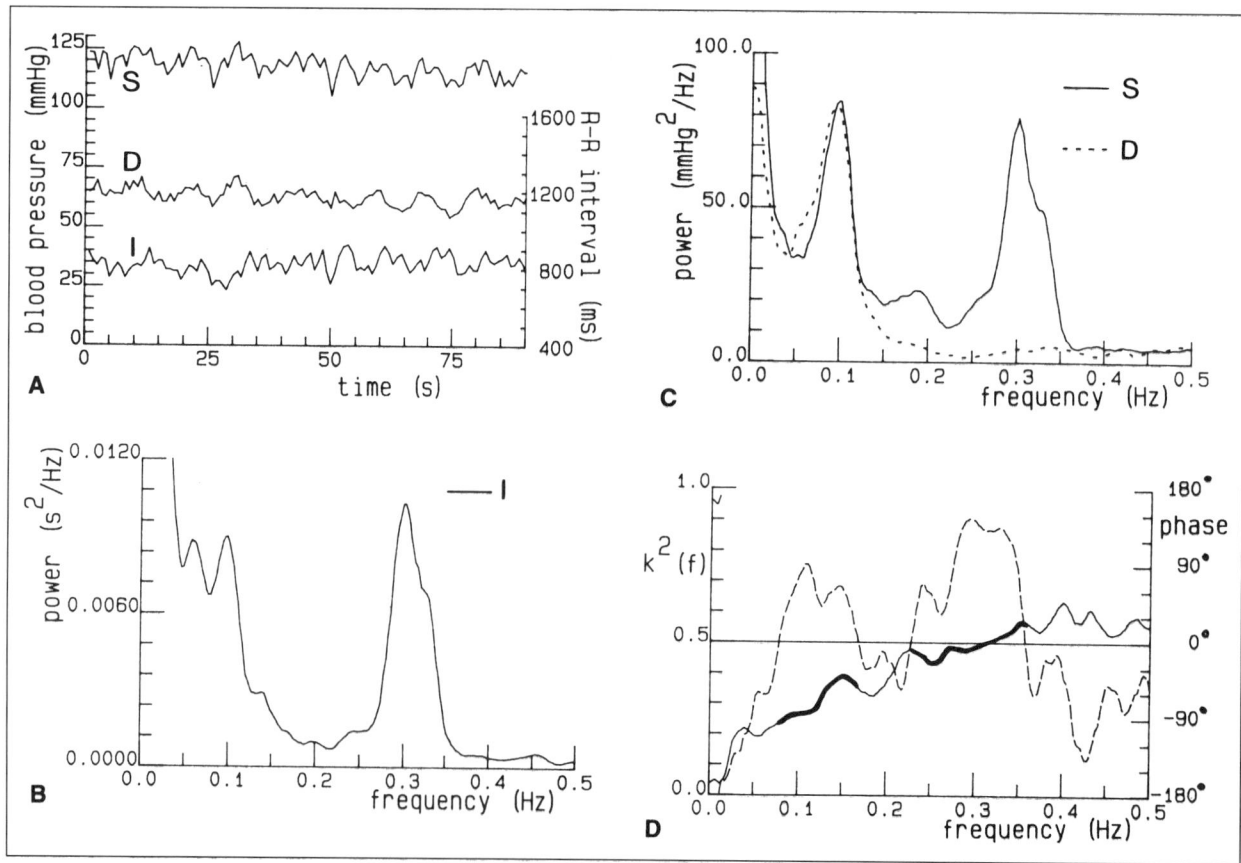

FIG. 9. A: Data set as in Fig. 2, subjected to spectral analysis in the remainder of this figure. **B:** Power spectrum of interval variability (950 beats; mean interval duration, 820 msec). **C:** Power spectra of systolic pressures (S) and diastolic pressures (D). **D:** Squared coherence spectrum [$k^2(f)$] (*broken line*, values between 0 and 1) and phase spectrum (*solid line*, values between −180° and +180°. If $k^2(f)$ is sufficiently large, the phase can be reliably estimated and is printed in a *heavy line*. From DeBoer et al. (13), with permission.

ging" becomes a matter of interpretation, not of mathematics. Obviously, the phase relationship between two sinusoids can only make sense if coherence is sufficiently high to be of statistical significance. In Fig. 9D, therefore, the phase curve is drawn in heavy lines in the regions where coherence is >0.5 (i.e., correlation >0.7) (14). Phase in other parts of the curve is insufficiently determined to warrant correct interpretation.

Regarding the underlying theory and the techniques for computing cross-spectra, readers are referred to the literature devoted to the topic (5,41). For the purposes of this chapter, it is sufficient to have a general understanding of the implications of phase and coherence between two related signals.

FREQUENCY ANALYSIS OF HEART RATE AND BLOOD PRESSURE VARIABILITY: PHYSIOLOGIC INTERPRETATION

As stated at the beginning of this chapter, the above excursion into the technical aspect of spectral analysis was undertaken to establish and then interpret rhythms in BP and HR recordings. Figure 9 provides an example of these rhythms that have been detected by spectral analysis. In this figure, there are clear-cut frequency bands in the spectra of systolic BP and heart period at ~0.3 Hz, and these are coupled to respiration. Both spectra also show a peak in the midfrequency region of 0.1 Hz, but this is less easily understood. It is, obviously, one of these slower waves that is not coupled to respiration, making it a Mayer wave. These waves may also be observed at still lower frequencies than 0.1 Hz; however, the resolution of the present spectra is insufficient to elaborate the low-frequency band much further. Different explanations for more or less rhythmic physiologic activity at these slow rates have been advanced, such as temperature regulation (27) or respiratory variability (54) stemming from the properties of the chemoreflex system.

To interpret the rhythms in BP and heart period at 0.1 and 0.3 Hz, the phase relationships between these two signals can be investigated, as analyzed in Fig. 9D. The phase is negative for most of the spectrum, indicating that the systolic BP change is occurring before the heart period change. The phase curve crosses the zero line at ~0.3 Hz; here, both signals are in phase. However, it must now be determined how both signals have been assigned to their places on the time-number or beat-number axis. Figure 10 shows the convention that is used to work out this problem: the systolic, mean, and diastolic BP values are assigned the same number as the duration of the heart period in which they occur. Actually, systolic pressure values precede the end of the heart period by a variable amount of time, depending on the HR. The lower the HR is, the longer is this time delay. Therefore, *in phase* means that respiratory changes in systolic BP may be followed by compensatory changes in the duration of the ongoing heart period. This interpretation is compatible with the delay that occurs between a change in baroreceptor afferent activity and vagally mediated heart period changes as it has been measured in humans (6). Base on this interpretation, we defend the idea that respiration influences BP first and then changes HR through a baroreceptor-mediated vagus nerve effect on the sinus node of the heart (14). However, this view is at variance with experimental results obtained in animals, notably in dogs (1). The emerging opinion on this issue is that this phenomenon represents a true species difference in that the respiratory cycle in dogs is accompanied

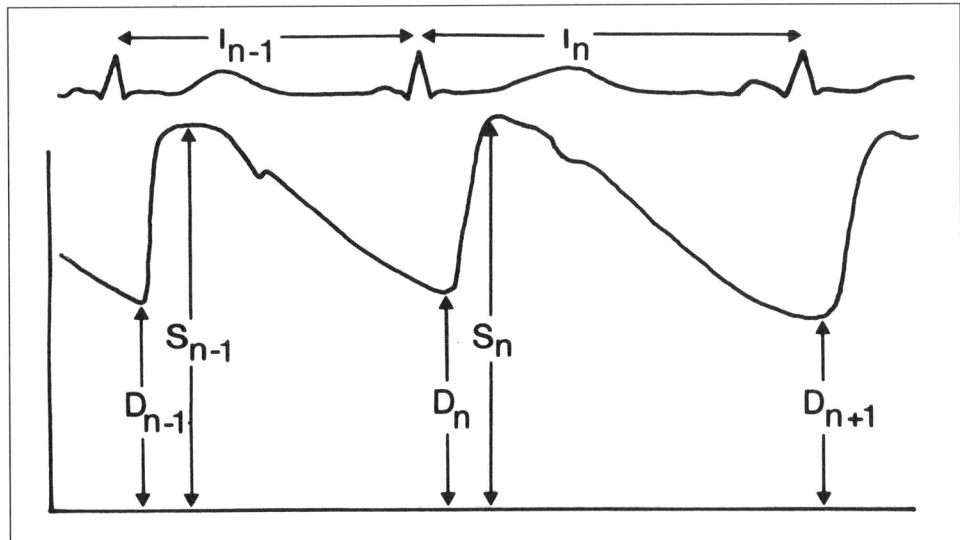

FIG. 10. Notation as used in our work. Systolic pressure (Sn) and diastolic pressure (Dn) occur during interval In. In the data set entered into spectral analysis programs, all events with index "n" are considered to have occurred at the same moment. Adapted from DeBoer (11), with permission.

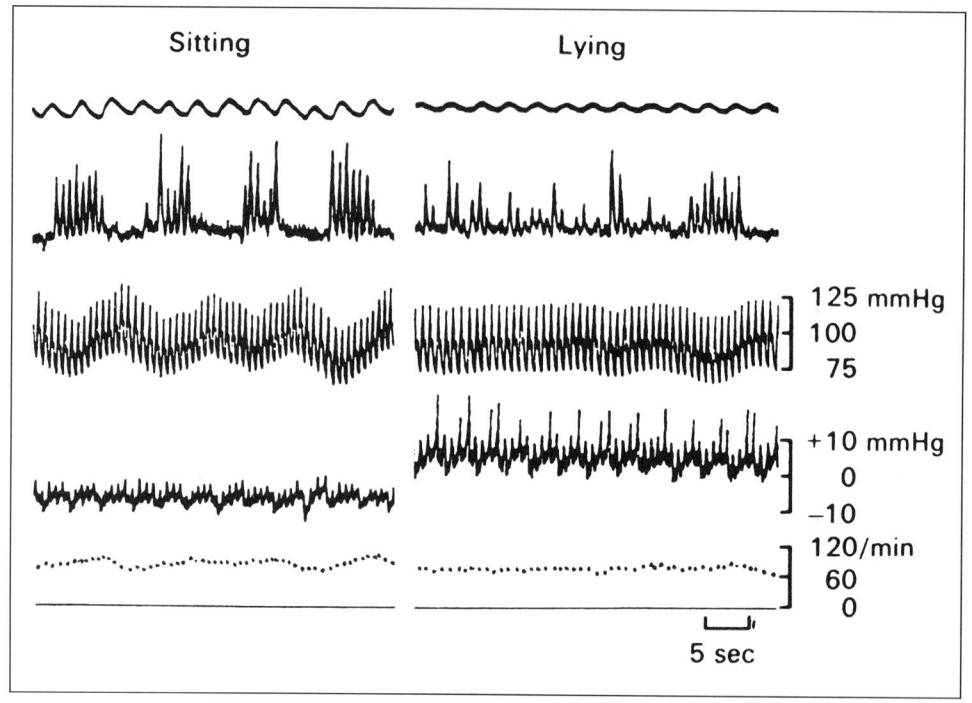

FIG. 11. Experimental records obtained in an awake human test subject in sitting and lying positions. Traces from *top to bottom*: trace 1, respiratory movement; trace 2, integrated muscle sympathetic activity; trace 3, intraarterial blood pressure; trace 4, central venous pressure; and trace 5, heart rate. Each upward deflection in the sympathetic activity represents a burst of action potentials in one or a few nerve fibers of the peroneal nerve at the fibular head. The nerve has been impaled by a percutaneous tungsten microelectrode. From Burke et al. (7), with permission.

by strong, centrally mediated vagus nerve effects on HR (1,4,15).

It is more difficult to find an explanation for the 0.1-Hz rhythm in BP and HR, as a 10-sec oscillator does not appear to exist. Periodicities are common phenomena in many physiologic systems, from contraction of parts of the gastrointestinal system to periodic changes in the local perfusion of many tissues (29). However, this global rhythm in both BP and HR, because of its frequency, can be caused only by neural mechanisms, as the liberation of hormones such as epinephrine or renin could produce only much slower rhythms.

When examining the phase relation between BP and heart period at 0.1 Hz (see Fig. 9D), the BP increments are noted to precede the prolongations in heart period by ~60°. In other words, this represents one-sixth of the cycle of 10 sec or 1.7 sec (ignoring the previously mentioned problem of the exact timing of the different phenomena in the cardiac cycle). Such a time delay is still compatible with a baroreflex action, now mainly acting through the sympathetic nervous system. The time delay from the sympathetic nerve activation to the ensuing change in HR is known to take ~1–2 sec (6). However, a parasympathetic contribution to this part of the baroreflex feedback cannot be ruled out by this reasoning. Moreover, studies in which test subjects received a muscarinic receptor blockade have shown that this intervention not only nullifies the HR variability at the respiratory frequency but also reduces the variability in the 0.1-Hz region (1,58). This demonstrates that parasympathetic activity contributes to HR variability over the entire spectrum, up to the respiratory frequency, while the sympathetic system's contribution is restricted to the lower frequencies.

Now that the 0.1-Hz rhythm in HR as a consequence of the underlying BP rhythm has been dealt with, the mechanism of BP variability will be discussed. The literature on the genesis of this rhythm is in uniform agreement that it must be due to generalized bursts of sympathetic vasomotor activity (31,34,46). Such generalized sympathetic outflow can be activated, both centrally in the brainstem and peripherally by disturbances in BP on the high- and low-pressure sides of the heart or by changes in the composition of the blood (pH, partial pressure of carbon dioxide, and oxygen saturation). All of these are signaled to the brainstem by afferent nerves and are known to reflexly alter sympathetic outflow. Such a multitude of different inputs, all impinging on one and the same output channel, would, at first sight, give rise to a BP pattern as noisy as the input activity itself. However, any change in vasomotor output activity that leads to a change in BP gives rise to feedback to the brainstem via the baroreceptor afferent nerves. By the same route, the baroreflex imposes its own timing properties on the eventual pattern of BP variability.

This effect requires explanation. If BP falls, stemming from a temporary lack of vasomotor activity, when someone stands or sits upright, the resulting decrease in baroreceptor afferent activity (from the high-pressure receptors and possibly also from the low-pressure receptors in the cardiopulmonary area) leads to a strong, synchronized increase in vasomotor activity. BP starts to rise ~2 sec later, switching off the sympathetic nerve activity induced by the baroreceptor reflex. However, the response in the vascular smooth muscle has only begun: BP continues to rise for a couple of seconds, although the baroreflex no longer prompts this action. Therefore, BP overshoots and then starts to fall, all without very much ongoing sympathetic nerve activity. Finally BP drops below some (baroreflex) activation level and the whole cycle is repeated. Such a pattern in sympathetic nerve activity has been observed in transcutaneous microneurographic studies done in healthy subjects. Figure 11 from Burke et al. (7) provides an example of this pattern. This represents a mechanism by which the baroreflex may impose a specific rhythm on more or less randomly occurring BP disturbances (14).

CARDIOVASCULAR CONTROL AS A WELL-DEFINED BUT POORLY PREDICTABLE SYSTEM: NOISE, PEAKS, AND FRACTALS

From daily practice, we know many systems that, on a detailed scale, are governed by simple and well-known laws of physics, yet the total system is made up of so many interacting subsystems that the overall behavior is poorly predictable. A good example is the weather: predictions over longer periods are bound to fail, and even tomorrow's weather forecast has limited value.

The cardiovascular control system is one in the ranks of more or less well-defined but poorly predictable systems. History of a person's HR and BP up till now can only help predict future HR and BP to a certain degree. Still, we know for a fact that the system will remain within reasonable boundaries set by physiology. Some diseases may reduce this unpredictability: it is not uncommon for patients in the coronary care unit to have very stable HR and BP over a long period after a myocardial infarction. In cardiology, an increasing number of publications indicate that 24-hr HR variability around the day of discharge is a good predictor for the eventual outcome of recovery (10,28,32). In addition, the presence or absence of high-frequency variability (vagus nerve activity) has predictive value, probably reflecting a good baroreceptor to HR reflex (16) (cf. the previous section on cross-spectral analysis of HR and BP variability). In view of the inherent ethical problems and technical difficulties, 24-hr BP_{BB} variability has not yet been studied in this context.

The complex of low frequencies (as observed in Fig. 9) has, formerly, been considered as unwanted noise rather than as a useful signal. In chaos analysis, one way to look at the overall aspect of a spectrum is by measuring power (variance) and frequency on logarithmic scales. Then, almost a straight line appears for HR variability spectra: there is a "1/f" relationship between the two. This relationship holds true for very long-lasting recordings (45): the longer the recording is, the more very low frequency power is found. Such behavior is known from many systems that can be described by fractals. Most of us will know fractals from the mind-boggling pictures produced by so-called "Mandelbrot sets": sets of simple drawing rules that may define outlines like tree branchings and coastal area formations [cf. Goldberger et al. (20)]. A property of fractals is their scaling phenomenon: when we increase the magnification of a fractal figure, we see more or less the same pattern as on the coarser scale. To a certain degree, this can be seen in HR recordings as well: the "jumpy" aspect of a 24-hr recording (Fig. 1) is not very much different from a recording on a much more detailed time scale, as in Fig. 2.

By chaos analysis, one can derive various measures from the signal to be analyzed, all indicating the level of inherent complexity of the signal and/or its degree of unpredictability (26). A frequently used measure is the *dimension* of the signal (be it fractal dimension or otherwise defined), which can be considered as the minimum number of independent underlying variables that are required to explain the signal as is. The lower the dimension is, the simpler is the signal. One of the publications along these lines analyzed the HR variability of aging men and women and asked in the title "Are women more complex than men?" (44). Alternatively, in diseased states as just described, one would expect the dimension to be lower as well (50).

FREQUENCY ANALYSIS OF HEART RATE AND BLOOD PRESSURE VARIABILITY: CLINICAL APPLICABILITY

The preceding description has shown what may be learned about BP regulation in normal, healthy subjects through frequency analysis of HR and BP variability. This technique has led to new insights into cardiovascular control and the interaction of the different mechanisms involved (1,4,14,42,47). Spectral analysis may also be used to study the involvement of the autonomic nervous system in the evolution of diseased states (9,30,35). The question, however, is whether these techniques have a role in the clinical neurophysiology laboratory.

Many reports on HR variability suggest that information on autonomic balance is extracted from the relative amounts of power in the respiratory band (parasympathetic activity) and 0.1-Hz band (sympathetic activity) [see, e.g., Akselrod et al. (2) and Pagani et al. (35)]. Chapter 24 by Freeman also hints that spectral analysis of HR variability is possibly superior to the use of simple statistical measures, such as standard deviation, maximal beat-to-beat change in the RR interval, and other, more complicated derived measures. Spectral analysis provides a comprehensive view of almost any variability measure that can be derived from a signal. Large, resting, beat-to-beat variations, for example, will show up as high-frequency variability on the order of the respiratory frequency or higher. The above explanation agrees with the conclusion reached by Freeman that such large short-term variations are proof of parasympathetic activity (excluding arrhythmias caused by cardiac disorders).

Is it possible to draw conclusions about the status of autonomic balance from the ratio of high-frequency to midfrequency power in the HR variability spectrum? It follows from the analysis already presented in this chapter that this claim is based on oversimplification: HR variability is, for the most part, the reflection of underlying BP variability operating by way of the baroreflex. If the causal BP variations are not taken into account, conclusions based on the HR variations alone may be spurious (56). This may also be true for the measurement of HR variability in the early diagnosis of autonomic neuropathy in diabetes, as has been proposed (9,51,60). Moreover, now that the noninvasive measurement of continuous BP has become easily available [with the Finapres device, i.e., photoplethysmographic BP recording (25)], neglecting the BP variability is no longer acceptable.

The next question is whether there is a clinical role for the spectral analysis of cardiovascular variability if beat-to-beat BP can be recorded. There is growing literature on this subject (21,36,37,39,60). Certain stresses, such as standing, induce an increase in the mean HR by increasing sympathetic and decreased parasympathetic outflow to the sinus node; at the same time, vasomotor activity is also increased. In the power spectrum, these changes are manifested as an overall decreased HR variability, specifically in the respiratory band (parasympathetic withdrawal) and an increased midfrequency variability (at ~0.1 Hz), most conspicuous in BP readings (39,60). In this respect, spectral analysis may help in the interpretation of observed changes in the pattern of BP and HR.

In many applications, spectral analysis has, for obvious reasons, been restricted to HR variability only. The statement in many such reports that high-frequency variability represents vagal, low frequency sympathetic outflow is incorrect. Low-frequency BP variability is sympathetically mediated, but, at that frequency HR, is under the combined control of vagus and sympathetics. This implies that the proportion of low-frequency to high-frequency variability cannot be used as a sure measure of *sympathovagal balance*.

When examining the current clinical applications of spectral analysis, two fields can be identified: on the one hand, suspected autonomic neuropathy or related problems, as in diabetes (51,59), and, on the other hand, general cardiovascular regulatory deficiencies, based on underlying conditions like congestive heart failure (10,28,32) or neonatal distress (3,43).

In the case of autonomic neuropathy, spectral analysis has mostly been applied to severe cases of mainly vagus nerve deficiency, where various HR-derived measures, including spectral analysis, are used to detect abnormalities. However, vigorous tests of the specificity and sensitivity of diagnosis by spectral analysis alone have, to my knowledge, not been undertaken. Two reports that came close to this (9,19) compared the classic battery of tests for diabetic autonomic neuropathy with newer spectral measures. Especially the effects on high-frequency power correlated well with tests like deep breathing (as expected). A more recent study (49) showed that in healthy humans all vagal nerve-related HR measures decline with age, including high-frequency spectral power.

The study of general cardiovascular regulatory properties by spectral analysis and related techniques (chaos analysis; cf. earlier in this chapter) has, thus far, produced less clear-cut results. HR variability analysis is, especially in cardiology, being used for risk stratification. However, the detected correlation between poor prognosis and low HR variability is still at the level of statistics more than at that of pathophysiology. In part, low HR variability can be due to low baroreflex sensitivity and, in the view of some authors this is the real underlying problem, correlating better with eventual outcome (16,17). Since baroreflex sensitivity is measured as the amount of heart period change per BP change (ms/mm Hg), it is still mainly the beneficial effects on the heart of vagus nerve activity that are being measured. However, this does not account for the correlation between low HR variability in all frequency areas and all-cause mortality in a 4-year follow-up study of 736 subjects who had a Holter-monitoring session as part of the Framingham study (53).

In clinical practice, diagnostic tests yield a result for one individual at one moment under standardized circumstances. In view of the above-described difficulties in the technique of spectral estimation, it is doubtful that power spectral analysis of spontaneous HR or BP variability, or both, will soon become routine clinical tests. In most studies, group averages and correlation techniques have been used, with the use of spectral analysis. The inherent variability of the method makes application to a specific case in one brief recording a hazardous approach. However, power spectral analysis may be of help in quantifying the induced variability in paced-breathing tests (38), where the pacing frequency may be set to emphasize the frequency bands of vagal or combined vagal–sympathetic branch of autonomic control of HR. Furthermore, HR variability in 24-hr Holter recordings may be analyzed by time–frequency analysis techniques as is discussed in Chapter 26. This analysis avoids the problem of variability in one spectrum of spontaneous HR variations by computing many spectra of slightly overlapping segments from a 24-hr recording. Apart from providing insight into the overall activity of the autonomic nervous system, this might also help to detect conspicuous low-frequency variability during sleep, indicative of periods of sleep apnea (55).

REFERENCES

1. Akselrod S, et al. Hemodynamic regulation: investigation by spectral analysis. *Am J Physiol* 1985;249:H867–H875.
2. Akselrod S, et al. Power spectrum analysis of heart rate fluctuation: a quantitative probe of beat-to-beat cardiovascular control. *Science* 1981;213:220–222.
3. Baldzer K, et al. Heart rate variability analysis in full-term infants: spectral indices for study of neonatal cardiorespiratory control. *Pediatr Res* 1989;26:188–195.
4. Baselli G, et al. Cardiovascular variability signals: towards the identification of a closed-loop model of the neural control mechanisms. *IEEE Trans Biomed Eng* 1988;35:1033–1046.
5. Bendat JS, Piersol AG. *Random data: analysis and measurement procedures.* New York: Wiley Interscience, 1971.
6. Borst C, Karemaker JM. Time delays in the human baroreceptor reflex. *J Auton Nerv Syst* 1983;9:399–409.
7. Burke D, Sundlof G, Wallin G. Postural effects on muscle nerve sympathetic activity in man. *J Physiol (Lond)* 1977;272:399–414.
8. Camm AJ, et al. Heart rate variability: standards of measurement, physiological interpretation, and clinical use [Review]. *Circulation* 1996;93:1043–1065.
9. Comi G, et al. Spectral analysis of short-term heart rate variability in diabetic patients. *J Auton Nerv Syst* 1990;30(Suppl):S45–S49.
10. Dambrink JH, et al. Association between reduced heart rate variability and left ventricular dilatation in patients with a first anterior myocardial infarction: CATS Investigators—Captopril and Thrombolysis Study. *Br Heart J* 1994;72:514–520.
11. DeBoer RW. *Beat-to-beat blood-pressure fluctuations and heart-rate variability in man: physiological relationships, analysis techniques and a simple model* [Thesis]. Amsterdam: University of Amsterdam, 1985.
12. DeBoer RW, Karemaker JM, Strackee J. Comparing spectra of a series of point events particularly for heart rate variability data. *IEEE Trans Biomed Eng* 1984;31:384–387.
13. DeBoer RW, Karemaker JM, Strackee J. Determination of baroreflex sensitivity by spectral analysis of spontaneous blood-pressure and heart-rate fluctuations in man. In: Lown B, Malliani A, Prosdocimi M, eds. *Neural mechanisms and cardiovascular disease.* Padova: Liviana, 1986:303–315.
14. DeBoer RW, Karemaker JM, Strackee J. Hemodynamic fluctuations and baroreflex sensitivity in humans: a beat-to-beat model. *Am J Physiol* 1987;253:H680–H689.
15. DeBoer RW, Karemaker JM, Strackee J. On the spectral analysis of blood pressure variability. *Am J Physiol* 1986;251:H685–H687.
16. De Ferrari GM, et al. Baroreflex sensitivity, but not heart rate variability, is reduced in patients with life-threatening ventricular arrhythmias long after myocardial infarction. *Am Heart J* 1995;130:473–480.
17. Farrell TG, et al. Prognostic value of baroreflex sensitivity testing after acute myocardial infarction. *Br Heart J* 1992;67:129–137.
18. Fernandez de Molina A, Perl ER. Sympathetic activity and the systemic circulation in the spinal cat. *J Physiol (Lond)* 1965;181:82–102.
19. Freeman R, et al. Spectral analysis of heart rate in diabetic autonomic neuropathy: a comparison with standard tests of autonomic function. *Arch Neurol* 1991;48:185–190.
20. Goldberger AL, Rigney DR, West BJ. Chaos and fractals in human physiology. *Sci Am* 1990;262:42–49.
21. Gordon D, et al. Heart-rate spectral analysis: a noninvasive probe of cardiovascular regulation in critically ill children with heart disease. *Pediatr Cardiol* 1988;9:69–77.
22. Hering E. *Sitzungsberichte der mathematisch-naturwissenschaftlichen classe der kaiserlichen akademie der wissenschaften LX.* Band II 1869;60:829–856.
23. Heymans C, Neil E. *Reflexogenic areas of the cardiovascular system.* London: J & A Churchill, 1958.
24. Hyndman BW, Kitney RI, Sayers BM. Spontaneous rhythms in physiological control systems. *Nature* 1971;233:339–341.
25. Imholz BP, et al. Continuous finger arterial pressure: utility in the cardiovascular laboratory. *Clin Auton Res* 1991;1:43–53.
26. Kaplan D, Glass L. *Understanding nonlinear dynamics.* New York: Springer-Verlag, 1995.
27. Kitney RI. An analysis of the thermoregulatory influences on heart-rate variability. In: Kitney RI, Rompelman O, eds. *The study of heart-rate variability.* Oxford: Clarendon, 1980:81–106.
28. Kleiger RE, et al. Decreased heart rate variability and its association with increased mortality after acute myocardial infarction. *Am J Cardiol* 1987;59:256–262.
29. Koepchen HP. History and studies of concepts in blood-pressure waves. In: Miyakawa K, Koepchen HP, Polosa C, eds. *Mechanisms of blood pressure waves.* Berlin: Springer-Verlag, 1984:3–23.
30. Lipsitz LA, et al. Spectral characteristics of heart rate variability before and during postural tilt: relations to aging and risk of syncope. *Circulation* 1990;81:1803–1810.
31. Lombardi F, et al. Spectral analysis of sympathetic discharge in decerebrate cats. *J Auton Nerv Syst* 1990;30(Suppl):S97–S99.
32. Malik M, Camm AJ. Significance of long term components of heart rate variability for the further prognosis after acute myocardial infarction. *Cardiovasc Res* 1990;24:793–803.
33. Mayer S. *Studien zur Physiologie des Herzens und der Blutgefässe;* vol 5: *Über spontane Blutdruckschwankungen.* Vienna: Sber. math.-naturw. Cl. Akad. Wiss., 1876;74:281–307.
34. Pagani M, et al. Power spectral analysis of heart rate and arterial pressure variabilities as a marker of sympatho-vagal interaction in man and conscious dog. *Circ Res* 1986;59:178–193.
35. Pagani M, et al. Power spectral density of heart rate variability as an index of sympatho-vagal interaction in normal and hypertensive subjects. *J Hypertens Suppl* 1984;2:S383–S385.
36. Pagani M, et al. Spectral analysis of R-R and arterial pressure variabilities to assess sympatho-vagal interaction during mental stress in humans. *J Hypertens Suppl* 1989;7:S14–S15.
37. Pagani M, et al. Sympathovagal interaction during mental stress: a study using spectral analysis of heart rate variability in healthy control subjects and patients with a prior myocardial infarction. *Circulation* 1991;83(Suppl 2):II-43–II-51.
38. Patwardhan AR, et al. Voluntary control of breathing does not alter vagal modulation of heart rate. *J Appl Physiol* 1995;78:2087–2094.
39. Pomeranz B, et al. Assessment of autonomic function in humans by heart rate spectral analysis. *Am J Physiol* 1985;248:H151–H153.
40. Preiss G, Polosa C. Patterns of sympathetic neuron activity associated with Mayer waves. *Am J Physiol* 1974;226:724–730.
41. Press WH, et al. *Numerical recipes: the art of scientific computing.* Cambridge: Cambridge University Press, 1987.
42. Robbe HW, et al. Assessment of baroreceptor reflex sensitivity by means of spectral analysis. *Hypertension* 1987;10:538–543.
43. Rother M, et al. Objective characterization and differentiation of sleep states in healthy newborns and newborns-at-risk by spectral analysis of heart rate and respiration rhythms. *Acta Physiol Hung* 1988;71:383–393.
44. Ryan SM, et al. Gender- and age-related differences in heart rate dynamics: are women more complex than men? *J Am Coll Cardiol* 1994;24:1700–1707.
45. Saul JP, et al. Analysis of long term heart rate variability: methods, 1/f scaling and implications. *Comp Cardiol* 1988;14:419–422.
46. Saul JP, et al. Heart rate and muscle sympathetic nerve variability during reflex changes of autonomic activity. *Am J Physiol* 1990;258:H713–H721.
47. Saul JP, et al. Transfer function analysis of the circulation: unique insights into cardiovascular regulation. *Am J Physiol* 1991;261:H1231–H1245.
48. Schweitzer A. Rhythmical fluctuations of the arterial blood pressure. *J Physiol (Lond)* 1945;104:25P(abst).
49. Sega S, Jager F, Kiauta T. A comparison of cardiovascular reflex tests and spectral analysis of heart rate variability in healthy subjects. *Clin Auton Res* 1993;3:175–182.
50. Signorini MG, et al. Non-linear dynamics of cardiovascular variability signals. *Methods Inf Med* 1994;33:81–84.
51. Thomaseth K, et al. Heart rate spectral analysis for assessing autonomic regulation in diabetic patients. *J Auton Nerv Syst* 1990;30(Suppl):S169–S171.

52. Traube L. Ueber periodische Thätigkeits-Aeusserungen des vasomotorischen und Hemmungs-Nervencentrums. *Centralbl Med Wiss* 1865;3:881–885.
53. Tsuji H, et al. Reduced heart rate variability and mortality risk in an elderly cohort: the Framingham Heart Study. *Circulation* 1994;90:878–883.
54. Van den Aardweg JG, Karemaker JM. Respiratory variability and associated cardiovascular changes in adults at rest [Review]. *Clin Physiol* 1991;11:95–118.
55. Van den Aardweg JG, van Steenwijk RP, Karemaker JM. A chemoreflex model of relation between blood pressure and heart rate in sleep apnea syndrome. *Am J Physiol* 1995;268:H2145–H2156.
56. Van Lieshout JJ, et al. Pitfalls in the assessment of cardiovascular reflexes in patients with sympathetic failure but intact vagal control. *Clin Sci (Colch)* 1989;76:523–528.
57. Van Montfrans GA. *Continuous ambulatory blood pressure registration in uncomplicated hypertension: cuff-responders and blood pressure variability* [Thesis]. Amsterdam: University of Amsterdam, 1984.
58. Weise F, Baltrusch K, Heydenreich F. Effect of low-dose atropine on heart rate fluctuations during orthostatic load: a spectral analysis. *J Auton Nerv Syst* 1989;26:223–230.
59. Weise F, Heydenreich F. A non-invasive approach to cardiac autonomic neuropathy in patients with diabetes mellitus. *Clin Physiol* 1990;10:137–145.
60. Weise F, Heydenreich F, Runge U. Contributions of sympathetic and vagal mechanisms to the genesis of heart rate fluctuations during orthostatic load: a spectral analysis. *J Auton Nerv Syst* 1987;21:127–134.

CHAPTER 26

Time–Frequency Analysis of Cardiovascular Function and Its Clinical Applications

Vera Novak, Peter Novak, and Phillip A. Low

1. Beat-to-beat rhythms in heart rate and blood pressure are divided into oscillations at respiratory frequencies (RFs) and slower nonrespiratory frequencies (NONRFs) with periods from 30 sec to 1 min.
2. The heart rate oscillations at RF match the actual breathing frequency. Their amplitude increases at larger tidal volumes and decreases at faster breathing rate. The maximum power is found at frequencies ~0.1 Hz (6 breaths/min). Respiratory oscillations in heart rate are a good estimate of cardiovagal activity.
3. The slow non-RF rhythms in blood pressure are related to vasomotor sympathetic activity. The slow rhythms in heart rate (<0.08 Hz) are influenced by a combination of the sympathetic, parasympathetic, and baroreceptor inputs. The amplitude of vasomotor blood pressure rhythms increases during sympathetic activation on assuming the upright posture (with tilt-up).
4. Mild orthostatic intolerance is characterized by lightheadedness, BP instability, and increased propensity to syncope. In the upright position, a transient blood pressure drop, mild tachycardia, and reduction in both respiratory and nonrespiratory rhythms in heart rate occur. Slow vasomotor rhythms disappear before the onset of vasodepressor syncope.
5. The subgroup of patients with florid postural orthostatic tachycardia syndrome, with a heart rate of >120 beats/min when upright, often suffer from a peripheral autonomic neuropathy with peripheral adrenergic and sudomotor failure. Spectral analysis shows a severe reduction of both respiratory and non-respiratory oscillations in RR interval (RRI), down to <30% of normal values. Sympathetic vasomotor rhythms are initially exaggerated on tilt-up. The increment of total peripheral resistance is abnormal, being either absent or exaggerated but poorly sustained.
6. An overall loss of rhythmicity affecting both RF and NONRF oscillations in RRI is a hallmark of effector failure (e.g., in heart failure) or central generator failure (brainstem damage). In contrast, vasomotor sympathetic blood pressure rhythms, which are generated by a medullary circuitry, remain present.
7. Spectral analysis of RRI in the peripheral neuropathies, such as diabetic neuropathy, correlates well with other indices of autonomic neuropathy. The reduction of respiratory powers in the heart rate correlates well with the severity of cardiovagal failure. Its role in clinical evaluation of clinical trials is not yet well defined.
8. Classic methods of spectral analysis like Fourier transform (FFT) or autoregressive modeling are adequate for the analysis of the stationary data, but are inadequate for the analysis of the rapid changes in signal structure, including the change from the supine rest to standing. Instead, time–frequency distributions are needed (like Wigner distribution, moving periodogram, dynamic autoregressive modeling, and wavelet transform).
9. Standardization is needed for spectral analysis in clinical trials and the clinical laboratory. The minimal duration of recording is 5–10 min. Respiration should always be recorded unless breathing frequency is paced. Data processing requires an optimal sampling rate of 250 Hz, the removal of bad points (artifacts, outliers, and extrasystoles), and a sufficiently broad-frequency band, including a cutoff frequency of <0.02 Hz.

V. Novak, P. Novak, and P. A. Low: Department of Neurology, Mayo Clinic and Foundation, Rochester, Minnesota 55905.

INTRODUCTION

In this chapter, we focus on a description and interpretation of the spontaneous oscillations in beat-to-beat heart rate, blood pressure, and respiration. Classic power-spectrum methods comprise fast Fourier transform (FFT) and the autoregressive model. Later in the chapter, we also discuss the advantages of the newer approach using time–frequency analysis. In the final section, we discuss the technical requirements needed for the standardization of spectral analysis for clinical purposes.

Briefly, Fourier power spectrum quantifies the proportion of one frequency relative to that of other frequencies in the signal. One spectrum is obtained from one data segment (Fig. 1). In the example presented in the Fig. 1, two frequencies are present in the signal (faster rhythm at 0.06 Hz and slower rhythm at 0.01 Hz). Two peaks corresponding to these frequencies can be seen in the Fourier spectrum. In contrast, the dynamic method of time–frequency analysis describes simultaneously both frequency and time components as well as a shift from the fast to the slower frequency. Numerous spectral estimations are obtained from the single time series, resulting in a time–frequency map. Time–frequency maps presented in our chapter were obtained by using the modified Wigner distribution (43).

Evaluation of heart rate variability as a diagnostic and prognostic tool is rapidly gaining attention in medicine. Results of power-spectrum analysis can be found in different medical specialties like cardiology, anesthesiology, cardiac

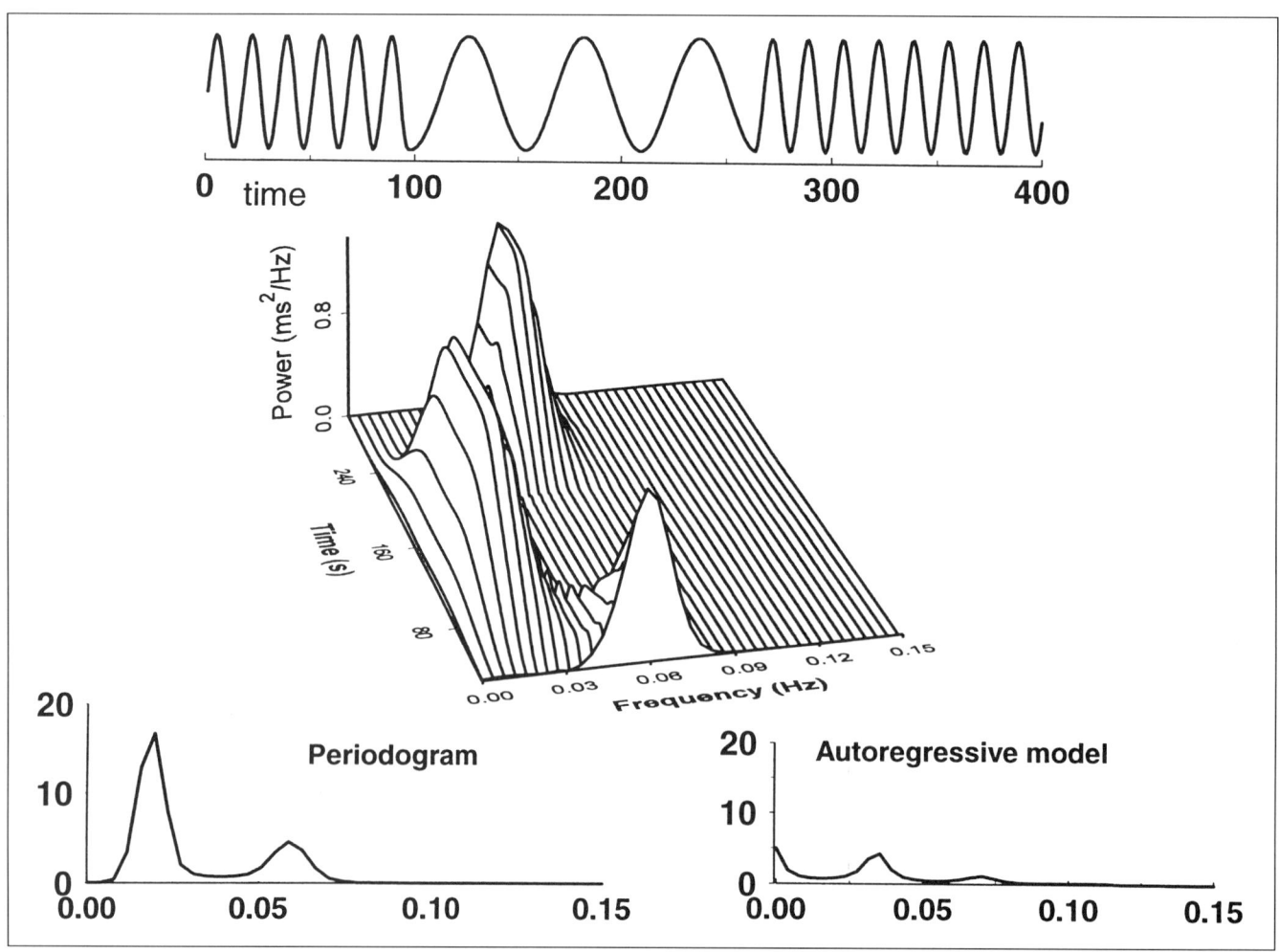

FIG. 1. Time series (*top*), Wigner map (*middle*), periodogram (*bottom left*), and autoregressive model (*bottom right*). An artificial signal is composed of the two frequencies, the faster at 0.06 Hz and slower at 0.01 Hz. In the global periodogram, both frequencies are represented accurately, but dynamic alterations, such as the change from the faster to the slower frequency, are not detected. A similar spectrum is obtained by using the autoregressive model, but an additional spurious harmonic faster frequency is present in the spectrum. The time–frequency distribution faithfully tracks the dynamic changes of the signal.

surgery, and neurology. The underlying interest in these studies is autonomic control of vital functions, crucial for patient well-being because the integrity of this regulation affects outcome. We will characterize the physiology and pathophysiology of the spontaneous slow and respiratory rhythms in heart rate and blood pressure. The slow oscillations at nonrespiratory frequencies (NONRFs) occur at frequencies between 0.01 to 0.15 Hz. These rhythms are independent of oscillations that are locked to the respiratory frequency (RF). It is generally accepted that the respiratory oscillations in RRI (RR interval) provide an accurate index of cardiovagal activity. The NONRF rhythms in blood pressure can serve as an indirect measure of the vasomotor sympathetic activity. The NONRF rhythms in heart rate reflect combined effects of sympathetic activity and baroreceptor feedback, but only partially reflect parasympathetic activity (2,3,20).

These rhythms represent primarily the peripheral response to central autonomic drive. The normal profile of cardiovascular rhythms changes in response to such variables as aging, a change of posture, and emotional state. Certain characteristic pathologic profiles can be identified, such as those of orthostatic intolerance, vasodepressor syncope, peripheral neuropathy, cardiac failure, and certain central nervous system (CNS) lesions.

CARDIOVASCULAR OSCILLATIONS DURING DEVELOPMENT AND AGING

Cardiovascular and other systems are continuously perturbed by two main rhythms, reflecting respiratory and vasomotor oscillations. Oscillations at RF are locked to the actual breathing frequency and can occur within the frequency range of 0.01–1.0 Hz. Both respiratory and vasomotor rhythms are present during early human development and can be detected even during fetal life from weeks 26 to 40 of gestation (51,63,64). During late gestation, between weeks 36 and 40, respiratory oscillations of RRI correspond to the fetal breathing movements (0.4–1.0 Hz) and are responsible for at least 20% of the total power. Low-frequency rhythms (~0.04 Hz) can also be identified. Spectral analysis of fetal heart rate by using the energy value and frequency in the faster (respiratory) frequency band enables the discrimination of fetal distress from the normal state. Typically, a loss of heart rate variability results in flat spectral maps that correlate with fetal distress and poor outcome (18,63).

After birth and during early childhood, relative sympathicotonia is often present. The breathing frequency is fast, and respiratory oscillations in RRI occur at frequencies of >0.4 Hz. Later on, during childhood and adult life, as the

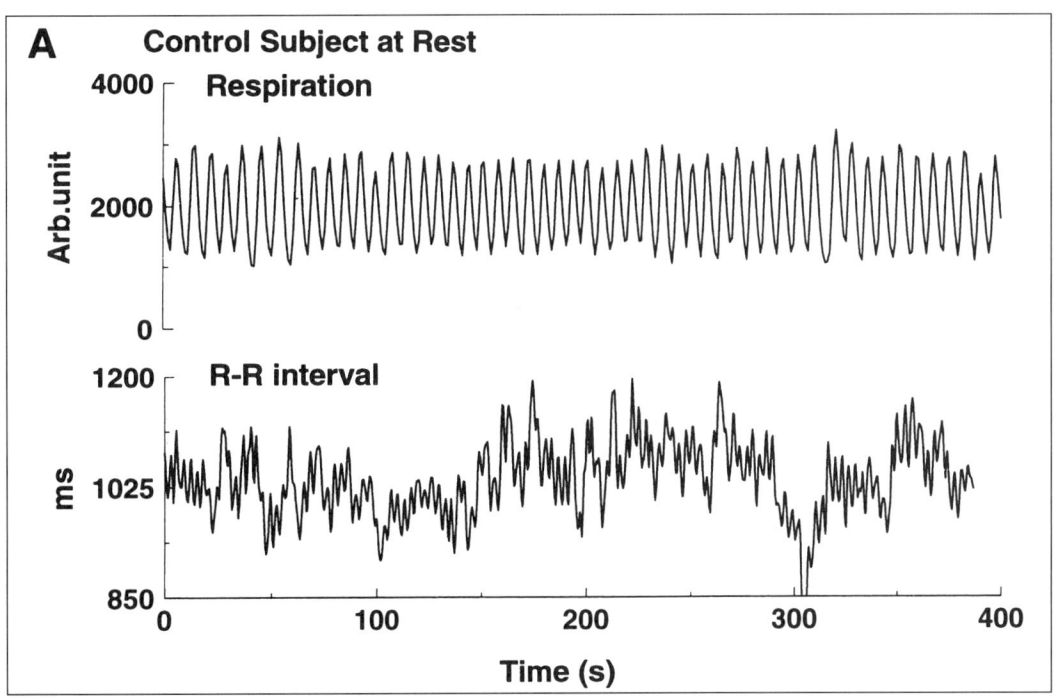

FIG. 2. A: Time series of respiration and RR intervals (RRIs) from a young healthy volunteer during rest while supine.

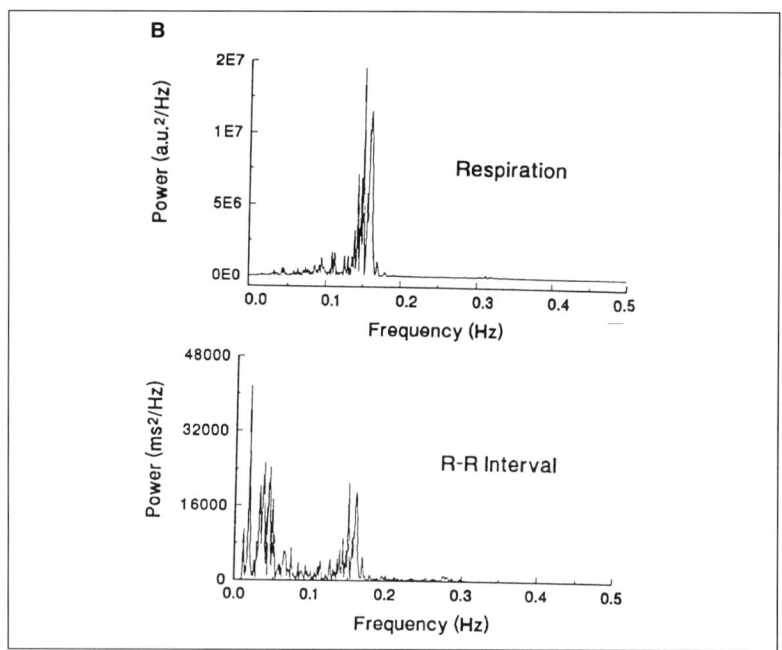

FIG. 2. B: The respiratory frequency remains stable, and the subject is breathing at a frequency of 0.15 Hz (9 breaths/min). The global periodogram of RRIs shows three distinct peaks (*bottom panel*). Thus, the occasional slowing of the nonrespiratory oscillations is represented as a distinct peak.

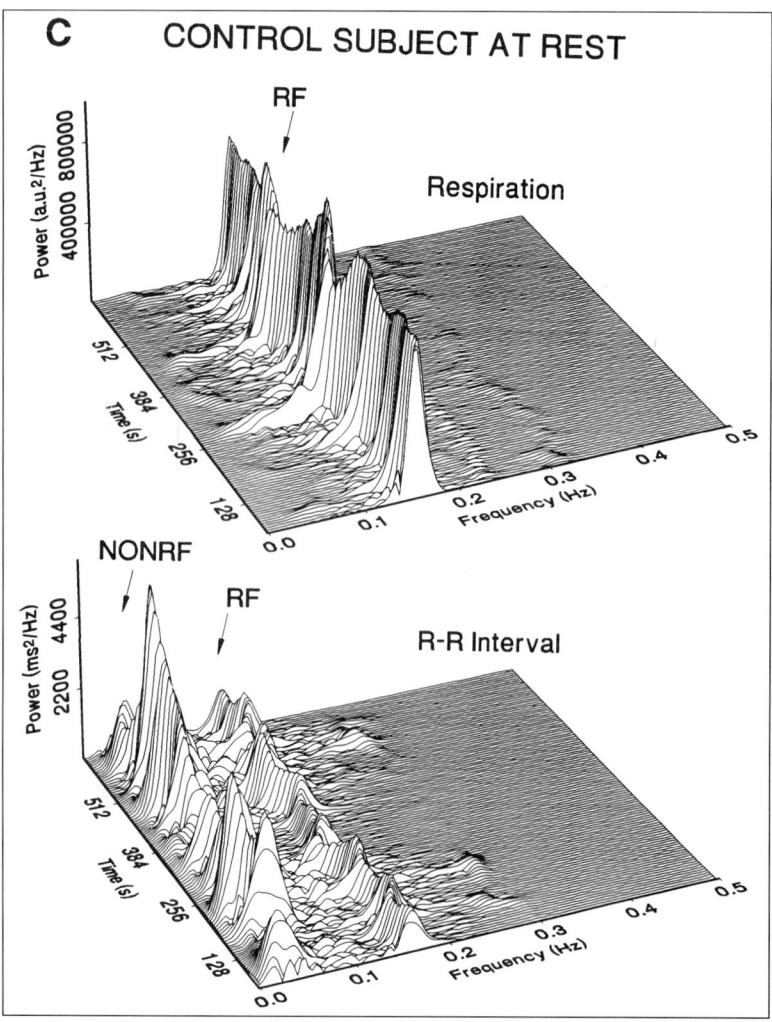

FIG. 2. C: Both RRI and respiratory variation are clearly represented on the time–frequency distribution. The respiratory oscillations are clearly represented in RRI and follow closely even a slight change of the breathing frequency. Slow nonrespiratory oscillations are also distinct.

breathing frequency slows, respiratory oscillations are present mainly in the 0.01- to 0.4-Hz range, with the median frequency at 0.2–0.3 Hz. During maturation of the autonomic nervous system in childhood and adolescence, sympathetic–parasympathetic balance becomes established. The maturation process is associated with development of the more complex dynamics of autonomic control, and different patterns of cardiovascular rhythms evolve. In general, children (aged 1–12 years) have greater heart rate variability and greater power at both low frequencies (0.01–0.05 Hz) and RFs (0.2–0.5 Hz) during supine rest than do adults. Respiratory power remains greater than in adults, even when standing. These results, as well as those of previous pharmacologic studies, suggest that sympathetic activity diminishes between 5 and 10 years of age, possibly associated with a slight decrease in parasympathetic activity as well (16,75).

The pattern of cardiovascular rhythms in young adults, between 20 to 40 years, is characterized by prominent RF and low-frequency oscillations in heart rate and blood pressure. Figure 2A shows data series of RRI and respiration obtained from a young adult during supine rest. From visual inspection of RRI signal, it is clear that oscillations are present at multiple frequencies. In the respiratory signal, only one dominant frequency is present. The global FFT spectrum shows one dominant frequency in the respiratory signal at 0.15 Hz (Fig. 2B). However, three peaks can be identified in the power spectrum of RRI, e.g., RF at 0.15 Hz and two peaks at NONRFs at 0.05 and 0.07 Hz. The dynamic time–frequency map (Fig. 2C) revealed that

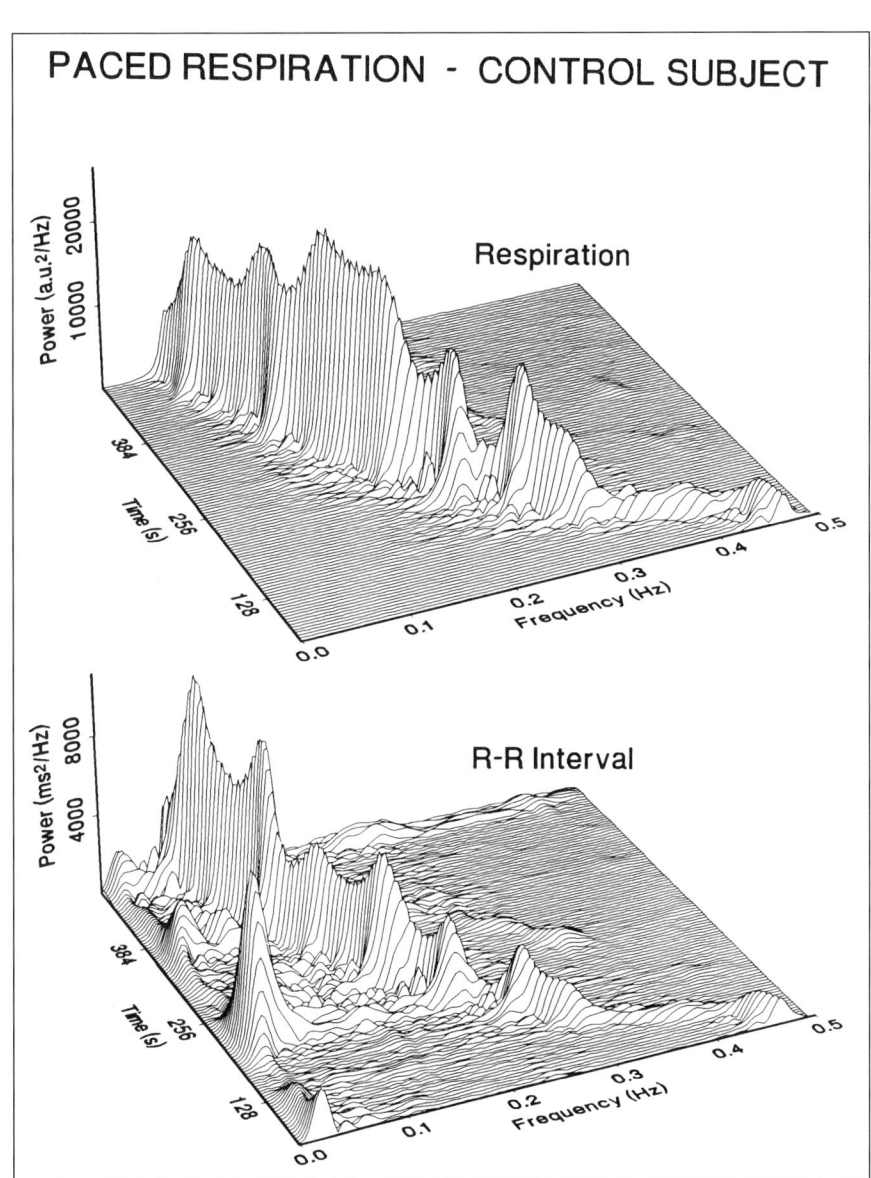

FIG. 3. In this study, the subject's respiration is paced. The breathing rate starts at fast frequencies (0.5 Hz; 120 breaths/min) and slows to 0.05 Hz (3 breaths/min). Note that respiratory oscillations in RR interval faithfully follow breathing rate over this wide range and that their amplitude largely increases at slower frequencies. (Reproduced from ref. 47).

there were indeed only two dominant rhythms in RRI. The first are respiratory oscillations at 0.15 Hz and follow even minor variations in RF. The second are nonrespiratory oscillations, present at a dominant frequency at 0.06 Hz and occasionally accelerating to faster frequencies. Occasional acceleration of the slow rhythm has been spuriously represented in the Fourier spectrum as an independent peak, since the global spectrum alone was not able to detect dynamics of faster changes. Thus, careful interpretation of data is needed because transient changes of the signal frequency may appear as an independent rhythm on the global spectra. The amplitude of respiratory oscillations in RRI is also proportional to the tidal volume and increases as breathing frequency slows. The maximal power is usually found at frequencies of 0.1 Hz (6 breaths/min). The tidal volume is also maximal at this frequency. Figure 3 demonstrates that, in normal young adults, respiratory oscillations in RRI closely follow the actual breathing frequency and amplitude. In this experiment, the subject was asked to synchronize his respiration with a tape playback. His breathing frequency started at 0.5 Hz (2 cycles/sec) and slowed to 0.07 Hz. This observation is clinically relevant, since, under normal conditions, respiratory oscillations can be present at very low frequencies during slow breathing, especially during sleep. Vasomotor rhythms occur mainly at frequencies of 0.01–0.1 Hz, with a dominant frequency at ~0.04 Hz. Multiple rhythms can be superimposed in the low-frequency range (0.01–0.08 Hz), resulting in a rich and complex pattern. These oscillations can be generated from the interaction of the multiple central generators within the brainstem. In addition, there is a significant contribution of the multiple feedback loops from both sympathetic and vagal portions of the baroreflex. The slow oscillations in RRI are partially dependent on the slow blood pressure rhythms, since a significant portion of slow RRI oscillations is generated in the baroreceptor feedback loop in response to the blood pressure alterations. The low-frequency oscillations in RRI are therefore not a reliable index of sympathetic activity, as was originally hoped (3), because of the multiple variables involved in their generation. These oscillations are also affected by variations in venous return, cardiac filling, and baroreflex feedback loop, and in cardiac sympathetic activity. In addition, muscle contraction, respiration, or responses to external stimuli can all contribute to the slow rhythms in this range.

Some questions exist as to the role of cardiac versus vasomotor sympathetic contributions to the slow rhythms. The distribution of the low-frequency powers in RRI suggests that these rhythms are partially generated by the blood pressure-mediated baroreflex loop and only partially through cardiac sympathetic activity (36). Moreover, comparison of positron-emission tomographic imaging of the heart with spectral analysis suggests that the low-frequency oscillations are not a specific index of cardiac sympathetic activity (12). In contrast to the nonspecificity of

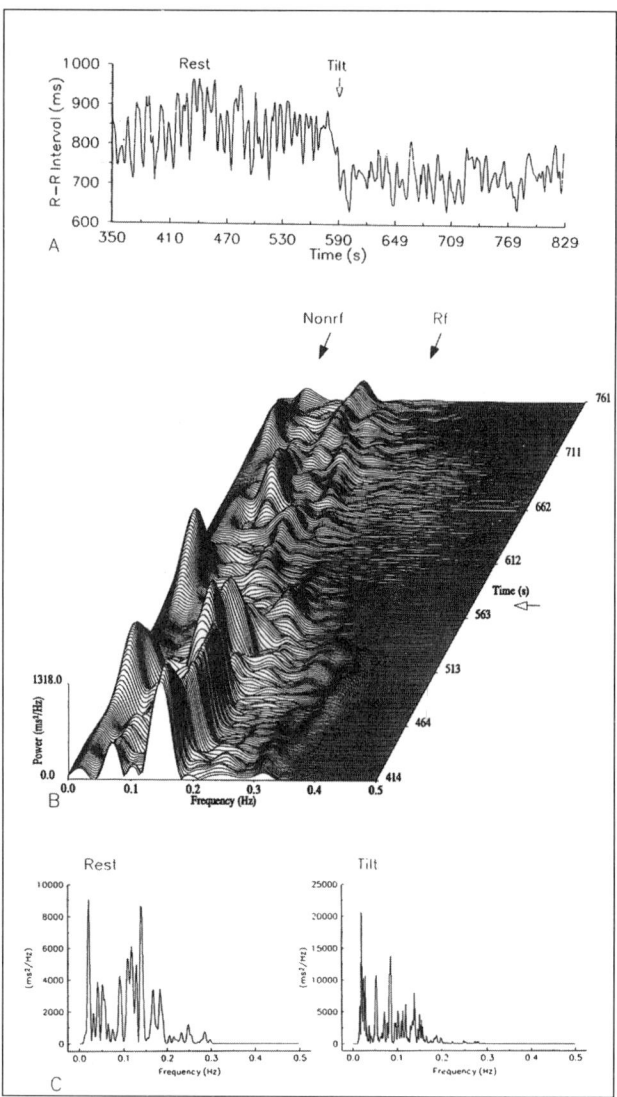

FIG. 4. Time series (*top*), time–frequency map (*middle*), and global spectrum (*bottom*). RR interval (RRI) from a young healthy volunteer during rest while supine, followed by upright tilt. Tilt-up (indicated by an *arrow*) is accompanied by a tachycardia and diminished respiratory oscillations in RRI. The nonrespiratory RRI oscillations at slow frequencies are regular and continuously present during the tilt. Their profile is less stable than when supine, and their frequency occasionally accelerated. The global spectrum shows two dominant peaks during rest. However, transient changes of the signal frequency are spuriously represented as additional peaks in the global spectrum. From Lepicovska et al. (32), with permission.

low-frequency oscillations in RRI, it has been well established that sympathetic vasomotor activity is well reflected in the slow blood pressure oscillations at frequencies of <0.08 Hz (36). These blood pressure rhythms are sensed by baroreceptors, which then contribute to the generation of slow heart rate variation. Slow heart rate rhythms serve to damp blood pressure oscillations generated by changes

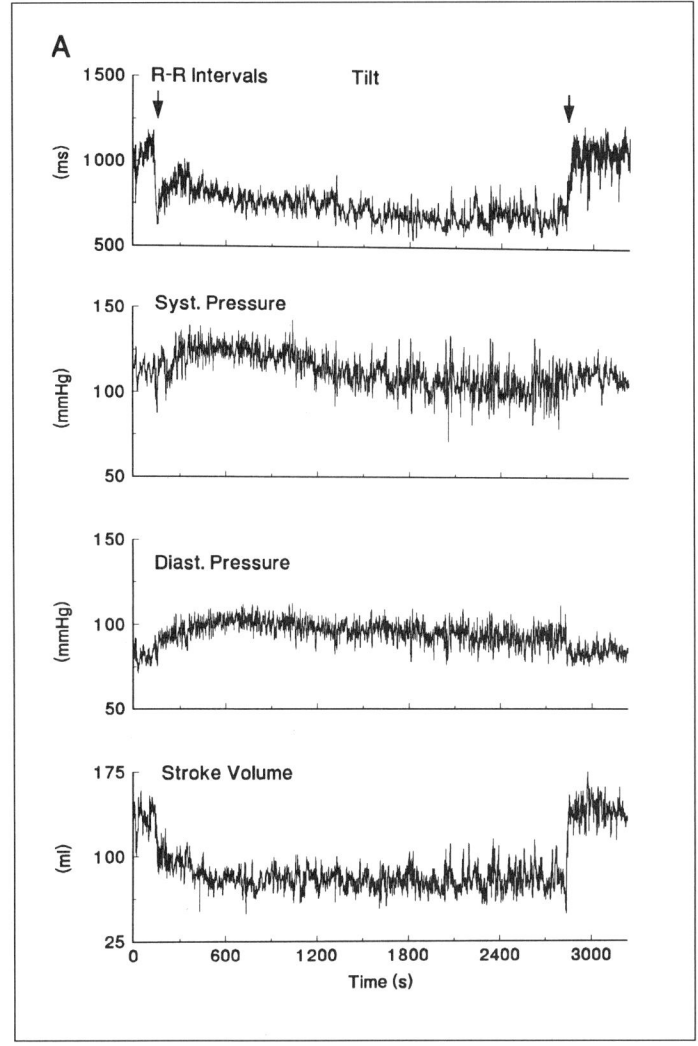

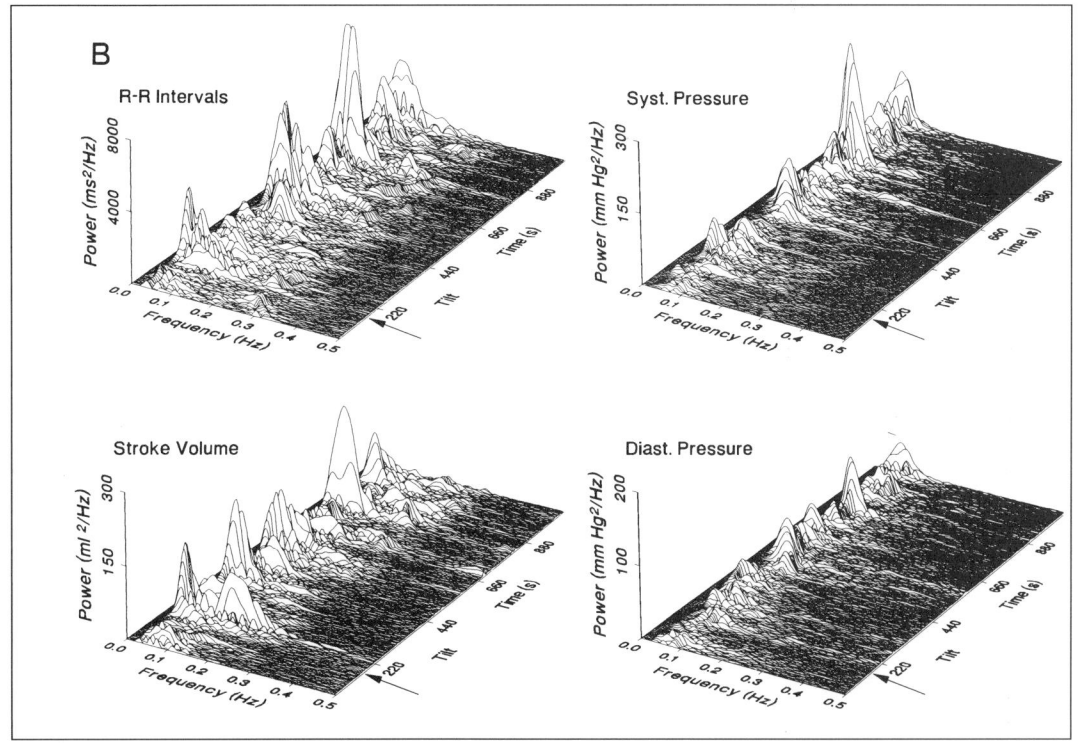

FIG. 5. Typical profile of cardiovascular signals from a young healthy volunteer in response to tilt-up: **(A)** time series, **(B)** corresponding time–frequency maps.

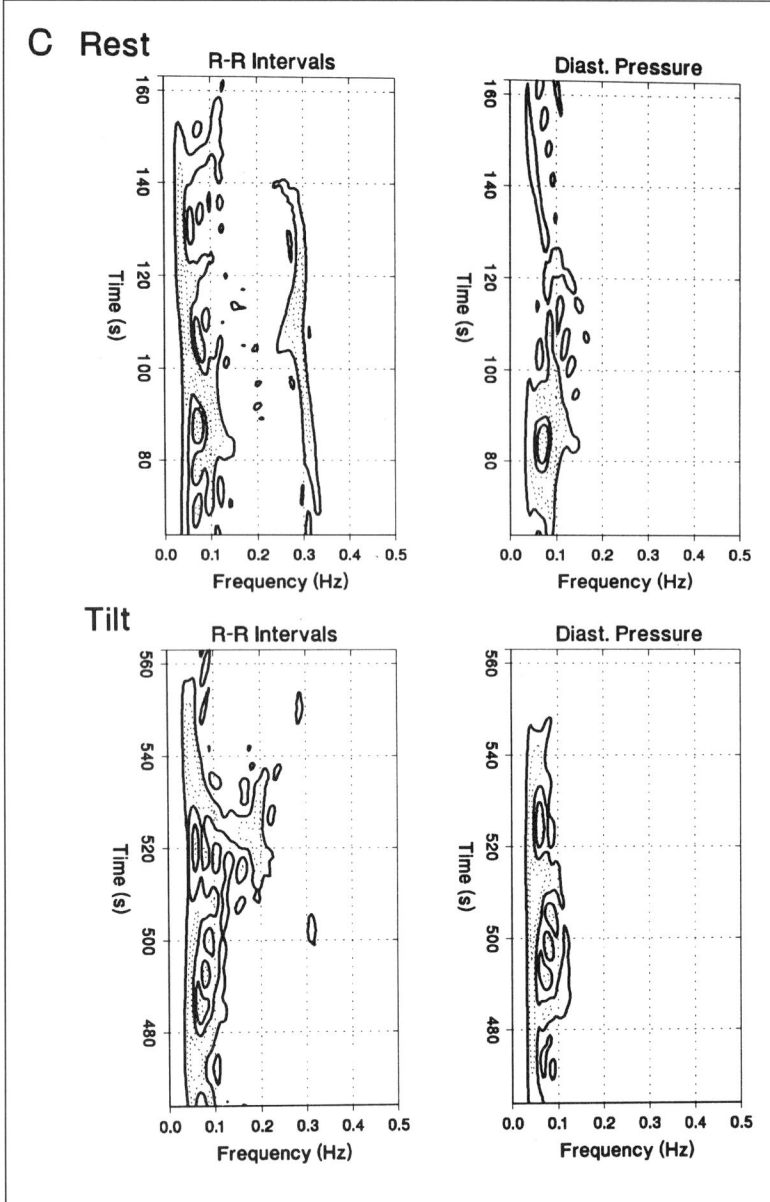

FIG. 5. (C) contour maps. In A, there is rapid cardioacceleration (RR intervals or RRIs), a mild increase of systolic pressure, an increase of diastolic pressure, and a 50% reduction of stroke volume. The corresponding time–frequency distributions (B) display clear profiles of nonrespiratory oscillations (0.05 Hz), which increase in amplitude with tilt-up (indicated by an *arrow*). The contour plot (C) constructed from these time–frequency distribution shows the greater complexity of the RRI profile, compared with the contours of diastolic pressure during both rest and tilt-up.

of the vasomotor tone. During standing, the dominant frequency of the slow blood pressure rhythms accelerates from 0.05 to 0.07–0.08 Hz, and their amplitude increases. Heart rate response to head-up tilt and detailed profiles of time–frequency maps and global spectra are presented in Fig. 4. It is important to note that the profile of both respiratory and nonrespiratory oscillations changes dynamically and dramatically after tilt-up. There is a marked reduction of RRI oscillations at RFs, while the slower rhythms remain preserved with a relatively unchanged amplitude. Another example of the normal cardiovascular responses to orthostasis in a young normal subject is presented in Fig. 5.

Figure 5A shows a typical normal cardiovascular profile during head-up tilt (cardioacceleration, diastolic pressure increment, and stroke volume reduction). Time–frequency maps in Fig. 5B reveal prominent slow frequency oscillations in all signals (RRI, stroke volume, and systolic and diastolic pressures). After tilt-up, slow oscillations are preserved, and their amplitude in systolic pressure and stroke volume increases. These changes are partially transferred to RRI. A detailed analysis of data segment extending from rest to tilt-up is presented as contour plots (Fig. 5C). It can be appreciated that the RRI plot has multiple slow rhythms and is more spread out than the blood pressure map. The

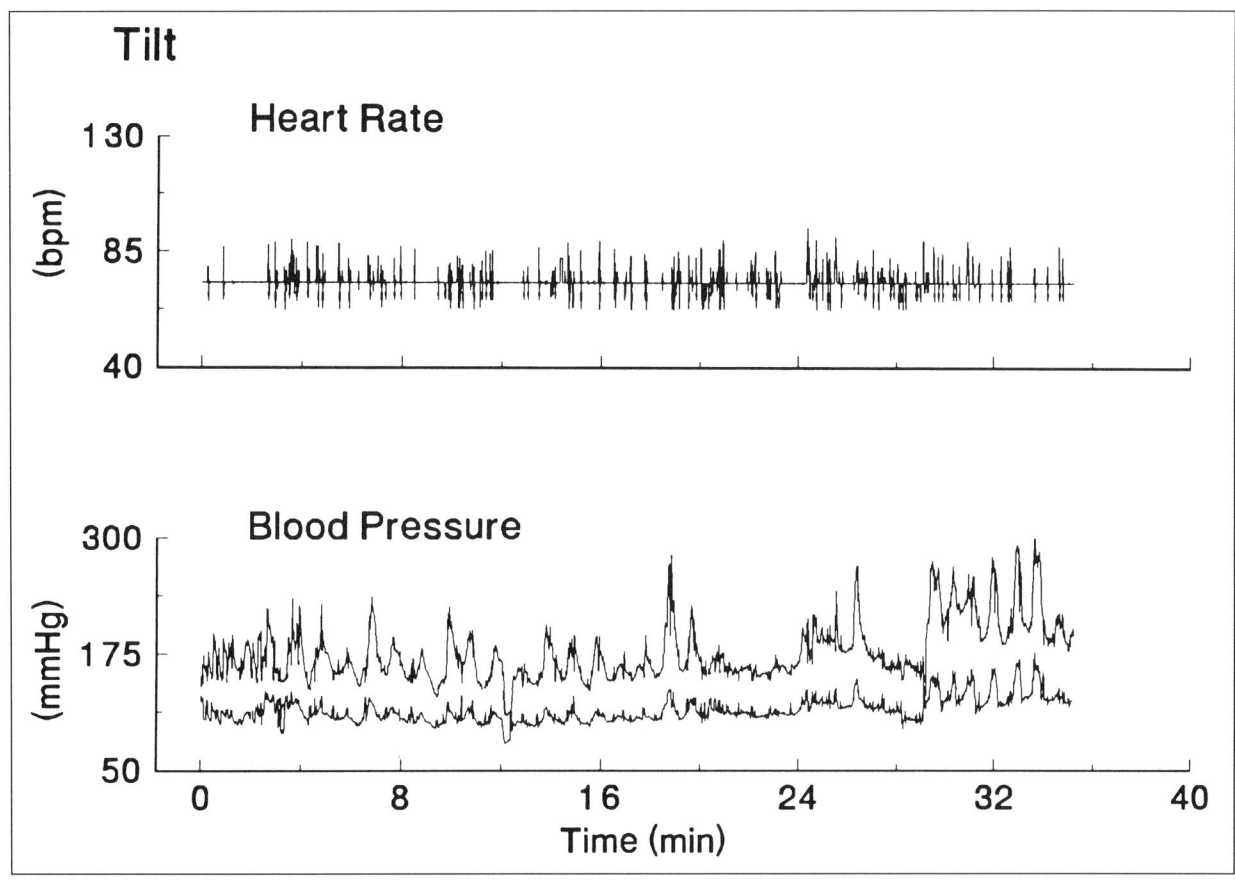

FIG. 6. The *top trace* shows heart rate during tilt-up. There is no cardioacceleration because heart rate is fixed by the pacemaker. Prominent slow-frequency oscillations can be seen on the *bottom trace* of BP_{BB}.

fact that slow vasomotor rhythms are independent of HR become obvious when HR variation is abolished (Fig. 6). In this example, heart rate was fixed by implantation of a pacemaker. Hence, there was no cardioacceleration during head-up tilt. However, slow blood pressure rhythms persisted and their amplitude was large during head-up tilt. This illustration further confirms that slow BP rhythms reflect sympathetic vasomotor drive, independent of HR.

The profile of cardiac and BP rhythms changes substantially with increasing age, beginning after 40 years and especially after 60 years of age. Briefly, heart rate variability is reduced, and the spectrum become simplified. Power-spectral analysis revealed a reduction in power at the mid-frequency range (0.08–0.12 Hz) of both systolic and diastolic blood pressures in the elderly in the standing position. Reduced heart rate variability is most pronounced in the range of respiratory oscillations (0.15– 0.40 Hz). Additionally, the profile of slow rhythms becomes simplified. These rhythms do remain clearly defined and are continuously present in patients who are both supine or upright. Figure 7, comprising data from a supine, healthy, elderly man (81 years old), illustrates the effect of aging on cardiovascular rhythms. There is reduction of power at respiratory oscillations in RRI, while the amplitude of vasomotor rhythms is well preserved. These results suggest that aging affects not only the magnitude of BP and pulse interval variability, but also causes a complex rearrangement of the dynamics of neurocardiovascular regulation. These changes might be also related to the reduced influence from the baroreceptors, which contribute to the generation of the slow heart rate oscillations (65,69).

There have been a few attempts to quantify the level of *complexity* of the signal by using its approximate entropy, a measure of regularity derived from nonlinear dynamics (*chaos* theory). Very little is known about the gender specificity of cardiovascular rhythms also. The reduction of heart rate variability is present in both sexes. However, spectral power, variability, and the overall complexity of heart rate dynamics were greater in women than in men (57).

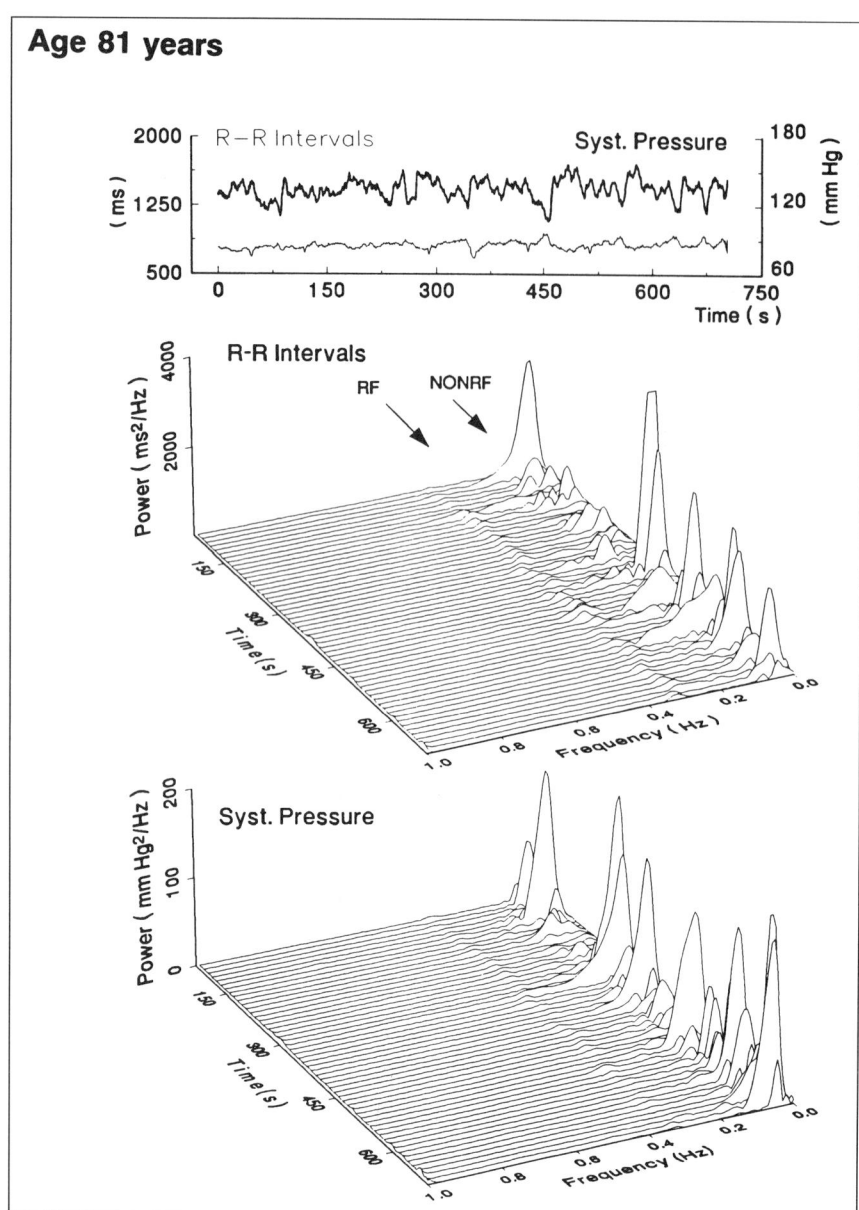

FIG. 7. The effect of aging on cardiovascular rhythms obtained from a supine 81-year-old man. The time series is shown in at the *top*. The time–frequency distributions reveal reduced respiratory oscillations in RR interval (*middle*). The profile of slower rhythms is simplified, but they remain distinct from respiratory oscillations. The profile of slow rhythms in blood pressure (*bottom*) is similar to that seen in young subjects.

CARDIOVASCULAR OSCILLATIONS IN DISEASE

Identification of the pathologic patterns of cardiovascular rhythms and the application of spectral analysis techniques to clinical practice have been challenges for both clinicians and researchers. A major limiting factor thus far has been the lack of a "gold standard" in terms of the length of recordings and technical parameters required for spectral analysis. Despite these limitations, frequency domain methods possess great potential with their high sensitivity, although their specificity might be limited. Studies have appeared mainly in three major fields: (a) Analyses of mainly short-term recordings and, recently, some long-term recordings of heart rate variability, have been used in a limited number of mainly cardiac diseases. Here, spectral analysis has been used to generate information to predict patient mortality or morbidity, typically in patients after myocardial infarction or heart failure. (b) Neurologic applications have been limited to a relatively small number of studies in patients following brain or spinal cord injury and to the evaluation of peripheral neuropathies. Of those, diabetic neuropathy has received considerable attention. (c) In the autonomic laboratories, frequency analysis has been successfully applied mainly to the evaluation of patients with orthostatic intolerance and especially of vasodepressor syncope.

Autonomic Dysfunction and Orthostatic Intolerance

In susceptive individuals, standing up often triggers numerous symptoms of orthostatic intolerance. These range from light-headedness, dizziness, headache, tiredness, unsteadiness, blurred vision, and nausea to syncope and orthostatic hypotension. Causes range from a number of benign disorders of reduced orthostatic tolerance to devastating degenerative diseases like the autonomic neuropathies and multiple-system atrophy (35). The normal response to head-up tilt (80°) has been thoroughly described. There is a rapid increase in heart rate of >15 beats/min and diastolic pressure within the first minute. Both parameters stabilize after that (see Figs. 4 and 5). Typically, respiratory oscillations in RRI that are of large amplitude in the supine position diminish rapidly and remain low during tilt-up. The NONRF oscillations in RRI have a similar distribution in the upright and supine positions, with two dominant frequencies present at 0.05 and 0.08 Hz. Their amplitudes remain unchanged or mildly increased (32,48). Typically, the NONRF oscillations in both systolic and diastolic pressures accelerate from 0.05 to 0.07 Hz and persist throughout the entire recording. Their amplitude also increases proportionally to the angle of tilt.

Mild orthostatic intolerance usually comprises relatively benign conditions without generalized autonomic failure. This group includes patients with the postural orthostatic tachycardia syndrome (POTS), neurally mediated syncope, deconditioning, and hypovolemia. The orthostatic response in patients with mild orthostatic intolerance (MOI) typically consists of a transient blood pressure drop with rapid recovery, and a HR increment of >30 but <120 beats/min. This group usually exhibits a mild reduction of respiratory and nonrespiratory oscillations in RRI (Fig. 8; MOI I). Nonrespiratory oscillations in blood pressure, an index of sympathetic vasomotor activity, typically surge in the first minute of the tilt and then decline to normal values. Very similar findings can be apparent in patients with a history of neurally mediated syncope with infrequent recurrence (<1/month), who do not experience syncope during tilt-table testing. In this group, diagnosis often cannot be confirmed by a tilt study, it syncope is not induced by tilt-up or after isoproterenol infusion (48). An abnormal profile of the vasomotor slow rhythms can be identified, however, and used to separate these patients from normal controls. The amplitude of NONRF oscillations in BP surges with tilt-up and exceeds normal control values, but low blood pressure rhythms remain present during tilt-up. Thus, an abnormal profile of vasomotor rhythms can serve as an additional diagnostic tool in neurally mediated syncope.

The profile of cardiovascular responses in patients who experience frequent syncopal episodes is often heterogeneous. One group comprises patients with high resting vagal tone. These patients have a low resting heart rate (<60 beats/min) and typically have excessive respiratory and nonrespiratory oscillations. A second group, mainly female, is characterized by a higher resting heart rate and larger increment (>30 beats/min) on tilt-up (58). Some studies have reported a reduction of heart rate variability in RRI (62) in patients with syncope induced after an isoproterenol infusion. A hyperadrenergic surge with a large increment in slow blood pressure oscillations is present shortly after tilt-up in both tilt-positive patients (when syncope was reproduced during the test) as well as tilt-negative patients (when syncope was not reproduced). In

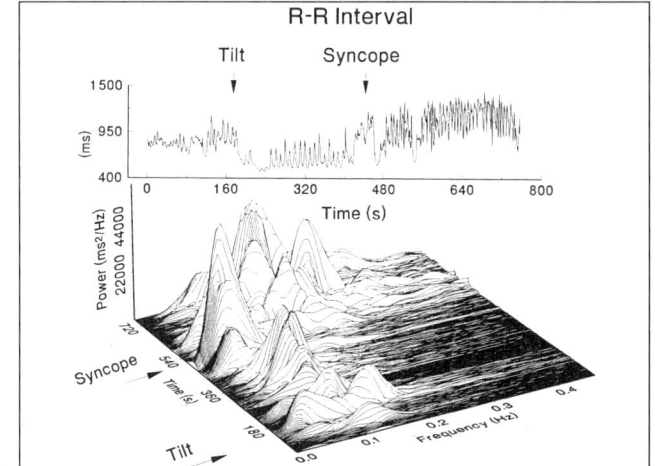 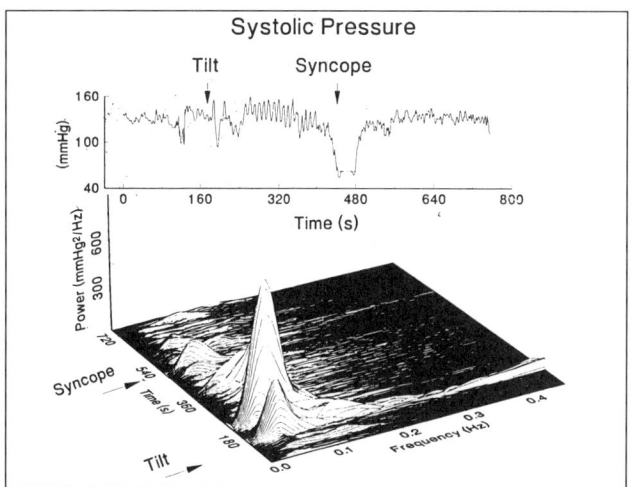

FIG. 9. Time series and time–frequency map of RR interval (RRI) (*left*) and of systolic pressure (*right*) in a 26-year-old patient during the supine rest, tilt-up, and syncope. The time–frequency map of the systolic pressure reveals a large increase of the slow sympathetically mediated rhythms with tilt-up, an increase that disappears shortly before the onset of syncope. Note the large increase in respiratory rhythms in RRI after syncope.

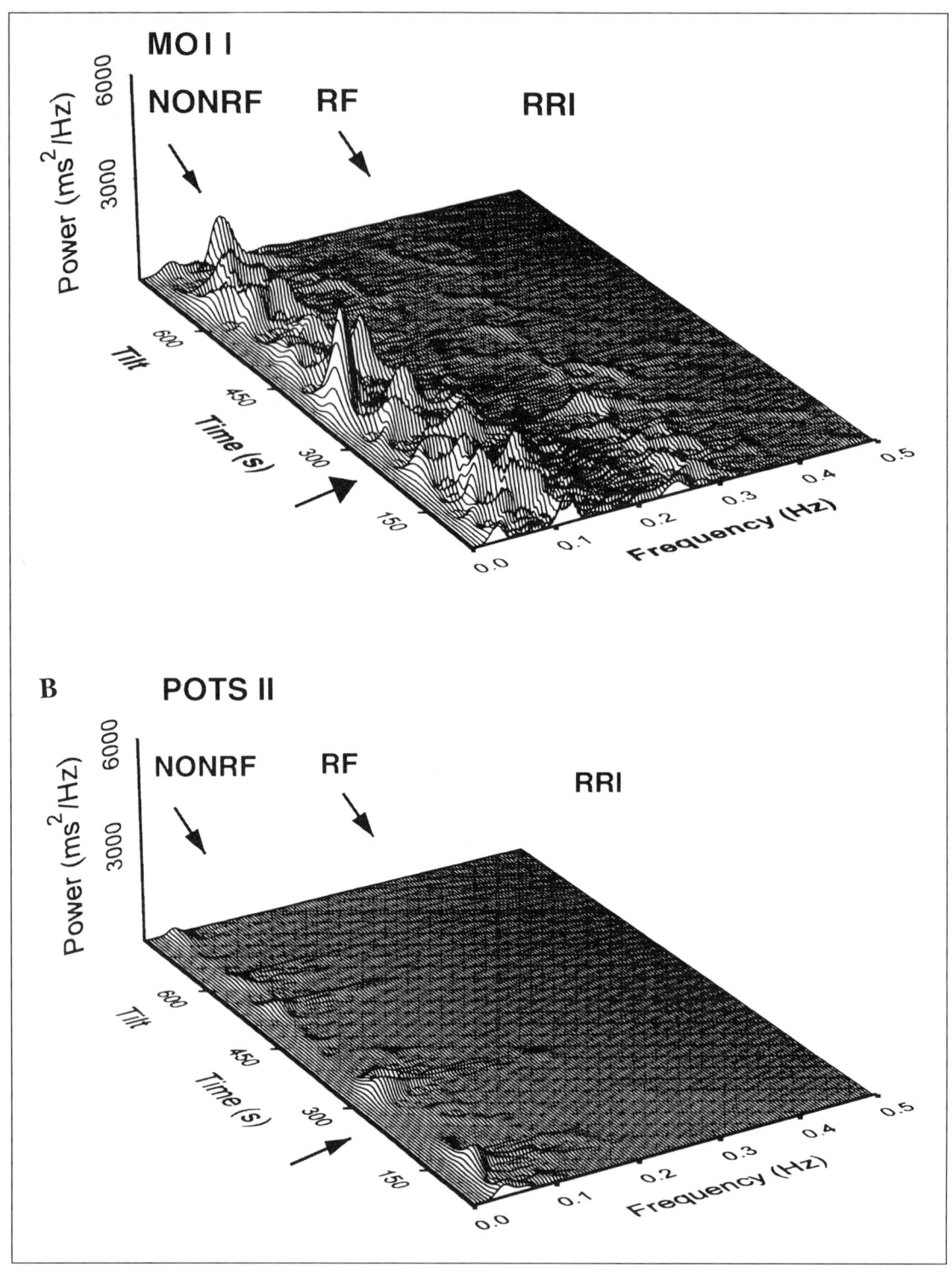

FIG. 8. Time–frequency maps of RR interval (RRI) in a young female with a mild postural intolerance (MOI I) and of another patient with severe orthostatic intolerance and severe postural tachycardia (POTS). During both rest and tilt-up, RRI oscillations are mildly reduced in MOI I. In POTS, both respiratory and nonrespiratory oscillations in RRI are blunted.

Tilt-up

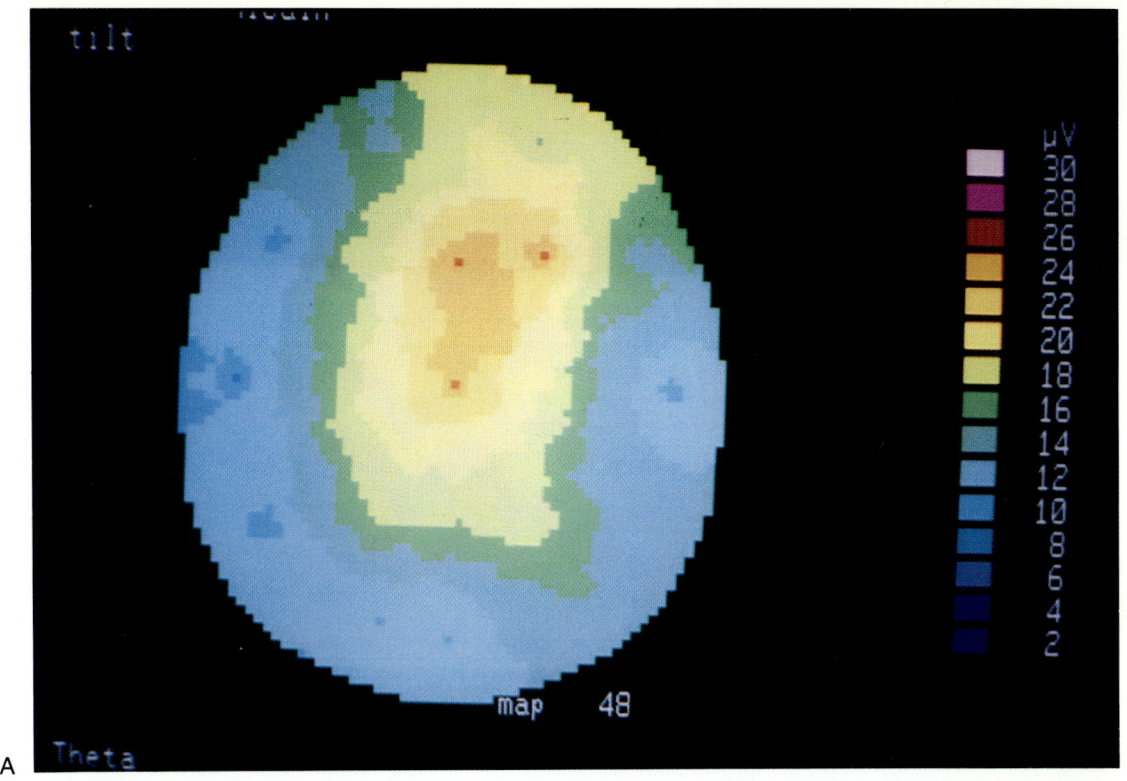

Presyncope

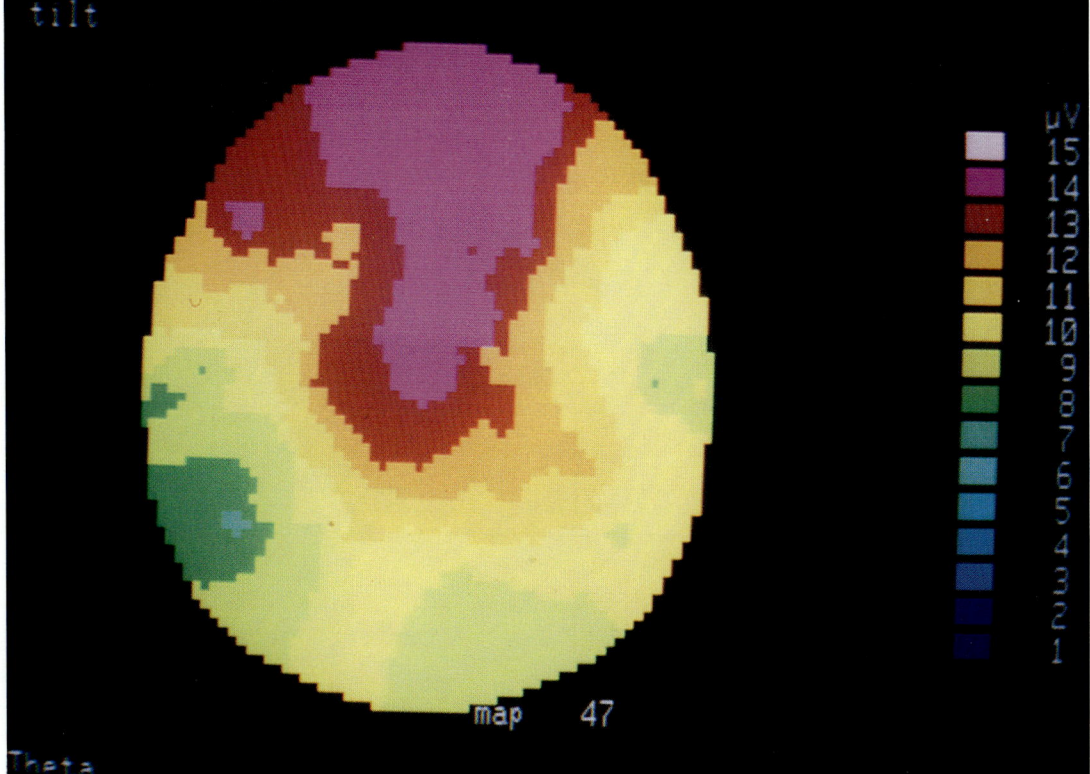

COLOR FIG. 3. On-line electroencephalographic mapping was performed during supine rest and tilt-up in a patient with recurrent syncope. The map of baseline theta activity shows a lower amplitude theta, mainly over the central areas. An increased amplitude of theta rhythm and its propagation to the frontal areas are seen shortly before syncope (red).

Tilt-up

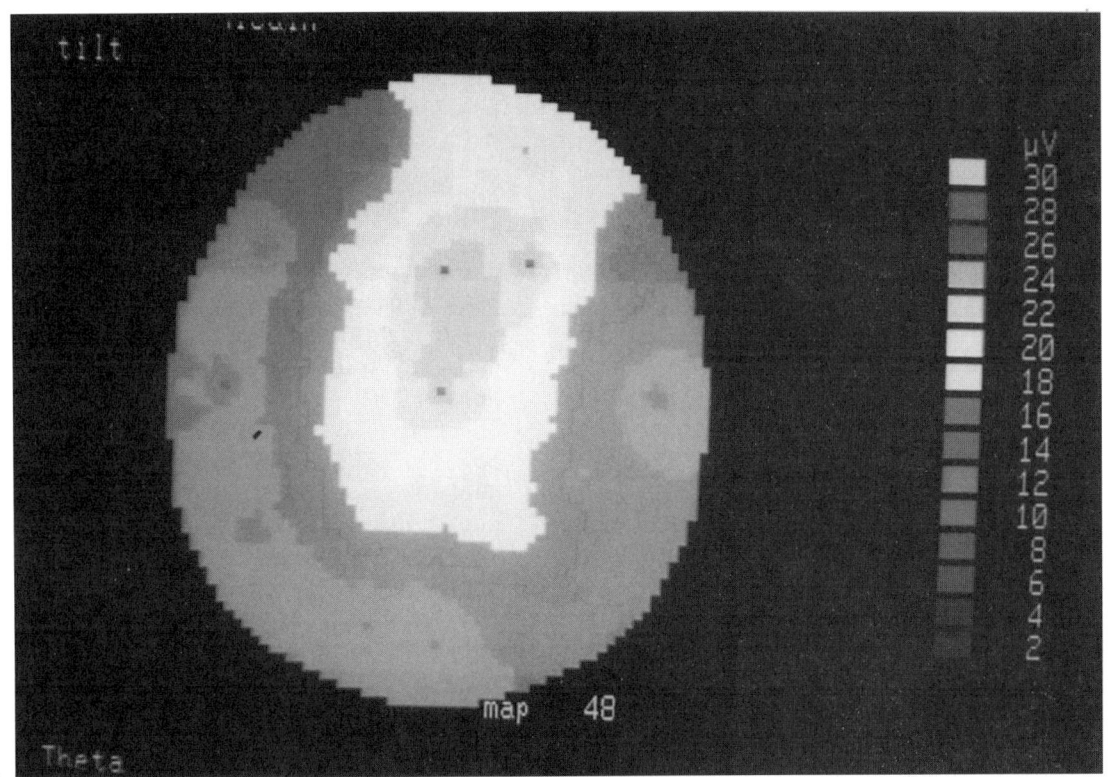

Presyncope

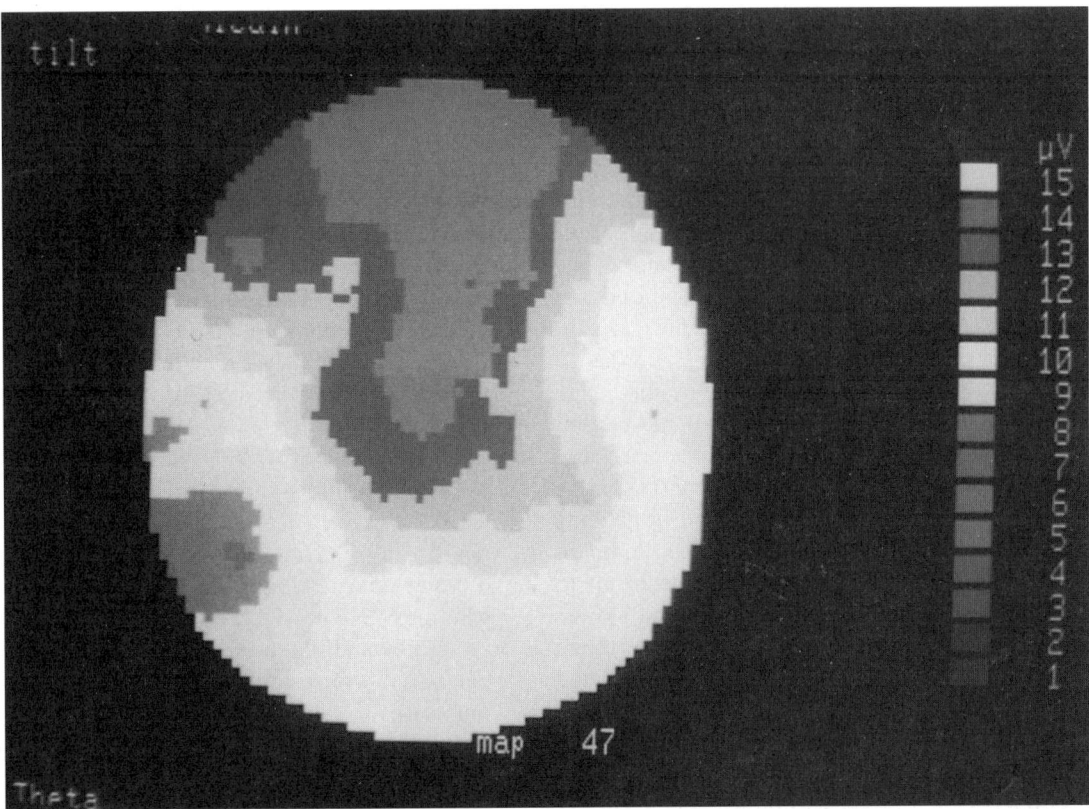

FIG. 10. On-line electroencephalographic mapping was performed during supine rest and tilt-up in a patient with recurrent syncope. The map of baseline theta activity shows a lower amplitude theta, mainly over the central areas. An increased amplitude of theta rhythm and its propagation to the frontal areas are seen shortly before syncope (*red*). *See color Fig. 3.*

syncope positive patients, however, these oscillations disappeared shortly after the tilt-up, the blood pressure profile becoming simplified, and this loss of slow blood pressure oscillations signals impending syncope (Fig. 9). Thus, the presence of slow blood pressure oscillations can be considered as another index of orthostatic compensation. This is particularly useful in the patients with less severe abnormalities or when vasodepressor syncope is not induced during tilt-table testing. We hypothesize that the disappearance of slow oscillations might reflect withdrawal of efferent sympathetic drive and an initiation of the central inhibitory vasodepressor reflex as an early trigger of syncope (68). Thus, a detailed analysis of the temporal profile of cardiovascular oscillations provides additional information in the evaluation of patients with orthostatic intolerance. In addition, at syncope, there is no significant reduction of cardiac output and stroke volume, which does not suggest diminished cardiac filling (45,60). These data do not support the widely held hypothesis that neurally mediated syncope is triggered once a threshold decrease in cardiac filling is reached.

The role of central triggers leading to the withdrawal of the sympathetic drive is not clear. Presyncope is associated with significant cerebral hypoperfusion, as indicated by transcranial blood flow studies (31,39). Furthermore, electroencephalographic (EEG) recordings of syncope are characterized by generalized EEG slowing and development of theta and delta rhythms (Fig. 10). On-line brain mapping has been performed during tilt-table testing in a patient with vasodepressor syncope (49). The amplitude of the theta rhythm increased progressively over the frontal areas before syncope (marked in red over the frontal areas). EEG amplitude is further modulated by slow rhythms at frequencies similar to the peripheral vasomotor rhythms, and it has been hypothesized that these rhythms might reflect the central component of autonomic modulation. The theory of slow amplitude modulation is discussed in detail in the Chapter 27. Briefly, these rhythms, in normal subjects, are present at frequencies of 0.03–0.06 Hz in the alpha and theta range over the scalp. They are prominent in the occipital leads in the alpha range and in the central leads in the theta range. During tilt-up, distribution and amplitude of the slow activity did not significantly change in orthostatically tolerant subjects. In contrast, in patients who experienced syncope during tilt, slowing of dominant alpha activity toward the theta range was observed *prior* to syncope. At the same time, the amplitude of the slower 0.06-Hz rhythm increased (49). We can only hypothesize that augmentation of the slow EEG rhythms is associated with central sympathetic inhibition.

About one-half of the patients with POTS suffer from more severe symptoms of orthostatic intolerance and are associated with a HR of >120 beats/min when upright, excessive blood pressure change, and progressive reductions of pulse pressure and total peripheral resistance in response to tilt-up. Some of these patients have a length-dependent autonomic neuropathy (61). According to this concept, peripheral adrenergic and cardiovagal efferents, having the longest postganglionic efferent fibers, would be the most affected, while cardiac sympathetic postganglionic fibers, being shorter, would be spared. Impairment of the sudomotor axon reflex volume on distal sites, mainly on the feet, and neuropathic distribution of anhidrosis on the thermoregulatory sweat test and skin potential recordings are often present (21). Indices of peripheral adrenergic dysfunction, which are manifested by an excessive early phase II during the Valsalva maneuver and attenuated late phase II, are also present (35,61). Our data showed that the magnitude of both respiratory and nonrespiratory oscillations in RRI is reduced to <30% of normal values (Fig. 8B). Figure 8B illustrates a dramatic reduction of spectral power in RRI, which affects both respiratory and nonrespiratory ranges during rest and tilt-up. Transfer from respiratory oscillations to RRI is attenuated in POTS, suggesting a decreased responsiveness to cardiopulmonary inhibitory reflexes, indicating additional cardiovagal efferent failure. That cardiovagal impairment is part of an autonomic neuropathy in POTS is suggested by the commonly associated gastrointestinal symptoms (possibly also indicating parasympathetic involvement), acral sweat loss (involvement of postganglionic sympathetic sudomotor fibers), and prominent vasomotor symptoms (peripheral adrenergic fibers). There are several lines of evidence for peripheral adrenergic impairment. First, NONRF power in both blood pressure and RRI is reduced. Second, nonrespiratory oscillations in RRI are paradoxically reduced during the tilt-up, while the sympathetically mediated nonrespiratory oscillations in blood pressure are preserved.

Peripheral Neuropathy

Autonomic evaluation in the frequency domain is increasingly being applied to the peripheral neuropathies. Much of the published data have been in diabetic neuropathy. There are several reasons for this. In diabetes, autonomic neuropathy is associated with a shortened life expectancy (see Chapter 37). Autonomic dysregulation has been suggested as a mechanism for sudden cardiac death. There have been active clinical treatment trials of diabetic neuropathy, and autonomic function has been one of the indices evaluated, since it has been suggested to be amenable to improvement. Much emphasis has been placed on tests of cardiovagal function, and "new" tests have usually been compared with established tests for its sensitivity. In the opinion of the authors, this is misplaced emphasis. The majority of tests of cardiovagal function have adequate sensitivity. Marginal differences in sensitivity are inadequate reasons for introducing a new test. The value of frequency analysis, well done, is in providing information that is lacking with other tests. First, it has the capability to provide an index of sympathovagal balance. In the evaluation of sympathovagal balance by conventional tests, sympathetic tests and vagal tests are performed on different systems, with the tests having very different sensitivities, and nonsimultaneously. It is possible in spectral analysis to choose simultaneously recorded and simultaneously processed data that index sympathetic and cardiovagal function (see below). Another advantage of frequency analysis is its ability to record dynamic alterations in autonomic function. Finally, although it requires patient relaxation, it does not require the performance of complicated autonomic maneuvers.

Autonomic data are greatly influenced by confounding variables. In the frequency domain, the quality of data, the algorithmic parameters, and the method chosen to analyze the data all significantly influence the results. Much of the published work on the peripheral neuropathies does not fulfill minimum requirements of adequate length of data, simultaneous recording of respiration, or satisfactory recording system, and many reports do not include the parameters of the program used to analyze the data. For this reason, at the end of this chapter, we summarize what we consider to be minimal requirements for an adequate study.

There is good agreement that diabetic neuropathy is associated with a reduction in power at all RFs and midfrequencies, and that there is a correlation between the severity of neuropathy and the loss of power (17,71,72,76, 77,79) Weise et al. (72) compared resting and standing midfrequency (0.05–0.15 Hz) and respiration-related (RF, power around respiration rate) heart rate variation in three groups of patients with insulin-dependent diabetes mellitus. There were diabetics without neuropathy (group 1), diabetics with peripheral neuropathy (group 2), and diabetics with peripheral and autonomic neuropathy (group 3). Heart rate variations were significantly lower in group 2 and group 3 diabetics than in controls, indicating a reduced parasympathetic nervous system influence on the heart. Standing midfrequency and RF spectral power has significantly lower in all diabetic groups than in controls, suggesting impairment of autonomic function in response to orthostatic stress even in group 1. The loss of power increases with age and, when compared with controls, the diabetic state appeared to aggravate the effect of aging (71). These authors considered that the increment in midfrequency power on standing up is an index of cardiac sympathetic activation—a conclusion that is questionable (see below).

Spectral power decreases with age (71) and is reproducible (77). Respiration was not included in the recordings by Ziegler et al. (77–79), who compared heart rate spectral analysis and vector analysis with standard tests of HR variation and BP responses in 261 diabetic patients aged 11–76 years and with various stages of peripheral neuropathy (79). The most frequently abnormal indices were the coefficient of variation, low-frequency and midfrequency power spectrum at rest, mean circular resultant, postural change in systolic BP, and the max./min. 30 : 15 ratio and Valsalva ratio. Spectral power is at least as sensitive as conventional tests of parasympathetic function in both chronic and recently diagnosed diabetes (79). Figure 11 presents an example of a patient (a 39-year-old man) with a 1-year history of insulin-dependent diabetes and diabetic neuropathy with orthostatic hypotension and postganglionic sudomotor failure and adrenergic failure. Time–frequency maps showed the obvious loss of variability, affecting both the low-frequency and the RF ranges. The blood pressure profile was also blunted, resulting in reduced amplitude of the slow rhythms. These findings would be suggestive of combined cardiovagal and peripheral adrenergic failure.

Chau et al. (10), who reported another method of measuring variability—fractal dimension (FD) of HR and BP—in 28 healthy subjects and in 64 diabetics, determined FD of heart rate (or systolic BP) by a relatively simple method. They measured the curve of 500 successive heart rates with a rule of length L, obtaining $N \times L$. The FD is the slope of the regression line of $\log(N)$ versus $\log(1/L)$ for different L. They found a lower FD of heart rate in diabetics than in healthy subjects ($p = 0.0002$) and a similar FD of systolic blood pressure in the two groups. In diabetic subjects, the FD of heart rate was negatively correlated with age ($r = -0.27$, $p = 0.03$), duration of diabetes ($r = -0.33$, $p = 0.0078$), and the grade of autonomic failure ($r = -0.43$, $p = 0.0007$). Spectral power was compared with vibratory threshold, and there were significant inverse correlations between the low-frequency and high-frequency components of the power-spectral analysis of heart rate variations and the vibratory perception thresholds (76).

Standard techniques measuring heart rate variability do not account for its dependence on the rate and depth of respiration or measure the time relationship between changes in lung volume and heart rate. To relate these parameters, Freeman et al. (17) studied transfer function analysis of respiratory sinus arrhythmia in controls and diabetics with varying degrees of autonomic dysfunction. Specifically, reduced supine vagal and increased supine sympathetic heart rate modulation was found with progression of the autonomic neuropathy. In response to postural change, the diabetics displayed impaired sympathetic heart rate modulation. The authors considered that transfer function analysis yields new insight into the sequence of changes that occur with diabetic autonomic neuropathy and provides an accurate, easily comprehensible measurement of respiration-related rate variability.

Long-term recordings provide information on the circadian distribution of heart rate variation. Significant abnormalities are seen, and it has been suggested that the high incidence of cardiovascular accidents in diabetic patients might be related to abnormalities of autonomic tone. Diabetics with or without signs of autonomic neuropathy showed decreased vagal activity (and hence a relatively higher sympathetic activity) during the night, coinciding in

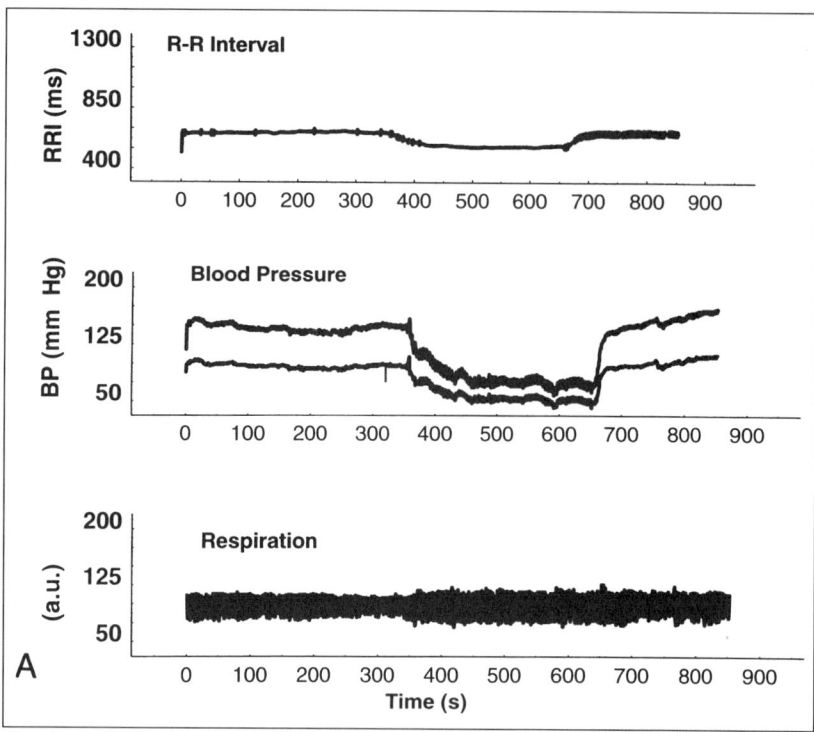
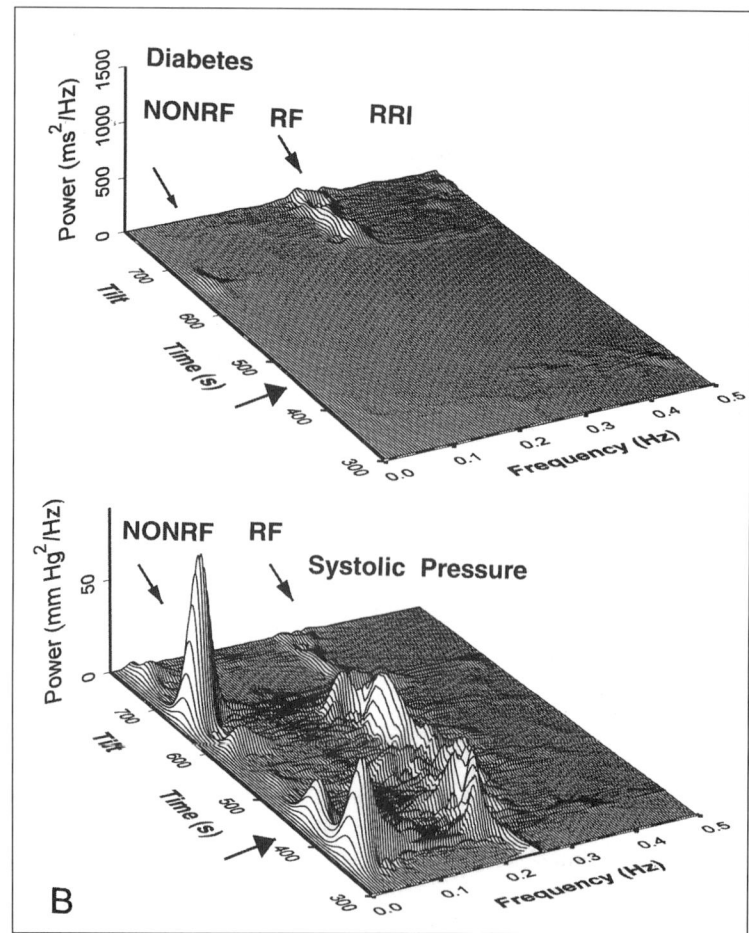

FIG. 11. Time series of RR interval (RRI) (*top*), blood pressure (*second*), respiration (*third*), and time–frequency maps of RRI (*top map*) and systolic pressure (*bottom map*) obtained during rest and with tilt-up of a 39-year-old man with insulin-dependent diabetes mellitus and orthostatic hypotension. The Wigner distribution clearly shows blunted RRI variability over the wide range of frequencies. Blood pressure nonrespiratory oscillations are also reduced.

time with a higher frequency of cardiovascular accidents (7). With regard to asymptomatic diabetic patients, however, controversy still exists as to whether vagal damage is followed by sympathetic involvement or whether they occur simultaneously.

Effector Failure

With end-organ failure, as in myocardial infarction and particularly with heart failure, the pattern of heart rate variability is dramatically changed. The amplitude of sympathetic vasomotor rhythms is diminished. More importantly, heart rate oscillations are lost and replaced by a noiselike profile. In a model of cardiac failure induced by rapid ventricular pacing in dogs, loss of rhythmicity appeared early during the 6-week pacing period and preceded clinical symptoms. As heart failure developed, low-frequency and high-frequency components were smeared out, and low-amplitude noisy oscillations were spread over the time–frequency maps. Vagally mediated respiratory rhythms in RRI disappeared, and the amplitude in the low-frequency range was drastically reduced. In contrast, respiratory and low-frequency rhythms in BP were consistently detectable (38) (Fig. 12). Their amplitude was also reduced, however, as can be expected in the hyperadrenergic state. In humans, augmented sympathetic efferent neural traffic was documented from peroneal nerve recordings and correlated with increased plasma norepinephrine levels (19). These findings provide additional evidence for peripheral sympathoexcitation during cardiac failure. Cardiac and pulmonary baroreceptors and mechanoreceptors, which are stimulated by chronically increased pulmonary pressure, would normally inhibit further norepinephrine release. Reduced activity of vagal afferents, however, resulted in a failure to reduce the sympathetic outflow (13,56,66). Withdrawal of cardiovagal efferent activity in the failing heart was further suggested from a diminished peak at RFs (>0.15 Hz) in RRI. In previous studies, an *increased power at slow frequencies from 0.01 to 0.15 Hz in RRI and BP and diminished respiratory peak in RRI* were proposed as an index of *sympathoexcitation* (8, 52). Kienzle et al. (27) have shown a negative correlation between spectral peaks in the low-frequency range and sympathetic efferent discharges and proposed that *decreased heart rate variability* was a marker of sympathoexcitation. In humans during orthostasis, a model of mild sympathoexcitation, the amplitude of low-frequency oscillations depends on the HR increment during standing. At a HR of <100 beats/min, the amplitude of low-frequency oscillations remains stable or mildly increases. However, at HR frequencies of >120 beats/min, as, i.e., in POTS, the amplitude of low-frequency oscillations diminishes (see below). Thus diminished amplitude but normal pattern of BP NONRF rhythms suggests sympathoexcitation and increase of tonic sympathetic activity. Thus, disappearance of vagally mediated rhythms might be a typical component of dysautonomia in heart failure. At the same time, the pattern of slow BP rhythms, originating presumably from upper medulla, did not deteriorate. The loss of oscillatory character of RRI rhythms (pattern simplification) is a hallmark of early effector failure. This has been also confirmed by studies using other methods, i.e., Poincare plots (RRI is plotted against the successive beat) (74). The patients with "complex" pattern or diffuse plots "had more severe cardiac failure than did patients with torpedo shape or regular pattern." The *torpedo shape* would represent a pattern with one or two oscillators, whereas the *complex pattern* would suggest a noiselike spectral profile.

Central Nervous System Lesions

Physiologic observations in animals, describing possible sources of generation of slow oscillations, have been supplemented by observations of humans with CNS lesions affecting the central autonomic network (5). Thus far, relatively few studies have focused on the relationship between central autonomic disorders and altered dynamics of cardiovascular control. Although the relationship between cardiovagal and vasomotor rhythms and respiration is well established at the periphery, less is known about the central effect of respiration on the EEG and the level of arousal. Experiments in cats showed that respiratory rhythms propagate both caudally to cardiomotor neurons and sympathetic neurons, and rostrally to the prefrontal cortex and limbic system (23,24).

Occasional synchrony between respiration and 0.1-Hz modulation of spectral powers in the alpha band in humans was described by Pfurtscheller (54). As we mentioned earlier in this chapter, the dominant EEG rhythms (alpha and theta) are, under normal conditions, further modulated by slower rhythms. This *amplitude EEG modulation* is reviewed in detail in Chapter 27. Slow modulation of the EEG was observed in healthy subjects at frequencies of 0.015–0.028 and 0.04–0.07 Hz and in the respiratory range of 0.09–0.15 Hz in the alpha and theta bands (40,41,44). Low-frequency RRI rhythms at frequencies similar to slow EEG rhythms were found in 60% of these subjects. It was hypothesized that these slow EEG rhythms are good candidates for representing sympathetic activity in the central autonomic network.

There is only limited information on central autonomic EEG rhythms in the neurodegenerative disorders. Alzheimer's disease is associated with neuronal loss in the areas associated with the central autonomic network, like the temporal and frontal lobes (59,73). A decreased cholinergic input to cortical neurons is associated with a slowing of background EEG activity and augmentation of powers in theta and delta frequencies (37). Spectral analysis of temporal re-

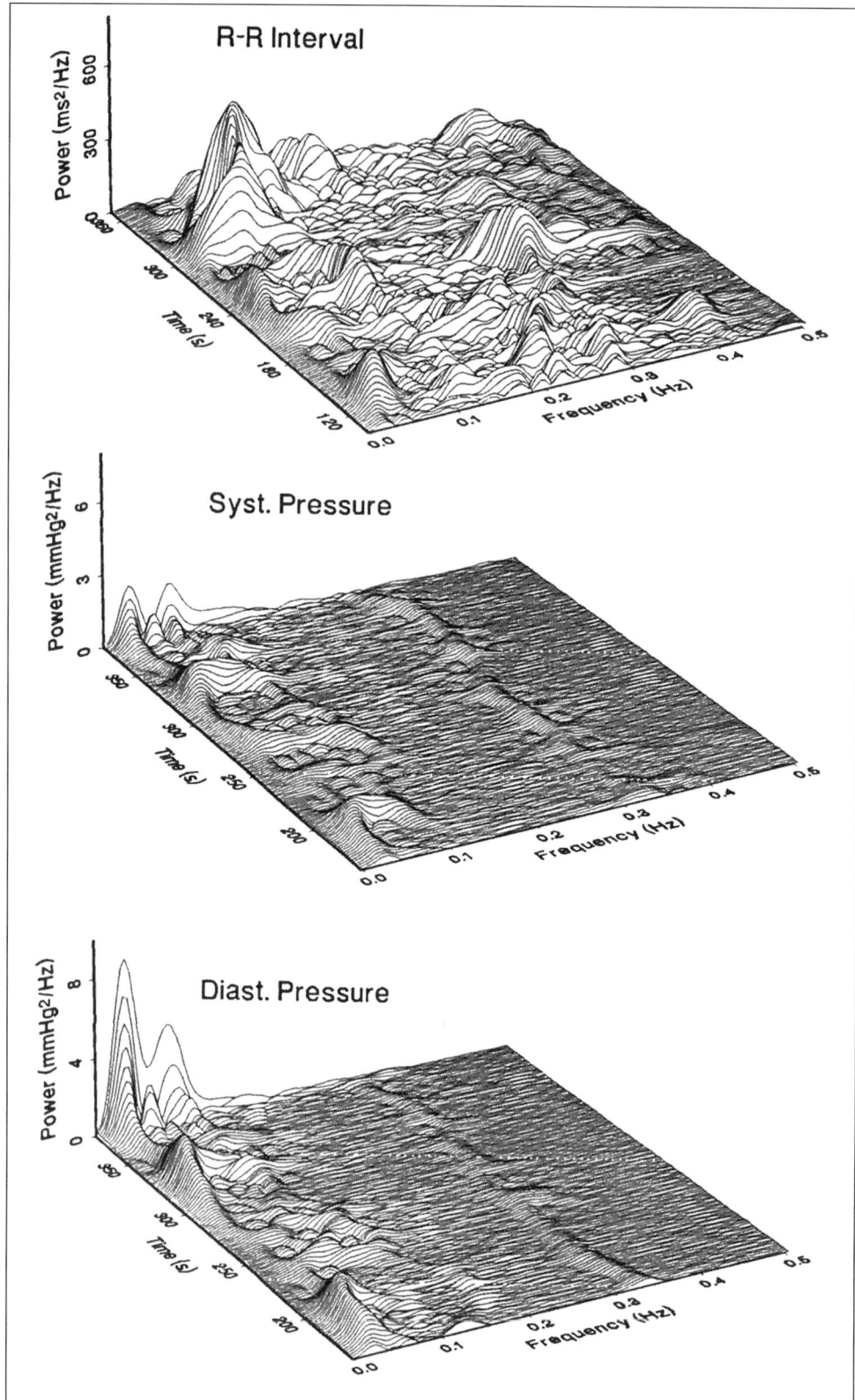

FIG. 12. Wigner distributions were computed from a dog with advanced-stage heart failure, which was induced by rapid ventricular pacing at 240 beats/min. The RR interval profile shows widespread noisy fluctuations of low amplitude, suggesting lost spontaneous rhythmicity. The systolic and diastolic pressure maps reveal the preservation of low-amplitude respiratory oscillations, mainly generated by the effect of respiration on venous return and cardiac contractility. The amplitude of sympathetically mediated low-frequency blood pressure rhythms is reduced, but their profile is preserved.

gions during rapid-eye-movement sleep showed prominent slowing of the EEG, with prevalence of theta rhythm especially in the temporal region and during wakefulness (53).

Dysautonomia in Alzheimer's disease usually does not progress to orthostatic hypotension, but mild-to-moderate impairment of cardiovascular regulation has been reported. Dysautonomia was associated with diminished amplitude of the respiratory oscillations in RRI (1). Orthostatic tolerance is also reduced in Alzheimer's disease compared with healthy elderly controls. Cardioacceleration on standing up is diminished, and systolic BP fell by >15 mmHg and diastolic pressure remained lower than in the controls (15). It has been reported that spontaneous hypotension in Alzheimer's disease can be present even in supine position. Simultaneous EEG and BP recordings showed that BP reductions were preceded by further slowing of EEG activity. Spontaneous hypotensive episodes in supine patients, with a BP decrement of >40 mmHg, were concomitant with augmentation of the slow EEG modulation of theta rhythm at 0.01–0.02 Hz (40). This general slowing was further potentiated by the BP fall. These repetitive spontaneous hypotensive episodes have been suggested to contribute to the progression of the disease (44). The hypotensive episodes occurred spontaneously and after hyperventilation, and were associated with corresponding low-frequency peaks in systolic BP. Theta activity and, in particular, slow modulation of theta activity increased in parallel with the systolic pressure falls.

In degenerative progressive autonomic disorders such as multiple-system atrophy (MSA), the impairment of cardiovascular regulation is profound (Fig. 14). Typically, both vagally and sympathetically mediated rhythms essentially disappear. Figure 14 depicts results from a 57-year-old woman with parkinsonism, progressive hypokinesia, non-responsiveness to levodopa Sinemet, and marked autonomic failure, including orthostatic hypotension and widespread anhidrosis. She was diagnosed as having MSA. Time–frequency maps during rest and tilt-up showed a severe loss of variability affecting both the parasympathetically mediated RRI respiratory oscillations as well as sympathetically mediated blood pressure rhythms. Further studies need to be done to evaluate whether spectral analy-

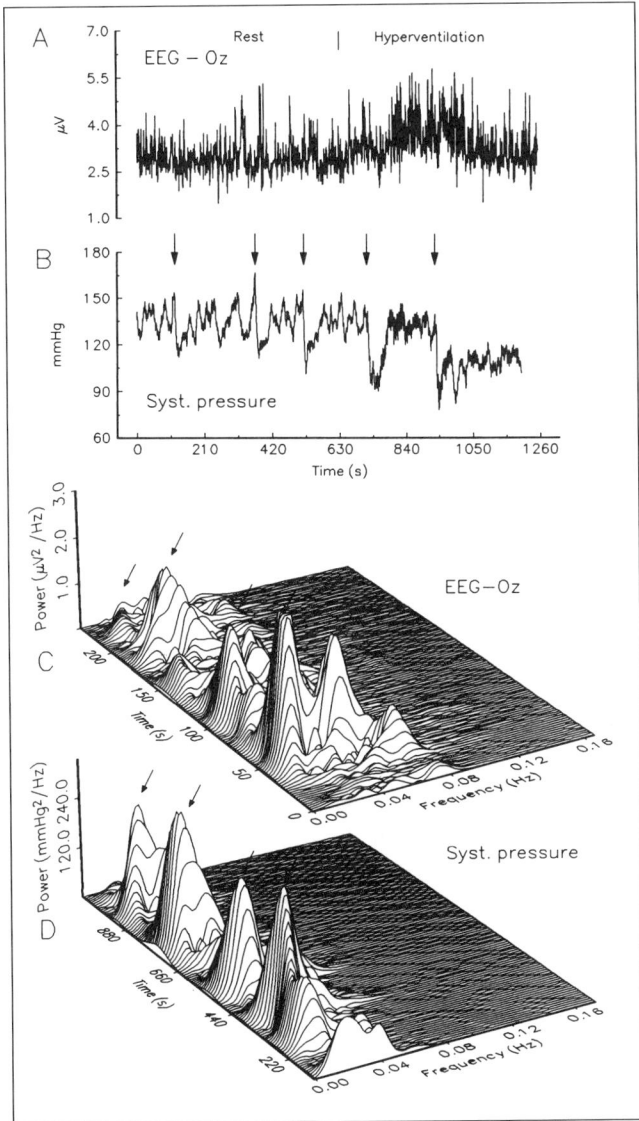

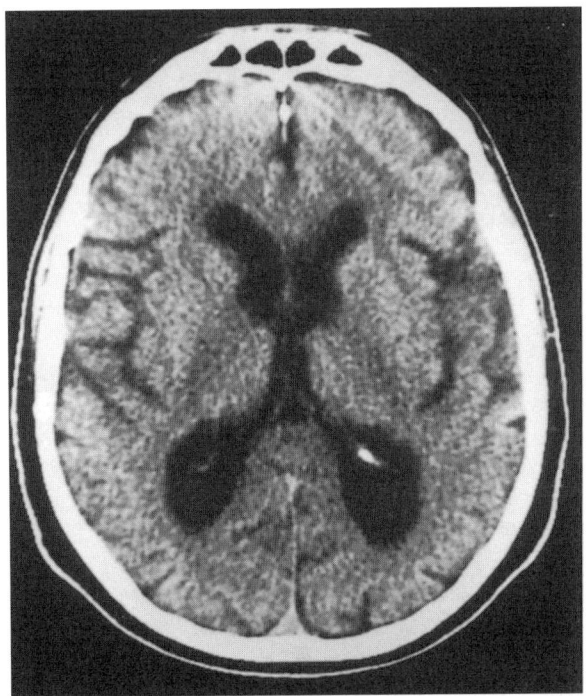

FIG. 13. Time series of electroencephalogram (EEG) **(A)** and systolic BP **(B)**, time–frequency maps of EEG **(C)** and systolic BP **(D)**, and magnetic resonance imaging (MRI) (*right*). This patient had Alzheimer's disease, with a 2-year history of progressive cognitive impairment. The MRI shows diffuse cortical and subcortical atrophy. Tracings of EEG theta activity and systolic pressure show EEG slowing concomitant with spontaneous falls in BP. From Novak et al. (44), with permission.

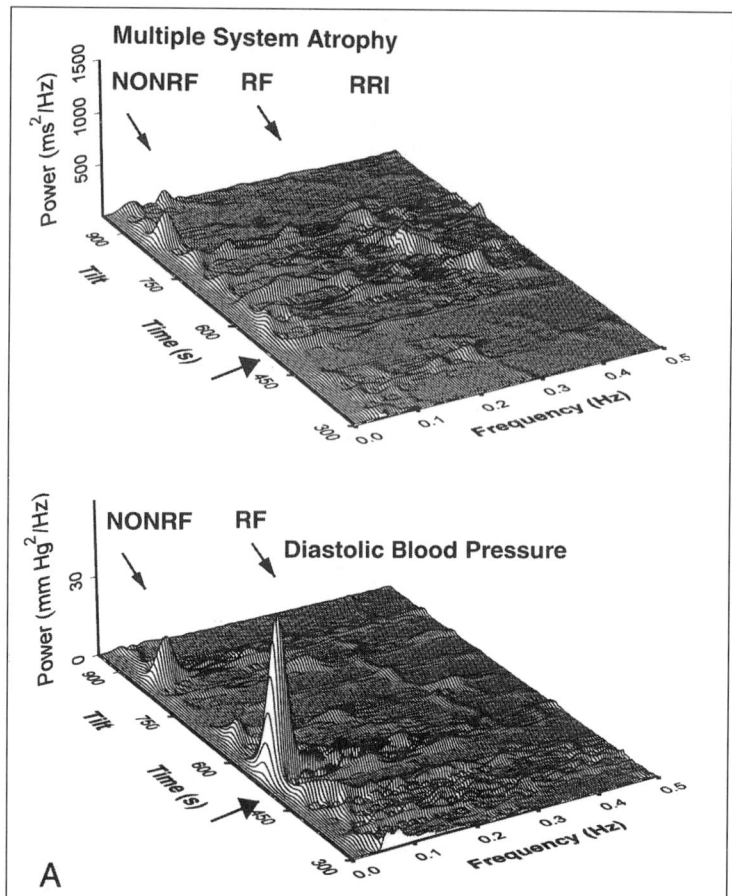
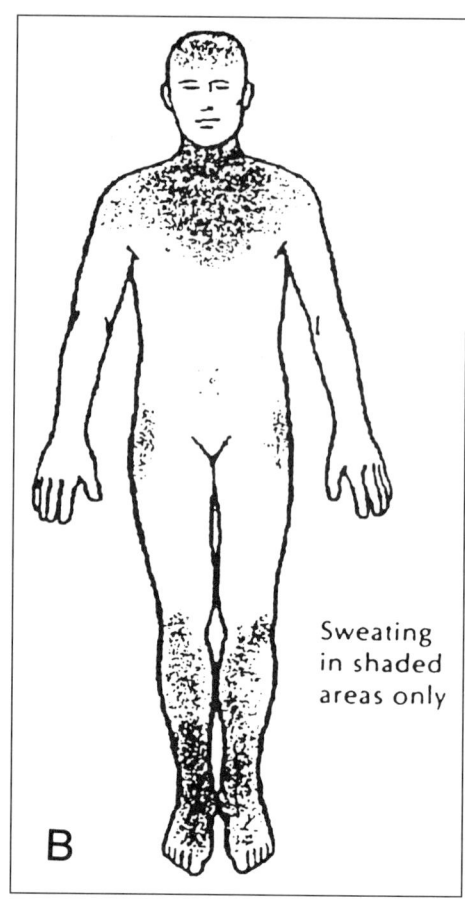

FIG. 14. Time–frequency maps **(left)** display a widespread loss of rhythmicity in RR interval and sympathetically mediated slow oscillations in blood pressure during rest and tilt-up. The thermoregulatory sweat test **(right)** reveals a widespread anhidrosis affecting >66% of the body surface.

sis can be used to separate patients with Parkinson's disease from early patients with MSA. Simultaneous recording of respiration can be helpful in the differential diagnosis because MSA patients often exhibit dysrhythmic breathing with irregular rate and amplitude. Some patients may develop central apnea or Cheyne–Stokes respiration, which typically worsens during the night (4,11). Loss of cardiovascular rhythms, both respiratory and low frequency, together with loss of slow BP oscillations, as well as abnormalities in the breathing pattern are indicators of brain stem involvement and may precede brain stem failure.

The activity of the sympathetic nervous system changes drastically after closed head injury. An early surge of sympathetic overactivity occurs within the first 2 weeks after the injury. An increase of heart rate correlates with this transitional stage, when heart rate variability is reduced as well, and can serve as an index of autonomic imbalance. This state of hyperactivity is important to recognize because it may damage the brain (22). Reduced HR variability in patients with brainstem lesions indicates vagal involvement, since it has an abnormal responses to infused atropine (70).

Several studies of patients with localized CNS lesions involving the brain or spinal cord injury have been conducted to evaluate the outcome in neurosurgical patients (14). In patients who are brain dead following brain stem hemorrhage, slow nonrespiratory oscillations in BP were preserved when both respiratory and nonrespiratory oscillations were abolished (46). One report using standard spectral analysis techniques described a very slow 0.002- to 0.01-Hz rhythm in blood pressure and RRI in brainstem-dead patients (28). Neuropathologic examinations of the medulla and spinal cord showed that the spinal cord, ventral and dorsal nerve roots, and the nucleus intermediolateralis below C3/C4 were largely intact. Unfortunately, all of these patients received dopamine and vasopressin in order to maintain BP. The intravenous infusion of these agents may artificially generate rhythmic nonneurogenic cardiovascular fluctuations that are simply related to the number of drops/min of solution infused. Nonrespiratory

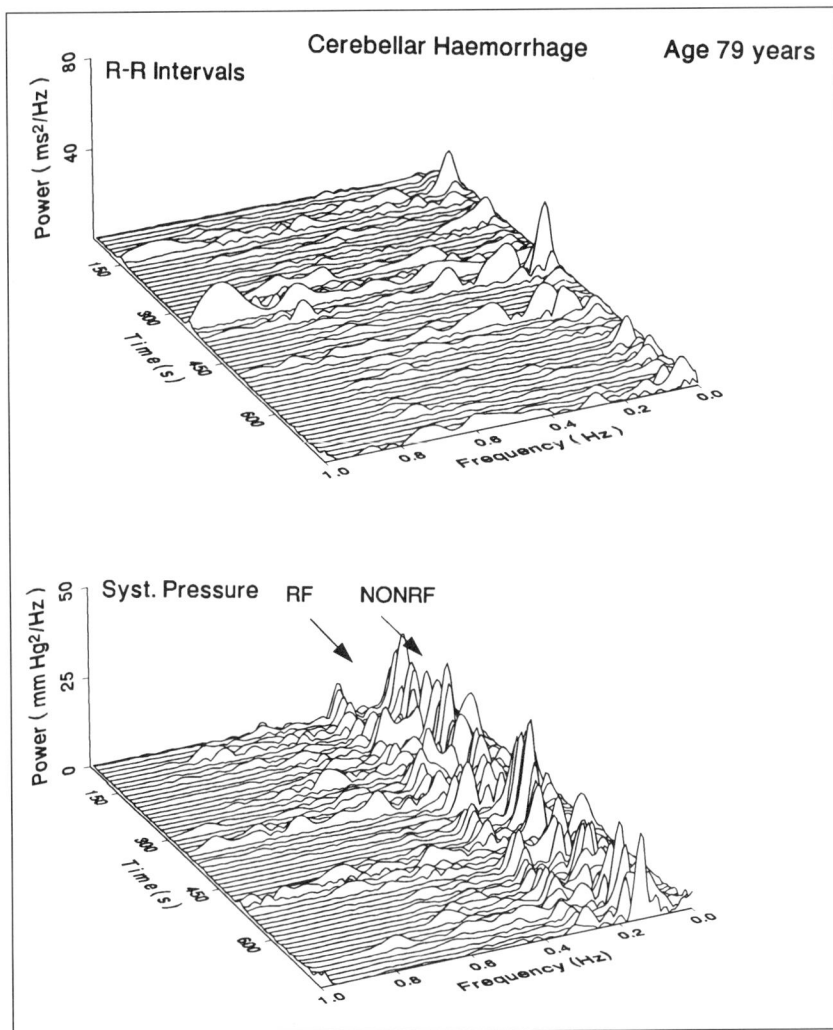
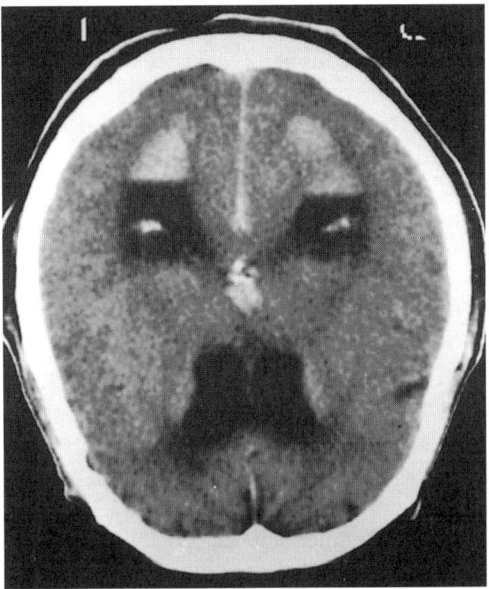

FIG. 15. A brain-dead patient, 79 years of age, following cerebellar hemorrhage. Magnetic resonance imaging **(right)** shows blood in the third and lateral ventricles. Time–frequency maps **(left)** reveal an almost complete loss of rhythmicity in RR interval. However, the sympathetically mediated rhythms remain well preserved.

RRI or blood pressure oscillations have not been observed in quadriplegic patients (25,26,30) following spinal injury, but similar rhythms have been observed in midcollicular decerebrated cats (33). The absence of these nonrespiratory oscillations in quadriplegic patients was attributed to interruption of supraspinal input to spinal sympathetic cardiomotor and vasomotor preganglionic neurons. In our study, nonrespiratory blood pressure fluctuations were observed in all five patients, although the time profile of these fluctuations was less regular than that of normal controls (46). Figure 15 illustrates the case of a 79-year-old women who had a large cerebellar hemorrhage, likely originating in the deep cerebellar nuclei and rupturing into and occluding the fourth ventricle, which caused an acute hydrocephalus. Note that hemorrhage has extended into the third and lateral ventricles. The patient was comatose, unresponsive, with no spontaneous respiration, and met criteria for brainstem death. RRI maps show a complete loss of rhythmicity at both RF and NONRF. In the systolic pressure map, we can see the mechanical oscillations at RF as well as a preserved low-frequency rhythm.

These data suggest that the spinal cord or caudal medulla may contain neural circuitry that can generate at least a portion of the nonrespiratory blood pressure rhythms and that integrity of the medulla further contributes to their generation.

Technical Guidelines

Spectral analysis of cardiovascular parameters is becoming an important tool in the evaluation of the autonomic nervous system. Therefore, it is crucially important to exclude confounding variables and to standardize an approach to clinical spectral analysis. Results of spectral analysis are greatly dependent on the quality of the data and the choice of parameters to analyze the data, described below, irrespective of whether one is using the classic

Fourier transformation, autoregressive modeling, moving periodogram, or time–frequency distributions. A recent review summarizing different methods of interpretation of both the time and the frequency domains has been published by the Task Force of the European Society of Cardiology and the North American Society of Pacing and Electrophysiology (67). In the time domain, standardization of statistical measures of evaluating heart rate variability have been recommended, especially regarding the minimal duration of recording. Acceptable methods of evaluating RRIs in terms of their variability and variability over time were defined as (a) standard deviation of RRIs (SDRR), (b) standard deviation of the average RRIs (SDARR), (c) heart rate variability triangular index (HRV), and (d) RMSSD square root of the mean squared differences of successive RRIs.

In the frequency domain, both FFT (autoregressive models) were recommended. However, there is a significant shortcoming of these standards in the frequency domain. The task force recommended the use of predetermined ranges, e.g., 0.04–0.15 Hz for the low-frequency power and 0.15–0.4 Hz for the high-frequency power. This recommendation is appropriate only when respiration is controlled at frequencies of >0.15 Hz. As we have clearly demonstrated, slow respiration can significantly affect spectral powers at frequencies of <0.15 Hz.

The following comprise minimum guidelines for an adequate spectral analysis:

Physiologic Variables

These need to be controlled. Resting recordings need to be done with a supine patient in a controlled environment for at least 10 min.

Respiration

This is one of the most important variables to control because it significantly affects results of spectral analysis. As was pointed out by Brown et al. (9), the effect of respiration on heart rate variability is dramatic but surprisingly often neglected. Ideally, RF and amplitude should be recorded routinely and included in the analysis of all data that undergo frequency analysis. Brown et al. (9) reviewed 147 articles reporting RRI power spectra in humans. Respiratory rate was measured only in 51% and tidal volume in 22%, and respiratory rate was controlled only in 37% and tidal volume in 11%. Slowing of respiration can greatly confound the results of spectral analysis. In normal subjects, respiration can entrain heart rate and blood pressure oscillations over a wide range of frequencies, from 0.01 to 0.5 Hz. Additionally, as the tidal volume is increased at slower frequencies, the amplitude of respiratory oscillations is increased almost tenfold (maximal at 0.07 Hz) compared with the values at 0.2 Hz. Hence, even a brief slowing of breathing frequency, by interacting with spectral power at slower frequencies, can greatly bias results. Slowing of respiration can result in a false-positive increase in low-frequency power, yielding a false-positive increase in low-frequency power (47). This can be falsely attributed to the augmentation of the sympathetic outflow. Once the actual breathing rate is known, detection of the *high-frequency powers* should be centered around the dominant breathing frequency and not at a default frequency.

Length of Recordings

As a general rule, the Fourier analysis requires a minimum of ~5 cycles of the slowest rhythm of interest (five consecutive slow waves) (6). Thus, if the very slow frequencies of interest have a period of ~1 min, then 5-min recording time should be viewed as a minimal. Because of the high variability of the spontaneous rhythms, longer, i.e., 10-min, recordings provide a reasonable compromise between resolution and physiologic variability. With Fourier methods, the spectral content can be only defined at harmonics of the fundamental frequency; hence, if a true component lies between two harmonics, its power will be divided.

Data Acquisition

During data acquisition, sampling rates need to be sufficiently high to provide good time resolution, especially for higher heart rates. Practically, a sampling rate of 250 Hz gives a time resolution of 4 ms, sufficient for heart rates of <240 beats/min. Acquired data need to be artifact free. In routine recordings, artifacts such as extrasystoles, movement, and muscle contraction are practically unavoidable and these "bad points" need to be removed. The most frequently used method is simply to replace the bad point by the previous value. In the case of an extrasystole, its RRI can be replaced by the mean of the preceding and following heartbeats. Most of the spectral methods still require equidistant data sampling. Since the time series of RRIs are not equidistant, data need to be resampled. The common method used for resampling is either polynomial or linear interpolation or *equidistant interpolation*. The latter simply means that two successive RRIs represent a trigonometric function, with the equidistant points on one side of this triangle and resampled RRIs on the axis. This allows equidistant data sampling at different rates and sufficient resolution. At a HR of <120 beats/min, resampling at 2 Hz provides adequate time and frequency resolution, whereas a HR of >120 beats/min usually requires more frequent sampling, i.e., at 4 Hz. Filtering and smoothing can significantly affect the spectral powers at the frequencies of interest. The setting of the parameters and of the low-pass filter needs to be such that the very slow frequencies (i.e., >0.02 Hz) are not excluded. The optimal setting would include at least 512 data points at the given resampling range or 256 points for a window in a moving periodogram setting. The filtering window commonly used is the Blackman window in the moving periodogram setting (50). Here, the spectrum is computed from data segments that shift along the signal with ~50% overlap.

CONCEPT OF TIME–FREQUENCY DISTRIBUTIONS

The major shortcoming of conventional methods is the requirement of data stationarity. Therefore, approaches such as the global periodogram or global Fourier transform methods are *not* suitable for the evaluation of transient changes. In fact, the majority of the physiologic phenomena—i.e., responses to postural change, mental arithmetic, and emotional stress, and responses to the autonomic function tests (tilt test, handgrip, cold pressure responses, or drug-infusion responses)—do not satisfy criteria for data stationarity. Indeed, it is often the transitional response that enables the autonomic physiologist to differentiate the abnormal from the normal reactions. New techniques from the class of time–frequency distributions that have been specially designed and tested to meet these needs include Wigner–Ville distribution, wavelet transform, and short-term Fourier transform and dynamic autoregressive modeling. Among these methods, Wigner–Ville distribution provides the most accurate estimate and the highest frequency resolution (29). In tilt studies, changes in cardiovascular signals evaluated by simultaneous time and frequency smoothing result in a modified Wigner distribution, which has been shown to provide a reliable estimate of spectral powers without generating undesirable cross-terms (43). The Wigner distribution decomposes signal expressed as a function of time into signal expressed as functions of both time and frequency. The modified Wigner distribution was demonstrated to be a good estimation method for short nonstationary time series, and its resolution was enhanced by independent time and frequency smoothing using a moving 128-event data window. The time–frequency distributions were computed with the same parameter set for all signals. The function used to calculate the modified Wigner distribution is

$$W_{zx}(n,m) = \tfrac{1}{2}N \sum_{k=0}^{N-1} |h(k)^2| * \sum_{p=-M+1}^{M-1} g(p)\, z(n+p+k) x^* (n+p-k) e^{-2i\pi km/N}$$

where n = frequency smoothing window and m = time smoothing window, $h(k)$ = window function with the length $2N - 1$ applied for frequency smoothing, $g(p)$ = window function with the length $2M - 1$ applied for time smoothing, and the *asterisk* denotes the complex conjugation.

To track even slight changes of the RF accurately, the cross-time–frequency distributions between respiration and, i.e., RRI, are calculated. Then, respiratory oscillations in RRI are determined at frequencies corresponding to the actual RF at given moment. The spectral powers are decomposed into respiratory and nonrespiratory components for each instant. The RF content is defined as the local maximum at the actual RF on the respiratory, RRI, systolic, and diastolic pressure time–frequency distributions. The remaining NONRF fluctuations are identified as the local maximum at all frequencies below the RF down to 0.01 Hz.

The periodogram computed from global time series has been used for comparisons with time–frequency analysis (50). Properties of Wigner distribution were compared with moving periodogram using two chirp signals. The frequency of chirp signal A increases, while the frequency of signal B slows. Signal C is a sum of A and B; thus, only two frequencies are present in signal C at the same time. Wigner distribution accurately depicted both frequencies from the signal, while moving periodogram was found to generate spurious frequencies (42). Figure 16 depicts comparisons between the modified Wigner distribution and the Fourier spectrum. The signal with decreasing frequency (a) was reversed, resulting in the signal b. Signal c is the sum of signals a and b. The time–frequency mapping of the signal c was performed with the following parameters: N = 128, M = 9, and $q(k)$ Gaussian window with $\alpha = 2.5$, $h(k) = 1$. For the Fourier analysis (e), the 128-point data window was multiplied by the Hanning window and the square of the 128-point FFT was taken. The data window was then shifted by one sample until the spectra of all remaining segments were obtained. Spurious peaks at 28 and 50 Hz at a time interval of 80–150 ms dominate in the Fourier analysis (e). There is also an error at the direct-current level (at 0 Hz). The real frequencies are suppressed and smeared out. Poor estimation of the Fourier spectrum is due to the time variation of the signal frequency within the data window. Time–frequency mapping follows the signal structure well, and the two main frequencies dominate on the Wigner plain.

The wavelet transform is a useful estimate of stationary signals, but different parameters need to be applied to the nonstationary data, and the frequency resolution is lower than in the Wigner–Ville distribution. Moreover, information about the change in the frequency band is needed prior to computation. Dynamic autoregressive modeling is one of the newer approaches, although it has been criticized for the great dependence of the estimation on the model used (55). These estimations are based either on the estimation of the autocorrelation function or on the linear prediction techniques. The method of forward–backward least squares, also called the modified covariance method, which is one of the most successful, is based on the minimalization of error using the least-squares method. As with FFT and short FFT, the shortcoming of this technique is mainly the variation in power when short data segments are used.

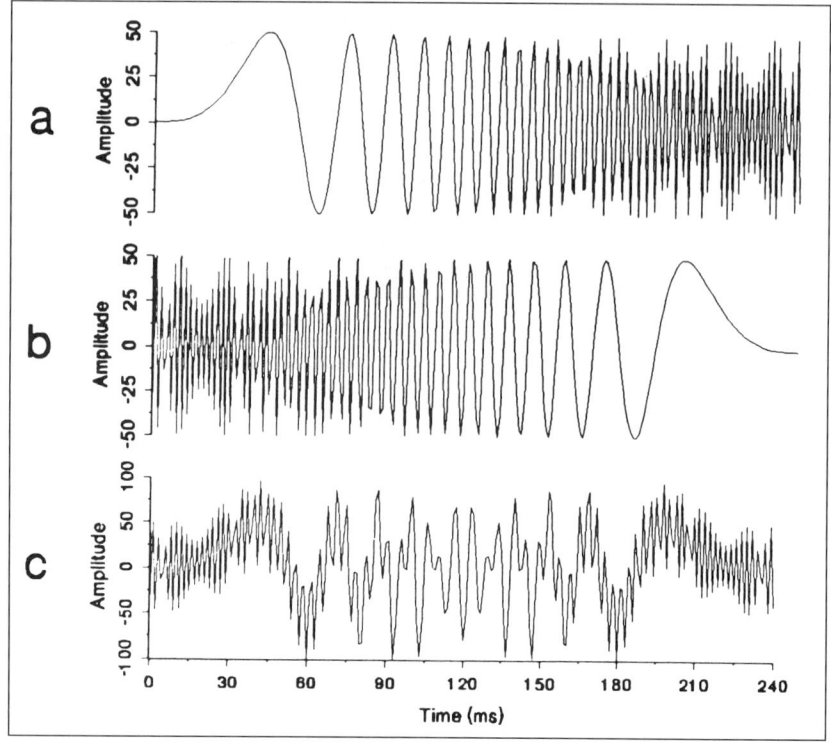
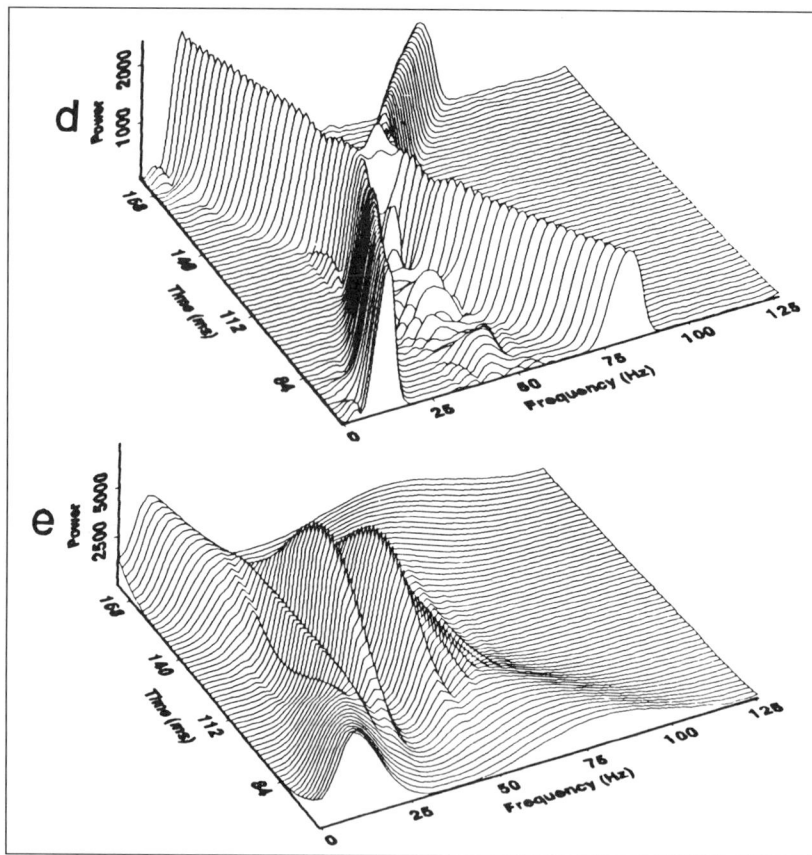

FIG. 16. Comparisons between the modified Wigner distribution and the Fourier spectrum. The signal in *a* shows a progressive change in frequency, and *b* is the reverse of *a*. The signal *c* is the sum of signals *a* and *b*. Spurious peaks dominate in the Fourier analysis (*e*). There is also an error at the direct-current level (at 0 Hz). The real frequencies are suppressed and smeared out. Poor estimation of the Fourier spectrum is due to the time variation of the signal frequency within the data window. The time–frequency map, in contrast, faithfully follows the signal structure, and the two main frequencies dominate on the Wigner plane. From Novak et al. (48), with permission.

Longer data segments provide a more reliable estimate. An additional drawback is that variation in power depends highly on the quality of the model estimate. Models of higher order tend to generate harmonic frequencies, whereas the frequency resolution is reduced in low-order models.

In conclusion, several methods currently are available for the evaluation of the stationary and nonstationary beat-to-beat cardiovascular data. Each technique has its strengths and limitations. It is most important that physicians who use spectral analysis to acquire and interpret data are aware of the requirements for adequate data recording, the limitations of the technique, and the boundaries in the interpretation of the results.

REFERENCES

1. Aharon-Peretz J, et al. Increased sympathetic and decreased parasympathetic cardiac innervation in patients with Alzheimer's disease. *Arch Neurol* 1992;49:919–922.
2. Akselrod S. Spectral analysis of fluctuations in cardiovascular parameters: a quantitative tool for the investigation of autonomic control. *Trends Pharmacol Sci* 1988;9:6–9.
3. Akselrod S, et al. Hemodynamic regulation: investigation by spectral analysis. *Am J Physiol* 1985;249:H867–H875.
4. Bannister R. *Autonomic failure*. Oxford: Oxford University Press, 1988.
5. Benarroch EE, et al. Central autonomic disorders. *J Clin Neurophysiol* 1993;10:39–50.
6. Bergland GD. A guided tour of the fast Fourier transform. *IEEE Spectrum* 1969;6:41–52.
7. Bernardi L, et al. Impaired circadian modulation of sympathovagal activity in diabetes: a possible explanation for altered temporal onset of cardiovascular disease. *Circulation* 1992;86:1443–1452.
8. Binkley PF, et al. Parasympathetic withdrawal is an integral component of autonomic imbalance in congestive heart failure: demonstration in human subjects and verification in a paced canine model of ventricular failure. *J Am Coll Cardiol* 1991;18:464–472.
9. Brown TE, et al. Important influence of respiration on human R-R interval power spectra is largely ignored. *J Appl Physiol* 1993;75:2310–2317.
10. Chau NP, et al. Fractal dimension of heart rate and blood pressure in healthy subjects and in diabetic subjects. *Blood Pressure* 1993;2:101–107.
11. Chokroverty S. Sleep and breathing in neurological disorders. In: Edelman NH, Santiago TV, eds. *Breathing disorders of sleep*. New York: Churchill Livingstone, 1986:225–264.
12. Claus D, et al. Investigation of parasympathetic and sympathetic cardiac innervation in diabetic neuropathy: heart rate variation versus meta-iodo-benzylguanidine measured by single photon emission computed tomography. *Clin Auton Res* 1994;4:117–123.
13. Cohn JN. Abnormalities of peripheral sympathetic nervous system control in congestive heart failure. *Circulation* 1990;82(Suppl 2):I-59–I-67.
14. Donchin Y, et al. Cardiac vagal tone predicts outcome in neurosurgical patients. *Crit Care Med* 1992;20:942–949.
15. Elmstahl S, et al. Autonomic cardiovascular responses to tilting in patients with Alzheimer's disease and in healthy elderly women. *Age Ageing* 1992;21:301–307.
16. Finley JP, et al. Heart rate variability in infants, children and young adults. *J Auton Nerv Syst* 1995;51:103–108.
17. Freeman R, et al. Transfer function analysis of respiratory sinus arrhythmia: a measure of autonomic function in diabetic neuropathy. *Muscle Nerve* 1995;18:74–84.
18. Groome LJ, et al. Spectral analysis of heart rate variability during quiet sleep in normal human fetuses between 36 and 40 weeks of gestation. *Early Hum Dev* 1994;38:1–9.
19. Hasking GJ, et al. Norepinephrine spillover to plasma in patients with congestive heart failure: evidence of increased overall and cardiorenal sympathetic nervous activity. *Circulation* 1986;73:615–621.
20. Hayano J, et al. Accuracy of assessment of cardiac vagal tone by heart rate variability in normal subjects. *Am J Cardiol* 1991;67:199–204.
21. Hoeldtke RD, et al. The orthostatic tachycardia syndrome: evaluation of autonomic function and treatment with octreotide and ergot alkaloids. *J Clin Endocrinol Metab* 1991;73:132–139.
22. Hortnagl H, et al. The activity of the sympathetic nervous system following severe head injury. *Intensive Care Med* 1980;6:169–177.
23. Hugelin A. Forebrain and midbrain influence on respiration. In: Cherniack NS, Widdicombe JG, eds. *Handbook of physiology*. Bethesda, MD: American Physiological Society, 1986:69–91.
24. Hukuhara T Jr, et al. Periodic variations of the electrocorticogram in relation to the respiratory rhythm and long-term periodic fluctuations of the renal sympathetic activity. In: Sieck GC, Gandevia SC, Cameron WE, eds. *Respiratory muscles and their neuromotor control*. New York: Alan R Liss, 1987:121–125.
25. Inoue K, et al. Power spectral analysis of blood pressure variability in traumatic quadriplegic humans. *Am J Physiol* 1991;260:H842–H847.
26. Inoue K, et al. Power spectral analysis of heart rate variability in traumatic quadriplegic humans. *Am J Physiol* 1990;258:H1722–H1726.
27. Kienzle MG, et al. Clinical, hemodynamic and sympathetic neural correlates of heart rate variability in congestive heart failure. *Am J Cardiol* 1992;69:761–767.
28. Kita Y, et al. Power spectral analysis of heart rate and arterial blood pressure oscillation in brain-dead patients. *J Auton Nerv Syst* 1993;44:101–107.
29. Kitney RI, et al. Techniques for studying short-term changes in cardiorespiratory data: II. In: Di Rienzo M, ed. *Computer analysis of cardiovascular signals*. IOS, 1995:41–52.
30. Koh J, et al. Human autonomic rhythms: vagal cardiac mechanisms in tetraplegic subjects. *J Physiol (Lond)* 1994;474:483–495.
31. Lagi A, et al. Cerebral autoregulation in orthostatic hypotension: a transcranial Doppler study. *Stroke* 1994;25:1771–1775.
32. Lepicovska V, et al. Time–frequency mapping in neurally mediated syncope. *Clin Auton Res* 1992;2:317–326.
33. Lombardi F, et al. Spectral analysis of sympathetic discharge in decerebrate cats. *J Auton Nerv Syst* 1990;30:S97–S100.
34. Low PA, et al. Postural tachycardia syndrome (POTS). *Neurology* 1995;45(Suppl 5):S19–S25.
35. Low PA, et al. Comparison of the postural tachycardia syndrome (POTS) with orthostatic hypotension due to autonomic failure. *J Auton Nerv Syst* 1994;50:181–188.
36. Madwed JB, et al. Heart rate response to hemorrhage-induced 0.05 Hz oscillations in arterial pressure in conscious dog. *Am J Physiol* 1991;260:H1248–H1253.
37. Mirra SS, et al. The Consortium to Establish a Registry of Alzheimer's Disease (CERAD). II. Standardization of the neuropathologic assessment of Alzheimer's disease. *Neurology* 1991;41:479–486.
38. Nadeau R, et al. Spectral estimations in heart failure in dogs. *IUPS* XXXII Glasgow 1993, also 173.6;85. 1993;32, Glasgow 85(abst).
39. Njemanze PC. Noninvasive circulation dysfunction and hemodynamic abnormalities in syncope during upright tilt test. *Can J Cardiol* 1993;9:238–242.
40. Novak P, et al. Increase of slow periodic modulation of EEG in a patient with Alzheimer's disease. *Physiol Res* 1992;41:293–297.
41. Novak P, et al. Slow modulation of EEG. *Neuroreport* 1992;3:189–192.
42. Novak P, et al. Time–frequency mapping of the entire QRS complex in normal subjects and in postmyocardial infarction patients. *J Electrocardiol* 1994;27:49–60.
43. Novak P, et al. Time/frequency mapping of the heart rate, blood pressure and respiratory signals. *Med Biol Eng Comput* 1993;31:103–110.
44. Novak P, et al. Time–frequency analysis of slow cortical activity and cardiovascular fluctuations in a case of Alzheimer's disease. *Clin Auton Res* 1994;4:141–148.
45. Novak V, et al. Hemodynamic profile of neurally-mediated syncope. *J Auton Nerv Syst* 1996;60:83–92.
46. Novak V, et al. Desynchronization of cardiovascular rhythms after severe brainstem injury. *Clin Auton Res* 1995;5:24–30.

47. Novak V, et al. Influence of respiration on heart rate and blood pressure fluctuations. *J Appl Physiol* 1993;74:617–626.
48. Novak V, et al. Slow cardiovascular rhythms at tilt and syncope. *J Clin Neurophysiol* 1995;12:64–71.
49. Novak V, et al. Topography of slow modulation of EEG in normal subjects during rest and head-up tilt. *Clin Auton Res* 1994;4:200 (abst).
50. Oppenheim AV, et al. *Digital signal processing.* Englewood Cliffs, NJ: Prentice Hall, 1985.
51. Oppenheimer LW, et al. Power spectral analysis of fetal heart rate. *Baillieres Clin Obstet Gynaecol* 1994;8:643–661.
52. Pagani M, et al. Power spectral analysis of heart rate and arterial pressure variabilities as a marker of sympatho-vagal interaction in man and conscious dog. *Circ Res* 1986;59:178–193.
53. Petit D, et al. Spectral analysis of the rapid eye movement sleep electroencephalogram in right and left temporal regions: a biological marker of Alzheimer's disease. *Ann Neurol* 1992;32:172-176.
54. Pfurtscheller G. Ultralangsame Schwankungen innerhalb der rhythmischen Aktivität im Alpha-Band und deren mögliche Ursachen. *Pflügers Arch* 1976;367:55–66.
55. Pola S, et al. Estimation of the power spectral density in nonstationary cardiovascular time series: assessing the role of the time–frequency representations (TFR). *IEEE Trans Biomed Eng* 1996;43: 46–59.
56. Porter TR, et al. Autonomic pathophysiology in heart failure patients: sympathetic–cholinergic interrelations. *J Clin Invest* 1990;85:1362–1371.
57. Ryan SM, et al. Gender- and age-related differences in heart rate dynamics: are women more complex than men? *J Am Coll Cardiol* 1994;24:1700–1707.
58. Sandroni P, et al. Early cardiovascular predictors of syncope. *Neurology* 1995;45:A396(abst).
59. Scheff SW, et al. Synapse loss in the temporal lobe in Alzheimer's disease. *Ann Neurol* 1993;33:190–199.
60. Schondorf R, et al. Echocardiographic measurements during neurally mediated syncope: no evidence of an "empty heart." *Clin Auton Res* 1994;4:196.(abst).
61. Schondorf R, et al. Idiopathic postural orthostatic tachycardia syndrome: an attenuated form of acute pandysautonomia? *Neurology* 1993;43:132–137.
62. Sheldon R, et al. Changes in heart rate variability during fainting. *Chaos* 1991;3:257–261.
63. Sibony O, et al. Quantification of the fetal heart rate variability by spectral analysis of fetal well-being and fetal distress. *Eur J Obstet Gynecol Reprod Biol* 1994;54:103–108.
64. Sibony O, et al. Spectral analysis of fetal heart rate in flat recordings. *Early Hum Dev* 1995;41:215–220.
65. Simpson DM, et al. Spectral analysis of heart rate indicates reduced baroreceptor-related heart rate variability in elderly persons. *J Gerontol* 1988;43:M21–M24.
66. Sopher SM, et al. Autonomic pathophysiology in heart failure: carotid baroreceptor-cardiac reflexes. *Am J Physiol* 1990;259:H689–H696.
67. Task Force of the European Society of Cardiology and the North American Society of Pacing and Electrophysiology. Heart rate variability: standards of measurements, physiological interpretation and clinical use. *Circulation* 1996;93:1043–1065.
68. Van Lieshout JJ, et al. The vasovagal response [Review]. *Clin Sci* 1991;81:575–586.
69. Veerman DP, et al. Effects of aging on blood pressure variability in resting conditions. *Hypertension* 1994;24:120–130.
70. Weis M, et al. Disorders of autonomic heart rate regulation in patients with brain stem lesions [in German]. *Nervenarzt* 1994;65:381–389.
71. Weise F, et al. Age-related changes of heart rate power spectra in a diabetic man during orthostasis. *Diabetes Res Clin Pract* 1991;11: 23–32.
72. Weise F, et al. Heart rate variability in diabetic patients during orthostatic load: a spectral analytic approach. *Klin Wochenschr* 1990;68: 26–32.
73. Wilcock GK. Recent research into dementia. *Age Ageing* 1988;17: 73–86.
74. Woo MA, et al. Complex heart rate variability and serum norepinephrine levels in patients with advanced heart failure. *J Am Coll Cardiol* 1994;23:565–569.
75. Yeragani VK, et al. Relationship between age and heart rate variability in supine and standing postures: a study of spectral analysis of heart rate. *Pediatr Cardiol* 1994;15:14–20.
76. Yoshioka K, et al. Relationship between diabetic autonomic neuropathy and peripheral neuropathy as assessed by power spectral analysis of heart rate variations and vibratory perception thresholds. *Diabetes Res Clin Pract* 1994;24:9–14.
77. Ziegler D, et al. Assessment of cardiovascular autonomic function: age-related normal ranges and reproducibility of spectral analysis, vector analysis, and standard tests of heart rate variation and blood pressure responses. *Diabetic Med* 1992;9:166–175.
78. Ziegler D, et al. Prevalence and clinical correlates of cardiovascular autonomic and peripheral diabetic neuropathy in patients attending diabetes centers: the Diacan Multicenter Study Group. *Diabetes Metab Rev* 1993;19:143–151.
79. Ziegler D, et al. Prevalence of cardiovascular autonomic dysfunction assessed by spectral analysis and standard tests of heart-rate variation in newly diagnosed IDDM patients. *Diabetes Care* 1992;15:908–911.

CHAPTER 27

Transcranial Doppler Evaluation in Disorders of Reduced Orthostatic Tolerance

Peter Novak, Vera Novak, Phillip A. Low, and George W. Petty

1. We describe a novel approach to evaluate central autonomic vascular regulation, using the simultaneous monitoring of electroencephalogram (EEG), transcranial Doppler (TCD), respiration, carbon dioxide heart rate, and blood pressure during autonomic testing.
2. The concept of amplitude modulation of EEG (AM-EEG) has been recently introduced. AM-EEG refers to the slow rhythms superimposed on the baseline EEG activity and occurs at three major frequencies: 0.02–0.03, 0.05–0.06, and 0.10–0.12 Hz in awake human subjects. We posit that these rhythms reflect the activity of the central autonomic network and propagate to the cortex from the brainstem autonomic centers.
3. Orthostatic hypotension in patients with multiple-system atrophy, pure autonomic failure, or peripheral neuropathy may or may not be associated with cerebral autoregulation failure.
4. In autoregulation failure, the profile of blood flow velocity passively follows the profile of blood pressure during the Valsalva maneuver and upright tilt.
5. A mildly abnormal profile of cerebral autoregulation can also be seen in the patients with mild orthostatic intolerance, postural tachycardia syndrome, or vasodepressor syncope.
6. The addition of the quantitative evaluation of the EEG and TCD to standard autonomic function tests significantly augments the value of autonomic testing, especially when novel methods of signal analysis are also used.

TECHNICAL ASPECTS OF TRANSCRANIAL DOPPLER, EEG, RESPIRATION, AND CARBON DIOXIDE MONITORING DURING AUTONOMIC TESTING

Transcranial Doppler

Transcranial Doppler (TCD) is a portable, noninvasive technology that assesses the intracranial circulation. Clinical applications include evaluations of conditions such as vasospasm, ischemic stroke and transient ischemic attack, arteriovenous malformations, head injury, and suspected brain death. It is also widely employed in intraoperative and postoperative monitoring of neurosurgical patients (46). Only recently has this technology been extended to the evaluation of patients with autonomic nervous system disease. The major advantage of TCD in autonomic evaluations is that it enables continuous and noninvasive monitoring of cerebral blood flow velocity (BFV) during physiologic tests like the Valsalva maneuver, tilt-table test, or deep breathing. This ability to detect autonomic stimulus-induced alterations in cerebral BFV offers promise of insights into the mechanisms of symptoms in patients with orthostatic intolerance or syncope.

TCD devices employ a pulsed, range-gated probe that emits a 2-MHz ultrasound signal focused by a plastic lens. The *lower frequency* ultrasound signal is needed to allow sound waves to penetrate the skull and brain tissues so that the main circle of Willis arteries at the base of the brain can be studied. This signal is reflected from erythrocytes within the vessel under investigation and sensed again by the probe. When the signal is received, it is converted using the piezoelectric material into electrical pulses that are then further processed by real-time fast Fourier techniques to obtain

---

P. Novak, V. Novak, P. A. Low, and G. W. Petty: Department of Neurology, Mayo Clinic and Foundation, Rochester, Minnesota 55905.

the measured frequency of the reflected signal. Doppler shift, a difference between the frequency of the emitted signal (2 MHz) and its echo (frequency of the reflected signal), is then used to calculate the velocity of blood flow (Fig. 1). The spectral analysis of BFVs is then presented as a waveform, similar to the blood pressure waveform.

The TCD ultrasound signal cannot be transmitted through all areas of the skull. Three main areas, so-called "ultrasound windows," have been identified and used for clinical evaluation. In the *transtemporal approach* (Fig. 2), the probe is placed over the temporal area, above the zygomatic arch, so that the signal is able to traverse the thin temporal bone. The *transorbital window* (Fig. 2) is insonated by placing the probe on the eye and directing the signal through the orbit. The *suboccipital approach* (Fig. 2) is used by placing the probe beneath the inion and directing the signal through the foramen magnum. The most convenient artery to insonate for the purpose of autonomic evaluation is the middle cerebral artery (MCA) M_1 segment (transtemporal window). Also, estimation of BFVs is a function of a cosine of the angle between the Doppler beam and the artery, so the most accurate BFVs are obtained from the MCA M_1 segment, since the angle of insonation of this vessel via the transtemporal approaches zero.

For autonomic studies, TCD monitoring has been modified to meet criteria for continuous stable and relatively long-duration monitoring during autonomic physiologic perturbations. Strict technical requirements must be satisfied with particular attention paid to the stable positioning of the probe. We typically insonate the left MCA. We begin insonation at the anterior temporal window and, in a zigzag trajectory, edge toward the posterior temporal window. The location with maximal velocity and thus the smallest angle of insonation is highlighted by a marker. We prefer the anterior window because of its higher signal quality and because it permits more flexibility in fixing the probe holder. The Doppler probe holder is made from Teflon (Multigon Industries, Yonkers, N.Y.) and allows three-dimensional manipulation of the probe, which can be fixed in any desired position by elastic straps and centered on the highlighted area over the temporal bone. Final adjustment of probe position is done just before starting autonomic tests. Proper fixing of the probe at a constant angle of insonation in the same patient is crucial for the comparisons of data

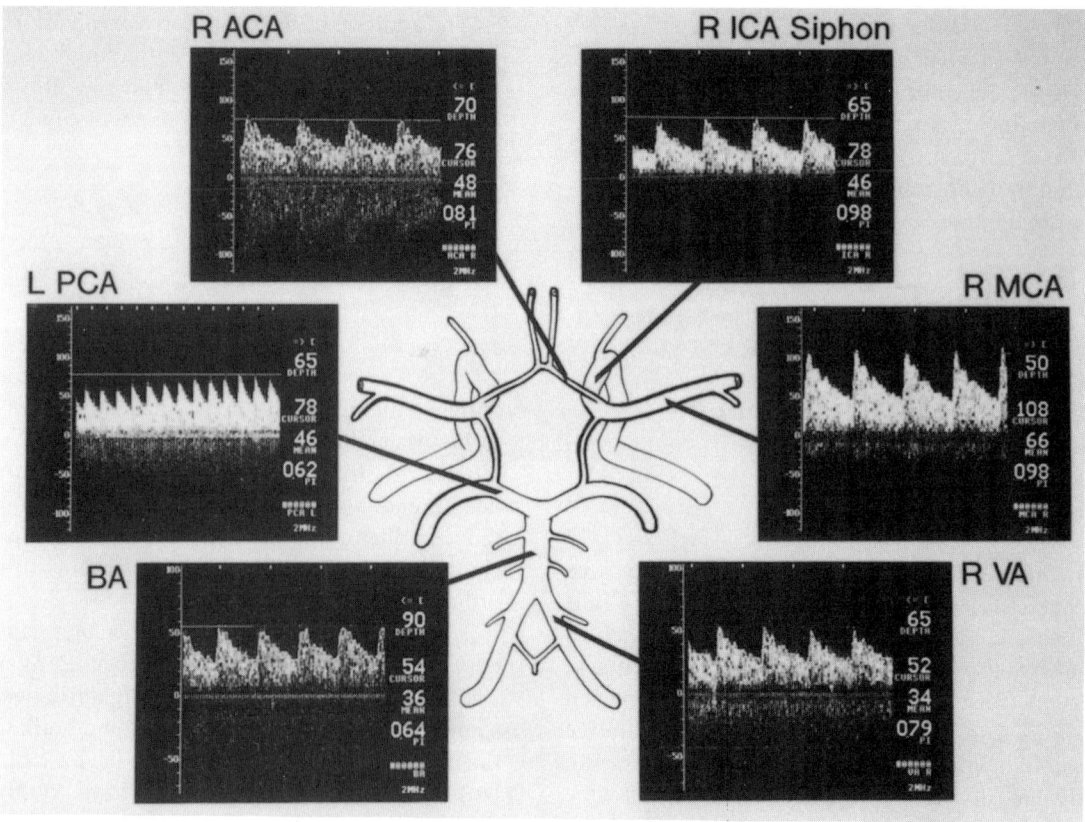

FIG. 1. Typical blood flow profile waveform from the anterior cerebral artery (ACA), middle cerebral artery (MCA), bifurcation (ACA/MCA), basilar artery, posterior basilar artery, and vertebral artery. From Petty et al. (46), with permission.

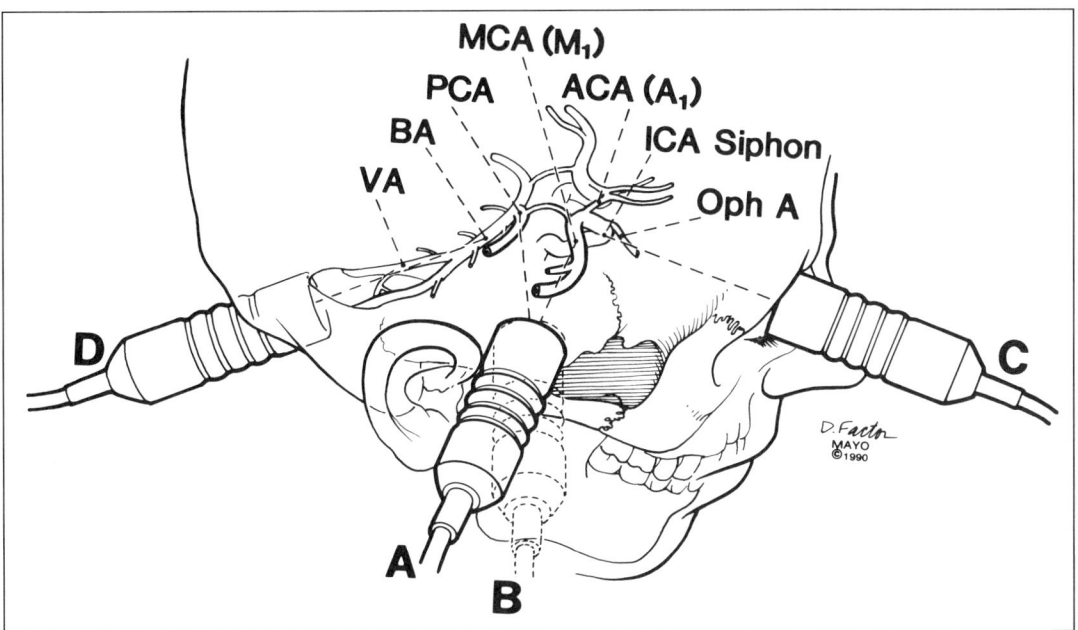

FIG. 2. Scheme of the insonation approaches used for transcranial Doppler (TCD) monitoring. The transtemporal approaches **A** and **B** are used to insonate MCA (middle cerebral artery) M_1, ACA (anterior cerebral artery) anterior segment A_1, and distal internal carotid artery (ICA) siphon and posterior cerebral artery (PCA) P_1 segments. The transorbital window is used for insonation of the ophthalmic artery and ICA siphon. The suboccipital window is used for insonation of vertebral arteries and basilar artery (BA). From Petty et al. (46), with permission.

from different maneuvers. The Doppler signal thus obtained is recorded on a computer for further signal processing.

Time Domain

The parameters of major interest are the maximal velocity or spectral envelope. These signals can be generated in real time by using commercially available hardware (add-in card in the Multigon TCD System), or off-line by simply saving data on the hard drive and processing them afterward. The maximal velocity is recorded on the proprietary computerized system. We routinely record other signals such as electroencephalogram (EEG) (six leads), CO_2, respiration, electrocardiogram, and BP. In the clinical setting, average or mean values of velocity are usually computed from several cardiac cycles. In the experimental setting, more instantaneous beat-to-beat analysis is usually required. Momentum statistics comprises detection of the systolic peak and diastolic trough, mean velocity, and derived parameters such as pulsatility index. Several indices have been proposed to evaluate central resistance. The most frequently used index, proposed by Gosling and King (17), is called the *pulsatility index* (PI), defined as $PI = (v_s - v_d)/V$, where v_s = the systolic velocity, v_d = diastolic velocity, and V = mean velocity (35). There is a preliminary report that the TCD signal can be described as a chaotic process (4) and thus estimation of fractal properties might be helpful (25). Our approach is to compute the Hurst coefficient (2,24), which gives a measure of self similarity and randomness of the signal.

Frequency Domain

Both Fourier and time–frequency distributions can be generated. These methods have been described in detail in the preceding chapter and will be described only briefly. For spectral analysis using fast Fourier transform of TCD signals, the same criteria are used as for the analysis of blood pressure. These include a requirement of stationary signal, removal of "bad points," equidistant data resampling, mean removal, and data filtering. Similarly, for application of the modified Wigner distribution or other methods of the time–frequency analysis, the approach outlined in the preceding chapter is necessary.

EEG Monitoring

In our laboratory, we use the standard 10–20 montage, using mainly monopolar recordings with the ears as a common reference. EEG monitoring during autonomic testing, especially tilt-up, is valuable for the detection of diffuse or focal cerebral hypoxia, or seizure activity in response to induced autonomic perturbations. Simultaneous monitoring of EEG during autonomic testing is useful in evaluating patients with the unexplained loss of consciousness, in the differential diagnosis between seizure and syncope. In the occasional patient with frequent loss of consciousness, pseudosyncope can be diagnosed when these episodes are associated with normal systemic cardiovascular parameters and a normal EEG. EEG monitoring also provides valuable information about the central response to acute or chronic hypoperfusion. Typically, the response is a global hypoxia, characterized by an EEG dominated by high-voltage slow-wave activity. Less frequently, focal ischemia, or even strokes, can occur (15,19).

Tilt-induced loss of consciousness is often associated with a few myoclonic jerks, recognized as being caused by cerebral hypoxia. However, syncope is sometimes associated with florid involuntary movements indistinguishable from seizures clinically. A simultaneous EEG recording can resolve this question. Recently, EEG, audiovisual, and autonomic recordings of tilt-induced syncope were presented (9). Patients with apparent florid seizures were found to have EEG changes of cerebral hypoxia but without EEG seizure activity.

Carbon Dioxide and Respiratory Monitoring

Although respiration has an important effect on autonomic testing, it is frequently not recorded or its influence is neglected (7). Monitoring of respiratory rate is essential in order to evaluate whether a patient's breathing pattern is normal. It will enable such important diagnoses as the hyperventilation syndrome, apneas, or irregular breathing. Monitoring of respiratory volume and rate is also important for the evaluation of respiratory and nonrespiratory oscillations in heart rate, blood pressure, or blood flow. Slow deep breaths or apneas greatly augment oscillations at slow frequencies and could lead to the spurious interpretation of increased sympathetic activity. Indeed, not only are abnormal respiratory patterns found in several autonomic disorders, but the prevalence of the sleep-related breathing disorders is also high in the general population (13). The disorders range from obstructive sleep apnea to central sleep apnea (Chapter 47). Disturbed breathing can result from an interaction of different factors, such as increased CO_2 threshold, decreased chemical drive, respiratory muscle failure, and impairment in the brainstem centers (13,45).

Patients suffering from obstructive or central sleep apnea present with frequent complaints of autonomic dysfunction and profound daytime fatigue, sleepiness, sleep attacks, and often depression. The major autonomic manifestation is sympathetic overactivity, characterized by the elevated levels of both daytime and nocturnal plasma norepinephrine, higher blood pressure during head-up tilt, and diminished cardiovagal indices (deep breathing and Valsalva ratio) (52). High sympathetic activity is found throughout the day and night. However, only nighttime urinary norepinephrine and averaged 24-hr blood pressure were found to correlate with the severity of the obstructive sleep apnea. Treatment with continuous positive-pressure breathing during the night improved not only the clinical symptoms, but daytime plasma norepinephrine fell by 50% and nighttime vanylmandelic acid and metanephrine by 32%–54% (21). It is now widely accepted that sleep disorders are causally related to daytime hypertension and can have severe cardiovascular consequences like arterial hypertension and arrhythmia (45). Patients with mild hypertension may be unaware of daytime apneas (42). However, overall reduction of cardiovagal activity is detectable in the autonomic laboratory as reduced heart rate variability at both respiratory and nonrespiratory frequencies. Transient increases of the amplitude of the nonrespiratory (<0.1 Hz) oscillations in heart rate, previously attributed to the spontaneous augmentation of sympathetic drive in these patients, are in fact related to the apneas. It is the augmentation of these nonrespiratory oscillations in blood pressure that is associated with elevated sympathetic vasomotor outflow in these patients (42).

As we briefly discussed in the preceding chapter, periodic breathing or apneas can be also found in the patients with multiple-system atrophy (MSA) and may be a harbinger of the onset of brainstem failure (11). Death often occurs at night and may be due to either obstructive or central sleep apnea; often the pattern is mixed. Sleep breathing disorders can also be a serious life-threatening complication in advanced multiple sclerosis and can lead to a severe respiratory insufficiency (22) and failure. ALthough the frequency of sleep-related breathing disorders in certain conditions (such as MSA) is well known, its prevalence in the general population of patients suffering from orthostatic hypotension and supine hypertension has not been well studied.

Monitoring of respiration is also useful in the evaluation of the milder forms of orthostatic intolerance. In the evaluation of patients with syncope, orthostatic weakness, or orthostatic tachycardia, it is important to determine whether the hyperventilation syndrome is present. Especially in young individuals with vasomotor overactivity, hyperventilation-induced cerebral vasoconstriction can trigger hypoperfusion and syncope (18,36), cerebral circulation dysfunction, and hemodynamic abnormalities in syncope during upright tilt.

Hyperventilatory response to upright position occurs in some patients with orthostatic tachycardia. Reduction of CO_2 triggers vasoconstriction of cerebral vessels, which contribute to symptoms of orthostatic intolerance.

INDICES OF THE CENTRAL AUTONOMIC FUNCTIONS

Amplitude Modulation of EEG

The concept of amplitude modulation of the EEG (AM-EEG) that has recently been introduced (39,40) is based on the observation that the brainstem neural network oscillates at frequencies of <0.5 Hz. Pfurtscheller (47) observed the occasional synchrony between respiration and alpha rhythm in human EEG. The spontaneous oscillations generated by the brainstem cardiovascular and respiratory network are well known and detectable in the heart rate and blood pressure. Here, two main oscillations are recognized (a) oscillations at respiratory frequencies, synchronized with the breathing frequency, and (b) oscillations at slower (<0.1 Hz) nonrespiratory frequencies. These rhythms reflect central modulation of the cardiovagal and vasomotor outflows, emphasizing the importance of the central autonomic network (3) (Chapter 2). The structures involved in the generation of slow oscillations in the cardiovascular system are likely in the brain stem autonomic centers (includes tractus solitarii, respiratory network, and the sympathetic nuclei in the ventrolateral medulla), but the medial reticular formation could also be involved. The medial brainstem reticular formation belongs to a common brainstem system for the integration of somatosensory and autonomic functions. All neurons are located in the medial two-thirds of the reticular formation of the lower brainstem. These neurons are modulated by inputs from baroreceptors, subject to respiratory modulation, and their activity can be correlated with rhythms of the electrocorticogram. The substrate essential for wake–sleep is located in the vicinity of the nucleus solitarius. These neurons are also responsible for generating rhythmic discharges (8,27,29).

Baseline EEG in normal healthy awake subjects is characterized by the presence of alpha spindles (8–12 Hz), beta rhythms (13–30 Hz) and, during deep relaxation, also by theta rhythm (5–7 Hz). There is no clear separation between the slower alpha and theta rhythms. The dominant EEG activity might shift continuously within the range of 8–12 Hz. AM-EEG has been recently reported (39,40) and is manifested in healthy subjects at frequencies of 0.02–0.03, 0.05–0.06, and 0.10–0.12 Hz. Another peak corresponding to the respiratory frequency was also frequently present.

Figure 3 demonstrates the technical concept of slow amplitude modulation. This concept have been known for many years in other areas, e.g., the physics of propagation of sound waves. In our example, we have generated two signals with constant frequency and amplitude. The signal at the top of the figure has the faster frequency, and the second signal, in the middle of the figure, has a slower frequency. Both signals have constant amplitudes. These two signals have been mixed together, resulting in the third signal with the spindlelike character. The faster frequency is preserved as the baseline frequency of the faster rhythm, and the envelope of spindles has the frequency of the slow rhythm. The envelope of these spindles is then what is technically called the *amplitude modulation* or AM.

In our approach, alpha and theta rhythms have been extracted from the raw EEG signal and constructed as independent time series. Data from 108 young healthy volun-

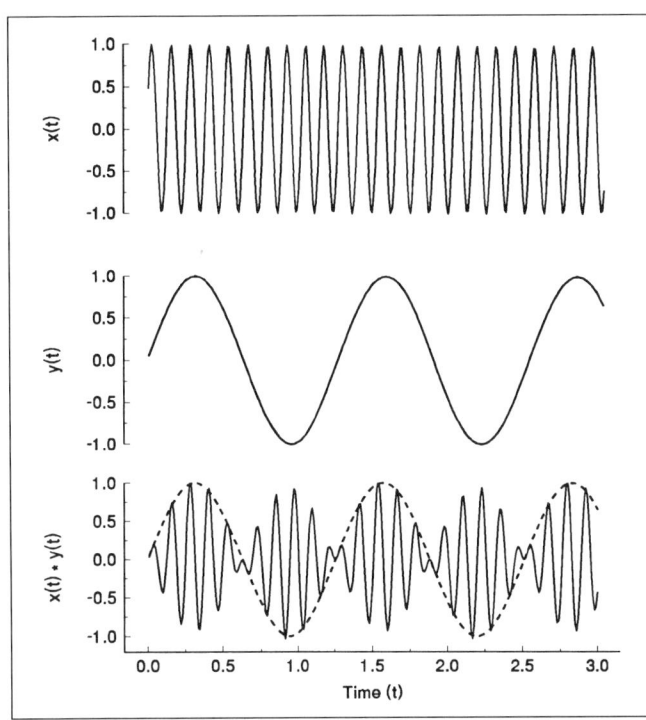

FIG. 3. The concept of the amplitude modulation. Artificial signal $x(t)$, which has a faster frequency, is mixed with signal $y(t)$, which has a slower frequency and similar amplitude. The resulting signal $x(t) \cdot y(t)$ has a spindlelike pattern. The slow modulation (*dashed line*) represents the envelope of these spindles.

teers were recorded using the 32-channel mapping system (Brain Imager IIs, Neuroscience) while the volunteers were resting supine with eyes closed. Data were recorded from the 28 channels with monopolar leads, and linked earlobes served as a common reference. Monopolar EEGs were recorded using the standard 10–20 system. The EEG signal was filtered at 40 Hz and digitized at a sampling frequency of 200 Hz with 12-bit resolution per channel. Fast Fourier transform (FFT) was calculated for 2.5-sec-long segments, multiplied by a Tukey window. The resulting spectrum was divided into theta (4.3–7.8 Hz), alpha (8.2–11.7 Hz), and beta I (12.1–16.0 Hz) and beta II (16.4–30.0 Hz) bands. The theta, alpha, beta I, and beta II band powers have been obtained as an integral over the band. The FFT of the next segment was then processed until all segments were evaluated. The theta, alpha, beta I, and beta II band powers were considered as time series with a sampling rate of 2.5 sec. The recordings of all leads were analyzed using Fourier transform, autoregressive model and, recently, Wigner distribution. The mean and baseline trends were removed by a third-order moving polynomial with a 65-sample window length. The frequencies above the Nyquist rate were filtered by a FIR filter. The frequency of the slow modulation was further analyzed by FFT and autoregressive modeling.

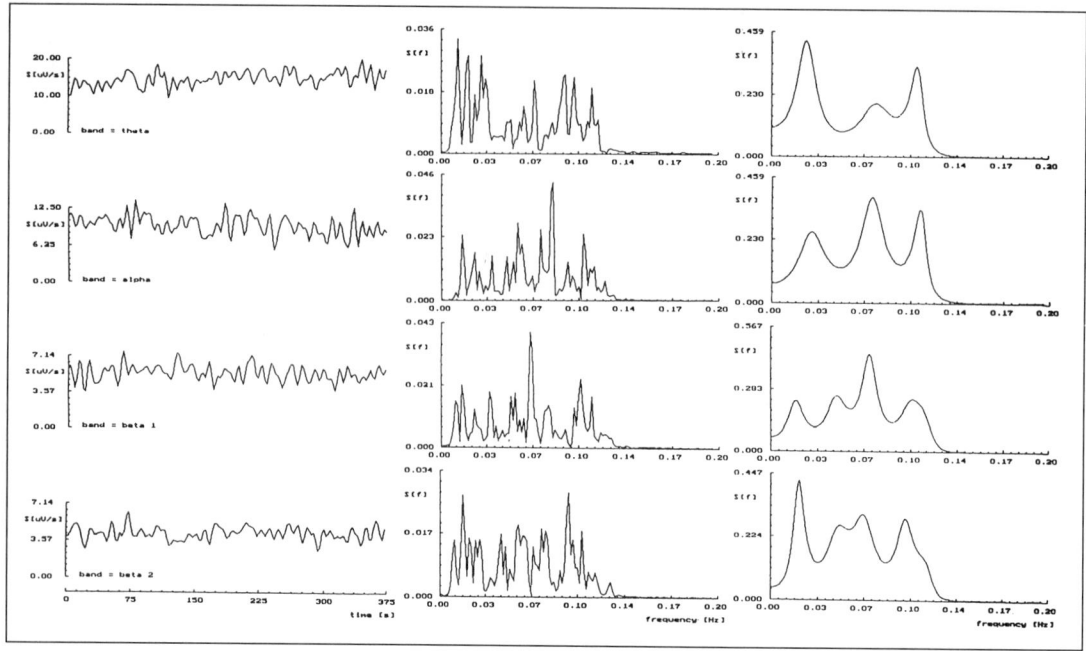

FIG. 4. The envelope slow modulation during supine rest in a young healthy subject from the C_z lead in the theta, alpha, beta I, and beta II bands. On the corresponding Fourier and autoregressive spectra, three peaks corresponding to the three amplitude modulation rhythms at frequencies of 0.03, 0.06, and 0.1 Hz are clearly present.

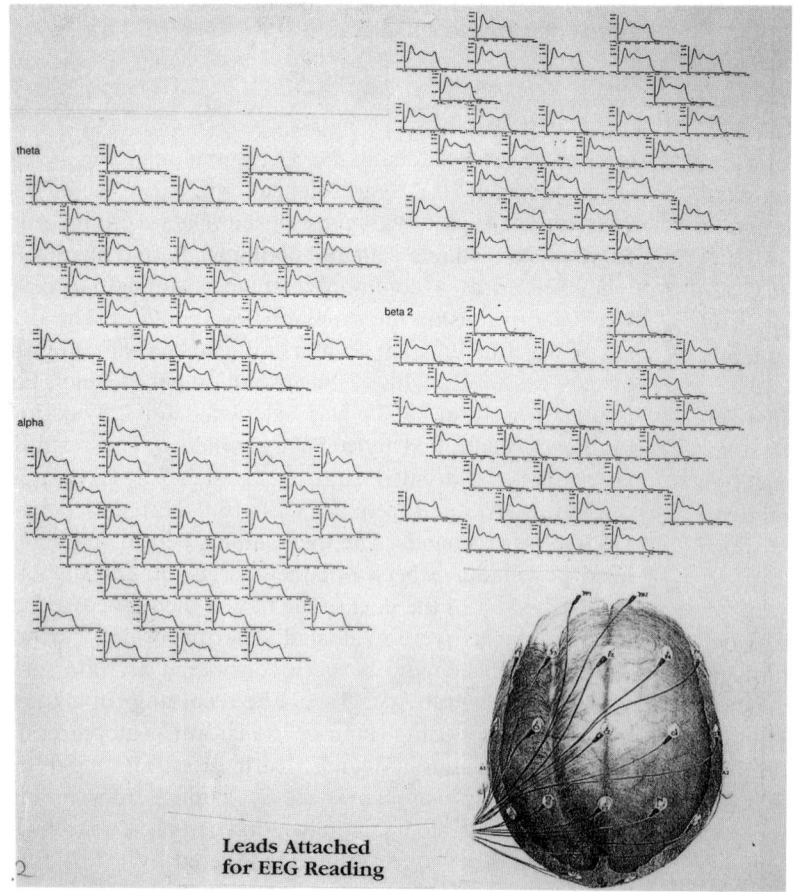

FIG. 5. Autoregressive spectra averaged over 108 healthy young subjects showing distribution of the slow amplitude modulation rhythms during supine rest with eyes closed. It is important to note that all three rhythms (0.02, 0.05, and 0.1 Hz) are present in all frequency bands alpha, theta, beta I, and beta II. The slow rhythm (0.02 Hz) is most prominent over the scalp.

TABLE 1. *Summary data of the three amplitude modulation rhythms*

band EED	1.rhythm				2.rhythm				3.rhythm			
	frequency [Hz]	sd	period [s]	sd	frequency [Hz]	sd	period [s]	sd	frequency [Hz]	sd	period [s]	sd
theta	0.0218	0.0003	45.9	0.6	0.0534	0.0016	18.1	0.1	0.1021	0.0012	9.8	0.1
alpha	0.0214	0.0007	46.7	1.5	0.0538	0.0009	18.6	0.3	0.1033	0.0014	9.7	0.1
beta1	0.0219	0.0005	45.7	1.0	0.0543	0.0014	18.4	0.5	0.1037	0.0008	9.6	0.1
beta2	0.0221	0.0009	45.3	1.8	0.0527	0.0020	18.9	0.7	0.1026	0.0010	9.8	0.1
mean	0.0219	0.0006	45.7	1.3	0.0536	0.0014	18.5	0.4	0.1030	0.0013	9.7	0.1
					frequency [Hz]		period [s]		frequency [Hz]		period [s]	
range					0.04–0.07		14.3–25		0.07–0.13		7.7–14.3	
R-R interval					0.066		15.1		0.102		9.8	
respiration									0.117		8.5	

Figure 4 shows time series constructed from baseline theta, alpha, beta I, and beta II band powers from a young subject resting with eyes closed, and corresponding FFT and autoregressive spectra recorded from the C_z (central midline) lead. It can be clearly appreciated using both methods of frequency analysis that three rhythms modulated the baseline EEG band powers at frequencies of 0.02–0.03, 0.05–0.06, and 0.10–0.12 Hz, and another peak corresponding to the respiratory frequency was also frequently present. A pilot study using 108 healthy young subjects has been conducted to evaluate the distribution and character of AM-EEG during the relaxed resting awake state. Mean values of the frequencies and their distribution for each band are presented in Table 1 and Fig. 5. There was a striking similarity between the frequencies of the AM-EEG in each range among the subjects. The domi-

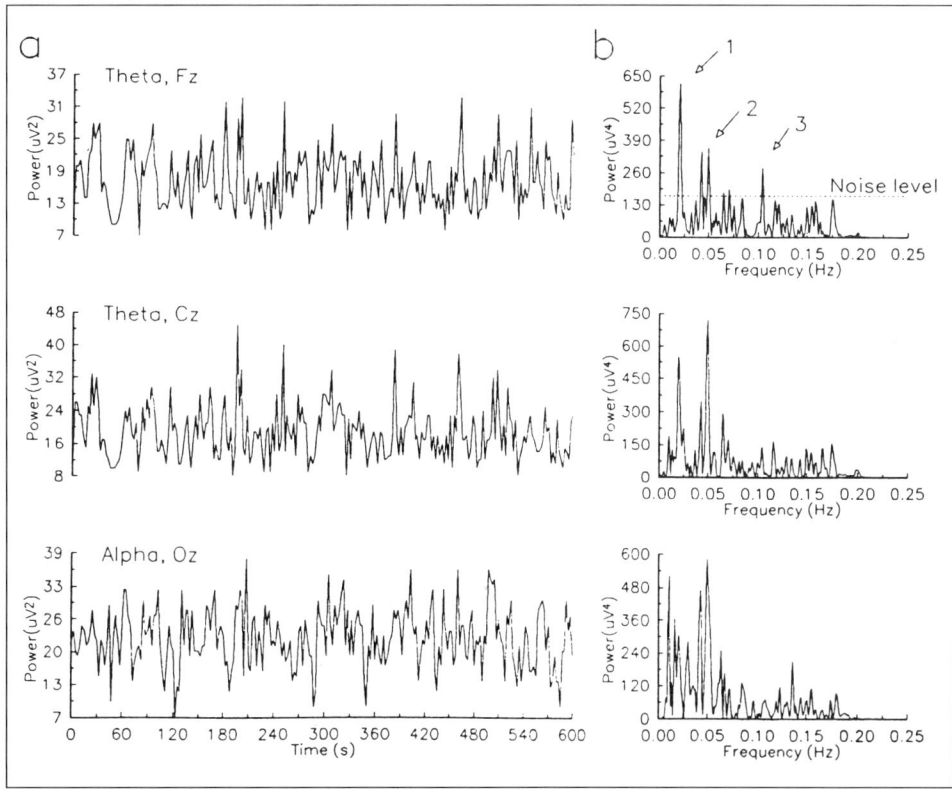

FIG. 6. Another example of the slow modulation in a young, healthy, supine subject. The envelope of the baseline theta and alpha rhythms is obvious to the naked eye. The EEG recorded from leads C_z and O_z is modulated by slow activity. Three dominant rhythms are clearly represented on the corresponding Fourier spectrum (*right*).

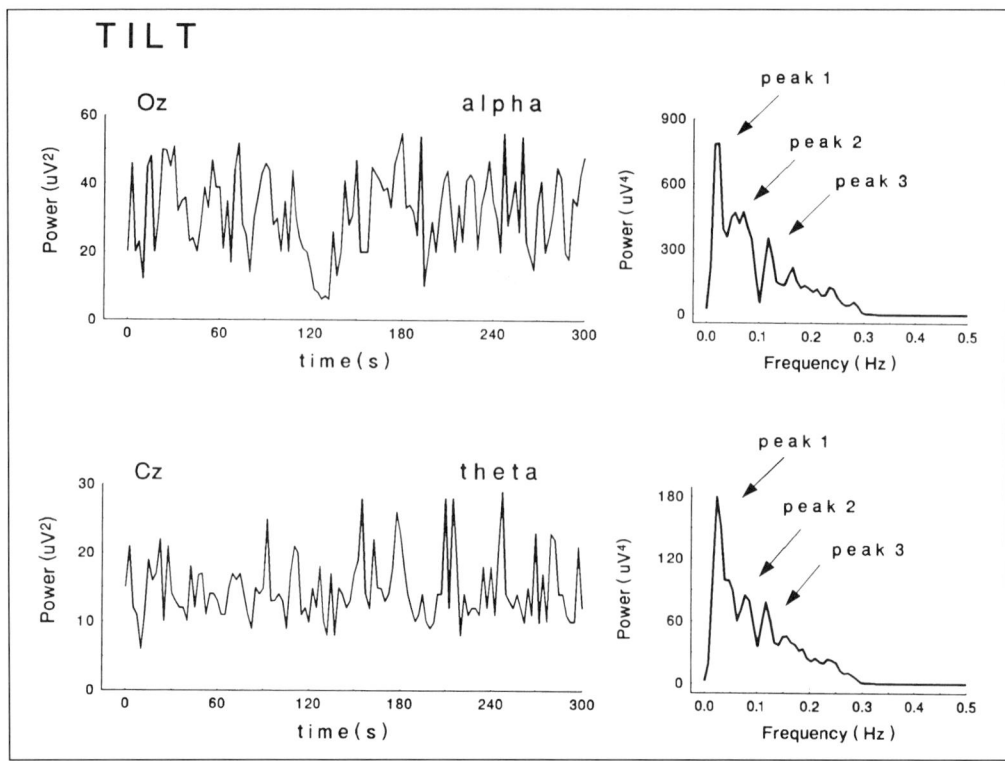

FIG. 7. The profile of the slow modulation in the monopolar C_z and O_z leads in the alpha and theta bands from a young orthostatically tolerant subject during the tilt-up.

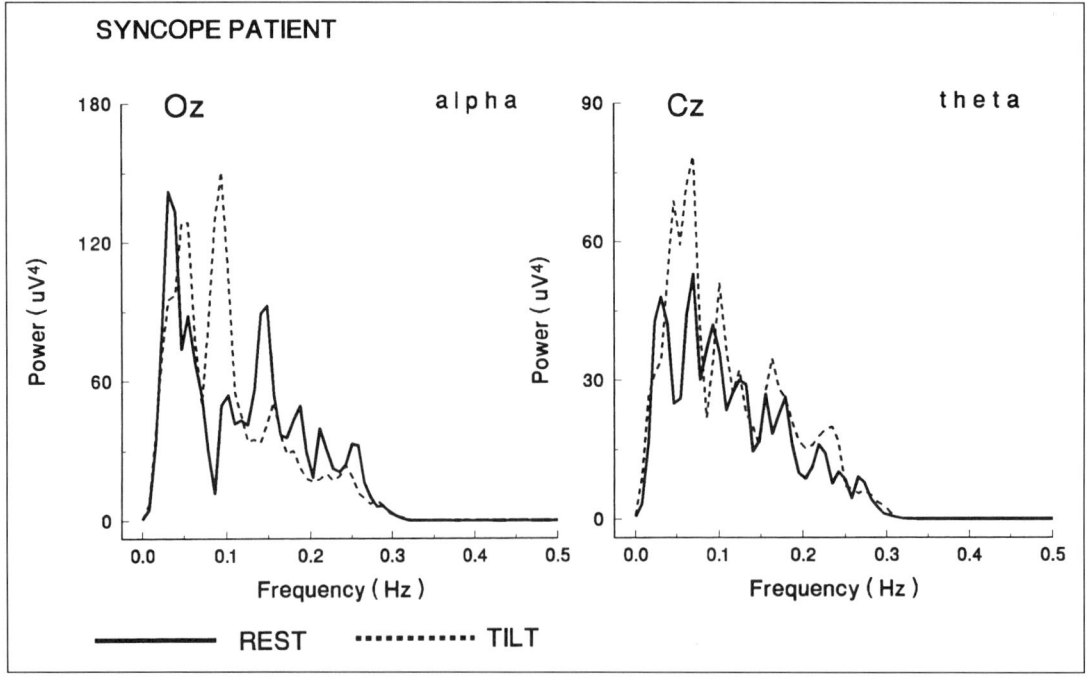

FIG. 8. Spectrum of slow modulation of the alpha and theta rhythms from the monopolar O_z and C_z leads during rest (*solid line*) and during tilt (*dotted line*) with the patient presyncopal. An increase in the amplitude of the 0.05-Hz rhythm in both alpha and theta bands is present during tilt-up and presyncope, corresponding to the generalized EEG slowing.

nant rhythm at slow frequencies (0.02–0.03 Hz) had a period of ~46 sec. The second dominant rhythm (0.05–0.06 Hz) had a period of 18–20 sec, and the fastest rhythm occurred at frequencies of 0.10–0.12 Hz, with a period of 10 sec (Fig. 6). FFT and autoregressive modeling were also calculated from simultaneously recorded heart rate and respiration. Dominant peaks at similar frequencies to that recorded by AM-EEG have been observed in the RR interval (0.04–0.07 and 0.07–0.13 Hz). These RR interval rhythms are generated by the combined influence of the sympathetic and baroreflex activity. Respiratory rate in our subjects was in the slower range at 0.12 Hz (8 breaths/min). The significance of the RR interval and respiratory rhythms is discussed in detail in the preceding chapter (40). The first and largest peak was detected in 98% of subjects, the second peak in 95%, and the third peak in 65%.

We have further studied the behavior of these rhythms under the physiologic perturbations of sympathetic activation with tilt-up (43) and hyperventilation (40). In normal subjects, in the alpha band, the two main slower AM-EEG rhythms were dominant during rest and were maintained during tilt-up. In the alpha band, the amplitude of the 0.025-Hz rhythms was larger in the posterior parietal and occipital leads ($p < 0.001$), while the amplitude of the 0.15-Hz rhythm was smaller in all leads. In the theta band, the 0.025-Hz rhythm was dominant and greater in the central leads ($p < 0.001$), as was the 0.054-Hz rhythm, while the 0.15-Hz rhythm was smaller in all leads ($p < 0.001$). There were no significant differences between resting and standing recordings in asymptomatic healthy subjects (Fig. 7) (50). Five patients experienced vasodepressor presyncope during head-up tilt, accompanied by a significant blood pressure fall. None of these patients actually lost consciousness. Figure 8 shows a power spectra from a patient who developed syncope. The recording shows changes evolving from supine rest to syncope. There was an increase in the amplitude of the second 0.1-Hz rhythm in the alpha band, and marked EEG slowing with prominent theta activity and an increment of the slow 0.025- and 0.05-Hz activity in the theta range.

These results have been confirmed by dynamic time–frequency mapping (38) in which the Wigner distribution was applied directly to the raw EEG signal, bypassing preprocessing using Fourier transform. We reasoned that, since EEG is a dynamic process, the requirement for signal stationarity (needed for Fourier spectrum) is hard to satisfy, and that the use of a dynamic method of nonlinear spectral estimations to determine slow EEG modulation would be a distinct improvement. We used modified Wigner distribution (41) and defined the instantaneous coherence (39), which specified the linear relationship between two signals based on the cross-Wigner distribution. Prior to the computation, the time series was converted to complex power series by using the Hilbert transform (44). The resulting analytical signal has a real part (the original data) and the imaginary part, comprising the original data sequence that had undergone a 90° phase shift. The analytical signal has the same amplitude and frequency content as the real data. For two discrete signals z and x, the smoothed discrete Wigner distribution is defined (41). The function used to calculate the modified Wigner distribution is

$$W_{zx}(n,m) = \tfrac{1}{2}N \sum_{k=-N+1}^{N-1} |h(k)|^2 \left(\sum_{p=M+1}^{M-1} g(p) z(n) + p + k \right) x^* (n + p - k)) e^{-2i\pi km/N}$$

where n = time index and m = frequency index, $h(k)$ = window function with the length $2N - 1$ applied for frequency smoothing, $g(p)$ = window function with the length $2M - 1$ applied for time smoothing, and *asterisk* denotes the complex conjugate. The auto Wigner distribution is computed with $z = x$. We have also defined the instantaneous coherence (ICoh) as

$$\text{ICoh}_{zx}(n,m) = \frac{W_{zx}^2(n,m)}{W_z(n,m) * W_x(n,m)}$$

The instantaneous coherence specifies the linear relationship between the two signals z and x for each frequency m at each time instant n. The Wigner distributions were computed with $N = 64$, $M = 9$, and $g(p) = 1$. The Gaussian window was used for the $h(k)$. Computational details can be found in Novak and Novak (41).

The results were similar to those of previous studies. Time–frequency Wigner distributions of theta and alpha activity showed two dominant rhythms. The frequencies of both rhythms were relatively stable, but their amplitude varied over time. High correlations ($r = 0.7$–0.8, $p < 0.01$) were found between the average magnitudes of both peaks of the theta Wigner distribution and the average theta powers as well as the average magnitudes of both peaks of the theta Wigner distributions. Similarly, the powers of alpha Wigner distributions displayed also a high centro-occipital coherence for both peaks ($r = 0.9$ and $r = 0.89$). During hyperventilation, the average theta power increased, while the average alpha power was nonsignificantly lower (Fig. 9). Hyperventilation increased the spectral power in the slow 0.02-Hz peak in both alpha and theta ranges, without a significant shift of either frequencies. Correlations between the average theta power and corresponding magnitudes of these peaks diminished. Both average alpha power and the amplitude of the slow peak diminished during hyperventilation. The subjects with a higher resting theta and alpha activity tended to have a higher amplitude of the slow modulation. The high centro-occipital coherence suggests that the same underlying process in these two regions is responsible for the slow oscillations. Hyperventilation reduces CO_2 and leads to the cerebral vasoconstriction with the resultant ischemia and hypoxia presumably responsible for the EEG slowing. The subjects with high resting theta and alpha activity might have more vasoactive

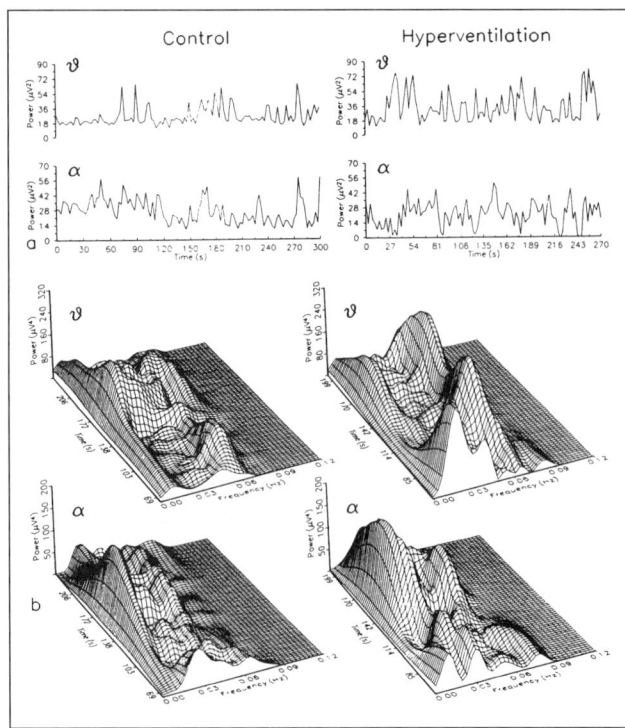

FIG. 9. Successive alpha and theta band powers **(a)** and corresponding Wigner distributions **(b)**. The *left panel* represents resting recordings, and the *right panel* represents hyperventilation. Increased power during hyperventilation is present at frequencies of 0.05 Hz in the theta band and at 0.02 Hz in the alpha band.

cerebral vessels, which react more vigorously to hyperventilation.

Further evidence supporting the existence of EEG rhythms at frequencies 0.1–1.0 Hz has been derived from animal studies by Steriade et al. (54,55,57). The experiments, which were performed on cats under different conditions, included deep anesthesia, deafferenting the cortex (states similar to the deep sleep), brainstem-isolated, undrugged, and cerveau isole preparations. Neocortical activity is characterized by three major oscillations at frequency ranges of ~0.3, 1–4, and 7–14 Hz. Similar recordings have also been made from various sites in the neocortex and thalamus in naturally sleeping cats (54,55). The cerveau isolé preparations displayed the major sleep patterns even in the absence of general anesthetics, although most of the studies were done with the cats under general anesthesia. Two types of slow rhythms were described (a) slow modulation at frequencies of 0.3–0.4 Hz found in 38% of neurons with delta rhythm and (b) spontaneous EEG recordings from the sleeping and anesthetized cats showing slowly recurring (0.3–0.9 Hz) sequences of slow waves (surface positive and depth negative) often followed by rapid activity of sleep spindles.

Spindle waves, which are generated in the thalamus, are also subject to modulation by thalamocortical feedback loops. Spindle waves are grouped in sequences lasting ~1.5–3.0 sec and recurring periodically, every 5–10 sec. As yet, there is no clear description of the intrinsic or synaptic origin of the slow rhythm separating the spindles. The spindles are a typical network product, which is driven and synchronized by the reticulothalamic thalamic nuclei. Both spindles and interspindle sequences (0.1–0.2 Hz) exist in the reticuloendothelium of thalamus even after disconnecting them from the cortical and dorsal thalamic inputs (56). The presence of slow rhythm after transection of corpus callosum in thalamically lesioned animals suggests that the thalamus is not essential for the generation of the slow rhythm. After transection of the cortical connections, the synchronization initially disappeared, but was restored again after 2– hr. As the loss of coherence was not permanent, it was suggested that intergyral pathways or corticothalamocortical loops may exert compensatory synchronization (1). Cortical cells and the cells from the reticular thalamic nucleus were hyperpolarized during the depth-positive EEG waves and were depolarized during the depth-negative EEG deflections. In many instances, the depolarization of these cells was associated with oscillations at the spindle frequency. Simultaneous intracellular recordings of the pairs of cortical cells, or cortical and thalamocortical cells, showed spontaneous transitions from less synchronized to more synchronized sleep EEG states with a marked simultaneous hyperpolarization coincident with an overt depth-positive wave. In 44% of thalamocortical cells, the slow (0.03–0.5 Hz) rhythm was apparent, and it could coexist with delta and spindle oscillations from the same neurons. It was recorded in 65% of reticular thalamic neurons: the rhythm consisted of prolonged depolarizations characterized as slowly recurring envelopes (57). It was therefore concluded that,in anesthetized cats, the low-frequency oscillatory states are characteristic of slow-wave sleep and also that synchronization results from a generalized inhibitory phenomenon. Moreover, it seems that EEG synchronization might be related to the active inhibition of the thalamocortical neurons (12). Neuronal recordings from the cardiovascular and respiratory neurons at the brainstem level showed a similar synchronization at the respiratory frequencies (28). In this study, spontaneous rhythms at a frequency of <0.08 Hz, typically at 0.05 Hz ("20-sec rhythm") and at 0.016 Hz ("1-min rhythm") were recorded from the brainstem cardiovascular and respiratory centers responsible for the blood pressure vasomotor regulation and from respiratory neurons (23). Viewing these studies together, it seems that neuronal synchronization may occur at deeper levels. Figure 10 shows the centers possibly involved in the synchronization phenomenon. We hypothesize that the original synchronization occurs at the brainstem level and propagates to the cortex via ascending/descending pathways. Several regions of the

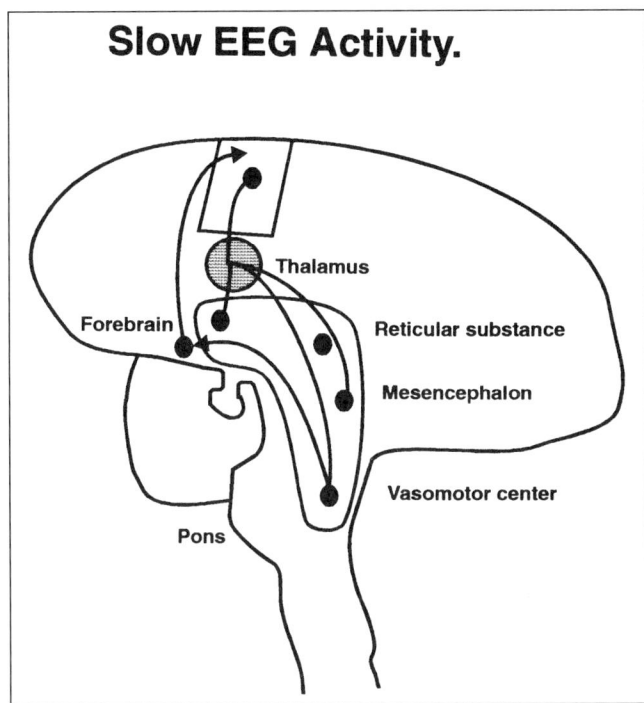

FIG. 10. Schematic representation of centers involved in generation of the slow amplitude modulation.

medulla are critical for the tonic and reflex control of the cardiovascular functions: the nucleus tractus solitarii is the first relay station for the afferents, and the ventrolateral medulla contains vasomotor, cardiovagal, and respiratory neurons.

CLINICAL APPLICATIONS OF TRANSCRANIAL DOPPLER AND EEG DURING ORTHOSTATIC INTOLERANCE

Symptoms of orthostatic intolerance due to reduced cerebral perfusion are present in many autonomic disorders and can be manifested as dizziness, light-headedness, weakness, dyspnea, sweating, or syncope. Cerebral hypoperfusion develops when cerebral autoregulation fails, and occurs in the context of a severe blood pressure reduction. This orthostatic hypotension is typically seen in generalized autonomic failure, as occurs in MSA and the autonomic neuropathies. Severe hypotension can be secondary to cardiac events such as arrhythmias or asystole, including that associated with malignant vasodepressor syncope. Cerebral hypoperfusion would not be expected to result from reduced stroke volume caused by the excessive heart rate in severe postural tachycardia syndrome (POTS) or the tachyarrhythmias alone, and symptoms can occur when additional cerebral mechanisms, such as paradoxical vasoconstriction, are superimposed. Since a patient's complaints can be vague and nonspecific, an objective indicator of reduced cerebral perfusion is needed.

There is an overall strong positive correlation between a fall in blood pressure or an excessive HR increment during the tilt test and symptoms of orthostatic intolerance. However, correlation between blood pressure and cerebral perfusion cannot be directly predicted from the blood pressure change alone, since the relationship between blood pressure and cerebral perfusion is nonlinear, due to cerebral autoregulation. The primary goal of cerebral autoregulation is to maintain cerebral perfusion constant during variation of blood pressure (59). Any BP reduction is counteracted by dilatation of small intracranial arterioles leading to a lower vascular resistance, preventing a fall in blood flow. Rapid increases of blood pressure are buffered by the elasticity of the aorta and central arteries, and the Windkessel effect results in the rapid release of systolic pressure and prevents perfusion collapse during diastole. The regulation of cerebral blood flow is complex and incompletely understood. It can, however, be operationally described clinically by three simplified concepts: (a) perfusion pressure (inflow pressure minus outflow pressure), (b) resistance, and (c) flow volume (35). In the cerebral circulation, the perfusion pressure is the difference between the arterial and intracranial pressures, since the venous pressure cannot be lower than the intracranial pressure. If cerebrovascular resistance was constant, then there would be a linear relationship between the flow and arterial pressure, a situation approximated in autoregulatory failure. The pressure flow relationship is modified by autoregulation, however, resulting in a nonlinear relationship.

The three levels of cerebral autoregulation control are metabolic, myogenic, and neurogenic: *metabolic autoregulation* is the response of arteriolar smooth muscle to changing cerebral metabolic microenvironment; *myogenic autoregulation* is defined as the smooth muscle response, which in turn depends on its intrinsic properties that adapt muscle tension to changes of vessel caliber and transmural tension; and *neurogenic autoregulation* is mediated by the sympathetic fibers.

Cerebral autoregulation ensures stable perfusion in spite of a wide range of blood pressure fluctuations. The autoregulated range is typically 70–140 mmHg. Cerebral autoregulation is ineffective when the blood pressure falls to <70 mmHg, and here the cerebral perfusion might be severely compromised (20,30). There is some controversy about whether autoregulation is mainly neurogenic or myogenic. Current evidence suggests that autoregulation is mainly myogenic, but neurogenic and metabolic mechanisms can modulate this response.

In a majority of patients with chronic orthostatic hypotension, mean blood pressure in the upright position is >60 mmHg, i.e., within the autoregulated range. Furthermore, patients with chronic orthostatic hypotension may have an expansion of their autoregulated range to lower BP (60). It would be important to evaluate autoregulatory status in these patients with chronic orthostatic hypotension. The term *autoregulatory failure* is used when the blood pressure-to-BFV relationship becomes linearized. This is manifested by a BFV recording that follows the blood pressure trace. Patients with lesser degrees of orthostatic intolerance may have a paradoxical response by intracranial vessels; in response to a fall in systemic blood and pulse pressure, cerebral arterioles constrict instead of dilating. TCD recordings enable this determination. Finally, TCD enables the recognition of impaired cerebral perfusion in a number of other circumstances. In acute stresses like vasodepressor syncope, hypoperfusion can result from a rapid BP fall to <40 mmHg. Its effect on the cerebral circulation cannot be predicted without knowledge of cerebral vasoregulation. Beat-to-beat TCD analysis can be used continuously during various provocative maneuvers, and this feature makes it an attractive tool for estimation of blood flow changes in syndromes of orthostatic intolerance.

There are several limitations of TCD recordings. TCD provides an indirect estimation of blood flow because it measures changes in BFV. In the absence of pathologic conditions that decrease arterial wall diameter (atherosclerosis or vasospasm), increased BFV is due to increased flow through dilated arterioles distal to the probe. However, an increase can also result from constriction of the insonated trunk. Available data suggest that the latter mechanism is unimportant except under extreme circumstances such as subarachnoid hemorrhage or injury of the vessel The MCA trunk appears to retain a stable diameter in response to changes induced in flow velocity (16).

Effect of the Valsalva Maneuver on Transcranial Doppler

As described earlier, we have adopted an approach where we monitor a comprehensive battery of indices of the central and peripheral circulation to study patients with orthostatic intolerance. Simultaneous monitoring of these indices enables us to undertake beat-to-beat analysis of BFV, BP, respiration, EEG and CO_2, and their interrelationships.

Figure 11 shows simultaneously recorded profiles of beat-to-beat BFVs of the MCA, HR, and BP in a normal control subject. Since the pathophysiology of the blood pressure profile during the Valsalva maneuver has been described in detail in Chapter 16, we will mention it only briefly. In normal subjects, the BFV profile is similar to the BP profile. Phase I of the Valsalva maneuver (expiratory pressure mechanically compresses the aorta and related structures, causing a rise in BP) is characterized by a small increase of BP and MCA BFV. Phase II is elicited by the reduction in preload secondary to continued expiratory pressure (compressing the vena cava) and results in an early (phase II_e) fall of both BP and BFV. This is followed a recovery in BP (phase II_l), due to arteriolar vasoconstriction. Typically, both early and late phase II can be identified in both systolic and diastolic BFV. Phase III corre-

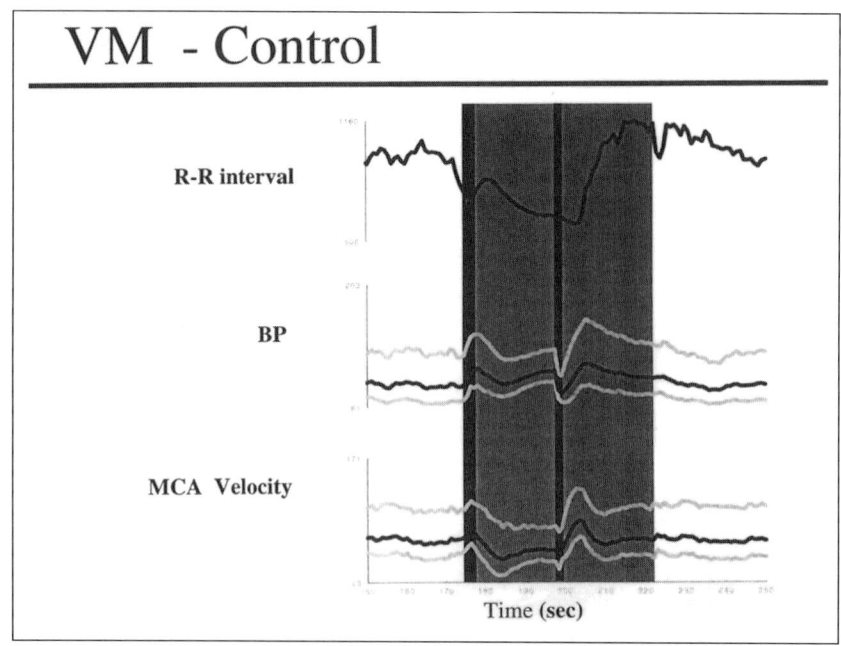

FIG. 11. Beat-to-beat profile of blood pressure and middle cerebral artery (MCA) velocity during Valsalva maneuver in a healthy control.

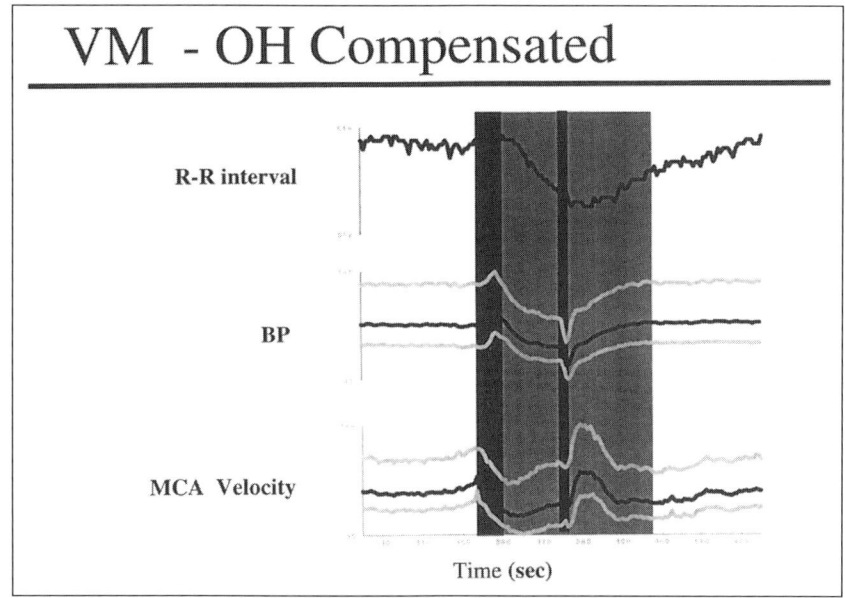

FIG. 12. Beat-to-beat profile of blood pressure and middle cerebral artery (MCA) velocity during Valsalva maneuver in a patient with orthostatic hypotension and normal cerebral autoregulation. The blood pressure profile during Valsalva maneuver was abnormal with reduced late phase II and phase IV. The profile of MCA velocity was normal.

sponds to the cessation of expiratory pressure at the end of maneuver and is also mechanically induced. It is characterized by a small dip in both BP and BFV. In phase IV, venous return to the heart and ensuing cardiac output has returned to normal, while the arteriolar bed remains constricted. In studies of normal human subjects who perform the maneuver while supine, phase IV may be due, in major part, to augmented cardiac contractility (48). Ejection of the normal or increased stroke volume results in a BP overshoot. Overshoot in phase IV can be also identified in the systolic and diastolic BFV, but its duration is briefer than in the periphery. The mechanism of this significantly re-

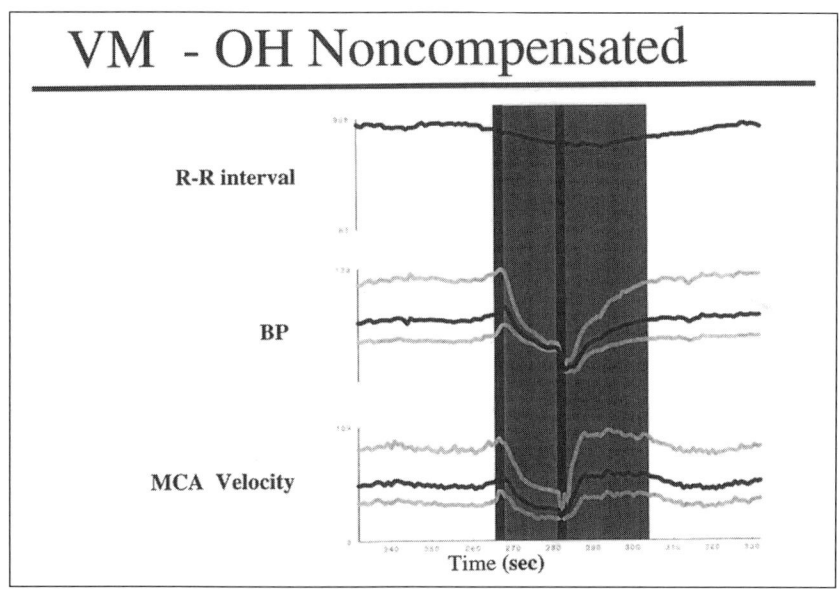

FIG. 13. Beat-to-beat profile of blood pressure and middle cerebral artery (MCA) velocity during Valsalva maneuver in a patient with orthostatic hypotension and abnormal cerebral autoregulation. The blood pressure profile during Valsalva maneuver was abnormal with reduced late phase II and phase IV. The profile of MCA velocity was abnormal.

duced duration of phase IV is uncertain. One possibility is that cerebral arteriolar smooth muscle has different properties than that of limb arterioles. Presumably, it maintains its tone after sympathetic withdrawal for a briefer duration. A alternative possibility is a different discharge pattern of central sympathetic activation.

Figure 12 is a representative recording from a patient with orthostatic hypotension and peripheral adrenergic failure, but preserved cerebral autoregulation. As it is typically seen in these patients, Valsalva maneuver induces a profound fall of BP in early phase II with little or no recovery in late phase II. The sympathetically mediated phase IV is also absent. In contrast, the BFV profile showed clearly defined phases and preserved late phase II and phase IV. Figure 13 is a representative recording from a patient with a suspected MSA and orthostatic hypotension but inadequate autoregulation. As in Fig. 13, the peripheral indices of the Valsalva maneuver were abnormal; they were characterized by pulse pressure collapse with absent late phase II and IV. In this case, cerebral autoregulation has also failed. In contrast with the recording in Fig. 11, BFV of MCA in Fig. 13 follows passively the systemic BP changes, indicating that the caliber of the small arterioles remained constant, i.e., no autoregulation was present. These examples illustrate how the application of TCD can help to distinguish between the preserved and failing cerebral autoregulation on a case-by-case basis.

Another typical abnormality of the Valsalva maneuver is seen in patients with POTS (Chapter 50). Symptoms include light-headedness, dizziness, syncope, headache, tiredness, unsteadiness, blurred vision, and nausea after assuming the upright position. It is preceded by an antecedent viral infection in ~50% of patients, and a length-dependent autonomic neuropathy is often present (32,58). Beat-to-beat responses to Valsalva maneuver are also abnormal, typically showing a reduced late phase II and augmented phase IV, i.e., reduced peripheral adrenergic and increase cardiac (β) adrenergic responses (48,49,51). Clinically, some symptoms during the Valsalva maneuver—such as dizziness, light-headedness, blurred vision, and presyncope—are suggestive of cerebral hypoperfusion. Figure 14A illustrates impaired cerebral blood flow responses in a 32-year-old woman with POTS and a mild postganglionic sudomotor impairment. In this patient, Valsalva maneuver evoked marked pulse pressure collapse with reduced or absent late phase II and dramatically increased phase IV. Pharmacologic dissection has suggested that the mechanism of the large phase IV in POTS patients is mainly that of β-adrenergic overactivity with some contribution of altered preload. The new finding is that cerebral autoregulation might also been altered in these patients. The profile of BFV was abnormal, with a profile similar to the blood pressure. Pulsatility was reduced, late phase II was absent or reduced, and phase IV overshoot was greatly exaggerated. The presence of cerebral hypoperfusion was also evident in the EEG (Fig. 14B), which showed generalized slowing and bursts of theta waves in the central and occipital leads. The patient complained of severe dizziness followed by headache, presumably reflecting the sequential effects of cerebral hypoxia followed by rebound hypertension after tilt-back to supine position.

Transcranial Doppler and Tilt

Cardiovascular functions in orthostatic intolerance have been studied in detail using time domain, frequency domain, and nonlinear approaches (Chapter 26). However, little information is available on central alterations in orthostatic intolerance. The limited studies thus far have focused mainly on the use of the EEG in the differential diagnosis between syncope and epilepsy.

Relatively few studies have been performed to evaluate cerebral autoregulation in the patients with autonomic failure, and the results have not been consistent. There are reports of both impaired and intact cerebral autoregulation in patients with MSA and pure autonomic failure (PAF). In the early studies using the measurements of arteriovenous oxygen differences, Caronna and Plum (10) reported intact autoregulation in three patients with MSA, but impaired autoregulation in a patient with PAF; these patients had preserved CO_2 reactivity. Meyer et al. (33), using the same method, found impaired autoregulation in all of their three patients with MSA but did confirm preserved CO_2 reactivity. Reduced cerebral blood flow, measured using the xenon-133 perfusion technique, was found in a patient with primary dysautonomia while sitting when compared with the supine position (37). In contrast, Nanda et al. (34) and Thomas and Bannister (60), using the xenon clearance method, reported intact cerebral autoregulation in all their PAF and MSA subjects. Brooks et al. (6), compared MCA velocity and xenon clearance methods in the patients with MSA and PAF during tilt. Tilt to 45° induced orthostatic hypotension in all patients and none of the controls. Their mean HR increased by 5%, while the mean BP fell by 20%. In normal controls, MCA velocity remained stable during the tilt. As measured by the xenon-133 washout method, there was a negligible change in the cerebral blood flow of these patients, but their MCA velocities dropped by 16%. It was concluded that cerebral autoregulation was likely preserved in the patients with MSA or PAF if the BP in the upright position remained within the autoregulatory range (>60 mmHg). However, simultaneous EEG and measurement of cerebral blood flow (xenon-133 method) in a patient with MSA suggested that the breaking point of autoregulation might be relatively higher, between 100 and 120 mmHg of the mean BP. At this point, EEG showed generalized slowing, which partially improved after 4 min in the upright position, and cerebral blood flow stabilized at a lower level (14). In a recent TCD study (26), impaired cerebral autoregulation was also reported in patients with autonomic failure. Hypotension was induced by active

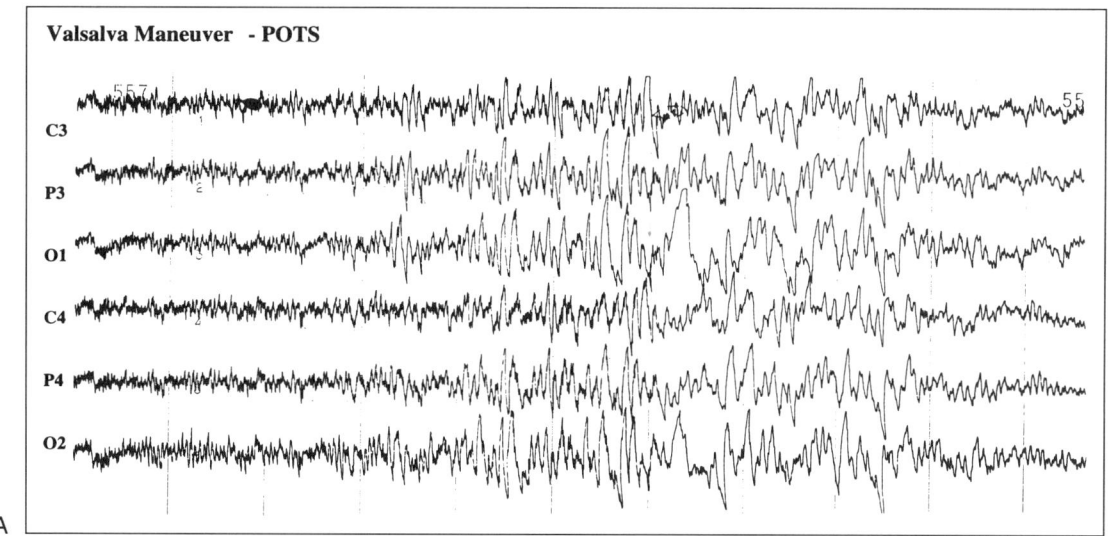

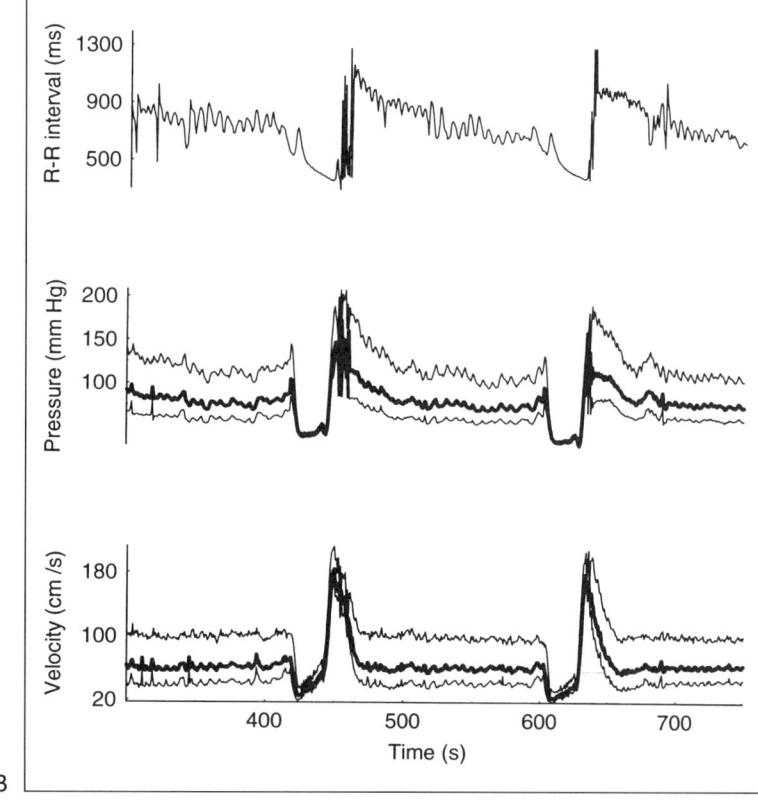

FIG. 14. **A:** Raw EEG data here and in following figures were obtained from monopolar recordings from the left and right central, parietal, and occipital areas (left: C3, P3, O1; and right: C4, P4, O2), with the earlobe as a reference. In a patient with postural tachycardia syndrome, Valsalva maneuver induced slowing of background EEG activity. **B:** Simultaneous profiles of blood pressure and blood flow velocity (BFV) during Valsalva maneuver were both abnormal. Both blood pressure and transcranial Doppler (TCD) showed reduced late phase II and exaggerated phase IV.

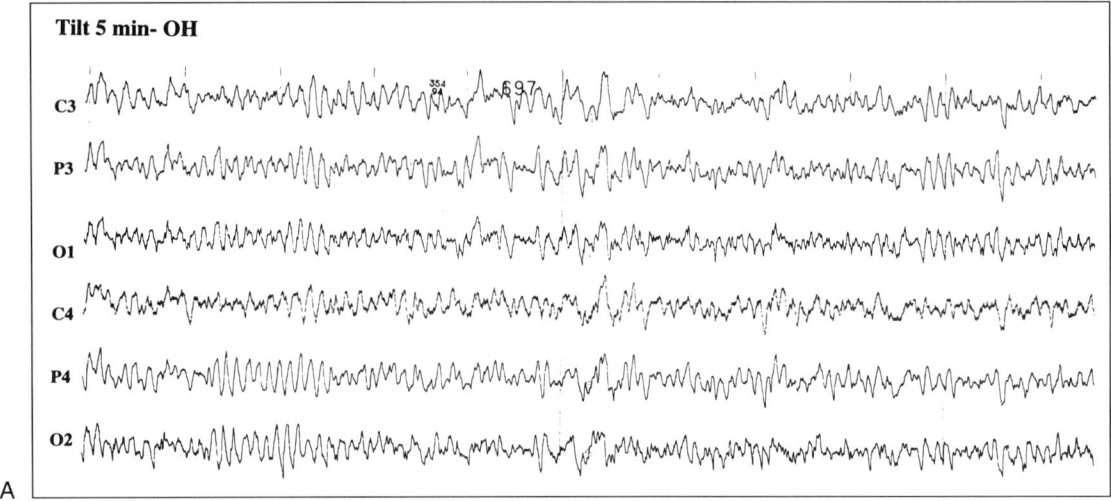

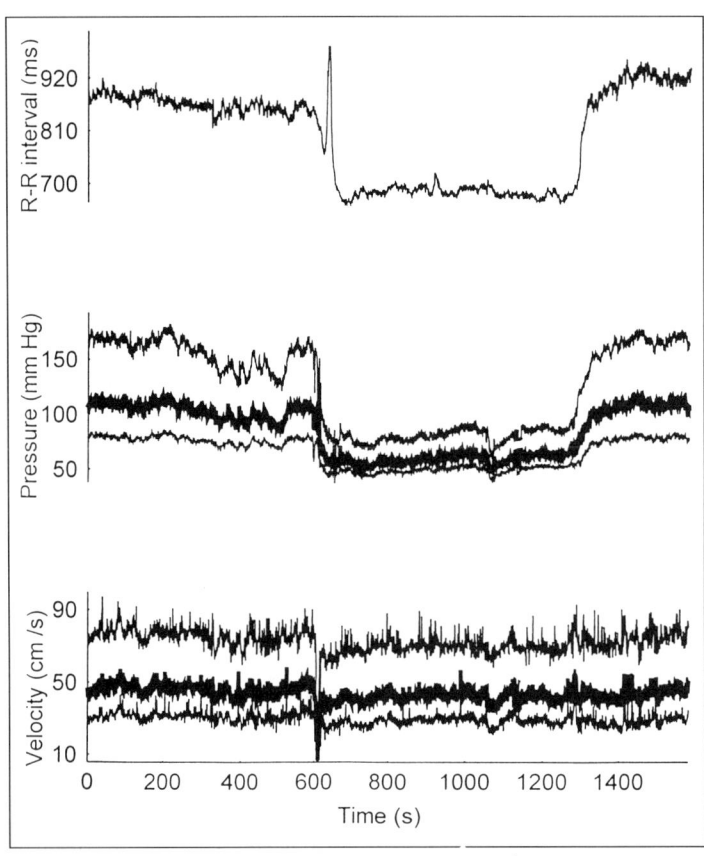

FIG. 15. A: EEG data (see the Fig. 14 legend) were obtained from a patient with orthostatic hypotension during the 5-min tilt. The EEG activity slowed to the theta range in all leads at the end of tilt. **B:** Simultaneous profiles of heart rate, blood pressure, and blood flow velocity (BFV) during the 5-min tilt revealed a mild tachycardia with the tilt-up and orthostatic hypotension. In contrast, middle cerebral artery (MCA) blood flow was preserved and remained stable during tilt, which is suggestive of preserved autoregulation.

limb hyperemia with the patients supine. In this group, mean velocity profile moved in a parallel fashion with systemic blood pressure (26). There is some suggestion that autoregulation is dynamic so that there can be rapid alterations in the autoregulated range (53). The combined use of TCD–EEG with BP recordings enables a more complete understanding of the effect of low BP on cerebral perfusion.

Figure 15 illustrates the case of a 62-year-old woman with widespread cardiovagal, peripheral adrenergic and postganglionic sudomotor failure. Pontocerebellar degeneration was suspected and magnetic resonance imaging showed brainstem and cerebellar atrophy. She had orthostatic gait ataxia and falls, but without a loss of consciousness. Tilt-up resulted in severe orthostatic hypotension with preserved cardiac tachycardic response, during which the patient was asymptomatic. Cerebral blood flow remained stable despite a severe reduction of BP (Fig. 15A). The EEG showed predominant alpha activity during rest and tilt-up (Fig. 15B). Occasional slowing into theta range was observed at the end of tilt. These findings indicate that evaluation of BFV provides important information about cerebral perfusion in orthostatic hypotension that is not available with blood pressure recordings alone.

As reviewed in detail in Chapter 37, diabetes mellitus is often associated with devastating autonomic neuropathy. Although, orthostatic hypotension is well recognized in diabetic autonomic neuropathy, little information is available on alterations of cerebral blood flow in diabetes. Since both macrovascular and microvascular disease are common in diabetes, and since a reduction in BP can cause focal (15) as well as global ischemia, the recording of cerebral perfusion during tilt-up is especially important. Figure 16 illustrates the case of a 29-year-old woman with insulin-dependent diabetes mellitus and a 6-month history of severe orthostatic hypotension, associated with dizziness, light-headedness, and blurred vision. Autonomic testing confirmed orthostatic hypotension with severe cardiovagal and moderate sudomotor failure. BP decreased to 70/54 mmHg at the end of 10 min of upright tilt. Concomitant recording of cerebral blood flow showed impaired autoregulation, indicated by a rapid decline of the mean BFV, mainly due to a fall of diastolic BFV, while the systolic BFV remained stable. Preservation of the systolic BFV can be explained by the increased cardiac contractility, since stroke volume did not decline. Cardiac output was mildly increased during tilt-up due to a mild compensatory tachycardia of 115 beats/min.

The last example in this series (Fig. 17) is the case of a 72-year-woman with widespread autonomic failure due to MSA. Autonomic evaluation revealed severe orthostatic hypotension, accompanied by a severe and progressive decline of systolic, diastolic, and mean BFV. BP progres-

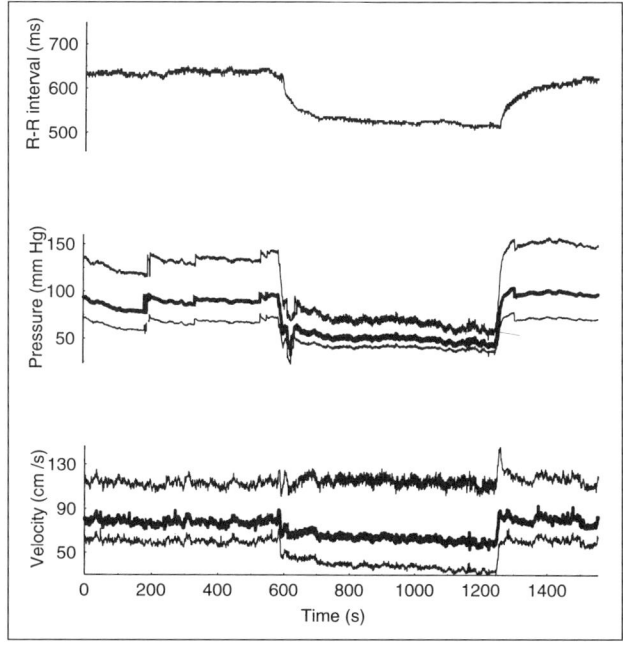

FIG. 16. The tilt-table test of this 29-year-old patient with autonomic neuropathy showed severe orthostatic hypotension with mild tachycardia. Concomitant recording of the cerebral blood flow showed impaired autoregulation, indicated by a rapid decline of the mean blood flow velocity (BFV), mainly due to a fall of diastolic BFV, while the systolic BFV remained stable.

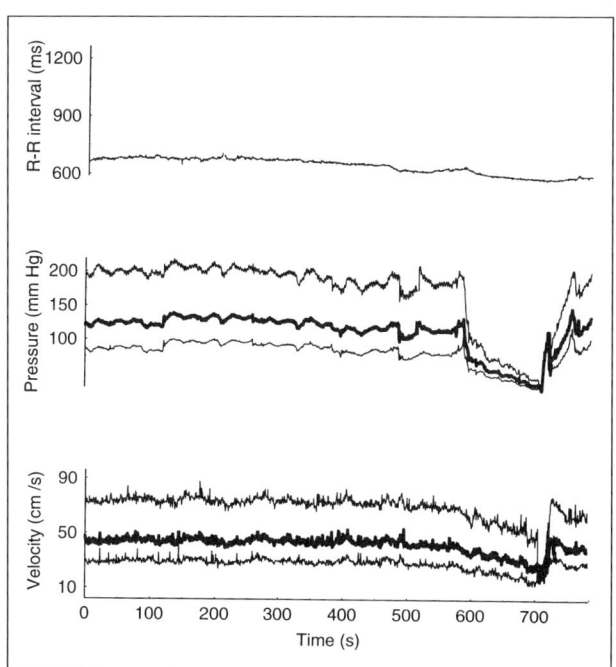

FIG. 17. The tilt-table test of this 72-year-old patient with multiple-system atrophy showed severe orthostatic hypotension with blunted cardiac response. Concomitant recording of cerebral blood flow showed autoregulatory failure, indicated by a gradual decline of the mean blood flow velocity (BFV) and systolic and diastolic BFV. The BFV was falling with the same pattern as blood pressure.

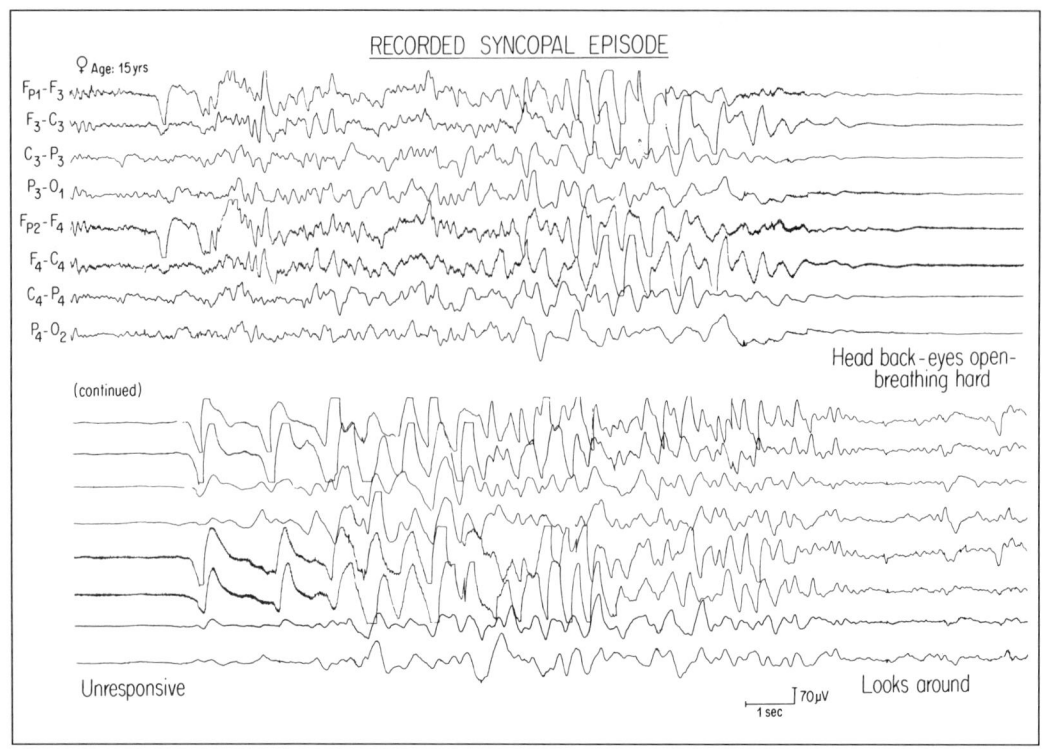

FIG. 18. EEG changes in a 15-year-old girl during vasodepressor syncope. Generalized EEG slowing develops with prominent theta and delta waves. The actual loss of consciousness is characterized by a flat EEG with no detectable dominant activity. Recovery from syncope and EEG silence is characterized by the reoccurrence of delta and theta activity, followed by restoration of the normal alpha activity. Courtesy of Dr. Barbara Westmoreland, Department of Neurology, Mayo Clinic, Rochester, MN.

sively declined to 75/52 mmHg by minute 4 of tilt (values similar to those of the previous case). The profile of MCA velocity showed more complete autoregulatory failure than did the previous case. MCA BFV did not compensate in this case and instead passively followed the blood pressure decline. Additionally, there was no cardioacceleration with tilt, and the patient became symptomatic after 4 min of tilt and thus needed to be returned to the supine position.

In a preliminary study, we evaluated a group of 13 patients with orthostatic hypotension and 13 control subjects. Five patients had diabetic neuropathy, four had autonomic neuropathy, and four had MSA or PAF. All patients presented with systolic/mean blood pressure reduction of >30/25 mmHg during tilt-up and had abnormal Valsalva maneuver responses. Only two patients had preserved cardiovagal indices, and four patients had preserved postganglionic sudomotor responses. Healthy controls showed a mild, but significant, drop in MCA velocity ($12.8 \pm 7.7\%$), $p < 0.001$), during 10 min of 80° head-up tilt. Eleven patients demonstrated preserved cerebral autoregulation, and the mean MCA velocity did not differ from that of controls. A small but significant reduction in mean MCA velocity was observed in these patients ($15.0 \pm 7.8\%$, $p < 0.001$). Two patients showed poor cerebral autoregulation with a progressive fall in the MCA (33.3% and 42.4%), which was significantly different from the patients with preserved autoregulation and from the normal controls. To a first approximation, patients with severe orthostatic hypotension who remain asymptomatic have preserved autoregulation, and those who are symptomatic have impaired autoregulation.

A more challenging problem is the autoregulatory status in patients with milder forms of orthostatic intolerance, such as POTS or recurrent vasodepressor syncope. The pathophysiology of vasodepressor syncope, which is detailed in Chapter 48, is incompletely understood. In brief, neurally mediated syncope comprises a reflex syncope that can be triggered by a number of peripheral or central inputs. The ultimate autonomic mechanism is one of an abrupt cessation of sympathetic outflow, resulting in a fall in BP. Bradycardia occurs, reflecting augmented efferent vagal activity, in response to a sudden cessation of the sympathetic tone. Ultimately, BP falls and cerebral blood flow becomes sufficiently impaired to result in cerebral hypoxia and loss of consciousness (61). Recent results using TCD studies with syncope or presyncope induced using the lower body negative pressure (LBNP) report that cerebral *vasoconstriction* occurs before the fall in blood pressure, instead of compensatory vasodilatation, as it would be predicted from the classic concept of autoregulation. In healthy humans, syncope induced by LBNP was preceded by a reduction in BFV and increased pulsatility prior to the onset of BP fall, suggestive of increased cerebrovascular resistance and small vessel constriction. However, the reduction in the mean velocity was only 15.5% below normal values, significantly less than that induced during hyperventilation (42%), and hyperventilation never triggered syncope in these subjects (31). In our observation, a 15% drop in the MCA velocity was also observed in normal asymptomatic healthy subjects during head-up tilt. Other reports confirming paradoxical cerebral vasoconstriction have appeared, and some workers have reported larger decrements in BFV. Syncope, induced by LBNP (5) or by head-up tilt (18,36), was preceded by cerebral vasoconstriction. The latter study was associated with a 44% reduction of mean BFV. However, none of these studies differentiated a passive decrease of BFV (failed autoregulation) or whether active vasoconstriction occurred abruptly. The EEG changes during syncope are those of cerebral hypoxia and hypoperfusion. Figure 18 shows the evolution of EEG changes in a 15-year-old girl during vasodepressor syncope. There is the development of generalized EEG slowing with prominent theta and delta waves. The actual loss of consciousness is characterized by a flat EEG with no detectable dominant activity. Recovery from syncope and EEG silence is characterized by the reoccurrence of delta and theta activity, followed by restoration of the normal alpha activity. Figure 19 shows recordings from a 21-year-old woman with a history of recurrent loss of consciousness triggered mainly by an upright position. Head-up tilt induced a mild tachycardia (120 beats/min) with a profound but transient BP fall to 60/40 mmHg that partially recovered in minute 2 of the tilt. MCA velocity (systolic, mean, and diastolic) declined by >40% and only gradually increased toward the end of tilt. Loss of consciousness occurred after 3 min of tilt with BP of 100/45 mmHg and normal values of BFV. With the tilt-induced BP fall, simultaneous recordings of EEG showed desychronization followed by theta and delta bursts, suggesting cerebral hypoperfusion. In contrast, the EEG during loss of consciousness was unrevealing with normal alpha spindles. This case illustrates perplexing discordance among BP, BFV, and EEG recordings.

In conclusion, symptomatic orthostatic intolerance is a manifestation of cerebral hypoperfusion, with some symptoms of sympathetic activation. Cardiovascular recordings provide important information on the regulation of the systemic circulation. To better understand the effect of peripheral autonomic failure on the patient, however, it is necessary to evaluate the dynamic cerebral responses to systemic hypotension. TCD and EEG provide reliable and dynamic recordings of the cerebral response. Evaluation of the cerebral response is focused on whether autoregulation is maintained, is expanded, or has failed. Additionally, the brain may play an active role in provoking syncope or symptoms by active paradoxical vasoconstriction. EEG enables an evaluation of cerebral hypoxic threshold, reactivity, and susceptibility to seizures. Finally, AM-EEG can be evaluated to gain insights into presumed brainstem autonomic rhythms.

REFERENCES

1. Amzica F, et al. Disconnection of intracortical synaptic linkages disrupts synchronization of a slow oscillation. *J Neurosci* 1995; 15:4658–4677.
2. Bassingthwaighte JB, et al. Evaluating rescaled ranged analysis for time series. *Ann Biomed Eng* 1994;22:432–444.
3. Benarroch EE, et al. Central autonomic disorders. *J Clin Neurophysiol* 1993;10:39–50.
4. Blaber A, et al. Complexity of cerebral blood flow in autonomic failure patients: effects of tilt and relationship to cerebral autoregulation. *Neurology* 1996;46:A312(abst).
5. Bondar RL, et al. Simultaneous cerebrovascular and cardiovascular responses during presyncope. *Stroke* 1995;26:1794–1800.
6. Brooks DJ, et al. The effect of orthostatic hypotension on cerebral blood flow and middle cerebral artery velocity in autonomic failure, with observations on the action of ephedrine. *J Neurol Neurosurg Psychiatry* 1989;52:962–966.
7. Brown TE, et al. Important influence of respiration on human R-R interval power spectra is largely ignored. *J Appl Physiol* 1993;75:2310–2317.

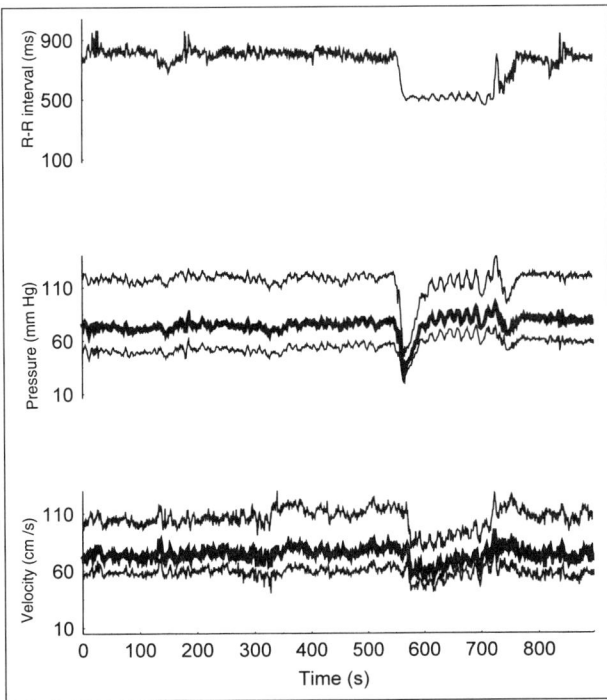

FIG. 19. Recordings from a 21-year-old woman with a history of recurrent loss of consciousness triggered mainly by an upright position. Head-up tilt induced a mild tachycardia (120 beats/min) with a transient blood pressure fall to 60/40 mm Hg, which partially recovered during the tilt. Blood flow velocity (BFV) declined by >40% and also gradually recovered to the end of tilt. Loss of consciousness occurred after 3 min of tilt, with blood pressure of 100/45 mm Hg and normal values of BFV.

8. Calaresu FR, et al. Medullary basal sympathetic tone [Review]. *Annu Rev Physiol* 1988;50:511–524.
9. Caro S, et al. Abnormal motor activity in autonomic failure: distinction from seizures. *Neurology* 1996;46:A224 (abst).
10. Caronna JJ, et al. Cerebrovascular regulation in preganglionic and postganglionic autonomic insufficiency. *Stroke* 1973;4:12–19.
11. Chokroverty S. Sleep apnea and respiratory disturbances in multiple system atrophy with autonomic failure. In: Bannister R, ed. *Autonomic failure*. Oxford: Oxford University Press, 1988:432–451.
12. Contreras D, et al. Cellular basis of EEG slow rhythms: a study of dynamic corticothalamic relationships. *J Neurosci* 1995;15:604–622.
13. De Backer WA. Central sleep apnoea, pathogenesis and treatment: an overview and perspective [Review]. *Eur Respir J* 1995;8:1372–1383.
14. Depresseux JC, et al. The autoregulation of cerebral blood flow, the cerebrovascular reactivity and their interaction in the Shy–Drager syndrome. *Eur Neurol* 1979;18: 295–301.
15. Dobkin BH. Orthostatic hypotension as a risk factor for symptomatic occlusive cerebrovascular disease. *Neurology* 1989;39:30–34.
16. Giller CA, et al. Cerebral arterial diameters during changes in blood pressure and carbon dioxide during craniotomy. *Neurosurgery* 1993; 32:737–742.
17. Gosling RG, et al. Arterial assessment by Doppler-shift ultrasound. *Proc R Soc Med* 1974;67:447–449.
18. Grubb BP, et al. Cerebral vasoconstriction during head-upright tilt-induced vasovagal syncope: a paradoxic and unexpected response. *Circulation* 1991;84:1157–1164.
19. Grubb BP, et al. Postpartum syncope. *PACE* 1995;18:1028–1031.
20. Harper AM. Autoregulation of cerebral blood flow: influence of the arterial blood pressure on the blood flow through the cerebral cortex. *J Neurol Neurosurg Psychiatry* 1966;29:398–403.
21. Hedner J, et al. Reduction in sympathetic activity after long-term CPAP treatment in sleep apnoea: cardiovascular implications. *Eur Respir J* 1995;8:222–229.
22. Howard RS, et al. Respiratory involvement in multiple sclerosis. *Brain* 1992;115:479–494.
23. Hukuhara T. Discharge properties of respiratory modulated brainstem reticular neurons, and their relation to slow arterial pressure fluctuations in rabbit. In: Miyakawa K, Koepchen HP, Polosa C, eds. *Mechanisms of blood pressure waves*. Berlin: Springer-Verlag, 1984:241–254.
24. Hurst HE. Long-term storage capacity of reservoirs. *Trans Am Soc Civ Eng* 1951;116:770–808.
25. Keunen RW, et al. Dynamical chaos determines the variability of transcranial Doppler signals. *Neurol Res* 1994;16:353–358.
26. Lagi A, et al. Cerebral autoregulation in orthostatic hypotension: a transcranial Doppler study. *Stroke* 1994;25:1771–1775.
27. Langhorst P, et al. Common brainstem system (CBS): a multifunctional "centre." In: Rother M, Zwiener U, eds. *Quantitative EEG analysis: clinical utility and new methods*. Jena: Jena University Press, 1993:228–239.
28. Langhorst P, et al. Oscillating neuronal network of the "common brainstem system." In: Miyakawa K, Koepchen HP, Polosa C, eds. *Mechanisms of blood pressure waves*. Berlin: Springer-Verlag, 1984: 257–275.
29. Langhorst P, et al. Dynamic characteristic of the "unspecific brain stem system." In: Koepchen HP, Hilton SM, Trzebski A. eds. *Central interaction between respiratory and cardiovascular control systems*. Berlin: Springer-Verlag, 1980:30–39.
30. Lassen NA. Control of cerebral circulation in health and disease [Review]. *Circ Res* 1974;34:749–760.
31. Levine BD, et al. Cerebral versus systemic hemodynamics during graded orthostatic stress in humans. *Circulation* 1994;90:298–306.
32. Low PA, et al. Comparison of the postural tachycardia syndrome (POTS) with orthostatic hypotension due to autonomic failure. *J Auton Nerv Syst* 1994;50:181–188.
33. Meyer JS, et al. Cerebral dysautoregulation in central neurogenic orthostatic hypotension (Shy–Drager syndrome). *Neurology* 1973;23: 262–273.
34. Nanda RN, et al. Cerebral blood flow in paraplegia. *Paraplegia* 1974;12:212–218.
35. Newell DW, et al. *Transcranial Doppler.* New York: Raven, 1992.
36. Njemanze PC. Transcranial Doppler evaluation of syncope: an application in aerospace physiology. *Aviat Space Environ Med* 1991; 62:569–572.
37. Nobili F, et al. Primary dysautonomia: cerebral blood flow and hemodynamic findings—case report. *Ital J Neurol Sci* 1990;11:283–288.
38. Novak P, et al. Increase of slow periodic modulation of EEG in a patient with Alzheimer's disease. *Physiol Res* 1992;41:293–297.
39. Novak P, et al. Slow modulation of EEG. *Neuroreport* 1992;3:189–192.
40. Novak P, et al. Periodic amplitude modulation of EEG. *Neurosci Lett* 1992;136:213–215.
41. Novak P, et al. Time/frequency mapping of the heart rate, blood pressure and respiratory signals. *Med Biol Eng Comput* 1993;31:103–110.
42. Novak V, et al. Altered breathing pattern of hypertensive patients. *Hypertension* 1994;23:104–113.
43. Novak V, et al. Topography of slow modulation of EEG in normal subjects during rest and head-up tilt. *Clin Auton Res* 1994;4:200 (abst).
44. Oppenheim AV, et al. *Digital signal processing*. Englewood Cliffs, NJ: Prentice Hall, 1985.
45. Peter JH, et al. Manifestations and consequences of obstructive sleep apnoea [Review]. *Eur Respir J* 1995;8:1572–1583.
46. Petty GW, et al. Transcranial Doppler ultrasonography: clinical applications in cerebrovascular disease [Review]. *Mayo Clin Proc* 1990;65:1350–1364.
47. Pfurtscheller G. Ultralangsame Schwankungen innerhalb der rhythmischen Aktivität im Alpha-Band und deren mögliche Ursachen. *Pflugers Arch* 1976;367:55–66.
48. Sandroni P, et al. Pharmacological dissection of components of the Valsalva maneuver in adrenergic failure. *J Appl Physiol* 1991;71: 1563–1567.
49. Sandroni P, et al. Postural tachycardia syndrome: mechanisms of blood pressure alterations during the Valsalva maneuver. *Neurology* 1996;46:A224(abst).
50. Schondorf R, et al. Echocardiographic measurements during neurally mediated syncope: no evidence of an "empty heart." *Clin Auton Res* 1994;4:196(abst).
51. Schondorf R, Low PA. Idiopathic postural orthostatic tachycardia syndrome: an attenuated form of acute pandysautonomia? *Neurology* 1993;43:132–137.
52. Sforza E, et al. Do autonomic cardiovascular reflexes predict the nocturnal rise in blood pressure in obstructive sleep apnea syndrome? *Blood Pressure* 1994;3:295–302.
53. Shinohara Y, et al. Cerebral hemodynamics in Shy–Drager syndrome: variability of cerebral blood flow dysautoregulation and the compensatory role of chemical control in dysautoregulation. *Stroke* 1978;9: 504–508.
54. Steriade M, et al. A novel slow (<1 Hz) oscillation of neocortical neurons *in vivo*: depolarizing and hyperpolarizing components. *J Neurosci* 1993;13:3252–3265.
55. Steriade M, et al. Intracellular analysis of relations between the slow (<1 Hz) neocortical oscillation and other sleep rhythms of the electroencephalogram. *J Neurosci* 1993;13:3266–3283.
56. Steriade M, et al. The deafferented reticular thalamic nucleus generates spindle rhythmicity. *J Neurophysiol* 1987;57:260–273.
57. Steriade M, et al. The slow (<1 Hz) oscillation in reticular thalamic and thalamocortical neurons: scenario of sleep rhythm generation in interacting thalamic and neocortical networks. *J Neurosci* 1993;13: 3284–3299.
58. Streeten DH, et al. Abnormal orthostatic changes in blood pressure and heart rate in subjects with intact sympathetic nervous function: evidence for excessive venous pooling. *J Lab Clin Med* 1988;111: 326–335.
59. Symon L. Pathological regulation in cerebral ischemia. In: Wood JH, ed. *Cerebral blood flow: physiologic and clinical aspects*. New York: McGraw-Hill, 1987:423–424.
60. Thomas DJ, et al. Preservation of autoregulation of cerebral blood flow in autonomic failure. *J Neurol Sci* 1980;44:205–212.
61. Van Lieshout JJ, et al. The vasovagal response [Review]. *Clin Sci* 1991;81:575–586.

CHAPTER 28

The Neuropathology of Autonomic Neuropathies

Phillip A. Low and Peter James Dyck

1. Sural nerve biopsy may be diagnostic in neuropathies caused by amyloidosis, Fabry's disease, Tangier disease, leprosy, necrotizing angiopathy, and sarcoidosis, and in certain inherited neuropathies.
2. The splanchnic outflow is critically important in the maintenance of postural normotension. Orthostatic hypotension seems to occur when >50% of preganglionic neurons are lost.
3. The most common variety of familial amyloid polyneuropathy is diagnosable by the finding of transthyretin in amyloid.
4. Diabetic autonomic neuropathy is characterized by widespread involvement of autonomic fibers, parasympathetic and sympathetic, preganglionic and postganglionic.
5. Proximal diabetic neuropathy is typically associated with generalized autonomic failure. Perivascular round cell infiltration is relatively common.
6. The autonomic lesion in Tangier disease appears to be restricted to the postganglionic sympathetic axon, with prominent lipid inclusions.
7. Acute panautonomic neuropathy is often characterized by a postganglionic neuropathy with perivascular round cell infiltration.
8. Multiple-system atrophy is characterized by a marked reduction of preganglionic autonomic neurons and a peripheral neuropathy occurring in from one in seven to one in five patients.
9. The Riley–Day syndrome is characterized by a reduction in small and intermediate neurons and a marked depletion of substance P in the substantia gelatinosa.

INTRODUCTION

The postganglionic sympathetic fibers, both adrenergic and sudomotor, are often affected in the axonal neuropathies. In certain inherited and immune-mediated neuropathies, these fibers are affected disproportionately. This chapter focuses on the histopathologic descriptions of a number of autonomic neuropathies. Particular emphasis is placed on studies using quantitative methodology.

COMPOSITION OF PERIPHERAL NERVE

Peripheral nerve comprises somatic motor, somatic sensory, and unmyelinated C (somatic and sympathetic) fibers. The composition and type of unmyelinated fibers may vary by nerve. For instance, Schmalbruch (71), reporting on the composition of the rat midsciatic nerve, found that myelinated fibers comprised 29% (motor 6% and sensory 23%) and unmyelinated fibers 71%, with a somatic–sympathetic C ratio of 2:1. The component nerves had a variable sympathetic composition (Table 1). The percent of unmyelinated fibers remained relatively constant within the component nerves, comprising 67%, 62%, and 80% for tibial, peroneal, and sural nerves, respectively. Greater variation is reported for the percent of sympathetic fibers within the "C" fiber population, being 41%, 4%, and 35% respectively for tibial, peroneal, and sural nerves.

Normal unmyelinated fibers are encased in Schwann cell cytoplasm and occur in clusters (Fig. 1). With acute fiber degeneration, there is cytoplasmic swelling, granular degeneration of microtubules and neurofilaments, and subsequent disappearance of the axolemma. Regeneration occurs within days and results in miniature regenerating axons. In a study of degeneration and regeneration following

P. A. Low and P. J. Dyck: Department of Neurology, Mayo Clinic, Rochester, Minnesota 55905.

TABLE 1. *Nerve composition of rat peripheral nerve fiber*

Nerve	Myelinated fibers		Unmyelinated fibers	
	Motor	Sensory	Sympathetic	Somatic
Tibial	1,000	3,500	3,700	5,400
Peroneal	600	1,300	110	3,000
Sural	—	1,100	1,500	2,800

crush, degeneration was far advanced by 4 days, regenerating fibers seen by 5 days, and miniature profiles persisted (Fig. 2), so that diameters had a mode of only 0.25 mm at 15 weeks (22).

The sympathetic component is difficult to identify and appears to comprise a small percent of total unmyelinated fibers. Methods of determining sympathetic fiber content have usually been indirect, such as the comparison of counts in sural nerve subjected to sympathectomy versus nonsympathectomized nerves (16). More direct methods such as the electron-microscopic identification of unmyelinated fibers with dense core particles is not only tedious but imprecise since many axons might not contain a core particle in the section studied. Immunogold localization of tyrosine hydroxylase in electron micrographs provides reliable visualization of adrenergic terminals but has not been applied to human peripheral nerve. Cruder estimates of the content of sympathetic adrenergic fibers can be made by the use of fluorescence microscopy (such as the glyoxylic acid method; Fig. 3), nerve norepinephrine content (16,20,73,83), or dopamine–β-hydroxylase (12) measurements.

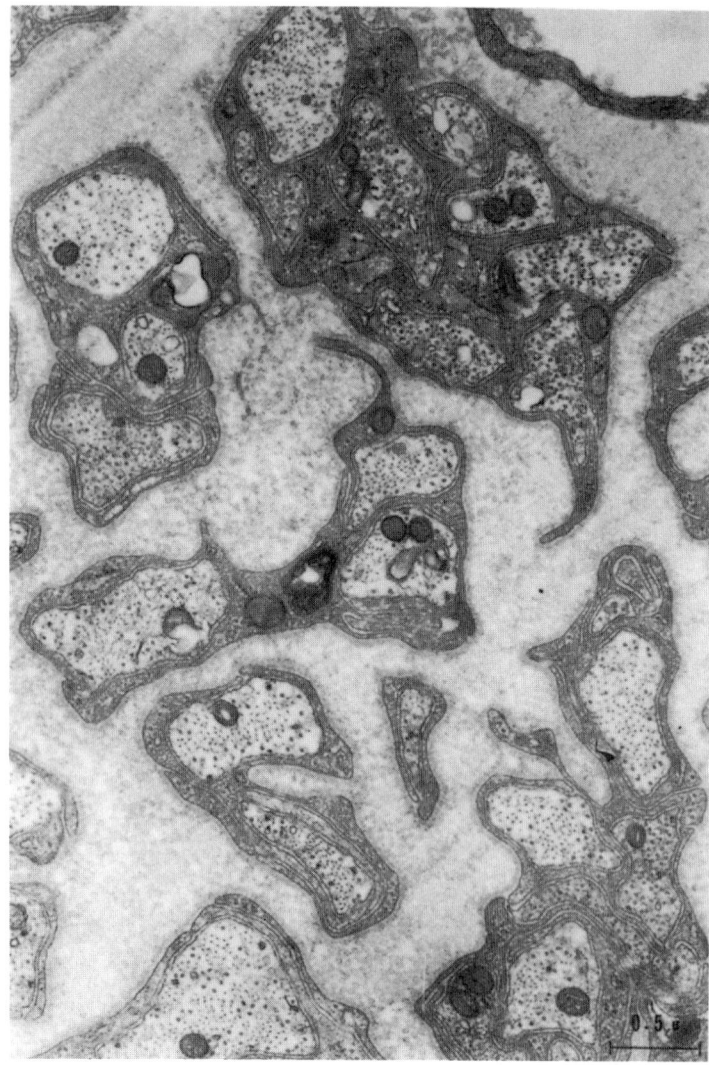

FIG. 1. Electron micrograph of a transverse section of rat cervical sympathetic chain showing the morphology of normal unmyelinated fibers. From Dyck and Hopkins (22), with permission.

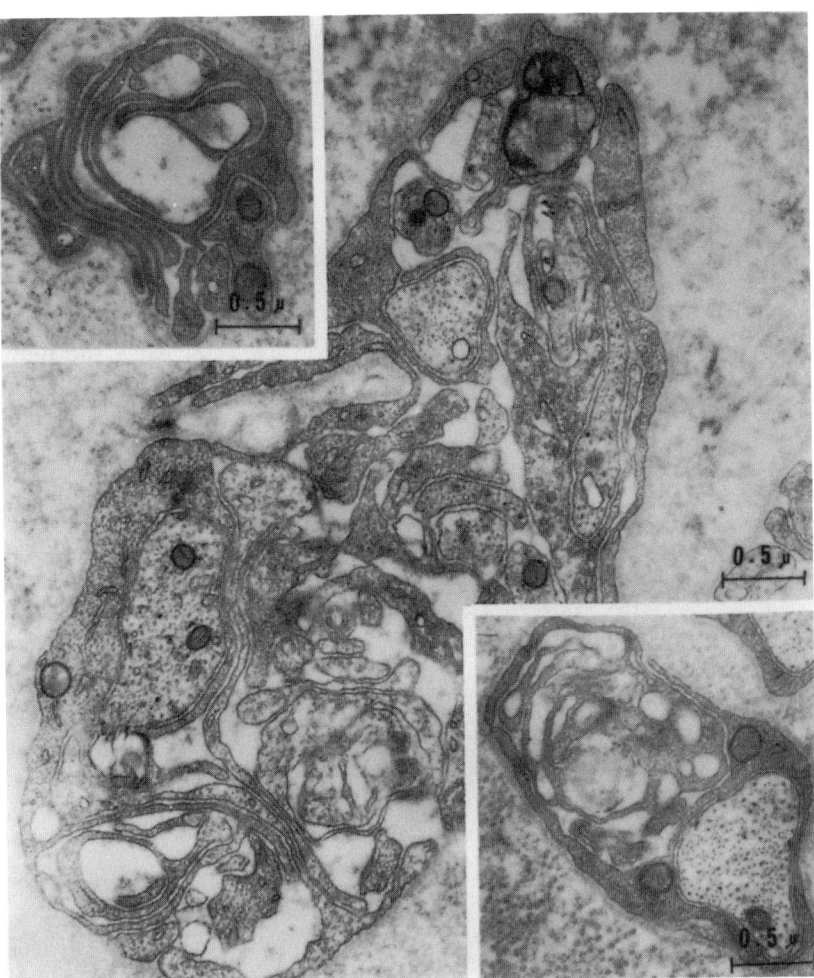

FIG. 2. Top left: At 69 hr after and distal to crush, a remnant of a previous unmyelinated fiber cluster showing stacks of Schwann cell processes with empty spaces and without unmyelinated fibers. **Center:** A remnant of a cluster of unmyelinated fibers that consists mainly of Schwann cell cytoplasmic processes, in fingerlike and curvilinear stacks, and containing two unmyelinated fibers showing stacks of cytoplasmic processes and one intact axis cylinder. **Bottom right:** Another example of an occasional normal unmyelinated fiber. From Dyck and Hopkins (22), with permission.

Skin Biopsies

Recently, unmyelinated fibers and their subtypes have been evaluated by using a number of antibodies. Kennedy and Wendelschafer-Crabb (44), using immunohistochemical procedures, found numerous nerve fibers in all cell layers of human epidermis. These nerves originate from nerve trunks in the dermis, enter the epidermis, and then divide distally to eventually end in small enlargements, near the surface of the skin and in deeper areas. Some endings may be external to stratum granulosum cells. Epidermal nerves appear to have a three-dimensional territorial distribution

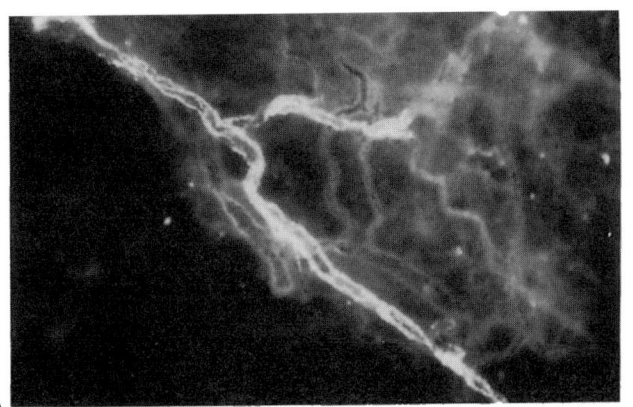 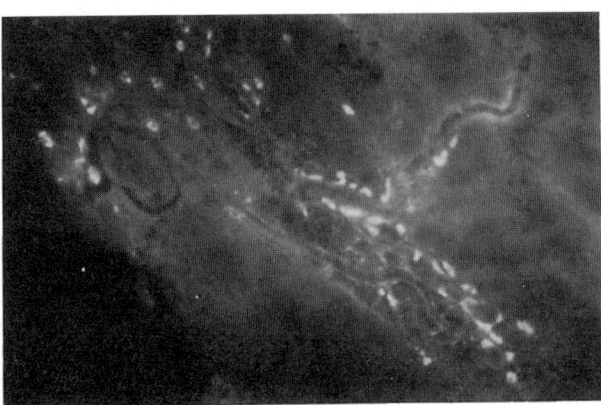

FIG. 3. Norepinephrine fluorescence of normal rat sciatic nerve sheath **(A)** and guanethidine-treated animals **(B)**. Only residual fluorescence (bottom) is in mast cells. Glyoxylic acid method.

in relationship to the skin's surface. The presence of epidermal nerve fibers was confirmed by electron-microscopic studies. The nerves are presumed to be sensory in nature. In a subsequent report, Kennedy et al. (45) detailed innervation and vasculature of human sweat glands by using immunohistochemistry and laser scanning confocal fluorescence microscopic study. Using these techniques, the three-dimensional distribution of up to three substances within a single specimen was investigated by collecting a series of optical sections for each of three fluorophores. Each sweat gland received several nerve fibers. These branched into delicate bands of one or more axons that ran longitudinal to the sweat tubule and then encircled the tubule. A heavy complement of capillaries was interwoven among the sweat tubules. Sweat ducts were accompanied from the sweat gland toward the skin surface by one or two longitudinally oriented nerve fibers and capillaries. Immunoreactive staining of nerves was heaviest with protein gene product (PGP)-9.5 antibody, but triple labeling showed that immunoreactivity to calcitonin gene-related peptide, vasoactive intestinal polypeptide, and synaptophysin was also present in the same axons. Substance P-immunoreactive axons were sparse in sweat glands but were present in other areas of the skin.

Skin biopsy specimens stained with the panaxonal marker anti-PGP-9.5 have been used to evaluate other sensory neuropathies (58). McCarthy et al. (58) used punch skin biopsies performed on the heel and leg of HIV-seronegative controls, HIV-seropositive individuals without neuropathy, and patients with sensory neuropathies, including HIV-seronegative and HIV-positive individuals. They evaluated the number of intraepidermal fibers per millimeter in at least three sections from each patient and reported that the immunostaining technique reliably demonstrated a dermal plexus of myelinated and unmyelinated fibers parallel to the surface of the skin. In the epidermis, unmyelinated fibers ascended vertically between the keratinocytes to reach the stratum corneum. The number of intraepidermal fibers per millimeter in the distal leg was significantly reduced ($p = 0.01$) in five HIV-infected patients with sensory neuropathies and in eight HIV-seronegative patients with sensory neuropathies. Four of five neurologically normal HIV-seropositive patients had reduced numbers of epidermal fibers, suggesting a subclinical neuropathy. Serial biopsies in one individual demonstrated the evolution of degenerating epidermal fibers after development of zalcitabine-induced sensory neuropathy. They concluded that this simple and repeatable technique is a reliable method for quantitation of small cutaneous sensory fibers in peripheral nerve disease.

Sural Nerve Biopsy in Autonomic Neuropathies

The nerve biopsy, well done and adequately interpreted, can be very useful in evaluation of the autonomic neu-

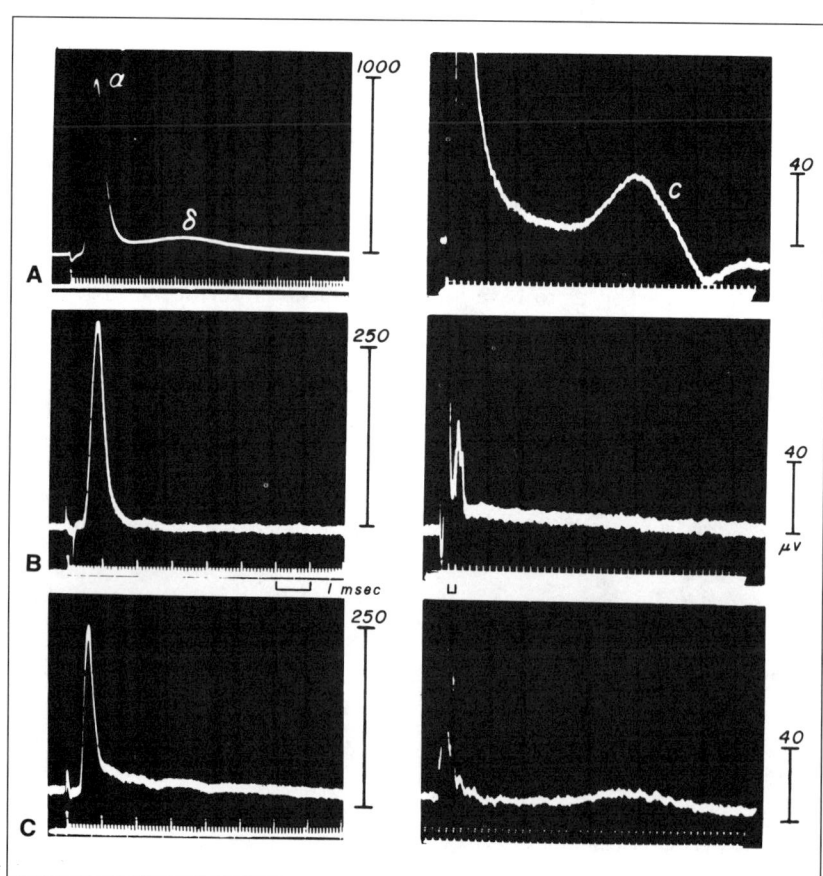

FIG. 4. Compound action potential of sural nerve *in vitro* showing Aα, Aδ, and C fiber potentials from a normal control **(top)** and from patients with amyloidosis **(middle and bottom)**, showing absence (middle) or reduction (bottom) of the C and reduction of Aδ (middle and bottom) potentials. From Dyck and Lambert (24), with permission.

TABLE 2. *Enzyme content and transport in human sural nerve biopsy samples*

Group[a]	n	Dopamine–β-hydroxylase (DBH)		Acetylcholinesterase (AChE)	
		Content (units/mg wet weight)	Average velocity (mm/hr)	Content (units/mg wet weight)	Average velocity (mm/hr)
Controls	20	104 ± 15	1.8 ± 0.1	27 ± 4	1.0 ± 0.1
HSN I	4	64 ± 26	1.1 ± 0.4*	—	—
HSN II	2	74	0.4	—	—
HMSN I	1	38	0.2	—	—
HMSN II	4	74 ± 18	0.7 ± 0.5**	—	—
HMSN III	9	106 ± 3	0.2 ± 0.1***	—	—
Diabetic neuropathy	10	56 ± 11*	0.6 ± 0.1***	7.5 ± 1.7***	0.5 ± 0.1**
Uremia	4	115 ± 14	0.9 ± 0.3	—	—
Sodium cyanate	2	91	2.0	—	—
Pandysautonomia	1	28	1.2	—	—

[a]HSN, hereditary sensory neuropathy; HMSN, hereditary motor and sensory neuropathy. Enzyme units are pmol octopamine produced per hour (DBH) and nmol acetylcholine hydrolyzed per hour (AChE). Modified from Brimijoin (11), with permission.
[b]*$p < 0.05$ versus control; **$p < 0.01$ versus control; ***$p < 0.001$ versus control.

ropathies. Unmyelinated fiber function can be evaluated by using measurements of the monophasic compound action potential of excised fascicles *in vitro*. The compound action potential is made up of Aα, Aδ, and "C" components (Fig. 4). The Aα component in sural nerve has a maximal velocity of 61 m/sec and a diameter of 11–12 mm (47) and conveys mainly touch pressure, two-point discrimination, joint position, and vibration sensations. The Aδ component has a peak conduction of 19 m/sec and mediates epicritic pain and cold sensation. The "C" component has a peak conduction velocity at 37°C of 1.1 m/sec and conveys protopathic pain, warmth, cold, and sympathetic adrenergic and sudomotor functions. A limitation of recording the "C" potential is the inability to separate autonomic from somatic "C" and adrenergic from sudomotor fibers.

Nerve norepinephrine or dopamine–β-hydroxylase activity can be used to determine the number of adrenergic fibers and to measure their redistribution (fast axonal flow). Another useful method is to demonstrate epineurial catecholamine fluorescence by the glyoxylic method. Sural nerve dopamine–β-hydroxylase content and transport velocity can be determined (11), which has been used to study a number of neuropathies in biopsied human sural nerves (Table 2). The method is impractical for routine use.

Tissue norepinephrine can be measured by using high-performance liquid chromatography and electrochemical detection (83), and values are available for rats. Experimental adrenergic neuropathy results in a dramatic reduction of norepinephrine content (Table 3). Norepinephrine content of autonomic ganglia and artery, relative to peripheral nerve, is ~20 and 3–4 times greater, respectively. The content of a parasympathetic nerve (vagus) is not different from that of somatic sensory (sural) or mixed nerve (peroneal or tibial), suggesting that most of the norepinephrine is in epineurium, as has been shown in fluorescence studies (20,68).

In human sural nerve, it is not possible to separate out the sympathetic from somatic "C" fibers reliably. Unmyelinated fibers are identifiable on electron microscopy although considerable difficulty may be encountered in differentiating Schwann cell processes from regenerating or small unmyelinated fibers. Adrenergic fibers are identifiable by the presence of dense core vesicles (81), although the paucity of these particles in the sample on view renders the differentiation difficult (79). Unmyelinated fiber pathology is recognizable in biopsied human nerves. Changes consist of the development of denervated bands of Bugner (79), collagen pockets, miniature profiles (Fig. 2) (61), a shift in unmyelinated fiber diameter histogram to a smaller diameter peak (61), and a reduction in fiber density (24, 60). The diameter distribution shift from a unimodal distribution to a bimodal distribution has been suggested to be a more sensitive index of unmyelinated fiber pathology than is unmyelinated fiber density (Fig. 5) (60).

Indications and Complications

Nerve biopsy (usually sural nerve biopsy) can provide important information and is sometimes diagnostic of certain types of neuropathy. For a detailed discussion, see Dyck et al. (26). The procedure does have significant mor-

TABLE 3. *Norepinephrine content (ng/mg wet weight) in rats*

Tissue	Guanethidine	Control
n	11	12
Superior cervical ganglion	1.66 ± 0.31	22.47 ± 2.06
Vagus nerve	0.20 ± 0.07	0.77 ± 0.16
Peroneal nerve	0.28 ± 0.16	1.45 ± 0.76
Sural nerve	0.32 ± 0.19	1.27 ± 0.25
Tibial nerve	0.09 ± 0.05	0.77 ± 0.18
Artery to tibial nerve	0.57 ± 0.43	3.61 ± 1.21

Guanethidine significantly reduced $p < 0.001$ for all groups. All data expressed as mean ±SEM.

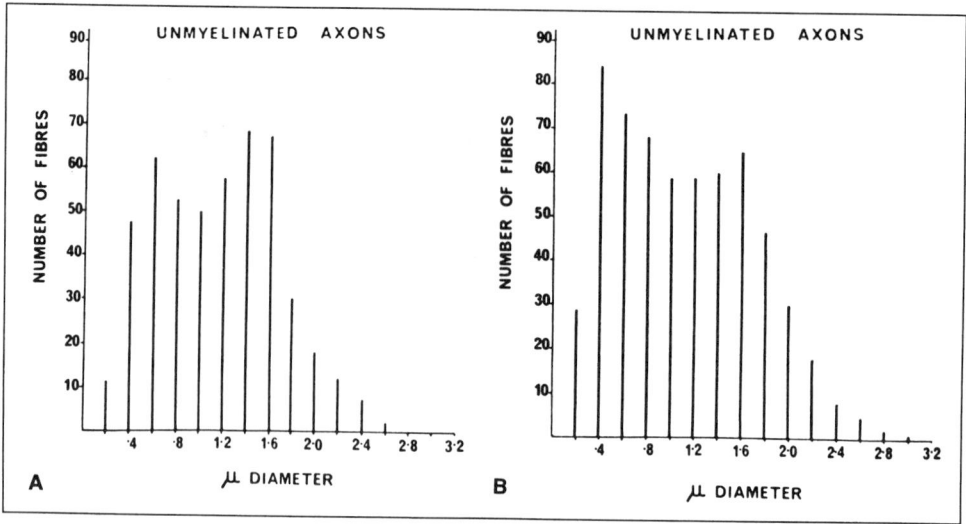

FIG. 5. Fiber size histograms of unmyelinated axons in the man of 34 (**left**) and the man of 59 (**right**). From Ochoa and Mair (61), with permission.

bidity: ~30%–40% of patients will complain of discomfort or uncomfortable numbness at 3 and 12 months after the biopsy (26). The procedure should be performed by a surgeon experienced with nerve biopsies and by a laboratory with personnel and facilities to prepare and interpret the tissue adequately. The minimum study should consist of specific stains for amyloid (Congo red or methyl violet) and myelin, single-teased-fiber evaluation, and tissue embedded in a plastic medium so that the nerve is available for electron microscopy should that be necessary.

Single-teased-fiber studies are necessary to define the nature of the pathologic process adequately. Longitudinal light-microscopic sections alone are inadequate. The type and severity of pathologic processes can be quantitated and graded by using the grading system of Dyck et al. (26). Single-teased-fiber studies can be done on autonomic preganglionic fibers (5) as has been done on rami communicantes and the greater splanchnic nerve (50,55) removed at autopsy. For living patients, autonomic fibers are not studied directly. However, patients with aggressive axonal degeneration tend to have more autonomic failure than do patients with a chronic demyelinating process (53).

The nerve biopsy may be diagnostic for the following neuropathies: (1) amyloid, (2) necrotizing vasculitis, (3) Fabry's disease, (4) Tangier disease, (5) neuroaxonal dystrophy, (6) leprosy, (7) hereditary motor and sensory neuropathy type III (Dejerine–Sottas disease), and (8) sarcoidosis. It may provide useful but not diagnostic information in acute panautonomic, chronic inflammatory demyelinating polyradiculoneuropathy (CIDP), and motor and sensory neuropathy type I (HMSN-I; hypertrophic Charcot–Marie–Tooth disease). In acute panautonomic neuropathy, norepinephrine should be reduced, and perivascular round cell infiltration may be present. The latter finding may be seen in CIDP. Large concentric arrays of Schwann cell processes may surround demyelinated or remyelinating axons in HMSN-I.

It is important that optimal research utilization be made of the limited available biopsy tissue. Research functions include the morphometric analysis of nerve fiber populations and of microvessels, and the use of antibodies to identify T-cell subtypes and components of nerve and microvessels. Molecular biologic techniques, including *in situ* hybridization studies, might identify key antigenic targets.

PATHOLOGY OF AUTONOMIC NEUROPATHIES

Splanchnic Outflow

In human subjects, postural hypotension depends more on splanchnic–mesenteric microvascular tone than on muscle arterioles (56). The main sympathetic nerve supply to the splanchnic–mesenteric bed is the greater splanchnic nerve, with its cell body in the intermediolateral column (mainly T4 to T9). Much research and clinical evidence supports the importance of the sympathetic outflow in the maintenance of postural normotension (48,55). Bilateral splanchnicectomy regularly results in orthostatic hypotension, whereas neither bilateral lumbar sympathectomy nor cardiac denervation cause orthostatic hypotension (55). Orthostatic hypotension regularly occurs in spinal cord lesions above T4 (decentralizing the splanchnic outflow) but is absent in lesions below T9.

We studied the splanchnic outflow in fresh autopsy material of 12 persons aged $4\frac{1}{2}$–79 years who had died free of autonomic disorders. The predominant cell type within the intermediolateral column had the staining characteristics of motor neurons with coarse and irregular Nissl substance. The nucleus was large and often eccentric, and neurons were oval, polygonal, or spindle or club shaped. The mean preganglionic cell counts in the intermediolateral column at T6, T7, and T8 spinal cord segments were 5,002, 5,004, and 4,654, respectively (51). There was no significant sex difference. Most cells ranged in diameter from 6 to 23 mm, with the major peak at 12–13 mm. There was a progressive reduction of preganglionic neuron numbers with age. In adults, 370 preganglionic neurons (8%) were lost per decade (51). No significant differences in neuron numbers were found among segments.

Morphometric studies were also done on the corresponding ventral spinal root (49) and autonomic rami (50). There was good concordance between intermediolateral column neurons and ventral spinal root preganglionic axon numbers (0.81) and with autonomic rami (0.95). The preganglionic axon numbers in ventral spinal root and rami underwent a similar attrition with age (8% and 5%, respectively).

We have reported morphometric studies on the splanchnic sympathetic outflow in multiple-system atrophy (MSA), pure autonomic failure (52), amyloid neuropathy, and Tangier disease (54), familial dysautonomia (25), and in diabetic autonomic neuropathy (48,55). Based on the correlation of orthostatic hypotension with preganglionic neuron attrition with age, and a loss in disorders where the brunt of the pathology falls on the preganglionic system, we suggested that orthostatic hypotension does not occur until an attrition of at least 50% of preganglionic neurons has occurred. This observation does not apply to disorders such as pure autonomic failure and the peripheral autonomic neuropathies where there is an additional postganglionic lesion.

Amyloid Neuropathy

The hallmarks of histopathologic analysis of amyloid neuropathy, familial and primary, are the selective loss of small myelinated and unmyelinated fibers, axonal degeneration, and amyloid deposits (23,78). Four patterns of amyloid deposition have been described (17): (a) a diffuse pattern of amyloid deposition, (b) globular deposits displacing nerve fibers, (c) vascular wall deposition, and (d) deposition among collagen as in carpal ligament causing compression neuropathy. Using immunohistochemistry approaches, the precursor proteins of amyloid deposits can now be recognized. Finding transthyretin in amyloid is diagnostic of familial amyloid polyneuropathy. Approximately 20 allelic mutations of transthyretin are recognized. The protein characteristic of primary amyloidosis is either κ or λ light chains, which can also be identified by immunohistochemistry. The pattern of selective loss of small and unmyelinated fibers is not always found but is especially common in some early cases of familial amyloid polyneuropathy and is responsible for dissociated sensory impairment (23) and reflected in the loss of C potential

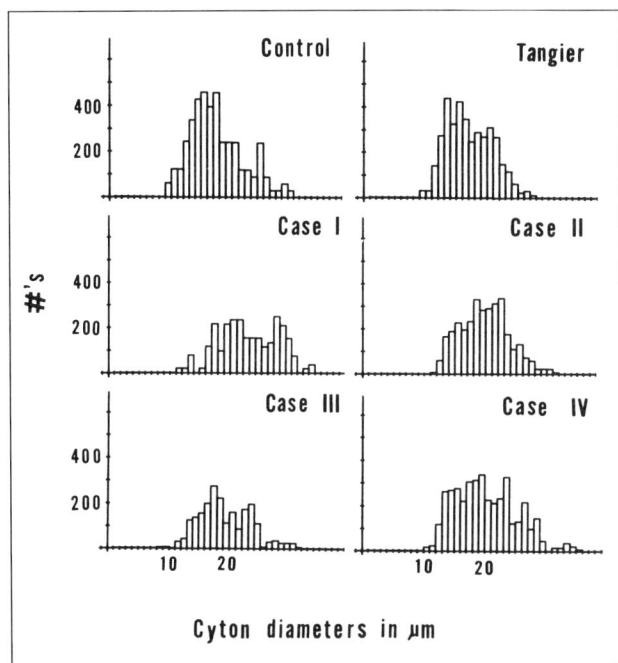

FIG. 6. Histograms of the T7 intermediolateral column neuron diameters of control, of Tangier disease, and of four patients with amyloid neuropathy. From Low et al. (54), with permission.

in the *in vitro* monophasic compound action potential (Fig. 2).

We performed a morphometric analysis of preganglionic sympathetic neurons at the T7 intermediolateral columns of four patients aged 41–67 who had died of amyloid neuropathy (54). These patients all had impairment of blood pressure control. Neuronal counts were reduced and ranged from 50% to 79% of control values. The diameter distribution was not different from that of controls (Fig. 6). Although the brunt of the pathology falls on the postganglionic axon, the preganglionic neuron is also involved and likely contributes to the orthostatic hypotension.

Diabetic Neuropathy

Limited studies have been done on the sympathetic nervous system of patients with diabetes. Abnormally large neurons containing periodic acid–Schiff-positive material have been described in sympathetic ganglia (6,21,39), as have swelling and degeneration of postganglionic dendritic processes (39). Duchen et al. (21) consistently found inflammatory changes in the autonomic ganglia at necropsy in five patients with insulin-dependent diabetes mellitus (IDDM) but not in somatic nerves. This finding is of particular interest in view of the recent finding of antisympathetic antibodies (13), and the frequent occurrence of iritis, an autoimmune disorder in IDDM patients with autonomic neuropathy (37). Since nerve growth factor and insulin

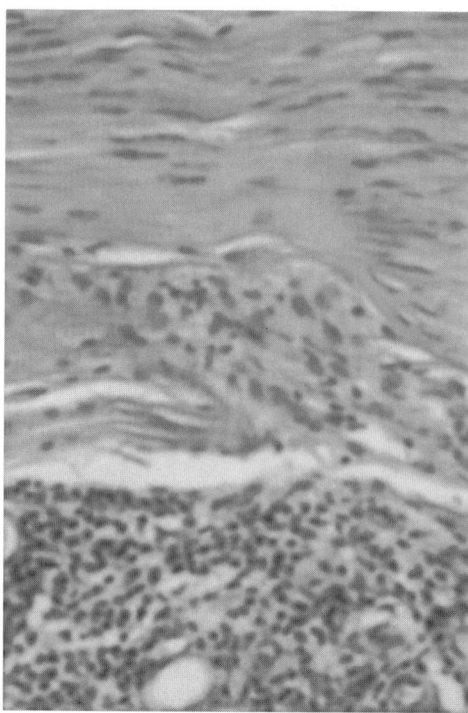

FIG. 7. Longitudinal paraffin section of sural nerve stained with hematoxylin–eosin (×300) from a patient with typical asymmetric proximal diabetic neuropathy. The *top one-third* of the frame is endoneurium. The *bottom one-third* shows a prominent epineurial perivascular mononuclear infiltrate. Courtesy of Dr. James and Peter Dyck.

share antigenic determinants (33,72), it has been suggested that insulin antibodies may cross-react with nerve growth factor and cause sympathetic nerve damage (37,38).

In a review of 44 diabetic patients with subacute diabetic proximal neuropathy who were seen over a 12-year period, the patients were middle aged or elderly, of either sex, with proximal muscle weakness associated with reduced or absent lower extremity reflexes. Electrophysiologically, the majority had some evidence of demyelination on nerve conduction but invariably accompanied by concomitant axonal degeneration. Cerebrospinal fluid protein was usually increased. Diffuse and significant autonomic failure was usually present. Sural nerve biopsy was done in nine patients, eight at the Mayo Clinic. Most had some suggestion of demyelination, although only two had evidence of an inflammatory infiltrate. In an ongoing study (J. Dyck and P. Dyck), perivascular round cell infiltration was found in the majority of patients with proximal diabetic neuropathy (Fig. 7). The investigators (P. J. B. Dyck et al., personal communication) have found that such epineurial infiltrates, sometimes involving the vessel wall, axonal degeneration, and focal and multifocal fiber loss, are typical pathologic findings of the sural nerve in this disorder. They consider that these pathologic findings are in keeping with an immune disorder of nutrient vessels to nerve.

Walsh (82) demonstrated that in control subjects the density and diameter distribution of myelinated fibers are similar in the splanchnic nerve to that in the sympathetic

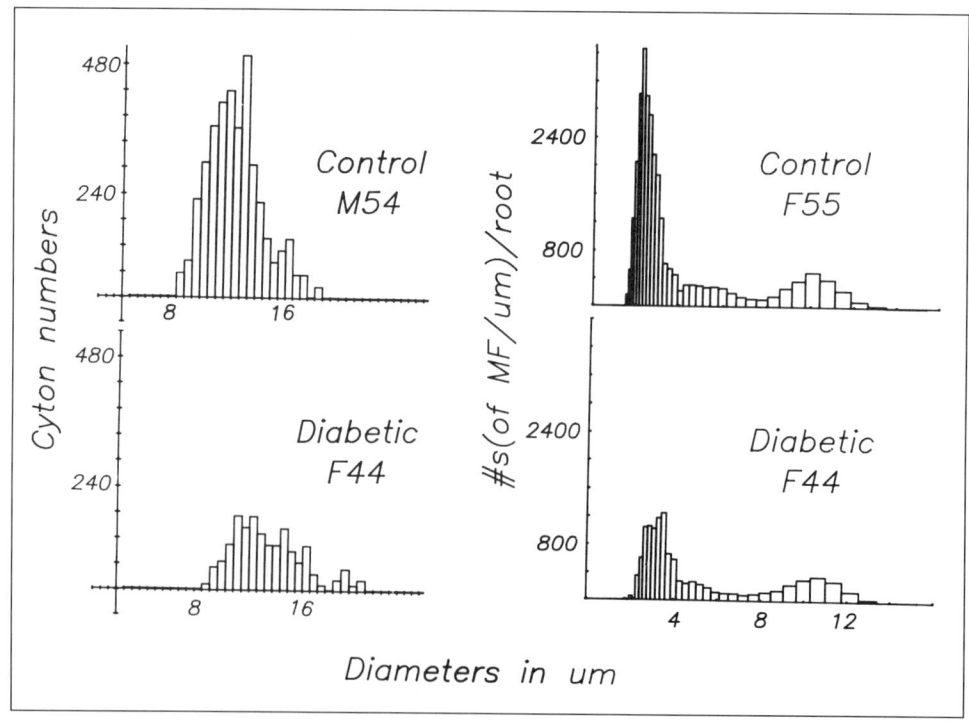

FIG. 8. Preganglionic autonomic neurons and myelinated fibers (MF) of the T7 intermediolateral column and corresponding ventral root of a control and a diabetic patient. From Low et al. (48), with permission.

trunk and white rami. Quantitative studies have been done on the greater splanchnic nerve of patients with diabetes, obtained at autopsy (55). The myelinated fiber density is reduced, and the predominant pathology on single-teased-fiber examination was that of demyelination (55). The intermediolateral column neuron counts are also reduced (Fig. 8) and abnormalities have been described in rami communicantes (5), consisting of an increased density and reduced internodal lengths suggestive of degeneration and regeneration. More pronounced changes of both demyelination and axonal loss have also been found (62). Budzilovich (14) described focal neuromatous lesions, consisting of bundles of unmyelinated axons and associated Schwann cells, suggestive of aberrant regeneration in diabetic rami.

Pathologic abnormalities have been consistently found in the vagus nerve in the limited studies done thus far (21,38,46). Severe loss of small myelinated axons was found in the vagus nerve (21,46), including the abdominal vagus (38), and esophagus (74). Guy et al. (38) performed quantitative studies of unmyelinated fibers from the abdominal vagus of a patient with severe gastroparesis. The density was markedly reduced, axons were of reduced diameter, and there were increased numbers of collagen pockets and denervated Schwann cell subunits indicative of unmyelinated fiber pathology.

Abnormalities have been found in other nerves, including the carotid sinus nerve (75). The distribution of sympathetic nerve fibers are reported to run parallel to the skin surface while somatic "C" fibers run perpendicular to the skin surface (84). Histologic studies of anhidrotic skin have demonstrated beading, thickening, and fragmentation of silver-stained postganglionic sympathetic axons adjacent to the sweat glands (30). Similar histologic/histochemical findings have been made in urinary bladder, corpora cavernosa, and heart (28,29,31). Erectile tissue from corpora cavernosa of impotent diabetic males have >80% depletion of vasoactive polypeptide (38). Acetylcholine and norepinephrine contents are also reduced (59).

Tangier Disease

The autonomic lesion in Tangier disease appears to be restricted to the postganglionic sympathetic axon. Low et al. (54) found normal intermediolateral column neuronal counts and normal preganglionic sympathetic neuron axons in the thoracic ventral spinal root of a 67-year-old woman who died of Tangier disease (Fig. 6). She had severe involvement of peripheral nerve unmyelinated fibers, with fiber loss and lipid inclusions, and clinically had severe impairment of pain perception (25) and widespread anhidrosis (Fig. 9).

Acute Panautonomic Neuropathy

Acute panautonomic neuropathy, idiopathic or paraneoplastic, has been associated with normal (86) or abnormal sural nerve biopsy findings. Abnormalities include perivascular round cell infiltration and loss of small myelinated and unmyelinated fibers (53). Appenzeller and Kornfeld (4) performed a sural nerve biopsy 12 years after the onset of the neuropathy and found an increased number of small unmyelinated fibers, suggestive of remyelination of unmyelinated fibers. Yokota et al. (85) attempted to segregate patients into postganglionic axonopathy and preganglionic demyelinating categories. Postganglionic lesions were characterized by a concordant reduction in skin potential and acetylcholinesterase histochemistry of sural nerve, whereas preganglionic lesions were associated with discrepancies between acetylcholinesterase-positive fiber density and sympathetic skin responses, and histologic and electrophysiologic evidence of demyelination.

In rabbits sensitized to extracted antigen from human sympathetic ganglion/nerve, transient mild abnormalities of vasomotor function develop (3). Regeneration of unmyelinated fibers in the paravertebral sympathetic chain and serum antibody to sympathetic antigens has been reported in this model (9). The association of antineuronal antibodies in the paraneoplastic autonomic neuropathy (see Chapters 38 and 41), the demonstration of antibodies in the experimental model, and the histologic findings of perivascular round cell infiltration (see Fig. 31-1) suggest an immunologically mediated process.

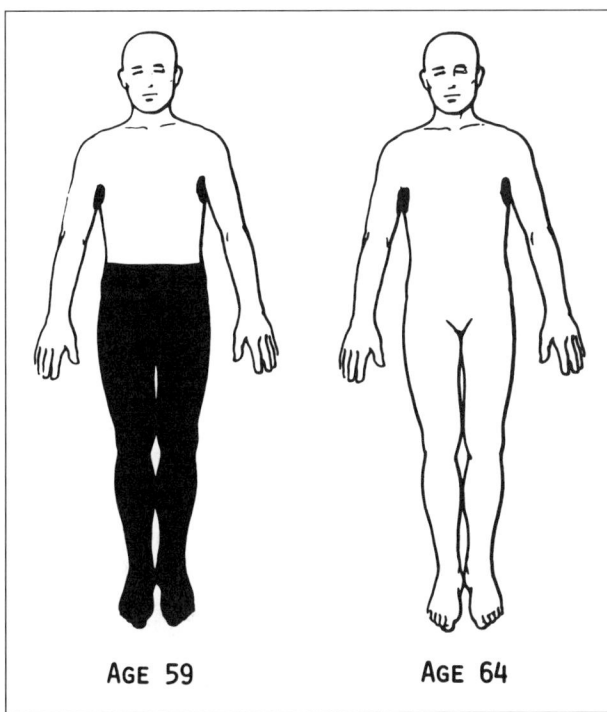

FIG. 9. Thermoregulatory sweat pattern of a patient with Tangier disease. Sweating is indicated as *shaded area*.

TABLE 4. *Neuron and axon counts of T7 splanchnic autonomic outflow*

Subjects[a]	ILC neurons[b]	Myelinated fibers		
		Small	Intermediate	Large
Patient 1 (MSA)	463	386	160	858
Patient 2 (MSA)	1,060	1,315	350	555
Patient 3 (PAF)	2,325	1,645	455	1,173
Controls[c]	3,459–5,873	2,935–6,315	345–868	1,219–1,438
Mean	4,506	3,983	573	1,332
SD	959	993	182	81

[b]ILC,
[a]MSA, multiple system atrophy; PAF, pure autonomic failure.
[c]Nine patients aged 35–79 years (mean, 58.1; SD, 18). From Low et al. (54), with permission.

Multiple-System Atrophy

The preganglionic sympathetic neurons counts are markedly reduced in MSA (8,42,43,52). In our study on two patients with MSA and one with pure autonomic failure, we measured preganglionic neuron sizes as well and related our neuron counts to axonal counts (Table 4). In the patients with MSA, the T7 preganglionic neuron numbers were 10% and 24% of age-matched controls. Their corresponding preganglionic axon numbers were 10% and 33% of controls. Abnormalities in the preganglionic axons were milder in the patient with pure autonomic failure. The preganglionic neurons and axons were 52% and 41% of normal. The diameter distributions of neurons and axons were not different from controls. Pathologic changes in the postganglionic neuron in autonomic ganglia has been described in MSA (76) but is usually absent.

A peripheral neuropathy occurs in from one of seven (18) to one of five (70) patients with MSA. In the majority of cases, the neuropathy is mild or asymptomatic and is overshadowed by autonomic failure. There is a loss of small myelinated and unmyelinated fibers in some patients with MSA (34,80).

Riley–Day Syndrome

This recessively inherited disorder of Ashkenazi Jews is characterized by dysautonomia and small-fiber-type sensory impairment and distal weakness. Pathologic findings in the central nervous system have been inconsistent; some studies have found abnormalities while others have not (19,27,32,66). The numbers of autonomic and dorsal root ganglia neurons were estimated by Pearson et al. (63, 65,66) and found to be markedly reduced.

Sural nerve studies by Aguayo et al. (1) found markedly reduced densities of unmyelinated fibers and a virtual absence of fibers 12 mm. On single-teased-fiber examination, they found reduced internodal lengths. The severe reduction in myelinated fibers was confirmed by Pearson et al. (67). In a detailed morphometric postmortem study of a patient with dysautonomia (25), the α-neurons and presumed γ-neurons, and sensory and preganglionic and postganglionic sympathetic neurons were studied at multiple levels. The studies demonstrated a selected depletion of small neurons. For the motor system, L5 α-motoneuron counts were normal (96% of controls) while γ-motoneurons were 11% of controls (Fig. 10). However, α-motoneuron axons are distally atrophic as evidenced by the reduced diameter

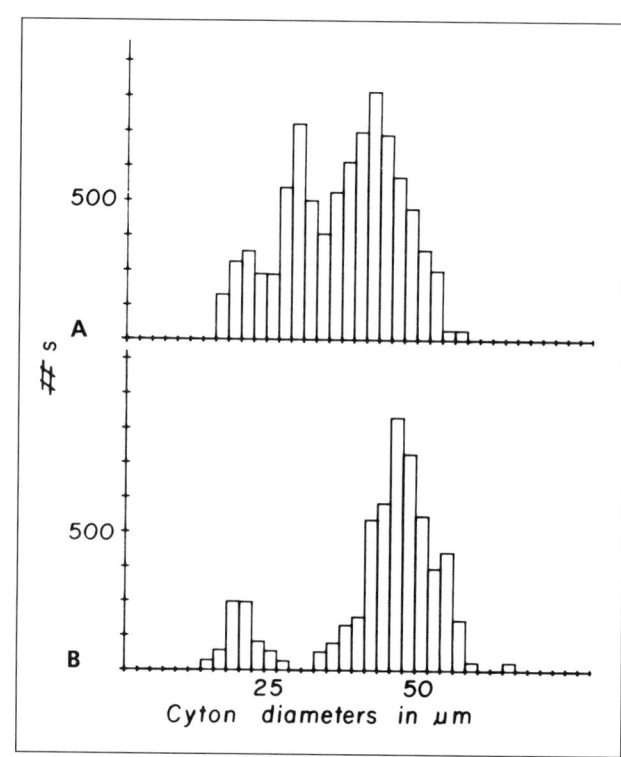

FIG. 10. Diameter histograms of cell bodies of L5 motoneuron columns in the L5 segment of a representative control **(top)** and of a dysautonomic patient **(bottom)**. In the control, three peaks are found: large (C_L), intermediate (C_I), and small (C_S). In the patient, only two peaks are found: large and small. Because C_I and A_I of ventral root are thought to be from γ-motoneurons, this is evidence of a preferential absence of γ-motoneurons in dysautonomia. From Dyck et al. (26a), with permission.

TABLE 5. *Number of T7 intermediolateral column cell bodies and their ventral root myelinated axons (A_s) in dysautonomia and in controls*

	Control	Dysautonomia (D)	D/C × 100
Neurons	5,004	1,652	33%
Axons			
A_L	1,357	1,218	90%
A_I	535	143	27%
A_s	4,198	863	21%
Total	6,090	2,224	37%

From Dyck et al. (22a), with permission.

distribution of nerve to peroneus brevis. The L5 dorsal root ganglion has a trimodal distribution in normals. The percentages of large, intermediate, and small neurons were 11%, 11%, and 4%, respectively. The T7 preganglionic and postganglionic sympathetic neurons were reduced to ~33% and ~15% of control, respectively (Table 5). Similar findings have been reported by other workers. There is marked depletion of substance P-containing axons in substantia gelatinosa of patients with dysautonomia and diminished pain sensitivity (64). Pearson and Pytel (66) found ~50% depletion of preganglionic neurons of T1–3 and an 80%–90% depletion of postganglionic sympathetic neurons of the superior cervical ganglia (66).

Porphyria

Dysautonomia—manifest as abdominal pain, constipation, tachycardia, hypertension, and orthostatic hypotension—is common in acute intermittent porphyria. Autonomic neurons are affected and may be unusually sensitive (69). The neuropathic lesion appears to be mainly a length-dependent axonal process (15). Cavanagh and Mellick (15) studied the limb nerves of four patients who died of porphyric neuropathy and found a proximodistal distribution of degenerating fibers, maximal distally. The distribution of deficits, however, is not strictly length dependent, since sensory and motor deficits may be especially prominent proximally, especially in muscles that are subject to much activity. Sural nerve biopsy specimens have typically shown both axonal degeneration and demyelination (2,77).

Evidence of autonomic involvement is available. Chromatolysis of celiac ganglion cells has been described (40), and prominent demyelination has been described in the vagus nerves of five patients who died of acute intermittent porphyria (35).

Guillain–Barré Syndrome

Dysautonomia, manifest as failure or overactivity, is relatively common in Guillain–Barré syndrome (see Chapter 36). Pathologic changes of autonomic structures have been described. Extensive inflammatory–demyelinating changes of sympathetic ganglia and vagus nerve and chromatolysis of intermediolateral column neurons have been described in fatal cases of Guillain–Barré syndrome (7,10,41,57).

Alcoholic Neuropathy

The postganglionic axon is affected as a part of this axonal neuropathy, and distal loss of unmyelinated fibers results in distal anhidrosis (55) and vasomotor changes. Cardiovagal function is relatively normal in mild alcoholic neuropathy, and orthostatic hypotension is absent. The greater splanchnic nerve has a normal density of preganglionic sympathetic axons (55). In more severely affected patients, cardiovagal function is impaired and pathologic changes are present in the vagus nerve (36) and the splanchnic system. The carotid sinus nerve is affected, with reduced density of myelinated fibers in chronic alcoholism (75).

CONCLUDING REMARKS

Neuropathologic studies of the autonomic nervous system to date are largely descriptive or at best quantitative. Future advances will likely be made on several fronts. These include the better targeting of the autonomic neuron by using antibodies to autonomic enzymes and antigens, molecular biologic methods with adequate amplification, and better correlation between autonomic function tests of the same tissue that is studied subsequently in the neuropathology laboratory.

REFERENCES

1. Aguayo AJ, et al. Peripheral nerve abnormalities in the Riley–Day syndrome: findings in a sural nerve biopsy. *Arch Neurol* 1971;24:106–116.
2. Anzil AP, Dozic S. Peripheral nerve changes in porphyric neuropathy: findings in a sural nerve biopsy. *Acta Neuropathol (Berl)* 1978;42:121–126.
3. Appenzeller O, et al. Experimental autonomic neuropathy: an immunologically induced disorder of reflex vasomotor function. *J Neurol Neurosurg Psychiatry* 1965;28:510–515.
4. Appenzeller O, Kornfeld M. Acute pandysautonomia: clinical and morphologic study. *Arch Neurol* 1973;29:334–339.
5. Appenzeller O, Ogin G. Myelinated fibres in the human paravertebral sympathetic chain: quantitative studies on white rami communicantes. *J Neurol Neurosurg Psychiatry* 1973;36:777–785.
6. Appenzeller O, Richardson EP Jr. The sympathetic chain in patients with diabetic and alcoholic polyneuropathy. *Neurology* 1966;16:1205–1209.
7. Asbury AK, et al. The inflammatory lesion in idiopathic polyneuritis: its role in pathogenesis. *Medicine (Baltimore)* 1969;48:173–215.
8. Bannister R, Oppenheimer DR. Degenerative diseases of the nervous system associated with autonomic failure. *Brain* 1972;95:457–474.
9. Becker W, et al. Experimental autonomic neuropathy: ultrastructure and immunohistochemical study of a disorder of reflex vasomotor function. *J Auton Nerv Syst* 1979;1:53–67.
10. Birchfield RI, Shaw C-M. Postural hypotension in the Guillain–Barré syndrome. *Arch Neurol* 1964;10:149–157.

11. Brimijoin S. The role of axonal transport in nerve disease. In: Dyck PJ, et al., eds. *Peripheral neuropathy*. Philadelphia: WB Saunders, 1984:477–493.
12. Brimijoin S, Dyck PJ. Axonal transport of dopamine–beta-hydroxylase and acetylcholinesterase in human peripheral neuropathy. *Exp Neurol* 1979;66:467–478.
13. Brown FM, et al. Anti-sympathetic nervous system autoantibodies: diminished catecholamines with orthostasis. *Diabetes* 1989;38:938–941.
14. Budzilovich GN. Peripheral sympathetic nervous system in diabetes mellitus. In: Anonymous, ed. *Proceedings of the sixth International Congress of Neuropathology*. Paris: Masson et Cie, 1970:275.
15. Cavanagh JB, Mellick RS. On the nature of the peripheral nerve lesions associated with acute intermittent porphyria. *J Neurol Neurosurg Psychiatry* 1965;28:320–327.
16. Chad D, et al. Sympathetic postganglionic unmyelinated axons in the rat peripheral nervous system. *Neurology* 1983;33:841–847.
17. Cohen AS, Rubinow A. Amyloid neuropathy. In: Dyck PJ, et al., eds. *Peripheral neuropathy*. Philadelphia: WB Saunders, 1984:1866–1898.
18. Cohen J, et al. Somatic and autonomic function in progressive autonomic failure and multiple system atrophy. *Ann Neurol* 1987;22:692–699.
19. Cohen P, Soloman NH. Familial dysautonomia: case report with autopsy. *J Pediatr* 1965;46:663–670.
20. Dhital K, et al. Adrenergic innervation of vasa and nervi nervorum of optic, sciatic, vagus and sympathetic nerve trunks in normal and streptozotocin-diabetic rats. *Brain Res* 1986;367:39–44.
21. Duchen LW, et al. Pathology of autonomic neuropathy in diabetes mellitus. *Ann Intern Med* 1980;92:301–303.
22. Dyck PJ, Hopkins AP. Electron microscopic observations on degeneration and regeneration of unmyelinated fibres. *Brain* 1972;95:233–234.
23. Dyck PJ, Lambert EH. Dissociated sensation in amyloidosis: compound action potentials, quantitative histologic and teased fibers, and electron microscopic studies of sural nerve biopsies. *Trans Am Neurol Assoc* 1968;93:112–115.
24. Dyck PJ, Lambert EH. Dissociated sensation in amyloidosis: compound action potential, quantitative histologic and teased-fiber, and electron microscopic studies of sural nerve biopsies. *Arch Neurol* 1969;20:490–507.
25. Dyck PJ, et al. Adult-onset of Tangier disease. 1. Morphometric and pathologic studies suggesting delayed degradation of neutral lipids after fiber degeneration. *J Neuropathol Exp Neurol* 1978;37:119–137.
26. Dyck PJ, et al. Pathologic alterations of the peripheral nervous system in humans. In: Dyck PJ, et al., eds. *Peripheral neuropathy*. Philadelphia: WB Saunders, 1984:760–870.
26a. Dyck PJ, et al. The number and sizes of reconstructed peripheral autonomic, sensory and motor neurons in a case of dysautonomia. *J Neuropathol Exp Neurol* 1978;37:741–755.
27. Engel GL, Aring CD. Hypothalamic attacks with thalamic lesion. I. Physiologic and psychologic considerations. *Arch Neurol Psychiatry* 1945;54:37–43.
28. Faerman I, et al. Autonomic nervous system and diabetes: histological and histochemical study of the autonomic nerve fibers of the urinary bladder in diabetic patients. *Diabetes* 1973;22:225–237.
29. Faerman I, et al. Autonomic neuropathy and painless myocardial infarction in diabetic patients: histologic evidence of their relationship. *Diabetes* 1977;26:1147–1158.
30. Faerman I, et al. Autonomic neuropathy in the skin: a histological study of the sympathetic nerve fibres in diabetic anhidrosis. *Diabetologia* 1982;22:96–99.
31. Faerman I, et al. Impotence and diabetes: histological studies of the autonomic nervous fibers of the corpora cavernosa in impotent diabetic males. *Diabetes* 1974;23:971–976.
32. Fogelson MH, et al. Spinal cord changes in familial dysautonomia. *Arch Neurol* 1967;17:103–108.
33. Frazier WA, et al. Nerve growth factor and insulin. *Science* 1972;176:482–488.
34. Galassi G, et al. Peripheral neuropathy in multiple system atrophy with autonomic failure. *Neurology* 1982;32:1116–1121.
35. Gibson JB, Goldberg A. The neuropathology of acute porphyria. *J Pathol Bacteriol* 1956;71:495–509.
36. Guo YP, et al. Pathological changes in the vagus nerve in diabetes and chronic alcoholism. *J Neurol Neurosurg Psychiatry* 1987;50:1449–1453.
37. Guy RJ, et al. Diabetic autonomic neuropathy and iritis: an association suggesting an immunological cause. *BMJ* 1984;289:343–345.
38. Guy RJ, et al. Diabetic gastroparesis from autonomic neuropathy: surgical considerations and changes in vagus nerve morphology. *J Neurol Neurosurg Psychiatry* 1984;47:686–691.
39. Hensley GT, Soergel KH. Neuropathologic findings in diabetic diarrhea. *Arch Pathol* 1968;85:587–597.
40. Hierons R. Changes in the nervous system in acute porphyria. *Brain* 1957;80:176–192.
41. Hodson AK, et al. Dysautonomia in Guillain–Barré syndrome with dorsal root ganglioneuropathy, wallerian degeneration, and fatal myocarditis. *Ann Neurol* 1984;15:88–95.
42. Johnson RH, et al. Autonomic failure with orthostatic hypotension due to intermediolateral column degeneration: a report of two cases with autopsies. *Q J Med* 1966;35:276–292.
43. Kennedy PG, Duchen LW. A quantitative study of intermediolateral column cells in motor neuron disease and the Shy–Drager syndrome. *J Neurol Neurosurg Psychiatry* 1985;48:1103–1106.
44. Kennedy WR, Wendelschafer-Crabb G. The innervation of human epidermis. *J Neurol Sci* 1993;115:184–190.
45. Kennedy WR, et al. Innervation and vasculature of human sweat glands: an immunohistochemistry–laser scanning confocal fluorescence microscopy study. *J Neurosci* 1994; 14:6825–6833.
46. Kristensson K, et al. Changes in the vagus nerve in diabetes mellitus. *Acta Pathol Microbiol Scand* 1971;79:684–685.
47. Lambert EH, Dyck PJ. Compound action potentials of sural nerve *in vitro* in peripheral neuropathy. In: Dyck PJ, et al., eds. *Peripheral neuropathy*. Philadelphia: WB Saunders, 1984:1130–1144.
48. Low PA. Quantitation of autonomic responses. In: Dyck PJ, et al., eds. *Peripheral neuropathy*. Philadelphia: WB Saunders, 1984:1139–1165.
49. Low PA, Dyck PJ. Splanchnic preganglionic neurons in man. II. Morphometry of myelinated fibers of T7 ventral spinal root. *Acta Neuropathol (Berl)* 1977;40:219–225.
50. Low PA, Dyck PJ. Splanchnic preganglionic neurons in man. III. Morphometry of myelinated fibers of rami communicantes. *J Neuropathol Exp Neurol* 1978;37:734–740.
51. Low PA, et al. Splanchnic preganglionic neurons in man. I. Morphometry of preganglionic cytons. *Acta Neuropathol (Berl)* 1977;40:55–61.
52. Low PA, et al. The splanchnic autonomic outflow in Shy–Drager syndrome and idiopathic orthostatic hypotension. *Ann Neurol* 1978;4:511–514.
53. Low PA, et al. Acute panautonomic neuropathy. *Ann Neurol* 1983;13:412–417.
54. Low PA, et al. The splanchnic autonomic outflow in amyloid neuropathy and Tangier disease. *Neurology* 1981;31:461–463.
55. Low PA, et al. The sympathetic nervous system in diabetic neuropathy: a clinical and pathological study. *Brain* 1975;98:341–356.
56. Mancia G, et al. Reflex cardiovascular regulation in humans. *J Cardiovasc Pharmacol* 1985;7(Suppl 3):S152–S159.
57. Matsuyama H, Haymaker W. Distribution of lesions in the Landry–Guillain–Barré syndrome, with emphasis on involvement of the sympathetic system. *Acta Neuropathol (Berl)* 1967;8:230–241.
58. McCarthy BG, et al. Cutaneous innervation in sensory neuropathies: evaluation by skin biopsy. *Neurology* 1995;45:1848–1855.
59. Melman A, Henry D. The possible role of the catecholamines of the corpora in penile erection. *J Urol* 1979;121:419–421.
60. Ochoa J. Recognition of unmyelinated fiber disease: morphologic criteria. *Muscle Nerve* 1978;1:375–387.
61. Ochoa J, Mair WGP. The normal sural nerve in man. II. Changes in the axons and Schwann cells due to ageing. *Acta Neuropathol (Berl)* 1969;13:217–239.
62. Olsson Y, Sourander P. Changes in the sympathetic nervous system in diabetes mellitus: a preliminary report. *J Neurovisc Relations* 1968; 31:86–95.
63. Pearson J, et al. Trophic functions of the neuron. V. Familial dysautonomia: current concepts of dysautonomia—neuropathological defects. *Ann NY Acad Sci* 1974;228:288–300.

64. Pearson J, et al. Depletion of substance P-containing axons in substantia gelatinosa of patients with diminished pain sensitivity. *Nature* 1982;295:61–63.
65. Pearson J, et al. Sensory, motor, and autonomic dysfunction: the nervous system in familial dysautonomia. *Neurology* 1971;21:486–493.
66. Pearson J, Pytel BA. Quantitative studies of sympathetic ganglia and spinal cord intermedio-lateral gray columns in familial dysautonomia. *J Neurol Sci* 1978;39:47–59.
67. Pearson J, et al. The sural nerve in familial dysautonomia. *J Neuropathol Exp Neurol* 1975;34:413–424.
68. Rechthand E, et al. Distribution of adrenergic innervation of blood vessels in peripheral nerve. *Brain Res* 1986;374:185–189.
69. Ridley A, et al. Tachycardia and the neuropathy of porphyria. *Lancet* 1968;2:708–710.
70. Sandroni P, et al. Autonomic involvement in extrapyramidal and cerebellar disorders. *Clin Auton Res* 1991;1:147–155.
71. Schmalbruch H. Fiber composition of the rat sciatic nerve. *Anat Rec* 1986;215:71–81.
72. Sebesan MN. Secondary structural and active site homologies between nerve growth factor and insulin. *J Theor Biol* 1980;83:469–476.
73. Shupeck M, et al. Comparison of nerve regeneration in vascularized and conventional grafts: nerve electrophysiology, norepinephrine, prostacyclin, malondialdehyde, and the blood–nerve barrier. *Brain Res* 1989;493:225–230.
74. Smith B. Neuropathology of the oesophagus in diabetes mellitus. *J Neurol Neurosurg Psychiatry* 1974;37:1151–1154.
75. Tamura N, et al. A morphometric study of the carotid sinus nerve in patients with diabetes mellitus and chronic alcoholism. *J Auton Nerv Syst* 1988;23:9–15.
76. Thapedi IM, et al. Shy–Drager syndrome: report of an autopsied case. *Neurology* 1971;21:26–32.
77. Thomas PK. The histopathology of peripheral neuropathy. *Nord Med* 1971;86:1442.
78. Thomas PK, King RH. Peripheral nerve changes in amyloid neuropathy. *Brain* 1974;97:395–406.
79. Thomas PK, Ocha J. Microscopic anatomy of peripheral nerve fibers. In: Dyck PJ, et al., eds. *Peripheral neuropathy.* Philadelphia: WB Saunders, 1984:39–96.
80. Tohgi H, et al. Selective loss of small myelinated and unmyelinated fibers in Shy–Drager syndrome. *Acta Neuropathol (Berl)* 1982;57:282–286.
81. Von Euler WS, Hillarp NA. Evidence for the presence of noradrenaline in submicroscopic structures of adrenergic axons. *Nature* 1956;177:44–45.
82. Walsh JC. *The peripheral nervous system in lymphoma and multiple myeloma* [Thesis]. Sydney: University of Sydney, 1972.
83. Ward KK, et al. Prostacyclin and noradrenaline in peripheral nerve of chronic experimental diabetes in rats. *Brain* 1989;112:197–208.
84. Winkleman RK. Cutaneous nerves. In: Zelickson AS, ed. *Ultrastructure of normal and abnormal skin.* Philadelphia: Lea and Febiger, 1967:202–227.
85. Yokota T, et al. Dysautonomia with acute sensory motor neuropathy: a new classification of acute autonomic neuropathy. *Arch Neurol* 1994;51:1022–1031.
86. Young RR, et al. Pure pan-dysautonomia with recovery: description and discussion of diagnostic criteria. *Brain* 1975;98:613–636.

CHAPTER 29

Development of an Autonomic Laboratory

Phillip A. Low and Irvin R. Zimmerman

---

1. The modular design of the noninvasive autonomic laboratory facilitates its development as an independent unit or as a component of an EMG, sleep, peripheral nerve research, or sensation laboratory.
2. The laboratory should be temperature controllable. The air vents must be baffled so that air flow is directed away from the patient for thermographic recordings. Humidity control is less critical.
3. The noninvasive tests can be performed by experienced technicians, but a supervising physician should be nearby. The physician should be involved with tilt studies. A full reflex screen in a busy laboratory is best performed by two technicians.
4. Technician training is critical. The technician must be: familiar with sudomotor, ECG, beat-to-beat BP, and blood flow recordings, computer literate, able to recognize the main ECG abnormalities, able to detect technical problems and their management, and trained in cardiopulmonary resuscitation.
5. The **autonomic reflex screen** comprises the distribution of QSART responses, heart rate responses to deep breathing, the Valsalva ratio, and beat-to-beat BP responses to the Valsalva maneuver and tilt.
6. The **sympathetic dysfunction** screen comprises telethermography or infrared thermometry, resting sweat output, and bilateral QSART recordings. All recordings in the sympathetic dysfunction screen are performed bilaterally and simultaneously.
7. Data acquisition and analysis requires a computer console consisting of a PC system with hard disk and suitable archiving, as well as the software and hardware necessary for the acquisition and analysis of data. The analog outputs from devices such as the infrared thermometer, the sudorometers, and the laser Doppler flowmeters are converted to digital data. The serial output data from the Finapres device are obtained by use of a serial communications channel. Heart rate is calculated from a QRS detection pulse obtained from the ECG monitor.
8. The software is written in C language. The program is user friendly and menu driven. A hierarchy of menu-selectable functions is provided to enable the operator to acquire the data, monitor the responses, save desired screens of data, and analyze the data off-line. Alternative programs can be developed with use of such programs as Visual Basic, Labtech Notebook, and Labview. Commercial packages are available for general autonomic data acquisition, display, and analysis.

INTRODUCTION

Since the founding of the Mayo Autonomic Reflex Laboratory in 1982, we have built two more such laboratories. Each plan and its implementation has been a learning experience. This chapter is an attempt to translate some of our experience into suggestions for persons planning such a laboratory. The specifics described below are not the only way to set up a laboratory, and the equipment we list is not endorsed by us. Since the last edition of this book, much has happened in the United States in autonomic testing. The Academy of Neurology has taken a proactive role, and its Therapeutics and Technology Committee has published a position paper on autonomic testing (*Clinical Autonomic Testing Report 1996*). It has also championed the application for and granting of three CPT codes (adrenergic, sudomotor, cardiovagal) for autonomic function tests. The American Autonomic Society, in conjunction with the American Academy of Neurology, has successfully completed a consensus document on the definition of orthostatic hypotension and that of multiple system atrophy and

---

P. A. Low: Department of Neurology I. R. Zimmerman: Department of Engineering Mayo Clinic, Rochester, MN 55905.

pure autonomic failure (1). It has also been agreed that there should be standardization of tests of autonomic function and expansion of autonomic function tests for clinical use. The latter involves the potential roles of transcranial Doppler (see Chapter 27) and electroencephalography (EEG) in monitoring brain activity and the increasing use of frequency analysis (see Chapters 25 and 26). The setting of standards for the training of clinicians and technicians is also evolving. There is greater integration of technician cross-training in electromyographic (EMG), EEG, sleep laboratory, and autonomic testing. This chapter discusses some of these changes.

MODELS OF AUTONOMIC LABORATORIES

Depending on one's background and needs, autonomic testing can be undertaken in a number of laboratory settings. There are at least five models of autonomic laboratories. In the following description, the setting up of a free-standing autonomic reflex laboratory is described. The components are explained in a modular fashion so that a laboratory that needs to implement a more limited range of tests can use a small number of modules. In the alternative models, the autonomic laboratory is a component of:

1. An EMG laboratory
2. A sleep laboratory
3. A peripheral nerve research laboratory
4. A sensation laboratory

A modular design is practical and reasonable. The models listed above are a natural evolution for many neurologists. It should be recognized that the clinical neurophysiologist is not trained to undertake tests of autonomic function. It should also be recognized that the value of the interpretation is only as good as the quality of the data. There are numerous pitfalls (see Chapter 30). There are large differences between autonomic research and clinical laboratory evaluation of autonomic function. Experienced investigators may be quite naive in the clinical autonomic laboratory without additional training.

THE AUTONOMIC LABORATORY

Space

The minimum space for a free-standing laboratory is about 12 × 20 feet. Optimally, there should also be two adjoining rooms about 10 × 10 feet each. We prefer a laboratory that is rectangular, with limited storage space. The air or nitrogen tanks are stored outside the laboratory so that these can be replaced without disturbing the smooth running of the laboratory. If there is a central supply, this can be piped in. Adequate space is essential next to the tilt table. This space is needed to permit a patient trolley for the transfer of ill patients onto the tilt-table. It is also needed for the performance of telethermographic recordings and for additional pieces of equipment as needed. The laboratory should be temperature controllable. Most laboratories can be temperature controlled by a thermostat with a heating unit around the incoming air duct. The air vents must be baffled so that air flow is directed away from the patient for thermographic recordings. Ideally, the telethermographic recordings should be taken in a different room that is about 20°C; the autonomic testing is performed at 23°C. Humidity control is less critical.

A small adjacent office is needed for the technician and clerk typist. Calls are taken and reports are generated and stored here. As the volume increases, it is preferable to have a separate physician office, with a one-way mirror looking into the laboratory. Alternatively, the physician could have a combined video monitor–computer to monitor the patient's study. This approach permits the physician to be in an adjacent office monitoring the patient during a tilt study. The cardiovascular parameters, including the electrocardiogram (ECG), can be evaluated, and the patient can be watched on the video monitor. The physician can determine whether changes in the duration of tilt are required and can intervene if necessary. This arrangement also fulfills the requirement that physicians actively participate in the evaluation of the patient.

Personnel

The noninvasive tests can be performed by two experienced technicians, but a supervising physician should be nearby. The physician, in particular, supervises the tilt. For prolonged tilt, physician supervision is recommended. A full reflex screen is best performed by two technicians. We have done some testing with a single technician, but efficiency and quality were not as good. Sudorometric recordings include skin preparation, loading of the capsules with acetylcholine, application of an exact constant current, and supervision of four sites simultaneously. The recording of resting sweat output is technically demanding and sometimes requires one technician to manually manage the capsule while the second works the controls. The tilt procedure is strenuous, and it is difficult to monitor a Finapres recording, check the ECG monitor, observe the patient for presyncopal symptoms, write down the results, and undertake manual recordings of blood pressure (BP).

Technician training is critical. The technician must be familiar with sudomotor, ECG, BP_{BB}, and blood flow recordings, must have a practical knowledge of computers, and must be able to recognize technical problems and their management. Technicians and physicians must be knowledgeable about electrical safety and trained in cardiopulmonary resuscitation. They must be able to recognize the main ECG abnormalities.

Tests

Two test batteries are used—the autonomic reflex screen and the screen for sympathetic dysfunction (the reflex sympathetic dystrophy [RSD] screen).

The *autonomic reflex screen* comprises: (1) QSART (quantitative sudomotor axon reflex test) (2–4); (2) orthostatic BP and heart rate (HR) responses to tilt; (3) HR response to deep breathing (HR_{DB}) (4); (4) the Valsalva ratio (4); and (5) beat-to-beat BP (BP_{BB}) to Valsalva maneuver, tilt, and deep breathing (see Chapter 15). When required, the salivation test (see Chapter 14) can be added.

The *sympathetic dysfunction* screen comprises: (1) telethermography or infrared thermometry; (2) resting sweat output; and (3) bilateral QSART recordings.

The sympathetic dysfunction screen differs from the reflex screen in that the recordings are performed bilaterally and simultaneously. Details of the tests are described in Chapter 16. The thermoregulatory sweat test is described in Chapter 19.

Equipment

The major pieces of equipment and their function are described below. Most of this equipment is used in Mayo Autonomic Reflex Laboratories. The suppliers and prices are listed in the Appendix. The mention of a particular brand does not constitute an endorsement of that brand over an alternative brand. The prices quoted are subject to change. The software, sudorometers, constant current generators, and sweat capsules are all designed and produced by Mayo. They may differ significantly from those that are available commercially.

Data Acquisition and Analysis

Computer

Several configurations are possible and practicable. In the previous edition, we gave details on the configuration we used. However, we recognize that that system is not the only one or even the best one. Therefore, we have modified this chapter to provide guidelines rather than specifics.

The computer configuration needed for the laboratory depends on the specific aims of the laboratory. If the laboratory is interested in acquiring information on HR and Finapres through its serial line, then the hardware and memory demands are quite modest. A system with modest memory (hard disk capacity of <500 MB) and speed (≤25 MHz) will suffice. If data acquisition includes the waveform (arterial and ECG), then memory and speed escalate. Hardware and memory costs have become modest, and most laboratories should use a Pentium PC system, >75 MHz, with a hard disk capacity in excess of 500 MB and a suitable archiving medium (either network or optical disk backup).

Data acquisition should be at 250 Hz. A higher rate is unwarranted and wasteful for the acquisition of BP, HR, and sweat response. In the research laboratory, a higher acquisition rate might be needed for certain signals (such as microneurography and EEG). When a large number of channels are used, it is often economical to have two boards, one running at a high rate and one at the standard 250 Hz.

Software and Hardware for Data Acquisition

There are a number of software approaches to meet the needs of an autonomic laboratory. We will briefly outline some of these options.

Current Mayo Autonomic Laboratory Configuration

The current configuration consists of standard data acquisition boards installed in the PC. These provide a 16-channel analog-to-digital converter, several serial communications controllers, digital input/output, and process interrupt inputs. Various analog outputs (i.e., infrared thermometer, the sudorometers, ECG, and arterial waveforms) are converted to digital data. The serial output data from the Finapres device are obtained by use of a serial communications channel. HR is calculated from a QRS detection pulse obtained from the ECG monitor. The acquisition board formats the acquired data and acquires data at 250 Hz. The additional channels can be used to acquire data from other units, such as the BoMed impedance cardiography unit, that is connected to a LaserJet printer.

The software is written in C language. The program is user friendly and menu driven. There is user-selectable control of channels to be displayed, gain, and choice of colors. A hierarchy of menu-selectable functions is provided to enable the operator to acquire the data, monitor the responses, save desired screens of data, and analyze the data off-line. The menus have been developed to accommodate commonly used tests, such as HR response to deep breathing, HR response to the Valsalva maneuver, HR response to tilt, and the QSART recordings. A hand-held operator control panel is provided to facilitate operator control of data acquisition. Functions such as rejecting or saving a screen and making a mark on the screen can be done closer to the patient, away from the computer keypad.

The program stores patient information as a separate text file with the extension "PID." Analog data (ECG and arterial waveforms) and digital data files are saved separately, with different extensions.

Off-line data analysis is menu selectable. Two illustrative examples follow.

If the QSART selection is made, a menu listing the individual recordings is displayed. When a particular sudorometer recording is selected, it is displayed and the user can adjust the gain and time axis. The area under the curve is accurately delineated by adjusting the cursor at both the beginning and end of the base of the curve. When digitization is selected, the sweat volume in liters per square centimeter is instantly displayed.

If a selection of HR and Finapres is chosen, the user-selected components of the acquired trace are displayed (mean, systolic, and diastolic BP; HR; expiratory pressure). The relevant ECG and arterial waveforms are simultaneously displayed.

Visual Basic

An integrated program to record the HR and BP parameters by way of the serial line of the Finapres device can be designed with the use of Visual Basic. The equipment block diagram is shown in Fig. 1. The analog ECG signal is detected and analyzed by a Cardiotach board (which has a resolution of 1 millisecond) and undergoes a pulse-to-time conversion; this is subsequently led into the PC. The HR from Finapres is derived from the digital arterial waveform and is output by way of a serial line of the PC. These data, together with systolic BP, diastolic BP, and mean BP, are input into a PC computer by use of the Visual Basic program. The display is user selectable.

A similar program has been developed to analyze sudorometric data (QSART or resting sweat output).

Labview or Labtech Notebook

We have not used these programs ourselves. However, they have been used successfully by programmers to acquire, display, and analyze HR, BP, and analog data.

Proprietary Programs

Several of these programs are available. There are three commercially available programs that have functions that meet many of the needs of the autonomic laboratory—the Medikro 9433 Transducer Interface Unit, CVMS (Cardiovascular Monitoring System), and ANAPRES v1.2. These systems all have general data acquisition capabilities, although they are not specifically designed to meet the needs of the clinical autonomic laboratory. The Medikro 9433 Transducer Interface Unit can be installed into IBM Think pad 755, 755C, 755CE, or 755CD models, substituting for the diskette drive.

Reflex Laboratory Tests

The focus of this section is on the specific equipment used in an autonomic reflex laboratory. Where practical, we will indicate commercially available equipment. The listing of commercial equipment is not intended to be comprehensive and is not meant to be a recommendation for a

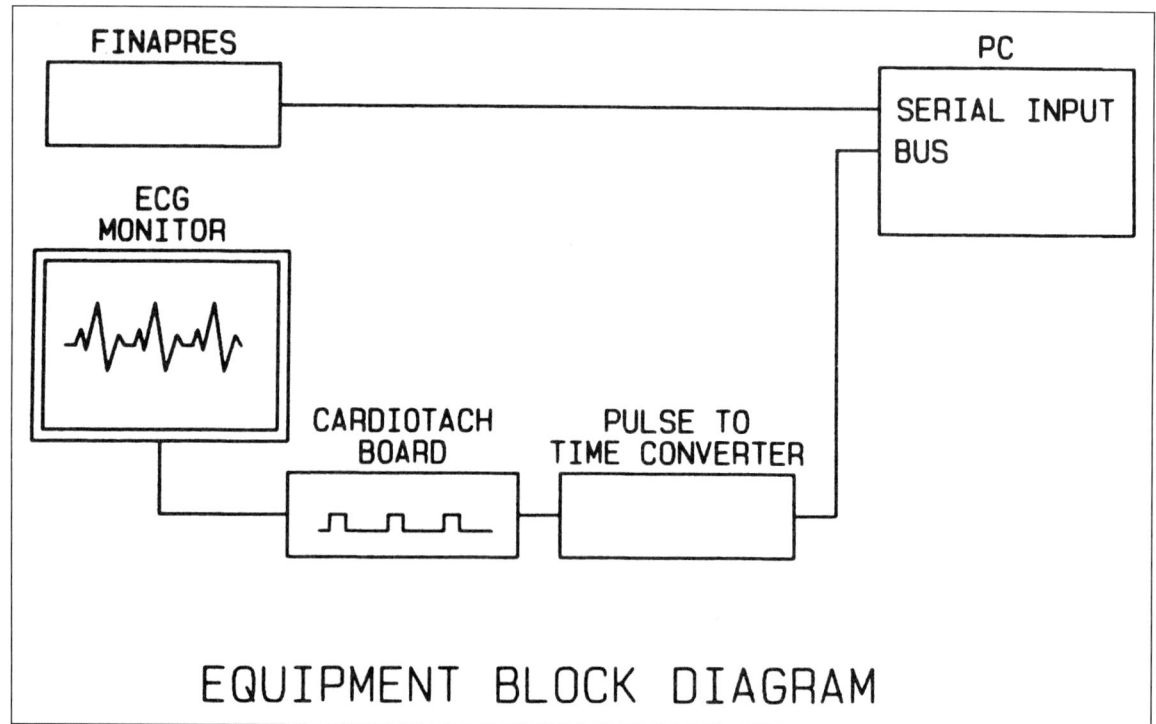

FIG. 1. Block diagram of data acquisition interface.

particular make. The underlying principles of the respective tests are covered in other chapters, as are the recommendations on testing.

Temperature Control

Control of Room Temperature

It is important that the room temperature be maintained at 23 ± 0.5°C. This is achieved by thermostatic control. The room temperature for the RSD screen is 20°C.

Infrared Heaters

Ceiling-mounted infrared heaters are needed to rapidly warm patients when necessary. We use a 1600-W infrared heater.

Infrared Thermometer

We use an infrared pyrometer with 0.1°C accuracy. This unit dynamically measures, in real time, infrared emittance from skin. Skin temperature may be asymmetrically altered in nerve lesions and in sympathetically maintained pain. This unit can be used alone in the sympathetic dysfunction screen or in conjunction with telethermography. We prefer it to thermography in recording temperature from the toe or finger pads. At these sites, the temperatures may be 10°C colder than the foot or palm and will be inaccurately displayed in a single frame of a thermogram.

Controller for Infrared Heat Lamp

Infrared lamps are connected to a temperature controller. The skin temperature is recorded with a skin probe, and the temperature set-point is maintained at 31.5°C by feedback control.

QSART (Quantitative Sudomotor Axon Reflex Test)

The following equipment is necessary to run QSART:

1. Sudorometers
2. Multicompartmental, calibration, sealed, and resting sweat capsules
3. Constant current generator
4. Source of nitrogen or air
5. Recording system (Data Acquisition Interface and computer)
6. Acetylcholine
7. Hamilton syringe for calibration
8. Temperature control (infrared lamps with controller)

Sudorometer

The Mayo sudorometer console consists of four sudorometers permitting dynamic recording of sweat output from four sites simultaneously. The details of the sudorometer system are shown in Fig. 2. The heart of each sudorometer is a Model 10-677 thermal conductivity cell (Gow-Mac). The single unit is available commercially (see Appendix).

Sweat Cells

Four types of sweat cells are available.

QSART Capsule: Used to measure axon reflex–mediated sweat output (see Fig. 2).

Sealed QSART Capsule: Dimensions are identical to those of QSART capsule, but compartments are sealed and used to provide a system baseline.

Calibration QSART Capsule: Modified from QSART capsule, with dimensions identical to those of the central compartment but with a broad rim to ensure a reliable seal. Used to run sudorometer calibrations.

Resting Sweat Output: Larger-dimension capsules used to measure resting sweat output. Diameter of the capsule is 5.31 cm^2.

Constant Current Generators

We build our own constant current generator unit consisting of four constant current generators with output varying from 0 to 3 mA. Single units are commercially available.

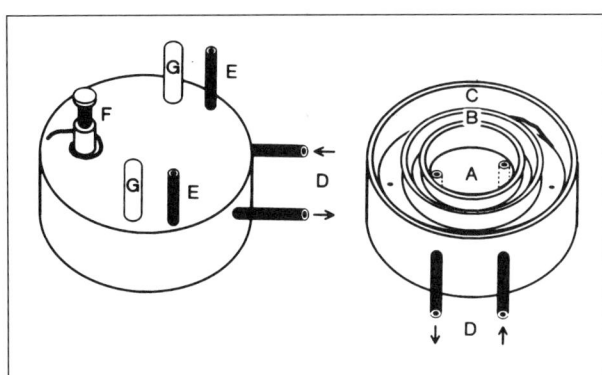

FIG. 2. Multicompartmental sweat capsule. Acetylcholine solution is loaded by way of **E**, iontophoresed by way of the anode (**F**), and connected to the stimulus compartment (**C**). The axon reflex–mediated sweat response is recorded from **A**. Gas flows through cannulae **D**. The capsule is attached to skin by way of attachment posts (**G**). (Reprinted with permission from Harati Y, Low PA. Autonomic peripheral neuropathies: diagnosis and clinical presentation. In: Appel SH [ed]. *Current Neurology.* Chicago: Year Book Medical Publishers. 1990;10:105–176.)

Calibration Syringe

For calibration we use a Hamilton syringe with a 10-μl capacity. Calibration is performed for 1, 2, and 5 μl in duplicate.

Heart Period Recordings

Electrocardiograph Monitor

We use a Model 101T IVY ECG monitor because of its superior QRS detection algorithm.

Valsalva Maneuver

For the Valsalva maneuver, a 60-ml plastic disposable syringe connected to a disposable cardboard mouthpiece is attached to a column of mercury. A small air leak is provided.

Skin Temperature Distribution

Skin temperature distribution has been detected satisfactorily with two methods. The first and less expensive method is the use of the infrared pyrometer connected by way of the DAI and autonomic reflex screen software to the computer, where the temperatures are displayed and analyzed. The temperatures of identical sites of the two limbs are graphed. An alternative textural display of temperatures and differences between sides is also available on the program.

An alternative and better method is the use of telethermography to display in a color-coded format the distribution of skin temperatures. We have an Agema Thermovision 870/TIC-8000 system (Agema, Secaucus, NJ) and a Teletherm Mark-1026 SC3 System (PM-100 Medical Research Group, Clearwater, FL).

A less expensive thermographic alternative is the use of liquid crystal thermography.

Vasomotor Testing

Noninvasive Blood Pressure Monitor

We use the Finapres Continuous NIBP (noninvasive blood pressure) Monitor for beat-to-beat recording of systolic arterial pressure, diastolic arterial pressure, and mean arterial pressure.

Tilt Table

The tilt table is designed and built by TRI W-G Incorporated. The table is constructed for tilt-up (to 80°) and tilt-back. For most studies it is preferable to provide a smooth tilt-up, over 10 to 20 sec. In the previous edition, we emphasized rapid tilt. We found that rapid movements were disturbing to the elderly and resulted in BP and HR alterations. An adjustable armrest is provided such that the Finapres device remains at heart level during all positions of tilt.

Laser Doppler Flowmeters

We use TSI Laserflo Blood Perfusion Monitors Model 403A. The device is used to record skin blood flow for skin vasomotor reflex, the venoarteriolar reflex, and neurogenic flare responses.

Cardiovascular Hemodynamic Studies Using Bioimpedance Methodology

This system provides noninvasive measurements using bioimpedance determination of physiologic and hemodynamic indices. The instrument will measure and display a total of 12 cardiodynamic parameters: cardiac output/cardiac index; HR; stroke volume/stroke index; peak flow/peak flow index; ejection fraction; end-diastolic volume/end-diastolic index; index of contractility; thoracic fluid index; acceleration index; ventricular ejection time; ejection ratio ("preload index"); and systolic time ratio.

REFERENCES

1. Anonymous consensus statement on the definition of orthostatic hypotension, pure autonomic failure, and multiple system atrophy. *Neurology* 1996;46:873–880.
2. Low PA et al. Quantitative sudomotor axon reflex test in normal and neuropathic subjects. *Ann Neurol* 1983;14:573–580.
3. Low PA et al. The effect of aging on cardiac autonomic and postganglionic sudomotor function. *Muscle Nerve* 1990;13:152–157.
4. Low PA, et al. Comparison of distal sympathetic with vagal function in diabetic neuropathy. *Muscle Nerve* 1986;9:592–596.

APPENDIX: COMMERCIALLY AVAILABLE EQUIPMENT

Listed below is commercially available equipment. Information on these systems was sent to us. This may not be the equipment used in the Mayo Laboratory, and their listing does not imply our endorsement.

SUDOROMETERS

Evaporative Water Loss Units with Flow Rate Regulator
Abrams Instruments Corp.
Lansing, MI 48910-3688 USA
Phone: 517-882-7211
Fax: 517-882-3136
Price: $8000 each
Capsules: $235 each
Function: Units for measuring sweat volume accurately and in real time

Alternatives:
Hydrograph AMU-3
Contact person: Dr. Junichi Sugenoya
Dept. of Physiology
Aichi Medical University
Nagakute 480-11 Japan
Price quote: Y3,500,000, but may be revised downward)

Multicompartmental Sweat Cells
Function: Unit for iontophoresis. Can be used separately for recording sweat output from skin. The multiple compartments permit separate studies of the afferent and efferent limbs of the axon reflex. The large sweat cell records resting sweat output.

Flow Regulator for Nitrogen Gas (CGA-120)
Price: About $200

Precision Flowmeter

Constant Current Generators
Function: Provide constant current stimulus to iontophorese acetylcholine into test site of skin.

a. Wescor Sweat Inducer 3600
Chemlab Scientific Instruments
Romford, United Kingdom
Develops 1.5 mA for 5 minutes. Used in general pediatrics as a sweat inducer for cystic fibrosis testing.

b. Model 360 Stimulus Isolator (standard battery operated)
Price: $595

Model 360A Stimulus Isolator (rechargeable)
Price: $895
World Precision Instruments Inc.
375 Quinnipiac Ave.
New Haven, CT 06513
Phone: (203) 469-8281
Fax: (203) 468-6207

Hamilton Syringes
(10-μl capacity Cat. No. 14-824 Fisher Scientific)
Function: Provide an accurate small volume of fluid to calibrate sudorometer.
Price: $20 each

SOFTWARE

For Finapres Output
Software is needed for display of heart rate recordings and beat-to-beat BP. Several software packages have been developed to handle information from Finapres.

a. Medikro 9433 Transducer Interface Unit
Medidro Oy
Phone: 358 71 2833000
Fax: 358-71-2833300

b. CVMS (Cardiovascular Monitoring System)
McPherson Scientific
PO Box 442
Heidelberg, Victoria 3084, Australia
Fax: 61-3-457-7039
Price $US 5950

c. ANAPRES v1.2
Notocord Systems
113 Chemin de Ronde
78290 Croissy-sur-Seine
Croissy, France
Phone: 33-1-34-800000
Fax: 33-1-34-801214

More Generic Systems

a. MacLab data acquisition of the MacIntosh
Contact Physiology Research Instruments
MacLab/4 $4875
Phone: 708-860-9700
Fax: 708-860-9775

b. Labtech Notebook ($1395) with LabMaster DMA ($1750)
Contact Physiology Research Instruments
Phone: 708-860-9700
Fax: 708-860-9775

c. Labview 2 (for MacIntosh computers)
National Instruments
6504 Bridge Point Parkway
Austin, TX 78730-5039
Phone: 512-794-0100 or 800-433-3488

Labview with windows (for PC)
National Instruments
6504 Bridge Point Parkway
Austin, TX 78730-5039
Phone: 512-794-0100 or 800-433-3488

MEASUREMENTS OF HEART RATE

Electrocardiograph Monitor
This monitor has the capability of detecting, displaying, and providing the heart rate input to a computer. We use the following:

Model 101T ECG Monitor
IVY Biomedical System Inc.
11 Business Park Drive
Branford, CT 06405
Price: $2400.00
Phone: 203-481-4183

Useful attachments:
Cable (part # 590170) $150.00
Leads (part # 590162) $ 59.00
Interconnect cable (part # 1564-01-01) $ 60.00

Alternatives:
Neurocard
Prama d.o.o.
Rueigajeva 31
SI-64000 Kranj, Slovenia
Phone/Fax: 386-61-342-074

Lifepak 8
Physio-control Inc.
Redmond, WA 98052

Hewlett Packard EKG monitor 78203A
(Andover, MA)
EKG monitor
Electronics for Medicine Inc.
Model PM-2

Hewlett-Packard 8020A heart rate monitor
HP 7834A

An alternative approach, suggested by Dr. Mike Pfeifer (and with which we have no experience), is:

Monitor One nDx
QMED Inc.
Suite 403
Clark, NJ 07066
Phone: 201-381-6880

Beat-to-Beat Measurements of Blood Pressure
There is a significant problem with BP_{BB} recordings. These require the Finapres

APPENDIX: COMMERCIALLY AVAILABLE EQUIPMENT (continued)

device. Ohmeda holds the license for this but has decided not to supply the device anymore. Because they hold the license, no other company, including the parent company, can supply the instrument.

The company's address is:
Noninvasive BP Monitor
Finapres Continuous NIBP Monitor
Model No. 2300
Ohmeda
355 Inverness Drive South
Englewood CO 80112-5810
Phone: 800-345-2700

Critikon Dinamap Vital Signs Monitor 1846SX/P
Johnson and Johnson Critikon Inc.
Tampa, FL

TILT TABLE
TRI W-G Incorporated
P.O. Box 905
Valley City, ND 58072
Phone: 701-845-3984
Attention: Duane Fast
Price: Variable, depending on design, typically $7000 to $12,000.
These tilt tables are well designed for autonomic testing.

The following company is developing a complete system for autonomic testing with the aim of duplicating the Mayo system.

WR Medical Electronics Company
123 North Second St.
Stillwater, MN 55082
(612) 430-1200

CHAPTER 30

Pitfalls in Autonomic Testing

Phillip A. Low

---

1. Noninvasive tests of autonomic function are easy to perform but difficult to interpret.
2. Noninvasiveness is often associated with *suboptimal instrumentation* and the monitoring of an inadequate number of parameters.
3. The applied *stimulus* may be several steps removed from the stimulus recognized by the receptor.
4. The *response* is usually an indirect effector response. The underlying reflex is often complex and modulated by multiple confounding inputs.
5. In a clinical laboratory environment, extraneous patient variables may also affect the test results.
6. The facts outlined above contribute to test results whose interpretation is valid only for a narrow range of conditions; extrapolations are hazardous.
7. Some popular tests have been poorly validated for general use, and suggested normal ranges are of doubtful value. Criteria based on sensitivity, specificity, reproducibility, and relevance are suggested as a means of evaluating new tests of autonomic function.
8. To define the site of a lesion, the tests compared must be of similar sensitivity and specificity.

INTRODUCTION

Numerous noninvasive tests of autonomic function have been introduced over the past 15 years. The tests are appealing because of their apparent simplicity, ease of performance, and straightforward interpretation. An important milestone in quantitative patient testing has been the development of autonomic testing laboratories, either free standing, extensions of established laboratories (e.g., electromyography, electroencephalography, or sleep), or integral components of peripheral nerve research laboratories (with sensation and electrophysiologic testing). However, there are certain pitfalls that are inherent to noninvasive testing and others that have evolved from the use of the tests. In this chapter, the focus will be on the limitations of these tests and some fallacies that have crept into the literature.

PITFALL OF OVERSIMPLIFYING ASSUMPTIONS

In most autonomic testing, a stimulus is applied, a response is recorded, and, as a result, the integrity of the reflex tested is deduced. It is important to realize that the applied stimulus and the true systems stimulus may be quite different. For example, three patients aged 30 to 35 years could perform identical standardized Valsalva maneuvers resulting in different Valsalva ratios (VR). Subject A could have a VR of 1.2, whereas the other two could exhibit normal but different VRs. Conventional wisdom suggests that VR measures vagal function (12,14) and, therefore, one patient could have vagal denervation and the other two could have different vagal responses. In fact, the results could mean something totally different. A reasonable approximation of the true stimulus to reflex bradycardia is the rate and magnitude of blood pressure (BP) reduction (phase II and III) and increment (phase IV), which are not usually measured. One patient could have an adrenergic neuropathy resulting in an inability to vasoconstrict the systemic arteriolar bed; therefore, phase IV would be reduced or absent. Even though this patient's vagus nerve is intact, VR is reduced because the true stimulus (δBP) is absent. Similarly, even though the other two patients generated the same expiratory pressure, phases II and IV may have been of a different size and may have developed at a different rate. Indeed, the problem is even more complex. The true stimulus may be impossible to quantitate (Fig. 1) (10) because multiple reflex adjustments occur during the

---

P. A. Low: Department of Neurology, Mayo Clinic, Rochester, Minnesota 55905.

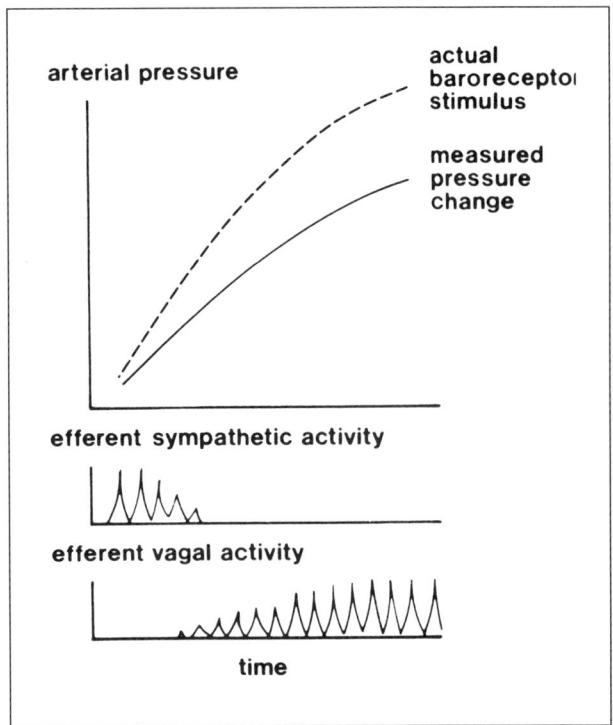

FIG. 1. Ongoing reflex adjustments reduce arterial pressure elevation that occurs during phase IV of the Valsalva maneuver. (Reprinted with permission from Eckberg D. Parasympathetic cardiovascular control in human disease: critical review of methods and results. *Am J Physiol* 1980; 239:H581–H593.)

maneuver. The arterial pressure changes encountered in phases II to III and IV are reasonable but depressed indices of the baroreceptor stimulus (10,21).

The measured responses may be more indirect than those in other neurophysiologic tests. For example, in nerve conduction studies, the stimulus is an electric shock and the measured response is a nerve action potential. The integrity of the nerve trunk can be reasonably deduced. Autonomic testing is more indirect; effector function is usually measured instead. For example, a patient with anhidrosis undergoing the thermoregulatory sweat test (25,26) is presumed to have an abnormality in his or her neural pathways. However, the response could reflect an abnormality of the effector (the eccrine sweat gland) or its modulators.

An additional problem with autonomic testing is the complexity of the underlying reflexes; this causes many simplifying assumptions to enter into the interpretation. For instance, in the heart rate (HR) response to deep breathing (HR_{DB}), the stimulus is forced respiration at a defined rate and the response is the HR. However, this reflex is quite complex. Although effector function is measured, this response is determined by afferent impulses along the vagus nerve, its cell station in the nucleus of the tractus solitarius (NTS), and its efferent pathway by way of the nucleus ambiguus and dorsomotor nucleus of the vagus down to the sinoatrial node. The NTS is the central processing unit, and it is here that multiple inputs from baroreceptor, chemoreceptor, sympathetic, and supranuclear afferents (see Chapter 3) that affect the response are received. BP alterations activate baroreceptors, which modify the response. Deep breathing causes hypocapnia, which attenuates the response (4). Inspiration and expiration result in an HR increase, followed by a decrease, but with different latencies and amplitudes (35). The characteristic latencies and amplitudes differ among individuals, so that a different amount of cancellation or summation occurs. Thus, caution should be exercised when basing the diagnosis of a vagal lesion solely on a reduced HR_{DB}.

The simplified assumptions and the indirect nature of many of the noninvasive tests mean that conclusions are valid only within certain tight constraints. Particular care is necessary when a battery of noninvasive tests is used to dissect the autonomic nervous system. Extrapolations beyond a test are quite hazardous.

STANDARDIZATION PITFALL

The simplicity of noninvasive tests has been oversold! Simple "bedside" noninvasive tests (9,13) with a recommended generic normal and abnormal range have been advertised. HR_{DB} is described as being abnormal if it falls below 10 beats per minute (bpm) (13). It is clear, however, that the response is age dependent (see Chapter 14). An HR_{DB} of 10 bpm is certainly abnormal in a 20-year-old but may be normal for an 80-year-old. Each laboratory must define its own paradigm and standardize its own range of normals by age and sex (53). Much more variability exists in autonomic testing than in nerve conduction studies, so a large group of controls, from whom percentiles can be derived, is needed. Even with a relatively large normative database, the derived equations may be an oversimplification. In a recent publication, Braune and colleagues (5) suggested that tests of cardiovagal function are of no value for subjects older than 60 years of age. Although the values for HR_{DB} and the VR are clearly reduced with age, a linear regression does not account for the flattening out of the curve beyond age 60, which is evident in Figures 5 and 6 of Braune's article (5). A sufficient database probably requires about 300 subjects.

The danger of the standardization pitfall has been appreciated by several investigators (28,32,33,39,52). Pfeifer and associates (39) recommended the use of intravenous propranolol before determining the HR_{DB}. Weinbery and Pfeifer also recommended the use of vector analysis (51), which minimizes sympathetic modulation.

PITFALL ASSOCIATED WITH BLACK-BOXING AUTONOMIC FUNCTION

Important applications of noninvasive quantitative tests include monitoring the course of the autonomic component of the neuropathy and the response to treatment. In most neuropathies, it is necessary to monitor motor and large sensory fibers (e.g., nerve conduction) and small sensory fibers (tests of thermal warming or cooling and pain), as well as autonomic function. Hence, the investigator is tempted to adopt one or two tests to generically evaluate autonomic function. There is reasonable concordance among tests. For example, HR tests of "cardiovagal" function correlate well with the quantitative sudomotor axon reflex test (QSART) (33), and there is good concordance between sympathetic skin response and QSART (34) and between TST and QSART (26,29) in the same subjects. Therefore, for epidemiologic and certain clinical studies, a limited representative test battery may suffice.

For individual patients, however, this black-box approach is inadequate. There is discordance between HR and QSART in about 1 of 6 patients (33). A dissociation between vasomotor and sudomotor function is also often encountered in patients (18). A more convincing argument is that these tests evaluate different parts of the autonomic neuraxis in different ways. They are complementary, not interchangeable. In the individual patient, precise rather than approximate information is needed.

PITFALL ASSOCIATED WITH DEDUCING SITE OF THE LESION

A loss of autonomic function may be due to a lesion of afferent, central (usually polysynaptic), preganglionic, or postganglionic pathways or effector sites. When one limb of an autonomic reflex arc is tested, deductions are often made about the integrity of the nontested limb and the site of the lesion. In contrast to the reliability of assessing function based on the part of the reflex arc tested, deduction by exclusion is less reliable. To illustrate, the conclusion that parasympathetic failure occurs before sympathetic failure in diabetic neuropathy (14,50) was based on the observation that HR_{DB} was impaired when indices of generalized autonomic failure such as orthostatic hypotension (OH), supine plasma norepinephrine, and BP response to sustained handgrip were unaffected. Whether the phenomenon is true or not is irrelevant. The conclusion is fallacious because the results of a sensitive test are being compared with those of relatively insensitive tests. HR_{DB} becomes abnormal when any lesion occurs within its long pathway, whereas the sympathetic tests do not become abnormal until the bulk of the peripheral vasculature has been denervated.

Similarly, some authors concluded that the lesion in diabetic OH was afferent (45) because the efferent limb, as determined by the presence of OH or the level of plasma norepinephrine, was unimpaired. When more sensitive tests of efferent function are used, such as the thermoregulatory sweat test or QSART, the efferent site is clearly affected.

The venoarteriolar reflex is a relatively insensitive test of postganglionic sympathetic adrenergic function (36), whereas QSART is a sensitive test of postganglionic sympathetic sudomotor function. A neuropathic patient may have an abnormal QSART and normal venoarteriolar reflex. However, it would be erroneous to conclude that the patient has a selective involvement of sudomotor function. In contrast, if a patient has a normal QSART and anhidrosis on TST, it would be more reasonable to conclude that the lesion is preganglionic because these tests have similar sensitivities (29).

INACCURACIES OF SOME COMMON OBSERVATIONS

Patients with sympathetically maintained pain (reflex sympathetic dystrophy, RSD) typically exhibit reduced skin temperature, excessive resting sweat output, and a QSART response of altered latency, volume, and morphology (Fig. 2) (26). It would be tempting to conclude that these conditions are indicative of increased sympathetic efferent traffic. However, this conclusion would go beyond the evidence. These conditions could be due to end-organ alterations (e.g., receptor upregulation or alteration in tissue microenvironment), which would increase effector gain. A related fallacy is the assumption that the demonstrated increased sympathetic effect is caused by pain. Some patients with increased sympathetic effect do not respond to

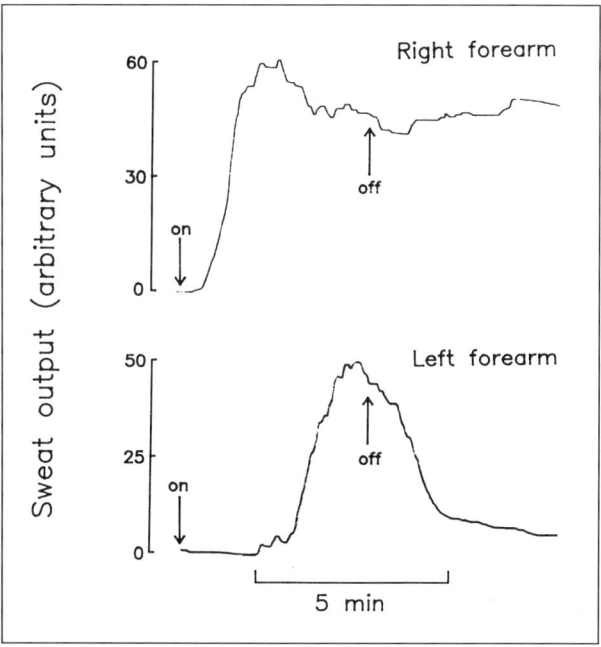

FIG. 2. QSART recordings from the painful (**top**) and normal (**bottom**) forearm of a patient with a pain syndrome. Short latency QSART response with persistent sweat activity (**top**) is due to augmented somatosympathetic activation.

sympathetic block but improve with blockade of somatic afferents. This observation and the demonstration of a very short QSART latency (from somatosympathetic activation) are suggestive of the fact that the increased sympathetic effect is due to a peripheral mechanism resulting in enhanced somatosympathetic activity. Sympathetic activity, in this instance, is a useful index but is not the cause. Not surprisingly, it will not respond to sympathetic block.

The VR is a commonly used test of autonomic function and has been proposed as a test of parasympathetic function (14). The ratio is derived from the maximal HR in response to phases II and III divided by the minimal HR following phase IV. There are two pitfalls encountered with the use of VR as an index of cardiovagal function. First, as discussed earlier, the true stimulus to reflex bradycardia is not the standardized forced expiratory pressure, as is usually assumed, but the baroreflex stimulus, approximated by BP undershoot/overshoot in phases II and IV (10). The latter occurs after the cessation of the maneuver. Within a few seconds, venous return and cardiac output return to normal, whereas sympathetically mediated peripheral vasoconstriction persists for 2 to 3 min. Normal cardiac output at a time when total peripheral resistance is still elevated results in the overshoot in BP. If widespread peripheral sympathetic denervation is present with intact cardiac autonomic innervation, as might occur in the length-dependent neuropathies, phase IV may be absent. VR may be reduced, not because of cardiovagal failure but because the stimulus to reflex bradycardia is absent. To summarize, VR is an index of cardiovagal function only if sympathetic innervation is intact.

A second pitfall is the fact that VR may remain normal even when the vagus nerve is denervated; this is another cause of misdiagnosis (32). Tachycardia during phases II and III is preserved and returns to baseline with cessation of the maneuver. Phase IV may be small (due to cardioacceleration). The patient may retain a low-normal VR.

SOME PROBLEMS WITH HEART RATE RECORDINGS

Heart Rate Versus Heart Period

The HR range, heart period (HP) range, and E:I (expiration to inspiration) ratio are three indices measured by different laboratories to evaluate the deep breathing response. The E:I ratio was described by Sundkvist and colleagues (47), who determined the ratio of the shortest RR interval during inspiration to the longest R-R interval during expiration and derived the E:I ratio. At the extremes of HR, the HR range, HP range, and E:I ratio yield markedly disparate results. A patient with a resting HR of 60 breaths/min has an HP of 1000 millisec. An increase of 10 bpm results in a relatively large HP reduction. In contrast, a patient with a resting HR of 120 bpm has an HP of 500 millisec. An increase of 10 bpm in this second patient results in a relatively small HP increase. With high sympathetic tone, respiratory sinus arrhythmia (RSA) is inhibited (39). Optimal testing would, therefore, require selective adrenergic blockade. In the clinical setting, nervous teenagers often have an attenuated HP range as a result of resting tachycardia. The use of HR instead of HP would more likely yield normal results in a nervous normal subject. A more satisfactory method would be that of analysis in the frequency domain (see Chapter 25).

Averaged Versus Nonaveraged Heart Rate Responses

Algorithms are available that display the averaged or unaveraged HP. The averaged algorithm is unacceptable. The premature beat, extrasystole, and artifact are buried in the averaged response. Instead, the unaveraged response should be displayed. The artifact is seen as a single large deflection and the premature beat is recognized by the ensuing compensatory pause. The patient with atrial fibrillation has a characteristic HR pattern reflecting the irregular pulse rate.

Factors Affecting Heart Rate Responses

Although HR_{DB} is a relatively reliable test of cardiovagal function, the HR range is affected by certain variables, sometimes significantly. Because of significant sympathetic–parasympathetic interactions (23), sympathetic activation depresses the cardiovagal response (39). This effect is especially prominent in nervous young children and young subjects. β-adrenergic blockade minimizes this inhibition (8,39). The administration of intravenous propranolol before the test has been recommended (39).

Another mode of increasing sympathetic tone is by way of somatosympathetic interactions. Intense somatic afferent activity, as might occur in the painful neuropathies or when the subject is exposed to the cold (as in the cold pressor test), can result in sympathetic activation and inhibition of parasympathetic function.

Cardiovagal function is markedly affected by age. HR_{DB} is linearly related to age (31). A similar age effect is present for the HR response to standing, and most studies have found an age effect for the VR. A linear regression of HR range against age was found to have a slope of 0.36 times age in years (see Chapter 14) (31). The use of a normal range without regard to age and conditions of testing is, therefore, unsatisfactory.

Most normal subjects have a maximal HR range at a respiratory rate of 6 breaths/min (2). Certain individuals exhibit markedly greater initial responses. Some of these subjects have a markedly attenuated HR range, but a normal range is revealed at a slightly different respiratory rate. These individuals do not have vagal failure. Mehlsen and associates (35) found that both inspiration and expiration are followed by a tachycardia–bradycardia sequence.

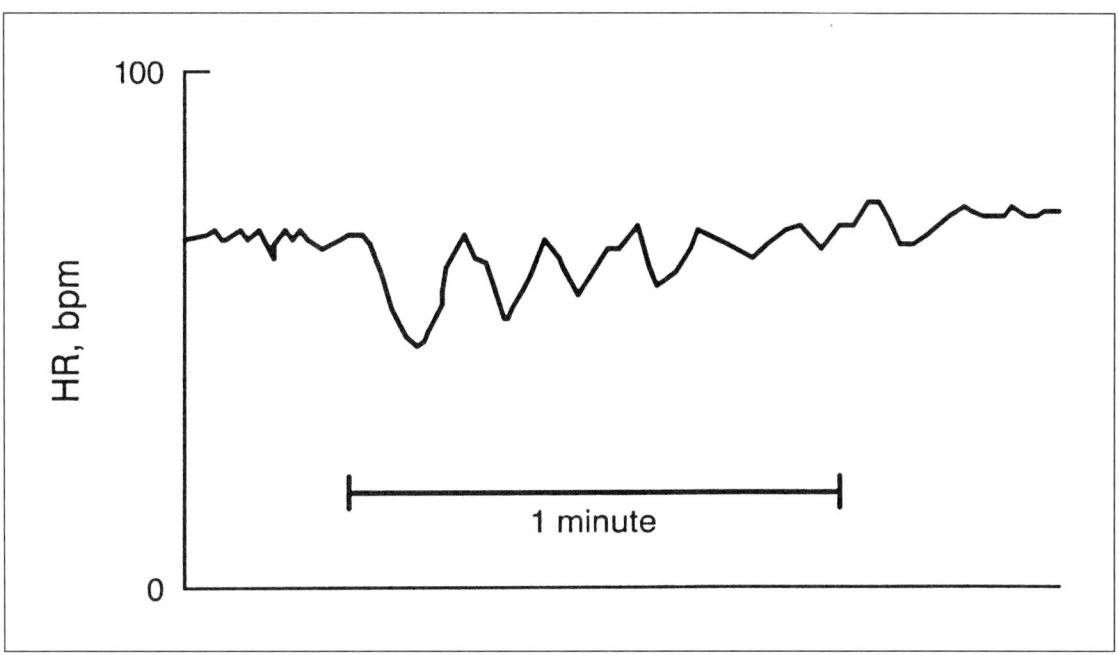

FIG. 3. Reduction in HR range with hypocapnia.

However, inspiration and expiration differ in two ways. The latencies to peak maximum and minimum HR are longer and the amplitude is smaller for expiration. A significant cancellation of the HR response occurs maximally at certain respiratory rates that are specific to the individual.

Although it is important to ensure that the patient breathes regularly, rhythmically, and deeply during HR_{DB}, continuing the procedure beyond 1 minute is inadvisable because the ensuing hypocapnia causes an increase in baseline HR and a depression of RSA (Fig. 3) (4).

It can be assumed that the HR recordings will be incorrect under certain important circumstances. The price paid for noninvasiveness includes the fact that the VR, as an index of cardiovagal function, is an example of oversimplification. It has been pointed out that the VR may be reduced in patients with intact vagus but impaired sympathetic function (32). To compound the interpretation, some patients with widespread sympathetic adrenergic failure may exhibit an entirely normal VR. These patients may have a brisk, vagally mediated cardioacceleration followed by cardiodeceleration, which results in a normal VR (49). The beat-to-beat HR and BP curves are, however, markedly abnormal, underlining the importance of looking at enough of the data when dealing with a complicated reflex. Similarly, the patient with cardiovagal failure may still retain a normal VR with cardioacceleration and deceleration being mediated by cardiac sympathetic function alone (32).

Pitfalls have been described in other commonly used tests of parasympathetic function. The 30:15 ratio on standing has been suggested as a test of vagal function. In a patient with widespread sympathetic failure with sparing of cardiovagal fibers, the response to standing consisted of a brisk and large cardioacceleration without cardiodeceleration so that the 30:15 ratio was altered. This patient had an entirely normal HR_{DB} and other evidence to indicate intact cardiovagal function. The absence of reflex bradycardia instead reflects the lack of a BP overshoot secondary to adrenergic failure (Fig. 4) (49).

In certain tests of sympathetic adrenergic function, such as the sustained handgrip and cold pressor tests, the variable of interest is the integrity of the sympathetic α-adrenergic system, sympathetic activation results in an increase in total peripheral resistance and a pressor response (46). However, a pressor response may occur in the presence of widespread α-adrenergic blockade with intact cardiac sympathetic and/or cardiovagal innervation. For example, α-adrenergic blockade results in an enhancement of the phase IV pressor response to the Valsalva maneuver in the supine subject (42), and the pressor response to sustained handgrip and mental stress may be intact in patients with severe OH (49). In the situations described above, reflex tachycardia is able to raise BP despite α-adrenergic blockade. Indeed, phase IV of the Valsalva maneuver is suppressed much more efficiently by propranolol or atropine than by phentolamine (42).

Pitfall Associated With Hypovolemia

Hypovolemia may result in orthostatic lightheadedness associated with a marked reduction in pulse pressure and significant tachycardia. These characteristics are easy to recognize. One mechanism of the postural orthostatic tachycardia syndrome (POTS) in patients with intact car-

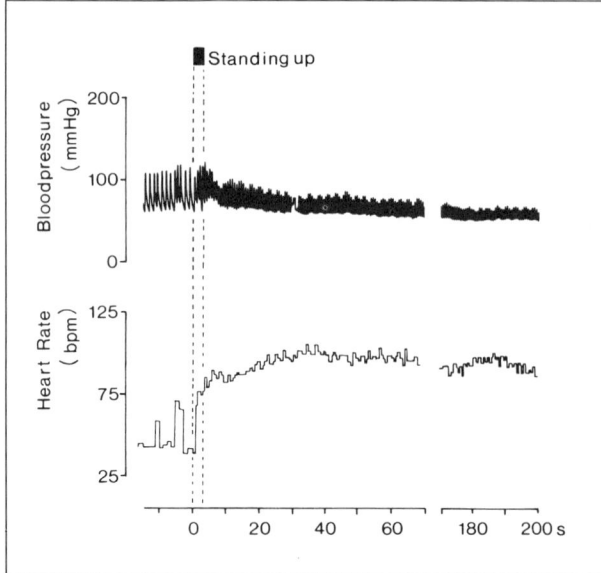

FIG. 4. Blood pressure and heart rate responses to standing. A progressive fall in blood pressure is accompanied by an instantaneous heart rate increment, indicating sympathetic denervation and intact cardiovagal function. (Reprinted with permission from van Lieshout JJ, Wieling W, Wesseling KH et al. Orthostatic hypotension caused by sympathectomies performed for hyperhidrosis. *Neth J Med* 1990;36:53–57.)

diovagal and cardiac sympathetic innervation is a smaller effective blood volume (see Chapter 49). However, the critical role of blood volume in tests of autonomic function is not well appreciated. The maintenance of postural normotension depends on neural reflexes, a normal blood volume, and humoral mechanisms (see Chapter 5). Patients with peripheral sympathetic denervation have lost the neural vasoconstrictor reflexes necessary for the dynamic redistribution of blood volume and flow. Their systemic circulation has been converted to a large-capacitance system that dampens BP oscillations. A capacitance system is exquisitely sensitive to volume changes. When the subject is mildly dehydrated, as with ingestion of diuretics, the effective plasma volume may be dramatically reduced. Patients with generalized autonomic failure will not be able to establish a tachycardiac response. Thus, relatively small changes in blood volume or tone may result in significant OH. In contrast to the patient with pure vagal failure in whom the BP oscillations accompanying RSA are accentuated, the hypovolemic patient with generalized autonomic failure exhibits markedly attenuated BP oscillations.

More subtle changes occur in patients who have preserved cardiac autonomic innervation, as might be found in some patients with length-dependent peripheral neuropathy. The lack of peripheral innervation results in a systemic capacitance system, as described above. However, these patients are able to produce a tachycardiac response on standing. Postural normotension is maintained by mounting a postural tachycardia. These patients are exquisitely sensitive to blood volume changes and are one cause of the POTS syndrome (see Chapter 49).

Position causes relatively minor changes in RSA (11) in normal subjects. However, standing results in the pooling of blood, which greatly accentuates the effective capacitance in patients with autonomic failure. A related problem is that of deconditioning, which occurs with bed rest exceeding a few days and with prolonged space flight. Plasma volume is reduced in these subjects. Other variables that must be controlled are discussed in Chapter 49.

PROBLEMS WITH FREQUENCY ANALYSIS

This issue is covered in greater detail in Chapter 26 and 27. Apart from the issues of standardization of the evaluation of autonomic function in the frequency domain, the biggest problem is the pitfall of failing to recognize the effect of respiration on low-frequency power. Standardization of the duration of recording, the choice of algorithms to filter the signal (detrending, bad-point removal, type and shape of filters), and the selection of methods of analysis is beyond the scope of this chapter (see Chapters 26 and 27) but is necessary. Of great importance is the influence of respiration on power spectra. Slowing of respiration can *greatly* influence power. As pointed out in Chapter 27, respiratory rate was measured in about half of the studies in which frequency analysis was undertaken. Respiration can entrain HR and BP oscillations over a wide range of frequencies, from 0.01 to 0.5 Hz. Additionally, if tidal volume is increased at slower frequencies, the amplitude of respiratory oscillations increases almost tenfold (maximal at 0.07 Hz) compared with the values at 0.2 Hz. Hence, even a short-lasting slowing of breathing frequency (or breath holding), by interacting with spectral power at slower frequencies, can greatly bias results. Slowing of respiration can result in a false-positive increase in low-frequency power (37). Related to the importance of respiration is the logical conclusion that once the actual breathing rate is known, detection of the high-frequency powers should be centered around the dominant breathing frequency and not at a default frequency.

PROBLEMS WITH THE NEUROGENIC FLARE RESPONSE

The neurogenic flare response can be recorded during QSART by use of a laser Doppler flowmeter embedded in the central compartment (A) of the sweat capsule (Chapter 29, Fig. 2) (38). This response has been recommended as a suitable quantitative test of polymodal C nociceptor function. Although good experimental evidence exists to suggest that the underlying neural substrate of the neurogenic flare response is the polymodal C nociceptor (24), there is inadequate validation for increased skin blood flow to be an index of polymodal C nociceptor status. A large number of compounds are involved in the neurogenic flare response (6).

Mast cells degranulate after antidromic stimulation of cutaneous nerves (19), and compound 48/80, a 5-hydroxytryptamine antagonist, suppresses the vasodilatation. A painful stimulus results in the release of SP, which causes vasodilatation and mast cell degranulation. Pain also results in the release of ATP, which causes vasodilatation directly and indirectly. The latter is mediated by mast cell degranulation and the synthesis of vasodilator prostaglandins (6). Tissue injury also results in the release of K- from cells, bradykinin from kallikrein activation, and prostaglandins (22). Somatostatin and vasoactive intestinal polypeptide (VIP), which are present in human skin, are also involved in vasodilatation (1). Histamine appears to play a key role as an amplifier of the neurogenic vasodilatory response (22).

The vasodilatory response following acetylcholine iontophoresis is considered to be of little value as a clinical test of polymodal C nociceptor integrity. Considerable variability exists in the response exhibited by control subjects. In addition, even with adequate warming of the subject (skin temperature $\geq 34°C$), the flare is smaller than that seen in patients with selective sympathetic adrenergic lesions. The problem may be related to competition between sympathetically mediated vasoconstriction and polymodal C nociceptor–mediated vasodilatation. In subjects with intact sympathetic neurons, vasoconstriction may overwhelm neurogenic vasodilatation. Finally, the flare is retained in many subjects with severe impairment of pain perception (3).

PROBLEMS WITH SKIN POTENTIAL RECORDINGS

The value of and problems with skin potential recordings are described in Chapter 17. From a clinical standpoint, there are three major problems. First, the test is not a quantitative test of peripheral nerve sympathetic sudomotor function, as has been suggested (20,44). The neural pathway consists of a somatosympathetic reflex with a long afferent pathway, suprabulbar connections, and a long efferent pathway containing central, preganglionic, and postganglionic sympathetic fibers with many modulatory influences. An abnormality anywhere along the extensive autonomic neuraxis will affect the response. Second, the test is subject to habituation and considerable moment-to-moment fluctuations in amplitude and waveform. Third, the response is consistently present on the palm and sole but is less so at other sites. In our laboratory, this test appears to be considerably less sensitive than QSART in the detection of distal small-fiber neuropathies.

PITFALLS IN EVALUATING SYSTEMIC ADRENERGIC FUNCTION

Perhaps the most distressing and dangerous manifestation of generalized autonomic failure is OH. OH without compensatory tachycardia is a manifestation of widespread sympathetic adrenergic failure. It is highly desirable to quantitate the distribution and severity of adrenergic failure. Such information is of prime importance in diagnosing the disorder, monitoring progression of the disorder, and determining the response to treatment of the disorder. The maintenance of postural normotension depends on the integrity of certain neural reflexes (cardiopulmonary and arterial baroreflexes and, perhaps, the venoarteriolar and vestibular reflexes; see Chapter 6), a normal effective blood volume, and intact humoral mechanisms (norepinephrine, renin–angiotensin, vasopressin, neuropeptide Y, and, perhaps, atriopeptin).

Problems arise in the quantitation of the neural reflexes. Humoral mechanisms can be measured, but blood volume, which is critical in the maintenance of postural normotension, is not measured as part of the clinical autonomic screen. As discussed earlier in this chapter, differences in orthostatic BP may reflect variations in effective plasma volume. Older individuals may develop severe OH while taking recommended doses of diuretics (7,54).

There are standardized isotopic methods for measuring plasma volume (see Chapter 49). However, these tests are cumbersome, expensive, and impractical for the laboratory. The lack of a simple noninvasive test that can be performed repeatedly is a serious shortcoming. Volume stress tests such as upright-tilt, lower body negative pressure, and trinitroglycerin (15,32) do not distinguish between adrenergic failure and hypovolemia.

To diagnose milder manifestations of adrenergic failure, it would be desirable to quantitate focal adrenergic failure and its distribution. It is possible to study regional adrenergic function by using invasive techniques such as the intra-arterial infusion of very low concentrations of direct- (i.e., phenylephrine) and indirect- (i.e., tyramine) acting agents (27,32,40). Because such methodology is too invasive for repeated clinical use, investigators have focused on tests that evaluate the regulation of skin blood flow. Candidate tests have included skin vasomotor reflexes, reflex heating, and the venoarteriolar reflex. The problem with all of these tests is the variability of skin blood flow, which presents itself as rhythmic oscillations as well as marked moment-to-moment variations caused by psychic influences and temperature. Skin vasoconstrictor reflexes are usually tested on the finger pads or toepads. Other sites are less satisfactory; the more proximal limb sites have dual innervation with vasodilator as well as vasoconstrictor fibers, whereas acral sites have purely vasoconstrictor fibers (see Chapter 16). The toepads have considerable sympathetic tone under ambient temperatures. Warming is necessary, and this creates another variable because vascular smooth muscle is temperature dependent *in vitro* (17) and *in vivo* (30). The vasoconstrictor response varies from moment to moment depending on resting blood flow and other factors that affect skin sympathetic activity.

Skin vasomotor reflexes are straightforward to perform on the finger pads and toe pads (30) and yield important semiquantitative information. The percentage of vasoconstriction in response to the Valsalva maneuver, inspiratory gasp, standing, and contralateral cold stimulus can be accurately quantitated. However, the response is also affected by competing influences on skin sympathetic activity. Hence, the test is regarded as semiquantitative, just as PASP is semiquantitative. The various tests have different afferent pathways but a final common pathway. Thus, it might be possible to test the afferent pathways. Their value in this regard is somewhat degraded by the variability problem.

Reflex heating results in reflex vasodilation (see Chapter 16), provided the subject is suitably warmed. It is theoretically possible to raise the central temperature to, for instance, 37°C and monitor the vasodilatation at several sites in a limb in response to this heat stimulus. The problem is that the rate and amount of vasodilatation depend on the sympathetic tone at different sites. Thus, the quantitative differences observed between sites may reflect tone rather than innervative changes. At a practical level, the test is time-consuming and lacking in sensitivity.

The venoarteriolar reflex (see Chapter 16) has been suggested as a test of postganglionic adrenergic function. Skin blood flow (measured with laser Doppler velocimetry) and the vasoconstrictor response to limb dependency have been suggested to be abnormal in patients with diabetic neuropathy (41). However, it has never been convincingly demonstrated that these tests can be used to diagnose the presence of diabetic neuropathy or other neuropathies with sensitivity and specificity. In the study by Rayman and colleagues (41), the resting skin blood flow was significantly greater in diabetics than in controls. When flow was increased by warming to a level similar to that in the diabetics, the difference in reflex vasoconstriction was no longer significant. We studied the reflex in diabetic and other neuropathies and found the response to be unreliable for the purpose of diagnosis (36).

PHOTOPLETHYSMOGRAPHIC MEASUREMENTS OF BEAT-TO-BEAT BLOOD PRESSURE

Photoplethysmographic measurements of beat-to-beat BP (PRBP) faithfully record BP_{BB} and, especially, its alterations (16,48,55). The BP pulse causes changes in tissue volume that are sensed by photoelectric sensors connected to an active servo-null system. This system generates a counterforce that exactly nulls the deforming force. The

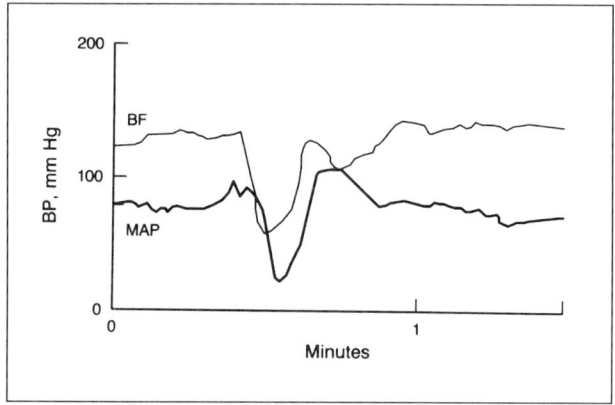

FIG. 5. The effect of inspiratory gasp on blood flow (BF) and mean arterial pressure (MAP), recorded with the Finapres device. Vasoconstriction results in an attenuation of the amplitude of the arterial waveform (not shown) and a reduction in Finapres-recorded MAP.

volume decrement associated with the vasoconstrictor reflex may alter tissue volume and the PRBP recording. However, comparisons between the noninvasive and intraarterial recordings appear to be satisfactory (16,48). We recently performed a detailed study of the Valsalva maneuver in normal subjects (3) and in patients with graded autonomic failure (42). The results are comparable to those obtained with intraarterial recordings (21).

Photoplethysmographic measurements of beat-to-beat BP are increasingly used in clinical laboratories and intensive care units. In laboratories, the effect of autonomic reflexes (such as the Valsalva maneuver, cold pressor test, tilt, and deep breathing) on PRBP constitutes a part of the clinical noninvasive evaluation of autonomic function. There are two problems. We previously documented powerful skin vasoconstrictor reflexes in the distal extremities of normal subjects. These are the skin vasomotor (30) and the venoarteriolar (36) reflexes, both of which affect PRBP (Fig. 5). Peripheral vasoconstriction may greatly dampen the transmitted arterial pulse wave. A substantial difference in BP between the upper arm and finger is often seen in patients in the standing position who have powerful vasoconstrictor reflexes. Figure 6 shows a 33-year-old female with orthostatic intolerance. Tilt-up results in intense vasoconstriction. Note that there was relatively good agreement between the Finapres recordings and the manual recordings (brachial) with the patient supine. With tilt up, Finapres reads much higher than the manual recordings. It is recommended that sphygmomanometric recordings also be taken in the supine and standing positions to avoid the erroneous diagnosis of orthostatic hypotension in these subjects. A second problem occurs during prolonged recording periods in excess of 1 hr. Local tissue turgidity increases and there is a gradual increase in recorded pressures.

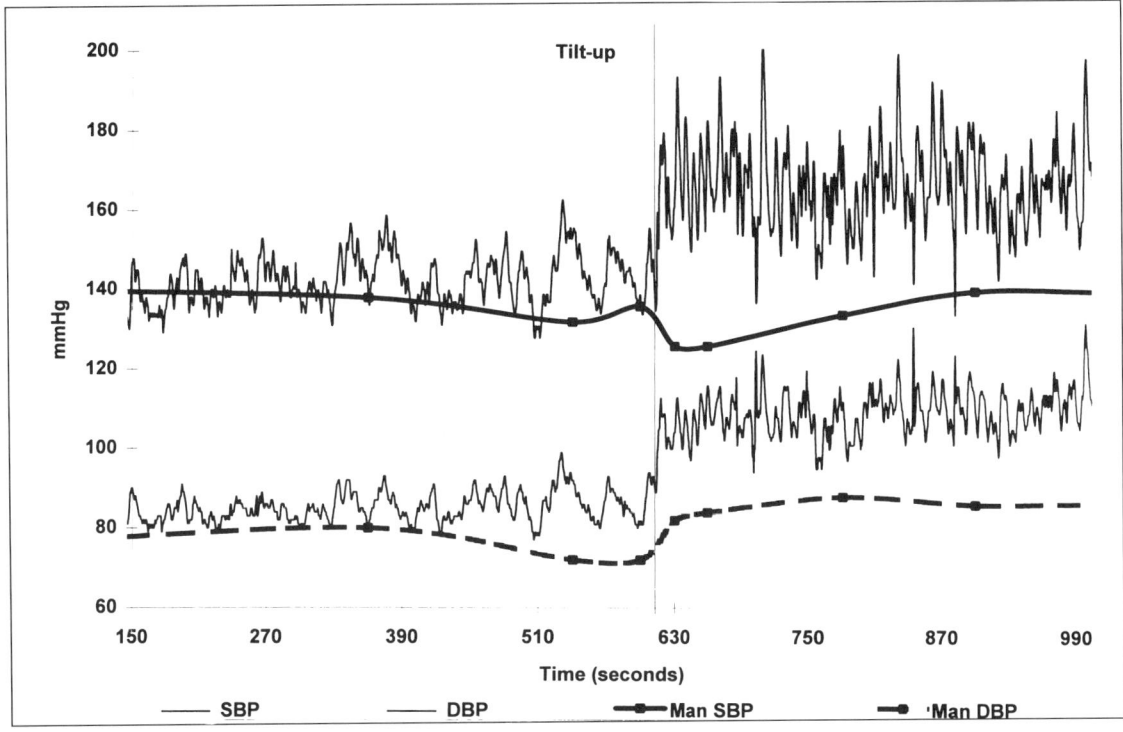

FIG. 6. Comparison of Finapres recordings of systolic blood pressure (*SBP*) and diastolic blood pressure (*DBP*) versus manual recordings (*Man SBP, Man DBP*) with the patient supine and in a tilt-up position. Tilt up causes the Finapres readings of systolic and diastolic blood pressure to be significantly higher than the manual (brachial) values.

PROBLEMS ASSOCIATED WITH THE AUTONOMIC STATUS OF THE PATIENT

Apart from disease-related autonomic dysfunction, the physical, emotional, and comfort state of the subject may profoundly affect tests of autonomic function, especially tests of complex systems.

The state of hydration may greatly affect the maintenance of postural normotension (see earlier). The hypovolemic subject may exhibit blunting of BP oscillations with the Valsalva maneuver. TST, the volume of sweat droplets, and the distribution of anhidrosis may be affected by dehydration. An increase in sweat threshold and areas of partial thermoregulatory failure, which may fail completely, occur as a result of dehydration. Another potent stimulus resulting in the inhibition of thermoregulatory sweating is cold. A cold compress totally inhibited the sweat response in a patient who had a headache. The next day, the test was repeated and a normal sweat pattern was obtained (P.A.L., personal observations).

Among the patients referred to the autonomic laboratory, a significant percentage are taking anticholinergics as tricyclic antidepressant medication for pain; for the management of extrapyramidal disorders; and, sometimes, as proprietary cold and cough medication. A formalized study of the effect of anticholinergic medication on autonomic function is not available. Our impression is that anticholinergic medication has a profound effect on the TST, a moderate effect on chemical sweating (QSART), and a mild effect on cardiovagal function.

Sympathetic activation due to full bladder, anxiety, or pain has a powerful effect on BP, HR, and cardiovagal function.

PITFALL IN THE VALIDATION OF TESTS

Tests of autonomic function must be sensitive, specific, and reproducible. One common mistake made in the introduction of new tests is the comparison (using patients with severe autonomic failure involving the system of interest) between the new test and an established one. For example, PASP might show good concordance with QSART for patients with severe sudomotor failure but not for those with moderate failure. A comparison of PASP with the thermoregulatory sweat test and sweat imprint counts (43) demonstrated that PASP lacked sensitivity in unselected patients.

For the establishment of a new test, the following are suggested as minimal criteria:

1. *Sensitivity*: The new test should be compared with an established test using a group of subjects whose abnor-

malities range from mild to severe. Confining the test to patients with severe autonomic failure will yield falsely good concordance.

2. *Specificity*: There should be few false positives.
3. *Reproducibility*: The test–retest agreement should be acceptable (e.g., coefficient of variability <20%).
4. *Test relevance*: The test should be physiologically relevant. Ideally, the test should evaluate the system of direct interest. For example, patients who have acral neuropathic pain should undergo a test of distal nerve function and not one of a distant nerve such as the vagus.

CONCLUSION

Noninvasive tests of autonomic function can be powerful when properly harnessed. They do have certain limitations. The laboratory personnel must have a clear knowledge of the test reflex (how complex?), the clinical procedure (applied and true stimulus, desired and recorded response), and the status of the patient (for interfering variables) to make a valid interpretation of the results.

REFERENCES

1. Anand P, Bloom SR, McGregor GP. Topical capsaicin pretreatment inhibits axon reflex vasodilatation caused by somatostatin and vasoactive intestinal polypeptide in human skin. *Br J Pharmacol* 1983; 78:665–669.
2. Angelone A, Coulter NA. Respiratory sinus arrhythmia: a frequency dependent phenomenon. *J Appl Physiol* 1964;19:479–482.
3. Benarroch EE, et al. Use of the photoplethysmographic technique to analyze the Valsalva maneuver in normal man. *Muscle Nerve* 1991; 14:1165–1172.
4. Borgdorff P. Respiratory fluctuations in pupil size. *Am J Physiol* 1975;228:1094–1102.
5. Braune S et al. Cardiovascular parameters: sensitivity to detect autonomic dysfunction and influence of age and sex in normal subjects. *Clin Auton Res* 1996;6:3–16.
6. Burnstock G. Autonomic neuroeffector junctions—reflex vasodilatation of the skin (review). *J Invest Dermatol* 1977;69:47–57.
7. Caird FI, et al. The cardiovascular system. In: Brocklehurst JC (ed). *Textbook of Geriatric Medicine and Gerontology*. Edinburgh: Churchill Livingstone.1985;230.
8. Coker R et al. Does the sympathetic nervous system influence sinus arrhythmia in man? Evidence from combined autonomic blockade. *J Physiol* 1984;356:459–464.
9. Dyrberg T et al. Prevalence of diabetic autonomic neuropathy measured by simple bedside tests. *Diabetologia* 1981;20:190–194.
10. Eckberg D. Parasympathetic cardiovascular control in human disease: critical review of methods and results. *Am J Physiol* 1980;239: H581–H593.
11. Eckberg DL, Orshan CR. Respiratory and baroreceptor reflex interactions in man. *J Clin Invest* 1977;59:780–785.
12. Ewing DJ et al. Vascular reflexes in diabetic autonomic neuropathy. *Lancet* 1973;2:1354–1356.
13. Ewing DJ, Clark BF. Diabetic autonomic neuropathy: a clinical viewpoint. In: Dyck PJ, Thomas PK, Asbury AK et al (eds). *Diabetic Neuropathy*. Philadelphia: WB Saunders.1987;66–88.
14. Ewing DJ et al. The value of cardiovascular autonomic function tests: 10 years experience in diabetes. *Diabetes Care* 1985;8:491–498.
15. Hume L et al. Provocation of postural hypotension by nitroglycerin in diabetic autonomic neuropathy. *Diabetes Care* 1980;3:27–30.
16. Imholz BP et al. Continuous non-invasive blood pressure monitoring: reliability of Finapres device during the Valsalva manoeuvre. *Cardiovasc Res* 1988;22:390–397.
17. Johnson JM et al. Regulation of the cutaneous circulation. *Fed Proc* 1986;45:2841–2850.
18. Johnson RH, Prout BJ. Dissociation of some sympathetic nervous functions. *Bibl Anat* 1967;9:349–354.
19. Kiernan JA. A pharmacological and histological investigation of the involvement of mast cells in cutaneous axon reflex vasodilatation. *Q J Exp Physiol* 1975;60:123–130.
20. Knezevic W, Bajada S. Peripheral autonomic surface potential. A quantitative technique for recording sympathetic conduction in man. *J Neurol Sci* 1985;67:239–251.
21. Korner PI, et al. Reflex and mechanical circulatory effects of graded Valsalva maneuvers in normal man. *J Appl Physiol* 1976;40:434–440.
22. Lembeck F. Mediators of vasodilatation in the skin. *Br J Dermatol* 1983;109(suppl 25):1–9.
23. Levy MN. Sympathetic–parasympathetic interactions in the heart (review). *Circ Res* 1971;29:437–445.
24. Lewis T, Pochin EE. The double pain response of the human skin to a single stimulus. *Clin Sci* 1937;3:67–76.
25. Low PA. Quantitation of autonomic responses. In: Dyck PJ, Thomas PK, Lambert EH, Bunge R (eds). *Peripheral Neuropathy*. Philadelphia: WB Saunders. 1984;1139–1165.
26. Low PA. Sudomotor function and dysfunction. In: Asbury AK, McKhann GM, McDonald WI (eds). *Diseases of the Nervous System*. Philadelphia: WB Saunders. 1986;596–605.
27. Low PA. Quantitation of autonomic function. In: Dyck PJ, Thomas PK, Griffin JW et al (eds). *Peripheral Neuropathy*. Philadelphia: WB Saunders. 1993;729–745.
28. Low PA et al. Quantitative sudomotor axon reflex test in normal and neuropathic subjects. *Ann Neurol* 1983;14:573–580.
29. Low PA, Fealey RD. Sudomotor neuropathy. In: Dyck PJ, Thomas PK, Winegrad A, Porte D (eds). *Diabetic Neuropathy*. Philadelphia: WB Saunders. 1987;140–145.
30. Low PA et al. Evaluation of skin vasomotor reflexes by using laser Doppler velocimetry. *Mayo Clin Proc* 1983;58:583–592.
31. Low PA et al. The effect of aging on cardiac autonomic and postganglionic sudomotor function. *Muscle Nerve* 1990;13:152–157.
32. Low PA et al. The sympathetic nervous system in diabetic neuropathy. A clinical and pathological study. *Brain* 1975;98:341–356.
33. Low PA, et al. Comparison of distal sympathetic with vagal function in diabetic neuropathy. *Muscle Nerve* 1986; 9:592–596.
34. Maselli RA et al. Comparison of sympathetic skin response with quantitative sudomotor axon reflex test in diabetic neuropathy. *Muscle Nerve* 1989;12:420–423.
35. Mehlsen J et al. Heart rate response to breathing: dependency upon breathing pattern. *Clin Physiol* 1987;7:115–124.
36. Moy S et al. The venoarteriolar reflex in diabetic and other neuropathies. *Neurology* 1989;39:1490–1492.
37. Novak V et al. Influence of respiration on heart rate and blood pressure fluctuations. *J Appl Physiol* 1993;74:617–626.
38. Parkhouse N, LeQuesne PM. Quantitative objective assessment of peripheral nociceptive C fibre function. *J Neurol Neurosurg Psychiatry* 1988;51:28–34.
39. Pfeifer MA et al. Quantitative evaluation of cardiac parasympathetic activity in normal and diabetic man. *Diabetes* 1982;31:339–345.
40. Polinsky RJ et al. Pharmacologic distinction of different orthostatic hypotension syndromes. *Neurology* 1981;31:1–7.
41. Rayman G, Hassan A, Tooke JE. Blood flow in the skin of the foot related to posture in diabetes mellitus. *Br Med J* 1986;292:87–90.
42. Sandroni P, et al. Pharmacological dissection of components of the Valsalva maneuver in adrenergic failure. *J Appl Physiol* 1991; 71:1563–1567.
43. Schondorf R, Gendron D. Evaluation of sudomotor function in patients with peripheral neuropathy (abstract). *Neurology* 1990;40 (suppl 1):386.
44. Shahani BT et al. Sympathetic skin response—a method of assessing unmyelinated axon dysfunction in peripheral neuropathies. *J Neurol Neurosurg Psychiatry* 1984;47:536–542.
45. Sharpey-Schafer EP, Taylor PJ. Absent circulatory reflexes in diabetic neuritis. *Lancet* 1960;i:559–562.
46. Shepherd JT, Vanhoutte PM. *The Human Cardiovascular System: Facts and Concepts*. New York: Raven Press. 1979.

47. Sundkvist G, et al. Respiratory influence on heart rate in diabetes mellitus. *Br Med J* 1979;1:924–925.
48. van Egmond J, et al. Invasive v. non-invasive measurement of arterial pressure. Comparison of two automatic methods and simultaneously measured direct intra-arterial pressure. *Br J Anaesth* 1985;57:434–444.
49. van Lieshout JJ et al. Pitfalls in the assessment of cardiovascular reflexes in patients with sympathetic failure but intact vagal control. *Clin Sci* 1989;76:523–528.
50. Weinberg CR, Pfeifer MA. Development of a predictive model for symptomatic neuropathy (SN) in diabetes. *Diabetes* 1986;35:873–880.
51. Weinberg CR, Pfeifer MA. An improved method for measuring heart-rate variability: assessment of cardiac autonomic function. *Biometrics* 1984;40:855–861.
52. Wieling W et al. Reflex control of heart rate in normal subjects in relation to age: a data base for cardiac vagal neuropathy. *Diabetologia* 1982;22:163–166.
53. Wieling W, van Lieshout JJ. The assessment of cardiovascular reflex activity: standardization is needed. *Diabetologia* 1990;33:182–183.
54. Wollner L, Spalding JMK. The autonomic nervous system. In: Brocklehurst JC (ed). *Textbook of Geriatric Medicine and Gerontology*. Edinburgh: Churchill Livingstone. 1985;449.
55. Yamakoshi K, et al. Indirect measurement of instantaneous arterial blood pressure in the human finger by the vascular unloading technique. *IEEE Trans Biomed Eng* 1980;27: 150–155.

CHAPTER 31

Experimental Models of Autonomic Neuropathy

Roger R. Tuck and Stephen Brimijoin

1. The autonomic nervous system has been investigated in animals with experimental diabetes mellitus, acrylamide-induced neuropathy, and experimental allergic neuritis. Histologic studies have confirmed that sympathetic and parasympathetic nerves are affected in these three experimental disorders.
2. In experimental diabetic neuropathy, physiologic studies have revealed impairment of autonomic control of the heart, blood vessels, alimentary canal, and urinary bladder.
3. In acrylamide-induced neuropathy, which is regarded as a model of toxic and nutritional neuropathies, impaired cardiovascular, bronchopulmonary, and esophageal reflexes result from damage to large-diameter, myelinated afferent vagal fibers or their mechanoreceptors (such as baroreceptors), or both, as well as from damage to efferent sympathetic vasomotor fibers.
4. In experimental allergic neuritis, which is a model of the Guillain-Barré syndrome, demyelination and axonal degeneration occur in the splanchnic and sympathetic nerves, and control of heart rate is impaired.
5. Study of these models has provided some insights into the autonomic disturbances that may affect humans with peripheral neuropathy.
6. Experimental sympathectomy has been produced with 6-hydroxydopamine, guanethidine, antibodies to nerve growth factor and to acetylcholinesterase, and extract of human sympathetic chain. In the first three of these cases, the postganglionic sympathetic fibers are affected. In contrast, sympathectomy induced by acetylcholinesterase antibodies selectively involves preganglionic fibers and the sympathetic nerve supply to the adrenal medulla.
7. Some of these experimental autonomic neuropathies have provided useful tools for studying the role of the sympathetic nervous system in vasomotor control and hypertension, and they may prove to be useful models of human disease.

EXPERIMENTAL DIABETIC AUTONOMIC NEUROPATHY

The autonomic nervous system of animals with diabetes mellitus induced by islet-cell toxins (streptozocin and alloxan) or with genetic diabetes (BB rat, diabetic Chinese hamster, and dystrophic mouse) has been studied in considerable detail. The clinical manifestations of autonomic neuropathy in these animals include poorly formed stools, colonic dilatation, and urinary retention (24, 88, 101).

Histopathology

In the sympathetic chains and Auerbach's plexuses of rats with streptozocin-induced diabetes, chromatolysis of ganglion cells and axonal degeneration are observed (65). Unmyelinated postganglionic sympathetic nerves of the mesentery, parotid gland, and choroid plexus of animals with streptozocin-induced diabetes exhibit dystrophic changes; these consist of focal swellings in which there are tubulovesicular and dense core profiles as well as lamellar

---

R. R. Tuck: Canberra Specialist Centre, Deakin, A.C.T., 2600.
S. Brimijoin: Department of Pharmacology, Mayo Clinic, Rochester, Minnesota 55905.

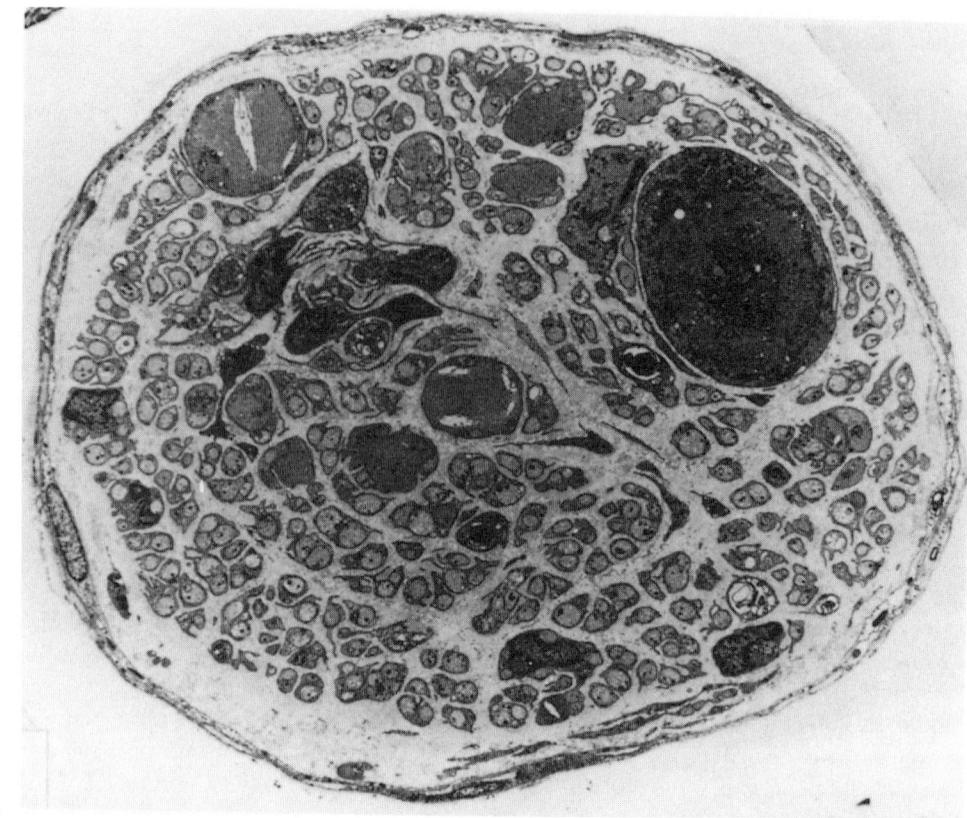

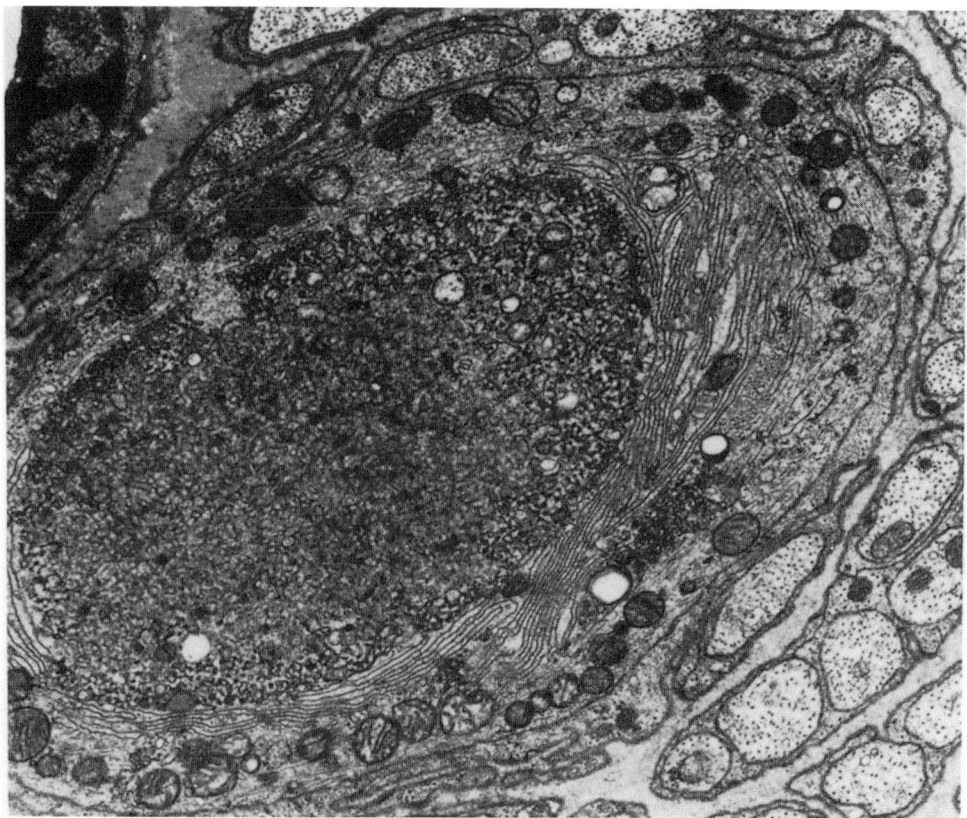

FIG. 1. A: Enlarged dystrophic axons in a paravascular ileal nerve fascicle of a rat with streptozocin-induced diabetes. x2300. **B:** Ultrastructure of dystrophic ileal mesenteric nerve of a diabetic rat, showing tubular rings, layered loops, and tubulovesicular profiles. x17,000. (From Schmidt and Plurad, ref. 89. Reprinted with permission.)

bodies (2,29,38,89,91,92) (Fig. 1). Similar abnormalities have been observed in sympathetic nerves in the diabetic BB rat (101,102,104) and in the diabetic Chinese hamster (25,26,87). Axonal dystrophy affects preganglionic as well as postganglionic sympathetic fibers in experimental diabetes (89) (Fig. 2).

Myelinated fibers in the vagus and pelvic parasympathetic nerves of animals with experimental diabetes contain increased amounts of glycogen. These fibers are reduced in caliber and density and have abnormally thin myelin sheaths (24,28,71,79,88,89,103) (Fig. 3).

Physiologic Studies

Cardiovascular System

Reduced spontaneous, respiration-related variations in heart rate (HR) are common in humans with diabetic autonomic neuropathy; they reflect disease of the vagus nerves (33). Similar observations have been made in the diabetic BB-Wistar rat, in which a significant reduction in HR variability appears as early as 8 weeks after the onset of diabetes (65). In short-term diabetic rats, there is evidence of an exaggerated HR response to vagal stimulation. Direct stimulation of the vagus nerves or baroreceptor stimulation causes a more marked bradycardia in short-term diabetic rats than in control rats (21,48,97). In animals that have been diabetic for long periods, the baroreceptor-HR reflex is significantly impaired (19,21), as in humans with diabetic autonomic neuropathy (11,62).

There is evidence of sympathetic denervation of the peripheral vasculature of the diabetic rat. The caudal artery and hindlimb vasoconstrictor response to sympathetic stimulation is reduced in rats with diabetes, resembling that observed in sympathectomized animals (41,67). In the rat hindlimb, the vasoconstrictor effect of norepinephrine is exaggerated because of denervation hypersensitivity (19,22,67). Denervation of blood vessels is likely to be a major contributing factor to the orthostatic hypotension that occurs frequently in patients with diabetic autonomic neuropathy (62).

Urinary Bladder

Reflex urinary bladder function is impaired both in rats with drug-induced diabetes and in the diabetic BB rat. In

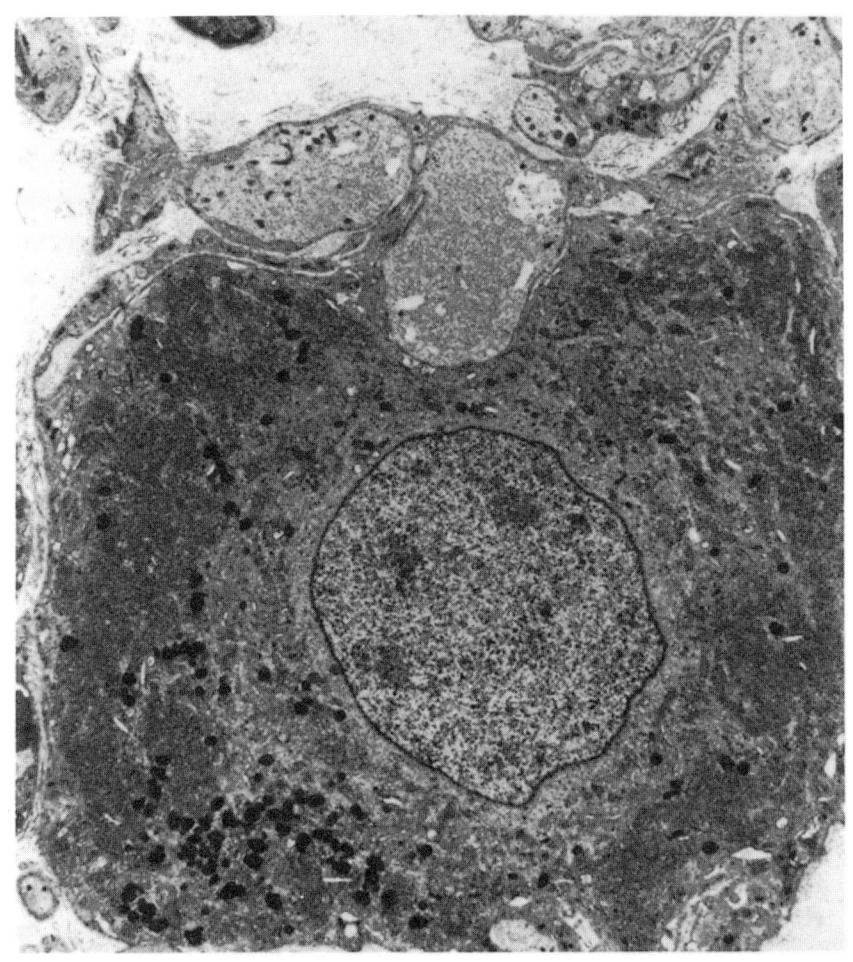

FIG. 2. Dystrophic axoneuropathy affecting two swollen presynaptic axons that are indenting a sympathetic neuron in the superior mesenteric ganglion of a diabetic rat. x3760. (From Schmidt and Plurad, ref. 89. Reprinted with permission.)

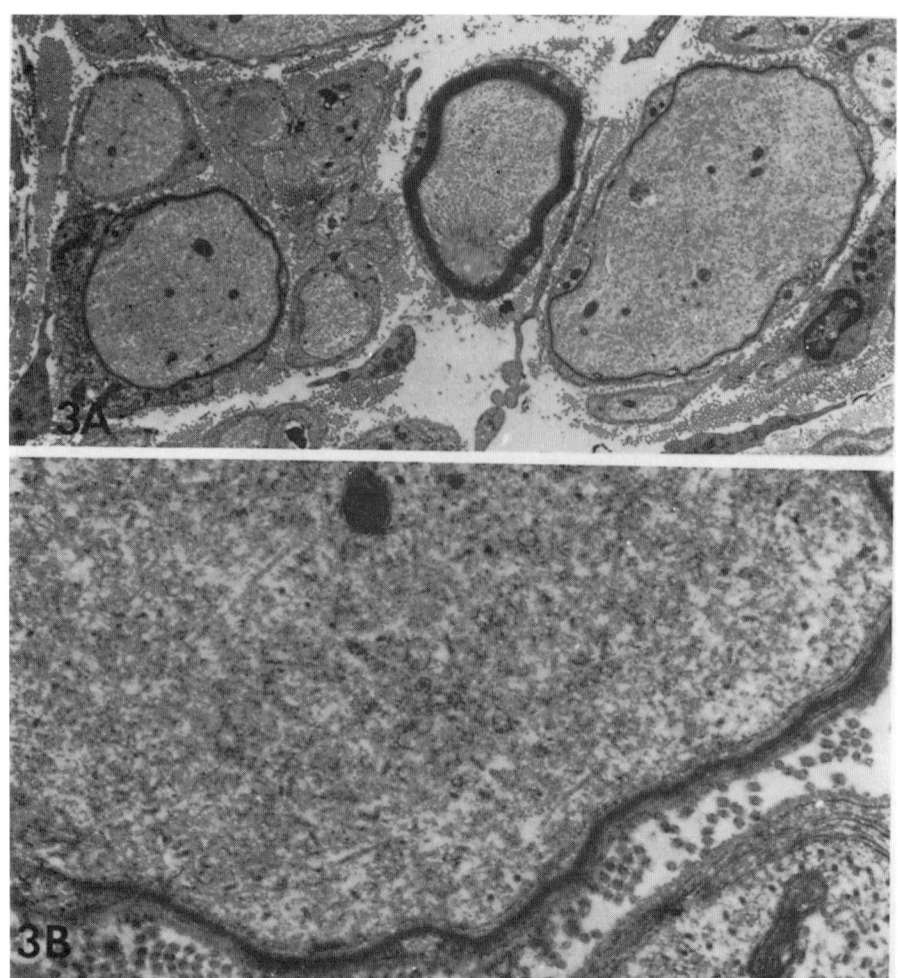

FIG. 3. Axoneuropathy affecting myelinated fibers in the mesenteric nerve of a rat with streptozocin-induced diabetes. **A:** Enlarged axons with thin myelin sheaths. x6400. **B:** Relatively unstructured axoplasm of a dilated myelinated fiber containing vascular elements and misaligned microtubules. x30,100. (From Schmidt and Plurad, ref. 89. Reprinted with permission.)

addition to hypertrophy of the bladder, there is an increase in the volume threshold above which reflex bladder contraction begins, and a decrease in the frequency of contractions that becomes greater as the duration of diabetes increases (56,71,72). These changes in bladder function have been attributed to an axonopathy involving the vesical afferents in the pelvic nerves and efferents in the hypogastric nerves (71).

Gastrointestinal Tract

In diabetic rats, secretion from the parotid gland during stimulation of the parasympathetic or sympathetic nerves is less than in control animals, but the secretion evoked directly by cholinergic or peptidergic agonists is unchanged. This pattern is consistent with an abnormality of the autonomic nerve supply to the gland (2). Decreased parotid salivary flow has been found in humans with diabetes (57).

The release of glucagon by the endocrine pancreas is affected in diabetic rats as it is in humans (73). Glucagon release in response to hypoglycemia is prevented by cholinergic-blocking but not adrenergic-blocking drugs, and glucagon release is provoked by cholinomimetic drugs (73). Rats with streptozocin-induced diabetes have no glucagon response to hypoglycemia, although the response to carbachol remains. These findings are in accord with histochemical changes in the pancreas showing loss of fibers in pancreatic parasympathetic nerves (29,63).

In the alimentary canal of the diabetic Chinese hamster, radiologic techniques have been used to demonstrate dilatation, hypomotility, delayed gastric emptying, and increased bowel transit time in association with ultrastructural degenerative changes in the myenteric plexus (27). Cholinergic neurotransmission in the longitudinal smooth muscle of the small intestine in the diabetic rat is defective, but the defect is partially corrected with insulin treatment (68).

ACRYLAMIDE AUTONOMIC NEUROPATHY

Animals treated with monomeric acrylamide have been used as models of autonomic involvement in axonal or dying-back neuropathies, such as the neuropathy of alcoholism. Post and McLeod (75–78) found a reduction in the density of large and small myelinated fibers in the splanchnic and vagus nerves of acrylamide-affected cats. The reduction in fiber density in the autonomic nerves is not as great as that in longer peripheral nerves. Axonal degeneration takes place in myelinated fibers of the splanchnic nerve (Fig. 4) and occasionally in myelinated fibers of the thoracic vagus in acrylamide-affected dogs (80). In severely poisoned cats, axonal degeneration occurs in unmyelinated fibers of the splanchnic nerves (75) (Fig. 5).

In acrylamide-treated rats, there is almost complete loss of sympathetic adrenergic axons from the blood vessels and parenchyma of the pineal gland, the nerve supply of which is made up of postganglionic sympathetic axons emanating from cell bodies in the superior cervical ganglia. The proximal, surviving parts of the sympathetic axons are swollen and contain neurofilaments and tubulovesicular bodies that may represent attempts at regeneration (90). The cell bodies in the superior cervical ganglia undergo changes resembling chromatolysis that may be caused by degeneration of the distal axons (95).

Physiologic Studies

Neurophysiology

Electrophysiologic studies of myelinated fibers of the vagus and splanchnic nerves of acrylamide-affected animals have revealed slowing of conduction velocity and decreased action-potential amplitude (75,77). However, the amplitude of the C-fiber action potential of the cervical sympathetic trunk of acrylamide-affected rats is normal (47).

Cardiovascular System

Rats treated with acrylamide have increased HR and blood pressure (BP) variability and significant increases in the mean resting levels of HR and BP, which may be a result of damage to arterial baroreceptors or their afferent fibers in the glossopharyngeal and vagus nerves (96). Acrylamide-treated dogs likewise show abnormally large changes in systemic arterial pressure and HR in response to

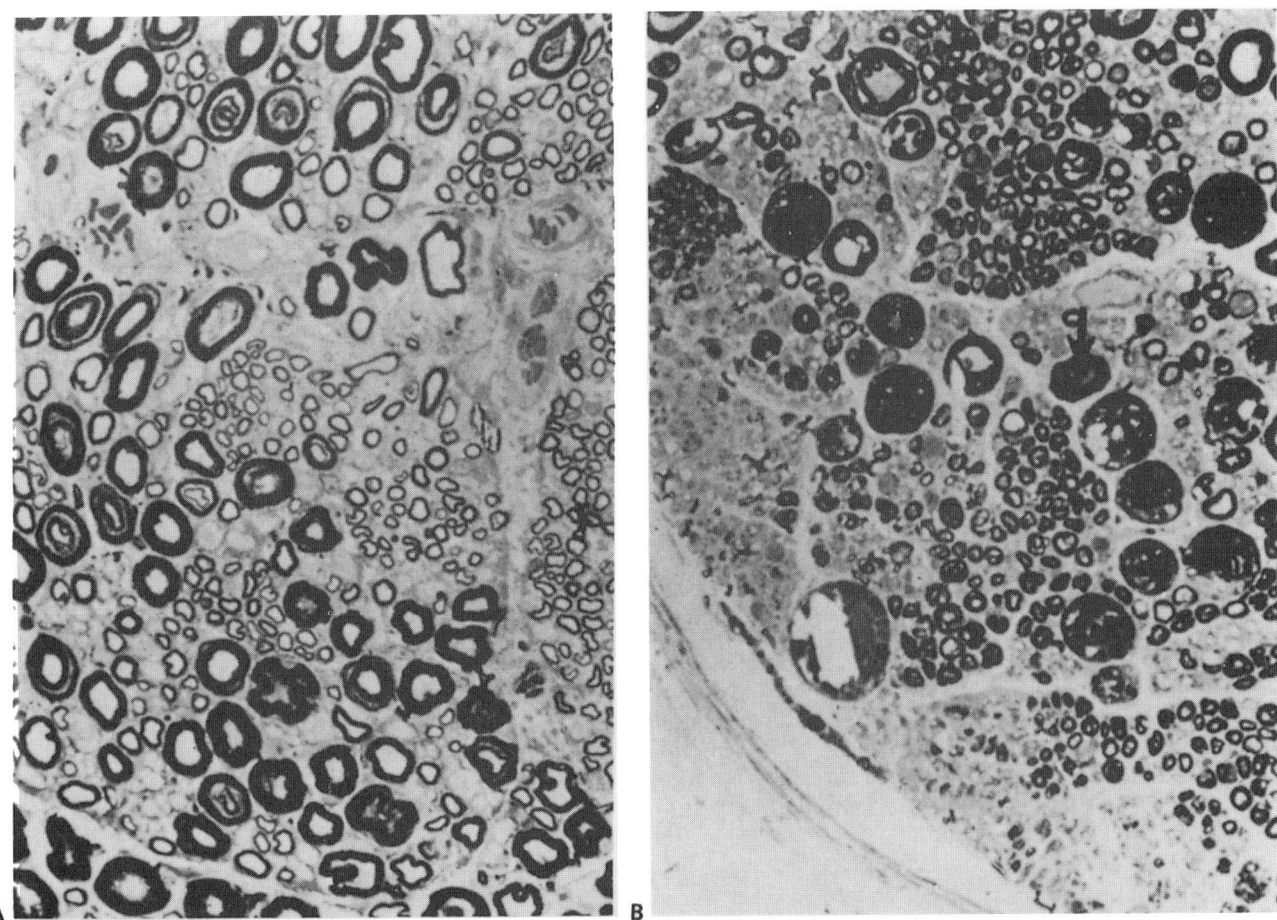

FIG. 4. Splanchnic nerve of cat. **A:** Normal. **B:** Severely poisoned with acrylamide, showing degeneration of some large-diameter myelinated fibers. x560. (From Post and McLeod, ref. 77. Reprinted with permission.)

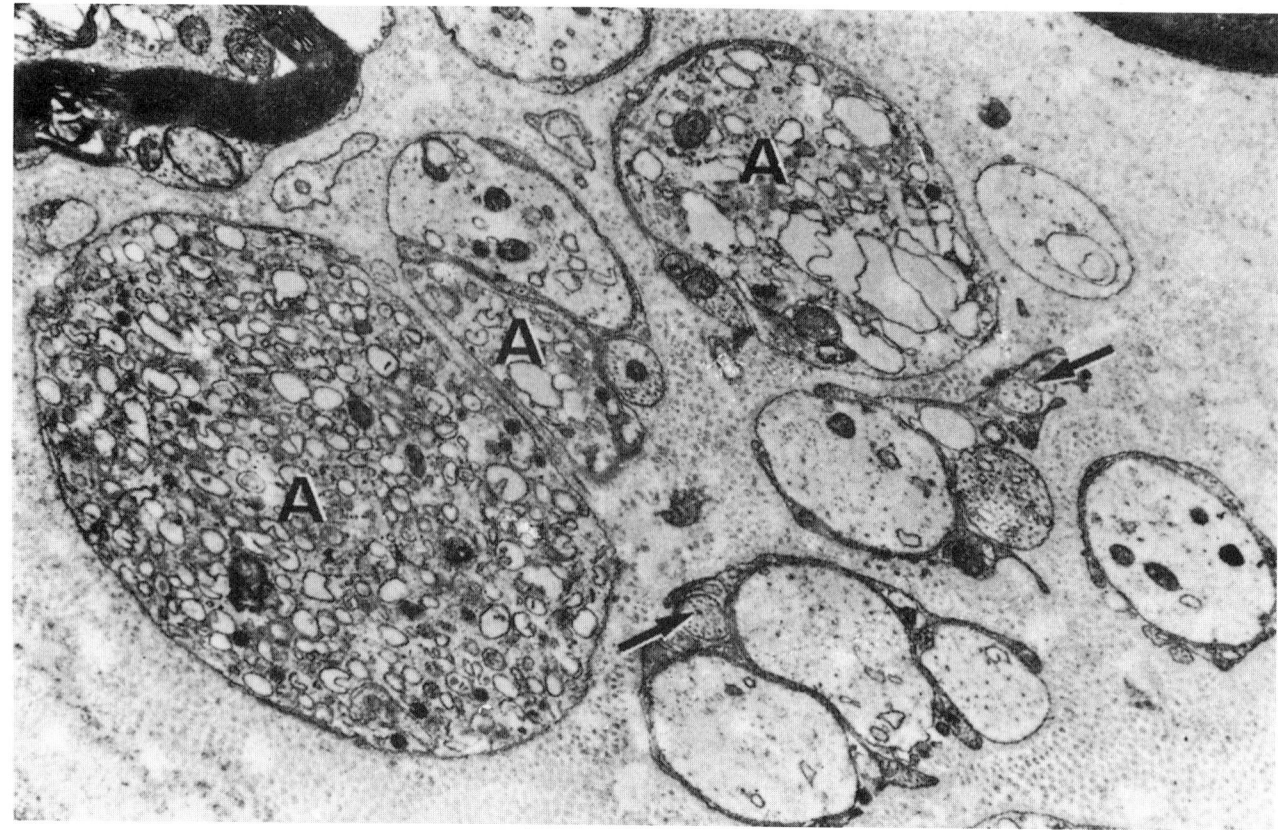

FIG. 5. Degenerating unmyelinated axons (*A*) in the splanchnic nerve of a severely acrylamide-poisoned cat. x17,700. (From Post and McLeod, ref. 77. Reprinted with permission.)

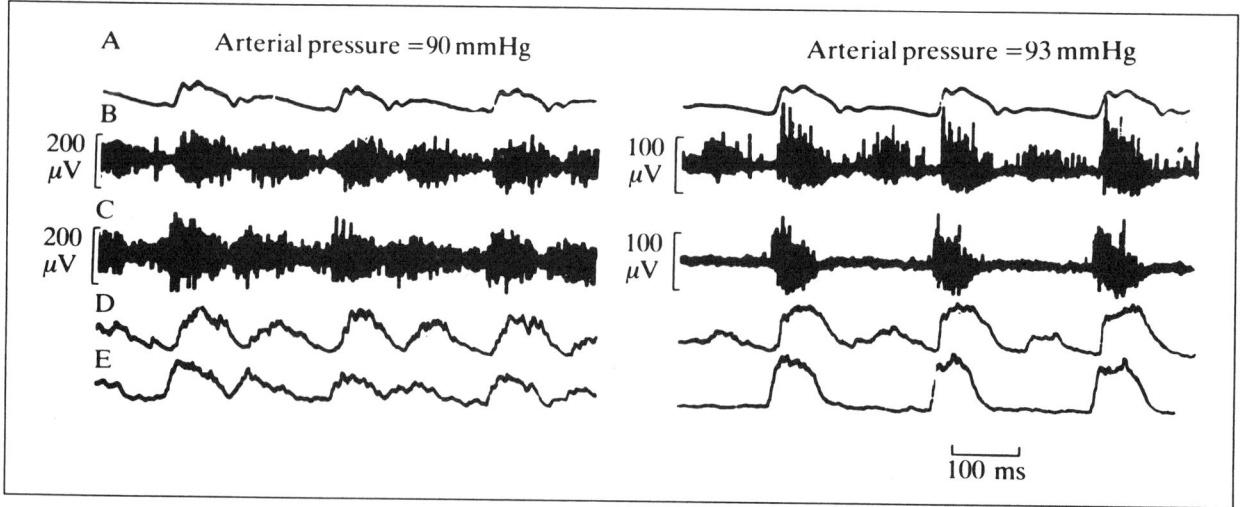

FIG. 6. Baroreceptor nerve activity in a control rabbit (*left*) and rabbit with acrylamide-induced neuropathy (*right*). There is very little activity during diastole in the acrylamide-affected animals. *A*, arterial blood pressure; *B*, carotid sinus nerve activity; *C*, depressor nerve activity; *D*, carotid sinus nerve neurogram; *E*, depressor nerve neurogram. (From Satchell, ref. 84. Reprinted with permission of Oxford University Press.)

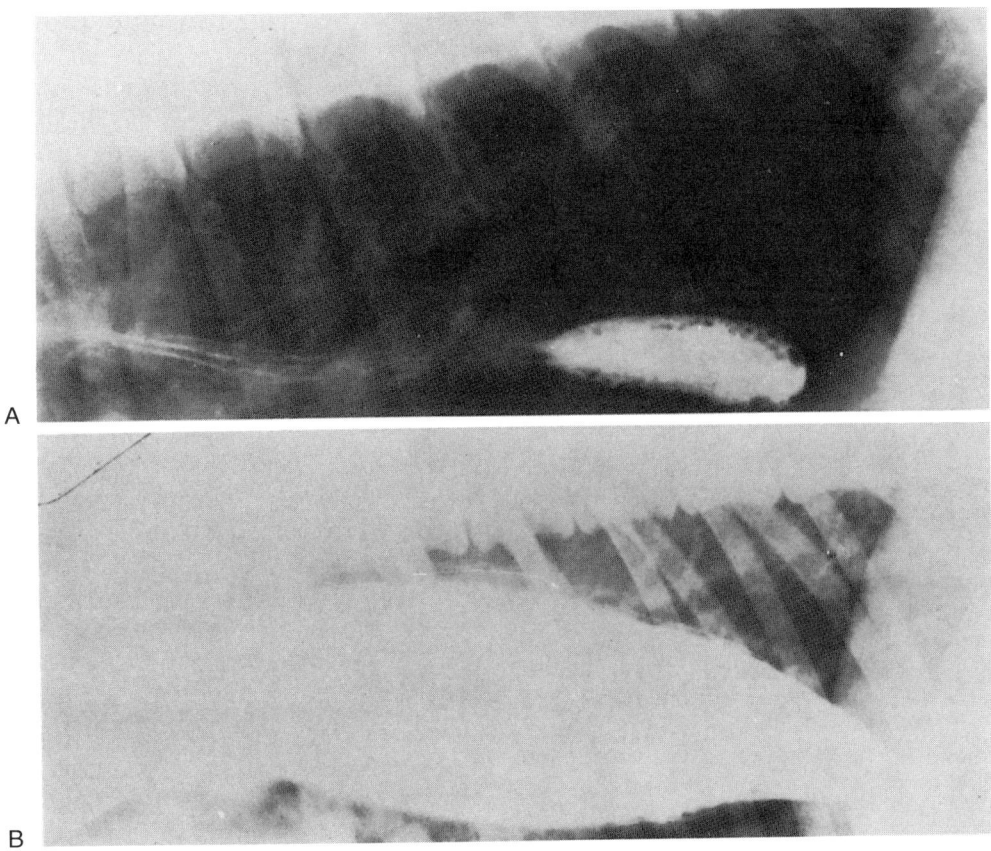

FIG. 7. Barium swallow radiologic examination of the lower thoracic esophagus in a control (**A**) and acrylamide-affected (**B**) dog. There is marked dilatation of the esophagus in the animal with acrylamide-induced neuropathy. (From Satchell and McLeod, ref. 85. Reprinted with permission.)

pressure changes in the isolated carotid sinus because the buffering effect of the vagally innervated intrathoracic baroreceptors is lost (81).

Recordings from the renal nerves of control dogs contain pulse-synchronous bursts of sympathetic activity that are not abolished when carotid sinus pressure is maintained at a constant level. In acrylamide-treated dogs, pulse-synchronous renal sympathetic activity is abolished by constant pressure in the carotid sinuses because of involvement of the intrathoracic baroreceptors or their afferent fibers, or both, in the vagus nerves (83). Additional evidence of abnormalities of both carotid sinus and intrathoracic baroreceptor function in rabbits with mild acrylamide-induced neuropathy has been found by making direct recordings from the glossopharyngeal and depressor nerves during alterations of intravascular volume (Fig. 6). Baroreceptor nerve activity is reduced during diastole, and the threshold for aortic arch baroreceptors is increased (84).

The decline in mesenteric vascular conductance that takes place following electrical stimulation of the splanchnic nerve or infusion of the indirectly acting sympathomimetic drug tyramine is much smaller in severely acrylamide-poisoned cats than in controls (78). Infusion of directly acting sympathomimetics, such as phenylephrine, evokes a much greater increase in vascular resistance in affected animals than in controls. These results are consistent with the damage of postganglionic, unmyelinated vasomotor fibers that has been described in the splanchnic nerves of severely poisoned animals (80).

Respiratory System

Respiratory reflexes that are subserved by afferent fibers in the vagus nerves are affected in experimental canine acrylamide-induced neuropathy. The sensitivity of the Hering-Breuer reflex is diminished (82). This reflex is mediated via slowly adapting lung stretch receptors, impulses from which are conveyed in relatively large, myelinated vagal afferent fibers (69). In acrylamide-induced neuropathy, the threshold of these receptors is increased, but the firing rate and number of functioning units is decreased (45). The cough reflex is impaired in dogs with acrylamide-induced neuropathy, probably because of degeneration of bronchopulmonary receptors or their myelinated vagal afferent nerve fibers (45). Impairment of the cough reflex in axonal neuropathies might explain the occurrence of aspiration pneumonia in patients with disorders such as alcoholic neuropathy (45). Functions that are controlled by smaller vagal myelinated and unmyelinated efferent fibers, such as sinus rhythm and bronchial smooth muscle tone, are relatively resistant to the toxic effects of acrylamide (44).

Gastrointestinal System

The vagal sensory innervation of the esophagus is also affected in canine acrylamide-induced neuropathy. A markedly dilated esophagus develops in some acrylamide-poisoned dogs (Fig. 7), and the dogs tend to regurgitate (85). The esophagus contracts when the vagus nerves are stimulated electrically (75), but abnormalities of the threshold and rate of firing of esophageal vagal afferents suggest a disorder of esophageal stretch receptors or of the distal segments of the esophageal sensory fibers (86).

EXPERIMENTAL ALLERGIC NEURITIS

The clinical, pathologic, and electrophysiologic features of experimental allergic neuritis (EAN), produced by injections of peripheral nerve tissue and adjuvants (100), closely resemble those of acute idiopathic polyneuritis in humans (Guillain-Barré syndrome) (8), in which the autonomic nervous system may be affected (12,61,64,74,98). Clinical signs of autonomic involvement in EAN are usually apparent only in severely affected animals, in some of which urinary and fecal incontinence develops in addition to limb weakness (55).

In EAN, the vagus and splanchnic nerves show lesions similar to but less severe than those found in the peripheral nerves (55,66,94,99) (Figs. 8 and 9). Affected nerves exhibit evidence of demyelination, remyelination, and axonal degeneration. Around small blood vessels, there are infiltrates of plasma cells, lymphocytes, mononuclear cells, and occasional polymorphonuclear cells. Degeneration of unmyelinated fibers has been found in the splanchnic nerves of rats with EAN but not in the cervical sympathetic nerves (66,99) (Fig. 10).

In vitro conduction studies of the vagus and splanchnic nerves of animals with EAN have revealed slowing of conduction and dispersion of the myelinated-fiber action potentials that are consistent with demyelination (94,99). The

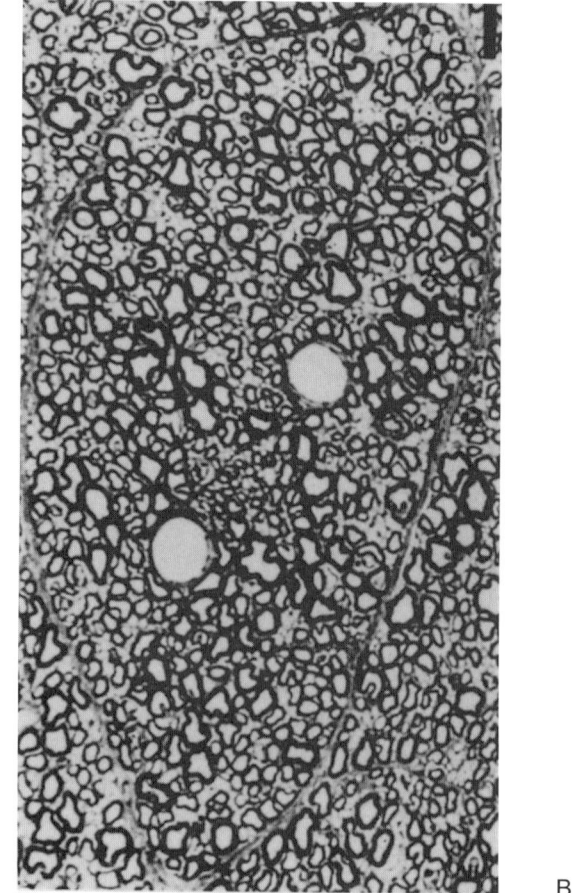 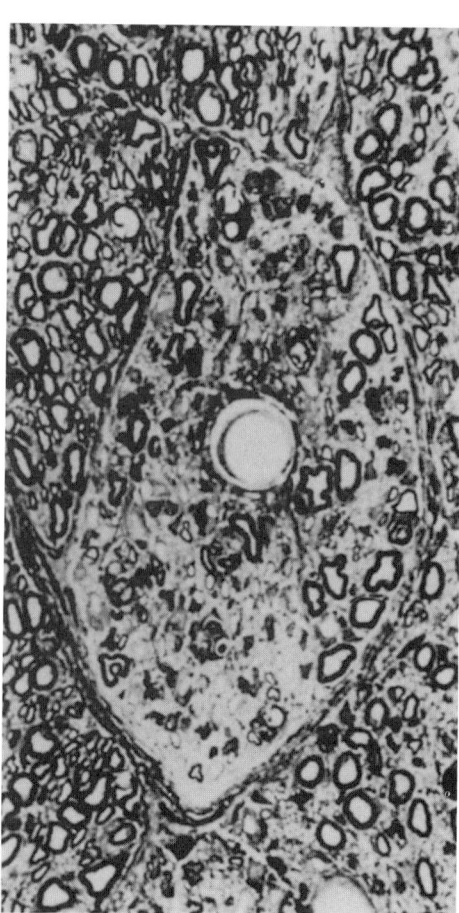

FIG. 8. Cervical vagus nerve from control guinea pig (**A**) and guinea pig with experimental allergic neuritis (**B**). In the latter, there is a loss of myelinated fibers in the center fascicle. Scale = 5 m. (From Tuck et al., ref. 99. Reprinted with permission of Oxford University Press.)

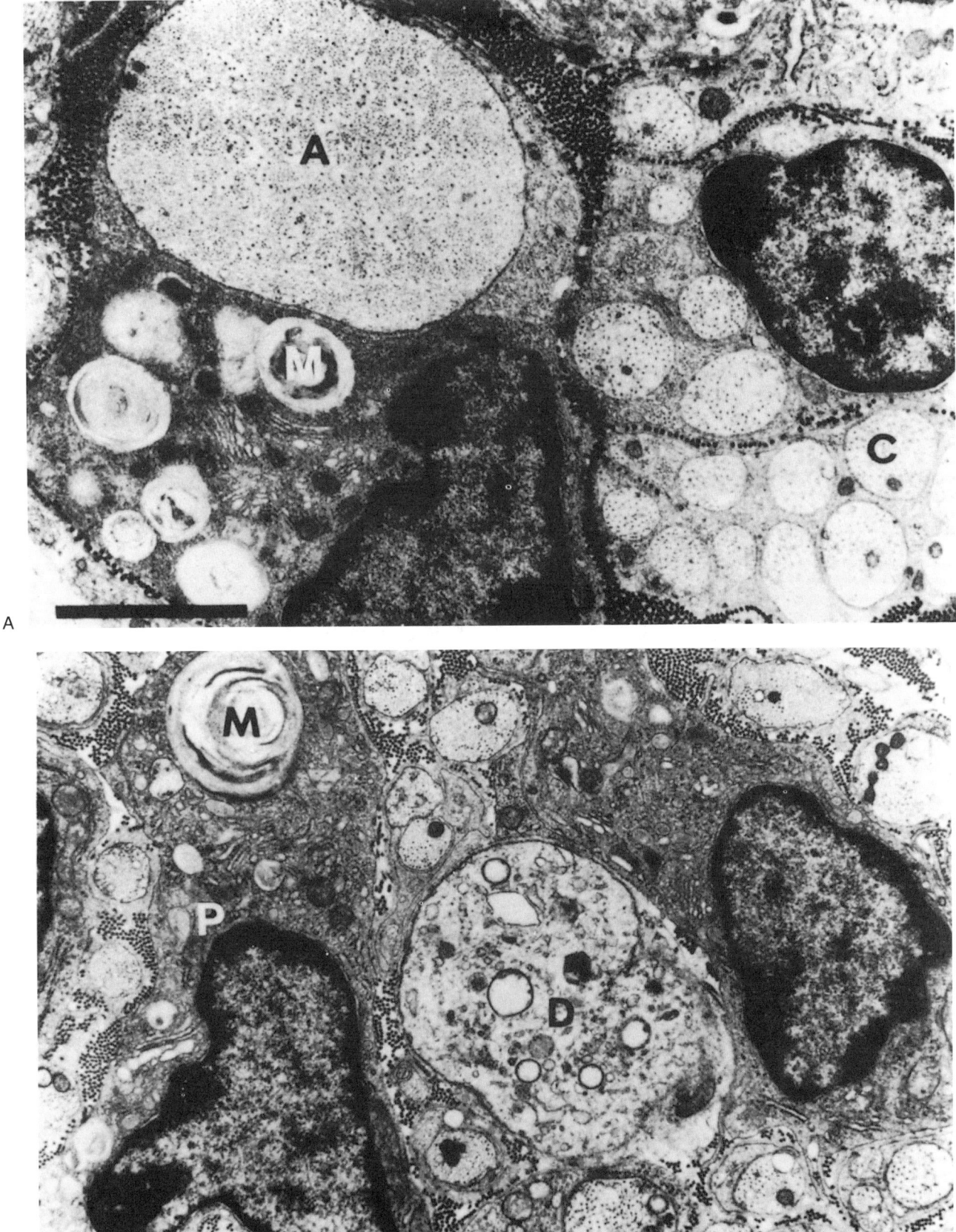

FIG. 9. A, B: Greater splanchnic nerve from a guinea pig with experimental allergic neuritis, showing demyelinated axons (A), degenerating axons (D), myelin debris (M), phagocytic cell (P), and unmyelinated axons (C). Scale = 5 m. (From Tuck et al., ref. 99. Reprinted with permission of Oxford University Press.)

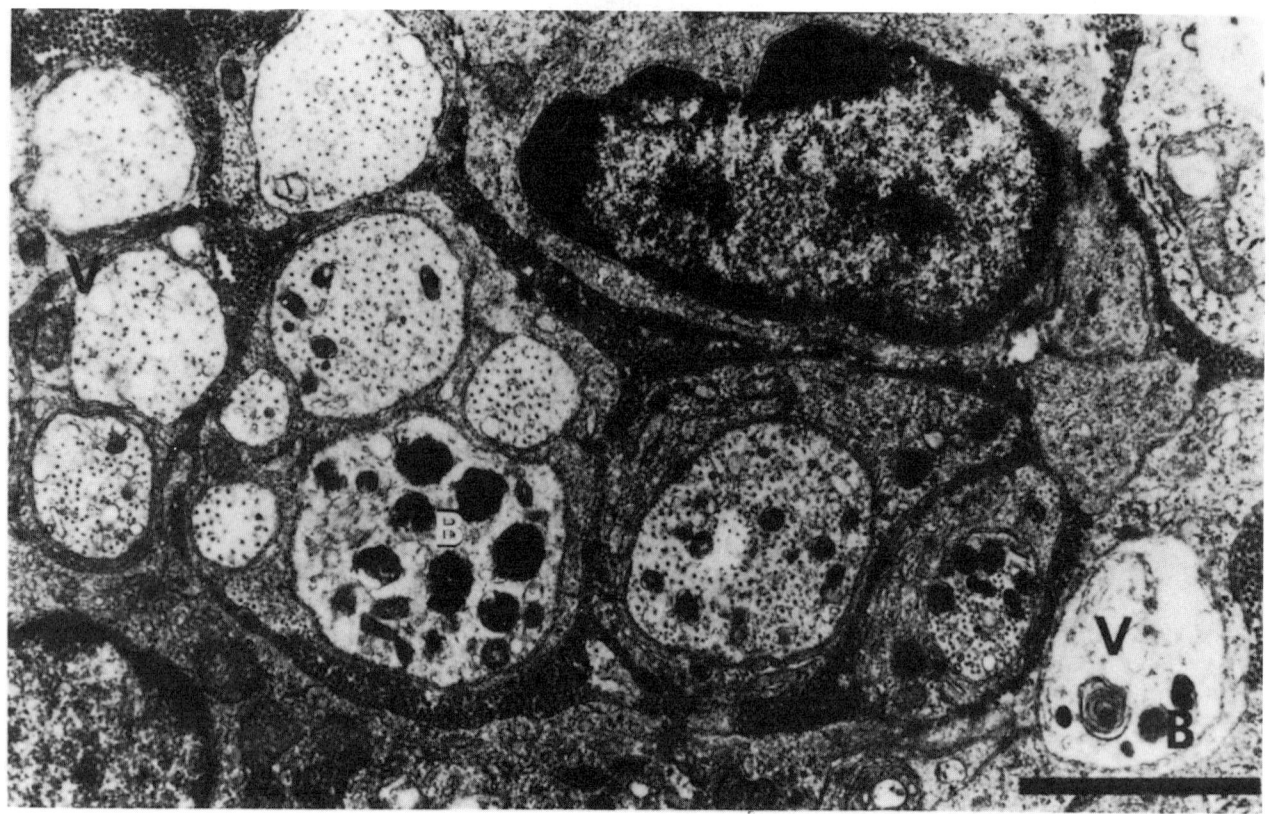

FIG. 10. Axonal degeneration affecting unmyelinated fibers in the greater splanchnic nerve of a guinea pig with experimental allergic neuritis. *B*, electron dense bodies; *V*, vesicles. Scale = 5 m. (From Tuck et al., ref. 99. Reprinted with permission of Oxford University Press.)

unmyelinated-fiber component of the compound nerve action potential is normal in the vagus but is reduced in amplitude in the splanchnic nerves of guinea pigs with EAN (99). Variation in RR interval is decreased in rats with EAN (94); the same abnormality has been observed in patients with acute idiopathic polyneuritis and reflects involvement of the cardiac parasympathetic fibers in the vagus nerves (77).

6-HYDROXYDOPAMINE SYMPATHECTOMY

Injection of 6-hydroxydopamine (6-OHDA) into rodents causes a widespread sympathectomy that is an experimental model of adrenergic neuronal damage. Treated animals exhibit ptosis, weight loss, diarrhea, hypotension, and decreased survival rates (23). Administration of 6-OHDA to adult rodents produces a short-lasting but extensive sympathectomy (34). In contrast, administration to newborn animals produces a less complete but permanent sympathectomy (35).

6-Hydroxydopamine selectively destroys postganglionic noradrenergic sympathetic nerves (23). In adult animals, only the terminal portion of the adrenergic axon is damaged. Rapid regeneration of this portion is responsible for the transient nature of 6-OHDA sympathectomy in mature animals (35). In newborn animals, recovery and regeneration are not possible because the nerve-cell bodies of postganglionic noradrenergic fibers are destroyed by 6-OHDA (3,4,70).

The results of physiologic studies of animals treated with 6-OHDA are consistent with a disorder affecting postganglionic noradrenergic sympathetic axons. Total sympathetic stimulation, selective stimulation of the sympathetic nerve supply to mesenteric blood vessels, and intravenously administered tyramine evoke much less vasoconstriction in treated animals than in controls (23,35). Contractions of the lower eyelid, the vas deferens, and the sympathetically innervated anococcygeus muscle in rodents are also diminished or abolished by 6-OHDA (33,34,35,36,37,39).

GUANETHIDINE-INDUCED SYMPATHECTOMY

Parenterally administered guanethidine generates almost complete sympathectomy in newborn and adult rats (3, 20,30), with little or no effect on parasympathetic, enteric, or peripheral nerves (42,43). Treatment of adult and immature rodents with guanethidine produces total or nearly total loss of sympathetic adrenergic nerve fibers (20,31). In the superior cervical ganglion, destruction of almost all

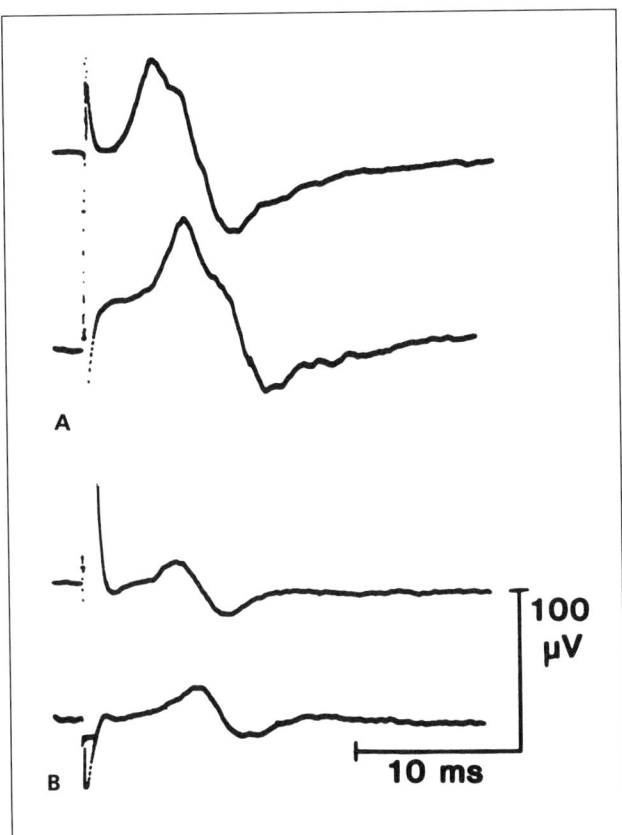

FIG. 11. C-fiber potentials recorded at two sites in vitro from unmyelinated cranial sympathetic chains of (**A**) a control rat and (**B**) a rat treated with guanethidine. The amplitude in the latter is less than half that in the control animal. (From Zochodne et al., ref. 109. Reprinted with permission.)

cell bodies is accompanied by an inflammatory cell infiltrate (20,49,109), and there is extensive degeneration of axons in the cervical sympathetic trunk (20,106). Surviving sympathetic ganglion cells contain damaged mitochondria and swollen endoplasmic reticulum (6,20,49). These effects are immunologically mediated (53), probably by natural killer cells (46).

Rats with guanethidine-induced sympathectomy have reduced survival, decreased weight gain, relatively low BP, ptosis, and diarrhea (10,50,109). Except in the brain, tissue concentrations of norepinephrine are reduced to as low as 2% of control levels (37,50). Vascular resistance is decreased in peripheral nerves, and smooth muscle contraction in blood vessels and the vas deferens in response to electrical stimulation of sympathetic nerves is impaired (32, 50,54,107). The pressor response to intravenously administered norepinephrine and neuropeptide Y is exaggerated, and that to tyramine is attenuated (10). The amplitude of the C-fiber action potential recorded from the cervical sympathetic trunk is diminished (Fig. 11), whereas that from the vagus is unaffected (109). These findings are all consistent with the selective destruction of adrenergic postganglionic nerve fibers that is seen in histologic studies.

SYMPATHECTOMY INDUCED BY ANTIBODIES TO NERVE GROWTH FACTOR

Nerve growth factor (NGF) is a protein that can be extracted from mouse sarcomas, snake venom, and mouse salivary glands, and it is present in trace amounts in the serum of mammals, including humans. Nerve growth factor promotes growth of embryonic sensory nerve cells and of sympathetic nerve cells of embryonic, newborn, and adult animals (58). The administration of antiserum specific for NGF to newborn animals results in irreversible and almost complete loss of sympathetic ganglia and axons (immunosympathectomy) (1,60). In adult animals, anti-NGF serum causes a reversible reduction in the size of sympathetic ganglia caused by neuronal shrinkage, along with temporary sympathetic denervation of peripheral tissues (1,5). There is loss of adrenergic nerve fibers and norepinephrine content from organs such as the heart and from vascular smooth muscle, but not from the vas deferens (13,40,59,106).

Immunosympathectomized rats and mice do not have decreased survival or other clinical abnormalities apart from enophthalmos, ptosis, and miosis (18,60). Increased mortality has been observed in rabbits (52) and guinea pigs (51) with raised levels of anti-NGF antibodies, presumably because a more pronounced immunosympathectomy is induced by active autoimmunity. The resting BP of immunosympathectomized animals is lower than normal and the pressor response to norepinephrine is exaggerated, consistent with sympathetic vasomotor denervation (18,105, 106). There is no vasoconstriction in response to electrical stimulation of the sympathetic nerve supply of the hindlimb blood vessels (18), nor is there contraction of the anococcygeus muscle when its adrenergic nerve supply is stimulated (39). The resting neurogram recorded from the sympathetic chains of immunosympathectomized rats is markedly reduced compared with that of controls, as is the magnitude of the response to asphyxia (17). However, even 12 months of NGF deprivation by repeated anti-NGF administration fails to produce the typical diabetic signs of neuroaxonal dystrophy in prevertebral ganglia or ileal mesenteric nerves (93).

SYMPATHECTOMY INDUCED BY ANTIBODIES TO ACETYLCHOLINESTERASE

A complement-dependent sympathectomy that selectively affects preganglionic sympathetic fibers has been reported recently (16) (Fig. 12). Monoclonal antibodies to acetylcholinesterase (AChE), injected intravenously into rats, produce signs of transient sympathetic overactivity (exophthalmos, piloerection, tachycardia, and hypertension) that are followed within hours by longer-lasting or even permanent signs of sympathetic failure (ptosis, bradycardia, and hypotension). Presynaptic electrical stimula-

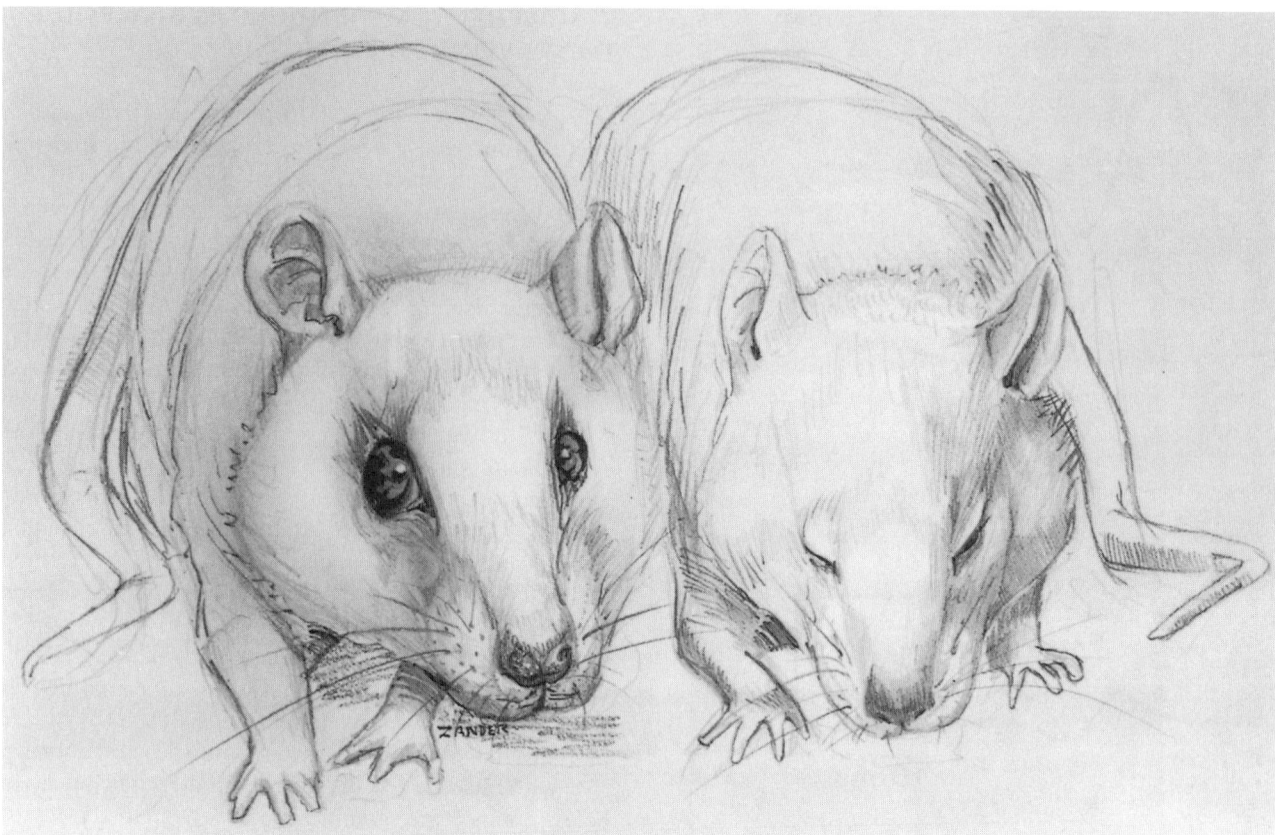

FIG. 12. Signs of autonomic dysfunction in experimental AChE autoimmunity. Severe eyelid drooping (*right*) appears within 4 hours of an intravenous injection of AChE antibodies and persists indefinitely, usually for the life of the rat. The rats retain grossly normal musculoskeletal function but exhibit long-lasting hypotension and bradycardia.

tion of the superior cervical ganglion of treated rats evokes no contraction of eyelid smooth muscle or action potentials in ganglionic neurons, but responses to direct electrical and pharmacologic stimulation of the ganglion are maintained.

In rats treated with AChE antibodies, there is a marked reduction in choline acetyltransferase (ChAT) activity in most sympathetic ganglia and in the adrenal medulla. Levels of total AChE activity are less severely reduced, but histochemistry reveals a nearly total loss of activity in the neuropil of the superior cervical ganglion and in the adrenal medulla. This change and the loss of ChAT activity both imply a selective loss of preganglionic fibers, which has been confirmed by electron microscopy.

Cholinergic motor and parasympathetic vagal fibers appear to be unaffected or only marginally affected in this model of preganglionic sympathectomy. Levels of ChAT in skeletal muscle and the cardiac atria are not diminished in treated animals, and electrical stimulation of the vagus nerves causes bradycardia and asystole with normal frequency-dependence.

Examination of the intermediolateral spinal cord reveals neuropathologic changes consistent with the irreversible sympathetic deficit induced by AChE antibodies (15). In particular, the thoracic intermediolateral spinal cord shows a loss of neurons immunopositive for ChAT or nitric oxide synthase. Neuronal loss is also seen in Nissl-stained preparations. The deficit develops slowly but approaches 70% at 4 months after antibody treatment. This feature resembles the spinal cord pathology in multiple-systems atrophy.

Global alteration of adrenergic function in the antibody-induced preganglionic sympathectomy includes a large decrease in stress-induced catecholamine release (14). However, as in patients with multiple-systems atrophy, there is little or no change in urinary excretion of noradrenaline, adrenaline, or catecholamine metabolites. This finding may imply that a large fraction of basal catecholamine output, both in rodents and humans, reflects transmitter release in the absence of nerve activity.

AUTONOMIC NEUROPATHY INDUCED BY SYMPATHETIC CHAIN ANTIGENS WITH ADJUVANT

Rabbits injected with a mixture of either emulsion or extract of human sympathetic chain and complete Freund's adjuvant have abnormal cutaneous vasomotor control characterized by an inability to increase earlobe temperature in response to direct heating of the skin of the back (7). This reflex is probably mediated by efferent sympathetic, cholinergic vasodilator fibers. The sympathetic chains and perivascular and sciatic nerves of treated animals contain infiltrates of lymphocytes and macrophages. There is no evidence of destruction of myelinated or unmyelinated nerve fibers, although there is a relative increase in the number of small unmyelinated fibers, consistent with regeneration (9). It is unlikely that the lesions in the sympathetic nerves cause the abnormalities of cutaneous blood flow, because similar but more severe changes are found in the sympathetic nerves in EAN, in which vasomotor control in the ear is normal (9). It has been suggested that this experimental disorder, called *experimental autonomic neuropathy*, may be a model of acute pandysautonomia. However, the lack of clinical evidence of a generalized autonomic disorder in these animals suggests that there is not a close analogy with the human disease.

REFERENCES

1. Aguayo AJ, et al. Effects of nerve growth factor antiserum on peripheral unmyelinated nerve fibers. *Acta Neuropathol (Berl)* 1972; 20:288–298.
2. Anderson LC, et al. Effects of streptozotocin-induced diabetes on sympathetic and parasympathetic stimulation of parotid salivary gland function in rats. *Diabetes* 1989;38:1381–1389.
3. Angeletti PU. Chemical sympathectomy in newborn animals. *Neuropharmacology* 1971;10:55–59.
4. Angeletti PU, et al. Sympathetic nerve cell destruction in newborn animals by 6-hydroxydopamine. *Proc Natl Acad Sci U S A* 1970; 65:114–121.
5. Angeletti PU, et al. Analysis of the effects of the antiserum to the nerve growth factor in adult mice. *Brain Res* 1971;27:343–355.
6. Angeletti PU, et al. Structural and ultrastructural changes in developing sympathetic ganglion induced by guanethidine. *Brain Res* 1972;43:515–525.
7. Appenzeller O, et al. Experimental autonomic neuropathy: an immunologically induced disorder of reflex vasomotor function. *J Neurol Neurosurg Psychiatry* 1965;28:510–515.
8. Arnason BGW, et al. Animal models of acute inflammatory polyradiculoneuropathy. In: Dyck PJ, et al., ed. *Peripheral Neuropathy*. 3rd ed. Philadelphia: WB Saunders; 1993:1466–1473.
9. Becker W, et al. Experimental autonomic neuropathy: ultrastructural and immunohistochemical study of a disorder of reflex vasomotor function. *J Auton Nerv Syst* 1979;1:53–67.
10. Benarroch EE, et al. Noradrenergic and neuropeptide Y mechanisms in guanethidine-sympathectomized rats. *Am J Physiol* 1990;259: R371–R375.
11. Bennett T, et al. Baroreflex sensitivity and responses to the Valsalva manoeuvre in subjects with diabetes mellitus. *J Neurol Neurosurg Psychiatry* 1976;39:178–183.
12. Birchfield RI, et al. Postural hypotension in the Guillain-Barré syndrome. *Arch Neurol* 1964;10:149–157.
13. Bjerre B, et al. A study of the de- and regenerative changes in the sympathetic nervous system of the adult mouse after treatment with the antiserum to nerve growth factor. *Brain Res* 1975;92:257–278.
14. Brimijoin S, et al. Catecholamine release and excretion in rats with immunologically induced preganglionic sympathectomy. *J Neurochem* 1994;62:2195–2204.
15. Brimijoin S, et al. Death of intermediolateral spinal cord neurons follows selective, complement-mediated destruction of their preganglionic sympathetic terminals by cholinesterase antibodies. *Neuroscience* 1993;54:201–223.
16. Brimijoin S, et al. Autoimmune preganglionic sympathectomy induced by acetylcholinesterase antibodies. *Proc Natl Acad Sci U S A* 1990;87:9630–9634.
17. Brody MJ. Electrical activity in sympathetic nerves of immunologically sympathectomized rats. *Proc Soc Exp Biol Med* 1963;114: 565–567.
18. Brody MJ. Cardiovascular responses following immunological sympathectomy. *Circ Res* 1964;15:161–167.
19. Brody MJ, et al. Vascular reactivity in experimental diabetes mellitus. *Circ Res* 1964;14:494–501.
20. Burnstock G, et al. A new method of destroying adrenergic nerves in adult animals using guanethidine. *Br J Pharmacol* 1971;43:295–301.
21. Chang KSK, et al. Alterations in the baroreceptor reflex control of heart rate in streptozotocin diabetic rats. *J Mol Cell Cardiol* 1986; 18:617–624.
22. Christlieb AR. Diabetes and hypertensive vascular disease: mechanisms and treatment. *Am J Cardiol* 1973;32:592–606.
23. Clark DWJ, et al. Long-lasting peripheral and central effects of 6-hydroxydopamine in rats. *Br J Pharmacol* 1972;44: 233–243.
24. Dail W, et al. Abnormalities in pelvic visceral nerves: a basis for neurogenic bladder in the diabetic Chinese hamster. *Invest Urol* 1977;15:161–166.
25. Diani A, et al. A study of the morphological changes in the small intestine of the spontaneously diabetic Chinese hamster. *Diabetologia* 1976;12:101–109.
26. Diani A, et al. Autonomic neuropathy associated with the small intestine and abdominal sympathetic trunk of the ketotic diabetic Chinese hamster. *Diabetes* 1978;27:435(abst).
27. Diani A, et al. Radiologic abnormalities and autonomic neuropathology in the digestive tract of the ketonuric diabetic Chinese hamster. *Diabetologia* 1979;17:33–40.
28. Diani A, et al. Morphometric analysis of the vagus nerve in nondiabetic and ketonuric diabetic Chinese hamsters. *J Comp Pathol* 1984; 94:495–504.
29. Diani AR, et al. Islet innervation of non-diabetic and diabetic Chinese hamsters. I. Acetylcholinesterase histochemistry and norepinephrine fluorescence. *J Neural Transm* 1983;56: 223–238.
30. Eranko L, et al. Effect of guanethidine on nerve cells and small intensely fluorescent cells in sympathetic ganglia of newborn and adult rats. *Acta Pharmacol Toxicol* 1971;30:403–416.
31. Eranko O, et al. Histochemical evidence of chemical sympathectomy by guanethidine in newborn rats. *Histochem J* 1971;3:451–456.
32. Evans B, et al. Long-lasting supersensitivity of the rat vas deferens to norepinephrine after chronic guanethidine administration. *J Pharmacol Exp Ther* 1973;185:60–69.
33. Ewing DJ, et al. Heart rate changes in diabetes mellitus. *Lancet* 1981;1:183–186.
34. Finch L, et al. Rapid recovery of vascular adrenergic nerves in the rat after chemical sympathectomy with 6-hydroxydopamine. *Br J Pharmacol* 1973;48:59–72.
35. Finch L, et al. A comparison of the effects of chemical sympathectomy by 6-hydroxydopamine in newborn and adult rats. *Br J Pharmacol* 1973;47:249–260.
36. Furness JB, et al. Cellular studies of sympathetic denervation produced by 6-hydroxydopamine in the vas deferens. *J Pharmacol Exp Ther* 1970;174:111–122.
37. Gannon BJ, et al. Prolonged effects of chronic guanethidine treatment on the sympathetic innervation of the genitalia of male rats. *Med J Aust* 1971;2:207–208.
38. Gartner J, et al. Experimental autonomic neuropathy in the choroid of streptozotocin diabetic rats. *Retina* 1989;9:49–58.
39. Gibson A, et al. The effect of immunosympathectomy and 6-hydroxydopamine on the responses of the rat anococcygeus to nerve stimulation and to some drugs. *Br J Pharmacol* 1973;47:261–267.
40. Hamberger BR, et al. Monoamines in immunosympathectomized rats. *Int J Neuropharmacol* 1965;4:91–95.
41. Hart JL, et al. Adrenergic nerve function and contractile activity of the caudal artery of the streptozotocin diabetic rat. *J Auton Nerv Syst* 1988;25:49–57.
42. Heath JW, et al. Degeneration of adrenergic neurons following guanethidine treatment: an ultrastructural study. *Virchows Arch B* 1972;11:182–197.
43. Heath JW, et al. Selectivity of neuronal degeneration produced by chronic guanethidine treatment. *J Neurocytol* 1977;6: 397–405.

44. Hersch M, et al. Breathing pattern, lung inflation reflex and airway tone in acrylamide neuropathy. *Respir Physiol* 1989;76:257–276.
45. Hersch MI. Abnormal pulmonary slowly adapting receptors in canine acrylamide neuropathy. *J Appl Physiol* 1986;60:376–384.
46. Hickey WF, et al. Exogenously induced, natural killer cell-mediated neuronal killing: a novel pathogenetic mechanism. *J Exp Med* 1992;176:811–817.
47. Hopkins AP, et al. Conduction in unmyelinated fibres in experimental neuropathy. *J Neurol Neurosurg Psychiatry* 1972;35:163–169.
48. Jackson CV, et al. Influence of short-term experimental diabetes on blood pressure and heart rate in response to norepinephrine and angiotensin II in the conscious rat. *J Cardiovasc Pharmacol* 1983;5:260–265.
49. Jensen-Holm J, et al. Ultrastructural changes in the rat superior cervical ganglion following prolonged guanethidine administration. *Acta Pharmacol Toxicol* 1971;30:308–320.
50. Johnson E, et al. Biochemical and functional evaluation of the sympathectomy produced by the administration of guanethidine to newborn rats. *J Pharmacol Exp Ther* 1975;193:503–512.
51. Johnson EM, et al. Dorsal root ganglion neurons are destroyed by exposure in utero to maternal antibody to nerve growth factor. *Science* 1980;210:916–918.
52. Johnson EM, et al. Effects of autoimmune NGF deprivation in the adult rabbit and offspring. *Brain Res* 1982;240:131–140.
53. Johnson EM, et al. Guanethidine-induced destruction of sympathetic neurons. *Int Rev Neurol* 1984;25:1–37.
54. Johnson EM, et al. Modification and characterization of the permanent sympathectomy produced by the administration of guanethidine to newborn rats. *Eur J Pharmacol* 1976;37:45–54.
55. Kalimo H, et al. Involvement of autonomic nervous system in experimental allergic neuritis. A light- and electron-microscope study. *J Neuroimmunol* 1982;2:9–19.
56. Kudlacz EM, et al. Diabetes and diuretic-induced alterations in function of rat urinary bladder. *Diabetes* 1988;37:949–955.
57. Lamey P-J, et al. The effects of diabetes and autonomic neuropathy on parotid salivary flow in man. *Diabet Med* 1986;3:537–540.
58. Levi-Montalcini A, et al. Nerve growth factor. *Physiol Rev* 1968;48:534–569.
59. Levi-Montalcini R, et al. Noradrenaline and monoamine oxidase content in immunosympathectomized animals. *Int J Neuropharmacol* 1962;1:161–164.
60. Levi-Montalcini R, et al. Immunosympathectomy. *Pharmacol Rev* 1966;18:619–628.
61. Lichtenfeld P. Autonomic dysfunction in the Guillain-Barré syndrome. *Am J Med* 1971;50:772–780.
62. Low PA, et al. The sympathetic nervous system in diabetic neuropathy—a clinical and pathological study. *Brain* 1975;98:341–356.
63. Luiten PGM, et al. Autonomic innervation of the pancreas in diabetic and non-diabetic rats. A new view on intraneural sympathetic structural organization. *J Auton Nerv Syst* 1986;15:33–44.
64. Matsuyama H, et al. Distribution of lesions in the Landry-Guillain-Barré syndrome with emphasis on involvement of the sympathetic system. *Acta Neuropathol (Berl)* 1967;8:230–241.
65. McEwen TAJ, et al. Microcomputer collection and analysis of RR-interval in the BB-rat. *Comp Biol Med* 1989;19:443–452.
66. Morey MK, et al. Autonomic nerves in experimental allergic neuritis in the rat. *Acta Neuropathol (Berl)* 1985;67.
67. Mueller SM, et al. Sympathetic and vascular dysfunction in early experimental juvenile diabetes mellitus. *Am J Physiol* 1982;243:H139–H144.
68. Nowak TV, et al. Evidence for abnormal cholinergic neuromuscular transmission in diabetic rat small intestine. *Gastroenterology* 1986;91:124–132.
69. Paintal AS. The conduction velocities of respiratory and cardiovascular afferent fibres in the vagus nerve. *J Physiol (Lond)* 1953;121:341–359.
70. Papka RE. The ultrastructure of adrenergic neurons in sympathetic ganglion of the newborn rabbit after treatment with 6-hydroxydopamine. *Am J Anat* 1973;137:447–466.
71. Paro M, et al. Autonomic neuropathy in BB rats and alterations in bladder function. *Diabetes* 1989;38:1023–1030.
72. Paro M, et al. Experimental diabetes in the rat: alterations in the vesical function. *J Auton Nerv Syst* 1987;21:59–66.
73. Patel DG. Role of sympathetic nervous system in glucagon response to insulin hypoglycemia in normal and diabetic rats. *Diabetes* 1984;33:1154–1159.
74. Persson A, et al. RR interval in Guillain-Barré syndrome: a test of autonomic dysfunction. *Acta Neurol Scand* 1983;67:294–300.
75. Post EJ. Unmyelinated nerve fibers in feline acrylamide neuropathy. *Acta Neuropathol (Berl)* 1978;42:19–24.
76. Post EJ, et al. Experimental autonomic neuropathy. *Proc Aust Assoc Neurol* 1973;10:109–115.
77. Post EJ, et al. Acrylamide autonomic neuropathy in the cat. Part 1. Neurophysiological and histological studies. *J Neurol Sci* 1977;33:353–374.
78. Post EJ, et al. Acrylamide autonomic neuropathy in the cat. Part 2. Effects on mesenteric vascular control. *J Neurol Sci* 1977;33:375–385.
79. Robertson D, et al. Diabetic neuropathy in the mutant mouse [C57 BL/ks (db/db)]. A morphometric study. *Diabetes* 1980;29:60–67.
80. Satchell PM, et al. Abnormalities in the vagus nerve in canine acrylamide neuropathy. *J Neurol Neursurg Psychiatry* 1982;45:609–619.
81. Satchell PM. Circulatory control in canine acrylamide neuropathy. *J Auton Nerv Syst* 1984;10:93–106.
82. Satchell PM. Reversible abnormalities of the Hering-Breuer reflex in acrylamide neuropathy. *J Neurol Neurosurg Psychiatry* 1985;48:670–675.
83. Satchell PM. Abnormalities of sympathetic vasomotor tone in distal axonal neuropathy. *J Neurol Sci* 1989;90:251–261.
84. Satchell PM. Baroreceptor dysfunction in acrylamide axonal neuropathy. *Brain* 1990;113:167–176.
85. Satchell PM, et al. Megaoesophagus due to acrylamide neuropathy. *J Neurol Neurosurg Psychiatry* 1981;44:906–913.
86. Satchell PM, et al. Abnormalities of oesophageal mechanoreceptors in canine acrylamide neuropathy. *J Neurol Neurosurg Psychiatry* 1984;47:692–698.
87. Schmidt RE, et al. Ultrastructural and immunohistochemical characterization of autonomic neuropathy in genetically diabetic Chinese hamsters. *Lab Invest* 1989;61:77–92.
88. Schmidt RE, et al. Experimental diabetic autonomic neuropathy. *Am J Pathol* 1981;103:210–225.
89. Schmidt RE, et al. Ultrastructural and biochemical characterization of autonomic neuropathy in rats with chronic streptozotocin diabetes. *J Neuropathol Exp Neurol* 1986;45:524–544.
90. Schmidt RE, et al. Acrylamide-induced sympathetic autonomic neuropathy resulting in pineal denervation. *Lab Invest* 1987;56:505–517.
91. Schmidt RE, et al. Experimental diabetic autonomic neuropathy. Characterization in streptozotocin-diabetic Sprague-Dawley rats. *Lab Invest* 1983;49:538–552.
92. Schmidt RE, et al. Axonal dystrophy in experimental diabetic autonomic neuropathy. *Diabetes* 1982;31:761–770.
93. Shroer JA, et al. Effect of chronic autoimmune nerve growth factor deprivation on sympathetic neuroaxonal dystrophy in rats. *Synapse* 1995;20:249–256.
94. Solders G, et al. Autonomic dysfunction in experimental allergic neuritis. *Acta Neurol Scand* 1985;72:18–25.
95. Sterman AB. Acrylamide-induced remodelling of perikarya in rat superior cervical ganglia. *Neuropathol Appl Neurobiol* 1984;10:221–234.
96. Sterman AB, et al. Autonomic cardiovascular dysfunction accompanies sensory-motor impairment during acrylamide intoxication. *Neurotoxicology* 1983;4:45–52.
97. Stuesse SL, et al. Vagal control of heart period in alloxan diabetic rats. *Life Sci* 1982;31:393–398.
98. Tuck RR, et al. Autonomic dysfunction in the Landry-Guillain-Barré syndrome. *J Neurol Neurosurg Psychiatry* 1982;44:983–990.
99. Tuck RR, et al. Autonomic neuropathy in experimental allergic neuritis. An electrophysiological and histological study. *Brain* 1981;104:187–208.
100. Waksman BH, et al. Allergic neuritis: an experimental disease of rabbits induced by the injection of peripheral nervous tissue and adjuvants. *J Exp Med* 1955;102:213–236.
101. Yagihashi S, et al. Diabetic autonomic neuropathy in the BB rat. Ultrastructural and morphometric changes in sympathetic nerves. *Diabetes* 1985;34:558–564.

102. Yagihashi S, et al. Diabetic autonomic neuropathy: the distribution of structural changes in sympathetic nerves in the BB rat. *Am J Pathol* 1985;121:138–147.
103. Yagihashi S, et al. Diabetic autonomic neuropathy in BB rat. Ultrastructural and morphometric changes in parasympathetic nerves. *Diabetes* 1986;35:733–743.
104. Yagihashi S, et al. Neuroaxonal and dendritic dystrophy in diabetic neuropathy. Classification and topographic distribution in the BB-rat. *J Neuropathol Exp Neurol* 1986;45:545–565.
105. Zaimis E. The immunosympathectomized animal: a valuable tool in physiological and pharmacological research. *J Physiol (Lond)* 1964;177:35–37.
106. Zaimis E, et al. Biochemical and functional changes in the sympathetic nervous system of rats treated with nerve growth factor antiserum. *Nature* 1972;206:1220–1222.
107. Zochodne DW, et al. Guanethidine-induced adrenergic sympathectomy augments endoneurial perfusion and lowers endoneurial microvascular resistance. *Brain Res* 1990;519:112–117.
108. Zochodne DW, et al. Adrenergic sympathectomy ablates unmyelinated fibers in the rat "preganglionic" cervical sympathetic trunk. *Brain Res* 1989;498:221–228.
109. Zochodne DW, et al. Guanethidine adrenergic neuropathy: an animal model of selective autonomic neuropathy. *Brain Res* 1988;461:10–16.

SECTION III
Clinical Disorders of Autonomic Function

CHAPTER 32

Central Disorders of Autonomic Function

Eduardo E. Benarroch

1. Stroke, seizures, or other disorders affecting the cortical autonomic areas or the amygdala can produce cardiac arrhythmias, some of them life-threatening. Strokes can also produce contralateral hyperhidrosis, Horner's syndrome, and uninhibited bladder. Complex partial seizures may manifest with sudomotor, vasomotor, gastrointestinal, or respiratory phenomena.
2. Hypothalamic disorders commonly produce hypothermia. Wernicke's encephalopathy should be suspected in alcoholic or malnourished patients presenting with hypothermia. Other causes include multiple sclerosis, head trauma, and toluene toxicity. Episodic hyperhidrosis with hypothermia may occur with agenesis of the corpus callosum or with other lesions affecting the anterior hypothalamus. Periodic hypothermia can also occur with no clear cause. The syndrome may respond to clonidine, cyproheptadine, or oxybutynin.
3. Severe head trauma with diffuse axonal injury, acute hydrocephalus complicating subarachnoid hemorrhage, or tumors in the region of the third ventricle may produce paroxysmal autonomic hyperactivity with tachycardia, hypertension, hyperhidrosis, hypo- or hyperthermia, and other manifestations of excessive sympathetic discharge. This syndrome may respond to bromocriptine, opioids, or drainage of the hydrocephalus.
4. The neuroleptic malignant syndrome consists of hyperthermia, rigidity, and autonomic hyperactivity and is most often triggered by high-potency antipsychotic agents. However, it can also occur in patients with Parkinson's disease upon discontinuation of L-DOPA therapy. Treatment includes discontinuation of the offending drug, fluid replacement, bromocriptine, and dantrolene. The serotonin syndrome is a combination of mental and behavioral changes, motor hyperactivity, and autonomic lability that occurs after the use of serotonin reuptake inhibitors or serotonin agonists alone or in combination with nonspecific monoamine oxidase inhibitors.
5. Fatal familial insomnia is an autosomal dominant prion disease that selectively affects the dorsomedial and anterior nuclei of the thalamus. Its manifestations are progressive intractable insomnia, motor dysfunction, and sympathetic hyperactivity.
6. Medullary lesions can produce baroreflex failure, neurogenic hypertension, orthostatic hypotension, syncope, sleep apnea, vomiting, and Horner's syndrome. Orthostatic hypotension or paroxysmal hypertension may be the major presenting manifestation of posterior fossa tumors. Syringobulbia can produce orthostatic hypotension, abnormal cardiovagal function, and baroreflex failure. Arnold-Chiari malformation can produce syncope, sleep apnea, and cardiorespiratory arrest. Transient ischemic attacks in the basilar artery territory may present with paroxysmal hypertension, before any focal neurologic deficit.
7. Spinal cord injury above the T5 level produces loss of basal sympathetic tone, which predisposes to orthostatic hypotension, poikilothermia, and cardiac arrest during tracheal suction. In chronic tetraplegics with lesions above the T5 level, stimulation of the bladder, bowel, or skin innervated by segments below the lesion may result in *autonomic dysreflexia*. Its most severe manifestation is hypertension.

continued on next page

E. E. Benarroch: Department of Neurology, Mayo Clinic, Rochester, Minnesota 55905

8. Multiple sclerosis produces prominent bladder, bowel, and sexual dysfunction, as well as subclinical abnormalities in cardiovascular sympathetic and parasympathetic function tests. Syringomyelia produces Horner's syndrome, sudomotor dysfunction, and vasomotor and trophic changes in the limbs.

9. Sympathetic hyperactivity in tetanus produces tachycardia, arrhythmias, labile hypertension, progressive and refractory hypotension, peripheral vasoconstriction, fever, and profuse sweating. The stiff-man syndrome may also manifest with hyperpyrexia, diaphoresis, hypertension, tachycardia, tachypnea, and pupillary dilatation associated with the muscle spasms.

INTRODUCTION

The areas of telencephalon, diencephalon, brain stem, and spinal cord that control autonomic function may be involved in neurodegenerative disorders such as multiple system atrophy, a stroke, tumors, inflammation, and other structural lesions. These secondary disorders may manifest with either autonomic failure or autonomic hyperactivity.

DISORDERS OF THE TELENCEPHALON

The insular, anterior cingulate, and ventromedial frontal cortices, together with the amygdala, participate in the high-level processing of autonomic responses associated with emotion (see Chapter 2). Seizures, stroke, or other disorders affecting these areas may produce severe arrhythmias and other autonomic manifestations.

Stroke

Ischemic stroke involving the insula and other regions of the frontal cortex can produce cardiac arrhythmias (5,14) that may explain cases of sudden death that occur early after stroke (83). In some studies, right hemispheric strokes were significantly associated with supraventricular tachycardia, whereas left hemispheric strokes were more frequently associated with ventricular arrhythmias (61). If confirmed, these observations would support a possible lateralized hemispheric influence on autonomic function (82).

Hemispheric infarctions in the territory of the middle cerebral artery, including the opercular cortex, may produce contralateral hyperhidrosis (56,58,60). This tends to occur in patients with severe hemiparesis and correlates with a poor prognosis for recovery (58,60). Horner's syndrome with hypohidrosis occurs with ipsilateral stroke involving the lateral tegmentum of the brain stem (25,58). Posterior cerebral artery territory infarction involving the hypothalamus and upper brain stem may produce the combination of ipsilateral Horner's syndrome and contralateral hyperhidrosis, referred to as hemiplegia vegetativa alterna.

Infarction in the territory of the anterior cerebral artery, involving the anterior cingulate and paracentral regions of the frontal lobe, can produce urinary incontinence due to involuntary bladder contractions and reflex relaxation of the external sphincter (uninhibited bladder) (8,54).

Seizures

Amygdalo-hippocampal, cingulate, opercular, anterior frontopolar, and orbitofrontal seizures can activate sympathetic or parasympathetic outflows. Autonomic manifestations of seizures are often misdiagnosed as a primary disorder of the target organ (37). They may occur during clinical auras, before the onset of any recognizable epileptiform discharges in the surface electroencephalogram (EEG) (29,69,103).

Arrhythmias are the most common autonomic manifestation of complex partial seizures, and some may be life-threatening. Many arrhythmias can be explained by increased sympathetic activity. Sinus tachycardia is the most common ictal arrhythmia (69). Other sympathetically mediated arrhythmias include transient atrial fibrillation, premature atrial and ventricular contractions, supraventricular or ventricular tachycardia, and ventricular fibrillation (9, 29,76). Vagally-mediated bradyarrhythmias are much less common than tachycardia, but ictal sinus bradycardia, sinus arrest, atrioventricular block, and prolonged asystole have been reported (23,29,50). Syncope due to cardiovagal hyperactivity during unilateral temporal seizures may be difficult to diagnose without simultaneous EEG–ECG (electrocardiogram) recordings (65). The precise temporal relationship between the onset of the seizure and cardiac arrhythmia (9,69) is best assessed with depth electrode recordings, because deep cortical or subcortical discharges triggering arrhythmias can be detected before changes in the surface EEG (37).

Patients with epilepsy have a higher than average incidence of sudden unexpected death (32,62). Both arrhythmias and neurogenic pulmonary edema are presumed causes (62,103). Most cases involve young men with a long history of seizures and occur in the setting of subtherapeutic levels of antiepileptic drugs (62). The effects of carbamazepine should be considered because it can produce severe bradycardia or complete cardiac block, even at "therapeutic" plasma levels (11,53).

Other cardiovascular manifestations of temporolimbic seizures include chest pain simulating angina pectoris

(29,76) and manifestations resembling a pheochromocytoma (15,72).

Temporolimbic discharges may activate thermoregulatory responses such as cutaneous vasodilatation with flushing, pallor, shivering, sweating, and piloerection (39,76). These manifestations are usually symmetric. Nevertheless, unilateral pilomotor seizures, although rare, may be important as a manifestation of tumors in the ipsilateral temporal lobe, particularly on the right side (39).

Unilateral mydriasis can occur with both ipsilateral and contralateral epileptic discharges (115), but miosis, accompanied or not by internal ophthalmoplegia and ptosis, is rare (92).

Ictal visceral sensations, referred to as "abdominal epilepsy," are more common in children than in adults (86). Recurrent ictal vomiting (ictus emeticus) has been documented by simultaneous EEG and video recordings (49,59) and appears to indicate involvement of the non-dominant temporal lobe by the seizure discharge (28,40). Respiratory manifestations are less common than other ictal autonomic manifestations in adults and include shortness of breath, coughing, choking, stridor, and apnea (37).

DISORDERS INVOLVING THE DIENCEPHALON

Disorders affecting the hypothalamus can produce disturbances of thermoregulation and other autonomic functions. These disturbances are commonly associated with alterations of osmotic balance, endocrine function, and state of alertness (19). Iatrogenic disorders such as the neuroleptic malignant syndrome (NMS) and the serotonin syndrome presumably involve the hypothalamus and its brain stem connections. Fatal familial insomnia affects primarily the thalamus, but it may affect autonomic connections between the diencephalon and other areas of the nervous system.

Hypothalamic disorders are commonly associated with disturbances in thermoregulation (6,19,57,70). Most commonly, chronic or progressing lesions (tumors, granulomas) cause hypothermia, whereas acute lesions may cause hypo- or hyperthermia (19,38,84,112). Hyperthermia with acute lesions generally occurs in the setting of autonomic hyperactivity (91,100). Hypothalamic thermoregulatory disorders can be subclinical, chronic, or paroxysmal. Poikilothermia may be a common manifestation of hypothalamic disorder (67). Abnormal circadian variation of temperature can occur with lesions involving the region of the suprachiasmatic nucleus (94).

Wernicke's Encephalopathy and Other Causes of Hypothermia

Continuous hypothermia has been described in association with several disorders affecting the hypothalamus or its connections, including Wernicke's encephalopathy (3, 1,87,108), head injury (88), multiple sclerosis (MS) (99), mesodiencephalic hematoma (38), and toluene toxicity (101). In patients presenting with hypothermia and a hypothalamic lesion, central hypothyroidism should first be excluded (70).

Wernicke's encephalopathy should be considered in alcoholic and other malnourished patients presenting with unexplained hypothermia (108) because hypothermia may be the initial presenting feature of the disease. Hypothermia occurs particularly in advanced cases and is commonly associated with stupor or coma, hypotension, and bradycardia (31,87,108). Immediate treatment with thiamine produces normalization of temperature and improvement of alertness within 3 to 4 days (108).

Episodic Hyperhidrosis and Hypothermia

Spontaneous periodic hypothermia of hypothalamic origin may occur as a manifestation of multiple structural and functional disorders (57). Episodic hyperhidrosis with hypothermia may occur during "diencephalic seizures" associated with lesions in the region of the third ventricle (84), or it may be the primary manifestation of agenesis of the corpus callosum (Shapiro syndrome) (64,95) or other structural lesions presumably affecting the hypothalamus or its connections (22). Spontaneous periodic hypothermia (57) occurs with no clear underlying structural or systemic cause (27,36,44).

The clinical features of the syndrome of episodic hyperhidrosis with hypothermia have been reviewed (57,64). Hypothermia and hyperhidrosis may be associated with pallor or vasodilatation, nausea, vomiting, lacrimation, salivation, and bradycardia. The episodes may last for minutes to hours and may be associated with impairment of neurologic function. Spontaneous remissions may last for several months to years (64).

Episodic hyperhidrosis and hypothermia may reflect a lowering of the thermoregulatory set-point (57) that is perhaps due to central monoaminergic dysfunction (2,93). Some of these patients respond to clonidine (27,57,109), cyproheptadine (2), naloxone (75), and peripheral muscarinic blockade with oxybutynin (63).

Paroxysmal Autonomic Hyperactivity: "Diencephalic Seizures"

In 1929, Penfield (84) coined the term "diencephalic epilepsy" to describe a syndrome of paroxysmal autonomic hyperactivity observed in a patient who had a tumor at the level of the foramen of Monro associated with hydrocephalus. He presented with periodic headache and episodes of increased arterial pressure, tachycardia, skin vasodilatation, diaphoresis, lacrimation, pupillary change, and transient shivering. Since this initial description, several cases of episodic autonomic paroxysms attributed to diencephalic dysfunction have been reported, usually in association with lesions near the third ventricle (91). The term diencephalic epilepsy is actually a misnomer, because the EEG fails to show ictal activity and the patients generally do not respond to anticonvulsants (91). Most cases of diencephalic autonomic paroxysms in clinical practice are due to severe closed head injury, usually associated with widespread axonal injury in the white matter. Autonomic paroxysms may be associated with decerebrate posturing and an episodic increase in intracranial pressure; they respond to treatment with bromocriptine and opioids (17).

Acute hydrocephalus, typically occurring after subarachnoid hemorrhage, may also produce paroxysms of autonomic hyperactivity (91). Subarachnoid hemorrhage is a typical example of an acute central nervous system lesion associated with massive sympathoexcitation. This results in a variety of serious complications, including myocardial contraction band necrosis, supraventricular and ventricular arrhythmias, acute hypertension, and cardiogenic pulmonary edema. Acute hydrocephalus producing autonomic hyperactivity may be associated with hyperthermia, muscle hypertonia, and an altered state of consciousness; this closely resembles NMS (100). All of these abnormalities may reverse completely after shunt treatment.

Neuroleptic Malignant Syndrome

Neuroleptic malignant syndrome is a life-threatening condition characterized by severe hyperthermia, rigidity, autonomic hyperactivity (hyperhidrosis, tachycardia, cardiac arrhythmias, fluctuating arterial pressure), and increased plasma levels of creatine kinase. It typically occurs 3 to 9 days after initiation or dosage increase of high-potency D2-dopamine receptor blocking antipsychotic agents, but it has also been reported after the use of clozapine (a D4 antagonist), metoclopramide, and other centrally active drugs (16,33). Patients with Parkinson's disease may develop an NMS-like syndrome upon discontinuation of L-DOPA therapy or substitution of a controlled-release tablet of L-DOPA/carbidopa.

The pathophysiology of NMS is not fully understood. A decrease of dopaminergic transmission in the basal ganglia and hypothalamus may result in both an increase in heat production through muscle contraction and impairment of heat-dissipation mechanisms (33). Necrosis in the anterior hypothalamic nuclei and lateral and tuberal hypothalamic areas has been described in a case of NMS (45).

Early recognition and management of NMS is essential for recovery. The treatment of NMS includes discontinuation of the drug, fluid replacement, oral administration of bromocriptine or levodopa/carbidopa, and intravenous infusion of dantrolene. Subcutaneous infusion of lisuride has been successfully used in patients unable to tolerate oral dopaminergic agents (16,33).

Serotonin Syndrome

The serotonin syndrome is the combination of mental and behavioral changes, motor hyperactivity, and autonomic lability that occurs after the use of potent serotomimetic agents alone or in combination with nonspecific monoamine oxidase inhibitors (MAOIs) (10,97). It can be produced by serotonin precursors, reuptake inhibitors (e.g., fluoxetine, sertraline, clomipramine, imipramine, nortriptyline, MAOIs [tranylcypromine, iproniazid]), or direct serotonin agonists (trazodone, buspirone). The manifestations of the serotonin syndrome vary among patients but include changes in mental status and behavior, motor abnormalities (e.g., myoclonus), and autonomic instability with low-grade fever, nausea, diarrhea, shivering, flushing, pupil dilatation, diaphoresis, tachycardia, blood pressure changes, and tachypnea (10,97). Treatment of the serotonin syndrome includes withdrawal of the causative agents, close observation with monitoring of vital signs, fluids, and antipyretic agents. This syndrome tends to have a short duration and to resolve spontaneously (10).

Fatal Familial Insomnia

Fatal familial insomnia (FFI) is an autosomal dominant prion disease linked to a mutation in the prion protein (PrP) gene (66). The manifestations of FFI are progressive intractable insomnia, dysautonomia, and motor dysfunction (66). Autonomic involvement consists of sympathetic hyperactivity manifested by hyperhidrosis, pyrexia, tachycardia, hypertension, and irregular breathing (66). An exaggerated background and stimulated sympathetic activity are noted, and there are preserved cardiovascular parasympathetic responses. The characteristic neuropathologic findings in FFI consist of severe atrophy of the anteroventral and dorsomedial nuclei of the thalamus (66). These nuclei are part of the "limbic" circuits connecting the amygdala, hypothalamus, hippocampus, and prefrontal cortex.

DISORDERS OF THE BRAIN STEM

Neuronal groups of the lower pons and medulla control vasomotor, cardiovagal, and respiratory functions and are functionally interactive. Cardiovascular manifestations of medullary lesions include baroreflex failure, neurogenic hypertension, orthostatic hypotension, syncope, sleep apnea, vomiting, and Horner's syndrome. Baroreflex failure is a typical manifestation of medullary lesions involving the nucleus of tractus solitarius (7,68). It manifests with acute fulminant hypertension or markedly fluctuating arterial pressure and heart rate; episodes of paroxysmal hypertension closely resemble those occurring in a pheochromocytoma (90). Acute neurogenic hypertension is a manifestation of medullary ischemia, like that occurring in the context of severe intracranial hypertension (i.e., the Cushing response) or vertebrobasilar disease (30). Orthostatic hypotension may occur as a manifestation of tumors or vascular lesions involving sympathoexcitatory neurons of the medulla. Central hypoventilation and sleep apnea (41) may occur with medullary damage from stroke (1,3,12), encephalitis, MS (46), syringobulbia (78), type I Arnold-Chiari malformation, and abnormal left vertebral artery loop.

Tumors

Orthostatic hypotension may be the major presenting manifestation of posterior fossa tumors; it may precede other progressive neurologic deficits by several years (47,102,105) or may develop after surgery for posterior fossa tumors (89). Paroxysmal hypertension resembling a pheochromocytoma has been reported in tumors involving the cerebellum or the cerebellopontine angle, including cerebellar astrocytoma, hemangioblastoma, and medulloblastoma (18,35). Brain stem tumors may present with intractable vomiting (4,113).

Syringobulbia and Arnold-Chiari Malformation

Syringobulbia may affect the NTS or its connections with cardiovagal and vasomotor neurons of the ventrolateral medulla. These patients may have orthostatic hypotension and abnormal indices of cardiovagal function (78) or abnormal fluctuations of blood pressure due to bilateral NTS lesions (68). Central hypoventilation and compromise of cardiovascular reflexes contribute to the risk of sudden death in these patients, particularly during sleep (78). Syringomyelia and syringobulbia can occur in association with the Arnold-Chiari malformation. Compression of the lower medulla by cerebellar tonsils (due to the Arnold-Chiari malformation) may produce syncope, sleep apnea, and cardiorespiratory arrest (43,111). Syncope in patients with the Arnold-Chiari malformation may result from compressive or vascular involvement of the lower medulla due to tonsillar impaction secondary to transient dissociation of intracranial and lumbar cerebrospinal fluid pressures during Valsalva-type maneuvers (24) or coughing.

Stroke

Transient ischemic attacks in the basilar artery territory may present with paroxysmal hypertension, before any focal neurologic deficit (74). Bilateral pontomedullary strokes can produce widespread cardiovascular, respiratory, gastrointestinal, bladder, and sudomotor dysfunction, with manifestations of both hyper- and hypoactivity (48,55). Lateral medullary infarctions (Wallenberg's syndrome) produce Horner's syndrome and, occasionally, more severe abnormalities, including profound bradycardia, supine hypotension, and central hypoventilation (81).

Inflammatory Disorders

Poliomyelitis involving the medullary reticular formation may produce hypertension (52,68). Tetanus can be associated with autonomic hyperactivity, probably as a result of disinhibition of preganglionic sympathetic and parasympathetic neurons (24,107,114). Baroreflex functions appear to be spared in tetanus (107). MS may affect the area surrounding the NTS and may result in fulminant neurogenic pulmonary edema (96).

DISORDERS OF THE SPINAL CORD

The spinal cord contains all the preganglionic sympathetic and sacral preganglionic parasympathetic neurons. Supraspinal autonomic pathways provide both tonic background excitation and coordination of activity of preganglionic neurons. Disruption of any of these mechanisms may result in orthostatic hypotension, massive sympathoexcitation, and disturbances in thermoregulation and in bladder, bowel, and sexual function.

Traumatic Spinal Cord Injury

Spinal cord injury, particularly above T5, is associated with severe cardiovascular dysfunction and disabling gastrointestinal, bladder, and sexual dysfunction. Tetraplegic patients with lesions above T5 have a reduction in their basal arterial pressure. This is due to hypoexcitability of preganglionic autonomic neurons isolated from tonic excitatory brain stem influences (71), as reflected by reduced skin and muscle sympathetic nerve discharge (98) and low basal plasma catecholamine levels (71). Supraspinal stimuli, such as emotion and mental arithmetic, fail to elicit an increase in sympathetic discharge (71).

Because of an interruption of hypoxia-triggered medullary sympathoexcitatory reflexes, mechanically ventilated tetraplegics with high cervical lesions above the phrenic motoneuron pool (C4-5) are prone to severe bradycardia and cardiac arrest during tracheal suction or other maneuvers that activate vagovagal reflexes (71).

In the absence of resting sympathetic tone, vasopressin and the renin-angiotensin-aldosterone system play an important role in the maintenance of supine arterial pressure. After several weeks or months, most patients are able to maintain blood pressure and remain asymptomatic while in a sitting posture because of compensatory activation of these humoral systems. The regular use of head-up tilt and mobilization often improves blood pressure control in chronic tetraplegic patients.

Disorders of thermoregulation and of gastrointestinal, bladder, and sexual function are discussed in detail in other chapters of this book.

In chronic tetraplegics with lesions above T5, stimulation of the skin, muscles, or viscera innervated by sements below the lesion may result in a massive reflex activation of sympathetic and sacral parasympathetic outflows; this is referred to as *autonomic dysreflexia* (42, 71,106). The basic mechanism is a diffuse, unpatterned activation of viscero- or somatosympathetic reflexes triggered by stimuli below the level of the lesion and lacking the normal supraspinal modulation. This results in a widespread constriction of resistance and capacitance vessels below the lesion, an elevation of cardiac output, and a rapid increase in arterial pressure.

Stimuli that trigger autonomic dysreflexia arise primarily from the bladder (e.g., insertion of a catheter, distention due to a plugged catheter, cystometry), bowel (fecal impaction, digital evacuation, enemas, insertion of a rectal tube, rectal prolapse, hemorrhoids, fissures, abscesses), and skin (deep pressure sores, burns, ingrown toenails). Autonomic dysreflexia may be a serious complication in pregnancy and labor (71,106,110).

The major symptoms of autonomic dysreflexia are pounding headache, chest oppression with a shivering or hot feeling, nausea, dyspnea, visual disturbance, anxiety, paresthesias, a desire to void, and restlessness. Vasodilation above the level of the lesion produces flushing of the face, chest, and upper arms and congestion of the nasopharyngeal mucosa. There may be excessive sweating above the anesthetic dermatome, piloerection, pallor in the abdomen and lower extremities, and pupil dilatation (106).

The cardiovascular manifestations of autonomic dysreflexia may be life-threatening. Severe hypertension is a prominent feature and may result in neurologic complications such as hypertensive encephalopathy or intracranial, subarachnoid, or retinal hemorrhage (34). The combined parasympathetic and sympathetic stimulation may cause potentially dangerous supraventricular and ventricular arrhythmias.

Management of autonomic dysreflexia consists first of determining and correcting any precipitating cause. Blood pressure can often be decreased by upright tilting of the head of the bed. However, hypotension induced by orthostatic challenge may itself trigger autonomic dysreflexia. Clonidine has been used prophylactically in autonomic dysreflexia. Nitrates and nifedipine may cause a marked decrease in arterial pressure in supine tetraplegics but are not useful when given prophylactically (71,106).

Multiple Sclerosis

Bladder, bowel, and sexual dysfunction are prominent autonomic manifestations of MS (13,21). The main mechanisms of bladder dysfunction are detrusor hyperreflexia and detrusor–sphincter dyssynergy (21). Several studies have shown subclinical abnormalities in cardiovascular sympathetic and parasympathetic function tests in patients with MS. These include reduced heart rate variability in response to deep breathing, exaggerated heart rate responses to tilt, subnormal increase in diastolic pressure during the handgrip maneuver, and attenuated blood pressure and heart rate responses to exercise during arm ergometry (20,77,80,85,104). Abnormal thermoregulatory sweating is often found in MS patients (51). Sympathetic dysfunction may affect immune regulation, including lymphocyte function, in MS patients (51).

Syringomyelia

Syringomyelia produces partial interruption of sympathetic output pathways in the intermediolateral cell columns of the spinal cord. Autonomic manifestations include Horner's syndrome, sudomotor dysfunction, and vasomotor and trophic changes in the limbs, especially the hands (79). Micturition and defecation may be affected in advanced stages. In general, patients with syringomyelia without bulbar involvement have an incomplete sympathetic vasomotor defect that does not commonly produce orthostatic hypotension. Cardiovagal function tests are typically normal in these patients (79).

Amyotrophic Lateral Sclerosis

Morphometric studies have shown a modest but significant loss of neurons in the sacral intermediolateral column in patients with amyotrophic lateral sclerosis (ALS). Patients with classical ALS often have abnormal sudomotor axon reflex responses in the foot and the heart rate responses to deep breathing (26).

Tetanus

Sympathetic hyperactivity in tetanus results from impaired release of gamma-aminobutyric acid (GABA) and glycine at inhibitory synapses on preganglionic autonomic neurons (114). It results in tachycardia, arrhythmias, labile hypertension, progressive and refractory hypotension, peripheral vasoconstriction, fever, and profuse sweating (114). Cardiovascular instability in tetanus, with alternating arterial hypertension and hypotension, is probably multifactorial (107).

Stiff-Man Syndrome

Stiff-man syndrome is an autoimmune disorder associated with autoantibodies against glutamic acid decarboxylase (GAD), and its clinical manifestations (rigidity, spasms) are thought to be due to impairment of GABAergic transmission in the spinal cord, brain stem, or both. Paroxysmal autonomic dysfunction with hyperpyrexia, diaphoresis, hypertension, tachycardia, tachypnea, and pupillary dilatation can occur in these patients; in general, it is associated with the muscle spasms. Autonomic manifestations may be prominent and result in sudden death (73).

REFERENCES

1. Armstrong E, et al. The effects of the somatostatin analogue, octreotide, on postural hypotension, before and after food ingestion, in primary autonomic failure. *Clin Auton Res* 1991;1:135—140.
2. Arroyo HA, et al. A syndrome of hyperhidrosis, hypothermia, and bradycardia possibly due to central monoaminergic dysfunction. *Neurology* 1990;40:556–557.
3. Askenasy JJ, et al. Sleep apnea as a feature of bulbar stroke. *Stroke* 1988;19:637–639.
4. Baker PC, et al. The neuroanatomy of vomiting in man: association of projectile vomiting with a solitary metastasis in the lateral tegmentum of the pons and the middle cerebellar peduncle. *J Neurol Neurosurg Psychiatry* 1985;48:1165–1168.
5. Barron SA, et al. Autonomic consequences of cerebral hemisphere infarction. *Stroke* 1994;25:113–116.
6. Bauer HG. Endocrine and other manifestations of hypothalamic disease: a survey of 60 cases, with autopsies. *J Clin Endocrinol* 1954; 14:13–31.
7. Biaggioni I et al. Baroreflex failure in a patient with central nervous system lesions involving the nucleus tractus solitarii. *Hypertension* 1994;23:491–495.
8. Blaivas JG. The neurophysiology of micturition: a clinical study of 550 patients. *J Urol* 1982;127:958–963.
9. Blumhardt LD, et al. Electrocardiographic accompaniments of temporal lobe epileptic seizures. *Lancet* 1986;1:1051–1056.
10. Bodner RA et al. Serotonin syndrome. *Neurology* 1995;45:219–223.
11. Boesen F et al. Cardiac conduction disturbances during carbamazepine therapy. *Acta Neurol Scand* 1983;68:49–52.
12. Bogousslavsky J et al. Respiratory failure and unilateral caudal brainstem infarction. *Ann Neurol* 1990;28:668–673.
13. Bradley WE. The diagnosis and treatment of patients with neurologic dysfunction of the urinary bladder. In: Low PA (ed). *Clinical Autonomic Disorders: Evaluation and Management.* Boston: Little, Brown and Company, 1993;573–588.
14. Brillman J. *Neurologic Clinics.* Philadelphia: WB Saunders. 1993.
15. Brown RW, et al. Sympathetic stimulation with temporal lobe epilepsy. *Med J Aust* 1973;2:274–276.
16. Buckley PF, et al. Neuroleptic malignant syndrome (editorial). *J Neurol Neurosurg Psychiatry* 1995;58:271–273.
17. Bullard DE. Diencephalic seizures: responsiveness to bromocriptine and morphine. *Ann Neurol* 1987;21:609–611.
18. Cameron SJ, et al. Cerebellar tumours presenting with clinical features of phaeochromocytoma. *Lancet* 1970;1:492–494.
19. Carmel PW. Vegetative dysfunctions of the hypothalamus. *Acta Neurochir* 1985;75:113–121.
20. Cartlidge NE. Autonomic function in multiple sclerosis. *Brain* 1972;95:661–664.
21. Chancellor MB, et al. Urological and sexual problems in multiple sclerosis. *Clin Neurosci* 1994;2:189–195.
22. Chaney RH, et al. Hypothalamic dysthermia in persons with brain damage. *Brain Inj* 1994;8:475–481.
23. Constantin L et al. Bradycardia and syncope as manifestations of partial epilepsy. *J Am Coll Cardiol* 1990;15:900–905.
24. Corbett JL, et al. Hypotension in tetanus. *Br Med J* 1973;3:423–428.
25. Cross SA. Autonomic disorders of the pupil, ciliary body, and lactimal apparatus. In: Low PA (ed). *Clinical Autonomic Disorders: Evaluation and Management.* Boston: Little, Brown and Company. 1993;263–277.
26. Daube JR et al. Classification of ALS by autonomic abnormalities. In: Tsubaki T, Yase Y (eds). *Amyotrophic Lateral Sclerosis.* Amsterdam: Elsevier Science Publishers. 1988;189–191.
27. De Plaen JL, et al. Paroxysmal hypertension and spontaneous periodic hypothermia. *Acta Clin Belg* 1992;47: 401–407.
28. Devinsky O et al. Ictus emeticus: further evidence of nondominant temporal involvement. *Neurology* 1995;45:1158–1160.
29. Devinsky O, et al. Cardiac manifestations of complex partial seizures. *Am J Med* 1986;80:195–202.
30. Dickinson CJ. Reappraisal of the Cushing reflex: the most powerful neural blood pressure stabilizing system (editorial). *Clin Sci* 1990; 79:543–550.
31. Donnan GA, et al. Coma and hypothermia in Wernicke's encephalopathy. *Aust N Z J Med* 1980;10:438–439.
32. Earnest MP et al. The sudden unexplained death syndrome in epilepsy: demographic, clinical, and postmortem features. *Epilepsia* 1992;33:310–316.
33. Ebadi M, et al. Pathogenesis and treatment of neuroleptic malignant syndrome. *Gen Pharmacol* 1990;21:367–86.
34. Eltorai I et al. Fatal cerebral hemorrhage due to autonomic dysreflexia in a tetraplegic patient: case report and review. *Paraplegia* 1992;30:355–360.
35. Evans CH, et al. Astrocytoma mimicking the features of pheochromocytoma. *N Engl J Med* 1972;286:1397–1399.
36. Fox RH et al. Spontaneous periodic hypothermia: diencephalic epilepsy. *Br Med J* 1973;2:693–695.
37. Freeman R, et al. Autonomic epilepsy (review). *Semin Neurol* 1995;15:158–166.
38. Gaymard G et al. Hypothermia in a mesodiencephalic haematoma (letter). *J Neurol Neurosurg Psychiatry* 1990;53:1014–1015.
39. Green JB. Pilomotor seizures. *Neurology* 1984;34:837–839.
40. Guerrini R et al. Occipitotemporal seizures with ictus emeticus induced by intermittent photic stimulation. *Neurology* 1994;44:253–259.
41. Guilleminault C et al. The impact of autonomic nervous system dysfunction on breathing during sleep. *Sleep* 1981;4:263–278.
42. Guttman L, et al. Effects of bladder distension on autonomic mechanisms after spinal cord injuries. *Brain* 1947;70:361–405.
43. Hampton F, et al. Syncope as a presenting feature of hindbrain herniation with syringomyelia. *J Neurol Neurosurg Psychiatry* 1982; 45:919–922.
44. Hines EA, et al. Intermittent hypothermia with disabling hyperhidrosis: report of a case with successful treatment. *Mayo Clin Proc* 1934;9:705.
45. Horn E et al. Hypothalamic pathology in the neuroleptic malignant syndrome. *Am J Psychiatry* 1988;145:617–620.
46. Howard RS et al. Respiratory involvement in multiple sclerosis. *Brain* 1992;115:479–494.
47. Hsu CY et al. Orthostatic hypotension with brainstem tumors. *Neurology* 1984;34:1137–1143.
48. Ito A, et al. Acute changes in blood pressure following vascular diseases in the brain stem. *Stroke* 1973;4:80–84.
49. Jacome DE, et al. Ictus emeticus. *Neurology* 1982;32:209–212.
50. Jacome DE, et al. Ictal bradycardia. *Am J Med Sci* 1988; 295:469–471.
51. Karaszewski JW et al. Sympathetic skin responses are decreased and lymphocyte beta-adrenergic receptors are increased in progressive multiple sclerosis. *Ann Neurol* 1990;27:366–372.
52. Kemp E. Arterial hypertension in poliomyelitis. *Acta Med Scand* 1957;157:109–118.
53. Kenneback G et al. Electrophysiologic effects and clinical hazards of carbamazepine treatment for neurologic disorders in patients with abnormalities of the cardiac conduction system. *Am Heart J* 1991;121:1421–1429.
54. Khan Z, et al. Neurologic basis of voiding disorders in patients with cerebrovascular accident. *Semin Neurol* 1988;8: 156–158.
55. Khurana RK. Autonomic dysfunction in pontomedullary stroke (abstr). *Ann Neurol* 1982;12:86.
56. Kim BS, et al. Contralateral hyperhidrosis after cerebral infarction. Clinicoanatomic correlations in five cases. *Stroke* 1995;26:896–899.
57. Kloos RT. Spontaneous periodic hypothermia (review). *Medicine* 1995;74:268–280.
58. Korpelainen JT, et al. Asymmetric sweating in stroke: a prospective quantitative study of patients with hemispheral brain infarction. *Neurology* 1993;43:1211–1214.
59. Kramer RE et al. Ictus emeticus: an electroclinical analysis. *Neurology* 1988;38:1048–1052.
60. Labar DR et al. Unilateral hyperhidrosis after cerebral infarction. *Neurology* 1988;38:1679–1682.
61. Lane RD et al. Supraventricular tachycardia in patients with right hemisphere strokes [see comments]. *Stroke* 1992;23:362–366.
62. Leestma JE et al. A prospective study on sudden unexpected death in epilepsy. *Ann Neurol* 1989;26:195–203.

63. LeWitt P. Hyperhidrosis and hypothermia responsive to oxybutynin. *Neurology* 1988;38:506–507.
64. LeWitt PA et al. Episodic hyperhidrosis, hypothermia, and agenesis of corpus callosum. *Neurology* 1983;33:1122–1129.
65. Liedholm LJ, et al. Cardiac arrest due to partial epileptic seizures. *Neurology* 1982;42:824–829.
66. Lugaresi E et al. Fatal familial insomnia and dysautonomia with selective degeneration of thalamic nuclei. *N Engl J Med* 1986;315: 997–1003.
67. MacKenzie MA et al. Sudomotor function in human poikilothermia. *Neurology* 1995;45:1602–1607.
68. Magnus O, et al. Cerebral mechanisms and neurogenic hypertension in man, with special reference to baroreceptor control. In: de Jong W, Provoost AP, Shapiro AP (eds). *Hypertension and Brain Mechanisms*. Amsterdam: Elsevier. 1977;47: 199–218.
69. Marshall DW, et al. Ictal tachycardia during temporal lobe seizures. *Mayo Clin Proc* 1983;58:443–446.
70. Martin JB, et al. Neurologic manifestations of hypothalamic disease. *Prog Brain Res* 1992;93:31–42.
71. Mathias CJ, et al. Autonomic disturbances in spinal cord lesions. In: Bannister R, Mathias CJ (eds). *Autonomic Failure*. Oxford: Oxford University Press. 1992;839–881.
72. Metz SA et al. Autonomic epilepsy: clonidine blockade of paroxysmal catecholamine release and flushing. *Ann Intern Med* 1978;88: 189–193.
73. Mitsumoto H et al. Sudden death and paroxysmal autonomic dysfunction in stiff-man syndrome. *J Neurol* 1991;238:91–96.
74. Montgomery BM. The basilar artery hypertensive syndrome. *Arch Intern Med* 1961;108:115–125.
75. Mooradian AD et al. Spontaneous periodic hypothermia. *Neurology* 1984;34:79–82.
76. Mulder DW, et al. Visceral epilepsy. *Arch Intern Med* 1954;93: 481–493.
77. Neubauer B, et al. Analysis of heart rate variations in patients with multiple sclerosis. A simple measure of autonomic nervous disturbances using an ordinary ECG. *J Neurol Neurosurg Psychiatry* 1978;41:417–419.
78. Nogues MA, et al. Risk of sudden death during sleep in syringomyelia and syringobulbia. *J Neurol Neurosurg Psychiatry* 1992;55:585–589.
79. Nogues MA et al. Cardiovascular reflexes in syringomyelia. *Brain* 1982;105:835–849.
80. Nordenbo AM, et al. Cardiovascular autonomic function in multiple sclerosis. *J Auton Nerv Syst* 1989;26:77–84.
81. Norrving B, et al. Lateral medullary infarction: prognosis in an unselected series. *Neurology* 1991;41:244–248.
82. Oppenheimer SM et al. Cardiovascular effects of human insular cortex stimulation. *Neurology* 1992;42:1727–1732.
83. Oppenheimer SM, et al. The cardiac consequences of stroke (review). *Neurol Clin* 1992;10:167–176.
84. Penfield W. Diencephalic autonomic epilepsy. *Arch Neurol* 1929;22: 358–374.
85. Pentland B, et al. Cardiovascular reflexes in multiple sclerosis. *Eur Neurol* 1987;26:46–50.
86. Peppercorn MA, et al. The spectrum of abdominal epilepsy in adults. *Am J Gastroenterol* 1989;84:1294–1296.
87. Philip G, et al. Hypothermia and Wernicke's encephalopathy. *Lancet* 1973;2:122–124.
88. Ratcliffe PJ, et al. Late onset post-traumatic hypothalamic hypothermia. *J Neurol Neurosurg Psychiatry* 1983;46:72–74.
89. Riedel G et al. Orthostatic hypotension following surgery on brainstem neoplasms: report of two cases. *Arch Phys Med Rehabil* 1974; 55:471–473.
90. Robertson D et al. The diagnosis and treatment of baroreflex failure. *N Engl J Med* 1993;329:1449–1455.
91. Ropper AH. Acute autonomic emergencies and autonomic storm. In: Low PA (ed). *Clinical Autonomic Disorders: Evaluation and Management*. Boston: Little, Brown and Company. 1993;747–760.
92. Rosenberg ML, Jabbari B. Miosis and internal ophthalmoplegia as a manifestation of partial seizures. *Neurology* 1991;41:737–739.
93. Sanfield JA et al. Altered norepinephrine metabolism in Shapiro's syndrome. *Arch Neurol* 1989;46:53–57.
94. Schwartz WJ, et al. A discrete lesion of ventral hypothalamus and optic chiasm that disturbed the daily temperature rhythm. *J Neurol* 1986;233:1–4.
95. Shapiro WR, et al. Spontaneous recurrent hypothermia accompanying agenesis of the corpus callosum. *Brain* 1969;92:423–436.
96. Simon RP, et al. Medullary lesion inducing pulmonary edema: a magnetic resonance imaging study. *Ann Neurol* 1991;30:727–730.
97. Sternbach H. The serotonin syndrome [see comments] (review). *Am J Psychiatry* 1991;148:705–713.
98. Stjernberg L, et al. Sympathetic activity in man after spinal cord injury. Outflow to muscle below the lesion. *Brain* 1986;109:695–715.
99. Sullivan F et al. Chronic hypothermia in multiple sclerosis. *J Neurol Neurosurg Psychiatry* 1987;50:813–815.
100. Talman WT, et al. A hyperthermic syndrome in two subjects with acute hydrocephalus. *Arch Neurol* 1988;45:1037–1040.
101. Teelucksingh S et al. Hypothalamic syndrome and central sleep apnoea associated with toluene exposure. *Q J Med* 1991;78:185–190.
102. Telerman Toppet N, et al. Orthostatic hypotension with lower brain stem glioma. *J Neurol Neurosurg Psychiatry* 1982;45:1147–1150.
103. Terrence CF Jr, et al. Unexpected, unexplained death in epileptic patients. *Neurology* 1975;25:594–598.
104. Thomaides TN et al. Physiological assessment of aspects of autonomic function in patients with secondary progressive multiple sclerosis. *J Neurol* 1993;240:139–143.
105. Thomas JE et al. Orthostatic hypotension as the presenting sign in craniopharyngioma. *Neurology* 1961;11:418–423.
106. Trop CS, et al. The evaluation of autonomic dysreflexia. *Semin Urol* 1992;10:95–101.
107. van Lieshout JJ et al. Cardiovascular instability and baroreflex activity in a patient with tetanus. *Clin Auton Res* 1991;1:5–8.
108. Victor M, et al. The Wernicke-Korsahoff syndrome and related neurologic disorders due to alcoholism and malnutrition. In: *Anonymous Contemporary Neurology Series*. Philadelphia: FA Davis. 1989.
109. Walker BR, et al. Clonidine therapy for Shapiro's syndrome. *Q J Med* 1992;82:235–245.
110. Wanner MB, et al. Pregnancy and autonomic hyperreflexia in patients with spinal cord lesions. *Paraplegia* 1987;25: 482–490.
111. Weig SG et al. Recurrent syncope as the presenting symptom of Arnold-Chiari malformation. *Neurology* 1991;41:1673–1674.
112. Wolf SM, et al. A syndrome of periodic hypothalamic discharge. *Am J Med* 1964;36:956–967.
113. Wood JR et al. Brainstem tumor presenting as an upper gut motility disorder. *Gastroenterology* 1985;89:1411–1414.
114. Wright DK et al. Autonomic nervous system dysfunction in severe tetanus: current prospectives. *Crit Care Med* 1989;17:371–375.
115. Zee DS, et al. Unilateral pupillary dilatation during adversive seizures. *Arch Neurol* 1974;30:403–405.

CHAPTER 33

Conditions of Reduced Gravity

Victor A. Convertino

1. Prolonged exposure to spaceflight or bed rest, by reducing gravity stress along the vertical axis, results in adaptation processes that involve many autonomic functions.
2. Reduced parasympathetic activation results in a higher baseline heart rate (HR).
3. Reduced sympathetic activation may contribute to underlying mechanisms that induce hypovolemia and increase responsiveness of cardiac and vascular β-adrenoreceptors.
4. Low-pressure baroreceptors appear to be reset to a lower operating point for central venous pressure, which in turn acts to maintain a lower blood volume and reduce cardiac filling and stroke volume.
5. The consequences of these alterations become most apparent on return to upright posture in normal gravity.
   a. Reduced cardiac filling is compounded by enhanced blood pooling in the lower extremities as a consequence of more compliant veins.
   b. Orthostatic tachycardia occurs but is partially inhibited by attenuated carotid-cardiac baroreflex response.
   c. Reflex vasoconstriction, controlled by low-pressure (cardiopulmonary) baroreceptors, is reduced, thereby attenuating the rise in systemic vascular resistance.
6. The impairment in venous pooling, baroreflex gain, and reflex vasoconstriction contributes to the orthostatic intolerance on standing in normal gravity that occurs after prolonged microgravity.

INTRODUCTION

The autonomic nervous system has evolved to provide moment-to-moment regulation of blood pressure (BP) through effective control of HR, stroke volume, and systemic peripheral resistance. This function is of critical importance in humans, who naturally assume and function in an upright posture in a gravity environment, in which adequate cerebral perfusion may be challenged by hydrostatic columns along the longitudinal axis of the body. However, the autonomic nervous system demonstrates great plasticity as it adapts its functions appropriately to redistribution of volumes and pressures within the cardiovascular system during chronic exposure to reduced gravity along the longitudinal axis of the body, as occurs during space travel or bed rest. In fact, the adaptations of the cardiovascular system to spaceflight and bed rest are so similar that head-down tilt has been used as an excellent analogue to investigate the effects of microgravity on the BP regulation system. Unfortunately, functioning at a low-gravity capacity can prove detrimental during a rapid return to normal upright posture.

Accumulating evidence suggests that exposure to low-gravity environments causes fundamental disturbances of autonomic homeostasis. This chapter presents an overview of alterations (disorders) in autonomic function associated with conditions of reduced gravity in humans. The discussion emphasizes the effects of spaceflight, as autonomic impairments caused by exposure to microgravity occur in otherwise healthy individuals. This approach provides the unique opportunity to study autonomic dysfunctions independent of disease. Because exposure to head-down tilt or horizontal bed rest produces physiologic alterations similar to those observed during spaceflight (13), the investigation of changes observed in these ground-based models also provides a novel insight into the effects of low gravity on autonomic function and a useful demonstration of the clinical consequences of confinement to bed rest.

V. A. Convertino: Physiology Research Branch, Clinical Sciences Division, Aerospace Medicine Directorate, Armstrong Laboratory, Brooks Air Force Base, Texas 78235.

ORTHOSTATIC HYPOTENSION AND INTOLERANCE

Spaceflight and bed rest cause little change in arterial pressure, compared with standing in earth's gravity, which suggests that BP regulation is preserved in low gravity. However, orthostatic hypotension commonly develops in individuals who stand on return from prolonged exposure to low gravity (4,9,17,46,52,77). Despite compensatory elevations in HR, about one third of astronauts who are tested immediately on return from spaceflight cannot tolerate 10 min of standing without presyncopal symptoms (47). Similar observations have been reported in subjects confined to bed rest (17,77). Astronauts and bedridden patients commonly experience orthostatic instability, manifested by dizziness, dimming of vision, discomfort or throbbing in the neck and shoulders, and, in some cases, frank syncope. The inability of cardiovascular mechanisms to provide adequate protection of BP in astronauts and bed-rested subjects during standing supports the notion that conditions of low gravity can induce significant disorders in autonomic function.

ALTERED AUTONOMIC BALANCE

Power spectral and time-series analyses of baseline RR intervals in subjects exposed to head-down bed rest indicate reductions in the high-frequency (0.25 Hz) spectrum and standard deviations of RR intervals (Fig. 1), suggesting a reduction in parasympathetic activity (27). Reduction in diurnal variation of HR and systolic and diastolic pressures (47) and attenuation of vagal baroreflex function (9, 17,16,35,38,39,45) in astronauts during spaceflight and subjects restricted to bed rest also support the notion that parasympathetic activity is reduced.

Although direct measurements of sympathetic nerve activity have not been conducted in individuals exposed to low gravity, reduction in plasma catecholamines during bed rest (20,24,49) and spaceflight (58,69) supports the hypothesis that reduced sympathetic stimulation and discharge might be expected with low-gravity environments. HR, which increases in response to sympathetic stimulation, would be expected to decrease if circulating catecholamines were low. The fact that HR during conditions of low gravity usually is not altered or increased is not nec-

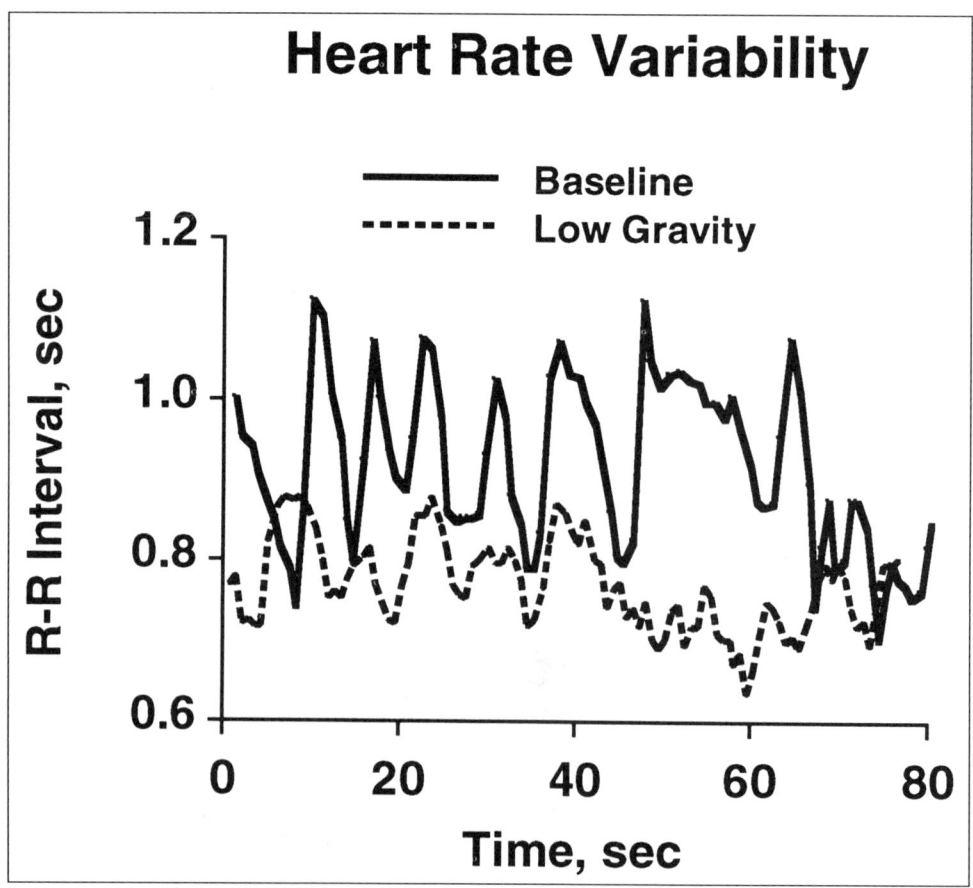

FIG. 1. Average (n = 8) variability of RR interval before and after exposure to low gravity. (Original data extracted from Crandall et al., ref. 28.)

essarily contradictory to lower sympathetic stimulation and discharge, but it probably reflects the concurrent reduction in baseline parasympathetic activity and elevated cardiac adrenoreceptor responsiveness (see below). Thus, current data suggest that exposure to low gravity causes reductions in both sympathetic and parasympathetic nerve activity.

INCREASED VENOUS COMPLIANCE

Increased compliance of the veins is associated with lower orthostatic tolerance (55), presumably because more blood is pooled in the lower extremities, resulting in lower cardiac filling (venous return) for a given pressure column. The notion that low gravity causes venous compliance to increase is supported by the observations that venous compliance is elevated in the legs early in spaceflight (56,76) and that increased venous pooling in the upright posture is associated with difficulty in maintaining BP after spaceflight (53). The underlying mechanisms for elevated venous compliance following exposure to low gravity are unclear, but multiple factors may be involved. After analysis of cross-sectional data, it was reported that the largest contributing predictor of high leg compliance is low cross-sectional area of muscle (18). Longitudinal reduction of leg muscle size in humans with the use of a low-gravity model (bed rest) increases venous compliance (21), supporting a causal relationship between loss in the muscle compartment surrounding the large veins and increased venous compliance. Muscle mass exerts mechanical compression on the veins, which acts to resist venous stretching and consequently reduces accumulation of blood at any particular venous pressure. Leg compliance appears to be less when a large muscle mass provides mechanical resistance to limit expansion of the veins. Therefore, an increase in venous compliance in low gravity seems reasonable, as a loss of muscle mass in the legs resulting from disuse in microgravity and bed rest is well established (8,10,36,76). Attenuation of autonomic activation of vascular smooth muscle, baseline contractile activity, or skeletal muscle and venosomatic reflexes (75), and other factors, such as vascular wall structure and fluid shifts of as much as 1 to 1.5 L from the legs to the circulation (3), can also contribute to an overall increase of venous compliance. Although not yet demonstrated, the possibility that low gravity may induce physiologically significant alterations in one or more of these other determinants of limb compliance cannot be ruled out. However, relationships derived from previous investigations (21) suggest that reduced muscle size is the primary cause of elevated limb compliance in subjects exposed to low gravity.

HYPOVOLEMIA

In addition to increased blood pooling in the lower extremities associated with more compliant veins, venous re-

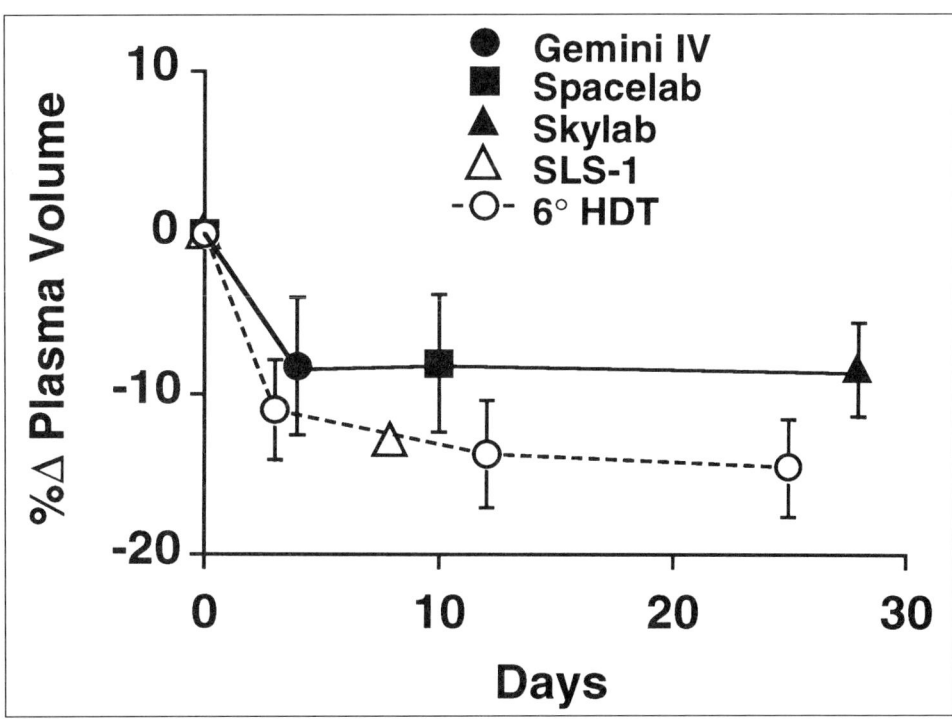

FIG. 2. Time course of percentage change (%Δ) in plasma volume during exposure to low gravity. (Modified from Convertino et al., ref. 13.)

turn and cardiac filling can be compromised during standing by reduction in total circulating blood volume. Reductions in plasma and blood volume of as much as 15%–20% induced by spaceflight and bed rest (1,4,12, 13,14,22) provide support to the hypothesis that exposure to low gravity alters homeostasis of blood volume. In the hypovolemia induced by low gravity, a rapid reduction during the initial days of exposure is followed by a new equilibrium at a lower volume (Fig. 2). Reduction in total circulating blood volume is related to increased tachycardia during standing after spaceflight (6,52,77), suggesting that vascular volume can be an important contributing factor to orthostatic hypotension and instability after spaceflight. Although the mechanisms are unclear, normal balance of fluid intake and output and normal renal function throughout exposure to low gravity suggest that reduction of plasma volume and failure for its maintenance at normal gravity levels during low gravity are not associated with clinical renal dysfunction (22). A rapid diuresis occurs within the initial 24 to 48 hrs of exposure (22,40), and its magnitude can account for the degree of plasma volume reduction. The diuresis can be partly explained by stimulation of pulmonary, atrial, and carotid mechanoreceptors with release of atrial natriuretic peptide (49) and a fall in antidiuretic hormone (ADH), renin, and aldosterone (30,40).

Central venous pressure (CVP) is reduced immediately on entry into low gravity (5) and remains low for the duration of exposure (14,20). Chronic reduction in CVP during low gravity may represent an alteration in autonomic functions associated with feedback regulation of blood volume (14). Evidence is compelling that the reduction in CVP observed during long exposure to low gravity represents a "resetting" of CVP to a lower operating point. Evidence to support this hypothesis includes the fact that fluid input fails to expand plasma volume effectively (77), similar volumes of fluid infusion induce similar volumes of urine excretion despite lower plasma volume in low gravity compared with normal gravity (33), and exposure to head-down tilt causes the cardiopulmonary baroreflex stimulus-response relationship to shift to the left, so that the response for peripheral vascular resistance occurs in a lower range of CVPs (20). Physiologically, these observations suggest that low gravity causes a resetting of volume control mechanism(s) to a lower operational range for CVP. Clinically, this change in autonomic function limits the capacity for replacement of plasma volume by simple drinking techniques.

Alterations in autonomic function during exposure to low gravity may have direct effects on blood volume regulation. It has been postulated that lower sympathetic stimulation and discharge in low gravity may contribute to the hypovolemia and anemia that accompany spaceflight (69). Renal denervation substantially increases renal sodium loss. Patients with the Bradbury-Eggleston syndrome, characterized by degeneration of peripheral autonomic nerves, particularly illustrate this natriuretic effect, which occurs while kidney production of dopamine is relatively normal (70). The expected effects of this neurohumoral alteration would fit the observation that the reduction in circulating plasma volume and sodium occurring in spaceflight and bed rest is accompanied by a reduction in plasma renin activity (30). Therefore, it is possible that a reduction in sympathetic activation and circulating norepinephrine in low gravity could result in increased renal sodium loss because the natriuretic effect of dopamine would be unopposed. This could contribute to the hypovolemia that seems to occur during the first few days of exposure to low gravity (Fig. 2). Although the central fluid shift seen with low gravity may have the most significant effect on reduced plasma volume, the specific role of renal sympathetic activity deserves further investigation.

In addition to a loss in plasma volume, the hypovolemia induced by prolonged exposure to low gravity can also be caused by a more gradual reduction in red cell mass (8,34,59), probably the result of a fall in erythropoietin levels (1,59). An association between the sympathetic nervous system and erythropoiesis has been supported by the observation that the reticulocyte response to acute bloodletting is greatly diminished after renal denervation (2,73). Intravenous administration of salbutamol (a β-adrenergic receptor agonist) increased serum erythropoietin (43), whereas beta blockers blunted the erythropoietin response to hypoxia (44). These experimental results provide compelling evidence that sympathetic stimulation, acting through β_2-adrenoreceptors, may modulate erythropoiesis through an increase in erythropoietin production. Thus, reduced sympathetic activity and reduced circulating norepinephrine associated with low gravity could represent an underlying mechanism for the anemia observed with spaceflight and bed rest.

Following space missions of less than 7 days in duration, ingestion of approximately 1L of isotonic saline solution reduced the HR response and maintained BP in astronauts during standing tests (6). This observation supports the hypothesis that body fluid loss is a primary mechanism of orthostatic compromise following spaceflight. However, when standing tests were conducted in bed-rested subjects or astronauts who had been exposed to low gravity for 1 week or longer, it became apparent that hypovolemia alone could not explain orthostatic compromise, as HR and BP responses during standing were similar in individuals who did and did not undergo fluid loading procedures (77,78). It has become apparent that alterations in autonomic functions associated with regulation of blood volume and pressure are induced by exposure to low gravity.

CARDIAC RHYTHM DISTURBANCES

Although HR may decrease during short-term exposure to low gravity (47), it usually increases during exposures of more than 1 week (17,19,20,23,27,53,55,71). The changing time course for HR may reflect a reduction in sympathetic activity during early exposure to low gravity, followed by a later reduction in parasympathetic activity. An exaggerated elevation in HR in subjects during standing after long-term exposure to low gravity is an appropriate response to a reduced stroke volume, representing an attempt to maintain cardiac output and arterial pressure. The underlying mechanism for this tachycardia probably includes a greater sympathetic response (77,79).

Although the incidence of cardiac dysrhythmias has not increased during space missions of less than 10 days (47), an increased incidence has been reported during both spaceflight and bed rest of longer than 2 weeks. Preventricular atrial contractions, supraventricular and ventricular contractions, and nodal bigeminy were reported in Apollo 15 crew members who had not experienced such dysrhythmias before flight (51). During provocative testing with adrenergic agonists, increased occurrence of junctional or nodal arrhythmias has been reported following head-down bed rest (24). This is particularly intriguing, considering that altered autonomic function was postulated as a possible mechanism underlying the changes in junctional rhythm frequently observed in astronauts during the U.S. Skylab missions (53). There were no junctional rhythms in eight subjects during adrenergic agonist infusion tests conducted before head-down bed rest. However, following 14 days of exposure to low gravity, isoproterenol induced junctional rhythms in three subjects, with preventricular contractions occurring in one and preatrial contractions in another. Phenylephrine infusion was associated with junctional rhythm for 2 min with one interpolated beat in one subject, junctional rhythm and preventricular contractions in one subject, bradycardia of 35 beats/min with erratic rhythm and escape beats in one subject, and preatrial contractions in one subject. These observations indicate that increased responsiveness of cardiac adrenoreceptors resulting from exposure and adaptation to microgravity may represent a mechanism for increased risk for cardiac arrhythmias during and after exposure to low gravity.

ENHANCED AORTIC-CARDIAC BAROREFLEX RESPONSIVENESS

During assumption of an upright posture, the distribution of blood in the lower extremities reduces cardiac filling and stroke volume. The defense of cardiac output is therefore supported by the ability of arterial baroreflexes to elevate HR and cardiac contractility. One mechanism that elicits a compensatory tachycardia during orthostatism involves the stimulation of aortic baroreceptors in response to hypotension. Aortic baroreceptors are critical to the regulation of BP, with a more prominent role than that of the carotid baroreflex in altering HR responses and muscle sympathetic nerve activity in humans (42).

Although the ability to investigate aortic-cardiac baroreflex function in humans is limited by the anatomic location of baroreceptors, the isolation of aortic baroreceptors has been attempted with the application of neck chambers and lower-body negative-pressure devices designed to "clamp" carotid and cardiopulmonary baroreceptor activity during selective pharmacologic stimulation (16,29). When these procedures are applied, it is clear that the HR response to aortic baroreceptor stimulation is enhanced following exposure to low gravity (29). Although this enhanced baroreflex responsiveness may reflect alteration in autonomic function, it appears that a primary underlying mechanism is the hypovolemia associated with exposure to low gravity, as normovolemia reverses the heightened response (16).

IMPAIRED CAROTID-CARDIAC BAROREFLEX FUNCTION

Another mechanism that elicits compensatory tachycardia during standing involves the stimulation of carotid baroreceptors in response to hypotension. Despite an increase in standing tachycardia after spaceflight and bed rest, standing HRs were lower in syncopal compared with nonsyncopal subjects following bed rest (17) and began to decline as the duration of spaceflight became longer than 10 to 12 days (64). These observations raised the possibility that low gravity causes impairment of cardioacceleratory reflexes elicited by carotid baroreceptors, as aortic baroreceptor stimulation was associated with enhanced chronotropic response (see above). Carotid baroreceptor reflex dysfunction has subsequently been demonstrated after bed rest (11,15,17,35,39) and spaceflight (45,64).

The changes in carotid-cardiac baroreflex function induced by exposure to low gravity are illustrated in Fig. 3. A prominent feature of adaptation to low gravity is a shift of the carotid-cardiac stimulus-response relationship downward and to the right, producing a lower gain (less maximal response slope). This indicates that for a given reduction in arterial pressure, there will be a smaller compensatory increase in HR (decrease in RR interval) after adaptation to low gravity. As there is little change in baseline mean arterial pressure, elevation in baseline HR places the operational point at a lower position, near the threshold on the response curve. This relocation of operational point on a less responsive part of the stimulus-response relationship further compromises the capacity of this reflex to increase HR in the face of an orthostatic challenge, such as simple standing. Acute alterations in plasma volume do not affect the carotid-cardiac baroreflex response (74), and the time course of changes in baroreflex function during bed rest do not parallel that of changes in plasma volume (11). These data suggest that unlike aortic-cardiac baroreflex function, impaired carotid-cardiac baroreflex function occurs during low gravity independently of plasma volume reduction.

These alterations in carotid-cardiac baroreflex can explain several clinical observations regarding the develop-

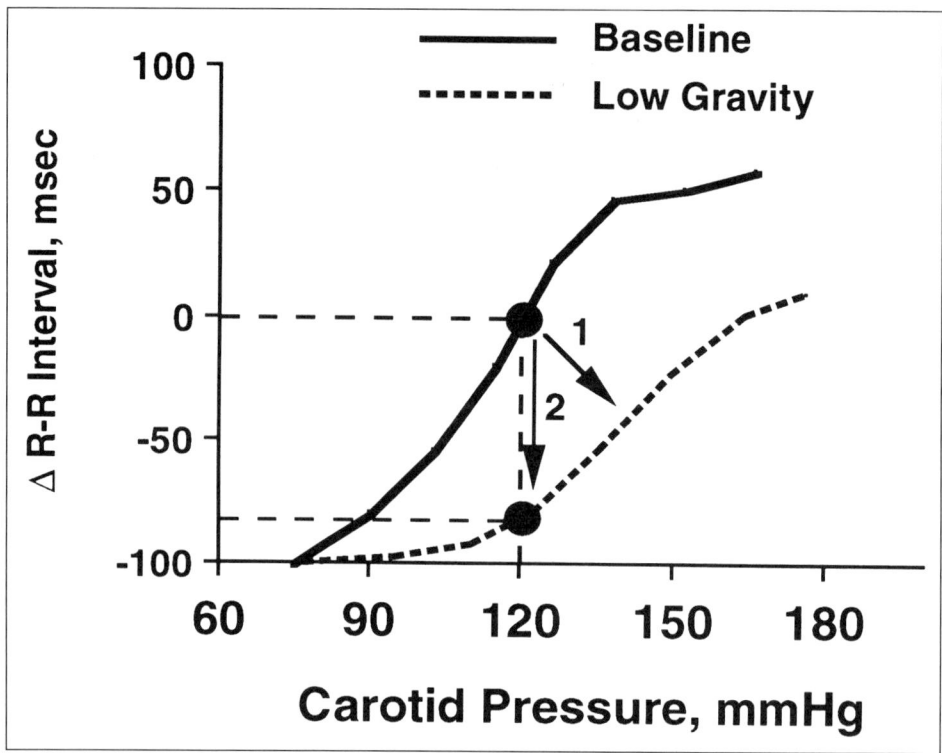

FIG. 3. Theoretical illustration of the carotid-cardiac stimulus-response baroreflex relationship at baseline and low gravity. *Circles* represent position of operational points. *Arrow (1)* represents shift to lesser responsiveness (maximum slope) and *arrow (2)* represents change in operational point (i.e., baseline RR interval and systolic BP).

ment of orthostatic hypotension and intolerance following long-term exposure to low gravity. The increase in standing HR following bed rest or spaceflight can be explained by hypovolemia that elicits an exaggerated cardiac response from aortic baroreceptor stimulation. However, individuals with pronounced orthostatic hypotension after bed rest have demonstrated less tachycardia during standing than subjects who maintain BP (17), and orthostatic instability after spaceflight was associated with a lower operational set point (46). These results are similar to those reported in carotid-denervated dogs (26). The observation that reduced maximal gain or lower operational point of the carotid-cardiac baroreflex stimulus-response relationship predicts orthostatic intolerance after bed rest or spaceflight (17,46) as well as in normal ambulatory conditions (61) supports the notion that impairment of this reflex function may represent a major autonomic disorder associated with low gravity.

REDUCED VASOCONSTRICTIVE RESERVE

Numerous investigators have reported that exposure to low gravity increases baseline peripheral vascular resistance (20,24,28,48). Reflex peripheral vasoconstriction induced by activation of cardiopulmonary baroreceptors in response to a reduction in CVP is a basic mechanism for elevating systemic vascular resistance and defending arterial BP during an orthostatic challenge. The stimulus-response relationship of this reflex is illustrated in Fig. 4. When hypovolemia is acutely induced in ambulatory subjects, forearm vascular resistance (FVR) is elevated, with an upward shift of the response curve in comparison with a normovolemic baseline state (74). Because the vascular system has a finite vasoconstrictive capacity, it is reasonable to interpret elevated FVR during hypovolemia as representing a reduction in the reserve capacity for further vasoconstriction. The increased slope, or gain, of the cardiopulmonary baroreflex response induced by hypovolemia demonstrates a more responsive peripheral vasoconstriction in a volume-depleted state than in a normovolemic state. This appears to be an appropriate adjustment to defend arterial BP. However, the increased cardiopulmonary baroreflex gain represents utilization of vasoconstrictive reserves, which, depending on the degree of hypovolemia, could significantly compromise the capacity to provide adequate vascular resistance during orthostatism. As hypovolemia occurs in low gravity, inadequate elevation of peripheral vascular resistance and maintenance of arterial pressure during standing immediately after bed rest and spaceflight can limit orthostatic function. This notion is supported by the observation that astronauts who could not complete a 10-min

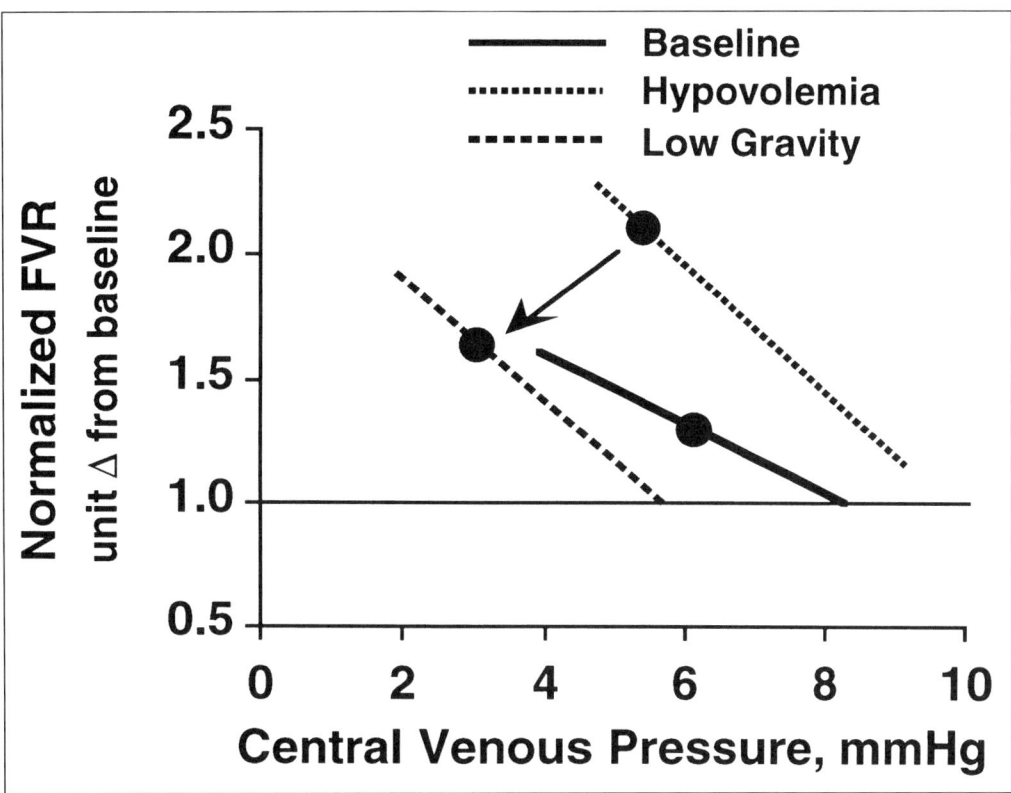

FIG. 4. Theoretical illustration of the cardiopulmonary-FVR stimulus-response baroreflex relationship under baseline, hypovolemic, and low-gravity conditions. *Circles* represent position of operational points.

stand test following their mission were unable to increase their systemic vascular resistance to the same degree as those who completed the test (4), and earlier onset of syncopal symptoms following bed rest was associated with less increase in vascular resistance from baseline levels (39).

As pointed out earlier, the hypovolemia induced by low gravity is associated with a reduction in CVP that reflects an appropriate autonomic resetting of low-pressure baroreceptors to defend the constancy of venous capacitance. As a result, there is a shift of the cardiopulmonary baroreflex stimulus-response relationship downward and to the left, so that the response for peripheral vascular resistance occurs in a lower range of CVPs (Fig. 4). This has two potentially compromising consequences. First, there is less vasoconstriction at a given level of hypovolemia and CVP following exposure to low gravity than in normal ambulatory conditions. Therefore, less vascular resistance can be developed in the face of low plasma volume and BP after exposure to low gravity. Second, lower CVP during orthostatic challenge at low gravity is associated with lower cardiac filling and stroke volume (20,29), factors that also limit appropriate BP regulation. Therefore, the adaptation of the cardiopulmonary baroreflex to low gravity can compromise the capacity to increase both cardiac output and peripheral vascular resistance, the two factors that dictate maintenance of arterial pressure during standing.

Finally, the integration of various baroreflex systems should be appreciated. There is evidence that cardiopulmonary baroreceptor unloading results in elevated sensitivity of aortic baroreceptors (2). Because low gravity reduces blood volume and CVP, reduced tonic inhibition of aortic baroreceptors associated with cardiopulmonary baroreceptor unloading may represent a primary mechanism that contributes to the accentuation of aortic-cardiac baroreflex gain observed with low gravity.

ADRENORECEPTOR HYPERSENSITIVITY

Following exposure to low gravity, elevations in plasma catecholamines during standing (77,79) and exercise (37), and increases in baseline urinary noradrenaline as well as its metabolites normetanephrine and adrenaline (57,60), are generally excessive. Such increases would suggest a high level of sympathetic activity and would be expected under conditions of hypovolemia and orthostatic hypotension. It has been postulated that orthostatic hypotension associated with exposure to low gravity may be partly attributable to adrenergic receptor hypersensitivity in the face of excessively high sympathetic activation (69).

If plasma norepinephrine becomes low during exposure to low gravity, the attenuated hormonal stimulation may

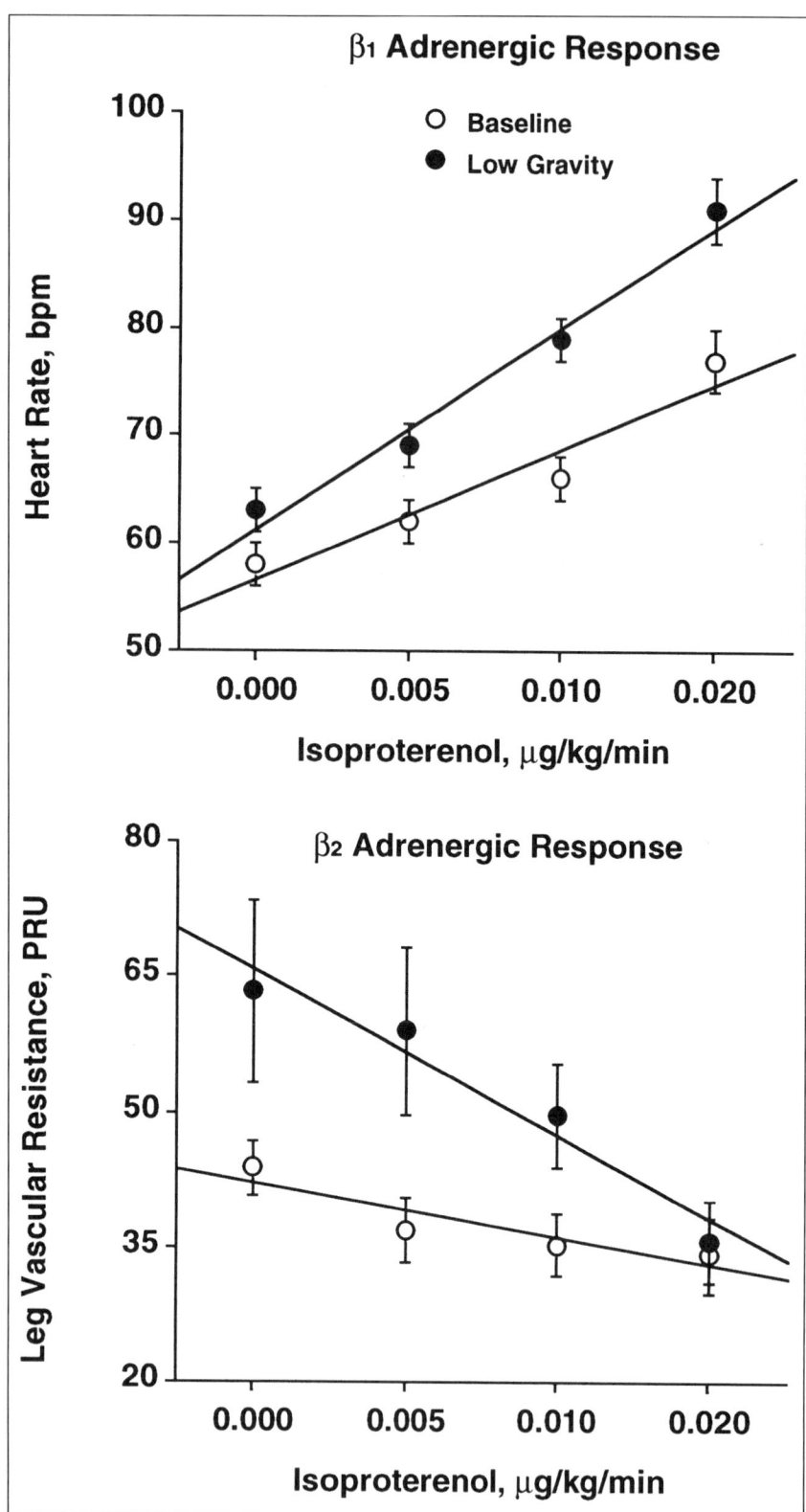

FIG. 5. Dose-response relationships for cardiac (β_1) and peripheral (β_2) resistance adrenergic responses. (Data modified from Convertino et al., ref. 24.)

lead to increased sensitivity of adrenoreceptors. Indeed, low gravity caused substantial increases in HR (Fig. 5, *top panel*) and vasodilator responses (Fig. 5, *bottom panel*) to a β-adrenergic agonist, but had little effect on the vasoconstrictive response to α-adrenergic stimulation (24), demonstrating that low gravity causes selective increases in β_1- and β_2-adrenergic responsiveness in healthy humans associated with reduced circulating norepinephrine; α_1-adrenergic vascular responses are not affected (24). The mechanism of increased β-adrenergic responsiveness in low gravity is associated with a dramatic reduction in total circulating norepinephrine. β-Adrenoreceptor activity was reduced in individuals with elevated plasma norepinephrine as a result of regular exposure to upright posture (41) and physical exercise (7), but was accentuated in patients with dysautonomia in which circulating catecholamines are absent or reduced (69,70). It is therefore possible that reduction of orthostatic and physical work stresses in a low-gravity environment could be responsible for chronically reduced secretion of norepinephrine, leading to increased responsiveness of β-adrenoreceptors and greater tachycardia and vasodilation in response to sympathomimetic stimulation.

With such alterations in adrenoreceptor function, a given adrenergic discharge would be expected to lead to excessive tachycardia. Tachycardia is a well-documented phenomenon associated with return to upright posture following exposure to low gravity. Therefore, in addition to hypovolemia, elevated catecholamines, and increased responsiveness of aortic baroreceptor stimulation, increased responsiveness of cardiac $β_1$-adrenergic receptors represents an additional mechanism that may contribute to orthostatically induced tachycardia following exposure to low gravity.

If $β_2$-adrenergic receptor sensitivity was relatively greater than α-adrenergic sensitivity, a normal vasoconstrictor response to upright posture might be transformed into a reduced vasopressor response that could have a significant effect on BP regulation. Because vascular $β_2$-adrenoreceptors elicit vasodilation (compared with vascular constriction mediated by $α_1$-adrenoreceptors), the overall effect of greater $β_2$ responsiveness in the absence of changes in $α_1$ responses could be reduced vasoconstriction, especially under a condition of increased sympathetic discharge during standing after exposure to low gravity. This hypothesis is supported by the observations that maximal contractile tension in isolated rat aorta evoked by norepinephrine, phenylephrine, and vasopressin was diminished by 14 days of head-down tilt (31), and that normal reductions in blood flow to inactive muscle and visceral tissue during exercise did not occur in rats exposed to head-down tilt (62). The potential to limit orthostatically induced elevations in peripheral resistance could compromise the capacity of the cardiovascular system to maintain adequate arterial BP and cerebral perfusion during standing.

Especially in the setting of hypovolemia, excessive adrenergic discharge observed on standing after exposure to low gravity might be ineffective in maintaining upright BP, and baroreceptor-mediated elevations in HR might be further enhanced. As excessive tachycardia is known to trigger the Bezold-Jarisch response, increased cardiac β-adrenoreceptor hypersensitivity may be an underlying mechanism for orthostatic hypotension and vasovagal syncope associated with low gravity. Although speculative, this possibility has practical implications for the development of possible treatments. For example, the use of a beta blocker before reambulation might reduce the potential for a vasovagal event. Combined with treatment to diminish volume losses, this might improve orthostatic stability at critical times following return from low-gravity conditions.

VESTIBULAR-AUTONOMIC INTERACTIONS

Although it is clear that a reduction in sympathetic activity can be important to the etiology of autonomic disorders associated with low gravity, the origin of this decrease is unknown. However, it has been recognized that the neurovestibular system is especially challenged by low-gravity environments (54) and is probably pivotal in the syndrome of space motion sickness (68). Based on observations that nausea and vomiting, primary features of space motion sickness, are closely linked to parasympathetic activation and concomitant sympathetic withdrawal (67,68), it is possible that disturbances in vestibular function may represent a potentially important explanation for reduced sympathetic activity in low gravity as well as contribute to hypovolemia by reducing fluid intake and increasing fluid loss through motion sickness.

It is also well documented that vestibular and/or oculomotor stimulation (nystagmus) can influence autonomic control of the cardiovascular system (32,63,65–68,72), under some conditions causing parasympathetic activation that results in bradycardia and hypotension (63,65–68,72). Specifically, there is some compelling evidence from measurements of HR and BP during head movements that stimulation of the receptors in the semicircular canals may increase parasympathetic nerve output, thereby inhibiting vagal withdrawal (67). If this is true, then cases of orthostatic hypotension with rapid head movements could, at least in part, be explained by inhibition of the vagally mediated carotid-cardiac baroreflex response, as attenuation of HR response from reflex stimulation of the carotid baroreceptors has been associated with orthostatic incompetence (9,17,26,37,39,61). This hypothesis was supported by a recent finding that head rotation about the body's vertical axis in normal ambulatory subjects reduces the cardiac reflex response to controlled stimulation of the carotid baroreceptors by approximately 30% (25). Attenuation of the cardiac response could not be explained by mechanical manipulation of the carotid baroreceptors, as the head was held stationary relative to the body during rotation. These results clearly demonstrate that vestibular stimulation associated with yaw rotation inhibits vagally mediated baroreflex control of HR responsiveness.

This change was virtually identical to the 31% loss of sensitivity reported in subjects following 12 to 25 days of exposure to a ground-based analogue of microgravity (17). Because the magnitude of carotid-cardiac baroreflex impairment after exposure to low gravity is associated with orthostatic incompetence and syncope (17), it is reasonable to speculate that the inhibition of HR response associated with vestibular stimulation might impair BP regulation in situations in which head movements are combined with orthostatic challenges during reambulation.

The inhibitory relationship between vestibular stimulation and carotid-cardiac baroreflex responsiveness has implications for the management of patients or astronauts with orthostatic hypotension. Disturbances in function of the labyrinth function are experienced by astronauts following spaceflight (54,68). It is possible that vestibular disturbances caused by adaptation to low gravity might contribute to orthostatic hypotension by exacerbating already impaired carotid-cardiac baroreflex function. Initial rehabilitation following prolonged confinement to bed rest or spaceflight should therefore include minimal yaw motions of the head. Development of countermeasures that enhance baroreflex responsiveness should be considered as an approach to minimize the effects of vestibular inhibition on cardiac function in orthostatic conditions.

CONCLUSION

Effects on autonomic functions and their interactions with mechanisms of BP regulation induced by low gravity are summarized in Fig. 6. Lower hydrostatic pressure gradients in the cardiovascular system act to reduce the overall reserve capacities of central (cardiac) and peripheral mechanisms associated with orthostatic function. During exposure to low gravity, an apparent reduction in parasympathetic activation associated with higher HR and reduced sympathetic activation may contribute to the underlying mechanisms for hypovolemia and increased responsiveness of cardiac and vascular β-adrenoreceptors. CVP is reduced and venous compliance of the lower extremities is increased during exposure to low gravity. The consequences of these alterations in normal autonomic function become most apparent on return to upright posture in normal gravity. Despite an enhanced aortic-cardiac baroreflex, orthostatic tachycardia can be inhibited by an attenuated

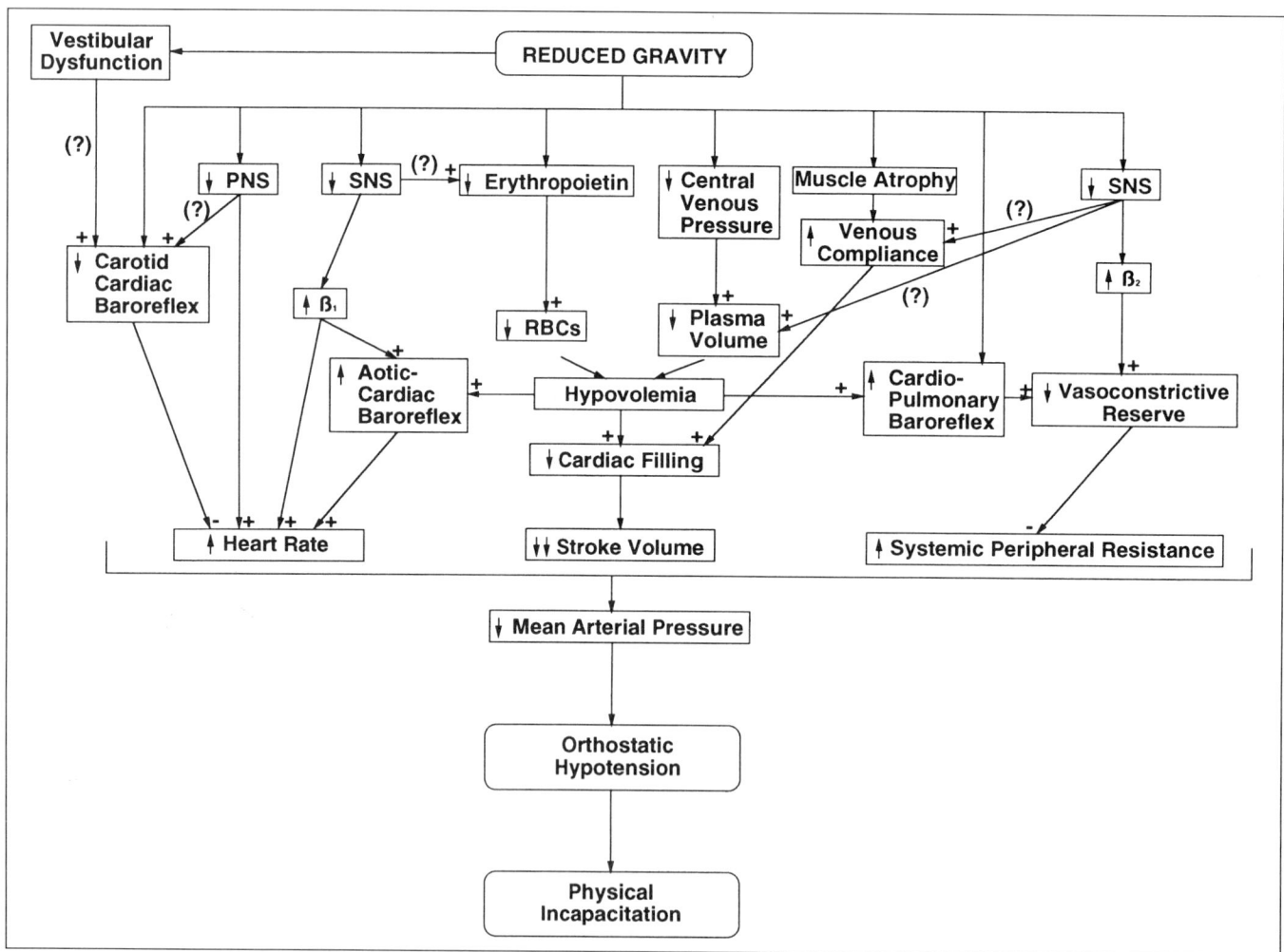

FIG. 6. The effects of low gravity on autonomic functions and interactions as they relate to mechanisms of arterial BP regulation during standing.

carotid-cardiac baroreflex response. Despite increased HR and cardiac contractility during standing, the combination of low central blood volume, reduced central filling pressure, and greater blood pooling can contribute to reduced venous return, lowered stroke volume, and cardiac output. Apparent enhancement of cardiac contractility must be associated with less blood volume and lower CVP. In the face of limited cardiac factors, the capacity to increase systemic peripheral resistance is limited by increased responsiveness of cardiopulmonary baroreflex and vascular β_2-adrenoreceptors, which act to reduce the reserve for vasoconstriction. Because mean arterial pressure is the product of HR, stroke volume, and systemic resistance, the dramatic reduction in stroke volume and attenuated HR and vasoconstrictive responses can lead to disabling orthostatic hypotension.

Effective development and application of treatments designed to prevent diminished orthostatic performance after adaptation to low gravity should include an understanding of changes in the physiologic mechanisms involved and an ability to reverse these changes. Therefore, future research should be aimed at investigations designed to apply treatments that can replace the physiologic stimulus lost by the reduction of gravity.

REFERENCES

1. Alfrey C. Regulation of red cell volume at microgravity. *Med Sci Sports Exerc* 1996;28(suppl):542–544.
2. Bishop VS, Malliani A, Thoren P. Cardiac mechanoreceptors. In: Shepherd JT, Abboud FM, eds. *Peripheral Circulation and Organ Blood Flow*. Bethesda, MD: American Physiological Society; 1983: 497–555 (*Handbook of Physiology: The Cardiovascular Systemy*; section 2, vol III).
3. Blomqvist CG, Stone HL. Cardiovascular adjustments to gravitational stress. In: Shepherd JT, Abboud FM, eds. *Peripheral Circulation and Organ Blood Flow*. Bethesda, MD: American Physiological Society; 1983:1025–1063 (*Handbook of Physiology: The Cardiovascular System*; part 2, vol III).
4. Buckey JC Jr, Lane LD, Levine BD, Watenpaugh DE, Wright SJ, Moore WE, Gaffney FA, Blomqvist CG. Orthostatic intolerance after spaceflight. *J Appl Physiol* 1996;81:7–18.
5. Buckey JC Jr, Gaffney FA, Lane LD, Levine BD, Watenpaugh DE, Wright SJ, Yancy CW, Meyer D, Blomqvist CG. Central venous pressure in space. *J Appl Physiol* 1996;81:19–25.
6. Bungo MW, Charles CB, Johnson PC Jr. Cardiovascular deconditioning during spaceflight and the use of saline as a countermeasure to orthostatic intolerance. *Aviat Space Environ Med* 1985;56:985–990.
7. Butler J, O'Brien M, O'Malley K, Kelly JG. Relationship of β-adrenoreceptor density to fitness in athletes. *Nature* 1982;298:60–62.
8. Convertino VA. Physiological adaptations to weightlessness: effects on exercise and work performance. *Exerc Sport Sci Rev* 1990;18:119–165.
9. Convertino VA. Carotid-cardiac baroreflex: relation with orthostatic hypotension following simulated microgravity and implications for development of countermeasures. *Acta Astronautica* 1991;23: 9–17.
10. Convertino VA. Neuromuscular aspects in development of exercise countermeasures. *Physiologist* 1991;34(Suppl):S125–S128.
11. Convertino VA. Effects of exercise and inactivity on intravascular volume and cardiovascular control mechanisms. *Acta Astronautica* 1992;27:123–129.
12. Convertino VA. Countermeasures against cardiovascular deconditioning. *J Gravitational Physiol* 1994;1:P125–P128.
13. Convertino VA. Exercise and adaptation to microgravity environments. In: Fregly MJ, Blatteis CM, eds. *The Gravitational Environment*. New York: Oxford University Press; 1995:815–843 (*Handbook of Physiology: Environmental Physiology*; section 4, vol II).
14. Convertino VA. Clinical aspects of the control of plasma volume at microgravity and during return to one gravity. *Med Sci Sports Exerc* 1996;28(suppl):545–552.
15. Convertino VA, Adams WC, Shea JD, Thompson CA, Hoffler GW. Impairment of carotid-cardiac vagal baroreflex in wheelchair-dependent quadriplegics. *Am J Physiol* 1991;260:R576–R580.
16. Convertino VA, Baumgartner N. Effects of hypovolemia on aortic baroreflex control of heart rate in humans. *Aviat Space Environ Med* 1995;66:491.
17. Convertino VA, Doerr DF, Eckberg DL, Fritsch JM, Vernikos-Danellis J. Headdown bedrest impairs vagal baroreflex responses and provokes orthostatic hypotension. *J Appl Physiol* 1990;68:1458–1464.
18. Convertino VA, Doerr DF, Flores JF, Hoffler GW, Buchanan P. Leg size and muscle functions associated with leg compliance. *J Appl Physiol* 1988;64:1017–1021.
19. Convertino VA, Doerr DF, Guell A, Marini JF. Effects of acute exercise on attenuated vagal baroreflex function during bedrest. *Aviat Space Environ Med* 1992;63:999–1003.
20. Convertino VA, Doerr DF, Ludwig DA, Vernikos J. Effect of simulated microgravity on cardiopulmonary baroreflex control of forearm vascular resistance. *Am J Physiol* 1994;266:R1962–R1969.
21. Convertino VA, Doerr DF, Stein SL. Changes in size and compliance of the calf following 30 days of simulated microgravity. *J Appl Physiol* 1989;66:1509–1512.
22. Convertino VA, Engelke KA, Ludwig DA, Doerr DF. Restoration of plasma volume after 16 days of head-down tilt induced by a single bout of maximal exercise. *Am J Physiol* 1996;270:R3–R10.
23. Convertino VA, Hoffler GW. Cardiovascular physiology: effects of microgravity. *J Fla Med Assoc* 1992;79:517–524.
24. Convertino VA, Polet JL, Engelke KA, Hoffler GW, Lane LD, Blomqvist CG. Increased β-adrenergic responsiveness induced by 14 days of exposure to simulated microgravity. *J Gravitational Physiol* 1995;2:P66–P67.
25. Convertino, VA, Previc FH, Ludwig DA, Engelken EJ. Effects of vestibular and oculomotor stimulation on responsiveness of the carotid-cardiac baroreflex. *Am J Physiol* (*in press*).
26. Cowley AW, Liard JF, Guyton AC. Role of the baroreceptor reflex in daily control of arterial pressure and other variables in dogs. *Circ Res* 1973;32:564–576.
27. Crandall CG, Engelke KA, Pawelczyk JA, Raven PB, Convertino VA. Power spectral and time-based analysis of heart rate variability following 15 days of simulated microgravity exposure in humans. *Aviat Space Environ Med* 1994;65:1105–1109.
28. Crandall CG, Johnson JM, Convertino VA, Raven PB, Engelke KA. Altered thermoregulatory responses after 15 days of head-down tilt. *J Appl Physiol* 1994;77:1863–1867.
29. Crandall CG, Engelke KA, Convertino VA, Raven PB. Aortic baroreflex control of heart rate following 15 days of simulated microgravity exposure. *J Appl Physiol* 1994;77:2134–2139.
30. Dallman MF, Vernikos J, Keil LC, O'Hara D, Convertino VA. Hormonal, fluid and electrolyte responses to 6° antiorthostatic bed rest in healthy male subjects. In: Usdin E., Lvetnansky R., Axelrod J., eds. *Stress: Role of Catecholamines and Other Neurotransmitters*. New York: Gordon and Breach Scientific Publications; 1984:1057–1077.
31. Delp MD, Holder-Brinkley T, Laughlin MH, Hasser EM. Vasoconstrictor properties of rat aorta are diminished by hindlimb unweighting. *J Appl Physiol* 1993;75:2620–2628.
32. Doba N, Reis DJ. Role of the cerebellum and vestibular apparatus in regulation of orthostatic reflexes in the cat. *Circ Res* 1974;34:9–18.
33. Drummer C, Heer M, Baisch F, Blomqvist CG, Lang RE, Maass H, Gerzer R. Diuresis and natriuresis following isotonic saline infusion in healthy young volunteers before, during and after HDT. *Acta Physiol Scand* 1992;144:101–111.
34. Dunn CD, Lange RD, Kimzey SL, Johnson PC, Leach CS. Serum erythropoietin titers during prolonged bed rest: relevance to the "anemia" of space flight. *Eur J Appl Physiol* 1984;52:178–182.
35. Eckberg DL, Fritsch JM. Influence of ten-day head-down bed rest on human carotid baroreceptor-cardiac reflex function. *Acta Physiol Scand* 1992;144:69–76.

36. Edgerton VR, Zhou M-Y, Ohira Y, Klitgaard H, Jiang B, Bell G, Harris B, Saltin B, Gollnick PD, Roy RR, Day MK, Greenisen M. Human fiber size and enzymatic propoerties after 5 and 11 days of spaceflight. *J Appl Physiol* 1995;78:1733–1739.
37. Engelke KA, Convertino VA. Catecholamine response to maximal exercise following 16 days of simulated microgravity. *Aviat Space Environ Med* 1996;67:243–247.
38. Engelke KA, Doerr DF, Convertino VA. A single bout of exhaustive exercise affects integrated baroreflex function after 16 days of head-down tilt. *Am J Physiol* 1995;269:R614–R620.
39. Engelke KA, Doerr DF, Convertino VA. Application of acute maximal exercise to protect orthostatic tolerance following 16 days of simulated microgravity. *Am J Physiol* 1996;271:R837–R847.
40. Epstein M. Renal, endocrine, and hemodynamic effects of water immersion in humans. In: Fregly MJ, Blatteis CM, eds. *The Gravitational Environment*. New York: Oxford University Press; 1995:845–853 (*Handbook of Physiology: Environmental Physiology*; section 1, vol III).
41. Feldman RD, Limbird LE, Nadeau J, Fitzgerald GA, Robertson D, Wood AJJ. Dynamic regulation of leukocyte beta-adrenergic receptor agonist interactions by physiological changes in circulating catecholamines. *J Clin Invest* 1983;72:164–170.
42. Ferguson DW, Abboud FM, Mark AL. Relative contribution of aortic and carotid baroreflexes to heart rate control in man during steady state and dynamic increase in arterial pressure. *J Clin Invest* 1985;76:2265–2274.
43. Fink GD, Fisher JW. Stimulation of erythropoiesis by beta-adrenergic agonists. II. Mechanism of action. *J Pharmacol Exp Ther* 1977;202:199–207.
44. Fink GD, Paulo LG, Fisher JW. Effects of beta-adrenergic blocking agents on erythropoietin production in rabbits exposed to hypoxia. *J Pharmacol Exp Ther* 1975;193:176–181.
45. Fritsch JM, Charles JB, Bennett BS, Jones MM, Wood DL. Short-duration spaceflight impairs human carotid baroreceptor-cardiac reflex responses. *J Appl Physiol* 1992;73:664–671.
46. Fritsch-Yelle JM, Charles JB, Jones MM, Beightol LA, Eckberg DL. Spaceflight alters autonomic regulation of arterial pressure in humans. *J Appl Physiol* 1994;77:1776–1783.
47. Fritsch-Yelle JM, Charles JB, Jones MM, Wood ML. Microgravity decreases heart rate and arterial pressure in humans. *J Appl Physiol* 1996;80:910–914.
48. Gabrielsen A, Norsk P, Videraek R, Hendriksen O. Effect of microgravity on forearm subcutaneous vascular resistance in humans. *J Appl Physiol* 1995;79:434–438.
49. Goldstein DS, Vernikos J, Holmes C, Convertino VA. Catecholaminergic effects of prolonged head-down bed rest. *J Appl Physiol* 1995;78:1023–1029.
50. Graham RM, Zisfein JB. Atrial natriuretic factor regulation and control in circulatory homeostasis. In: Fozzard HA, Haber E, Jennings RB, Katz AM, Morgan HE, eds. *The Heart and Cardiovascular System. Scientific Foundation*. New York: Raven Press; 1986:1559–1572.
51. Hawkins WR, Zieglschmid JF. Clinical aspects of crew health. In: Johnston RS, Dietlein LF, Berry CA, eds. *Biomedical Results of Apollo*. Washington, DC: BioTechnology; 1975:43–81.
52. Hoffler GW. Cardiovascular studies of U.S. space crews: an overview and perspective. In: Hwang NHC, Normann NA, eds. *Cardiovascular Flow Dynamics and Measurements*. Baltimore: University Park Press; 1977:335–363.
53. Hoffler GW, Johnson RL, Nicogossian AE, Bergman SA Jr, Jackson MM. Vectorcardiographic results from Skylab medical experiment MO92: lower body negative pressure. In: Johnston RS, Dietlein LF, eds. *Biomedical Results from Skylab*. Washington, DC: NASA; 1977:313–323 (NASA Special Report SP-377).
54. Homick JL, Reschke MF, Miller EF. The effects of prolonged exposure to weightlessness on postural equilibrium. In: Johnston RS, Dietlein LF, eds. *Biomedical Results from Skylab*. Washington, DC: NASA; 1977:104–112 (NASA Special Report SP-377).
55. Johnson RL, Hoffler GW, Nicogossian AE, Bergman SA Jr, Jackson MM. Lower body negative pressure: third manned Skylab mission. In: Johnston RS, Dietlein LF, eds. *Biomedical Results from Skylab*. Washington, DC: NASA; 1977:284–312 (NASA Special Report SP-377).
56. Klein KE, Wegmann HM, Kuklinski P. Athletic endurance training—advantage for spaceflight? The significance of physical fitness for selection and training of Spacelab crews. *Aviat Space Environ Med* 1977;48:215–222.
57. Kvetnansky R, Noskov VB, Blazicek P, Gharib C, Popova IA, Gauquelin G, et al. Activity of the sympathoadrenal system in cosmonauts during 25-day space flight on station Mir. *Acta Astronautica* 1991;23:109–116.
58. Leach CS, Altchuler SI, Cintron-Trevino NM. The endocrine and metabolic responses to space flight. *Med Sci Sports Exerc* 1983;15:432–440.
59. Leach CS, Johnson PC. Influence of spaceflight on erythrokinetics in man. *Science* 1984;225:216–218.
60. Leach CS, Rambaut PC. Endocrine responses in long-duration manned space flight. *Acta Astronautica* 1975;2:115–127.
61. Ludwig DA, Convertino VA. Predicting orthostatic intolerance: physics or physiology? *Aviat Space Environ Med* 1994;65:404–411.
62. McDonald KS, Delp MD, Fitts RH. Effect of hindlimb unweighting on tissue blood flow in the rat. *J Appl Physiol* 1992;72:2210–2218.
63. Milot JA, Jacob JL, Blanc VF, Hardy JF. The oculocardiac reflex in strabismus surgery. *Can J Ophthalmol* 1983;18:314–317.
64. Nicogossian AE, Charles CB, Bungo MW, Leach-Huntoon CS. Cardiovascular function in space flight. *Acta Astronautica* 1991;24:323–328.
65. Norre ME, Degroote M. Influence of caloric and rotation testing upon blood pressure and pulse rate. In: Claussen C-F, Kirtane MV, Schlitter K, eds. *Vertigo, Nausea, Tinnitus and Hypoacusia in Metabolic Disorders*. New York: Excerpta Medica; 1988:139–142.
66. Patil NP, Schneider D, Claussen C-F, Popivanova C. Cardiac reactions in neuro-otological patients during vestibular stimulation. In: Claussen C-F, Kirtane MV, Schlitter K, eds. *Vertigo, Nausea, Tinnitus and Hypoacusia in Metabolic Disorders*. New York: Excerpta Medica; 1988:149–154.
67. Previc FH. Do the organs of the labyrinth differentially influence the sympathetic and parasympathetic systems? *Neurosci Biobehav Rev* 1993;17:397–404.
68. Previc FH. Autonomic disturbances resulting from exposure to unusual gravitational environments. In: Yates BJ, Miller AD, eds. *Vestibular Autonomic Regulation*. Boca Raton, FL: CRC Press; 1996:175–196.
69. Robertson D, Convertino VA, Vernikos J. The sympathetic nervous system and the physiologic consequences of spaceflight: a hypothesis. *Am J Med Sci* 1994;308:126–132.
70. Robertson D, Perry SE, Hollister AS, Robertson RM, Biaggioni I. Dopamine-β-hydroxylase deficiency: a genetic disorder of cardiovascular regulation. *Hypertension* 1991;18:1–8.
71. Smith RF, Stanton K, Stoop D, Janusz W, King P. Quantitative electrocardiography during extended spaceflight: the second Skylab mission. *Aviat Space Environ Med* 1976;47:353–359.
72. Spiegel EA. Effect of labyrinthine reflexes on the vegetative nervous system. *Arch Otolaryngol* 1946;44:61–71.
73. Takaru F, Hirashima K, Okinaka S. Effect of bilateral section of the splanchnic nerve on erythropoiesis. *Nature* 1961;191:500–501.
74. Thompson CA, Tatro DL, Ludwig DA, Convertino VA. Baroreflex responses to acute changes in blood volume in man. *Am J Physiol* 1990;259:R792–R798.
75. Thompson FJ, Yates BJ, Franzen O, Wald JR. Lumbar spinal cord responses to limb vein distention. *J Auton Nerv Syst* 1983;9:531–546.
76. Thornton WE, Hoffler GW. Hemodynamic studies of the legs under weightlessness. In: Johnson RS, Dietlein, LF, eds. *Biomedical Results from Skylab*. Washington, DC: NASA; 1977:324–329 (NASA Special Report SP-377).
77. Vernikos J, Convertino VA. Advantages and disadvantages of fludrocortisone or saline load in preventing post-spaceflight orthostatic hypotension. *Acta Astronautica* 1994;33:259–266.
78. White RJ, Leonard JI, Srinivasan RS, Charles JB. Mathematical modeling of acute and chronic cardiovascular changes during extended duration orbitor (EDO) flights. *Acta Astronautica* 1991;23:41–51.
79. Whitson PA, Charles JB, Williams WJ, Cintron NM. Changes in sympathoadrenal response to standing in humans after spaceflight. *J Appl Physiol* 1995;79:428–433.

CHAPTER 34

Autonomic Disorders of the Pupil, Ciliary Body, and Lacrimal Apparatus

Shelley Ann Cross

1. Failed parasympathetic control of pupillary function may arise when prenuclear (supranuclear), nuclear or axonal (cell body outflow), or postganglionic lesions occur. Prenuclear lesions include Argyll Robertson pupils and spastic miosis. Nuclear and axonal lesions include third-nerve palsies that result in internal, external, or complete ophthalmoplegia. Postganglionic lesions cause tonic pupils, of which Adie's pupil is one type.
2. Failed sympathetic control of pupillary function results in Horner's syndrome. This may involve the first-order neuron (central), the second-order neuron (preganglionic), or the third-order neuron (postganglionic). It may be either congenital or acquired.
3. Irritative lesions of the sympathetic innervation to the eye may precipitate oculosympathetic spasm. Irritative lesions of the parasympathetic innervation may cause periodic miosis or elliptic pupil.
4. Numerous exogenous substances, acting either topically or systemically, affect pupil size and reactivity. Agents that dilate the pupils are either parasympatholytic or sympathomimetic. Agents that constrict the pupils are either parasympathomimetic or sympatholytic.
5. Anisocoria and light-near dissociation can be evaluated based on the details of their clinical features and the results of selected pharmacologic maneuvers with topical agents.
6. Objective measures of pupillary function include the edge-light pupil cycle time and pupillography.
7. Lesions that affect the tearing apparatus may be parasympathetic or sympathetic, but parasympathetic input predominates. They may be prenuclear (supranuclear), nuclear or axonal (cell body or outflow), or postganglionic. A classic example of an outflow disorder is the syndrome of crocodile tears. This syndrome is caused by aberrant regeneration of taste fibers into empty sudomotor pathways.
8. Keratoconjunctivitis sicca is a condition of dry eyes that results from decreased tear production, and is a measure of autonomic innervation to the eye. It can be evaluated using Schirmer's test, assessment of tear osmolarity, inspection of the cornea for evidence of dryness, and determination of the chemical constituents of tears.
9. Numerous diseases, by interrupting the pathways of the autonomic nervous system at prenuclear, nuclear, axonal, postganglionic, or neuromuscular junction levels, affect the functions of the pupil, ciliary muscle, and lacrimal glands.

PARASYMPATHETIC DEFICIENCIES

The various parasympathetic deficiencies are described below and summarized in Table 1. Figure 1 is a flow chart for evaluation of anisocoria including pharmacologic testing.

S. A. Cross: Department of Neurology, Mayo Clinic, Rochester, Minnesota 55905.

Argyll Robertson Pupils

In 1869, Douglas Argyll Robertson published two articles that described five cases of tabes dorsalis. The characteristic ocular findings included the following: (a) the retinas were sensitive to light; (b) the pupils did not respond to light; (c) the pupils constricted normally during accommodation and convergence; (d) the pupils constricted with

TABLE 1. *Parasympathetic deficiencies*

Argyll-Robertson pupils
1. Very small pupils
2. Unresponsive to light
3. Constrict normally during accommodation and convergence
4. Constrict with physostigmine
5. Dilate poorly with Atropine

Light-near dissociation
1. Large pupils
2. Do not constrict to light
3. React well to near stimuli

Spastic miosis
1. Partial or total loss of both light and near reactions

Internal and external ophthalmoplegia
1. Fixed and dilated pupils

Aberrant regeneration involving the pupil
1. Pupils constrict with gaze in certain directions
2. Segmental contractions of the iris
3. Pupillary unrest in pupils which do not react to light

Tonic pupil
1. Poor pupillary constriction to light
2. Regional palsy of the iris sphincter
3. Paralysis of accommodation
4. Cholinergic supersensitivity of the denervated pupillary constrictor
5. Strong and tonic response to near
6. Tonic redilatation after constriction to near stimuli

Adies pupil
1. A subset of tonic pupil
2. Associated with reduced or absent deep tendon reflexes

physostigmine but dilated poorly with atropine; and (e) the pupils were very small (58). When it was finally understood that tabetic general paresis and central nervous system lues were all manifestations of central nervous system syphilis, the Argyll Robertson pupil was regarded as being virtually pathognomonic of neurosyphilis.

One of the hallmarks of the syndrome is that the pupils are smaller than those observed for a normal subject in darkness. The pupils are also irregular. Large pupils in conjunction with the other features of light-near dissociation are more often associated with diseases other than syphilis. As Argyll Robertson pupils develop, the light reflex is first impaired and then completely lost. The near response is usually somewhat impaired, but dissociation between light and near responses remains. Usually both pupils are affected, but sometimes there is asymmetric or even unilateral involvement. Patients may or may not have prompt pupillary dilation in response to psychosensory stimulation. Some patients exhibit associated atrophy of the iris, although atrophy can occur in patients with syphilis who do not have Argyll Robertson pupils. As long as this atrophy is not present, Argyll Robertson pupils dilate in response to administration of atropine and cocaine and constrict well in response to miotics.

Although the location of the lesion that results in the Argyll Robertson pupil has been disputed, the rostral midbrain is the most likely place (58). A variety of lines of evidence support this conclusion. The oculomotor light-reflex fibers enter the Edinger-Westphal nucleus on its dorsal aspect; the fibers for near vision enter this nucleus slightly more ventrally and hence could be spared in a dorsal lesion. Bilateral loss of the light reflex, with an intact near response, is often seen in patients with dorsal midbrain lesions, such as pinealomas. There is experimental evidence in animals of intact accommodation and abolished light reflexes when the brachia of the superior colliculi have been cut bilaterally (27). Neuropathologic studies in patients who have died of tabes or general paresis show marked diffuse ependymitis and subependymal gliosis in the periaqueductal gray region. Besides the injury to the light-reflex fibers from the pretectal area, the supranuclear inhibitory pathways may be compromised. The absence of this descending inhibition causes permanent spasticity in the motor system of the pupil, that is, spastic paralysis.

The complete syndrome of Argyll Robertson pupils has been observed in a number of diseases other than neurosyphilis, including viral encephalitis, multiple sclerosis, degenerative diseases of the nervous system, systemic inflammatory illnesses, tumors, diabetes, and chronic alcoholism (29,35,42,58).

Light-Near Dissociation

Features of the syndrome of light-near dissociation typically consist of large pupils that do not constrict in response to light but do react well to near stimuli. One underlying cause for this is a lesion in the area of the posterior commissure. Supranuclear vertical gaze palsies and convergence retraction nystagmus on upward gaze are associated anomalies. Other pupillary findings in patients with midbrain lesions include fixed dilated pupils and pupils that react poorly to both light and near stimuli. These are caused by damage to afferents that extend to the visceral oculomotor nuclei, or by damage to the nuclei and their efferents. Minimally reactive or unreactive pupils may precede the development of supranuclear gaze palsies and convergence retraction nystagmus (58). Other types of light-near dissociation are discussed later in this chapter.

Spastic Miosis

Spastic miosis is characterized by partial or total loss of both light and near reactions. The pupils do not dilate in darkness, but they do dilate in response to topically administered anticholinergic agents. They therefore possess all the features of Argyll Robertson pupils except for the dis-

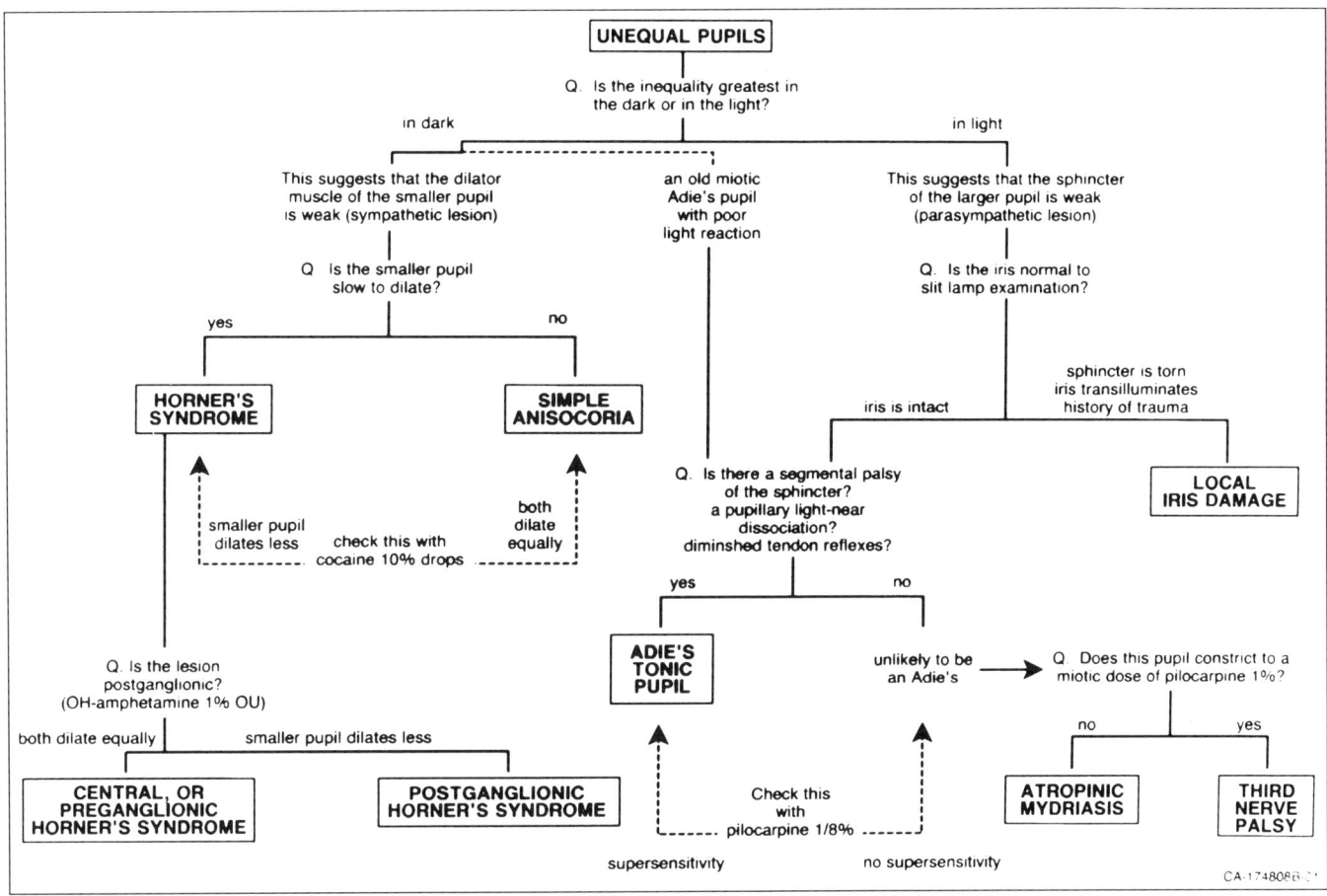

FIG. 1. Flow chart for the evaluation of anisocoria.

sociation between light and near reactions. These small pupils are seen in patients with atherosclerosis, degenerative disease, and long-standing diabetes. The lesion is possibly located in the midbrain where excitatory and inhibitory light impulses converge on the Edinger-Westphal nucleus (58).

Internal and External Ophthalmoplegia

Lesions of the parasympathetic outflow pathway abolish pupillary constriction. In this condition, the pupils are fixed and dilated. Accommodation may also be lost. This combined loss of both pupillary constriction and accommodation is called *internal ophthalmoplegia*. It is distinct from *external ophthalmoplegia*, in which the extraocular muscles are paralyzed although the pupillary and accommodative responses are intact, and from *complete ophthalmoplegia*, in which both groups of muscles are involved. Isolated iris paralysis should prompt a search for a pathologic lesion along this outflow pathway.

If the nuclei themselves are involved, rarely does the lesion produce only isolated dilated pupils. Because the parasympathetic fibers lie superficially within the third nerve, inflammatory lesions such as meningitis may involve them preferentially. Inflammatory and infectious lesions may also involve the ciliary ganglion, the postganglionic fibers, or both. Illnesses causing such lesions include leprosy, herpes zoster, varicella, measles, diphtheria, scarlet fever, pertussis, and influenza.

Intracranial aneurysms can cause a fixed and dilated pupil, but they almost always produce paralysis of the extraocular muscles as well. Temporal arteritis can also cause similar findings (43). There is a variant of ophthalmoplegic migraine that elicits transient pupillary dilation, blurred vision, and headaches (58). These patients probably have increased sympathetic activity rather than parasympathetic weakness. Unilateral dilation of the pupil in a comatose patient is a sign of transtentorial herniation of the hippocampal gyrus.

Aberrant Regeneration Involving the Pupil

Traumatic lesions of the third nerve may result in aberrant regeneration, and this misdirected regrowth can involve axons destined for the ciliary ganglion. Somatic motor axons can grow into the nerve sheaths leading to the ganglion, and this causes the pupils to constrict when the patient is asked to look in a certain direction. There may be segmental contractions of the iris in response to light or eye movements and abnormal pupillary unrest in patients whose pupils do not react to light. Observation with the aid of magnification helps assess these clinical findings. Pupillary constriction can occur in association with gaze in any direction that requires functioning of the third nerve, but it is most often seen with attempted adduction. For this reason, aberrant regeneration can be confused with the Argyll Robertson pupil (58).

Tonic Pupil

The postganglionic parasympathetic fibers may be damaged, causing a syndrome that involves poor pupillary constriction to light, regional palsy of the iris sphincter, paralysis of accommodation, cholinergic supersensitivity of the denervated muscle, a strong and tonic response to a near stimulus, and slow and tonic redilation after constriction to a near stimulus. These pupils are termed *tonic*. Tonic pupils may arise from local inflammatory disease in the ciliary ganglion (4), or they may be part of a generalized neuropathic process such as autonomic neuropathy (55), congenital syphilis (53), or Guillain-Barré syndrome; they may also be part of the Adie's tonic pupil syndrome (9,34).

Adie's Pupil

In Adie's tonic pupil syndrome, tonic pupils are associated with reduced or absent deep tendon reflexes, but no other nervous system disease. The syndrome occurs sporadically in otherwise healthy individuals, who are usually between the ages of 20 and 50 years; 70% of those affected are women. The onset is usually unilateral, but the second pupil can eventually become involved. The patients generally complain of a difference in the size of their pupils, problems adapting to the dark, photophobia, and difficulty focusing. The symptoms generally gradually disappear, because the pupils tend to get smaller with time and the ciliary muscle becomes reinnervated. Adie's syndrome usually arises acutely and can be mistaken for a pharmacologically induced mydriasis and cycloplegia. Vermiform movements of the iris probably represent physiologic hippus occurring in certain sectors of the iris sphincter that are still reactive.

The etiology of Adie's syndrome is unknown, but it probably results from a systemic infection with a neurotropic virus. The ganglionic parasympathetic fibers that have their cell bodies in the ciliary ganglion are affected by the lesion. In pathologic studies, the ciliary ganglion is almost devoid of cells. Both the spinal cord and spinal roots have been implicated as the site of the lesion causing the areflexia. The number of nerve cell bodies in the dorsal root ganglia is reduced, and the axons of the posterior columns secondarily degenerate (46).

The question has been raised as to why the light reflex is much more severely impaired than the near reflex. To answer this question, one must realize that once damage has occurred in the autonomic nervous system, regeneration of injured fibers is extremely active. Collateral fibers can even sprout from undamaged axons, and aberrant regeneration is the rule. The fibers to the iris sphincter constitute a small percentage of the total number of postganglionic neurons, as most of the axons supply the ciliary muscle. When the ganglion is injured, there is therefore a greater chance for the cells serving accommodation to survive, and when collateral fibers sprout, there is a greater probability for these to arise from axons of accommodation. These sprouting fibers innervate the ciliary muscle and the iris, so the pupil constricts in response to a near stimulus. This may also explain why the pupil becomes smaller with time (36).

Both the iris sphincter and the ciliary muscle are supersensitive to acetylcholine, and when stimulated, their response is strong and tonic, whereas their relaxation is slow and sustained. The Adie's pupil can be diagnosed by this denervation supersensitivity. A 2.5% solution of methacholine chloride (Mecholyl) produces intense miosis, whereas 15% concentrations are needed to obtain even a slight response in a normal pupil. A 0.1% solution of pilocarpine possesses an even stronger miotic action. Adie's pupils react normally to cocaine and epinephrine, thus showing that the sympathetic nervous system is intact.

Use of a weak solution of pilocarpine to treat patients with uncomfortable photophobia has been advocated. Because of the denervation supersensitivity of the ciliary muscle, however, pilocarpine can cause excessive uncomfortable spasm. Astigmatism, which is induced by irregular muscular contraction in the ciliary muscle that distorts the lens, develops in some patients with Adie's syndrome. When necessary, this can be corrected with lenses.

SYMPATHETIC DEFICIENCY

Horner's Syndrome

When the sympathetic outflow to the eye is interrupted, Horner's syndrome results (Table 2). Complete paralysis of this outflow to the head causes moderate miosis, ptosis, and facial anhidrosis. In addition, ocular hypotony, a decrease in the amplitude of accommodation, and pigmentary abnormalities in the iris may be seen. Pupillary reactions to light and near vision are normal. The pupil is small because the dilator muscle is paretic. In bright light, the pupils may appear equal, but when examined in dim light, there is obvious anisocoria. This is the opposite of what occurs in essential anisocoria, a simple nonpathologic variation in the

TABLE 2. *Sympathetic deficiencies: Horner's syndrome*

1. Miosis more apparent in dim light
2. Ptosis
3. Facial anhydrosis
4. Ocular hypotomy
5. Decreased amplitude of accommodation
6. Failure to acquire iris pigment (Congenital Horner's syndrome)
7. Loss of iris pigment (Acquired Horner's syndrome)

size of pupils that is less prominent in the dark and more obvious in the light. In the presence of intense sympathetic outflow brought about by stress or excitement, the denervated Horner's pupil can become paradoxically enlarged owing to denervation supersensitivity to circulating catecholamines. The paralysis of the dilator muscle in Horner's syndrome can be demonstrated, in that a Horner's pupil dilates more slowly in darkness than does a normal pupil. Ptosis occurs because of paralysis of Muller's muscle, a sympathetically innervated muscle in the upper lid. Similar smooth muscle fibers in the lower lid are also denervated, causing elevation of the lower lid and further narrowing of the palpebral fissure. The patient appears to have enophthalmos, but this is apparent rather than real.

Ipsilateral impairment of sweating and vasoconstriction on the face and neck are characteristic of a preganglionic Horner's syndrome. After an acute denervation injury, the skin temperature rises on the side of the lesion because of the loss of vasomotor control. Later, the skin may have a lower temperature and be paler because of supersensitivity of the denervated blood vessels, with resultant vasoconstriction to circulating α-adrenergic amines. Paradoxic sweating and flushing can be a late development in patients following cervical sympathectomy and cervical injuries. Apparently, some axons in the vagus nerve pass through the superior cervical ganglion, and by collateral sprouting they establish anomalous vagal connections with postganglionic sympathetic neurons going to the head and neck. The patient may have sudomotor and pilomotor activity, as well as flushing that is reflexively linked to vagus nerve function (58).

The sympathetic innervation of the eye plays a role in aqueous humor dynamics. Patients with postganglionic Horner's syndrome have decreased intraocular pressure, lowered aqueous humor production, and normal outflow. This hypotony, however, is neither a constant nor permanent feature of Horner's syndrome. Parasympathetic innervation can also affect aqueous humor dynamics, and glaucomatous eyes may show parasympathetic denervation as well.

In patients with congenital Horner's syndrome, heterochromia iridis, with the affected iris remaining blue, is a common finding. It is caused by failure of pigment development. The sympathetic nervous system may influence iris pigmentation by delivering norepinephrine or other melanin precursors to the melanocytes; by inducing tyrosinase activity, the rate-limiting enzyme in melanin synthesis; by activating prostaglandins that enhance melanin synthesis; and by releasing other melanotropic substances (47). Iris depigmentation can also occur after sympathetic nervous system injury in adults.

Congenital Horner's Syndrome

Congenital Horner's syndrome is uncommon. Many of the cases are caused by brachial plexus injuries sustained at birth, but some have been reported in association with congenital tumors, viral infections, fibromuscular dysplasia of the internal carotid artery, and prenatal or neonatal trauma to the neck. High-forceps deliveries, which cause stretching of the sympathetic plexus in the carotid sheath, may result in a postganglionic Horner's lesion. Some patients have lesions that can be pharmacologically localized to the superior cervical ganglion, possibly resulting from abnormal embryologic development of the ganglion, damage to its vascular supply, or transsynaptic degeneration from a preganglionic injury. The preganglionic pathway is usually injured during trauma to the brachial plexus or by surgery in the thoracic region. Pharmacologic testing may suggest a postganglionic lesion, probably indicating transsynaptic degeneration (59). Congenital Horner's syndrome has been reported in association with facial hemiatrophy, or Möbius' syndrome, and with congenital abnormalities of the cervical vertebrae (58).

Acquired Horner's Syndrome

Acquired Horner's syndrome may be central, preganglionic, or postganglionic (48). In the central type of Horner's syndrome, the lesion is in the first-order neuron somewhere between its origin in the hypothalamus and its termination in the spinal center of Budge-Waller. Many of these central lesions are secondary to brain stem infarction, particularly the lateral medullary syndrome of Wallenberg; cerebral infarction and hemorrhage; tumor; syringomyelia; multiple sclerosis; trauma; or chronic infection. In some patients with cervical cord lesions, the Horner's syndrome appears to affect one eye and then the other in alternating fashion. This probably represents intermittent interruption of the sympathetic outflow down the cervical cord, first on one side and then on the other, or intermittent irritation of the ciliospinal center of Budge-Waller by, for example, fluid in a syrinx (15).

Preganglionic Horner's syndrome affects the second-order neuron from its origin in the spinal center of Budge-Waller to its termination in the superior cervical ganglion. It is caused by lesions of the high thoracic and low cervical regions, particularly trauma and tumor. If cervical sympathetic pathways are interrupted in the lower neck, where fibers are bundled together, the complete syndrome is likely to ensue. When the axons leaving the spinal center of Budge are involved, the lesion may be less complete, because the fibers are somewhat dispersed. The syndrome has been seen with fracture dislocations of the cervical spine; traction on the brachial plexus; surgical trauma to the thorax or neck, including cervical fusions; carotid artery or jugular vein puncture; extradural thoracic anesthesia; radical thyroid surgery; and anesthesia given by the lumbar epidural route. A variety of tumors may invade the lung apex and mediastinum and produce a Horner's syndrome, including lung and breast carcinoma, sarcoma, lymphoma, and tumors of the vertebral column and the meninges. As the sympathetic fibers exit the intervertebral foramina, they can be injured by osteophytes, meningitis, or pressure from a thoracic aneurysm (58).

Postganglionic Horner's syndrome involves the final neuron in the sympathetic pathway, between its origin in the superior cervical ganglion and its termination in sympathetically innervated smooth muscle. Lesions affecting this neuron may be extracranial, in the carotid artery of the neck, or intracranial, in the sympathetic chain at the base of the skull, carotid canal, middle ear, or cavernous sinus.

Tumors and other lesions in the cavernous sinus may produce a Horner's syndrome in association with ophthalmoplegia and a deficit in the first division of the fifth nerve. In cases in which the third nerve is also involved, the Horner's syndrome may be masked by the ptosis and mydriasis of the third-nerve lesion. A small pupil can be secondary to primary aberrant third-nerve regeneration, rather than a true Horner's syndrome.

Inflammatory conditions such as otitis media, herpetic geniculate neuralgia, meningitis, sinusitis, herpes zoster, and Tolosa-Hunt syndrome can all be associated with Horner's syndrome. Blunt and penetrating trauma can also be responsible. Horner's syndrome is prominent during cluster headaches and may be present in migraine as well. Abnormalities of the carotid artery, including aneurysms, fibromuscular hyperplasia, atherosclerosis, and occlusion, can all result in a Horner's syndrome by interrupting the vasa nervorum or stretching the sympathetic fibers themselves.

When Horner's syndrome is acquired in childhood, it is often associated with serious disease, including spinal cord tumor, traumatic brachial plexus palsy, intrathoracic aneurysm, embryonal cell carcinoma, neuroblastoma, rhabdomyosarcoma, and thrombosis of the internal carotid artery. It is sometimes part of a generalized peripheral or autonomic neuropathy that may be caused by diabetes, the Miller-Fisher variant of Guillain-Barré syndrome, or multiple-system atrophy (58).

It can be difficult to distinguish between simple anisocoria and Horner's syndrome, as a benign difference in the size of the pupils is seen in about 20% of the normal population. The pupillary inequality in Horner's syndrome is more obvious in darkness, and that of essential anisocoria is less obvious. In addition, pharmacologic maneuvers can be helpful in making this distinction. The neurotransmitter released by the third-order neuron at the neuromuscular junction in the sympathetic nervous system is norepinephrine. Release of this substance acts on the iris dilator muscle to dilate the pupil. Cocaine prevents the reuptake of norepinephrine into the nerve terminal and therefore causes the normal pupil to dilate. With complete interruption of the sympathetic pathway, however, no physiologic release of norepinephrine occurs and cocaine has nothing to act on, so the pupil dilates poorly or not at all. This is true for a Horner's syndrome, no matter where the lesion is located. A 10% solution of cocaine is generally preferred, because it acts more quickly than do the more dilute solutions. One drop is placed in each eye and the procedure is repeated 5 min later. The pupils are evaluated in dim light every 15 min for 45 min to assess the extent and speed of pupillary dilation. Cocaine is painful when applied to the cornea, but it is preferable to avoid pretreatment with an anesthetic for fear of damaging the corneal epithelium and influencing the outcome of the test.

Once Horner's syndrome has been confirmed, the location—central, preganglionic, or postganglionic—must be determined. Associated neurologic signs and symptoms can be extremely useful in establishing this. Pharmacologic testing is also helpful. Hydroxyamphetamine hydrobromide (Paredrine) and tyramine hydrochloride appear to be the best agents for distinguishing postganglionic from preganglionic or central lesions. Their primary mode of action is the release of norepinephrine from the nerve terminals of postganglionic sympathetic neurons. If the postganglionic neuron has been injured, norepinephrine will not be available for release and these substances will not dilate the pupil. A drop of 1% Paredrine is instilled in each eye, and the procedure is repeated 5 min later. About 45 min later, the pupils are evaluated in a darkened room. Occasionally, patients appear to have a preganglionic lesion clinically, but they show poor mydriasis when tested with Paredrine and supersensitivity to 1% phenylephrine. The reason for this probably involves transsynaptic degeneration of the postganglionic neuron. This test, therefore, can be difficult to interpret in patients with congenital Horner's syndrome or in newborns with acquired Horner's syndrome. Unfortunately, Paredrine has recently become unavailable.

A second type of pharmacologic test that can differentiate between postganglionic and preganglionic Horner's syndrome involves the use of very dilute concentrations of epinephrine or norepinephrine. Neither of these agents, in dilute solution, dilates a normal pupil, but they do dilate a postganglionic Horner's pupil because of the denervation supersensitivity of the iris dilator muscle. A 1% solution of phenylephrine hydrochloride may be used for this test. Because it is essential that approximately equal amounts of the drug reach the iris dilator in each eye, there must be absolutely no mechanical or pharmacologic disruption of the corneal epithelium before the test. Disturbance of the epithelium might cause increased permeability and thus allow enough of the drug to enter the eye to dilate a normal pupil. At least 24 to 48 hrs should elapse after cocaine testing before Paredrine or phenylephrine is used.

AUTONOMIC IRRITATION

Sympathetic Irritation or Oculosympathetic Spasm

The converse of a Horner's syndrome is sympathetic irritation or oculosympathetic spasm (Table 3). This consists of irritation of the sympathetic pathway, resulting in intermittent or constant ipsilateral pupillary dilation, sometimes associated with facial flushing and hyperhidrosis. It can be caused by chronic cervical spinal cord disease, such as syringomyelia (30), and it has been described in patients with malignant lung tumors, puncture of the internal carotid artery, pulmonary infections, or pneumothorax, or who have undergone thyroidectomy (58). It has been postulated that the large pupils seen in some patients with migraine may be the result of sympathetic irritation (12). Sometimes the pupils are large and irregular, suggesting sympathetic spasm that affects the iris. Thompson and Zackon (57) reported on 26 of these patients with what they termed "tadpole-shaped pupils" caused by segmental spasm of the iris dilator muscle. Eleven had Horner's syndrome, four had Adie's pupil, and eight had definite or probable migraine. Central sympathetic discharges may occur during or after seizures and can evoke transient pupillary dilation. This usually occurs after *petit mal* seizures but can be seen with partial motor seizures as well. The mechanism may involve sympathetic irritation and parasympathetic interruption (32,58).

Parasympathetic Irritation

Periodic miosis with conjunctival hyperemia and increased accommodation may be associated with cluster headache (11).

TABLE 3. *Autonomic irritation*

Sympathetic irritation or oculosympathetic spasm
1. Pupillary dilitation, intermittent or constant
2. Facial flushing
3. Hyperhidrosis
Parasympathetic Irritation
1. Miosis, generally periodic
2. Conjunctival hyperemia
3. Increased accommodation

EXOGENOUS SUBSTANCES AFFECTING PUPILLARY SIZE AND REACTIVITY

A number of topical agents dilate or constrict the pupil, but there are wide individual variations in the sensitivity to these drugs. The emotional and physical state of the patient may also affect the size of the pupils. If there is denervation hypersensitivity, the exact location and completeness of the lesion may affect the result of a test using drops. Whenever possible, one pupil should be used as an internal control.

Pupillary Dilators

Agents that dilate the pupil either prevent the functioning of the iris sphincter or stimulate the dilator.

Parasympatholytic Agents

Parasympatholytic (anticholinergic) agents act directly on the iris sphincter and ciliary muscles to block the action of the acetylcholine released by the postganglionic sympathetic neurons. They produce both mydriasis and cycloplegia. All cycloplegic agents produce mydriasis, but not all mydriatic agents produce cycloplegia. Atropine and scopolamine are naturally occurring alkaloids found in the deadly nightshade, henbane, jimsonweed, and moonflower plants; they block parasympathetic activity by competing with acetylcholine at the neuromuscular junction, thereby preventing depolarization. Most cases of mydriasis and cycloplegia occur after topical absorption of these agents, although mydriasis can arise after systemic administration. The mydriasis and cycloplegia may continue for from 10 days to 3 weeks. Scopolamine, in concentrations of 0.25%–0.5%, is similar to atropine in its action, but the effects are of shorter duration, lasting up to 7 days. Homatropine and eucatropine are synthetic anticholinergic agents that cause mydriasis and cycloplegia.

Tropicamide (Mydriacyl, 0.5%–1%) is a synthetic anticholinergic agent that produces transient mydriasis and cycloplegia, with an onset of action in 15 to 30 min and a duration of action of 30 min to 4 hrs. Cyclopentolate (Cycologyl, 0.5%–2%) is another synthetic agent with very little mydriatic but greater cycloplegic effect. Its onset of action is 20 to 45 min, and its duration of action is 3 to 24 hrs.

The parasympathetic pathway can be interrupted by blocking the release of acetylcholine, as with botulinum toxin, and by interfering with the synthesis of acetylcholine, as with hemicholinum. Systemic doses of these drugs are also effective.

All the above-mentioned parasympatholytic agents result in a dilated nonreactive pupil. There are two other instances of large, unreactive pupils having a similar appearance—an acute tonic pupil (Adie's pupil), and an early third-nerve palsy presenting with pupillary dilation but no other signs. These are discussed on page 443 and 444.

Sympathomimetic Agents

Sympathomimetic agents produce mydriasis by stimulating the iris dilator directly, by causing release of norepinephrine at the nerve terminal, or by blocking the reuptake of norepinephrine. Epinephrine (0.25%–4%) directly stimulates the receptor sites on the iris dilator. It is not a very effective dilator of the normal pupil, but it dilates a denervated, and therefore hypersensitive, iris. Dipivalyl-epinephrine (Propine, 0.1%) produces similar effects. Phenylephrine hydrochloride (Neo-Synephrine, 0.125%–10%) has a variable mydriatic effect, depending on the concentration used. It is used in a concentration of 2.5% for general ophthalmologic examinations and in a concentration of 1% to evaluate patients with Horner's syndrome for the denervation hypersensitivity consistent with a postganglionic lesion. Because of its possible side effects of elevated blood pressure and stimulation of the cardiac system, it should be used with caution in older people. It is contraindicated in patients with untreated angle-closure glaucoma and patients taking monoamine oxidase inhibitors or tricyclic antidepressants. Hydroxyamphetamine hydrobromide (Paredrine, 1%) is a synthetic sympathomimetic agent that releases norepinephrine from sympathetic nerve endings and causes pupillary dilation without cycloplegia. It produces very little central nervous system stimulation and is an excellent drug for diagnosing a postganglionic Horner's syndrome. Dopamine (10%) eye drops produce marked pupillary dilation, probably by releasing norepinephrine from adrenergic nerve endings (52).

Cocaine (2%–10%) can be used as a topical anesthetic and a mydriatic. It produces accumulation of norepinephrine at the receptor sites by interfering with reuptake by the presynaptic nerve terminal.

Epinephrine, norepinephrine, phenylephrine, and cocaine are all bound in significant amounts by the melanin pigment in the iris, and patients with heavily pigmented irides respond with less mydriasis than those with lightly colored eyes. The recovery from the effects of mydriatics on pupil size and accommodation occurs within 5 to 7 hrs in most patients (41). Recovery takes longer in subjects with darkly pigmented irides.

Pupillary Constrictors

A number of topical agents produce pupillary constriction, either by stimulating the iris sphincter or blocking the iris dilator.

Parasympathomimetic Agents

Parasympathomimetic agents cause miosis and spasm of accommodation. Some drugs are direct cholinergic agents, and others inhibit acetylcholinesterase and thereby potentiate the action of acetylcholine. For some drugs, both mechanisms operate simultaneously.

Pilocarpine and methacholine (Mecholyl) are chemically similar to acetylcholine. They depolarize muscle, causing miosis and spasm of accommodation. The most common pilocarpine solutions are 0.5%–2%. Weaker solutions of 0.1% and 0.125% can be used to test for parasympathetic denervation hypersensitivity.

Physostigmine (Eserine, 0.25%–0.5%) is an anticholinesterase agent that causes ciliary irritability and conjunctival hyperemia, but it is used despite these properties. Neostigmine (3.0%–5.0%) causes miosis that lasts 12 to 36 hrs.

Organophosphate esters inhibit the action of acetylcholinesterase, forming irreversible complexes with this enzyme and producing miosis that lasts for days to weeks. These agents are used as insecticides and also cause severe generalized neurologic toxicity.

Sympatholytic Agents

Sympatholytic agents either interfere with the normal release of norepinephrine from the sympathetic nerve terminals or block α- or β-adrenergic receptors on the iris dilator. Guanethidine (Ismelin) and reserpine increase the rate of release of norepinephrine from nerve endings and deplete norepinephrine stores. When applied to the eye, they produce a Horner's syndrome, with ptosis, miosis, and hypersensitivity to adrenergic drugs. The effects of guanethidine last 1 to 2 days, and those of reserpine last 1 to 2 weeks.

There is very little β-adrenergic activity in the iris. Therefore, drugs that act exclusively on β-adrenergic receptors do not affect the pupil. Timolol maleate (Timoptic) does not affect pupillary size or reactivity.

Histamine directly affects the iris sphincter muscle and can constrict the pupil. Prostaglandins produce ocular inflammation and miosis when given topically. Irritation of the trigeminal nerve by topical agents such as nitrogen mustard can cause the release of substance P, which in turn acts on a specific receptor in the iris sphincter to cause pupillary constriction.

Agents That Act Systemically and Affect Pupillary Size

A wide variety of agents, when absorbed systemically, act on the sympathetic and parasympathetic nervous systems and on the dilator and sphincter muscles to influence the size of the pupil. Their effects can be predicted from their general effects on autonomic function.

A number of systemic agents produce pupillary dilation. Atropine, when given topically, produces mydriasis, but intravenously administered atropine in doses of 0.4 mg to 0.6 mg does not affect pupil size (16). Scopolamine, administered in the form of transdermal patches and acting by way of systemic absorption, has been implicated in mydriasis. It is much more likely, however, that patients contaminate their fingers with the scopolamine, with the resulting direct application of the agent to the eye causing the pupillary dilation.

Doses of atropine (1.2 mg) or glycopyrrolate (0.6 mg), when given to patients under general anesthesia, cause mydriasis. Mydriasis is also a feature of barracuda meat poisoning. Low serum levels of calcium can impair acetylcholine release at the parasympathetic nerve endings on the iris and result in fixed large pupils. Phenhydramine hydrochloride (Benadryl) overdose may cause anisocoria with poorly reactive pupils. Glutethimide (Doriden) characteristically produces midposition pupils at 4 mm to 8 mm that are sometimes unequal and fixed to light. Levodopa produces transient pupillary dilation by releasing norepinephrine.

The injection of lidocaine through the pterygopalatine fossa and the inferior orbital fissure can transiently dilate a pupil and render it unreactive. High concentrations of magnesium, by blocking the release of acetylcholine, can produce bilateral fixed dilated pupils. Nalorphine (Nalline) is a systemic narcotic antagonist that reverses the effects of morphine, including miosis. The tricyclic antidepressants produce a dose-related mydriasis. The anticholinergic agent trihexyphenidyl hydrochloride (Artane) causes large, poorly reactive pupils. These effects must be kept in mind when treating patients with these agents, as they may lose accommodative as well as pupillary function and hence may have difficulty focusing at close range. Such patients may benefit from reading glasses.

Systemic agents that produce pupillary constriction include adrenergic blocking agents, such as reserpine and methyldopa, as well as heroin and other narcotics. Lidocaine produces a high incidence of transient pupillary constriction, probably through pharmocologic blockade of sympathetic outflow in the high-thoracic region when it is given as extradural thoracic analgesia.

DIAGNOSTIC TESTS

Evaluation of Anisocoria

The first step in the evaluation of pupillary anisocoria is assessment of the pupillary light reaction (Fig. 2). If one

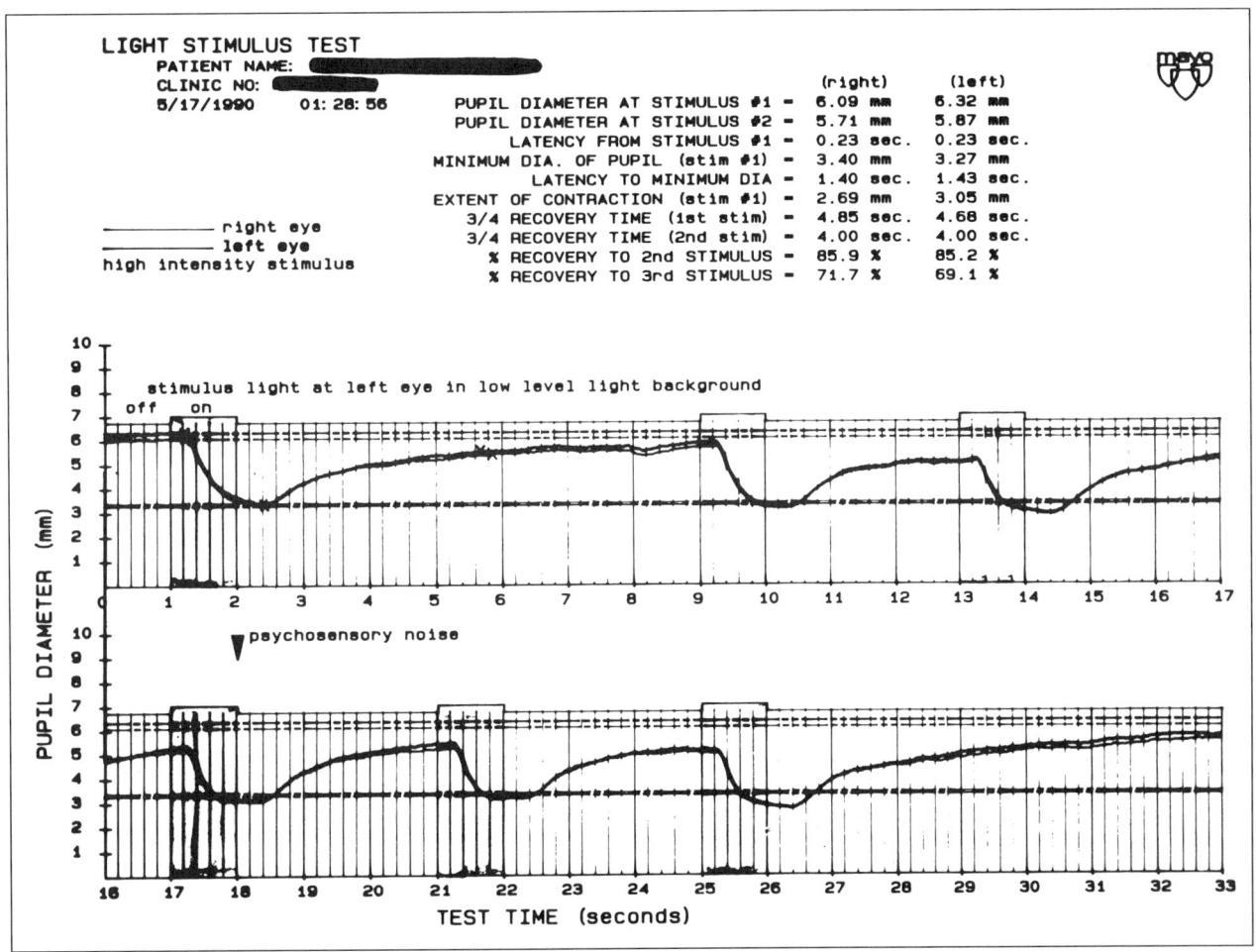

FIG. 2. Normal pupillogram showing direct pupillary constriction of the left eye and consensual response of the right eye to light stimulus shown periodically in the left eye. The pupils are equal in size and react equally to the light stimulus.

pupil reacts poorly or not at all, this constitutes the abnormal pupil. The problem will be more obvious in light than in darkness, because the difficulty stems from impaired pupillary constriction. A poorly reactive pupil may be caused by trauma, pharmacologic agents, ciliary ganglion damage, or third-nerve damage. The clinical examination, consisting of slit lamp examination of the iris, and pharmacologic tests using 0.1% or 0.125% pilocarpine to look for denervation hypersensitivity and 0.5%–1% pilocarpine to test for pharmacologic blockade, can help differentiate between these causes. A dilated pupil that does not constrict maximally to 1% pilocarpine can be assumed to be dilated by a pharmacologic agent.

If unequal pupils react equally well to light stimulation, the anisocoria will be more prominent in darkness, and the differential diagnosis is between a Horner's syndrome and benign simple central anisocoria. If the smaller pupil is slow to dilate in darkness or is associated with ipsilateral ptosis, Horner's syndrome should be considered. Failure of the pupil to dilate in response to a 10% cocaine solution can confirm this diagnosis. Further pharmacologic testing can be done to localize the lesion. If both pupils dilate equally in the dark, no ptosis is present, and testing with cocaine is negative for Horner's syndrome, then simple benign anisocoria can be diagnosed. Examination of old photographs, such as a driver's license, with magnification usually discloses a long-standing anisocoria (10).

Evaluation of Light-Near Dissociation

There are several entities that produce pupillary light-near dissociation. In most cases, the light reflex is abnormal and the near response remains intact. All cases involve damage to either the afferent or the efferent pathways responsible for pupillary constriction.

When there is severe unilateral or asymmetric damage to the afferent fibers in the visual sensory system, such as occurs with optic neuropathy or retinopathy, light-near dissociation arises. The light response is sluggish, but the near response is brisk. Damage in the dorsal mesencephalon of the brain stem can produce a Parinaud's syndrome, in which large pupils are virtually unreactive to light but normally reactive to a near stimulus. When the cause is neurosyphilis, the damage in the dorsal mesencephalon is so specific that the pupils exhibit the features of Argyll Robertson syndrome—they are small and irregular with no light reaction, but with a normal or near-normal response to convergence and accommodation.

Aberrant third-nerve regeneration produces light-near dissociation. Another cause is damage to the ciliary ganglion, resulting in Adie's tonic pupil. In this condition, the light response is very poor and delayed, and the near response may be preserved, although it is usually slow and tonic. A careful history and examination can usually help determine the exact nature of the light-near dissociation.

Edge-Light Pupil Cycle Time

In 1944, Stern described how repeated regular oscillation of the pupil could be elicited using a slit lamp (38). A spot of light was directed through the pupil at the edge of the iris. This light stimulated the retina, resulting in contraction of the iris, which in turn blocked the projection of light onto the retina, so that redilation of the pupil followed. The cycle repeated itself indefinitely. In 1978, Miller and Thompson (39), who were looking for a reliable way to quantitate the light reflex, resurrected this technique and refined it. They demonstrated the stability and reproducibility of this measurement and applied it to the evaluation of optic nerve disorders.

The uncertainty about what is actually being measured has limited the usefulness of the test. The initial assumption was that the cycles are generated by the afferent and efferent limbs of the light reflex arc. The afferent limb involves stimulation of the retina and optic nerve, with impulses passing along the optic tracts to the midbrain. The efferent limb is the parasympathetic outflow for pupillary constriction from the Edinger-Westphal nucleus. It was thought that sympathetic influences on the pupil were unimportant in the reflex (56).

Contraction and dilation of the pupil, however, are controlled by both components of the autonomic nervous system. Contraction is largely the result of parasympathetic activation of the sphincter. The sympathetic system, however, furnishes an underlying tone, causing inhibition of the dilator. Conversely, dilation of the pupil occurs by means of sympathetic stimulation of the dilator and parasympathetic inhibition of the constrictor (19,40). Finally, mechanical factors in the iris, including atrophy, play a role in changes in pupil size.

The edge-light pupil cycle time is a sensitive measure of an abnormality in the parasympathetic efferent limb of the pupillary reflex arc. Patients with abnormal cardiovascular reflexes tend to have pupils that cycle slowly, although this is not always the case, as they can also be slow in the presence of normal cardiovascular reflexes (38).

The pupil cycle time is also prolonged in abnormalities of the sympathetic nervous system. In Horner's syndrome, whether the lesion is central, preganglionic, or postganglionic, the tonic sympathetic effect that tends to dilate the pupils is lost, and redilation is slowed. The edge-light pupil cycle time is thereby prolonged (6).

The edge-light pupil cycle time is also prolonged when lesions involve both the sympathetic and parasympathetic nervous systems, and when the afferent limb of the light reflex arc is damaged. Miller and Thompson (39) measured the edge-light pupil cycle time and found it to be clearly abnormal in patients with optic neuritis. Akai, however, using a thin beam of light from a streak retinoscope and an infrared television pupillometer, could not reproduce these results (56). The amount of light entering the eye has in general not been well controlled. This technique must undergo further investigation before it can be used reliably.

Pupillography

Pupillography uses infrared photography to measure changes in pupil size under different conditions, as specified by the examiner. With an infrared source, the pupils are measured in darkness. The eyes are scanned by a television camera, and the pupillary diameter (or, in some machines, the pupillary area) is measured from the image on the monitor. Light flashes from a bright source are small enough so that they are unaffected by the iris margin. The brightness can be varied by placing neutral-density filters in front of the light source. Output is shown in analogue form for display or in digital form for computer analysis (Table 2).

PATHOLOGIC CONDITIONS OF TEAR SECRETION

Central Abnormalities of Tear Secretion

Patients with pseudobulbar palsy may have inappropriate and unexpected spells of crying accompanied by tearing. Excessive lacrimation can also be associated with photophobia caused by meningitis or encephalitis.

Abnormalities of tear secretion are seldom recognized in patients with brain stem lesions. Tearing may be absent in the congenital absence of brain stem nuclei, as in Möbius' syndrome. Involvement of the superior salivary nucleus by vascular disease or other lesions is characterized by a peripheral type of seventh-nerve palsy and an associated dry-eye condition stemming from involvement of the lacrimal nucleus. The production of saliva from the submaxillary gland is also reduced. The superior salivary nucleus is close to the rostral end of the vestibular nucleus, and patients with lesions there often have vertical or rotatory nystagmus accompanying decreased salivation.

Peripheral Abnormalities of Tear Secretion

A variety of abnormalities of tear secretion are associated with extra-axial lesions. The secretory fibers to the lacrimal gland leave the brain stem with the nervus intermedius adjacent to the seventh and eighth cranial nerves in the cerebellopontine angle and internal auditory meatus (see Chapter 11). Tumors involving these nerves can produce loss of hearing, vestibular palsy, facial palsy, loss of taste, hyperacusis, and dry eye. A peripheral facial palsy associated with reduced reflex tearing suggests a lesion in the petrous bone or cerebellopontine angle. Tumors in the internal auditory meatus may cause, as a very early sign, decreased tearing in the ipsilateral eye. Lesions of the greater superficial petrosal nerve in the floor of the middle fossa or near the gasserian ganglion can result in reduced tears ipsilaterally. The fifth and seventh cranial nerves are often affected. A number of primary and metastatic tumors, sphenoid sinus disease, middle fossa fractures, alcohol injections, and surgery on the fifth nerve to treat neuralgia can cause this complication. The finding of reduced tear secretion ipsilaterally indicates that the lesion is in the middle fossa and generally extradural in location, as the greater superficial petrosal nerve is situated outside the dura mater in this region.

Lesions in the sphenopalatine ganglion can reduce tear secretion and cause dryness in the nasal mucosa and sensory disturbances in the area supplied by the maxillary division of the fifth cranial nerve. Damage to the zygomaticotemporal nerve produces postganglionic denervation of the lacrimal gland. The usual cause is trauma to the posterior lateral orbital wall. A postganglionic parasympathetic lesion of the fibers to the lacrimal gland provokes denervation hypersensitivity. This hypersensitivity, however, can also occur in the presence of preganglionic lesions, and therefore testing for denervation hypersensitivity is not helpful in these cases.

Crocodile Tears

The term *crocodile tears* (*gustolacrimal reflex*) denotes an abnormality characterized by unilateral profuse tearing in response to the stimulation of the taste receptors, usually occurring after a facial palsy. It can be congenital, in which case it is associated with congenital sixth-nerve palsy, and probably represents a centrally mediated abnormality acquired because of a peripheral lesion. It can also be acquired in the initial stages of a facial palsy, without a facial palsy, or as a result of facial palsy. Sometimes chewing and sucking motions evoke the lacrimation. The mechanism is probably one of ephaptic transmission occurring between efferent and afferent autonomic axons in the proximal trunk of the facial nerve (see Chapter 11).

When the gustolacrimal reflex occurs after a seventh-nerve palsy or section of the greater superficial petrosal nerve, it is thought that collateral axons sprout from the glossopharyngeal preganglionic salivary nucleus, where the tympanic branch forms an anastomosis with the greater superficial petrosal nerve. These sprouts reinnervate the sphenopalatine ganglion and the lacrimal gland and become collaterals from intact fibers that normally supply the otic ganglion and the parotid gland. Salivary axons could therefore circumvent a superficial petrosal nerve that has been cut. Sectioning of the ninth cranial nerve in the posterior fossa can relieve the problem of crocodile tears in some patients.

Effects of Drugs on Tearing

Drugs can induce tearing by irritating the corneal epithelium or by a direct parasympathomimetic action, as is seen with the administration of pilocarpine or methacholine. A few drugs, such as psychotropic drugs and practolol, can reduce tear secretion.

Keratoconjunctivitis Sicca

Keratoconjunctivitis sicca is a condition in which dry eyes result from decreased tear production (21). The clinical manifestations include a chronic conjunctivitis with injection, discomfort, and photophobia. Paradoxically, patients with dry eyes often complain that their eyes water. In point of fact, the eyes are dry and become irritated, and then reflex tear production produces "watering." Examination of the tear film with a slit lamp reveals mucin formation, indicating decreased water content in the tears. The application of rose bengal, which stains devitalized cells and mucin, reveals punctate staining and erosions. The time for tear film breakup, or interval between a blink and the first randomly distributed dry spot on the cornea, is less than the lower limit of normal, which is 10 sec.

Schirmer's test has been used as a quantitative measure of tear production. It can be performed with or without topical anesthesia. When done without anesthesia, care should be taken that the strips do not touch the cornea. In this method, standard sterile strips of filter paper are used. The rounded wick end of the strip is bent at 90° and inserted over the eyelid border at the junction of the middle and nasal thirds of the lower eyelid margin. After 5 min, the strips are removed and the length of the wetting from the 90° bend in the strip is measured. A length of 15 mm is the standard minimum for tear production. The test is 100% specific when a cutoff of 3 mm of wetting at 5 min is used, but 10% of patients with dry eyes are missed because of insensitivity (3).

The test has been performed with topical anesthetic (31). In this method, the *cul-de-sac* is dried after the anesthetic is applied, as the anesthetic inhibits initial reflex tearing. When the accuracy of this test was evaluated, abnormally low values were obtained in 15% of normal volunteers (25).

The usefulness of Schirmer's test is limited by false-negative responses. Patients should be treated for dry eyes if they are symptomatic and if the slit lamp examination is positive, regardless of the result of Schirmer's test (3).

Another quantitative assessment of tear production is tear osmolarity. In this method, basal tears are collected and their freezing point measured with a nanoliter osmometer. This test is 84% specific and 76% sensitive in cases of dry eyes that show a tear osmolarity of greater than 312 mOsm/L (3).

There is considerable overlap between patients with dry eyes and normal patients in regard to basal tear volume, results of Schirmer's test, and rose bengal staining pattern, as well as in results of two other tests—concentrations of lysozyme and lactoferrin in basal and reflex tear samples. These last two tests are actually the most sensitive, with a 96% rate of accurate detection, but they are cumbersome and therefore not frequently performed.

The mainstay of treatment for dry eyes is artificial tears and lubricating inserts, but because of their brief retention time, other modalities are often also employed. Surgical closure of the puncta, mucinolytic agents, and hydrophilic bandage contact lenses may be used in conjunction with artificial tear application (13).

DISTURBANCES OF AUTONOMIC FUNCTION AFFECTING PUPILLARY SIZE AND REACTIVITY, ACCOMMODATION, AND LACRIMATION

The Riley-Day syndrome, which is characterized by autonomic instability, impaired pain and taste sensation, hyperreflexia, fever, seizures, and attacks of vomiting, is also associated with dry eyes and corneal ulceration. Crying elicits a reduced quantity of tears in these patients. Children with Riley-Day syndrome produce copious amounts of tears after a parenteral dose of methacholine, which suggests a parasympathetic denervation hypersensitivity of the lacrimal gland (58). A number of congenital neuropathies, such as congenital familial sensory neuropathy with anhidrosis and the neural crest syndromes, are associated with abnormal innervation of the pupil (5).

Multiple-system atrophy (the Shy-Drager syndrome), which is characterized by orthostatic hypotension, anhidrosis, urinary incontinence, and sexual impotence, also is associated with ocular signs, including anisocoria, iris atrophy, convergence insufficiency, and nystagmus. Some patients with this syndrome have decreased tear production, decreased corneal sensation, methacholine-induced miosis, and sometimes ocular sympathetic and parasympathetic insufficiency with alternating Horner's syndrome, cholinergic sensitivity, decreased lacrimation, and corneal hypoesthesia (59).

In the syndrome of acute panautonomic neuropathy, characterized by orthostatic hypotension, fixed cardiac rate, decreased salivation, anhidrosis, atony of the bladder, diarrhea, constipation, impotence, and abnormal skin flushing, there are associated pupillary abnormalities, including mydriasis, poor or absent constriction to light and near stimuli, and irregularity of the pupillary margin. The findings represent both parasympathetic and sympathetic postganglionic denervation with denervation hypersensitivity of both the iris sphincter and the iris dilator muscles. Causes include infections and immune processes. Many patients experience partial or complete recovery (22,54).

In the Fisher variant of Landry-Guillain-Barré syndrome, patients are seen with dilated, poorly reactive or unreactive pupils, suggesting ciliary ganglion involvement. Results of pharmacologic testing in these patients have suggested both postganglionic parasympathetic blockade and sympathetic involvement. An acute painful third-nerve palsy involving the pupil in a patient with chronic inflammatory demyelinating polyneuropathy has been reported (1).

Patients with mixed somatic and autonomic neuropathies may have ocular autonomic findings. In diabetic patients, the dark-adapted pupil size may be reduced, indicating failure of sympathetically mediated dilation (23). This small pupil is associated with cardiac vagal dysfunction and somatic sensory loss (49,50). However, increased pupillary light-reflex latencies are encountered even more often than reduced pupil size in darkness in diabetic patients, whether or not they have cardiovascular reflex abnormalities. This suggests that parasympathetic defects may occur earlier and in milder cases of the disease than the sympathetic abnormalities (26,33). Overall, parasympathetic abnormalities in the context of diabetes may not be as severe as the sympathetic ones (19). According to Barron et al. (2), who measured heart rate variability and heart rate variability during deep breathing by techniques of power spectral analysis, and parasympathetic pupillary denervation by the maximal velocity of pupillary constriction, heart rate abnormalities are twice as common. This may be so because the neuropathy may be nerve length-dependent (2).

Alcoholic patients with evidence of cardiac vagal neuropathy tend to have greater resting pupillary diameters and heightened responses to methacholine than do either control subjects or alcoholic patients without vagal neuropathy. Ocular parasympathetic abnormalities are common when such patients manifest other evidence of parasympathetic dysfunction (55).

Charcot-Marie-Tooth disease has autonomic as well as somatic features, including regulation of skin temperature independent of body temperature, abnormal autonomic adaption, and impaired sweating in the lower extremities. In addition, there may be findings that indicate both sympathetic and parasympathetic involvement of the eye. Tear production is decreased, and it is markedly increased after the administration of neostigmine or epinephrine. The pupils may be small, with no dilation in dim light and no response to pilocarpine or homatropine, suggesting postganglionic sympathetic involvement (25). The pupils of some patients show a positive response to the methacholine test, suggesting parasympathetic denervation (28). There may also be iris atrophy. Patients with larger denervated pupils sometimes obtain relief from photophobia with 0.025% pilocarpine (28).

The ocular findings associated with myasthenia gravis are many and varied. With regard to the pupil, however, the contractility abnormalities are usually subtle, but complete internal ophthalmoplegia responding to auticholinesterase drugs has been reported (20). Pupil cycle times are prolonged (60), either because of abnormalities at the neuromuscular junction (34), in the nicotinic receptors of the ciliary ganglion (5), or both. The pupillary reaction to light may be fatigued when the pupil is exercised at its maximal intrinsic rate (14).

Autonomic involvement is also a component of the Lambert-Eaton myasthenic syndrome, with about two thirds of patients manifesting abnormal pupillary responses to light, decreased reflex tear production, and parasympathetic and sympathetic denervation hypersensitivity of the iris musculature (8). Accommodation, sweating, and salivation can also be affected (44).

There is controversy about whether there are sympathetic nervous system abnormalities in patients with myotonic dystrophy (51). Dark-adapted pupil size during sympathetic blockade with 1% tropicamide has been reported to be abnormally small, suggesting a sympathetic defect (5).

The pupil may be atonic after cataract surgery (17).

Based on cardiac and pupillary supersensitivity to anticholinergics reported in persons with Down syndrome, and the neuropathologic and neurochemical similarities between Down syndrome and Alzheimer's disease, Scinto and colleagues (45) tested 19 patients with clinically diagnosed or suspected Alzheimer's disease and 32 controls; a dilute solution of tropicamide (0.01%), which blocks the action of acetycholine, was applied to one eye and sterile water to the other. They found that the pupils of the subjects with Alzheimer's disease dilated in response to this dilute agent, suggesting that patients with Alzheimer's disease could potentially be identified by sensitivity to anticholinergic agents applied to the eye. This report spawned similar studies to determine whether dilute pilocarpine, a directly acting parasympathomimetic agent, would produce the same response (18,24).

Critics pointed out the wide variability in pupillary dilation in response to tropicamide related to corneal integrity (drugs are absorbed faster when the cornea has been damaged), eye color (dark eyes dilate more slowly), and age of the patient. Loupe et al. (37) attempted to reproduce the results, but could not do so. They also looked at whether administration of tacrine affected the results. They attempted to control for several pitfalls in pupillary drug studies, including varying concentrations of the drug, corneal permeability, and inaccurate measurements of pupillary size resulting from irregularities of shape (measuring pupil area as well as diameter). The issue of possible pupillary hypersensitivity to dilute anticholinergics has not yet been settled. Considering the great interest this topic has generated, further studies will no doubt be forthcoming.

REFERENCES

1. Arroyo JG, et al. Acute, painful, pupil-involving third nerve palsy in chronic inflammatory demyelinating polyneuropathy. *Neurology* 1995;45:846–847.
2. Barron SA, et al. Parasympathetic autonomic neuropathy in diabetes mellitus: the heart is denervated more often than the pupil. *Electromyogr Clin Neurophysiol* 1994;34:467–469.
3. Baum J. Discussion of Farris RL, Stuchell RN, Mandel ID. Basal and reflex human tear analysis. *Ophthalmology* 1981;88:862.

4. Bell TAG. Adie's tonic pupil in a patient with carcinomatous neuromyopathy. *Arch Ophthalmol* 1986;104:331–332.
5. Bird TD, et al. Autonomic nervous system function in genetic neuromuscular disorders. Hereditary motor-sensory neuropathy and myotonic dystrophy. *Arch Neurol* 1984;41:43–46.
6. Blumen SC, et al. The pupil cycle time in Horner's syndrome. *J Clin Neuroophthalmol* 1986;6:232–234.
7. Bryant RC. Asymmetrical pupillary slowing and degree of severity in myasthenia gravis. *Ann Neurol* 1980;7:288–289.
8. Clark CV, et al. Ocular autonomic nerve function in Lambert-Eaton myasthenic syndrome. *Eye* 1990;4:473–481.
9. Currie J, et al. Tonic pupil with giant cell arteritis. *Br J Ophthalmol* 1984;68:135–138.
10. Czarnecki J, et al. The analysis of anisocoria: the use of photography in clinical evaluation of unequal pupils. *Can J Ophthalmol* 1979;14:297–302.
11. Drummond PD. Autonomic disturbance in cluster headache. *Brain* 1988;111:1199–1209.
12. Drummond PD. Disturbances in ocular sympathetic function and facial blood flow in unilateral migraine headache. *J Neurol Neurosurg Psychiatry* 1990;53:121–125.
13. Duke-Elder S. *System of Ophthalmology.* 1965;8:128–136 (part 1).
14. Dutton GN, et al. Pupillary fatigue in myasthenia gravis. *Trans Ophthalmol Soc U K* 1982;102:510–513.
15. Freeman LW, et al. The significance of temporary and alternating ptosis, miosis, and anhidrosis. *J Neurosurg* 1955;12:584–590.
16. Goetting MG, et al. Systemic atropine administration during cardiac arrest does not cause fixed and dilated pupils. *Ann Emerg Med* 1991;20:55–57.
17. Golnick KC, et al. Atonic pupil after cataract surgery. *J Cataract Refract Surg* 1995;21:170–175.
18. Hannannel M, et al. Parasympathetic function of the eye in dementia of the Alzheimer's type. *Neurology* 1995;45(Suppl 4):A356.
19. Heller PH, et al. Autonomic components of the human pupillary light reflex. *Invest Ophthalmol Vis Sci* 1990; 31:156–162.
20. Herishanu Y, et al. Internal ophthalmoplegia in myasthenia gravis. *Ophthalmologica* 1971;163:302–305.
21. Holly FJ. Tear physiology and dry eyes. *Surv Ophthalmol* 1977;22:69–84.
22. Hopkins IJ, et al. Subacute cholinergic dysautonomia in childhood. *Clin Exp Neurol* 1981;17:147–151.
23. Hreidarsson AB. Pupil motility in long-term diabetes. *Diabetologia* 1979;17:145–150.
24. Idiaquez J. Cholinergic supersensitivity of the iris in Alzheimer's Disease. *J Neurol Neurosurg Psychiatry* 1994;57:1544–1545.
25. Jammes JL. The autonomic nervous system in peroneal muscular atrophy. *Arch Neurol* 1972;27:213–220.
26. Karavanski K, et al. Pupil size in diabetes. *Arch Dis Child* 1994;71:511–515.
27. Karplus JP, et al. Weber die bahn des pupillarreflexes (die reflectorische pupillenstarre). *Pflugers Arch Ges Physiol Menschen Tiere* 1913;149:115–155.
28. Keltner JL, et al. Myotonic pupils in Charcot-Marie-Tooth. Successful relief of symptoms with 0.025% pilocarpine. *Arch Ophthalmol* 1975;93:1141–1148.
29. Kirkham TH, et al. Monocular elevator paresis. Argyll Robertson pupils and sarcoidosis. *Can J Ophthalmol* 1976;11:330–335.
30. Kline LB, et al. Oculosympathetic spasm with cervical spinal cord injury. *Arch Neurol* 1984;41:61–64.
31. Lamberts DN, et al. Schirmer test after topical anesthesia and tear meniscus height in normal eyes. *Arch Ophthalmol* 1979;97:1082.
32. Lance JW. Pupillary dilatation and arm weakness as negative ictal phenomena. *J Neurol Neurosurg Psychiatry* 1995;58:261–262.
33. Lanting P, et al. Assessment of pupillary light reflex latency and darkness adapted pupil size in control subjects and in diabetic patients with and without cardiovascular autonomic neuropathy. *J Neurol Neurosurg Psychiatry* 1990;53:912–914.
34. Lepore FE, et al. Pupillary dysfunction in myasthenia gravis. *Ann Neurol* 1979;6:29–33.
35. Loewenfeld IE. The Argyll Robertson pupil 1869–1969: a critical survey of the literature. *Surv Ophthalmol* 1969;14:199–299 (reprinted with references in Schwarz B, ed. *Syphilis and the Eye.* Baltimore: Williams & Wilkins; 1970:300–559).
36. Loewenfeld IE, et al. Mechanism of tonic pupil. *Ann Neurol* 1981; 10:275–276.
37. Loupe DN, et al. Pupillary response to tropicamide in patients with Alzheimer's disease. *Ophthalmology* 1996;103:495–503.
38. Martyn CN, et al. Pupil cycle time: a simple way of measuring an autonomic reflex. *J Neurol Neurosurg Psychiatry* 1986;49:771–774.
39. Miller SD, et al. Pupil cycle time in optic neuritis. *Am J Ophthalmol* 1978;85:635–642.
40. Milton JG, et al. Evaluation of pupil constriction and dilation from cycling measurements. *Vision Res* 1990;30:515–525.
41. Paggiarino DA, et al. The effects on pupil size and accommodation of sympathetic and parasympatholytic agents. *Ann Ophthalmol* 1993; 25:244–253.
42. Poole, CJM. Argyll Robertson pupils due to neurosarcoidosis: evidence for site of lesion. *Br Med J* 1984;289:356.
43. Rabinowich L, et al. Parasympathetic pupillary involvement in biopsy-proven temporal arteritis. *Ann Ophthalmol* 1988;20:400–402.
44. Rubenstein AE, et al. Cholinergic dysautonomia and Eaton-Lambert syndrome. *Neurology* 1979;29:720–723.
45. Scinto LF, et al. A potential noninvasive neurobiological test for Alzheimer's disease. *Science* 1994;266:1051–1054.
46. Selhorst JB, et al. The neuropathy of the Holmes-Adie syndrome. *Ann Neurol* 1984;16:138.
47. Simon D, et al. Heterochromia pardus: implications of the spotted pale iris. *Neuroophthalmology* 1982;2:279–291.
48. Smith PG, et al. Topographic analysis of Horner's syndrome. *Otolaryngol Head Neck Surg* 1986;94:451–457.
49. Smith SA, et al. Evidence for a neuropathic aetiology in the small pupil of diabetes mellitus. *Br J Ophthalmol* 1983;67:89–93.
50. Smith SA, et al. Assessment of pupillary function in diabetic neuropathy. *Diabetic Neuropathy.* Philadelphia: WB Saunders; 1987; 134–139.
51. Spaide R. Decreased sympathetic stimulation to the pupils in two patients with myotonic dystrophy. *Ann Ophthalmol* 1984;16:685–686.
52. Spiers ASD, et al. Action of dopamine on the human iris. *Br Med J* 1969;4:333–335.
53. Sundaram MBM. Pupillary abnormalities in congenital neurosyphilis. *Can J Neurol Sci* 1985;12:134–135.
54. Takayama H, et al. A case of postganglionic cholinergic dysautonomia. *J Neurol Neurosurg Psychiatry* 1987;50:915–918.
55. Tan E, et al. Parasympathetic denervation of the iris in alcoholics with vagal neuropathy. *J Neurol Neurosurg Psychiatry* 1984;47:61–64.
56. Thompson HS. The pupil cycle time (Editorial). *J Clin Neuroophthalmol* 1987;7:38–39.
57. Thompson HS, et al. Tadpole-shaped pupils caused by segmental spasm of the iris dilator muscle. *Am J Ophthalmol* 1983;96:467–477.
58. Walshe, Hoyt. In: Miller, ed. *Clinical Neuroophthalmology.* Baltimore: Williams & Wilkins; 1985 (chapter 31).
59. Weinstein JM, et al. Congenital Horner's syndrome. *Arch Ophthalmol* 1980;98:1074–1078.
60. Yamazaki A, et al. Abnormal pupillary responses in myasthenia gravis. A pupillographic study. *Br J Ophthalmol* 1976;60:575–580.

CHAPTER 35

Autonomic Disorders Associated with Spinal Cord Injury

Yadollah Harati

1. Spinal cord injuries are relatively common, and their impact is devastating.
2. The site and extent (complete or incomplete) of a lesion are important. A lesion above T5 is much more serious than one below T5. The syndrome of "autonomic dysreflexia" occurs exclusively in patients with cervical and high-thoracic spinal cord lesions.
3. During a period of "spinal shock," which lasts a few days to a few weeks, supraspinal excitatory activities are lost, reflexes and muscle tone are markedly diminished, and blood pressure is low. Marked orthostatic hypotension is the rule, and blood pressure is mainly regulated by posture and volume.
4. Autonomic dysreflexia typically first occurs about 6 months after injury. It is characterized by a massively disordered autonomic response to a stimulus below the lesion and is seen in patients with spinal cord injuries above the level of splanchnic outflow. The syndrome is caused by altered supraspinal influences and the activation of sympathetic efferent nerves at the spinal level, independent of the brain.
5. By far the two most important stimuli that elicit autonomic hyperreflexia are bladder and bowel distention.
6. The typical clinical presentation of autonomic dysreflexia consists of sudden and paroxysmal headache, hypertension, bradycardia, and hyperhidrosis. Piloerection and pallor are also frequently observed below the level of the spinal cord lesion.
7. Prevention of the acute dysreflexic episode involves bladder and bowel training, optimal skin care, and avoidance of environmental precipitants. Education of the patient and family in recognizing the symptoms of autonomic dysreflexia and understanding their treatment is of utmost importance.
8. The acute management of autonomic dysreflexia consists of the removal of the provoking stimulus (in most cases a distended bladder or fecal impaction); physical measures, including elevation of the head of the bed; removal of constricting clothing and abdominal binders; and close monitoring of blood pressure.
9. Severe hypertension can be treated with such agents as nifedipine, phenoxybenzamine, prazosin, mecamylamine, and nitrates. Mecamylamine or nifedipine, taken before the onset of a provoking stimulus (e.g., a diagnostic procedure), can be effective in preventing an attack. The most commonly used agents for an acute attack are short-acting calcium channel blockers.
10. Careful urogenital management is important. Care of the bladder to ensure adequate emptying is critical.

INTRODUCTION

Approximately 12,000 spinal cord injuries caused by motor vehicle accidents (47%), falls (21%), athletic events (14%), and acts of violence (14%) are encountered annually in the United States, and about 200,000 patients with such injuries are currently living (28). Many of these injuries occur in young male individuals between the ages of 15 and 30. Cervical lesions constitute the majority of cases (53%), followed by thoracic (35%) and lumbosacral (10%) lesions (36). Paraplegia and quadriplegia resulting from

---

Y. Harati: Department of Neurology, Baylor College of Medicine, Houston, Texas 77030.

these injuries require both immediate and long-term specialized, extensive multidisciplinary care, of which recognition and management of acute and chronic dysautonomias occupy an important segment. With the development of such an approach, the U.S. mortality rate from spinal cord injuries declined from 80% in patients injured during World War I to about 40% in patients injured during World War II, and still further to 25% in patients injured during the Korean War and a minimal rate in patients injured during the Vietnam War (3,11). The specialized regional treatment units at the Veterans Affairs medical centers in the United States have played an important and leading role in the management and understanding of spinal cord injuries.

Although most serious and complicated autonomic dysfunctions are usually encountered in traumatic spinal cord injuries, other conditions, such as syringomyelia, multiple sclerosis, spinal cord compression from tumors, cervical spondylosis, and transverse myelitis, may also cause variable degrees of dysautonomias. For example, cervical spondylosis may cause Horner's syndrome, and orthostatic hypotension or hyperhidrosis may occur in syringomyelia. The discussion in this chapter largely concerns traumatic spinal cord lesions, the most frequently occurring spinal cord disorders in which problems related to dysautonomia develop.

In evaluating a patient with a spinal cord lesion and dysautonomia, four important principles must be considered:

1. With a spinal cord injury, there is an *interruption of the autonomic pathways* from the brain stem and hypothalamus to the intermediolateral cell column of the spinal cord, and the brain can no longer control the sympathetic outflow below the level of the lesion. This results in the loss of tonic background excitation of the intermediolateral cells, diminution or loss of modulation of segmental spinal autonomic reflexes, and disorganization of the autonomic responses.
2. *Recent* injuries to the spinal cord cause different autonomic dysfunctions than do *chronic* injuries.
3. The *site* of lesion, above or below T-5, is an important determinant of the presence of serious, chronic autonomic abnormalities. The syndrome of autonomic dysreflexia (see below) exclusively occurs in patients with cervical and high-thoracic spinal cord lesions.
4. The *extent* of injury, whether complete or incomplete, may influence the type and severity of autonomic dysfunction.

CLINICAL MANIFESTATIONS

Cardiovascular

Immediately following an acute spinal cord injury, a period of "spinal shock" or hypoexcitability develops, during which supraspinal excitatory activities are lost and reflexes and muscle tone are markedly diminished (25). Loss of sympathetic outflow results in decreased peripheral vasoconstriction and cardiac chronotropic activity. Although there is usually a low baseline HR and supine BP and low levels of plasma noradrenaline and adrenaline in spinal shock (10,24), marked orthostatic hypotension is the rule. Systolic blood pressure in the quadriplegic patient is usually less than 100 mmHg, with a pulse rate of about 60 to 65/min. Because during this stage of injury blood pressure is mainly regulated by posture and volume, great care should be taken to avoid raising the head above the horizontal level when a patient is removed from the scene of the accident or must be moved in the hospital during the early stages of evaluation and rehabilitation. Peripheral vasodilation, decreased cardiac output, bradycardia, and venous pooling all contribute to the low blood pressure seen in this stage of injury. Plasma noradrenaline levels do not rise with head-up postural change (23). Orthostatic hypotension in the first few weeks after injury is even more significant, as autoregulation of cerebral blood flow may be impaired during this period (40), resulting in loss of consciousness in sitting or upright positions. The ability to autoregulate the cerebral blood flow, however, gradually returns to normal. Any volume loss (e.g., during administration of diuretics) may result in significant supine or orthostatic low BP. Activation of renin-angiotensin-aldosterone system, by inducing vasoconstriction and volume expansion, helps to raise the blood pressure; drugs that affect angiotensin-converting enzyme or aldosterone may cause significant supine hypotension (26).

Interruption of the efferent sympathetic pathway also impairs the responses of the baroreceptor reflex arc to the effect of raised intrathoracic pressure (Valsalva maneuver), and BP may fall precipitously with no immediate recovery being observed (39). However, because of intercostal muscle paralysis, significant intrathoracic pressure is rarely achieved or maintained in a tetraplegic patient.

Vasodilation in the extremities often causes a warm feeling of the skin; venous pooling and diminished venous return result in edema of the distal limbs and a bluish discoloration. The Lewis cutaneous response below the lesion is exaggerated. Loss of sympathetic tone also results in passive engorgement of the penis (pseudopriapism). Such engorgement, seen shortly after an acute spinal cord injury, signifies a very serious disruption of the spinal cord (2).

Stimuli to the upper part of the body (e.g., cold or pain) or mental stress (e.g., mental arithmetic), which normally evoke an increase in BP and HR response, have no effect in tetraplegics.

The duration of spinal shock may be from a few days to a few weeks, after which isolated spinal function returns to result in different autonomic symptoms, especially autonomic dysreflexia.

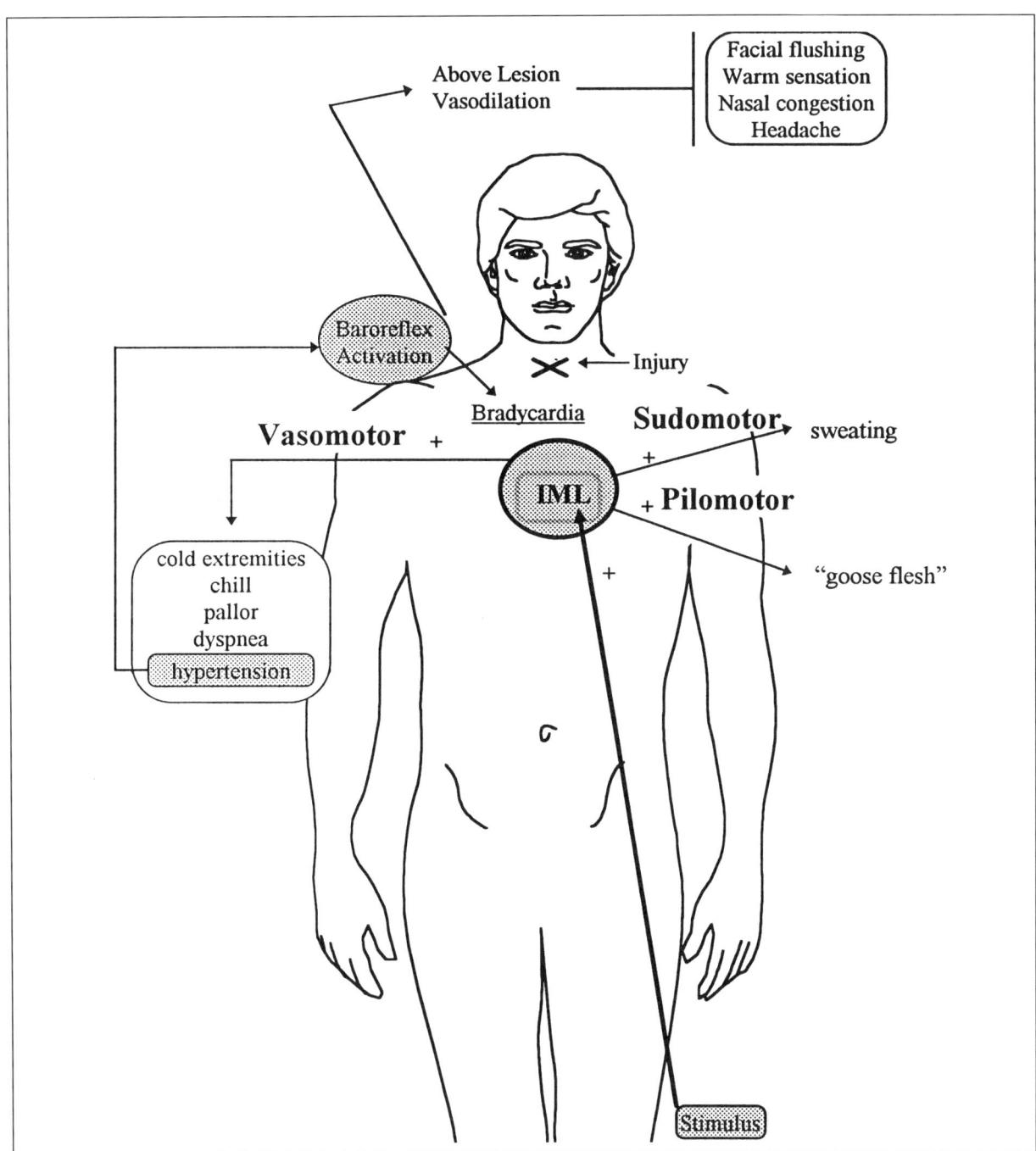

FIG. 1. Impulses produced by noxious, proprioceptive, or other sensory stimuli are carried by fibers which synapse within the spinal cord at various levels and ascend the spinal cord until blocked at the level of injury. Excitation of interneurons within the spinal cord activate IML cells at multiple levels, resulting in widespread sympathetic adrenergic and cholinergic activities (vasomotor, sudomotor and pilomotor). Hypertension, resulting from the increased vasomotor activation, stimulates carotid and aortic baroreceptors which, in turn, regulate central sympathetic inhibitory pathways and parasympathetic activity. Since due to injury the supraspinal inhibitory pathways are unable to reach pre-ganglionic sympathetic fibers below the injury, the sympathetic reflex continues, resulting in persistent hypertension. Above the injury, however, these pathways can modulate the sympathetic activity and vasodilation of the head and neck occurs. Baroreflex activities of the vagus nerve and its effect on the sinoatrial node results in bradycardia. However, correction of hypertension by bradycardia is minimal, and tachycardia may persist unless the offending stimulus is removed.

Autonomic Dysreflexia

This important autonomic complication of spinal cord injury, occurring 2 months to 15 years after injury (usually 6 months), is defined as an acute syndrome of a massively disordered autonomic response to a specific stimulus that is seen in patients with spinal cord injuries above the level of splanchnic outflow (1,6,8,9,13,17,21,37,38). Its early descriptions were in 1860 by Hilton (15) and in 1890 by Bowlby (5). It is also known as *autonomic hyperreflexia, sympathetic hyperreflexia, spinal poikilopoiesis, paroxysmal neurogenic hypertension, paroxysmal hypertension, autonomic reflex, autonomic spasticity, mass reflex,* and the *neurovegetative syndrome*. Head and Riddoch (14), investigating spinal cord injuries during World War I, were the first to recognize that only stimuli arising below the level of spinal cord injury produced the phenomenon, and they postulated the occurrence of a "mass reflex" to account for their observation. It is now abundantly clear that the syndrome occurs because of altered supraspinal influences and the activation of sympathetic efferent nerves at the spinal level, independent of the brain. Although the true incidence of autonomic dysreflexia is unknown, it is estimated to be present in 30%–85% of quadriplegics (4,17,20,21). According to Braddon and Rocco (6), a total of 11 deaths caused by autonomic dysreflexia were reported between 1970 and 1981 in the United States. A syndrome similar to human autonomic dysreflexia has been reproduced in animals with chronic spinal cord injury (19,32,33).

In 1956, Kurnick (20) provided a detailed account of the mechanism for the development of autonomic dysreflexia. Any noxious stimulus, even one that appears innocuous, can provoke the attack (Table 1). The two major stimuli that elicit autonomic hyperreflexia are bladder and bowel distention. In fact, urogenital stimulation accounts for hyperreflexia 75%–82% of the time, whereas stimulation of the lower gastrointestinal tract is responsible for 13%–19% of the episodes (17,21).

The typical clinical presentation of autonomic dysreflexia consists of sudden and paroxysmal headache, hypertension, bradycardia, and hyperhidrosis (8,9,26) (Table 2). Piloerection and pallor below the level of the spinal cord lesion are also frequently observed. Less commonly reported symptoms are also listed in Table 2.

Hypertension with systolic pressure as high as 300 mm Hg and vasospasm may cause myocardial failure, visual disturbances, hypertensive encephalopathy and seizure, and retinal or intracerebral hemorrhage. Headache, which is of pounding quality, may result from passive dilation of cerebral blood vessels (29), as digital compression of the carotid arteries sometimes diminishes the intensity of the headache. Elevated plasma level of prostaglandin E2

TABLE 1. *Stimuli associated with the development of autonomic dysreflexia in spinal cord-injured patients*

Common stimuli
  Distended bladder
  Distended bowel
  Skin breakdown or pressure
  Urinary tract infection
Others
  Urogenital diagnostic procedures
  Surgical procedures
  Pregnancy/delivery
  Digital stimulation
  Electroejaculation
  Intermittent catheterization
  Extracorporeal shock-wave lithotripsy
  Enemas
  Anal fissure
  Cutaneous stimulation
  Burns
  Deep vein thrombosis
  Fracture site manipulation
  Acute abdomen
  Exophageal reflux
  Radiologic procedures
  Functional electrical stimulation
  Position changes
  Immersion of lower limbs in cold water
  Range-of-motion exercises
  Tight clothing
  Ingrown toenails
  Coitus
  Orthostatic hypotension
  Medication (decongestants, sympathomimetics, and vasoconstrictors)

TABLE 2. *Symptoms of autonomic dysreflexia*

Common symptoms
  Hypertension
  Headache
  Diaphoresis above the level of spinal cord lesion
  Bradycardia
  Piloerection (goose flesh) and pallor below the level of lesion
Others
  Nausea
  Confusion
  Extreme anxiety
  Impending sense of doom
  Malaise
  Respiratory distress
  Conjunctival congestion
  Nasal congestion
  Mydriasis
  Cardiac arrhythmia (tachycardia or, less commonly, bradycardia)
  Patchy erythema above the neck
  Visual disturbances
  Metallic taste
  Penile erection
  Increased spasticity

during an attack of hyperreflexia may also play an important role in the pathogenesis of headaches (29). Milder forms of autonomic dysreflexia are manifested as sweating, an increase in spasticity, and goose pimples, with or without any significant rise in blood pressure or fall in pulse rate.

It is generally agreed that during episodes of autonomic hyperreflexia, plasma levels of noradrenaline and dopamine-β-hydroxylase are raised from the low basal level (24,27,29). Although plasma noradrenaline rises acutely (24), there is a delay in the rise of plasma dopamine-β-hydroxylase (27). As there is no significant elevation of urinary metabolites of adrenaline (13,20), expected with stimulation of the adrenal glands, the raised level of noradrenaline is thought to be exclusively caused by stimulation of sympathetic adrenergic nerve terminals and not of the adrenals. The modest elevation of noradrenaline above the normal level is disproportionate to the marked hypertension observed in autonomic dysreflexia and is, perhaps, best explained by the increased activity of α-adrenergic receptors (22). No elevation in plasma renin has been found during or after an episode of autonomic dysreflexia (13, 23,31).

The differential diagnosis of autonomic dysreflexia includes tumors of the posterior fossa, pheochromocytoma, and pre-eclampsia.

Management of Autonomic Dysreflexia

Management includes prevention of acute dysreflexic episodes, treatment of acute and recurrent hyperreflexia, and preoperative preparation of at-risk spinal cord-injured patients (6,8,26,38).

Prevention of acute dysreflexic episodes is the combined responsibility of physicians, ancillary medical staff, patient, and caregivers. It involves bladder and bowel training, optimal skin care, and avoidance of environmental precipitants.

Education of patients and their families in recognizing the symptoms of autonomic dysreflexia and understanding their treatment is of the utmost importance.

In acute management of autonomic dysreflexia, the only definitive treatment is removal of the stimulus, which, in most cases, is a distended bladder or fecal impaction. If a cause for dysreflexia cannot be identified immediately, physical measures are usually highly effective, including elevation of the head of the bed or vertical tilt. Constricting clothing and abdominal binders that increase caval pressure should be removed. Blood pressure should be frequently monitored during an attack, as pressure changes can be rapid and profound. Autonomic hyperreflexia not associated with the usual stimuli may indicate serious visceral disease, and an intense effort must be made to identify a cause.

Depending on the severity of hypertension, pharmacologic agents may be utilized at any time (6). Short-acting antihypertensive agents are most efficacious. Agents used most frequently include nifedipine, phenoxybenzamine, prazosin, mecamylamine, and nitrates. Mecamylamine or nifedipine, administered before the onset of a provoking stimulus (e.g., a diagnostic procedure), can be effective in preventing an attack (12). The most commonly used agents for an acute attack are short-acting calcium channel blockers (6).

Thermoregulatory

Patients with acute cervical spinal cord injuries may have marked disturbances of temperature control. These arise from an imbalance of two important thermoregulatory mechanisms: the ability to prevent heat loss, and active thermogenesis through shivering. Loss of peripheral sympathetic tone results in vasodilation and a warm feeling of the skin, but also an uncontrollable passive loss of heat below the level of the spinal lesion, which can result in hypothermia, especially in temperate climates. In addition, because of motor paralysis, active thermogenesis by shivering cannot occur below the level of the lesion. Shivering by muscles innervated from above the level of the lesion may not suffice to increase metabolism. The profound core hypothermia must be continuously monitored by measurement of rectal temperature, and the warm feeling of the extremities should not mislead examiners to assume that the patient is feeling uncomfortably warm. If such patients are left uncovered to facilitate an examination, the resulting profound hypothermia may have drastic systemic and metabolic consequences. Fortunately, these patients exhibit a rapid response to passive rewarming with a blanket, a warm drink, or an infusion of warm saline solution, possibly because the peripheral vasculature is already dilated. Patients with a spinal cord lesion below the cervical level are at lesser risk, because the sympathetic activity subserving sweat glands and blood vessels in normally innervated regions is retained.

When environmental temperature is elevated or an infection is present, hyperthermia may occur in chronic quadriplegics. Impaired thermoregulatory sweating and vasodilation below the lesion are responsible for the rise of core body temperature. Avoidance of exposure to heat is important in preventing marked hyperthermia and heat stroke in quadriplegics. Infections must be treated and antipyretic drugs administered to treat hyperthermia secondary to infection.

Urogenital

During spinal shock in a patient with a spinal cord lesion above the conus medullaris, the bladder is completely paralyzed, causing distention, urinary retention, and overflow (34). After the spinal shock has ended and detrusor muscle contraction has returned, the bladder usually empties spontaneously or in response to external stimuli (neurogenic bladder). Once it starts to empty, it continues to do so. Simple maneuvers, such as the application of abdominal pressure, pulling the pubic hair, tapping the suprapubic abdominal wall, hitting the thigh, or digital stimulation of the external rectal sphincter are usually sufficient to initiate a response. In some patients, a flaccid bladder may persist, even in the chronic stages of injury. Crede's maneuver is needed to ensure complete emptying of the bladder. If urine is retained, bladder and kidney infection may follow. If the lesion is above the midthoracic region, a full bladder may cause autonomic dysreflexia, including sweating, piloerection, and headache, which may alert the patient to a full bladder.

Passive penile engorgement and priapism, which normally resolve within days, occur during spinal shock (2). In chronic complete injury, manipulation of the genitalia results in penile erection, as the isolated spinal reflex activity has returned. Ejaculation, dependent on the sympathetic nerve supply, is usually retrograde, because the function of the internal urethral sphincter, which prevents seminal fluid from flowing back to the bladder, is usually impaired. Ejaculation is not associated with orgasm. With electroejaculation, collection of seminal fluid for artificial insemination is now possible. Pretreatment with nifedipine may prevent autonomic dysreflexia during electroejaculation (35). Spermatogenesis, however, may be considerably reduced in paraplegics.

In female patients with quadriplegia and paraplegia, a period of anovulation usually follows an acute cord injury, but menses soon return. At one time pregnancy was considered to be contraindicated in these patients. However, it is now recognized that women with spinal cord injuries can conceive and carry to term (16). Pregnancy is not without risks, however, as it often exacerbates other conditions complicating spinal cord injury. The problem of autonomic dysreflexia requires special attention (16,18). Spontaneous vaginal delivery is frequently possible in these patients, and cesarean section is rarely required (7). The pregnancies of women with spinal cord injuries are considered to be high-risk pregnancies, and these patients must be cared for in specialized obstetric units.

REFERENCES

1. Ascoli R. The neurovegetative syndrome of vesical distention in paraplegics: prevention and therapy. *Paraplegia* 1971;9:82.
2. Bedbrook GM. *The Care and Management of Spinal Cord Injuries*. New York: Springer-Verlag;1981.
3. Borges PM, et al. The urologic status of the Vietnam War paraplegic: a 15-year prospective follow-up. *J Urol* 1982;127:710.
4. Bors E. The challenge of quadriplegia; some personal observations in series of 233 cases. *Bull Los Angeles Neurol Soc* 1956;21:105.
5. Bowlby AA. The reflexes in cases of injury to the spinal cord. *Lancet* 1890;1:1071.
6. Braddon RL, et al. Autonomic dysreflexia. A survey of current treatment. *Am J Phys Med Rehabil* 1991;70:234–241.
7. Brian JE Jr, et al. Autonomic hyperreflexia, cesarean section and anesthesia. A case report. *J Reprod Med* 1988;33:645–648.
8. Colachis SC 3rd. Autonomic hyperreflexia with spinal cord injury. *J Am Paraplegia Soc* 1992;15:171–186.
9. Comarr AE. Autonomic dysreflexia (hyperreflexia). *J Am Paraplegia Soc* 1984;7:53.
10. Debarge O, et al. Plasma catecholamines in tetraplegics. *Paraplegia* 1974; 12:44–49.
11. Donnelly J, et al. Present urologic status of the World War II paraplegic: 25-year follow-up: comparison with the status of the 20-year Korean War paraplegic and the 5-year Vietnam paraplegic. *J Urol* 1972;108:558.
12. Dykstra DD, et al. The effect of nifedipine on cystoscopy-induced autonomic hyperreflexia in patients with high spinal cord injuries. *J Urol* 1987;138:1155–1157.
13. Frankel HL. Cardiovascular aspects of autonomic dysreflexia since Guttman and Whitteridge (1947). *Paraplegia* 1979;17: 46–51.
14. Head H, et al. The autonomic bladder, excessive sweating and some other reflex conditions in gross injuries of the spinal cord. *Brain* 1917;40:188.
15. Hilton J. Pain and the therapeutic influence of mechanical and physiological rest in accidents and surgical diseases. *Lancet* 1860;2:401.
16. Hughes SJ, et al. Management of the pregnant woman with spinal cord injuries. *Br J Obstet Gynaecol* 1991;98:513–518.
17. Kewalramani LS. Autonomic dysreflexia in traumatic myelopathy. *Am J Phys Med* 1980;59:1–21.
18. Kobayashi A, et al. Autonomic hyperreflexia during labour. *Can J Anaesth* 1995;42:1134–1136.
19. Krassioukov AV, et al. Episodic hypertension due to autonomic dysreflexia in acute and chronic spinal cord-injured rats. *Am J Physiol* 1995;268:H2077–H2083.
20. Kurnick NB. Autonomic hyperreflexia and its control in patients with spinal cord lesions. *Ann Intern Med* 1956;44:678–686.
21. Lindan R, et al. Incidence and clinical features of autonomic dysreflexia in patients with spinal cord injury. *Paraplegia* 1980;18:285–292.
22. Mathias CJ. Role of sympathetic efferent nerves in blood pressure regulation and in hypertension. *Hypertension* 1991;18:III22–III30.
23. Mathias CJ, et al. Plasma catecholamines, plasma renin activity and plasma aldosterone in tetraplegic man, horizontal and tilted. *Clin Sci Mol Med* 1975;49:291–299.
24. Mathias CJ, et al. Plasma catecholamines during paroxysmal neurogenic hypertension in quadriplegic man. *Circ Res* 1976;39:204–208.
25. Mathias CJ, et al. Clinical manifestations of malfunctioning sympathetic mechanisms in tetraplegia. *J Auton Nerv Syst* 1983;7: 303–312.
26. Mathias CJ, et al. Autonomic disturbances in spinal cord lesions. In: Bannister R, Mathias CJ, eds. *Autonomic Failure*. Oxford: Oxford University Press; 1992.
27. Mathias CJ, et al. Dopamine-β-hydroxylase release during hypertension from sympathetic nervous overactivity in man. *Cardiovasc Res* 1976;10:176–181.
28. Maynard F, et al. The prevention and management of urinary infections among people with spinal cord injuries. *J Am Paraplegia Soc* 1992;15:194.
29. Naftchi NE, et al. Hypertensive crises in quadriplegic patients. Changes in cardiac output, blood volume, serum dopamine-β-hydroxylase activity, and arterial PGE_2. *Circulation* 1978;57:336–341.
30. Naftchi NE, et al. Relationship between serum dopamine-β-hydroxylase activity, catecholamine metabolism, and hemodynamic changes during paroxysmal hypertension in quadriplegia. *Circ Res* 1974;35: 850–861.
31. Nanninga JB, et al. Effect of autonomic hyperreflexia on plasma renin. *Urology* 1976;7:638.
32. Osborn JW, et al. Chronic cervical spinal cord injury and autonomic hyperreflexia in rats. *Am J Physiol* 1990;258:R169–174.
33. Rivas DA, et al. Autonomic dysreflexia in a rat model. Spinal cord injury and the effect of pharmacologic agents. *Neurourol Urodyn* 1995;14:141–152.

34. Selzman AA, et al. Urologic complications of spinal cord injury. *Urol Clin North Am* 1993;20:453–464.
35. Steinberger RE, et al. Nifedipine pretreatment for autonomic dysreflexia during electroejaculation. *Urology* 1990;36:228–231.
36. Stover SL, et al. *Spinal Cord Injury: The Facts and Figures*. Birmingham: University of Alabama; 1986.
37. Trop CS, et al. Autonomic dysreflexia and its urological implications: a review. *J Urol* 1991;146:1461–1469.
38. Trop CS, et al. The evaluation of autonomic dysreflexia. *Semin Urol* 1992;10:95–101.
39. van Lieshout JJ, et al. Singing-induced hypotension: a complication of high spinal cord lesion. *Neth J Med* 1991;38:75–79.
40. Yamamoto M, et al. Effect of differential spinal cord transection on human cerebral blood flow. *J Neurol Sci* 1980; 47:395–406.

CHAPTER 36

Autonomic Neuropathies

Phillip A. Low and James G. McLeod

1. The acute autonomic neuropathies comprise acute panautonomic neuropathy (idiopathic or paraneoplastic), acute cholinergic neuropathy, Guillain-Barré syndrome, botulism, porphyria, and drug-induced or toxic autonomic neuropathies.
2. Acute panautonomic neuropathy is characterized by acute or subacute onset of widespread and severe sympathetic and parasympathetic failure with relative or complete sparing of somatic nerve fibers.
3. Acute cholinergic neuropathy is probably a restricted expression of acute panautonomic neuropathy with abnormalities confined to the postganglionic cholinergic neuron. Patients have alacrima, xerostomia, anhidrosis, constipation, urinary retention, and blurred vision but do not have orthostatic hypotension.
4. Guillain-Barré syndrome is characterized by acute onset of an ascending, predominantly motor polyradiculoneuropathy with increased cerobrospinal fluid (CSF) protein and autonomic overactivity/underactivity.
5. Botulism is manifested as the acute development of cholinergic neuropathy, ptosis, and bulbar weakness following the ingestion of home-canned foods contaminated by *Clostridium botulinum* spores.
6. Dysautonomia is common in acute intermittent porphyria, and autonomic overactivity predominates over autonomic failure, although both are present and often coexistent. Symptoms of sympathetic overactivity include abdominal colic, hypertension, and tachycardia.
7. Drugs causing acute autonomic neuropathies are cisplatinum, vincristine, Vacor, amiodarone, and perhexilene.
8. Toxic acute autonomic neuropathies may be caused by heavy metals such as thallium, arsenic, or mercury, and by organic solvents such as acrylamide.
9. Amyloid neuropathy is diagnosed by the combination of small-fiber-type sensory loss, autonomic failure, and the finding of amyloid deposits in tissue. Prognosis is significantly worse with the development of autonomic failure. Familial amyloid polyneuropathy is dominantly inherited, and is usually the consequence of a point mutation in the transthyretin (prealbumin) gene, encoded on human chromosome 18.
10. Sensory neuronopathy with autonomic failure may be idiopathic or paraneopastic, or it may be associated with Sjögren's syndrome, pyridoxine overdose, cisplatinum administration, monoclonal gammopathy, or Vacor intoxication.

INTRODUCTION

Autonomic neuropathy is the term used to describe autonomic disturbances resulting from diseases of the peripheral autonomic nervous system. Because autonomic fibers innervate all organ systems, the manifestations of dysautonomia are protean. The clinical evaluation of autonomic function is described in Chapter 1 and the laboratory evaluation in Chapter 16. In this chapter, a classification of the autonomic neuropathies is provided, followed by a description of the individual neuropathies. Certain specific aspects of treatment are covered in this chapter, but the management of common autonomic symptoms, such as orthostatic hypotension and bowel/bladder symptoms, are covered in the individual chapters on these topics.

In the peripheral neuropathies, certain characteristic patterns, based on the temporal pattern, or gestalt, of symptoms and signs, are important in the approach to management (159). Typical patterns include those of small-fiber

---

P. A. Low: Department of Neurology, Mayo Clinic, Rochester, Minnesota 55905.

J. G. McLeod: Department of Medicine, University of Sydney, Sydney, NSW 2006, Australia.

neuropathy, polyradiculoneuropathy, and sensory neuronopathy. Also, certain characteristic patterns of autonomic neuropathies are important in the differential diagnosis (Table 1). In some cases, the unique autonomic gestalt may render a precise diagnosis possible.

The present classification is modified from that of a previous publication (152). In the previous classification, the autonomic neuropathies were divided into two categories: autonomic failure as the sole or major manifestation of a neuropathy, and a second major category of autonomic failure as part of a peripheral neuropathy. The first category is more characteristic, less common, and can be subdivided into combined sympathetic and parasympathetic, pure cholinergic, and restricted dysautonomias. A major modification in this chapter is the inclusion of a separate category of *acute* autonomic neuropathies.

ACUTE AUTONOMIC NEUROPATHIES

Perspective

There is a spectrum of acute autonomic neuropathies. At one extreme is acute panautonomic neuropathy (idiopathic or paraneoplastic), characterized by widespread and severe

TABLE 1. *Classification of autonomic neuropathies*

ACUTE AUTONOMIC NEUROPATHIES

Acute panautonomic neuropathy (pandysautonomia)
Acute paraneoplastic autonomic neuropathy (Chapter 41)
Acute cholinergic neuropathy
Guillain-Barré syndrome
Botulism
Porphyria
Drug-induced acute autonomic neuropathies
   Cisplatin
   Vincristine
   Vacor
   Amiodarone
   Perhexilene
   Paclitaxel (Taxol)
Toxic acute autonomic neuropathies
   Heavy metals
   Organic solvents
   Acrylamide
   Hexacarbons

CHRONIC PERIPHERAL AUTONOMIC NEUROPATHIES

Distal sympathetic neuropathies
   Distal small fiber neuropathy
   Other peripheral neuropathies
Pure cholinergic neuropathies
   Lambert-Eaton myasthenic syndrome (LEMS) (Chapter 41)
   Chronic idiopathic anhidrosis
   Adie's syndrome
   Chágas' disease
Pure adrenergic neuropathy
Combined adrenergic and sensory neuropeptide-deficient neuropathy
Combined sympathetic and parasympathetic failure
  Autonomic dysfunction clinically important
   Amyloid neuropathy
    Sporadic systemic amyloid neuropathy
    Multiple myeloma-associated amyloid neuropathy
    Familial amyloidotic polyneuropathy (FAP)
   Diabetic autonomic neuropathy (Chapter 37)
   Chronic autonomic including parautonomic neuropathy
   Chronic paraneoplastic autonomic including panautonomic neuropathy
   Sensory neuronopathy with autonomic failure
   Pure autonomic failure (Chapter 42)
   Familial dysautonomia

Combined sympathetic and parasympathetic failure
  Autonomic dysfunction usually clinically unimportant
   Hereditary neuropathies
    Hereditary motor and sensory neuropathies
    Friedreich's ataxia
    Hereditary sensory neuropathy
    Adrenomyeloneuropathy
    Fabry's disease
   Connective tissue diseases
    Rheumatoid arthritis
    Systemic lupus erythematosus and mixed connective tissue diseases
    Sjögren's syndrome
   Infections
    Leprosy
    AIDS (Chapter 52)
    Diphtheria
    Lyme disease
   Immune-mediated
    Chronic inflammatory demyelinating polyradiculoneuropathy (CIDP)
   Metabolic
    Uremia
    Liver disease
   Nutritional deficiencies
    Subacute combined degeneration
    Alcoholic neuropathy
   Dysautonomia of old age (Chapter 14)
   Amyotrophic lateral sclerosis (ALS)
   Inflammatory bowel disease
   Multiple symmetric lipomatosis (Madelung's disease)
Paroxysmal or intermittent acral dysautonomia
   Paroxysmal hyperhidrosis (Chapter 59)
   Raynaud's syndrome (Chapter 59)
   Erythromelalgia
Disorders of reduced orthostatic tolerance (Chapters 48 and 49)
   Vasovagal syncope
   Prolonged bed rest
   Dysautonomia sometimes associated with mitral valve prolapse
   Postural orthostatic tachycardia syndrome (POTS)
   Prolonged weightlessness (Chapter 33)
   Postexercise syncope

sympathetic and parasympathetic failure. Guillain-Barré syndrome is at the other end of the spectrum, in which the somatic nervous system is primarily affected. Pure acute panautonomic neuropathies are relatively rare. Most acute autonomic neuropathies have some minor somatic features. Some cases of acute autonomic neuropathy have quite florid somatic involvement (14,40,65,75). Dysautonomia may be restricted to the cholinergic system (acute cholinergic neuropathy). There are other forms of restricted acute autonomic neuropathy. Some cases occur after viral infection and may be manifested as the postural orthostatic tachycardia syndrome (236) (Chapter 49). Other cases are manifested as neurogenic motility disorders (Chapter 45). Many of these cases are misdiagnosed as functional or psychiatric complaints, as the symptoms and signs are not especially dramatic and may be missed during a bedside evaluation.

There are several reasons to suspect that many of the acute autonomic neuropathies are immune-mediated. There is considerable overlap among the disorders. Some degree of autonomic involvement occurs in the majority of patients with Guillain-Barré syndrome. Some degree of somatic involvement is present in the majority of patients with autonomic neuropathies, such as acute panautonomic neuropathy (14,65,189). Indeed, all cases of acute panautonomic neuropathy have had some evidence of somatic involvement, including the case of Young et al. (277). Acute panautonomic neuropathy may be associated with CSF albuminocytologic dissociation (247,277). The sural nerve biopsy may show perivascular round cell infiltration.

There is also strong evidence of immune-mediated mechanisms in the paraneoplastic neuropathies, including the Lambert-Eaton myasthenic syndrome (LEMS) (Chapter 41).

In the following description of the autonomic neuropathies, minor or insignificant sensory impairment is accepted within acute panautonomic neuropathy. Clinically significant sensory neuropathy is best designated *acute panautonomic neuropathy with sensory neuro(no)pathy*. The other entities cause less confusion.

Acute Panautonomic Neuropathy (Pandysautonomia)

Clinical Features

The core features of acute panautonomic neuropathy are as follows: (a) acute or subacute onset; (b) widespread and severe sympathetic and parasympathetic failure; and (c) relative or complete sparing of somatic nerve fibers. The syndrome of acute panautonomic neuropathy (acute pandysautonomia; acute autonomic neuropathy) is rare but highly distinctive (9,14,65,155,190,247,275,277). Acute autonomic neuropathies with more restricted expression of dysautonomia are more common. The acute or subacute onset of combined sympathetic and parasympathetic failure develops in previously healthy individuals. Widespread sympathetic failure is manifested as severe orthostatic hypotension, anhidrosis, and parasympathetic failure, as indicated by dry eyes, dry mouth, and disturbances of bowel, bladder, and sexual function. Abdominal pain, often colicky, is very common, and gastrointestinal symptoms, such as early satiety, bloating, nausea, vomiting, pain, diarrhea, or alternating constipation and diarrhea, may persist for years. Patients usually have a fixed heart rate and pupils.

The original case described by Young et al. (277) was remarkable for the relative "purity" of autonomic involvement and remarkable recovery experienced by the patient. In actuality, mild sensory impairment is common. For instance, the patient reported by Young et al. (277) had loss of pain and a negative flare response, indicating a lesion of somatic C fibers. Most of the later cases in the literature, including the cases seen at the Mayo Clinic (9,65,155), showed only partial improvement. There may be an antecedent viral infection, such as herpes simplex (190), infectious mononucleosis (75), or rubella (247), or a febrile, presumed viral infection (65,159,252). The frequency of such an infection is unknown but appears to be less than in Guillain-Barré syndrome. Somatic involvement is insignificant, but minor paresthesias or itching is common, and there may be some degree of small-fiber involvement. Occasionally, acute autonomic failure is associated with acute and severe neuropathic pain. We evaluated the natural history, electrophysiologic characteristics, spectrum of autonomic involvement, pathology, and laboratory features in 27 patients with idiopathic autonomic neuropathy who were followed for a mean of 32 months (246). The typical features of idiopathic autonomic neuropathy included the absence of an associated disease, frequent history of preceding infection (about 50%), and acute or subacute onset with a monophasic course. The spectrum of autonomic involvement ranged from panautonomic to selective adrenergic or cholinergic failure. There is infrequent involvement of somatic nerve fibers as assessed by routine nerve conduction studies. Pathologic features included the presence of a small inflammatory mononuclear cell infiltrate in the epineurium. Recovery tended to be gradual and was frequently incomplete. The acute onset, frequent antecedent viral infection, selectivity of involvement by fiber type and autonomic level, and presence of perivascular mononuclear cell infiltration suggest that the underlying mechanism is likely to be immune-mediated.

Neurologic examination confirms the presence of orthostatic hypotension, fixed HR, and fixed dilated pupils. The skin is dry and there is usually urinary retention. Strength and sensation are normal. Occasionally, there may be some distal impairment of pain and temperature perception. The site of the lesion is peripheral and postganglionic, although involvement of preganglionic or central sites has been reported (202).

Investigations

Results of nerve conduction studies are normal. The motor unit potential is usually normal, although infrequent distal fibrillation potentials or minor abnormalities suggestive of chronic partial denervation may be occasionally seen

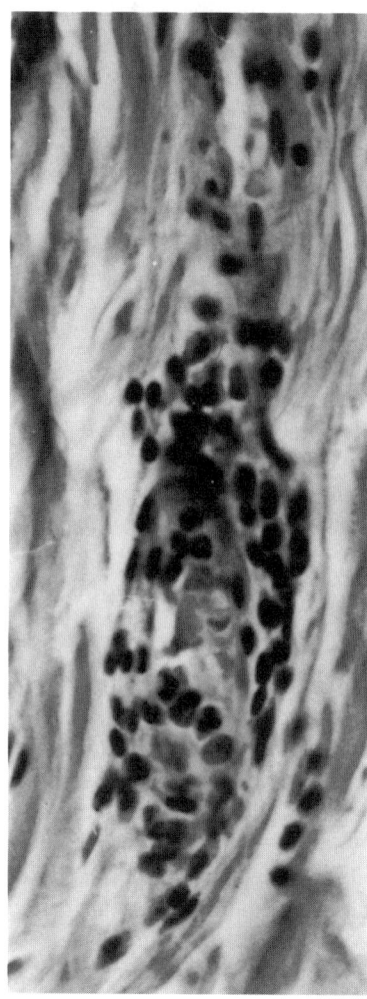

FIG. 1. Perivascular round cell infiltration in a sural nerve of a patient with acute pandysautonomia.

and do not negate the diagnosis. Computer-assisted sensory examination may occasionally show impairment of temperature or pain perception (159). Sural nerve biopsy may show perivascular round cell infiltration (Fig. 1), and the C potential may be reduced or absent (Fig. 2).

Results of the autonomic reflex screen and thermoregulatory sweat test (TST) are markedly abnormal. The TST shows widespread anhidrosis. Typically, there is greater than 70% total body anhidrosis (155). Results of the quantitative sudomotor axon reflex test (QSART) are diffusely abnormal, indicating widespread postganglionic sympathetic denervation. Widespread adrenergic failure is found, manifested as orthostatic hypotension with a fixed HR and BP_{BB} recordings to the Valsalva maneuver (VM) showing a phase II drop in mean blood pressure of >40 mm Hg with a loss of late phase II and IV. Salivation is usually reduced, and the Schirmer test confirms reduced tear secretion. Gastrointestinal motility is markedly abnormal (155), and cystometrogram shows detrusor denervation. Supine plasma norepinephrine is reduced and fails to rise on standing.

The sural nerve biopsy findings are described in Chapter 28. In brief, the biopsy results may be negative (277), or there may be a reduction of unmyelinated and small myelinated fibers and an absence of the C potential on in vitro compound nerve action potential recordings (155). In a chronic case, an increased number of miniature fibers suggestive of regeneration of unmyelinated fibers was seen (14). Some of these features are illustrated in Table 2.

Differential Diagnosis

The diagnosis is restricted to a diffuse autonomic neuropathy. Although minor sensory symptoms do not negate the diagnosis, the neuropathy is best designated *acute panautonomic neuropathy with sensory neuropathy* when a distinct sensory neuropathy is evident. The main differential diagnoses are paraneoplastic pandysautonomia, the acute cholinergic neuropathies, and Guillain-Barré syndrome. It may be indistinguishable from paraneoplastic dysautonomia until a neoplasm is found (see below). The acute cholinergic neuropathies are not associated with adrenergic failure, and therefore such patients do not have significant orthostatic hypotension. A problem may occur in the bedridden patient with acute cholinergic neuropathy who is dehydrated or severely deconditioned. Because cardiovagal function is impaired, cardioacceleration is impaired, so that some orthostatic hypotension can be seen. The severe motor paresis of Guillain-Barré syndrome provides a clear separation from panautonomic neuropathy. Infrequently, widespread, severe autonomic failure associated with only moderate somatic involvement is seen in Guillain-Barré syndrome, and the separation of the two disorders is then an academic exercise. The temporal pattern separates acute panautonomic neuropathy from the chronic dysautonomias.

Etiology or Mechanisms

The disorder is unknown but is likely to be immune-mediated. The evidence is based on the sural nerve biopsy finding of perivascular round cell infiltration (Fig. 1), the occasional antecedent viral infection, the selectivity of involvement by fiber type and autonomic level, and the cases that seem to be intermediate between Guillain-Barré syndrome and pandysautonomia.

Course and Prognosis

Little information is available on the course and prognosis of panautonomic neuropathy. The Mayo experience, based on a review of 27 cases (246), suggests that there is a range of outcomes. Approximately one in three cases makes a good functional improvement, and about one in three makes a partial recovery but is left with substantial deficits, including debilitating orthostatic hypotension. The remaining third do not improve. The overall impres-

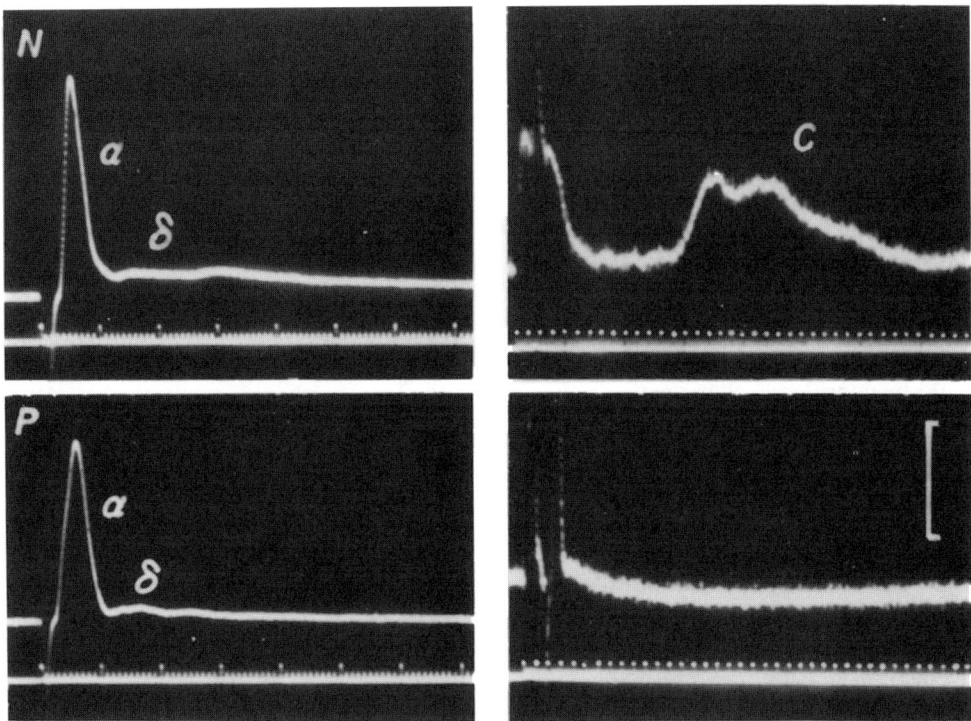

FIG. 2. Compound action potential of a fascicle of sural nerve from (*P*) a patient with pandysautonomia and (*N*) a normal control with comparable α and δ potentials. *Vertical bar* represents 0.5 mV and 100 V for the records on the *left* and *right*, respectively. Temperature was 37°C. (From Low PA, Dyck PJ, Lambert EH, Brimijoin WS, Trautman JC, Malagelada JR, Fealey RD, Barrétt DM. Acute panautonomic neuropathy. *Ann Neurol* 1983;13:412–417. Reproduced with permission.)

TABLE 2. *Results of autonomic tests in two patients*

Test	Patient 1 response 1976		Patient 1 response 1981		Patient 2 response		Expected response
Pupillary response to dilute pilocarpine	Marked and sustained R pupillary constriction		No response		Marked and sustained R & L pupillary constriction		No response
Pupillography	Left	Right	Left	Right	Left	Right	
Light stimulus							
Latency	0.39 sec	0.35 sec	Prolonged	Prolonged	0.4 sec	0.4 sec	0.2–0.3 sec
Amplitude	0.55 mm	0.80 mm	Minimal	Minimal	0.35 mm	0.75 mm	2.5–4.0 mm
Redilation to psychosensory stimulus	Reduced	Reduced	Reduced	Reduced	Absent	Absent	Prompt
Schirmer's test (5 min)	13 mm	14 mm	>15 mm	>15 mm	Not done	Not done	≥15 mm
Valsalva ratio	1.02		1.20		Not done		≥1.5 mm
MAP rise (25 μg IV phenylephrine)	35 mm Hg		10 mm Hg		Not done		No response
Pl. NE (standing/ supine, pg/ml)	Not done		20/19		61/17		(200–1700)/70–750)
Sweat test							
Thermal	Absent sweating		Islands of heavy sweating		Patchy areas of hypohidrosis		Diffuse and profuse sweating
Intradermal methacholine (1:1000)	Marked reduction		Reduced		Not done		Sweating about 5 cm around injection site

From Low et al., ref. 155. Reprinted with permission.
MAP, mean arterial pressure; Pl. NE, plasma norepinephrine.

sion is that panautonomic neuropathy runs a chronic debilitating course with significant residual deficits in the majority of patients. Patients seem to improve substantially during the first year, after which the rate of improvement is slower during the subsequent 4 years.

Management

Treatment, which is mainly supportive, consists of management of orthostatic hypotension and bowel and bladder symptoms (see respective chapters). There is suggestive evidence of an immune-mediated process, so that treatment with prednisone, plasma exchange, or intravenous gamma globulin could be considered. Some patients seem to improve more rapidly on these treatments, although the reports remain anecdotal. Heathfield et al. (98) reported on a patient who had acute panautonomic neuropathy with severe postural hypotension and fixed dilated pupils who responded within 36 hours of receiving intravenous gamma globulin. Two weeks later the autonomic failure recurred but again responded to treatment with intravenous gamma globulin. Smit et al. (240) reported on a patient with well-documented improvement following intravenous immunoglobulin. If this treatment is used, it is important to quantitate the neurologic and autonomic status before and during treatment. We administer 50 mg of prednisone daily for 2 weeks followed by a taper over 2 weeks. Plasma exchange is given as three exchanges a week for 2 weeks. Intravenous gamma globulin is given at 0.4 g/kg for two infusions (over 4 hours) and then at 0.2 g/kg for 4 further infusions. The six infusions are given over 2 weeks.

The following example illustrates some of the points made above.

In November 1986, a febrile illness developed in a white woman, age 40 years, with sore throat and myalgias. This was followed within 2 weeks by persistent severe burning pains in the hands, feet, and face. Severe orthostatic presyncope and syncope developed. In April 1987, because of severe pain and orthostatic symptoms, she was started on 60 mg of prednisone daily; improvement of pain and burning was dramatic. In January 1987, she was seen at the Mayo Clinic. She reported orthostatic dizziness, dyspnea, palpitations, tiredness and tremulousness, dry skin, and constipation.

On examination, generalized areflexia with distal hypesthesia was found. Results of electrophysiologic studies were completely normal, as was computer-assisted sensory examination for touch/pressure, vibration, and thermal cooling. Supine BP was 130/70 mm HG, and HR was 76 beats/min. Standing BP was 102/79 mm Hg and was associated with a rise in HR to 126 beats/min.

Findings of autonomic tests included a Valsalva ratio (VR) of 1.70 (>1.5) and an HR response to deep breathing of 15 beats/min (>18). Finapres recording of the VM demonstrated an excessive phase II and reduced phase IV. QSART findings were normal over the forearm and absent in all three sites over the lower extremity. Thermoregulatory sweat test showed complete anhidrosis of the lower extremities and patchy anhidrosis over the trunk and arms.

The case illustrates the development of an acute autonomic neuropathy (*forme fruste* of acute panautonomic neuropathy) with minor somatic involvement (areflexia and pain) and pain as a major manifestation, and the response to prednisone.

Acute Paraneoplastic Autonomic Neuropathy (Chapter 41)

Acute Cholinergic Neuropathy

This disorder is probably a restricted expression of acute panautonomic neuropathy, with abnormalities confined to the postganglionic cholinergic neuron (95,106,108,129, 250,259). Patients have alacrima, xerostomia, anhidrosis, constipation, urinary retention, and blurred vision, but they do not have orthostatic hypotension. Gastrointestinal problems are very common, with ileus during the early stages and abdominal pain, gastroparesis, and constipation during the chronic phase. In some patients, motility abnormalities may dominate the clinical picture (19). Abnormalities in muscle biopsy consisting of excess lipid accumulation, z-line and myofilamentous disorganization, and honeycomb formation were described in one case (1). Kirby et al. (129) reported the loss of cholinergic fibers to detrusor muscle in their case. The possibility that some cases of acute cholinergic neuropathy are actually botulism type B has been raised (118).

Guillain-Barré Syndrome

Core Features

1. Acute onset
2. Ascending, predominantly motor polyradiculoneuropathy
3. Autonomic overactivity/underactivity

Clinical Features

Autonomic dysfunction, mainly cardiovascular, manifested as tachycardia and orthostatic hypotension alternating with hypertension, is relatively common in some series, occurring in one third to two thirds of patients (148,238,254). Compared with the somatic deficit, which is usually severe, autonomic clinical involvement when present in patients with Guillain-Barré syndrome is usually mild. Early publications have emphasized that urinary retention is characteristically absent, and bladder or bowel involvement has been suggested as a reason to exclude the diagnosis of Guillain-Barré syndrome (205). Most bedridden patients do not have urinary retention, indicating that parasympathetic control to the bladder is largely spared. However, some series have reported that urinary sphincter impairment is common. Hewer et al. (101) reported that 21 of 35 cases requiring assisted ventilation were either incontinent or required catheterization. In many series, urinary retention occurs in about one third of patients (135,148,165,254,273).

Some patients with Guillain-Barré syndrome have life-threatening dysautonomia, occurring most frequently in the acute evolving phase of the disease. It tends to correlate with the severity of somatic involvement, being especially common in patients with respiratory failure (148), although the relationship between autonomic and somatic impairment is inconsistent (256). Dysautonomia seems to be associated with increased mortality (148).

Orthostatic hypotension and anhidrosis are well described (26,148,238,254,256). Parasympathetic abnormalities may occur. Cardiovagal failure, manifested as resting tachycardia (31,86,148,238,254,256), is most common in patients with more severe cases of Guillain-Barré syndrome (254). More widespread vagal failure may also occur, manifested as gastrointestinal atony or iridoplegia, and it may perhaps be responsible for the inappropriate secretion of antidiuretic hormone (237).

Less common but very distressing are episodes of autonomic hyperactivity. There may be excessive acral sweating, vasoconstriction, and color changes. Even more distressing is sustained or paroxysmal and fluctuating hypertension (48,180,254), tachyarrhythmias (37,214), and bradyarrythmias (37,59,67).

The hypertension may be caused by denervation supersensitivity with normal or increased catecholamines (220, 261). The episodes of hypertension, often associated with headaches, may closely mimic pheochromocytoma. The mechanisms of hypertension may be similar in the two conditions. In pheochromocytoma, there is an increase in circulating catecholamines. In Guillain-Barré syndrome, levels of catecholamines may be normal or only mildly increased, but there is denervation supersensitivity, so that the effect is the same. Another mechanism is increased levels of renin in patients who have hypertension associated with Guillain-Barré syndrome (142). A third mechanism is baroreceptor denervation, which results in episodic BP increases similar to those seen in tetraplegics. Sinus tachycardia may occur in more than 50% of patients with severe Guillain-Barré syndrome (84,148). In some cases, the mechanism is vagal failure, but patients with tachycardia who have intact vagal function have been described, and a myocarditis may be responsible in some of these latter cases (97,229).

Less common or less troublesome autonomic symptoms include constipation (148,254), rectal incontinence (254), gastroparesis (43,148), ileus, sexual impairment (89), and pupillary abnormalities (213,274).

Investigations

The diagnosis of Guillain-Barré syndrome is based on clinical criteria, and a uniform set of criteria has been suggested (16). Results of tests of autonomic function are often abnormal. Orthostatic hypotension may be present (148,238,254,256). The mechanism of orthostatic hypotension is multifactorial. The patients are bedridden, and prolonged bed rest may result in reduced orthostatic tolerance (242). Efferent sympathetic denervation is often present as suggested by an abnormal TST (256), denervation supersensitivity to phenylephrine (26), and reduced pressor response to sustained handgrip and cold immersion (238). These autonomic tests depend on reflex pathways with somatic afferents and sympathetic efferents. In our experience, both afferent and efferent lesions are usually present. Other abnormal test findings include a blocked Valsalva response (26,270) and impaired cardiovagal function (74, 211), anhidrosis (256), vasomotor abnormalities (15,256), and an excessive pressor response to directly acting alpha agonists (26). There has been microneurographic evidence of muscle sympathetic efferent hyperactivity during the phase when BP and HR are increased (64). The abnormalities were ascribed to lesions of the afferent limb.

Abnormalities of cardiac rhythm include sinus tachycardia and bradyarrhythmias. Heart block or even asystole has been described and may necessitate placement of a cardiac pacemaker (59,67,188). Sinus arrest may follow vigorous vagal stimulation—for example, with tracheal suction (254).

Heart rate response to deep breathing is abnormal in about one fourth to one third of patients (74,211,238) and may return to normal with recovery from the neuropathy (211). Baroreflex gain, derived from the heart period response to BP increase secondary to a directly acting alpha agonist (256), is reduced in about half of patients. Pathologic changes of autonomic structures have been described (Chapter 28).

Treatment

Severe or progressive Guillain-Barré syndrome is treated with plasma exchange or intravenous gamma globulin (13, 258), whereas mild or improving Guillain-Barré syndrome is treated with supportive measures alone. The management of acute dysautonomic symptoms is covered in Chapter 57. Patients with autonomic instability require close monitoring of HR and BP. Paroxysmal hypertension is difficult to treat as it is usually very brief, may alternate with hypotension, and may be supersensitive to hypotensive and other agents (47). For these patients, the use of hypotensive agents is usually best avoided. When sustained hypertension develops, combined α- and β-adrenergic blockade has been suggested, and bradyarrythmias are probably best treated by the use of a demand pacemaker.

Beyond the intensive care unit, the management of autonomic failure continues to be important. Meticulous attention should be paid to maintaining an adequate blood volume, as the denervated vascular bed is extremely sensitive to volume depletion. Also important is the need to prevent deconditioning. The head of the bed should be elevated about 10 inches at all times, and the patient should be mobilized as soon as possible to prevent the reduced orthostatic tolerance of prolonged bed rest. Monitoring of heart period response to deep breathing has been suggested. The treatment of hypertension associated with Guillain-Barré syndrome is covered in Chapter 57. Treatment of orthostatic hypotension is described later.

Botulism

Clinical Features

Core features are the acute development of cholinergic neuropathy, ptosis, and bulbar weakness following the ingestion of home-canned foods contaminated by *Clostridium botulinum* spores. Symptoms of nausea and vomiting are common. Neurologic symptoms are ptosis, extraocular muscle palsy, paralysis of other cranial nerve-supplied musculature, dyspnea that may progress to apnea, and generalized neuromuscular paralysis (195,212). Autonomic symptoms consist of severe cholinergic failure, with anhidrosis, dry eyes and mouth, paralytic ileus, and urinary retention (195). Gastrointestinal symptoms, including paralytic ileus and gastric dilatation, are relatively common (42,195). Orthostatic hypotension may also occur (263), and fluctuations in BP and vasomotor tone have been noted (150). Typically, symptoms begin 12 to 36 hrs after the ingestion of contaminated food. The syndrome of inappropriate secretion of antidiuretic hormone may also be observed (150,228).

The frequency, severity, and duration of autonomic failure may relate to the type of botulism. Jenzer et al. (118) described nine cases of botulism B characterized by prominent cholinergic failure, especially blurred vision and dry mouth, without significant weakness. These patients had no evidence of neuromuscular transmission failure. The symptoms persisted for months, and there was a favorable response to guanidine but not antitoxin. Type B appears to be milder than type A, neuromuscular deficit is less constant (118,134), and autonomic dysfunction is more consistently present. Autonomic failure is not consistently present in type A (35,66,227).

Investigations

Results of cardiovascular HR tests of autonomic function are abnormal, suggesting cardiovagal impairment, and orthostatic hypotension may be present (263). Orthostatic hypotension disappears before parasympathetic function recovers, and the neuromuscular transmission deficit disappears last of all (263). Electrodiagnostic findings may be relatively nonspecific (212). Findings include low-amplitude and short-duration motor unit potentials and low compound muscle action potential amplitudes, which may undergo a modest increment with rapid repetitive stimulation (91,212). Normal neuromuscular transmission does not exclude the diagnosis of botulism, as autonomic failure can occur without neuromuscular transmission deficit in some cases of botulism B (118). Single-fiber electromyographic studies may reveal increased jitter and impulse blocking (44). Esophageal manometry may demonstrate marked reduction in peristaltic amplitude (195). Schirmer test may confirm impaired tear secretion, and salivation is reduced, as demonstrated by the recording of salivary secretion using salivary duct cannulation (118).

Diagnosis and Management

The diagnosis is clinical. It can be confirmed by identification of the toxin in the food or serum (212). If available, contaminated food can be suspended in saline solution and injected intraperitoneally in mice. In the event of botulism infection, the animal dies within 24 hrs (the mouse test). Management is mainly supportive, consisting of early tracheostomy and ventilatory support in patients with respiratory failure. The role of antitoxins is uncertain. They do not seem to be effective in botulism type B. Guanidine may be effective in some cases (35,118) but not others (66).

Porphyria

Dysautonomia is common in acute intermittent porphyria, and autonomic overactivity predominates over autonomic failure, although both are present and often coexistent. Symptoms of sympathetic overactivity include abdominal colic, hypertension, and tachycardia (82,222) (see also Chapter 56). Porphyria is consistently associated with obstinate constipation (221). Postural hypotension may occur in acute intermittent and variegate porphyria, although hypertension is more common and may precede the manifestation of peripheral neuropathy (235). Persistent tachycardia may be an early feature of an attack and may also precede the onset of neuropathy. Other clinical features of autonomic neuropathy include abdominal pain, nausea and vomiting, constipation, diarrhea, bladder distention, and disorder of sweating—both anhidrosis and hyperhidrosis (221,235).

Autonomic function studies have demonstrated abnormalities of sympathetic and parasympathetic function (141,245). There is pathologic evidence of involvement of brain stem and spinal cord neurons, and of the vagus and sympathetic nerves (80,210). Management is described in Chapters 56 and 57.

Drug-Induced Acute Autonomic Neuropathies

Cisplatin

Cisplatin (*cis*-dichlorodiammineplatinum) is a cell-cycle-nonspecific cytotoxic agent. It is neurotoxic; side effects include ototoxicity, retrobulbar neuritis, and peripheral neuropathy. Neuropathy when present has usually developed in patients who have received a cumulative dose of 210 to 825 mg/m^2, corresponding to about three or four courses of therapy (92,224). Although a paraneoplastic neuropathy associated with the carcinoma may be responsible for autonomic failure, the temporal relationship to cisplatinum administration suggests a cause-and-effect relationship. For instance, in the cases reported, patients had bronchogenic carcinoma but no evidence of autonomic failure until treatment with cisplatinum, after which progressive orthostatic hypotension, dry mouth, and poikilothermia developed.

Vincristine

Vincristine, used in the treatment of lymphoma, leukemia, and some other malignancies, causes an axonal peripheral neuropathy (174). It is a very useful antineoplastic drug, lacking the usual emetic effects and myelotoxicity of most anticancer drugs, but its usefulness is limited by its neurotoxicity. The neurotoxicity is dose-related and cumulative with repeated dosing, such that the drug needs to be stopped after a cumulative dose of 30 to 50 mg (143). The autonomic complications are recognized but inadequately studied. Autonomic symptoms include postural hypotension, constipation, abdominal pain, paralytic ileus, and urinary retention (93,143,144,174). Published accounts of autonomic function studies in patients with vincristine-induced autonomic neuropathy are limited but have described abnormalities of postganglionic sympathetic efferent function and abnormal Valsalva responses in patients with postural hypotension (93). Heart rate response to deep breathing was impaired during the induction phase (104). The preganglionic axons of the greater splanchnic nerve were reported to be normal in a single case report (268).

Autonomic dysfunction may develop within days of commencement of vincristine therapy. The mechanism of action is not clear, although there is some evidence in humans and other mammals that the primary site of damage is the unmyelinated noradrenergic fibers of the sympathetic nervous system. However, the symptoms in humans of constipation, paralytic ileus, and bladder disturbances indicate that parasympathetic fibers are also affected. Ultrastructurally, Vinca alkaloids disrupt microtubules and cause an increase in neurofilaments and the appearance of paracrystalline structures in axons (144). Unmyelinated fibers are more susceptible to the neurotoxin than myelinated fibers.

Vacor

Vacor (N-3-pyridylmethyl-N'-p-nitrophenyl urea; PNU) is a rodenticide that antagonizes nicotinamide metabolism. Ingestion is usually deliberate (suicidal or homicidal) or accidental. Quantities ingested have usually been between 0.39 g and 7 g. Ingestion results in acute hyperglycemic ketoacidosis and a combined somatic and autonomic neuropathy. The mortality rate following Vacor ingestion is high. Autonomic manifestations include orthostatic hypotension and gastrointestinal hypomotility (120,147,179,215). Parenteral nicotinamide, especially if administered early, may be beneficial (120).

Amiodarone

Amiodarone, an antiarrhythmic agent, causes a sensorimotor neuropathy that occurs in about 10% of patients in most series (8,166,207). Sural nerve neuropathologic changes, which involve both unmyelinated and myelinated fibers, include fiber loss, mixed demyelination, and axonal degeneration; lamellated lysosomal inclusions are characteristic (114,209). In an experimental study, inclusions were absent from neural tissue protected by the blood-nerve and blood-brain barriers. Of neural tissues situated outside these barriers, autonomic ganglia were the most affected, with large accumulations of lysosomal bodies in nerve cells and processes; these inclusions were associated with evidence of degenerative changes (41). No significant changes were seen in peripheral nerves (114). However, in a study of three patients with neuropathy, high serum levels were present, and sural nerve concentration was 80 times that of serum concentration in one patient (72). Autonomic failure with severe orthostatic hypotension may occur (163), but detailed autonomic studies have not been published. Abatement of neuropathy occurs with cessation of the drug.

Perhexiline Maleate

Perhexiline maleate, used in the treatment of angina pectoris, may cause a peripheral neuropathy. Fraser et al. (73) described three patients in whom autonomic neuropathy developed, manifested by postural hypotension and an abnormal Valsalva ratio following perhexiline maleate treatment.

Taxol

Paclitaxel (Taxol; Bristol-Myers Squibb, Princeton, New Jersey) is a novel antitubulin chemotherapeutic agent. The dose-limiting toxicity of paclitaxel is reported to be peripheral neuropathy at the dose level of 300 mg/m^2 (234). Paclitaxel causes a sensory neuropathy in at least 10% of patients. Neuropathy tends to develop when the cumulative dose exceeds 600 mg/m^2 (103), but a wider range of cumulative doses (50 to 750 mg/m^2) and dose levels (10 to 115 mg/m^2) has been reported (191). Autonomic neuropathy is not usually a feature but has been reported. Jerian et al. (119) described two patients with autonomic failure, including orthostatic hypotension. One patient was a diabetic. The patients did not have symptoms of autonomic dysfunction before paclitaxel therapy. Severe orthostatic hypotension developed in both following completion of a 24-hr infusion of paclitaxel at 170 to 250 mg/m^2. Noninvasive autonomic tests performed in one patient demonstrated both impaired cardiovagal and adrenergic function (tilt test, sustained handgrip).

Toxic Acute Autonomic Neuropathies

Heavy Metal Poisoning

There have been very few cases of heavy metal poisoning in which autonomic function has been adequately studied. In thallium poisoning, tachycardia and hypertension have been reported in association with peripheral neuropathy (20). In arsenic poisoning, excessive sweating and impairment of sweating in the extremities have been described (83,145). Subacute or chronic inorganic mercury poisoning is the cause of acrodynia; it occurs mainly in children and includes among its manifestations tachycardia; hypertension; pain and redness of the fingers, toes, and ears (hence the name *pink disease*); and profuse sweating (269). Treatment with ganglion-blocking agents and chelation has been recommended (29). Subclinical impairment of cardiovagal function with environmental exposure to heavy metals has been reported (184).

Organic Solvents

Autonomic function has been shown to be disturbed in some workers with prolonged chronic occupational exposure to a variety of organic solvents containing mainly aliphatic, aromatic, and other hydrocarbons, alcohols, ketones, esters, and ethers, as well as exposure to carbon disulfide and toluene. They had significant impairment of HR variation with respiration and Valsalva ratio compared with controls. The most severely affected patients were those exposed to carbon disulfide. Some of the patients had clinical and electrophysiologic evidence of peripheral neuropathy (168).

Hexacarbon neuropathy occurs through industrial exposure or through inhalant abuse. Inhalation of *n*-hexane and methyl-*n*-butyl-ketone may result in a rapidly progressive polyneuropathy associated with autonomic features of excessive or impaired sweating, vasomotor alterations of the extremities, postural hypotension, and impotence (4).

Acrylamide

Acrylamide is neurotoxic in its soluble monomeric form, in which it is manufactured and distributed. After transformation to a polymer, it is used in industry as a flocculator for separating solids from aqueous solutions. It is also used in the preparation of grouts for the sealing of pipes and subterranean tunnels. The major toxic effect in humans is a predominantly sensory polyneuropathy, often preceded by blue color and excessive sweating of the extremities resulting from a disturbance of sympathetic function (17,143). Other autonomic disturbances in humans are rarely seen, although they have been studied extensively in experimental animals. In the latter, degeneration of preganglionic and postganglionic sympathetic and parasympathetic fibers has been demonstrated associated with impaired vasomotor tone (216,217).

CHRONIC PERIPHERAL AUTONOMIC NEUROPATHIES

Distal Sympathetic Neuropathies

Distal Small-Fiber Neuropathy (see also Chapter 50)

Clinical Features

Distal small-fiber neuropathy is characterized by distal dysesthesias and postganglionic sympathetic dysfunction in the absence of significant somatic neuropathy. Symptoms include superficial burning and a deeper aching pain. The pain is most common in the sole and toe pads, with later involvement of the dorsum. Troublesome allodynia, in which light touch or firm pressure (as with weight bearing) causes pain, is common. Sympathetic dysfunction is manifested as vasomotor changes; also common are pallor (sometimes alternating with rubor that is associated with accentuation of pain, referred to as *erythromelalgia*), cyanosis, and mottling. Sudomotor dysfunction, manifested commonly as excessive sweating or anhidrosis, is also common.

Distal small-fiber neuropathy may be a manifestation of conditions such as diabetes and inherited and immune-mediated neuropathies. However, the majority of cases of distal small-fiber neuropathy are idiopathic and run a benign course.

The neurologic examination in idiopathic distal small-fiber neuropathy is usually unremarkable. Strength is normal. Sensation may be mildly impaired, especially for sharp-dull discrimination and temperature perception. Sometimes it is normal. Reflexes are usually normal. Electromyography and nerve conduction studies are unremarkable. Occasionally the medial plantar sensory action potential is reduced, or minimal motor unit changes or occasional fibrillation potentials are seen. The most sensitive diagnostic test is QSART or TST showing distal anhidrosis (243).

Idiopathic distal small-fiber neuropathy is distinguishable from the distal sympathetic failure associated with chronic neuropathies by the dearth of somatic motor and sensory findings and the lack of electrophysiologic abnormalities. It can be differentiated from the generalized small-fiber neuropathies (i.e., diabetic, amyloid acute panautonomic) by the absence of orthostatic hypotension or other manifestations of generalized autonomic failure.

Investigations

Most patients with distal small-fiber neuropathy have abnormalities of QSART in the distal lower extremities

(244). The diagnostic yield is enhanced if multiple recording sites are used (see Chapter 15). The QSART shows normal sweat volume in the forearm and anhidrosis in the lower extremities, maximal distally (Fig. 3). Routine electromyography is usually unhelpful, although recordings of medial plantar nerve may show abnormalities in some patients. The peripheral autonomic surface potential (PASP) is positive in a minority of patients (62). Computer-assisted sensory examination for small-fiber function may be helpful (116). Jamal et al. (116) found abnormalities in sensory testing in 25 of 25 patients. However, the actual sensitivity in uncertain, as these patients were selected into the study on the basis of examinations indicating impaired sensory function.

Other Peripheral Neuropathies

Most chronic peripheral neuropathies are associated with some distal axonal degeneration. In general, the demyelinating neuropathies, such as chronic inflammatory demyelinating polyradiculoneuropathy and monoclonal gammopathy-associated neuropathies, are associated with a lesser degree of postganglionic autonomic failure than the axonal neuropathies, such as arsenical neuropathies (244). The neuropathies with prominent diffuse autonomic failure are covered separately.

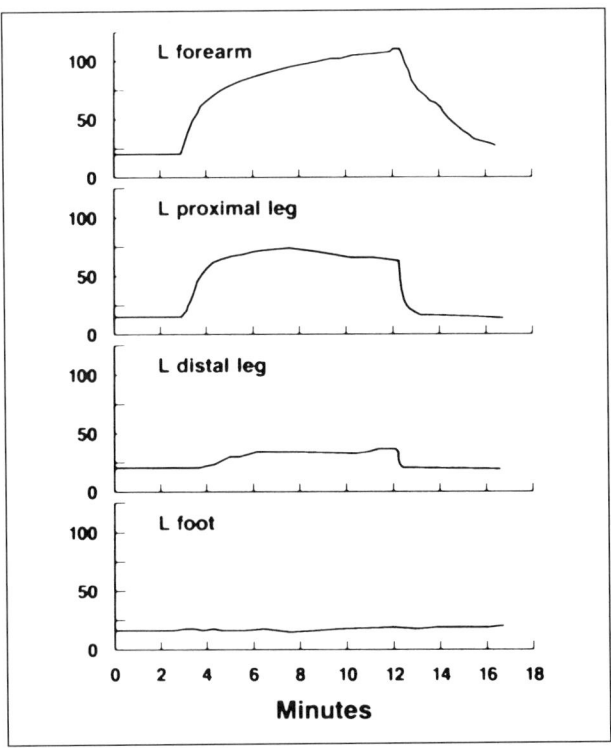

FIG. 3. QSART distribution in a patient with distal small-fiber neuropathy. There is distal anhidrosis.

Pure Cholinergic Neuropathies

Lambert-Eaton Myasthenic Syndrome (Chapter 37)

Chronic Idiopathic Anhidrosis

Clinical Features

The core feature is acquired widespread anhidrosis in the absence of generalized adrenergic and cardiovagal failure. These patients have total or subtotal anhidrosis and are heat-intolerant, becoming hot, flushed, dizzy, dyspneic, and weak when the ambient temperature is high or when they exercise. Distal vasomotor changes may be present, but orthostatic hypotension, or other evidence of generalized adrenergic failure, and symptomatic somatic neuropathy are absent. Pupillary abnormalities may be present. It is important to distinguish the entity from the progressive autonomic failures, such as multiple-system atrophy and pure autonomic failure. Chronic idiopathic anhidrosis probably comprises a heterogenous group of disorders with restricted autonomic failure. Some cases are associated with a small-fiber neuropathy (246). It is important to recognize, as it is relatively common and often confused with the more malignant autonomic disorders. In some cases, there is evidence for an immunologic mechanism (246). Segmental anhidrosis with Adie's pupil (Ross syndrome) is well recognized (225) and is often one type of chronic idiopathic anhidrosis, although rare cases of Ross syndrome are associated with more widespread autonomic failure.

The prognosis appears to be distinctly better than in other forms of progressive autonomic neuropathy. The sweating deficit may remain stable, progress, or infrequently regress. Adrenergic failure does not subsequently develop in the great majority of patients.

Investigations

These patients have widespread anhidrosis on TST (Chapter 19). The majority of cases are associated with postganglionic impairment, as usually indicated by QSART. Some cases may be preganglionic (157). Orthostatic hypotension is absent, and cardiovascular HR tests, supine and standing plasma norepinephrine levels, and BP_{BB} responses to tilt and the VM show no evidence of autonomic failure.

Treatment

Treatment is focused on the avoidance of heat stress. These patients should live in an air-conditioned environment. Some patients seem to have an altered comfort zone, setting their home thermostats to relatively lower temperatures (often slightly above 60°F). They should avoid vigorous exercise in a hot environment, as they are more prone to heat injury, including heat exhaustion and heat stroke.

Adie's Syndrome

The tonic pupil (Chapter 20) is an abnormal pupil caused by a postganglionic parasympathetic lesion. It is usually large and does not react to a brief light stimulus. Because of denervation supersensitivity, it constricts on instillation of dilute pilocarpine (0.125%) or methacholine (2.5%), in contrast to a normal pupil, which is unaffected. The pupillary abnormality is usually unilateral and may occur in isolation. *Adie's syndrome* denotes the combination of a tonic pupil with other neurologic manifestations. The best-known combination is tonic pupil(s) with areflexia (123, 164,271), and the term *Adie's syndrome* is usually applied to this combination. Widespread sympathetic failure is uncommon but is well documented (121,123). Another combination is tonic pupil and segmental anhidrosis, sometimes referred to as *Ross syndrome* (225). This syndrome is important to recognize, as the widespread anhidrosis does not indicate a progressive autonomic disorder (157). Yet another combination is tonic pupil(s) with chronic inflammatory demyelinating polyradiculoneuropathy (CIDP). Experience is limited with this disorder. It is the impression of the authors that these patients have a less favorable prognosis than those who have CIDP without tonic pupil. Another combination is tonic pupil(s) with a sensory neuronopathy as part of Sjögren's syndrome. These patients have widespread autonomic failure with anhidrosis, orthostatic hypotension, impairment of cardiovagal function, and keratoconjunctivitis sicca and xerostomia (87,158). Adie's pupil may also occur as part of the autonomic paraneoplastic neuropathy (see above). The site of the lesion is likely in the ciliary ganglion, and degenerative changes have been described in autopsy tissue (96).

Chagas' Disease

Chagas' disease causes combined parasympathetic and sympathetic neuropathy, but because the parasympathetic component predominates, it is covered in this section. Chagas' disease is caused by *Trypanosoma cruzi*, an intracellular protozoan. *T. cruzi* is found only in the Americas, from the southern United States to southern Argentina. Acute Chagas' disease is rare in the United States, and chronic Chagas' disease, which develops years to decades after primary infection, is currently seen in increasing numbers in Latin American immigrants, especially those from Salvador, Nicaragua, and Mexico. The most commonly affected organs are the heart, in which biventricular cardiomegaly and conduction defects occur, and the gastrointestinal tract (133).

Autonomic syndromes are manifested as a chronic cholinergic neuropathy. The dysautonomia has been briefly reviewed (94,123). Megaesophagus, megaduodenum, and megacolon develop, and patients describe progressively worsening dysphagia and constipation. Other parts of the gastrointestinal and urinary tracts, the gall bladder, and the salivary glands may be affected (69,132). Results of cardiovascular autonomic tests may be abnormal. Findings include orthostatic hypotension and abnormalities of baroreflex and HR response to standing and Valsalva maneuver (6,77,162,208,241). Plasma norepinephrine may be reduced (112). Cardiac nerves undergo degeneration (5,162). Multifocal inflammatory lesions associated with demyelination are present in the peripheral nervous system in humans and in the murine experimental model (231). There is evidence that the destruction of the peripheral and sympathetic nervous systems has an autoimmune basis, T lymphocytes and possibly humoral factors being responsible for an attack on neural elements. Antigenic determinants may be shared by the parasite and host. A recent placebo-controlled clinical trial of mixed gangliosides has demonstrated improved control of BP, possibly the consequence of an indirect neurotropic effect (113).

The disease may be transmitted in endemic areas in South America by the bite of a reduviid bug. Transmission may also occur via blood transfusions, a more likely mode of infection within the United States. The diagnosis of chronic Chagas' disease is made by detecting antibodies to *T. cruzi* using complement fixation, immunofluorescence, or enzyme-linked immunosorbent assay (ELISA). A false-positive test may occur in cases of leishmaniasis. When the result of one test is positive, it is usually confirmed by two additional tests (130).

Pure Adrenergic Neuropathy

Pure adrenergic neuropathy is uncommon. It may occur as part of an unusual immune-mediated acute or chronic autonomic adrenergic neuropathy. Pure autonomic failure and multiple-system atrophy may also occur as a pure adrenergic failure, with orthostatic hypotension but normal results on TSTs and tests of cardiovagal function. The combination is uncommon, occurring in fewer than 10% of patients with multiple-system atrophy and pure autonomic failure.

Another pure adrenergic neuropathy is an adrenergic neuropathy caused by an inherited absence of the enzyme dopamine-β-hydroxylase (24,167,223). Patients have an inability to convert dopamine to norepinephrine. The disorder is characterized by early onset of severe orthostatic hypotension, an absence of plasma norepinephrine, and excessive levels of dopamine. The disorder responds to treatment with levodopa, which can be converted to norepinephrine.

Combined Adrenergic/Sensory Neuropeptide-Deficient Neuropathy

Anand et al. (7) described a 30-year-old woman with long-standing orthostatic lightheadedness; she was found to have a severe orthostatic hypotension and a reduced skin axon reflex flare response. Autonomic tests indicated selective impairment of adrenergic sympathetic function. Plasma noradrenaline, adrenaline, dopamine, and dopamine-β-hydroxylase were undetectable. Skin biopsy specimens showed loss of tyrosine hydroxylase and neuropeptide Y (markers of adrenergic sympathetic fibers) and of substance P and calcitonin gene-related peptide (sensory neuropeptides). A sural nerve biopsy specimen showed severe depletion of unmyelinated fibers. The constellation of losses were compatible with nerve growth factor (NGF) deprivation, which was confirmed on assay. It has been suggested that this new syndrome may be a consequence of a loss of trophic action of NGF.

Combined Sympathetic and Parasympathetic Failure

Autonomic Dysfunction Clinically Important

Amyloid Neuropathy

Biochemistry and Classification

Amyloid consists mainly of protein with some glycosaminoglycan. It has a fibrillary structure. The property of birefringence is a consequence of its beta configuration. It stains selectively with Congo red stain or methyl violet, and when viewed under the polarizing microscope, it exhibits a characteristic, green birefringence (23).

Chemically, there are three types of amyloid (39). The AL type, consisting of monoclonal immunoglobulin kappa or lambda light chains, is associated with multiple myeloma. The AA type, consisting of amyloid A subunit protein, is secondary amyloid and is seen in inflammatory diseases such as osteomyelitis, tuberculosis, and bronchiectasis. The AH type, with transthyretin (prealbumin) as the subunit protein, is responsible for familial amyloid polyneuropathy (FAP).

Sporadic Systemic Amyloid Neuropathy

Core features
1. Small-fiber-type sensory loss
2. Autonomic failure
3. Amyloid deposits in tissue

Clinical features

Sporadic systemic amyloid neuropathy is characterized by the onset in middle to old age of a generalized small-fiber neuropathy with a predominant loss of pain and temperature perception (56), autonomic failure, and weight loss. The diagnosis is confirmed by the demonstration of amyloid deposits in tissues. Autonomic failure is an early and prominent cause of symptoms. Orthostatic hypotension with presyncope and syncope is common (140,196) and is of serious prognostic significance (139). Dysphagia is common and caused by amyloid infiltration of the lower esophagus (226). Diarrhea, constipation, or constipation alternating with diarrhea are common and are caused by infiltration of the myenteric (Auerbach) and submucosal (Meissner) plexuses. At a later stage, vomiting and abdominal distention may be a problem. Impotence is common in male patients. Anhidrosis is usually widespread.

Nonautonomic features include a sensory, often painful neuropathy, that begins in the lower extremities. Pain and temperature perception is characteristically affected (56), but a dissociated pattern of sensory loss is not always present. Weight loss is consistently present and macroglossia is common. Renal involvement with the nephrotic syndrome may occur.

Investigations

Nerve conduction studies confirm the presence of an axonal neuropathy. Nerve biopsy confirms the presence of amyloid deposits. There is a perivascular deposition of a homogeneous, glassy material that is congophilic and exhibits apple-green birefringence when viewed under polarized light. The nerve has a predominant loss of small and unmyelinated fibers. The neuropathology of amyloidosis is described in more detail in Chapter 28. The C potential is absent on the compound nerve action potential. Peripheral vasomotor and sudomotor control is impaired (154). Skin vasoconstrictor reflexes are impaired, indicating a lesion of sympathetic adrenergic fibers (Fig. 4). The pattern of sudomotor impairment (more widespread thermoregulatory sweat impairment than postganglionic impairment) suggests a preganglionic sympathetic component in addition

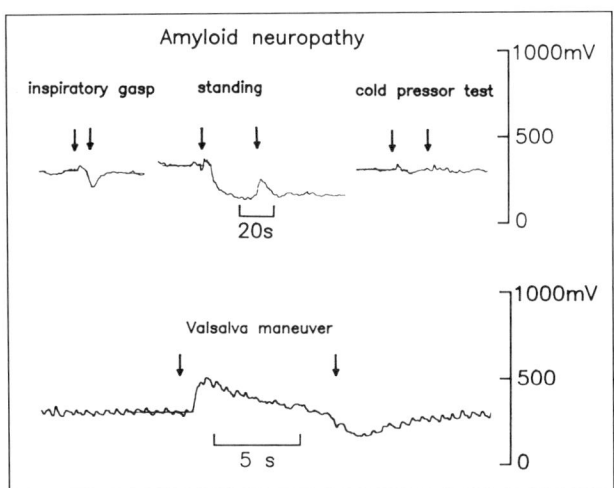

FIG. 4. Skin blood flow responses recorded with laser Doppler flowmetry. The responses to inspiratory gasp, cold pressor test, and Valsalva maneuver are reduced, and there is a passive reduction in flow secondary to a fall in BP on standing. *Arrows* indiate onset and cessation of the autonomic maneuver. (From Low PA, Neumann C, Dyck PJ, Fealey RD, Tuck RR. Evaluation of skin vasomotor reflexes by using laser Doppler velocimetry. *Mayo Clin Proc* 1983; 58:583–592. Reprinted with permission.)

to postganglionic failure, in keeping with the known loss of preganglionic neurons in this disease (156). Orthostatic hypotension is present in most patients, caused by an impairment of sympathetic innervation to the arterioles and the splanchnic and mesenteric veins (156). Compounding mechanisms are the hypovolemia associated with diarrhea, cardiovagal impairment, and cardiomyopathy with reduced cardiac contractility. Heart period responses to deep breathing and to VM are much reduced. Cardiac abnormalities in sporadic and familial amyloid polyneuropathy are similar and include the sick sinus syndrome (204) and atrioventricular conduction abnormalities. These are common and are a consequence of direct amyloid infiltration (61). Amyloidosis may mimic achalasia of the lower esophageal sphincter. Esophageal manometry has occasionally demonstrated a hypertensive sphincter with failure of relaxation after swallow (182). More often, the lower esophageal sphincter pressure is decreased and heartburn is common (226).

Diagnosis

The diagnosis is made from the gestalt of a small-fiber and autonomic neuropathy, with confirmation of amyloid deposition in tissue by nerve, rectal, or subcutaneous fat biopsy. Results of conjunctival biopsy are positive in at least 80% of patients (232). Amyloid may also be identified in muscle biopsy specimens, where it is present in perivascular sites and intramuscular nerve bundles (137). The prognosis is poor. The neuropathy progresses relentlessly despite all attempted treatments. The clinical and laboratory features based on 229 patients with primary systemic amyloidosis seen at the Mayo Clinic has recently been reported. Median survival from the time of diagnosis for patients with peripheral neuropathy, carpal tunnel syndrome, orthostatic hypotension, and cardiac failure was 60, 45, 9.5 and 6.5 months, respectively (139). Poor prognostic indices were appreciable weight loss, congestive cardiac failure, and presence of light chains in the urine.

Multiple Myeloma-Associated Amyloid Neuropathy Autonomic impairment is much less common in amyloidosis associated with multiple myeloma than in sporadic systemic amyloidosis or FAP. A small-fiber-type neuropathy similar to that of FAP I has been described in three patients with multiple myeloma (262). Amyloid infiltration of peripheral nerve is also uncommon, occurring in perhaps only 15% of cases (264).

Familial Amyloid Polyneuropathy All forms of FAP are dominantly inherited. Prognosis for life tends to be better than in primary systemic amyloidosis. The clinical features and course have been best studied for FAP I. Age of onset is relatively young, between 20 and 40 years. Patients usually die of cardiac or renal failure or of inanition 10 to 15 years after onset. As in primary systemic amyloidosis, autonomic failure is a prominent manifestation of the neuropathy. The autonomic features of FAP I are similar to those of primary systemic amyloidosis.

The AH type of systemic amyloidosis is usually the consequence of a point mutation in the transthyretin (prealbumin) gene, encoded on human chromosome 18 (267). Transthyretin is a single polypeptide chain of 127 amino acid residues (124). The genomic structure has been determined (233,255). The most common point mutation is at position 30, where methionine substitutes for valine, and it has been responsible for most cases of inherited amyloid polyneuropathy seen in the United States (12,23). However, at least seven different mutations of the transthyretin gene have been described (53,54,115,186,198,266). The clinical classification of FAP was previously based on the pattern of neuropathy. FAP I, or Portuguese or Andrade (also Swedish, Japanese, English, Greek) type, was most common, beginning in the lower extremity and associated with autonomic failure. FAP II, or Indiana type, typically began with involvement of the upper extremity. FAP III, or Iowa type, began with neuropathy of the lower extremity, renal amyloidosis, and gastric ulcers. FAP IV, or Finnish type, was characterized by lattice corneal dystrophy and cranial neuropathy. The clinical classification has been supplanted by a chemical classification. FAPs I, II and IV are caused by transthyretin-containing deposits. Recently, the amyloid protein of FAP IV has been shown by N-terminal amino acid sequence analysis to be a fragment of the inner region of human gelsolin that contains an asparagine-for-aspartic acid substitution at position 15, corresponding to residue 187 of the secreted protein (169). FAP III has been reported to be caused by deposits containing apolipoprotein A_1 (192,257).

Diagnosis

The pattern of dominant inheritance and onset in young adulthood, coupled with orthostatic hypotension and a dissociated pattern of sensory loss with relatively selective loss of pain and temperature perception, is suggestive of FAP. The electrophysiologic and autonomic features of the most common variety, FAP I, are very similar to those of primary systemic amyloidosis. The gene carrier in FAP is determined by isolatiion of DNA from peripheral leukocytes followed by digestion with specific restriction endonucleases that detect the various mutations, or by direct visualization after amplification (23,193). Rapid detection of variant transthyretin (containing the methionine-for-valine substitution) at position 30 can be measured using radioimmunoassay based on a nonapeptide (positions 22–30) derived from variant transthyretin (187).

Management

There is no proven treatment of the primary process. Symptoms of autonomic failure are managed along the lines described in the respective chapters for the relevant organ systems. Recently, liver transplantation has been reported to halt progression and possibly to decrease neuropathy. Holmgren et al. (105) reported clinical outcome after 1 to 2 years of transplantation in patients with the

Met-30 variant of the plasma protein transthyretin. They reported that three of the first four patients felt better, had improved ability to walk and better bowel function, but no objective improvement in neuropathy. It was their opinion that transplantation prevents the inexorable progression.

Diabetic Autonomic Neuropathy (Chapter 37)

Chronic Idiopathic and Paraneoplastic Panautonomic Neuropathy

Chronic Paraneoplastic Autonomic Neuropathy, Including Pandysautonomic Neuropathy

Chronic pandysautonomia, idiopathic or paraneoplastic, refers to the slowly evolving form of panautonomic neuropathy. The difference between acute and chronic panautonomic neuropathy is akin to the difference between Guillain-Barré syndrome and CIDP. A reasonable working criterion for separation is to consider an autonomic neuropathy evolving over 4 weeks or less as acute and over 4 weeks or more as chronic. The autonomic involvement is usually diffuse, but in comparison with the acute syndrome, the distribution of autonomic deficits is restricted in the majority of patients with chronic panautonomic neuropathy. Separation from pure autonomic failure can be made based on the wider distribution of autonomic deficits and the presence of somatic involvement.

Sensory Neuronopathy with Autonomic Failure

Sensory neuronopathy has several causes, and it may be associated with autonomic failure. Sensory neuronopathy with autonomic failure may be idiopathic or paraneoplastic, or it may be associated with Sjögren's syndrome, pyridoxine overdose, cisplatinum administration, monoclonal gammopathy, or Vacor intoxication.

Idiopathic sensory neuronopathy (40,197,203) is characterized by severe sensory impairment, especially of proprioception and vibration sense, so that these patients have a sensory ataxia with positive rombergism, and they often have pseudoathetosis. The distribution of sensory loss often involves most of the body surface. The patients are areflexic, and sensory action potentials are absent on nerve conduction studies. Appreciable recovery tends not to occur. The dorsal root ganglion and its extensions centrally (dorsal root and columns) are devastated (203), and peripheral sensory nerves show axonal degeneration (40,197, 203). Degeneration of neurons and nerves in the sympathetic trunk, myenteric plexus, and vagus nerve have been described (203). These cases of dysautonomia are probably variants of a related inflammatory immune process. Inflammatory round cell infiltration may be seen in acute panautonomic neuropathy (Fig. 1), and cases intermediate between the different categories are seen. For instance, Nass and Chutorian (189) described an acute self-limited syndrome in childhood dominated by positive sensory symptoms (pruritus, burning dysesthesia) and autonomic symptoms (hypertension, tachycardia, piloerection) with recovery. Although positive symptoms dominated the clinical picture in these three cases, all patients did have some evidence of sensory and autonomic failure. Autonomic neuropathy has also been reported in patients with evidence of autoimmune disease (88).

Primary Sjögren's syndrome is often associated with neuropathy. There are several neuropathic patterns. The most characteristic pattern consists of a subacute or chronic asymmetric sensory neuronopathy with initial involvement of the upper extremity, predominant loss of vibration and position sense, Adie's pupil, trigeminal sensory loss, and combined sympathetic and parasympathetic failure (87, 158). However, the most common clinical pattern is probably a distal sensory or sensorimotor neuropathy. Other patterns are sensory neuronopathy, mononeuropathy multiplex, chronic inflammatory demyelinating polyradiculoneuropathy, and multiple cranial neuropathies (10,11,71, 87,126,176,265).

We have previously described six cases of Sjögren's syndrome to illustrate the spectrum of autonomic neuropathies (173). All cases had keratoconjunctivitis sicca, xerostomia, and neuropathy and autonomic failure, but in different combinations. Autonomic function was studied by the TST, postural evaluation of BP, neuro-ophthalmologic evaluation, and autonomic reflex testing. All patients had widespread and multifocal anhidrosis on TST. QSART indicated that the anhidrosis was postganglionic. Salivation was reduced in three of the six patients. Four patients with clinical Adie's pupils had denervation supersensitivity to dilute pilocarpine, sectorial contractions, and a slow and tonic response to accommodation. Cardiac parasympathetic function was impaired in all five patients tested. The pattern of sensory involvement was multifocal in all patients. Sural nerve biopsy performed in three patients showed perivascular mononuclear infiltration and changes suggestive but not diagnostic of necrotizing angiopathy.

The patterns of neuropathy in our patients were heterogeneous. Four of six patients had sensory neuronopathy with pseudoathetosis and positive rombergism. Three of six patients had facial involvement, Adie's pupils, orthostatic hypotension, and were female. One patient had a pure cholinergic autonomic neuropathy with normal adrenergic indices and electromyography. One patient had a sensorimotor neuropathy, total-body anhidrosis, and LEMS.

Raynaud's phenomenon is relatively common, occurring in one third of patients with Sjögren's syndrome (239), and it may precede sicca syndrome in 42%. Clinical sequelae are swollen hands and small soft tissue calcifications on x-rays. Autonomic failure is common, with Adie's pupils, fixed tachycardia and orthostatic hypotension, and anhidrosis (79,87,250). The peripheral autonomic surface potential may be absent in these patients with autonomic neuropathy (79).

Autonomic failure may also be secondary to central nervous system involvement, which occurs in 25% of patients with primary Sjögren's syndrome (2). An abnormal electroencephalograph was reported in 48% (102), and visual evoked potentials were abnormal in 12% (102). An abnormal Minnesota Multiphasic Personality Inventory was found in 33 of 43, with depression commonly present (102). Magnetic resonance imaging is much more sensitive than computed tomography in detecting focal lesions (3).

Laboratory confirmation of Sjögren's syndrome is essential. Keratoconjunctivitis sicca is confirmed by the Schirmer and rose bengal tests. Salivation can be quantitated (Chapter 15). Labial biopsy of minor salivary glands demonstrating perivascular round cell infiltration is necessary to confirm the diagnosis.

Immune findings include antibodies to Ro (SS-A), La (SS-B), and rheumatoid factor. There is a significant association between vasculitis and antibody to the extractable nuclear antigens (such as Ro and La [25]). Some laboratories have reported that the detection of terminal complement complexes (SC5b-9) by ELISA is more sensitive than circulating immune complex or complement assays (3).

Cutaneous vasculitis is a frequent extraglandular manifestation of primary Sjögren's syndrome. Two types have been described. The first is leukocytoclastic angiitis, found in association with high titers of anti-Ro (SS-A) and anti-La (SS-B) antibodies and rheumatoid factor, hypergammaglobulinemia, and hypocomplementemia. The second type is a mononuclear inflammatory vasculopathy found in association with low titers of anti-Ro and normal levels of complement, gamma globulin, and rheumatoid factor. Both types are associated with peripheral and central lesions that appear to be a vasculopathy.

In patients with central nervous system vasculitis, CSF findings consist of an increase of immunoglobulin G indices, oligoclonal bands, and mild pleocytosis (2).

A review of 11 sural nerve biopsy specimens at Mayo Clinic has been reported (176). All specimens showed perivascular inflammatory infiltrates. The histologic changes in 2 of 11 biopsies were considered to be diagnostic of necrotizing vasculitis, and in 6 of 11 strongly suggestive. Axonal degeneration was the predominant change. Pathologic studies of six cutaneous nerve biopsy specimens showed perivascular round cell infiltration without necrotizing arteritis (87). Biopsy specimens of thoracic dorsal root ganglion in three patients showed lymphocytic infiltration with degeneration of dorsal root ganglion cells (87).

Cisplatinum chemotherapy may be associated with sensory neuronopathy and an autonomic neuropathy. Vacor poisoning may result in a sensory neuronopathy, diabetes, and autonomic failure. These two entities have been described earlier in this chapter. Pyridoxine neuropathy is associated with a sensory neuronopathy, but autonomic failure does not seem to be a prominent feature in this disorder.

Pure Autonomic Failure

Pure autonomic failure is covered in detail in Chapter 42.

Familial Dysautonomia (Hereditary Sensory and Autonomic Neuropathy Type III; Riley-Day Syndrome)

This recessively inherited neuropathy affects especially Ashkenazi Jews and has an onset in infancy. It is an autonomic and sensory-motor neuropathy. These patients lack fungiform papillae of the tongue and have defective control of lacrimation, temperature, sweating, and BP (161).

Clinical Features

The disorder is present at birth; characteristically the infant fails to thrive, sucks poorly, and has episodes of unexplained fever. Alacrima, blotching of the skin, and corneal insensitivity are present. Hypertension and postural hypotension have been documented, as has excessive and erratic sweating. Gastrointestinal symptoms are prominent in infancy and early childhood. There is also involvement of lower motor and sensory neurons, as suggested by hyporeflexia and kyphoscoliosis. Pain and temperature perception are more severely affected than is tactile sensation. Charcot joints resulting from insensitivity to pain have been described.

Laboratory Findings

There is mild slowing of motor conduction velocity. Neuropathologic findings are described in Chapter 28. There is distinct degeneration of all three populations, with a somewhat selective involvement of small neurons (autonomic, small sensory, gamma motoneurons). Homovanillic acid excretion is increased, and vanillylmandelic acid secretion is reduced. Levels of dopamine-β-hydroxylase, the enzyme that converts dopamine to norepinephrine, are significantly reduced in the serum of patients with dysautonomia (272).

Course and Prognosis

Life expectancy is markedly shortened. Only occasional patients have lived to the age of 30 years.

Combined Sympathetic and Parasympathetic Failure

Autonomic Dysfunction Usually Clinically Unimportant

Most neuropathies in this category are not associated with substantial autonomic involvement, and many have not been subjected to detailed autonomic studies.

Hereditary Neuropathies

Hereditary Motor and Sensory Neuropathy (Charcot-Marie-Tooth Disease) Autonomic function is impaired in hereditary motor and sensory neuropathies (HMSN) of the type associated with widespread demyelination (HMSN type I; hypertrophic Charcot-Marie-Tooth disease) or with predominantly axonal neuropathy (HMSN type II; neuronal Charcot-Marie-Tooth disease), but it is confined to distal vasomotor dysfunction, manifested as coldness, discoloration, and anhidrosis (117) and pupillary abnormalities (27,117, 128). Impaired cardiovascular reflexes have been found by some workers (27,32), but not by others (110). Widespread adrenergic failure is not a feature of the disease.

Friedreich's Ataxia Patients with Friedreich's ataxia have had detailed autonomic studies. Results of autonomic function studies, including sweat tests, are normal, with no evidence of postural hypotension or impairment of baroreflex function (109). These negative findings are consistent with the predominantly large-fiber involvement in the disease.

Hereditary Sensory Neuropathy Apart from HMSN type III, the autonomic nervous system may be affected in HSAN type IV (55,248), in which there is a marked loss of small myelinated and unmyelinated fibers (249), and HSAN type V, in which there is a marked reduction of small-diameter myelinated fibers but unmyelinated fibers are normal (153).

Adrenomyeloneuropathy Adrenomyeloneuropathy may be associated with orthostatic hypotension. These patients have a reduced plasma volume because of adrenal failure and in addition have involvement of long tracts and peripheral sympathetic neurons. Detailed studies have not been reported.

Fabry's Disease This is an inborn error of glycosphingolipid metabolism, transmitted by an X-linked recessive gene, that results in a deficiency of α-galactosidase and is characterized biochemically by an accumulation of neutral glycosphingolipids, mainly ceramide trihexoside. Clinically it is characterized by the development in young boys of a painful neuropathy, with episodic exacerbations of pain, angiokeratomas of the skin, and telangiectasia of conjunctiva, nail bed, and oral mucosa. Vascular disease develops prematurely, and patients have strokes, hypertension, and myocardial infarction in their mid to late 40s. They typically die of renal, cardiac, or cerebral complications of vascular disease.

There is lipid accumulation in sympathetic ganglion cells and degeneration of unmyelinated fibers (30,201). Cable et al. (33) performed clinical autonomic testing in 10 patients with Fabry's disease and found reduced neurogenic flare response and sudomotor function in all patients. Pupilloconstriction to pilocarpine, suggestive of parasympathetic denervation supersensitivity, and reduced tear and saliva secretion were noted in about half the patients. BP and HR and plasma norepinephrine responses to tilt were intact. Heterozygous female patients may exhibit an attenuated form of the disease, usually manifested as corneal opacities, but may occasionally have symptomatic orthostatic hypotension and sympathetic and parasympathetic failure (185). The expressive level of the enzyme may vary significantly in heterozygous female patients because the gene encoding α-galactosidase undergoes random X-inactivation (49). The pain responds to carbamazepine, but autonomic dysfunction may be exacerbated, with ileus, urinary retention, and gastrointestinal dysfunction (70).

Connective Tissue Diseases

Rheumatoid Arthritis Impairment of sweating on the extremities is relatively common in rheumatoid arthritis and is probably related in most cases to damage of postganglionic sympathetic efferent fibers in the peripheral nerves (22). In addition, there may be vagal nerve involvement, as the HR rate response to standing, the Valsalva maneuver, and respiration may be impaired, particularly in patients with peripheral neuropathy (57). Rarely, autonomic neuropathy may be seen with secondary (AA type) amyloidosis, and extensive amyloid deposits throughout the autonomic nervous system have been described, associated with disabling orthostatic hypotension (172).

Systemic Lupus Erythematosus and Mixed Connective Tissue Diseases Autonomic neuropathy has been reported as a complication of systemic lupus erythematosus (81, 171) and mixed connective tissue diseases (88).

Infections

Leprosy Leprosy, one of the most common causes of peripheral neuropathy, may be associated with autonomic disturbances. Loss of sweating over hypopigmented and hypesthetic skin is common. In addition, cardiac denervation, postural hypotension (127,219), widespread sweating impairment, and impaired response to the cold pressor test, even in the absence of other features of peripheral neuropathy (76), have been described.

AIDS (Chapter 52)

Diphtheria Diphtheritic neuropathy can be associated with some impairment of cardiovagal function, but orthostatic hypotension is usually absent (107).

Immune-Mediated Disorder: Chronic Inflammatory Demyelinating Polyradiculoneuropathy

In CIDP, postural hypotension and other symptoms of autonomic nervous system dysfunction are very uncommon (111). These findings are in contrast to those in acute inflammatory neuropathy, in which the more severe disturbances of autonomic function are presumed to be related to acute conduction block and possibly more extensive involvement of unmyelinated fibers in the acute stages. CIDP is also associated with relatively less acral postganglionic sudomotor failure than is distal small-fiber neuropathy (244).

Metabolic Disorders

Uremia Impairment of autonomic function is common in patients with terminal uremia, and disturbances of sympathetic and parasympathetic function and impaired baroreflex gain have been demonstrated (63,194). Improvement follows renal transplantation. Persistent hypotension in patients on chronic hemodialysis can be an important clinical problem and has been investigated to determine whether it is caused by some central mechanism (194).

Liver Disease Clinical autonomic neuropathy is not a feature of liver disease. However, Hendrickse et al. (99), who prospectively evaluated 60 patients (33 male, 27 female) with initially well-preserved hepatic function during the ensuing 4 years, reported that the severity of liver disease and of vagal neuropathy were independent predictors of mortality.

Nutritional Deficiencies

Subacute Combined Degeneration Orthostatic hypotension may be an initial manifestation of avitaminosis B_{12} neuropathy, although most cases are not associated with orthostatic hypotension. The pathologic changes are those of axonal degeneration. Postural hypotension may be caused by a combination of central mechanisms as well as damage to peripheral autonomic nerves (170).

Alcoholic Neuropathy Postural hypotension is common in patients with Wernicke's encephalopathy and is probably the result of impaired sympathetic outflow at central or peripheral levels. Clinical manifestations of autonomic dysfunction are unusual in uncomplicated alcoholic peripheral neuropathy (52,160), although postural hypotension may occur in patients who are severely affected (199). These findings indicate that peripheral sympathetic vasomotor control is relatively well preserved in alcoholics until the peripheral neuropathy reaches an advanced stage, even though sweat tests indicate that there is early involvement of sympathetic efferent fibers (160). Duncan et al. (52) have provided definite evidence of vagal damage in chronic alcoholics by demonstrating impaired HR responses to Valsalva maneuver, deep breathing, change in posture, neck suction, and atropine. Novak and Victor (199) reported hoarseness and weakness of the voice and dysphagia as clinical manifestations of vagal neuropathy in patients with severe alcoholic neuropathy. Other possible manifestations of disordered parasympathetic function in alcoholics include impaired esophageal motility, abnormal pupillary reflexes, and impotence. Alcoholics with vagal neuropathy have an increased mortality rate (122). Morphometric studies have demonstrated a significant reduction in the density of myelinated fibers in the distal parts of the vagus (90) and carotid sinus nerves in chronic alcoholics (251), but the splanchnic nerves are relatively spared (160).

Alcoholic neuropathy is a dying-back neuropathy identical to that of beriberi (199). The most distal parts of the longest fibers in the vagus nerve are affected, but the shorter and more proximal myelinated fibers of the sympathetic system are not affected until later in the illness, when the peripheral neuropathy is severe. The absence of postural hypotension and the relatively normal baroreflex function are consistent with a lack of pathology in the splanchnic nerves, as postural hypotension is more likely to occur if the splanchnic outflow is involved.

Dysautonomia of Old Age (Chapter 14)

Amyotrophic Lateral Sclerosis

Autonomic symptoms are not a prominent feature in amyotrophic lateral sclerosis (ALS). Asymptomatic autonomic failure as indicated by abnormal results of tests of autonomic function is often present (21,28,36,149,230,253). Abnormalities have been described in the peripheral autonomic surface potential (21), cardiovascular HR tests (36,149), and QSART (149). Chida et al. (36) reported that resting norepinephrine is increased and respiratory sinus arrhythmia is reduced in ALS. Pharmacologically, HR increase to atropine is reduced (30 ± 7.2 vs. 48 ± 1.9), and the response to phentolamine (-30 ± 4.1 vs. -15 ± 1.5) is increased. The response to phenylephrine is unchanged. They suggested that the combination of increased norepinephrine and increased response to phentolamine indicates subclinical hyperfunction of the sympathetic nervous system. In the study by Litchy et al. (149) of unselected patients with ALS, abnormalities on autonomic testing were found in 40% of patients. These consisted of abnormalities of cardiovagal function or postganglionic sudomotor function without symptomatic autonomic failure.

Multiple Symmetric Lipomatosis (Madelung's Disease)

Multiple symmetric lipomatosis (MSL) is characterized by a typical neck and shoulder distribution of subcutaneous lipomata and is often associated with polyneuropathy (60). Enzi et al. (60) reviewed 33 male patients affected by MSL and reported a high prevalence of somatic and autonomic neuropathies. In 84% of the patients, clinical examination revealed signs or symptoms of neural disturbances, ranging from a vibratory sensory loss to severely incapacitating trophic ulcers or Charcot's arthropathy. Electrodiagnostic investigations demonstrated a significant reduction of motor and sensory conduction velocity in the peroneal and sural nerves. Morphometric studies of nerve and muscle biopsy specimens from five patients with MSL revealed a significant reduction in myelinated fiber density (4435 ± 593 fibers/mm$_2$ in MSL vs. 7660 ± 800 in controls; $p < .05$), a selective reduction in the diameter of large fibers of 7 to 10 µm, and signs of chronic denervation-reinnervation processes. Bedside tests for autonomic neuropathy were abnormal in 15 of 20 patients studied. Fedele et al. (68) reported on cardiovascular reflex tests (VR, HRDB; 30:15 ratio) and sustained handgrip and orthostatic BP recordings in 13 patients. Because the majority of patients were alcoholics, they compared these recordings with those of controls and alcoholics without MSL. Mean values of VR and DB were significantly ($p < .001$) lower in patients with MSL than in controls and heavy drinkers. No significant differences were observed in the three groups in sympathetic tests. Klopstock et al. (131) reported evidence of a mitochondrial defect in muscle. In muscle biopsy specimens, the most prominent feature was pathologic subsarcolemmal aggregates of mitochondria. Biochemical analysis of respiratory chain enzymes revealed a moderate but significant decrease of cytochrome c oxidase activity in comparison with age-matched controls. In one patient, Southern blot analysis showed multiple deletions of mitochondrial DNA.

Paroxysmal or Intermittent Dysautonomia

Dysautonomia may be paroxysmal, as in certain acute peripheral autonomic storms (Chapters 56 and 59) and central autonomic disorders (Chapter 32). These paroxysmal or intermittent disorders may sometimes be acral and relatively less dramatic, presenting as vasomotor disorders of the hands or feet. Patients with mild neuropathy may have intermittent coldness of the extremities. The disorders that are better characterized include Raynaud's phenomenon, paroxysmal hyperhidrosis (Chapter 59), acrodynia, and erythromelalgia, characterized by prominent changes in skin color.

Paroxysmal Hyperhidrosis (Chapter 59)

Raynaud's Syndrome (Chapter 59)

Erythromelalgia

Erythromelalgia refers to acral erythema on warming associated with an intense burning sensation. The condition is classified as primary (idiopathic) or secondary (to other diseases) (177). It is associated with myeloproliferative disorders, especially thrombocythemia (177,178), and use of certain drugs, including verapamil (50), nicardipine (146), bromocriptine (58), pergolide (181), and mercury. It has also been described in the collagen vascular disorders (51,177), Raynaud's syndrome, pernicious anemia (175), and thrombotic thrombocytopenic purpura (276), and in association with cancer (138), infectious mononucleosis (38), vasculitis (51), and pregnancy (78). Many of these patients have a small-fiber neuropathy. In a preliminary analysis of cases studied in the Mayo Autonomic Laboratory, 21 of 27 patients had evidence of a small-fiber neuropathy. The condition occurs in other neuropathies, including diabetes (260) and hereditary sensory neuropathy (100). Some patients have marked accentuation of the erythema and pain with warming of the feet. The mechanism of erythema and pain has in some cases been shown to be activation of neurogenic flare by a polymodal "C" nociceptor axon reflex; hence the term *ABC syndrome (angry backfiring "C" nociceptor)* (200). These patients often obtain marked relief of symptoms with cold soaks. Some patients with erythromelalgia report significant relief of symptoms with acetylsalicylic acid, reported to control symptoms in 70% of cases, or ibuprofen. Other treatments are less consistently beneficial. Some respond to the local application of capsaicin cream (183). Other treatments claiming varying degrees of success have included amitriptyline (100), beta blockers (18), clonazepam (136), sodium nitroprusside (206), piroxicam (34), and biofeedback (218). Aggressive therapy has also been attempted, including epidural infusions (46), stereotactic surgery (125), and spinal cord stimulation (85).

Disorders of Reduced Orthostatic Tolerance (Chapters 48 and 49)

CONCLUSION

The management of the autonomic neuropathies has improved significantly in the past decade. Several evolving areas of promise include the following: (a) improved understanding of pathogenesis, resulting in more logical treatment; (b) improved noninvasive measurements of autonomic function in both quantitative and dynamic terms (151); (c) recognition of the existence of transient autonomic failure, such as transient adrenergic failure secondary to hypoglycemia (45) and transient gastroparesis secondary to hyperglycemia.

REFERENCES

1. Afifi AK, et al. Postganglionic cholinergic dysautonomia: report of muscle findings in 1 case. *Eur Neurol* 1982;21:8–21.
2. Alexander EL, et al. Primary Sjögren's syndrome with central nervous system disease mimicking multiple sclerosis. *Ann Intern Med* 1986;104:323–330.
3. Alexander EL, et al. Serum complement activation in central nervous system disease in Sjögren's syndrome. *Am J Med* 1988;85:513–518.
4. Altenkirch H, et al. Toxic polyneuropathies after sniffing a glue thinner. *J Neurol* 1977;214:137–152.
5. Amorim DS, et al. Effects of acute elevation in blood pressure and of atropine on heart rate in Chagas' disease. A preliminary report. *Circulation* 1968;38:289–294.
6. Amorim DS, et al. Chagas' heart disease as an experimental model for studies of cardiac autonomic function in man. *Mayo Clin Proc* 1982;57(Suppl):46–60.
7. Anand P, et al. New autonomic and sensory neuropathy with loss of adrenergic sympathetic function and sensory neuropeptides (see comments). *Lancet* 1991;337:1253–1254.
8. Anastasiou-Nana MI, et al. High incidence of clinical and subclinical toxicity associated with amiodarone treatment of refractory tachyarrhythmias. *Can J Cardiol* 1986;2:138–145.
9. Andersen O, et al. Subacute dysautonomia with incomplete recovery. *Acta Neurol Scand* 1972;48:510–519.

10. Andonopoulos AP, et al. Neurologic involvement in primary Sjögren's syndrome: a preliminary report. *J Autoimmun* 1989;2:485–488.
11. Andonopoulos AP, et al. The spectrum of neurological involvement in Sjögren's syndrome. *Br J Rheumatol* 1990;29:21–23.
12. Andrade C. A peculiar form of peripheral neuropathy: familial atypical generalized amyloidosis with special involvement of peripheral nerves. *Brain* 1952;75:408–427.
13. Anonymous. Plasmapheresis and acute Guillain-Barré syndrome. The Guillain-Barré Syndrome Study Group. *Neurology* 1985;35:1096–1104.
14. Appenzeller O, Kornfeld M. Acute pandysautonomia. Clinical and morphologic study. *Arch Neurol* 1973;29:334–339.
15. Appenzeller O, Marshall J. Vasomotor disturbance in Landry-Guillain-Barré syndrome. *Arch Neurol* 1963;9:368–372.
16. Asbury AK, et al. Criteria for diagnosis of Guillain-Barré syndrome. *Ann Neurol* 1978;3:565–566.
17. Auld RB, Bedwell SF. Peripheral neuropathy with sympathetic overactivity from industrial contact with acrylamide. *Can Med Assoc J* 1967;96:652–654.
18. Bada JL. Treatment of erythromelalgia with propranolol (Letter). *Lancet* 1977;2:412.
19. Balm R, et al. Visceral dysautonomia in a subset of patients with idiopathic chronic intestinal pseudo-obstruction. *Gastroenterology* 1990;98:A324(abst).
20. Bank WJ, et al. Thallium poisoning. *Arch Neurol* 1972;26:456–464.
21. Barron SA, et al. Sympathetic cholinergic dysfunction in amyotrophic lateral sclerosis. *Acta Neurol Scand* 1987;75: 62–63.
22. Bennett PH, Scott JT. Autonomic neuropathy in rheumatoid arthritis. *Ann Rheum Dis* 1965;24:161–168.
23. Benson MD. Familial amyloidotic polyneuropathy. *Trends Neurosci* 1989;12:88–92.
24. Biaggioni I, et al. Dopamine-beta-hydroxylase deficiency in humans. *Neurology* 1990;40:370–373.
25. Binder A, et al. Sjögren's syndrome: a study of its neurological complications. *Br J Rheumatol* 1988;27:275–280.
26. Birchfield RI, Shaw C-M. Postural hypotension in the Guillain-Barré syndrome. *Arch Neurol* 1964;10:149–157.
27. Bird TD, et al. Autonomic nervous system function in genetic neuromuscular disorders. Hereditary motor-sensory neuropathy and myotonic dystrophy. *Arch Neurol* 1984;41:43–46.
28. Bogucki A, Salvesen R. Sympathetic iris function in amyotrophic lateral sclerosis. *J Neurol* 1987;234:185–186.
29. Bower BD. Pink disease: autonomic disorder and its treatment with ganglion blocking agents. *Q J Med* 1954;23:215–230.
30. Brady RO. Fabry disease. In: Dyck PJ, Thomas PK, Lambert EH, Bunge R, eds. *Peripheral Neuropathy*. Philadelphia: WB Saunders; 1984:1717–1727.
31. Bredin CP. Guillain-Barré syndrome: the unsolved cardiovascular problems. *Ir J Med Sci* 1977;146:273–279.
32. Brooks AP. Abnormal vascular reflexes in Charcot-Marie-Tooth disease. *J Neurol Neurosurg Psychiatry* 1980;43:348–350.
33. Cable WJ, et al. Fabry disease: impaired autonomic function. *Neurology* 1982;32:498–502.
34. Calderone DC, Finzi E. Treatment of primary erythromelalgia with piroxicam. *J Am Acad Dermatol* 1991;24:145–146.
35. Cherington M, Ryan DW. Treatment of botulism and guanidine. *N Engl J Med* 1970;282:195–197.
36. Chida K, et al. Alteration in autonomic function and cardiovascular regulation in amyotrophic lateral sclerosis. *J Neurol* 1989;236:127–130.
37. Clark E, et al. Landry-Guillain-Barré syndrome: cardiovascular complications. *Br Med J* 1954;2:1504–1507.
38. Clayton C, Faden H. Erythromelalgia in a twenty-year-old with infectious mononucleosis. *Pediatr Infect Dis J* 1993;12:101–102.
39. Cohen AS. Amyloidosis. In: Wilson JD, Braunwald E, Isselbacher KJ, Petersdorf RG, Martin JB, Fauci AS, Root RK, eds. *Harrison's Principles of Internal Medicine*. New York: McGraw-Hill; 1991:1417–1421.
40. Colan RV, et al. Acute autonomic and sensory neuropathy. *Ann Neurol* 1980;8:441–444.
41. Costa-Jussa FR, Jacobs JM. The pathology of amiodarone neurotoxicity. I. Experimental studies with reference to changes in other tissues. *Brain* 1985;108:735–752.
42. Critchley EM, Mitchell JD. Human botulism. *Br J Hosp Med* 1990;43:290–292.
43. Crozier RE, Ainley AB. The Guillain-Barré syndrome. *N Engl J Med* 1955;252:83–88.
44. Cruz-Martinez A, et al. Electrophysiologic study in benign human botulism type B. *Muscle Nerve* 1985;8:580–585.
45. Cryer PE. Iatrogenic hypoglycemia as a cause of hypoglycemia-associated autonomic failure in IDDM. A vicious cycle. *Diabetes* 1992;41:255–260.
46. D'Angelo R, et al. Continuous epidural infusion of bupivacaine and fentanyl for erythromelalgia in an adolescent. *Anesth Analg* 1992;74:142–144.
47. Dalos NP, et al. Cardiovascular autonomic dysfunction in Guillain-Barré syndrome. Therapeutic implications of Swan-Ganz monitoring. *Arch Neurol* 1988;45:115–117.
48. Davidson DL, Jellinek EH. Hypertension and papilloedema in the Guillain-Barré syndrome. *J Neurol Neurosurg Psychiatry* 1977;40:144–148.
49. Desnick RJ, Astrin KH, Bishop DF. Fabry disease: molecular genetics of the inherited nephropathy (Review). *Adv Nephrol* 1989;18:113–127.
50. Drenth JP, et al. Verapamil-induced secondary erythromelalgia (Review). *Br J Dermatol* 1992;127:292–294.
51. Drenth JP, et al. Secondary erythermalgia associated with an autoimmune disorder of undetermined significance. *Dermatology* 1995;232–234.
52. Duncan G, et al. Evidence of vagal neuropathy in chronic alcoholics. *Lancet* 1980;2:1053–1057.
53. Dwulet FE, Benson MD. Primary structure of an amyloid prealbumin and its plasma precursor in a heroedofamilial polyneuropathy of Swedish origin. *Proc Natl Acad Sci U S A* 1984;81:694–698.
54. Dwulet FE, Benson MD. Characterization of a transthyretin (prealbumin) variant associated with familial amyloidotic polyneuropathy type II (Indiana/Swiss). *J Clin Invest* 1986;78:880–888.
55. Dyck PJ. Neuronal atrophy affecting peripheral sensory neurons. In: Dyck PJ, Thomas PK, Lambert EH, Bunge R, eds. *Peripheral Neuropathy*. Philadelphia: WB Saunders; 1984:1557–1599.
56. Dyck PJ, Lambert EH. Dissociated sensation in amyloidosis. Compound action potential, quantitative histologic and teased-fiber, and electron microscopic studies of sural nerve biopsies. *Arch Neurol* 1969;20:490–507.
57. Edmonds ME, et al. Autonomic neuropathy in rheumatoid arthritis. *Br Med J* 1979;2:173–175.
58. Eisler T, et al. Erythromelalgia-like eruption in parkinsonian patients treated with bromocriptine. *Neurology* 1981;31:1368–1370.
59. Emmons PR, Blume WT, DuShane JW. Cardiac monitoring and demand pacemaker in Guillain-Barré syndrome. *Arch Neurol* 1975;32:59–61.
60. Enzi G, et al. Sensory, motor, and autonomic neuropathy in patients with multiple symmetric lipomatosis. *Medicine* 1985;64:388–393.
61. Eriksson P, et al. Cardiac arrhythmias in familial amyloid polyneuropathy during anaesthesia. *Acta Anaesthesiol Scand* 1986;30:317–320.
62. Evans BA, et al. The peripheral autonomic surface potential in suspected small fiber peripheral neuropathy. *Muscle Nerve* 1988;11:982(abst).
63. Ewing DJ, Winney R. Autonomic function in patients with chronic renal failure on intermittent hemodialysis. *Nephron* 1975;15:424–429.
64. Fagius J, Wallin BG. Microneurographic evidence of excessive sympathetic outflow in the Guillain-Barré syndrome. *Brain* 1983;106:589–600.
65. Fagius J, et al. Acute pandysautonomia and severe sensory deficit with poor recovery. A clinical, neurophysiological and pathological case study. *J Neurol Neurosurg Psychiatry* 1983;46:725–733.
66. Faich GA, et al. Failure of guanidine therapy in botulism A. *N Engl J Med* 1971;285:773–776.
67. Favre H, et al. Use of demand pacemaker in a case of Guillain-Barré syndrome. *Lancet* 1970;1:1062–1063.
68. Fedele D, et al. Impairment of cardiovascular autonomic reflexes in multiple symmetric lipomatosis. *J Auton Nerv Syst* 1984;11:181–188.
69. Ferreira-Santos R. Megacolon and megarectum in Chagas' disease. *Proc R Soc Med* 1961;54:1047–1053.

70. Filling-Katz MR, et al. Carbamazepine in Fabry's disease: effective analgesia with dose-dependent exacerbation of autonomic dysfunction. *Neurology* 1989;39:598–600.
71. Font J, et al. Pure sensory neuropathy in patients with primary Sjögren's syndrome: clinical, immunological, and electromyographic findings. *Ann Rheum Dis* 1990;49:775–778.
72. Fraser AG, et al. Peripheral neuropathy during long-term high-dose amiodarone therapy. *J Neurol Neurosurg Psychiatry* 1985;48:576–578.
73. Fraser DM, et al. Peripheral and autonomic neuropathy after treatment with perhexiline maleate. *Br Med J* 1977;2:675–676.
74. Frison JC, et al. Heart rate variations in the Guillain-Barré syndrome. *Br Med J* 1980;281:649.
75. Fujii N, et al. Acute autonomic and sensory neuropathy associated with elevated Epstein-Barr virus antibody titre (Letter). *J Neurol Neurosurg Psychiatry* 1982;45:656–657.
76. Gadoth N, et al. Somatosensory and autonomic neuropathy as the only manifestation of long-standing leprosy. *J Neurol Sci* 1979;43:471–477.
77. Gallo L Jr, et al. Abnormal heart rate responses during exercise in patients with Chagas' disease. *Cardiology* 1975;60:147–162.
78. Garrett SJ, Robinson JK. Erythromelalgia and pregnancy. *Arch Dermatol* 1990;126:157–158.
79. Gemignani F, et al. Polyneuropathy in Sjögren's syndrome. A case of prevalently autonomic neuropathy with tonic pupil and hypohidrosis (Review). *Funct Neurol* 1988;3:337–348.
80. Gibson JB, Goldberg A. The neuropathology of acute porphyria. *J Pathol Bacteriol* 1956;71:495–509.
81. Gledhill RF, Dessein PH. Autonomic neuropathy in systemic lupus erythematosus (Letter). *J Neurol Neurosurg Psychiatry* 1988;51:1238–1240.
82. Goldberg A. Acute intermittent porphyria. A study of 50 cases. *Q J Med* 1959;28:183–209.
83. Goldstein NP, et al. Metal neuropathy. In: Dyck PJ, Thomas PK, Lambert EH, eds. *Peripheral Neuropathy*. Philadelphia: WB Saunders; 1975:1227–1262.
84. Goulon M, et al. Dysautonomia in acute primary polyradiculoneuritis (in French). *Rev Neurol (Paris)* 1975;131:95–119.
85. Graziotti PJ, Goucke CR. Control of intractable pain in erythromelalgia by using spinal cord stimulation. *J Pain Symptom Manage* 1993;8:502–504.
86. Greenland P, Griggs RC. Arrhythmic complications in the Guillain-Barré syndrome. *Arch Intern Med* 1980;140:1053–1055.
87. Griffin JW, et al. Ataxic sensory neuropathy and dorsal root ganglionitis associated with Sjögren's syndrome. *Ann Neurol* 1990;27:304–315.
88. Gudesblatt M, et al. Autonomic neuropathy associated with autoimmune disease. *Neurology* 1985;35:261–264.
89. Guillain G. Radiculoneuritis with acellular hyperalbuminosis of the cerebrospinal fluid. *Arch Neurol Psychiatry* 1936;36:975–990.
90. Guo YP, et al. Pathological changes in the vagus nerve in diabetes and chronic alcoholism. *J Neurol Neurosurg Psychiatry* 1987;50:1449–1453.
91. Guttmann L, et al. Neuromuscular junction in human botulism. *Neurology* 1973;23:424–425.
92. Hadley D, Herr HW. Peripheral neuropathy associated with *cis*-dichlorodiammineplatinum (II) treatment. *Cancer* 1979;44:2026–2028.
93. Hancock BW, Naysmith A. Vincristine-induced autonomic neuropathy. *Br Med J* 1975;3:207.
94. Harati Y, Low PA. Autonomic peripheral neuropathies: diagnosis and clinical presentation. In: Appel SH, ed. *Current Neurology*. Chicago: Year Book; 1990:105–176.
95. Harik SI, et al. Postganglionic cholinergic dysautonomia. *Ann Neurol* 1977;1:393–396.
96. Harriman DGF, Garland HG. The pathology of Adie's syndrome. *Brain* 1968;91:401–418.
97. Haymaker W, Kernohan JW. Landry-Guillain-Barré syndrome: clinicopathologic report of 50 fatal cases and a critique of the literature. *Medicine* 1949;28:59–141.
98. Heathfield MT, et al. Idiopathic dysautonomia treated with intravenous gammaglobulin. *Lancet* 1996;347:28–29.
99. Hendrickse MT, et al. Natural history of autonomic neuropathy in chronic liver disease (see comments). *Lancet* 1992;339:1462–1464.
100. Herskovitz S, et al. Erythromelalgia: association with hereditary sensory neuropathy and response to amitriptyline. *Neurology* 1993;43:621–622.
101. Hewer RL, et al. Acute polyneuritis requiring artificial respiration. *Q J Med* 1968;37:479–491.
102. Hietaharju A, et al. Nervous system manifestations in Sjögren's syndrome. *Acta Neurol Scand* 1990;81:144–152.
103. Hilkens PH, et al. Peripheral neurotoxicity induced by docetaxel (see comments). *Neurology* 1996;46:104–108.
104. Hirvonen HE, et al. Vincristine treatment of acute lymphoblastic leukemia induces transient autonomic cardioneuropathy. *Cancer* 1989;64:801–805.
105. Holmgren G, et al. Clinical improvement and amyloid regression after liver transplantation in hereditary transthyretin amyloidosis. *Lancet* 1993;341:1113–1116.
106. Hopkins A, et al. Autonomic neuropathy of acute onset. *Lancet* 1974;1:769–771.
107. Idiaquez J. Autonomic dysfunction in diphtheritic neuropathy. *J Neurol Neurosurg Psychiatry* 1992;55:159–161.
108. Inamdar S, et al. Acquired postganglionic cholinergic dysautonomia: case report and review of the literature. *Pediatrics* 1982;70:976–978.
109. Ingall TJ, McLeod JG. Autonomic function in Friedreich's ataxia. *J Neurol Neurosurg Psychiatry* 1991;54:162–164.
110. Ingall TJ, McLeod JG. Autonomic function in hereditary motor and sensory neuropathy (Charcot-Marie-Tooth disease) (see comments). *Muscle Nerve* 1991;14:1080–1083.
111. Ingall TJ, et al. Autonomic function and unmyelinated fibers in chronic inflammatory demyelinating polyradiculoneuropathy. *Muscle Nerve* 1990;13:70–76.
112. Iosa D, et al. Plasma norepinephrine in Chagas' cardioneuromyopathy: a marker of progressive dysautonomia. *Am Heart J* 1989;117:882–887.
113. Iosa D, et al. Chagas' cardioneuropathy: effect of ganglioside treatment in chronic dysautonomic patients—a randomized double-blind parallel placebo-controlled study. *Am Heart J* 1991;122:775–785.
114. Jacobs JM, Costa-Jussà FR. The pathology of amiodarone neurotoxicity. II. Peripheral neuropathy in man. *Brain* 1985;108:753–769.
115. Jacobson DR, et al. Is senile symetric amyloidosis a recessive disease? *Arthritis Rheum* 1988;31:S124(abst).
116. Jamal GA, et al. The neurophysiologic investigation of small fiber neuropathies. *Muscle Nerve* 1987;10:537–545.
117. Jammes JL. The autonomic nervous system in peroneal muscular atrophy. *Arch Neurol* 1972;27:213–220.
118. Jenzer G, et al. Autonomic dysfunction in botulism B: a clinical report. *Neurology* 1975;25:150–153.
119. Jerian SM, et al. Incapacitating autonomic neuropathy precipitated by Taxol. *Gynecol Oncol* 1993;51:277–280.
120. Johnson D, et al. Accidental ingestion of Vacor rodenticide: the systems and sequelae in a 25-month-old child. *Am J Dis Child* 1980;134:161–164.
121. Johnson RH, et al. Orthostatic hypotension and the Holmes-Adie syndrome. A study of two patients with afferent baroreceptor block. *J Neurol Neurosurg Psychiatry* 1971;34:562–570.
122. Johnson RH, Robinson BJ. Mortality in alcoholics with autonomic neuropathy. *J Neurol Neurosurg Psychiatry* 1988;51:476–480.
123. Johnson RH, Spalding JMK. *Disorders of the Autonomic Nervous System*. Philadelphia: FA Davis; 1974.
124. Kanda Y, et al. The amino acid sequence of human plasma prealbumin. *J Biol Chem* 1974;249:6796–6805.
125. Kandel EI. Stereotactic surgery of erythromelalgia. *Stereotact Funct Neurosurg* 1990;54/55:96–100.
126. Kaplan JG, et al. Invited review: peripheral neuropathy in Sjögren's syndrome (Review). *Muscle Nerve* 1990;13:570–579.
127. Khattri HN, et al. Cardiac dysautonomia in leprosy. *Int J Lepr Other Mycobact Dis* 1978;46:172–174.
128. Kilimov N. Charcot-Marie-Tooth neural muscular atrophy with pupillary anomalies. *Eur Neurol* 1973;10:292–300.
129. Kirby RS, et al. Bladder dysfunction in distal autonomic neuropathy of acute onset. *J Neurol Neurosurg Psychiatry* 1985;48:762–767.
130. Kirchoff LV. Trypanosomiasis. In: Wilson J, et al, eds. *Harrison's Principles of Internal Medicine*. New York: McGraw Hill; 1991.
131. Klopstock T, et al. Multiple symmetric lipomatosis: Abnormalities in complex IV and multiple deletions in mitochondrial DNA. *Neurology* 1994;44:862–866.

132. Koberle F. Enteromegaly and cardiomegaly in Chagas' disease. *Gut* 1963;4:399–405.
133. Koberle F. Chagas' disease and Chagas' syndromes. *Adv Parasitol* 1968;6:63–116.
134. Koenig MG, et al. Type B botulism in man. *Am J Med* 1967;42:208–219.
135. Kogan BA, et al. Urinary retention secondary to Landry-Guillain-Barré syndrome. *J Urol* 1981;126:643–644.
136. Kraus A. Erythromelalgia in a patient with systemic lupus erythematosus treated with clonazepam (see comments). *J Rheumatol* 1990;17:120.
137. Kudo M, Griggs RC. Diagnosis usefulness of intramuscular nerve bundles. *Arch Pathol Lab Med* 1982;106:355–359.
138. Kurzrock R, Cohen PR. Paraneoplastic erythromelalgia (Review). *Clin Dermatol* 1993;11:73–82.
139. Kyle RA, Greipp PR. Amyloidosis: clinical and laboratory features in 229 cases. *Mayo Clin Proc* 1983;58:665–683.
140. Kyle RA, et al. Orthostatic hypotension as a clue to primary systemic amyloidosis. *Circulation* 1966;34:883–888.
141. Laiwah AC, et al. Autonomic neuropathy in acute intermittent porphyria. *J Neurol Neurosurg Psychiatry* 1095;48:1025–1030.
142. Laufer J, et al. Raised plasma renin activity in the hypertension of the Guillain-Barré syndrome. *Br Med J Clin Res Ed* 1981;282:1272–1273.
143. Legha SS. Vincristine neurotoxicity. Pathophysiology and management. *Med Toxicol* 1986;1:421–427.
144. LeQuesne PM. Neuropathy due to drugs. In: Dyck PJ, Thomas PK, Lambert EH, Bunge R, eds. *Peripheral Neuropathy*. Philadelphia: WB Saunders; 1984:2162–2179.
145. LeQuesne PM, McLeod JG. Peripheral neuropathy following a single exposure to arsenic. *J Neurol Sci* 1977;32:437–451.
146. Levesque H, et al. Erythromelalgia induced by nicardipine (inverse Raynaud's phenomenon?). *Br Med J* 1989;298:1252–1253.
147. LeWitt PA. Neurotoxicity of the rat poison Vacor. A clinical study of 12 cases. *N Engl J Med* 1980;302:73–77.
148. Lichtenfeld P. Autonomic dysfunction in the Guillain-Barré syndrome. *Am J Med* 1971;50:772–780.
149. Litchy WJ, et al. Autonomic abnormalities in amyotrophic lateral sclerosis. *Neurology* 1987;37(Suppl 1):162(abst).
150. Long SS, et al. Clinical, laboratory, and environmental features of infant botulism in southeastern Pennsylvania. *Pediatrics* 1985;75:935–941.
151. Low PA. Sudomotor function and dysfunction. In: Asbury AK, McKhann GM, McDonald WI, eds. *Diseases of the Nervous System*. Philadelphia: WB Saunders; 1986:596–605.
152. Low PA. Autonomic neuropathy. *Semin Neurol* 1978;7:49–57.
153. Low PA, et al. Congenital sensory neuropathy with selective loss of small myelinated fibers. *Ann Neurol* 1978; 3:179–182.
154. Low PA, et al. Quantitative sudomotor axon reflex test in normal and neuropathic subjects. *Ann Neurol* 1983;14:573–580.
155. Low PA, et al. Acute panautonomic neuropathy. *Ann Neurol* 1983; 13:412–417.
156. Low PA, et al. The splanchnic autonomic outflow in amyloid neuropathy and Tangier disease. *Neurology* 1981;31:461–463.
157. Low PA, et al. Chronic idiopathic anhidrosis. *Ann Neurol* 1985; 18:344–348.
158. Low PA, et al. The autonomic neuropathies of Sjögren's syndrome. *Neurology* 1988;38(Suppl 1):104(abst).
159. Low PA, Stevens JC. Peripheral neuropathies including autonomic neuropathies. In: Spittell JA, ed. *Clinical Medicine*. Hargerstown: Harper & Row; 1985.
160. Low PA, et al. The sympathetic nervous system in alcoholic neuropathy. A clinical and pathological study. *Brain* 1975;98:357–364.
161. Mahloudji M, et al. Clinical neurological aspects of familial dysautonomia. *J Neurol Sci* 1970;11:383–395.
162. Manco JC, et al. Degeneration of the cardiac nerves in Chagas' disease. *Circulation* 1969;40:879–885.
163. Manolis AS, et al. Atypical pulmonary and neurologic complications of amiodarone in the same patient. Report of a case and review of the literature. *Arch Intern Med* 1987;147:1805–1809.
164. Markus C. Notes on a peculiar pupil phenomenon in cases of partial iridoplegia. *Trans Ophthalmol Soc U K* 1906;26:50–56.
165. Marshall J. The Landry-Guillain-Barré syndrome. *Brain* 1963;86:55–66.
166. Martinez-Arizala A, et al. Amiodarone neuropathy. *Neurology* 1983;33:643–645.
167. Mathias CJ, et al. Clinical autonomic and therapeutic observations in two siblings with postural hypotension and sympathetic failure due to an inability to synthesize noradrenaline from dopamine because of a deficiency of dopamine beta hydroxylase. *Q J Med* 1990;75:617–633.
168. Matikainen E, Juntunen J. Autonomic nervous system dysfunction in workers exposed to organic solvents. *J Neurol Neurosurg Psychiatry* 1985;48:1021–1024.
169. Maury CP, Baumann M. Isolation and characterization of cardiac amyloid in familial amyloid neuropathy type IV (Finnish): relation of the amyloid protein to variant gelsolin. *Biochim Biophys Acta* 1990;1096:84–86.
170. McCombe PA, McLeod JG. The peripheral neuropathy of vitamin B_{12} deficiency. *J Neurol Sci* 1984;66:117–126.
171. McCombe PA, et al. Peripheral sensorimotor and autonomic neuropathy associated with systemic lupus erythematosus. Clinical, pathological and immunological features. *Brain* 1987;110:533–549.
172. McGill NW, et al. Severe autonomic neuropathy in amyloidosis secondary to rheumatoid arthritis. *Aust N Z J Med* 1986;16:705–707.
173. McLeod JG, et al. Charcot-Marie-Tooth disease with Leber optic atrophy. *Neurology* 1978;28:179–184.
174. McLeod JG, Penny R. Vincristine neuropathy: an electrophysiological and histological study. *J Neurol Neurosurg Psychiatry* 1969; 32:297–304.
175. Mehle AL, et al. Erythromelalgia. *Int J Dermatol* 1990;29:567–570.
176. Mellgren SI, et al. Peripheral neuropathy in primary Sjögren's syndrome. *Neurology* 1989;39:390–394.
177. Michiels JJ, et al. Classification and diagnosis of erythromelalgia and erythermalgia (Review). *Int J Dermatol* 1995;34:97–100.
178. Michiels JJ, ten Kate FJ. Erythromelalgia in thrombocythemia of various myeloproliferative disorders (see comments). *Am J Hematol* 1992;39:131–136.
179. Miller LV, et al. Diabetes mellitus and autonomic dysfunction after Vacor rodenticide ingestion. *Diabetes Care* 1978; 1:73–76.
180. Mitchell PL, Meilman E. The mechanism of hypertension in the Guillain-Barré syndrome. *Am J Med* 1967;42:986–995.
181. Monk BE, et al. Erythromelalgia following pergolide administration. *Br J Dermatol* 1984;111:97–99.
182. Morita K, et al. Familial amyloidotic polyneuropathy in Hokkaido: a case report. *Jpn J Med* 1990;29:61–65.
183. Muhiddin KA, et al. The use of capsaicin cream in a case of erythromelalgia. *Postgrad Med J* 1994;70:841–843.
184. Murata K, Araki S. Autonomic nervous system dysfunction in workers exposed to lead, zinc, and copper in relation to peripheral nerve conduction: a study of R-R interval variability. *Am J Ind Med* 1991;20:663–671.
185. Mutoh T, et al. Severe orthostatic hypotension in a female carrier of Fabry's disease. *Arch Neurol* 1988;45:468–472.
186. Nakazato M, et al. Revised analysis of amino acid replacement in a prealbumin variant (SKO-III) associated with familial amyloidotic polyneuropathy of Jewish origin. *Biochem Biophys Res Commun* 1984;123:921–928.
187. Nakazato M, et al. Diagnostic radioimmunoassay for familial amyloidotic polyneuropathy before clinical onset. *J Clin Invest* 1986; 77:1699–1703.
188. Narayan D, et al. Bradycardia and asystole requiring permanent pacemaker in Guillain-Barré syndrome. *Am Heart J* 1984;108:426–428.
189. Nass R, Chutorian A. Dysaesthesias and dysautonomia: a self-limited syndrome of painful dysaesthesias and autonomic dysfunction in childhood. *J Neurol Neurosurg Psychiatry* 1982;45:162–165.
190. Neville BG, Sladen GE. Acute autonomic neuropathy following primary herpes simplex infection. *J Neurol Neurosurg Psychiatry* 1984;47:648–650.
191. New PZ, et al. Peripheral neuropathy secondary to docetaxel (Taxotere) (see comments). *Neurology* 1996;46:108–111.
192. Nichols WC, et al. Variant apolipoprotein AI as a major constituent of a human hereditary amyloid. *Biochem Biophys Res Commun* 1988;156:762–768.
193. Nichols WC, et al. Enzymatic amplification of prealbumin genomic sequences and potential use in diagnosis of hereditary amyloidosis. *Am J Hum Genet* 1987;41:A230.

194. Nies AS, et al. Hemodialysis hypotension is not the result of uremic peripheral autonomic neuropathy. *J Lab Clin Med* 1979;94:395–402.
195. Nix WA, et al. Reversible esophageal motor dysfunction in botulism. *Muscle Nerve* 1985;8:791–795.
196. Nordborg C, et al. Involvement of the autonomic nervous system in primary and secondary amyloidosis. *Acta Neurol Scand* 1983;49:31–38.
197. Nordborg C, et al. Involvement of the autonomic nervous system in primary and secondary amyloidosis. *Acta Neurol Scand* 1973;49:31–38.
198. Nordlie M, et al. A new prealbumin variant in familial amyloid cardiomyopathy of Danish origin. *Scand J Immunol* 1988;27:119–122.
199. Novak DJ, Victor M. The vagus and sympathetic nerves in alcoholic polyneuropathy. *Arch Neurol* 1974;30:273–284.
200. Ochoa J. The newly recognized painful ABC syndrome: thermographic aspects. *Thermology* 1986;2:65–107.
201. Ohnishi A, Dyck PJ. Loss of small peripheral sensory neurons in Fabry disease. Histologic and morphometric evaluation of cutaneous nerves, spinal ganglia, and posterior columns. *Arch Neurol* 1974;31:120–127.
202. Okada F, Shintomi Y. The central sites of the autonomic nervous system may also be disturbed in some cases with acute pandysautonomia (Letter). *Arch Neurol* 1990;47:127–128.
203. Okajima T, et al. Chronic sensory and autonomic neuropathy. *Neurology* 1983;33:1061–1064.
204. Olofsson B-O, et al. The sick sinus syndrome in familial amyloidosis with polyneuropathy. *Int J Cardiol* 1983;4:71–73.
205. Osler LD, Siddell AD. The Guillain-Barré syndrome: the need for exact diagnostic criteria. *N Engl J Med* 1960;262:964–969.
206. Ozsoylu S, et al. Successful treatment of erythromelalgia with sodium nitroprusside. *J Pediatr* 1979;94:619–621.
207. Palakurthy PR, et al. Unusual neurotoxicity associated with amiodarone therapy. *Arch Intern Med* 1987;147:881–884.
208. Palmero HA, et al. Prevalence of slow heart rates in chronic Chagas' disease. *Am J Trop Med Hyg* 1981;30:1179–1182.
209. Pellissier JF, et al. Peripheral neuropathy induced by amiodarone chlorhydrate. A clinicopathological study. *J Neurol Sci* 1984;63:251–266.
210. Perlroth MG, et al. Acute intermittent porphyria. New morphologic and biochemical findings. *Am J Med* 1966;41:149–162.
211. Persson A, Solders G. R-R variations in Guillain-Barré syndrome: a test of autonomic dysfunction. *Acta Neurol Scand* 1983;67:294–300.
212. Pickett JB. AAEE case report #16: botulism. *Muscle Nerve* 1988;11:1201–1205.
213. Pinckney C. Acute infective polyneuritis with a report of five cases. *Br Med J* 1936;2:333–355.
214. Polk BV. Cardiopulmonary complications of Guillain-Barré syndrome. *Heart Lung* 1976;5:967–970.
215. Pont A, et al. Diabetes mellitus and neuropathy following Vacor ingestion in man. *Arch Intern Med* 1979;139:185–187.
216. Post EJ, McLeod JG. Acrylamide autonomic neuropathy in the cat. Part 1. Neurophysiological and histological studies. *J Neurol Sci* 1977;33:353–374.
217. Post EJ, McLeod JG. Acrylamide autonomic neuropathy in the cat. Part 2. Effects on mesenteric vascular control. *J Neurol Sci* 1977;33:375–385.
218. Putt AM. Erythromelalgia—a case for biofeedback. *Nurs Clin North Am* 1978;13:625–630.
219. Radhakrishnan K, et al. Orthostatic hypotension in lepromatous leprosy. *Neurology* 1978;26:25–27.
220. Richards AM, et al. Severe hypertension and raised haematocrit: unusual presentation of Guillain-Barré syndrome. *Postgrad Med J* 1985;61:53–55.
221. Ridley A. Porphyric neuropathy. In: Dyck PJ, Thomas PK, Lambert EH, Bunge R, eds. *Peripheral Neuropathy*. Philadelphia: WB Saunders; 1984:1704–1706.
222. Ridley A, et al. Tachycardia and the neuropathy of porphyria. *Lancet* 1968;2:708–710.
223. Robertson D, et al. Isolated failure of autonomic noradrenergic neurotransmission. Evidence for impaired beta-hydroxylation of dopamine. *N Engl J Med* 1986;314:1494–1497.
224. Rosenfeld CS, Broder LE. Cisplatin-induced autonomic neuropathy. *Cancer Treat Rep* 1984;68:659–660.
225. Ross AT. Progressive selective sudomotor denervation—a case with co-existing Adie's syndrome. *Neurology* 1958;8:809–817.
226. Rubinow A, et al. Esophageal manometry in systemic amyloidosis. A study of 30 patients. *Am J Med* 1983;75:951–956.
227. Ryan DW, Cherington M. Human type A botulism. *JAMA* 1971;216:513–514.
228. Ryan PJ. Infant botulism—the first reported case from Queensland. *Med J Aust* 1987;146:105–106.
229. Sabin AB, Aring CD. Visceral lesions in infectious polyneuritis (infectious neuronitis, acute polyneuritis with facial diplegia, Guillain-Barré syndrome, Landry's paralysis). *Am J Pathol* 1941;17:469–482.
230. Sachs C, et al. Autonomic function in amyotrophic lateral sclerosis: a study of cardiovascular responses. *Acta Neurol Scand* 1985;71:373–378.
231. Said G, et al. Neuropathy associated with experimental Chagas' disease. *Ann Neurol* 1985;18:676–683.
232. Sandgren O, Hofer PA. Conjunctival involvement in familial amyloidotic polyneuropathy. *Acta Ophthalmol* 1990;68:292–296.
233. Sasaki H, et al. Structure of the chromosomal gene for human serum prealbumin. *Gene* 1985;37:191–197.
234. Schiller JH, et al. A phase I trial of 3-hour infusions of paclitaxel (Taxol) with or without granulocyte colony-stimulating factor. *Semin Oncol* 1994;21:9–14.
235. Schirger A, et al. Orthostatic hypotension in association with acute exacerbations of porphyria. *Mayo Clin Proc* 1962;37:7(abst).
236. Schondorf R, Low PA. Idiopathic postural tachycardia syndrome. *Ann Neurol* 1990;28:271(abst).
237. Share L, Levy MN. Cardiovascular receptors and blood titer of antidiuretic hormone. *Am J Physiol* 1962;203:425–428.
238. Singh NK, et al. Assessment of autonomic dysfunction in Guillain-Barré syndrome and its prognostic implications. *Acta Neurol Scand* 1987;75:101–105.
239. Skopouli FN, et al. Raynaud's phenomenon in primary Sjögren's syndrome. *J Rheumatol* 1990;17:618–620.
240. Smit AAJ, et al. An unusual recovery in a patient with acute pandysautonomia after intravenous immunoglobulin therapy. *Clin Auton Res* 1995;5:323A(abst).
241. Sousa AC, et al. Cardiac parasympathetic impairment in gastrointestinal Chagas' disease (Letter). *Lancet* 1987;1:985.
242. Stevens PM. Cardiovascular dynamics during orthostasis and the influence of intravascular instrumentation. *Am J Cardiol* 1966;17:211–218.
243. Stewart JD, et al. Small-fiber peripheral neuropathy: diagnostic value of sweat tests and autonomic cardiovascular reflexes. *Ann Neurol* 1989;26:145A(abst).
244. Stewart JD, et al. Distal small fiber neuropathy: results of tests of sweating and autonomic cardiovascular reflexes. *Muscle Nerve* 1992;15:661–665.
245. Stewart PM, Hensley WJ. An acute attack of variegate porphyria complicated by severe autonomic neuropathy. *Aust N Z J Med* 1981;11:82–83.
246. Suarez GA, et al. Idiopathic autonomic neuropathy: clinical, neurophysiologic, and follow-up studies on 27 patients. *Neurology* 1994;44:1675–1682.
247. Summers Q, Harris A. Autonomic neuropathy after rubella infection. *Med J Aust* 1987;147:353–355.
248. Swanson AG. Congenital insensitivity to pain with anhidrosis. A unique syndrome in two male siblings. *Arch Neurol* 1963;8:299–306.
249. Swanson AG, et al. Autonomic changes in congenital insensitivity to pain: absence of small primary sensory neurons in ganglia, roots, and Lissauer's tract. *Arch Neurol* 1965;12:12–18.
250. Takayama H, et al. A case of postganglionic cholinergic dysautonomia. *J Neurol Neurosurg Psychiatry* 1987;50:915–918.
251. Tamura N, et al. A morphometric study of the carotid sinus nerve in patients with diabetes mellitus and chronic alcoholism. *J Auton Nerv Syst* 1988;23:9–15.
252. Thomashefsky AJ, et al. Acute autonomic neuropathy. *Neurology* 1972;22:251–255.
253. Toyokura Y. Amyotrophic lateral sclerosis. A clinical and pathological study on the "negative features" of the disease (author's translation; in Japanese). *Nippon Naika Gakkai Zasshi* 1977;66:751–762.

254. Truax BT. Autonomic disturbances in Guillain-Barré syndrome. *Neurology* 1984;4:462–468.
255. Tsuzuki T, et al. Structure of the human prealbumin gene. *J Biol Chem* 1985;260:12224–12227.
256. Tuck RR, McLeod JG. Autonomic dysfunction in Guillain-Barré syndrome. *J Neurol Neurosurg Psychiatry* 1981;44:983–990.
257. Van Allen MW, et al. Inherited predisposition to generalized amyloidosis. Clinical and pathological study of a family with neuropathy, nephropathy, and peptic ulcer. *Neurology* 1969; 19:10–25.
258. van der Meche FGA, Schmitz PIM, The Dutch Guillain-Barré Study Group. A randomized trial comparing intravenous immune globulin and plasma exchange in Guillain-Barré syndrome. *N Engl J Med* 1992;326:1123–1129.
259. Vassallo M, et al. Gastrointestinal motor dysfunction in acquired selective cholinergic dysautonomia associated with infectious mononucleosis. *Gastroenterology* 1991;100:252–258.
260. Vendrell J, et al. Erythromelalgia associated with acute diabetic neuropathy: an unusual condition. *Diabetes Res* 1988;7:149–151.
261. Ventura HO, et al. Norepinephrine-induced hypertension in Guillain-Barré syndrome. *J Hypertens* 1986;4:265–267.
262. Verghese JP, et al. Amyloid neuropathy in multiple myeloma and other plasma cell dyscrasias. A hypothesis of the pathogenesis of amyloid neuropathies. *J Neurol Sci* 1983;59:237–246.
263. Vita G, et al. Cardiovascular-reflex testing and single-fiber electromyography in botulism. A longitudinal study. *Arch Neurol* 1987;44:202–206.
264. Vital C, et al. Amyloid neuropathy and multiple myeloma. Ultrastructural and immunopathological study of two cases. *Eur Neurol* 1983;22:106–112.
265. Vrethem M, et al. Neuropathy and myopathy in primary Sjögren's syndrome: neurophysiological, immunological and muscle biopsy results. *Acta Neurol Scand* 1990;82:126–131.
266. Wallace MR, et al. Biochemical and molecular genetic characterization of a new variant prealbumin associated with hereditary amyloidosis. *J Clin Invest* 1986;78:6–12.
267. Wallace MR, et al. Localization of the human prealbumin gene to chromosome 18. *Biochem Biophys Res Commun* 1985;129:753–758.
268. Walsh JC. *The peripheral nervous system in lymphoma and multiple myeloma* (Thesis). Sydney: University of Sydney; 1972.
269. Warkany J, Hubbard DM. Mercury in urine of children with acrodynia. *Lancet* 1948;1:829–830.
270. Watson WE. Some circulatory responses to Valsalva's manoeuvre in patients with polyneuritis and spinal cord disease. *J Neurol Neurosurg Psychiatry* 1962;25:19–23.
271. Weber FP. Dr. Markus's original case of Markus's syndrome ("myotonic pupil" with absence of patellar and Achilles reflexes) shown twenty-seven and a half years ago. *Proc R Soc Med* 1933;26:530–531.
272. Weinshilboum RM, Axelrod J. Reduced plasma dopamine beta-hydroxylase activity in familial dysautonomia. *N Engl J Med* 1971; 285:938–942.
273. Wheeler JS Jr, et al. The urodynamic aspects of the Guillain-Barré syndrome. *J Urol* 1984;131:917–919.
274. Williams D, et al. Landry-Guillain-Barré syndrome with abnormal pupils and normal eye movements: a case report. *Neurology* 1979; 29:1033–1040.
275. Yahr MD, Frontera AT. Acute autonomic neuropathy. Its occurrence in infectious mononucleosis. *Arch Neurol* 1975;32:132–133.
276. Yosipovitch G, Krause I, Blickstein D. Erythromelalgia in a patient with thrombotic thrombocytopenic purpura. *J Am Acad Dermatol* 1992;26:825–827.
277. Young RR, et al. Pure pan-dysautonomia with recovery. Description and discussion of diagnostic criteria. *Brain* 1975;98:613–636.

CHAPTER 37

Diabetic Autonomic Neuropathy

Jannik Hilsted and Phillip A. Low

1. The true prevalence of diabetic autonomic neuropathy is not known, and depends on the diagnostic criteria. Clinical autonomic failure increases with the duration of diabetes and the age of the subject.
2. There are several types of diabetic neuropathy. Distal sensory and sensorimotor neuropathy is the most common.
3. Reduction of plasma norepinephrine provides an index of sympathetic adrenergic neuropathy but is relatively insensitive. The suggestion that neuropeptide Y or plasma dihydroxyphenylglycol may be more sensitive needs to be validated.
4. Cardiac parasympathetic impairment, evaluated as heart rate (HR) response to deep breathing, Valsalva maneuver (VM), and standing up, is recognized very early. Pancreatic polypeptide response may be impaired even earlier.
5. Orthostatic hypotension occurs later than cardiovagal impairment. In most series it affects 10%–30% of patients with diabetic neuropathy.
6. The physiologic response to exercise is impaired. These patients exhibit a reduced aerobic capacity, maximal HR, and in some cases a reduction in blood pressure (BP).
7. Cardiovascular risks include silent myocardial infarction, decreased longevity, and increased cardiovascular complications with general anesthesia, especially in patients with prolonged QT intervals.
8. The concept of functional autonomic failure has evolved. After a hypoglycemic insult, transiently impaired pancreatic polypeptide and epinephrine responses may develop in patients with insulin-dependent diabetes mellitus.
9. Abnormal results of the quantitative sudomotor axon reflex text (QSART) at the distal foot occurs with approximately the same frequency as abnormalities of cardiovagal function in cases of diabetic neuropathy.
10. Baroreflex indices such as the heart period range and mean gain are more sensitive indices of baroreflex abnormalities than the Valsalva ratio.
11. An exaggerated pressor response indicating denervation hypersensitivity, seen when denervation of postganglionic sympathetic fibers is widespread, occurs in about 25% of patients with diabetic neuropathy.
12. Pupillary abnormalities suggestive of sympathetic or parasympathetic impairment are a common manifestation of autonomic involvement.
13. Gastric motor abnormalities occur in 20%–30% of diabetic patients but are usually asymptomatic. Nausea, early satiety, postprandial bloating, and diffuse epigastric pain are the most frequent symptoms when present.
14. Diabetic diarrhea tends to appear in patients with established neuropathy. It may occur nocturnally and paroxysmally and be very troublesome.
15. Diabetic cystopathy may be asymptomatic or manifested as increased residual urine volume, overflow incontinence, and secondary infections, which may ultimately lead to pyelonephritis and uremia.
16. Erectile failure is common and increases with duration of diabetes. It is caused by a combination of vascular disease and autonomic failure.

J. Hilsted: Department of Internal Medicine and Endocrinology, Hvidovre Hospital, DK-2650 Hvidovre, Denmark.

P. A. Low: Department of Neurology, Mayo Clinic, Rochester, Minnesota 55905.

INTRODUCTION

Autonomic dysfunction was recognized in diabetic patients long before the discovery of insulin (46). However, the first comprehensive description of autonomic failure in diabetic patients did not emerge until 1945, when Rundles (175) described symptoms of end-organ failure possibly caused by autonomic dysfunction in 125 diabetic patients. With increases in longevity following the availability of insulin, autonomic complications took on greater importance. In the last two decades, the availability of quantitative and noninvasive tests of autonomic function has resulted in a better characterization of the distribution, sites, and severity of autonomic dysfunction. Considerable information has been obtained regarding the frequency of autonomic abnormalities, and prevalence data are now available. Treatment trials are becoming relatively common.

PREVALENCE

Diabetic neuropathy is the most common generalized neuropathy in developed countries, but its incidence and prevalence are unclear. Much of the uncertainty relates to methodologic problems, such as diagnostic criteria, sensitivity of diagnostic test(s), case ascertainment, selection, and referral bias (152). Incidence (new cases in a defined population during a specified period of time) is more difficult to determine accurately than is the cross-sectional index of prevalence (proportion of persons with the condition at some specified time). Prevalence of diabetic autonomic neuropathy varies greatly in the literature. Clinical autonomic failure varies with duration of diabetes and age of the subject. The prevalence is much greater if autonomic test results rather than clinical features are used as diagnostic criteria. Clinical autonomic failure is described in the section below on natural history. Some of the available data based on autonomic test results are summarized in Table 1. The data are of some interest because they reflect what is seen in clinical centers, but they are epidemiologically unacceptable, as the studies are not population-based and the tests are of variable sensitivity and evaluate different components of the autonomic neuraxis.

In the Rochester Diabetic Study, now in its 12th year, Dyck et al. (52) enrolled 380 of 870 diabetic patients in Rochester, Minnesota (Table 2). The prevalence of diabetes was 1.3% (National Diabetes Data Group criteria). Of the 380 enrolled patients, 102 (26.8%) had insulin-dependent diabetes mellitus (IDDM) and 278 (73.2%) had non-insulin-dependent diabetes mellitus (NIDDM). Of patients with IDDM, 66% had some form of neuropathy, but symptomatic degrees of polyneuropathy occurred in only 15% of IDDM and 13% of NIDDM patients. The more severe stage of polyneuropathy, in which patients were unable to walk on their heels and also had distal sensory and autonomic deficits (stage 2b), occurred even less frequently

TABLE 1. *Frequency of autonomic abnormalities by cardiovascular tests*

Author (ref.)	No. Diabetics	Autonomic tests	Percent abnormal	Comments
Ewing et al. (68)	37	VR	62	symptomatic patients
Ewing et al. (75)	42	HR_{var}	52	asymptomatic
Ewing et al. (74)	543	VM HR_{DB} ST	40	unselected
Canal et al. (33)	105	VM	36	unselected
Hilsted and Jensen (105)	126	HR_{DB}	40	higher % with increasing duration and neuropathy
Sundkvist et al. (194)	41	E:I ratio	56	impaired vibration;
			82	absent ankle jerks
Mackay et al. (142)	287	HR_{DB} ST	97	symptomatic;
			30	neuropathy;
			7	asymptomatic
Dyrberg et al. (54)	75	HR_{DB}	27	grouped by duration;
		VM	17	worse with duration
Smith and Smith (190)	67	HR_{var}	43	patients had retinopathy;
		HR_{DB}	52	abnormalities related to
		VR	6	degree of retinopathy
Masaoka et al. (148)	218	HR_{DB}	82	symptomatic;
			64	neuropathic;
			36	asymptomatic
Low et al. (140)	73	HR_{DB}	67	55% had combined
		VR	67	abnormalities
Dyck et al. (52)	380	HR_{DB} VR	66	see text

HR_{DB}, heart rate range to deep breathing; VR, Valsalva ratio; HR_{var}, resting heart rate variability; VM, Valsalva maneuver; ST, standing; E:I ratio,

TABLE 2. *Comparison of IDDM with NIDDM*

Parameter	IDDM, %	NIDDM, %
Prevalence of neuropathy		
Total	66	59
Symptomatic	15	13
Type of neuropathy		
Polyneuropathy	54	45
Carpal tunnel syndrome	33	35
Visceral autonomic	7	5
Others	3	3

From Dyck et al., ref. 52.
IDDM, insulin-dependent diabetes mellitus; NIDDM, non-insulin-dependent diabetes mellitus.

(6% of IDDM and 1% of NIDDM patients). The frequencies of individual types were as follows: polyneuropathy, 54%; asymptomatic carpal tunnel syndrome, 22%; symptomatic carpal tunnel syndrome, 11%; visceral autonomic neuropathy, 7%; other varieties, 3%. Among NIDDM patients, 59% had various neuropathies; the respective percentages were 45%, 29%, 6%, 5%, and 3%. Approximately 10% of diabetic patients had neurologic deficits attributable to nondiabetic causes. Among laboratory tests, abnormalities of nerve conduction in two or more nerves and abnormalities on autonomic function tests (decreased heart beat response to deep breathing or the Valsalva ratio) or on CASS (composite autonomic scoring scale) were the most sensitive and objective and were especially suitable for the detection of subclinical neuropathy (51).

CLASSIFICATION

Diabetic neuropathy is heterogenous by clinical pattern and perhaps by etiopathogenesis. The suggested classification in Table 3 provides a working model; the painful neuropathies are classified in Table 4. In a strict sense, the great majority of diabetic neuropathies are asymmetric according to results of sensitive tests such as bilateral nerve conduction studies, QSART, and thermoregulatory sweat tests (TSTs) (80,138). For practical purposes, asymmetry is accepted only when major clinical motor, sensory, or autonomic asymmetry is seen, usually the result of unilateral involvement of major nerves.

Distal sensory and sensorimotor neuropathy is the most common type of diabetic neuropathy. Sensory deficits are manifested as loss of vibratory perception and hypesthesia, or positive symptoms of paresthesias or pain may predominate, but some motor involvement is usually present, at least electrophysiologically (137,198). The Achilles tendon reflex is often reduced. When sensory deficits, mediated by large myelinated fibers, are overrepresented, the term *large-fiber-type neuropathy* is suggested. Proprioceptive and vibratory perception are particularly impaired. When deficits are severe, the term *diabetic pseudotabes* is sometimes used. These patients have pseudoathetosis, rombergism, and walk with a stamping gait. Patients with small-fiber neuropathy have disproportionate involvement of small myelinated and unmyelinated fibers, both somatic and sympathetic. Typically, they have orthostatic hypotension and other evidence of autonomic failure, and disproportionate impairment of pain and temperature perception. Pain may be present (137,211).

Diabetic distal small-fiber neuropathy (192,211) is a more restricted variety of small-fiber neuropathy. The primary complaint is distal pain manifested as burning or hyperalgesia. Pain and temperature perception may be disproportionately impaired, and QSART is impaired distally (Chapter 50). *Insulin neuropathy* refers to an uncommon neuropathy that develops within 1 month of the institution of aggressive insulin therapy (34).

The asymmetric neuropathies are caused by involvement of nerve trunks as mononeuropathy, mononeuropathy multiplex, or radiculopathies. The pattern of chronic inflammatory demyelinating polyradiculoneuropathy (CIDP) may be symmetric or asymmetric and therefore appears in both categories. Proximal diabetic neuropathy clinically appears to be a hybrid of diabetic radiculoplexopathy and CIDP, with a course that more closely resembles the former.

TABLE 3. *Classification of diabetic neuropathy*

Symmetric neuropathy
  Distal sensory and sensorimotor neuropathy
  Large-fiber type of diabetic neuropathy
  Small-fiber type of diabetic neuropathy
  Distal small-fiber neuropathy
  "Insulin" neuropathy
  Proximal diabetic neuropathy
  Chronic inflammatory demyelinating radiculopathy (CIDP)

Asymmetric neuropathy
  Mononeuropathy
  Mononeuropathy multiplex
  Radiculopathies
  Lumbar plexopathy or radiculoplexopathy
  CIDP

TABLE 4. *Types of painful diabetic neuropathy*

Acute painful diabetic neuropathy
  Acute lumbar radiculoplexopathy
  Acute thoracic radiculopathy
  Acute distal sensory neuropathy
  Insulin neuropathy
  Acute small-fiber neuropathy (panautonomic)

Chronic painful diabetic neuropathy
  Distal small-fiber neuropathy
  Small-fiber type of diabetic neuropathy
  Diabetic sensory neuropathy
  Proximal diabetic neuropathy

Acute Diabetic Painful Neuropathies

The acute diabetic painful neuropathies should be differentiated from the chronic ones, as the clinical features, etiopathogenesis, response to treatment, and prognosis may all be different.

Acute Painful Diabetic Neuropathy

One category of acute painful diabetic neuropathy has an acute onset, and it clears within approximately six months (8).

Small fibers either are unmyelinated or are small (<5 μm) myelinated nerve fibers that mediate autonomic and certain sensory functions. Autonomic fibers to blood vessels are responsible for vasoconstriction, and those to sweat glands control sudomotor function. Small-fiber sensory functions mainly mediate pain and temperature sensation. Distal small-fiber neuropathy is characterized by predominantly positive symptoms related to mediation by small myelinated and unmyelinated fibers. Patients have cold feet that are sometimes discolored. Sweating may be increased early and lost later. Patients complain of burning, prickling, and aching and may exhibit allodynia and hyperalgesia. They do not have widespread sensory impairment or generalized autonomic failure.

Diabetic Radiculopathies

Diabetic radiculopathies are electrophysiologically common (15), but most are not painful. One subgroup, however, can be painful, and affected patients have an acute onset, typically in the thoracic or lumbar region. The radiculopathy is characterized by the acute onset of pain that is typically aching, but sometimes sharp or burning, over the thorax or abdomen. The distribution is most often unilateral and involves one or two roots (60). Sensory loss is variable and weakness can occur, resulting in an abdominal bulge when the lower thoracic dermatomes are involved. A useful diagnostic test is the TST, which accurately depicts the bandlike distribution of anhidrosis, sometimes with perilesional hyperhidrosis (79).

Diabetic Lumbosacral Radiculoplexopathies

The next category comprises the diabetic radiculoplexopathies (especially lumbar or lumbosacral). The entity is acute or subacute in onset, with thigh pain that is usually deep and dull and associated with significant weight loss (58). Weakness develops as pain recedes. The affected muscles are weak, and hyporeflexia or areflexia is present. The lesion is unilateral in the majority of cases. The whole process is monophasic, with recovery taking place within 3 to 18 months (36). Electromyographically, there is active denervation of affected muscles, increased femoral nerve latency, and denervation of paraspinal muscles (193).

Acute Insulin Neuritis

Infrequently, an acute painful neuropathy develops within 1 month of institution of tight glycemic control with insulin therapy in a diabetic patient who previously did not have a neuropathy (34,56,89,154). The neuropathy is usually a distal sensory polyneuropathy, although it may be more acute and severe. Occasional patients may have several episodes of worsening of diabetic symptoms with tight control, and this observation has infrequently been an obstacle to the attainment of euglycemia. Recent experimental studies provide some insight into the mechanism of insulin neuritis. Insulin administration reproducibly causes acute endoneurial hypoxia, by increasing arteriovenous flow in nerves and reducing nutritive flow of normal nerves (123). The diabetic state confers resistance to this effect. Within one month of commencement of insulin treatment, such susceptibility to the endoneurial hypoxic effect of insulin recurs (123). Endoneurial hypoxia has been demonstrated in experimental and human diabetic neuropathy (157,199). We have suggested that diabetic nerve fibers survive under these hypoxic conditions because of the greatly increased energy substrate stores in experimental and human diabetes (53,139), coupled with the low energy requirements of peripheral nerve (139). Anaerobic metabolism suffices under these circumstance. Insulin treatment causes transient hypoxia in normal but not diabetic nerves (123). With continued insulin treatment, energy substrates are normalized and the susceptibility to insulin-induced endoneurial hypoxia returns in diabetic nerves. The hypoxic tissues with normal energy substrates fare poorly, because anaerobic metabolism is inefficient (139), and there may be sufficient hypoxia to result in fiber degeneration.

From the standpoint of management, the benefits of a chronic nearly euglycemic state clearly outweigh those of hyperglycemia (1). It is prudent to titrate glycemic control to nerve function gradually in these patients. The outlook for recovery of function is generally good, and sensory function, including pain, tends to stabilize during a period months.

Diabetic Small-Fiber Neuropathy

Generalized small-fiber neuropathy is uncommon, but the manifestations are dramatic. These patients have generalized small-fiber dysfunction. The best known causes of small-fiber neuropathy are as follows:

1. Diabetes
2. Amyloid
3. Acute panautonomic neuropathy (acute pandysautonomia)
4. Acute paraneoplastic panautonomic neuropathy

Diabetic small-fiber neuropathy has many features in common with acute panautonomic neuropathy. It may follow a viral or a bacterial infection. Patients have selective or disproportionate small-fiber dysfunction, both autonomic and sensory, manifested as a mix of lost function and exaggerated or altered function (of remaining fibers). In some patients without antecedent neuropathy, the onset of small-fiber manifestations occurs abruptly in relative isolation. The onset may on occasion be sufficiently acute or subacute to resemble acute panautonomic neuropathy. Infrequently, this pattern occurs in relative isolation, with preserved reflexes and normal results of conventional electrophysiologic studies. Patients have severe dysautonomia with postural hypotension, impairment of bowel and bladder control, and impotence. They often have a feeling of bloat in the abdomen and watery diarrhea, which is often nocturnal and tends to appear episodically. The selective involvement of autonomic fibers is suggestive of an immune-mediated mechanism.

Sensory symptoms consist of a combination of a loss of sensation (of pain and temperature discrimination) and spontaneous pain.

Chronic Diabetic Painful Neuropathies

Chronic Distal Painful Neuropathy

Pain is a feature in about 5%–10% of patients with diabetic neuropathy. Overall, the most common type of painful diabetic neuropathy occurs in patients with distal sensory neuropathy (more accurately, sensorimotor neuropathy). Most patients who have had diabetes for longer than ten years have electrophysiologic evidence of a neuropathy. Many of these patients have clinical evidence of neuropathy, with distal loss of perception of vibration >touch >pain/temperature (i.e., large-fiber >small-fiber impairment). Strength is typically normal and ankle reflexes are reduced. About 10% of these patients have significant small-fiber dysfunction, which may be manifested as pain.

Distal Small-Fiber Neuropathy

Distal small-fiber neuropathy has been defined above. It is perhaps the most common type of neuropathy seen by neurologists specializing in the treatment of pain. The patient describes burning or aching feet. Examination may show allodynia and some blunting of pain and temperature perception. Often the changes are relatively minor. Results of electromyography are essentially normal. Results of sensation tests may be normal or may show some impairment of thermal cooling or warming. The most sensitive tests are quantitative tests of sudomotor function. These show an acral loss of sweating.

TABLE 5. *Clinical features of neuropathy in 44 diabetic patients*

Parameter	Number	%
Antecedent neuropathy	19	43
Pain	28	64
Reduced/absent tendon reflexes		
Knee	42	95
Ankle	44	100
Sensory loss	40	91
Upper and lower extremities	16	36
Lower extremity only	24	55
Weakness		
Lower extremity	44	100
Upper extremity	12	27
Cerebrospinal fluid (n = 26)		
Percentage abnormal		100
Mean value (mg/dL)	92.5 ± 29.7	
Percentage >100 mg/dL		42
Percentage <70 mg/dL		27

From Low et al., ref. 136.

There are a number of causes of small-fiber neuropathy, although most cases are idiopathic. Diabetes is a known cause, and small-fiber neuropathy may be associated with inherited sensory neuropathy and immune-mediated neuropathy.

Proximal Diabetic Neuropathy

In some patients with diabetes, a diabetic neuropathy of subacute onset progresses to involve both lower extremities proximally (42,193). Motor function is affected more than sensory loss, but pain may be a prominent feature. These patients have some features resembling those of CIDP, with proximal >distal weakness, areflexia, increased cerebrospinal fluid protein, and slowing of nerve conduction velocity (203). In many patients, pain is diffuse or radicular. As in CIDP, patients respond to immunotherapy with prednisone, plasma exchange, or intravenous gamma globulin.

We recently reviewed the Mayo Clinic experience of proximal diabetic neuropathy (136). Forty-four diabetic patients with subacute diabetic proximal neuropathy were seen during a 12-year period. The majority of patients were middle-aged or elderly, of either sex, and had proximal muscle weakness associated with reduced or absent reflexes in the lower extremity (Table 5). Electrophysiologically, the majority had some evidence of demyelination on nerve conduction, but invariably this was accompanied by axonal degeneration. Cerebrospinal fluid protein was usually increased.

Diffuse and significant autonomic failure was usually present. Table 6 summarizes the CASS, which quantitates the combined sudomotor, adrenergic, and cardiovagal autonomic deficits, correcting for the confounding effects of age and sex (132). CASS (Chapter 15) has a range of 0 (no deficit) to 10 (maximal deficit). It also has subscores for

TABLE 6. *CASS and subscores in proximal diabetic neuropathy*

Parameter	Mean ± SD
CASS	7.8 ± 2.2
CASS-sudomotor	2.3 ± 1.0
CASS-cardiovagal	2.1 ± 1.0
CASS-adrenergic	3.4 ± 1.0

sudomotor (0–3), cardiovagal (0–3), and adrenergic deficits (0–4). A value of 7.8 indicates severe and generalized autonomic failure.

In most cases (n = 4; 57%), sural nerve biopsy indicated some degree of demyelination, although only 2 patients (29%) had evidence of an inflammatory infiltrate. Approximately 75% (9 of 12) of patients treated for an immune-mediated neuropathy (prednisone, intravenous immunoglobulin, plasma exchange) improved, but 58% (18 of 29) of untreated patients with follow-up also eventually improved, although much more slowly. Improvement was usually incomplete. We suggest that the entity of subacute proximal diabetic motor neuropathy is a more extensive and severe form of lumbosacral radiculoplexopathy, with some features suggestive of an immune-mediated etiology. It differs from CIDP in that the majority of cases have a more restricted distribution, and it appears to be monophasic and self-limiting. Treatment with immunotherapy may be warranted in the more severe and progressive cases.

INVOLVEMENT BY SYSTEM

Biochemical and Neurophysiologic Markers of Autonomic Neuropathy in Diabetes

Sympathetic Neuropathy

The neurotransmitter of the peripheral sympathetic nervous system is norepinephrine (39). It is released from presynaptic vesicles on sympathetic stimulation. Most of the released norepinephrine is inactivated by a reuptake mechanism in the terminals; 10%–20% spills over into the systemic circulation and can be measured in peripheral blood. The double enzymatic technique for measuring catecholamines became established in the early 1970s (64); the best indicator of sympathetic nerve activity in humans was therefore the plasma level of norepinephrine (127), because establishing methods for direct measurement of sympathetic nerve activity (see below) proved difficult. The assumption that plasma norepinephrine is a reliable marker of sympathetic neuropathy is based on a number of premises, the most important ones being that norepinephrine secretion and the fraction of norepinephrine spilling into the circulation are constant, and that clearance of norepinephrine is constant within and between subjects. These assumptions are not always correct (96). Because clearance is a function of sympathetic neuronal integrity, concerns arose that changes in norepinephrine clearance in patients with diabetic autonomic neuropathy might reflect the disease process itself rather than sympathetic nerve activity, so that plasma norepinephrine would be an inaccurate index of sympathetic function in these patients (100). However, the concern proved to be largely theoretical, as simultaneous measurements of rates of plasma norepinephrine appearance and clearance showed plasma norepinephrine clearance to be identical in diabetic patients with and without autonomic neuropathy, whereas the appearance rate was significantly reduced in patients with diabetic autonomic neuropathy (48). Thus, for the majority of patients, plasma catecholamine kinetics are no more sensitive than supine plasma norepinephrine determinations in the diagnosis of diabetic autonomic neuropathy.

The biochemical precursors of norepinephrine (dopamine and dopa) are not very sensitive to changes in activity of the sympathetic nervous system and are not useful as markers of sympathetic neuropathy (55). Plasma dihydroxyphenylglycol has been reported to be a more sensitive marker of autonomic neuropathy than plasma norepinephrine (38). This observation needs to be confirmed in larger numbers of patients with different degrees of adrenergic failure. Neuropeptide Y is released with norepinephrine on sympathetic nerve stimulation (6). Because reuptake of neuropeptide Y does not occur, it is potentially a better marker of sympathetic adrenergic neuropathy. Neuropeptide Y and norepinephrine in nerve are reduced to a similar degree in experimental autonomic neuropathy (21). Plasma measurements of norepinephrine and neuropeptide Y to compare their sensitivity and specificity have not been reported in any clinical studies involving significant numbers of subjects.

Parasympathetic Neuropathy

Unlike the sympathetic neurotransmitter, the parasympathetic neurotransmitter (acetylcholine) cannot be measured in peripheral venous blood, primarily because of the ubiquitous presence and high intrinsic activity of cholinesterase. Therefore, measurement of plasma acetylcholine concentrations are not a useful index of cholinergic function. Other biochemical markers of parasympathetic neuropathy are indirect. Pancreatic polypeptide is secreted from the polypeptide cells of the human pancreas on vagal stimulation (185). Other stimuli, notably circulating catecholamines and to a small extent sympathetic nerve stimulation, may also induce an increase in secretion of pancreatic polypeptide (104,106). It has been shown that the secretion of pancreatic polypeptide in response to hypoglycemia and to a mixed meal depends solely on vagal stimulation (atropine and surgical vagotomy completely abolish these responses) (185). Therefore, both these stimuli have been applied to determine the functional state of the parasympathetic nervous system in diabetes (98,107, 141). It has consistently been shown that the pancreatic polypeptide response to these stimuli is blunted even in patients with diabetes of short duration who have no other measurable signs of neuropathy, including abnormal results of cardiovascular reflex tests (170). Perhaps impairment of cholinergic innervation to the gut precedes cardiovagal impairment, and it is conceivable that the blunted pancreatic polypeptide response to one of these two stimuli may be the first evidence of parasympathetic neuropathy in diabetic patients.

Microneurography

Direct measurement of sympathetic nerve action potentials is now possible (77) (Chapter 18). Microneurography can be used to measure muscle and skin sympathetic activity, but is time-consuming and technically demanding and requires a very cooperative patient. The method has been applied in diabetic patients with signs of peripheral somatic neuropathy, in whom both amplitude and frequency of spontaneous action potentials were decreased (76). The method is not practical as a clinical test of autonomic function.

Cardiovascular Reflexes in Diabetes

Although the basis of the various cardiovascular heart rate (HR) tests has been known for a long time, the tests were not applied clinically in large numbers of diabetic patients until the 1970s (68,138,209). The most widely used test is the HR response to deep breathing (HR_{DB}) (17,23,54,68,86,94,105,121,140,165,186,194,196,197,209,

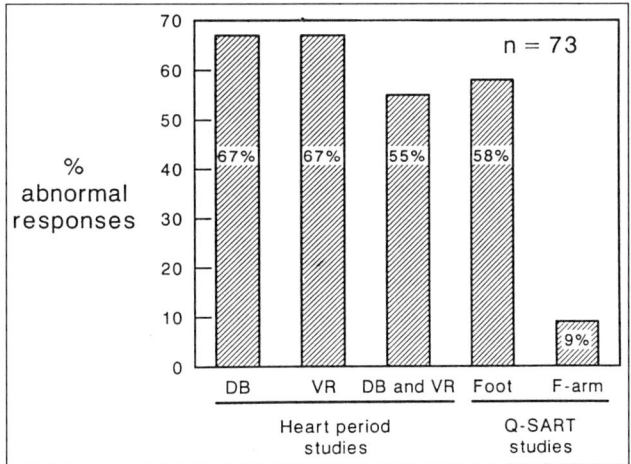

FIG. 1. The frequency of abnormalities detected with HR_{DB}, VR, and QSART. (From Low et al., ref. 140. Reprinted with permission.)

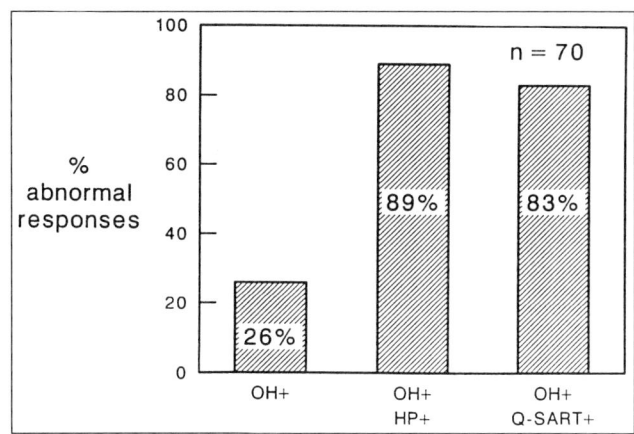

FIG. 2. Concordance of tests of cardiovagal function with QSART. (From Low et al., ref. 140. Reprinted with permission.)

214) (Chapters 15, 24, and 26). The next most commonly used and validated tests are the HR responses to the Valsalva maneuver (Valsalva ratio; VR) (11,22,24,54,73,138, 140,166,187), and to standing up (30:15 ratio) (70). The sensitivity of HR_{DB} and VR are similar (Fig. 1), and there is reasonable concordance with QSART (Fig. 2). The prevalence of abnormalities in autonomic function tests is reportedly greater in NIDDM than in IDDM (17,54,94, 142,156,158).

Other tests of cardiovagal function used to study diabetic subjects include the HR responses to apneic face immersion and mental stress (25), and to coughing (35).

If the HR is monitored during a 24-hr period, the major fluctuations in rate seen in normal subjects may be absent in patients with diabetic autonomic neuropathy. In a study of 21 normal subjects and 64 diabetics (67), diabetics had a higher mean resting HR. With increasing autonomic failure, there was a greater reduction in diurnal HR variation.

More recently, HR changes in the frequency domain have been studied (Chapters 25,26). The high-frequency heart period component is a quantitative assessment of respiratory sinus arrhythmia and indicative of cardiovagal activity exclusively (5,124). It is most pronounced in supine subjects and is decreased relative to the low-frequency component during upright tilt (161). The low-frequency oscillation is present in the supine position and enhanced during upright tilt (124,161). Power spectral analysis makes it possible to analyze the sympathetic-parasympathetic balance simultaneously and has recently been used to study diabetic autonomic neuropathy. Sympathetic and parasympathetic involvement appeared to be similar in degree (161). The high-frequency power was found to be a significant predictor of the expiratory-inspiratory ratio, HR_{DB}, the 30:15 ratio, and the VR. The low-frequency power was a modest or poor predictor of blood pressure (BP) response to sustained handgrip or orthostatic hypotension (87). The approach is of interest for research purposes but is not likely to evolve into a "bedside test" similar to the cardiovascular HR tests. A related approach is the use of spectral analysis to describe the relationship between HR fluctuations and respiration (28).

Some controversy exists concerning the prevalence of abnormal autonomic test results at the time of diagnosis. Pfeifer et al. (166) reported the majority of patients to have have impaired HR_{DB} at the time of diagnosis. They studied 17 patients with IDDM and 17 with NIDDM within 12 and 24 months of diagnosis, respectively. Most other workers report a lower prevalence. It is well recognized that some diabetic patients have asymptomatic abnormalities of cardiovascular HR tests within 2 years of diabetes (17,72). The prevalence of abnormal cardiovascular HR tests in asymptomatic subjects varies (Table 1). The higher percentage is more concordant with the experience of the authors.

Many factors affect cardiovascular HR tests (see Chapters 14, 15, 24, and 30). The prevalence of positive results and degree of severity, best studied for HR_{DB}, increase with duration of diabetes (54,69,94,142,195). In a large study of 237 diabetics studied 3 months or more apart, Ewing et al. (74) found that 71% were unchanged, 26% had deteriorated, and 3% had improved. The experience of Mackay et al. (142) and Sampson et al. (179), who found a reduction of about one beat per minute per year, is probably representative.

Cardiovascular HR tests are indirect tests of autonomic function, modulated by sympathetic activity and other variables (Chapter 30). The good correlation of well-studied tests such as HR_{DB} with other tests of neuropathy suggest that in the majority of patients, an abnormal test result does indicate autonomic failure. For the individual subject some uncertainty persists, and attempts to overcome this by using multiple tests, five for example (74), may provide a false sense of security. On balance, the tests are useful and reliable indirect indicators of autonomic function.

Orthostatic Hypotension

Orthostatic hypotension is the most dramatic clinical manifestation of autonomic neuropathy. Although orthostatic hypotension is relatively common in some reported studies (135,138,174,175,201), the frequency reflects referral bias. We found orthostatic hypotension in 43% of 16 patients (138) and 26% of 73 patients (135). Mulder et al. (155) found orthostatic hypotension in 18 of 103 unselected patients with diabetes, of whom 43 had polyneuropathy. Veglio et al. (201) reported orthostatic intolerance in 34% of 221 patients with NIDDM. In some studies clinical failure is very uncommon. For instance, Young et al. (213), in a study of teenagers, did not find any symptoms of autonomic failure. The prevalence of symptomatic orthostatic hypotension is less than 1% in population-based studies (163) (ongoing Rochester diabetic study).

The mechanism of diabetic orthostatic hypotension involves degeneration of the sympathetic preganglionic and postganglionic fibers supplying the splanchnic mesenteric bed (108,138). Autonomic denervation of the muscular resistance bed is also present, but in humans sustained postural normotension depends to a greater degree on the splanchnic system, whereas innervation of skeletal muscle is more important in moment-to-moment adjustments (146). Plasma volume, cardioacceleration, and central blood volume are normal or nearly normal in diabetic orthostatic hypotension (108). Subcutaneous vasoconstrictor function is impaired (108,133,138,172).

Limited information is available on recording of the splanchnic mesenteric bed in patients with diabetic neuropathy. It is possible to measure superior mesenteric arterial flow using a duplex scanner (Chapter 15). Normal subject undergo a two- to threefold increase in superior mesenteric flow with a meal, and splanchnic capacitance falls with tilt-up. Patients with neurogenic orthostatic hypotension are reported to undergo a normal increase in capacity postprandially, and hypotension develops because of failure of arteriolar vasoconstriction in muscle (126). Some workers have reported similar responses to tilt and a meal in diabetic neuropathic patients in comparison with controls and conclude that the splanchnic bed may be less important than was assumed (169).

Exercise

In healthy subjects, physical exercise induces major cardiovascular changes, in large part mediated by the activity of the autonomic nervous system. The involvement of the autonomic nervous system is very important for the physiologic adaptation to exercise (173). In diabetic autonomic neuropathy, the physiologic response to exercise has been shown to be clearly abnormal. These patients display a decrease in aerobic capacity, a decrease in maximal HR, an impaired tachycardic HR response to exercise, even at an intensity equivalent to everyday activities, and, in some cases, a decrease in BP during exercise (101–103). These findings can be explained by and are generally compatible with widespread autonomic denervation of both the sympathetic and parasympathetic nervous system (98). Undoubtedly, the reduction in physical capacity in diabetic patients with autonomic neuropathy contributes to incapacity in cases of long duration.

General Anesthesia

Unexpected cardiovascular complications in association with general anesthesia have been reported in patients with longstanding diabetes (125,162). It has been suggested that these complications are a consequence of cardiovascular neuropathy, which renders the patient unable to adapt to preoperative and postoperative changes in blood volume.

Recently, this notion has been confirmed by a study in which the cardiovascular reflexes of diabetic patients were investigated preoperatively. Patients who had abnormal results on cardiovascular reflex tests had a significantly higher incidence of arrhythmias and unexplained BP reduction in the preoperative and postoperative period (30). Thus, special attention should be given during general anesthesia to cardiovascular monitoring of diabetic patients whose cardiovascular HR tests indicate impaired reflexes.

Hormonal and Metabolic Aspects

Autonomic neuropathy may affect the intermediary metabolism in diabetic patients through several mechanisms: (a) Glycogen stores (i.e., in the liver) are directly controlled by sympathetic nerves, as are fat depots; (b) the secretion of carbohydrate- and fat-mobilizing hormones is at least in part regulated by autonomic nerve function; (c) autonomic neuropathy may affect cardiovascular function and thereby alter the pattern of blood flow to several organs, resulting in an altered extraction of metabolic substrates.

Hormonal Secretion and Metabolic Function in Diabetic Autonomic Neuropathy

In addition to its role as a neurotransmitter, norepinephrine also functions as a hormone, with lipolytic and glycogenolytic actions. The norepinephrine responses to a number of stimuli (i.e., exercise and standing) (102,108) are diminished in diabetic autonomic neuropathy, resulting in reduced substrate mobilization. Epinephrine, which is secreted from the adrenal medulla on activation of its sympathetic supply, has potent lipolytic, glycogenolytic, and ketogenic properties. During hypoglycemia, the epinephrine response is diminished in patients with diabetic autonomic neuropathy (106). The epinephrine response to exercise is also diminished (102,103). The orthostatic increase in plasma epinephrine is relatively small in normal subjects. Although it may be decreased in diabetic autonomic neuropathy, it is better preserved than the norepinephrine response.

Glucagon is secreted from the α cells of the pancreas in response to a number of stimuli, such as exercise, hypoglycemia, and protein intake. The secretion of glucagon is, to some extent, regulated by autonomic nerves, in addition to changes in blood concentrations of glucose and amino acids (112). Glucagon secretion in response to hypoglycemia is severely reduced in diabetes mellitus (90), and in diabetic autonomic neuropathy there is no glucagon response at all (106,143). The underlying pathogenic mechanism has not yet been established. The glucagon secretory defect during insulin-induced hypoglycemia is not caused by atrophy of the α cells, as glucagon is secreted in response to other stimuli (i.e., exercise and amino acid intake) (143).

Growth hormone and cortisol are secreted in response to various types of stress. Increased activity in afferent sympathetic nerves may elicit growth hormone and cortisol secretion, and lesions of these nerves may be responsible for the reduced cortisol and growth hormone secretion during exercise in patients with diabetic neuropathy (102). During hypoglycemia, growth hormone and cortisol secretion is elicited by stimulation of central glucoreceptors. The secretion of these hormones is not affected to any great extent by the presence of diabetic autonomic neuropathy (106).

PP is secreted from D cells in the human pancreas. The secretion is purely neurogenic; increases in both parasympathetic and sympathetic activity increase PP secretion. During hypoglycemia, PP is secreted through increased vagal activity. In diabetic patients with autonomic neuropathy, the PP response is absent (107,129). It is conceivable that PP secretion during hypoglycemia is the most sensitive test for autonomic neuropathy in diabetes, in that the PP response to hypoglycemia is somewhat reduced in patients with IDDM who have no other measurable signs of neuropathy, suggesting that vagal nerves supplying the pancreatic D cells may be damaged very early in such cases (129). PP is also released by a vagal mechanism in response to a mixed meal. During exercise, PP is secreted to adrenergic stimulation; in exercise there is no PP response in patients with autonomic neuropathy. Somatostatin is secreted from endocrine cells in the brain and in the gastrointestinal tract. The factors regulating somatostatin secretion are poorly defined, but it is now evident that neural regulation is significant in the regulation of somatostatin secretion during hypoglycemia. In humans, the somatostatin response to hypoglycemia is eliminated by vagotomy, and in diabetic patients with autonomic neuropathy the somatostatin response was absent, probably because of vagal neuropathy (107).

The above-mentioned observations indicate that the hormonal secretion pattern is altered to a significant extent by the presence of autonomic neuropathy in diabetic patients, and such hormonal dysfunction might be expected to result in metabolic maladaptation. However, no experimental data suggest that metabolic functions in patients with autonomic neuropathy are different from those of patients without neuropathy (99). A relatively small number of metabolic studies have been performed in patients with autonomic neuropathy, and the studies have been done only during hypoglycemia and exercise.

In normal humans, glucose counterregulation after hypoglycemia depends on the secretion of glucagon and epinephrine. If secretion of one of these hormones is impaired, glucose counterregulation is not detectably affected if the other hormone is released in sufficient amounts. If the secretion of both hormones is impaired or if the actions of both hormones are blocked, glucose counterregulation is abolished (44).

Surprisingly, glucose counterregulation has been found to be similar in patients with and without autonomic neuropathy (84,106). The mobilization of free fatty acids was found even to be enhanced in patients with diabetic autonomic neuropathy (106). These observations led to the hypothesis that the sensitivity of hepatic glycogenolysis and adipose lipolysis to circulating epinephrine is greater in diabetic patients with autonomic neuropathy than in patients without neuropathy (106). This was documented by epinephrine infusion in such subjects, during which the response of glucose, glucose appearance rate in plasma, and levels of lactate and free fatty acids were significantly greater in patients with diabetic autonomic neuropathy than in patients without neuropathy (109). The mechanism for this increase in β-adrenergic sensitivity may be altered kinetic properties of infused epinephrine, changes in adrenergic receptor systems, or both. Indeed, the kinetic properties of infused epinephrine actually are different in diabetic patients with autonomic neuropathy than in control subjects (49). The mean sojourn (residence) time is increased in diabetic patients with autonomic neuropathy, probably resulting in increased cellular effects of a given amount of infused epinephrine. Adrenergic receptor systems have been studied in blood cells in diabetic patients with and without autonomic neuropathy. No changes been found in mononuclear leukocyte and platelet adrenergic receptor systems (50). However, in a small subset of diabetic patients with autonomic neuropathy, target tissue (adipose tissue) receptor systems have been shown to have an increased activity (160). Thus, changes in kinetic properties of catecholamines, changes in receptor systems, and postreceptor abnormalities could all possibly account for the increase in β-adrenergic sensitivity in these patients.

Thus, the reduced secretion of several hormones in patients with diabetic autonomic neuropathy is probably a consequence of defective autonomic nerve function. Metabolic functions are less affected. The preservation of metabolic responses may at least in part be attributable to the development of increased β-adrenergic sensitivity in patients with diabetic autonomic neuropathy. In everyday life, insulin availability probably plays a major role in metabolic functions in diabetic patients, a factor that further limits the significance of their altered patterns of hormonal secretion (99).

Functional Autonomic Failure

The concept of functional autonomic failure caused by hypoglycemia or hyperglycemia is a new and evolving concept of transient autonomic failure affecting patients with IDDM. One such entity is hypoglycemia-associated autonomic failure (HAAF) in IDDM (45). Following a hypoglycemic insult, the gastrointestinal parasympathetic (PP) and sympathetic (epinephrine) responses are impaired. The problem is compounded by cosegregation of the clinical syndromes of defective glucose counterregulation, hypoglycemia unawareness, and elevated glycemic threshold for symptoms; thus, a vicious cycle of hypoglycemia causing HAAF, with impaired counterregulation and hypoglycemia unawareness, further exacerbates hypoglycemia (45). Defective counterregulation, which is the combined impairment of glucagon and epinephrine responses to hypoglycemia, results in a 25-fold greater risk for severe iatrogenic hypoglycemia (29,210). HAAF appears to be distinct from classic diabetic neuropathy in that the two do not necessarily cosegregate, and the impaired epinephrine response is specific to hypoglycemia (45). Another example of functional autonomic failure is the impairment of gastric emptying with severe hyperglycemia.

Sudomotor Function

The best-known test of sudomotor function in diabetic neuropathy is the TST (Chapter 19). The most sensitive test of distal postganglionic sudomotor function is the QSART, which measures the distal ends of the postganglionic axon (Chapters 15, 23, and 29). QSART impairment at the distal foot occurs at approximately the same frequency as abnormalities of cardiovagal function in diabetic neuropathy (140) (Fig. 1), but abnormalities of sudomotor function manifested as increased resting sweat activity or persistent sweat activity following axon reflex activation occurs more commonly than vagal abnormalities. Several alternative methods of studying sudomotor function in diabetes have been described. The most intensively studied has been the sweat imprint following the iontophoresis of pilocarpine (122). Alternative methods of quantitating distal sudomotor function include the sweat drop method (176) and gravimetric method. Sudometric methods of varying levels of sophistication have been recently used (14,122,131). The peripheral autonomic skin potential is discussed in Chapter 17.

Vasomotor Function

No completely satisfactory noninvasive quantitative test of vasomotor function is available. Tests of vasomotor function in diabetic neuropathy are discussed according to the following categories: baroreflex gain, denervation supersensitivity, and peripheral reflexes.

Baroreflexes

Baroreflexes are activated when a change in BP (especially pulse pressure) or blood volume occurs (Chapters 4, 5, 6, 15, and 44). Baroreceptor function may be assessed by measuring the HR response to alterations in BP (Chap-

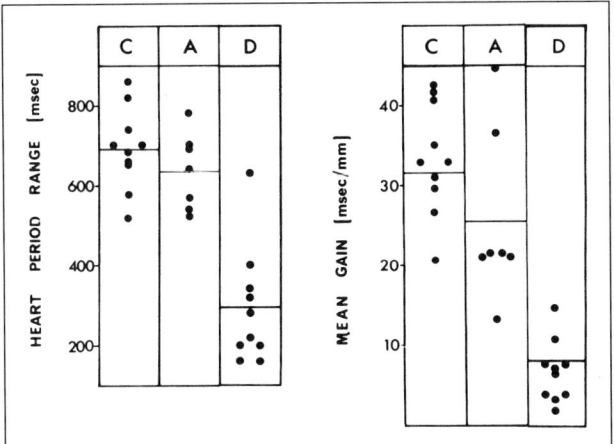

FIG. 3. Heart period range and mean gain in control subjects, alcoholics, and patients with diabetic neuropathy. (From Low PA, Walsh JC, Huang CY, McLeod JG. The autonomic nervous system in alcoholic and diabetic neuropathy. *Proc Aust Assoc Neurol* 1975;12:145–150. Reprinted with permission.)

ter 15). The heart period range and mean gain are more sensitive indices of baroreflex function than is the VR, and values are usually abnormal in diabetic neuropathy (Fig. 3). Stimulus-response curves may be abnormal when the VR is still normal (138). Instead of inducing BP changes with pharmacologic agents, it is possible to relate HR to BP during the Valsalva maneuver. The latency of the HR and BP responses has been suggested as an index of baroreflex gain (85). Although this approach may correlate with baroreflex gain, the relationship is indirect, as it assumes a predictable relationship between HR and BP when it fact this relationship is nonlinear.

Denervation Supersensitivity

An exaggerated pressor response indicating denervation hypersensitivity may be seen in cases of widespread denervation of postganglionic sympathetic fibers, and it occurs in about 25% of patients with diabetic neuropathy (138) (Fig. 4). Exaggerated pressor responses occur to norepinephrine and other agents, such as angiotensin and phenylephrine, that act directly on α receptors. The most important common mechanisms of denervation supersensitivity are increases in receptor density and affinity, and the efficacy of receptor-effector coupling or other postreceptor events.

Peripheral Reflexes

Skin vasomotor reflexes are often impaired in diabetic neuropathy, indicating sympathetic vasoconstrictor failure (133) (Chapter 14). The venoarteriolar reflex (Chapter 15) is mediated by the postganglionic adrenergic neuron. This reflex was first evaluated in diabetic patients by Hilsted (97). Recently, Rayman et al. (172) measured the venoarteriolar reflex in the feet of patients with diabetes and found it to be decreased in those who had diabetic neuropathy. We studied the venoarteriolar reflex, QSART, and HR responses to deep breathing and VM in 40 controls, 49 diabetic subjects, and 29 patients with other neuropathies. The mean vasoconstrictor response was greater in controls than in diabetic or other patients with neuropathies, but there were marked overlaps between groups (Fig. 5). The venoarteriolar reflex appeared to be of lower specificity and much lower sensitivity than other tests of autonomic function. We concluded that the venoarteriolar reflex, although impaired in the neuropathies, was of little value as

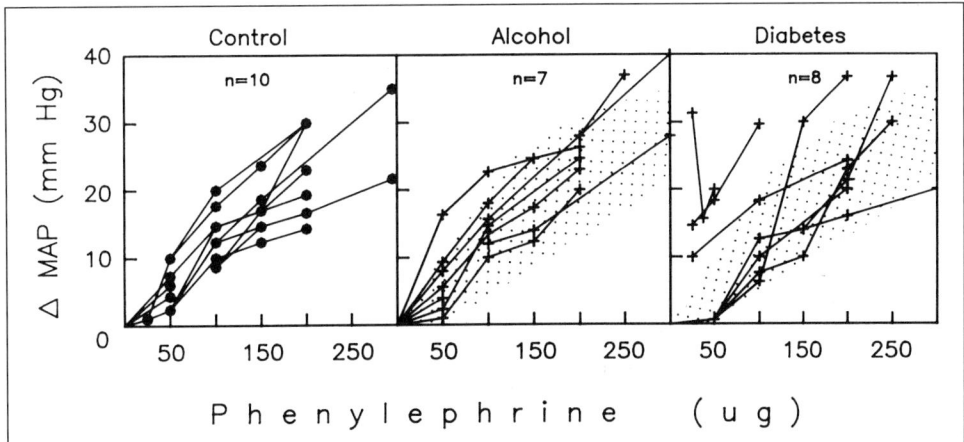

FIG. 4. The change in mean arterial pressure (δ*MAP*) with graded doses of intravenous phenylephrine in control and diabetic subjects. *Shaded area* indicates control range. (From Low PA, Walsh JC, Huang CY, McLeod JG. The autonomic nervous system in alcoholic and diabetic neuropathy. *Proc Aust Assoc Neurol* 1975;12:145–150. Reprinted with permission.)

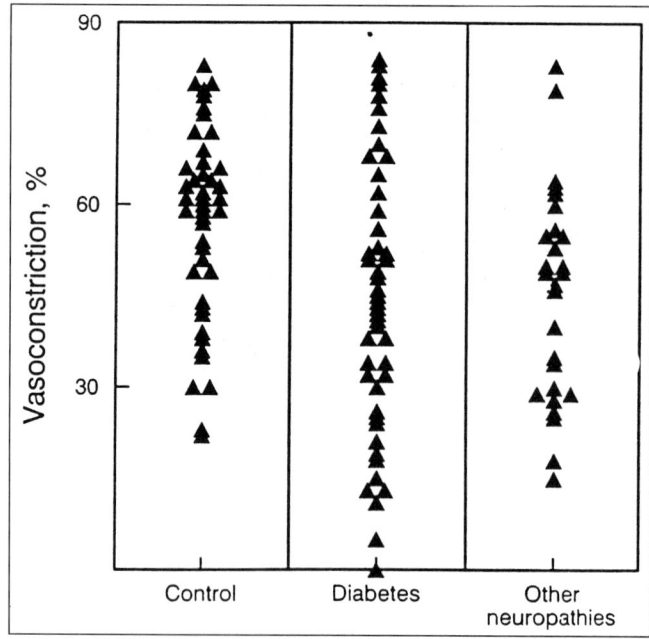

FIG. 5. The venoarteriolar reflex in controls, patients with diabetic neuropathy, and patients with other neuropathies. (From Moy S, Opfer-Gehrking TL, Proper CJ, Low PA. The venoarteriolar reflex in diabetic and other neuropathies. *Neurology* 1989;39:1490–1492. Reprinted with permission.)

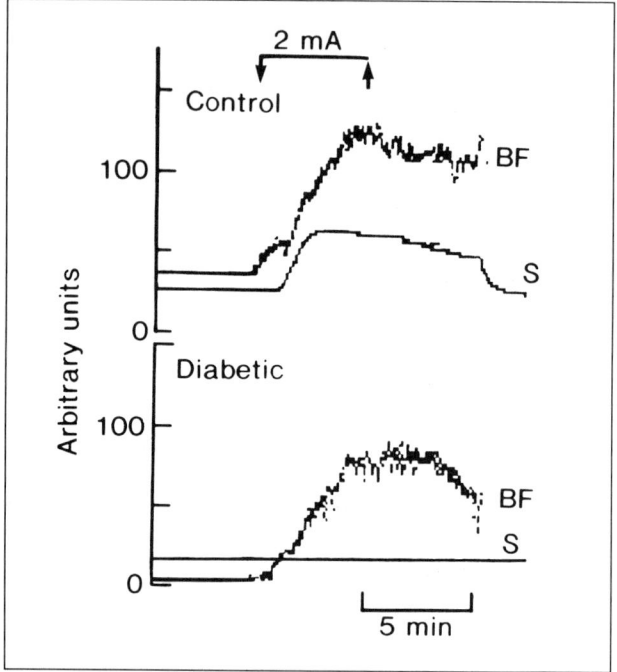

FIG. 6. Simultaneous recordings of blood flow (*BF*) and sudomotor QSART (*S*) responses to the iontophoresis of acetylcholine in a normal subject (*upper panel*) and an age-matched and sex-matched diabetic patient (*lower panel*). (From Benarroch and Low, ref. 20. Reprinted with permission.)

a clinical test and is a less reliable test of autonomic function than the QSART or HR_{DB} or the VM.

The neurogenic flare response (Chapter 15) is also reported to be diminished in neuropathic diabetic patients (9,164). The advantage of the test is that a laser flow probe can be installed in the recording compartment of the multicompartmental sweat cell during QSART and the sudomotor and blood flow responses simultaneously recorded. Unfortunately, the flare response has a much lower sensitivity and specificity than QSART and is not likely to detect the majority of patients with impairment of polymodal C nociceptor function (20). The flare response is often preserved when QSART is abolished (Fig. 6).

Pupillary Function

Recently there has been increased interest in nonpharmacologic pupillometric evaluation. Tests have included infrared recording of the dark-adapted pupil diameter, light-reflex amplitude, light-reflex latency, velocity of redilation, and pupil cycle time. Dark-adapted pupil size has been suggested to be a good quantitative measure of sympathetic function (114,165,191), especially following parasympathetic blockade (165). The test has high sensitivity, specificity, and reproducibility. Pupil diameter is measured using an infrared pupillometer or a simple polaroid pupillometer (188). The absolute size of pupil diameter can be measured from photographic enlargements, or pupil diameter percent can be determined ([horizontal pupil diameter/ horizontal iris diameter] $\times$ 100). Pupil diameter is greatly age-dependent (188).

The magnitude of the light reflex is rather variable, being affected by the initial size of the pupil, and is independent of age. The test appears to lack the sensitivity of dark-adapted pupil size and pupil cycle time.

The time course of pupilloconstriction has been used to evaluate diabetic autonomic neuropathy (165,191). The latency and maximal velocity of pupilloconstriction are affected by the amplitude of the response (189). These workers suggest that the velocity of redilation may be preferable as a test and provides a reliable index of sympathetic function (189).

Pupil cycle time, another index of parasympathetic function (147), is the frequency of oscillations of the pupil in response to a light stimulus. This frequency is reduced in diabetic autonomic neuropathy (147). Its utility as a test is uncertain.

Gastrointestinal Neuropathy

Diabetic neuropathy may affect any organ in the gastrointestinal tract. Although gastric atony and diabetic diarrhea are well-known, these clinical symptoms are relatively rare. Lesser degrees of autonomic failure are often detectable when motility studies are performed (Chapters 12 and 45).

Disorders of the Esophagus

Clinical symptoms of esophageal disease are extremely rare in diabetes. Motor dysfunction, characterized by an absent or markedly decreased primary peristaltic wave with delayed esophageal emptying, has been described in long-term diabetic patients (204). Decreased pressure of the lower esophageal sphincter and gastroesophageal reflux have been reported in selected diabetic patients with autonomic neuropathy (111). Neuropathologic findings consist of degeneration or absence of the extrinsic and intrinsic parasympathetic fibers of the esophagus. No evidence has been found, however, for denervation hypersensitivity of the esophageal muscle in diabetic patients with autonomic neuropathy (128).

Gastric Neuropathy

The most striking symptom of gastric involvement in diabetic neuropathy is atony and delayed gastric emptying. Generally, gastric motor abnormalities occur in 20%–30% of diabetic patients, often without clinical manifestations (119). Nausea, early satiety, postprandial bloating, and diffuse epigastric pain are the most frequent complaints. There is a relatively poor concordance between symptoms and gastroparesis. For instance, almost 60% of patients attending a diabetes clinic had such symptoms, but fewer than 10% were found to have gastroparesis, whereas up to 25% of brittle diabetic patients had gastroparesis, and these patients were often asymptomatic (4). Weight loss is common in some studies but not others (4,212), and a gastric splash may be elicited (212). In advanced cases, protracted vomiting is encountered (92). The methods generally employed in the diagnosis of gastric atony in diabetes were previously confined to barium meal examination. Abnormalities include gastric dilatation, delayed emptying, decreased peristalsis, a patulous pylorus, and an atonic duodenal bulb (110,119). In recent years, several methods have been developed for scintigraphic measurements of gastrointestinal transit (4,91,206) (Chapters 12 and 45).

The etiology of gastroparesis is incompletely known. Vagal function is impaired pathologically (95,130), and functionally as gastric acid secretion to hypoglycemia (113) and sham feeding (82). Motility studies suggest that sympathetic function may also be impaired (31). Other mechanisms, such as hyperglycemia *per se*, may also affect gastric emptying (10).

Intestinal Neuropathy

The most prominent symptom of intestinal neuropathy is diabetic diarrhea. Diabetic diarrhea can be sudden, explosive, paroxysmal, nocturnal, seasonal, uncontrollable, and often embarrassing (13). Surprisingly, it does not lead to severe malnutrition and tends to be self-limiting. Although several mechanisms have been postulated to be operative in the pathophysiology of this condition, diarrhea is essentially unexplained in diabetic neuropathy (144). Clinical signs of autonomic neuropathy are a common finding in these patients, and most patients with diarrhea have had such symptoms for a long period before the development of diarrhea. The usual causes of prolonged diarrhea must always be excluded in these patients. Chronic pancreatitis, gluten intolerance, and infections should be considered among the etiologic possibilities in patients with diabetic diarrhea. Thus, the diagnosis of diabetic diarrhea is one of exclusion. The patients usually experience profuse watery diarrhea that often persists for several days. Fecal incontinence is not uncommon. Although the pathogenesis of diabetic diarrhea with or without steatorrhea has not been clearly established, several mechanisms involving autonomic neuropathy, bacterial overgrowth, and pancreatic exocrine insufficiency as well as intestinal mucosal ischemia have been postulated as pathogenic factors. Radiologic transit studies have demonstrated both increased and decreased transit times in these patients (182). By means of the breath hydrogen test, it has been shown that small-bowel transit time in diabetic patients with autonomic neuropathy is significantly longer than transit time in patients without complications (180,181).

In the majority of patients with diabetic diarrhea, the intestinal mucosa functions in a normal manner despite significant steatorrhea (26). The absorption of xylose and of sodium and water is usually normal (208). In patients with grossly prolonged transit time, bacterial overgrowth within the intestinal lumen is a plausible explanation of diarrhea. This may represent a situation analogous to the blind-loop syndrome. Bacterial overgrowth results in deconjugation of bile salts, with defective micellar formation and fat malabsorption. Deconjugated bile salts are not actively reabsorbed by the distal ileum, and excessive amounts are discharged into the colon, where they may impair the absorption of water (180,181). It has also been claimed that a specific defect of small-bowel bile salts exists in patients with diabetic diarrhea (153).

Intestinal mucosal ischemia resulting from microangiopathy has been postulated as a cause of diabetic diarrhea. However, to date no specific lesion of the small-intestinal microvasculature has been demonstrated in diabetic patients. Other potential mechanisms, such as hypersecretion of gastrointestinal hormones, are attractive, but these have not been studied in any systematic fashion in patients with diabetic diarrhea.

Whenever bacterial overgrowth is demonstrated, antibiotic treatment is required. For the treatment of diarrhea sometimes seen in diabetic autonomic neuropathy, 250 to 500 mg of tetracycline as a single dose at onset of the diarrheal attack may abort symptoms dramatically in about half of cases (144). Recently, it has been demonstrated that erythromycin is sometimes effective in diabetic diarrhea. This drug also acts as a motilin agonist. Cholestyramine may be tried; it has been used to treat diarrhea after vagotomy, but its effectiveness has been questioned. Clonidine improves fluid absorption in experimental diabetes and has been reported to reduce diabetic diarrhea in humans (81).

Fecal incontinence is a most disturbing symptom of diabetic rectal neuropathy. It creates awkward situations for patients, who have to use pads. Function is evaluated using anorectal manometry, which quantitates maximal basal sphincter pressure and the rectoanal reflex. The rectal wall is distended with an inflated balloon, causing reflex relaxation of the internal anal sphincter.

Constipation is the most prominent colonic manifestation of gastrointestinal neuropathy in diabetes (120). This may be caused by extensive denervation of the colon, as denervation of the lower intestinal tract in the experimental animal resulted in obstipation (16).

Enck et al. (63) compared the frequency of gastrointestinal symptoms in 190 diabetic patients and 180 nondiabetic healthy subjects serving as (matched) controls. They compared IDDM with NIDDM patients. There were no differences in prevalence of symptoms that could be referred to the upper and lower gastrointestinal tract in type 1 diabetic patients in comparison with controls. NIDDM patients had significantly more constipation and nausea than normal subjects.

Diabetic Cystopathy

The prevalence of diabetic cystopathy varies in different studies from 20%–80% of patients with IDDM. Like many other complications of long-term diabetes, diabetic cystopathy is related to the duration of the disease. The majority of patients with diabetic cystopathy have prominent signs of other complications of long-term diabetes (88). The clinical symptoms of diabetic cystopathy include increased residual urine volume, overflow incontinence, and secondary infections, which may ultimately lead to pyelonephritis and uremia.

Intravenous urography demonstrates a large bladder with hydroureters. A large amount of residual urine remains after an attempt to void. A residual urine volume in excess of 100 mL is abnormal. In addition, vesicourethral reflux is found in a large percentage of patients (88).

One of the most important parameters in the diabetic neurogenic bladder is the volume of residual urine (62). The volume of residual urine is probably a determinant of urologic complications in diabetes, although the exact volume that induces these complications has not been precisely established. On cystometry, bladder filling is normally associated with a gradual increase in intravesical pressure; the first awareness of bladder fullness occurs somewhere between 100 and 200 mL, and discomfort occurs between 300 to 500 mL. In diabetic cystopathy, a bladder filling to between 300 and 500 mL results in only a slight rise in intravesical pressure. When asked to void, the voluntary voiding spike of between 40 and 80 mL of water seen in normal subjects is absent. An areflexic and atonic pattern with absence of sensation of bladder fullness and a marked increase in bladder capacity is found in the diabetic neurogenic bladder. Bladder capacities of more than 2 L are not uncommonly encountered in these patients. Results of the bethanechol test, in which 5 mg of this muscarinic agonist is administered subcutaneously and the cystometrogram then repeated, are considered positive if intravesical pressure rises >20 cm H_2O above the pre-bethanechol value. A positive test result indicates denervation supersensitivity caused by postganglionic efferent denervation. The sensitivity and specificity of the test are not known.

Uroflowmetry, which provides a quantitative measurement of urine flow, is useful in differentiating among the various causes of a voiding dysfunction. Maximal flow, average flow, flow patterns, and flow duration are obtained by this method. In diabetics, two patterns have been observed: In the first, there is a low peak flow and a prolonged duration of voiding; in the second group, a prolonged intermittent flow pattern is seen, resulting from the need for abdominal straining to void. This pattern is very often seen in patients with diabetic neurogenic bladder. Normally, a peak flow of approximately 30 mL/s is expected; in patients with neurogenic bladder, peak flow values of 10 mL/s are not uncommon (207). Evoked potential studies are also available and are described elsewhere (7) (Chapter 10).

Impotence

Impotence in diabetic male patients is well recognized (57,174,175) and common, being often the first manifestation of autonomic failure. It is initially partial and becomes complete within 1 to 2 years (150). The mechanism of impotence is likely to be a combination of autonomic neuropathy and accelerated atherosclerotic involvement of the internal pudendal artery. Penile systolic BP (118) and penile pulse amplitude (12) are decreased. Erection requires a normal function of the nerves innervating the vascular bed in the corpora cavernosa, as well as an intrinsic capacity of the vessels to dilate. Impotence in diabetic men may be related in part to impaired neurogenic and endothelium-mediated relaxation of penile smooth muscle (178). In addition to the role of neuropathy and angiopathy in long-term diabetes, the quality of metabolic control also has an influence on erectile function (3).

In addition to autonomic failure, somatic sensory impairment may contribute to erectile failure. Patients may have impaired perception of touch and pressure and reduced perception of testicular pain (76). Histopathologic alterations of autonomic fibers to the corpora cavernosa have been reported (185). Tissue concentrations of vasoactive intestinal peptide (93) and norepinephrine (151) have been described for human corpora cavernosa in diabetic impotence. Once established, diabetic impotence is usually irreversible (150). Diabetic neuropathic impotence is usually associated with an intact libido, although this may be lost later (78).

The mechanism of ejaculation is detailed in Chapter 11. Retrograde ejaculation may uncommonly occur in diabetic patients with selective sympathetic failure (61). The patient has the sensation of ejaculation but no ejaculate appears. When the patient voids, urine may appear milky, and spermatozoa are seen in urine. Lesser degrees of ejaculatory failure are much more common (78). Decreased volume of ejaculate may be caused by parasympathetic failure.

There have been fewer studies of sexual function in female patients. Orgasmic failure has been reported, but most studies suggest that the female sexual response in either intact (59,116) or only mildly impaired (200). Studies of female sexual dysfunction using vaginal plethysmography to measure lubrication and vaginal flushing hold promise but are not well established.

NATURAL HISTORY OF DIABETIC AUTONOMIC NEUROPATHY

Information on the natural history of diabetic autonomic neuropathy is limited, as previous studies have not been population-based and have not used approaches of known sensitivity, specificity, and reproducibility. The two best studies to date are those of Pirart (167,168) and Palumbo et al. (163). The first was based on more than 4000 diabetic patients who attended hospital clinics in Brussels. However, the study was not population-based and did not focus on autonomic neuropathy. The second was population-based, but the data regarding neuropathy were abstracted from medical records and autonomic neuropathy was not a specific focus. Palumbo et al. (163) reported a cumulative incidence of neuropathy of 4% in 5 years and 15% in 15 years of follow-up of 995 adult-onset diabetic patients in Olmsted County. Clinical autonomic neuropathy was seen in only 0.3%.

The ongoing NIH-funded Rochester Diabetic Neuropathy Study, now in its 12th year, is population-based; it utilizes autonomic, sensory, pathologic, and electrophysiologic tests of well-validated sensitivity and specificity and is beginning to generate important new information. A cohort of 380 diabetic patients from Rochester, Minnesota, are being studied prospectively. Initial results have shown that within a 2-year period results of autonomic function tests deteriorated as follows:

IDDM: HR_{DB}, 2.05 beats/min ($p = .005$); VR, 0.03 ($p = .568$); QSART (foot), 0.17 L ($p = .073$).

NIDDM: HR_{DB}, 1.56 beats/min ($p < .001$); VR, 0.02 ($p = .293$); QSART (foot), 0.10 L ($p = .075$).

Clinical or laboratory evidence of autonomic neuropathy is usually not evident at the inception of the diabetic state and is usually absent in the first 10 years, although this has been questioned (see section on cardiovascular reflexes in diabetes). After 10 to 15 years, measurable signs of autonomic neuropathy develop in about 30% of insulin-treated diabetic patients (66). Clinical autonomic failure is less common, occurring in about 5% of the diabetic population, but the frequency is extremely variable, reflecting the referral and selection bias of study populations. The symptoms increase with duration and severity of peripheral neuropathy and with age (27,41,66,71,74,142,158). Common symptoms are orthostatic lightheadedness, impotence (57), retrograde ejaculation (61), diarrhea (144), bladder problems, and sudomotor dysfunction, including gustatory sweating. The type of symptoms reported has also greatly varied. For instance, Rundles (174,175) reviewed the clinical features of 125 cases and found constipation (42%) >bladder complaints (26%) >diarrhea (22%) >sudomotor failure in the feet (10%) >orthostatic syncope (6%). Aagenaes (2) emphasized hypoglycemia unawareness (7%), although this is not related to classic autonomic failure (106,177). Fernandez-Castaner et al. (83) and Canal et al. (33) reported prevalences of 29% and 28%, respectively. Impotence is very common and increases with increasing age and duration of diabetes. An overall prevalence of 35% is representative of reported prevalences and increases with age (148) and duration (149,150) of diabetes. It is probably caused by a combination of autonomic failure and vascular disease (57,61,202). Once abnormal tests results are present, they progressively worsen, with rare exceptions.

Although it is generally agreed that autonomic failure causes significant morbidity, there is greater controversy regarding its impact on mortality. Ewing et al. (70) reported a mortality rate of 50% at $2\frac{1}{2}$ years in patients with symptomatic autonomic neuropathy. However, these patients had long-standing clinical autonomic neuropathy and died of renal failure. Other subsequent studies have found a somewhat better prognosis. Sampson et al. (179), in a 10- to 15-year follow-up of 111 patients, found a better prognosis. The 10-year survival of patients with clinical autonomic neuropathy (73%) was significantly worse than that of patient with abnormal HR variability (90%). The latter had a normal 10-year survival. Worsening in RR interval variability of patients with isolated cardiovascular reflex abnormalities at the beginning of the study did occur, with a decline of 1.02 beats/year. This latter study excluded patients with renal failure and with clinical features of autonomic failure for longer than 2 years when first seen. A reduction of about one beat per year in RR variability has been found in other studies, including the Rochester Diabetic Study (see above). Similar results were reported in a small retrospective study (35 patients with and the same number without cardiovascular autonomic failure) by Rathmann et al. (171). They reported an estimated 8-year survival rate in patients with autonomic neuropathy of

77%, compared with 97% in those with normal autonomic function ($p < .05$). Deaths were mainly caused by macrovascular diseases or were sudden unexpected deaths.

QT lengthening in diabetes has been reported to be associated with a poorer prognosis and has been suggested to be associated with sudden deaths (18,19,37,65). A prolonged QT interval is associated with sudden death in other diseases (184,205). In the congenital "long QT syndrome," in which sudden death sometimes occurs, it has been postulated that there is underactivity of the right stellate ganglion and overactivity of the left stellate ganglion, resulting in QT lengthening and increased myocardial irritability, which may lead to sustained ventricular arrhythmias (184). QT lengthening is associated with autonomic RR interval abnormalities (19) and increases with duration of diabetes (65,117), but not in normal subjects.

PATHOGENESIS

The pathogenesis of diabetic autonomic neuropathy is not completely known. Hyperglycemia is clearly important. The pattern of autonomic involvement of acute onset with relative sparing of somatic fibers seen in some patients with acute diabetic autonomic neuropathy, and the presence of antibodies to sympathetic neurons (Chapter 38), suggest the involvement of immune mechanisms in at least this subset. Genetic, metabolic, ischemic (134), and growth factors may also be involved. A detailed description of pathogenesis is beyond the scope of this book.

TREATMENT

Treatment of diabetic neuropathy can be considered under three broad categories: prevention, treatment of established neuropathy, and treatment of complications.

Prevention of Diabetic Neuropathy

Until the cause and cure of diabetic neuropathy become known, prevention is based on certain assumptions. The principle of the optimal maintenance of euglycemia and normal lipid levels and weight is reasonable and based on the likely pivotal importance of persistent hyperglycemia. The Diabetes Control and Complications Trial (DCCT), which studied 1441 patients with IDDM for 10 years, has been completed. This is an outstanding study in several respects; 99% of patients completed the study, and 98% and 97% of patients in the conventional and tight control limbs, respectively, were able to abide by the study treatment requirements. Glycosylated hemoglobin was significantly reduced in the experimental group, although only 5% achieved values that fell within the control range. The patients with multiple insulin injections by year 3 had a significantly reduced rate of development of all three complications (neuropathy, retinopathy, and nephropathy). The development of clinical neuropathy was reduced by 60%. Of importance is the progressive divergence of the conventional and stringent control groups. The main complication with tight control was a threefold increase in hypoglycemic complications.

In view of the accumulating evidence for microvascular ischemia, the prevention of microangiopathy is desirable and is likely to be optimally effective when combined with control of hyperglycemia. A detailed description is premature and beyond the scope of this chapter. Possible avenues include the following: (a) maintenance of euglycemia, with normalization of risk factors such as smoking and hypertension and maintenance of ideal weight and adequate exercise regimens; (b) avoidance of hyperinsulinemia, which, with exogenous insulin, may be atherogenic, especially to microvessels (reviewed in ref. 134); (c) consideration of vasodilator therapy alone (43) or combined with prostaglandins (prostaglandin E_1; prostacyclin analogs), which have also a platelet antiaggregant effect; (d) administration of efamol, as a reduction in n-6 essential fatty acids may be important in etiopathogenesis (115). Other possibilities include the use of aldose reductase inhibitors, growth factors, α-lipoic acid (215), and methylcobalamin. A detailed description of these approaches is beyond the scope of this chapter.

Treatment of Established Neuropathy

The general measures to be employed involve prevention of the complications of reduced sensation (Table 7) and include the following: (a) avoidance of abuse of joints with impaired sensation, especially deep sensation, which is important to prevent the development of neuropathic joints; (b) avoidance of trauma to skin, necessary to prevent ulceration; (c) avoidance of cold and heat injury.

Measures focused on autonomic failure include the avoidance of bladder infection and the treatment of ortho-

TABLE 7. *Treatment of established neuropathy*

Preventing complications of reduced sensation
    Avoiding abuse of joints
    Avoiding trauma to skin
    Avoiding cold and heat injury
Treating the consequences of autonomic failure
    Avoiding bladder infection
    Treating orthostatic hypotension
    Treating diarrhea
    Treating gastroparesis
    Treating impotence
    Treating pain
    Treating specific subsets of neuropathy

static hypotension, diarrhea, gastroparesis, impotence, and pain. Treatment of these symptoms is covered in the respective chapters. In addition, the treatment of specific subsets of neuropathy may need to be individualized. The treatment of specific aspects of autonomic failure is covered in the respective chapters.

The treatment of orthostatic hypotension is described in Chapter 55. Plasma volume expansion by 9-α-fludrohydrocortisone (Florinef) is important and has been shown to have an effect on BP measurements (32,183). However, fludrocortisone in high doses is potentially dangerous, as cardiac dysfunction resulting from diabetic angiopathy may be present. Cardiac decompensation and stroke have been reported in patients treated with fludrocortisone for diabetic orthostatic hypotension (40). Plasma expansion by an increase in salt intake or the use of prostaglandin inhibitors (such as ibuprofen or indomethacin) may sometimes be effective (159), as might be the Jobst stocking and behavioral modification (159). Finally, beta blockers with intrinsic sympathomimetic activity have been suggested for the treatment of orthostatic hypotension (145); this treatment has not, however, been confirmed in more systematic studies (47).

The treatment of symptomatic upper gastrointestinal symptoms in diabetic autonomic neuropathy is unsatisfactory (see also Chapter 45). Antiemetics may provide temporal relief of nausea. Small meals are generally encouraged. Ten milligrams of metoclopramide taken three times daily $\frac{1}{2}$ to 1 hr before meals may be helpful and is the mainstay of treatment, being more effective than other cholinergic agents, such as bethanecol. It is a dopamine antagonist with central antiemetic effects. Involuntary movements may occur at higher doses. Extrapyramidal side effects, such as acute dystonic reactions and tardive dyskinesia, may also occur at higher doses.

Treatment of the neurogenic bladder is detailed in Chapter 46. In diabetes, behavior modification with scheduled voiding and instruction in double or triple voiding techniques to compensate for the lack of desire to void are very important and will help diminish the amount of residual urine. The use of a small-diameter urethral catheter may be necessary for varying periods of time during treatment of the hypotonic bladder. Patients are instructed to do self-catheterization, and this is found to be a more efficient way of reducing the residual urinary volume than is pharmacologic treatment with bethanechol and phenoxybenzamine. Finally, in patients with a dilated bladder, a transurethral resection of the prostate may be required to reduce resistance to flow at the bladder neck and prostatic area; sometimes this may be all that is needed to decrease or abolish the presence of residual urine.

As for any patients with impotence, psychologic factors are important, and careful counseling of patients and their partners is an important aspect of treatment. In selected cases, the use of a penile prosthesis has been used with success. In recent years, self-injection with papaverine or prostaglandin E in the corpora cavernosa has been shown to be effective.

REFERENCES

1. The effect of intensive treatment of diabetes on the development and progression of long-term complications in insulin-dependent diabetes mellitus. The Diabetes Control and Complications Trial Research Group. *N Engl J Med* 1993;329:977–986.
2. Aagenaes *Neurovascular Examinations on the Lower Extremities in Young Diabetics, with Special Reference to the Autonomic Neuropathy.* Copenhagen: C Hamburgers Bogtrykkeri A/S; 1962.
3. Abelson D. Diagnostic value of the penile pulse and blood pressure: a Doppler study of impotence in diabetics. *J Urol* 1975;113:636–639.
4. Achem-Karam SR, et al. Plasma motilin concentration and interdigestive migrating motor complex in diabetic gastroparesis: effect of metoclopramide. *Gastroenterology* 1985;88:492–499.
5. Akselrod S, et al. Hemodynamic regulation: investigation by spectral analysis. *Am J Physiol* 1985;249:H867–H875.
6. Allen JM, Bloom SR. Neuropeptide Y: a putative neurotransmitter. *Neurochem Int* 1986;8:1–8.
7. Andersen JT, Bradley WE. Early detection of diabetic visceral neuropathy. An electrophysiologic study of bladder and urethral innervation. *Diabetes* 1976;25:1100–1105.
8. Archer AG, et al. The natural history of acute painful neuropathy in diabetes mellitus. *J Neurol Neurosurg Psychiatry* 1983;46:491–499.
9. Aronin N, et al. Diminished flare response in neuropathic diabetic patients. Comparison of effects of substance P, histamine, and capsaicin. *Diabetes* 1987;36:1139–1143.
10. Aylett P. Gastric emptying and changes in the blood sugar level as affected by glucagon and insulin. *Clin Sci* 1962;22:171–178.
11. Baldwa VS, Ewing DJ. Heart rate response to Valsalva manoeuvre. Reproducibility in normals, and relation to variation in resting heart rate in diabetics. *Br Heart J* 1977;39:641–644.
12. Bancroft J, et al. Assessment of erectile function in diabetic and non-diabetic impotence by simultaneous recording of penile diameter and penile arterial pulse. *J Psychosom Res* 1985;29:315–324.
13. Barnett JL, Vinik AI. Gastrointestinal disturbances. In: Lebovitz AE, ed. *Therapy for Diabetes Mellitus and Related Disorders.* Alexandria, VA: American Diabetes Association; 1991:279–287.
14. Baser SM, et al. Sudomotor function in autonomic failure. *Neurology* 1991;41:1564–1566.
15. Bastron JA, Thomas JE. Diabetic polyradiculopathy: clinical and electromyographic findings in 105 patients. *Mayo Clin Proc* 1981;56:725–732.
16. Battle WM, et al. Colonic dysfunction in diabetes mellitus. *Gastroenterology* 1980;79:1217–1221.
17. Bellavere F, et al. Evidence of early impairment of parasympathetic reflexes in insulin-dependent diabetics without autonomic symptoms. *Diabete Metab* 1985;11:152–156.
18. Bellavere F, et al. Analysis of QT versus RR ECG interval variations in diabetic patients shows a longer QT period in subjects with autonomic neuropathy. *Diabetologia* 1984;27:255(abst).
19. Bellavere F, et al. Prolonged QT period in diabetic autonomic neuropathy: a possible role in sudden cardiac death?. *Br Heart J* 1988;59:379–383.
20. Benarroch EE, Low PA. The acetylcholine-induced flare response in evaluation of small fiber dysfunction. *Ann Neurol* 1991;29:590–595.
21. Benarroch EE, et al. Noradrenergic and neuropeptide Y mechanisms in guanethidine-sympathectomized rats. *Am J Physiol* 1990;259:R371–R375.
22. Bennett T, et al. Assessment of methods for estimating autonomic nervous control of the heart in patients with diabetes mellitus. *Diabetes* 1978;27:1167–1174.
23. Bennett T, et al. Assessment of vagal control of the heart in diabetes. Measures of R-R interval variation under different conditions. *Br Heart J* 1977;39:25–28.

24. Bennett T, et al. Baroreflex sensitivity and responses to the Valsalva manoeuvre in subjects with diabetes mellitus. *J Neurol Neurosurg Psychiatry* 1976;39:178–183.
25. Bennett T, et al. Cardiovascular reflex responses to apnoeic face immersion and mental stress in diabetic subjects. *Cardiovasc Res* 1976;10:192–199.
26. Berge KG, et al. The intestinal tract in diabetic diarrhea. *Diabetes* 1956;5:289–294.
27. Bergstrom B, et al. Autonomic nerve function tests. Reference values in healthy subjects. *Clin Physiol* 1986;6:523–528.
28. Bernardi L, et al. Cross-correlation of heart rate and respiration versus deep breathing. Assessment of new test of cardiac autonomic function in diabetes. *Diabetes* 1989;38:589–596.
29. Bolli GB, et al. A reliable and reproducible test for adequate glucose counterregulation in type I diabetes mellitus. *Diabetes* 1984;33:732–737.
30. Burgos LG, et al. Increased intraoperative cardiovascular morbidity in diabetics with autonomic neuropathy. *Anesthesiology* 1989;70:591–597.
31. Camilleri M, Malagelada JR. Abnormal intestinal motility in diabetics with the gastroparesis syndrome. *Eur J Clin Invest* 1984;14:420–427.
32. Campbell IW, et al. Therapeutic experience with fludrocortisone in diabetic postural hypotension. *Br Med J* 1976;1:872–874.
33. Canal N, et al. The relationship between peripheral and autonomic neuropathy in insulin-dependent diabetes: a clinical and instrumental evaluation. In: Canal N, Pozza G, eds. *Peripheral Neuropathies*. Amsterdam: Elsevier North-Holland; 1978:247–255.
34. Caravati CM. Insulin neuritis. A case report. *Va Med Mo* 1933;59:745–746.
35. Cardone C, et al. Cough test to assess cardiovascular autonomic reflexes in diabetes. *Diabetes Care* 1990;13:719–724.
36. Casey EB, Harrison MJ. Diabetic amyotrophy: a follow-up study. *Br Med J* 1972;1:656–659.
37. Chambers JB, et al. QT prolongation on the electrocardiogram in diabetic autonomic neuropathy (see comments). *Diabet Med* 1990;7:105–110.
38. Christensen NJ, et al. Plasma dihydroxyphenylglycol (DHPG) as an index of diabetic autonomic neuropathy. *Clin Physiol* 1988;8:577–580.
39. Christensen NJ, et al. *The Sympathoadrenal System*. Copenhagen: Munksgaard; 1986.
40. Christensen NJ, Hilsted J. Treatment of orthostatic hypotension (Review). *Clin Physiol* 1985;5(Suppl 5):94–96.
41. Clarke BF, et al. Diabetic autonomic neuropathy (Review). *Diabetologia* 1979;17:195–212.
42. Cornblath DR, et al. Demyelinating motor neuropathy in patients with diabetic polyneuropathy. *Ann Neurol* 1987;22:126(abst).
43. Cotter MA, et al. Effects of chronic alpha-adrenoceptor blockade on nerve function and vascular supply in diabetic rats. *Diabetologia* 1990;33:A92(abst).
44. Cryer PE. Glucose counterregulation in man (Review). *Diabetes* 1981;30:261–264.
45. Cryer PE. Iatrogenic hypoglycemia as a cause of hypoglycemia-associated autonomic failure in IDDM. A vicious cycle. *Diabetes* 1992;41:255–260.
46. De Calvi M. *Recherches sur les Accidents Diabétiques et Essai d'une Théorie Générale du Diabète*. Paris: P Asselin; 1864.
47. Dejgaard A, Hilsted J. No effect of pindolol on postural hypotension in type 1 (insulin-dependent) diabetic patients with autonomic neuropathy. A randomised double-blind controlled study. *Diabetologia* 1988;31:281–284.
48. Dejgaard A, et al. Noradrenaline and isoproterenol kinetics in diabetic patients with and without autonomic neuropathy. *Diabetologia* 1986;29:773–777.
49. Dejgaard A, et al. Plasma adrenaline kinetics in type 1 (insulin-dependent) diabetic patients with and without autonomic neuropathy. *Diabetologia* 1989;32:810–813.
50. Dejgaard A, et al. Adrenergic receptors are a fallible index of adrenergic denervation hypersensitivity. *Scand J Clin Lab Invest* 1991;51:659–666.
51. Dyck PJ, et al. The Rochester Diabetic Neuropathy Study: reassessment of tests and criteria for diagnosis and staged severity. *Neurology* 1992;42:1164–1170.
52. Dyck PJ, et al. The prevalence by staged severity of various types of diabetic neuropathy, retinopathy, and nephropathy in a population-based cohort: the Rochester Diabetic Neuropathy Study. *Neurology* 1993;43:817–824.
53. Dyck PJ, et al. Nerve glucose, fructose, sorbitol, myo-inositol, and fiber degeneration and regeneration in diabetic neuropathy. *N Engl J Med* 1988;319:542–548.
54. Dyrberg T, et al. Prevalence of diabetic autonomic neuropathy measured by simple bedside tests. *Diabetologia* 1981;20:190–194.
55. Eldrup E, et al. Plasma dihydroxyphenylalanine (DOPA) is independent of sympathetic activity in humans. *Eur J Clin Invest* 1989;19:514–517.
56. Ellenberg M. Diabetic neuropathy precipitating after institution of diabetic control. *Am J Med Sci* 1958;236:466–471.
57. Ellenberg M. Impotence in diabetes: the neurologic factor. *Ann Intern Med* 1971;75:213–219.
58. Ellenberg M. Diabetic neuropathic cachexia. *Diabetes* 1974;23:418–423.
59. Ellenberg M. Sexual aspects of the female diabetic. *Mt Sinai J Med* 1977;44:495–500.
60. Ellenberg M. Diabetic truncal mononeuropathy—a new clinical syndrome. *Diabetes Care* 1978;1:10–13.
61. Ellenberg M, Weber H. Retrograde ejaculation in diabetic neuropathy. *Ann Intern Med* 1966;65:1237–1246.
62. Ellenberg M, Weber H. The incipient asymptomatic diabetic bladder. *Diabetes* 1967;16:331–335.
63. Enck P, et al. Prevalence of gastrointestinal symptoms in diabetic patients and non-diabetic subjects. *Z Gastroenterol* 1994;32:637–641.
64. Engelman K, Portnoy B. A sensitive double-isotope derivative assay for norepinephrine and epinephrine. Normal resting human plasma levels. *Circ Res* 1970;26:53–57.
65. Ewing DJ, et al. Autonomic neuropathy, QT interval lengthening, and unexpected deaths in male diabetic patients. *Diabetologia* 1991;34:182–185.
66. Ewing DJ, et al. Cardiac autonomic neuropathy in diabetes: comparison of measures of R-R interval variation. *Diabetologia* 1981;21:18–24.
67. Ewing DJ, et al. Abnormalities of ambulatory 24-hour heart rate in diabetes mellitus. *Diabetes* 1983;32:101–105.
68. Ewing DJ, et al. Vascular reflexes in diabetic autonomic neuropathy. *Lancet* 1973;2:1354–1356.
69. Ewing DJ, et al. The natural history of diabetic autonomic neuropathy. *Q J Med* 1980;49:95–108.
70. Ewing DJ, et al. Immediate heart rate response to standing: simple test of autonomic neuropathy in diabetes. *Br Med J* 1978;1:145–147.
71. Ewing DJ, Clarke BF. Diagnosis and management of diabetic autonomic neuropathy (Review). *Br Med J Clin Res Ed* 1982;285:916–918.
72. Ewing DJ, Clarke BF. Diabetic autonomic neuropathy: present insights and future prospects (Review). *Diabetes Care* 1986;9:648–665.
73. Ewing DJ, et al. Cardiovascular responses to sustained handgrip in normal subjects and in patients with diabetes mellitus: a test of autonomic function. *Clin Sci Mol Med* 1974;46:295–306.
74. Ewing DJ, et al. The value of cardiovascular autonomic function tests: 10 years' experience in diabetes. *Diabetes Care* 1985;8:491–498.
75. Ewing DJ, Winney R. Autonomic function in patients with chronic renal failure on intermittent haemodialysis. *Nephron* 1975;15:424–429.
76. Fagius J. Sympathetic reflex latencies and conduction velocoties in diabetic polyneuropathy. *Clin Physiol* 1985;5(Suppl):49–53.
77. Fagius J, et al. Sympathetic outflow in man after anaesthesia of the glossopharyngeal and vagus nerves. *Brain* 1985;108:423–438.
78. Fairburn CG, et al. The clinical features of diabetic impotence: a preliminary study. *Br J Psychiatry* 1982;140:447–452.
79. Fealey RD. The thermoregulatory sweat test. In: Low PA, ed. *Clinical Autonomic Disorders: Evaluation and Management*. Boston: Little, Brown; 1993:217–229.
80. Fealey RD, et al. Thermoregulatory sweating abnormalities in diabetes mellitus. *Mayo Clin Proc* 1989;64:617–628.
81. Fedorak RN, et al. Treatment of diabetic diarrhea with clonidine. *Ann Intern Med* 1985;102:197–199.

82. Feldman M, et al. Abnormal gastric function in long-standing, insulin-dependent diabetic patients. *Gastroenterology* 1979;77:12–17.
83. Fernandez-Castaner M, et al. Prevalence and clinical aspects of cardiovascular vegetative neuropathy in a diabetic population. *Med Clin* 1985;84:215–218.
84. Fernandez-Castaner M, et al. Somatostatin and counterregulatory hormone responses to hypoglycaemia in diabetics with and without autonomic neuropathy. *Diabete Metab* 1985;11:81–86.
85. Ferrer MT, et al. Baroreflexes in patients with diabetes mellitus. *Neurology* 1991;41:1462–1466.
86. Fraser DM, et al. Peripheral and autonomic nerve function in newly diagnosed diabetes mellitus. *Diabetes* 1977;26:546–550.
87. Freeman R, et al. Spectral analysis of heart rate in diabetic autonomic neuropathy. A comparison with standard tests of autonomic function. *Arch Neurol* 1991;48:185–190.
88. Frimodt-Moller C. Diabetic cystopathy. A clinical study of the frequency of bladder. *Dan Med Bull* 1976;23:267–279.
89. Garland H. Diabetic amyotrophy. *Br Med J* 1955;2:1287–1290.
90. Gerich JE, et al. Lack of glucagon response to hypoglycemia in diabetes: evidence for an intrinsic pancreatic alpha cell defect. *Science* 1973;182:171–173.
91. Gilbey SG, Watkins PJ. Measurement by epigastric impedance of gastric emptying in diabetic autonomic neuropathy. *Diabet Med* 1987;4:122–126.
92. Goyal RK, Spiro HM. Gastrointestinal manifestations of diabetes mellitus (Review). *Med Clin North Am* 1971;55:1031–1044.
93. Gu J, et al. Decrease of vasoactive intestinal polypeptide (VIP) in the penises from impotent men. *Lancet* 1984;2:315–318.
94. Gundersen HJ, Neubauer B. A long-term diabetic autonomic nervous abnormality. Reduced variations in resting heart rate measured by a simple and sensitive method. *Diabetologia* 1977;13:137–140.
95. Guy RJ, et al. Diabetic gastroparesis from autonomic neuropathy: surgical considerations and changes in vagus nerve morphology. *J Neurol Neurosurg Psychiatry* 1984;47:686–691.
96. Henriksen JH, Christensen NJ. Plasma norepinephrine in humans: limitations in assessment of whole body norepinephrine kinetics and plasma clearance. *Am J Physiol* 1989;257:E743–750.
97. Hilsted J. Decreased sympathetic vasomotor tone in diabetic orthostatic hypotension. *Diabetes* 1979;28:970–973.
98. Hilsted J. Pathophysiology in diabetic autonomic neuropathy: cardiovascular, hormonal, and metabolic studies (Review). *Diabetes* 1982;31:730–737.
99. Hilsted J. Hormonal and metabolic dysfunction in diabetic autonomic neuropathy. *Fidia Res Ser* 1987;10:273–278.
100. Hilsted J, et al. Whole body clearance of norepinephrine. The significance of arterial sampling and of surgical stress. *J Clin Invest* 1983;71:500–505.
101. Hilsted J, et al. Impaired cardiovascular responses to graded exercise in diabetic autonomic neuropathy. *Diabetes* 1979;28:313–319.
102. Hilsted J, et al. Impaired responses of catecholamines, growth hormone, and cortisol to graded exercise in diabetic autonomic neuropathy. *Diabetes* 1980;29:257–262.
103. Hilsted J, et al. Haemodynamic changes during graded exercise in patients with diabetic autonomic neuropathy. *Diabetologia* 1982;22:318–323.
104. Hilsted J, et al. Hormonal and metabolic responses to exercise in insulin-dependent diabetics with and without autonomic neuropathy and in normal subjects. *Int J Sports Med* 1981;2:216–219.
105. Hilsted J, Jensen SB. A simple test for autonomic neuropathy in juvenile diabetics. *Acta Med Scand* 1979;205:385–387.
106. Hilsted J, et al. Hormonal, metabolic, and cardiovascular responses to hypoglycemia in diabetic autonomic neuropathy. *Diabetes* 1981;30:626–633.
107. Hilsted J, et al. No response of pancreatic hormones to hypoglycemia in diabetic autonomic neuropathy. *J Clin Endocrinol Metab* 1982;54:815–819.
108. Hilsted J, et al. Hemodynamics in diabetic orthostatic hypotension. *J Clin Invest* 1981;68:1427–1434.
109. Hilsted J, et al. Metabolic and cardiovascular responses to epinephrine in diabetic autonomic neuropathy. *N Engl J Med* 1987;317:421–426.
110. Hodges FJ, et al. Roentgenologic study of small intestine. 2. Dysfunction associated with neurologic disease. *Radiology* 1947;49:659–673.
111. Hollis JB, et al. Esophageal function in diabetes mellitus and its relation to peripheral neuropathy. *Gastroenterology* 1977;73:1098–1102.
112. Holst JJ. Neural regulation of pancreatic hormone secretion (Review). *Clin Physiol* 1985;5(Suppl 5):34–42.
113. Hosking DJ, et al. Vagal impairment of gastric secretion in diabetic autonomic neuropathy. *Br Med J* 1975;2:588–590.
114. Hreidarsson AB. Pupil size in insulin-dependent diabetes. Relationship to duration, metabolic control, and long-term manifestations. *Diabetes* 1982;31:442–448.
115. Jamal GA, et al. Gamma-linolenic acid in diabetic neuropathy (Letter). *Lancet* 1986;1:1098.
116. Jensen SB. Diabetic sexual dysfunction: a comparative study of 160 insulin-treated diabetic men and women and an age-matched control group. *Arch Sex Behav* 1981;10:493–504.
117. Jermendy G, et al. QT interval in diabetic autonomic neuropathy (Letter; Comment). *Diabet Med* 1990;7:750.
118. Karacan I. Diagnosis of erectile impotence in diabetes mellitus. An objective and specific method. *Ann Intern Med* 1980;92:334–337.
119. Kassander P. Asymptomatic gastric retention in diabetics (gastroparesis diabeticorum). *Ann Intern Med* 1958;48:797–812.
120. Katz LA, Spiro HM. Gastrointestinal manifestations of diabetes. *N Engl J Med* 1966;275:1350–1361.
121. Kennedy WR, Navarro X. Sympathetic sudomotor function in diabetic neuropathy. *Arch Neurol* 1989;46:1182–1186.
122. Kennedy WR, et al. Quantitation of the sweating deficit in diabetes mellitus. *Ann Neurol* 1984;15:482–488.
123. Kihara M, et al. Hypoxic effect of exogenous insulin on normal and diabetic peripheral nerve. *Am J Physiol* 1994;266:E980–E985.
124. Kitney RI, et al. Transient interactions between blood pressure, respiration and heart rate in man. *J Biomed Eng* 1985;7:217–224.
125. Knuttgen D, et al. Diabetic autonomic neuropathy: abnormal cardiovascular reactions under general anesthesia. *Klin Wochenschr* 1990;68:1168–1172.
126. Kooner JS, et al. Relationship between splanchnic vasodilation and postprandial hypotension in patients with primary autonomic failure. *J Hypertens Suppl* 1989;7:S40–S41.
127. Kopin I. *Catecholamine Metabolism (and the Biochemical Assessment of Sympathetic Activity)*. London: WB Saunders; 1977 (*Clinics in Endocrinology and Metabolism*).
128. Kramer P, Ingelfinger FJ. Esophageal sensitivity to mecholyl in cardiospasms. *Gastroenterology* 1968;54(Suppl):771–773.
129. Krarup T, et al. Impaired response of pancreatic polypeptide to hypoglycaemia: an early sign of autonomic neuropathy in diabetics. *Br Med J* 1979;2:1544–1546.
130. Kristensson K, et al. Changes in the vagus nerve in diabetes mellitus. *Acta Pathol Microbiol Scand* 1971;79:684–685.
131. Levy DM, et al. Assessment of basal and stimulated sweating in diabetes using a direct-reading computerized sudorometer. *Diabet Med* 1991;8:S78–S81.
132. Low PA. Composite autonomic scoring scale for laboratory quantification of generalized autonomic failure. *Mayo Clin Proc* 1993;68:748–752.
133. Low PA, et al. Quantitative sudomotor axon reflex test in normal and neuropathic subjects. *Ann Neurol* 1983;14:573–580.
134. Low PA, et al. Nerve blood flow and oxygen delivery in normal, diabetic, and ischemic neuropathy. *Int Rev Neurobiol* 1989;31:355–438.
135. Low PA, et al. The effect of aging on cardiac autonomic and postganglionic sudomotor function. *Muscle Nerve* 1990;13:152–157.
136. Low PA, et al. Subacute diabetic proximal motor neuropathy. *Neurology* 1996;46:A447(abst).
137. Low PA, Stevens JC. Peripheral neuropathies including autonomic neuropathies. In: Spittell JA, ed. *Clinical Medicine*. Hargerstown: Harper & Row; 1985.
138. Low PA, et al. The sympathetic nervous system in diabetic neuropathy. A clinical and pathological study. *Brain* 1975;98:341–356.
139. Low PA, et al. Ischemic conduction failure and energy metabolism in experimental diabetic neuropathy. *Am J Physiol* 1985;248:E457–E462.
140. Low PA, et al. Comparison of distal sympathetic with vagal function in diabetic neuropathy. *Muscle Nerve* 1986;9:592–596.
141. Lugari R, et al. Diabetic autonomic neuropathy and impaired human pancreatic polypeptide secretion in response to food. *J Clin Endocrinol Metab* 1987;64:279–282.

142. Mackay JD, et al. Diabetic autonomic neuropathy. The diagnostic value of heart rate monitoring. *Diabetologia* 1980;18:471–478.
143. Maher TD, et al. Lack of glucagon response to hypoglycemia in diabetic autonomic neuropathy. *Diabetes* 1977;26:196–200.
144. Malins JM, French JM. Diabetic diarrhoea. *Q J Med* 1957;26:467–480.
145. Man in't Veld AJ, Schalekamp MA. Pindolol acts as beta-adrenoceptor agonist in orthostatic hypotension: therapeutic implications. *Br Med J Clin Res Ed* 1981;282:929–931.
146. Mancia G, et al. Reflex cardiovascular regulation in humans. *J Cardiovasc Pharmacol* 1985;7(Suppl 3):S152–S159.
147. Martyn CN, Ewing DJ. Pupil cycle time—a simple way of measuring an autonomic reflex. *J Neurol Neurosurg Psychiatry* 1986;49:771–774.
148. Masaoka S, et al. Heart rate variability in diabetes: relationship to age and duration of the disease. *Diabetes Care* 1985;8:64–68.
149. McCulloch DK, et al. The prevalence of diabetic impotence. *Diabetologia* 1980;18:279–283.
150. McCulloch DK, et al. The natural history of impotence in diabetic men. *Diabetologia* 1984;26:437–440.
151. Melman A, Henry D. The possible role of the catecholamines of the corpora in penile erection. *J Urol* 1979;121:419–421.
152. Melton LJ, Dyck PJ. Epidemiology. In: Dyck PJ, Thomas PK, Asbury AK, Winegrad AI, Porte D, eds. *Diabetic Neuropathy*. Philadelphia: WB Saunders; 1987:27–35.
153. Molloy AM, Tomkin GH. Altered bile in diabetic diarrhoea. *Br Med J* 1978;2:1462–1463.
154. Mulder DW, et al. Hyperinsulin neuropathy. *Neurology* 1956;6:627–635.
155. Mulder DW, et al. The neuropathies associated with diabetes mellitus: a clinical and electromyographic study of 103 unselected diabetic patients. *Neurology* 1961;11:275–284.
156. Murray A, et al. RR interval variations in young male diabetics. *Br Heart J* 1985;37:882–885.
157. Newrick PG, et al. Sural nerve oxygen tension in diabetes. *Br Med J* 1986;293:1053–1054.
158. O'Brien IA, et al. The prevalence of autonomic neuropathy in insulin-dependent diabetes mellitus: a controlled study based on heart rate variability. *Q J Med* 1986;61:957–967.
159. Onrot J, et al. Management of chronic orthostatic hypotension (Review). *Am J Med* 1986;80:454–464.
160. Ostman J, et al. Increased lipolytic sensitivity to catecholamines in diabetics with severe autonomic neuropathy. *Diabetes Res Clin Pract* 1988;5(Suppl 1):S89(abst).
161. Pagani M, et al. Spectral analysis of heart rate variability in the assessment of autonomic diabetic neuropathy. *J Auton Nerv Syst* 1988;23:143–153.
162. Page MM, Watkins PJ. Cardiorespiratory arrest and diabetic autonomic neuropathy. *Lancet* 1978;1:14–16.
163. Palumbo PJ, et al. Neurologic complications of diabetes mellitus: transient ischemic attack, stroke, and peripheral neuropathy. *Adv Neurol* 1978;19:593–601.
164. Parkhouse N, LeQuesne PM. Quantitative objective assessment of peripheral nociceptive C fibre function. *J Neurol Neurosurg Psychiatry* 1988;51:28–34.
165. Pfeifer MA, et al. Quantitative evaluation of cardiac parasympathetic activity in normal and diabetic man. *Diabetes* 1982;31:339–345.
166. Pfeifer MA, et al. Autonomic neural dysfunction in recently diagnosed diabetic subjects. *Diabetes Care* 1984;7:447–453.
167. Pirart J. Diabetic neuropathy: a metabolic or a vascular disease? *Diabetes* 1965;14:1–9.
168. Pirart J. Diabetes mellitus and its degenerative complications: a prospective study of 4400 patients observed between 1947 and 1973. Part 1. *Diabetes Care* 1978;1:168–188.
169. Purewal TS, et al. The splanchnic circulation and postural hypotension in diabetic autonomic neuropathy. *Diabet Med* 1995;12:513–522.
170. Rasmussen MH, et al. Impaired pancreatic polypeptide response to a meal in type 1 diabetic patients: vagal neuropathy or islet cell dysfunction? *J Cardiovasc Pharmacol* 1993;21:863–868.
171. Rathmann W, et al. Mortality in diabetic patients with cardiovascular autonomic neuropathy. *Diabet Med* 1993;10:820–824.
172. Rayman G, Hassan A, Tooke JE. Blood flow in the skin of the foot related to posture in diabetes mellitus. *Br Med J* 1986;292: 87–90.
173. Rowell LB. Human cardiovascular adjustments to exercise and thermal stress (Review). *Physiol Rev* 1974;54:75–159.
174. Rundles RW. Diabetic neuropathy. In: Anonymous *Analytical Reviews of General Medicine, Neurology and Pediatrics*. Baltimore: Williams & Wilkins; 1945:11–60.
175. Rundles RW. Diabetic neuropathy. General review with report of 125 cases. *Medicine* 1945;24:111–160.
176. Ryder RE, et al. Acetylcholine sweat spot test for autonomic denervation. *Lancet* 1988;1:1303–1305.
177. Ryder RE, et al. Unawareness of hypoglycaemia and inadequate hypoglycaemic counterregulation: no causal relation with diabetic autonomic neuropathy (see comments). *Br Med J* 1990;301:783–787.
178. Saenz de Tejada I, et al. Impaired neurogenic and endothelium-mediated relaxation of penile smooth muscle from diabetic men with impotence. *N Engl J Med* 1989;320:1025–1030.
179. Sampson MJ, et al. Progression of diabetic autonomic neuropathy over a decade in insulin-dependent diabetics. *Q J Med* 1990;75: 635–646.
180. Scarpello JH, et al. Small intestinal transit in diabetics. *Br Med J* 1976;2:1225–1226.
181. Scarpello JH, et al. The ^{14}C-glycocholate test in diabetic diarrhoea. *Br Med J* 1976;2:673–675.
182. Scarpello JH, Sladen GE. Diabetes and the gut (Review). *Gut* 1978;19:1153–1162.
183. Schmid PG, et al. Effect of 9-alpha-fluorohydrocortisone on forearm vascular responses to norepinephrine. *Circulation* 1966;34: 620–626.
184. Schwartz PJ. Idiopathic long QT syndrome: progress and questions. *Am Heart J* 1985;109:399–411.
185. Schwartz TW, et al. Vagal, cholinergic regulation of pancreatic polypeptide secretion. *J Clin Invest* 1978;61:781–789.
186. Smith SA. Reduced sinus arrhythmia in diabetic autonomic neuropathy: diagnostic value of an age-related normal range. *Br Med J* 1982;285:1599–1601.
187. Smith SA. Diagnostic value of the Valsalva ratio reduction in diabetic autonomic neuropathy: use of an age-related normal range. *Diabet Med* 1984;1:295–297.
188. Smith SA, Dewhirst RR. A simple diagnostic test for pupillary abnormality in diabetic autonomic neuropathy. *Diabet Med* 1986;3: 38–41.
189. Smith SA, Smith SE. Assessment of pupillary function in diabetic neuropathy. In: Dyck PJ, Thomas PK, Asbury AK, Winegrad AI, Porte D, eds. *Diabetic Neuropathy*. Philadelphia: WB Saunders; 1987:134–139.
190. Smith SE, Smith SA. Heart rate variability in healthy subjects measured with a bedside computer-based technique. *Clin Sci* 1981;61: 379–383.
191. Smith SE, et al. Pupillary signs in diabetic autonomic neuropathy. *Br Med J* 1978;2:924–927.
192. Stewart JD, et al. Small-fiber peripheral neuropathy: diagnostic value of sweat tests and autonomic cardiovascular reflexes. *Ann Neurol* 1989;26:145A(abst).
193. Subramony SH, Wilbourn AJ. Diabetic proximal neuropathy. Clinical and electromyographic studies. *J Neurol Sci* 1982;53:293–304.
194. Sundkvist G, et al. Respiratory influence on heart rate in diabetes mellitus. *Br Med J* 1979;1:924–925.
195. Sundkvist G, Lilja B. Autonomic neuropathy in diabetes mellitus: a follow-up study. *Diabetes Care* 1985;8:129–133.
196. Sundkvist G, et al. Deep breathing, Valsalva, and tilt table tests in diabetics with and without symptoms of autonomic neuropathy. *Acta Med Scand* 1982;211:369–373.
197. Tackmann W, et al. Autonomic disturbances in relation to sensorimotor peripheral neuropathy in diabetes mellitus. *J Neurol* 1981; 224:273–281.
198. Thomas PK, Eliasson SG. Diabetic neuropathy. In: Dyck PJ, Thomas PK, Lambert EH, Bunge R, eds. *Peripheral Neuropathy*. Philadelphia: WB Saunders; 1984:1773–1810.
199. Tuck RR, et al. Endoneurial blood flow and oxygen tension in the sciatic nerves of rats with experimental diabetic neuropathy. *Brain* 1984;107:935–950.
200. Tyrer G, et al. Sexual responsiveness in diabetic women. *Diabetologia* 1983;24:166–171.

201. Veglio M, et al. Autonomic neuropathy in non-insulin-dependent diabetic patients: correlation with age, sex, duration and metabolic control of diabetes. *Diabete Metab* 1990;16:200–206.
202. Virag R, et al. Is impotence an arterial disorder? A study of arterial risk factors in 440 impotent men. *Lancet* 1985;1:181–184.
203. Vital C, et al. Acute inflammatory demyelinating polyneuropathy in a diabetic patient: predominance of vesicular disruption in myelin sheaths. *Acta Neuropathol* 1985;67:337–340.
204. Vix VA. Esophageal motility in diabetes mellitus. *Radiology* 1969;92:363–364.
205. Vlay SC, et al. Documented sudden cardiac death in prolonged QT syndrome. *Arch Intern Med* 1984;144:833–835.
206. Vogelberg KH, et al. Sonographic examination of gastric motility in diabetics with autonomic neuropathy. *Diabetes Res* 1987;5:175–179.
207. Webster GD, Older RA. Value of subtracted bladder pressure measurement in routine urodynamics. *Urology* 1980;16:656–660.
208. Whalen GE, et al. Diabetic diarrhea. A clinical and pathophysiological study. *Gastroenterology* 1969;56:1021–1032.
209. Wheeler T, Watkins PJ. Cardiac denervation in diabetes. *Br Med J* 1973;4:584–586.
210. White NH, et al. Identification of type I diabetic patients at increased risk for hypoglycemia during intensive therapy. *N Engl J Med* 1983;308:485–491.
211. Willner C, Low PA. Pharmacologic approaches to the neuropathic pain. In: Dyck PJ, Thomas PK, Griffin JW, Low PA, Poduslo JF, eds. *Peripheral Neuropathy*. Philadelphia: WB Saunders; 1993: 1709–1720.
212. Wooten RL, Merriwether TW. Diabetic gastric atony. A clinical study. *JAMA* 1961;176:1082–1087.
213. Young RJ, et al. Nerve function and metabolic control in teenage diabetics. *Diabetes* 1983;32:142–147.
214. Young RJ, et al. Variable relationship between peripheral somatic and autonomic neuropathy in patients with different syndromes of diabetic polyneuropathy. *Diabetes* 1986;35:192–197.
215. Ziegler D, et al. Treatment of symptomatic diabetic peripheral neuropathy with the anti-oxidant α-lipoic acid. A 3-week multicentre randomized controlled trial (ALADIN Study). *Diabetologia* 1995; 38:1425–1433.

CHAPTER 38

Immune Mechanisms in Diabetic Autonomic and Related Neuropathies

Steven L. Rabinowe

---

1. There is strong evidence that type I diabetes mellitus is an autoimmune disorder associated with antibody and cell-mediated immunity that is directed against islet cells of the pancreas.
2. The antigenic similarities between islet cells and the nervous system have generated interest in the possible involvement of immune factors in the pathogenesis of diabetic neuropathy.
3. Antineuronal antibodies have been demonstrated in diabetic subjects and their first-degree relatives. The presence of antibodies directed against autonomic nervous system structures is associated with changes in autonomic function.
4. Type I diabetes often occurs as a component of the type II polyglandular autoimmune syndrome, which consists of several associated autoimmune glandular and nonglandular disorders, including myasthenia gravis and Parkinson's disease. Evidence is accumulating that suggests that many patients have "polyneuroendocrine" autoimmunity
5. Preliminary observations suggest that glycoconjugate antigens are targets in diabetes as well as in other neurologic diseases.

INTRODUCTION

A large body of evidence suggests that type I diabetes mellitus is an autoimmune disorder associated with antibody- and cell-mediated immunity directed against islet cells of the pancreas. There are many antigenic similarities between islet cells and the nervous system (e.g., specific gangliosides, sulfatides, and glutamic acid decarboxylase). This has generated interest in examining the role of immunologic factors in the pathogenesis of "diabetic" neuropathy (15,17,47,87,157,174).

Many studies have suggested a role for metabolic and vascular factors in the generation of diabetic neuropathy (44,53,62,63,169,188,192). However, the extent to which neuropathy in diabetic subjects is an associated disorder or genetically determined has not been established (105). The frequent lack of correlation between the degree of blood sugar control and the presence of neuropathic symptoms has been appreciated for some time. Antineuronal antibodies have been demonstrated in a number of conditions affecting the nervous system, such as IgM, IgG, and IgA paraproteinemias, stiff-man syndrome, Guillain-Barré syndrome, chronic inflammatory demyelinating polyradiculoneuropathy (CIDP), Parkinson's disease, multiple sclerosis, and systemic lupus erythematosus (6–8,16,19,31,36, 49,50,73,74,78,79,82,98,99,111,126,131,133,143,147,157, 171,172). Recent evidence has also demonstrated antineuronal antibodies in diabetic subjects and their first-degree relatives (22). The degree to which antineuronal antibodies are pathogenic in neuropathy is the subject of considerable debate.

Antineuronal antibodies have been reported in patients with different types of neuropathy, as previously noted. In some instances, correlations exist between the presence of antibodies against neuronal structures and physiologic dysfunction. In addition, antibody titer may be diminished with immunosuppressive therapy. Although clearly an important marker of disease in many neurologic diseases, direct evidence showing the ability of these antibodies to

---

S. L. Rabinowe: Department of Medicine, Sinai Hospital, Detroit, Michigan 48235.

Dr. Rabinowe's research in this discipline is supported by a generous grant from the Thomas Foundation and by Mt. Sinai Hospital of Detroit.

cause clinical pathology is limited. Two research groups have demonstrated that intraneural injection of cats with anti-MAG (myelin-associated glycoprotein) antibodies can lead to demyelination (72,184). This differs from paraprotein-associated neuropathy in the finding of cell-mediated immunologic damage. It has been suggested that this may result from acute as opposed to chronic exposure to antineuronal antibodies. Immunization of rabbits with the glycolipid sulfate-3-glucuronyl paragloboside (SGPG) has been reported to cause a demyelinating neuropathy (96). This glycoconjugate is a target antigen in human antineuronal autoimmunity. Antiganglioside antibodies have caused pathologic changes in neural tissue of rats and in tissue culture (152,153). Antiganglioside antibodies have been shown to bind to the nodes of Ranvier in peripheral nerves. Antisulfatide antibodies appear to bind to myelin (115).

A recent study of serum from an individual with acute sensory neuropathy demonstrated the presence of high-titer monoclonal IgM recognizing B-series gangliosides GD2, GD1b, GT1b, and GQ1b. *In vitro*, the IgM fraction was cytotoxic to rat dorsal root ganglion neurons. This cytotoxicity was blocked by preabsorption with ganglioside GD1b (121).

Studies of complement-fixing immunoglobulins from type I diabetic subjects have been shown to be toxic when incubated with neuroblastoma cells *in vitro* (127,128).

Antineuronal antibodies can antedate the presence of clinical type I diabetes (20,135). This suggests that they may play a primary role and are not restricted to the secondary effects of hyperglycemia-mediated nerve damage. Studies also indicate that antineuronal antibodies may be found after trauma and are not unique to seemingly spontaneous "autoimmune" disorders. This does not eliminate a potential role as a secondary cause of significant tissue damage. Studies of class II major histocompatibility complex (MHC) genes in CIDP suggest that genetic factors may be important in the chronicity of the immune response directed against the nervous system (1,159).

Type I diabetes is also found as a component of the type II polyglandular autoimmune syndrome (117,136). This syndrome consists of several associated "autoimmune" glandular and nonglandular disorders. The syndrome is defined by two or more of the component diseases in the same subject. They include myasthenia gravis and a more recently demonstrated link with Parkinson's disease (131). Several studies have linked polyglandular disease to antibody- and cell-mediated immunity directed against nervous system structures (9,30). The clinical neuropathies seen in diabetic patients bear striking similarities to those seen as more isolated clinical events in the absence of a metabolic disorder. This chapter examines the evidence for a link between autoimmunity and neuropathy in diabetes mellitus (48). It also examines the similarities with other neurologic disorders, including autonomic neuropathy, Parkinson's disease, myasthenia gravis, Lambert-Eaton syndrome, stiff-man syndrome, acquired neuromyotonia (Isaacs' syndrome), and POEMS (polyneuropathy, organomegaly, endocrinopathy, monoclonal gammopathy [M protein], skin changes) syndrome.

THE IMMUNE SYSTEM: EFFECTS OF GLYCOSYLATION AND VASCULAR DISEASE

Glycosylation of proteins occurs in proportion to the average glucose concentration (25). Glycosylation of myelin has been demonstrated in diabetic rodents (177). Glycosylated myelin proteins are recognized by receptors, and macrophage-mediated attack may occur (29,32,178). Capillary leak of plasma proteins has been demonstrated in diabetic individuals (166). Increased IgG and IgM have been demonstrated in diabetic peripheral nerves as a result of trapping or specific deposition (26). Either mechanism may make the nerve more susceptible to immunologic attack. Complement-fixing antibodies directed against sciatic nerve have been demonstrated in diabetic individuals (141).

Pittenger and colleagues (127,128) recently described the toxic effects of complement-fixing autoantibodies from type I diabetic subjects when incubated with neuroblastoma cells *in vitro*. The immunoglobulins specifically inhibited neuronal growth in culture and bound to a membrane-bound antigen.

PATHOLOGY OF DIABETIC AUTONOMIC NEUROPATHY

Duchen and associates (42) published a study of the pathology of the autonomic system in five diabetic subjects. All had premortem evidence of clinical autonomic dysfunction. The clinical problems included signs of cardiac denervation, orthostatic hypotension, bladder dysfunction, impotence, and diarrhea. The authors noted the presence of inflammatory cell infiltrates, which included lymphocytes, macrophages, and plasma cells, in association with unmyelinated autonomic nerve bundles and sympathetic ganglia. The inflammation appeared to be an early process and not secondary to degenerating neurons. The vagus nerve and sympathetic trunks showed a severe loss of myelinated fibers. Fibrosis was noted in the vagus nerve. One previous study of the autonomic nervous system noted discarding samples of ganglia with inflammatory infiltrates before the analysis of samples. Two recent controlled studies focused on the pathology of the adrenal medulla in diabetic subjects at autopsy (21,23). The presence of lymphocytic infiltrates ("adrenal medullitis") was noted in 20% of the type I diabetic subjects. The cellular infiltrate was demonstrated using the monoclonal antibody UCHL1, which recognizes predominantly T lymphocytes (21,155). An additional 19% of the type I diabetic subjects had moderate to severe fibrosis of the adrenal medulla with severe loss of adrenal medullary tissue. Therefore, about

40% of the type I diabetic subjects had a significant pathologic defect.

A recent case report of an individual with the type II polyglandular autoimmune syndrome consisting of type I diabetes, hypothyroidism, and hypopituitarism noted inflammatory infiltrates in both sensory and sympathetic ganglia (180).

CIRCULATING T CELLS

Increased numbers of class II antigen-positive (activated) T lymphocytes have been reported in the circulation and pancreatic islets of new-onset type I diabetic subjects (87). Similar abnormalities are seen in patients with polyglandular autoimmune illness (87,137). Gilbey and coworkers (58,59) have demonstrated the presence of increased numbers of activated T cells in patients with long-standing type I diabetes with severe symptomatic autonomic neuropathy as compared with uncomplicated subjects. These defects are seen in individuals without proteinuria, which argues against nephropathy being the cause of the abnormality. This suggests a role for cell-mediated autoimmunity in diabetic autonomic neuropathy; however, any definitive answer regarding the role of this arm of the immune system will require analysis of T-cell receptors and the antigen specificity of the activated T cells.

ANTIBODY-MEDIATED IMMUNITY

Adrenal Medullary Autoantibodies

The first description of anti-adrenal medullary antibodies in islet cell antibody (ICA)-positive children was published by Schopfer and colleagues (150). Adrenal medullary antibodies were described in 40% of the subjects, with 28% capable of fixing complement (complement-fixing adrenal medullary antibodies, CF-ADM antibodies; Fig. 1). The percentage of CF-ADM antibodies in patients with recent-onset type I diabetes has been confirmed and their association with ICAs demonstrated (20). Subsequent studies have shown that anti-adrenal medullary antibodies are present in individuals before the onset of clinical type I diabetes. Cross-sectional studies of CF-ADM antibodies in type I diabetic subjects have shown that about 20% of subjects with diabetes of less than 16 years' duration have the antibodies. The prevalence drops to about 3% after 16 years of type I diabetes (Fig. 2). After 6 years' duration of type I diabetes, many subjects lack ICAs but are positive for CF-ADM antibodies.

Anti-adrenal medullary antibodies are of the IgG class. Some investigators have subdivided the antibodies into a homogeneous or spotty immunofluorescent pattern. The antigens involved in adrenal medullary antibody binding are not known but are under investigation. Preliminary evi-

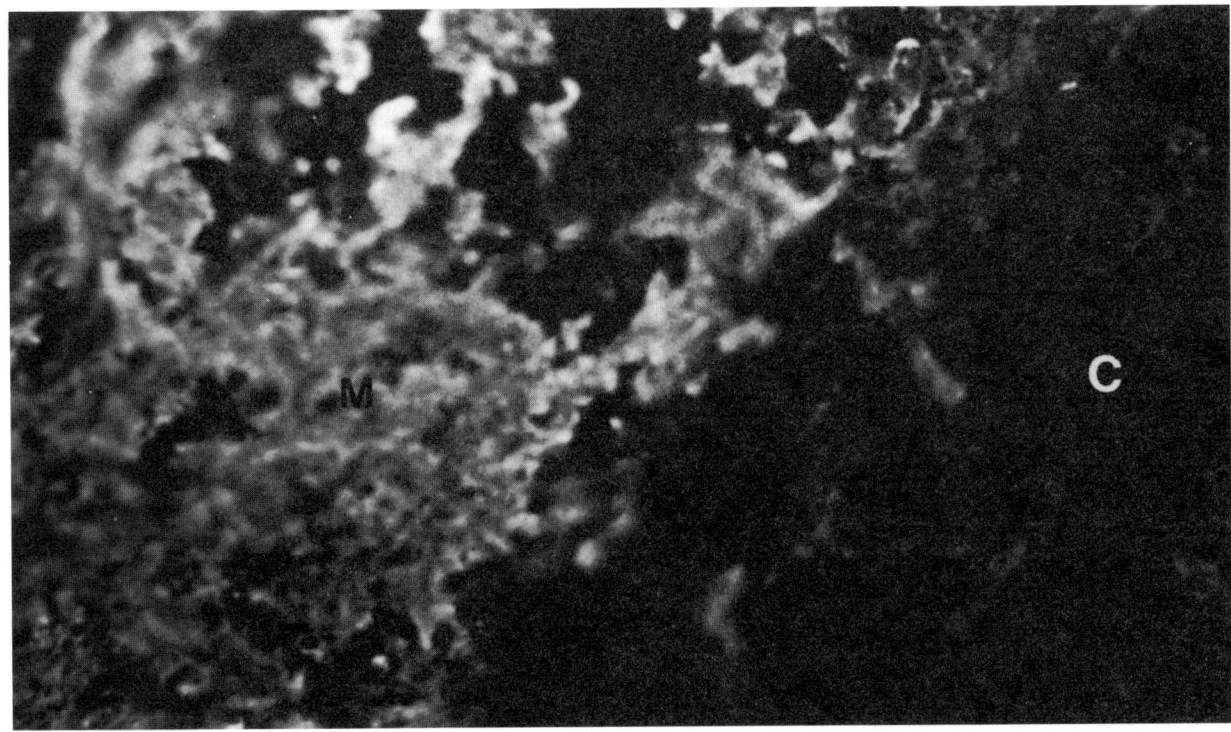

FIG. 1. Anti-adrenal medullary antibody staining of adrenal medulla (*M*) with a nonstaining adrenal cortex (*C*).

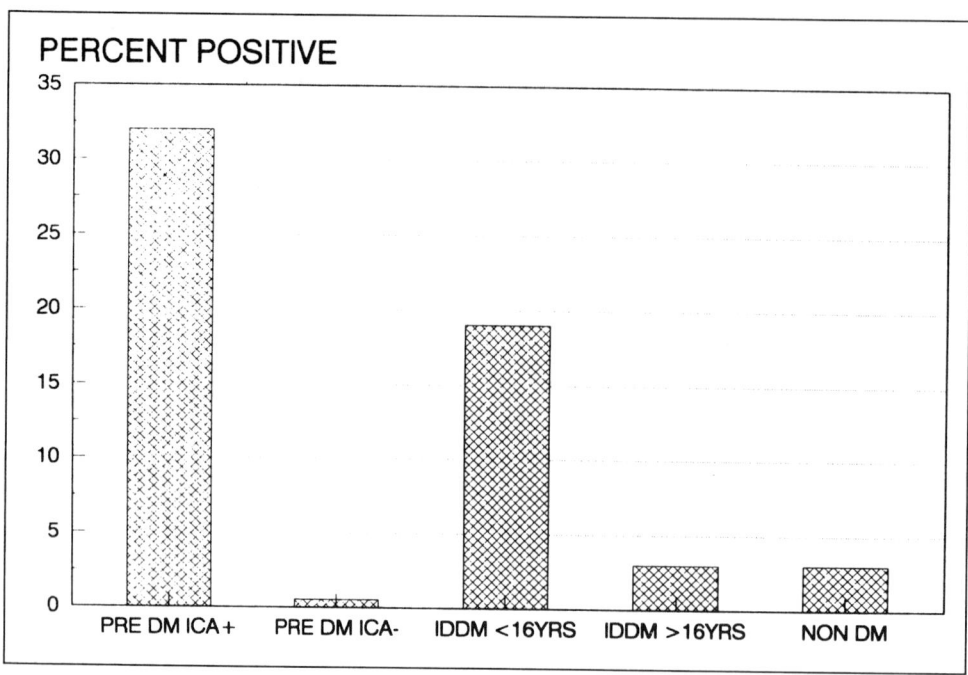

FIG. 2. Anti-adrenal medullary antibodies are present in islet cell antibody—positive prediabetic individuals (*PRE DM*) and are related to duration of type I diabetes (*IDDM*; insulin-dependent diabetes mellitus).

dence suggests that the antigens include peptides and glycolipids containing sialic acid residues (83).

Anti-Sympathetic Ganglia Antibodies

Circulating antibodies directed against sympathetic ganglia have been identified using the complement fixation technique on cryostat sections (Fig. 3). These antibodies antedate the development of clinical type I diabetes and are not restricted to ICA-positive individuals (134,135). In one study, 52% of the ICA-positive subjects at high risk for the development of type I diabetes had complement-fixing anti-sympathetic ganglia (CF-SG) antibodies. Forty-four percent of ICA-negative subjects with either an impaired glucose tolerance or impaired first-phase insulin release (1- to 3-minute values) during an intravenous glucose tolerance test (IVGTT) were positive for CF-SG antibodies. About 27% of the subjects with type I diabetes for less than 20 years are positive for CF-SG antibodies, and this percentage drops to about 10% after 20 years' duration of diabetes (Fig. 4).

Anti-Vagus Nerve Antibodies

Circulating autoantibodies directed against the vagus nerve (CF-V) have also been detected in pre-type I diabetes and in subjects with type I diabetes (Fig. 5) (135). About 14% of ICA-positive subjects at high risk of developing type I diabetes were found to have vagus nerve antibodies. About 10% of individuals with overt type I diabetes have vagus nerve antibodies, and no relationship to duration of diabetes has been found.

Autonomic Antibody Correlations in Type I Diabetes

Many type I diabetic subjects have abnormalities of both sympathetic and parasympathetic function. Similarly, one would expect that if the antibodies directed against these nerve structures are markers of and/or involved in disease pathogenesis, correlations would exist between the antibodies. These correlations have been documented. In ICA-positive type I diabetics (<1 year in duration), anti-adrenal medullary (CF-ADM) antibodies and anti-sympathetic ganglia antibodies (CF-SG) correlated with $r = 0.7$, $P < 0.02$. In a study of all type I diabetics regardless of duration, the anti-adrenal medullary and anti-sympathetic ganglia antibodies correlated with $r = 0.5$, $P < 0.0001$. During the first 16 years of type I diabetes, vagus nerve antibodies (CF-V) correlated with anti-adrenal medullary antibodies ($r = 0.61$, $P < 0.0001$). The vagus nerve antibodies also correlated with sympathetic ganglia antibodies ($r = 0.39$, $P < 0.05$). As would be expected from clinical studies of autonomic dysfunction, a minority of diabetic subjects have antibodies directed against only one component of the autonomic nervous system.

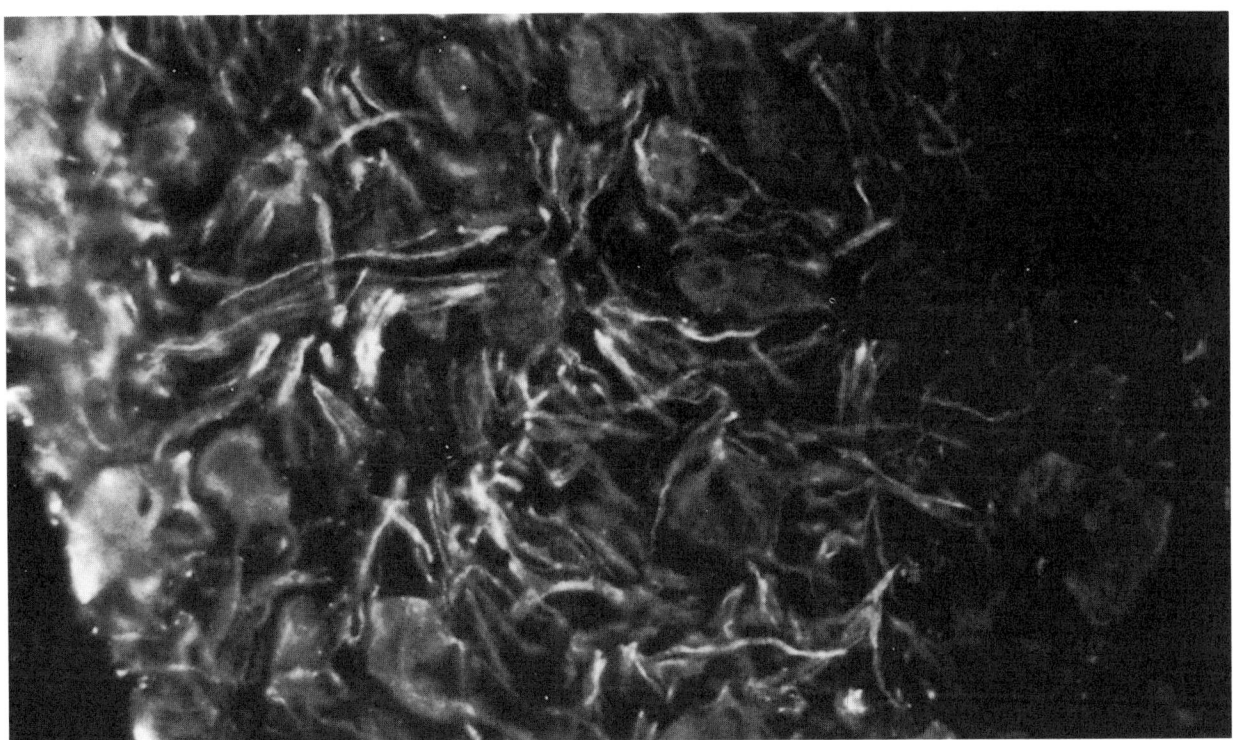

FIG. 3. Anti-sympathetic ganglia antibody staining by immunofluorescence with sera from a type I diabetic individual.

Family Studies and the Genetics of Autonomic Autoantibodies

A recent study of autonomic antibodies in the first-degree relatives of type I diabetics showed no association with HLA-DR3 or -DR4 on chromosome 6 (22). However, a striking familial aggregation of these antibodies was noted, with almost 50% of first-degree relatives (multiplex families) of type I diabetics being positive as compared with less than 3% of healthy population controls. In addi-

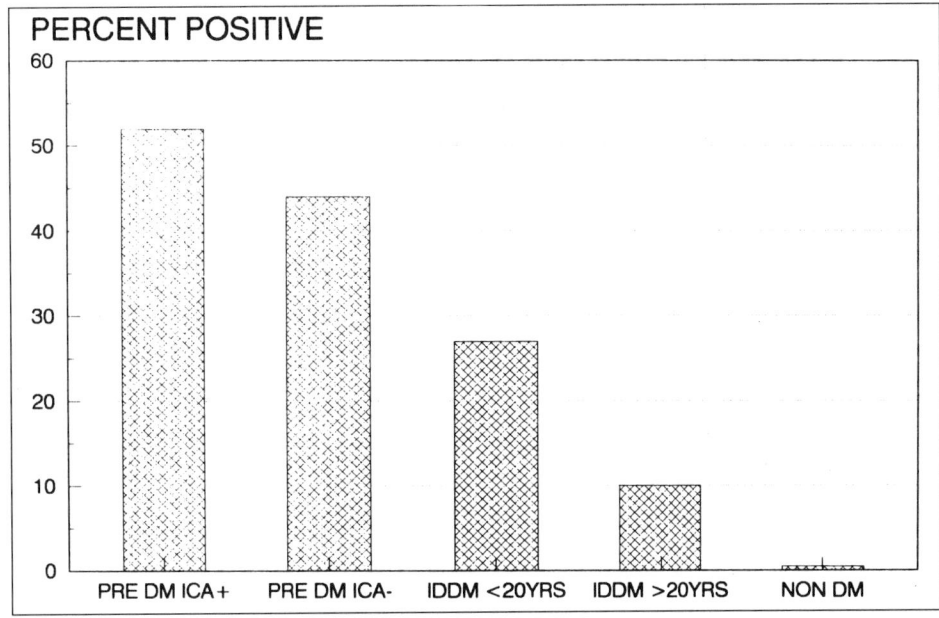

FIG. 4. Anti-sympathetic ganglia antibodies are present in prediabetic individuals (*PRE DM*) and are related to duration of type I diabetes (*IDDM*).

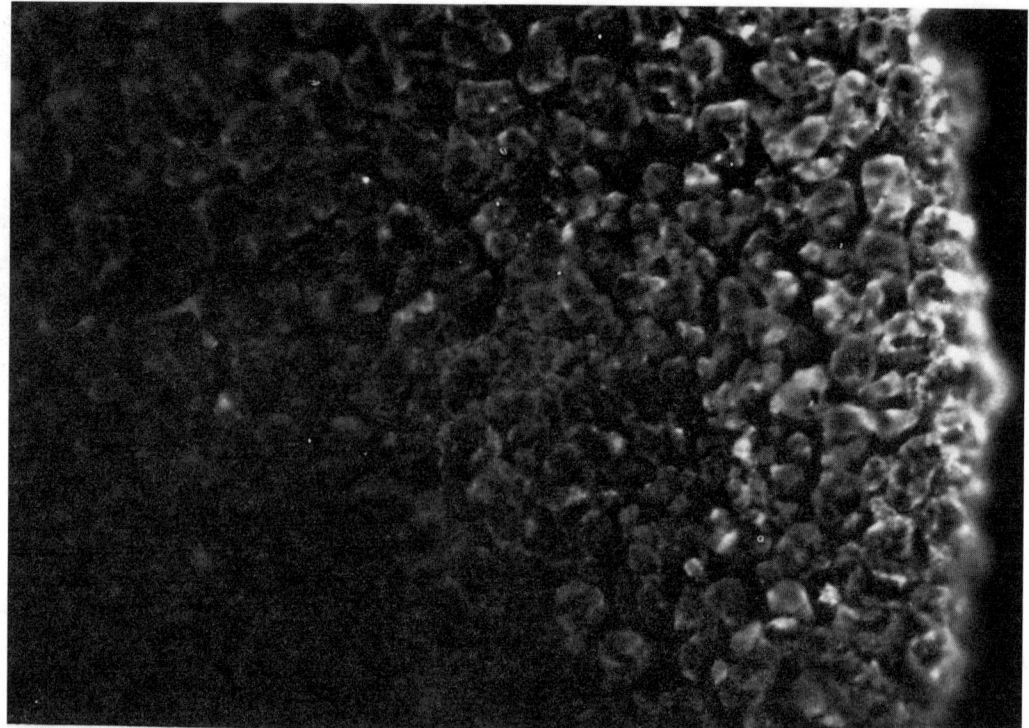

FIG. 5. Anti-vagus nerve antibody staining by immunofluorescence with sera from a type I diabetic individual.

tion, subclinical deficits of autonomic function were detected in some autonomic antibody-positive relatives without diabetes.

COMPLEMENT ACTIVATION AND IMMUNE COMPLEXES

Circulating immune complexes have been reported in diabetics with autonomic dysfunction (58). Changes in circulating C3d (a breakdown product of C3 found with complement activation) were also found in association with diabetic autonomic neuropathy. Low C4 levels were not noted in these subjects. Low levels of C4 occur in up to 25% of type I diabetics, and this was confirmed in uncomplicated subjects (112).

AUTONOMIC NERVOUS SYSTEM ANTIBODIES IN TYPE II DIABETES

Several investigators have documented the presence of anti-ICAs in subjects with clinical type II diabetes mellitus (64). This has led to the suggestion that our clinical classification scheme is imprecise and that some subjects with "type II" diabetes may have a slower immune process directed against pancreatic islet cells. Similarly, recent studies have documented the presence of complement-fixing anti-adrenal medullary, anti-sympathetic ganglia, and anti-vagus nerve antibodies in some patients with type II diabetes mellitus (162). Abnormal expiratory/inspiratory (E/I) ratios have been associated with anti-vagus nerve antibodies (CF-V) in type II diabetic subjects.

AUTONOMIC AUTOANTIBODIES AND PATHOPHYSIOLOGY

Postural Blood Pressure

Orthostatic hypotension is one of the hallmarks of severe autonomic dysfunction in subjects with type I diabetes mellitus. This may be due to an abnormality in the sympathetic nervous system. Therefore, studies have been performed to delineate any relationship between anti-sympathetic ganglia antibodies and orthostatic changes in blood pressure. In a cross-sectional study, 70% of subjects with postural blood pressures in the lower normal range were positive, versus 20% of subjects in the upper normal range (n = 24, $P < 0.03$). At the time of the blood pressure study, none of the patients with orthostatic hypotension had anti-sympathetic ganglia antibodies. One subject, however, had serum available from 9 and 10 years' duration of diabetes and had antibodies (CF-SG) detectable at those time points. The group that was negative for anti-sympathetic ganglia antibodies had a mean rise in systolic blood pressure of 5.6 mmHg, and the positive group had a fall of -2.9 mmHg (Fig. 6). This information, coupled with data on anti-sympa-

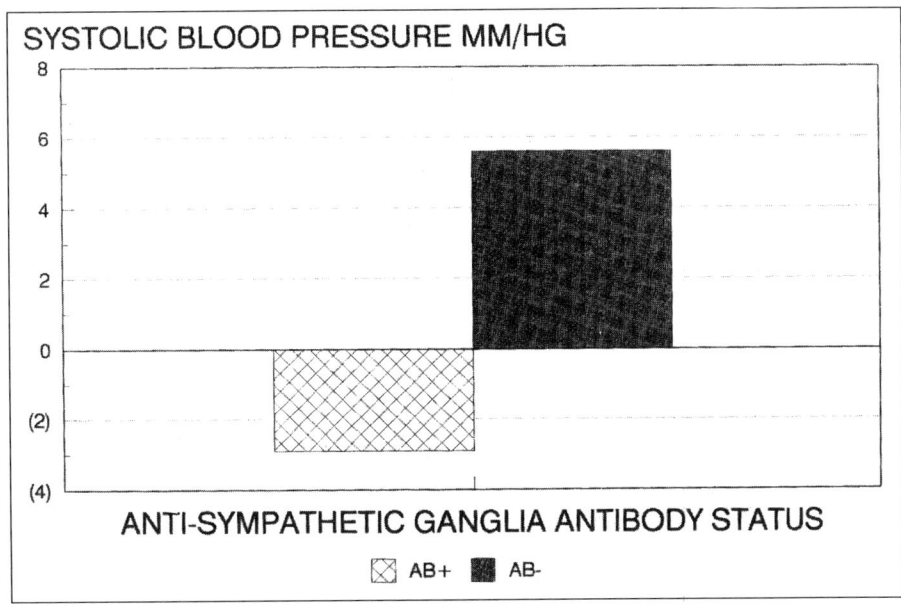

FIG. 6. Type I diabetic individuals who are positive for anti-sympathetic ganglia antibodies have a mean fall in systolic blood pressure with orthostasis, whereas antibody-negative subjects have a rise in blood.

thetic ganglia antibodies and duration of diabetes, suggests that the antibodies are present during the "active" phase of tissue destruction and are subsequently lost (134,138).

Postural Catecholamines

Studies of orthostatic hypotension in type I diabetic subjects have demonstrated individuals with abnormally low catecholamine responses during postural maneuvers. The reason for this catecholamine deficit has not been completely defined.

A study has been performed to evaluate whether subjects with CF-ADM antibodies and/or CF-SG antibodies have a decreased catecholamine response to change in posture (18).

Longitudinally collected sera were evaluated for the presence of CF-ADM and CF-SG antibodies, and subjects were typed as positive or negative on any date. Postural

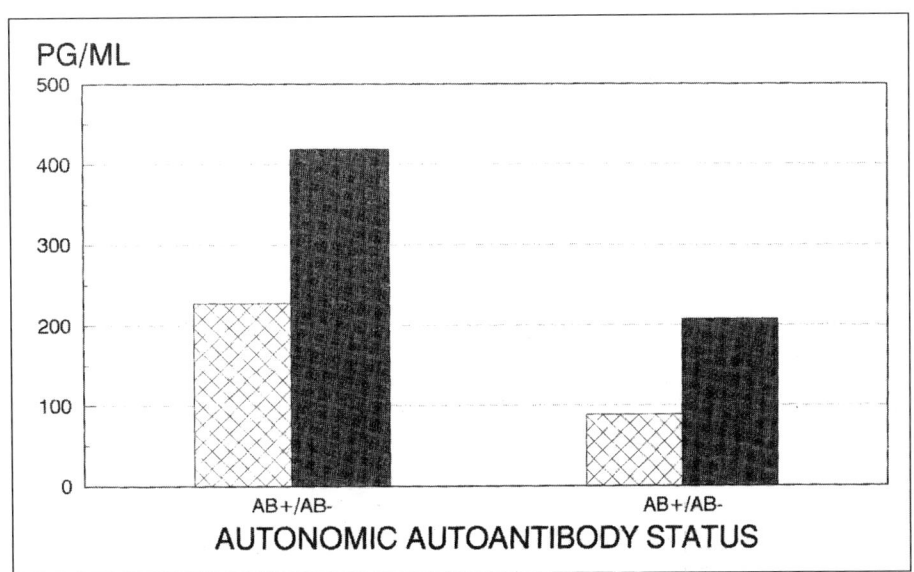

FIG. 7. Norepinephrine levels after 5 minutes of standing and at 5 min minus basal in antibody-positive and -negative subjects.

catecholamine studies were performed in seven type I diabetic subjects 19 to 41 years of age who had a duration of disease of 5 to 21 years. Baseline mean norepinephrine and epinephrine values were not significantly different in the supine position. However, after 5 minutes of standing, the mean norepinephrine values were 227 pg/ml (Ab+) and 419 pg/ml (Ab−) ($P<0.03$). Similarly, epinephrine levels were 35 pg/ml (Ab+) and 101 pg/ml (Ab−) at 5 min ($P<0.03$) (Fig. 7). The data also showed a difference when expressed as 5 min minus basal catecholamine levels. This suggests that CF-ADM and CF-SG antibodies are associated with a decreased catecholamine response to change in posture.

Parasympathetic Function and Anti-Vagus Nerve Antibodies

Autonomic Brake Index

Evaluations of heart rate variation during paced breathing or postural tilt have been used in studies of cardiovascular autonomic dysfunction (13,52,161). An abnormally low "brake index" has been described in diabetic subjects with abnormal vital capacity tests, suggesting a link with vagal dysfunction. The index is calculated according to the equation $C - B/A \times 100$, where A is the RR interval at rest in a supine position, B is the shortest RR interval after active tilting, and C is the longest RR interval after B. Because of its link with vagal dysfunction, the brake index was studied in type I diabetic subjects with vagus nerve autoantibodies (135). Brake indices ranged from 12.7 to 17.3 (mean, 15.1) in subjects with vagus nerve antibodies. Subjects with adrenal medullary antibodies had brake indices ranging from 26.9 to 45.1 (mean, 32.9), and subjects with sympathetic ganglia antibodies had brake indices ranging from 14.7 to 51.3 (mean, 37.3). Type I diabetic subjects with adrenergic nervous system antibodies had higher brake indices than did those with vagus nerve antibodies.

Data from Zanone and colleagues (190) on patients with symptomatic autonomic neuropathy showed similar results.

NEURONAL AND ISLET ANTIGENS

Antibodies directed against neuronal and islet antigens may be directed against proteins and/or glycolipids (35,132). The glycolipid antigens have included both gangliosides and sulfatide molecules (158,164). Gangliosides are sialic acid–containing sphingolipids (89,165). The sialic acid of gangliosides and the sulfate group of sulfatides appear to be important in antibody binding. Carbohydrate structures of glycolipids and glycoproteins may be cellular-differentiation antigens, tumor-associated antigens, portions of receptor systems, and nerve cell adhesion molecules (N-CAM) (46,69,101,183).

A glycolipid with mobility on thin-layer chromatography between GM1 and GM2 gangliosides has been implicated as a target antigen in islet cell antibody binding (34,116,132). A number of other "autoimmune" diseases have been associated with antiganglioside antibodies. In subjects with systemic lupus erythematosus, antibodies have been reported against ganglioside GM1 and the asialo structure (asialo GM1) (50,73). Recent data indicate that these antibodies exist in diabetic subjects with peripheral neuropathy (138,140). In multiple sclerosis, antibodies have been reported against a number of neuronal glycolipids (GM1, GM2, GM4, galactosylcerebroside, and digalactosyl diglyceride) (7,50,74,147,171). In a similar fashion, antibodies directed against glycoproteins and glycolipids have been reported in Graves' thyroid disease, autoimmune hemolytic anemia, Behçet's disease, and acquired immunodeficiency syndrome (41,54,81,95,185, 187). Antibodies directed against gangliosides and a neutral Forssman-like glycolipid have been reported in subjects with the Guillain-Barré syndrome (98). A multicenter study has shown plasmapheresis to be an effective therapy in the Guillain-Barré syndrome (66). In cases of paraprotein-associated polyneuropathy, antibodies may bind to MAGs and to gangliosides (16,78,111,133). Glycoproteins of the immune system, MAGs, and other neuronal glycoproteins have amino acid sequence homologies (101,183). Both N-CAM (a neuronal adhesion molecule) and MAG are members of the immunoglobulin gene superfamily (182).

Most studies of autonomic autoantibodies in diabetes have been performed by complement fixation using sera of patients with indirect immunofluorescent detection techniques. A few studies have begun to explore the biochemistry of the antigenic targets in diabetics. Itoh and associates (84) described two patterns of complement-fixing adrenal medullary antibodies in type I and type II diabetic subjects. These were termed homogeneous immunofluorescence and spotty pattern immunofluorescence. The homogeneous pattern antibodies were significantly higher in patients with type I diabetes of short duration. Both types of antibody were of the IgG class, consistent with the determination of other investigators. The epitope for the homogeneous pattern was likely to be a glycoconjugate because the binding of the antibody was abolished after periodate oxidation. The antigen was also chloroform–methanol extractable and may have been a glycolipid. The spotty-type pattern was considered to be a peptide because it was trypsin sensitive. Preliminary data are available on the nature of some of these antigenic targets. Anti-ganglioside GT1b IgG antibodies have been described in diabetes mellitus, and their presence has been associated with complement-fixing anti-adrenal medullary and anti-sympathetic ganglia antibodies. They are also associated with changes in orthostatic blood pressure (138). GT1b is a known constituent of adrenal medulla and sympathetic ganglia. In addition, IgG autoantibodies directed against a chromogranin A peptide have been associated with complement-fixing adrenal medullary antibodies (139). Antilactose series glycolipid LM1 and ganglioside GD3 IgG antibodies have also been associated with complement-fixing antibodies to the vagus nerve (140). Both LM1 and GD3 are present in relatively high quantities in the vagus nerve substrates used in the indirect immunofluorescence reactions. Although not associated with autonomic dysfunction in diabetic patients, antisulfatide antibodies are increased in patients with new-onset diabetes and in some diabetics of longer disease duration. In individuals with longer disease duration, these antibodies are associated with altered peripheral nerve conduction (125).

An immunologic picture is emerging in a wide range of illnesses from multiple sclerosis to type I diabetes mellitus. Adhesion molecules are involved in the migration of systemic immune responses into the target tissue(s). Adhesion molecules are upregulated through cytokines such as tumor necrosis factor-alpha. Circulating adhesion molecules may reflect acute inflammatory episodes and may also modulate inflammatory responses over time. Cytokines released by TH1 cells lead to the activation of macrophages and microglia to synthesize and release abundant amounts of inflammatory mediators, which may include components of the complement system, oxygen radicals, and nitric oxide metabolites.

T cells respond to peptide antigen(s), and humoral immune responses may target peptide and/or glycolipid antigens, as noted. The terminal complement complex or membrane attack complex can penetrate the target cell membrane and damage cells by pore formation. Although C3a, C5a, and the terminal complement complex stimulate phospholipase A_2 and transmethylation, they inhibit acyltransferase. Eicosanoids are produced that can amplify inflammatory responses. Activation of pericellular macrophages and/or microglia may start a positive feedback loop of injury (71).

NEURONAL AUTOIMMUNITY AND GANGLIOSIDE THERAPY

Recent evidence that several of the neuronal antibody targets are gangliosides suggests a possible role for ganglioside therapy in diabetic neuropathy (10,138,140). Gangliosides are located in the outer leaflet of the cell membrane bilayer (56). *In vitro* evidence suggests that gangliosides augment neurite outgrowth (144). Animal and human studies have suggested that gangliosides may stimulate the growth of neurons and promote the regeneration of damaged nervous tissue. Studies in animal models and humans with diabetic neuropathy suggest a possible beneficial effect. Although speculative, beneficial effects might result from blocked neuronal antibody binding, insertion into a damaged membrane, and/or the induction of tolerance (152).

STIFF-MAN SYNDROME AND GLUTAMIC ACID DECARBOXYLASE

Stiff-man syndrome is a rare neurologic disorder characterized by muscle rigidity and painful spasms (61,113). Continuous motor unit activity is noted at rest on electromyography. The continuous alpha motor activity is linked to a defect in gamma-aminobutyric acid (GABA) inhibitory systems (14). Early reports linked the disorder with type I diabetes, hyperthyroidism, and hypopituitarism in some individuals (33,40,57,75,108,160,181). The enzyme glutamic acid decarboxylase (GAD) is found in the GABA-ergic portions of the nervous system and is enriched in the islets of Langerhans (174). Recent evidence has shown that antibodies directed against this enzyme are present in subjects with stiff-man syndrome, type I diabetes mellitus, and polyglandular autoimmune disease (70, 156,157,173). The antibody titer appears to be greater in patients with stiff-man syndrome by at least a factor of 10 when compared with diabetic subjects. Antibodies against the cloned 65 and 67K forms of GAD (which derive from two genes) have been reported in type I diabetics, and patients differentially recognize the two forms of the enzyme (170). Epitope mapping with sera from type I diabetic subjects has revealed different patterns of recognition. A report has shown that eight of nine subjects with "diabetic" neuropathy had anti-GAD antibodies several years after the onset of diabetes (90). Two recent studies have examined that question in detail (163,191). Both studies showed no association between glutamic acid decarboxylase antibodies and either autonomic neuropathy symptoms or function. In addition, one study examined the question of whether these antibodies were associated with complement-fixing antibodies to autonomic structures in the patients. No association was found.

IMMUNOSUPPRESSION

If autoimmunity is of pathogenic importance in diabetic subjects, immunosuppressive regimens would be expected to be of use in the clinical setting. Very little information is available on this subject. A pilot study of immunosuppressive therapy has been reported in two subjects with autonomic nervous system autoantibodies and autonomic neuropathy. Plasmapheresis and prednisone were used in one subject, and azathioprine and prednisone in the second. An improvement in the E/I ratio and response to Valsalva maneuver was noted in conjunction with a fall in autonomic antibody titer (60,91).

IRITIS AND DIABETIC AUTONOMIC NEUROPATHY

Iritis is believed to have an immunologic cause with immune complexes in the circulation (38,76,186). It is also frequently associated with other immunologically mediated disorders. Guy and colleagues (68) found an association between iritis and severe autonomic neuropathy in diabetic subjects. Other researchers have questioned the association (109).

A possible mechanism was suggested by Guy and coworkers (68). The hypothesis is that insulin antibodies may cross-react with nerve growth factor, leading to sympathetic nerve damage. In experimental systems, nerve growth factor has been shown to be important for the growth and survival of sympathetic nerves. Structural similarities exist between nerve growth factor and insulin in amino acid sequences and the predicted secondary and tertiary structure. Therefore, it is further postulated that with similar antigenic determinants on nerve growth factor and insulin, insulin antibodies might cross-react and lead to sympathetic damage. Sympathetic denervation has been shown to lead to a rapid increase in nerve growth factor in the iris. This might then be a target for immune complex formation in the iris. Although this approach remains an interesting hypothesis, a recent investigation has failed to find antibodies to nerve growth factor in individuals with diabetic autonomic neuropathy (189).

NEURONAL AUTOIMMUNITY AND ANIMAL MODELS OF DIABETES

The NOD mouse and BB rat have been useful models of type I diabetes mellitus and have been of special importance in unraveling the immunogenetics of the disorder (77). The NOD mouse develops gastroparesis and a proximal muscle disorder, although complete studies of neuropathy are lacking in this model. Antineuronal antibodies have been detected in more than 90% of NOD mice and in over 50% of NOD mice crossed with Balb/cJ (F1). These antibodies are not found in the NON (nondiabetic) control strain, Balb/cJ, and C3H/SnJ, suggesting that the NOD mouse may be a valuable model of antineuronal antibodies in human disease (39).

POLYNEUROENDOCRINE AUTOIMMUNITY AND PARKINSON'S DISEASE

Emile and associates (49,131) have reported an increased frequency of gastric parietal cell antibodies and reticulin autoantibodies in patients with Parkinson's disease. They also noted the presence of islet cell antibodies in 7.8% of 115 subjects studied. In recent studies from our group, clinical diseases of the polyglandular autoimmune syndrome type II were noted in 6 of 36 subjects. The clinically overt polyglandular diseases included hypothyroidism, premature menopause, pernicious anemia, Addison's disease, and Graves' disease. An additional five subjects were noted to have serologic evidence of polyglandular autoimmunity (19). Barbeau and Pourcher (11) previously suggested that a higher frequency of hypothyroidism and hyperthyroidism is found in Parkinson's disease subjects with an age of onset less than 40 years.

Emile and colleagues noted the presence of anti-sympathetic ganglia antibodies in 66% of subjects with Parkinson's disease as opposed to 20% of controls. Antibodies directed against the adrenal medulla were noted in 44% of subjects. The authors used fluorescein conjugated anti-immunoglobulin (IgG, A, M) antibodies and detected antibodies with a titer between $\frac{1}{4}$ and $\frac{1}{50}$. Using the complement fixation technique, our group found sympathetic ganglia antibodies in 17% of Parkinson's subjects and none of the controls. Anti-adrenal medullary antibodies were present in 23%. In addition, antibodies reacting with the substantia nigra were found in 42% of Parkinson's disease subjects as opposed to none of the controls (stroke patients, patients with Alzheimer's disease, and normal subjects). A pathology study has documented a striking decrease in the catecholamine content of adrenal glands from patients with Parkinson's disease as compared with age-matched controls (28). The cause of this decrease was not elucidated. Longitudinal follow-up of Parkinson's disease subjects and the molecular nature of the antibody targets will be required to determine the significance of these findings.

Recent research from FIDIA Research Laboratories has demonstrated that a complement-dependent humoral immune response in iodiopathic parkinsonian patients is toxic to rat mesencephalic dopaminergic neurons in culture (37).

NONDIABETIC NEURONAL AUTOIMMUNITY IN POLYGLANDULAR ILLNESS

Several pathology studies have suggested the presence of antineuronal autoimmunity in nondiabetic polyglandular diseases. A *New England Journal of Medicine* case report of a subject with autoimmune oophoritis and thyroid autoimmunity demonstrated the presence of a lymphocytic infiltrate surrounding the nerve in the hilus of the ovary (30). After this single report, a study from Australia documented perineural lymphocytic infiltrates in 20% of autoimmune oophoritis subjects (9). Taylor and associates (167) reported the pathology of a subject with Hashimoto's thyroiditis and an excessive catecholamine output. No evidence of a pheochromocytoma was found at autopsy; however, a striking lymphocytic infiltrate was noted in the adrenal medulla and sympathetic ganglia. This subject had no history of diabetes mellitus but was noted to have a lymphocytic infiltrate of the pancreatic islets.

As previously noted, a recent case report of an individual with the type II polyglandular autoimmune syndrome consisting of type I diabetes, hypothyroidism, and hypopituitarism demonstrated that the patient had inflammatory infiltrates in both sensory and sympathetic ganglia (127, 128).

Myasthenia gravis is an HLA-B8-DR3–associated illness that may be part of the type II polyglandular autoimmune syndrome, as previously noted. The disorder may also occur in isolation without diabetes or other "glandular" autoimmunity (2,124). The major functional abnormality stems from a loss of acetylcholine receptors. Anti-acetylcholine receptor antibodies are known to be present and are thought to reduce receptor number by cross-linking and complement-fixation mechanisms (4,51,104,146). Immunotherapy has included the use of steroids, thymectomy, azathioprine, and, more recently, cyclosporin A (65,88, 107,110,122,123,149,152).

LAMBERT-EATON SYNDROME

The Lambert-Eaton syndrome is a myasthenic disorder often associated with small-cell carcinoma of the lung. The disorder has also been reported in association with several autoimmune diseases, including hypothyroidism, hyperthyroidism, pernicious anemia, and Sjögren's syndrome (67). One report has linked combined features of myasthenia gravis and Lambert-Eaton syndrome in the same subjects (100). In Lambert-Eaton syndrome, an insufficient number of acetylcholine quanta are released at the motor nerve terminal in response to a neural impulse (102,145). The autoimmune nature of this deficiency is well established (24,67,93,94,100,103,114,118–120,179). IgG antibodies react with voltage-dependent calcium channels and block their function (92). In subjects with combined features of myasthenia gravis and Lambert-Eaton syndrome, antibodies reacting with gangliosides GT1b, GD1a, and sialylparagloboside have also been reported. Gangliosides have also been implicated as having a role in presynaptic neurotransmitter release. Similarly, IgG antibodies directed against GT1b have recently been reported in subjects with type I diabetes mellitus and are associated with the presence of anti-sympathetic ganglia (CF-SG) and anti-adrenal medullary (CF-ADM) antibodies. They have also been related to changes in mean arterial and diastolic blood pressure with orthostasis (138).

ACQUIRED NEUROMYOTONIA (ISAACS' SYNDROME)

Isaacs reported an acquired neuromyotonia in 1961. The syndrome consists of an increasingly incapacitating muscle stiffness and weakness associated with muscle fasciculation and continuous muscle fiber activity. Studies of neuromuscular blockade have suggested a peripheral nerve abnormality. The disorder is clinically distinct from the stiff-man syndrome, which is a disorder of the central nervous system associated with high-titer antibodies to GAD (see earlier). Isaacs' syndrome may be associated with neoplastic disease. Therefore, there is similarity to Lambert-Eaton syndrome, in which autoimmune mechanisms have been implicated. A recent study has shown that IgG antibodies from Isaacs' syndrome patients enhanced *in vitro* resistance to d-tubocurarine at the neuromuscular junction of phrenic nerve diaphragm preparations (154). A reduction in functional potassium channels may cause an increase in neurotransmitter release. The reported patient had high-titer thyroid microsomal antibodies and had an improvement in the neurologic disorder in response to plasmapheresis. A separate report from Japan has demonstrated creatine kinase complexed with IgA in the muscle fiber membrane and motor endplate.

POEMS SYNDROME

POEMS syndrome consists of a plasma cell dyscrasia associated with polyneuropathy, organomegaly, endocrinopathy, M protein, and skin changes (3,12,80,85,148). Fifty percent of subjects have diabetes mellitus that is responsive to small insulin doses. About 70% of subjects have primary gonadal failure. Sclerotic bone lesions may be found. Radiotherapy of the bone lesions may lead to temporary normalization of the blood sugar. Patients have a severe progressive sensorimotor polyneuropathy, lymphadenopathy, hepatosplenomegaly, and hyperpigmentation. Circulating light-chain immunoglobulins are found.

CHRONIC INFLAMMATORY POLYNEUROPATHY

Inflammatory neuropathy can be found in isolation or associated with a systemic illness (43,175). Diabetes mellitus, uremia, lymphoma, and carcinoma have been found to be clinically associated (176). The neuropathy can be further divided clinically according to acute or chronic time course, and it can have predominantly motor, predominantly sensory, or mixed forms. Autonomic dysfunction is often associated with all types. CIDP is a chronic progressive nonviral form of Guillain-Barré syndrome. Two investigations suggest that it may be diabetes associated and has an HLA association (A1, B8, and Dw3) (1,159). One group failed to find an HLA association (55). Type I diabetes mellitus is also HLA associated. Humoral immune mechanisms are believed to be operative in some chronic inflammatory neuropathies. Autoantibodies directed against the monosialoganglioside GM1 have been reported in some patients (126). A recent report from our group has found autoantibodies directed against GM1 in diabetic subjects (5). Immunosuppression with prednisone or cyclophosphamide has been reported to improve subjects with CIDP that is associated with a decrease in the titer of anti-GM1 antibodies. Individual subjects with CIDP have been reported to also have components of the type II polyglandular autoimmune syndrome (type I diabetes mellitus, Hashimoto's thyroiditis, and myasthenia gravis) (97,130, 142).

The presence of class II MHC antigens is important in the presentation of antigens to the T cells of the immune system. Schwann cells do not express class II antigen under normal conditions (27,129). Class II antigen expression has been reported on Schwann cells in subjects with CIDP and to a lesser extent in hereditary motor and sensory neuropathy (HMSN) (106). A few cases of diabetic and toxic neuropathies have been studied, and nerve tissues express class II antigen. Areas of cellular proliferation in an onion bulb fashion appear to be associated with more intense class II antigen staining. It is not possible to assess the importance of these findings in disease processes in man with our current limited knowledge.

HEREDITARY MOTOR AND SENSORY NEUROPATHY

Hereditary neuropathies are a diverse group of disorders (168). Some are related to known metabolic defects or amyloid deposition, but many are idiopathic. Nerve pathology in HMSN type I (Charcot-Marie-Tooth disease) may be strikingly similar to that found in diabetic subjects. Dyck and associates (45) have reported that some subjects have features similar to those in CIDP and may improve with corticosteroid therapy. It is not clear whether CIDP and HMSN are associated or whether a common mechanism is involved in the etiopathogenesis. Similar to the idiopathic hereditary neuropathies, a recent report suggests that autonomic autoantibodies and subclinical autonomic dysfunction are inherited in nondiabetic family members of type I diabetics (22). This association strengthens the notion of an inflammatory component in the etiology of autonomic disease.

CONCLUSION

Several nervous system disorders are believed to be caused by immunologic damage to neuronal tissue. There is now substantial interest in humoral immune mechanisms directed against neuronal antigens. Direct evidence of the ability of these antibodies to cause neurologic disease is limited (72,96,184). Diabetic neuropathy has only recently been linked to clinical, morphologic, serologic, and cellular observations of an immune process directed against neuronal targets. Documented associations between neurologic "autoimmune" syndromes and polyglandular autoimmune disease strengthen this argument. The antigenic target molecules in diabetic neuropathy are being explored, and evidence suggests a similarity with nondiabetic neurologic disease. New investigations should focus on both peptide and glycolipid target antigens. The role of cell adhesion molecules, lymphokines, and mediators of cell damage, such as the complement attack complex, oxygen radicals, and nitric oxide metabolites, should be investigated. Both T cell–mediated responses to peptide antigens and complement-fixing antibody responses to peptide and/or glycolipid antigens are likely to be of importance.

The accumulating evidence suggests that many patients have "polyneuroendocrine" autoimmunity.

REFERENCES

1. Adams D, et al. HLA antigens in chronic relapsing idiopathic inflammatory polyneuropathy. *J Neurol Neurosurg Psychiatry* 1979; 42:184–186.
2. Almon RR, et al. Serum globulin in myasthenia gravis: inhibition of alpha-bungarotoxin binding to acetylcholine receptors. *Science* 1974;186:55–57.
3. Amiel K, et al. Dyscrasie plasmocytaire avec arteriopathie, polyneuropathie, syndrome endocrine. *Ann Med Interne (Paris)* 1975; 126:745–749.
4. Appel SH, et al. Acetylcholine receptor antibodies in myasthenia gravis. *N Engl J Med* 1975;293:760–761.
5. Arioglu E, et al. Diabetic neuropathy: anti-GM1 and asialo GM1 antibodies. *Diabetes* 1991;40(suppl 1):330A.
6. Armati PJ, Pollard JD. Cytotoxic response of serum from patients with chronic inflammatory demyelinating polyradiculoneuropathy (CIDP). *Acta Neurol Scand* 1987;76:24–27.
7. Arnon R, et al. Anti-ganglioside antibodies in multiple sclerosis. *J Neurol Sci* 1980;46:179–186.
8. Baba H, et al. Anti-GM1 ganglioside antibodies with differing fine specificities in patients with multifocal motor neuropathy. *J Neuroimmunol* 1989;25:143–150.
9. Bannatyne P, et al. Autoimmune oophoritis: a clinicopathologic assessment of 12 cases. *Int J Gynecol Pathol* 1990;9:191–207.
10. Bassi S, et al. Electromyographic study of diabetic and alcoholic poly-neuropathic patients treated with gangliosides. *Muscle Nerve* 1982;5:351–356.
11. Barbeau A, Pourcher E. New data on the genetics of Parkinson's disease. *Can J Neurol Sci* 1982;9:60–63.
12. Bardwick PA, et al. Plasma cell dyscrasia with polyneuropathy, organomegaly, endocrinopathy, M protein and skin changes: the POEMS syndrome. *Medicine* 1980;59:311–322.
13. Bergstrom B, et al. Autonomic neuropathy in type I diabetes: influence of duration and other diabetes complications. *Acta Med Scand* 1987;222:147–154.
14. Boiardi A, et al. Neurological and pharmacological evaluation of a case of stiff-man syndrome. *J Neurol* 1980; 223:127–133.
15. Bottazzo GF, et al. Islet cell antibodies in diabetes mellitus with autoimmune polyendocrine diseases. *Lancet* 1974;ii:1279–1283.
16. Braun PE, et al. Myelin associated glycoprotein is the antigen for a monoclonal IgM in polyneuropathy. *J Neurochem* 1987;39:1261–1265.
17. Brogren C-H, Anderson P. BB Wistar rat monoclonal autoantibodies. Program of the Juvenile Diabetes Foundation Workshop on the spontaneously diabetic BB rat, Banff. *Metabolism* 1983;32(suppl 1):165.
18. Brown FM, et al. Anti-sympathetic nervous system autoantibodies: diminished catecholamines with orthostasis. *Diabetes* 1989;38: 938–941.
19. Brown FM, et al. Polyneuroendocrine autoimmunity and Parkinson's disease (abstr). *Clin Res* 1989;37:356A.
20. Brown FM, et al. Anti-adrenal medullary antibodies in insulin dependent diabetes and patients at high risk of developing insulin dependent diabetes. *Diabetes Care* 1987;11: 30–33.
21. Brown FM, et al. Adrenal medullitis in type I diabetes mellitus. *J Clin Endocrinol Metab* 1990; 71:1491–1495.
22. Brown FM, et al. Inheritance of anti-autonomic nervous system autoantibodies in type I diabetes (abstr). *Diabetes* 1990;39(suppl 1):497.
23. Brown FM, et al. Adrenal medullary fibrosis in IDDM of long duration. *Diabetes Care* 1989; 12:494–497.
24. Brown JW, et al. Sjögren's syndrome with myopathic and myasthenic features. *Bull Los Angeles Neurol Soc* 1968; 33:9–20.
25. Brownlee M, et al. Nonenzymatic glycosylation and the pathogenesis of diabetic complications. *Ann Intern Med* 1985;101:527–537.
26. Brownlee M, et al. Trapped immunoglobulins on peripheral nerve myelin from patients with diabetes mellitus. *Diabetes* 1986;35: 999–1003.

27. Cadoni A, et al. Schwann cell expression of HLA-DR antigen in peripheral neuropathies. *Lancet* 1986;2:1282–1283.
28. Carmichael SW, et al. Decreased catecholamines in the adrenal medulla of patients with parkinsonism. *N Engl J Med* 1988;318:254.
29. Carson KA, et al. Peripheral neuropathy in mouse hereditary diabetes mellitus. *Neuropathol Appl Neurobiol* 1980; 6:361–374.
30. Case Records of the Massachusetts General Hospital. Case 46-1987. *N Engl J Med* 1987;317:1270–1278.
31. Chou DKH, et al. Structure of sulfated glucuronyl glycolipids in the nervous system reacting with HNK-1 antibody and IgM paraproteins in some neuropathy patients. *J Biol Chem* 1986;261: 11717–11725.
32. Clements RS Jr. New trends in the etiopathogenesis of diabetic neuropathy. In: Andreani D, Crepaldi G, Di Mario U, Pozza G (eds). *Diabetic Complications: Early Diagnosis and Treatment*. Chichester, England: John Wiley & Sons. 1987;115–122.
33. Cohen L. Stiff-man syndrome: two patients treated with diazepam. *JAMA* 1966;195:222–224.
34. Colman PG, et al. "Cytoplasmic" islet cell antibodies: evidence that the target antigen is a sialoglycoconjugate. *Diabetes* 1985;34:617–619.
35. Colman PG, et al. Binding of cytoplasmic islet cell antibodies is blocked by human pancreatic glycolipid extracts. *Diabetes* 1988;37: 645–652.
36. Daikas MC, Engel WK. Chronic relapsing (dysimmune) polyneuropathy: pathogenesis and treatment. *Ann Neurol* 1981;9(suppl): 134–135.
37. Defazio G, et al. Parkinsonian serum carries complement-dependent toxicity for rat dopaminergic neurons in culture. *Brain Res* 1994; 633:206–212.
38. Dernouchamps JP, et al. Immune complexes in the aqueous humor and serum. *Am J Ophthalmol* 1977;84:24–31.
39. Dotta F, Rabinowe SL. Type I diabetes: anti-neuronal antibodies in the NOD mouse (abstr). *Clin Res* 1990;38:366A.
40. Drake ME Jr. Stiff-man syndrome and dementia. *Am J Med* 1983; 74:1085–1087.
41. Drexhage HA, et al. The multiplicity of stimulating and blocking autoantibodies in relation to thyroid and extrathyroidal tissues. In: Doniach D, Bottazzo GF (eds). *Bailliere's Clinical Immunology and Allergy: Endocrine and Other Organ-Oriented Autoimmune Disorders*. London: Bailliere Tindall. 1987;125– 140.
42. Duchen LW, et al. Pathology of autonomic neuropathy in diabetes mellitus. *Ann Intern Med* 1980; 92:301–303.
43. Dyck PJ, et al. Chronic inflammatory polyradiculoneuropathy. *Mayo Clin Proc* 1975;50:621–637.
44. Dyck PJ, et al. Human diabetic endoneurial sorbitol, fructose, and myo-inositol related to sural nerve morphometry. *Ann Neurol* 1980;8:590–596.
45. Dyck PJ, et al. Prednisone-responsive hereditary motor and sensory neuropathy. *Mayo Clin Proc* 1982;57: 239–246.
46. Edelman GM. CAMs and Igs: cell adhesion and the evolutionary origins of immunity. *Immunol Rev* 1987;100:11–45.
47. Eisenbarth GS. Type I diabetes mellitus. A chronic autoimmune disease. *N Engl J Med* 1986;314:1360–1368.
48. Eisenbarth GS, et al. Type I diabetes as a chronic autoimmune disease. *J Diabetes Complications* 1988; 2: 54–58.
49. Emile J, et al. Maladie de Parkinson, dysautonomie et auto-anticorps diriges contre les neurones sympathetiques. *Rev Neurol (Paris)* 1980;136: 221–233.
50. Endo T, et al. Antibodies to glycosphingolipids in patients with multiple sclerosis and SLE. *J Immunol* 1984;132:1793–1797.
51. Engel AG, Arahata K. The membrane attack complex of complement at the endplate in myasthenia gravis. In: Drachman DB (ed). *Myasthenia Gravis: Biology and Treatment. Ann NY Acad Sci* 1987; 505:326–332.
52. Ewing DJ, et al. Immediate heart rate response to standing: simple test for autonomic neuropathy in diabetes. *Br Med J* 1978;1: 145–147.
53. Fagius J, Jameson S. Effects of aldose reductase inhibitor treatment in diabetic polyneuropathy: a clinical and neurophysiological study. *J Neurol Neurosurg Psychiatry* 1981;44:991–1001.
54. Feizi T, Handler N. Autoantibodies and disease. In: Elkeles RS, Tavill AS (eds). *Biochemical Aspects of Human Disease*. Oxford: Blackwell Scientific. 1983;656–692.
55. Feeney DJ, et al. HLA antigens in chronic inflammatory demyelinating polyneuropathy. *J Neurol Neurosurg Psychiatry* 1990;53: 170–172.
56. Fong JW, et al. Gangliosides of peripheral nerve myelin. *J Neurochem* 1976;26:157–162.
57. George TM, et al. Resolution of stiff-man syndrome with cortisol replacement in a patient with deficiencies of ACTH, growth hormone, and prolactin. *N Engl J Med* 1984;310:1511–1513.
58. Gilbey SG, et al. Diabetes and autonomic neuropathy: an immunologic association? *Diabet Med* 1986;3:241–245.
59. Gilbey SG, et al. Cell-mediated immunity and symptomatic diabetic autonomic neuropathy. *Diabet Med* 1988;5:845–848.
60. Goncalves E, et al. Pilot study of immunosuppressive therapy in diabetic neuropathy associated with neuronal auto-antibodies (abstr). *Diabetes* 1990; 39(suppl 1):778.
61. Gordon EE, et al. A critical survey of stiff-man syndrome. *Am J Med* 1967;42:582–599.
62. Graf RJ, et al. Nerve conduction abnormalities in untreated maturity onset diabetes: relation to levels of fasting plasma glucose and glycosylated hemoglobin. *Ann Intern Med* 1979;90:298–303.
63. Gregersen G. Diabetic neuropathy: influence of age, sex, metabolic control and duration of diabetes on motor conduction velocity. *Neurology* 1967;17:972–980.
64. Groop LC, et al. Islet cell antibodies identify latent type I diabetes in patients aged 35–75 years at diagnosis. *Diabetes* 1986;35:237–241.
65. Goulon M, et al. Preliminary results in myasthenia gravis treated with cyclosporin. In: Drachman DB (ed). *Myasthenia Gravis: Biology and Treatment. Ann NY Acad Sci* 1987; 505:857–860.
66. Guillain-Barré Study Group. Plasmapheresis and acute Guillain-Barré Syndrome. *Neurology* 1985;35:1096–1104.
67. Gutmann L, et al. The Eaton-Lambert syndrome and autoimmune disorders. *Am J Med* 1972;53: 354–356.
68. Guy RJC, et al. Diabetic autonomic neuropathy and iritis: an association suggesting an immunological cause. *Br Med J* 1984;289: 343–345.
69. Hakomori S-I. Glycosphingolipids in cellular interaction, differentiation, and oncogenesis. *Annu Rev Biochem* 1981;50:733–764.
70. Harding AE, et al. Plasma exchange and immunosuppression in the stiff man syndrome. *Lancet* 1989;2:915.
71. Hartung HP, et al. Circulating adhesion molecules and inflammatory mediators. *Neurology* 1995; 45(suppl 6):s22–s32.
72. Hays AP, et al. Experimental demyelination of nerve induced by serum of patients with neuropathy and an anti-MAG IgM M-protein. *Neurology* 1987;37:242–256.
73. Hirano T, et al. Anti-glycolipid autoantibody detected in the sera from systemic lupus erythematosus patients. *J Clin Invest* 1980;66: 1437–1440.
74. Hirsch HE, Parks ME. Serological reactions against glycolipid-sensitized liposomes in multiple sclerosis. *Nature* 1976;264:785–787.
75. Howard FM Jr. A new and effective drug in the treatment of the "stiff-man" syndrome: preliminary report. *Mayo Clin Proc* 1963;38: 203–212.
76. Howes EL, McKay DG. Circulating immune complexes. Effects on ocular vascular permeability in the rabbit. *Arch Ophthalmol* 1975; 93:365–370.
77. Ikegami H, et al. Immunogenetics and immunopathogenesis of the NOD mouse. In: Eisenbarth GS (ed). *Immunotherapy of Diabetes and Selected Autoimmune Diseases*. Boca Raton, FL: CRC Press. 1989;23–33.
78. Ilyas AA, et al. IgM in a human neuropathy related to paraproteinemia binds to a carbohydrate determinant in the myelin-associated glycoprotein and to a ganglioside. *Proc Natl Acad Sci U S A* 1984; 81:1225–1229.
79. Ilyas AA, et al. Serum antibodies to gangliosides in Guillain-Barré syndrome. *Ann Neurol* 1988;23:440– 447.
80. Imawari M, et al. Syndrome of plasma cell dyscrasia, polyneuropathy and endocrine disturbances. *Ann Intern Med* 1974;81:490–493.
81. Inaba G, Aoyama J. Anti-glycolipid antibodies in neuro-Behçet's syndrome. In: Inaba G (ed). *Behçet's Disease: Pathogenetic Mechanism and Clinical Future*. Tokyo: University of Tokyo Press. 1981; 145–152.
82. Ito H, Latov N. Monoclonal IgM in two patients with motor neuron disease bind to the carbohydrate antigens Gal(beta 1-3)GalNAc and Gal(beta 1-3)GlcNAc. *J Neuroimmunol* 1988;19:245–253.

83. Itoh N, et al. Two types of autoantibodies to adrenal medullary cells in patients with insulin dependent diabetes mellitus (IDDM). *Diabetes* 1991;40(suppl 1):225A.
84. Itoh N, et al. Two types of autoantibodies to adrenal medullary cells in type I (insulin dependent) diabetic patients: prevalence, properties and implications. *J Autoimmun* 1991; 4(5):807–818.
85. Iwashita H, et al. Polyneuropathy, skin hyperpigmentation, edema and hypertrichosis in localized osteosclerotic myeloma. *Neurology* 1977;27:675–681.
86. Jackson RA, et al. Ia+ T cells in new onset Graves' disease. *J Clin Endocrinol Metab* 1984;59:197–190.
87. Jackson RA, et al. Increased circulating Ia-antigen bearing T cells in type I diabetes mellitus. *N Engl J Med* 1982;306:785–788.
88. Johns TR. Long-term corticosteroid treatment of myasthenia gravis. In: Drachman DB (ed). *Myasthenia Gravis: Biology and Treatment*. *Ann NY Acad Sci* 1987;505:569–583.
89. Kamoshita S, et al. Infantile Niemann-Pick disease. A chemical study with isolation and characterization of membranous cytoplasmic bodies and myelin. *Am J Dis Child* 1969; 117:379–394.
90. Kaufman DL, et al. Glutamate decarboxylase (GAD) autoantibodies (GAD Ab) in insulin dependent diabetes mellitus. *Diabetes* 1991; 40(suppl 1):2A.
91. Kennedy WR, et al. Effects of pancreatic transplantation on diabetic neuropathy. *N Engl J Med* 1990;322:1031–1037.
92. Kim YI. Passively transferred Lambert-Eaton syndrome in mice receiving purified IgG. *Muscle Nerve* 1986;9:523–530.
93. Kim YI, Neher E. IgG from patients with Lambert-Eaton syndrome blocks voltage-dependent calcium channels. *Science* 1988;239:405–408.
94. Kissel P, et al. Myasthenia and thyrotoxicosis. In: Walton JN, Canal N, Scarlato G (eds). *Muscle Diseases*. Amsterdam: Excerpta Medica. 1970;464.
95. Kohn LD, et al. Autoimmune thyroid disease studied with monoclonal antibodies to the thyrotropin receptor. In: Haynes BF, Eisenbarth GS (eds). *Monoclonal Antibodies—Probes for the Study of Autoimmunity and Immunodeficiency*. Orlando: Academic Press. 1983; 221–258.
96. Kohriyama T, et al. Preparation and characterization of antibodies against a sulfated glucuronic acid-containing glycosphingolipid. *J Neurochem* 1988;51:869–877.
97. Korn-Lubetzki I, Abramsky O. Acute and chronic demyelinating inflammatory polyradiculoneuropathy: association with autoimmune diseases and lymphocyte response to human neuritogenic protein. *Arch Neurol* 1986;43:604–608.
98. Koski CL, et al. Anti-peripheral nerve myelin antibodies in Guillain-Barré syndrome bind a neutral glycolipid of peripheral myelin and cross-react with Forssman antigen. *J Clin Invest* 1989;84:280–287.
99. Koski CL, et al. Clinical correlations with anti-peripheral nerve myelin antibodies in Guillain-Barré syndrome. *Ann Neurol* 1986; 19:573–577.
100. Kusunoki S, et al. Combined features of myasthenia gravis and Eaton-Lambert syndrome: anti-ganglioside antibodies in serum. *J Neurol Sci* 1988;87:61–66.
101. Lai C, et al. Neural protein 1B236/MAG defines a subgroup of the immunoglobulin superfamily. *Immunol Rev* 1988;100:129–151.
102. Lambert EH, et al. Clinical physiology of the neuromuscular junction. In: Paul WM, Daniel EE, Kay CM, Monockton G (eds). *Muscle*. Oxford: Pergamon Press. 1965;487.
103. Lang B, et al. Autoimmune aetiology for myasthenic (Eaton-Lambert) syndrome. *Lancet* 1981;2:224–226.
104. Lindstom JM, et al. Antibody to acetylcholine receptor in myasthenia gravis: prevalence, clinical correlates and diagnostic value. *Neurology* 1976;26:1054–1059.
105. Locke S, Tarsey D. The nervous system and diabetes. In: Marble A, Krall LP, Bradley RF et al (eds). *Joslin's Diabetes Mellitus, 12th ed*. Philadelphia: Lea & Febiger. 1985;665–685.
106. Mancardi GL, et al. HLA-DR Schwann cell reactivity in peripheral neuropathies of different origins. *Neurology* 1988;38:848–851.140.
107. Mann JD, et al. Long-term administration of corticosteroids in myasthenia gravis. *Neurology* 1976;26:729–740.
108. Martinelli P, et al. Stiff-man syndrome associated with nocturnal myoclonus and epilepsy. *J Neurol Neurosurg Psychiatry* 1978;41:458–462.
109. Martyn CN, et al. Is there a link between iritis and diabetic autonomic neuropathy? *Br Med J* 292:934.
110. Matell G. Immunosuppressive drugs: azathioprine in the treatment of myasthenia gravis. In: Drachman DB (ed). *Myasthenia Gravis: Biology and Treatment*. *Ann NY Acad Sci* 1987;505:588–594.
111. McCleod JG, Pollard JD. Peripheral neuropathy associated with paraproteinemia. *Handbook of Clinical Neurology* 1987;51:429–444.
112. McCluskey J, et al. HLA and complement allotypes in type 1 (insulin-dependent) diabetes. *Diabetologia* 1983; 24:162–165.
113. Moersch FP, Woltman HW. Progressive fluctuating muscular rigidity and spasm (stiff-man syndrome): report of a case and some observations in 13 other cases. *Mayo Clin Proc* 1956;31:421–427.
114. Mori M, Takamori M. Hyperthyroidism and myasthenia gravis with features of Eaton-Lambert syndrome. *Neurology* 1976;26:882–887.
115. Nardelli E, et al. Pattern of nervous tissue immunostaining by human anti-glycolipid antibodies. *J Neurol Sci* 1994;122(2):220–227.
116. Nayak RC, et al. Cytoplasmic islet cell antibodies: evidence that the target antigen is a sialoglycoconjugate. *Diabetes* 1985;34:617–619.
117. Neufeld M, et al. Two types of autoimmune Addison's disease associated with different polyglandular autoimmune (PGA) syndromes. *Medicine* 1981;60:355–362.
118. Norris FH. Neuromuscular transmission in thyroid disease. *Ann Intern Med* 1966;64:81–86.
119. Oh SJ. The Lambert-Eaton syndrome in ocular myasthenia gravis. *Arch Neurol* 1974;31:183–186.
120. Oh SJ, et al. Overlap myasthenic syndrome: combined myasthenia gravis and Eaton-Lambert syndrome. *Neurology* 37:1411–1414.
121. Ohsawa T, et al. Anti-B-series ganglioside-recognizing autoantibodies in an acute sensory neuropathy patient cause cell death of rat dorsal root ganglion neurons. *Neurosci Lett* 1993;157(2):167–170.
122. Olanow CW, et al. A prospective study of thymectomy and the acetylcholine receptor antibodies in human myasthenia gravis. *Ann Surg* 1982;196:113–121.
123. Olanow CW, et al. Thymectomy as primary therapy in myasthenia gravis. In: Drachman DB (ed). *Myasthenia Gravis: Biology and Treatment*. *Ann NY Acad Sci* 1987; 505:595–606.
124. Osserman KE, Genkins G. Studies in myasthenia gravis. Review of a 20 year experience in over 1200 patients. *Mt Sinai J Med* 1971; 38:497–534.
125. Pack BA, et al. In: Baba S, Kaneko T (eds). *Diabetes 1994*. The Netherlands: Elsevier Science B.V. 1995;1113–1118.
126. Pestronk A, et al. A treatable multifocal motor neuropathy with antibodies to GM1 ganglioside. *Ann Neurol* 1988;24:73–78.
127. Pittenger GL, et al. The toxic effects of serum from patients with type I diabetes mellitus on mouse neuroblastoma cells: a new mechanism for development of diabetic autonomic neuropathy. *Diabet Med* 1993;10:925–932.
128. Pittenger GL, et al. The neuronal toxic factor in serum of type I diabetic patients is a complement-fixing autoantibody. *Diabet Med* 1995;12:380–386.
129. Pollard JD, et al. Class II antigen expression and T lymphocyte subsets in chronic inflammatory demyelinating polyneuropathy. *J Neuroimmunol* 1986;13:123–134.
130. Potz G, Neundorfer B. Polyradicular neuritis and Hashimoto thyroiditis. *J Neurol* 1975;210:283–289.
131. Pouplard A, Emile J. Autoimmunity in Parkinson's disease. *Adv Neurol* 1984;40:307–312.
132. Quarles RH. Antibodies to complex carbohydrates that may mediate neuropathy. *PNEI* 1989;2:109–119.
133. Quarles RH, et al. Antibodies to glycolipids in demyelinating diseases of the human peripheral nervous system. *Chem Phys Lipids* 1986;42:235–248.
134. Rabinowe SL, et al. Anti-sympathetic ganglia antibodies and postural blood pressure in IDDM subjects of varying duration and patients at high risk of developing IDDM. *Diabetes Care* 1989; 12:1–6.
135. Rabinowe SL, et al. Complement fixing antibodies to sympathetic and parasympathetic tissues in IDDM: the autonomic brake index and heart rate variation. *Diabetes Care* 1990;13:1084–1088.
136. Rabinowe SL, Eisenbarth GS. Polyglandular autoimmunity. *Adv Intern Med* 1986;31:293–307.
137. Rabinowe SL, et al. Ia+ T lymphocytes in recently diagnosed idiopathic Addison's disease. *Am J Med* 1984;77:597–601.

138. Rabinowe SL, et al. Anti-ganglioside GT1b IgG antibodies in type I diabetes: orthostatic blood pressure and autonomic autoantibodies. *Clin Res* 1991;39:364A.
139. Rabinowe SL, Myerov A. Chromogranin A IgG autoantibodies in type I diabetes: association with adrenal medullary autoimmunity (abstr). *Clin Res* 1992;
140. Rabinowe SL, et al. Anti-ganglioside LM1 IgG antibodies in diabetes mellitus: relationship to complement fixing anti-neuronal antibodies. *International Diabetes Federation Satellite Meeting on Controversies in Etiology and Treatment of Diabetic Neuropathy 1991.*
141. Rabinowe SL, et al. Complement fixing autoantibodies to the sympathetic nervous system and sciatic nerve in type I diabetes mellitus (XIII Congress of the International Diabetes Federation). *Diabetes Res Clin Pract* 1988;5:55–76.
142. Regev I, et al. Acute polyneuropathy combined with myasthenia gravis. *Acta Neurol Scand* 1982;65:681–682.
143. Rizzuto N, Simonati A. Chronic inflammatory demyelinating polyneuropathy. *Int J Tissue React* 1985;7:521–526.
144. Roisen FJ, et al. Ganglioside stimulation of axonal sprouting *in vitro*. *Science* 1981;214:577–578.
145. Rooke ED, et al. Myasthenia and malignant intrathoracic tumors. *Med Clin North Am* 1960;44:977–988.
146. Roses AD. Myasthenia gravis. In: Eisenbarth GS (ed). *Immunotherapy of Diabetes and Selected Autoimmune Diseases*. Boca Raton, FL: CRC Press. 1989;189–196.
147. Ryberg B. Multiple specificities of antibrain antibodies in multiple sclerosis and chronic myelopathy. *J Neurol Sci* 1978;38:357–382.
148. Saihan EM, et al. A new syndrome with pigmentation, scleroderma, gynecomastia, Raynaud's phenomenon, and peripheral neuropathy. *Br J Dermatol* 1978;99:437–440.
149. Schalke B, et al. Cyclosporin A treatment of myasthenia gravis: initial results of a double-blind trial of cyclosporin A versus azathioprine. In: Drachman DB (ed). *Myasthenia Gravis: Biology and Treatment. Ann NY Acad Sci* 1987;505:872–875.
150. Schopfer K, et al. Anti-glucagon cell and anti-adrenal medullary cell antibodies in islet cell autoantibody positive diabetic children. *N Engl J Med* 1984;310:1536–1537.
151. Schwartz M, et al. Antibodies to gangliosides and myelin autoantigens are produced in mice following sciatic nerve injury. *J Neurochem* 1982;38:1192–1195.
152. Schwartz M, Spirman N. Sprouting from chicken embryo dorsal root ganglia induced by nerve growth factors is specifically inhibited by affinity purified anti-ganglioside antibodies. *Proc Natl Acad Sci USA* 1982;79:6080–6083.
153. Schwerer B, et al. Ganglioside GM1, a molecular target for immunological and toxin attacks: similarity of neuropathological lesions induced by ganglioside antiserum and cholera toxin. *Acta Neuropathol* 1986;72:55–61.
154. Sinha S, et al. Autoimmune aetiology for acquired neuromyotonia (Isaacs' syndrome). *Lancet* 1991;338:75–77.
155. Smith SH, et al. Functional subsets of human helper-inducer cells defined by a new monoclonal antibody, UCHL1. *Immunology* 1986;58:63–70.
156. Solimena M, et al. Autoantibodies to GABA-ergic neurons and pancreatic beta cells in stiff-man syndrome. *N Engl J Med* 1990;322:1555–1560.
157. Solimena M, et al. Autoantibodies to glutamic acid decarboxylase in a patient with stiff-man syndrome, epilepsy, and type I diabetes mellitus. *N Engl J Med* 1988;318:1012–1020.
158. Spitalnik SL, et al. An islet cell specific human monoclonal autoantibody from a patient with type I diabetes recognizes a monosialoganglioside. *International Research Symposium: "The Immunology of Diabetes."* American Diabetes Association, Woods Hole, MA, Oct 27–30, 1987.
159. Stewart GJ, et al. HLA antigens in the Landry-Guillain-Barré syndrome and chronic relapsing polyneuritis. *Ann Neurol* 1978;4:285–289.
160. Stuart FS, et al. The stiff-man syndrome: report of a case. *Arthritis Rheum* 1960;3:229–232.
161. Sundkvist G, et al. Abnormal diastolic blood pressure and heart rate reactions to tilting in diabetes mellitus. *Diabetologia* 1980;19:433–438.
162. Sundkvist G, et al. Autonomic nerve antibodies and autonomic nerve function in type I and type 2 diabetic patients. *J Intern Med* 1991;229:505–510.
163. Sundkvist G, et al. Glutamic acid decarboxylase antibodies, autonomic nerve antibodies and autonomic neuropathy in diabetic patients. *Diabetologia* 1994;37(3):293–299.
164. Suzuki K. Formation and turnover of myelin ganglioside. *J Neurochem* 1970;17:209–213.
165. Svennerholm L. Chromatographic separation of human brain gangliosides. *J Neurochem* 1963;10:613–623.
166. Takekazn O, et al. Increased endoneurial albumin in diabetic polyneuropathy. *Neurology* 35:1790–1791.
167. Taylor HC, et al. Clonidine suppression test for pheochromocytoma: examples of misleading results. *J Clin Endocrinol Metab* 1986;63:238–242.
168. Thomas PK. Inherited neuropathies. *Mayo Clin Proc* 1983;58:476–480.
169. Timperley WR, et al. Small vessel disease in progressive diabetic neuropathy with good metabolic control. *J Clin Pathol* 1985;38:1030–1038.
170. Tobin AJ, et al. Autoantibodies in insulin-dependent diabetes mellitus. Patients differentially recognize two forms of glutamate decarboxylase, which derive from two genes. *Diabetes* 1991;40(suppl 1):2A.
171. Uhlig H, Dernick R. Monoclonal autoantibodies derived from multiple sclerosis patients and control persons and their reactivities with antigens of the central nervous system. *Autoimmunity* 1989;5:87–99.
172. van Doorn PA, et al. Clinical significance of antibodies against peripheral nerve tissue in inflammatory polyneuropathy. *Neurology* 1987;37:1796–1802.
173. Vicari AM, et al. Plasmapheresis in the treatment of stiff man syndrome. *N Engl J Med* 1989;320:1499.
174. Vincent SR, et al. Immunohistochemical studies of the GABA system in the pancreas. *Neuroendocrinology* 1983; 36:197–204.
175. Vital C, et al. Acute inflammatory demyelinating polyneuropathy in a diabetic patient: predominance of vesicular disruption in myelin sheaths. *Acta Neuropathol (Berl)* 1985;67:337–340.
176. Vital C, et al. Relapsing inflammatory demyelinating polyneuropathy in a diabetic patient. *Acta Neuropathol (Berl)* 1986;71:94–99.
177. Vlassara H, et al. Excessive nonenzymatic glycosylation of peripheral and central nervous system components in diabetic rats. *Diabetes* 1983;32:670–674.
178. Vlassara H, et al. Recognition and uptake of human diabetic peripheral nerve myelin by macrophages. *Diabetes* 1985;34:553–557.
179. Vroom FQ, Engel WK. Nonneoplastic steroid responsive Lambert-Eaton myasthenic syndrome (abstr). *Neurology* 1969;19:281.
180. Watkins PJ, et al. Severe sensory-autonomic neuropathy and endocrinopathy in insulin-dependent diabetes. *Q J Med* 1995;88:794–804.
181. Whelan JL. Baclofen in treatment of the "stiff-man" syndrome. *Arch Neurol* 1980;37:600–601.
182. Williams AF. A year in the life of the immunoglobulin superfamily. *Immunol Today* 1987;8:298–303.
183. Williams AF, Barclay NA. The immunoglobulin superfamily-domains for cell surface recognition. *Annu Rev Immunol* 1988;6:381–405.
184. Willison HJ, et al. Demyelination induced by intraneural injection of human anti-myelin associated glycoprotein antibodies. *Muscle Nerve* 1988;11:1169–1176.
185. Witkin SS, et al. Induction of antibody to asialo GM1 by spermatozoa and its occurrence in the sera of homosexual men with the acquired immune deficiency syndrome (AIDS). *Clin Exp Immunol* 1983;54:346–350.
186. Wong VG, et al. Endogenous immune uveitis: the role of serum sickness. *Arch Ophthalmol* 1971;85:93–102.
187. Yasuda T, et al. Antiglycolipid antibodies in Behçet's disease. In: Inaba G (ed). *Behçet's Disease: Pathogenetic Mechanism and Clinical Future*. Tokyo: University of Tokyo Press. 1981;413–420.
188. Young RJ, et al. A controlled trial of sorbinil, an aldose reductase inhibitor, in chronic painful diabetic neuropathy. *Diabetes* 1983;32:938–942.

189. Zanone MM, et al. An investigation of antibodies to nerve growth factor in diabetic autonomic neuropathy. *Diabet Med* 1994;11(4): 378–383.
190. Zanone MM, et al. Autoantibodies to nervous tissue structures are associated with autonomic neuropathy in type I (insulin dependent) diabetes mellitus. *Diabetologia* 1993;36 (6):564–569.
191. Zanone MM, et al. High prevalence of autoantibodies to glutamic acid decarboxylase in long-standing IDDM is not a marker of symptomatic autonomic neuropathy. *Diabetes* 1994;43(9):1146–1151.
192. Zimmerman BR. Aldose reductase inhibitors. In: Dyck PJ, Thomas PK, Asbury AK (eds). *Diabetic Neuropathy*. Philadelphia: WB Saunders. 1987;190–193.

CHAPTER 39

Familial Dysautonomia

Felicia B. Axelrod

---

1. Familial dysautonomia is a recessively inherited disorder confined to Ashkenazi Jews. The carrier rate is 1 in 30, and the disease frequency is 1 in 3600.
2. The genetic defect occurs in the long arm of chromosome 9 (q31). Prenatal diagnosis and carrier detection are possible in affected families. The genetic error probably affects the maintenance as well as development of the neuronal population, because there is clinical and objective evidence of progression with time.
3. Clinical features reflect widespread involvement of sensory and autonomic neurons. Sensory loss is manifested by hypotonia and impairment of pain and temperature perception. Autonomic features include dysphagia, vomiting crises, lability of blood pressure (BP), orthostatic hypotension without compensatory tachycardia, and vasomotor and sudomotor dysfunction. Central dysfunction is manifested by emotional lability and ataxia.
4. Diagnosis is based on the presence of five "cardinal" features: alacrima, absence of fungiform papillae, depression of patellar reflexes, absence of axon flare to intradermal histamine, and Ashkenazi Jewish background.
5. Pathologic alterations consist of a loss of both preganglionic and postganglionic sympathetic and parasympathetic neurons; sensory neurons are similarly affected.
6. Treatment is preventive, symptomatic, and supportive.
7. Prognosis has greatly improved with supportive treatment. About 40% of known patients are now over the age of 20 years. Causes of death are predominantly pulmonary failure and renal failure. Unexplained sudden death also occurs.

INTRODUCTION

Familial dysautonomia (FD) is an inherited neurologic disease that affects the development and survival of unmyelinated sensory and autonomic neurons. Following its original description in 1949 (51), FD was commonly referred to as the *Riley-Day syndrome* in acknowledgment of the authors of that report. In time it was recognized that FD is one of a group of disorders, the hereditary sensory and autonomic neuropathies (HSANs) (6), each of which is probably caused by a different error in neurodevelopment. Although all the HSANs are generally characterized by widespread sensory dysfunction and variable autonomic dysfunction, they can be distinguished by specific and consistent neuropathologic lesions (6,42), allowing for classification and precise nomenclature. Each of the HSANs is believed to be genetically distinct, but until the individual genetic errors have been identified, diagnosis depends on clinical and biochemical evaluation, with pathologic examination further serving to confirm differences. FD appears to be the most common of this uncommon group of disorders. Studies have shown that patients with FD are genetically and pathologically homogenous (18,22,38,42). Thus, the FD population can serve as an excellent model to make possible further understanding of the mechanisms involved in autonomic dysfunction.

Pervasive autonomic dysfunction results in protean functional abnormalities and a myriad of clinical manifestations (7) (Table 1). Signs of the disorder are present from birth (10) and neurologic function slowly deteriorates with age (8), so that symptoms and problems vary with time. The cardiovascular perturbations are particularly troublesome in the adult years (13). The disease process cannot be arrested. Treatment is preventive, symptomatic, and supportive (2,3,5). It must be directed toward specific problems that can vary considerably among patients and within the same patient at different ages.

F. B. Axelrod: Department of Neurology, New York University School of Medicine, New York, New York 10016.

TABLE 1. *Clinical manifestations of familial dysautonomia*

System	Affected area	Functional abnormalities
Nervous	Sensory	Decreased pain perception
		Decreased temperature appreciation
		Depressed deep tendon reflexes
		Decreased corneal reflex
		Deficient taste discrimination
	Motor	Hypotonia
		Ataxic gait
	Autonomic	Excessive sweating
		Blotching of skin
		Cold, mottled extremities
Gastrointestinal	Oropharynx	Feeding difficulties
		Drooling
	Esophagus and stomach (dysmotility)	Misdirected swallows
		Gastroesophageal reflux
		Episodic vomiting
	Bowel (dysmotility)	Constipation
Respiratory	Peripheral receptors (insensitivity to hypoxia and hypercapnia)	Problems with high altitudes, air travel, and underwater swimming
	Aspiration	Repeated pneumonias
		Bronchiectasis and atelectasis
		Hyperreactive airways
Blood pressure	Orthostatic hypotension	Dizzy spells
		Syncope
		Difficulty with anesthetics
	Hypertension	Headaches
Skeletal	Spine	High frequency of curvature
	Joints	Aseptic necrosis
		Neuropathic joints
	Long bones	Unrecognized fractures
Optic	Cornea	Excessive dryness
		Ulcerations
	Optic nerve	Pallor of disc
Renal	Glomeruli	Progressive ischemic sclerosis
		Rising BUN and creatinine with age

GENETICS

Familial Dysautonomia is an autosomal recessive disorder that currently appears to be confined to individuals of Ashkenazi Jewish extraction (22,38). In this population, the carrier rate has been estimated to be 1 in 30, with a disease frequency of 1 in 3600 live births (35). By means of genetic linkage, the gene has been localized to the distal long arm of chromosome 9 (q31), with sufficient DNA markers to permit prenatal diagnosis and carrier identification for families in which a member has been affected (18). On the basis of high levels of linkage disequilibrium, the FD gene is thought to be in close proximity to markers D9S58 and D9S1677, with 97% of FD chromosomes being carriers of allele 12 of the latter marker (53). Although penetrance is complete, expression of the disease varies markedly even among siblings, suggesting the presence of modifying genes.

DIAGNOSTIC CRITERIA

As the specific genetic mutation has not yet been identified, diagnosis of FD is based on the clinical recognition of both sensory and autonomic dysfunction. The diagnosis is made according to the presence of five "cardinal" criteria: alacrima, absence of fungiform papillae (58) (Fig. 1), depression of patellar reflexes, lack of an axon flare following intradermal histamine (54) (Fig. 2), and intraocular hypersensitivity to parasympathomimetic agents (pilocarpine 0.0625%) (57) in an individual of Ashkenazi Jewish extraction. Further supportive evidence is provided by findings of decreased response to pain and temperature, orthostatic hypotension, periodic erythematous blotching of the skin, and increased sweating. In addition, cinesophagrams may reveal delay in cricopharyngeal closure, tertiary contractions of the esophagus, gastroesophageal reflux, and delayed gastric emptying. Sural nerve biopsy is rarely re-

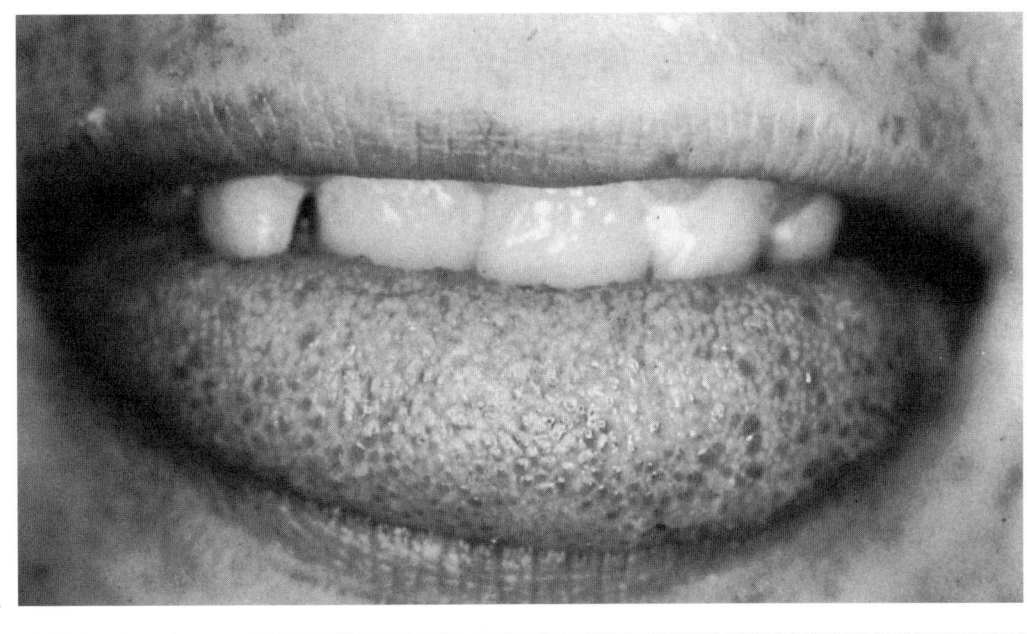
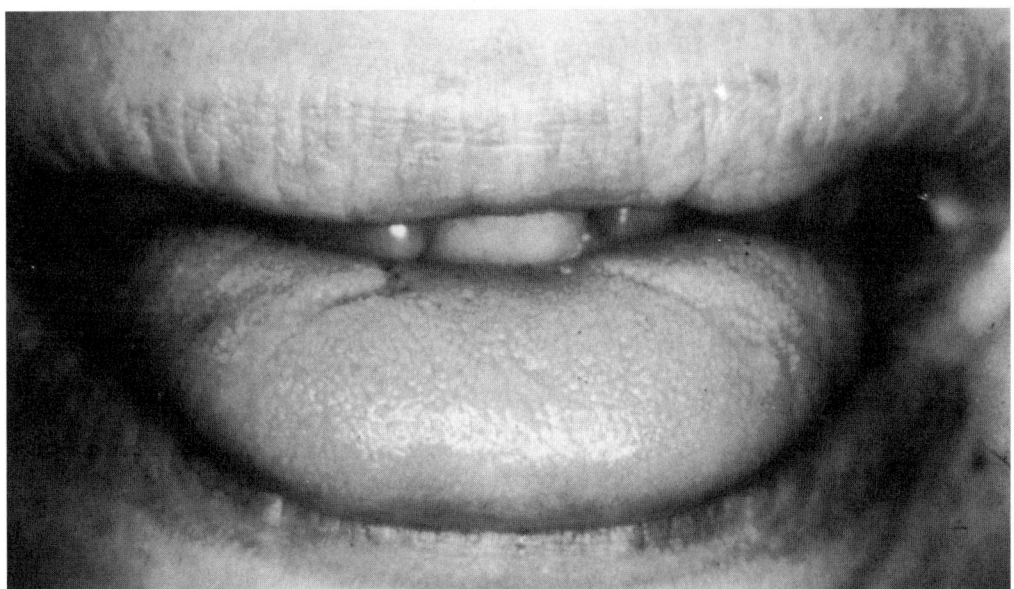

FIG. 1. A: Normal tongue with fungiform papillae present on the tip. **B:** Tongue of a dysautonomic patient.

quired unless one of the five cardinal criteria is not present or the patient is not of Jewish extraction.

Other problems frequently experienced by individuals with FD include excessive sweating, dysphagia and vomiting, aspiration and frequent pneumonia, speech and motor incoordination, lability of BP (episodic hypertension and postural hypotension), poor growth, and scoliosis. However, affected individuals usually are of normal intelligence (60).

In early childhood, the symptoms may be fairly nonspecific, such as poor feeding, delayed development milestones, failure to thrive, and recurrent respiratory illness. It is unusual for the diagnosis to be made after 5 years of age. Cardiovascular perturbations, such as easy fatigability, poor posture, and dizzy spells, are more likely to occur patients who are past adolescence. Cardiovascular instability and ataxic gait worsen with time, and some patients have succumbed to renal failure or sudden cardiac arrests (4). Nonetheless, patients with FD can function independently if treatment is begun early and major disabilities are avoided.

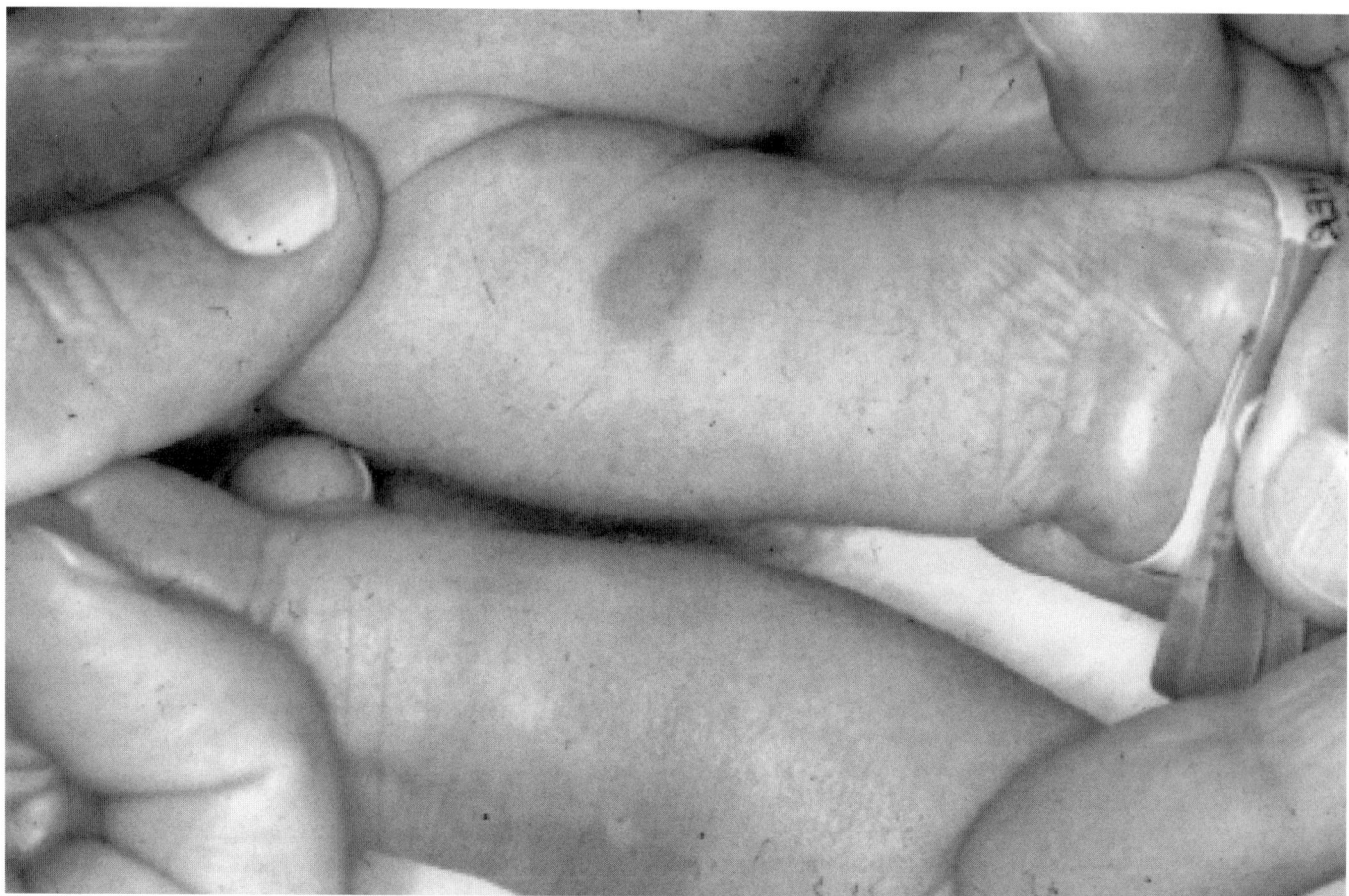

FIG. 2. A: Normal result of histamine test. Reaction displays diffuse axon flare around a central wheal.

NEUROPATHOLOGY

Although Riley et al. originally described FD as "central autonomic dysfunction with absent lacrimation" (51), and although the clinical evidence for central autonomic dysfunction is increasing, pathologic confirmation of central defects remains elusive. To date, neuropathologic examinations have demonstrated only lesions in the peripheral autonomic nervous system and the peripheral sensory system (1,31,40,41,43,44). The overall picture is one of diminished neuronal populations in the sensory and autonomic systems, consistent with a developmental arrest (Fig. 3).

Sympathetic Nervous System

In adult patients with FD, the mean volume of superior cervical sympathetic ganglia is reduced to 34% of normal, reflecting an actual, severe decrease in number of neurons. The anatomic defect in the ganglion cells extends to preganglionic neurons, as the intermediolateral gray columns of the spinal cord also contain low numbers of neurons (40).

Tyrosine hydroxylase, as measured by immunocytochemical techniques, can identify catecholaminergic neurons that produce dopamine (45). Although clinical, anatomic, biochemical, and pharmacologic data indicate diminution in the numbers of sympathetic neurons in FD, staining for tyrosine hydroxylase is enhanced in FD neurons from sympathetic ganglia (46).

Ultrastructural study of peripheral blood vessels has demonstrated the absence of autonomic nerve terminals (31). Lack of innervation is consistent with postural hypotension and denervation hypersensitivity, as demonstrated by exaggerated responses to sympathomimetic and parasympathomimetic agents (55,59).

Parasympathetic Nervous System

Although patients with FD do not produce overflow tears, pharmacologic evidence suggests denervation supersensitivity in effector tissues normally supplied by postganglionic parasympathetic nerve terminals (57). The sphenopalatine ganglia are consistently reduced in size, with low total neuronal counts, but the neuronal popula-

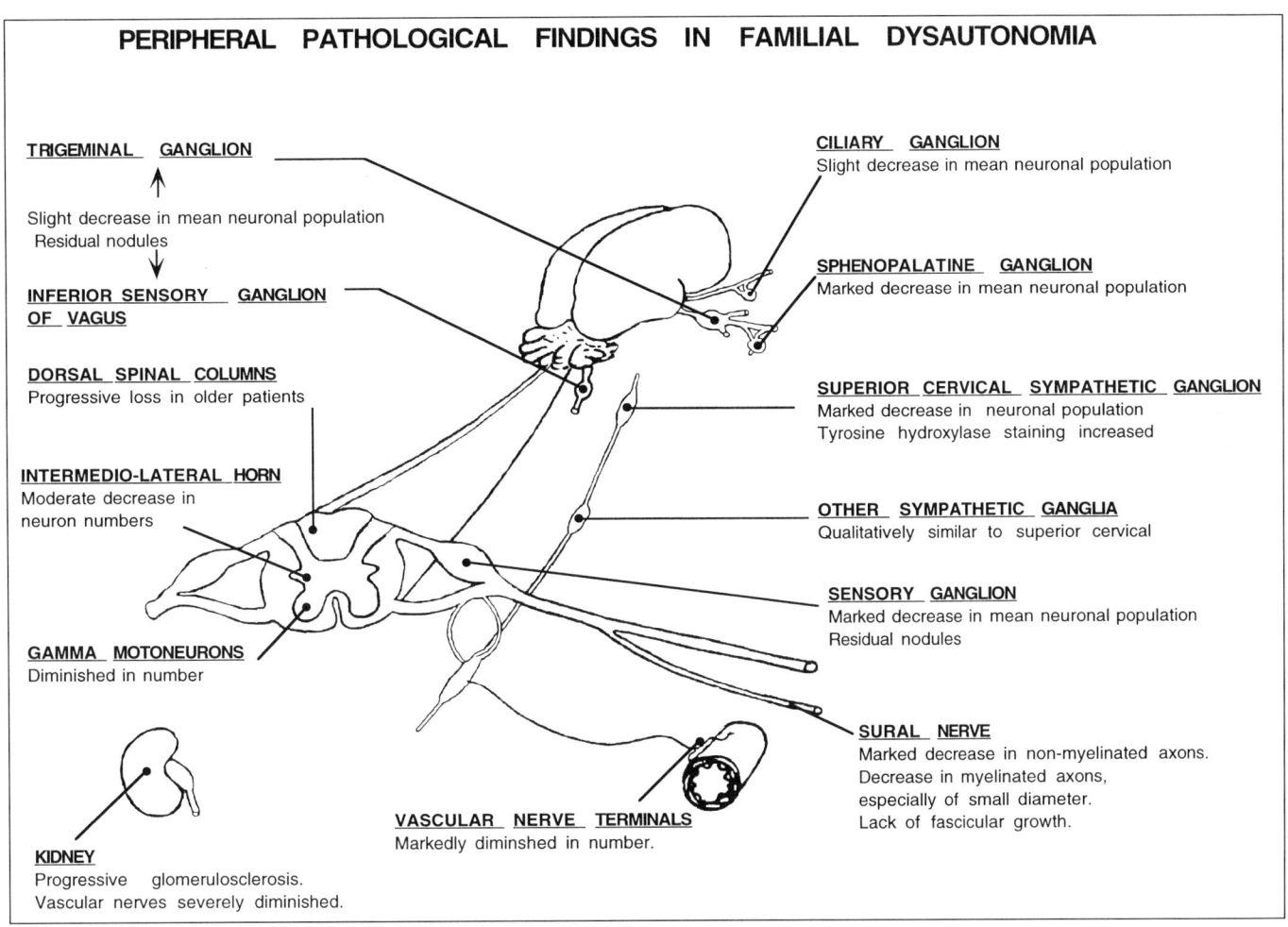

FIG. 3. Peripheral pathologic findings in FD.

tion is only questionably reduced in other parasympathetic ganglia, such as the ciliary ganglia (41). The paucity of neurons in the sphenopalatine ganglion would explain the supersensitivity of the lacrimal gland to infused methacholine (59), and may account for cerebral vascular disregulation, as direct activation of the sphenopalatine ganglia has been shown to modify cerebral blood flow (28).

Sensory Nervous System: Sural Nerve

The sural nerve is reduced in area and contains markedly diminished numbers of nonmyelinated axons and of small-diameter myelinated axons (1,42–44). Catecholamine-containing fibers are missing (31). Even in the youngest subjects, extensive pathology has been evident, as might be expected from the fact that clinical symptoms are present at birth. The sural nerve findings are sufficiently characteristic in FD to be a basis for differentiating it from other sensory neuropathies (6).

Spinal Cord

Intrauterine development and postnatal maintenance of dorsal root ganglion neurons are abnormal (44). The dorsal root ganglia are grossly reduced in size as a consequence of decreased neuronal population. Within the spinal cord, lateral root entry zones and Lissauer's tracts are severely depleted of axons (24). As evidence of slowly progressive degeneration, there is a definite trend with increasing age toward further depletion of the number of neurons in dorsal root ganglia and an increase in the abnormal numbers of residual nodules of Nageotte in the dorsal root ganglia. In addition, loss of myelinated axons in the dorsal column becomes evident in older patients. Neuronal depletion in dorsal root ganglia and the progressive pattern of cord changes correlate well with the clinical observations of worsening pain and diminishing sense of vibration with age (8).

Diminution of primary substance P axons in the substantia gelatinosa of the spinal cord and medulla has been demonstrated using immunohistochemistry (48). Because substance P may be involved in sensory neuron synaptic transmission, the immunoreactive findings support the electron microscopic findings.

NEUROCHEMICAL AND PHARMACOLOGIC ABNORMALITIES

Consistent with the decrease in the sympathetic neuronal population, synthesis of norepinephrine and excretion of catabolites are reduced (30). Dopamine products continue to be excreted in normal amounts, resulting in abnormal ratios of 3-methoxy-4-hydroxymandelic acid (VMA) to 3-methoxy-4-hydroxyphenylacetic acid (HVA). Patients with FD, like most other patients with neurogenic orthostatic hypotension, do not have an appropriate increase in plasma levels of norepinephrine and dopamine-β-hydroxylase on standing; their supine plasma levels of norepinephrine are normal or elevated (16,62). In addition, these patients appear to have a distinctive pattern of plasma levels of catechols (16) (Fig. 4). Regardless of posture, plasma levels of dihydroxyphenylalanine (DOPA) are disproportionately high and plasma levels of dihydroxyphenylglycol (DHPG) are low, resulting in elevated plasma ratios of DOPA to DHPG (Fig. 5), which are not seen in other disorders associated with neurogenic orthostatic hypotension (29). The low levels of DHPG could be a consequence of either decreased availability of axoplasmic norepinephrine or decreased sequential activity of monoamine oxidase and aldehydic reductase on norepinephrine. The high plasma levels of DOPA are consistent with the description of Pearson et al. (46) of large amounts of tyrosine hydroxylase in the superior cervical ganglia by monoclonal antibody stains. While upright, patients with FD have a remarkably strong correlation between BP and plasma levels of dopamine (16), suggesting that dopamine may be a pressor agent in these patients.

During emotional crises, plasma levels of norepinephrine and dopamine are markedly elevated, and vomiting usually coincides with the high dopamine levels. Elevated norepinephrine is attributed to peripheral conversion of dopamine by dopamine-β-hydroxylase. Diazepam sedates patients in crises and relieves vomiting (2), possibly by enhancing τ-aminobutyric acid (GABA) and damping the release of dopamine.

Supine early morning plasma renin activity is elevated in subjects with FD, and the release of renin and aldosterone is not coordinated (50). In FD patients with supine hypertension, an increase in plasma atrial natriuretic peptide has also been demonstrated (14). The combination of these factors may serve to explain the exaggerated nocturnal urinary volume and increased excretion of salt in some cases of FD (34).

As neuropathologic findings suggest that FD might result from arrested neurodevelopment, trophic substances essential to the development of sensory and sympathetic neurons have been investigated. Nerve growth factor (NGF) has been one candidate. Cultured fibroblasts from FD patients produce slightly less radioimmunoassayable NGF than do those of healthy controls (52). By means of cloned DNA probes, the structural gene regions that encode for β-NGF and the β-NGF receptor were excluded as possible causes of FD (19,20). However, it is still possible that the genetic error in FD involves other genes that potentiate β-NGF action.

CLINICAL FEATURES AND MANAGEMENT

Widespread clinical manifestations are the consequence of two important developmental features. FD is caused by a combined deficit of sensory and autonomic neurons, and the disorder affects both central and peripheral autonomic pathways.

Sensory System

Peripheral involvement of the sensory system is manifested by a diminished, but not absent, response to painful stimuli. Lower extremities are more affected than upper, and there is usually sparing of palms, soles of feet, neck, and genital areas (7). In fact, the spared areas can be exquisitely sensitive. Temperature appreciation, as documented by sympathetic skin responses and thermotest readings to both hot and cold stimuli, is also affected. As with diminished pain perception, the trunk and lower extremities are more affected (32), and losses are greater in older individuals than in younger. Patellar reflexes are depressed. In older patients, sense of vibration and joint position eventually become abnormal and rombergism may be noted. Visceral sensation is intact, so patients are able to perceive discomfort during pleuritic or peritoneal irritation.

Peripheral sensory deprivation has been suggested as an explanation for the frequent special mannerisms of the FD child, such as repeated rubbing of the nose, grinding of the teeth, or picking at the fingers to the point of mutilation. Masturbation is common in all children at various stages of development, but it may be prolonged or exaggerated in FD children, as it may be a compensation for sensory deprivation rather than solely a search for sexual stimulation. Insensitivity to pain can also result in unrecognized fractures and inadvertent trauma to joints, causing Charcot joints and aseptic necrosis (21,37). Because of spinal curvature, which can be early and pernicious in its course (61), extreme care must be taken in fitting of braces to avoid development of decubitus ulcers from pressure on insensitive skin.

Central sensory deficits are manifested by decreased pain perception along the branches of the trigeminal nerve and the sensory branch of the facial nerve; corneal reflexes are diminished. Taste is deficient, especially recognition of sweet, which corresponds to the absence of fungiform papillae on the tip of the tongue (56,58). Defects in taste reflect diminution of neurons in the geniculate ganglion. Although speech is frequently characterized as dysarthric and nasal, hearing is normal.

The frequent finding of hypotonia, especially in infants and young children, is thought to be caused by the combi-

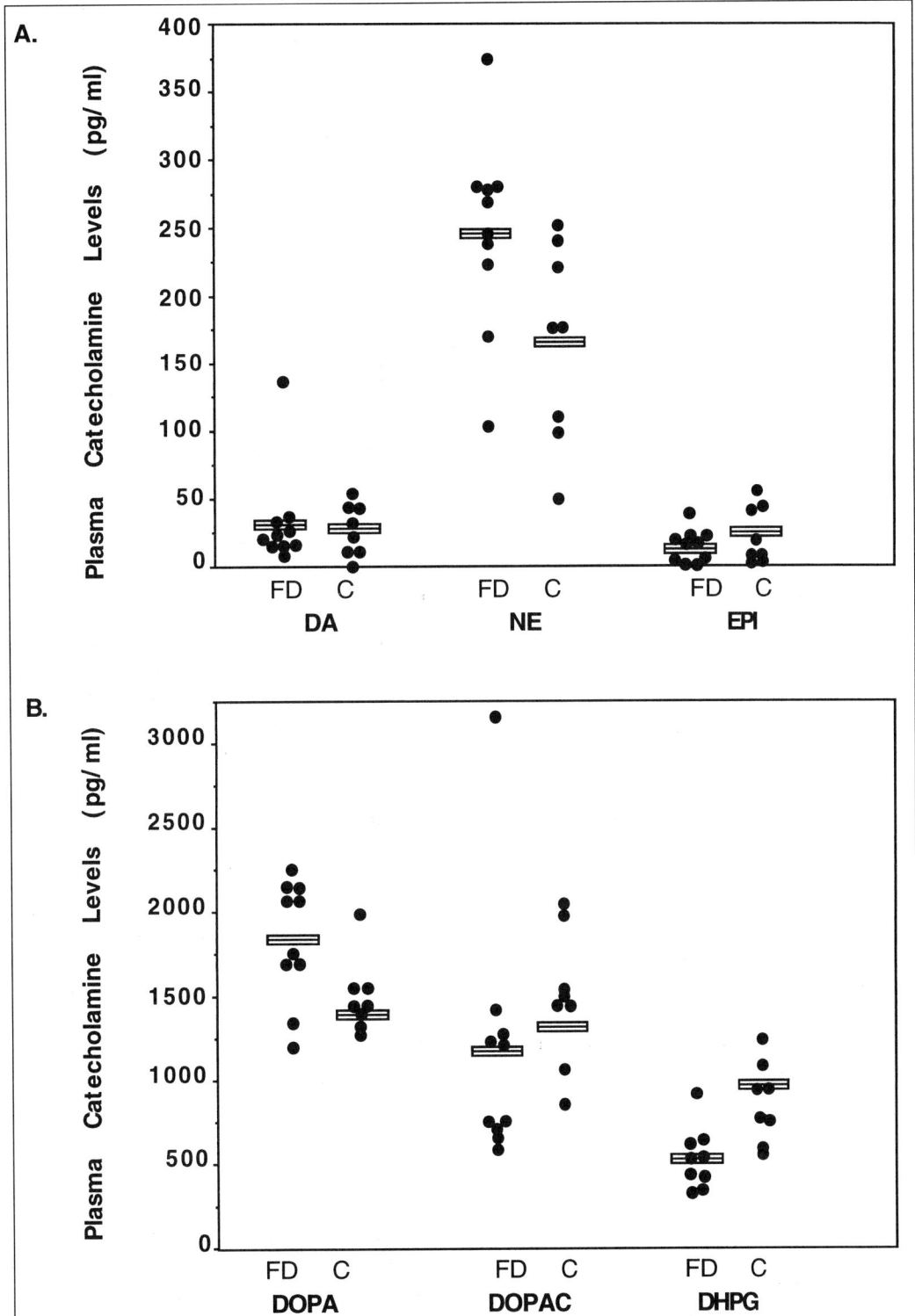

FIG. 4. Supine catechol values for 10 FD and 8 control subjects. Values for FD subjects are averages from two to three testing sessions. Control values are absolute values. *Horizontal bars* are means. **A:** Catecholamines. *DA*, dopamine; *NE*, norepinephrine; *EPI*, epinephrine. **B:** Catechol metabolites. *DOPA*, dihydroxyphenylalanine; *DOPAC*, dihydroxyphenylacetic acid; *DHPG*, dihydroxyphenylglycol.

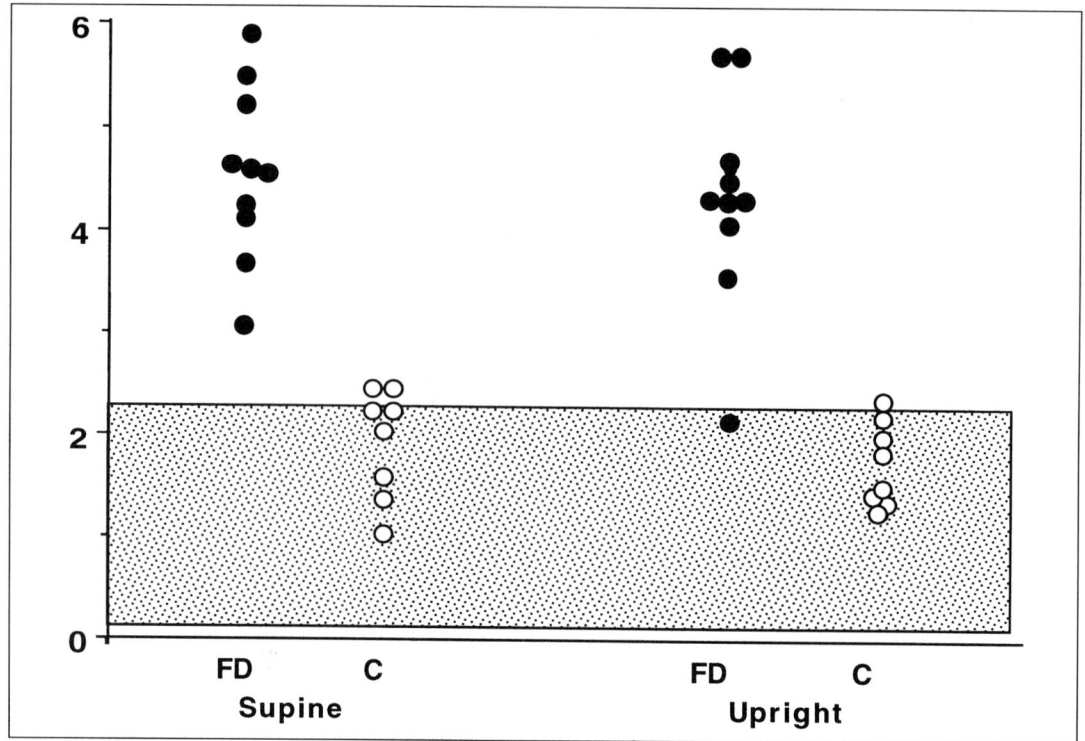

FIG. 5. Ratios of DOPA to DHPG for 9 FD and 8 control subjects. One FD subject was not included as DHPG values were not available. Values for FD subjects (●) are averages from two to three testing sessions. Control values (○) are absolute values. *Gray area* indicates reported normal range of this ratio in plasma (0.13–2.28). (From Goldstein et al., ref. 29.)

nation of central deficits and decreased tone of stretch receptors (24). In older patients, magnetic resonance imaging frequently shows generalized atrophy that affects the cerebellum. This may contribute to the broad-based and mildly ataxic gait that is associated with special difficulties in performing rapid movements or turning. Many patients walk listing forward, with a compensatory increased stiffness in the shoulders and neck that leads to protracted shoulders. Some adult patients have to use walkers or wheelchairs when outside the home.

Autonomic Dysfunction

Autonomic dysfunction becomes apparent during the examination, especially if the patient is agitated; excessive sweating and blotching can then be noted. Distal vasoconstriction in the peripheral skin causes cold, red hands; livid feet when they are dependent (cutis marmorata); and hypertension. In addition, autonomic dysfunction is so generalized that other systems are affected.

Gastrointestinal System

Oropharyngeal incoordination is one of the most frequent early signs (10). Dysphagia, with particular difficulty in avoiding misdirection of liquids, is commonly treated by insertion of a gastrostomy (2). The gastrostomy assures a route to maintain adequate hydration and avoids aspiration.

Esophageal dysmotility and *gastroesophageal reflux* are also common and increase the risk for aspiration. When medical management with prokinetic agents, H_2 antagonists, thickening of feeds, and positioning is not successful, then surgical intervention (fundoplication) is performed (9,12). Failure of medical management would be indicated by persistence of pneumonia, hematemesis, or apnea.

Vomiting crises occur in approximately 40% of patients with FD. The crises are a systemic reaction to stress, either physical or emotional. In addition to treatment of the precipitating cause, the crises are managed with a combination of intravenous or rectally administered diazepam (0.2 mg/kg every 3 hrs with a maximum dose of 10 mg) and chloral hydrate rectal suppositories (30 mg/kg every 6 hrs with a maximum dose of 2 g) and avoidance of dehydration and aspiration (2).

Respiratory System

A major cause of lung infections is *aspiration*. Therefore, many respiratory problems can be avoided when gastrointestinal dysfunction is well managed. Lung function in older patients may be compromised by the development of restrictive lung disease secondary to spinal curvature. However, a major problem for the FD patient is abnormal respiratory control, as the *ventilatory response to hypercapnia and hypoxia* is not normal. Filler et al. (26) demonstrated that rebreathing 12% oxygen for a period of min caused dramatic falls in oxygen saturation, resulting in extreme cyanosis, syncope, and even convulsions. When Edelman et al. (25) reinvestigated respiratory control, they noted that the response to hypercapnia was normalized if patients were kept hyperoxic; however, the hyperoxic state produced profound cardiovascular effects. Hypoxia in FD patients causes the heart rate (HR) and blood pressure (BP) to fall, which is the opposite of the normal response. This reaction is presumed to be a consequence of sympathetic insufficiency and secondary decreased circulation to the respiratory center. Clinical manifestations of abnormal respiratory control responses include drowning during underwater swimming, syncope and convulsions during air travel and travel at high altitudes, and a low threshold for cyanosis and decerebrate posturing during breath holding.

Lability of Blood Pressure

Cardiovascular irregularities are prominent in patients with FD. As a result of pathologic abnormalities of the sensory and autonomic systems, with wider sympathetic than parasympathetic involvement, the FD patient is unable to mount appropriate cardiovascular or catecholamine responses to physical stress, including change of position or exercise (7,13,62). Postural hypotension without compensatory tachycardia can be quite striking, especially in the adult population. In one study with tilt, mean BP decreased by ≥24 mmHg at 5 min in all FD subjects (17). However, when patients are agitated or in the supine position, BP is often in the hypertensive range. Postural hypotension can be treated with standard methods, such as adequate hydration, exercise of the lower extremities, elastic stockings, fludrocortisone, and midodrine (15). Hypertension is usually transitory, so treatment should be directed at factors precipitating the hypertension, such as anxiety or visceral pain. Diazepam and clonidine have been found to be particularly effective (2).

Although all FD subjects have abnormal orthostatic BP and HR responses, electrocardiographic and HR variability responses vary. Electrocardiographic changes are frequently noted, such as prolongation of the corrected QT interval and failure to shorten with exercise, as well as prolongation of the tQRS on signal-averaged electrocardiogram (17,27). Prolongation of the tQRS appears to be a sensitive but not specific indicator of autonomic dysfunction. Prolongation of QTc may be an ominous sign. Heart rate variability data suggest that patients with FD have abnormalities of parasympathetic, as well as sympathetic, tone. Heart rate variability is decreased (36). Frequency domain analyses of adults with FD reveal that mid- and high-frequency band areas are significantly decreased in the supine, but not upright, position. On time domain analysis, the pNN50 is frequently significantly decreased in FD subjects (17).

General anesthesia has caused profound hypotension and cardiac arrest (33). With greater attention to stabilization of the vascular bed by hydrating patients before surgery and titrating the anesthetic, the risk for these problems has been greatly reduced (11).

Renal Problems

Renal function appears to deteriorate with advancing age, as indicated by slowly rising serum urea and creatinine (47). Pathologic studies reveal excess glomerulosclerosis. On ultrastructural examination of renal biopsy specimens, vascular innervation is deficient in dysautonomic patients in comparison with controls. Although the cause of progressive renal disease is not certain, increasing evidence implicates abnormal renal hemodynamics as a major factor. Both hypotension and hypertension can result in inadequate renal perfusion and ischemic loss of glomerular and tubular integrity.

Doppler study of the renal arteries is a noninvasive method of evaluating renal blood flow characteristics (39). From the waveform of pulsed Doppler-derived renal artery blood flow velocity, a ratio can be obtained of peak systolic velocity (point A) to end diastolic velocity (point B). This ratio of A to B can serve as an index of renal arterial vascular resistance or impedance to pulsatile flow. With Doppler technology and the A-to-B ratio, renal perfusion in FD subjects has been shown to decrease during standing and after exercise (13). This perturbation in renal hemodynamics may result in ischemic damage, with eventual development of renal insufficiency.

FD patients are also susceptible to other problems that may result in hypoperfusion, such as dehydration if a gastrostomy has not been inserted to ensure adequate hydration, or vasoconstriction of renal vessels as a result of sympathetic supersensitivity during vomiting crises.

Ophthalmic Problems

Corneal hypesthesia and alacrima predispose the cornea to neurotrophic ulcerations from undetected trauma and excessive dryness. Special caution is required during febrile episodes, in dry climates, and on windy days. Corneal complications have been decreasing with regular use of artificial tear solutions and maintenance of normal body hydration. In addition, cautery of the tear duct puncta has been used in refractory situations. Cautery of the puncta inhibits drainage from the lacrimal bed. Tarsorrhaphy has been reserved for unresponsive and chronic cases. Soft contact lenses are also beneficial in promoting corneal healing. Corneal transplants have had limited success.

Reproduction

Sexual maturation is frequently delayed, but primary and secondary sex characteristics eventually develop in both sexes (7). Women with dysautonomia have conceived and delivered normal infants (49). Although pregnancies were tolerated well, BP lability was marked at delivery because of major hemodynamic shifts. One male patient has fathered seven children. All offspring of FD patients have been phenotypically normal despite their obligatory heterozygous state.

Intelligence and Emotion

Although intelligence generally falls within the normal range (60), autonomic instability delays attainment of developmental milestones and modifies emotional reactivity (23). The degree of autonomic dysfunction and lability influences ability to function and personality. Young children with FD can be frustrated by their inability to communicate needs or ideas verbally. As a result, some children exhibit breath holding, which may be severe enough to produce cyanosis and syncope. Occasionally, stiffening and decerebrate positioning are also observed, mainly during the first 5 years of life. It has occurred at least one time in 63% of patients. Breath holding usually stops by the age of 5 years as the ability to express needs improves. Special education is often required, as these individuals tend to be literal-minded and have difficulty with extrapolation, conceptual thinking, and self-motivation. The latter problem may be a result of chronic illness. Visual intelligence skills exceed auditory skills, but verbal performance on standardized intelligence tests is more accurate than motor performance because of mild incoordination defects.

A personality change is associated with the FD "dysautonomic crisis." In addition to experiencing hypertension, tachycardia, excessive sweating, erythematous skin blotching, and nausea, the patient becomes extremely irritable, withdrawn, and negative. Mutilation activity may increase, sleep may be difficult, and major problems in oral coordination may result in an inability to swallow saliva and reluctance or inability to speak. The massive systemic reaction suggests that the patient in FD crisis is experiencing central autonomic dysfunction, consistent with the response of patients in crisis to centrally acting agents, such as diazepam.

The repercussions of literal thinking, lack of flexibility, and fear of being ill can prevent normal emotional maturation in the adolescent years and even lead to phobias (23). However, despite lags in physical and emotional development, many adult patients have been able to achieve independent function.

PROGNOSIS

At present, about 40% of the known population with FD is over 20 years of age. Thus, FD can no longer be considered a disease exclusively of childhood. With greater understanding of the disorder and development of treatment programs, survival statistics have markedly improved, so that increasing numbers of patients are reaching adulthood. Survival statistics before 1960 reveal that 50% of patients died before 5 years of age (22). Current survival statistics indicate that a newborn with FD has a 50% probability of reaching 30 years of age (4).

Causes of death are still predominantly pulmonary, indicating that more aggressive treatment is still needed in this area. Another large group has succumbed to unexplained death, which may have been the result of unopposed vagal stimulation. A few adult patients have died of renal failure.

REFERENCES

1. Aguayo AJ, et al. Peripheral nerve abnormalities in the Riley-Day syndrome, findings in sural nerve biopsy. *Arch Neurol* 1971;24: 106–116.
2. Axelrod FB. Familial dysautonomia. In: Burg FD, Ingelfinger JR, Wald ER, eds. *Gellis and Kagen's Current Pediatric Therapy*. 14th ed. Philadelphia: WB Saunders; 1993:92–94.
3. Axelrod FB. Familial dysautonomia. In: Chernick V, ed. *Kendig's Disorders of the Respiratory Tract in Children*. 5th ed. Philadelphia: WB Saunders; 1990:916–919.
4. Axelrod FB, Abularrage JJ. Familial dysautonomia. A prospective study of survival. *J Pediatr* 1982;101:234–236.
5. Axelrod FB, D'Amico R. Familial dysautonomia. In: Fraunfelder FT, Hampton RF, eds. *Current Ocular Therapy*. 4th ed. Philadelphia: WB Saunders; 1995:413–415.
6. Axelrod FB, Pearson J. Congenital sensory neuropathies. Diagnostic distinction from familial dysautonomia. *Am J Dis Child* 1984;138: 947–954.
7. Axelrod FB, et al. Familial dysautonomia: diagnosis, pathogenesis and management. In: Schulman I, ed. *Advances in Pediatrics*. Chicago: Year Book; 1974:75–96 (vol 21).
8. Axelrod FB, et al. Progressive sensory loss in familial dysautonomia. *Pediatrics* 1981;65:517–522.
9. Axelrod FB, et al. Gastroesophageal fundoplication and gastrostomy in familial dysautonomia. *Ann Surg* 1982;195:253–258.
10. Axelrod FB, et al. Neonatal recognition of familial dysautonomia. *J Pediatr* 1987;110:946–948.
11. Axelrod FB, et al. Anesthesia in familial dysautonomia. *Anesthesiology* 1988;68: 631–635.
12. Axelrod FB, et al. Fundoplication and gastrostomy in familial dysautonomia. *J Pediatr* 1991;118:388–394.
13. Axelrod FB, et al. The effects of postural change and exercise on renal haemodynamics in familial dysautonomia. *Clin Auton Res* 1993; 3:195–200.
14. Axelrod FB, et al. Atrial natriuretic peptide and catecholamine response to orthostatic hypotension and treatments in familial dysautonomia. *Clin Auton Res* 1994;4:311–318.
15. Axelrod FB, et al. Preliminary observations on the use of midodrine in treating orthostatic hypotension in familial dysautonomia. *J Auton Nerv Syst* 1995;55:29–35.
16. Axelrod FB, et al. Pattern of plasma catechols in familial dysautonomia. *Clin Auton Res* 1996;6:205–209.

17. Axelrod FB, et al. Electrocardiographic measures and heart rate variability in patients with familial dysautonomia. *Am J Cardiol* 1996; 88:133–140.
18. Blumenfeld A, et al. Localization of the gene for familial dysautonomia on chromosome 9 and definition of DNA markers for genetic diagnosis. *Nat Genet* 1993;4:160–164.
19. Breakefield XO, et al. Structural gene for beta-nerve growth factor not defective in familial dysautonomia. *Proc Natl Acad Sci U S A* 1984;81:4213–4216.
20. Breakefield XO, et al. DNA polymorphisms for the nerve growth factor receptor gene exclude its role in familial dysautonomia. *Mol Biol Med* 1986;3:483–494.
21. Brunt PW. Unusual case of Charcot joints in early adolescence (Riley-Day syndrome). *Br Med J* 1967;4:277.
22. Brunt PW, McKusick VA. Familial dysautonomia. A report of genetic and clinical studies with a review of the literature. *Medicine* 1970; 48:343–374.
23. Clayson D, et al. Personality development and familial dysautonomia. *Pediatrics* 1980;65:269–274.
24. Dyck PJ, et al. The number and sizes of reconstructed peripheral autonomic sensory and motoneurons in a case of dysautonomia. *J Neuropath Exp Neurol* 1978;27:744.
25. Edelman NH, et al. The effects of abnormal sympathetic nervous function upon the ventilatory response to hypoxia. *J Clin Invest* 1970; 49;1153–1165.
26. Filler J, et al. Respiratory control in familial dysautonomia. *J Pediatr* 1965;66;509–516.
27. Glickstein JS, et al. Abnormalities of the corrected QT interval in familial dysautonomia: an indicator of autonomic dysfunction. *J Pediatr* 1993;122:925–928.
28. Goadsby PJ. Sphenopalatine ganglion stimulation increases regional cerebral blood flow independent of glucose utilization in the cat. *Brain Res* 1990;506:145–148.
29. Goldstein DS, et al. Patterns of plasma levels of catecholamines in neurogenic orthostatic hypotension. *Ann Neurol* 1989;26:558–563.
30. Goodall G, et al. Decreased noradrenaline synthesis in FD. *J Clin Invest* 1971;50:2734–2740.
31. Grover-Johnson N, Pearson J. Deficient vascular innervation in familial dysautonomia, an explanation for vasomotor instability. *Neuropathol Appl Neurobiol* 1976;2:217–224.
32. Hilz MJ, et al. Sympathetic skin response (SSR) to thermal stimulation in familial dysautonomia—an objective indicator of sensory small-fibre neuropathy. Rochester, MN: *American Autonomic Society Proceedings*, October 21–23, 1994.
33. Kritchman MM, et al. Experiences with general anesthesia in patients with familial dysautonomia. JAMA 1959;170:259–533.
34. Laundau H, et al. Salt conservation in familial dysautonomia. *Isr J Med Sci* 1977;13:278–282.
35. Maayan C, et al. Incidence of familial dysautonomia in Israel 1977–1981. *Clin Genet* 1987;32:106–108.
36. Maayan C, et al. Evaluation of autonomic dysfunction in familial dysautonomia by power spectral analysis. *J Auton Nerv Syst* 1987; 21:51–58.
37. Mitnick J, et al. Aseptic necrosis in familial dysautonomia. *Radiology* 1982;142:89–91.
38. Moses SW, et al. A clinical genetic and biochemical study of familial dysautonomia. *Isr J Med Sci* 1967;3:358–371.
39. Norris CS, Barnes RW. Renal artery flow analysis: a sensitive measure of experimental and clinical renovascular resistance. *J Surg Res* 1984;36:230–236.
40. Pearson J, Pytel B. Quantitative studies of sympathetic ganglia and spinal cord intermedio-lateral gray columns in familial dysautonomia. *J Neurol Sci* 1978;39:47–59.
41. Pearson J, Pytel B. Quantitative studies of ciliary and sphenopalatine ganglia in familial dysautonomia. *J Neurol Sci* 1978;39:123–130.
42. Pearson J, et al. Current concepts of dysautonomia: neurological defects. *Ann N Y Acad Sci* 1974;228:288–300.
43. Pearson J, et al. The sural nerve in familial dysautonomia. *J Neuropathol Exp Neurol* 1975;34:413–424.
44. Pearson J, et al. Quantitative studies of dorsal root ganglia and neuropathologic observations on spinal cords in familial dysautonomia. *J Neurol Sci* 1978;35:77–97.
45. Pearson J, et al. Tyrosine hydroxylase immunohistochemistry in human brain. *Brain Res* 1979;165:333–337.
46. Pearson J, et al. Tyrosine hydroxylase immunohistoreactivity in familial dysautonomia. *Science* 1979;206:71–72.
47. Pearson J, et al. Renal disease in familial dysautonomia. *Kidney Int* 1980;17:102–112.
48. Pearson J, et al. Depletion of substance P-containing axons in substantia gelatinosa of patients with diminished pain sensitivity. *Nature* 1982;295:61–63.
49. Porges RF, et al. Pregnancy in familial dysautonomia. *Am J Obstet Gynecol* 1978;132:485–488.
50. Rabinowitz D, et al. Plasma renin activity and aldosterone in familial dysautonomia. *Metabolism* 1974;23:1–5.
51. Riley CM, et al. Central autonomic dysfunction with defective lacrimation. Report of 5 cases. *Pediatrics* 1949;3:468–477.
52. Schwartz J, Breakefield X. Altered nerve growth factor in fibroblasts from patients with familial dysautonomia. *Proc Natl Acad Sci U S A* 1980;77:1154–1158.
53. Slaugenhaupt SA, et al. Isolation of candidate genes and physical mapping in the familial dysautonomia region of chromosome 9q31. *American Society of Human Genetics Annual Meeting*, 1994.
54. Smith AA, Dancis J. Response to intradermal histamine in familial dysautonomia—a diagnostic test. *J Pediatr* 1963;63:889–894.
55. Smith AA, Dancis J. Exaggerated response to infused norepinephrine in familial dysautonomia. *N Engl J Med* 1964;270:704–707.
56. Smith AA, Dancis J. Taste discrimination in familial dysautonomia. *Pediatrics* 1964;33:441–443.
57. Smith AA, et al. Ocular responses to autonomic drugs in familial dysautonomia. *Invest Ophthalmol* 1965;4:358–361.
58. Smith AA, et al. Absence of taste bud papillae in familial dysautonomia. Science 1965;147:1040–1041.
59. Smith AA, et al. Responses to infused methacholine in familial dysautonomia. *Pediatrics* 1965;36:225–230.
60. Welton W, et al. Intellectual development in familial dysautonomia. *Pediatrics* 1979;63:708–712.
61. Yaslow W, et al. Orthopedic defects in familial dysautonomia. *J Bone Joint Surg* 1971;53:1541–1550.
62. Ziegler MG, et al. Deficient sympathetic nervous system response in familial dysautonomia. *N Engl J Med* 1976;294:630–633.

CHAPTER 40

Reflex Sympathetic Dystrophy

Peter R. Wilson

1. Complex regional pain syndrome type I, or "reflex sympathetic dystrophy," is defined by the IASP Task Force as "a syndrome that usually develops after an initiating noxious event, is not limited to the distribution of a single peripheral nerve, and is apparently disproportionate to the inciting event. It is associated at some point with evidence of edema, changes in skin blood flow, abnormal sudomotor activity in the region of the pain, or allodynia or hyperalgesia."
2. Complex regional pain syndrome type II (causalgia) is defined as "burning pain, allodynia, and hyperpathia usually in the hand or foot after partial injury of a nerve or one of its major branches." Complex regional pain syndrome type II will not be discussed in this context.
3. Sympathetically maintained pain may be found in both of these conditions. This pain appears to be maintained by sympathetic efferent activity or by circulating catecholamines. Sympathetically independent pain may occur in conjunction with sympathetically maintained pain, or it may occur alone.
4. The sympathetic nervous system may be involved in the pathophysiologic mechanisms, but definitive evidence is not yet available.
5. The diagnosis of complex regional pain syndrome type I can be made using a combined clinical probability score together with a laboratory score.
6. Three stages have been proposed: an initial, acute hyperemic (hot) stage; a second, ischemic (cold) stage; and a final, dystrophic stage, in which sympathetic and somatic changes may be minimal but significant atrophy is present.
7. The pain of complex regional pain syndrome type I/reflex sympathetic dystrophy is typically described as burning in nature, spontaneous and continuous, and severe (7+/10), but it may have other sensory characteristics.
8. Allodynia, hyperpathia, or both are typically present, and exacerbate the "background" pain. The allodynia (perception of pain from a stimulus that is normally not noxious) may be produced by touch, temperature, pressure, or joint movement in the affected area, alone or in combination.
9. Autonomic manifestations include swelling, vasomotor changes, and sudomotor changes.
10. Fewer than 5% of patients have a tremor or dystonia.
11. Some of the response to treatment could be a placebo effect.

INTRODUCTION

Neuropathic pain syndromes present difficult diagnostic and therapeutic challenges. In many cases the fundamental mechanisms are unknown, and therapy is often empiric. The situation becomes even more difficult when the sympathetic nervous system is involved in addition to the somatosensory system. It may be impossible to determine whether the sympathetic changes are the result of the somatosensory malfunction, or whether primary autonomic pathology is present. This situation becomes most perplexing in the states now known as *complex regional pain syndrome (CRPS) type I*, formerly known as *reflex sympathetic dystrophy (RSD)*, and *CRPS type II*, formerly referred to as *causalgia* (13).

As defined by the IASP Task Force, CRPS type I/RSD is "a syndrome that usually develops after an initiating noxious event, is not limited to the distribution of a single peripheral nerve, and is apparently disproportionate to the inciting event. It is associated at some point with evidence of edema, changes in skin blood flow, abnormal sudomotor activity in the region of the pain, or allodynia or hyperalgesia."

CRPS type II (causalgia) is defined as "burning pain, allodynia, and hyperpathia usually in the hand or foot after

---

P. R. Wilson: Department of Anesthesiology, Mayo Clinic, Rochester, Minnesota 55905.

partial injury of a nerve or one of its major branches." CRPS type II will not be discussed in this context.

It has also been noted that sympathetically maintained pain (SMP) may be found in both of these conditions. This pain appears to be maintained by sympathetic efferent activity or by circulating catecholamines. Sympathetically independent pain (SIP) may occur in conjunction with SMP, or may occur alone. This is a critical concept, as many previous definitions of RSD relied on the presence of SMP, and diagnostic criteria were often weighted in favor of conditions exhibiting SMP. Consequently, evaluation of the previous literature is rendered virtually worthless in the light of the new concepts. There are no articles previously published with valid criteria for the condition, properly controlled interventions, or valid and objective outcome measures.

MECHANISMS

The role of the sympathetic nervous system in pain states has been an enigma since its original description more than 150 years ago. Jänig (7) has recently reviewed the subject, and he suggests from his own work, and that of others, that two general mechanisms exist for involvement of the sympathetic system in pain.

1. Responses to tissue damage involve both generalized and local reactions. Generalized reactions include "fight or flight," defense, and quiescent reactions; they are organized in the mesencephalon, hypothalamus, and suprahypothalamic structures of the brain. Local reactions include somatosympathetic, viscerosympathetic, and viscerovisceral reactions; these are mediated by the adrenocortical and somatomotor systems.
2. Peripheral responses to tissue damage may include hyperalgesia, allodynia, diffuse burning pain, and changes in blood flow and sweating, motor control, and the integrity of the bones, joints, muscles, subcutaneous tissue, and skin. Some of these changes may be responsive to alterations in sympathetic activity (by neural blockade, receptor blockade, or transmitter depletion).

Unfortunately, these explanations do not account for the fact that CRPS type I/RSD may develop as a result of minor trauma, or even in the absence of any identifiable trauma. Conversely, CRPS type I/RSD does not develop in most cases of either major or minor trauma. Attempts to define predisposing factors, such as psychologic status (3,4), have been unsuccessful.

CLINICAL CHARACTERISTICS

A consensus does not appear to have been reached with respect to the clinical characteristics of CRPS type I/RSD. It is agreed that symptoms and signs vary in frequency and severity. Several attempts have been made in retrospective studies and on *a priori* grounds to define diagnostic criteria using the three major symptom complexes: sensory, autonomic, and motor abnormalities. In some schemes, a single study, such as a three-phase bone scan (9) or sympathetic blockade (1), is used. More recently, schemes of greater complexity have been devised (3,6,8). Few prospective studies have been done to date (4,15).

Questions regarding the general applicability of studies have been raised. Baron et al. (2) reviewed the symptomatology in their patients (Table 1). Low et al. reviewed the experience of another institution (11), with a prospective component (Table 2). Questions also have been raised regarding whether the conditions are similar in adults and children (16). The question of the existence of clinical stages has not been resolved with prospective studies and therefore cannot be discussed. Various authors have proposed an initial, acute hyperemic (hot) stage; a second, ischemic (cold) stage; and a final, dystrophic stage, in which sympathetic and somatic changes may be minimal but significant atrophy has developed.

Pain

CRPS type I/RSD is by definition a pain syndrome. However, the pain varies greatly, both within and between individuals. It is typically described as burning in nature, spontaneous and continuous, and severe (7+/10). However, it may have other sensory characteristics (dull or sharp) and be evoked by physical or emotional stimuli on an intermittent basis. The patient may carry the affected extremity in a protective posture, with evidence of extreme pain behavior. On the other hand, there may be some use of the extremity, with little evidence of pain behavior.

Allodynia/Hyperpathia

Allodynia, hyperpathia, or both are typically present and exacerbate the "background" pain. Allodynia (perception of pain from a stimulus that is normally not noxious) may be produced by touch, temperature, pressure, or joint

TABLE 1. *Putative diagnostic criteria for RSD*

Clinical symptoms and signs
  Burning pain
  Hyperpathia/allodynia
  Temperature/color changes
  Edema
  Hair/nail growth changes

Laboratory results
  Thermometry/thermography
  Bone x-ray
  3-phase bone scan
  Quantitative sweat test
  Response to sympathetic blockade

Interpretation
  >6 Probable RSD
  3–5 Possible RSD
  <3 Unlikely RSD

TABLE 2. *Reflex sympathetic dystrophy probability scoring system*

Parameter[a]	Definite	Probable	Possible	Not RSD/SMP
Allodynia				
Touch (a)				
Pressure (b)	3/3	2/3	1/3	0/3
Movement (c)				
Vasomotor				
History (a)				
Examination (b)	4/4	≥2/4	≤1/4	0/4
Swelling				
History (a)				
Examination (b)				

From Low et al., ref. 11.
RSD, reflex sympathetic dystrophy; SMP, sympathetically maintained pain.
[a]Grading depends on a combination of (a) and (b).

movement in the affected area, alone or in combination. Insufficient data are available to determine whether the allodynia represents sympathetic overactivity, or whether it is a central or peripheral phenomenon. It is not necessarily alleviated by sympathetic blockade.

Autonomic Symptoms

Most patients have a history of swelling (edema) occurring at some stage; this is evident in fewer at the time of examination. The extent of the swelling has never been quantified in any group. The character of the edema (pitting, brawny) has also never been adequately described, although some believe that its features provide evidence of different stages of the condition.

Vasomotor changes are commonly described by patients: redness, blueness, and blotchiness in variable combinations. There may be an associated increase, decrease, or both in perceived temperature of the extremity, particularly the digits.

Sudomotor (sweating) changes (usually increased) are noted by a minority of patients.

Integumentary changes are also seen in a minority—increases or decreases in hair, skin, or nail thickness.

Motor Changes

Strength and range of joints are apparently normal in most patients. A few patients (<5%) have evidence of tremor or dystonia.

DIAGNOSTIC CRITERIA

Clinical

Complete clinical evaluation of the patient is essential, because the diagnosis of CRPS type I/RSD cannot be made in the presence of conditions that would otherwise account for the degree of pain and dysfunction.

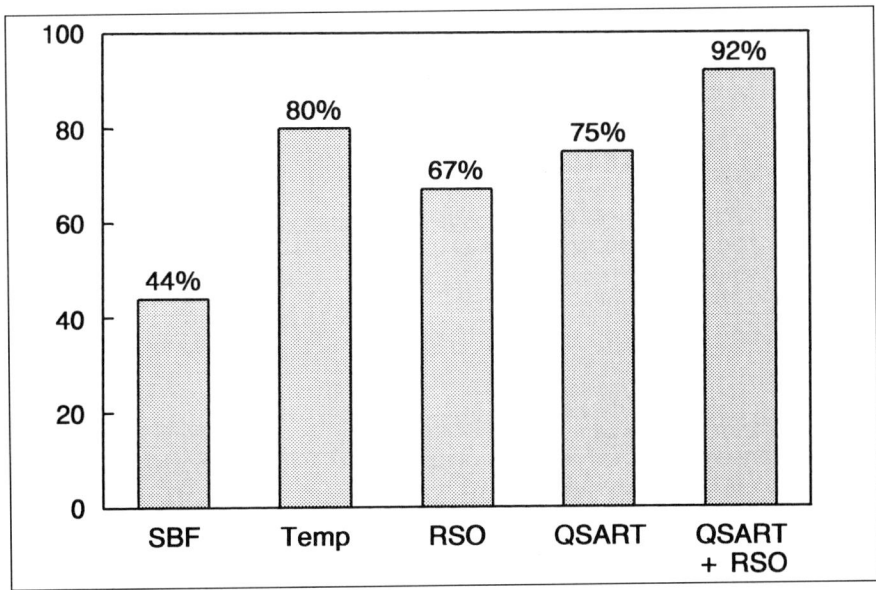

FIG. 1. Frequency percent of abnormalities in SBF (skin blood flow), Temp (skin temperature), RSO (resting sweat output), QSART (quantitative sudomotor axon reflex test), and combined QSART and RSO.

In the absence of prospective, controlled studies with objective outcome measures, it is impossible to provide anything but a collective clinical "best guess" with respect to diagnostic criteria for CRPS type I/RSD.

CRPS type I/RSD is a dynamic condition, so the clinical and laboratory findings may change from one period to another. In view of this observation, attempts to produce diagnostic criteria must incorporate information from both the history and examination, in addition to results of laboratory testing. Consequently, Low et al. suggested a probability score that gives equal weight to history and examination (Table 2). Clinical findings were compared with

TABLE 3. *Algorithm for diagnosis of complex regional pain syndrome (CRPS)*

Pain
The diagnosis of CRPS cannot be made in the absence of pain; it is a pain syndrome. However, the characteristics of the pain may vary with the initiating event and other factors. The pain is often described as burning and might be spontaneous or evoked in the context of hyperalgesia or allodynia. Both spontaneous and evoked pain can occur together.

History
Develops after an initiating noxious event or immobilization
Unilateral extremity onset (rarely spreads to another extremity)
Symptom onset usually within a month
Exclusion criteria
    Identifiable major nerve lesion (CRPS II)
    Existence of anatomic, physiologic, or psychological conditions that would otherwise account for the degree of pain and dysfunction

Symptoms (Patient Report)
A. Pain (spontaneous or evoked)
    Burning
    Aching, throbbing
B. Hyperalgesia or allodynia (at some time in the disease course) to mechanical stimuli (light touch or deep pressure), to thermal stimulation, or to joint motion
C. Associated symptoms (minor)
    Swelling
    Temperature or color: asymmetry and instability
    Sweating: asymmetry and instability
    Trophic changes: hair, nails, skin

Signs (Observed)
Hyperalgesia or allodynia (light touch, deep pressure, joint movement, cold)
Edema (if unilateral and other causes excluded)
Vasomotor changes: color, temperature instability, asymmetry
Sudomotor changes
Trophic changes in skin, joints, nails, hair
Impaired motor function (may include components of dystonia and tremor)

Criteria Required for Diagnosis of CRPS I
History of pain
    Plus allodynia, hyperalgesia, or hyperesthesia
    Plus two other signs from the above list
Characteristics of spontaneous pain
    Sympathetically maintained pain (SMP)
    Sympathetically independent pain (SIP)
    Combined SMP + SIP

Criteria for Diagnosis of Sympathetic Dysfunction
Noninvasive tests
    Surface temperature asymmetry by ≥1°C, either spontaneous or in response to provocative testing
    Resting or evoked sudomotor asymmetry
Invasive tests
    Sympathetic ganglion block (if equivocal, up to three may be required); will usually be considered adequate only if there is demonstrated inhibition of sympathetic mediated vasoconstriction of the involved extremity
    Systemic alpha-adrenergic antagonists, placebo controlled
    Neuraxial blockade above the lesion may provide useful information
Tests of unknown pathophysiologic significance
    Three-phase bone scan
    Radiographic patchy demineralization
    Tourniquet ischemia test
    Measurements of cutaneous blood flow with laser Doppler, percutaneous oxygen partial pressure differences, and computer-assisted sensory examination are interesting but evolving technologies that require further study.
    Somatosensory-evoked potential measurement is not of demonstrated utility.
    Regional sympathetic blockade is not recommended for diagnostic use because of multiple physiologic actions that confound interpretation.

CRPS, complex regional pain syndrome. (Adapted from 17.)

laboratory evaluations of vasomotor status (skin temperature), resting sweat output, and the quantitative sudomotor reflex test (QSART). This study showed excellent correlation within four clusters:

1. Vasomotor cluster: skin color and temperature, swelling by history and examination, sweating by history and examination
2. Pain cluster: shooting pain, dull pain, burning pain, type of injury
3. Motor function: motor strength, joint movement, contractures, activities of daily living
4. Allodynia in response to light touch, pressure, movement, cold

Not all centers have the capability to estimate resting sweat output or the QSART, and alternative criteria needed to be developed for the diagnosis. This has been attempted in a Dahlem format (17), and formal testing will be required to confirm or refute the hypothesis. The principles appear in Table 3. It will be seen that this scheme attempts for the first time to exclude SMP as an absolute requirement for the diagnosis. Pain is an essential component of the syndrome, but the characteristics are recognized as variable. Pain and sensory changes are essential components of the diagnosis. Unfortunately, pain, allodynia, and hyperpathia are subjective evaluations in the usual clinical setting. Changes related to autonomic dysfunction can also rarely be measured in the clinical setting, and the signs of autonomic dysfunction are difficult to measure clinically (10). The roles of dystonia and tremor are regarded as minor, because of the difficulty in quantifying these phenomena and also because it is difficult to assess whether they represent a basic pathophysiologic mechanism or rather voluntary or involuntary guarding or other protective activity in the affected extremity.

Laboratory

Clinical autonomic testing has been discussed by Low (Chapter 15). Other indirect tests of autonomic function include measurement of skin blood flow (laser Doppler) and three-phase bone scan and bone mineral density. However, the role of these tests in the diagnosis of CRPS type I/RSD is not clear.

Placebo

Placebo responses—a beneficial effect from pharmacologically inactive interventions or a response beyond that normally expected of active treatment—are elicited in virtually all medical treatments. The phenomenon is a particular problem when a report of pain reduction is required for the diagnosis of a particular condition or as a measure of the efficacy of a particular treatment. This subject has been exhaustively explored by Price et al. (14). They conclude that placebo effects are well established in a group of patients with documented organic pathology. Therefore, the presence of a placebo effect cannot provide any information about the veracity, severity, or psychogenic origin of the pain complaint. In addition to these observations, Fine et al. have shown that the placebo effect related to certain intravenous infusions may be delayed and prolonged, casting further doubt on the specificity and sensitivity of, for example, the phentolamine test.

DIFFERENTIAL DIAGNOSIS

More than 100 etiologic factors have been published as initiating causes of CRPS type I/RSD, so the differential diagnosis must encompass all types of neuropathic pain syndromes as well as orthopedic, vascular, and metabolic syndromes. It is essential in many cases to determine the underlying pathology, as CRPS type I/RSD is usually a response to an anatomic or physiologic insult to peripheral tissue. If any underlying cause is not treated, it is unlikely that merely treating the symptoms of CRPS type I/RSD will cause the condition to resolve.

It may be helpful to determine the relative contributions of SMP and SIP. If this is clarified, it should help direct therapy. For example, there is no point in continuing to block the sympathetic system if pain is independent of it.

TREATMENT

In the absence of valid outcome studies, treatment recommendations can be based only on clinical assumptions and impressions. Although many of these might seem logical, there is little evidence for their efficacy and safety. Indeed, more than 60 treatment modalities are described in the literature, but not a single one has been formally tested.

Etiologic Factors

It is a *sine qua non* of medical treatment that the underlying pathology must be treated to relieve the symptoms of that pathology. Unfortunately, in some cases of CRPS type I/RSD, the underlying pathologic processes cannot be determined. In such cases, it is reasonable to treat the symptoms, which can be profound and, if left untreated, lead to permanent tissue damage, chronic pain, and impairment.

Pain

Sympathetically Maintained Pain

Reduction of sympathetic efferent activity to the extremity (by local or regional sympathetic blockade), or generalized reduction in sympathetic tone (with α-adrenergic blockers) should reduce SMP, allowing more effective rehabilitation efforts. There is some anecdotal evidence that both transcutaneous and spinal electrical stimulation can reduce pain and improve peripheral blood flow in certain cases.

Sympathetically Independent Pain

Spontaneous or evoked pain in the affected extremity produces adverse effects directly on the person and indirectly on the extremity. The extremity is protected from any physical contact because of allodynia and hyperpathia. It develops the changes of disuse—loss of strength and endurance, reduction in joint mobility, atrophy of all tissues, reduced blood flow, and sensory and autonomic changes. Reducing SIP with analgesics or somatic nerve blocks may allow more aggressive efforts at physical therapy and improve function.

Autonomic Changes

It is usually assumed that the autonomic changes will resolve with successful treatment of the underlying pathology and reversal of the effects of disuse and pain. However, there are cases in which the autonomic changes (such as vasoconstriction) are so severe that they have to be treated separately. In such cases, appropriate monitoring is essential.

Motor Changes

There is no specific treatment for the motor abnormalities of CRPS type I/RSD, but is has been long assumed that with treatment of other aspects of the condition, these symptoms will also abate.

Disuse

Immobilization has been reported as a cause of CRPS type I/RSD. Conversely, physical therapy and rehabilitation have been shown to be effective in many case studies. Normal use, retraining, and re-education appear to be necessary to reverse the changes of the condition. Unfortunately, no guidelines are available for physical therapy. Patient and clinician have to find a level and rate of rehabilitation that will restore normal function without reinjuring the limb. It should be remembered that the clinical manifestations of "repetitive strain injury" and "cumulative trauma" may resemble those of CRPS type I/RSD. In these cases, aggressive physical rehabilitation may aggravate the problem.

PREVENTION

No data are available to support any preventive measures for this condition. It is extremely rare when the total number of minor injuries inflicted on a population is considered. However, some authors suggest that a genetic predisposition to the condition may exist. It has also been suggested that a past history of CRPS type I/RSD predisposes a patient to a recurrence of the condition if there should be further injury, surgery, or immobilization. The size of the populations required to test prevention hypotheses would be so large that the research cannot be done at this time. However, it would seem prudent to treat a patient who has had CRPS type I/RSD in the past as being at high risk and try to pre-empt putative causative factors. This might mean that prevention of postoperative pain, perhaps with regional anesthesia, and of overactivity of the sympathetic system, by regional or systemic methods, would be indicated. It would also be prudent to supervise all aspects of the rehabilitation process closely.

CONCLUSION

CRPS type I/RSD is a symptom complex that represents an exaggerated response to injury or tissue damage. The amplification of the normal responses probably occurs both in the periphery and the central nervous system. Diagnostic criteria are still under discussion. Treatment modalities are therefore still directed at symptoms, as the pathophysiology is not known. The pain of the condition may be sympathetically maintained or sympathetically independent (or both), and sympathetic blockade is therefore useful in the former category. Treatment modalities must be directed towards optimizing both comfort and function of the affected extremity. Such treatment programs might occur in a multidisciplinary setting.

REFERENCES

1. Arner S. Intravenous phentolamine test: diagnostic and prognostic use in reflex sympathetic dystrophy. *Pain* 1991;46:17–22.
2. Baron R, Blumberg H, Jänig W. Clinical characteristic of patients with complex regional pain syndrome in Germany with special emphasis on vasomotor function. In: Jänig W, Stanton-Hicks M, eds. *Reflex Sympathetic Dystrophy: A Reappraisal*. Seattle: IASP Press; 1996:25–48 (*Progress in Pain Research and Management*; vol 6).
3. Blumberg H. Clinical and pathophysiological aspects of reflex sympathetic dystrophy and sympathetically maintained pain. In: Jänig W, Schmidt RF, eds. *Reflex Sympathetic Dystrophy. Pathophysiological Mechanisms and Clinical Implications*. Weinheim; VCH Verlagsgesellschaft; 1992:372–375.
4. Chelimsky TC, et al. The value of autonomic testing in reflex sympathetic dystrophy. *Mayo Clin Proc* 1995;70:1029–1040.
5. Covington EC. Psychological issues in reflex sympathetic dystrophy. In: Jänig W, Stanton-Hicks M, eds. *Reflex Sympathetic Dystrophy: A Reappraisal*. Seattle: IASP Press; 1996:191–215 (*Progress in Pain Research and Management*; vol 6).
6. Gibbons JJ, Wilson PR. RSD score: criteria for the diagnosis of reflex sympathetic dystrophy and causalgia. *Clin J Pain* 1992;8:260–263.
7. Jänig W. The puzzle of "reflex sympathetic dystrophy": mechanisms, hypotheses, open questions. In: Jänig W, Stanton-Hicks M, eds. *Reflex Sympathetic Dystrophy: A Reappraisal*. Seattle: IASP Press; 1996:1–24 (*Progress in Pain Research and Management*; vol 6).

8. Jänig W, et al. The reflex sympathetic dystrophy syndrome. Consensus statement and general recommendations for diagnosis and clinical research. In: Bond MR, Charlton JE, Woolf CJ, eds. *Pain Research and Clinical Management. Proceedings of the VIth World Congress on Pain*. Amsterdam: Elsevier; 1991:372–375 (vol 4).
9. Kozin F, et al. Bone scintigraphy in the reflex sympathetic dystrophy syndrome. *Radiology* 1981;138:437–443.
10. Low PA. Pitfalls in autonomic testing. In: Low PA, ed. *Clinical Autonomic Disorders*. Boston: Little, Brown; 1993:355–365.
11. Low PA, et al. Clinical characteristics of patients with reflex sympathetic dystrophy (sympathetically maintained pain) in the USA. In: Jänig W, Stanton-Hicks M, eds. *Reflex Sympathetic Dystrophy: A Reappraisal*. Seattle: IASP Press; 1996:49–66 (*Progress in Pain Research and Management*; vol 6).
12. Merskey H. Regional pain is rarely hysterical. *Arch Neurol* 1988; 45:915–918.
13. Merskey H, Bogduk N, eds. *Classification of Chronic Pain*. 2nd ed. Seattle: IASP Press; 1994.
14. Price DD, et al. The challenge and the problems of placebo in assessment of sympathetically maintained pain. In: Jänig W, Stanton-Hicks M, eds. *Reflex Sympathetic Dystrophy: A Reappraisal*. Seattle: IASP Press; 1996:173–190 (*Progress in Pain Research and Management*; vol 6).
15. Veldman PHJM, et al. Signs and symptoms of reflex sympathetic dystrophy: prospective study of 829 patients. *Lancet* 1993;342:1012–1616.
16. Wilder RT. Reflex sympathetic dystrophy in children and adolescents: differences from adults. In: Jänig W, Stanton-Hicks M, eds. *Reflex Sympathetic Dystrophy: A Reappraisal*. Seattle: IASP Press; 1996:67–77 (*Progress in Pain Research and Management*; vol 6).
17. Wilson PR, et al. Diagnostic algorithm for complex regional pain syndromes. In: Jänig W, Stanton-Hicks M, eds. *Reflex Sympathetic Dystrophy: A Reappraisal*. Seattle: IASP Press; 1996:93–105 (*Progress in Pain Research and Management*; vol 6).

CHAPTER 41

Paraneoplastic Autonomic Dysfunction

Ramesh K. Khurana

1. There are three well-described paraneoplastic syndromes of autonomic dysfunction that are associated with somatic abnormalities. These are: Lambert-Eaton myasthenic syndrome (LEMS), subacute sensory neuronopathy, and enteric neuronopathy. Rarely, paraneoplastic autonomic dysfunction occurs without significant somatic involvement.
2. Eighty percent of patients with LEMS have autonomic symptoms. Dry mouth and impotence are common. Autonomic assessment shows widespread sympathetic and parasympathetic impairment. Early detection of the tumor is critical, and management of this tumor constitutes a specific treatment. Guanidine hydrochloride and 3,4-diaminopyridine can provide symptomatic relief.
3. Subacute sensory neuronopathy is characterized by the abrupt onset of dysesthesias, lancinating pain, and a prominent proprioceptive deficit. It may be associated with widespread autonomic dysfunction, including orthostatic hypotension. The presence of anti-Hu antibody in the serum of these patients helps confirm the diagnosis.
4. Enteric neuronopathy presents with features of intestinal pseudo-obstruction, and the patients usually have clinical and laboratory evidence of widespread autonomic dysfunction. Somatic involvement is variable. The presence of antibodies to the enteric neurons may help in the early diagnosis.
5. Autonomic neuropathy usually presents without manifesting any somatic neurologic dysfunction. Affected patients suffer a subacute onset of postural dizziness, gastrointestinal symptoms, and genitourinary complaints. Autonomic assessment reveals patchy but widespread abnormalities.
6. These paraneoplastic syndromes are presumably rare but disabling entities. The clinical recognition of these syndromes is, however, very important. Use of recently available serologic tests may lead to an early diagnosis and treatment of the underlying neoplasm may significantly reduce morbidity.

INTRODUCTION

Paraneoplastic neurologic syndromes (PNSs) or the "remote effects" of cancer, which are not attributable to the direct effects of the tumor or its metastases, occur in less than 1% of unselected patients with cancer (4). The practical importance of these syndromes, however, far exceeds their frequency because: (1) they may be the earliest indication that a patient has cancer; (2) they may be more disabling than the tumor itself; and (3) they may simulate metastatic disease or other disorders (28), thus leading to the use of inappropriate and inadequate treatment. Recent data suggest that treatment in some cases can improve the quality of life (50), and successful treatment of the associated neoplasm may even result in neurologic improvement (30). It is now possible to confirm suspected cases of PNS by serologic tests (41,63).

PNSs have varied clinical manifestations and can occur in the setting of any neoplasm, but they occur most often in patients with small-cell lung cancer (SCLC). PNSs can affect the somatic or the autonomic components of the nervous system, or both. There are several reports describing somatic neurologic involvement. This disorder can affect the brain, cranial nerves, spinal cord, dorsal root ganglia, peripheral nerves, neuromuscular junction, or skeletal muscle. Reports of autonomic dysfunction in PNS are infrequent. Affected patients may present with a spectrum of dysautonomia, ranging from panautonomic neuropathy (pandysautonomia) (10) to the relatively selective or predominant involvement of an organ (e.g., the gastrointesti-

---

R.K. Khurana: Department of Neurology, University of Maryland, Baltimore, Maryland 21201; Department of Neurology, The Johns Hopkins University School of Medicine, Baltimore, Maryland, 21287.

nal tract) (11) or the pupils (47). Somatic and autonomic abnormalities often occur in varying combinations. Three of these syndromes, Lambert-Eaton myasthenic syndrome (LEMS) (30), subacute sensory neuropathy (SSN) (74), and enteric neuronopathy (62), present with characteristic diagnostic features, whereas the features in other syndromes are nonspecific and still in the process of being delineated. This chapter reviews the subject of paraneoplastic autonomic dysfunction, with a special emphasis on LEMS because it led the way in the formulation of the modern concepts of PNS in terms of immune dysfunction and scientific approaches to treatment.

LAMBERT-EATON MYASTHENIC SYNDROME

LEMS is an acquired presynaptic disorder of neuromuscular transmission that involves a reduction in the nerve-stimulated quantal release of acetylcholine. A review of the clinical and electrophysiologic features in 50 consecutive cases revealed that neoplasms existed in half of the cases. SCLC occurred in 21 of 25 tumor cases. Of these 21 cases with SCLC, the tumor was diagnosed within 2 years of the occurrence of LEMS in 20 cases and within 3.8 years in 1 case (53). Although it is seen most often in patients with SCLC, LEMS has been described in association with lymphosarcoma and with carcinoma of the breast, colon, stomach, prostate, bladder, kidney, and gallbladder (22). Clinically, LEMS is characterized by proximal muscle weakness in 100% of the cases, reduced or absent muscle stretch reflexes in 92%, dysautonomia in 74%, and ptosis in 54%. Weakness and easy fatigability are the early symptoms. Pelvic and shoulder girdle muscles are predominantly affected, whereas extraocular and bulbar muscles are relatively spared (53). The transient improvement in strength, muscle stretch reflexes, and the electrophysiologic component after a few seconds of exercise is a characteristic feature. The electrophysiologic defect observed at the neuromuscular junction, as originally described by Lambert and colleagues in 1956 (36), consists of a reduced amplitude of the compound muscle action potentials (CMAP) as evoked by a supramaximal stimulus, postexercise facilitation of the CMAP, a decremental response at 2- to 5-Hz repetitive nerve stimulation, and an incremental response at 20- to 50-Hz stimulation (35). In a recent study, 2 of 50 patients showed no incremental response to maximum voluntary contraction, and 1 lacked an incremental response to a high-frequency electrical stimulation (53).

In 1989, Oh (52) published a description of two additional patterns of electrophysiologic abnormalities in patients with LEMS. One pattern consists of a low normal initial CMAP with a decremental response at low rates and no change at high rates of stimulation. An incremental response could be obtained in such patients using prolonged 4-second stimulation. The second pattern displays a low initial CMAP but decremental responses at low and high rates of stimulation. Oh attributed this second pattern to a more severe presynaptic block and lack of compensation for the depleted supply of immediately available acetylcholine.

Dry mouth was described as a feature of myasthenic syndrome (23,25) even before the classic electrophysiologic defect was recognized. Rooke and associates (58) observed the frequent occurrence of dry mouth and impotence in these patients. Subsequently, several authors added further observations to the spectrum of autonomic dysfunction, including decreased lacrimation (6), tonic pupils and orthostatic hypotension (5), and defective esophageal peristalsis, sluggish intestinal motility, and difficulty with micturition (24). My colleagues and I (30) noted autonomic symptoms in all of our six patients with LEMS. The symptoms included dry mouth in five patients, orthostatic lightheadedness in four, impotence in three of four male patients, and urinary difficulty in three patients. Constipation, decreased sweating, and dry eyes were uncommon. O'Neill and co-workers (53) reported autonomic symptoms in 64% of their patients with cancer and in 96% of those patients in whom cancer was not detected. Overall, 80% of their patients exhibited autonomic symptoms. Their patients frequently complained of dry mouth (74%) and impotence (41% of the males). Constipation (18%), blurred vision (8%), and impaired sweating (4%) were less common.

Symptoms of autonomic dysfunction are often described, but the results of formal autonomic testing have only recently been reported in a few cases. Clark and colleagues (12) studied the pupil cycle time, denervation supersensitivity of the iris musculature to 2.5% methacholine and 0.5% phenylephrine, and the results of Schirmer's test in 7 patients with LEMS and 50 age-matched control subjects. Abnormalities in the pupil cycle time and reflex lacrimation were noted in 69% of their patients. The cholinergic and adrenergic supersensitivity of the pupils was demonstrated in 57% of their patients. All 7 patients had an abnormality relating to the pupils or tear production, or both. This study showed the existence of both sympathetic and parasympathetic abnormalities in patients with LEMS, but it was limited to ocular autonomic functions. Review of the literature has revealed 8 additional cases (Tables 1 through 3) in whom more extensive investigations were performed (22,30,48,49,60,69). Of these 8 patients, 3 had SCLC and 1 had a malignant thymoma. No cancer was detected in 4. A battery of 5 to 12 tests was used to assess autonomic function in one to five organs. Orthostatic challenge and the Valsalva maneuver, the most common tests, were used to assess the integrity of the baroreceptor reflex arc. The cold pressor test, which is used to assess sympathetic function, was performed in 4 patients. The pilocarpine test, Schirmer's test, salivation test, and atropine test were used to evaluate parasympathetic functions in almost half the patients. The sweat test, a test of sympathetic cholinergic function, was used in 4 patients. Tests used in a battery varied from one study to another, rendering comparison difficult.

TABLE 1. *A summary of demographic and clinical features of patients with Lambert-Eaton myasthenic syndrome[a]*

Author	Patient No.	Age (yr)	Sex	Tumor	Comments
Rubenstein, 1979 (60)	1	47	F	ND	—
Mamdani et al., 1985 (48)	2	59	M	SCLC	Autonomic function improved along with tumor regression after treatment
Tabbaa et al., 1986 (69)	3	42	M	Malignant thymoma	Elevated acetylcholine receptor antibody titers: improvement in autonomic functions after removal of thymoma
Khurana et al., 1988 (30)	4	59	M	SCLC	Regression of tumor after chemotherapy Partial improvement of autonomic functions
	5	58	F	ND	—
Heath et al., 1988 (22)	6	59	M	ND	—
	7	72	M	ND	—
Manji et al., 1990 (49)	8	67	M	SCLC	Inappropriate antidiuretic hormone syndrome; autonomic dysfunction improved after chemotherapy

[a]For the autonomic function tests performed on each patient, refer to Tables 2 and 3.
ND, not detected; SCLC, small-cell lung cancer.

TABLE 2. *Results of sympathetic function tests*

Organs	Test	Patient No. 1	2	3	4	5	6	7	8
Eyes	Cocaine test	N	—	—	—	—	—	—	—
	Epinephrine test	—	A	—	—	—	—	—	—
Cardiovascular system	Orthostatic challenge	N	A	—	A	A	N	N	A
	Mental arithmetic test	—	A	—	A	A	—	—	—
	Cold pressor test	N	?A	A	—	—	—	—	A
	Valsalva's maneuver, (systolic overshoot)	—	A	A	A	A	—	—	A
	Handgrip test	—	—	—	—	—	A	N	—
	Norepinephrine infusion test	N	—	—	A	A	—	—	—
	Phenylephrine infusion test	—	A	—	—	—	—	—	—
Skin	Sweat test[a]	A	—	A	A	A	—	—	—

[a]Sudomotor pathway is cholinergic at the postganglionic level.
—, not reported; A, abnormal; N, normal.

TABLE 3. *Results of parasympathetic function tests*

Organs	Test	Patient No. 1	2	3	4	5	6	7	8
Eyes	Pilocarpine test	A	N	—	A	N	—	—	—
	Pupil cycle time	—	—	—	—	—	A	N	—
Lacrimal glands	Schirmer's test	A	A	—	A	N	—	—	—
Salivary glands	Parotid duct cannulation	A	A	—	A	A	—	—	—
Cardiovascular system	Valsalva's maneuver (ratio)	—	A	—	A	A	A	A	A
	Carotid sinus massage	N	—	—	—	—	—	—	—
	Oculocardiac reflex	N	—	—	—	—	—	—	—
	Cold face test	—	—	—	A	N	—	—	—
	Sinus arrhythmia	—	A	—	—	—	A	A	A
	Atropine	—	A	—	A	A	—	—	A
Esophagus	Barium swallow	—	—	—	A	—	—	—	—
Stomach	Barium swallow	—	—	—	A	—	—	—	—
	Endoscopy	—	—	—	A	—	—	—	—

—, not reported; A, abnormal; N, normal.

Dilute pilocarpine-induced miosis was noted in 3 of the 5 patients studied. Results of tests of salivation and sweating were abnormal in all 4 patients tested. Lacrimation was diminished in 3 of the 4 patients studied. Tachycardia in response to atropine administration was subnormal in all 4 cases evaluated. Thus, parasympathetic dysfunction affecting one or more organs was evident in all patients. Orthostatic challenge was abnormal in 4 of the 7 patients studied. Systolic blood pressure overshoot in response to the Valsalva maneuver was diminished in the 5 patients who were evaluated. Results of the mental arithmetic test, which was performed in 3 patients, were abnormal in all 3. Therefore, sympathetic insufficiency was documented by a few tests in 6 of the 8 patients. Only 2 patients (Nos. 1 and 7; see Table 2) showed normal responses. Patient 7 underwent only orthostatic challenge and handgrip tests. Patient 1 had a predominantly cholinergic dysautonomia, indicating that a presynaptic cholinergic defect involved the neuromuscular junction and autonomic effector organs. Patients 2 and 4 had widespread cholinergic and adrenergic involvement, suggesting that their synaptic defect may have been more generalized and may have involved transmitters other than acetylcholine (29). Other investigators have incriminated a coexisting neuropathy as the source of these findings (48).

Treatment of the tumor with chemotherapy or surgery has brought about substantial improvement in autonomic functions. Patient 4 (see Table 1) reported abatement of autonomic symptoms within 5 days of chemotherapy, suggesting a synaptic and possibly immune-mediated abnormality that was easily reversed. The usual therapeutic response, however, is slow, with objective clinical improvement commencing a few weeks after initiation of the tumor therapy. In all 4 cases with tumor, LEMS, and dysautonomia reported in the literature, tumor regression was associated with improvement in autonomic functions. Patient 3 was of particular interest because autonomic dysfunction accompanied the presynaptic as well as the postsynaptic abnormalities of the neuromuscular junction. The syndrome of inappropriate antidiuretic hormone and the autonomic insufficiency occurred together in Patient 8. Both conditions abated after chemotherapy. Five months later, the development of the clinical and electrophysiologic features of LEMS heralded a recurrence of the tumor, but without autonomic impairment; this suggested reversal of the sequence of LEMS and autonomic dysfunction. The authors, however, did not perform electrophysiologic studies at the time of the initial onset of the disorder, which raises the possibility that subclinical symptoms of LEMS could have gone unrecognized.

Pathogenesis

LEMS is considered a paraneoplastic autoimmune disorder. Because the immune response in a paraneoplastic disorder is not strictly autoimmune, the term antionconeural immune response has recently been proposed to apply in such instances (18). In the past, the evidence for autoimmunity was circumstantial. It consisted of its association with other autoimmune disorders (20), the occurrence of organ-specific antibodies against, for example, thyroid and gastric parietal cells (4), a higher incidence of histocompatibility antigens HLA-B8 and DR-w3 (55), clinical improvement with long-term prednisone therapy (68), and benefit obtained from plasma exchange and immunosuppressive drugs (14). Ishikawa and associates (26) noted a defect in neuromuscular transmission when extracts from a small-cell carcinoma in a patient with LEMS were added to the bathing solution of a frog nerve–muscle preparation. This suggested that the tumor extract contained a neuromuscular blocking agent. Vincent and co-workers (72) reported results from an experiment using athymic nude mice bearing human SCLC tumors derived from LEMS patients. The neuromuscular transmission in these mice was found to be normal.

The availability of a passive-transfer animal model and ultrastructural freeze-fracture studies opened avenues for more direct documentation of immune dysfunction. The disorder was passively transferred to laboratory mice by injection of plasma, crude immunoglobulins, or purified immunoglobulin G (IgG). Electrophysiologic and morphologic studies on these animals established it as a valid animal model of the human disorder (55) and provided evidence of a circulating immunoglobulin that was responsible for the production of the presynaptic neuromuscular defect. The Muscle Research Laboratory at the Mayo Clinic reported ultrastructural changes in the freeze-fracture preparations of biopsied human intercostal muscle (16). The density of the active zones and large intramembrane particles was measured, and the density of the active zones and active zone particles was noted to be markedly reduced, whereas the remaining active zone particles were found to be disorganized and clustered. It was assumed that active zone particles represented voltage-sensitive calcium channels (VSCCs), and the physiologic defect in LEMS was attributed to loss of VSCCs.

In a passive-transfer animal model, immunostaining substantiated the localization of LEMS IgG to the active zones at the presynaptic membrane. The earliest effect of LEMS IgG appears to be clustering of particles, followed by a progressive disorganization of their arrangement and a decrease in their number. These findings are consistent with the cross-linking of active zone particles by divalent autoantibodies (16,72). Several authors have studied the effects of LEMS IgG on VSCC of different cell types. Roberts and colleagues (57) demonstrated that LEMS IgG from patients with and without tumors impaired VSCC activity in a cultured SCLC cell line.

Kim and Neher (31) used a patch-clamp technique to study the effects of LEMS IgG on VSCC in bovine chromaffin cells. They demonstrated an approximately 40% reduction in VSCC, providing evidence for the reaction of IgG antibodies with calcium channels. Furthermore, they showed that antibody-induced dysfunction occurred in an all-or-none fashion, without any change in the kinetics of unblocked channels, and they demonstrated that the blocking effect of LEMS IgG on calcium-channel currents was dose dependent. LEMS IgG has been shown to reduce VSCC in SCLC cell lines, anterior pituitary cells, adrenal chromaffin cells, and neuroblastoma and glioma hybrid cells (16). L-type calcium channels in mouse ventricular muscle appear to be exempt, however, indicating that this antibody binds a specific channel determinant.

In 27 of 52 patients with LEMS, Lennon and Lambert (39) reported autoantibodies by radioimmunoassay. These autoantibodies bound specifically to VSCC extracted from SCLC cell lines obtained from LEMS patients, and bound specifically to that component of the VSCC complex that could be blocked by w-conotoxin. Similar findings were demonstrated with the neuronal cell line IMR32 (64). These two reports implicate VSCC as the antigen that initiates the autoimmunizing stimulus in a subset of patients with LEMS, and they further delineate the biochemical nature of the antigen. These studies describe a probable radioimmunoassay for LEMS antibodies. This is an important accomplishment, because LEMS precedes the diagnosis of tumor by several months. Sher and associates (63) monitored a patient with this antibody for 13 months, from the diagnosis of LEMS to the time the tumor was detected. A surgical specimen of this patient's tumor showed a high level of 125I-w-conotoxin binding sites, thus demonstrating both antigen and antibody in the same patient. In brief, the antigen source as well as the antibody have been demonstrated in LEMS patients (33). It is evident that the impaired release of acetylcholine from the presynaptic nerve terminals is mediated by antibody injury to the VSCC.

The molecular identity of the candidate antigen, a target of LEMS autoantibodies, is still not certain. According to recent studies, the binding of LEMS autoantibodies to synaptotagmin or syntaxin may indirectly impair neuromuscular transmission (70). Synaptotagmin, the synaptic vesicle membrane protein, and syntaxin, the nerve terminal membrane protein, are both presumed to be involved in docking and/or coupling the synaptic vesicles to the calcium channels for vesicle exocytosis. Hajela and Atchison (21), however, found no reactive component against synaptotagmin or syntaxin when they exposed, using western blot analysis of rat and human brain membrane proteins and pure recombinant synaptotagmin and syntaxin to LEMS sera.

The calcium channels consist of five subunits (α_1, α_2, β, Γ, and Ω) and several known types, including T, L, N, and P. The α_1 subunit, the central ion-channel component, contains the voltage sensor, antagonist binding site, and cation pore. The β subunit participates in the activation and inactivation of the channel. The typing of calcium channels is based on their electrophysiologic and pharmacologic properties. The calcium-channel subunit or calcium-channel type responsible for impaired neurotransmission in LEMS patients is not known. Rosenfeld and co-workers (59) used a high-titer LEMS serum to isolate a complementary DNA clone from a human brain expression library. The encoded antigen showed homology to the β subunit of the calcium channel. They found that 43% of LEMS sera recognized this protein, which suggests that this reactivity was specific for a subgroup of LEMS patients. The β subunit should not be a logical target of immune system response because of its intracellular and cytoplasmic orientation. It is postulated that β-subunit antibodies result from epitope spreading.

LEMS sera contain IgG antibodies to P-, Q-, and sometimes N-type voltage-sensitive calcium channels that have been implicated in impaired neuromuscular transmission. Lennon and colleagues (38) found anti–P/Q-type antibodies in 100% of patients with LEMS and cancer and in 91% of patients with LEMS but without cancer. Antibodies against N-type calcium channels were found in 73% of patients with LEMS and cancer. Motomura and associates (51) found anti–P-type antibodies in 85% of patients with LEMS. On the basis of the high frequency of P/Q-type antibodies, it is postulated that antibodies of this specificity have a role in the pathophysiology of LEMS. Furthermore, it is thought that patients with both anti–P/Q-type and anti-N antibodies are more likely to have cancer.

There is evidence of some heterogeneity in LEMS patients in terms of electrophysiologic defects and autonomic dysfunction. It is possible that a variety of calcium channels in tumor provoke IgG antibodies against a multitude of calcium-channel proteins. Different patients thus develop IgGs with different specificity toward calcium channel types, with a consequent variability in the clinical, electrophysiologic, and autonomic manifestations of LEMS.

Clinically, LEMS patients manifest a rather widespread involvement of the autonomic nervous system in that both cholinergic and adrenergic functions are affected. There are a few immunologic or ultrastructural studies that focus on the autonomic nerve terminals. Review of the literature has revealed three studies that focused on the end-organs (31,37): the cardiac ventricular muscle and the vas deferens innervated by the postganglionic nerves and the adrenal chromaffin cells innervated by the preganglionic nerves. LEMS IgG did not interfere with L-type calcium-channel currents in mouse ventricular muscle. Interestingly, w-conotoxin, which blocks the nerve-evoked quantal release of acetylcholine at the neuromuscular junction, also did not block the cardiac calcium channels, suggesting antigenic differences between cardiac and motor nerve calcium channels (37). These antigenic differences, however, may or may not apply to other species. LEMS IgG causes the functional loss of L-type calcium channels in bovine adrenal chromaffin cells (30), which are widely used as a model of sympathetic neurons. Recently, Waterman and co-workers (73) recorded (*in vitro*) contractions of the vas deferens in response to electrical stimulation. They demonstrated that LEMS IgG reduced sympathetic transmission in the mouse vas deferens through functional inactivation of P- or P- and Q-type voltage-sensitive calcium channels. Further studies of the calcium channels at the autonomic nerve terminals will be of value.

Treatment

In LEMS patients with neoplasms, the aim of treatment should be to eradicate the underlying tumor. In LEMS patients without tumors, treatment is directed toward the enhancement of cholinergic function and immunosuppression.

There are several reports of partial or complete remission of the autonomic and somatic neurologic deficits after treatment of the associated neoplasms. My colleagues and I (30) reported on four patients with SCLC and LEMS. In one patient, autonomic symptoms began to abate within 5 days of chemotherapy. This patient showed a remarkable decrease in the neurologic deficit after treatment of this tumor. Three other patients also experienced improvement and survived from 3 to 13 years. In another recent report, 7 of the 11 patients surviving for more than 2 months after tumor therapy showed substantial long-term neurologic improvement (9). One of these patients was in complete remission 7 years later.

Plasmapheresis, prednisone, plasmapheresis with prednisone, and other immunosuppressive drug regimens have been used in patients with LEMS who have no detectable tumor process. These treatments have been of variable benefit (14,68). Because some of the patients may harbor an occult neoplasm, immunosuppression may have adverse effects on the tumor. In a recent study, Chalk and associates (9) described patients who had undergone plasma exchange in conjunction with immunosuppressive drugs and antineoplastic therapy. No obvious adverse effect on oncologic outcome was observed in any of these patients. Immunosuppression, however, should be used with caution in patients with disease of less than four years' duration (53).

Antiacetylcholinesterase agents, guanidine hydrochloride, 4-aminopyridine, and 3,4-diaminopyridine have been used to enhance neuromuscular transmission for the purpose of symptomatic relief. Acetylcholinesterase inhibitors are of limited benefit, but they may potentiate the effects of 3,4-diaminopyridine (45). Guanidine inhibits the binding and uptake of calcium into subcellular organelles such as mitochondria, thereby increasing the free intracellular calcium level and facilitating acetylcholine release. It is given orally in dosages of 15 to 35 mg/kg per day. Side effects include paresthesias of the fingers and toes, unsteadiness, dose-related confusion, flushing, and tachycardia (35). Hematologic side effects occur in 20% of the patients, and the development of neutropenia and aplastic anemia may limit the use of this drug. Recently, guanidine-induced neutropenia was successfully reversed with low-dose alternate-day therapy (66). Patients on guanidine also need to be observed for possible renal or hepatic dysfunction.

Aminopyridines increase the quantal release of acetylcholine by blocking voltage-dependent potassium conductance, thus prolonging depolarization at the nerve terminal and enhancing voltage-dependent calcium influx. In short, they increase the efficiency of existing channels. The development of seizures, agitation, confusion, or ataxia precludes the clinical use of 4-aminopyridine. 3,4-Diaminopyridine is preferred because it crosses the blood–brain barrier less readily and is 6 to 10 times more potent in bringing about acetylcholine release at the neuromuscular junction (45). McEvoy and co-workers (50) performed a double-blind, placebo-controlled trial of 3,4-diaminopyridine in 12 patients with LEMS. The oral administration of 20 to 100 mg per day in divided doses produced electrophysiologic and motor improvement. There was also moderate improvement in autonomic function. There was subjective improvement in erectile function and dryness of the mouth. There was objective improvement in sweat production over the forearms and in the Valsalva ratio, but salivation and the orthostatic blood pressure response were unaffected. Perioral and acral paresthesias, lightheadedness, epigastric distress, and difficulty sleeping were noted as side effects. Only one patient had a seizure. Rhinorrhea, tearing, blurred vision, and frequent micturition and defecation were occasionally observed. Lundh and colleagues (46) recommended a daily dose ranging from 18 to 48 mg but not exceeding 60 mg. Central nervous system side effects were infrequent, but a case of persistent chorea was observed. In a few patients, the development of drug tolerance was reversed by withholding the drug for a few weeks. 3,4-Diaminopyridine has been safely used for up to 10 years and is the current drug of choice (45,50), where available.

Drugs that adversely affect the neuromuscular transmission should be avoided. A patient with LEMS and SCLC sustained respiratory failure after verapamil administration, with reversal of symptoms once verapamil treatment was stopped. Because LEMS is a disorder of calcium channels, calcium-channel blockers should be avoided (34).

SUBACUTE SENSORY NEURONOPATHY

In 1948, Denny-Brown (15) described two patients who had "primary sensory neuropathy with muscular changes associated with carcinoma." He observed the salient pathologic features of severe neuronal loss in the dorsal root ganglia, perivascular inflammatory infiltrates, and degeneration of the posterior roots and posterior columns. SSN is somewhat abrupt in onset, subacute in progression, and strongly associated with SCLC (32). Dysesthesias, paresthesias, lancinating pains, and numbness affect the extremities, face, and tongue. Loss of joint and position sense, sensory ataxia, and areflexia are also common. Motor strength as well as bowel and bladder functions are usually preserved. Myelopathy, brain-stem dysfunction, cerebellar degeneration, and dementia may occur in some patients (19). Electrophysiologic studies demonstrate absent or low-amplitude sensory nerve action potentials. Cerebrospinal fluid (CSF) shows mild pleocytosis, elevated protein levels, and oligoclonal bands (4).

Antineuronal nuclear antibody (anti-Hu) has been identified in patients with SCLC and SSN. It has also been found in patients with encephalomyelitis, cerebellar degeneration, and autonomic neuropathy, but not in patients with SCLC without neurologic symptoms, indicating that it is highly specific for the paraneoplastic disorder rather than the underlying cancer. Anti-Hu is a polyclonal, complement-fixing IgG present in serum and CSF. It is restricted to neurons in the dorsal root ganglia, trigeminal ganglia, and central nervous system. It has been found on the surface and in the nucleus of dorsal root ganglia neurons, suggesting that antibodies can be imbibed by the neurons. The target of the antibodies is an antigen protein with a molecular weight of 35 to 40 kd, which has been detected in both the primary and metastatic form of SCLC, and in SCLC cell lines prepared from patients with or without neurologic symptoms. The tumor antigen is identical to the brain nuclear antigen except for the absence of the 38-kd band (3,7,19).

Denny-Brown (15) observed a dilated stomach, megacolon, and enlarged rectum in one of his patients at postmortem examination. In a clinical study, tonic pupils were reported in two patients (47). The tonic pupils were an isolated autonomic finding in one patient; the second patient also showed orthostatic hypotension without any change in heart rate. In a report of two patients with SSN and positive anti-Hu antibodies, one patient suffered orthostatic hypotension (32). Andersen and co-workers (3) reviewed the clinical features observed in 14 patients positive for anti-Hu antibody, and some form of autonomic dysfunction was noted in 4. These studies suggest that autonomic dysfunction in patients with SSN may be more common than is customarily reported (3).

Generalized autonomic dysfunction has been reported in three patients. In the first case, a 31-year-old patient with testicular seminoma and embryonal carcinoma experienced the acute onset of autonomic dysfunction (32). Microneurography revealed a lack of muscle and skin afferent activity, with no sympathetic nerve activity. Postural hypotension, absent galvanic skin response, and absence of sweating pointed to sympathetic impairment. The combination of dilated pupils that were supersensitive to dilute pilocarpine, a diminished Valsalva ratio, dry mouth, diminished lacrimation, bladder paresis, and absence of penile erection was consistent with parasympathetic insufficiency (17). In another report, three patients with anti-Hu antibody were stated to have autonomic dysfunction. Of these three, one had encephalopathy, ataxia, sensory loss, hyporeflexia, and degeneration of the dorsal root ganglia and autonomic ganglia neurons. This patient had abnormal responses to the Valsalva maneuver, fecal and urinary retention, and incontinence indicative of parasympathetic dysfunction. Sympathetic dysfunction was evident from the marked orthostatic hypotension. I observed a third case in a 74-year-old woman with lancinating pains, dysesthesias, and proprioceptive and pyramidal signs who happened to complain of dry mouth during evaluation. Subsequent autonomic assessment revealed pilocarpine-induced pupillary miosis, diminished salivation, diminished Valsalva ratio, constipation, orthostatic hypotension with subnormal tachycardia, diminished systolic overshoot, supersensitivity to dilute norepinephrine, and abnormal sweat test results. Imaging studies of her chest and a subsequent biopsy revealed SCLC. Treatment of the SCLC partially alleviated the somatic and autonomic symptoms.

These three patients, all of whom were evaluated in sufficient detail, exhibited widespread autonomic dysfunction. In our patient, the diagnosis of a paraneoplastic disorder was not entertained until the patient complained of dry mouth. The availability of serum markers for paraneoplastic dysfunction should make it possible to evaluate these patients in the early stages of the illness and to observe for any specific pattern of autonomic involvement at various stages of the illness. Furthermore, early treatment of the tumor may stabilize or diminish the neurologic deficit.

ENTERIC NEURONOPATHY

Intestinal pseudo-obstruction is a recently recognized paraneoplastic syndrome. Because neurons of the enteric nervous system are the target of immune attack, and loss of these neurons is a salient pathologic feature, enteric neuronopathy seems to be a more apt designation. Gastrointestinal dysfunction as a presenting manifestation of a paraneoplastic disorder has been reported in a few patients. It is most commonly associated with SCLC, but it has also been observed in association with pulmonary carcinoid and undifferentiated epithelioma. Gastrointestinal symptoms usually precede discovery of the tumor but may follow diagnosis of the initial or recurrent tumor (11,42,43). The acute onset of progressive constipation, crampy abdominal pain, and vomiting point to the diagnosis of acute bowel obstruction. Such patients usually undergo exploratory laparotomy with negative findings before the diagnosis of pseudo-obstruction is entertained. Endoscopy reveals normal-appearing mucosa and no evidence of obstruction. Radiologic and electrophysiologic investigations reveal delayed gastric emptying, gastrointestinal dysmotility, and hypomotility, coupled with absent interdigestive migratory motor complexes. Loss of myenteric plexus neurons, vacuolations of the neuronal cytoplasm, infiltration of the plasma cells and lymphocytes with a preponderance of T cells, and fragmentation and degeneration of axons are the salient pathologic features (40).

Pseudo-obstruction of the bowel may be the only manifestation in some patients (1,13). In others, autonomic impairment of other organs has also been observed. Chinn and Schuffler (11) noted autonomic insufficiency in two of seven patients with pseudo-obstruction of the bowel. There is no specific pattern of autonomic impairment in this disorder, however. In one study, one patient had orthostatic hypotension, sweating abnormalities, and impaired ejaculation, but normal cardiovascular and vagal reflexes (67). A second patient had Adie's pupil, orthostatic hypotension, a diminished Valsalva ratio, and sinus arrhythmia with normal catecholamine levels (67). Somatic neurologic involvement ranges from none (1,13,67) to severe (43,62). Schuffler and associates (62) described a patient who had extrapyramidal dysfunction and ataxia that mimicked multiple-system atrophy (Shy-Drager syndrome).

The gastrointestinal dysfunction is usually refractory to treatment with cholinergic drugs or motility-promoting agents. Surgical intervention is also usually not beneficial. However, symptoms occasionally remit spontaneously (11). Sodhi and co-workers (67) published their observations in three patients treated for cancer with either chemotherapy or radiation. Resolution of the motility disorder was noted in two of the patients several months after the start of treatment.

In a previous immunologic study, antibodies directed against the myenteric plexus were not detected in tissue from a patient with pseudo-obstruction or in tissue from a normal individual (13). However, Sakai and colleagues (61) identified a gene encoding an autoantigen recognized by paraneoplastic anti-Purkinje cell antibodies in a patient with uterine cancer. A transcript of the gene was detected not only in the cerebellum but also in the intestine. Similarly, IgG from a 72-year-old patient with subacute cerebellar degeneration and ovarian carcinoma stained mouse myenteric plexus neurons (2). There are, however, no clinical reports of pseudo-obstruction of the bowels seen in association with paraneoplastic cerebellar degeneration. Lennon and associates (40,41) demonstrated IgG antibodies that were reactive with neurons of the myenteric and submucosal plexus of the jejunum and stomach. This seems to be a promising development and should help in the early diagnosis of pseudo-obstruction.

AUTONOMIC NEUROPATHY

Autonomic neuropathy is characterized by autonomic dysfunction in association with no (10) or minimal (56) somatic neurologic involvement. Peripheral neuropathy has been noted in an occasional patient (65). It has also been seen in association with inappropriate antidiuretic hormone secretion (8,27) and diminished aldosterone secretion (71). Autonomic neuropathy is usually associated with SCLC, but it can occur in the context of adenocarcinoma of the pancreas (71) or Hodgkin's disease (44). It is usually diagnosed several months before discovery of malignancy (10). It is considered a paraneoplastic disorder because of its temporal association with a malignancy and because patients occasionally experience recovery of autonomic function after treatment of their tumor (44,54).

Autonomic neuropathy is characterized by the subacute onset of postural dizziness, gastrointestinal symptoms, impotence, urinary retention, and dry mouth. Laboratory assessment of sympathetic functions reveals orthostatic hypotension with a subnormal rise in heart rate. Occasionally, tachycardia accompanies the orthostatic hypotension (44). The results of the thermoregulatory sweat test are often abnormal, but patients with normal sweating patterns have been reported (8,54,65). Involvement of the bowel, bladder, heart, pupils, and penile erection reflect parasympathetic dysfunction. The results of the Valsalva maneuver and atropine test are usually abnormal, but Van Lieshout and co-workers (44) demonstrated intact vagal function in a patient with orthostatic hypotension and Hodgkin's disease.

Autonomic neuropathy causes progressive disability, but improvement has been observed both during (44) and after (54) treatment of the tumor. Therefore, a paraneoplastic cause should be considered in the differential diagnosis of a patient with autonomic dysfunction of subacute onset, and such patients should be evaluated for malignancy, especially SCLC. Further research into the pathogenesis and immune dysfunction of the disorder may yield a serologic marker that can be used in the diagnosis of this paraneoplastic disorder.

REFERENCES

1. Ahmed MN, Carpenter S. Autonomic neuropathy and carcinoma of the lung. *Can Med Assoc J* 1975;113:410–412.
2. Altermatt HJ, et al. Paraneoplastic cerebellar autoantibodies associated with gynecologic cancer bind to myenteric plexus neurons. *Ann Neurol* 1991;29:687–688.
3. Andersen NE et al. Autoantibodies in paraneoplastic syndromes associated with small-cell lung cancer. *Neurology* 1988;38:1391–1398.
4. Andersen NE, et al. Autoimmune pathogenesis of paraneoplastic neurological syndromes. *Crit Rev Neurobiol* 1987;3:245–299.
5. Beallo A. Bilateral tonic pupils, ptosis and myasthenic syndrome associated with oat cell carcinoma of the lung. *Trans Pac Coast Otoophthalmol Soc* 1965;31:89–102.
6. Brown JC, Johns RJ. Diagnostic difficulties encountered in the myasthenic syndrome sometimes associated with carcinoma. *J Neurol Neurosurg Psychiatry* 1974;37:1214–1224.
7. Budde-Steffen C et al. Expression of an antigen in small-cell lung carcinoma lines detected by antibodies from patients with paraneoplastic dorsal root ganglionopathy. *Cancer Res* 1988;48:430–434.
8. Carr-Locke DL. Autonomic neuropathy and inappropriate secretion of antidiuretic hormone occurrence in a patient with bronchogenic carcinoma. *JAMA* 1979;241:2298.
9. Chalk CH et al. Response of the Lambert-Eaton myasthenic syndrome to treatment of associated small-cell lung carcinoma. *Neurology* 1990;40:1552–1556.
10. Chiappa KH, Young RR. A case of paracarcinomatous pandysautonomia. *Neurology* 1973;23:423.

11. Chinn JS, Schuffler MD. Paraneoplastic visceral neuropathy as a cause of severe gastrointestinal motor dysfunction. *Gastroenterology* 1988;95:1279–1286.
12. Clark CV, et al. Ocular autonomic nerve function in Lambert-Eaton myasthenic syndrome. *Eye* 1990;4:473–481.
13. Colombel JF et al. Paraneoplastic intestinal pseudo-obstruction as the presenting feature of small-cell lung cancer. *Gastroenterol Clin Biol* 1988;12:394–396.
14. Dau PC, Denys M. Plasmapheresis and immunosuppressive drug therapy in the Lambert-Eaton syndrome. *Ann Neurol* 1982;11:570–575.
15. Denny-Brown D. Primary sensory neuropathy with muscular changes associated with carcinoma. *J Neurol Neurosurg Psychiatry* 1948;11: 73–87.
16. Engel AG et al. Motor nerve terminal calcium channels in Lambert-Eaton myasthenic syndrome. *Ann N Y Acad Sci* 1989;560:278–290.
17. Fagius J, et al. Acute pandysautonomia and severe sensory deficit with poor recovery. A clinical, neurophysiological and pathological case study. *J Neurol Neurosurg Psychiatry* 1983;46:725–733.
18. Furneaux HM et al. Selective expression of Purkinje-cell antigens in tumor tissue from patients with paraneoplastic cerebellar degeneration. *N Engl J Med* 1990;322:1844–1851.
19. Grous F et al. Sensory neuronopathy and small cell lung cancer: antineuronal antibody that also reacts with the tumor. *Am J Med* 1986; 80:45–52.
20. Guttman L et al. The Eaton-Lambert syndrome and autoimmune disorders. *Am J Med* 1972;53:354–356.
21. Hajela RK, Atchison WD. The protein synaptotagmin and syntaxin are not general targets of Lambert-Eaton myasthenic syndrome autoantibody. *J Neurochem* 1995;64:1245–1251.
22. Heath JP, et al. Abnormalities of autonomic function in the Lambert-Eaton myasthenic syndrome. *J Neurol Neurosurg Psychiatry* 1988; 51:436–439.
23. Heathfield KWG, Williams JRB. Peripheral neuropathy and myopathy associated with bronchogenic carcinoma. *Brain* 1954;77:122–137.
24. Henriksson KG et al. Clinical, neurophysiological and morphological findings in Eaton-Lambert syndrome. *Acta Neurol Scand* 1977; 56:117–140.
25. Henson RA, et al. Carcinomatous neuropathy and myopathy. A clinical and pathological study. *Brain* 1954;77:82–121.
26. Ishikawa I et al. A neuromuscular transmission block produced by a cancer tissue extract derived from a patient with the myasthenic syndrome. *Neurology* 1977;27:140–143.
27. Ivy HK. Renal sodium loss and bronchogenic carcinoma. *Arch Intern Med* 1961;108:47–55.
28. Khurana RK. Dysautonomia associated with small cell lung cancer. *Neurology* 1988;38(suppl 1):306.
29. Khurana RK, et al. Dysautonomia in Eaton-Lambert syndrome. *Ann Neurol* 1988;14:123.
30. Khurana RK, et al. Autonomic dysfunction in Lambert-Eaton myasthenic syndrome. *J Neurol Sci* 1988;85:77–86.
31. Kim YI, Neher E. IgG from patients with Lambert-Eaton syndrome blocks voltage-dependent calcium channels. *Science* 1988;239:405–408.
32. Kimmel DW, et al. Subacute sensory neuronopathy associated with small cell lung carcinoma: diagnosis aided by autoimmune serology. *Mayo Clin Proc* 1988;63:29–32.
33. Kornguth SE. Neuronal protein and paraneoplastic syndromes. *N Engl J Med* 1989;321:1607–1608.
34. Krendel DA, Hopkins LC. Adverse effect of verapamil in a patient with the Lambert-Eaton syndrome. *Muscle Nerve* 1986;9:519–522.
35. Kula RW. Neuromuscular disorders associated with systemic neoplastic diseases. In: Vinken PJ, Bruyn GW, Ringel SP (eds). *Handbook of Clinical Neurology, Vol 41*. Amsterdam: North-Holland Publishing Company. 1979;317–403.
36. Lambert EH, et al. Defect of neuromuscular conduction associated with malignant neoplasms. *Am J Physiol* 1956;187:612–613.
37. Lang B, et al. The effect of Lambert-Eaton myasthenic syndrome antibody on slow action potentials in mouse cardiac ventricle. *Proc R Soc Lond (Biol)* 1988;235:103–110.
38. Lennon VA, et al. Calcium-channel antibodies in the Lambert-Eaton syndrome and other paraneoplastic syndromes. *N Engl J Med* 1995; 332:1467–1474.
39. Lennon VA, Lambert EH. Autoantibodies bind solubilized calcium channel-W-conotoxin complexes from small cell lung carcinoma: a diagnostic aid for Lambert-Eaton myasthenic syndrome. *Mayo Clin Proc* 1989;64:1498–1506.
40. Lennon VA, et al. Enteric neuronal autoantibodies in pseudo-obstruction with small-cell lung carcinoma. *Gastroenterology* 1991;100:1–6.
41. Lennon VA et al. Enteric neuronal autobodies in pseudoobstruction with small-cell lung carcinoma. *Gastroenterology* 1991;100:137–142.
42. Lhermitte F et al. Paralysis of digestive tract with lesions of myenteric plexus: a new paraneoplastic syndrome. *Rev Neurol (Paris)* 1980;136:825–836.
43. Lhermitte F et al. Paralysie du tube digestif avec lesions des plexus myenteriques et cancer. Un nouveau syndrome paraneoplastique possible. *Presse Med* 1981;10:253.
44. Van Lieshout JJ et al. Acute dysautonomia associated with Hodgkin's disease. *J Neurol Neurosurg Psychiatry* 1986;49:830–832.
45. Lundh H, et al. Current therapy of the Lambert-Eaton myasthenic syndrome. In: Aquilonius SM, Gillberg PG (eds). *Progress in Brain Research, Vol 84*. Amsterdam: Elsevier Science Publishers. 1990; 163–170.
46. Lundh H, et al. Practical aspects of 3-4 diaminopyridine treatment of the Lambert-Eaton myasthenic syndrome. *Acta Neurol Scand* 1993;88:136–140.
47. Maitland CG et al. Paraneoplastic tonic pupils. *J Clin Neuroophthalmol* 1985;5:99–104.
48. Mamdani MB, et al. Autonomic dysfunction and Eaton-Lambert syndrome. *J Auton Nerv Syst* 1985;12:315–320.
49. Manji H, et al. Lambert-Eaton syndrome: autonomic neuropathy and inappropriate antidiuretic hormone secretion in a patient with small cell carcinoma of the lung. *J Neurol* 1990;237:324–325.
50. McEvoy KM et al. Diaminopyridine in the treatment of Lambert-Eaton myasthenic syndrome. *N Engl J Med* 1989;321:1567–1571.
51. Motomura M, et al. An improved diagnostic assay for Lambert-Eaton myasthenic syndrome. *J Neurol Neurosurg Psychiatry* 1995;58: 85–87.
52. Oh SJ. Diverse electrophysiological spectrum of the Lambert-Eaton myasthenic syndrome. *Muscle Nerve* 1989;12:464–469.
53. O'Neill JH, et al. The Lambert-Eaton myasthenic syndrome: a review of 50 cases. *Brain* 1988;3:577–596.
54. Park DM et al. Orthostatic hypotension in bronchial carcinoma. *Br Med J* 1972;3:510–511.
55. Pascuzzi RM, Kim YI. Lambert-Eaton syndrome. *Semin Neurol* 1990;10:35–41.
56. Quinlan CD. Autonomic neuropathy in carcinoma of the lung. *J Ir Med Assoc* 1971;64:430–431.
57. Roberts A et al. Paraneoplastic myasthenic syndrome IgG inhibits Ca^{2+} flux in a human small cell carcinoma line. *Nature* 1985;317: 737–739.
58. Rooke ED et al. Myasthenia and malignant intrathoracic tumor. *Med Clin North Am* 1960;44:977–988.
59. Rosenfeld MR, et al. Cloning and characterization of a Lambert-Eaton myasthenic syndrome antigen. *Ann Neurol* 1993;33:113–120.
60. Rubenstein AE, et al. Cholinergic dysautonomia and Eaton-Lambert syndrome. *Neurology* 1979;29:720–723.
61. Sakai K et al. Isolation of a complementary DNA clone encoding an autoantigen recognized by an antineuronal cell antibody from a patient with paraneoplastic cerebellar degeneration. *Ann Neurol* 1990; 28:692–698.
62. Schuffler MD et al. Intestinal pseudo-obstruction as the presenting manifestation of small-cell carcinoma of the lung. A paraneoplastic neuropathy of the gastrointestinal tract. *Ann Intern Med* 1983;98: 129–134.
63. Sher E et al. Calcium channel autoantibody and non-small-cell lung cancer in patients with Lambert-Eaton syndrome. *Lancet* 1990; 335:413.
64. Sher E et al. Specificity of calcium channel autoantibodies in Lambert-Eaton myasthenic syndrome. *Lancet* 1989;2:640–643.
65. Siemsen JK, Meister L. Bronchogenic carcinoma associated with severe orthostatic hypotension. *Ann Intern Med* 1963;58:669–676.
66. Silbert PL, et al. Successful alternate day guanidine therapy following guanidine-induced neutropenia in the Lambert-Eaton myasthenic syndrome. *Muscle Nerve* 1990;13:360–361.

67. Sodhi N et al. Autonomic function and motility in intestinal pseudo-obstruction caused by paraneoplastic syndrome. *Dig Dis Sci* 1989;34:1937–1942.
68. Streib EW, Rothner AD. Eaton-Lambert myasthenic syndrome: long-term treatment of three patients with prednisone. *Ann Neurol* 1981;10:448–453.
69. Tabbaa MA, et al. Malignant thymoma with dysautonomic and disordered neuromuscular transmission. *Arch Neurol* 1986;43:955–957.
70. Takamori M, et al. Synaptotagmin can cause an immune-mediated model of Lambert-Eaton myasthenic syndrome in rats. *Ann Neurol* 1994;35:74–80.
71. Thomas JP, Sheilds R. Associated autonomic dysfunction and carcinoma of the pancreas. *Br Med J* 1970;4:32.
72. Vincent A, et al. Autoimmunity to the voltage gated calcium channel underlies the Lambert-Eaton myasthenic syndrome, a paraneoplastic disorder. *Trends Neurosci* 1989;12:496–502.
73. Waterman SA, et al. Lambert-Eaton myasthenic syndrome autoantibodies inhibit neurotransmission from postganglionic sympathetic neurons by blocking voltage-gated calcium channels. *Neurology* 1996;46:A223–A224.
74. Wiley RG et al. Autonomic insufficiency in the paraneoplastic neuropathy of oat cell carcinoma. *Neurology* 1988;38(suppl 1):115.

CHAPTER 42

Multiple System Atrophy and Pure Autonomic Failure

Phillip A. Low and Sir Roger Bannister

1. Multiple-system atrophy (MSA), because of involvement of multiple systems of the central nervous system, is quite distinct clinically from pure autonomic failure in which the central nervous system is unaffected.
2. Striatonigral, olivopontocerebellar, and pyramidal forms of MSA exist.
3. Key magnetic resonance imaging findings in patients with MSA consist of cerebellar atrophy and changes in the posterolateral putamen that reflect a loss of neurons. The changes are typically manifested as T2 hypodensity or linear lateral hyperdensities.
4. A characteristic finding on positron emission tomography is reduced uptake of F-dopa in the caudate and putamen.
5. The natural history of pure autonomic failure is one of slow progression over some 10 to 15 years, whereas MSA patients usually do not survive more than 6 to 8 years from the time of diagnosis.
6. Treatment of orthostatic hypotension with fludrocortisone, head-up tilt, vasoactive agents, or DDAVP may be partially effective.

HISTORY

Shy and Drager (145) were the first to describe other neurologic features with autonomic failure, the syndrome now called multiple system atrophy (MSA). It is appropriate to quote from their original description. "The full syndrome comprises the following features: orthostatic hypotension, urinary and rectal incontinence, loss of sweating, iris atrophy, external ocular palsies, rigidity, tremor, loss of associated movements, impotence, the findings of an atonic bladder and loss of rectal sphincter tone, fasciculations, wasting of distal muscles, evidence of a neuropathic lesion in the electromyogram (EMG) that suggests involvement of the anterior horn cells, and the finding of a neuropathic lesion in the muscle biopsy. The date of onset is usually in the 5th to 7th decade of life."

At this stage, olivopontocerebellar atrophy (OPCA) had not been linked with autonomic failure. Although Shy and Drager noted degeneration of the intermediolateral cell column in their pathologic report, credit for first specifically linking this finding with the presenting features of postural hypotension rests with Johnson and colleagues (67).

The first cases of pure autonomic failure (PAF) were described by Bradbury and Eggleston (23) as "idiopathic orthostatic hypotension" because of their presenting features. This term is misleading because it stresses only one feature of autonomic failure and ignores the more usually associated neurologic disturbances of bladder and sexual function and sweating. The term pure autonomic failure is now accepted generally for this syndrome.

MULTIPLE SYSTEM ATROPHY

Definition

A Consensus Panel convened by the American Autonomic Society and co-sponsored by the American Academy of Neurology defined MSA as "a sporadic, progressive, adult onset disorder characterized by autonomic dysfunction, parkinsonism, and ataxia in any combination. The features of this disorder include: (a) Parkinsonism (bradykinesia with rigidity or tremor or both), usually with a poor or unsustained motor response to chronic levodopa

---

P. A. Low: Department of Neurology, Mayo Clinic, Rochester, Minnesota 55905.
R. G. Bannister: Autonomic Department, The National Hospital for Neurology and Neurosurgery, Queen Square, London WC1.

therapy. (b) Cerebellar or corticospinal signs. (c) Orthostatic hypotension, impotence, urinary incontinence or retention, usually preceding or within 2 years after the onset of the motor symptoms. Characteristically, these features cannot be explained by medications or other disorders. Parkinsonian and cerebellar features commonly occur in combination. However, certain features may predominate. When parkinsonian features predominate, the term striatonigral degeneration is often used. When cerebellar features predominate, sporadic OPCA is often used. When autonomic failure predominates, the term Shy-Drager syndrome is often used. These manifestations may occur in various combinations and evolve with time."

Prevalence

Multiple system atrophy has increased in importance with the recognition that it occurs much more frequently than had previously been suspected. At the National Hospital Parkinson's Disease Brain Bank, which accepts for research purposes the brains of patients who were managed as having Parkinson's disease or parkinsonian-like syndromes, about one fifth of the brains prove to have the pathologic changes typical of MSA. Clearly, there are several factors in the selection of such cases that are likely to distort the true incidence of this disorder. The clinical diagnosis of Parkinson's disease might have included patients with parkinsonism. Most cases were not diagnosed by movement disorder or autonomic neurologists. The prevalence of MSA does appear to have been underestimated. The prevalence of MSA in the population may be on the order of 5 to 15 per 100,000 (44).

Clinical Features

Age of onset is in late middle age to old age. The two largest series (n > 50 in each) indicate a median age of onset of 53 years (range, 33 to 76 years; n=100) (168) and a mean of 60.3 years (SD 9.3; n=73) (139). The male-to-female ratio is 2:1 (139,168). Patients with MSA present most commonly with symptoms of autonomic failure and parkinsonism. There are usually features that suggest that the patient does not have Parkinson's disease. Three differences distinguish MSA from Parkinson's disease. These are the atypical nature of the parkinsonian features, the involvement beyond the extrapyramidal system, and the characteristic autonomic features. Among the extrapyramidal symptoms, rigidity, bradykinesia, and ataxia predominate over tremor, which is usually absent or minimal (139,168). The response to levodopa is often absent, poor, or poorly sustained. Wenning and associates (168) reported that 29% had a good or excellent levodopa response at some stage, although only 13% maintained this response. Orofacial and choreodystonic movements are side effects of treatment at this stage, although the characteristic change is the absence of this response, and they generally do not suffer an on–off type phenomenon. Wenning and associates reported dyskinesias in 53% of treated patients. Sandroni and co-workers (139) reported lower values for both levodopa response and dyskinesias. Dyskinesias correlated well with levodopa response and occurred in 16% of patients with MSA. Much of the difference relates to criteria for MSA. Many of the cases accepted by Wenning and colleagues (168) would have been defined as nonspecific MSA (n=75) or, less likely, parkinsonism-plus (n=54) in the Mayo series. Levodopa aggravates orthostatic hypotension and may provoke orthostatic symptoms. Mild pyramidal signs may be present. Some patients may have additional cerebellar or bulbar involvement. These features raise the possibility of more widespread involvement of the central nervous system (CNS) and hence the possible diagnosis of MSA. Following the recommendation of the Consensus Conference, terms such as parkinsonism-plus and nonspecific MSA should be discarded.

The diagnosis of MSA is made by the presence of autonomic failure. Orthostatic hypotension is the rule; it is present at first evaluation or within a year of development of parkinsonism. Orthostatic hypotension in patients with MSA is usually less severe than that seen in patients with PAF. Symptoms of orthostatic hypotension consist of lightheadedness, tiredness, ataxia (which worsens in proportion to the severity of fall in blood pressure), blurred vision, and retrocollic aching. In about half the patients the most common symptom or observation is orthostatic impairment of mentation (92). These patients may look dazed and may have trouble concentrating or thinking clearly. Symptoms are often worse on arising, especially after excessive nocturia (101); blood pressure falls after a meal (Fig. 1); and orthostatic hypotension may be aggravated. Symptoms may also worsen with exercise (148), with the duration of standing, and with a rise in core temperature (92).

In a study on early morning orthostatic hypotension, Mathias and associates (101) recorded day and night urine volume, morning and evening body weight, and supine and sitting blood pressure in five patients with chronic autonomic failure. All had nocturnal polyuria, overnight weight loss, and a pronounced postural fall in blood pressure, with the lowest levels in the morning. Desmopressin (2 to 4 µg given intramuscularly or by nasal insufflation at 8 PM) reduced nocturnal polyuria, diminished overnight weight loss, raised supine blood pressure, and reduced the postural fall, especially in the morning. The excessive nocturia might be related to an abnormal circadian rhythm of plasma antidiuretic hormone, which is paradoxically higher during the day than at night in these patients (116).

Patients with chronic orthostatic hypotension may be remarkably tolerant of very low orthostatic blood pressures, developing no symptoms, especially when the condition becomes chronic. This improvement in orthostatic tolerance appears to be related to an expansion of the autoregulated range of lower blood pressures (27,157). Within this

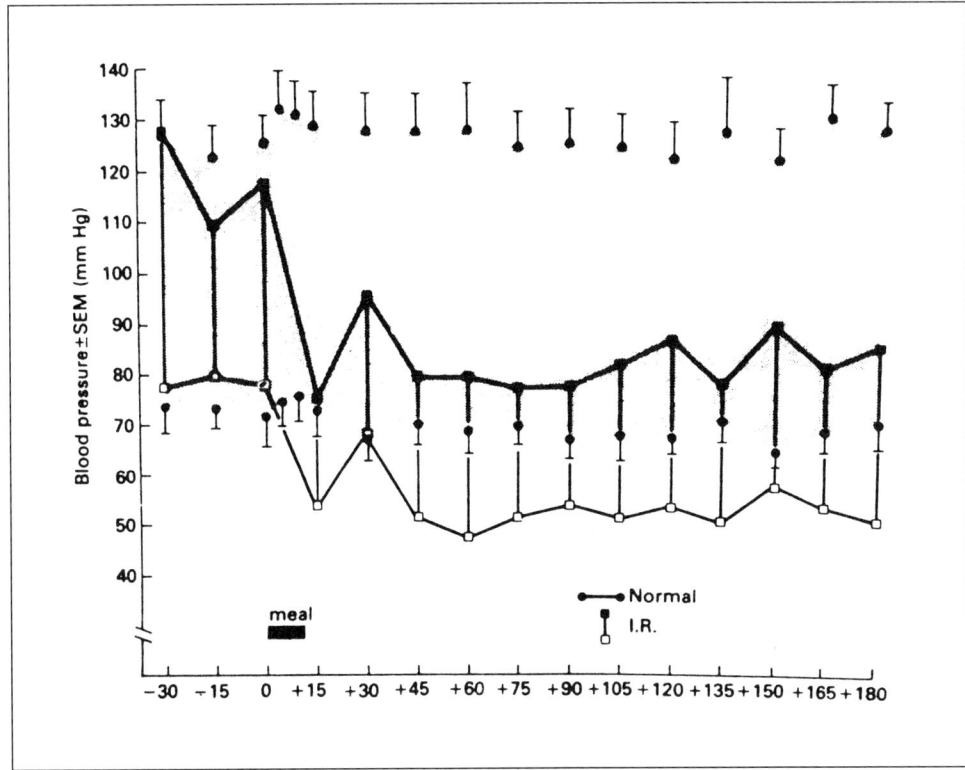

FIG. 1. Supine systolic and diastolic blood pressure before and after a standard meal in a group of normal subjects (*stippled area, with + SEM bars*) and in a patient (*I.R.*) with autonomic failure. Blood pressure in the normal subjects does not change after a meal. In the patient with autonomic failure there is a rapid fall in blood pressure to levels around 80/50 mmHg; these levels remain low in the supine position over the 3-hour observation period. (Reprinted with permission from Mathias CJ, Bannister R. Postcibal hypotension in autonomic disorders. In: Bannister R, Mathias C (eds). *Autonomic Failure*. Oxford: Oxford University Press. 1992; 489–509.)

range, cerebral blood flow remains constant in the face of changing systemic blood pressure by a change in cerebral arteriolar tone. Thomas and Bannister (157) demonstrated that cerebral blood flow was maintained in response to head-up tilt down to a systolic pressure of 60 mmHg. Recent studies have combined transcranial Doppler (TCD) with cerebral blood flow recordings. Flow velocity, measured by TCD, becomes reduced when cerebral arteriolar tone increases. It was demonstrated that blood flow was maintained by a change in cerebral arteriolar tone (27). Cerebral autoregulation in MSA may be a more dynamic process than originally conceived, and could change from day to day (144). With severe orthostatic hypotension, autoregulation fails, and reversal of flow at the end-diastolic phase on the Doppler flow image during duplex ultrasonography occurs, as has been demonstrated for both the common carotid and vertebral arteries (178). This reversal can be corrected when effectively treated by pressor agents.

Normal circadian blood pressure (BP) rhythm is characterized by a nocturnal fall and a diurnal rise and has been suggested to be mediated mainly by the circadian rhythm of sympathetic tone (62,63) and by the effects of recumbency. Ambulant BP recordings, initially with intra-arterial recordings and subsequently with noninvasive measurements, have demonstrated a consistent circadian trend in BP that was the inverse of the normal pattern in widespread autonomic failure, with the highest pressures at night and the lowest in the morning. These recordings of low BP seem to correlate with symptoms of orthostatic hypotension (62,63,95,160). Increased α-receptor number and decreased cyclic AMP production, which occur in PAF, contribute to supine hypertension, and an increase in α-receptor number may also contribute to the supine hypertension of MSA (69), analogous to the situation in essential hypertension.

The BP response to exercise is impaired in both MSA and PAF (73). With exercise, BP increases in normal subjects, but paradoxically it falls markedly in patients with MSA and PAF, with a delayed recovery. The fall in BP is largely due to a fall in systemic vascular resistance.

The brain bears the brunt of the ischemic effects of orthostatic hypotension. Rarely, other regions are affected. Severe angina associated with orthostatic hypotension has been reported. This patient had angina in association with normal coronary arteries (146). Vertigo is not uncommon (92) and is presumed to be due to ischemia of the vestibular end organ. Electronystagmographic abnormalities were reported in three patients with MSA with normal brain stem evoked potentials (114). Rarely, MSA is associated with Meniere's syndrome (58).

Although symptoms of orthostatic hypotension have attracted the most attention, cholinergic dysfunction is an integral part of the disorder (35,72,139). Symptoms include constipation, impotence, nocturia, hesitancy in micturition, anhidrosis, and xerostomia. Constipation is the rule and can be refractory to treatment. Rectal incontinence can also occur and is often accompanied by urologic symptoms. Bladder symptoms may mimic prostatism. Patients have frequency, nocturia, hesitancy, poor stream, and difficulty in bladder emptying. Many of these patients present to the neurologist after a failure of transurethral prostatic resection to relieve their urologic symptoms. Micturition is increasingly defective, with overflow incontinence due to uninhibited detrusor activity and sphincter weakness. In the male, sexual function is lost early in the disease, with failure of erection first and then failure of ejaculation. Cystometry/mictometry, if performed, will be abnormal in patients with impotence or urologic symptoms (133). With progression of the symptoms, incontinence and/or retention develops.

Genitourinary dysfunction is common in MSA. This is detailed under Urologic Evaluation. Symptoms may simulate outflow obstruction or stress incontinence (17).

Dysarthria is common in MSA (15,55) and may be due to cerebellar, striatal, or mixed dysfunction (88). Abductor paralysis of the vocal cords is reported to be relatively common (55,172). The sequence of involvement is typically increased snoring followed by episodes of inspiratory and expiratory stridor and, sometimes, sleep apnea. Respiratory failure or sleep apnea can be relieved by tracheostomy. This complication can occur in some patients with relatively early disease and uncommonly antedates autonomic failure (16,98); therefore, its presence should be sought. Voice alterations in patients with MSA might be distinguishable from those of Parkinson's disease. Hanson and co-workers (55) found that laryngeal stridor, hoarseness, intermittent glottal fry, and slow speech rate were found to be discriminating symptoms of MSA.

Electromyographic evidence of denervation of the posterior cricoarytenoid muscle, the sole abductors of the cords, is consistently found; the interarytenoid muscle or cricopharyngeal sphincter can also be involved (54). Clinical and pathologic findings have been reported in three cases of MSA with laryngeal stridor severe enough to require tracheostomy (9). Histologic studies showed a marked atrophy of the posterior cricoarytenoid muscles suggestive of denervation (9,54); despite this finding, no clear evidence of any motor cell loss in the nucleus ambiguus was obtained.

Multiple system atrophy is associated with obstructive (upper airways) disease and central apnea, both of which can be life threatening. Nocturnal snoring and sleep apnea are common and are related to obstruction of the upper airways (108). Patients can die suddenly during sleep (108).

Chokroverty and colleagues (33) reported a tilt-table polygraphic study in four patients with MSA who developed periodic apnea in the erect posture. One patient had reduced hypercapnic ventilatory response with necropsy findings of neuronal loss, and astrocytosis in the pontine tegmentum suggested dysfunctional respiratory neurons in the brain stem. One patient had Cheyne-Stokes respiration during the late stage of the illness.

Marked muscular wasting, often with fasciculations with electromyographic and pathologic confirmation of anterior horn disease, but without sensory loss, can occur in MSA (107). Ocular assessment shows restricted conjugate movements, although the restriction is less than those seen in progressive supranuclear palsy. The pupils may show alternating anisocoria.

Cognition is unimpaired in most MSA patients. However, about 20% of patients have mild cognitive impairment (139). Psychiatric manifestations are less common and are probably nonspecific, consisting of depression and anxiety. In general, they reflect an exaggeration of the patient's premorbid state.

Types of Multiple System Atrophy

The following three principal forms of motor disturbance occur in MSA but are entirely absent in PAF.

Striatonigral Degeneration

The term striatonigral degeneration was first used by Adams and associates (3) to describe patients with a parkinsonian syndrome possessing special pathologic features. Many physicians consider the disorder clinically indistinguishable from Parkinson's disease. In hindsight, these patients, especially if autonomic defects had been sought and found, could have been classified as having MSA. In this disease, there is a predominance of rigidity without much tremor, which is associated with progressive loss of facial expression and limb akinesia. The limbs show rigidity on examination, without the classic "cogwheel" or "lead pipe" rigidity of Parkinson's disease. The facial expression is often less affected than that in patients with Parkinson's disease. Patients have difficulty in standing, walking, or turning, and difficulty feeding themselves. Salivation is reduced. As a result of akinesia, the speech becomes faint and slurred. The gait becomes slow and clumsy, superficially resembling that seen in patients with Parkinson's disease, and there is an attitude of stooping and often extreme cervical flexion, which makes forward gaze difficult.

Olivopontocerebellar Atrophy

In the olivopontocerebellar form of MSA, not included in Shy and Drager's original clinical description of only two cases, there is a prominent disturbance of gait with truncal ataxia that frequently makes it impossible for the patient to stand without support. In addition, there is marked slurring of speech with irregularity of speed of diction. There may also be a mild or moderate intention tremor affecting the arms and legs. This form of MSA is distinct from familial OPCA, in which the associated clinical features may include optic atrophy, retinitis pigmentosa, chorea, cataracts, and areflexia (56). Neuropathy is more consistently present in familial OPCA.

Pyramidal Lesion

In both striatonigral degeneration and OPCA there may be a pyramidal increase in tone together with impaired rapid hand and foot movements and exaggerated deep tendon reflexes and bilateral extensor planter responses. It is difficult to detect a pyramidal disturbance of tone in the presence of the extrapyramidal disturbance. Primitive reflexes, such as the palmomental reflex, may also be present.

Peripheral Neuropathy

There is reasonably good agreement on the frequency of electrophysiologic generalized neuropathy in MSA. Cohen and colleagues (35) found electrophysiologic evidence of neuropathy in 7 of 36 patients with MSA (19%). Sandroni and associates (139) reported a figure of 23% in 75 patients with MSA. Pramstaller and co-workers (127) reported a frequency of 18% mixed sensorimotor axonal neuropathy. Another 23% showed EMG evidence of chronic partial denervation. Clinically, the neuropathy is usually subclinical or mild, but it is occasionally moderately severe. The pathologic alterations are uncertain. Reports have been few and contradictory. One sural nerve biopsy was reported to show a marked reduction in large myelinated fibers with complete sparing of unmyelinated fibers (47), whereas another reported a selective loss of small nerve fibers (161). Our own experience is that the neuropathy is a low-grade axonal polyneuropathy with nonspecific sural nerve changes. In 10 patients with chronic autonomic failure, the sympathetic perivascular nerve plexuses from quadriceps muscle biopsy specimens were studied by catecholamine fluorescence and electron microscopy. There was almost complete absence of catecholamine fluorescence and fewer than the normal numbers of small granular (noradrenergic) vesicles in all nerves studied. The most marked depletion of noradrenergic vesicles was seen in 2 of the patients with PAF (8).

Postprandial Hypotension

In patients with autonomic failure, ingestion of food can sometimes substantially lower BP (37). In one patient with autonomic failure, BP fell rapidly to 80/50 mmHg after food ingestion and remained low for up to 3 hrs, even while the patient was in the supine position (Fig. 1). Postcibal hypotension can be a major clinical problem for patients with autonomic failure. Glucose appears to be the major factor in food; lipid has a smaller, slower hypotensive effect, with a minimal change caused by protein alone. The hypotensive effect of glucose does not result from its osmolality, because an isocaloric, isosmotic, and isovolemic solution of glucose causes only minimal changes in BP. Insulin probably has a role in the hypotension induced by carbohydrate ingestion, but neurotensin, which has vasodilatory effects, and other vasoactive intestinal polypeptides may contribute to the vasodepressive effect of food in these patients (37,99).

Insulin has a hypotensive effect that appears to be independent of hypoglycemia (100). An associated problem in patients with generalized autonomic failure is the absence of sympathetic manifestations of hypoglycemia. Insulin is known to open up arteriovenous shunts in peripheral nerve (74). The increase in splanchnic–mesenteric capacitance is not different in patients with autonomic failure when compared with normals; the fall in BP is due to the loss of compensatory mechanisms (82). The hypotension is prevented by the peptide release inhibitor octreotide, with no change in cardiac index or in peripheral blood flow, suggesting an effect on the splanchnic vasculature, probably through inhibiting release of vasodilatory pancreatic and gut peptides (Fig. 2) (131).

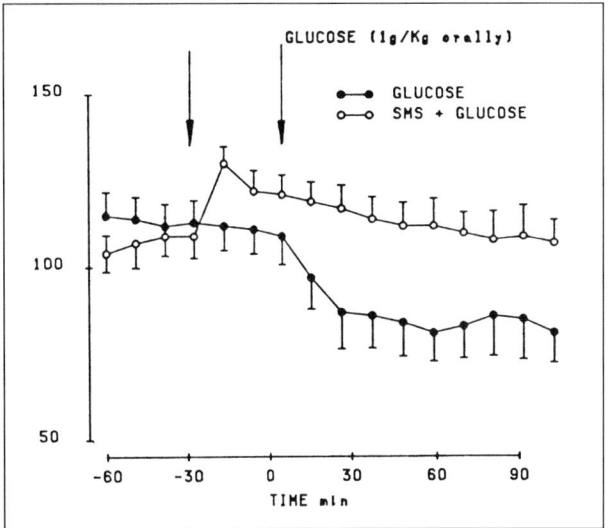

FIG. 2. Mean arterial blood pressure (MAP) in seven patients with chronic autonomic failure following oral glucose given after pretreatment with either placebo (○) or the somatostatin analogue SMS 201-995 (octreotide), 50 μg subcutaneously (●) given 30 minutes (↓) before the glucose. In the placebo cases, glucose caused a substantial fall in blood pressure. The reverse was seen after pretreatment with SMS 201-995.

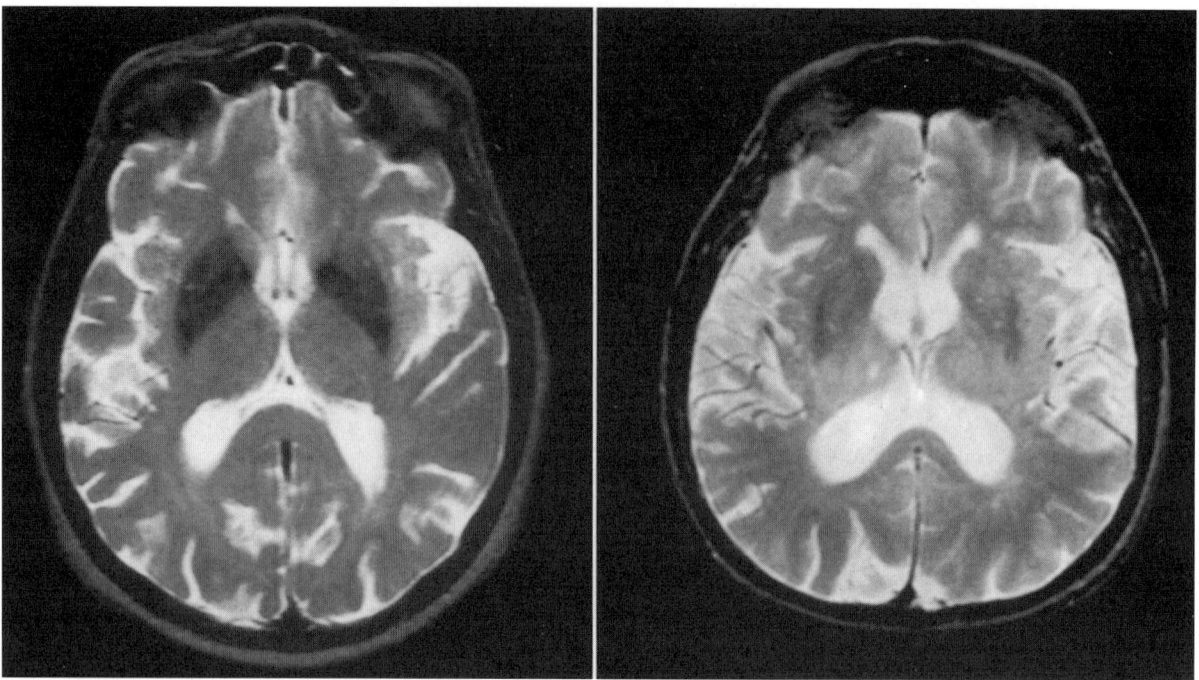

FIG. 3. T2-weighted magnetic resonance images of two different subjects acquired with essentially identical pulse sequence parameters. The image on the left is from a 66-year-old woman with MSA (MRI courtesy of Dr. Joseph Jankovich, Baylor College of Medicine, Houston, Texas), and the image on the right is from a neurologically normal 72-year-old woman (MRI courtesy of Dr. Clifford Jack, Department of Diagnostic Radiology, Mayo Clinic, Rochester, MN). The signal intensity of the lenticular nuclei of the MSA patient is significantly less than that of the neurologically normal subject.

CLINICAL FEATURES OF PURE AUTONOMIC FAILURE

The age of onset of PAF is typically middle age. Most cases are diagnosed between the ages of 50 and 70 years (158). In the series of 26 cases by Cohen and colleagues (35), ages ranged from 51 to 80 years (mean, 67 years), with a mean duration of symptoms of about 3 years. The symptoms of PAF are insidious in their onset, with mild symptoms concealed for years because of autonomic compensatory mechanisms. Patients may start with symptoms of vague orthostatic weakness, postural dizziness, or faintness that can very easily be overlooked or result in erroneous referral to a psychiatrist rather than a neurologist. The crux of the diagnosis is the demonstration of postural hypotension on standing, which is still often overlooked by physicians as a useful test. Some patients with autonomic failure first have bladder symptoms or impotence or defective sweating, not postural hypotension. Constipation is common (124), but other gastrointestinal symptoms are uncommon. Horner's syndrome can occur (124). These symptoms of PAF are similar for the autonomic failure associated with MSA described above. There are some subtle differences in the orthostatic hypotension of PAF when compared with MSA. The orthostatic hypotension tends to be more pronounced, and the symptoms tend to be more prominent, probably because of the greater mobility of patients with PAF. Postprandial orthostatic hypotension tends to be more severe.

INVESTIGATION

Magnetic Resonance Imaging

The two most characteristic findings in MSA are putamen hypointensity (Fig. 3) and slit-like lateral putamen hyperintensity on T2-weighted images studied in a high-field-strength system. The putamen hypodensity, especially along its lateral and posterior portions (45,119), correlates with rigidity (29) and with neuronal loss in these nuclei reported on postmortem examinations. Other changes in MSA include cerebellar and pontine atrophy (2,45,141). Stern and associates (153) reported, in a prospective study, that moderate to severe putaminal hypointensity distinguished MSA from Parkinson's disease but did not distinguish among the different system atrophies and degenerations. A less common finding is an anterior globose hyperintensity (79), which occurs in about half of patients, and least common is a T1 hypointensity. Lang and co-workers (86) related the "slit-like void signal" observed in the putamen to pathologic alterations in three patients with MSA. They reported that the magnetic resonance imaging (MRI) change is typical of striatonigral de-

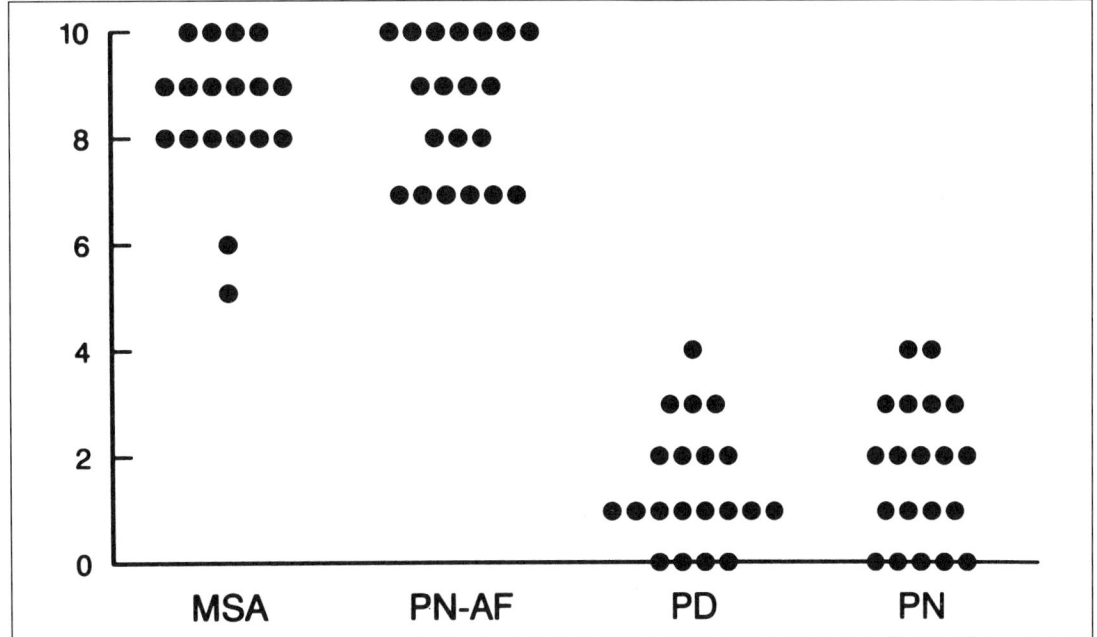

FIG 4. Composite autonomic scoring scale (CASS) results for patients with multiple system atrophy (*MSA*), peripheral neuropathy and autonomic failure (*PN-AF*), Parkinson's disease (*PD*), and peripheral neuropathy but no autonomic symptoms (*PN*). (Reprinted with permission from Low PA. Composite autonomic scoring scale for laboratory quantification of generalized autonomic failure. *Mayo Clin Proc* 1993; 68: 748–752.)

generation, and that their histochemical studies support the concept that increased iron deposition in the putamen is responsible for this MRI picture. The MRI changes are helpful in distinguishing MSA from Parkinson's disease. The test is useful, but a negative study does not exclude the diagnosis of MSA. It does not appear to reliably distinguish between MSA and progressive supranuclear palsy (141, 142).

Positron Emission Tomography

F-Dopa is a positron-emitting tracer analogue of levodopa. When administered intravenously, it is transported across the blood–brain barrier and stored as F-dopamine in caudate and putamen synaptosomes. With positron emission tomography (PET), the kinetics of F-dopa uptake in patients with MSA have been studied. There is reasonable correlation of the results of PET with functional impairment. Those patients with clinical evidence of striatonigral degeneration showed significantly reduced influx rate constants (K) for the uptake of F-dopa into the caudate and putamen (26). A short duration of disease, or mild parkinsonism, is associated with a normal PET scan, whereas increased severity and duration of parkinsonism is associated with reduced [18F]6-fluoro-1-dopa uptake, suggesting impaired nigrostriatal dopaminergic function (19).

[18F]-dopa and S-11C-nomifensine (NMF) are positron emitting tracers whose caudate and putamen uptakes reflect striatal dopamine storage capacity and the integrity of dopamine reuptake sites, respectively. Both MSA and Parkinson's disease patients showed a parallel decline of striatal dopamine storage capacity and reuptake site integrity, probably reflecting a loss of nigrostriatal nerve terminals (28). Caudate function was relatively preserved in Parkinson's disease compared with MSA. Most PAF patients have an intact nigrostriatal dopaminergic system. Benzodiazepine binding was largely preserved in the cerebral hemispheres, basal ganglia, thalamus, cerebellum, and brain stem in patients with either striatonigral or OPCA MSA (49).

Autonomic Function Tests

Detailed studies have been performed in the clinical autonomic laboratory (where the focus has been on the severity and distribution of autonomic failure) and in the research laboratory (where the emphasis has been on pathophysiologic mechanisms) (5,35,72,84,85,89,171). Cardiovascular reflex responses to standing and to the Valsalva maneuver are typically preserved in patients with Parkinson's disease but are grossly defective or absent in patients with MSA (171). Cohen and associates (35) evaluated 62 consecutive patients who presented to the Mayo Autonomic Reflex Laboratory; 26 patients had PAF and 36 patients had MSA. Patients were well matched in age (67 versus 66 years), duration (39 versus 36 months), and severity of autonomic failure. Postganglionic sudomotor and vasomotor functions were studied with the quantitative sudomotor axon reflex test and supine plasma norepinephrine. The distribution and severity of autonomic failure were assessed by the percent of anterior surface anhidrosis on the thermoregulatory sweat test, by heart rate responses to deep breathing (HR_{DB}) and the Valsalva maneuver, and by BP recordings. Severe and widespread anhidrosis was found in both PAF and MSA patients; 91% and 97% of body surface area, respectively, was anhidrotic. Postganglionic sudomotor failure occurred at the forearm in 50% of PAF and MSA patients and at the foot in 69% and 66% of PAF and MSA patients, respectively. However, postganglionic sudomotor function was preserved in some MSA patients with anhidrosis on the thermoregulatory sweat test, indicating a preganglionic lesion. Vagal abnormalities were found in 77% and 81% of PAF and MSA patients. We recently developed the composite autonomic scoring scale (CASS) that corrects for the confounding effects of age and gender and evaluates adrenergic function in greater detail (90). This scale assigns autonomic failure a score ranging from 0 (normal) to 10 (maximal impairment), with subscores for sudomotor, cardiovagal, and adrenergic deficits. Using CASS, we compared the scores in MSA and Parkinson's disease. MSA had a CASS of 8.5 ± 1.3 (SD), which is significantly higher ($P<0.001$) than that for Parkinson's disease (1.5 ± 1.1; Fig. 4).

Sympathetic skin responses were abnormal in most patients with MSA, sporadic OPCA, and striatonigral degeneration, whereas sympathetic skin responses were normal in patients with familial OPCA, sporadic cerebellar atrophy, and familial cerebellar atrophy (177).

Baser and associates (14) measured sweat production evoked by the sympathetic skin response to electrical stimulation and by intradermal methacholine in patients with either MSA or PAF and in normal subjects. Patients with PAF and MSA produced significantly less sweat than controls. The authors found that the sympathetic skin response was less sensitive than the sweat test and that it can occur in the absence of normal sweat gland function.

Cholinergic function is also impaired in patients with MSA (72). A battery of 12 tests was used to assess cholinergic function. Six tests demonstrated pupillary, lacrimal, salivary, urinary bladder, sexual, and sudomotor dysfunction in most patients. Cardiac vagal function as studied by the HR_{DB}, the response to the Valsalva maneuver, the cold face test, and the atropine test was affected in all patients. Esophageal motility was abnormal in six patients. Cholinergic dysfunction in MSA patients was widespread but of variable severity and distribution. Subcutaneous administration of the parasympathomimetic agent bethanechol demonstrated hyper-responsiveness of lacrimal, salivary, esophageal, bowel, bladder, and sudomotor functions. It was suggested that MSA was primarily a preganglionic cholinergic disorder with trans-synaptic degeneration accounting for the development of postganglionic cholinergic as well as adrenergic dysfunction.

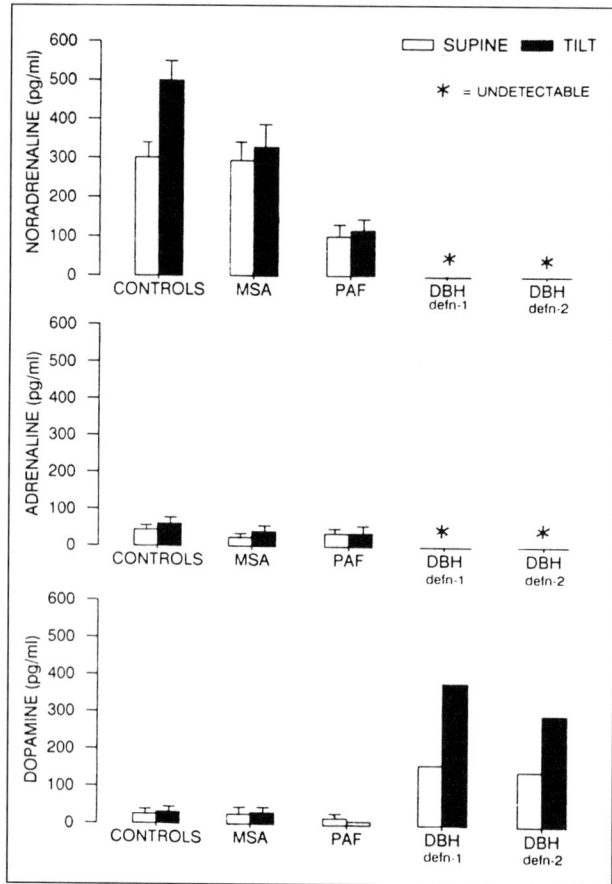

FIG. 5. Mean levels (+SEM) of plasma norepinephrine, adrenaline, and dopamine in 10 normal subjects, 12 patients with MSA, and 8 patients with PAF. Individual values on the first occasion in Patients 5 and 6 (1 and 2, respectively, in figure) with dopamine β-hydroxylase (DBH) deficiency are indicated. The asterisk indicates undetectable levels, which were below 5 pg/ml for norepinephrine and adrenaline and 20 pg/ml for dopamine. (Reprinted with permission from Mathias CJ, Bannister R. Dopamine beta-hydroxylase deficiency and other genetically determined autonomic disorders: A. Clinical features. In: Bannister R, Mathias C (eds). *Autonomic Failure, 3rd ed.* Oxford: Oxford University Press. 1992.)

Plasma Norepinephrine

The plasma norepinephrine level is an important but relatively insensitive measure of sympathetic efferent function. Patients with PAF almost always have a much lower resting level than do patients with MSA, but neither show a rise on head-up tilt or standing because of the block of baroreceptor pathways. Figure 5 compares the plasma norepinephrine values in normal subjects, patients with autonomic failure, and patients with the congenital disorder of dopamine β-hydroxylase deficiency. Table 1 shows the plasma norepinephrine levels in a group of patients with autonomic failure from the National Hospital for Neurology and Neurosurgery (United Kingdom) and the National Institutes of Health (United States). The Mayo data are

TABLE 1. *Plasma norepinephrine in autonomic failure*

Disorder	United Kingdom	United States
Pure autonomic failure		
Number	19	20
Supine (pg/ml)	119 + 19	76 + 18
Tilt (pg/ml)	135 + 21	[a]
Autonomic failure and multiple system atrophy		
Number	15	37
Supine (pg/ml)	279 + 38	265 + 21
Tilt (pg/ml)	334 + 50	[a]

[a]No values because standing was attempted for 5 minutes; many patients were unable to stand for this long, so measurements were unreliable and were not taken. (Reproduced with permission) from Bonnister R, Mathias C, Polinsky R. Autonomic failure: A comparison between UK and US experience. In: Bannister R (ed). *Autonomic Failure*. Oxford: Oxford University Press. 1988; 281–288.)

similar. Supine plasma free norepinephrine values were significantly reduced in PAF ($P<0.001$), but not MSA, patients (35). Standing plasma norepinephrine values were reduced in both PAF ($P<0.001$) and MSA ($P<0.001$) patients.

Sleep Laboratory Recordings

Several types of sleep abnormalities have been described in the sleep laboratory. Guilleminault and colleagues (53) reported sleep apnea, both obstructive and central in type, as well as disturbances of the respiratory oscillator in 10 patients with MSA. The observed respiratory irregularities were not associated with the usual cardiac response, because of autonomic failure. Other abnormalities include a reduction in total sleep time, increased sleep latency and awakening periods during the night, and reductions of rapid eye movement (REM) and non–rapid eye movement (NREM) sleep (97). In contrast to a reduction in BP during all sleep stages, the arterial BP of MSA patients rises progressively during NREM sleep stages, and these patients show a further increase in REM sleep with sudden phasic swings of systemic arterial pressure (34,97,164). These patients may also have REM sleep behaviors, described as wild, dream-enacting behaviors during REM sleep with a loss of the usual atonia of submental muscles (143). A disinhibited locomotor system during sleep appears to be responsible for this REM parasomnia. Pathologic changes in the brain stem in regions responsible for respiratory rhythmogenesis are mild or absent (32).

Evoked Potentials

Patients with MSA have abnormal brain stem potentials, in contrast to normal findings in patients with Parkinson's disease and PAF (128). Prasher and Bannister (128) surmised that the most likely involved area was the superior olivary complex. A subsequent study supports this notion. Uematsu and associates (165) related brain stem auditory evoked responses to computed tomography (CT) findings of pontine atrophy in 11 patients with MSA and 10 patients with olivopontocerebellar atrophy. The prolongation of I to III interpeak latencies in 6 patients with MSA and in 6 patients with olivopontocerebellar atrophy correlated well with the degree of the pontine atrophy estimated from the CT scan. In addition, prolongation of I to III interpeak latency was noted in patients with the striatonigral but not the OPCA pattern of involvement.

Urologic Evaluation

Patients with PAF and MSA have well-defined abnormalities on EMG cystometry. Three abnormalities have been described (76,138,170). First, almost all patients have profound urethral dysfunction due to poor proximal urethral sphincter tone, which causes bladder neck incompetence. In addition, the function of the striated component of the urethral sphincter is impaired, presumably due to degeneration of Onuf's nucleus; this affects at least 90% of patients (76,127,138). Second, there is loss of the ability to initiate a voluntary micturition reflex (detrusor areflexia); this affects about two thirds of patients (138). This may reflect the degeneration of neurons in pontine and medullary nuclei and in the sacral intermediolateral columns. In addition, these studies have demonstrated a significant reduction in the density of acetylcholinesterase-containing nerves in bladder muscle. The third abnormality is involuntary detrusor contractions in response to bladder filling (detrusor hyperreflexia), which affects about one in three patients (138). These may be the result of a loss of inhibitory influences from the corpus striatum and substantia nigra.

Urodynamic studies (42), especially urethral sphincter EMG (43), are reported to differentiate MSA from Parkinson's disease (42). MSA patients have detrusor hyperreflexia with a reduction of maximal cystometric capacity. In a recent study, Pramstaller and co-workers (127) reported that 90% of patients with MSA had an abnormal sphincter EMG; the test appears to be highly sensitive and specific for differentiating MSA from Parkinson's disease. Similar evidence of denervation can be obtained from an anal sphincter EMG (137). EMG of the anal sphincter muscles will differentiate amyotrophic lateral sclerosis (ALS) from Shy-Drager syndrome. In 30 patients with ALS, EMG of the external sphincter muscle was essentially normal, with no signs of denervation. In 8 cases of Shy-Drager syndrome, however, motor unit potentials of the anal sphincter had highly polyphasic forms of long duration and high amplitude (137).

Diagnosis of MSA

The definition of MSA given by the Consensus Panel (1), described earlier, is reasonable. In summary, the diagnosis of MSA is based on the clinical features of CNS involvement of the systems described above coupled with the presence of clinical autonomic failure. Autonomic features that are useful in the clinical setting are the early onset of orthostatic hypotension and bowel and bladder involvement. There are certain clinical features that help differentiate the parkinsonism of MSA from Parkinson's disease. These include the relative absence of tremor, the poor response to levodopa, the absence of levodopa-induced dyskinesias, and the aggravation of orthostatic hypotension by levodopa. When autonomic laboratory evaluation is available, patients with MSA show a characteristic pattern of involvement. They have severe and widespread impairment of sudomotor, adrenergic (both peripheral and cardiac), and cardiovagal function. When a thermoregulatory sweat test is performed, these patients have >40% (typically >60%) anterior surface anhidrosis, in contrast to patients with Parkinson's disease, who have <40% anhidrosis. The severity and distribution of autonomic failure are much milder in Parkinson's disease. The CASS score in MSA exceeds 7, whereas the score is <5 in Parkinson's disease (see Fig. 4). There is some evidence that patients with a worse autonomic failure score will progress more rapidly (139).

The charge to the autonomic clinician is to make the diagnosis of MSA using the criteria discussed above. The next step is to evaluate the distribution and severity of autonomic failure, because some believe that patients who fulfill the diagnosis of MSA will have a range of outlooks. In the largest retrospective review of patients studied at the Mayo Autonomic Reflex Laboratory, where all patients were evaluated with a similar panel of tests, including quantitative sudomotor testing, the severity and distribution of autonomic failure at presentation predicted the rate of progression. Patients with the striatonigral form of MSA with severe autonomic failure (often designated Shy-Drager syndrome) who had orthostatic hypotension at the onset of the illness have a poor prognosis, whereas patients with less severe involvement, with orthostatic hypotension developing years after the neurologic disorder, may progress less rapidly (139).

Diagnosis of PAF

The major emphasis in PAF publications has been a comparison between PAF and MSA. This comparison is necessary because of the importance of differentiating two conditions with different prognoses (see later) and because they provide models of postganglionic versus preganglionic autonomic disease. The Consensus Panel definition is reasonable but incomplete, resulting in the designation of all autonomic failures that do not have CNS involvement. This definition also does not differentiate idiopathic peripheral autonomic neuropathies from PAF. In practice, there a necessary second step, which involves differentiating PAF from the idiopathic autonomic neuropathies (IANs). Systematic prospective evaluation of non-CNS causes of orthostatic hypotension has not been reported. Some suggestions on the differential diagnosis of PAF from IAN are shown in Table 2. The onset of PAF is insidious, but it is acute or subacute in IAN and follows a viral infection in 50% of cases (154). The onset in IAN usually consists of a constellation of autonomic symptoms, including gastrointestinal failure, pain and distention, retention of urine, and cardiovascular failure. The cases with restricted autonomic failure are more problematic. Helpful differentiating points are the presence of some sensory symptoms (although the EMG is typically normal or only mildly abnormal), the prominence of ab-

TABLE 2. *Differentiation of pure autonomic failure, autonomic neuropathy, and multiple system atrophy*

Parameter	PAF	Autonomic Neuropathy	MSA
Onset	Insidious	Acute or subacute	Insidious
First symptom	Orthostatic hypotension	Constellation of Signs	Orthostatic hypotension or bladder involvement
Gastrointestinal symptoms	Absent, except constipation	Usually present	Uncommon
CNS involvement	Absent	Absent	Present
Somatic neuropathy	Absent	Often present but mild	Present in 14%–20%
Pain	Absent	Often present	Absent
Autonomic system review	Limited involvement	Widespread involvement	Relatively widespread involvement
Progression	Slowly progressive	? nonprogressive	Inexorably progressive
Prognosis	Good 10%–>MSA	Good	Bad
Lesion	Mainly postganglionic	Postganglionic, somatic	Mainly preganglionic; central
Supine plasma norepinephrine	Reduced	Reduced	Normal
EMG	Normal	±Abnormal	Usually normal

PAF, pure autonomic failure; MSA, multiple system atrophy; CNS, central nervous system; EMG, electromyography.

dominal colic, involvement of the pupil, and the antecedent viral infection.

Pharmacologic Tests

Pharmacologic tests of sympathetic function make use of Cannon's law of denervation supersensitivity (7). Trendelenburg (162a) showed experimentally that, after complete postganglionic section, there was supersensitivity to the neurotransmitter norepinephrine, if this was given intravenously, but a lack of response to tyramine. Polinsky and colleagues (124), in a classic pharmacologic dissection study of MSA versus PAF, defined the distinctive differences. Greater-than-normal slopes of the stimulus–response curves in patients with MSA and PAF were found and considered consistent with deficient reflex modulation (13, 124). Patients with PAF showed a shift to the left of the plasma norepinephrine–BP curves. This indicated the "denervation supersensitivity" observed previously by Trendelenburg, which is due to an increase in the density of postsynaptic α-receptors. This was consistent with the deficient plasma norepinephrine response to tyramine in these patients.

Patients with PAF and MSA may complain of feeling lightheaded after alcohol ingestion, particularly when assuming the upright posture. Alcohol has been shown to lower supine BP and dilate the superior mesenteric artery with no change in muscle or cutaneous blood flow in these patients (31).

As expected, spectral analysis of the RR interval and systolic BP demonstrates a marked reduction in power of all frequencies and in the baroreflex gain in PAF (46). Kingwell and associates (75) related spectral analysis to microneurography and norepinephrine measurements. They concluded that the heart rate variation at 0.1 Hz depends on other factors in addition to cardiac sympathetic nerve firing rates, including multiple neural reflexes, cardiac adrenergic receptor sensitivity, postsynaptic signal transduction, and electrochemical coupling, and is not directly related to cardiac norepinephrine spillover, which is a more direct measure of the sympathetic nerve firing rate.

Despite severe and widespread denervation, the plasma renin response to standing can remain intact, suggesting that plasma renin activity can be independent of sympathetic nervous activity and may be mediated by renal baroreceptors (102). However, generalized autonomic failure is usually associated with a loss of the renin mechanism (13,20).

The adrenal medullary response to hypoglycemia in patients with orthostatic hypotension appears to be impaired (123,140). There does not seem to be a difference between PAF and MSA in their deficient epinephrine response. The glucose counter-regulatory factors (e.g., glucagon, epinephrine, growth hormone, cortisol, and norepinephrine) to insulin-induced hypoglycemia also appear to be reduced in MSA (140).

Afferent and Central Pathways

Although detailed studies are available on the dissection of efferent pathways, studies on afferent or central pathways have been more indirect. The strategy has been to use a number of non-neural afferent stimuli that stimulate portions of the central neuraxis, such as the hypothalamus or pituitary, and to measure their products. These include growth hormone, prolactin and vasopressin (which can be stimulated by alterations in osmolarity), clonidine, and hypoglycemia.

The diurnal variation of growth hormone secretion is impaired in MSA patients (57), as is its response to clonidine (37). Patients with multiple system atrophy have normal values that fail to rise in response to clonidine (37). Konagaya and associates (80) evaluated the serum growth hormone and prolactin responses to dopaminergic stimulation or dopamine receptor blockade in nine patients with MSA. The impaired responses suggested pituitary dopaminergic involvement.

Patients with MSA have a severely blunted response of plasma arginine vasopressin (AVP) to the stimulus of head-up tilt (70,129,174). The rise in AVP with upright posture is modulated by central dopamine and opioid receptors. Patients with MSA may have depletion of brain dopamine and opioid peptides (129). In contrast, the increment in AVP in response to tilt-up is normal in PAF (70), indicating normal functioning of the efferent connections from the osmoreceptors within the hypothalamus.

Patients with MSA have intact plasma epinephrine responses to nicotinic adrenal stimulation with arecoline, whereas PAF patients lack this response; both conditions are associated with an impaired adrenocorticotropic hormone (ACTH) response (120). The lack of this response in patients with pure autonomic failure is consistent with peripheral sympathetic dysfunction. The appearance and exacerbation of tremor, vertigo, and pathologic affect in the MSA group suggest that some central cholinergic receptors remain functional.

Plasma β-endorphin and ACTH responses during insulin-induced hypoglycemia are significantly impaired in patients with MSA, in contrast to the normal levels found in PAF patients (121). The strong correlation between β-endorphin and ACTH levels is consistent with their common origin.

Cerebrospinal fluid (CSF) 3-methoxy-4-hydroxyphenylglycol (MHPG) is reduced in both MSA and PAF patients (122). However, only PAF is associated with a reduced plasma MHPG. In MSA, the abnormal function of the central noradrenergic pathways seems to cause the low CSF MHPG levels. In orthostatic hypotension, the decreased CSF MHPG results from the diminished plasma MHPG levels. It is possible to correct CSF MHPG levels for the contribution from plasma-free MHPG to provide an index of central norepinephrine metabolism.

Neurochemistry of MSA and PAF

The neurochemistry of MSA and PAF is described in **Chapter 44**.

PATHOLOGIC DIAGNOSIS

Pathology of Multiple System Atrophy and PAF

The neuropathology of MSA consists of neuronal cell loss and gliosis, without Lewy bodies or neurofibrillary tangles, in multiple pigmented nuclei (12,38,145). Cell populations that are severely and nearly always affected are:

Substantia nigra and putamen
Inferior olives
Pontine nuclei
Cerebellar Purkinje cells
Onuf's nucleus
Locus ceruleus
Intermediolateral column cells

There have been a number of pathologic studies of autonomic failure (67,115,151). Brain stem abnormalities have also been noted, with loss of pigment in the melanin-containing nuclei that are derived from the basal plate of the primitive neural tube, including the dorsal nucleus of the vagus, the locus ceruleus (162), and the nucleus tractus solitarius. Neurochemically, a common feature is a profound depletion in dopamine and noradrenaline from brain regions that are normally rich in these catecholamines. Central cholinergic systems appear to be involved also, but to a variable degree (151). Cell populations that are commonly but less severely affected are the caudate, pallidum, pyramidal tract, and vestibular nuclear complex (38,155). Cells that are only sometimes affected are the thalamus, subthalamic nucleus, cerebral cortex, Edinger-Westphal nucleus, dentate nucleus, arcuate nucleus, Clarke's nucleus, sympathetic ganglia, sensory ganglia, and peripheral nerve (38).

Parkinson's disease, in contrast, has a more restricted neuropathology, with neuronal loss in the substantia nigra and Lewy bodies in pigmented nuclei, and in autonomic neurons including intermediolateral column and postganglionic neurons (65), where the depletion is modest, in keeping with the minor or mild autonomic failure (4,139).

Pure autonomic failure is unassociated with substantial CNS involvement and is likely to be a postganglionic disorder. A modest reduction in intermediolateral column neurons has been reported (93,115).

Spinal Cord

In almost all patients carefully studied, MSA has been associated with at least a 75% reduction in the number of sympathetic preganglionic neurons in the intermediolateral cell columns of the spinal cord (12,71,93). Correction for age is important because there is a 5% to 8% attrition rate of preganglionic neurons per decade from the third decade onward (91). Ventral spinal root axons segregate into distinct groups of large, intermediate, and small myelinated axons, corresponding to alpha, gamma, and preganglionic axons. Axonal loss occurs predominantly in thin, myelinated fibers that correspond mainly to autonomic preganglionic axons (93,150). Intermediate and large myelinated fibers, mainly gamma and alpha axons, are also involved, but to a lesser degree. Neuronal and axonal loss is more prominent in caudal segments and less prominent in rostral segments. Axonal degeneration in single teased fibers is seen frequently in ventral spinal roots (150).

There are three groups of sacral motor neurons: the posterolateral motor neuron column (PL), inferior intermediolateral nucleus (IML), and cell group X of Onuf (Onuf). Morphometry disclosed a marked depletion of IML, Onuf, and somatic motor neurons in MSA patients (81). In contrast, in ALS patients there is a severe loss of somatic motor neurons, a modest reduction of IML neurons, and a normal or only modest reduction in Onuf's neucleus (81,96).

In MSA, small-sized myelinated fibers of the thoracic corticospinal tract appear to be markedly reduced, whereas large-sized myelinated fibers remain well preserved (149).

Some reduction in intermediolateral cell counts has been reported in PAF (93,115,166). The changes tend to be much milder than those of MSA, merging with the effects of aging. Low and associates (93) reported intermediolateral column neuron and corresponding axon counts and morphometry in two patients with MSA and one with PAF. The intermediolateral column (ILC) neuron cell body counts were reduced to 17% of control levels in MSA and 52% of control levels in PAF. The B fiber counts in the corresponding ventral spinal root were reduced to 21% and 41% of control levels in MSA and PAF, respectively.

Ganglionic Changes in Autonomic Failure

Matthews (104) has found differences in the ganglionic pathology between patients with PAF and those with MSA. In the latter, the neurons of the sympathetic ganglia were not severely reduced in number and did not appear grossly abnormal. There was evidence to suggest a severe deficiency of preganglionic endings on the ganglia, and possibly overdriving of surviving endings. In PAF, on the other hand, the packing density of ganglionic neurons was severely reduced, in one instance up to 25% of the number reported for normal ganglia, although the surviving ganglia did not appear to be grossly abnormal pathologically.

Nosology

Nosologic disorders are typically clinically distinct, and there is considerable homogeneity. Patients who present with apparent Parkinson's disease may develop MSA, although this is rare. Autonomic function tests are quite different in the two disorders (139). Patients with typical features of Parkinson's disease occasionally have additional neurologic involvement (such as corticospinal tract involvement, cerebellar signs, or some evidence of autonomic failure). These patients have autonomic findings that are intermediate in severity between MSA and Parkinson's disease. About 10% of patients with apparent PAF may develop MSA (159). The polar groups are distinct, but occasional cases are more difficult to classify. The criteria recommended in the Consensus Statement (1) represent a significant step forward. For instance, most of the cases in the study by Sandroni and co-workers (139) that are designated nonspecific multisystem degeneration would be accepted as MSA. In the British Parkinsonism Study, in which a neuropathologic "gold standard" was used, about 20% of patients with clinical Parkinson's disease had the neuropathologic features of MSA (130). However, as discussed earlier, the premortem evaluation was variable. Evaluation by neurologists using the criteria recommended by the Consensus Panel (1) would probably have significantly reduced the high figure of 20%. Infrequently, the neuropathologic features merge. For instance, Parkinson's disease itself has pathologic alterations beyond the nigrastriatum (66), and Lewy bodies can be seen in some cases of MSA (130). Transitional changes where features of Parkinson's disease with Lewy bodies in the substantia nigra and locus ceruleus and striatonigral degeneration and olivopontocerebellar atrophy were evident in both cases (147).

The simplest interpretation of these observations is that the two forms of autonomic failure, PAF and MSA, result from the loss of ganglionic and preganglionic neurons, respectively. The lesser loss of intermediolateral column cells in PAF could be a retrograde neuronal death consequent to target deprivation. The possibility cannot be excluded that the loss of intermediolateral neurons in MSA itself might be due to disruption of the retrograde trophic influences imposed on them by ganglionic neurons.

Pathogenetic Mechanisms

Argyrophilic cytoplasmic inclusions of oligodendrocytes have been described in cases of MSA (Fig. 6) with phenotypes of sporadic olivopontocerebellar atrophy, striatonigral degeneration, and the Shy-Drager syndrome (36,117,118). This subject was recently reviewed (36).

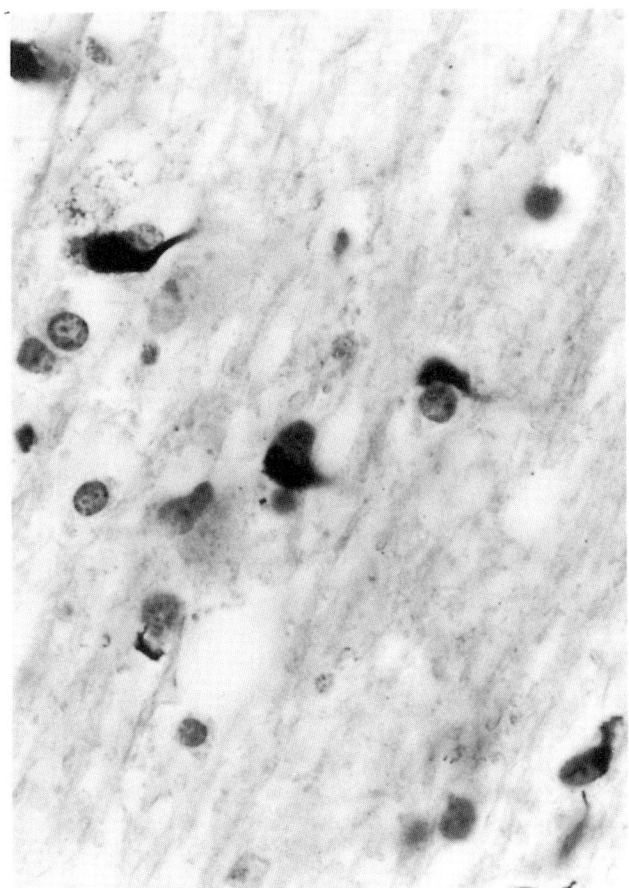

FIG. 6. Glial cytoplasmic inclusions in a patient with MSA (Gallyas stain, × 1500). (Courtesy of Dr. Joseph Parisi, Department of Laboratory Medicine and Pathology, Mayo Clinic, Rochester, Minnesota)

The oligodendroglial cytoplasmic inclusions are immunolabeled with antiubiquitin antibodies. Ultrastructurally, they appear as granule-associated filaments. More recently, similar argyrophilic inclusion bodies were reported in the cytoplasm of neurons and in both oligodendroglial and neuronal nuclei of MSA brains. Neuronal and oligodendroglial cytoplasmic inclusions have identical ultrastructural characteristics but different antigenic properties. Oligodendroglial cytoplasmic inclusions are reported to be recognized by anti-ubiquitin, anti-α- and anti-β-tubulin, and anti-τ antibodies, whereas neuronal cytoplasmic inclusions are recognized only by anti-ubiquitin antibodies (118). The chemical nature of the inclusions is largely unknown. Fractions containing glial cytoplasmic inclusion–bearing cells contain a 32-kd and a 40-kd protein, both of which are specifically recognized by anti-ubiquitin and anti-α B-crystallin antibodies; neither of these was found in the same fraction derived from control brains (156). These immunochemical results suggest that ubiquitinated α B-crystallin is present in glial cytoplasmic inclusions from the brains of patients with MSA. The significance of inclusions remains controversial: they could be a primary event in the course of the degenerative process or merely an epiphenomenon of some disordered cytoskeletal metabolism (36).

The current opinion is that these inclusions are present in all cases of MSA but are not specific to MSA (39). These workers found inclusions in all 56 brains with MSA; 3 of • with corticobasal degeneration and 2 of 18 with PSP. They have also been found in 2 of 22 patients with hereditary OPCA (50,109) and in a patient with chromosome 17–linked dementia (147).

Antibodies in human CSF against specific brain regions *in vitro* have been detected in patients with a variety of neurodegenerative disorders. These studies suggest that specific CSF antibodies may be markers of system-specific degeneration. Thus, a CSF antibody in Alzheimer's disease reacts against rat cholinergic septal neurons (105), and a CSF antibody in patients with Parkinson's disease reacts against dopaminergic neurons of the rat substantia nigra/ventral tegmental area (30). Polinsky and co-workers (125) reported that CSF immunoreactivity to rat locus ceruleus occurred in a significantly greater number of samples from MSA patients compared with control subjects or patients with PAF. Other brain regions infrequently showed immunoreactivity. These findings suggest that degeneration in MSA may release antigen(s) that induce antibodies against locus ceruleus neurons. Less specific immunologic alterations, representing antibody attachment to degenerating fibers, have been described (176).

In a study of 60 patients with MSA, their relatives, and an identical number of controls, MSA patients had significantly more potential exposures to metal dusts and fumes, plastic monomers and additives, organic solvents, and pesticides than did the control population (112). These findings were interpreted as possibly consistent with the hypothesis that MSA develops as a result of a genetically determined selective vulnerability in the nervous system to environmental insults or toxins.

There is no clear evidence of inherited MSA or of HLA association. In an original work on PAF, 16 patients with PAF had a frequency of the HLA antigen Aw32 that was 13 times more common than that in healthy controls (11); this was not confirmed in a subsequent study in either MSA or PAF (111).

TREATMENT OF AUTONOMIC FAILURE

The management of orthostatic hypotension in MSA and PAF is covered in detail in Chapter 55. We will summarize treatments specifically applied to MSA and PAF. Reports of benefits in MSA and PAF must be treated with caution. There have been few randomized placebo-controlled clinical trials. Most reports of benefits should be treated as anecdotal.

L-DOPS

DL-threo-3,4-dihydroxyphenylserine (DL-threo-DOPS) is a norepinephrine precursor that is currently unavailable in the United States. Anecdotal reports of its efficacy in reducing orthostatic hypotension have appeared (136), and the improvement is reported to be associated with an increase in muscle sympathetic nerve activity induced by tilt-up (68) and improved cerebral blood flow (103). Both the D- and L-enantiomers can be measured in human plasma and urine (21). The drug has been claimed to be beneficial in reducing L-dopa–related orthostatic hypotension (179).

Beta-Receptor Agonists

In a single case report, prenalterol, a selective β_1-adrenoreceptor agonist, was reported to improve supine and standing BP and relieve symptoms (52). Hemodynamically, prenalterol resulted in a substantial increase in standing cardiac output, primarily because of its chronotropic effects. Prenalterol additionally stimulates the renin–aldosterone system and restores the normal diurnal pattern of water and sodium excretion. One reported problem is the development of complex ventricular ectopic beats that occurs at higher doses (52).

Monoamine Oxidase Inhibitors With Tyramine

The combination of monoamine oxidase inhibitors with tyramine (110) or other amines (40) can increase BP in patients with MSA and PAF. Most experts now consider this combination unacceptable. These patients can develop hypertensive crises with certain foods such as cheese.

Indomethacin

Indomethacin and related nonsteroidal anti-inflammatory drugs are reported to improve BP (51,78), possibly by inhibiting vasodilator prostaglandins (51,78,163). All reports were uncontrolled reports of a small number of patients. An increase of 20 to 30 mmHg diastolic BP is typical for doses of 75 to 150 mg/day (51,78), but some authors have not observed a rise in standing BP (41). Clinical experience shows that indomethacin and ibuprofen have similar efficacies and that the benefits are modest in MSA and PAF. In one study, the drug increased the pressor supersensitivity to intravenous noradrenaline and angiotensin II while reducing supine plasma renin activity to 50% (41).

Ibopamine

Ibopamine, a dopaminergic prodrug with weak agonist activity on α- and β-adrenoreceptors, has been studied in three patients with PAF (132). Orthostatic tolerance was reported to improve as early as 10 to 30 minutes after administration of ibopamine and lasted 20 to 50 min. α-Adrenoreceptor blockade with phentolamine abolished the effect of ibopamine. Ibopamine appeared to be potent but had highly variable interindividual pharmacokinetics.

Beta-Blockers

Although β-blockers have been used in the treatment of MSA (24), their efficacy is questionable. Xamoterol, a cardioselective $β_1$-adrenoreceptor partial agonist, has been reported to be effective for postural hypotension (113,169). Xamoterol is reported to lessen the total number of symptomatic episodes of orthostatic hypotension over 24 hrs (169). However, episodes of severe hypertension (defined as a systolic intra-arterial BP above 200 mmHg) were more frequent with xamoterol (169), and the rise in BP was greater at night (113).

Dopamine Agonists

Dopamine agonists can be used in MSA in an attempt to ameliorate the extrapyramidal features of the disease. L-dopa has a central hypotensive effect and a peripheral vasoconstrictor effect. The use of L-dopa can result in a modest improvement in orthostatic hypotension, especially if it is combined with a volume expander or a vasoconstrictor (6,152). Lisuride, an ergolene derivative with dopamine receptor agonist properties, has been used in the treatment of MSA (87). A modest reduction in orthostatic hypotension occurred in two patients.

The use of Sinemet in MSA is reasonable if there is an increase in mobility or speech. Benefits tend to be modest and are usually obtainable with relatively small doses. Most patients do not need doses in excess of 25/250 t.i.d. The directly acting dopamine agonists and pergolide do not appear to confer any extra benefits (83).

Midodrine

Midodrine, a peripheral α-adrenergic agonist, causes veno- and arteriolar vasoconstriction. It is almost completely absorbed after oral administration and undergoes enzymatic hydrolysis to form its pharmacologically active metabolite, des-glymidodrine (106). It does not cross the blood–brain barrier. Comparative studies have clinically shown midodrine to be at least as effective as other sympathomimetic agents (norfenefrine, etilefrine, dimetofrine, and ephedrine) and dihydroergotamine in this regard. Jankovic and colleagues (64) reported the findings of a recent multicenter study of the safety and efficacy of midodrine therapy in 97 patients with neurogenic orthostatic hypotension. These included 18 patients with MSA and 20 with PAF. After 1 week of placebo therapy, the patients were randomized into four groups for a 4-week study: placebo, 2.5 mg, 5 mg, or 10 mg three times daily. These patients demonstrated a 27% ± 8% (22 mmHg) increase in standing systolic BP for the 10-mg dose. Fainting symptoms, blurred vision, energy level, standing time, and depressed feelings were also significantly improved even at lower doses ($P<0.05$ or less). Side effects were mild. Midodrine was considered an effective and safe agent for the treatment of neurogenic orthostatic hypotension (48,64).

In a double-blind, randomized, dose–response study (175), 15 patients with neurogenic orthostatic hypotension (consisting of PAF, MSA, and autonomic neuropathies—5 males, 10 females; mean age, 63 years) were randomized to a single-oral-dose, four-way crossover study of placebo and midodrine (2.5, 10, and 20 mg). BP was measured repeatedly supine and standing for 6 hrs. A global symptom relief score was given by the investigator and patient separately. Midodrine resulted in a log-linear, dose-dependent improvement in 1-hr postdose BP ($P<0.01$). Global symptom relief (both patient and investigator) favored midodrine 10 and 20 mg compared with placebo ($P<0.05$). The blood level of a single dose of midodrine was sustained for about 2 hrs, and that of des-glymidodrine was sustained for about 4 hours. Midodrine 10 mg and 20 mg resulted in supine hypertension in 20% and 47% of patients. The 10-mg dose of midodrine appeared to be both efficacious and safe in the treatment of orthostatic hypotension, and a t.i.d. regimen is supported by the study.

A randomized, double-blind, multicenter study comparing midodrine with placebo has been completed for neurogenic orthostatic hypotension (92). We compared midodrine 10 mg t.i.d. with placebo in patients with symptomatic neurogenic orthostatic hypotension (orthostatic hypotension). One hundred and seventy patients (M=F=85) with orthostatic hypotension were randomized to midodrine 10 mg t.i.d. or placebo in a 6-week study. The study consisted of a single blind run-in and washout at weeks 1, 5, and 6, with an intervening double-blind period (weeks 2 to 4). There were 40 patients with MSA and 37 with PAF. The primary end points were improved standing systolic BP, improved symptoms of lightheadedness, and a global symptom relief score (by the investigator and patient separately). Midodrine resulted in a significant improvement in standing systolic BP by the end of the first week, an improvement in symptoms by the end of the second week, and global symptom relief (both patient and investigator) at all evaluated time points. The main side effects were pilomotor reactions, bladder dysfunction, and supine hypertension. The 10-mg t.i.d. dose of midodrine appeared to be both efficacious and safe in the treatment of neurogenic orthostatic hypotension.

Vasopressin

Vasopressin, administered either as a nasal spray or intravenously, improves orthostatic BP (77). Two sprays are administered intranasally. Patients with PAF may have a supersensitive pressor response to arginine vasopressin (173).

The use of vasopressin analogues to reduce nocturnal diuresis was reported by Mathias and associates (101). Desmopressin (DDAVP) is a vasopressin-like substance that specifically acts on the V2-receptors on the renal tubules, which are responsible for the antidiuretic effect of vasopressin. It has virtually no effect on the V1 receptors, which are responsible for the vasoconstriction induced by vasopressin. Intramuscular DDAVP injection prevents nocturnal polyuria, induces overnight weight loss, and raises the supine BP in the morning, thus easing the symptoms resulting from postural hypotension (101). Studies of intranasally administered DDAVP indicate that it also is effective. Doses between 5 and 40 mcg, given at bedtime as a single dose, are of benefit in preventing both nocturia and morning postural hypotension. DDAVP can, however, cause hyponatremia. Therefore, it must be used cautiously, with monitoring of osmolality and plasma sodium levels on a 6-week basis.

Octreotide

The somatostatin analogue octreotide reduces splanchnic capacitance and reduces orthostatic hypotension in patients with PAF and MSA (60). Octreotide requires subcutaneous administration. Some patients in whom octreotide failed to stabilize upright BP had a satisfactory response to the drug after pretreatment with dihydroergotamine (60). Side effects are usually nausea or abdominal cramps after moderate doses (>1.0 µg/kg). The pressor response is not accompanied by an increase in the plasma norepinephrine level (167).

Sympathetic Neural Prosthesis

Polinsky and co-workers (126) reported on a prototype electromechanical analogue of the sympathetic division of the baroreceptor reflex arc that was used to maintain BP automatically in two patients with neurogenic orthostatic hypotension. The device prevented significant and sustained reductions in mean BP when the patients were tilted up to 85°. Upon achieving the preset mean BP, the device maintained this pressure with a standard error of less than 2 mmHg. Similar results were obtained when the patients were walking. The device did not cause supine hypertension during the trials.

Nonpharmacologic Approaches

Nonpharmacologic approaches have included the use of compression garments (see Chapter 56), an antigravity suit (25), postural training (59), and physical countermaneuvers. Drug therapy, combined with isometric exercises performed on a tilt table (whose angle was gradually increased during 3 weeks), made it possible for a patient with severe orthostatic hypotension to walk (59). Physical countermaneuvers will increase standing BP and standing time, largely by an increase in peripheral resistance (22).

Urologic Treatment

The most effective treatment for incontinence is clean intermittent catheterization. Anticholinergic medication is reserved for the discussion of detrusor hyperreflexia.

Fludrocortisone

Another line of treatment that is usually helpful is oral fludrocortisone. In a smaller dose (0.1 mg) than is necessary to increase blood volume, fludrocortisone appears to increase the sensitivity of blood vessels to very small amounts of norepinephrine, which may still be capable of being released in autonomic failure (40). A study was undertaken to assess a standard sodium intake. In this study, the body weight of the subjects did not change during the 14 days when the drug was given, so there is no reason to believe that the results are an effect of the change in blood volume. Larger doses of fludrocortisone (0.2 to 0.4 mg) increase blood volume, usually with a delay of about 1 to 2 weeks. A significant problem is supine hypertension. Many patients are thought to respond better to a small dose of fludrocortisone combined with the judicious use of vasopressor drugs. This combination better sustains BP at periods of greatest need, and by avoiding vasopressors after 6 PM, supine hypertension can be minimized.

Anesthetic Management

There are particular problems associated with anesthesia in patients with generalized autonomic failure. The choice between local, regional, and general anesthesia is less important than careful preoperative evaluation and careful operative control of blood volume, BP, and posture. Anesthesia may be associated with profound hypotension, and some of the signs of anesthesia may be absent (94). The response to cardiac depressant drugs and the reduction of circulating blood volume may be exaggerated because of the absence of compensatory mechanisms. The response to vasoactive agents is unpredictable.

Adequate cardiovascular monitoring and the maintenance of BP with intravenous fluids are essential (18, 61,94). Sympathomimetic drugs, if used at all, should be administered in very dilute solutions to avoid hypertension from denervation hypersensitivity (18). Certain anesthetics might be more hypotensive than others. A profound fall in

TABLE 3. *Clinical features of pure autonomic failure and multiple system atrophy based on two large programs*

	PAF		MSA	
	UK	NIH (US)	UK	NIH (US)
N	24	22	73	44
Age (years)	58 ± 10 (38–78)	47 ± 3 (25–68)	54 ± 10 (34–74)	51 ± 1 (25–67)
Duration (years)	9 ± 1 (2–16)	14 ± 2 (5–31)	3 ± 2 (1–8)	8 ± 1 (2–15)
Orthostatic hypotension (%)	92	73	74	30
Urinary symptoms (%)	27	0	52	18
Impotence (males, %)	94	55	83	48

PAF, pure autonomic failure; MSA, multiple system atrophy; UK, United Kingdom; NIH, National Institutes of Health. (Modified from Bannister R, Mathias C, Polinsky R. Autonomic failure: A comparison between UK and US experience. In: Bannister R (ed). *Autonomic Failure*. Oxford: Oxford University Press. 1988; 281–288.)

arterial pressure during anesthesia induced with thiopentone has been demonstrated (134), whereas anesthesia induced with ketamine, maintained with nitrous oxide in oxygen, and supplemented with fentanyl, diazepam, and suxamethonium did not cause a fall in arterial pressure. In the postoperative period, orthostatic hypotension may be severe, and its control requires volume expansion, postural training by graduated elevation of the head of the bed, and the careful use of vasoconstrictors.

PROGRESSION OF PURE AUTONOMIC FAILURE

Studies of PAF have almost invariably compared PAF with MSA. Information on the clinical features, progression, and outcome is actually quite limited. Some patients with PAF have continued relatively symptom free for many years, with standing BP levels around 80 mmHg. The natural history of PAF is that of a slow progression taking place over some 10 to 15 years. A comparison of the course of PAF with that of MSA in two large programs is summarized in Table 3. Some cases may be nonprogressive (158).

Prognosis of Multiple System Atrophy

Most patients with classic MSA do not survive longer than 7 years from the time of diagnosis of the disease. Wenning and colleagues (168), however, reported a median survival of 9.5 years, calculated by Kaplan-Meier analysis. Similar results have been reported (135), and the sporadic OPCA variety has been suggested to have a longer survival than the striatonigral variety (135). The differences in survival by different investigators likely relate to the criteria used to define MSA. Patients with MSA have a downhill course marked by increasing rigidity, urinary incontinence, and sometimes profound stridor, which may require tracheostomy. The extrapyramidal features rarely respond to levodopa (the form of levodopa with a dopamine decarboxylase inhibitor), probably because the central defect of norepinephrine and dopamine prevents the achievement of effective levels of dopamine. Death in MSA patients is frequently due, after about 6 years on average, to respiratory obstruction or failure after worsening movement disorder, akinesia, and bladder disorder. With the appreciation of a spectrum of severities, an attempt has been made to relate the severity and distribution of autonomic and nonautonomic involvement to outcome. We reviewed the clinical and autonomic features of all patients with extrapyramidal and cerebellar disorders studied in the Mayo Autonomic Reflex Laboratory from 1983 to 1989 (139). The orthostatic BP reduction, percentage of anhidrosis on thermoregulatory sweat test, quantitative sudomotor axon reflex test, and forearm response and heart rate response to deep breathing strongly regressed with severity of clinical involvement. The severity and distribution of autonomic failure at the time of first evaluation were predictive of a greater rate of progression 2 years later. Saito and associates (135) came to the same conclusion. They determined that the earlier and the more severe the involvement of the autonomic nervous system, and to a lesser extent the striatonigral system, the poorer the prognosis.

REFERENCES

1. Consensus statement on the definition of orthostatic hypotension, pure autonomic failure, and multiple system atrophy. *Neurology* 1996;46:1470.
2. Abe S et al. Evaluation of the brainstem with high-resolution CT in cerebellar atrophic processes. *Am J Neuroradiol* 1983;4:446–449.
3. Adams RD, et al. Striato-nigral degeneration. *J Neuropathol Exp Neurol* 1964;23:584–608.
4. Aminoff MJ, Wilcox CS. Assessment of autonomic function in patients with a parkinsonian syndrome. *Br Med J* 1971;4:80–84.
5. Aminoff MJ, et al. Autonomic defects in paralysis agitans and in the Shy-Drager syndrome. *Acta Neurol Scand* 1972;51(suppl):105–107.
6. Aminoff MJ et al. Levodopa therapy for parkinsonism in the Shy-Drager syndrome. *J Neurol Neurosurg Psychiatry* 1973;36:350–353.
7. Bannister R, et al. An assessment of various methods of treatment of idiopathic orthostatic hypotension. *Q J Med* 1969;38:377–395.
8. Bannister R et al. Adrenergic innervation in autonomic failure. *Neurology* 1981;31:1501–1506.
9. Bannister R et al. Laryngeal abductor paralysis in multiple system atrophy. A report on three necropsied cases, with observations on the laryngeal muscles and the nuclei ambigui. *Brain* 1981;104:351–368.

10. Bannister R, et al. Autonomic failure: a comparison between UK and US experience. In: Bannister R (ed). *Autonomic Failure.* Oxford: Oxford University Press. 1988;281–288.
11. Bannister R, et al. Genetic control of progressive autonomic failure: evidence for an association with an HLA antigen. *Lancet* 1983;1:1017.
12. Bannister R, Oppenheimer DR. Degenerative diseases of the nervous system associated with autonomic failure. *Brain* 1972;95:457–474.
13. Baser SM et al. Beta-receptor sensitivity in autonomic failure. *Neurology* 1991;41:1107–1112.
14. Baser SM et al. Sudomotor function in autonomic failure. *Neurology* 1991;41:1564–1566.
15. Bassich CJ, et al. Speech symptoms associated with early signs of Shy-Drager syndrome. *J Neurol Neurosurg Psychiatry* 1984;47:995–1001.
16. Bawa R, et al. Bilateral vocal cord paralysis with Shy-Drager syndrome. Review. *Otolaryngol Head Neck Surg* 1993;109:911–914.
17. Beck RO, et al. Genitourinary dysfunction in multiple system atrophy: clinical features and treatment in 62 cases. *J Urol* 1994;151:1336–1341.
18. Bevan DR. Shy-Drager syndrome. A review and a description of the anaesthetic management. *Anaesthesia* 1979;34:866–873.
19. Bhatt MH et al. Positron emission tomography in Shy-Drager syndrome. *Ann Neurol* 1990;28:101–103.
20. Biaggioni I et al. Hyporeninemic normoaldosteronism in severe autonomic failure. *J Clin Endocrinol Metab* 1993;76:580–586.
21. Boomsma F et al. Determination of D,L-threo-3,4-dihydroxyphenylserine and of the D- and L-enantiomers in human plasma and urine. *J Chromatogr* 1988;427:219–227.
22. Bouvette CM et al. Role of physical countermaneuvers in the management of orthostatic hypotension: efficacy and biofeedback augmentation (abstr). *Mayo Clin Proc* 1996;
23. Bradbury S, Eggleston C. Postural hypotension: a report of three cases. *Am Heart J* 1925;1:7386.
24. Brevetti G et al. Effective treatment of orthostatic hypotension by propranolol in the Shy-Drager syndrome. *Am Heart J* 1981;102:938–941.
25. Brook WH. Postural hypotension and the anti-gravity suit (review). *Aust Fam Physician* 1994;23:1948–1949.
26. Brooks DJ. Special investigations in multiple system atrophy: A. Positron emission tomography (PET) studies. In: Bannister R, Mathias C (eds). *Autonomic Failure.* Oxford: Oxford University Press. 1992;548–552.
27. Brooks DJ et al. The effect of orthostatic hypotension on cerebral blood flow and middle cerebral artery velocity in autonomic failure, with observations on the action of ephedrine. *J Neurol Neurosurg Psychiatry* 1989;52:962–966.
28. Brooks DJ et al. The relationship between locomotor disability, autonomic dysfunction, and the integrity of the striatal dopaminergic system in patients with multiple system atrophy, pure autonomic failure, and Parkinson's disease, studied with PET. *Brain* 1990;113:1539–1552.
29. Brown RT et al. MRI in autonomic failure. *J Neurol Neurosurg Psychiatry* 1987;50:913–914.
30. Carvey PM et al. The potential use of a dopamine neuron antibody and a striatal-derived neurotrophic factor as diagnostic markers in Parkinson's disease (review). *Neurology* 1991;41:53–58.
31. Chaudhuri KR et al. Alcohol ingestion lowers supine blood pressure, causes splanchnic vasodilatation and worsens postural hypotension in primary autonomic failure. *J Neurol* 1994;241:145–152.
32. Chester CS et al. Pathophysiological findings in a patient with Shy-Drager and alveolar hypoventilation syndromes. *Chest* 1988;94:212–214.
33. Chokroverty S, et al. Periodic respiration in erect posture in Shy-Drager syndrome. *J Neurol Neurosurg Psychiatry* 1978;41:980–986.
34. Coccagna G et al. Sleep-related respiratory and haemodynamic changes in Shy-Drager syndrome: a case report. *J Neurol* 1985;232:310–313.
35. Cohen J et al. Somatic and autonomic function in progressive autonomic failure and multiple system atrophy. *Ann Neurol* 1987;22:692–699.
36. Costa C, Duyckaerts C. Oligodendroglial and neuronal inclusions in multiple system atrophy. *Curr Opin Neurol* 1993;6:865–871.
37. da Costa DF et al. Growth hormone response to clonidine is impaired in patients with central sympathetic degeneration. *Clin Exp Hypertens* 1984;6:1843–1846.
38. Daniel SE. The neuropathology and neurochemistry of multiple system atrophy. In: Bannister R, Mathias C (eds). *Autonomic Failure.* Oxford: Oxford University Press. 1992;564–585.
39. Daniel SE, et al. Glial cytoplasmic inclusions are not exclusive to multiple system atrophy (letter). *J Neurol Neurosurg Psychiatry* 1995;58:262.
40. Davies B et al. The pressor actions of noradrenaline, angiotensin II and saralasin in chronic autonomic failure treated with fludrocortisone. *Br J Clin Pharmacol* 1979;8:253–260.
41. Davies IB et al. The pressor actions of noradrenaline and angiotensin II in chronic autonomic failure treated with indomethacin. *Br J Clin Pharmacol* 1980;10:223–229.
42. De Marinis M et al. Evaluation of vesico-urethral and sweating function in disorders presenting with parkinsonism. *Clin Auton Res* 1993;3:125–130.
43. Eardley I et al. The value of urethral sphincter electromyography in the differential diagnosis of parkinsonism. *Br J Urol* 1989;64:360–362.
44. Fearnley JM, Lees AJ. Striatonigral degeneration. A clinicopathological study. *Brain* 1990;113:1823–1842.
45. Fulham MJ et al. Computed tomography, magnetic resonance imaging and positron emission tomography with [18F]fluorodeoxyglucose in multiple system atrophy and pure autonomic failure. *Clin Auton Res* 1991;1:27–36.
46. Furlan R et al. Pure autonomic failure: complex abnormalities in the neural mechanisms regulating the cardiovascular system. *J Auton Nerv Syst* 1995;51:223–235.
47. Galassi G et al. Peripheral neuropathy in multiple system atrophy with autonomic failure. *Neurology* 1982;32:1116–1121.
48. Gilden JL. Midodrine in neurogenic orthostatic hypotension. A new treatment. *Int Angiol* 1993;12:125–131.
49. Gilman S et al. Benzodiazepine receptor binding in cerebellar degenerations studied with positron emission tomography. *Ann Neurol* 1995;38:176–185.
50. Gilman S, Quinn NP. The relationship of multiple system atrophy to sporadic olivopontocerebellar atrophy and other forms of idiopathic late-onset cerebellar atrophy. *Neurology* 1996;46:1197–1199.
51. Goldberg MR, et al. Prostacyclin biosynthesis and platelet function in autonomic dysfunction. *Neurology* 1985;35:120–123.
52. Goovaerts J et al. Prenalterol in the treatment of orthostatic hypotension in Shy-Drager syndrome. *Acta Cardiol* 1984;39:147–155.
53. Guilleminault C et al. The impact of autonomic nervous system dysfunction on breathing during sleep. *Sleep* 1981;4:263–278.
54. Guindi GM et al. Pathology of the intrinsic muscles of the larynx. *Clin Otolaryngol* 1981;6:101–109.
55. Hanson DG, et al. Vocal cord paresis in Shy-Drager syndrome. *Ann Otol Rhinol Laryngol* 1983;92:85–90.
56. Harding AE. "Idiopathic" late onset cerebellar ataxia. A clinical and genetic study of 36 cases. *J Neurol Sci* 1981;51:259–271.
57. Hasen J, et al. Hypothalamic dysfunction in a case of idiopathic orthostatic hypotension (Shy-Drager syndrome). *Am J Med Sci* 1982;283:36–40.
58. Hinton AE, et al. Shy-Drager syndrome presenting as Meniere's disease. *Am J Otol* 1993;14:407–408.
59. Hoeldtke RD, et al. Treatment of orthostatic hypotension: interaction of pressor drugs and tilt table conditioning. *Arch Phys Med Rehabil* 1988;69:895–898.
60. Hoeldtke RD, Israel BC. Treatment of orthostatic hypotension with octreotide. *J Clin Endocrinol Metab* 1989;68:1051–1059.
61. Hutchinson RC, Sugden JC. Anaesthesia for Shy-Drager syndrome. *Anaesthesia* 1984;39:1229–1231.
62. Imai Y et al. Circadian blood pressure variations under different pathophysiological conditions. *J Hypertens Suppl* 1990;8:S125–S132.
63. Imai Y et al. Does ambulatory blood pressure monitoring improve the diagnosis of secondary hypertension? *J Hypertens Suppl* 1990;8:S71–S75.

64. Jankovic J et al. Neurogenic orthostatic hypotension: a double-blind placebo-controlled study with midodrine. *Am J Med* 1993;95:38–48.
65. Jellinger K. Pathology of Parkinson's disease. In: Marsden CD, Fahn S (eds). *Movement Disorders*. London: Butterworth. 1989; 124–165.
66. Jellinger K. Pathology of Parkinson's disease. Changes other than the nigrostriatal pathway. *Mol Chem Neuropathol* 1991;14:153–197.
67. Johnson RH et al. Autonomic failure with orthostatic hypotension due to intermediolateral column degeneration. A report of two cases with autopsies. *Q J Med* 1966;35:276–292.
68. Kachi T et al. Effect of L-threo-3,4-dihydroxyphenylserine on muscle sympathetic nerve activities in Shy-Drager syndrome. *Neurology* 1988;38:1091–1094.
69. Kafka MS et al. Alpha-adrenergic receptors in orthostatic hypotension syndromes. *Neurology* 1984;34:1121–1125.
70. Kaufmann H et al. Hypotension-induced vasopressin release distinguishes between pure autonomic failure and multiple system atrophy with autonomic failure. *Neurology* 1992;42:590–593.
71. Kennedy PG, Duchen LW. A quantitative study of intermediolateral column cells in motor neuron disease and the Shy-Drager syndrome. *J Neurol Neurosurg Psychiatry* 1985;48:1103–1106.
72. Khurana RK. Cholinergic dysfunction in Shy-Drager syndrome: effect of the parasympathomimetic agent, bethanechol. *Clin Auton Res* 1994;4:5–13.
73. Kihara M, Low PA. Impaired vasoreactivity to nitric oxide in experimental diabetic neuropathy. *Exp Neurol* 1995;132:180–185.
74. Kihara M et al. Hypoxic effect of exogenous insulin on normal and diabetic peripheral nerve. *Am J Physiol* 1994;266:E980–E985.
75. Kingwell BA et al. Heart rate spectral analysis, cardiac norepinephrine spillover, and muscle sympathetic nerve activity during human sympathetic nervous activation and failure. *Circulation* 1994;90:234–240.
76. Kirby R et al. Urethro-vesicular dysfunction in progressive autonomic failure with multiple system atrophy. *J Neurol Neurosurg Psychiatry* 1986;49:554–562.
77. Kochar MS. Hemodynamic effects of lysine-vasopressin in orthostatic hypotension. *Am J Kidney Dis* 1985;6:49–52.
78. Kochar MS, Itskovitz HD. Treatment of idiopathic orthostatic hypotension (Shy-Drager syndrome) with indomethacin. *Lancet* 1978; 1:1011–1014.
79. Konagaya M, et al. Clinical and magnetic resonance imaging study of extrapyramidal symptoms in multiple system atrophy. *J Neurol Neurosurg Psychiatry* 1994;57:1528–1531.
80. Konagaya Y, et al. Tuberoinfundibular dopaminergic system and anterior pituitary dopamine receptor in Shy-Drager syndrome. *J Neurol Sci* 1985;67:93–103.
81. Konno H et al. Shy-Drager syndrome and amyotrophic lateral sclerosis. Cytoarchitectonic and morphometric studies of sacral autonomic neurons. *J Neurol Sci* 1986;73:193–204.
82. Kooner JS et al. Relationship between splanchnic vasodilation and postprandial hypotension in patients with primary autonomic failure. *J Hypertens Suppl* 1989;7:S40–S41.
83. Kurlan R et al. Long-term experience with pergolide therapy of advanced parkinsonism. *Neurology* 1985;35:738–742.
84. Kuroiwa Y, et al. Postural hypotension and low R-R interval variability in parkinsonism, spino-cerebellar degeneration, and Shy-Drager syndrome. *Neurology* 1983;33:463–467.
85. Kuroiwa Y, et al. Measurement of blood pressure and heart-rate variation while resting supine and standing for the evaluation of autonomic dysfunction. *J Neurol* 1987;235:65–68.
86. Lang AE et al. Striatonigral degeneration: iron deposition in putamen correlates with the slit-like void signal of magnetic resonance imaging. *Can J Neurol Sci* 1994;21:311–318.
87. Lees AJ, Bannister R. The use of lisuride in the treatment of multiple system atrophy with autonomic failure (Shy-Drager syndrome). *J Neurol Neurosurg Psychiatry* 1981;44:347–351.
88. Linebaugh C. The dysarthrias of Shy-Drager syndrome. *J Speech Hear Disord* 1979;44:55–60.
89. Low PA. Autonomic nervous system function. *J Clin Neurophysiol* 1993;10:14–27.
90. Low PA. Composite autonomic scoring scale for laboratory quantification of generalized autonomic failure. *Mayo Clin Proc* 1993; 68:748–752.
91. Low PA, et al. Splanchnic preganglionic neurons in man. I. Morphometry of preganglionic cytons. *Acta Neuropathol* 1977;40:55–61.
92. Low PA et al. Prospective evaluation of clinical characteristics of orthostatic hypotension. *Mayo Clin Proc* 1995;70:617–622.
93. Low PA, et al. The splanchnic autonomic outflow in Shy-Drager syndrome and idiopathic orthostatic hypotension. *Ann Neurol* 1978; 4:511–514.
94. Malan MD, Crago RR. Anaesthetic consideration in idiopathic orthostatic hypotension and the Shy-Drager syndrome. *Can Anaesth Soc J* 1979;26:322–327.
95. Mann S et al. Circadian variation of blood pressure in autonomic failure. *Circulation* 1983;68:477–483.
96. Mannen T et al. The Onuf's nucleus and the external anal sphincter muscles in amyotrophic lateral sclerosis and Shy-Drager syndrome. *Acta Neuropathol* 1982;58:255–260.
97. Martinelli P et al. Changes in systemic arterial pressure during sleep in Shy-Drager syndrome. *Sleep* 1981;4:139–146.
98. Martinovits G et al. Vocal cord paralysis as a presenting sign in the Shy-Drager syndrome. *J Laryngol Otol* 1988;102:280–281.
99. Mathias CJ, Bannister R. Postcibal hypotension in autonomic disorders. In: Bannister R, Mathias C (eds). *Autonomic Failure*. Oxford: Oxford University Press. 1992;489–509.
100. Mathias CJ et al. Hypotensive and sedative effects of insulin in autonomic failure. *Br Med J Clin Res Ed* 1987;295:161–163.
101. Mathias CJ et al. The effect of desmopressin on nocturnal polyuria, overnight weight loss, and morning postural hypotension in patients with autonomic failure. *Br Med J Clin Res Ed* 1986;293:353–354.
102. Mathias CJ, et al. Postural changes in plasma renin activity and responses to vasoactive drugs in a case of Shy-Drager syndrome. *J Neurol Neurosurg Psychiatry* 1977;40:138–143.
103. Matsubara S et al. Shy-Drager syndrome. Effect of fludrocortisone and L-threo-3,4-dihydroxyphenylserine on the blood pressure and regional cerebral blood flow. *J Neurol Neurosurg Psychiatry* 1990; 53:994–997.
104. Matthews MR. Autonomic ganglia in multiple system atrophy and pure autonomic failure. In: Bannister R, Mathias CJ (eds). *Autonomic Failure: A Textbook of Clinical Disorders of the Autonomic Nervous System*. Oxford: Oxford Medical Publishers. 1992;593–621.
105. McRae-Degueurce A et al. Antibodies in cerebrospinal fluid of some Alzheimer disease patients recognize cholinergic neurons in the rat central nervous system. *Proc Natl Acad Sci U S A* 1987;84:9214–9218.
106. McTavish D, Goa KL. Midodrine. A review of its pharmacological properties and therapeutic use in orthostatic hypotension and secondary hypotensive disorders. *Drugs* 1989;38:757–777.
107. Montagna P et al. Amyotrophy in Shy-Drager syndrome. *Acta Neurol Belg* 1983;83:142–157.
108. Munschauer FE et al. Abnormal respiration and sudden death during sleep in multiple system atrophy with autonomic failure. *Neurology* 1990;40:677–679.
109. Nakazato Y et al. Oligodendroglial microtubular tangles in olivopontocerebellar atrophy. *J Neuropathol Exp Neurol* 1990;49:521–530.
110. Nanda RN, et al. Treatment of neurogenic orthostatic hypotension with a monoamine oxidase inhibitor and tyramine. *Lancet* 1976;2:1164–1167.
111. Nee LE, et al. HLA in autonomic failure. *Arch Neurol* 1989;46:758–759.
112. Nee LE et al. Environmental–occupational risk factors and familial associations in multiple system atrophy: a preliminary investigation. *Clin Auton Res* 1991;1:9–13.
113. Obara A et al. Effect of xamoterol in Shy-Drager syndrome. *Circulation* 1992;85:606–611.
114. Ohashi N et al. Otoneurological manifestations of the Shy-Drager syndrome. *Eur Arch Otorhinolaryngol* 1991;248:150–152.
115. Oppenheimer DR. Lateral horn cells in progressive autonomic failure. *J Neurol Sci* 1980;46:393–404.

116. Ozawa T et al. Shy-Drager syndrome with abnormal circadian rhythm of plasma antidiuretic hormone secretion and urinary excretion. *Intern Med* 1993;32:225–227.
117. Papp MI, et al. Glial cytoplasmic inclusions in the CNS of patients with multiple system atrophy (striatonigral degeneration, olivopontocerebellar atrophy and Shy-Drager syndrome). *J Neurol Sci* 1989; 94:79–100.
118. Papp MI, Lantos PL. Accumulation of tubular structures in oligodendroglial and neuronal cells as the basic alteration in multiple system atrophy. *J Neurol Sci* 1992;107:172–182.
119. Pastakia B et al. Multiple system atrophy (Shy-Drager syndrome): MR imaging. *Radiology* 1986;159:499–502.
120. Polinsky RJ et al. Central and peripheral effects of arecoline in patients with autonomic failure. *J Neurol Neurosurg Psychiatry* 1991; 54:807–812.
121. Polinsky RJ et al. Beta-endorphin, ACTH, and catecholamine responses in chronic autonomic failure. *Ann Neurol* 1987;21:573–577.
122. Polinsky RJ, Jimerson DC, Kopin IJ. Chronic autonomic failure: CSF and plasma 3-methoxy-4-hydroxyphenylglycol. *Neurology* 1984;34:979–983.
123. Polinsky RJ et al. The adrenal medullary response to hypoglycemia in patients with orthostatic hypotension. *J Clin Endocrinol Metab* 1980;51:1401–1406.
124. Polinsky RJ et al. Pharmacologic distinction of different orthostatic hypotension syndromes. *Neurology* 1981;31:1–7.
125. Polinsky RJ et al. Antibody in the CSF of patients with multiple system atrophy reacts specifically with rat locus ceruleus. *J Neurol Sci* 1991;106:96–104.
126. Polinsky RJ, et al. Sympathetic neural prosthesis for managing orthostatic hypotension. *Lancet* 1983;1:901–904.
127. Pramstaller PP et al. Nerve conduction studies, skeletal muscle EMG, and sphincter EMG in multiple system atrophy. *J Neurol Neurosurg Psychiatry* 1995;58:618–621.
128. Prasher D, Bannister R. Brain stem auditory evoked potentials in patients with multiple system atrophy with progressive autonomic failure (Shy-Drager syndrome). *J Neurol Neurosurg Psychiatry* 1986; 49:278–289.
129. Puritz R et al. Blood pressure and vasopressin in progressive autonomic failure. Response to postural stimulation, L-dopa and naloxone. *Brain* 1983;106:503–511.
130. Quinn N. Multiple system atrophy—the nature of the beast. *J Neurol Neurosurg Psychiatry* 1989;(suppl):78–89.
131. Raimbach SJ et al. Prevention of glucose-induced hypotension by the somatostatin analogue octreotide (SMS 201-995) in chronic autonomic failure: haemodynamic and hormonal changes. *Clin Sci* 1989;77:623–628.
132. Rensma PL et al. Effects of ibopamine on postural hypotension in pure autonomic failure. *J Cardiovasc Pharmacol* 1993;21:863–868.
133. Rydin E, et al. Cystometry and mictometry as tools in diagnosing neurogenic impotence. *Acta Neurol Scand* 1981;63:181–188.
134. Saarnivaara L, et al. Ketamine anaesthesia for a patient with the Shy-Drager syndrome. *Acta Anaesthesiol Scand* 1983;27:123–125.
135. Saito Y et al. Survival of patients with multiple system atrophy. *Intern Med* 1994;33:321–325.
136. Sakoda S et al. Treatment of orthostatic hypotension in Shy-Drager syndrome with DL-threo-3,4-dihydroxyphenylserine: a case report. *Eur Neurol* 1985;24:330–334.
137. Sakuta M, et al. Anal muscle electromyograms differ in amyotrophic lateral sclerosis and Shy-Drager syndrome. *Neurology* 1978; 28:1289–1293.
138. Salinas JM et al. Urological evaluation in the Shy Drager syndrome. *J Urol* 1986;135:741–743.
139. Sandroni P et al. Autonomic involvement in extrapyramidal and cerebellar disorders. *Clin Auton Res* 1991;1:147–155.
140. Sasaki K et al. Pituitary-adrenocortical system in patients with Shy-Drager syndrome. *Horm Metab Res* 1983;15:143–146.
141. Savoiardo M et al. Magnetic resonance imaging in progressive supranuclear palsy and other parkinsonian disorders. *J Neural Transm Suppl* 1994;42:93–110.
142. Savoiardo M et al. MR imaging in progressive supranuclear palsy and Shy-Drager syndrome. *J Comput Assist Tomogr* 1989;13:555–560.
143. Sforza E et al. REM sleep behavioral disorders. *Eur Neurol* 1988; 28:295–300.
144. Shinohara Y, et al. Cerebral hemodynamics in Shy-Drager syndrome: variability of cerebral blood flow dysautoregulation and the compensatory role of chemical control in dysautoregulation. *Stroke* 1978;9:504–508.
145. Shy GM, Drager GA. A neurological syndrome associated with orthostatic hypotension. *Arch Neurol* 1960;3:511–527.
146. Silverberg R et al. Angina pectoris with normal coronary arteries in Shy-Drager syndrome. *J Neurol Neurosurg Psychiatry* 1979;42: 910–913.
147. Sima AA, et al. Shy-Drager syndrome: the transitional variant. *Clin Neuropathol* 1987;6:49–54.
148. Smith GD et al. Abnormal cardiovascular and catecholamine responses to supine exercise in human subjects with sympathetic dysfunction. *J Physiol* 1995;484:255–265.
149. Sobue G et al. Size-dependent myelinated fiber loss in the corticospinal tract in Shy-Drager syndrome and amyotrophic lateral sclerosis. *Neurology* 1987;37:529–532.
150. Sobue G et al. Shy-Drager syndrome: neuronal loss depends on size, function, and topography in ventral spinal outflow. *Neurology* 1986;36:404–407.
151. Spokes EG, et al. Multiple system atrophy with autonomic failure: clinical, histological and neurochemical observations on four cases. *J Neurol Sci* 1979;43:59–82.
152. Steiner JA et al. L-dopa and the Shy-Drager syndrome. *Med J Aust* 1974;2:133–136.
153. Stern MB et al. Magnetic resonance imaging in Parkinson's disease and parkinsonian syndromes. *Neurology* 1989;39:1524–1526.
154. Suarez GA et al. Idiopathic autonomic neuropathy: clinical, neurophysiologic, and follow-up studies on 27 patients. *Neurology* 1994;44:1675–1682.
155. Sung JH, et al. Pathology of Shy-Drager syndrome. *J Neuropathol Exp Neurol* 1979;38:353–368.
156. Tamaoka A et al. Ubiquitinated alpha B-crystallin in glial cytoplasmic inclusions from the brain of a patient with multiple system atrophy. *J Neurol Sci* 1995;129:192–198.
157. Thomas DJ, Bannister R. Preservation of autoregulation of cerebral blood flow in autonomic failure. *J Neurol Sci* 1980;44:205–212.
158. Thomas JE, Schirger A. Neurologic manifestations in idiopathic orthostatic hypotension. *Arch Neurol* 1963;8:204–208.
159. Thomas JE, Schirger A. Idiopathic orthostatic hypotension. A study of its natural history in 57 neurologically affected persons. *Arch Neurol* 1970;22:289–293.
160. Tochikubo O, et al. Relationship between 24-hour arterial pressure and heart rate variation in normotensives, hypertensives and patients with Shy-Drager syndrome. *Jpn Circ J* 1987;51:485–494.
161. Tohgi H et al. Selective loss of small myelinated and unmyelinated fibers in Shy-Drager syndrome. *Acta Neuropathol* 1982;57:282–286.
162. Tomonaga M. Neuropathology of the locus ceruleus: a semi-quantitative study. *J Neurol* 1983;230:231–240.
162a. Trendelenburg U. Mechanisms of supersensitivity and subsensitivity to sympathomimetic amines. *Pharmacol Rev* 1966;8:629–640.
163. Tsuda Y et al. Hemodynamics in Shy-Drager syndrome and treatment with indomethacin. *Eur Neurol* 1983;22:421–427.
164. Tulen JH et al. Sleep patterns and blood pressure variability in patients with pure autonomic failure. *Clin Auton Res* 1991;1:309–315.
165. Uematsu D, Hamada J, Gotoh F. Brainstem auditory evoked responses and CT findings in multiple system atrophy. *J Neurol Sci* 1987;77:161–171.
166. van Ingelghem E, van Zandijcke M, Lammens M. Pure autonomic failure: a new case with clinical, biochemical, and necropsy data. *J Neurol Neurosurg Psychiatry* 1994;57:745–747.
167. Weiss M, Shaeffer Z, Eisenstein Z. Postural hypotension: pressor effect of octreotide not mediated by norepinephrine. *South Med J* 1990;83:1315–1317.
168. Wenning GK et al. Clinical features and natural history of multiple system atrophy. An analysis of 100 cases. *Brain* 1994;117:835–845.
169. West JN et al. Xamoterol in the treatment of orthostatic hypotension associated with multiple system atrophy (Shy-Drager syndrome). *Q J Med* 1990;74:209–213.
170. Wheeler JSJ, Canning JR. Voiding dysfunction in Shy-Drager syndrome. *J Urol* 1985;134:362–363.

171. Wilcox CS, Aminoff MJ. Blood pressure responses to noradrenaline and dopamine infusions in Parkinson's disease and the Shy-Drager syndrome. *Br J Clin Pharmacol* 1976;3:207–214.
172. Williams A, et al. Vocal cord paralysis in the Shy-Drager syndrome. *J Neurol Neurosurg Psychiatry* 1979;42:151–153.
173. Williams TD et al. Pressor effect of arginine vasopressin in progressive autonomic failure. *Clin Sci* 1986;71:173–178.
174. Williams TD, et a. Vasopressin secretion in progressive autonomic failure: evidence for defective afferent cardiovascular pathways. *J Neurol Neurosurg Psychiatry* 1985;48:225–228.
175. Wright A et al. Double-blind, randomized dose-response study of midodrine in patients with neurogenic orthostatic hypotension (abstr). *Neurology* 1995;45(suppl):A396.
176. Yamada T, et a. Complement-activated oligodendroglia: a new pathologic entity identified by immunostaining with antibodies to human complement proteins C3d and C4d. *Neurosci Lett* 1990;112:161–166.
177. Yokota T et al. Sympathetic skin response in patients with cerebellar degeneration. *Arch Neurol* 1993;50:422–427.
178. Yonehara T et al. Detection of reverse flow by duplex ultrasonography in orthostatic hypotension. *Stroke* 1994;25:2407–2411.
179. Yoshida M, et a. L-threo-3,4-dihydroxyphenylserine treatment for gait apraxia in parkinsonian patients. *Kurume Med J* 1989;36:67–74.

CHAPTER 43

Other Extrapyramidal Disorders

Michael J. Aminoff

---

1. Autonomic dysfunction may be associated with clinical parkinsonism or with a more widespread neurologic disturbance in which extrapyramidal features are sometimes associated with pyramidal or cerebellar deficits. It may be associated with olivopontocerebellar atrophy (OPCA) or striatonigral degeneration, which are considered different manifestations of multiple-system atrophy (MSA).
2. Dysautonomia may occur not only as one feature of MSA, but also in Lewy body disease. Among patients with Lewy body disease, some have clinical evidence of Parkinson's disease, whereas others have neither clinical nor pathologic evidence of this disorder.
3. In the classic form of Parkinson's disease, many symptoms suggest autonomic dysfunction. However, cardiovascular reflexes are generally intact, although there may be mild postural hypotension or increased sensitivity to infused norepinephrine, suggesting a subtle autonomic disturbance caused by a central rather than a peripheral lesion.
4. In striatonigral degeneration, there may be gross dysautonomia, as in MSA, but the incidence of subclinical dysautonomia is unknown, because the neurologic disorder is diagnosed properly only at autopsy. Dopaminergic therapy may improve the resting blood pressure (BP) and reduce any postural hypotension, presumably because the central depressor effects of dopamine on BP cannot be manifested and only the peripheral pressor responses occur.
5. In patients with OPCA, dysautonomia may reflect cell loss in the intermediolateral columns of the cord, involvement of brain stem centers mediating cardiovascular reflexes and respiratory function, or an associated peripheral neuropathy. When the dysautonomia is prominent, the condition is designated MSA. In many other patients with typical OPCA, however, investigations reveal subclinical dysautonomia and respiratory abnormalities.
6. In progressive supranuclear palsy, there may be minor changes in autonomic function of dubious clinical relevance. Similarly, symptoms of autonomic dysfunction are common in Huntington's disease, but cardiovascular reflexes are not disturbed. There may, however, be a significantly greater decline in BP with changes in posture than that seen in normal subjects, suggesting that suprabulbar structures (e.g., the caudate nuclei) influence postural vasoregulatory mechanisms.

INTRODUCTION

Autonomic dysfunction may occur in isolation (pure autonomic failure or idiopathic orthostatic hypotension) or in the context of disease of the peripheral or central nervous system. This chapter considers its association with certain extrapyramidal disorders.

Autonomic dysfunction may be associated with parkinsonism or be part of a more widespread neurologic disturbance that may include, but not be limited to, parkinsonism. There is a male preponderance among such cases, and patients are usually in middle or later life. The cause is unknown. Early dysautonomic symptoms include impotence (in men), urinary incontinence, and other disturbances of sphincter function. Postural or postprandial hypotension is sometimes disabling, and impaired thermoregulatory sweating may be life-threatening for patients in hot climates. Dryness of the mouth is occasionally a conspicuous problem (24), laryngeal stridor and disorders of phonation may result from vocal cord paralysis (10), and bilateral vocal cord involvement may lead to respiratory failure, necessitating tracheostomy (22). Other respiratory abnormalities include sudden inspiratory gasping and, in some patients, sleep apnea. The ophthalmic findings can include iris atrophy, pupillary inequalities, Horner's syndrome, ab-

---

M. J. Aminoff: Department of Neurology, University of California Medical Center, San Francisco, California 94143.

normal pupillary responses to instilled drugs, and disturbances of ocular movements. The disorder tends to progress through the course of years and ultimately leads to severe incapacity.

Although the somatic neurologic manifestations often suggest parkinsonism, symptoms and signs respond poorly or not at all to treatment with levodopa. Some patients exhibit a conspicuous cerebellar syndrome. Pyramidal and lower motor neuron signs may also be present to a variable extent. Clinical and electrophysiologic evidence of peripheral neuropathy is found occasionally (17). Intellectual function is generally preserved or only mildly impaired. There may be an interval of several years between the development of autonomic dysfunction and the onset of somatic neurologic disturbances (47).

It is difficult to define the various extrapyramidal syndromes associated with impaired autonomic function. In 1960, Shy and Drager (43) were the first to emphasize that marked postural hypotension is sometimes caused by a primary degenerative disorder of the central nervous system. They described two patients with dysautonomia who had coexisting somatic neurologic deficits. At autopsy in one of their patients, pathologic changes were noted to be especially conspicuous in the caudate nuclei, substantia nigra, cerebellum, dorsal nuclei of the vagus, and spinal cord. Shortly thereafter, Adams et al. (1) reported on three patients with akinesia, rigidity, and a mild tremor, which were accompanied by pyramidal deficits in one patient and by a cerebellar disturbance in another. There was clear evidence of dysautonomia in two of these patients. Autopsy revealed pathologic changes in the substantia nigra and striatum, as well as in the olives and cerebellum. Johnson et al. (23) subsequently described two patients with autonomic failure, one of whom also had cerebellar, pyramidal, and extrapyramidal disturbances. At autopsy in this patient, abnormalities suggestive of OPCA were noted, with additional changes in the brain stem and spinal cord. In other cases reported at about the same time (19,32,42), the pathologic findings also suggested OPCA, but there were additional features typical of striatonigral degeneration. Graham and Oppenheimer (19) therefore suggested that OPCA and striatonigral degeneration were different manifestations of a single entity, which was designated *MSA*.

This term has not met with universal acceptance, however, and is applied differently by various authors. Some diagnose MSA only when there is striatonigral degeneration or OPCA in association with autonomic failure; others use the term to refer to the somatic neurologic disorder, even when there is no clinical evidence of autonomic dysfunction. Not surprisingly, then, the literature on MSA has become more confusing through the years. Some patients with dysautonomia are said to have parkinsonism or typical Parkinson's disease, whereas the clinical or pathologic features in others are said to be indicative of OPCA, striatonigral degeneration, Shy-Drager syndrome, or MSA, often without further clarification. Indeed, in some instances the same authors use these different designations interchangeably!

In his summary of the neuropathology of autonomic failure, Oppenheimer (33) pointed out that there were 56 cases of progressive autonomic failure published in the European and American literature that contained an adequate description of the pathologic findings. He found that these cases were clearly divisible into two groups: one with Lewy bodies in the substantia nigra, locus ceruleus, and elsewhere in the nervous system, and a second group that was properly designated as MSA. Some patients in the former group had clinical and pathologic evidence of Parkinson's disease, whereas others had neither clinical parkinsonism nor loss of pigmented cells. In the group of patients with MSA, there was always some degree of nigral cell damage, and in most—but not all—cases, there were clinical signs of parkinsonism before death.

Oppenheimer (33) has shown a correlation between the occurrence of autonomic failure and loss of cells from the lateral horns in the spinal cord. By contrast, a quantitative study in three patients with uncomplicated Parkinson's disease showed no difference from control subjects. In patients with MSA but no clinical evidence of autonomic failure, the number of cells in the lateral horns was considerably reduced, overlapping with that in patients with autonomic failure.

Although patients with MSA may present with a somatic deficit that suggests either OPCA or striatonigral degeneration, there are certain clinical differences between those patients who present with these somatic neurologic features and subsequently go on (often after an interval of a year or more) to exhibit symptoms and signs of dysautonomia, and those who present with autonomic dysfunction that is accompanied or followed by the development of a somatic neurologic disturbance. In particular, the latter patients (who are more properly regarded as having MSA) tend to suffer a more rapidly progressive course and have less severe loss of cells in the intermediolateral cell columns of the spinal cord (13).

The autonomic failure associated with Lewy body disease or MSA represents a degenerative disorder with an uncertain cause. It generally is not familial, although Lewis (26) reported on an unusual family in which four members had postural hypotension, parkinsonism, pyramidal deficits, and cerebellar ataxia, together with other, more atypical features, such as pes cavus and foot drop. The familial disorder described by Rosenberg (39) as a motor system degeneration exhibited an autosomal dominant mode of inheritance and occurred typically in patients of Portuguese ancestry. Although this disorder is frequently called *striatonigral degeneration*, the parkinsonian signs are relatively mild, and there are pathologic differences between it and the disorder of the same name associated with autonomic dysfunction (36). Among its clinical features are ophthalmoparesis, slowed saccadic eye movements, lid retraction, fasciculations involving the face and tongue, dystonia, spasticity, and extrapyramidal deficits. There is degeneration of the cerebellum and thoracic cord, and also of the striatum, substantia nigra, basis pontis, oculomotor nuclei, and peripheral nerves. The olives are spared, however, in contrast to the olives in dominant OPCA. The extrapyramidal symptoms may respond in some measure to treatment with dopaminergic medication.

The discussion that follows is directed at extrapyramidal disorders in which the somatic neurologic manifestations are sufficiently distinct to permit a clinical diagnosis to be made with some confidence. No attempt is made to survey the literature relating to that form of MSA (OPCA combined with striatonigral and corticospinal degeneration) associated with gross autonomic failure, which is considered in Chapter 42.

PARKINSON'S DISEASE

In his description of the disease that now bears his name, James Parkinson referred to several symptoms of autonomic dysfunction. Since that time, disturbances of salivation, sweating, and bladder and bowel function have been repeatedly emphasized, as have a low resting BP and the occurrence of postural hypotension.

It is widely held that BP in patients with Parkinson's disease tends to be low (9,50), and some investigators have suggested that this accounts for an allegedly reduced incidence of myocardial infarction or cerebrovascular disease in these patients (9). In fact, however, there is little or no evidence to support such statements. My colleagues and I (5) compared the casual systolic and diastolic BP of 411 patients with Parkinson's disease (none of whom were receiving dopaminergic agents) with those of a representative sample of the general population. Comparisons were also made among various subgroups of patients, depending on whether tremor, rigidity, or bradykinesia was the most conspicuous neurologic disturbance, and also on the severity of the extrapyramidal deficit. No significant differences in BP were found between patients with Parkinson's disease and the normal (nonparkinsonian) population.

The prevalence of postural hypotension is unclear, because orthostatic changes in BP are not necessarily symptomatic, certain antiparkinsonian drugs may cause them, and it may not be possible to distinguish Parkinson's disease from other neurologic disorders possessing conspicuous extrapyramidal features, such as striatonigral degeneration.

Gross et al. (20) studied the BP response to Valsalva's maneuver and postural tilt in 20 patients with Parkinson's disease, none of whom had dysautonomic symptoms. They found the efficiency of reflex vasoconstriction, as determined from Valsalva's maneuver, to be the same for both patients and age-matched control subjects, as was also the efficiency of reflex tachycardia. The average supine mean BP values in the patients with parkinsonism did not differ significantly from control values. The mean maximum percentage fall in the mean BP on tilting was, however, significantly higher in the parkinsonian patients, although the maximum percentage increase in heart rate (HR) did not differ between patients and controls. This postural drop in BP could not be ascribed to inactivity, because most patients were relatively active and had only mild disease, and it was not caused by dopaminergic medication, as none of the patients were receiving it. It was therefore attributed to a lesion in the upper brain stem that did not disrupt the pathways subserving Valsalva's maneuver but nevertheless affected the postural control of BP.

Wilcox and I (3) had earlier reached a similar conclusion, finding that cardiovascular reflexes were intact in patients with idiopathic Parkinson's disease. Our investigations revealed an increased sensitivity to infused norepinephrine, which we attributed to a reduction in the impulse traffic at sympathetic nerve terminals. This, in turn, was ascribed to a reduction in the descending vasoregulatory traffic from supraspinal centers not directly involved in the circulatory reflexes. The subsequent work of Mathias et al. (29) confirmed that the pressor responses to norepinephrine are enhanced in patients with central lesions, such as cervical cord transection. Wilcox and I also noted patchy impairment of thermoregulatory sweating and disturbed bladder function in our patients with Parkinson's disease.

The findings of these two groups and of Reid and Calne (38) conflict with those of Appenzeller and Goss (6), who tested autonomic function in patients with Parkinson's disease by evaluating thermoregulatory sweating, reflex vasodilation in the pulp of the digits, and the cardiovascular responses to Valsalva's maneuver and sudden head-up tilt. They found that only one patient showed a significant drop in mean BP following head-up tilt. By contrast, Valsalva's maneuver revealed that all patients had marked deficits in the BP overshoot that occurs on release of the forced expiration, unrelated to treatment with levodopa; in some patients, the baroreceptor reflex responses were completely blocked. In many patients, there was also an almost complete absence of sweating on the trunk and limbs, with compensatory hyperhidrosis on the face. These results were interpreted to indicate a failure in baroreceptor and thermoregulatory function. However, these authors compared the responses of parkinsonian patients with those expected in normal subjects, without fully taking into account the possibility of an age-related effect on baroreceptor function. Appenzeller and Goss (6) also found that reflex vasodilation failed to occur in response to an increase in body temperature, and they attributed this to lesions in the central or efferent structures subserving the response, in particular to degenerative changes in the hypothalamus and the paravertebral sympathetic ganglia.

More recently, Goetz et al. (18) studied autonomic function in 32 patients with Parkinson's disease, both before and after they had taken their regular dopaminergic medication. Before medication, when their motor disability was greatest, the patients had higher resting pulse rates, a greater postural decline in BP, and reduced responses to Valsalva's maneuver and cold pressor stimuli compared with controls, although their responses were within the normal range. Thermoregulatory sweating seemed increased in the head and neck, but this was not assessed with quantitative techniques. There was no change in the cardiovascular reflexes after medication. In their recent study, Bagheri et al. (7) compared lacrimal secretion using Schirmer's test in patients with Parkinson's disease (receiving dopaminergic therapy but not anticholinergic agents or amantadine) and normal controls. Resting tear secretion was significantly reduced in patients with stage 3 or 4 disease (Hoehn and Yahr scale), but not in patients with milder disease or in the controls. This was tentatively attributed to peripheral parasympathetic dysfunction, although no other studies were performed to provide support for this view.

These various studies suggest that the cardiovascular reflexes in patients with Parkinson's disease are generally preserved, although responses may be somewhat reduced compared with those of controls and there may be other evidence of a subtle disturbance of cardiovascular control. The findings in other recent studies agree with this view. It has been suggested that the BP response to food ingestion may be used to unmask a latent autonomic deficit. Thomaides et al. (46) investigated the effect of a balanced liquid meal on BP and HR in the supine position and after head-up tilt in patients with Parkinson's disease, MSA, or pure autonomic failure and in healthy controls. There was a postprandial fall in supine BP in all groups of patients but not in the controls; the decline was least in the patients with Parkinson's disease. Head-up tilt did not lower BP in controls or patients with Parkinson's disease, but it did so in those with MSA or pure autonomic failure. In none of the patients with Parkinson's disease was there clear evidence of sympathetic dysfunction—there was no postural hypotension, a normal plasma epinephrine response to head-up tilt, and normal responses to a series of tests of autonomic function, as well as no unmasking of postural hypotension postprandially. The results of this study conflict to some degree with the earlier but somewhat similar study of Micieli et al. (30), who examined the 24-hr pattern of BP, HR, and urinary catecholamine excretion and the response of BP and plasma catecholamine to 60° head-up tilt in 13 patients with untreated Parkinson's disease and in age-matched healthy control subjects. Seven of the 13 patients with Parkinson's disease showed a fall in postprandial supine systolic BP that exceeded the maximal decrease in controls. There was a significant relationship between degree of postprandial hypotension and 24-hr mean level of dopamine excretion. Eight patients also showed postural hypotension during the tilt test and postprandially.

Two other studies merit brief attention. van Dijk et al. (48) found no significant difference in HR variability or the response to Valsalva's maneuver between 67 patients with Parkinson's disease and a group of healthy, age-matched controls. There was, however, a mild difference in the BP response to standing and sustained handgrip, especially in patients who were older, had more advanced disease, or were taking antiparkinsonian medication. Magalhaes et al. (28) undertook a retrospective analysis of the medical records for evidence of autonomic dysfunction in patients with autopsy evidence of Parkinson's disease or MSA. The validity of such studies clearly depends on the quality of the records, and some symptoms regarded as evidence of autonomic dysfunction—such as bladder dysfunction or constipation—could have been related to other factors (prostatic hypertrophy and physical inactivity, respectively), whereas others—such as postural hypotension—might have arisen for many different reasons, including the use of certain medications. Accordingly, this study, which suggests that autonomic dysfunction is a feature of Parkinson's disease, is best discounted for methodologic reasons.

From the various studies discussed above, there is no agreement concerning the extent of autonomic involvement in Parkinson's disease, but the findings suggest that there is some impairment of cardiovascular responses in certain patients with Parkinson's disease.

Sandroni et al. (41) recently evaluated autonomic function in the context of Parkinson's disease and other neurodegenerative disorders. They divided patients into several diagnostic categories: classic Parkinson's disease, parkinsonism plus signs indicating more widespread involvement, MSA, familial degenerative central nervous system syndromes, and certain other categories (including nonspecific sporadic multisystem degeneration without conspicuous orthostatic hypotension). The autonomic involvement was mild or absent in patients with Parkinson's disease, in that frequency of anhidrosis was <40%, postural hypotension was absent or mild, and cardiovascular reflexes were normal or only mildly abnormal.

Pathologic studies in patients with Parkinson's disease have shown that Lewy bodies may be present in the sympathetic ganglia (37). Thus, on theoretical grounds, dysautonomia in this condition could relate to a central or peripheral disorder. As already indicated, the results of early studies (3,20) suggested that a central disorder was responsible, and the more recent work of Sachs et al. (40) confirms this. These authors studied the cardiovascular responses of 20 patients with Parkinson's disease who had been off carbidopa-levodopa (Sinemet) for 24 hrs, and again approximately 1 hr after treatment. They compared these findings to those in a control group of 15 healthy subjects. Measurements of autonomic function included evaluation of respiratory sinus arrhythmia, the Valsalva ratio, the response to contralateral isometric handgrip, the response of HR and BP to 60° head-up tilt, and the dive reflex response (i.e., the reduction in HR that occurs during immersion of the face in ice water for 10 seconds). The vagally mediated responses to Valsalva's maneuver and the dive reflex test were normal, but sinus arrhythmia, which is also mediated by the vagus nerve, was reduced. These findings suggest that a central rather than a peripheral lesion caused the reduced HR responses to respiration. There was no significant orthostatic drop in BP, in accord with the work of Wilcox and me (3) and of Reid and Calne (38), but the HR, BP, and contralateral forearm blood flow responses to isometric handgrip were significantly reduced. This also was attributed to a central disorder, and in particular to a reduced central command or reduced stimulation of peripheral receptors.

MULTIPLE-SYSTEM ATROPHY (STRIATONIGRAL DEGENERATION)

As indicated earlier, striatonigral degeneration with an associated dysautonomia is one of the disorders subsumed under the designation *MSA*, and is referred to by some as the *Shy-Drager syndrome*. Its clinical features have been discussed earlier in this chapter and in Chapter 42.

The clinical disorder is sometimes impossible to distinguish from Parkinson's disease, although bradykinesia and rigidity are often much more conspicuous than any associated tremor. Moreover, symptoms tend to have a symmetric onset, the course of the disorder is more rapidly progressive, and patients generally respond poorly to levodopa (15); there may also be atypical features, such as pyramidal deficits or cerebellar signs, to suggest the correct diagnosis. The designation *parkinsonism-plus syndrome* is occasionally applied to patients when the clinical deficit is atypical for classic Parkinson's disease but is insufficient to establish a diagnosis of striatonigral degeneration. Unlike patients with classic Parkinson's disease or pure autonomic failure (without associated somatic deficits), however, patients with striatonigral degeneration typically have abnormal brain stem auditory evoked potentials (35). The most common abnormality is a reduced amplitude of wave V relative to wave I, and absence of enhancement of wave V with binaural stimulation, presumably reflecting a pontine and midbrain defect.

The dysautonomia of striatonigral degeneration cannot be distinguished from that occurring in MSA (see Chapter 42). When autonomic failure is conspicuous, it is characterized by marked postural hypotension; impaired or absent cardiovascular responses to deep breathing, Valsalva's maneuver, mental arithmetic, and other stress tests; impaired thermoregulatory sweating (which may reflect a disorder that is predominantly preganglionic, postganglionic, or both); and a normal or low supine plasma level of norepinephrine, with a reduced norepinephrine response to standing. The incidence of subclinical dysautonomia is unknown, because the diagnosis of striatonigral degeneration can often be made only at autopsy.

Cerebral dopamine and norepinephrine stores are depleted, and there is variable involvement of the central cholinergic systems in patients with striatonigral degeneration (44). Despite this, levodopa treatment brings about little or no improvement, and may even cause deterioration in the somatic neurologic disturbance (4,25). This is also the case with bromocriptine (49) and lisuride (25). Dopaminergic therapy, either with levodopa or a dopamine receptor agonist, may actually improve the resting BP and reduce the degree of postural hypotension (4,45,49). Levodopa is converted in the body to dopamine, which has a central depressor and a peripheral pressor effect on BP. In patients with a lesion in the central autonomic pathways, the central effects of dopamine on the BP cannot be manifested, however, and a pressor response results.

OLIVOPONTOCEREBELLAR ATROPHY

There can be no doubt that OPCA embraces a heterogeneous group of disorders, but despite ambiguity, this nosologic label remains in widespread clinical use.

Some authors, such as Quinn (36), have attempted to distinguish between familial (dominantly inherited) and sporadic cases, for somewhat uncertain reasons, as the two may be indistinguishable both clinically and pathologically. Moreover, dominantly inherited OPCA may itself represent four or more distinct disorders, based on its biochemical characteristics (34). The extent to which autonomic dysfunction occurs in any or all of these disorders is unclear. Other authors distinguish OPCA from MSA when it has a familial basis and somatic neurologic manifestations precede gross autonomic dysfunction by several years. In fact, however, evidence of subclinical dysautonomia may be detected by tests of autonomic function in a number of patients with either familial or sporadic OPCA.

Caplan (12) has summarized the clinical features of sporadic OPCA. Typically, an ataxic gait, the earliest manifestation of the disorder, worsens until the patient is bedridden or confined to a chair. The disorder is slowly progressive, and as it advances, pyramidal and extrapyramidal (especially parkinsonian) disturbances also develop. In some instances, however, parkinsonian deficits dominate the clinical picture. The upper limbs are usually less involved than the lower extremities. Ocular motility may be disturbed, or there may be a supranuclear ophthalmoplegia. Speech is typically dysarthric, often with a somewhat nasal quality, and may eventually become soft and hoarse. Autonomic disturbances are relatively frequent, and the most common complaint is a disturbance of micturition (urinary frequency, incontinence, or both), which occurs particularly early in OPCA, in contrast to the other cerebellar degenerative disorders. There may also be severe constipation or, less commonly, fecal incontinence. Dysphagia may lead to aspiration pneumonia. Postural hypotension is sometimes conspicuous. Imaging studies show cerebellar and brain stem atrophy.

The brain stem centers mediating the cardiovascular reflex responses or those involved in regulating respiration are closely related anatomically to the sites of pathologic involvement in OPCA, suggesting that autonomic function may be compromised at this level in many patients. In other patients, the dysautonomia may stem from spinal cord involvement, with loss of cells in the lateral columns. As already indicated, OPCA can be one manifestation of MSA, in which context there are usually additional clinical or pathologic features to indicate more widespread involvement. Such patients have abnormal cardiovascular reflexes, with postural hypotension, abnormal responses to Valsalva's maneuver, reduced sinus arrhythmia and cardiovascular responses to stress, and hypohidrosis or anhidrosis. Plasma norepinephrine responses to standing are also typically diminished. However, not all patients with OPCA manifest symptoms of autonomic dysfunction, and even detailed laboratory investigations in some patients fail to reveal any signs of dysautonomia. Finally, in a few patients with OPCA, autonomic dysfunction may be linked to peripheral nerve involvement.

In patients presenting with typical OPCA, the incidence of clinical or subclinical autonomic dysfunction has been studied by several authors, but difficulties with nomenclature complicate interpretation of the findings. For example, Miyazaki (31) studied 45 patients with "cerebellar degeneration" and included under this designation patients with parenchymatous cerebellar degeneration, OPCA, and MSA. Attention was directed at the incidence of significant postural hypotension, defined as a decline in systolic pressure of >21 mmHg or in pulse pressure of >16 mmHg on arising to an erect position from a supine position. Twenty patients were found to have abnormal postural hypotension, three had "borderline" hypotension, and 22 had no abnormality. Of the 20 patients with significant postural hypotension, four were regarded as having MSA because autonomic symptoms, rather than cerebellar disturbances, were the initial complaint. Among the patients with postural hypotension, urinary incontinence was present in 85%, pyramidal signs in 40%, and extrapyramidal deficits and dementia in 35% each. By contrast, among the 22 patients with no postural hypotension, none had urinary incontinence or extrapyramidal disturbances; only five (23%) had pyramidal disturbances and two (9%) had dementia.

Chokroverty et al. (14) studied 10 men with OPCA that had been diagnosed on clinical grounds. The disorder had a familial basis in three (with dominant inheritance in two and a recessive inheritance in one), and was sporadic in the remaining seven. Two patients had associated extrapyramidal findings. Among these 10 patients, four had symptomatic postural hypotension, with a decline in systolic pressure of between 20 and 50 mmHg and in diastolic pressure of between 4 and 22 mmHg on head-up tilt; two others had a fixed HR despite the abrupt change in posture. One patient (who also had significant postural hypotension) had an abnormal response to Valsalva's maneuver, suggesting a lesion affecting the baroreceptor reflex arc. The cardiovascular responses to the cold pressor and mental arithmetic tests were abnormal in four patients, indicating a lesion in the central or efferent sympathetic pathways. Three patients had an abnormal response to head-up tilt but normal responses to the Valsalva maneuver, mental arithmetic, and the cold pressor test, suggesting a very discrete central lesion that, by its location, affected only certain autonomic responses. There was low supine plasma renin activity in three patients and failure of plasma renin activity to rise appropriately in five patients despite normal urinary sodium excretion; these findings suggest a reduced impulse traffic from supraspinal centers that produces inadequate stimulation of the renal sympathetic nerves. Similarly, a normal resting plasma norepinephrine level failed to rise adequately when one patient assumed an erect position, again implying sympathetic dysfunction with reduced impulse traffic at the sympathetic nerve endings. Thus, certain patients with OPCA exhibit defective autonomic function, although the precise site of the lesion is unclear and may vary in different patients.

One of the patients in the series of Chokroverty et al. (14) subsequently underwent postmortem examination. There were "no substantial changes" in the intermediolateral cell columns of the spinal cord, but quantitative studies were not performed and, in any event, this particular patient had neither clinical nor laboratory evidence of autonomic dysfunction.

The BP response to head-up tilt and the sympathetic skin response were found to be normal by Yokota et al. (51) in patients with familial OPCA as well as in patients with sporadic or familial cerebellar atrophy, whereas abnormalities were found in 22 of 24 patients with the sporadic variety of OPCA, of whom 19 also had orthostatic hypotension. These authors therefore believe that the marked difference in the incidence of dysautonomia between familial and sporadic cases of OPCA justifies their distinction, as proposed by Quinn (36).

Respiratory abnormalities occur in some patients with OPCA. Central, obstructive, or mixed sleep apnea may occur, and this is not necessarily related to other disturbances of autonomic function (14). In one case, the respiratory abnormality suggested a lesion at the pontomedullary level, with cluster breathing during sleep and wakefulness, but without altered respiratory chemoreceptor control (27). In occasional patients, cholinergic dysfunction may be especially conspicuous, with sexual and sphincter disturbances, anhidrosis, and xerostomia (24).

There is no specific treatment of the autonomic dysfunction associated with OPCA; management is similar to that for dysautonomia occurring in other circumstances.

PROGRESSIVE SUPRANUCLEAR PALSY

Progressive supranuclear palsy, which is characterized clinically by conspicuous supranuclear ophthalmoplegia associated with axial dystonia, rigidity, bradykinesia, pseudobulbar palsy, cognitive disturbances, and postural instability, may occasionally be accompanied by disturbances of bladder or bowel function. However, the associated pathologic changes noted in central autonomic nervous system structures led Gutrecht (21) to evaluate nine patients with this disorder using noninvasive studies of cardiovascular reflex function. In these patients he found a drop in BP on standing for 1 min that was significantly greater than that in control, age-matched subjects. More particularly, an orthostatic decline in BP occurred in five of the nine patients he studied, but its magnitude did not usually exceed that sometimes observed in normal subjects. The change in HR after standing, as indicated by the 30:15 ratio on rising to the erect position, was also abnormal in the patient group. There were no differences between patients and controls in response to Valsalva's maneuver, HR changes with deep breathing, pressor effects of sustained handgrip, and response to the cold pressor test. The severity of the somatic disorder did not appear to influence the results of the autonomic studies. Thus, Gutrecht found only minor changes, the significance of which is unclear.

Sandroni et al. (41) also studied autonomic function in a group of patients with progressive supranuclear palsy and found only minor abnormalities of dubious clinical relevance. In particular, there was insignificant orthostatic hypotension, and disturbances of sweating were uncommon and mild compared with those seen in conjunction with other extrapyramidal and cerebellar system disorders.

HUNTINGTON'S DISEASE

A variety of autonomic disturbances may arise in patients with Huntington's disease. Disturbances of swallowing and respiration may lead to aspiration pneumonia (11), and sphincter control is sometimes impaired. Hyperhidrosis of the hands and feet may occur, as may sialorrhea, hypogenitalism, polyuria, and polydipsia. Induction of general anesthesia with thiopentone produced prolonged apnea in one patient (16). Disturbances of BP regulation are uncommon, although postural hypotension may occur in response to neuroleptic medication given to control the dyskinesia or behavioral disturbance.

The caudate nuclei have been implicated in the postural regulation of BP. Barbeau et al. (8), for example, suggested that the caudate nuclei monitor BP through a feedback system, thereby modulating vasomotor centers in the brain stem and hypothalamus. The effect on cardiovascular reflexes of a defect involving the caudate nucleus was therefore investigated by Gross and me (2) in a study of 11 patients with Huntington's disease. We found no significant abnormality in either the resting BP or the baroreceptor reflex responses, compared with the findings in 13 control subjects. Nevertheless, there was a significantly greater fall in BP when patients were tilted abruptly to a 60° head-up position, compared with the findings in controls, and this could not be ascribed to either patient inactivity or medication. The effect of tilt on BP was expressed as a percentage of the reduction that occurred in the mean BP (diastolic plus one-third pulse pressure). In control subjects, this postural reduction in mean BP ranged from 5%–24% (mean, 13.5%); in the patients with Huntington's disease, it ranged from 10%–36% (mean, 23.4%). These findings were taken to suggest that suprabulbar structures, including the caudate nuclei, influence postural vasoregulatory mechanisms without affecting baroreceptor reflexes, and that in patients with Huntington's disease, there may be a defect in the postural vasoregulatory mechanisms, even though the resting BP and responses to Valsalva's maneuver are normal.

REFERENCES

1. Adams RD, et al. Dégénérescences nigro-striées et cerebello-nigro-striées. *Psychiatr Neurol* 1961;142:219–259.
2. Aminoff MJ, Gross M. Vasoregulatory activity in patients with Huntington's chorea. *J Neurol Sci* 1974;21:33–38.
3. Aminoff MJ, Wilcox CS. Assessment of autonomic function in patients with a parkinsonian syndrome. *Br Med J* 1971;4:80–84.
4. Aminoff MJ, et al. Levodopa therapy for parkinsonism in the Shy-Drager syndrome. *J Neurol Neurosurg Psychiatry* 1973;36:350–353.
5. Aminoff MJ, et al. Arterial blood pressure in patients with Parkinson's disease. *J Neurol Neurosurg Psychiatry* 1975;38:73–77.
6. Appenzeller O, Goss JE. Autonomic deficits in Parkinson's syndrome. *Arch Neurol* 1971;24:50–57.
7. Bagheri H, et al. Lacrimation in Parkinson's disease. *Clin Neuropharmacol* 1994;17:89–91.
8. Barbeau A, et al. Renin, dopamine and Parkinson's disease. In: Barbeau A, McDowell FH, eds. L-*Dopa and Parkinsonism*. Philadelphia: FA Davis; 1970:286–293.
9. Barbeau A, et al. Adverse clinical side effects of levodopa therapy. In: McDowell FH, Markham CH, eds. *Recent Advances in Parkinson's Disease*. Oxford: Blackwell; 1971:203–237.
10. Bassich CJ, et al. Speech symptoms associated with early signs of Shy Drager syndrome. *J Neurol Neurosurg Psychiatry* 1984;47:995–1001.
11. Bruyn GW. Huntington's chorea. Historical, clinical and laboratory synopsis. In: Vinken PJ, Bruyn GW, eds. *Diseases of Basal Ganglia*. Amsterdam: Elsevier North-Holland; 1968:298–378 (*Handbook of Clinical Neurology*; vol 6).
12. Caplan LR. Clinical features of sporadic (Dejerine-Thomas) olivopontocerebellar atrophy. *Adv Neurol* 1984;41:217–224.
13. Chokroverty S. Autonomic dysfunction in olivopontocerebellar atrophy. *Adv Neurol* 1984;41:105–141.
14. Chokroverty S, et al. Autonomic dysfunction and sleep apnea in olivopontocerebellar degeneration. *Arch Neurol* 1984;41:926–931.
15. Colosimo C, et al. Some specific clinical features differentiate multiple system atrophy (striatonigral variety) from Parkinson's disease. *Arch Neurol* 1995;52:294–298.
16. Davies DD. Abnormal response to anaesthesia in a case of Huntington's chorea. *Br J Anaesth* 1966;38:490–491.
17. Galassi G, et al. Peripheral neuropathy in multiple system atrophy with autonomic failure. *Neurology* 1982;32:1116–1121.
18. Goetz CG, et al. Autonomic dysfunction in Parkinson's disease. *Neurology* 1986;36:73–75.
19. Graham JG, Oppenheimer DR. Orthostatic hypotension and nicotine sensitivity in a case of multiple system atrophy. *J Neurol Neurosurg Psychiatry* 1969;32:28–34.
20. Gross M, et al. Orthostatic hypotension in Parkinson's disease. *Lancet* 1972;1:174–176.
21. Gutrecht JA. Autonomic cardiovascular reflexes in progressive supranuclear palsy. *J Auton Nerv Syst* 1992;39:29–35.
22. Israel RH, Marino JM. Upper airway obstruction in the Shy-Drager syndrome. *Ann Neurol* 1977;2:83.
23. Johnson RH, et al. Autonomic failure with orthostatic hypotension due to intermediolateral column degeneration: a report of two cases with autopsies. *Q J Med* 1966;35:276–292.

24. Khurana RK, et al. Shy-Drager syndrome: diagnosis and treatment of cholinergic dysfunction. *Neurology* 1980;30:805–809.
25. Lees AJ, Bannister R. The use of lisuride in the treatment of multiple system atrophy with autonomic failure (Shy-Drager syndrome). *J Neurol Neurosurg Psychiatry* 1981;44:347–351.
26. Lewis P. Familial orthostatic hypotension. *Brain* 1964;87:719–728.
27. Lockwood AH. Shy-Drager syndrome with abnormal respirations and antidiuretic hormone release. *Arch Neurol* 1976;33:292–295.
28. Magalhaes M, et al. Autonomic dysfunction in pathologically confirmed multiple system atrophy and idiopathic Parkinson's disease—a retrospective comparison. *Acta Neurol Scand* 1995;91:98–102.
29. Mathias CJ, et al. Enhanced pressor response to noradrenaline in patients with cervical spinal cord transection. *Brain* 1976;99:757–770.
30. Micieli G, et al. Postprandial and orthostatic hypotension in Parkinson's disease. *Neurology* 1987;37:386–393.
31. Miyazaki M. Shy-Drager syndrome: a nosological entity? The problem of orthostatic hypotension. In: Sobue I, ed. *Spinocerebellar Degenerations*. Baltimore: University Park Press; 1980:35–43.
32. Nick J, et al. Hypotension orthostatique idiopathique avec syndrome neurologique complexe à prédominance extra-pyramidale. *Rev Neurol (Paris)* 1967;116:213–227.
33. Oppenheimer D. Neuropathology and neurochemistry of autonomic failure. In: Bannister R, ed. *Autonomic Failure*. 2nd ed. Oxford: Oxford University Press; 1988:451–463.
34. Perry TL. Four biochemically different types of dominantly inherited olivopontocerebellar atrophy. *Adv Neurol* 1984;41:205–216.
35. Prasher D, Bannister R. Brain stem auditory evoked potentials in patients with multiple system atrophy with progressive autonomic failure (Shy-Drager syndrome). *J Neurol Neurosurg Psychiatry* 1986; 49:278–289.
36. Quinn N. Multiple system atrophy—the nature of the beast. *J Neurol Neurosurg Psychiatry* 1989; (Suppl):78–89.
37. Rajput AH, Rozdilsky B. Dysautonomia in parkinsonism: a clinicopathological study. *J Neurol Neurosurg Psychiatry* 1976;39:1092–1100.
38. Reid JL, Caine DB. Cardiovascular effects of levodopa in parkinsonism. *Adv Neurol* 1973;3:223–232.
39. Rosenberg RN. Joseph disease: an autosomal dominant motor system degeneration. *Adv Neurol* 1984;41:179–193.
40. Sachs C, et al. Autonomic cardiovascular responses in parkinsonism: effect of levodopa with dopa-decarboxylase inhibition. *Acta Neurol Scand* 1985;71:37–42.
41. Sandroni P, et al. Autonomic involvement in extrapyramidal and cerebellar disorders. *Clin Auton Res* 1991;1:147–155.
42. Schwarz GA. The orthostatic hypotension syndrome of Shy-Drager. *Arch Neurol* 1967;16:123–139.
43. Shy GM, Drager GA. A neurological syndrome associated with orthostatic hypotension. *Arch Neurol* 1960;2:511–527.
44. Spokes EGS, et al. Multiple system atrophy with autonomic failure. *J Neurol Sci* 1979;43:59–82.
45. Steiner JA, et al. L-Dopa and the Shy-Drager syndrome. *Med J Aust* 1974;2:133–136.
46. Thomaides T, et al. Cardiovascular and hormonal responses to liquid food challenge in idiopathic Parkinson's disease, multiple system atrophy, and pure autonomic failure. *Neurology* 1993;43:900–904.
47. Thomas JE, Schirger A. Idiopathic orthostatic hypotension. *Arch Neurol* 1970;22:289–293.
48. van Dijk JG, et al. Autonomic nervous system dysfunction in Parkinson's disease: relationships with age, medication, duration, and severity. *J Neurol Neurosurg Psychiatry* 1993;56:1090–1095.
49. Williams AC, et al. Actions of bromocriptine in the Shy-Drager and Steele-Richardson-Olszewski syndromes. In: Fuxe K, Caine DB, eds. *Dopaminergic Ergots and Motor Control*. Oxford: Pergamon Press; 1979:271–283.
50. Yahr MD. General discussion on clinical effects of L-dopa upon blood pressure. In: Barbeau A, McDowell FH, eds. *L-Dopa and Parkinsonism*. Philadelphia: FA Davis; 1970:266–268.
51. Yokota T, et al. Sympathetic skin response in patients with cerebellar degeneration. *Arch Neurol* 1993;50:422–427.

CHAPTER 44

Neurochemical and Pharmacologic Abnormalities in Chronic Autonomic Failure Syndromes

Ronald J. Polinsky

---

1. The cardiovascular responses to adrenergic drugs vary in different forms of autonomic failure according to the site of the lesion. The denervation in pure autonomic failure (PAF) can be distinguished pharmacologically from the decentralization in multiple-system atrophy (MSA).
2. Impaired adrenal medullary function can result from central and peripheral lesions in the autonomic nervous system. Severe adrenergic insufficiency does not alter the sequence, magnitude, and temporal profile of other counterregulatory hormones.
3. Neurotransmitter and neuropeptide measurements can provide biochemical evidence of pandysautonomia in patients with PAF and MSA.
4. Low levels of neurotransmitters in the cerebrospinal fluid (CSF) reflect central involvement of the monoaminergic and cholinergic systems in patients with MSA.
5. Abnormal peptide responses in patients with autonomic failure are generally manifestations of impaired control stemming from lesions in the neurotransmitter pathways that modulate release of these substances.
6. The abnormal pattern of melatonin excretion in MSA is consistent with dysfunction in the central pathways involved in mediating circadian rhythms.

INTRODUCTION

The principles of chemical neurotransmission provide a foundation for developing clinical research strategies to investigate patients with autonomic nervous system disorders. Substantial advances in our knowledge of neuronal function, combined with technologic progress, has facilitated a more refined approach to elucidating the neurochemical changes and neuropharmacologic abnormalities that result from lesions of the autonomic nervous system in humans. Current methods for assessing specific aspects of neurotransmitter metabolism and function contrast sharply with the state of the art nearly three decades ago, when Luft and von Euler (22) reported decreased urinary excretion of catecholamines in patients with orthostatic hypotension. In addition, the importance of neuropeptides and the relationship of the autonomic nervous system to other hormonal and peptide control systems in the regulation of numerous homeostatic mechanisms are being increasingly recognized.

Several approaches have proved to be extremely valuable in clinical studies of neurotransmitters and neuropeptides. In general, the levels of these substances or their metabolites, or both, in the plasma, urine, and CSF under resting conditions reflect basal activity, whereas changes in response to various physiologic and pharmacologic stimuli serve as indices of functional integrity. Two laboratory methods enable neurochemical measurements that possess the sensitivity and specificity necessary for detection in the picogram range. Neurotransmitters and their metabolites can be quantified using various methods, following chromatographic separation. Although gas chromatography–mass spectrometry has some advantages, high-performance liquid chromatography (HPLC) coupled with electrochemical detection is currently used in most laboratories. HPLC is

R. J. Polinsky: Department of Human Pharmacology, Sandoz Research Institute, East Hanover, New Jersey 07936.

well suited for small numbers of samples and permits the simultaneous analysis of various related compounds. Radioimmunoassay is the primary method for measuring hormonal and peptide levels. This technique depends critically on adequate preliminary preparation, which separates the compound of interest from other interfering substances, and on the availability of selective antibodies.

In addition to the technical limitations of these analytic methods, a variety of other factors may affect the results, confound their interpretation, or influence the validity of conclusions based on these approaches. The conditions under which samples are obtained constitute a major consideration in clinical investigations, because the autonomic nervous system responds rapidly to changes in the internal or external milieu. The time of day, position of the patient, level of activity, food intake, and clinical setting are examples of variables that require control. Physical and emotional stress should be minimized to achieve a consistent state of basal activity; the importance of this factor is highlighted by the need to wait at least 15 min following needle insertion before catecholamine levels can be sampled (19). The type of preservative as well as handling and storage of specimens can also affect the results of neurotransmitter and neuropeptide measurements. The origin of neurochemicals and their metabolites from various biologic compartments must be taken into account to justify use of their levels as indices of the activity within specific neuronal systems. Drugs can serve as pharmacologic probes to assess central and peripheral responses of various pathways. The value of this approach is limited by the specificity of the agents employed for this purpose. Furthermore, interactions between central and peripheral mechanisms as well as multiple neurotransmitter systems may complicate the interpretation of neuroendocrine responses.

Despite technical and clinical limitations, neurochemical measurements and pharmacologic responses can distinguish between different forms of autonomic failure. Neuropharmacologic investigations may also yield insights that can suggest opportunities for rational therapeutic interventions. This chapter focuses on achievements of the last decade made in the understanding of neurotransmitter metabolism and neuropeptide function in patients with PAF and MSA. These disorders serve as models to study the respective consequences of peripheral and central autonomic lesions in humans. In a number of instances, the observations made in patients with autonomic failure have shed light on normal physiologic, biochemical, and pharmacologic mechanisms, because specific responses can be studied in the absence of neurotransmitters or other relevant mechanisms.

NEUROTRANSMITTERS

Monoamines are among the most important chemical mediators of neurotransmission in the nervous system. Norepinephrine plays a particularly crucial role, because it is released at most postganglionic sympathetic nerve endings. Although release of epinephrine is primarily confined to the adrenal medulla, this essential stress hormone is carried to distant sites in the body through the bloodstream to effect metabolic and circulatory homeostasis despite provocative stimuli that may threaten survival. Dopamine and serotonin are present throughout the body, but their roles as central nervous system neurotransmitters have been more intensely investigated. Dopamine is best known for its function within the extrapyramidal system, whereas the distribution of serotonin in primitive brain regions is consistent with its influence on the control of wakefulness and vegetative functions. Acetylcholine mediates neurotransmission in many central and peripheral pathways; of particular relevance to autonomic function are its roles in parasympathetic nerve endings, sympathetic ganglia, and the hypothalamus. Each of these classic neurotransmitters will be discussed separately; however, interactions occur at many levels of the neuraxis, making it difficult to separate their individual effects in a clinical context.

Norepinephrine

Peripheral noradrenergic function has been studied in depth in patients with autonomic failure because the sympathetic nervous system provides the critical efferent element of the baroreflex arc. Sympathetic responses to postural stimuli are clinically relevant, in that orthostatic hypotension generally becomes the most disabling symptom of autonomic dysfunction. In normal subjects, supine plasma norepinephrine levels (usually about 200 pg/mL) double on standing (53). This increment in the plasma norepinephrine level reflects the increase in sympathetic nerve activity required to counteract the effect of blood pooling in the lower extremities induced by gravity. Patients with PAF generally have low supine plasma norepinephrine levels (often less than 75 pg/mL), whereas patients with MSA accompanied by autonomic failure have normal or slightly elevated levels (6,31,53). In neither group of patients does the plasma norepinephrine level increase in response to assuming an upright position. These neurochemical abnormalities differ between peripheral and central forms of autonomic failure. In PAF, the low basal plasma norepinephrine level is consistent with primary postganglionic involvement; in MSA, the sympathetic neurons are relatively intact but are not activated appropriately. The lack of a postural increment reflects the presence of a lesion in the baroreflex arc in both conditions.

The pattern of norepinephrine metabolite concentrations in plasma and urine provides further confirmation of this pathophysiologic distinction. Most released norepinephrine is cleared from the synaptic cleft by an active uptake process. Intraneuronal norepinephrine metabolism results in the formation of deaminated metabolites. Normetanephrine is produced from the O-methylation of norepinephrine that escapes neuronal uptake and "spills over" into the circulation; a portion of this metabolite is conjugated and excreted in the urine. Plasma levels of dihydroxyphenylalanine, a catecholamine precursor, and dihydroxyphenylglycol, a deaminated norepinephrine metabolite, are low in patients with PAF, consistent with a functional decrease in the number of sympathetic noradrenergic neurons (12). Low levels of urinary norepinephrine metabolites in PAF contrast with the selective reduction of normetanephrine in MSA (18). This latter finding reflects a decreased activation of relatively intact postganglionic neurons.

Several other aspects of peripheral noradrenergic function further clarify the pathophysiologic differences between central and peripheral lesions in the sympathetic nervous system. Newly synthesized norepinephrine is stored in dense-core vesicles within sympathetic nerve endings. This intraneuronal norepinephrine can be released in response to indirectly acting sympathomimetic drugs, such as tyramine. The plasma norepinephrine increment following the intravenous administration of tyramine is significantly smaller than normal in patients with PAF, consistent with an abnormality in the neuronal stores or the uptake of norepinephrine, or both (31). In patients with MSA, a normal tyramine-induced increment in norepinephrine levels provides further evidence of the functional integrity of postganglionic neurons.

Neuronal uptake can be assessed in humans by examining the kinetic disposition of radiolabeled catecholamines. In this strategy, the decline in plasma catecholamine radioactivity is measured after the labeled compounds have been infused at a constant rate to achieve steady-state conditions. At this point (after a minimum of three half-lives has elapsed for the compound of interest), the various processes that affect the plasma norepinephrine concentration are at equilibrium, so that the sum of exit rates from the circulation equals the infusion rate.

Quantitative analysis permits calculation of the clearance and endogenous secretion rate for norepinephrine. Comparison between the results obtained using norepinephrine and isoproterenol can indicate the degree to which neuronal uptake is affected, as isoproterenol is cleared solely by extraneuronal mechanisms. Clearance of norepinephrine is reduced only in patients with PAF (10, 33), consistent with the primary involvement of postganglionic sympathetic neurons in this disorder. The deficit in neuronal uptake is striking in PAF, because the rates of removal for norepinephrine and isoproterenol are very similar (33) (Fig. 1). The clearance of norepinephrine plays an

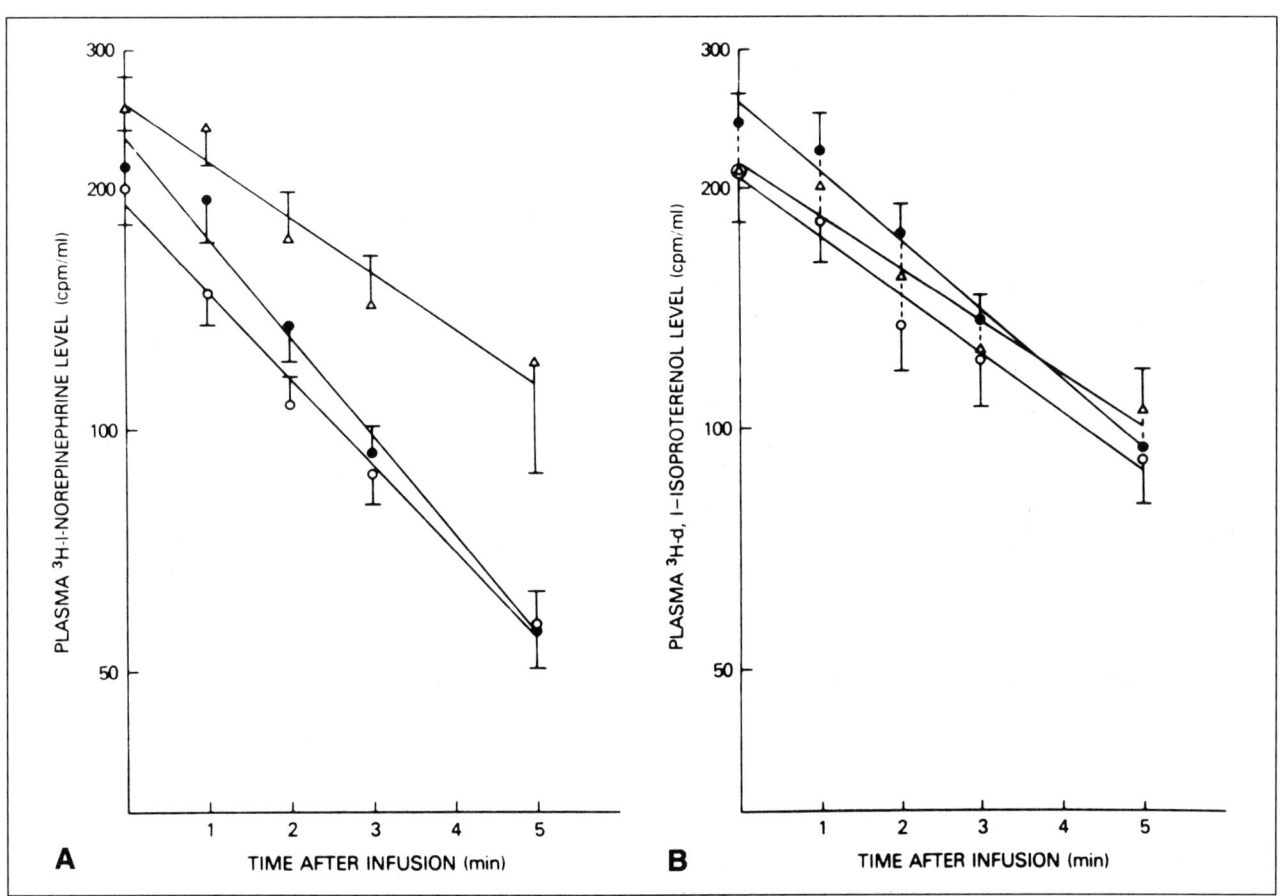

FIG. 1. The decline in radiolabeled plasma catecholamine levels (A, norepinephrine; B, isoproterenol) following infusion to steady-state levels in normal subjects (●) and patients with autonomic failure (○, MSA; △, PAF).

important role in determining the plasma level; thus, the normal levels observed in the patients with PAF studied by Esler et al. (10) presumably resulted from the delayed removal of catecholamines from plasma. Low plasma norepinephrine levels, despite reduced clearance, in patients with PAF may reflect greater involvement of the postganglionic neurons. Diminished clearance of catecholamines could also contribute to the prolonged pressor effect of injected sympathomimetic amines (2).

Impaired baroreflex control of blood pressure (BP) alters pressor responsivity. As observed in animal studies, the site and nature of the lesion determine the pharmacologic characteristics of the cardiovascular consequences (47). In the event of denervation, the BP response to norepinephrine is enhanced and the effects of indirectly acting sympathomimetics are diminished. In contrast, decentralization produces a more modest change in pressor responsiveness; the nonspecific increase in BP responses resulting from defective baroreflex modulation is not attended by a reduction in neuronal norepinephrine stores.

PAF and MSA can be distinguished on the basis of BP responses to various pressor drugs (31). Both disorders exhibit an exaggerated BP response to angiotensin, a nonadrenergic pressor agent. Although the response to norepinephrine is enhanced in both PAF and MSA, only patients with PAF exhibit a shift to the left in their BP-plasma norepinephrine dose-response curve. The decreased threshold in patients with PAF is a manifestation of true noradrenergic receptor supersensitivity, resulting from denervation caused by primary involvement of the postganglionic sympathetic neurons. The slope of this response is increased in patients with PAF because the lesion interrupts baroreflex control in addition to producing denervation. Although the response to tyramine is not totally absent, as in the experimental situation, the small norepinephrine increment suggests that neuronal stores may be reduced. Enhanced chronotropic and depressor effects of isoproterenol provide evidence of similar changes in cardiovascular functions controlled through β-adrenergic mechanisms (3). The in vitro observation of an increased number and affinity of α-adrenergic receptors on platelets (14) and the lack of catecholamine histofluorescence in skeletal muscle vessel walls (16) in PAF also support the existence of a primary defect in the postganglionic sympathetic neurons, which has been postulated in this disorder on the basis of neuropharmacologic findings (Table 1). Direct electrophysiologic measurements of sympathetic nerve activity in patients with PAF and MSA have confirmed this pathophysiologic distinction, which was suspected on the basis of neurochemical measurements and pharmacologic responses (9).

It is more difficult to assess central noradrenergic function, because limited access to the appropriate biologic compartments precludes direct measurements of brain metabolism. As mentioned earlier, norepinephrine is an important neurotransmitter in the central nervous system. Ascending and descending pathways originate from brain stem centers involved in various aspects of vegetative control. The locus ceruleus is one of the major noradrenergic nuclei in the brain; its connections with the hypothalamus and other higher brain regions highlight its key role in autonomic function.

Investigation of central neurotransmitter function is facilitated by the measurement of CSF levels of neurotransmitters and their metabolites. Although norepinephrine is present in CSF, its origin has not been clearly established. The predominant norepinephrine metabolite in the central nervous system is 3-methoxy-4-hydroxyphenylglycol (MHPG). Almost all MHPG in the CSF is unconjugated; because free MHPG easily crosses the blood-brain barrier, a portion of the MHPG in CSF is derived from peripheral norepinephrine metabolism. Thus, a correction for this contribution must be made to evaluate central noradrenergic function with this method (17).

A simple two-compartment kinetic model explains the relationships required for deriving an index of central norepinephrine metabolism (Fig. 2). By means of this model, it can be seen that a portion of the free MHPG in plasma must be subtracted from the total MHPG in CSF to arrive at the component generated by central norepinephrine metabolism. The fraction of plasma MHPG for this correction is yielded by the ratio of entry and exit constants for MHPG crossing into the central compartment. Theoretically, the exit constant should be slightly greater than the entry constant because of the bulk flow of the CSF. This ratio was determined empirically to be 0.9 by measuring the relationship between the CSF and plasma MHPG levels in normal subjects and patients with pheochromocytoma

TABLE 1. *Manifestations of peripheral noradrenergic involvement in pure autonomic failure*

Test	Result	Interpretation
Plasma NE	Low	Decrease in number or function of postganglionic sympathetic neurons
Plasma DHPG	Low	
Urinary NE metabolites	All reduced	
NE response to tyramine	Decreased	Reduced NE stores and/or defective neuronal uptake
Clearance of NE	Diminished	Impaired neuronal uptake
Cardiovascular responses to catecholamines	Leftward Shift	Denervation supersensitivity
Plasma NE response to acetylcholine	Absent	Ganglionic stimulation ineffective because of impaired function of noradrenergic neurons

NE, norepinephrine; DHPG, dihydroxyphenylglycol.

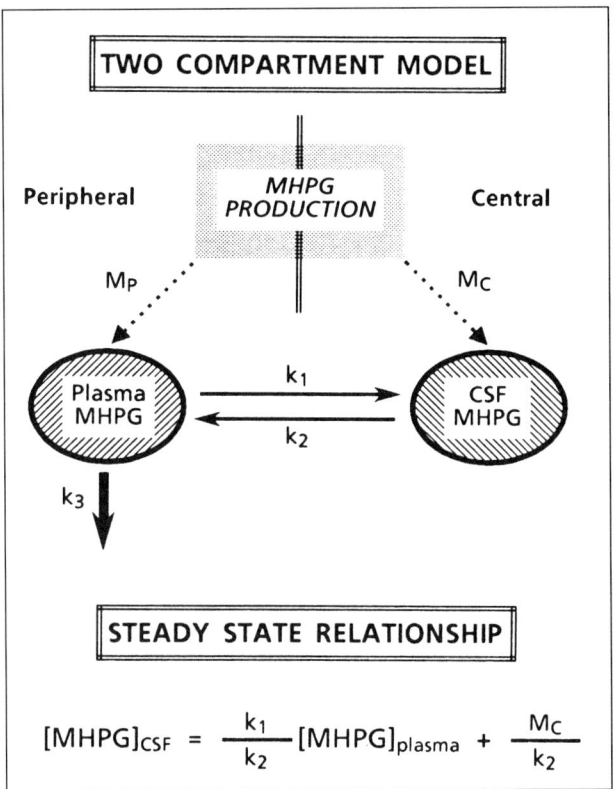

FIG. 2. A kinetic model illustrating the relationship between plasma and CSF levels of 3-methoxy-4-hydroxyphenylglycol (MHPG).

(17). Large amounts of norepinephrine and its metabolites are produced by this tumor; because this tumor is not under neural control, the elevation in the CSF level of MHPG results from the diffusion of free MHPG in plasma derived from a peripheral source.

The paradoxic observation of low levels of MHPG in the CSF of patients with PAF can be explained in view of the above correction method (28). Patients with PAF have low plasma norepinephrine levels, and consequently their plasma MHPG level reflects a small plasma contribution; the central norepinephrine metabolism appears to be normal. In contrast, the normal plasma MHPG concentrations in patients with MSA contribute a normal proportion of this metabolite to the total CSF level. Hence, the component of CSF MHPG derived from central norepinephrine metabolism is reduced. Neuropathologic studies in patients with MSA have confirmed degeneration in brain areas innervated by noradrenergic pathways, and neurochemical analyses have revealed a low norepinephrine content in the locus ceruleus, hypothalamus, and septal nuclei in patients with MSA (44).

Epinephrine

Although epinephrine certainly affects cardiovascular function, its role in metabolism has been more intensively investigated (11). Despite the importance of the adrenal medulla in protecting against severely stressful stimuli, there have been few studies in patients with autonomic failure. Insulin-induced hypoglycemia is a useful method for eliciting a variety of endocrine and autonomic responses (Table 2). To understand the changes caused by autonomic dysfunction, it is necessary first to describe the normal response. Plasma glucose levels drop precipitously within minutes of intravenous administration of insulin. Following the nadir, which occurs approximately 30 minutes after an insulin bolus, there is a biphasic glucose recovery curve (29), in which a brief rapid rise in the glucose level precedes a slower rate of recovery toward euglycemia (Fig. 3). Plasma catecholamine levels, primarily epinephrine and to a lesser extent norepinephrine, increase dramatically in conjunction with the hypoglycemia. This response is analogous to that induced by a bolus injection of epinephrine given when the glucose concentration drops below a critical level. The relationship between the epinephrine concentration and the rapid phase of glucose recovery is underscored by the absence of this phase in patients with adrenergic insufficiency, who lack catecholamine responses to hypoglycemia (29,30).

Most patients with MSA or PAF have deficient catecholamine responses (29). This abnormality has no localizing value, as diminished or absent responses have also been observed following sympathectomy, splanchnectomy, and adrenalectomy. The administration of arecoline, a cholinergic agonist, increases the plasma epinephrine level in normal subjects and patients with MSA after pretreatment with glycopyrrolate to block the peripheral muscarinic effects (41). Failure to increase the epinephrine level in response to direct cholinergic stimulation in patients with PAF suggests that the absence of catecholamine responses during hypoglycemia results from peripheral dysfunction. In contrast, the lesion responsible for preventing the hypoglycemic response in patients with MSA appears to be located centrally. Although the adrenal medulla may be critically important in the body's response to crisis situations, the absence of catecholamine responses does

TABLE 2. *Hormonal and peptide responses to insulin-induced hypoglycemia in patients with autonomic failure*

Hormone/Peptide	PAF	MSA
Adrenal		
Epinephrine	Decreased	Decreased
Cortisol	Normal	Normal
Gastrointestinal		
Glucagon	Normal	Normal
Pancreatic polypeptide	Decreased	Decreased
Gastrin	Increased	Decreased
Pituitary		
Growth hormone	Normal	Normal
β-Endorphin	Normal	Decreased
ACTH	Normal	Decreased

PAE, pure autonomic failure; MSA, multiple-system atrophy; ACTH, adrenocorticotropic hormone.

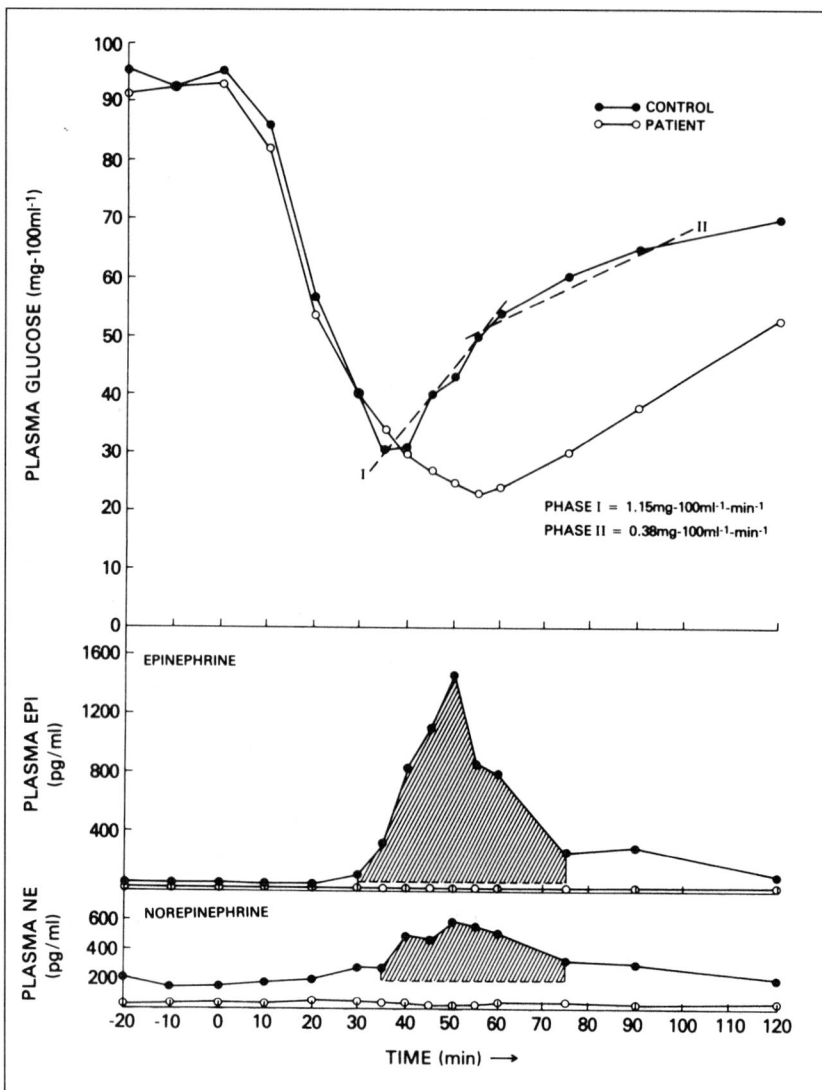

FIG. 3. Plasma glucose and catecholamine responses to insulin hypoglycemia in a normal subject and a patient with adrenergic insufficiency. *NE*, nonepinephrine; *EPI*, epinephrine.

not impair glucose homeostasis. Adrenergic insufficiency does not alter the sequence, magnitude, or temporal profile of other counterregulatory hormones (30).

Dopamine

Dopamine, a monoamine, is present in a variety of organs in the body, but plasma levels have not been systematically evaluated in patients with autonomic failure. Deficiency of dopamine β-hydroxylase is a rare cause of sympathetic dysfunction and is characterized by the inability to synthesize norepinephrine and epinephrine (4,23). The enzymatic block leads to the buildup of dopamine in the plasma and CSF (5). In affected patients, dopamine is released in response to sympathetic activation. Localization of the neurotransmitter in noradrenergic neurons is supported by tyramine release and clonidine suppression. Furthermore, BP is increased following the administration of metyrosine, suggesting that the elevated dopamine levels in plasma contribute to the occurrence of orthostatic hypotension (4).

Central dopaminergic pathways mediate many important functions. Of particular relevance to MSA is the nigrostriatal system, because its involvement produces parkinsonism in the context of several involuntary movement disorders. Central dopamine turnover can be gauged by measurement of CSF levels of homovanillic acid (HVA). Fortunately, interpretation of these results is less complicated than that for MHPG, because acidic compounds do not readily cross the blood-brain barrier. There is a rostral-caudal concentration gradient in the CSF for HVA, so a standardized method for collecting aliquots must be employed. In patients with MSA, the level of HVA in CSF is reduced to approximately half that observed in normal subjects (36). Dopaminergic receptors apparently remain functional in patients with MSA, as bromocriptine administration elicits decreases in the CSF level of HVA

(50). Consistent with the therapeutic benefit of antiparkinsonian medications, treatment with levodopa-carbidopa (Sinemet) increases the CSF level of HVA (36). It is interesting that patients with MSA who do not manifest parkinsonian features have low CSF levels of HVA. This might be explained by the existence of a threshold phenomenon or by the involvement of dopamine systems unrelated to motor control. Normal levels of HVA in the CSF of patients with PAF are in keeping with involvement limited to peripheral pathways.

Serotonin

Despite the presence of serotonin in tissues throughout the body, clinical investigations have focused on its role as a central nervous system neurotransmitter. Distribution of this monoamine within the brain and spinal cord is consistent with its importance in mediating vigilance and vegetative control. The major metabolite of serotonin, 5-hydroxyindoleacetic acid (5-HIAA), is removed from the CSF by an active transport system that can be blocked by probenecid. Similar to the pattern seen for HVA, there is no peripheral contribution of 5-HIAA to the CSF level, which makes interpretation of the CSF levels of these acid metabolites straightforward. The level of 5-HIAA in CSF is low in patients with MSA (36); this probably results from reduced turnover rather than from a transport deficit, as probenecid elevates the CSF levels of HVA and 5-HIAA in these patients. Low CSF levels of 5-HIAA in patients with MSA may reflect involvement of the serotonergic pathways in the spinal cord. The spinal cord contribution to the CSF level of 5-HIAA appears to be larger than that for HVA, as there is a less substantial rostral-caudal gradient for 5-HIAA. Although no consistent changes have been observed in the brains of patients with MSA obtained post mortem, regional reductions in serotonin concentration do occur in patients with Parkinson's disease. Central nervous system serotonergic function is apparently normal in patients with PAF, in that the CSF levels of 5-HIAA are normal in this disorder (36).

Acetylcholine

The evaluation of cholinergic function in the periphery is limited to the use of pharmacologic strategies. A somewhat more indirect approach involves assessment of the peptide responses that are under cholinergic control, which is discussed later in this chapter. Although it is possible to measure levels of acetylcholine, a number of factors (i.e., metabolism and lability) confound correlation with physiologic and pharmacologic responses. Ganglionic cholinergic (nicotinic) neurotransmission can be studied by measuring the plasma norepinephrine response to the intravenous infusion of acetylcholine after blocking peripheral muscarinic effects with glycopyrrolate (40). This is particularly relevant to MSA, as the number of neurons is reduced in the intermediolateral cell column, the site of origin for cholinergic neurons that innervate the sympathetic ganglia. In normal subjects, the plasma norepinephrine level increases in proportion to the rate of acetylcholine administration. Patients with PAF do not manifest an increment in the plasma norepinephrine level during acetylcholine infusion. Two response patterns occur in patients with MSA: (a) no response; and (b) a greater-than-normal increase in the plasma norepinephrine concentration at low doses, followed by a reduction to preinfusion norepinephrine levels with increasing infusion rates of acetylcholine. This latter response pattern is consistent with ganglionic supersensitivity, as the plasma norepinephrine response is exaggerated at low infusion rates. Depolarization blockade could produce the decrement observed with higher doses. Those patients with MSA who did not respond to the acetylcholine might have had peripheral involvement, which can occur in MSA; however, extreme supersensitivity could also prevent the response at lower doses. The lack of a norepinephrine response in patients with PAF is consistent with a primarily postganglionic noradrenergic dysfunction, as suggested by the results of numerous studies discussed earlier in this chapter.

Two approaches have been employed to investigate central cholinergic pathways. Acetylcholinesterase (AChE) activity is detectable in CSF; several neuropharmacologic and neurophysiologic lines of evidence point toward a neuronal source of the enzyme. Low AChE activity in the CSF from patients with MSA is consistent with central cholinergic involvement (38). However, the low enzyme activities do not correlate with low levels of monoamine metabolites in these patients. It therefore appears that these various transmitter systems are independently affected by the degenerative process. Because there are a number of cholinergic pathways with widespread innervation in the nervous system, it would be difficult to attribute this neurochemical abnormality to a specific lesion. Normal AChE activity in patients with PAF demonstrates that autonomic dysfunction alone does not alter the CSF levels of the enzyme.

The interaction between neurotransmitters and pituitary peptide release permits use of a neuroendocrine strategy to investigate cholinergic function in the hypothalamopituitary axis. A provocative drug must cross the blood-brain barrier or stimulate a response in an area that is relatively accessible. In addition, peripheral effects should be blocked to facilitate interpretation. The pituitary release of adrenocorticotropic hormone (ACTH) is modulated by a cholinergic mechanism in the hypothalamus. Following pretreatment with glycopyrrolate, arecoline failed to increase plasma ACTH levels in patients with PAF and MSA (41). Although these results might suggest a central cholinergic involvement in both disorders, this paradox highlights the need to consider interactions among various neurotransmitter systems. Findings from animal studies indicate that a β-adrenergic mechanism also appears to participate in mediating ACTH release. Intravenously administered isoproterenol increases the plasma ACTH level, even in rats that have undergone sectioning of the pituitary stalk or that have lesions of the median eminence (25). This effect of isoproterenol is blocked by propranolol. As mentioned earlier, patients with MSA but not PAF show an increase in their plasma epinephrine levels following arecoline administration (41). As epinephrine crosses the blood-brain barrier in the hypothalamic area, adrenal medullary activity could furnish the β-adrenergic stimulation required to release ACTH. Thus, in patients with PAF, the plasma ACTH cannot increase because the peripheral epinephrine increment is lacking. Although patients with MSA release epinephrine, the inability to increase the ACTH in response to arecoline likely results from degeneration in the hypothalamus. Neuropathologic and neurochemical studies have confirmed cholinergic involvement in several brain regions, including the hypothalamus (44).

NEUROPEPTIDES AND OTHER NEUROHUMORAL SUBSTANCES

The domain of control is amplified for the autonomic nervous system through its interaction with other peptide and hormonal control systems. These substances resemble true hormones, although many peptides serve as transmitters or modulators within the nervous system. The need for transport to target organs is consistent with the role of such peptides in the continuous regulation of secondary mechanisms critical for homeostasis; in contrast, responses of the autonomic nervous system occur immediately. Myriad peptides have been described in the last decade, but the specific function of many of these substances has not been determined. Three general classes of peptides are discussed here: (a) peptides related to cardiovascular control; (b) gastrointestinal peptides; and (c) peptides involved in pituitary responses. Melatonin is also included in this review because of its relationship to the neurologic control of circadian rhythms. This review is limited to substances that have been studied in patients with autonomic failure.

Cardiovascular Control

A vast array of substances has been associated with BP control (Table 3). The modulation of neurotransmitter function by neuropeptides provides an avenue for interaction among the various systems that relate to BP control. These interactions may be complex, making clinical investigation very difficult. However, relatively few peptides have been examined in the context of autonomic failure, despite their importance in cardiovascular regulation.

Activation of the renin-angiotensin system by decreases in blood volume, renal perfusion pressure, or plasma sodium content is consistent with its primary role in the ongoing maintenance of BP. Renin is synthesized, stored, and released by juxtaglomerular cells in the walls of afferent renal arterioles. A series of enzymatic reactions, initiated by the action of renin on angiotensinogen, leads to the formation of angiotensin II, the main hormone of this system. Autonomic influences are mediated by adrenergic receptors: α_1-adrenergic activation causes vasoconstriction in the renal bed, while renin secretion is modulated by β_1-adrenergic receptors located on juxtaglomerular cells. Hence, it is not surprising that patients with autonomic dysfunction exhibit abnormalities in the handling of sodium and water. Nocturnal diuresis in patients with MSA and PAF is characterized by excessive excretion of salt and water (48). The low supine levels of plasma renin activity in these patients do not respond to salt restriction, upright posture, or the infusion of isoproterenol (1,3,48,49). As mentioned earlier, patients with autonomic failure manifest exaggerated pressor responses to angiotensin (31). Although it is conceivable that low renin activity might produce an increase in angiotensin receptor sensitivity, the mechanism of this abnormal BP responsivity appears to involve defective baroreflex modulation.

More than three decades ago, atrium-specific granules were identified and later shown to contain atrial natriuretic peptide (ANP), which has extremely potent diuretic and natriuretic properties. This peptide is primarily released in response to atrial distention (13). The sympathetic nervous system may modulate release, as denervation abolishes the ANP response to volume expansion (27). In addition, sympathetic stimulation appears to accentuate ANP release. Autonomic dysfunction does not inhibit ANP release in humans. Plasma ANP levels fluctuate with systemic BP in patients who have autonomic failure as part of the Guillain-Barré syndrome (43). In patients with MSA and PAF, plasma levels of ANP respond appropriately to postural and fluid volume changes (15). Therefore, it does not appear likely that ANP is involved in causing the excessive nocturnal fluid loss seen in this disorder, because the plasma (15) and urinary (37) levels are lower at night, when the diuresis occurs.

Gastrointestinal Peptides

The anatomic distribution and localization of gastrointestinal peptides reflect their physiologic role. Some pep-

TABLE 3. *Neurotransmitters and neuropeptides involved in cardiovascular regulation[a]*

Acetylcholine	Neurotensin
Adrenocorticotropic hormone	**Norepinephrine**
Angiotensin	**Opioids**
Dopamine	Oxytocin
Epinephrine	**Serotonin**
γ-Aminobutyric acid	**Somatostatin**
Glutamic acid	**Substance P**
Histamine	Thyrotropin-releasing hormone
Natriuretic peptides	
Neuropeptide Y	**Vasopressin**

[a]Bold print indicates those that have been studied in autonomic failure.

tides are secreted from specific organs; these substances typically function as hormones. Other peptides are released from cells within their target organs, so that the local effects determine the major function of these substances. Gastrointestinal function may be dramatically altered in disorders of autonomic failure. Gastrointestinal peptides are pathophysiologically significant in understanding a variety of clinical phenomena observed in such patients. In addition, interaction between the autonomic nervous system and various gastrointestinal peptides permits the use of peptide responses to assess the functional integrity of gastrointestinal innervation.

Glucagon is an example of a gastrointestinal peptide. It is released from clusters of cells within the pancreas and functions primarily as a hyperglycemic hormone. Sympathectomy or adrenalectomy does not alter the glucagon response to hypoglycemia. Although patients with severe adrenergic insufficiency have normal basal levels and glucagon responses to hypoglycemia (30), diminished responses to insulin have been observed in some patients with MSA (21,42). The low plasma norepinephrine levels in the group studied by Sasaki et al. (42) suggest that their patients with MSA might have had peripheral sympathetic dysfunction.

Pancreatic polypeptide (PP) serves as a valuable biochemical index of parasympathetic nervous system activity, although its exact function has not been clearly established. Muscarinic anticholinergic drugs and truncal vagotomy block the PP response to hypoglycemia, consistent with control by a vagal, cholinergic mechanism. In normal subjects, plasma PP levels rise dramatically during hypoglycemia (32). Most patients with PAF and MSA have deficient PP responses to insulin-induced hypoglycemia. This abnormality provides biochemical evidence for the existence of pandysautonomia in these disorders. Insulin-induced hypoglycemia can also be used to assess sympathetic, parasympathetic, and adrenal medullary function in conjunction with measurement of catecholamine responses.

Gastrin increases antral motility and stomach acid production through its local effects on the gastric mucosa. The impact of autonomic nervous system innervation on gastrin release is complex. Basal gastrin levels are elevated after vagotomy, although vagal stimulation heightens release of the peptide. Other factors that affect gastrin release (e.g., distention and high stomach pH) presumably predominate following section of the vagus. The gastrin response to hypoglycemia persists even after highly selective vagotomy. An adrenergic influence has been suggested as an explanation for this apparent paradox; gastrin can be released by β-adrenergic stimulation, and there appears to be a correlation between epinephrine and gastrin responses during hypoglycemia. Basal gastrin levels are elevated in patients with PAF, presumably because these patients have peripheral vagal involvement (35). Differences in β-adrenergic receptor sensitivity may explain the greater-than-normal and less-than-normal gastrin increments during hypoglycemia observed in patients with PAF and MSA, respectively. As discussed previously, both groups of patients show diminished epinephrine responses to hypoglycemia, but only patients with PAF have supersensitive adrenergic pressor responses. In fact, only patients with PAF manifest an exaggerated gastrin response to intravenously administered isoproterenol (39), consistent with a supersensitive β-adrenergic-mediated release of this peptide.

Pituitary Responses

A variety of endocrine mechanisms in the body are activated by pituitary peptides, which are released through neural innervation or secretion of releasing factors from the hypothalamus. The hypothalamopituitary axis serves as the endocrine equivalent of the sympathetic nervous system, and also originates in the hypothalamus. Whereas the posterior pituitary is primarily concerned with the regulation of fluid balance, anterior pituitary hormones serve as messengers to activate diverse processes with long-term species survival value, including metabolism, growth, and protective responses against stress.

Growth hormone is released by the anterior pituitary following stimulation by many factors that also activate the sympathetic nervous system. Although patients with severe adrenergic insufficiency have normal growth hormone responses to insulin-induced hypoglycemia (30), Sasaki et al. (42) found the response to be absent in four patients with MSA. Normal growth hormone responses in patients who lack catecholamine responses to hypoglycemia serve to minimize the duration of low blood glucose levels by activating counterregulatory mechanisms. Clonidine, an α_2-adrenoceptor agonist, stimulates growth hormone release in patients with PAF but not MSA. This observation is consistent with lesions in the central pathways that modulate release of this pituitary peptide in MSA (7,46).

Two other anterior pituitary peptides, β-endorphin and ACTH, are derived from a common precursor. Insulin evokes an increase in the plasma levels of these peptides only if hypoglycemia develops. Pharmacologic studies suggest that release of β-endorphin and ACTH is mediated by a central cholinergic pathway. These peptide responses to hypoglycemia are virtually absent in patients with MSA (34). Normal β-endorphin and ACTH responses in patients with PAF are consistent with the normal function of this central cholinergic mechanism. Arecoline has been used as a pharmacologic probe to assess central cholinergic function. Curiously, patients with MSA and PAF do not show an increase in their plasma ACTH levels after arecoline administration (41) (Fig. 4). As discussed earlier, these paradoxic findings highlight the need to consider interactions among the various neurotransmitter systems. A central cholinergic involvement in MSA is supported by the observation of reduced choline acetyltransferase activity in postmortem brain tissue from patients with MSA (44).

Vasopressin, also known as *antidiuretic hormone*, is a potent vasoconstrictor, but its primary hormonal function relates to water conservation. Water deprivation and extra-

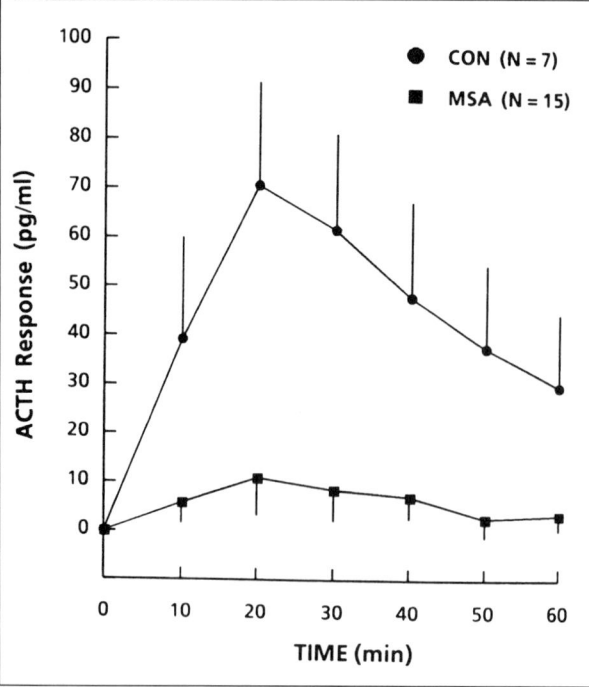

FIG. 4. The plasma ACTH response to arecoline administration in normal subjects (*CON*) and patients with multiple-system atrophy (*MSA*). Plasma ACTH levels in patients with pure autonomic failure also fail to increase in response to arecoline.

cellular fluid volume depletion can cause changes in serum osmolality and activate thoracic stretch receptors. Either of these two stimuli can elicit release of vasopressin from the posterior pituitary (20). Patients with autonomic failure lack the brisk rise in plasma vasopressin (52) observed in normal subjects (8). Preservation of the response to saline solution implicates an afferent lesion (51). In addition, suppression of vasopressin by levodopa or naloxone does not occur in patients with MSA, presumably as a result of central nervous system lesions. Like the pressor response to angiotensin, the pressor response to vasopressin is enhanced (26), but this nonspecific change reflects inadequate baroreflex function rather than receptor supersensitivity. Of clinical relevance, a synthetic analog of vasopressin may represent a useful therapeutic modality in some patients with orthostatic hypotension (24).

Melatonin

Circadian rhythms occur in many species but are most apparent in the periodic release of various hormones seen in humans. These cycles often correspond to patterns of light and sleep, but their functional significance is not entirely clear. The pineal gland is closely linked to the "biologic clock." The rhythmic secretion of melatonin is controlled by an endogenous circadian oscillator in the suprachiasmatic nucleus. Environmental light strongly influences the diurnal cycle, and this effect is mediated through retinohypothalamic projections. Interaction with the sympathetic nervous system occurs at the level of the thoracic intermediolateral cell column, which is innervated by fibers from the medial forebrain bundle and midbrain reticular formation. The superior cervical ganglion, with preganglionic input from the intermediolateral cell column, distributes ascending fibers that innervate the pineal gland. The activity of these noradrenergic synapses is increased at night; the pineal gland responds to β-adrenergic stimulation by increasing the synthesis and release of melatonin.

Although the function of melatonin is not known, determination of the secretion pattern can be of value in distinguishing between central and peripheral sympathetic nervous system lesions in humans. Relatively little melatonin is released during the day in normal subjects. Tetsuo et al. (45) demonstrated a diurnal pattern for the release of 6-hydroxymelatonin, the conjugated melatonin metabolite excreted in the urine. Urinary levels of 6-hydroxymelatonin can be used to evaluate pineal activity; differences in the diurnal pattern reflect localization of the lesion or lesions in patients with autonomic failure. The amount of 6-hydroxymelatonin excreted is low in patients with PAF, but the circadian rhythm is preserved, with most of the metabolite appearing during the night. In contrast, many patients with MSA excrete as much 6-hydroxymelatonin during the day as at night. Disruption of the cyclic pattern in patients with MSA probably stems from involvement of the central nervous system pathways that mediate the timing of melatonin synthesis and release. In patients with PAF, the low levels of melatonin excreted despite a normal pattern is consistent with reduced pineal stimulation, an expected result of postganglionic dysfunction.

CONCLUSION

Central and peripheral forms of autonomic failure are characterized by distinct differences in pathophysiologic characteristics that can be evaluated through neurochemical measurements and pharmacologic responses. The investigation of patients with autonomic dysfunction has shed light on the processes of normal function and metabolism. Neuropharmacologic approaches not only clarify the pathophysiologic nature of these disorders, but also point out directions for the development of rational pharmacotherapy. Current methods need refinement and new strategies must be developed that keep pace with new technology, so that our understanding of these degenerative neurologic disorders, for which there are no adequate animal models, will continue to increase.

REFERENCES

1. Bannister R, et al. Cardiovascular reflexes and biochemical responses in progressive autonomic failure. *Brain* 1977;100:327–344.
2. Bannister R, et al. Defective cardiovascular reflexes and supersensitivity to sympathomimetic drugs in autonomic failure. *Brain* 1979;102:163–176.

3. Baser SM, et al. Beta-receptor sensitivity in autonomic failure. *Neurology* 1991;41:1107–1112.
4. Biaggioni I, et al. Dopamine in dopamine-β-hydroxylase deficiency. *N Engl J Med* 1987;317:1415–1416.
5. Biaggioni I, et al. Dopamine-β-hydroxylase deficiency in humans. *Neurology* 1990;40:370–373.
6. Cohen J, et al. Somatic and autonomic function in progressive autonomic failure and multiple system atrophy. *Ann Neurol* 1987;22:692–699.
7. da Costa DF, et al. Growth hormone response to clonidine is impaired in patients with central sympathetic degeneration. *Clin Exp Hypertens* 1984;6:1843–1846.
8. Davis R, et al. The response of arginine vasopressin and plasma renin to postural change in normal man, with observations on syncope. *Clin Sci Mol Med* 1976;51:267–274.
9. Dotson R, et al. Sympathetic neural outflow directly recorded in patients with primary autonomic failure: clinical observations, microneurography, and histopathology. *Neurology* 1990;40:1079–1085.
10. Esler M, et al. Norepinephrine kinetics in patients with idiopathic autonomic insufficiency. *Circ Res* 1980;46(Suppl 1):147–148.
11. Garber AJ, et al. The role of adrenergic mechanisms in the substrate and hormonal response to insulin-induced hypoglycemia in man. *J Clin Invest* 1976;58:7–15.
12. Goldstein DS, et al. Patterns of plasma levels of catechols in neurogenic orthostatic hypotension. *Ann Neurol* 1989;26:558–563.
13. Hollister AS, et al. Sodium loading and posture modulate human atrial natriuretic factor plasma levels. *Hypertension* 1986;8(Suppl 2):106–111.
14. Kafka MS, et al. Alpha-adrenergic receptors in orthostatic hypotension syndromes. *Neurology* 1984;34:1121–1125.
15. Kaufmann H, et al. Atrial natriuretic factor in human autonomic failure. *Neurology* 1990;40:1115–1119.
16. Kontos HA, et al. Norepinephrine depletion in idiopathic orthostatic hypotension. *Ann Intern Med* 1975;82:336–341.
17. Kopin IJ, et al. Relationship between plasma and cerebrospinal fluid levels of 3-methoxy-4-hydroxyphenylglycol. *Science* 1983;219:73–75.
18. Kopin IJ, et al. Urinary catecholamine metabolites distinguish different types of sympathetic neuronal dysfunction in patients with orthostatic hypotension. *J Clin Endocrinol Metab* 1983;57:632–637.
19. Lake CR, et alJ. Use of plasma norepinephrine for evaluation of sympathetic neuronal function in man. *Life Sci* 1976;18:1315–1326.
20. Lightman SL, Williams TDM. Hypothalamic function in autonomic failure. In: Bannister R, ed. *Autonomic Failure*. London: Oxford University Press; 1988:381–392.
21. Long RG, et al. Pancreatic hormone release in Chagas' disease and the Shy-Drager syndrome. *Gut* 1979;20:A921.
22. Luft F, von Euler U. Two cases of postural hypotension showing a deficiency in release of norepinephrine and epinephrine. *J Clin Invest* 1953;32:1065–1069.
23. Man in't Veld AJ, et al. Congenital dopamine-β-hydroxylase deficiency: a novel orthostatic syndrome. *Lancet* 1987;1:183–187.
24. Mathias CJ, et al. Desmopressin reduces nocturnal polyuria, reverses overnight weight loss and improves morning postural hypotension in autonomic failure. *Br Med J* 1986;293:353–354.
25. Mezey E, et al. β-Adrenergic mechanism of insulin-induced adrenocorticotrophin release from the anterior pituitary. *Science* 1984;226:1085–1087.
26. Möhring J, et al. Greatly enhanced pressor response to antidiuretic hormone in patients with impaired cardiovascular reflexes due to idiopathic orthostatic hypotension. *J Cardiovasc Pharmacol* 1980;2:367–376.
27. Petterson A, et al. Effect of blood volume expansion and sympathetic denervation on plasma levels of atrial natriuretic factor (ANF) in the rat. *Acta Physiol Scand* 1985;124:309–311.
28. Polinsky RJ, et al. Chronic autonomic failure: CSF and plasma 3-methoxy-4-hydroxyphenylglycol. *Neurology* 1984;34:979–983.
29. Polinsky RJ, et al. The adrenal medullary response to hypoglycemia in patients with orthostatic hypotension. *J Clin Endocrinol Metab* 1980;51:1401–1406.
30. Polinsky RJ, et al. Hormonal responses to hypoglycemia in orthostatic hypotension patients with adrenergic insufficiency. *Life Sci* 1981;29:417–425.
31. Polinsky RJ, et al. Pharmacologic distinction of different orthostatic hypotension syndromes. *Neurology* 1981;31:1–7.
32. Polinsky RJ, et al. Pancreatic polypeptide responses to hypoglycemia in chronic autonomic failure. *J Clin Endocrinol Metab* 1982;54:48–52.
33. Polinsky RJ, et al. Decreased sympathetic neuronal uptake in idiopathic orthostatic hypotension. *Ann Neurol* 1985;18:48–53.
34. Polinsky RJ, et al. Beta-endorphin, ACTH, and catecholamine responses in chronic autonomic failure. *Ann Neurol* 1987;21:573–577.
35. Polinsky RJ, et al. Gastrin responses in patients with adrenergic insufficiency. *J Neurol Neurosurg Psychiatry* 1988;51:67–71.
36. Polinsky RJ, et al. Low lumbar CSF levels of homovanillic acid and 5-hydroxyindoleacetic acid in multiple system atrophy with autonomic failure. *J Neurol Neurosurg Psychiatry* 1988;51:914–919.
37. Polinsky RJ, et al. Atrial natriuretic peptide in autonomic failure. *Neurology (India)* 1989;37(Suppl):148.
38. Polinsky RJ, et al. CSF acetylcholinesterase levels are reduced in multiple system atrophy with autonomic failure. *Neurology* 1989;39:40–44.
39. Polinsky RJ, et al. Plasma gastrin responses to isoproterenol in patients with autonomic failure. *J Auton Nerv Syst* 1989;27:88–89.
40. Polinsky RJ, et al. Ganglionic responsivity in patients with autonomic failure. *Clin Auton Res* 1991;1:83.
41. Polinsky RJ, et al. Central and peripheral effects of arecoline in patients with autonomic failure. *J Neurol Neurosurg Psychiatry* 1991;54:807–812.
42. Sasaki K, et al. Hormonal response to insulin-induced hypoglycemia in patients with Shy-Drager syndrome. *Metabolism* 1983;32:977–981.
43. Saxenhofer H, et al. Atrial natriuretic factor in the Landry-Guillain-Barré syndrome. *N Engl J Med* 1988;319:448.
44. Spokes EGS, et al. Multiple system atrophy with autonomic failure: clinical, histological and neurochemical observations on four cases. *J Neurol Sci* 1979;43:59–82.
45. Tetsuo M, et al. Urinary 6-hydroxymelatonin excretion in patients with orthostatic hypotension. *J Clin Endocrinol Metab* 1981;53:607–610.
46. Thomaides TN, et al. Growth hormone response to clonidine in central and peripheral primary autonomic failure. *Lancet* 1992;340:263–266.
47. Trendelenburg U. Supersensitivity and subsensitivity to sympathomimetic amines. *Pharmacol Rev* 1963;15:225–276.
48. Wilcox CS, et al. Comparison of the renin response to dopamine and noradrenaline in normal subjects and patients with autonomic insufficiency. *Clin Sci Mol Med* 1974;46:481–488.
49. Wilcox CS, et al. Sodium homeostasis in patients with autonomic failure. *Clin Sci Mol Med* 1977;53:321–328.
50. Williams AC, et al. Actions of bromocriptine in the Shy-Drager and Steele-Richardson-Olszewski syndromes. In: Fuxe K, Calne DB, eds. *Dopaminergic Ergots and Motor Control*. New York: Pergamon Press; 1979:271–283.
51. Williams TDM, et al. Vasopressin secretion in progressive autonomic failure: evidence for defective afferent cardiovascular pathways. *J Neurol Neurosurg Psychiatry* 1985;48:225–228.
52. Zerbe RL, et al. Vasopressin response to orthostatic hypotension: etiologic and clinical implications. *Am J Med* 1983;74:265–271.
53. Ziegler MG, et al. The sympathetic-nervous-system defect in primary orthostatic hypotension. *N Engl J Med* 1977;296:293–297.

CHAPTER 45

Gastrointestinal Dysfunction: Approach to Management

Charlene M. Prather and Michael Camilleri

---

1. Gastrointestinal dysfunction may result from neurologic disease.
2. Neurologic disorders affect extrinsic autonomic nerve control or the enteric nervous system (the "little brain" in the digestive tract).
3. Pathophysiologic studies identify neuropathic and myopathic disorders in the upper gut (gastroparesis, intestinal pseudo-obstruction) and differentiate colonic inertia from disordered defecation in patients with constipation or incontinence.
4. Autonomic function tests identify disturbances of extrinsic neurologic control of viscera.
5. These strategies help select treatment for patients with gastrointestinal motor dysfunction secondary to neurologic disease. The principles of treatment are: restoration of hydration and nutrition, suppression of bacterial overgrowth, stimulation of motility, and decompression.

INTRODUCTION

The autonomic nervous system is intimately involved in the modulation of normal gastrointestinal function through the extrinsic neural supply and the enteric nervous system of the gastrointestinal tract. Disorders of the nervous system affecting gastrointestinal tract function are manifested primarily as abnormalities in motor (rather than absorptive or secretory) functions of digestive processes. The focus of this chapter will be on the normal neural–gut interactions, the common clinical manifestations of gut dysmotility encountered in neurologic disorders, and a discussion of the principles of diagnosis and treatment of neurologic diseases affecting the gut.

INTERACTIONS BETWEEN THE EXTRINSIC NERVOUS SYSTEM AND THE GUT

Normal motility and transit through the gastrointestinal tract result from an intricately balanced series of control mechanisms (see Fig. 12-2): the electrical and contractile properties of the smooth muscle cell, control by the intrinsic nervous system through chemical transmitters such as acetylcholine and gastrointestinal neuropeptides, and extrinsic neural pathways (sympathetic and parasympathetic). The neuropeptides may act as circulating hormones or may act at the site of their release (paracrine) (see Chapter 12).

The electrical properties of the smooth muscle of the gut are the result of transmembrane fluxes of ions; as in other excitable tissues, these fluxes alter the membrane potential and result in muscle contraction once the threshold potential is exceeded. Infiltrative or degenerative processes that affect the excitability of the smooth muscle cells of the gut prevent the development of normal contractions and result in disorders of gastrointestinal motility.

The intrinsic, or enteric, nervous system contains about 100 million neurons, approximately the number present in the spinal cord. This integrative system is separate from the sympathetic and parasympathetic portions of the autonomic nervous system. It has sensory mechanoreceptors and chemoreceptors, interneurons that process sensory input and control effector (motor and sensory) units, and motor neurons that serve as the primary effector cells involved in the development of motor function in the gut. Preprogrammed synaptic circuits serve to integrate motor function in different regions and thereby control the coordi-

---

C. M. Prather: Department of Gastroenterology, Mayo Medical School, Rochester, Minnesota 55905. M. Camilleri: Department of Gastroenterology, Mayo Clinic, Rochester, Minnesota 55905.

nated behavior of the entire gastrointestinal tract, such as the peristaltic reflex. The synaptic pathways in the gut wall are capable of autonomous adjustment in response to sensory input; they can also be modulated by the extrinsic nervous system, such as excitation by vagal preganglionic fibers, or inhibition by sympathetic pathways.

The vagus is composed of preganglionic cholinergic fibers (see Fig. 12-2) that synapse with preprogrammed circuits in ganglionated enteric plexuses. These enteric neurons include myenteric cholinergic neurons, which excite effector cells such as smooth muscle cells to produce contraction or excite surface epithelial cells to absorb or secrete fluids and electrolytes. The concept of programmed circuits, motor or secretory, controlled by command vagal preganglionic or sympathetic postganglionic fibers is consistent with the disparity between the number of extrinsic nerve fibers and the millions of enteric plexus neurons. Thus, there are about 40,000 preganglionic vagal fibers at the level of the diaphragm and 100 million neurons of the enteric nervous system (see Fig. 12-1). The sympathetic supply inactivates neural circuits that generate motor activity while allowing continuous activity of intrinsic inhibitory innervation by the enteric nerves. Extrinsic vagal fibers also synapse with nonadrenergic inhibitory intramural neurons in the gut. This presynaptic inhibition is mediated by several transmitters, including serotonin, opioid peptides, acetylcholine, and histamine, as well as sympathetic noradrenergic fibers. Loss of the sympathetic inhibitory supply ("the brake") results in excessive or uncoordinated phasic pressure activity in the gut (26).

The extrinsic innervation of the gut is considered in greater detail in Chapter 12. In summary, it consists of the parasympathetic vagal and sacral nerves (S-2, S-3, and S-4) and the sympathetic outflow from the intermediolateral column of the spinal cord, between the levels of the fifth thoracic and third lumbar segments. The sympathetic nerves synapse in the celiac, superior mesenteric, and inferior mesenteric ganglia; sympathetic fibers follow the respective arterial trunks.

Extrinsic nerves are intimately involved in the control of the striated muscle portions of the esophagus and the external anal sphincter. Although the smooth muscle portion of the gut can function fairly normally without the extrinsic nerves, the latter modulate the intrinsic neural circuits, integrate activity in widely separated regions of the gastrointestinal tract, and exert control in certain regions (i.e., the stomach and distal portion of the colon) more so than in others (e.g., the small bowel).

COMMON GASTROINTESTINAL SYNDROMES IN NEUROLOGIC DISORDERS

Dysphagia

Dysphagia is the sensation of difficult swallowing. Table 1 lists common causes of dysphagia encountered in clinical

TABLE 1. *Common causes of dysphagia in clinical practice*

Type	Cause
Transfer dysphagia	Brain stem lesion (*e.g.,* amyotrophic lateral sclerosis, parkinsonism)
	Glossopharyngeal or vagal injury (*e.g.,* thyroid cancer or surgery)
	Neuromuscular dysfunction (*e.g.,* myasthenia gravis)
Esophageal dysphagia	Mechanical (*e.g.,* benign or malignant stricture)
	Motor (*e.g.,* achalasia)

practice. Oropharyngeal dysfunction results in "transfer dysphagia" or an inability to propel the food bolus from the mouth to the esophagus (30). Neuromuscular dysphagia is encountered in diseases of the pharyngeal skeletal muscles, such as lower motor neuron (e.g., bulbar polio) or muscular (e.g., amyotrophic lateral sclerosis) diseases. These are manifested as difficulty in initiating a swallow. Dysphagia may also result from esophageal smooth muscle disorders; peristalsis is abnormal and may be due to neural or muscle dysfunction. The lower esophageal sphincter may fail to relax, as in achalasia, or the smooth muscle cells may degenerate or lose their excitability, as in systemic sclerosis.

Dysphagia that is restricted to solids suggests a mechanical cause due to a narrowed lumen that fails to allow the bolus to pass. Dysphagia restricted primarily to liquids is suggestive of oropharyngeal disease or achalasia, whereas dysphagia restricted to both liquids and solids may indicate neuromuscular dysphagia.

The physical examination may show evidence of coexisting disease such as neuromuscular abnormalities of the oropharynx. The clinician must check dentition, assess movement of the uvula for IX or X nerve palsy, check the jaw jerk (increased in pseudobulbar palsy), and palpate the cheek to exclude thyroid lesions or lymphadenopathy.

Videofluoroscopy is an essential part of the evaluation because it identifies transfer dysphagia and strictures and may show the characteristic dilatation with beaking of the esophagogastric junction typical of achalasia. A video examination also demonstrates barium penetration of the airway, which is an indicator of the risk of aspiration pneumonia. Pharyngoesophageal motility studies, preferably with solid-state pressure transducers, complement the diagnosis of pharyngoesophageal incoordination. Specific diseases and their evaluation and treatment will be covered separately later. Nutritional support and prevention of pulmonary aspiration are predominant considerations in planning therapy. Figure 1 is a practical algorithm for the management of patients with transfer dysphagia.

Gastroparesis

Gastric motor dysfunction is characterized typically as delayed gastric emptying that causes nausea, vomiting,

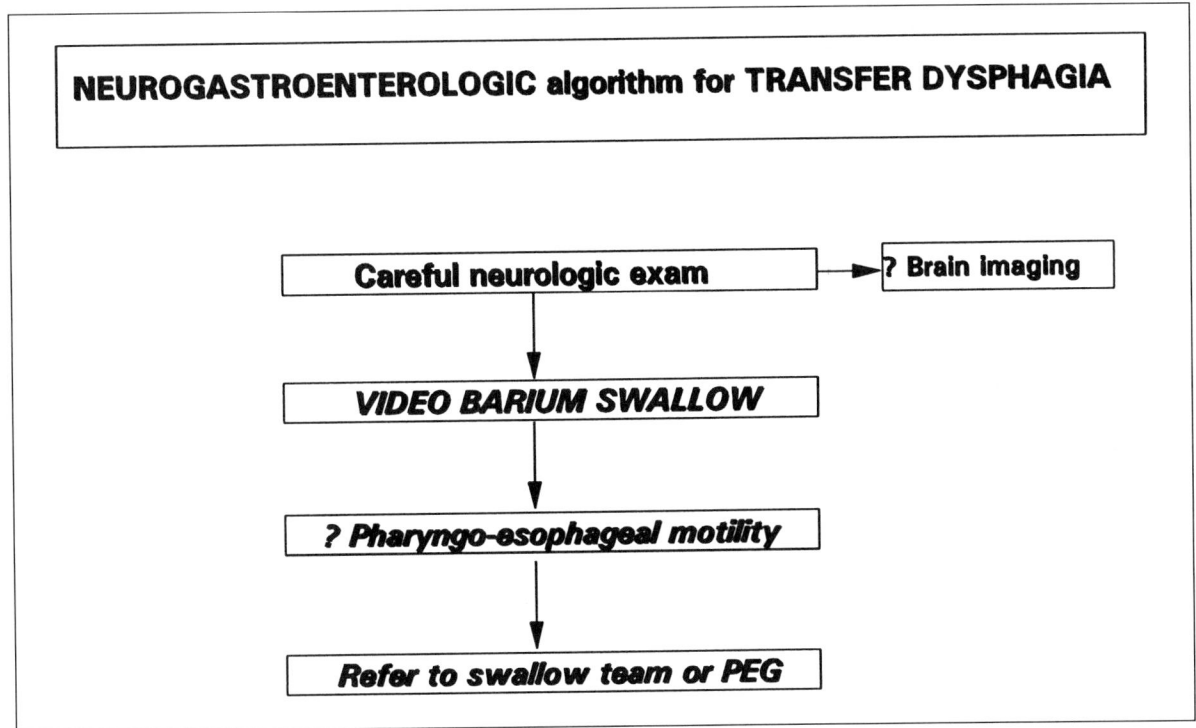

FIG. 1. Algorithm for the management of transfer dysphagia in patients with a suspected or proven neurologic disorder.

early satiety, anorexia, upper abdominal fullness, bloating, and, rarely, pain. Table 2 lists common causes of gastroparesis in clinical practice. Gastroparesis is a common gastrointestinal manifestation of autonomic neuropathies such as diabetes mellitus (13,34). Recurrent postprandial emesis may result in weight loss, malnutrition, and aggravation of glycemic control in patients with diabetes mellitus. Iatrogenic gastroparesis is induced by numerous medications, most commonly narcotic analgesics, tricyclic antidepressants, and dopaminergic agents. On physical examination there may be a succussion splash. It is important to rule out obstructing lesions (such as a pyloric channel ulcer) by a barium study or endoscopic examination. A scintigraphic study may be used to confirm the impaired emptying of solids from the stomach. Gastric stasis may result from abnormal motility of the stomach or small bowel, and these disturbances can be assessed by manometry or solid-state pressure transducers placed in the distal stomach and small bowel (Fig. 2). Figure 3 is an algorithm for diagnostic evaluation of patients with suspected upper gut dysmotility.

Prokinetic agents, antiemetics, and a more easily digestible diet (low in fat and fiber) may be beneficial in the treatment of gastroparesis. The most commonly used prokinetic medications are the $5HT_4$ agonists metoclopramide and cisapride. Metoclopramide also has antidopaminergic and antiemetic activity and is seldom used orally because of potential side effects, such as tardive dyskinesia and hyperprolactinemia. The usual oral dose of cisapride is 20 mg t.i.d., $\frac{1}{2}$ hr before meals and at bedtime. Antiemetics can be combined with prokinetics. The motilin agonist erythromycin is very effective in relieving acute gastric stasis when given at a dose of 3 mg/kg intravenously every 8 hours. The antidopaminergic agent domperidone (10 mg–20 mg t.i.d.) is not yet approved for use in the United States. There is evidence that all three agents provide symptomatic and objective benefit in the treatment of gastroparesis. Vagal dysfunction appears to negatively affect symptom improvement in gastroparesis and pseudo-obstruction. Nutritional support is an important component of management and is achieved with low-fat, low-fiber oral supplements and, rarely, by infusion of formula via a jejunal feeding tube.

TABLE 2. *Common causes of gastroparesis*

Type	Cause
Idiopathic	Suspected myenteric or intrinsic neuropathy
Autonomic neuropathy	Diabetes mellitus, amyloidosis, paraneoplastic, vagotomy
Infiltrative myopathy	Duchenne's muscular dystrophy, amyloidosis, scleroderma, dermatomyositis
Iatrogenic	Vagotomy, medications

Chronic Intestinal Pseudo-Obstruction

Chronic intestinal pseudo-obstruction is a syndrome characterized by nausea, vomiting, early satiety, abdominal

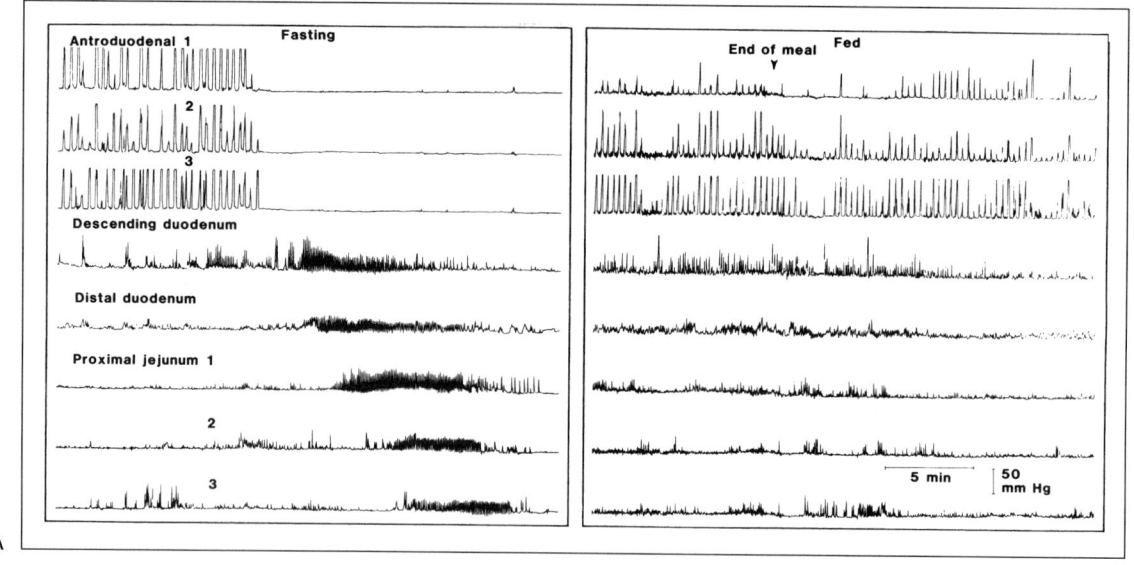

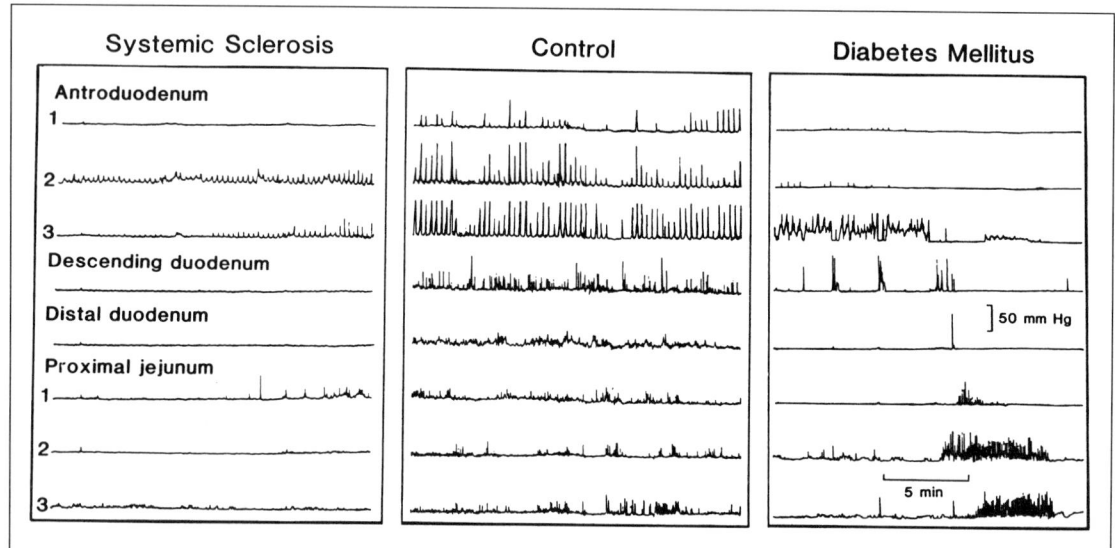

FIG. 2. (A) Tracing showing normal upper gastrointestinal motility in the fasting and fed states. The fasting tracing shows phase III of the interdigestive migrating motor complex. (Reprinted with permission from Malagelada J-R, Camilleri M, Stanghellini V. *Manometric Diagnosis of Gastrointestinal Motility Disorders.* New York: Thieme. 1986.) **(B)** Manometric tracings showing the myopathic pattern of intestinal pseudo-obstruction due to systemic sclerosis (*left panel*). Note the low amplitude of phasic pressure activity compared with the control (*middle panel*).

A manometric example of neuropathic intestinal pseudo-obstruction in diabetes mellitus. Note the absence of antral contractions and the persistence of cyclical fasting-type motility in the postprandial period (*right panel*). (Reprinted with permission from Camilleri M. Medical treatment of chronic intestinal pseudo-obstruction. *Practical Gastroenterology* 1991;15:10–22.)

discomfort, weight loss, and altered bowel movements that are the consequence of abnormal intestinal motility rather than mechanical obstruction. The syndrome can be regarded as an extension of gastroparesis with more prominent distention, a variable change in bowel habits, and sometimes, air–fluid levels or dilated intestinal loops on x-ray of the abdomen. The syndrome may result from a number of diseases extrinsic to the gut (e.g., disorders at any level of the brain–neural axis) (Fig. 4) or from an isolated dysfunction of neurons in the myenteric plexus (13).

The pathophysiologic features of these diseases can be broadly subdivided into a myopathic variety (e.g., infiltrative amyloidosis, hollow visceral myopathy, or muscular dystrophy) and a neuropathic variety (Tables 3 and 4).

Symptoms that suggest an underlying disease process should be sought. Postural dizziness, difficulties in visual accommodation, and sweating abnormalities suggest an autonomic neuropathy; urinary symptoms suggest genitourinary involvement by a generalized visceral neuromyopathic disorder. Patients should be questioned about the

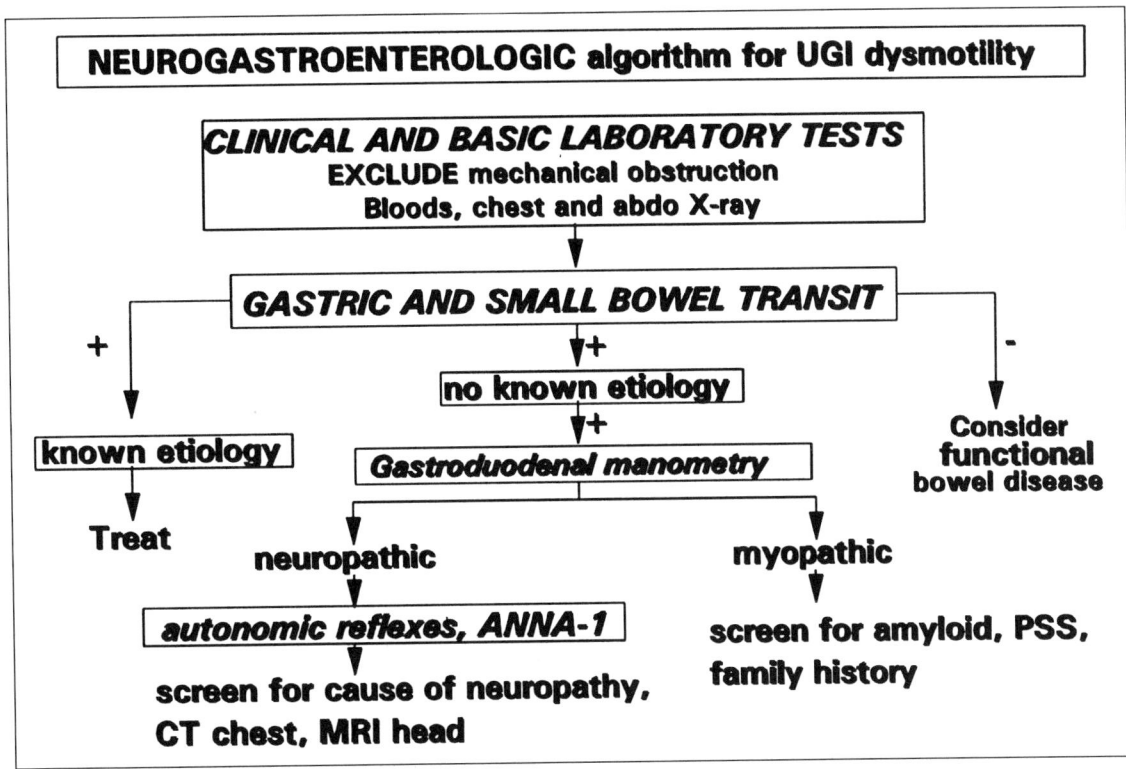

FIG. 3. Algorithm for the management of patients with upper gastrointestinal symptoms suggestive of a motility disorder. Note the need for a combined neurologic and gastroenterologic strategy.

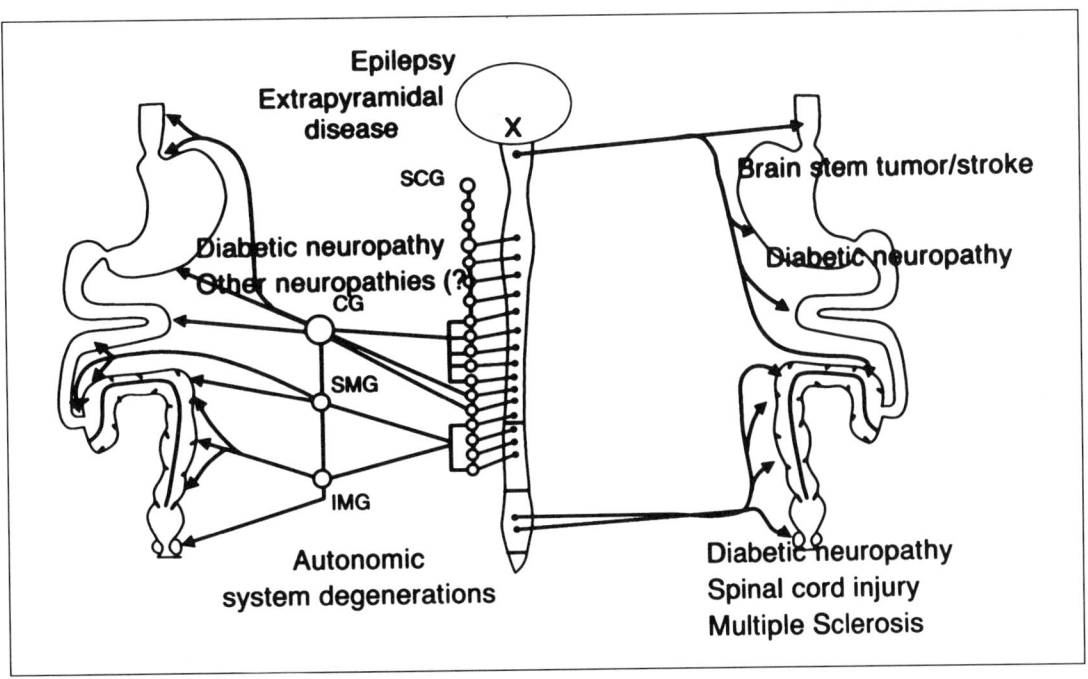

FIG. 4. Neurologic disorders known to affect gastrointestinal motility. Note involvement of sympathetic pathways (*left side*) and craniosacral parasympathetic pathways (*right side*). CG, celiac ganglion; SCG, superior cervical ganglion; SMG, superior mesenteric ganglion; IMG, inferior mesenteric ganglion.

TABLE 3. *Extrinsic neurologic disorders presenting with gastrointestinal dysmotility*

Anatomic Location	Examples
Brain	Parkinsonism
Brain stem	Stroke, tumor
Autonomic system	Selective or pandysautonomia, IOH
Spinal cord	Transection, spinal shock, multiple sclerosis
Spinal roots	Guillain-Barré syndrome
Peripheral nerve	Diabetic, amyloid neuropathy

IOH, idiopathic orthostatic hypotension.

TABLE 4. *Examples of acute and chronic neuropathies resulting in gastrointestinal dysmotility*

Acute	Chronic
Botulism	Diabetic neuropathy
Guillain-Barré syndrome	Paraneoplastic syndrome
	Amyloid neuropathy
	Chronic sensory and autonomic neuropathy
	Drug-induced neuropathy (*i.e.*, vincristine)

use of atropine-like drugs, phenothiazines, antihypertensive agents such as clonidine, and tricyclic antidepressants. A neurologic examination should be performed, and the physical examination should include a test of pupillary reflexes, measurement of blood pressure with the patient lying and standing, and a search for abdominal distention or a succussion splash.

Plain and barium radiologic studies are nonspecific, with dilatation of the small intestine a feature common to all types of chronic intestinal pseudo-obstruction. They are important, however, in ruling out mechanical obstruction. Motility studies are helpful to differentiate myopathic from neuropathic processes. If the motility tracing is suggestive of a neuropathic process, assessment of autonomic function and radiologic and serologic tests should be performed to identify the cause of the autonomic neuropathy (see later). Figure 3 is an algorithm for the management of patients with suspected upper gut dysmotility.

The goals of treatment of chronic intestinal pseudo-obstruction include the restoration of hydration and nutrition, stimulation of normal intestinal propulsion with agents similar to those used in gastroparesis, and suppression of bacterial overgrowth. There is little evidence that any of the prokinetics, other than cisapride, have any long-term, worthwhile benefit. Hence, cisapride is the drug of first choice. The antibiotics usually used for suppressing bacterial overgrowth are metronidazole (500 mg b.i.d.), doxycycline (100 mg t.i.d.), and ciprofloxacin (500 mg b.i.d.). These are usually administered for 7 to 10 days each month, although some patients with infiltrative or myopathic processes and severe dilatation and stasis may require chronic treatment. In such patients, new-onset diarrhea or rectal bleeding might result from pseudomembranous colitis, which requires cessation of the antibiotic and use of an alternative, such as oral vancomycin.

Constipation

Constipation is a common complaint and may be perceived by the patient as infrequent, incomplete evacuation or excessively hard stools. Most causes of constipation are easily identifiable and correctable, such as lack of exercise, too little fiber in the diet, and ignoring the urge to defecate. When these causes are excluded, constipation may be due to obstructing lesions, altered colonic motility, or disordered defecation (33). The management of intractable constipation has been reviewed elsewhere (10). Common neurologic disorders presenting with constipation are spinal cord transection, parkinsonism, and multiple sclerosis. Constipation is also common among patients with diabetes mellitus. Whether this is due to hyperglycemia, autonomic neuropathy, medications, or inadequate fiber intake is unclear.

Continence is maintained predominantly by the acute angle between the rectum and anal canal and by the function of the anal sphincters. The puborectalis sling serves to maintain the acute angle; during defecation, its relaxation results in a more obtuse rectoanal angle, descent of the pelvic floor, and facilitation of the passage of stool (Fig. 5). As the volume of stool in the sigmoid increases, contractions are triggered, thereby moving the contents into the rectum. Rectal distention induces inhibition of the internal anal sphincter, the so-called rectoanal inhibitory reflex. When it is the appropriate time to defecate, a sitting position is assumed, and this further lessens the acuteness of the anorectal angle. An increase in intrarectal and intra-abdominal pressure induced by straining causes reflex relaxation of the external anal sphincter, internal anal sphincter, and puborectalis muscles. This causes the pelvic floor to descend and the fecal bolus to be expelled (10,33).

Patients who complain of constipation use this term to describe a variety of disturbances. A clear description of the patient's symptoms must be elicited. The presence of blood in the stool necessitates further tests to exclude colonic mucosal lesions, such as polyps, or perianal conditions, such as hemorrhoids. The coexistence of a history of incontinence, a necessity for finger evacuation of the rectum, or a lack of rectal sensation also suggests neural dysfunction of the defecation mechanism.

Anatomic abnormalities such as tumors, megacolon, megarectum, or volvulus can be effectively ruled out by a barium enema and proctoscopy or by colonoscopy. Exclusion of these disorders, which are amenable to surgical treatment, is essential, even if the patient suffers an underlying neurologic disorder that could contribute to constipation. Figure 6 is a practical algorithm for the evaluation of patients with suspected lower gut dysmotility.

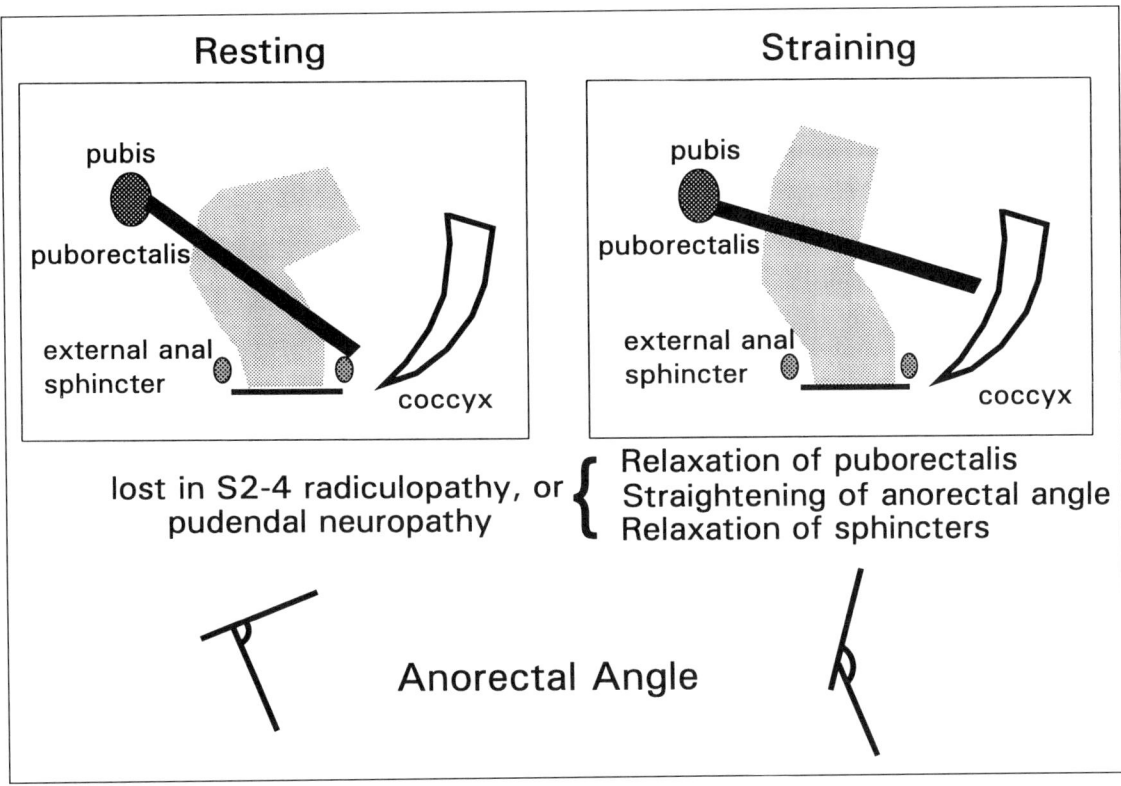

FIG 5. Illustration of the dynamics involved in the process of defecation. Straightening of the rectoanal angle and relaxation of the external anal sphincter are essential to facilitate defecation. Colonic contractions and increased abdominal pressure by a Valsalva maneuver propel the colonic or rectal content aborally. (Reprinted with permission from Camilleri M, Thompson WG, Fleshman JW, Pemberton JH. Clinical management of intractable constipation. *Ann Intern Med* 1994;121:520–528.)

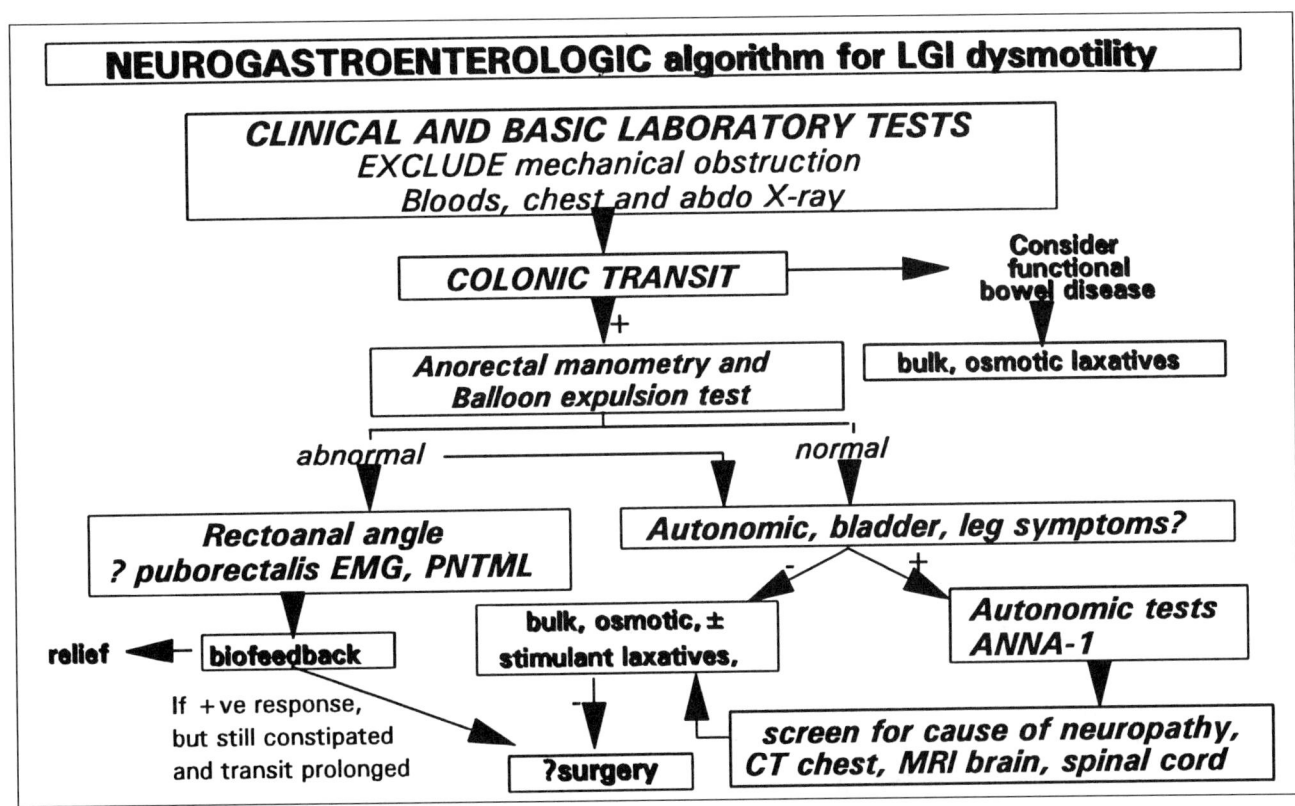

FIG. 6. Algorithm for the management of patients with lower gastrointestinal motility disorders includes evaluation of transit, defecatory dynamics, and neurologic function.

Colon transit studies with radiopaque markers (28) or radioscintigraphy (42) will detect abnormally prolonged transit; however, pelvic floor dysfunction may result in outlet obstruction and secondarily prolonged colonic transit. Hence, anorectal manometry, evaluation of rectal emptying by means of a screening balloon expulsion test and rectal sensation, and measurement of the anorectal angle are useful in assessing patients with disorders of defecation. These tests are reviewed elsewhere (48). Sphincter electromyography (EMG) or estimation of pudendal nerve terminal motor latency is sometimes needed to demonstrate sphincter denervation. Endoanal ultrasonography may be useful to exclude a surgically remediable sphincter defect, which is commonly found in multiparous women.

Most constipated patients respond well to fiber supplementation in the diet (at least 15 g/day), bulking agents such as psyllium, osmotic laxatives such as magnesium salts (two tablets of milk of magnesia up to four times a day) or lactulose (15 mL–30 mL t.i.d.), or stool softeners such as docusate (two tablets b.i.d.). Colonic inertia, which occurs frequently in wheelchair- or bed-bound patients, may require the addition of stimulant cathartics, such as bisacodyl orally or by suppository, or prokinetic medications, such as cisapride. Cisapride is rarely useful at usual therapeutic doses (20 mg q.i.d.). Patients with spinal cord injuries usually respond to a combination of bulk laxatives, digital stimulation, and scheduled enemas every 1 to 2 days. Recently, computer-assisted sacral anterior root stimulation has been advocated to simulate the sequence of sigmoid and rectal contractions and sphincter relaxation and, hence, to induce the dynamic events occurring during defecation (24). Dorsal rhizotomy must be performed to prevent sympathetic hyperreflexia syndrome. Surgery (i.e., colostomy or subtotal colectomy with ileorectostomy) is reserved for patients with intractable colonic inertia or for the correction of abnormalities such as rectal prolapse, rectocele, or painful perianal conditions resulting from the chronic constipation (e.g., anal fissure). It is essential to ensure that pelvic floor and anal sphincter function are normal before performing operations in patients with neurologic disorders. In extreme cases, patients with disorders of defecation may fail all treatment, including biofeedback (3), and require a defunctioning ileostomy or colostomy.

Fecal Incontinence

Major incontinence with loss of formed stool is frequently due to progressive neurologic damage to the pelvic nerves. This results in denervation of the pelvic floor musculature and the external and internal anal sphincters (33). In evaluating such patients, it is important to first exclude overflow incontinence due to fecal impaction. Similarly, overuse of laxatives or other medications, such as magnesium-containing antacids, may result in reversible incontinence.

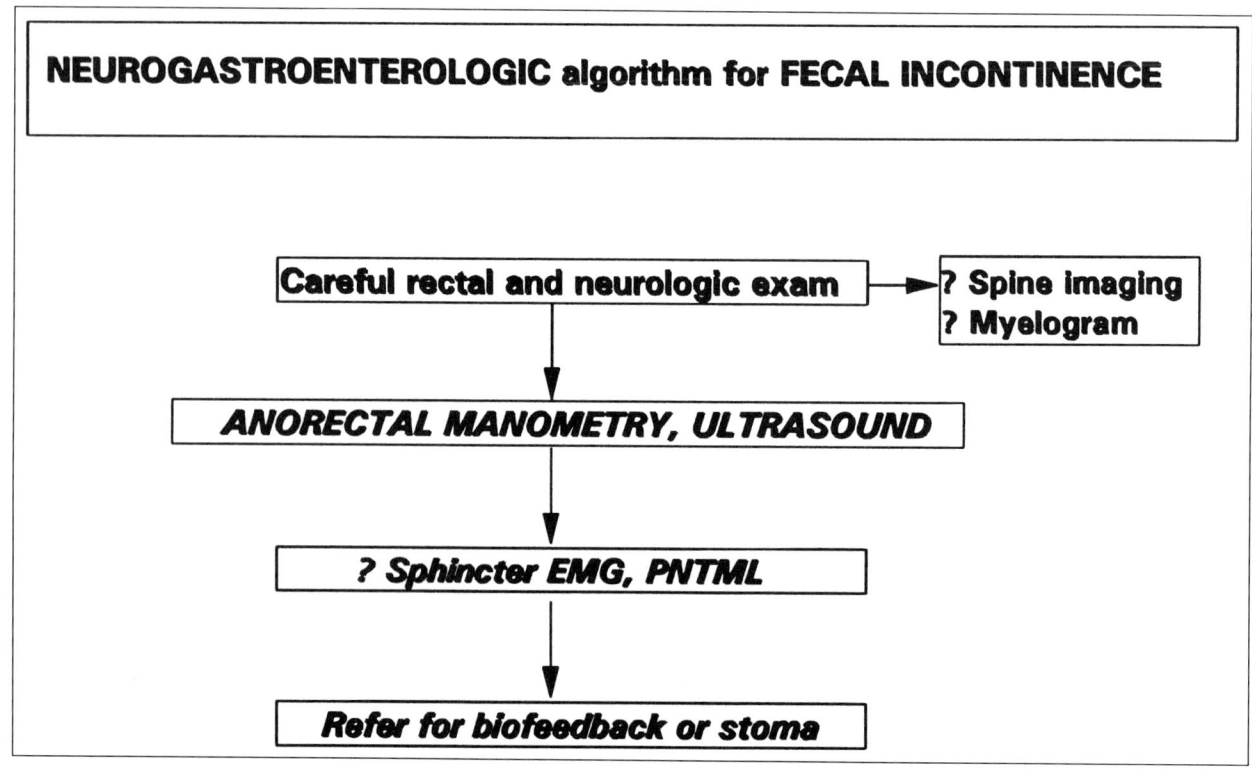

FIG 7. Algorithm for the practical management of fecal incontinence.

Examination of the incontinent patient should include inspection of the anus with and without straining to detect rectal prolapse, a digital rectal examination, and proctoscopy with barium enema or a colonoscopy to exclude mucosal lesions. If these fail to identify the cause of incontinence, further testing of the defecation dynamics is necessary, including anorectal manometry, rectal sensation and balloon expulsion, assessment of the anorectal angle, and defecating proctogram. External anal sphincter and puborectalis muscle EMG and pudendal nerve conduction studies are sometimes necessary. The management strategy is summarized in Figure 7. Initial treatment for patients with denervation-induced incontinence includes care of the perianal skin and use of incontinence pads. A "spinal" bowel regimen is useful to "control" the time of defecation and to try to avoid incontinence at other times. Biofeedback training is rarely helpful. Recent data suggest that magnetoelectric stimulation may be used to assess the function of lumbosacral motor roots and hence determine which patients have residual innervation sufficient for a response to biofeedback training (3).

EXTRINSIC NEUROLOGIC DISORDERS CAUSING GUT DYSMOTILITY

The intimate inter-relationships among the three levels of control of gut motility (see earlier) often render determination of the predominant disturbance difficult (see Fig. 4). In many instances, however, it is possible to distinguish the following: disorders that affect the gut muscle ("myopathic disorders"); disorders of the myenteric plexus, usually in the form of an idiopathic, chronic intestinal pseudo-obstruction; and diseases of the extrinsic pathways that supply the gut. Nevertheless, some diseases affect both intrinsic and extrinsic neural control (6). This review concentrates on diseases of extrinsic control. Diseases affecting smooth muscle and the enteric nervous system are reviewed elsewhere (6,17).

BRAIN DISEASES

Cerebrovascular Accident

Cerebrovascular accident patients may have significant dysphagia as a result of cranial nerve involvement; this may result in complications of malnutrition or aspiration. Evaluations of the swallowing mechanism with videofluoroscopy may demonstrate transfer dysphagia or aspiration. Placement of a percutaneous gastrostomy is usually the most effective method for providing nutrition without interfering with rehabilitation; feedings can be given in the form of boluses or by nighttime infusion. Not infrequently, patients subsequently recover sufficient oropharyngeal coordination for the gastrostomy to be removed without compromising nutrition or risking aspiration (35).

Parkinsonism

Patients with prolonged Parkinson's disease or progressive supranuclear palsy may also have oropharyngeal dysfunction with impaired swallowing (15). Shy-Drager syndrome, or multiple system atrophy, is discussed later. Patients may have mild to moderate malnutrition, and moderate dysphagia may be diagnosed by videofluoroscopy. In the absence of severe malnutrition or significant aspiration, conservative treatment will suffice. This consists of paying attention to the consistency of food (thickened liquids) and ensuring that the caloric content of meals is adequate. Feeding through a percutaneous gastrostomy is an appropriate alternative for severe symptoms.

Constipation is common in patients with parkinsonism and may be the result of colonic inertia or pelvic floor dysfunction (21). There is evidence of myenteric neural injury in the colon of patients with parkinsonism (37). Gastrointestinal hypomotility, generalized hypokinesia, autonomic dysfunction, and the effects of various anticholinergic and dopamine agonist medications may all play a role. The bioavailability of other medications can be considerably altered by the effects of parkinsonism on gut transit.

Head Injury

Immediately after moderate to severe head injury, most patients develop transient slow gastric emptying. The underlying mechanism is unknown, although a correlation exists between the severity of injury, increased intracranial pressure, and the severity of the gastric stasis. These patients are often intolerant of enteral feeding and require parenteral nutrition to meet their increased metabolic demands. In practice, enteral nutrition can often be reintroduced within 2 to 3 weeks as the gastroparesis resolves (32).

Amyotrophic Lateral Sclerosis

Patients with amyotrophic lateral sclerosis and progressive bulbar palsy have predominant weakness of the muscles supplied by the IX and X cranial nerves (17). Dysphagia is a frequent complaint, and patients may have respiratory difficulty while eating as a result of aspiration or respiratory muscle fatigue. Patients require a greater time to finish meals and may become malnourished or dehydrated.

Physical examination will show the cranial nerve palsies and muscle fasciculations. Videofluoroscopic barium swallow of liquids and solids will evaluate the swallowing mechanism and determine whether aspiration occurs.

For patients with significant dysphagia and weight loss or aspiration, oral feedings are replaced by feedings through a nasogastric tube or a percutaneously placed gastrostomy tube. Surgical procedures may be helpful in se-

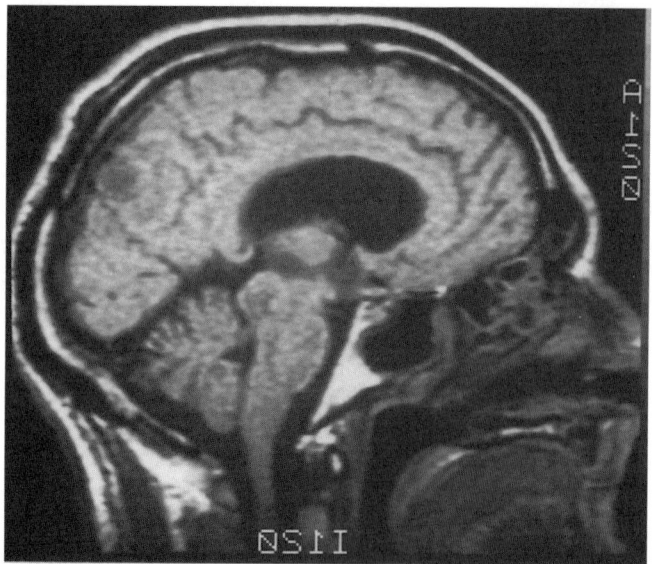

FIG. 8. Magnetic resonance imaging of the head showing lesions in the midbrain and parietal cortex in a patient with small-cell carcinoma of the lung who presented with unexplained vomiting of recent onset.

lected cases; cervical esophagostomy or cricopharyngeal myotomy can be performed if there is significant cricopharyngeal muscle dysfunction.

Postpolio Dysphagia

Individuals with postpolio syndrome often have symptoms of dysphagia (34). This usually occurs when bulbar involvement was present during the initial attack of poliomyelitis. These patients develop complications from aspiration, and esophageal motor function should be evaluated even in the absence of symptoms during swallowing. Videofluoroscopy is useful for screening and monitoring progression of disease. Attention to the position of the patient during swallowing and alteration of food consistency to semisolid food can decrease the incidence of choking and aspiration (17).

Brain Stem tumors

Brain stem lesions can present with isolated gastrointestinal motor dysfunction (50) (Fig. 8). In the absence of increased intracranial pressure, these symptoms are probably due to direct tumor effect in the medulla. Objective evidence of motor dysfunction can be documented by manometric or radionuclide studies of the stomach and small bowel (Fig. 9). The presence of autonomic neuropathy, particularly if preganglionic sympathetic nerves are involved, necessitates a search for a structural lesion in the central nervous system, such as a tumor. Magnetic resonance imaging is preferable for detecting brain stem lesions (51).

AUTONOMIC SYSTEM DEGENERATIONS

Pandysautonomia or Selective Dysautonomias

Pandysautonomias are characterized by preganglionic or postganglionic lesions affecting both sympathetic and parasympathetic nerves. Gastrointestinal involvement, which is manifested as vomiting, paralytic ileus, constipation, or a chronic pseudo-obstruction syndrome (44), has been reported in acute, subacute, and congenital pandysautonomia (5). Motor disturbances of the gut have been noted in the esophagus, the stomach, and the small bowel. There are also reports of individuals with selective cholinergic dys-

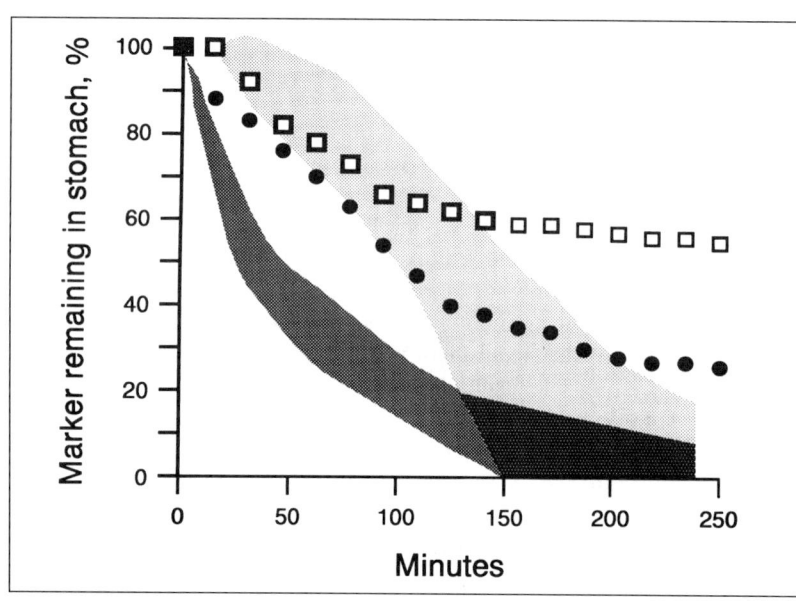

FIG 9. Scintigraphic study of delayed emptying of solids (□) and liquids (●) from the stomach. Normal data are shown by hatched areas: vertical, solids; horizontal, liquids).

function and disorders of gastrointestinal motor activity. A postmononucleosis selective cholinergic dysautonomia has been described (47).

Idiopathic Orthostatic Hypotension

Idiopathic orthostatic hypotension is sometimes associated with motor dysfunction of the gut, such as esophageal dysmotility, gastric stasis, alteration in bowel movements, and fecal incontinence (8,46). Cardiovascular and sudomotor abnormalities usually precede gut involvement. The precise level of the lesion along the neural axis and the appearance of the neurons of the myenteric plexus are as yet unclear.

Shy-Drager Syndrome

In the original description of the Shy-Drager syndrome (36), constipation and fecal incontinence were included among the classic features of the disorder. Other reports have documented a substantial reduction in fasting and postprandial antral and small-bowel motility. Abnormal esophageal motility has been demonstrated by videofluoroscopy and by frequent simultaneous low-amplitude peristaltic waves during esophageal manometry (reviewed in reference 5).

SPINAL CORD LESIONS

Spinal Cord Injury

During the acute phase after spinal cord injury, ileus is a frequent finding, but it is rarely prolonged. In the chronic phase, on the other hand, disorders of upper gastrointestinal motility are uncommon, but impaired gastric emptying or small-bowel transit has been described (19). Colonic and anorectal dysfunction are common and are probably a result of interruption of supraspinal control of the sacral parasympathetic supply to the colon, pelvic floor, and anal sphincters (43,45). There is a decrease in colonic compliance and an absence of postprandial colonic motor and myoelectric activity in patients with thoracic spinal cord injury (27).

The loss of voluntary control of defecation may be the most significant disturbance in patients who rely on reflex rectal stimulation for stool evacuation. Loss of control of the external anal sphincter is often distressing; fecal incontinence is the most common gastrointestinal problem in spinal cord injury patients.

The usual management for irregular bowel function is a combination of bulk agents and scheduled enemas. Stimulation of the sacral anterior roots may restore normal function of the pelvic colon and anorectal sphincters in these patients (24).

Multiple Sclerosis

Severe constipation is a frequent accompaniment of urinary bladder dysfunction in patients with advanced multiple sclerosis (49). The increases in intracolonic pressure that occur in response to a volume stimulus in patients with multiple sclerosis are excessive in comparison with the responses in healthy control subjects. In one study, colonic transit of radiopaque markers was prolonged in 14 of 16 patients with multiple sclerosis and urinary bladder involvement. In that series, 10 patients also had evidence of fecal incontinence, and 5 had spontaneous rectal contractions. The studies performed to date have not been sufficiently detailed to assess the relative contributions of the disturbances in the sympathetic and parasympathetic nervous systems. Nonetheless, pelvic colon dysfunction is probably due to impaired function of the supraspinal or descending pathways that control the sacral parasympathetic outflow. Further studies need to address the mechanism of impaired gut transit in multiple sclerosis that, as with spinal cord injury, results in motility disturbances in the lower gut more often than in the upper gut (11).

PERIPHERAL NEUROPATHY

Acute Peripheral Neuropathy

Autonomic dysfunction associated with certain acute viral infections may result in nausea, vomiting, abdominal cramps, constipation, or a clinical picture of pseudo-obstruction, as shown by a review of several individual case reports (see reference 13). Thus, in the Guillain-Barré syndrome, visceral involvement may include gastric dilation or adynamic ileus. Persistent gastrointestinal motor disturbances can also occur in association with infections such as herpes zoster, Epstein-Barr virus, or botulism B. Whether these infections result in an intrinsic or extrinsic neuropathy that affects the motor function of the gut is uncertain. Some investigators have shown that chronic intestinal pseudo-obstruction may result from cytomegalovirus infection of the myenteric plexus (40). We recently demonstrated that infectious mononucleosis induced selective cholinergic dysautonomia (47) with gastrointestinal dysfunction that developed within 1 week of the onset of the viral illness. It is conceivable that different viruses affect different levels of gut neural control but result in the same clinical picture.

Chronic Peripheral Neuropathy

Chronic peripheral neuropathy is the most commonly encountered extrinsic neurologic disorder that results in gastrointestinal motor dysfunction.

Diabetes Mellitus

Diabetic autonomic neuropathy of the gut has been studied extensively (16). Gastrointestinal symptoms are common in patients with type I diabetes who are seen in tertiary care centers, but in a community sample they are no more prevalent than they are in controls (18). Nevertheless, constipation and laxative use are more common in random samples of patients with type I diabetes mellitus than in age- and sex-matched community controls from Olmsted County, Minnesota (25). Gastric emptying of digestible or nondigestible solids is abnormal in patients with diabetes mellitus and gastrointestinal symptoms ("gastroparesis"); however, the pathogenesis and treatment of this relatively common disorder are incompletely understood. Studies in humans have demonstrated a paucity of antral contractions in the distal portion of the stomach during fasting postprandially; small-bowel motility may also be abnormal (1).

Constipation is a common, although often unreported, symptom in patients with diabetes, but little is known about its pathogenesis. Streptozocin-treated rats develop abnormal colonic compliance and selective deficiencies of certain neurotransmitters (i.e., calcitonin gene-related peptide) in the myenteric plexus. However, there are no human data to explain this frequent symptom. In contrast, diarrhea or fecal incontinence (or both) may result from several mechanisms: dysfunction of the anorectal sphincter or abnormal rectal sensation, osmotic diarrhea from bacterial overgrowth due to small-bowel stasis, or rapid transit from uncoordinated small-bowel motor activity. Rarely, an associated gluten-sensitive enteropathy or pancreatic exocrine insufficiency is present. These associated conditions should be sought because they are potentially reversible. The underlying mechanism must be identified if the appropriate treatment is to be provided.

Histopathologic studies of the vagus nerve have revealed reductions in unmyelinated axons; surviving axons are usually of small caliber. In patients with diabetic diarrhea, there are giant sympathetic neurons and dendritic swelling of the postganglionic neurons in prevertebral and paravertebral sympathetic ganglia, and there is reduced fiber density in the splanchnic nerves (14,23).

Peripheral cholinergic agonists (such as metoclopramide, bethanechol, and cisapride) and α_2-adrenergic agonists (such as clonidine) have been used to treat diabetic gut neuropathy. All available therapeutic options have resulted in only transient relief. Pancreas transplantation is reported to restore normal gastric emptying in patients with diabetic gastroparesis (29). Long-term results are awaited.

Amyloid Neuropathy

Amyloid neuropathy may lead to diarrhea and steatorrhea. In contrast, some patients with amyloidosis have infiltration of gut smooth muscle that commonly leads to a myopathic pseudo-obstruction or constipation. Patients with amyloid neuropathy demonstrate uncoordinated, nonpropagated contractions in the small bowel. These features are similar to the intestinal myoelectric disturbances observed in animals that have been subjected to ganglionectomy (26). Familial amyloidosis may also affect the gut.

Manometric studies and monitoring of the acute effects of cholinomimetic agents can distinguish between neuropathic (uncoordinated but normal-amplitude pressure activity) and myopathic (low-amplitude pressure activity) types of amyloid gastroenteropathy. These strategies may identify the patients (e.g., those with neuropathic disorders) who are more likely to respond to prokinetic agents.

Paraneoplastic Neuropathy

Autonomic neuropathy and gastrointestinal symptoms have been reported in association with small-cell carcinoma of the lung (>95% of cases) or pulmonary carcinoid (12). In the largest series (seven patients), all patients suffered constipation, six had gastroparesis, four had esophageal dysmotility suggestive of spasm or achalasia, and two had other evidence of autonomic neuropathy that affected bladder and blood pressure control (12). The myenteric plexus is infiltrated with lymphocytes and plasma cells, suggesting an immune ganglionitis. Our group has detected a circulating IgG antibody directed against enteric neuronal nuclei (22), which suggests that the enteric neurons are the major target of this paraneoplastic phenomenon. However, some patients also have evidence of extrinsic visceral neuropathies (38). The chest x-ray is often negative in these patients; hence, a chest computed tomography scan is indicated when the syndrome is suspected clinically in middle-aged smokers with recent onset of nausea, vomiting, or feeding intolerance.

Chronic Sensory and Autonomic Neuropathy of Unknown Cause

This is a rare, nonfamilial form of slowly progressive neuropathy affecting various autonomic functions (31). Patients may have only a chronic autonomic disturbance manifesting for many years as a gastrointestinal dysfunction before any involvement of the sensory nerves becomes apparent. In most patients, however, cardiovascular or sweating abnormalities precede involvement of the gut. This condition is important because it suggests that autonomic dysfunction may be the cause of functional gastrointestinal motor disorders, including the common problem of irritable bowel syndrome (6), as shown in Figure 10.

Other investigators have reported familial cases of intestinal pseudo-obstruction with degeneration of the myenteric plexus and evidence of sensory or motor neuropathies (or both) affecting peripheral or cranial nerves (20).

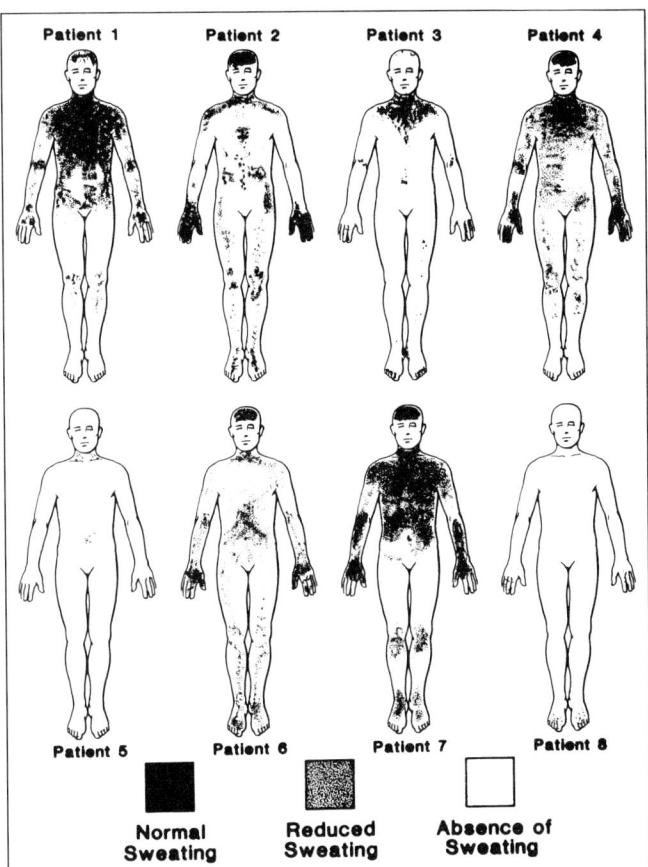

FIG. 10. Thermoregulatory sweat test showing impaired sweating in eight patients whose gastrointestinal symptoms of several years' duration was attributed to irritable bowel syndrome. (Reprinted with permission from Camilleri M et al. Idiopathic autonomic denervation in eight patients presenting with functional gastrointestinal disease: a causal association? *Dig Dis Sci* 1990;35:609–616).

dysfunction. A strategy is necessary in the diagnostic evaluation of disordered gastrointestinal function and its cause. It is here that the paths of the neurologist (with an interest in the autonomic nervous system) and the gastroenterologist cross, as shown in the algorithms in Figs. 1, 3, 6, and 7. Patients should undergo further testing, particularly if they have clinical features suggestive of autonomic or peripheral nerve dysfunction. The algorithms in Figs. 1, 3, 6, and 7 summarize the practical evaluation of patients with dysmotilities at several levels of the gastrointestinal tract.

The first steps in the history and physical examination should identify evidence of a generalized neurologic disorder; the physician should thoroughly evaluate all systems and inquire about the past medical history and family history. It is essential to record the use of all medications, because they may influence gut motility.

Gastrointestinal motility and transit measurements help the clinician to confirm the disturbance in the motor function of the gut and to distinguish between neuropathic and myopathic disorders. Indirect tests of autonomic function are useful for identifying the presence of other types of visceral denervation and for localizing the anatomic level of the disturbance in extrinsic neural control (5). The close concordance between abdominal vagal dysfunction and cardiovagal neuropathy in patients with diabetes (4) suggests that these tests may provide a good evaluation of the overall function of the autonomic supply to the viscera, including the gastrointestinal tract. Table 5 lists the autonomic investigations, the normal values at the Mayo Clinic, and the interpretations of abnormal tests (5). The pros and cons of autonomic tests in the setting of a gastroenterologic practice are reviewed elsewhere (7).

When a defect of the sympathetic nervous system has been identified, such as in the thermoregulatory sweat test (see Fig. 10), the effect of the intravenous administration of edrophonium on norepinephrine levels may provide further assessment of the integrity of postganglionic sympathetic nerves (Fig. 11). Similarly, dysfunction of the abdominal vagus nerve suggested by cardiac reflexes can be confirmed by means of the plasma pancreatic polypeptide response to either modified sham feeding ("chew and spit" technique) or hypoglycemia. This test, however, is rarely necessary in clinical practice because cardiac autonomic responses are easier, less expensive, and probably more sensitive indicators of abdominal vagal dysfunction.

Screening of a patient with visceral autonomic neuropathy must include tests that identify occult causes of the neuropathy, such as lung tumors, porphyria, or amyloidosis. Imaging of the brain and spinal cord becomes essential, particularly when the thermoregulatory sweat test is abnormal but tests of postganglionic nerves (e.g., the quantitative sudomotor axon reflex test and plasma norepinephrine response to edrophonium) are normal (38).

Porphyria

Gastrointestinal involvement is common in porphyria and usually presents with symptoms of abdominal pain, nausea, vomiting, and constipation (2,41). Patients with porphyria have a polyneuritis characterized by demyelination of peripheral and autonomic nerves; dilation and impaired motor function may be seen in any part of the intestinal tract and are likely the result of autonomic dysfunction. Effects of porphyria on the enteric nervous system have not yet been described.

IDENTIFICATION OF EXTRINSIC NEUROLOGIC DISEASE IN PATIENTS WITH FUNCTIONAL GASTROINTESTINAL SYMPTOMS

Patients with lesions at virtually any level of the nervous system may have symptoms of gastrointestinal motor

TABLE 5. *Interpretation of results of autonomic function tests*

Test of Autonomic Function	Normal Value	Abnormal Result Implies Dysfunction Of:
Pupillary tests		
Response to light		
Latency	0.2–0.3 sec	P
Constriction	2–4 mm	P
Pharmacologic tests		
0.125% Pilocarpine	0–0.5 mm constriction	P
0.1% Epinephrine	No change	pg, S
5% Cocaine	>1.5 mm dilation	S
Blood Pressure Reduction on tilt to 80°		
Systolic	<25 mmHg	S
Diastolic	<15 mmHg	S
Valsalva ratio	>1.5	S or P
Pulse rate change with		
deep breathing	Age related, 6–18 beats/min	P
Thermoregulatory sweat test		
(% surface area of anhidrosis)	M: 0%; F: <3%	S
Quantitative sudomotor axon reflex test		
Sweat output (μl/cm³)		
Forearm	M: 0.76–5.51; F: 0.34–1.33	
Foot	M: 0.92–5.73; F: 0.25–1.95	
Latency (min)		
Forearm	M: 1–2.4; F: 0.9–1.9	
Foot	M: 1–2.7; F: 1–2.8	
Plasma norepinephrine		
Patient supine	70–750 pg/mL	pg, S
Patient standing	200–1700 pg/mL	S
Response to I.V. edrophonium	>35% increase above baseline within 2–8 minutes	pg, S

P, parasympathetic system; S, sympathetic system; pg, postganglionic system; M, male; F, female.

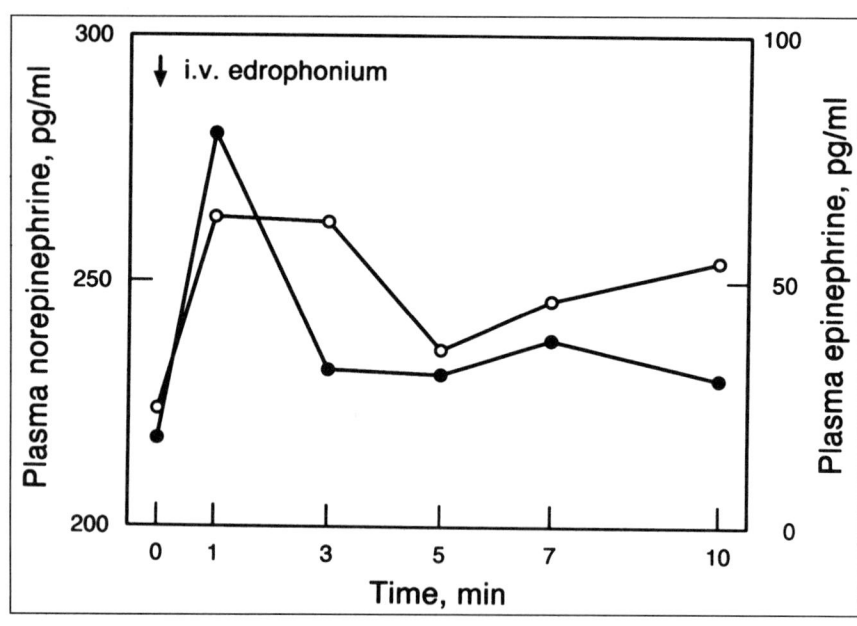

FIG. 11. Plasma norepinephrine (○) and epinephrine (●) response to 1 mg of intravenous edrophonium. Note the prompt rise in both catecholamine levels, suggesting normal postganglionic sympathetic pathways. (Reprinted with permission from Sodhi N, Camilleri M et al. Autonomic function and motility in intestinal pseudoobstruction caused by paraneoplastic syndrome. *Dig Dis Sci* 1989; 34:1937–1942.)

SUMMARY AND CONCLUSIONS

Gastrointestinal motor dysfunction results when extrinsic nerves are disturbed and are unable to modulate the autonomous motor functions of the digestive tract. The latter depend on the "little brain in the gut" or the enteric nervous system and the automaticity of the smooth muscles themselves. Disorders at all anatomic levels of the extrinsic neural control have been reported in association with gut motor dysfunction and illustrate the important role of the extrinsic pathways. Although much emphasis has been placed on dysphagia and constipation as a result of these neurologic disorders, more recent studies have highlighted incontinence, vomiting, and abdominal distention in the symptomatology of such patients. Strategies that evaluate the physiologic functions of the digestive tract and the function of the extrinsic neural control provide means for selecting rational therapies for these patients, including biofeedback training (e.g., dysphagia, incontinence), prokinetic agents (neuropathic forms of gastroparesis or intestinal pseudo-obstruction or colonic inertia), and nutritional support using the enteral or parenteral route. Electrical or magnetic stimulation (e.g., constipation in paraplegics) provides an exciting new method to alleviate symptoms. Electrical pacing of the stomach may also be feasible in the foreseeable future.

REFERENCES

1. Battle WM, et al. Gastrointestinal-motility dysfunction in amyloidosis. *N Engl J Med* 1979;301:24–25.
2. Berlin L, Cotton R. Gastro-intestinal manifestations of porphyria. *Am J Dig Dis* 1950;17:110–114.
3. Bielefeldt K, et al. Diagnosis and treatment of fecal incontinence. *Dig Dis Sci* 1990;8:179–188.
4. Buysschaert M, et al. Gastric acid and pancreatic polypeptide responses to sham feeding are impaired in diabetic subjects with autonomic neuropathy. *Diabetes* 1985;34:1181–1185.
5. Camilleri M. Disorders of gastrointestinal motility in neurologic diseases. *Mayo Clin Proc* 1990;65:825–846.
6. Camilleri M, Fealey RD. Idiopathic autonomic denervation in eight patients presenting with functional gastrointestinal disease: a causal association? *Dig Dis Sci* 1990;35:609–616.
7. Camilleri M, Ford MJ. Functional gastrointestinal disease and the autonomic nervous system: a way ahead? *Gastroenterology* 1994;106:1114–1118.
8. Camilleri M, Malagelada J-R. Abnormal intestinal motility in diabetics with gastroparesis. *Eur J Clin Invest* 1984;14:420–427.
9. Camilleri M, et al. Gastrointestinal motility disturbances in patients with orthostatic hypotension. *Gastroenterology* 1985;88:1852–1859.
10. Camilleri M, et al. Clinical management of intractable constipation. *Ann Intern Med* 1994;121:520–528.
11. Caruana BJ, et al. Anorectal sensory and motor function in neurogenic fecal incontinence. Comparison between multiple sclerosis and diabetes mellitus. *Gastroenterology* 1991;100:465–470.
12. Chinn JS, Schuffler MD. Paraneoplastic visceral neuropathy is a cause of severe gastrointestinal motor dysfunction in patients with lung cancer. *Gastroenterology* 1987;92:1345.
13. Colemont L, Camilleri M. Chronic intestinal pseudo-obstruction: diagnosis and treatment. *Mayo Clin Proc* 1989;64:60–70.
14. Duchen LW, et al. Pathology of autonomic neuropathy in diabetes mellitus. *Ann Intern Med* 1980;92:301–303.
15. Edwards LL, et al. Gastrointestinal symptoms in Parkinson's disease. *Mov Disord* 1991;6:151–156.
16. Feldman M, Schiller LR. Disorders of gastrointestinal motility associated with diabetes mellitus. *Ann Intern Med* 1983;98:378–384.
17. Hillel AD, Miller RM. Management of bulbar symptoms in amyotrophic lateral sclerosis. *Adv Exp Med Biol* 1987;209:201–221.
18. Janatuinen E, et al. Gastrointestinal symptoms in middle-aged diabetic patients. *Scand J Gastroenterol* 1993;28:427–432.
19. Keshavarzian A, et al. Delayed colonic transit in spinal cord injured patients measured by indium-111 Amberlite scintigraphy. *Am J Gastroenterol* 1995;90:1295–1300.
20. Krishnamurthy S, Schuffler MD. Pathology of neuromuscular disorders of the small intestine and colon. *Gastroenterology* 1987;93:610–639.
21. Kupsky WJ, et al. Parkinson's disease and megacolon: concentric hyaline inclusions (Lewy bodies) enteric ganglion cells. *Neurology* 1987;37:1253–1255.
22. Lennon VA, et al. Enteric neuronal autoantibodies in pseudoobstruction with small-cell lung carcinoma. *Gastroenterology* 1991;100:137–142.
23. Low PA, et al. The sympathetic nervous system in diabetic neuropathy: a clinical and pathological study. *Brain* 1975;98:341–356.
24. MacDonagh RP, et al. Control of defecation in patients with spinal injuries by stimulation of sacral anterior nerve roots. *Br Med J* 1990;300:1494–1497.
25. Maleki D, Camilleri M, Zinsmeister AR et al. Prevalence of gastrointestinal symptoms in insulin- (IDDM) and noninsulin-dependent diabetes mellitus (NIDDM) in a U.S. community (abstr). *Dig Dis Sci* 1996;A1:1990.
26. Marlett JA, Code CF. Effects of celiac and superior mesenteric ganglionectomy on interdigestive myoelectric complex in dogs. *Am J Physiol* 1979;237:E432–E436.
27. Meshkinpour H, et al. Colonic compliance in patients with spinal cord injury. *Arch Phys Med Rehabil* 1983;64:111–112.
28. Metcalf AM, et al. Simplified assessment of segmental colonic transit. *Gastroenterology* 1987;92:40–47.
29. Murat A, et al. Amélioration de la neuropathie péiphérique et de la vidange gastrique aprés transplantation simultanée rénale et pancréatique. *Diabete Metab* 1990;16:419–420.
30. Nelson JB, Richter JE. Upper esophageal motility disorders. In: Ouyang A (ed). *Gastroenterology Clinics of North America, Vol. 18.* Philadelphia: WB Saunders. 1989;195–222.
31. Okajima T, et al. Chronic sensory and autonomic neuropathy. *Neurology* 1983;33:1061–1064.
32. Ott L, et al. Altered gastric emptying in the head-injured patient: relationship to feeding intolerance. *J Neurosurg* 1991;74:738–742.
33. Pemberton JH, Phillips SF. Constipation and diarrhea. In: Moody FG (ed). *Surgical Treatment of Digestive Diseases, 2nd ed.* Chicago: Year Book Medical Publishers. 1990;39–52.
34. Read NW, Houghton LA. Physiology of gastric emptying and pathophysiology of gastroparesis. In: Ouyang A (ed). *Gastroenterology Clinics of North America, Vol. 18.* Philadelphia: WB Saunders. 1989;359–374.
35. Reynolds BJ, Eliasson SG. Colonic pseudoobstruction in patients with stroke. *Ann Neurol* 1977;1:305.
36. Shy GM, Drager GA. A neurological syndrome associated with orthostatic hypotension: a clinical-pathologic study. *Arch Neurol* 1960;2:511–527.
37. Singaram C, et al. Dopaminergic defect of enteric nervous system in Parkinson's disease patients with chronic constipation. *Lancet* 1995;346:861–864.
38. Sodhi N, et al. Autonomic function and motility in intestinal pseudoobstruction caused by paraneoplastic syndrome. *Dig Dis Sci* 1989;34:1937–1942.
39. Sonies BC, Dalakas MC. Dysphagia in patients with the post-polio syndrome. *N Engl J Med* 1991;324:1162–1167.
40. Sonsino E, et al. Intestinal pseudoobstruction related to cytomegalovirus infection of the myenteric plexus (letter to the editor). *N Engl J Med* 1984;311:196–197.
41. Stein JA, Tschudy DP. Acute intermittent porphyria. *Medicine* 1970;49:1–16.
42. Stivland T, et al. Scintigraphic measurement of regional gut transit in idiopathic constipation. *Gastroenterology* 1991;101:107–115.
43. Stone JM, et al. Chronic gastrointestinal problems in spinal cord injury patients: a prospective analysis. *Am J Gastroenterol* 1990;85:114–119.

44. Suarez GA, et al. Idiopathic autonomic neuropathy: clinical, neurophysiologic, and follow-up studies on 27 patients. *Neurology* 1994;44:1675–1682.
45. Sun WM, et al. Anorectal function in incontinent patients with cerebrospinal disease. *Gastroenterology* 1990;99:1372–1379.
46. Thatcher BS, et al. Altered gastroesophageal motility in patients with idiopathic orthostatic hypotension. *Cleve Clin J Med* 1987;54:77–82.
47. Vassallo M, et al. Gastrointestinal motor dysfunction in acquired selective cholinergic dysautonomia associated with infectious mononucleosis. *Gastroenterology* 1991;100:252–258.
48. Wald A. Colonic transit and anorectal manometry in chronic idiopathic constipation. *Arch Intern Med* 1986;146:1713–1716.
49. Weber J, et al. Radiopaque marker transit and anorectal manometry in 16 patients with multiple sclerosis and urinary bladder dysfunction. *Dis Colon Rectum* 1987;30:95–100.
50. Weber J, et al. Effect of brainstem lesion on colonic and anorectal motility: study of three patients. *Dig Dis Sci* 1985;30:419–425.
51. Wood JR, et al. Brainstem tumor presenting as an upper gut motility disorder. *Gastroenterology* 1985;89:1411–1414.

CHAPTER 46

The Diagnosis and Treatment of Urinary Bladder Dysfunction

Claire C. Yang and William E. Bradley

---

1. The diagnosis of neurologic urinary bladder dysfunction in patients with neurologic disease is established by integrating neuroanatomic findings, derived from the history and neurologic examination, with the results of bladder function tests.
2. In cystometry, which is a bladder function test useful for evaluating patients with neurologic disease, bladder pressure and bladder filling volume are recorded concurrently. The filling medium may be either water or carbon dioxide. The cystometric examination may demonstrate such abnormalities as detrusor hyperreflexia, hyporeflexia, or areflexia in patients with bladder dysfunction caused by neurologic disease. Other pertinent information can be obtained from external sphincter electromyography, cystourethrography, and measurement of urinary flow rate and postvoid residual volume.
3. Electrodiagnostic studies of bladder innervation include latency measurements of the urethroanal reflexes and cortical evoked responses. These studies help to define the integrity of the central and peripheral innervation of the bladder and urinary sphincters.
4. Treatment of the neurogenic bladder focuses on bypassing the neurologic deficit. In most cases, a combination of behavioral modifications and pharmacotherapy allows the patient adequate reservoir function of the lower urinary tract. Clean intermittent self-catheterization allows for continent urinary drainage without the sequelae of chronic catheterization. Surgical procedures are indicated in carefully selected patients.

INTRODUCTION

The evaluation and treatment of the patient with neurologic disease and urinary bladder dysfunction is challenging to both neurologists and urologists. A careful history of voiding symptoms and a general physical and neurologic examination are the foundation of the evaluation of neurologic voiding dysfunction. The history and examination are supplemented by laboratory procedures that analyze the different components of voiding, after which a treatment plan can be selected from a broad range of therapeutic strategies. However, the neurologic deficit frequently imposes limits on management goals; therefore, the results of treatment of neurologic bladder dysfunction may be modest.

Customarily, the neurologist and urologist cooperate in the care of these patients. However, practitioners from each specialty approach the patient with different concepts and assumptions. The neurologist is concerned with the accurate diagnosis of neurologic disease, based on a clinical assessment of the neuroanatomic deficit. The urologist accepts the neurologic diagnosis in a defined context and focuses on end-organ dysfunction. The challenge of neurourology is to combine the disparate approaches to diagnosis and management, in an effort to gain new understanding of neurologic dysfunction of the urinary bladder.

DIAGNOSIS

Patient History

A wide range of neurologic diseases is associated with urinary bladder dysfunction. These include multiple sclerosis (20,24,54), Parkinson's disease (3,59), dementia, stroke (78), spinal cord disease (38), and neurologic disease associated with diabetes mellitus (21,23). Moreover, as patients with neurologic disease age, superimposed

---

C. C. Yang: Department of Urology, University of Washington, Seattle, Washington 98195.

W. E. Bradley: Departments of Urology and Neurology, University of Washington, Seattle, Washington 98195.

symptoms of benign prostatic hyperplasia (31) and female stress incontinence (45) may develop.

A careful history should elicit information on the sensation of bladder filling, frequency of voiding, difficulty in initiation of voiding, capacity for suppressing the urge to void, and the presence or absence of urinary incontinence. Dysuria, or painful voiding, can be associated with infection or inflammation. However, asymptomatic bacteriuria is common in patients with neurologic disease. Stress urinary incontinence in female patients is manifested by sudden involuntary loss of urine induced by increases in intra-abdominal pressure (i.e., coughing, laughing, lifting heavy objects). Benign prostatic hyperplasia can be associated with a diminished urinary stream and difficulty in bladder evacuation.

Questions concerning the functioning of other pelvic organs can be enlightening in determining the site of a neurologic lesion (i.e., presence of fecal incontinence or disturbances of sexual function, such as impotence or anorgasmia). Patient should be asked about their medications, including anticholinergic and other agents. Many over-the-counter preparations, such as cold medicines, antihistamines, diet pills, and herbal remedies, contain ingredients that may affect urinary function. Any history of previous operative procedures on the lower urinary tract, such as sphincterotomy, transurethral resection of the prostate, urethropexy, or any pelvic or spinal operations, should be documented.

An important part of the history is the voiding diary, which charts the amount and type of fluid consumed, time of consumption, amount of urine voided, time of voiding, and associated symptoms. Patients can complete this diary at home during several days and return with it at the next office visit. Patients also should be questioned about their level of function in activities of daily living and the availability of familial or community support, especially if they are disabled in any way by a neurologic disorder. This information is critical in planning optimal bladder management.

General Physical Examination

The general physical examination of the patient with neurogenic bladder dysfunction includes examination of the abdomen, genitalia, and rectum. Palpation and percussion of the abdomen may reveal a lower abdominal mass arising from the pelvis, which may be an overly distended bladder. In female patients, a pelvic examination is done to assess the presence and position of the uterus, which may affect voiding symptoms. The rectal examination in male patients is performed to determine rectal contents and consistency of the prostate gland.

Neurologic Examination

The findings revealed by the neurologic examination indicate the nature and degree of the neuroanatomic deficit, and the extent to which patients can participate in their own care. The neurourologic examination, performed by the urologist, consists of testing genital and perineal sensation, anal sphincter tone, and voluntary contraction of the pelvic floor muscles and anal sphincter, all of which can be absent or impaired in lower motor neuron injury. The bulbocavernosus reflex and anal wink reflex, when present, indicate intact sacral reflex arcs; these reflexes are exaggerated in corticospinal tract disruption. Dementia precludes patient compliance with a drug regimen and understanding of voiding schedules. Rigidity, tremor, and postural instability in patients with Parkinson's disease impede the use of self-help procedures, such as intermittent self-catheterization (36,50). These patients demonstrate detrusor hyperreflexia on cystometry. Corticospinal tract interruption, resulting in hyperactive deep tendon reflexes and extensor plantar responses, can be manifested by spasticity of the external urinary sphincter and detrusor hyperreflexia. A transverse myelitic syndrome, characterized by a well-defined sensory level, is also associated with sphincter spasticity and bladder hyperactivity. Interruption of the roots of the cauda equina, indicated in part by a lax anal sphincter, is associated with detrusor areflexia. Peripheral neuropathy in patients with diabetes mellitus can be accompanied by impaired bladder sensation and detrusor areflexia.

Laboratory Evaluation

The laboratory evaluation is outlined in Table 1. Once the history and neurologic examination have been completed, urinalysis and urine culture can be performed.

TABLE 1. *Laboratory evaluation of urinary bladder function in neurologic disease*

General
   Urine analysis and culture
   Blood urea nitrogen and creatinine
   Upper urinary tract imaging
      Renal ultrasound
      Excretory urography
      Retrograde pyelography
   Lower urinary tract imaging
      Voiding cystourethrogram
      Cystourethroscopy
Bladder function assessment
   Cystometry
   Ambulatory cystometry
Urethral function assessment
   Uroflowmetry
   Urethral pressure profile
   Sphincter electromyography
Videourodynamics
Innervation studies
   Cortical evoked responses
   Urethroanal reflex
   Bulbocavernosus reflex

Asymptomatic or symptomatic bacteriuria can be present in patients with chronic indwelling catheters or condom drainage, and in patients who perform intermittent self-catheterization. Serum studies should include blood urea nitrogen and creatinine levels, and if these are elevated, or if any other indication of renal impairment is revealed by the patient's history or physical examination, then imaging of the upper urinary tract is indicated. A baseline renal ultrasonogram should be obtained in all patients with a neurogenic bladder, and contrast studies, such as an excretory urogram, which provide better imaging of the collecting system, should be performed periodically (i.e., every 3 years). If the serum creatinine level is greater than 1.5 mg/dL, or if the patient has a contrast allergy, then retrograde pyelography is safer. If there is radiographic evidence of hydronephrosis or calyectasis, a voiding cystourethrogram may be needed to exclude the possibility of vesicoureteral reflux.

When possible, a urinary flow rate and postvoid residual volume measurement should be obtained. A commercially available portable ultrasonographic machine can be used to obtain an estimate of residual volume noninvasively (29). Cystoscopy is performed to evaluate possible structural abnormalities or as part of an evaluation for hematuria.

Abnormal bladder function is difficult to assess without a conceptual understanding of normal function. The micturition cycle involves two phases: (a) bladder filling and urine storage, and (b) bladder emptying.

Bladder filling requires the following:

1. Accommodation of increasing volumes at low intravesical pressure and appropriate sensation.
2. Closure of the bladder outlet at rest and during increases in intra-abdominal pressure.
3. Absence of involuntary bladder contractions.

Bladder emptying requires the following:

1. Coordinated contractions of the bladder of adequate magnitude and duration.
2. Lowering of resistance at sphincters.
3. Absence of obstruction.

Bladder dysfunction can therefore be clinically identified as a problem of filling or emptying, or a combination of both; the site of dysfunction may be at the bladder, urethra, or both. Neurologic disease can interfere with all or some of these elements of normal bladder function.

Laboratory evaluation continues with the assessment of detrusor muscle function and an estimation of urethral control, and studies of innervation.

Detrusor function studies include the following:

1. Cystometry (19).
2. Ambulatory cystometry (14).

Urethral function studies include the following:

1. Uroflowmetry, or the measurement of urine flow (72).
2. Sphincter electromyography (EMG) (25), which consists of EMG recording of the activity in either the anal or external urinary sphincter in conjunction with the cystometrogram.
3. Urethral pressure profile (7).

Synchronous examination of pressure and flow (combined detrusor and urethral studies) with simultaneous radiographic examination of bladder filling and emptying is known as *videourodynamics* (17,45). It provides an integrated assessment of lower urinary tract function.

Cystometry

Carefully performed cystometry represents a valuable test of detrusor muscle function. Detrusor reflex contraction and its voluntary control are two of the most important aspects of voiding (27).

The cystometrogram is simple to perform with a modern cystometer. A urethral catheter is introduced after the patient has voided, so that the residual urine volume can be measured. Increased residual urine volume can be observed in a wide variety of syndromes involving impaired voiding. Although this test lacks specificity, it can give an overall indication of the efficiency of bladder function.

Cystometry can be performed with either carbon dioxide insufflation or water infusion (26,55) (Fig. 1). Carbon dioxide insufflation using rapid inflow rates may facilitate the appearance of a detrusor contraction. Additional maneuvers can be performed to provoke reflex induction, such as sitting, standing, and walking in place (4,8). Water is usually introduced at lower inflow rates than is carbon dioxide, and it is used when evaluation of voiding is necessary. The intravesical pressure is monitored continuously using a transducer calibrated in centimeters of water. Pressure is recorded on the y-axis; volume is recorded on the x-axis. A pressure transducer can be introduced into the rectum to measure increases in intra-abdominal pressure. Because intravesical pressure is a reflection of both detrusor and intra-abdominal pressure, intrarectal pressure subtracted from intravesical pressure yields the true pressure generated by the detrusor.

Normal findings on cystometry include an initial sensation of bladder filling at a low filling volume and maintenance of a low intravesical pressure during the accumulation of urine. This is expressed as bladder compliance ($\Delta V/\Delta P$). As bladder capacity is approached, the sensation of bladder filling becomes more prominent, followed by an intense urgency to void when the bladder reaches capacity. The patient is permitted to void, and this event coincides with an abrupt rise in the intravesical pressure, from a low to a high filling pressure. When the rise evoked by detrusor reflex contraction is at or near peak amplitude, the patient is asked to suppress the detrusor reflex contraction, usually by tightening the anal sphincter or the perineum, or both. In normal subjects, this prompts a rapid decline in intraves-

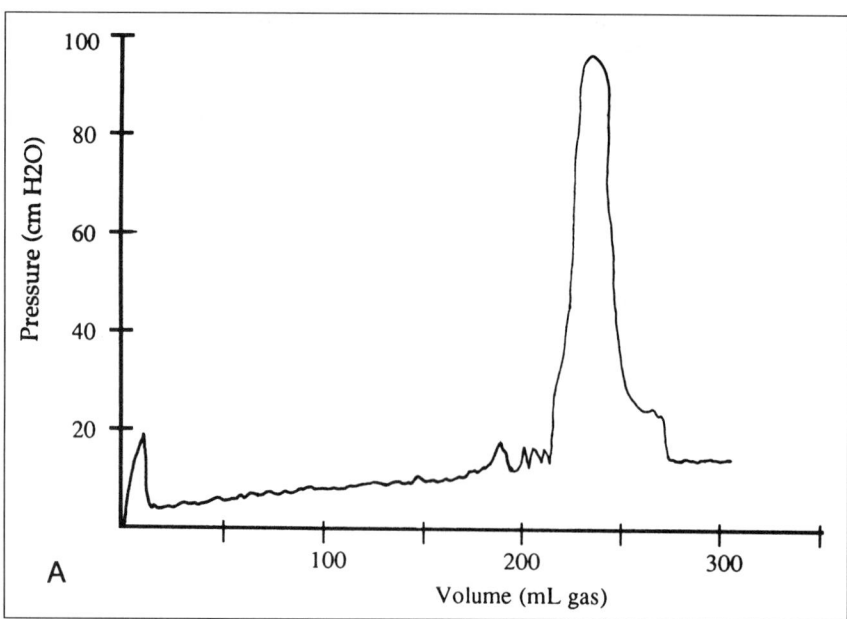
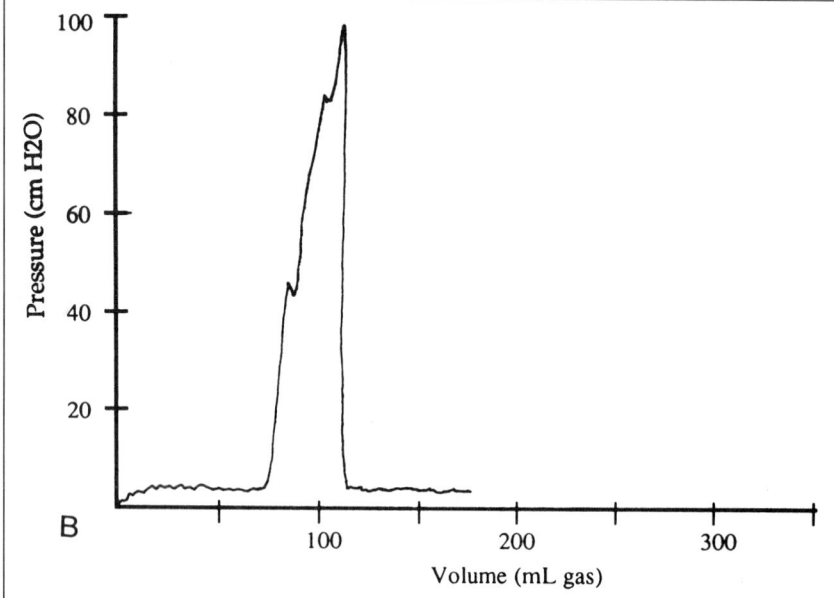
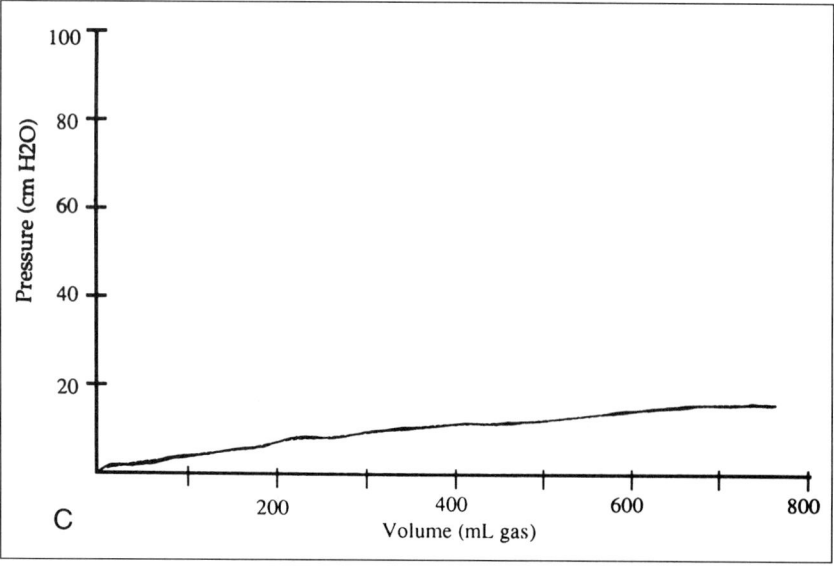

Fig. 1. Gas (CO2) cystometrograms **(A)** Normal study. As the bladder fills, there is little change in pressure. When a detrusor contraction occurs at capacity, the patient suppresses the reflex at the peak of the contraction, resulting in a rapid decline in intravesical pressure. The ability to generate a detrusor contraction and subsequently suppress it confirms the neurologic integrity of the detrusor reflex. **(B)** Detrusor hyperreflexia. A detrusor contraction occurs at low capacity and cannot be suppressed. **(C)** Detrusor areflexia. The bladder fills to large capacity and no contraction occurs.

ical pressure. A caveat is that a patient may not be able to cooperate with the command to suppress or may be malingering. Voiding studies are obtained after the bladder is refilled, and then the patient is allowed to empty to completion without suppressing the detrusor reflex. A high voiding pressure with a concomitant low urinary flow rate is pathognomonic for obstruction of the bladder outlet. In some normal individuals, a detrusor reflex contraction may not appear because embarrassment or discomfort leads to reflex suppression.

An overactive detrusor contraction is a detrusor reflex contraction that cannot be suppressed voluntarily. Detrusor hyperreflexia is defined as bladder overactivity caused by impairment or interruption of supraspinal or spinal bladder pathways (1). The ability to delineate this impairment depends on findings from the neurologic examination, supplemented by results of laboratory tests, including electrodiagnostic studies. Detrusor areflexia is defined as an absence of detrusor reflex contraction during cystometry. Absence of this response following provocative maneuvers, such as standing or walking in place, can indicate a cauda equina injury or autonomic neuropathy. These can be confirmed by laboratory studies that assess innervation. Detrusor hypocontractility is a condition in which the bladder can generate a contraction, but with insufficient magnitude or duration, or both, to empty the bladder.

Ambulatory cystometry is a technique that permits the continuous evaluation of detrusor reflex function during an extended period of time (14,43) (Fig. 2). The method permits nocturnal recording of bladder activity, measurement of the effect of pharmacologic agents, and monitoring of bladder function during activities of daily living. Further studies are needed to evaluate the clinical utility of this technique.

Testing of Urethral Function

The most basic assessment of urethral function is uroflowmetry (37,75). Measurement of urinary flow rate is obtained when the patient voids into either an electromagnetic flowmeter or the more rugged gravity-type of flowmeter. The information acquired includes average flow rate, maximal flow rate, voiding time, and volume voided (Fig. 3). Uroflowmetry may be used to define urinary obstruction in male patients caused by urethral stricture, benign prostatic hyperplasia, or detrusor-sphincter dyssyner-

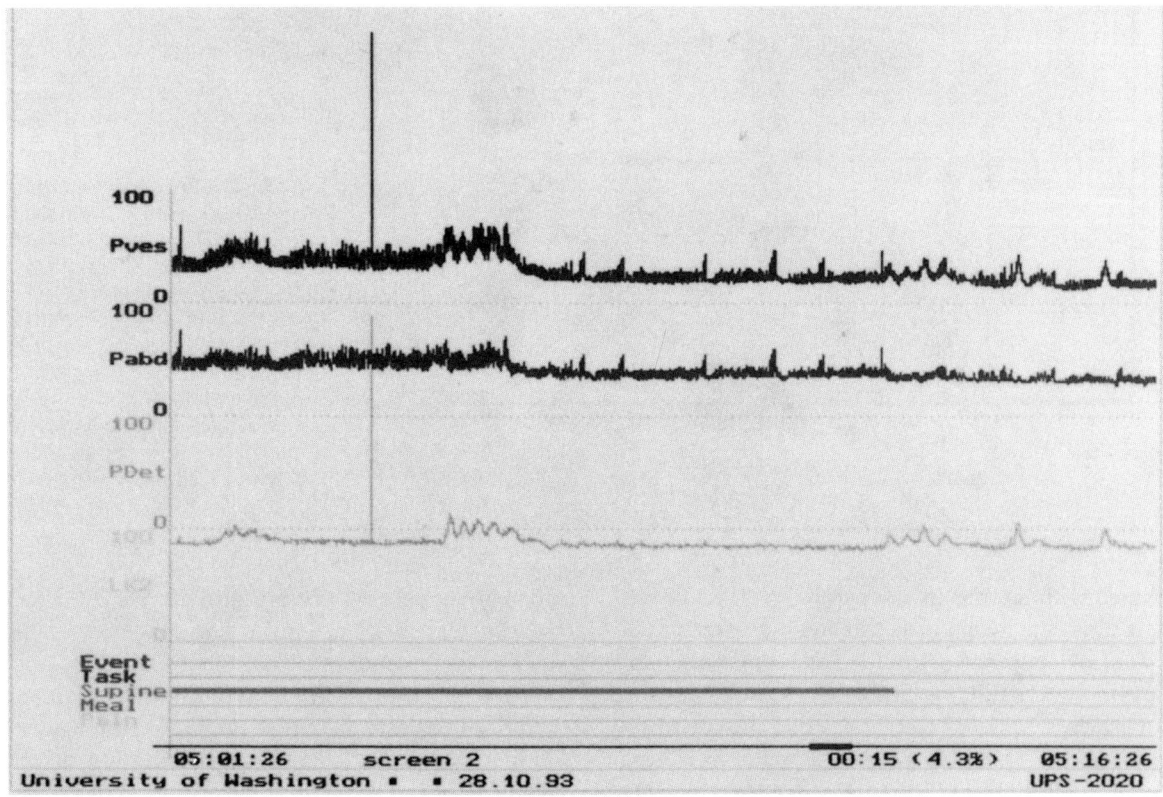

Fig. 2. Ambulatory cystometry. Tracing demonstrates 15 min of continuous cystometric monitoring in a quadripalegic man. Note waves of spontaneous bladder contractions. Pves = intravesical pressure, Pabd = abdominal pressure, PDet = Pves-Pabd or true detrusor pressure. (Largevertical lines are artefact.)

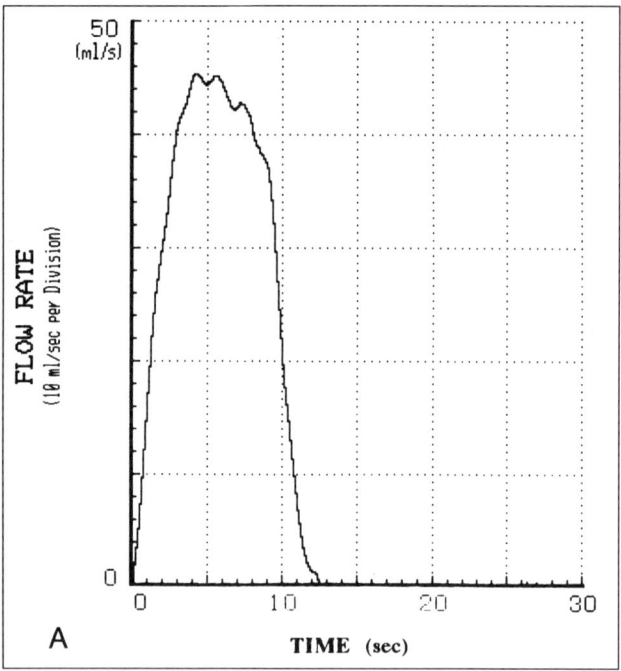
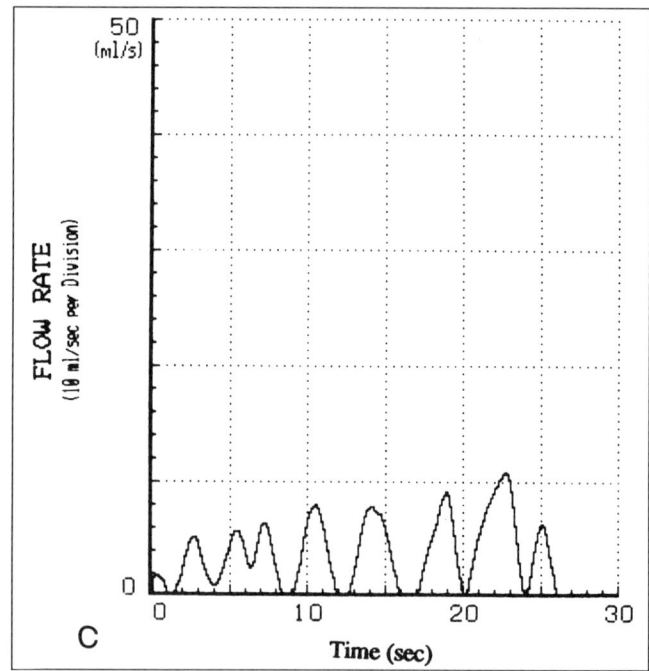
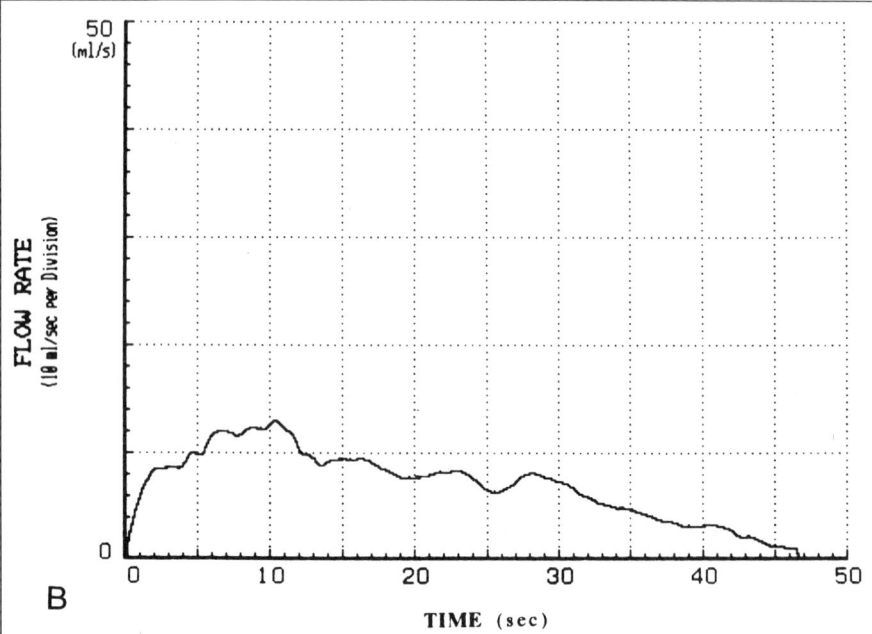

Fig. 3. Uroflowmetry. **(A)** Normal study, 34-year-old woman. Voided volume = 425 mL. **(B)** Infravesical obstruction, 61-year-old man. Peak flow rate < 15 mL/sec and voiding time is prolonged. Voided volume = 332 mL. **(C)** "Strain" pattern, 33-year-old man following pelvic injury. The flow curve is interrupted, typical of patients who use abdominal straining to void, suggesting inadequate detrusor function. Voided volume = 125 mL.

gia. Combined with the results of cystometry, the test can differentiate between an abnormal flow rate caused by obstruction and an abnormal flow rate resulting from impaired detrusor contractility.

Urethral function can also be evaluated with the urethral pressure profile. In this test, a catheter is withdrawn from the bladder at a constant velocity while the bladder is being perfused with water or carbon dioxide (7,9). As the catheter is withdrawn through the urethra, the pressure is continuously measured through perforations in the catheter. A curve obtained by plotting urethral pressure measured in centimeters of water on the y-axis against urethral length measured in centimeters on the x-axis. Three critical values obtained are maximal urethral pressure, functional urethral length, and maximal urethral closure pressure. The functional urethral length is that portion of the urethral length along which the urethral pressure exceeds the intravesical pressure. The maximal urethral closure pressure is obtained by subtracting the intravesical pressure from the maximal urethral pressure.

In women, the urethral pressure profile resembles a single curve (Fig. 4). A normal urethral pressure profile in male patients consists of a double hump: an initial increase produced by the prostate gland, followed by a second and higher increase in pressure produced by the external urethral sphincter. In patients with benign prostatic hyperplasia, the functional length of the prostatic portion of the profile is accentuated. In women with stress incontinence, the amplitude of the maximal urethral closure pressure is lowered, and the functional urethral length is decreased.

Urethral function can be assessed by sphincter EMG (19,25), usually done in conjunction with cystometry, uroflowmetry (72), and measurement of the urethral pressure profile (7). Sphincter EMG is performed by recording activity from one of several sites, using several different methods. EMG activity can be recorded from either the external urethral sphincter or the anal sphincter. In most patients, it is easier to record from the anal sphincter, and it can be safely assumed that responses to bladder filling and emptying are similar for both sphincters. Types of recording electrodes include EMG needles, ring electrodes mounted on an anal or urinary catheter, or cutaneous surface electrodes. The ring electrodes are placed on the catheter in close apposition to the sphincter muscle. The EMG signals are amplified and the output fed to the recorder, which is operating at the same time as the cystometrograph.

The normal sphincter pattern consists of an increase in the amplitude of the EMG signals with increased bladder filling. On detrusor reflex contraction, there may be either sphincter quiescence, if voiding is permitted, or enhanced EMG activity, if the patient is instructed to suppress the detrusor reflex. In patients with lesions of the corticospinal tract, voluntary control of sphincter contraction and relaxation is lost. The combined cystometric and sphincter EMG record demonstrates the pattern of detrusor-sphincter dyssynergia (5), in which failure of the sphincter to relax during detrusor reflex contraction is often associated with increased sphincter activity, with resultant obstruction to urinary flow.

In patients with a cauda equina injury and a lax external urinary sphincter, the sphincter EMG record reveals a lack of response to bladder filling and an absence of voluntary contraction or relaxation.

Videourodynamic Studies

The videourodynamics study, a comprehensive assessment of both bladder and urethral function, has become part of the routine evaluation of patients with complex neurogenic urinary dysfunction. It combines functional studies of the lower urinary tract with simultaneous fluoroscopic imaging (17,42). Cystometry, urethral pressure monitoring, measurement of urinary flow rate, sphincter EMG, and cystourethrography together provide a dynamic real-time evaluation of the micturition reflex (Fig. 5).

First, a urinary flow rate is obtained. The bladder is then catheterized with a double- or triple-lumen urodynamic catheter for intravesical and urethral pressure measurements; at the same time a postvoid residual volume is obtained. Abdominal pressure is monitored through a separate rectal catheter, and EMG electrodes are placed on the perineum or perianally. Radiographic contrast is used as the medium for cystometry, and fluoroscopic images are obtained throughout the filling and voiding portions of the study and recorded on videotape, with the corresponding manometric data from the bladder and urethra.

These studies and the supportive facilities require significant time and expense, and the results can be full of arti-

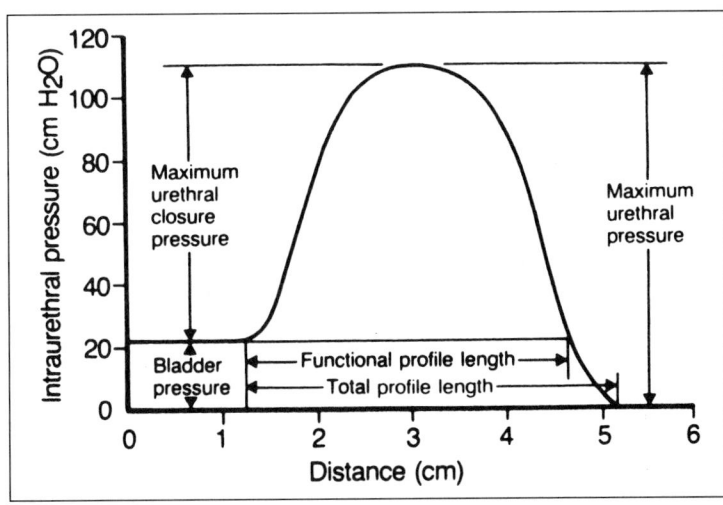

Fig. 4. Urethral pressure profile, normal female. (See text for explanation of terms.)

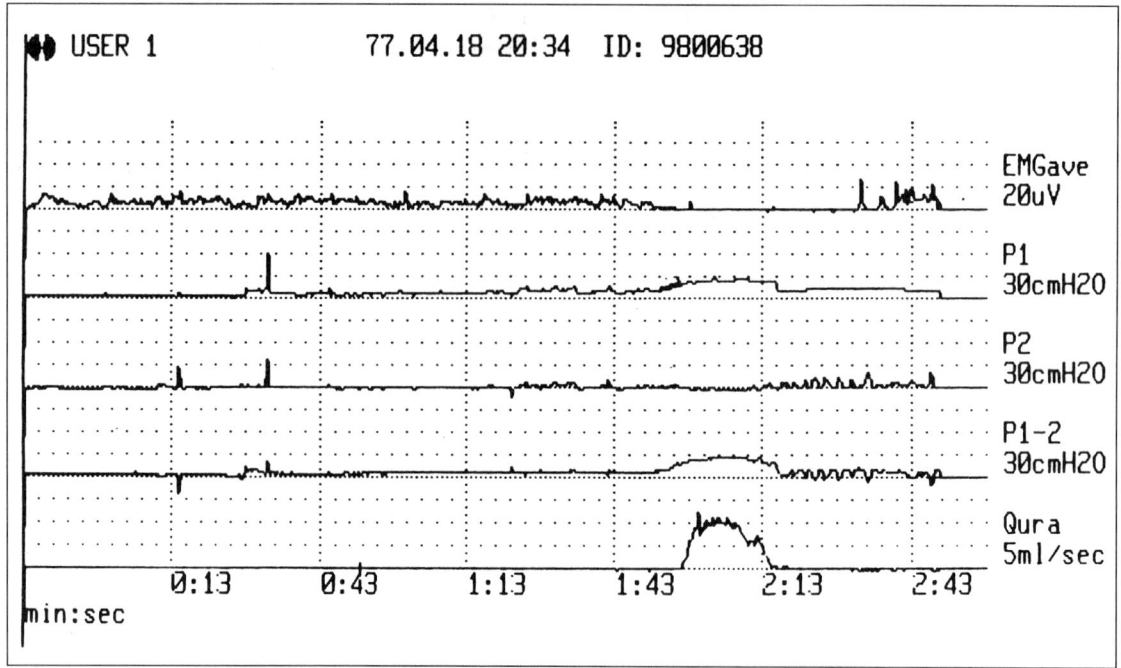

Fig. 5. Videourodynamics, normal study. During filling, there is good bladder compliance and no uninhibites detrusor contractions. with voiding, urethral sphincter activity is quiescent (as noted on EMG tracing) with the generation of a contraction. Urine flow begins soon thereafter. The study is accompanied by real-time fluoroscopic imaging of the bladder and sphincter. EMGave = integrated sphincter electromyography, P1 = intravesical pressure, P2 = abdominal pressure, P1-P2 = true detrusor pressure, Qura = urinary flow rate.

facts. However, coordination of multiple components of evaluation of the lower tract makes videourodynamics a valuable tool in the diagnosis of the neurogenic bladder.

Innervation Studies

The neuroanatomic pathways of the genitourinary system can be evaluated with electrodiagnostic studies. They can identify the presence of neuropathy, delineate the connections of the pelvic and pudendal nuclei in the sacral spinal cord, and define spinal cord and cerebral connections to the urinary tract. Studies measuring the function of the bladder and urethra (i.e., cystometry, urethral pressure profile) combined with data obtained from electrodiagnostic studies can provide an accurate assessment of the neurologic integrity of the system.

The following electrodiagnostic tests are used in the urinary tract:

Bladder: The latency of the pelvic nerve cortical evoked response can reveal the integrity of the autonomic pathway between the bladder and the cortex. However, stimulation of the bladder wall with successful recording from the cortex has not yet been demonstrated in humans. Cortical representation of the visceral afferents from the bladder neck can be achieved by stimulating electrodes on a urethral catheter (67). All these responses can theoretically be measured in the spine, but the small electrical response in this area makes reception difficult. Sacral reflex pathways between the bladder and other pelvic structures have yet to be electrically identified in humans.

Urethra: Sacral reflex pathways can be measured with the urethroanal evoked response (64). The urethroanal evoked response is elicited by stimulating the urethra with ring electrodes mounted on a urethral catheter and measuring the response in the anal sphincter, either with a needle or surface or anal plug electrodes (Fig. 6).

Because of technical limitations in accessing the individual nerves to the bladder and urethra, electrodiagnostic testing of adjacent nerves provides analogous information on the innervation of the pelvic viscera. The pudendal cortical evoked response from the dorsal nerve of the clitoris/penis demonstrates the integrity of the innervation from the sacral segments to the cortex (Fig. 7). Transcutaneous stimulation of this branch of the pudendal nerve results in a cortical response at the C_{z2} position (International 10-20 System). The bulbocavernosus reflex latency is obtained in men by transcutaneously stimulating the dorsal nerve of the penis and recording the response in the

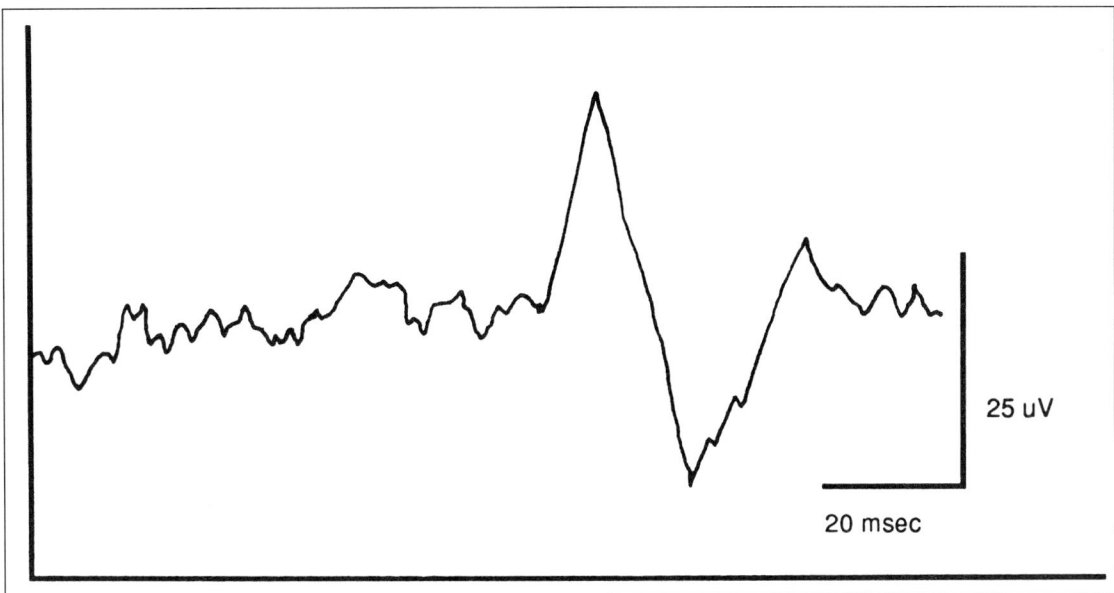

Fig. 6. Urethroanal evoked response. Response in anal sphincter evoked by stimulation of proximal urethra.

bulbocavernosus muscle using bipolar EMG electrodes or cutaneous surface electrodes (35). The equivalent reflex is elicited in women by stimulating the dorsal nerve of the clitoris and measuring anal sphincter contraction. Both these tests define the integrity of sacral reflex arcs.

Neurologic and Laboratory Findings in Neurologic Dysfunction of the Urinary Bladder

Diseases of the Brain

Cerebrovascular Disease

Urinary bladder dysfunction is not a significant problem in patients who have transient ischemic attacks but may occur in the context of occlusive cerebrovascular disease (78). Infarction of the frontal cortex or its pathways subserving control of the urinary bladder results in frequency, urgency, urge incontinence, and detrusor hyperreflexia. In the acute stage of a stroke, detrusor areflexia is evident, and this is followed by detrusor hyperreflexia on recovery of activity in the deep tendon reflexes.

Parkinson's Disease

The incidence of bladder dysfunction in patients with Parkinson's disease is high, with estimates ranging from 25%–85% (2,59). The presence of bradykinesia and dementia often is associated with urinary incontinence. Typically, the patient with Parkinson's disease demonstrates a hyperreflexic, hypocontractile bladder on cystometry (3).

The hypocontractility may arise from the use of anticholinergic therapy for parkinsonism. Men who have benign prostatic hyperplasia may also demonstrate obstruction during voiding; however, the results of transurethral prostatectomy in this situation are poor, with patients remaining unable to empty their bladders and concomitantly experiencing incontinence.

Brain Tumor

Urinary bladder dysfunction may be observed in patients with brain tumors in the superomedial portion of the frontal lobe (11), although bladder dysfunction is rarely an initial symptom in patients with brain tumors. Symptoms include frequency, urge, and urge incontinence. Detrusor hyperreflexia is evident on cystometric evaluation.

Dementia

The precise incidence of urinary bladder dysfunction in patients with dementia is unknown. Many neurologists believe urinary incontinence is a late manifestation of the disease and that it may be the result of the patient's inability to acknowledge the need for social continence. Frequently, bladder dysfunction may be exacerbated by medications, immobility, and inattentiveness to bladder hygiene by caregivers. There have been no reports of the results of cystometric studies in patients with dementia.

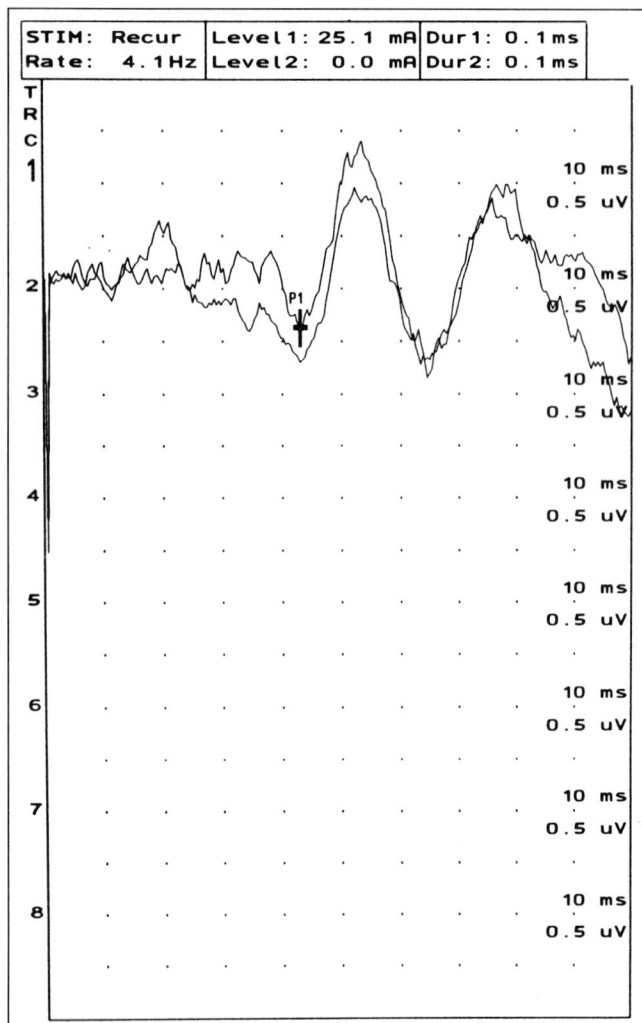

Fig. 7. Pudendal cortical evoked response, normal 28-year-old man. Recorded at scalp from stimulation of the dorsal nerve of the penis, latency = 42 msec.

Diseases Affecting the Brain and Spinal Cord

Multiple Sclerosis

In multiple sclerosis, plaques in the periventricular white matter of the brain stem and in the spinal cord frequently involve the tracts that innervate the urinary bladder (6). Frequency, urge, and urge incontinence are common symptoms in patients with multiple sclerosis, and they are occasionally the initial manifestations of the disease. The clinical neurologic course of exacerbation and remission can be associated with a progressive worsening of urinary tract dysfunction. The incidence of urinary tract dysfunction varies with the time course of the disease, but it can occur in up to 90% of affected patients. Severe, low-threshold detrusor hyperreflexia is revealed by cystometry in the majority of patients with urinary complaints; reports of bladder areflexia range from 1%–40%. Detrusor sphincter dyssynergia is present in 30%–65% of patients with detrusor hyperreflexia and is associated with generalized spastic paraparesis. The urethral pressure profile can be abnormal, showing a high pressure associated with spasticity of the external urinary sphincter. There may be an increase in latency of the bulbocavernosus and urethroanal reflexes in patients with demyelination of the conus medullaris (77). The latency of the pudendal cortical evoked response may also be increased (46).

Damage to the upper urinary tract is a rare occurrence in patients with multiple sclerosis, contrary to popular belief (20). Hydronephrosis and vesicoureteral reflux caused by poor bladder compliance, high-pressure voiding, or both can lead to sequelae, the most worrisome of which is renal insufficiency. Urinary tract infections are frequent in patients with multiple sclerosis, as is chronic bacteriuria.

Amyotrophic Lateral Sclerosis

Patients with amyotrophic lateral sclerosis occasionally report urinary bladder difficulty, with frequency and urge incontinence. These patients exhibit brisk deep tendon reflexes in the lower extremities with extensor plantar responses; detrusor hyperreflexia is revealed by cystometric examination. It can be concluded from this finding that the cerebrocortical areas affected by the pathologic process of amyotrophic lateral sclerosis include those responsible for control of the urinary bladder. The external urinary sphincter is spared the effects of amyotrophic lateral sclerosis until late in the disease (30).

Spinal Cord Injury

Urinary bladder dysfunction resulting from spinal cord injury is extensively documented in the literature (18,38).

In spinal cord-injured patients, the clinical level of the neurologic deficit can predict the results of bladder function testing. Lesions may be classified according to whether they are located above the conus or at the level of the conus or cauda equina.

During the period of spinal shock after injury, urinary retention and detrusor areflexia are revealed by cystometry. With the recovery of reflex function, one of several voiding patterns may develop, depending on the site of neurologic injury. These patterns generally persist after stabilization of the initial injury, but in some cases bladder and sphincter function may change because of other factors. The severity of injury and degree of urinary tract dysfunction are interrelated.

Supraconus Spinal Injury

After recovery from spinal shock, the bladder demonstrates hyperreflexia and incomplete emptying on cystometry. Sphincter EMG commonly shows detrusor-sphincter dyssynergia. Because of chronic infection and detrusor fibrosis, bladder compliance may decrease, eventually leading to renal insufficiency resulting from hydronephrosis. The pudendal cortical evoked potential is absent, and the urethroanal and bulbocavernosus reflex latencies are normal.

Autonomic dysreflexia is common in patients with injury at or above T-6, and overdistention of the bladder may induce severe hypertension accompanied by headache, dizziness, and sweating above the level of injury.

Lesions of the Conus Medullaris and Cauda Equina

Urinary retention and straining to void are seen in patients with lesions of the conus medullaris or cauda equina. A lax anal sphincter is revealed on neurologic examination, and the cystometrogram shows detrusor areflexia. Sphincter EMG activity is depressed or absent. Denervation potentials are evident on needle EMG examination of the anal sphincter. The urethroanal and bulbocavernosus reflex latencies are prolonged or absent (22).

Spinal Cord Disease

Cervical Spondylosis with Myelopathy

Frequency, urge, and urge incontinence are seen in patients who have cervical spondylosis and myelopathy associated with bladder dysfunction. Such patients exhibit signs of long-tract involvement, including impairment of vibration and position sense, brisk reflexes in the lower extremities, and possibly extensor plantar responses. Cystometric examination demonstrates detrusor hyperreflexia but rarely show evidence of detrusor-sphincter dyssynergia. There is an accompanying increase in the latency of the pudendal cortical evoked response in these patients (Fig. 8).

Spinovascular Disease

Spinovascular disease may arise following repair of an aortic aneurysm or as a consequence of diabetic angiopathy or collagen vascular disease (58). Cystometric findings are similar to those noted in patients with traumatic spinal cord injury.

Spinal Cord Tumors

Spinal cord tumors can cause symptoms in the lower urinary tract, depending on their location. The most common spinal cord tumor, resulting from extradural spinal cord metastasis, evokes bladder problems when spinal cord compression becomes clinically evident. Intradural and intramedullary spinal cord tumors are infrequently associated with urinary tract symptoms. Detrusor hyperreflexia is a cystometric finding encountered in patients with extramedullary, extradural tumors. When the spinal cord is compressed, the latency of the pudendal cortical evoked response increases and detrusor-sphincter dyssynergia may be present.

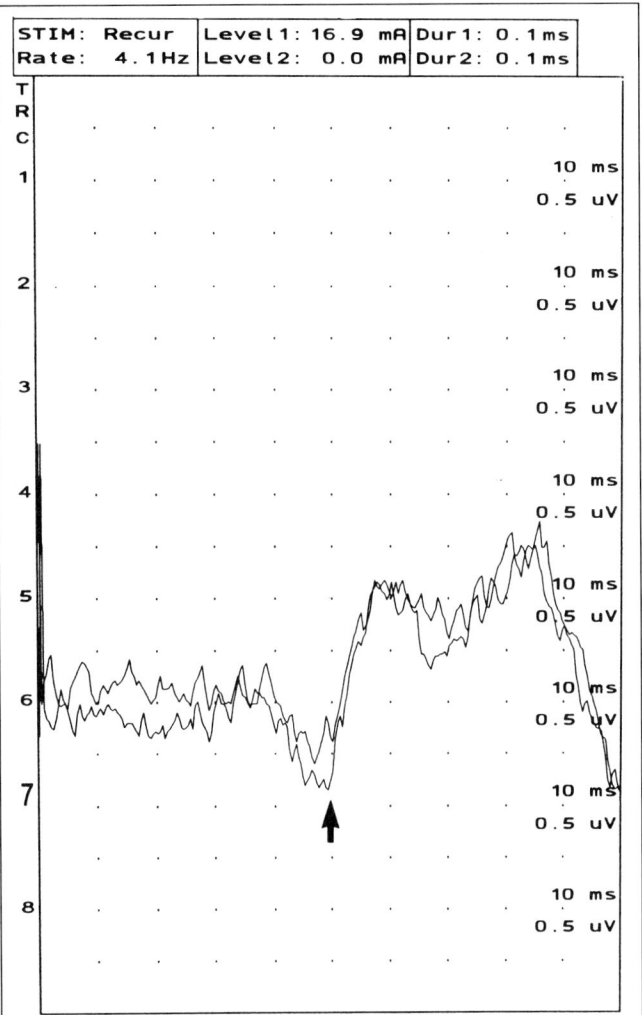

Fig. 8. Pudendal cortical evoked response, 60-year-old man with cervical spondylosis and myelopathy. The latency is delayed at 49 msec. This man presented with urinary frequency, urgency, and erectile dysfunction.

Diseases of the Nervous System Affecting Peripheral Innervation of the Urinary Bladder

The following conditions can affect peripheral innervation of the urinary bladder:

1. Autonomic neuropathy
2. Traumatic injury
3. Lumbar spinal stenosis
4. Sacral agenesis
5. Myelodysplasia
6. Herpes zoster
7. Cauda equina tumors

8. Spinal arachnoiditis
9. Guillain-Barré syndrome

In many cases, symptoms and findings are similar to those seen in victims of traumatic injury to the cauda equina (39,45). Initiating urination is difficult, residual urine volume is increased, and impaired sensation and detrusor areflexia are noted on cystometric examination. The anal sphincter is lax, and sphincter EMG activity is diminished during bladder filling. The latencies of the bulbocavernosus or urethroanal reflexes may be increased or the responses absent.

Autonomic Neuropathy

Of all the forms of neurologic disease, autonomic neuropathy probably most frequently causes urinary bladder dysfunction (21,45). The various origins of autonomic neuropathy are described in earlier chapters.

The precise incidence of urinary bladder dysfunction in patients with diabetes mellitus is unknown. This may in part be a consequence of the pathophysiologic process of diabetes. Because the initial neuropathic changes are confined to vesical afferents, bladder dysfunction remains asymptomatic. Clinically, the bladder volume gradually increases, and the patient voids less frequently because of impaired sensation. Initial cystometric examinations show an increased threshold for the first sensation of bladder filling with a normal detrusor reflex contraction and a retained ability to suppress the detrusor reflex contraction voluntarily.

As the disease progresses, impairment of bladder sensation is greater, with subsequent detrusor areflexia caused by chronic overdistention; as a result, bladder capacity is increased and residual urine volume is large. Uroflow rates are decreased, and abdominal straining is required to initiate and maintain the urinary stream. Findings from neuropathologic studies suggest that the disease may be confined to bladder afferents and affects the autonomic innervation at a late stage. Neurologic examination usually discloses evidence of a peripheral neuropathy. The latency of the bulbocavernosus reflex is increased.

Summary of Diagnosis

Urinary tract dysfunction in patients with neurologic disease is very common, and the diagnosis depends on correlating findings obtained through a thorough history, neurologic examination, and laboratory studies. Unfortunately, the neurologist frequently may fail to ask pertinent questions regarding voiding function, and the urologist may fail to recognize the signs and symptoms of neurologic disease. Collaboration between the disciplines would bring about a greater understanding of the neuroanatomic findings and the effect of the neurologic deficit on laboratory results. Furthermore, a larger number of electrodiagnostic studies of bladder innervation would be done in these patients, thus increasing our knowledge of human pathophysiology.

THERAPY OF NEUROLOGIC DYSFUNCTION OF THE URINARY BLADDER

The therapeutic alternatives for patients with neurogenic bladder dysfunction are extensive, and they include both medical and surgical approaches (Table 2). Except in occasional cases, the neurologic injury causing voiding dysfunction is not reversible. Treatment is therefore based largely on maneuvers to bypass the neurologic injury, and is directed at providing a low-pressure lower urinary tract, a measure of continence, and a method of urine drainage appropriate to the patient's level of function. This section outlines therapeutic possibilities; most treatment regimens include a combination of two or more techniques.

Medical Treatment

Behavioral Therapy

One of the most important and perhaps least appreciated of the treatment modalities is behavioral modification. These maneuvers include timed voiding, as in diabetic patients with insensate bladders; fluid restriction in spinal cord-injured patients with nocturnal incontinence resulting from large urine volumes; suprapubic tapping to induce reflex bladder contractions; avoidance of caffeinated beverages; and biofeedback/physical therapy, in which reflex detrusor activity is suppressed by evoking contraction of

TABLE 2. *Therapy of neurologic dysfunction of the urinary bladder*

Medical treatment
  Behavioral therapy
  Clean intermittent catheterization
  Urine collection devices
    Condom catheters
    Indwelling catheters
    Diapers and pads
  Pharmacotherapy
    Cholinergic agonists
    Anticholinergic agents
    Antiadrenergic agents
    Adrenergic agonists
    Calcium-channel blocking agents
    Muscle relaxants
    Estrogens
Surgical treatment
  Operations on the detrusor muscle
    Denervation procedures for control of detrusor hyperreflexia
    Augmentation cystoplasty/continent urinary diversion
    Ileal conduit
  Operations on the urethra
    Sphincterotomy
    Prostatectomy
    Artificial urinary sphincter

the pelvic floor musculature (28,48,60). The latter maneuver is primarily used in patients with stress urinary incontinence. Behavioral modifications can be used alone to treat minor problems of voiding dysfunction, usually related to continence, or in conjunction with other medical and surgical therapies.

Clean Intermittent Catheterization

Clean intermittent catheterization (CIC), introduced by Lapides et al. in 1972 (50), is now a frequently used and valuable tool in neurogenic bladder hygiene. The technique is based on the concept that efficient bladder emptying is important, even if it entails introduction of bacteria into the urinary system, and that the pitfalls of continuous catheterization can be bypassed with intermittent catheterization. The advantages of this strategy also include the maintenance of low bladder pressure, total evacuation of bladder contents, and voluntary control of urine drainage. Patients are encouraged to use the catheter according to a schedule that allows drainage of urine volumes between 450 mL and 500 mL or less, which is the normal adult bladder capacity. In patients with reflex bladder activity, CIC is used in combination with anticholinergic medications. Most patients can perform CIC, provided that they have adequate cognitive ability and manual dexterity/physical agility to position themselves for catheterization. Young children are able to perform intermittent catheterization on their own. The use of a mirror can assist female patients in learning the technique. Catheter care requires cleaning the reusable catheters with soap and water after each use, followed by air drying.

Complications are few, but these include occasional urinary tract infections, urinary tract trauma (usually during the learning curve), and formation of bladder stones, commonly a result of introducing small foreign bodies, such as lint or hair, into the bladder. Bacteriuria and pyuria are common and generally should not be treated unless the patient is experiencing symptoms, such as fever, dysuria/pain, incontinence, or increased spasticity. Studies have shown no overall benefit from suppressive antibiotics in patients who perform CIC (57). Frequent urinary tract infections (versus colonization or bacteriuria) can be caused by improper catheterization technique or may be a sign of another problem, such as urolithiasis.

Urine Collection Devices

Condom catheters are often used for urine collection in patients who are unable to do self-catheterization. They have a theoretical advantage of not being indwelling, but they are nonetheless associated with chronic bacteriuria as a consequence of the high concentration of organisms at the urethral meatus (41). For the catheters to be used most effectively, the bladder must be able to empty reasonably well at low pressures, as after sphincterotomy. Skin laceration and urethral obstruction occur when the condom catheter is applied too tightly to the penis. Some patients have difficulty in retaining the condom because of inadequate penile length or redundant foreskin. In such cases, surgical placement of a penile prosthesis can aid in management of the catheter. Condom catheters are not reusable and should be changed once a day, with careful attention to penile skin care.

Indwelling catheters, either urethral or suprapubic, are frequently used in patients with neurologic disease, particularly those who are unable to care for themselves. Although the complications of continuous catheterization are well known, a large number of patients tolerate them well and demonstrate no significant increase in upper urinary tract pathology in comparison with patients using other methods of bladder management (33). Appropriate care includes changing the catheter at least monthly, securing the catheter to avoid unnecessary movement or traction, and having a one-way valve on the drainage bag to prevent drained urine from refluxing; in addition, copious fluid intake is required to minimize accumulation of sediment in the bladder. The risk for bladder cancer may be increased in patients who have been continuously catheterized for many years. An annual cystoscopic examination is recommended for patients who have had an indwelling catheter for more than 10 years, although the data to support this screening measure are limited (15)

Diapers and other protective undergarments are used in patients with uncontrollable urinary incontinence related to dementia or in patients in whom trauma from an indwelling catheter is likely. Smaller-sized pads are available to protect clothing for patients with a lesser degree of incontinence.

Pharmacotherapy

Many patients with neurogenic bladder dysfunction are on regimens that include pharmacologic agents. Whether dysfunction is the result of failure to store urine or failure to empty urine, medications can aid in voiding symptomatology. Drugs can be administered orally, parenterally, or intravesically. However, although many patients benefit from drug treatment, medications cannot recreate a normal micturition reflex in the neurologically impaired urinary tract.

The following classes of drugs are most commonly used in the treatment of patients who have neurologic disease associated with bladder dysfunction.

Cholinergic Agonists

The evidence in humans that the peripheral innervation of the urinary detrusor is cholinergically mediated is convincing. Hence, bethanechol, a cholinergic agonist (79), has been employed extensively for the treatment of detrusor areflexia in such conditions as diabetic autonomic neuropathy. An oral dosage of several hundred milligrams a day has been suggested from its use in the clinical setting.

However, the lack of data on drug metabolism, the absence of randomized trials, and the impression that bethanechol is relatively ineffective in resuscitating an impaired detrusor reflex (12) have discouraged continued use of the drug.

Anticholinergic Agents

Anticholinergic agents have long been used for the suppression of detrusor hyperreflexia. The prototype of this group of agents is propantheline bromide (13), and the usual adult oral dosage is 15 to 30 mg every 4 to 6 hrs. Hyoscyamine sulfate (0.125 mg every 4 hrs) is another related agent. Oxybutynin chloride (5 mg three times daily, orally or intravesically), dicyclomine hydrochloride (20 mg three times daily), and flavoxate hydrochloride (100 mg to 200 mg three to four times daily) are agents with anticholinergic properties that also are reported to possess independent musculotropic relaxant effects and local anesthetic activity. All these drugs increase residual urine volume, so CIC by the patient may also need to be instituted.

Other medications with anticholinergic properties used to promote urine storage include tricyclic antidepressants, such as imipramine and doxepin (53).

Adrenergic Blocking Agents

Adrenergic antagonists have been prescribed for the treatment of voiding dysfunction caused by bladder outlet obstruction. Phenoxybenzamine was the first reported effective α-adrenergic-receptor antagonist, used to promote voiding in patients with increased tonus of urethral smooth muscle (49). The drug is not as commonly used now because of the availability of more selective α_1-adrenergic antagonists (prazosin, terazosin, and doxazosin), which have fewer side effects. This class of drugs has also been employed in the treatment of autonomic dysreflexia (32) and is used in the general population for the treatment of bladder outlet obstruction caused by benign prostatic hyperplasia (51). Postural hypotension, the most common side effect, is seen during commencement of treatment.

The β-adrenergic blocker propranolol has been used to increase urethral resistance, but without significant effect. The rationale was that β-adrenergic blockers might be able to potentiate an α-adrenergic effect, resulting in increased tonus of the bladder neck and urethra, but this has not been proved clinically (34).

Adrenergic Agonists

Treatment of stress urinary incontinence with sympathomimetic agents has been used to increase tonus of the urethra and bladder neck. Phenylpropanolamine (50 to 75 mg twice a day), ephedrine (25 to 50 mg three to four times daily), and pseudoephedrine (30 to 60 mg twice a day) are the most commonly prescribed. As with all sympathomimetic agents, they should be used with caution in persons with cardiac disease, hypertension, or hyperthyroidism.

Calcium Channel Blockers

Calcium channel blockers have been employed to improve urinary bladder function (10). These agents include nifedipine, terodiline, and verapamil. At the present time, only terodiline, which possesses additional antimuscarinic properties, holds promise. In oral doses of 25 to 50 mg two times daily, terodiline has been reported to be effective in the treatment of idiopathic detrusor overactivity (76). There have been reports associating this drug with cardiac arrhythmias (74). Further studies in patients with neurologic disease will help define the effectiveness of this agent.

Muscle Relaxants

Skeletal muscle relaxants such as diazepam, baclofen, and dantrolene have been reported to be effective in the treatment of detrusor-sphincter dyssynergia, although sphincterotomy appears to be a more effective treatment for this problem. The doses required to achieve a therapeutic effect on the external urethral sphincter often are intolerable to the patient (i.e., excessive drowsiness).

Estrogen

Estrogen is used in women for the treatment of stress incontinence (56,66). The mechanism of activity is in part a result of potentiation of α-adrenergic tone within the urethra (68).

Surgical Treatment

Operative measures for the treatment of neurogenic voiding dysfunction are generally reserved for those patients with stable neurologic disease in whom conservative medical management has failed. Patient selection and patient education are critical to the success of any operation.

Operations on the Detrusor Muscle

Denervation Procedures for Control of Detrusor Hyperreflexia

The operative approaches used for denervation in the control of detrusor hyperreflexia include section of the sacral nerve roots, carried out by the neurosurgeon, and section of the peripheral innervation of the urinary detrusor, performed by the urologist (61–63). When these procedures are performed in patients with detrusor hyperreflexia whose neurologic reflex control is already impaired, the postoperative goal is to increase the detrusor reflex threshold at the

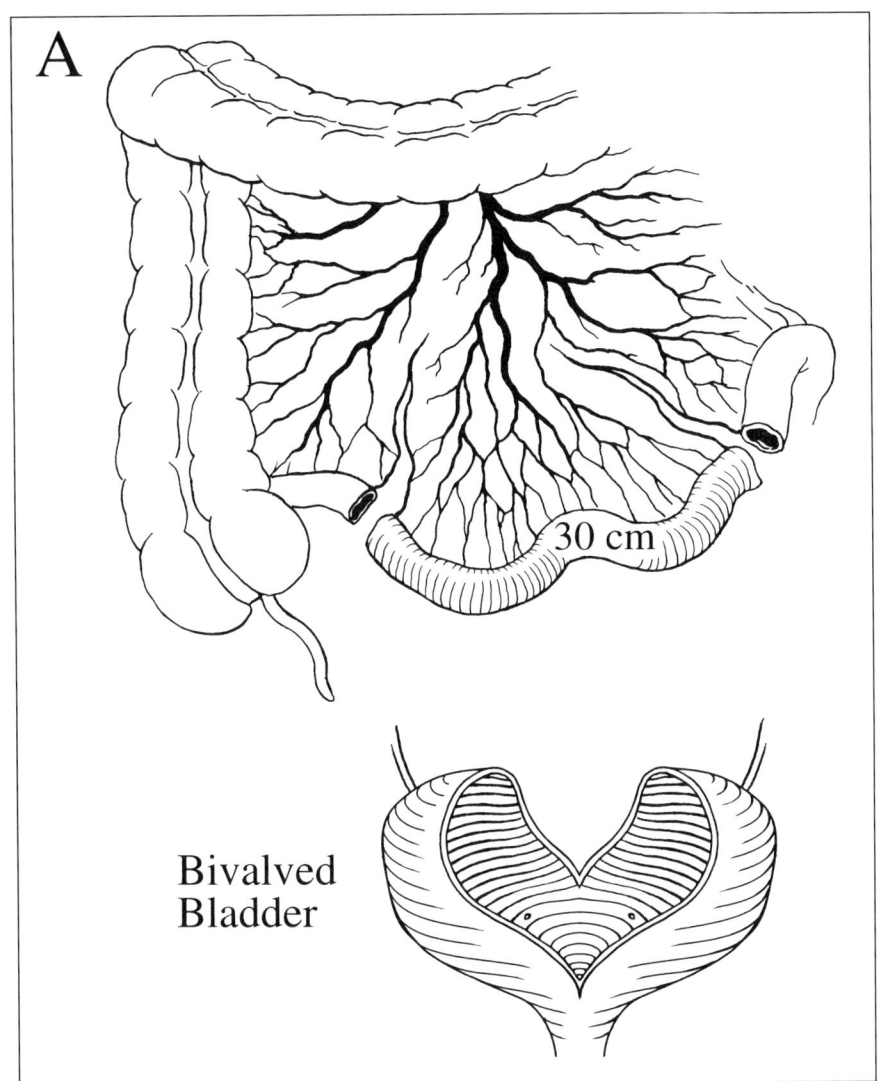
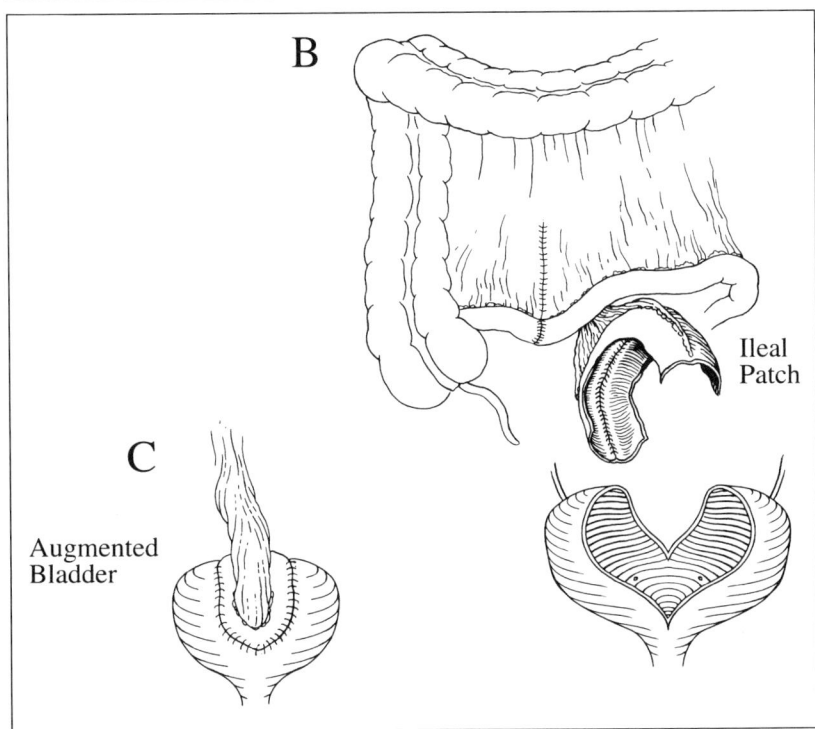

Fig. 9. Augmentation cystoplasty. (A) A segment of distal ileum is isolated from the GI tract, based on the terminal branches of the superior mesenteric artery. The bladder is bivalved from near the anterior bladder neck to the trigone posteriorly. (B) The ileal segment is opened into an inverted U-shaped patch. (C) The patch is sewn onto the opened bladder.

expense of bladder emptying. Because of disappointing results, this technique is used infrequently for bladder management. Other denervation procedures for the treatment of detrusor hyperreflexia include supratrigonal transection of the detrusor muscle, ganglionectomy, and bladder hyperdistention (45). These operations are rarely performed.

Augmentation Cystoplasty

Bladder augmentation is used when medical therapy is unable to effect a low-pressure reservoir of adequate capacity, as in cases of detrusor hyperreflexia that is refractory to pharmacotherapy or poor bladder compliance caused by fibrosis. The standard technique consists of dividing the bladder into two parts and suturing a detubularized segment of bowel onto the bladder (Fig. 9). In this manner, bladder capacity and compliance are increased. In most cases, patients must perform intermittent catheterization, as the bladder's ability to generate a coordinated detrusor reflex of adequate magnitude and duration is compromised by the operation. A continent stoma that can be catheterized is created on the abdominal wall in women who are unable to access their urethra easily.

The complications of this treatment include those of any major bowel operation (i.e., peritonitis, bowel obstruction or perforation, and anastomotic leak). Urinary tract infections, the presence of mucus in the urine (which may impede drainage of urine), and long-term diarrhea are infrequent sequelae.

Ileal Conduit

A last-resort measure to bypass a bladder that is not amenable to medical or surgical management is the creation of an ileal conduit, whereby the ureters are sewn onto a segment of distal ileum and brought to the skin (Fig. 10). Urine collects in a urostomy bag affixed to the stoma.

Operations on the Urethra

Sphincterotomy

Sphincterotomy is frequently used for the treatment of detrusor-sphincter dyssynergia in patients with supraconus spinal cord injuries (47,65). In this procedure, the external urinary sphincter is incised, with or without bladder neck incision or resection. The patient subsequently requires a condom catheter for urine collection. Patients who undergo sphincterotomy require continued follow-up, as a significant percentage require a repeated operation (80). Stimulation of trigger points by finger tapping of the skin of the anterior abdominal wall may be done to facilitate emptying in these patients. An intraurethral stainless steel mesh stent, placed at the level of the external urinary sphincter, is currently being evaluated in the treatment of external sphincter dyssynergia (71).

Prostatectomy

A prostatectomy can be performed in patients with neurologic urinary bladder dysfunction as a method of decreasing outlet resistance. However, the results are frequently unsatisfactory (52,73).

Artificial Urinary Sphincter

An artificial urinary sphincter device has been in use since 1973 for the control of urinary incontinence in patients with neurologic bladder dysfunction (69,70). This method was introduced by Scott et al. (69.70) and has since been successfully and progressively improved for the treatment of patients with myelodysplasia, spinal cord injury, and multiple sclerosis, as well as other disease states resulting in incontinence.

The device consists of an inflatable cuff, reservoir, pump, and control assembly (Fig. 11). The prosthesis is coated with Silastic and implanted near the bladder with the cuff placed around the bladder neck. The pump is located in the labia or scrotum, which makes it accessible for external manual manipulation. By squeezing the pump, fluid is expelled from the cuff into the balloon reservoir, and this permits voiding. Fluid from the reservoir is then automatically and gradually transferred from the reservoir to the cuff during an interval of several minutes, with voiding occurring during the interval.

Postoperative complications that have been observed for this method include urethral necrosis (40,44) and deterioration of the upper urinary tract (16). The method continues to offer promise, but careful preoperative selection is imperative.

Summary of Treatment

There are no easy methods to evaluate or treat patients with neurologic disease and urinary dysfunction. In some cases, the therapeutic options are limited and expectations must be modest, especially if the patient is cognitively impaired. Therefore, the assessment of neurologic disease is an important factor in understanding the nature of bladder dysfunction as well as in deciding what approach to take in therapy. A collaborative effort between the neurologist, who has the ability to translate the nervous system disease process into neuroanatomic and neurophysiologic changes in bladder function, and the urologist, who has the knowledge and techniques to manage the lower urinary tract, would result in a better understanding of neurourologic problems. Productive research and improved patient care would emerge from this fusion of disciplines.

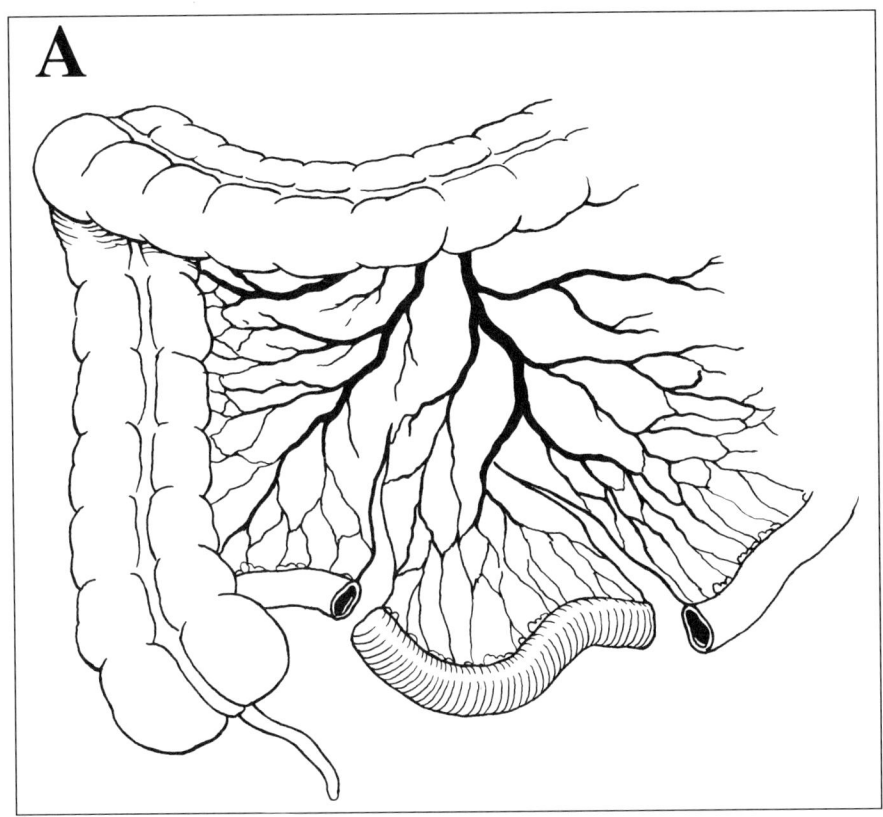
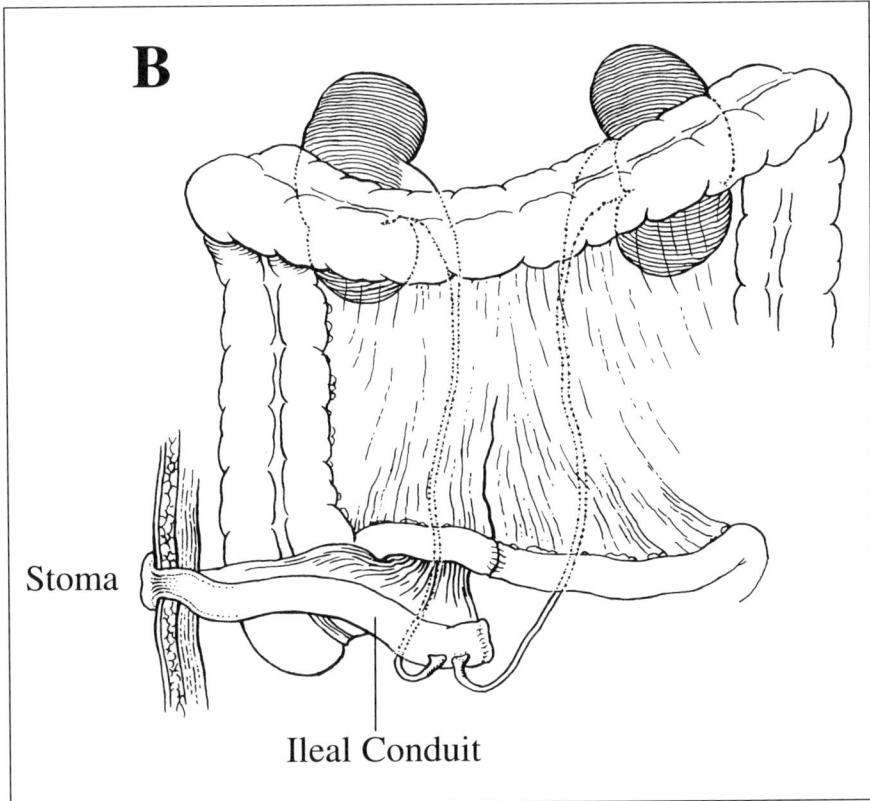

Fig. 10. Ileal conduit. **(A)** A 15 cm segment of distal ileum is taken for creation of the conduit. **(B)** The ureters are anastomosed to the segment and urine is drained to the skin.

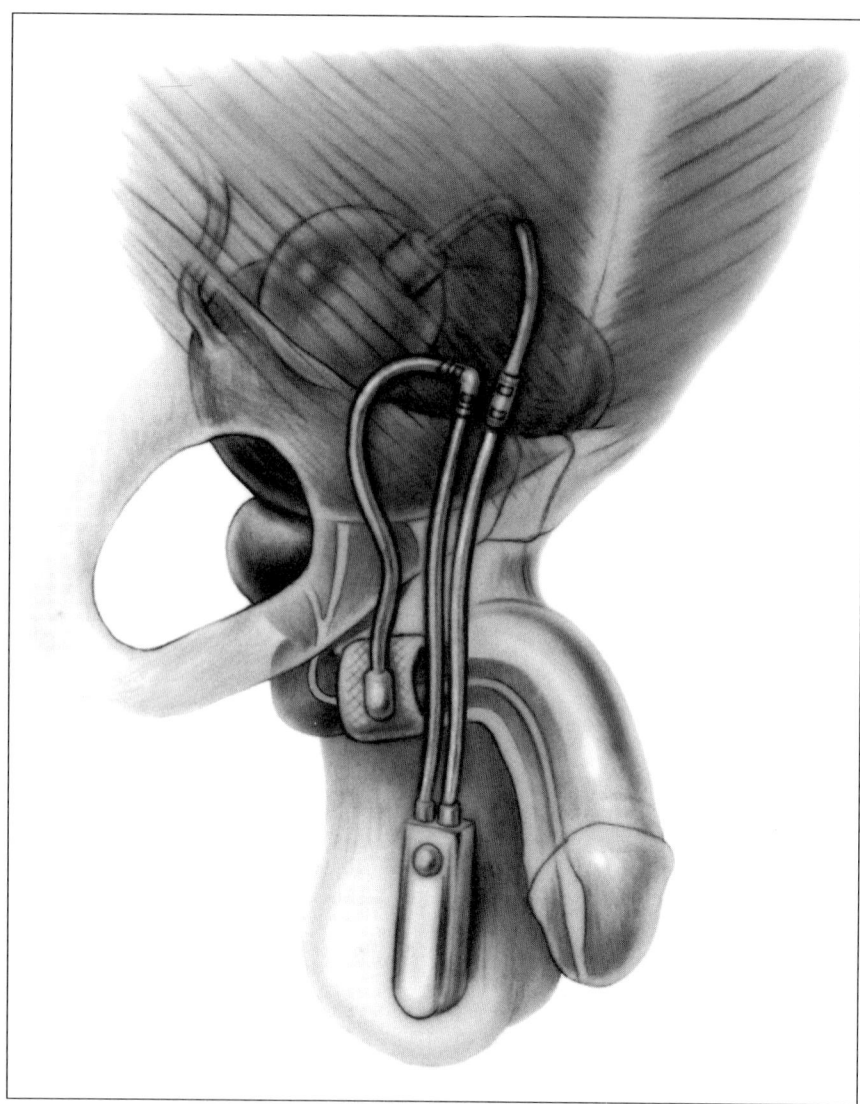

Fig. 11. Artificial urinary sphincter in male. The cuff is placed around the bulbous urethra and is connected to the pump placed in the scrotum. The pressure-regulating balloon (resevoir) is placed in the retropubic space and is connected to the pump. The mechanism is activated by manually squeezing the pump, which deflates the cuff and allows urine to pass through the urethra. The placement of the prosthesis is modified in women by placing the cuff around the bladder neck and the pump in the labia.

REFERENCES

1. Abrams P, et al. Standardization of terminology of lower urinary tract function. *Neurourol Urodyn* 1988;7:403–477.
2. Andersen JT. Disturbances of bladder and urethral function in Parkinson's disease. *Int Urol Nephrol* 1985;17:35–41.
3. Andersen JT, Bradley WE. Cystometric, sphincter and electromyographic abnormalities in Parkinson's disease. *J Urol* 1976;116: 75–78.
4. Andersen JT, Bradley WE. Postural detrusor hyperreflexia. *J Urol* 1976;116:228–230.
5. Andersen JT, Bradley WE. The syndrome of detrusor-sphincter dyssynergia. *J Urol* 1976;116:493–495.
6. Andersen JT, Bradley WE. Bladder and urethral innervation in multiple sclerosis. *Br J Urol* 1976;48:239–243.
7. Andersen JT, Bradley WE. The urethral closure pressure profile. *Br J Urol* 1976;48:341–345.
8. Andersen JT, Bradley WE. Cystometry: detrusor reflex activation, classification and terminology. *J Urol* 1977;118:623–625.
9. Andersen JT, et al. The urethral electromyographic and gas pressure profile. *Scand J Urol Nephrol* 1976;10:185–188.
10. Andersson K-E, Forman A. Effects of calcium channel blockers on urinary tract smooth muscle. *Acta Pharmacol Toxicol* 1986;58(Suppl II):193–200.
11. Andrew T, Nathan PW. Lesions of the anterior frontal lobes and disturbances of micturition and defecation. *Brain* 1964;87:233–262.
12. Barrett DM. The effect of oral bethanechol chloride on voiding in female patients with excessive residual urine: a randomized double-blind study. *J Urol* 1981;126:640–642.
13. Benson GW, et al. Bladder muscle contractility: comparative effects and mechanisms of action of atropine, propantheline, flavoxate and imipramine. *Urology* 1977;9:31–35.
14. Bhatia NN, et al. Urodynamics: continuous monitoring. *J Urol* 1982; 128:963–968.
15. Bickel A, et al. Bladder cancer in spinal cord injury patients. *J Urol* 1991;146:1240–1242.
16. Bitsch M, et al. Upper urinary tract deterioration after implantation of artificial urinary sphincter. *Scand J Urol Nephrol* 1990;24:31–34.
17. Blaivas JG, Fisher DM. Combined radiographic and urodynamic monitoring: advances in technique. *J Urol* 1981;125:693–694.
18. Bors E, Comarr AE. *Neurological Urology: Physiology of Micturition, Its Neurological Disorders and Sequelae.* Baltimore: University Park Press; 1971.
19. Bradley WE. Cystometry and sphincter electromyography. *Mayo Clin Proc* 1976;51:329–335.
20. Bradley WE. Urinary bladder dysfunction in multiple sclerosis. *Neurology* 1978;28(Pt 2):52–58.
21. Bradley WE. Diagnosis of urinary bladder dysfunction in diabetes mellitus. *Ann Intern Med* 1980;92:323–326.

22. Bradley WE, Andersen JT. Neuromuscular dysfunction of lower urinary tract in patients with lesions of the cauda equina and conus medullaris. *J Urol* 1976;116:620–621.
23. Bradley WE, Lin JT. Assessment of diabetic sexual dysfunction and cystopathy. In: Dyck PJ, et al, eds. *Diabetic Neuropathy*. Philadelphia: WB Saunders; 1987:146–154.
24. Bradley WE, et al. Cystometric and sphincter abnormalities in multiple sclerosis. *Neurology* 1973;23:1131–1139.
25. Bradley WE, et al. Sphincter electromyography. *Urol Clin North Am* 1974;1:69–80.
26. Bradley WE, Timm GW. Cystometry: III. Cystometers. *Urology* 1975;5:843–848.
27. Bradley WE, Timm GW. Cystometry: VI. Interpretation. *Urology* 1976;7:231–235.
28. Burgio KL, et al. Urinary incontinence in the elderly: bladder-sphincter biofeedback and toileting skills training. *Ann Intern Med* 1985;103:507–515.
29. Cardenas DD, et al. Residual urine measurements in patients with spinal cord injury: measurement with a portable ultrasound instrument. *Arch Phys Med Rehabil* 1988;69:514–516.
30. Carvalho M, et al. Involvement of the external anal sphincter in amyotrophic lateral sclerosis. *Muscle Nerve* 1995;18:848–853.
31. Chalfin SA, Bradley WE. The etiology of detrusor hyperreflexia in patients with intravesical obstruction. *J Urol* 1982;127:938–942.
32. Chancellor MB, et al. Prospective evaluation of terazosin for the treatment of autonomic dysreflexia. *J Urol* 1994;151:111–113.
33. Chao R, Clowers D, Mayo ME. Fate of upper tracts in patients with indwelling catheters after spinal cord injury. *Urology* 1993;42:259–262.
34. Donker PJ, van der Sluis C. Action of β-adrenergic blocking agents on the urethral pressure profile. *Urol Int* 1976;31:6–12.
35. Dick H, et al. Pudendal sexual reflexes. *Urology* 1974;3:376–379.
36. Diokno AC, et al. Fate of patients started on clean intermittent self-catheterization therapy 10 years ago. *J Urol* 1983;129:1120–1122.
37. Drach GW, et al. Male peak urinary flow rate: relationships to volume voided and age. *J Urol* 1979;122:210–214.
38. Fam BA, et al. Experience in the urologic management of 120 early spinal cord injury patients. *J Urol* 1978;119:485–487.
39. Fanciullacci F, et al. Clinical, urodynamic and neurophysiological findings in patients with neuropathic bladder due to a lumbar intervertebral disc protrusion. *Paraplegia* 1989;27:354–358.
40. Fishman IJ, et al. Experience with the artificial urinary sphincter model AS800 in 148 patients. *J Urol* 1989;141:307–310.
41. Golji H. Complications of external condom drainage. *Paraplegia* 1987;19:189–197.
42. Griffiths DJ. Urodynamic assessment of bladder function. *Br J Urol* 1977;49:29–36.
43. Griffiths CJ, et al. Ambulatory monitoring of bladder and detrusor pressure during natural filling. *J Urol* 1989;142:180–184.
44. Gundian JC, et al. Mayo Clinic experience with use of AMS800 artificial urinary sphincter for urinary incontinence following radical prostatectomy. *J Urol* 1989;142:1459–1461.
45. Hald T, Bradley WE. *The Urinary Bladder: Neurology and Dynamics*. Baltimore: Williams & Wilkins; 1982.
46. Haldeman S, et al. Colonometry, cystometry and evoked potentials in multiple sclerosis. *Arch Neurol* 1982;39:698–701.
47. Herr HW, et al. External sphincterotomy in traumatic neurogenic bladder dysfunction. *J Urol* 1975;113:32–34.
48. Kegel AH. Physiologic therapy for urinary stress incontinence. *JAMA* 1951;146:915–917.
49. Krane RJ, Olsson CA. Phenoxybenzamine in neurogenic bladder dysfunction. II. Clinical considerations. *J Urol* 1973;110:653–656.
50. Lapides J, et al. Clean, intermittent self-catheterization in the treatment of urinary tract disease. *J Urol* 1972;107:458–461.
51. Lepor H, et al. The safety, efficacy, and compliance of terazosin therapy for benign prostatic hyperplasia. *J Urol* 1992;147:1554–1557.
52. Lim SK, Marshall VR. Results of prostatectomy in patients following a cerebrovascular accident. *Br J Urol* 1982;54:186–189.
53. Lose G, Jørgensen L, Thunedborg P. Doxepin in the treatment of female detrusor overactivity: a randomized double-blind crossover study. *J Urol* 1989;142:1024–1026.
54. Mayo ME, Chetner MP. Lower urinary tract dysfunction in multiple sclerosis. *Urology* 1992;34:67–70.
55. Merrill DC, et al. Air cystometry II. A clinical evaluation of normal adults. *J Urol* 1972;108:85–88.
56. Miodrag A, et al. Sex hormones and the female urinary tract. *Drugs* 1988;36:491–504.
57. Mohler JL, et al. Suppression and treatment of urinary tract infection in patients with an intermittently catheterized neurogenic bladder. *J Urol* 1987;138:336–340.
58. Murayama N, et al. Disturbances of micturition in patients with a spinal arteriovenous malformation. *Paraplegia* 1989;27:212–216.
59. Murnaghan GF. Neurogenic disorders of the bladder in parkinsonism. *Br J Urol* 1961;33:403–409.
60. Pollock DD, Liberman RP. Behavior therapy of incontinence in demented inpatients. *Gerontologist* 1974;14:488–491.
61. Rockswold GL, et al. Differential sacral rhizotomy in the treatment of neurogenic bladder dysfunction. *J Neurosurg* 1973;38:748–754.
62. Rockswold GL, et al. Effect of sacral nerve blocks on the function of the urinary bladder in humans. *J Neurosurg* 1974;40:83–89.
63. Rockswold GL, et al. Re-evaluation of differential sacral rhizotomy for neurological bladder disease. *J Neurosurg* 1978;48:773–778.
64. Rockswold GL, et al. Electrophysiological technique for evaluating lesions of the conus medullaris and cauda equina. *J Neurosurg* 1976;45:321–326.
65. Ross JC, et al. Division of the external sphincter in the treatment of the neurogenic bladder: a ten-year review. *Br J Surg* 1967;54:627–628.
66. Rud T. The effect of estrogens and gestagens on the urethral pressure profile in urinary continent and stress incontinent women. *Acta Obstet Gynecol Scand* 1980;59:265–270.
67. Sarica Y, Karacan I. Cerebral responses evoked by stimulation of the vesico-urethral junction in normal subjects. *Electroencephalogr Clin Neurophysiol* 1986;65:440–446.
68. Schreiter F, et al. Estrogenic sensitivity of α-receptors in the urethra musculature. *Urol Int* 1976;31:13–19.
69. Scott FB, et al. Treatment of urinary incontinence by implantable prosthetic sphincter. *Urology* 1973;1:252–259.
70. Scott FB, et al. Treatment of urinary incontinence by an implantable prosthetic urinary sphincter. *J Urol* 1974;112:75–80.
71. Shaw FJR, et al. Permanent external striated sphincter stents in patients with spinal injuries. *Br J Urol* 1990;66:297–302.
72. Siroky MB, et al. The flow rate nomogram: II. Clinical correlation. *J Urol* 1980;123:208–210.
73. Staskin DS, et al. Post-prostatectomy continence in the parkinsonian patient: the significance of poor voluntary sphincter control. *J Urol* 1988;140:117–118.
74. Stewart DA, et al. Terodiline causes polymorphic ventricular tachycardia due to reduced heart rate and prolongation of QT interval. *Eur J Clin Pharmacol* 1992;42:577–580.
75. Susset JG, et al. Critical evaluation of uroflowmeters and analysis of normal curves. *J Urol* 1973;109:874–878.
76. Tapp A, et al. Terodiline: a dose-titrated, multicenter study of the treatment of idiopathic detrusor instability in women. *J Urol* 1989;142:1027–1031.
77. Taylor MC, et al. The conus demyelination syndrome in multiple sclerosis. *Acta Neurol Scand* 1984;69:80–89.
78. Tsuchida S, et al. Urodynamic studies in hemiplegic patients after cerebrovascular accident. *Urology* 1983;21:315–318.
79. Wein AJ, et al. The effects of bethanechol chloride on urodynamic parameters in normal women and in women with significant residual urine volumes. *J Urol* 1980;124:397–399.
80. Yang CC, Mayo ME. External urethral sphincterotomy: long-term follow-up. *Neurourol Urodyn* 1995;14:25–31.

CHAPTER 47

Sleep Apnea and Autonomic Failure

Sudhansu Chokroverty

---

1. Medullary respiratory neurons that possess inherent rhythmicity comprise a dorsal group that is mainly inspiratory and a ventral group that has combined inspiratory and expiratory properties. These neurons are influenced by the pneumotaxic center in the rostral pons and apneustic center in the lower pons, as well as other central and peripheral inputs.
2. Non-rapid-eye-movement (NREM) sleep predominates, and its four stages are characterized by an increasing degree and amount of slowing of the electroencephalographic (EEG) recording. Autonomic indices, including blood pressure (BP), heart rate (HR), thermoregulatory set point, and respiratory chemosensitivity, are reduced.
3. Rapid-eye-movement (REM), or paradoxical, sleep is associated with phasic irregularities of eye movements, HR, BP, and respiration. Erection occurs during this phase.
4. Patients with multiple-system atrophy (MSA) commonly have sleep apnea, hypopnea, respiratory dysrhythmia, or nocturnal stridor. Central mechanisms predominate, but there may also be an obstructive component.
5. Abnormalities noted in familial dysautonomia (FD) include sleep apnea, severe breath holding, respiratory dysrhythmias, prolonged onset of REM sleep, and reduced total REM sleep.
6. The peripheral neuropathies, especially diabetic neuropathy, may be associated with sleep apnea; central, obstructive, or mixed patterns have been observed.
7. Important investigations of the disorder include polysomnographic studies, multiple sleep latency test, respiratory function tests, and laryngeal electromyography (EMG).
8. Drugs used in the treatment of sleep apnea include protriptyline, medroxyprogesterone, and acetazolamide. Mechanisms of action include alerting properties or an increase in ventilatory drive.
9. Nasal continuous positive airway pressure is effective for treating obstructive apnea.
10. Tracheostomy may be useful, especially in the treatment of stridor.

INTRODUCTION

Sleep-related respiratory disturbances have been described recently in many patients with autonomic failure. There has also been a growing and parallel awareness of the importance of autonomic dysfunction as a cause of human diseases, as well as of the interaction of sleep and breathing in normal and pathologic conditions. Progress in understanding the nature of the central autonomic network and respiratory physiology and anatomy, and new knowledge of the anatomy and physiology of mammalian sleep, have clearly shown that the autonomic nervous system, sleep, and breathing are closely interrelated. To understand the subject of sleep apnea in the context of autonomic failure, a brief description of the anatomy and physiology of these interdependent entities is essential. This is provided at the beginning of the chapter, after which the diagnosis and treatment of sleep-related breathing disorders, specifically sleep apnea in patients with autonomic failure, are discussed.

ANATOMY OF THE CENTRAL AUTONOMIC NETWORK, SLEEP, AND BREATHING

Work done during the past 20 years has clearly shown the existence of a central autonomic network in the brain stem with ascending and descending projections (28,60) that are often reciprocally connected (Figs. 1 and 2). The nucleus tractus solitarii (NTS) in the medulla is the most

---

S. Chokroverty: Department of Neurology, New York Medical College, Valhalla, New York, Department of Neurology, Robert Wood Johnson Medical School, New Brunswick, New Jersey 08903.

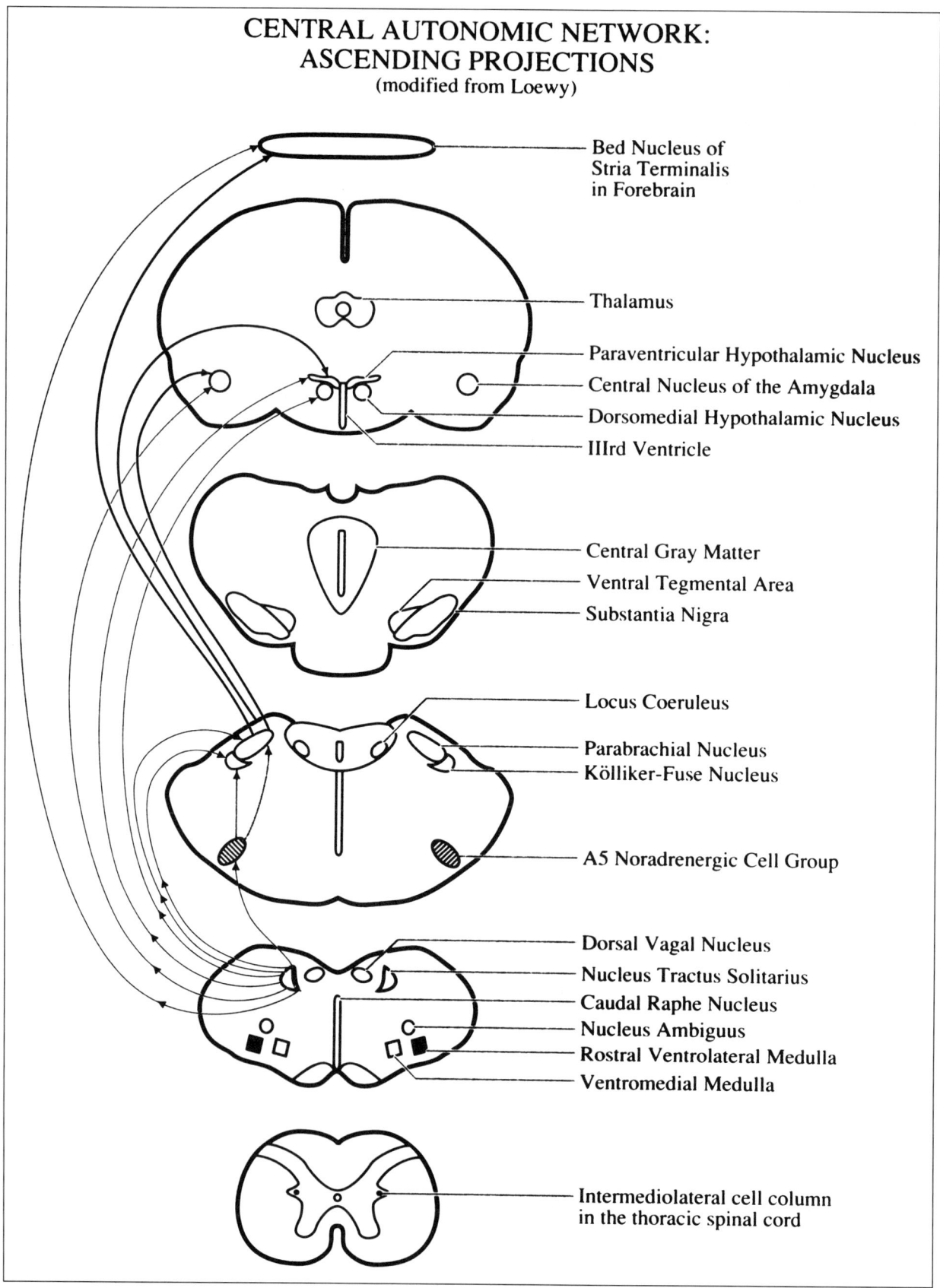

FIG. 1. The ascending projections of the central autonomic network. (Modified from Lowey and Spyer, ref. 60, with permission from Chokroverty, ref. 28, and the American Academy of Neurology.)

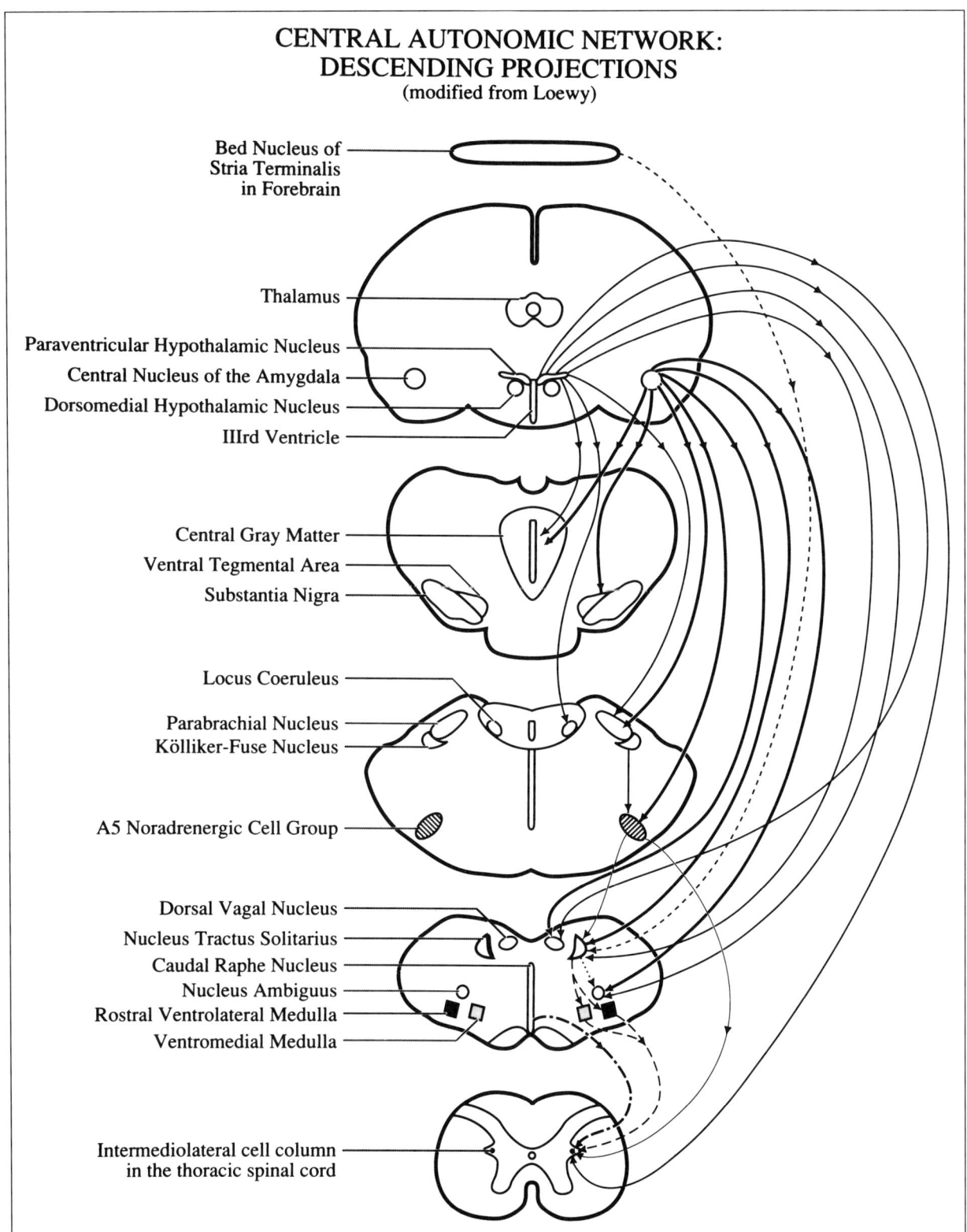

FIG. 2. The descending projections of the central autonomic network. (Modified from Lowey and Spyer, ref. 60, with permission from Chokroverty, ref. 28, and the American Academy of Neurology.)

crucial structure of the central autonomic network; through its ascending and descending projections, it regulates the central autonomic network. The NTS, which is located in the dorsomedial region of the medulla ventral to the dorsal vagal nucleus, receives important afferents from the cardiovascular and respiratory tracts that are necessary for the autonomic control of cardiac rhythm, circulation, and respiration. The NTS sends efferents as ascending projections to the supramedullary area, including the hypothalamic and limbic regions, as well as descending projections to the ventral medulla, which in turn sends efferents to the intermediolateral neurons of the spinal cord (28,60). The final common pathways from the NTS use the vagus nerve and sympathetic fibers from the intermediolateral neurons of the spinal cord to orchestrate the central autonomic network and integrate various autonomic functions. Lower brain stem hypnogenic neurons and central respiratory neurons are also located in the NTS (28). Thus, autonomic control of vital cardiorespiratory and other functions during sleep are integrated in the region of the NTS.

CONTROL OF BREATHING IN SLEEP AND WAKEFULNESS

Normal human respiration depends on three controlling systems: (a) the metabolic and autonomic, or automatic, system (6,64); (b) a voluntary or behavioral system (74); and (c) a reticular arousal system (50,62) that is responsible for the wakefulness stimulus, which exerts a tonic influence on the brain stem respiratory neurons. The autonomic respiratory neurons are located in the medulla (6,64,70,71,88), and these in turn are influenced by two groups of upper brain stem respiratory neurons (20): (a) the pneumotaxic center, located in the rostral pons in the region of the parabrachial and Kölliker-Fuse nuclei; and (b) the apneustic center, located in the dorsolateral region of the lower pons. These upper brain stem neurons and the medullary respiratory neurons are also influenced by structures in the forebrain, hypothalamus, and limbic regions throughout the central autonomic network (28,60).

The medullary respiratory neurons, which possess inherent rhythmicity, comprise two principal nuclear groups (20,24,27,63): (a) the dorsal respiratory neurons, located in the NTS; and (b) the ventral group of neurons, located in the region of the nucleus ambiguus and nucleus retroambigualis (Fig. 3). The dorsal neurons are predominantly but not exclusively inspiratory, and the ventral group consists of both inspiratory and expiratory neurons. Fibers from these respiratory premotor neurons cross through the medullary reticular formation as the reticulospinal tracts and travel to the contralateral phrenic and intercostal nerves; they are responsible for controlling breathing during sleep and wakefulness (6,64,68,74). The parasympa-

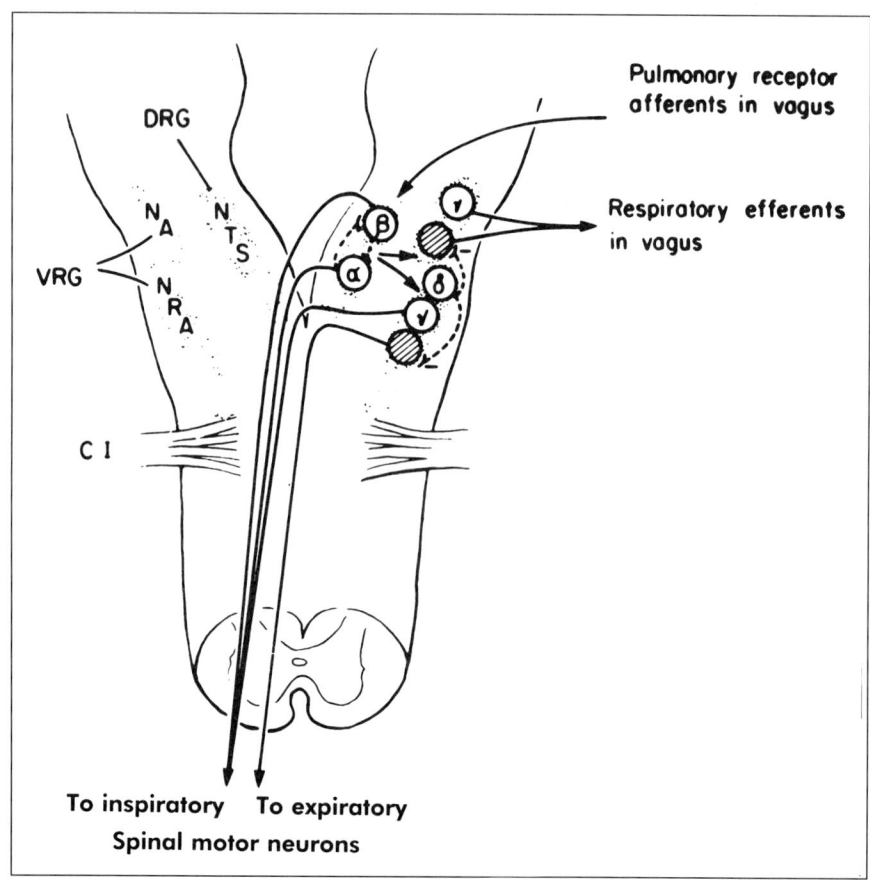

FIG. 3. Medullary respiratory neurons. *DRG*, dorsal respiratory group; *VRG*, ventral respiratory group; *NTS*, nucleus tractus solitarius; *NA*, nucleus ambiguus; *NRA*, nucleus retroambigualis; *CI*, first cervical root; α, β, τ, δ, inspiratory cell types; ○, inspiratory cells; ⦸, expiratory cells. (From Berger et al., ref. 6, with permission.)

thetic afferents from the peripheral respiratory tracts, the carotid and aortic body peripheral chemoreceptors, the central chemoreceptors on the ventral surface of the medulla, and the supramedullary (forebrain, midbrain, and pontine regions) and reticular activating system all influence the medullary respiratory neurons to regulate the rate, rhythm, and amplitude of breathing (20,24,27,64).

The voluntary or behavioral breathing system controls respiration during wakefulness but is nonfunctional during sleep, except during part of REM sleep (70). Although the exact anatomic origin and pathways of the voluntary respiratory system are not known, it is believed that the fibers originate in the cerebral cortex (forebrain and limbic system) (74) and descend partly to the autonomic medullary controlling system, but mostly with the corticospinal tracts to spinal respiratory motor neurons, where the fibers are finally integrated with the reticulospinal fibers originating from the autonomic medullary respiratory neurons (6,27, 68,74).

OVERVIEW OF SLEEP

Sleep Stages

Sleep is not a homogeneous state. It has two separate and distinct aspects that are based on EEG, behavioral, and physiologic characteristics: non-REM (slow-wave) sleep and REM (paradoxical) sleep (27,69,77,98). Non-REM sleep accounts for 75%–80% of sleep time in adult human beings, and REM sleep accounts for 20%–25% of sleep time.

Based on EEG criteria, there are four stages of non-REM sleep. EEG findings during stage I of non-REM sleep consist of a general disorganization of the background rhythm, diminution of the alpha rhythm, and the appearance of low-voltage theta (4 to 7 Hz) and beta ($>$13 Hz) rhythms. Stage II is characterized by sleep spindles (12 to 14 Hz) and K complexes. In accordance with the standard sleep-scoring criteria, the duration of the spindles and K complexes must be $\geq$0.5 second. In stage II sleep, $<$20% of the EEG recording consists of high-voltage ($>$75 μV) slow waves (0.5 to 2 Hz), and in stage III sleep, $\geq$20% but not $>$50% of the EEG recording is made up of delta waves with a frequency of $\leq$2 Hz and an amplitude of $>$75 μV. In stage IV non-REM sleep, $>$50% of the EEG recording contains waves with a frequency of $\leq$2 Hz and an amplitude of $>$75 μV.

REM sleep begins 60 to 90 min after sleep onset and recurs in a cyclic manner every 90 to 110 min throughout the night, for a total of about four to six cycles in normal individuals. Based on EEG, EMG, and eye movement criteria, REM sleep can be divided into two stages: tonic and phasic (69,75). A desynchronized EEG, hypotonia of the axial muscles, and depression of monosynaptic and polysynaptic reflexes are characteristic of the tonic stage. The phasic stage is discontinuous and superimposed on the tonic stage. The phasic events comprise bursts of rapid eye movements, myoclonic twitchings of the facial and limb muscles, irregularities of HR and respiration with variable BP, spontaneous activity of the middle ear muscles, and tongue movements (22,27). The EEG during REM sleep is characterized by low-voltage, fast activities mixed with a small amount of theta rhythm and sometimes "sawtooth" waves.

Theories of Sleep

Evidence obtained from ablation and stimulation experiments, single-unit recordings, and human pathologic observations indicate that non-REM or synchronized sleep results from a combination of two factors: activation of hypnogenic neurons in the anterior hypothalamus and the preoptic region as well as the NTS in the medulla, coupled with inhibition of the ascending reticular activating system (4,5,10,11,36,46,54,66,91). A popular recent theory for REM sleep suggests that there are anatomically distributed and neurochemically interconnected REM "on" and "off" cells in the brain stem (47,48). REM "on" cells are thought to be located in the laterodorsal and peduculo-pantine tegmental nucleus. REM "off" cells are thought to be located in the locus ceruleus, raphe nuclei (dorsal raphe nucleus, raphe pontis, and raphe magnus), and peribrachial region in the pons. A reciprocal interaction between the REM "on" and "off" cells in the brain stem precipitates REM sleep. The REM-promoting neurons are cholinergic and the REM-inhibiting neurons are aminergic; interaction or oscillation between these two groups of neurons generates the cycle of REM and non-REM sleep (47,53,54,100).

ALTERATIONS IN AUTONOMIC FUNCTIONS DURING SLEEP

Most of the autonomic alterations that occur during normal sleep involve the cardiovascular and respiratory systems (28,60).

Cardiovascular Changes

In non-REM sleep, the HR slows, BP falls, and cardiac output decreases. In REM sleep, there is a further slowing of the HR and fall in BP resulting from a marked decrease in peripheral resistance. During phasic REM, BP and HR are unstable because of phasic vagal inhibition and sympathetic activation caused by alterations in the brain stem neural activity. In humans, HR and BP fluctuate during REM sleep. The parasympathetic activity predominates during sleep, with an additional reduction in sympathetic activity during REM sleep.

Respiratory Changes

In non-REM sleep, respiration is completely under metabolic control and involves the medullary respiratory and hypothalamic neurons (28,32,70,71,88,92). The activity of the respiratory neurons in the pons and medulla is decreased during both non-REM and REM sleep. Because of decreased sensitivity of the respiratory neurons to carbon dioxide, inhibition of the reticular activating system, and alteration of the metabolic control of the respiratory neurons during sleep, the tidal volume, minute ventilation, and alveolar ventilation decrease (14,15,19,32,70,71,88,92). The diminished alveolar ventilation causes the arterial carbon dioxide tension to rise, and the arterial oxygen tension and oxygen saturation to decrease (14,15,32,70,71,88,92). These blood gas changes are noted despite a fall in oxygen consumption and carbon dioxide production during sleep (93). Both the hypercapnic (8,34,40) and hypoxic (7,33,94) ventilatory responses are decreased during REM and non-REM sleep, with a more marked decrease during REM sleep (20,26,27,70–72,88,92). This decrement results from a combination of factors: (a) a decreasing number of functional medullary respiratory neurons during sleep; (b) decreased sensitivity of the central chemoreceptors subserving medullary respiratory neurons; and (c) increased resistance in the upper airway (49,85,96).

In REM sleep, respiration becomes rapid and irregular (70,71). Both the tonic and phasic activities in the intercostal and upper-airway muscles decrease, with phasic activities maintained in the diaphragm but tonic activity in the diaphragm reduced (35,70–72,88). The resulting hypotonia of the muscles dilating the upper airway causes upper-airway resistance to increase during sleep (49,85,96). The arousal responses are also decreased, particularly during REM sleep (72). The voluntary respiratory control system may be active during some of REM sleep (70).

Even in normal individuals, respiration is vulnerable during sleep, in that mild respiratory irregularities and brief apneic episodes with an apnea index of <5 may occur in normal individuals. In disease states, apnea may become pathologically significant.

This brief review of the anatomy and physiology of the autonomic nervous system, sleep, and respiration underscores the close interrelationship of the respiratory, central autonomic, and hypnogenic neurons, which creates a delicate balance between the autonomic and respiratory neurons and the neuronal systems controlling sleep and wakefulness.

SLEEP APNEA IN CLINICAL AUTONOMIC FAILURE

Autonomic failure can be broadly classified into two categories: primary autonomic failure, in which no obvious known cause is found, and secondary autonomic failure, which results from a variety of lesions in the central and peripheral nervous system, from general medical disorders, or from drugs or other causes (25,28). Respiratory disturbances, particularly sleep apnea, have been described extensively for the best-known form primary autonomic failure—MSA with progressive autonomic failure, also known as the *Shy-Drager syndrome*. Sleep apnea has also been described in association with several cases of FD, a recessively inherited disease with autonomic failure, and in some cases of acquired dysautonomia and polyneuropathies, particularly diabetic neuropathy associated with autonomic neuropathy.

Sleep Apnea in Multiple-System Atrophy (Shy-Drager Syndrome)

MSA is a multisystem neurodegenerative disease (23–25,31,83) presenting initially with progressive autonomic failure. This is followed about 2 to 6 years later by progressively worsening somatic neurologic manifestations. Somatic features consist of a varying combination of pyramidal, extrapyramidal, upper motoneuronal, and lower motoneuronal dysfunctions, including bulbar deficits. Most commonly, affected patients manifest a parkinsonian-cerebellar or cerebellar-parkinsonian syndrome. At this stage of the illness, patients frequently manifest sleep and respiratory disturbances. Occasionally, in the initial stage of the illness, the patients may exhibit dysrhythmic breathing. A variety of sleep disturbances occur along with the respiratory disturbances, such as increased sleep latencies, an increased number of awakenings after sleep onset, and reduced total sleep, slow-wave sleep, and REM sleep times (99).

Several sleep-related respiratory dysrhythmias have been described in patients with MSA (24–27) (Fig. 4). The most common types are sleep apnea and sleep hypopnea, dysrhythmic breathing, and nocturnal stridor. The other respiratory disturbances that have been described for this condition include apneustic breathing, inspiratory gasps, and transient sudden respiratory arrest.

An analysis of the pattern of breathing has revealed the existence of three types of sleep apnea (29): central, upper-airway obstructive, and mixed. Normal individuals may have a few episodes of sleep apnea, particularly central apnea, at the onset of non-REM and during REM sleep. In pathologic conditions, sleep apnea is defined as follows: the duration of an episode should be at least 10 seconds, the apnea index (number of episodes of apnea per hour of sleep) should be at least 5, and the patient should have at least 30 episodes during 7 hours of all-night sleep (41).

Central apnea is characterized by cessation of air flow with no respiratory effort; both diaphragmatic and intercostal muscle activities and air exchange through the nose or mouth are absent. In upper-airway obstructive apnea, there is a lack of air exchange through the nose or mouth, as detected by oronasal thermistors, the diaphragmatic and intercostal muscle activities are preserved. Mixed apnea is manifested as an initial cessation of air flow with no respiratory effort (central apnea) followed by a period of upper-airway obstructive apnea. Rarely, the pattern may be re-

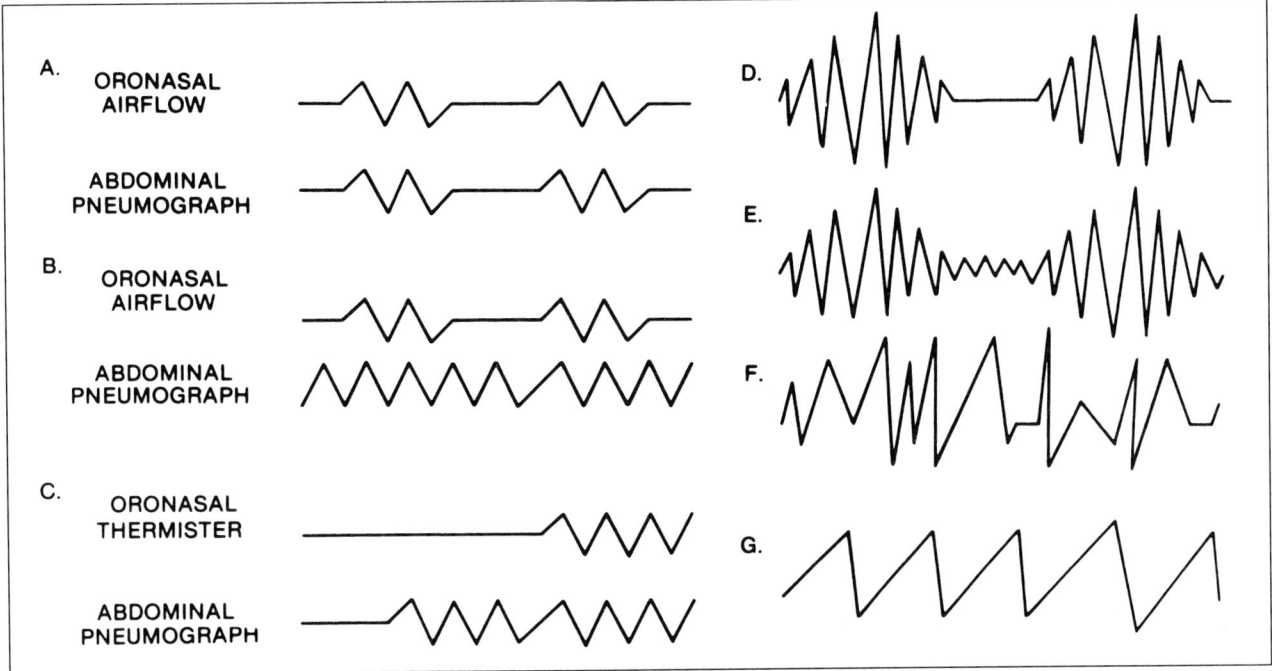

FIG. 4. Sleep-related respiratory dysrhythmias in MSA. *A*, central apnea; *B*, upper-airway obstructive apnea; *C*, mixed apnea; *D*, Cheyne-Stokes pattern; *E*, Cheyne-Stokes variant breathing; *F*, dysrhythmic breathing; *G*, apneustic breathing. (From Chokroverty, ref. 26, with permission of Oxford University Press.)

versed, with an initial period of obstructive apnea followed by central apnea.

Sleep-related hypopnea is characterized by decreased air flow at the mouth and nose and decreased chest movement. This brings about a reduction in the tidal volume, such that the amplitude of the oronasal thermistor or pneumographic signal is reduced by one-half the value recorded during the preceding or following respiratory cycles. The respiratory disturbance index, or apnea-hypopnea index, is defined as the number of episodes of apnea (central, obstructive, or mixed) plus the number of episodes of hypopnea occurring per hr of sleep. To be considered significant, this index should be at least 5.

A survey of the literature reveals many reports of sleep apnea and hypopnea, dysrhythmic breathing, and nocturnal stridor causing severe breathing difficulties in patients with MSA. The patient described by Lockwood (59) had cluster breathing with periods of apnea lasting up to 20 sec during wakefulness and up to 40 sec during sleep. Based on the normal hypercapnic ventilatory response in this patient and the pathologic findings of gliosis in the reticular formation near the pontomedullary respiratory neurons, Lockwood hypothesized that, at least in this patient, the neurons responsible for respiratory rhythmicity function independently from the medullary chemoreceptors controlling ventilation. The patient of Lehrman et al. (58) had approximately 450 episodes of predominantly obstructive apnea at night. The patients of Briskin et al. (12) had a high apnea index, and 70% of the apneic episodes were of the upper-airway obstructive type. Their patients had daytime hypersomnolence, and sleep scoring showed very little non-REM sleep stages III and IV and almost a total absence of REM sleep. Guilleminault et al. (43) also described a predominantly upper-airway obstructive type of apnea during sleep in patients with MSA, with a dissociation between the HR and respiratory response. The apneic episodes described by McNicholas et al. (62) in two patients were mostly central, but occasionally the episodes were characterized by transient occlusion of the upper airway or transient uncoupling of the intercostal and diaphragmatic muscle activities, taking the form of transient upper-airway obstructive apnea. The authors described dysrhythmic breathing as the most prominent finding and suggested that there was a defect in the autonomic respiratory rhythm generator in the brain stem of patients with MSA.

In our study of patients with MSA, we noted periodic episodes of central apnea in the upright position in four patients, with a Cheyne-Stokes type of respiration in one patient during the late stage of the illness (30). An impaired hypercapnic ventilatory response in one patient, along with findings of neuronal loss and gliosis in the pontine tegmentum at autopsy, suggested involvement of the respiratory neurons in the brain stem. In my recent studies (26,27) conducted in 10 patients with MSA, seven patients had central, two had upper-airway obstructive, and three had mixed apnea (Fig. 5) during non-REM sleep stages I and II and REM sleep. Four of these patients had several episodes

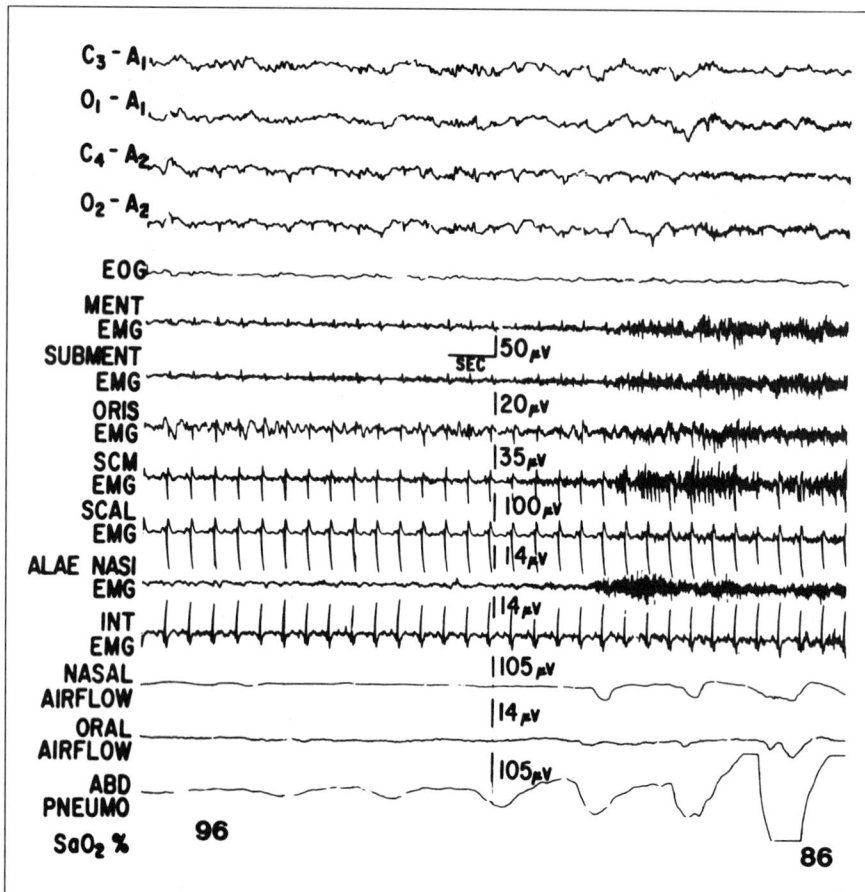

FIG. 5. Polygraphic recording in a patient with MSA. Only a portion of an episode of mixed apnea accompanied by oxygen desaturation during stage II non-REM sleep is shown. Top four channels refer to electroencephalogram. EOG, electro-oculogram. Channels 6 to 12 from the top represent electromyograms of mentalis (MENT), submental (SUBMENT), orbicularis oris (ORIS), sternomastoid (SCM), scalenus anticus (SCAL), and alae nasi and intercostal (INT) muscles. ABD PNEUMO, abdominal pneumogram; $SaO_2\%$, oxygen saturation. (From Chokroverty, ref. 26, with permission of Oxford University Press.)

of central apnea during relaxed wakefulness, as if the respiratory center "forgot" to breathe. There was no HR variation during respiratory cyclic changes that would suggest cardiac autonomic denervation in these patients. This finding contrasts with the bradyarrhythmia-tachyarrhythmia seen during apneic-eupneic cycles in patients with the usual sleep apnea syndrome. Overnight polysomnographic studies in two of these patients with MSA showed marked sleep disturbances that took the form of reduced non-REM sleep stages III and IV and REM sleep, frequent arousals after sleep onset, excessive body movements, and snoring associated with mild to moderate oxygen desaturation. Impairment of the hypercapnic ventilatory response and the mouth occlusion pressure ($P_{0.1}$) response in one of these patients suggested a defect in the metabolic respiratory control system. On the other hand, a normal hypercapnic and hypoxic ventilatory response in another patient in the presence of an abnormal respiratory pattern suggested that chemoreceptor control and the respiratory pattern generator are subserved by different populations of neurons. In our series, the most prominent finding of dysrhythmic breathing in eight of 10 patients during sleep and in four patients also during wakefulness implies that this type of respiratory dysrhythmia is very common in patients with MSA, as was previously suggested by McNicholas et al. (62). Dysrhythmic breathing associated with episodes of upper-airway obstructive apnea was also described by Munschauer et al. (67) in patients with MSA.

An important respiratory dysrhythmia in patients with MSA is laryngeal abductor paralysis, which causes laryngeal stridor, excessive snoring, and upper-airway obstruction during sleep (1,3,42,51,55,61,97). The nocturnal stridor can be either inspiratory or expiratory, or both. Tracheostomy relieved the stridor in these patients. Bannister et al. (3) found marked atrophy of the posterior cricoarytenoid muscles in three patients at postmortem examination. The quantitative cell count in the nucleus ambiguus, however, was normal, suggesting that a biochemical defect rather than a morphologic denervation of the laryngeal muscles is responsible in some of these patients.

In addition to sleep apnea and sleep hypopnea, several other respiratory dysrhythmias have been described in patients with MSA (Fig. 2): (a) inspiratory gasps, manifested by a short inspiratory time and a relatively prolonged expiratory time (2,27); (b) apneustic breathing, characterized by prolonged inspiration and an increased inspiratory-to-expiratory ratio (2,17); and (c) Cheyne-Stokes and Cheyne-Stokes variant breathing, characterized by cyclic changes in breathing with a crescendo-decrescendo sequence separated by episodes of central apnea (Cheyne-Stokes breathing) or hypopnea (Cheyne-Stokes variant pattern of breathing) (25,27,30). Chester et al. (21) described a patient with MSA who exhibited alveolar hypoventilation; on postmortem examination, no lesions were found in the brain stem respiratory neurons. These authors proposed a peripheral mechanism to account for the abnormal breathing in this patient.

Sleep Apnea and Autonomic Dysfunction in Olivopontocerebellar Atrophy

Olivopontocerebellar atrophy (OPCA) is a systemic neuronal degeneration affecting primarily the neurons of the inferior olives and the pontine, arcuate, and lateral reticular nuclei. The proximity of the baroreceptors and respiratory and hypnogenic neurons (6,11) to central autonomic neurons, which are known to be degenerated in OPCA (35a,68a), makes it logical to expect dysfunction of the autonomic and respiratory control mechanisms to occur along with the somatic structural deficits in OPCA. It should be noted that there are striking similarities in clinical and morphologic findings between the Shy-Drager syndrome and classic OPCA (68a). However, the severity and initial presentation of dysautonomic manifestations, the shorter duration of the illness, and the finding of severe loss of neurons of the intermediolateral cell column of the thoracic spinal cord separate the Shy-Drager syndrome from the usual cases of OPCA (28a).

Chokroverty et al. (28a) found evidence of autonomic dysfunction in nine of 10 patients with OPCA. These autonomic deficits, manifested by orthostatic hypotension, an insufficient increase in HR in the erect position and during the cold pressor test, an impaired Valsalva response, abnormal findings on cold pressor and mental arithmetic tests, plasma renin abnormalities, and a low supine plasma norepinephrine level and insufficient rise in plasma norepinephrine in the erect position, suggest a defective central control of the sympathetic nervous system. The exact site of the central lesion remains speculative. In one patient at postmortem examination, the authors (28a) found severe degeneration of the fastigial nucleus, making this the most likely site of a lesion causing autonomic deficit. In five of the nine patients with autonomic deficits, the authors also documented sleep apnea (central and obstructive) on polysomnographic study. They concluded that both sleep apnea and autonomic deficits in some patients with OPCA may result from degenerative lesions in the cerebellum, particularly those involving the fastigial nucleus and the brain stem, where respiratory, hypnogenic, and autonomic control mechanism are closely interrelated. It should be noted that patients with sporadic OPCA and dysautonomia will now be classified under the term "multiple system atrophy" (31a).

Sleep Apnea in Familial Dysautonomia

FD, or Riley-Day syndrome, is another condition associated with autonomic failure. It has been confined to the Jewish population and is inherited in a recessive manner (13). In addition to a variety of dysautonomic manifestations, patients exhibit cardiovascular, skeletal, renal, neuromuscular, and respiratory abnormalities. The dysautonomic manifestations include fluctuations in BP (postural hypotension and paroxysmal hypertension), defective lacrimation, impaired sweating, and vasomotor instability. They also show relative insensitivity to pain, absent muscle stretch reflexes, and a characteristic lack of fungiform papillae of the tongue. The clinical manifestations are usually present in childhood. Most of the patients display a mild respiratory and sleep disorder that is associated with episodes of both central and obstructive apnea (38).

Gadoth et al. (38) performed polysomnographic recordings in 13 patients with FD to investigate the role of the autonomic nervous system in the sleep and breathing disorders associated with this condition. All their patients had apnea, with an average of 73.5 episodes per night (11 had central and two had obstructive apnea during sleep). The REM sleep latency was prolonged, with a decreased REM sleep time in some patients. The adult patients also had increased sleep latency. All patients had orthostatic hypotension and evidence of cardiac dysautonomia. Cardiac responses during apneas were absent, indicating cardiac autonomic denervation.

Besides sleep apnea, patients with FD may exhibit other types of respiratory dysrhythmia. They often have severe breath-holding spells as a consequence of defective responses of the central respiratory neurons to changes in carbon dioxide arterial tension.

Guilleminault et al. (43) described two adolescent girls with FD who exhibited respiratory irregularities; one had esophageal reflux during sleep that caused frequent awakenings. These authors concluded that the sleep and breathing disturbances in this condition, as in MSA, are easily explained by the fact that the peripheral respiratory receptors and central respiratory and lower brain stem hypnogenic neurons are intimately linked by the autonomic nervous system.

McNicholas et al. (62) also found an irregular pattern of breathing in one patient with FD that was similar to that noted in patients with MSA.

The sleep disturbances encountered in FD, which result mostly from respiratory dysrhythmia, include increased arousals and awakenings after sleep onset, prolonged latency of sleep onset, difficulty in waking up in the morning, prolonged onset of REM sleep, and reduced total REM sleep time (99).

Sleep Apnea in Acquired Dysautonomia

Frank et al. (37) described a 6-year-old girl with evidence of dysautonomia who had had a subacute onset of hypoventilation and apnea during sleep. An all-night polysomnographic study revealed frequent episodes of obstructive and central apnea but no HR variation, indicating cardiac autonomic denervation. She died during sleep 2 years after onset of the illness. Postmortem findings included a ganglioneuroma that originated in the lumbar sympathetic ganglia and complete loss of neurons with gliosis in the Edinger-Westphal nuclei. Loss of neurons with gliosis in the locus ceruleus and the reticular formation of the brain stem was also observed. Polysomnographic study in this patient had revealed an absence of bradycardia-tachycardia during episodes of apnea and cynea unlike those noted in other patients who had sleep apnea syndrome but without autonomic dysfunction. This case is an example of an acquired nonprogressive dysautonomia syndrome.

Sleep Apnea in Autonomic Neuropathies

Autonomic neuropathies have been described in the context of many neurologic and medical disorders, but the sleep and respiratory functions have not been studied well for most of these conditions. However, disturbances of sleep and respiration have been reported in many patients with diabetic polyneuropathies associated with autonomic neuropathy, as well as in some patients with autonomic failure associated with amyloidosis and Guillain-Barré syndrome.

Rees et al. (78) monitored respiration during sleep using a magnetometer and thermistor in eight diabetic patients with autonomic neuropathy and eight without autonomic neuropathy. They found that 30 or more apneic episodes occurred during sleep at night in three patients with diabetic autonomic neuropathy; two patients showed mainly central and one predominantly obstructive apnea. None of these patients had excessive daytime somnolence or breathing complaints. These authors did not find any sleep-related respiratory dysrhythmias in the patients without autonomic neuropathy. They suggested that the cardiorespiratory arrests reported in some diabetic patients may be related to sleep-related apnea and autonomic failure.

In two of the four patients with juvenile diabetic autonomic neuropathies studied by Guilleminault et al. (43), obstructive sleep apnea was noted along with dissociation between the HR and the respiratory response. In addition, one patient had episodes of central apnea, and one patient had respiratory dysrhythmia associated with esophageal reflux during sleep.

Mondini and Guilleminault (65) found an abnormal breathing pattern during sleep in five of 12 patients with type I diabetes (1 with obstructive apnea, two with central apnea, and three with an irregular pattern of breathing). They also noted obstructive sleep apnea in one of seven patients with type II diabetes. All three patients with type I disease and apnea had evidence of an autonomic neuropathy.

In contrast to the findings in the above studies, Catterall et al. (18) found no significant difference in frequency of apnea between eight diabetic patients with autonomic neuropathy and age- and weight-matched diabetic patients without autonomic neuropathy.

Autonomic Dysfunction and Obstructive Sleep Apnea Syndrome

In our series of 18 patients with primary obstructive sleep apnea syndrome (OSAS), Sharp and I (29) found no evidence of an autonomic deficit in four patients assessed with special cardiovascular autonomic tests, and these patients also did not have dysautonomic symptoms. There are, however, isolated reports (44b,89a) of mild alterations of both sympathetic and parasympathetic divisions of the autonomic nervous system in patients with OSAS.

Micieli et al. (63a) found evidence of mild hypofunction of both sympathetic and parasympathetic divisions of the autonomic nervous system in five of 13 cases with OSAS on autonomic cardiovascular testing (i.e., tilt-table test, Valsalva's maneuver, handgrip, deep breathing, standing up), and in eight of 13 cases on pupillometric study. The authors suggested that the autonomic deficit in OSAS is secondary to hypoxemia or hypercapnia associated with sleep apnea rather than to any neurogenic alterations.

Veale et al (90a) performed autonomic cardiovascular tests in 33 patients with OSAS. They found abnormal responses in patients with severe OSAS (those with a respiratory disturbance index of more than 30) and concluded that these were probably secondary to hypoxemia.

Most reports emphasize hyperactivity of the sympathetic nervous system causing increased plasma norepinephrine levels (15a,35b) and urinary excretion of catecholamines attributed to hypoxemia associated with apneic episodes (36a). Tracheostomy can reverse the catecholamine abnormalities in these patients (36a). Physiologic studies by Hedner et al. (44a), Carlson et al. (15a) and Watanabe et al. (91b) demonstrated enhanced muscle sympathetic nerve activity during wakefulness and sleep in patients with OSAS. Waravdekar et al. (91a) recorded muscle sympathetic nerve activity during wakefulness via peroneal microneurography in seven patients with OSAS before and 1 month after therapy with nasal continuous positive airway pressure. They found a direct linear relationship between decrease in muscle sympathetic nerve activity and average hours of continuous positive airway pressure per night. Thus, an effective reduction in apnea index with continuous positive airway pressure therapy resulted in diminution of the high level of sympathetic tone present during resting wakefulness in patients with OSAS. The mechanism of sympathetic hyperactivity and its reduction by continuous positive airway pressure remains undetermined at present.

Cardiac arrhythmias, often noted in patients with OSAS, result from alterations in the autonomic nervous system (69a). Bradytachyarrhythmias (i.e., relative bradycardia during apnea and relative tachycardia immediately on resumption of normal breathing), sinus pauses, partial heart block, ventricular ectopic beats, and ventricular tachycardia have been documented in patients with OSAS (69a). Those with severe oxygen desaturation (<60%) are highly vulnerable to these arrhythmias.

Diagnosis of Sleep Apnea in Autonomic Failure

Clinical Diagnosis

The diagnosis of primary or secondary autonomic failure should first be based on the presence of a combination of characteristic clinical manifestations that document autonomic dysfunction, and then on the exclusion of other causes of dysautonomia and somatic neurologic disorders. A high degree of suspicion should direct the physician's attention to the possibility of sleep apnea in such disorders. A thorough history and physical examination, including otolaryngologic examination to detect laryngeal and oropharyngeal muscle weakness, should precede laboratory assessment. The clinical features of sleep-disordered breathing may include daytime hypersomnolence; fatigue; early morning headache; frequent arousals at night related to repeated episodes of apnea or hypopnea, causing severe sleep disturbances; and intellectual deterioration. It is important to recognize alveolar hypoventilation during sleep, as affected patients may die of sleep apnea. Furthermore, because of episodic or prolonged hypoxemia, hypercapnia, and respiratory acidosis in sleep, pulmonary hypertension, cor pulmonale, congestive cardiac failure, and sometimes cardiac arrhythmias may develop.

Laboratory Assessment

Polysomnographic Study

Polysomnographic study are required in patients with suspected sleep-disordered breathing. To assess the severity of the sleep-disordered breathing and accurately document sleep architecture, all-night recordings should be obtained. Sleep may adversely affect respiration, and respiratory dysrhythmia may adversely affect sleep; both these alterations may change the natural course of the illness, and therefore the sleep architecture should be studied (24). To assess the circadian variation in sleep and respiration, 24-hr ambulatory cassette recording is available.

The polysomnographic study should include simultaneous recordings of multiple channels of the EEG, EMGs of the orofacial muscles, electro-oculogram, and electrocardiogram; respiratory monitoring; and continuous determination of oxygen saturation by oximeter (29). Monitoring of respiration should include measurements of respiratory effort and air flow (57,73). Respiratory effort may be determined by recording rib cage and abdominal movements, intercostal and diaphragmatic EMGs, and pleural pressures. The following methods are available for detecting rib cage and abdominal movements: strain gauge (e.g., abdominal pneumobelt, thoracic and abdominal strain gauges), magne-

tometers, and respiratory inductive plethysmography (e.g., Respitrace). The most commonly used methods are strain gauge and Respitrace. Pleural pressures, which most accurately reflect respiratory effort, may be determined by measuring pressure within the esophagus pressure with an esophageal balloon. Intercostal and diaphragmatic EMGs are recorded by surface electrodes. An esophageal electrode can accurately detect the diaphragmatic EMG activities. Oronasal thermistors are the most commonly used method for detecting air flow. Laryngeal sound recordings may be obtained by placing a microphone over the neck.

It is important to record multiple channels of the EEG to identify accurately different sleep stages and their relationship to respiration. The EEG may reveal focal and diffuse neurologic lesions and seizure disorders that may sometimes be associated with sleep apnea. An electro-oculogram and EMGs of orofacial muscles are necessary to define REM sleep accurately and document upper-airway hypotonia. The recording should include REM sleep, which is usually observed in all-night rather than daytime recordings, because most severe breathing abnormalities are often manifested during this stage.

Multiple Sleep Latency Test

The multiple sleep latency test is an objective standardized test that measures the level of daytime sleepiness (16). It consists of four or five 20-min daytime recordings of at least an EEG, EMG, and electro-oculogram at 2-hr intervals. The endpoint of the test consists of one of the following: (a) 20 min of wakefulness; (b) one epoch for clinical purposes and three continuous epochs of stage I non-REM sleep for research purposes; or (c) one epoch of stage II non-REM or REM sleep. Scoring of the multiple sleep latency test includes measurement of either the average latency of sleep onset (time to the first epoch of sleep) or the REM latency (time from sleep onset to the first onset of REM sleep). A decreased sleep latency indicates pathologic sleepiness and an increased sleep latency indicates decreased sleepiness. A latency of sleep onset of <5 minutes indicates pathologic sleepiness. Patients are encouraged to remain awake between the recordings, and the tests must follow a standardized protocol to ensure valid results.

Respiratory Function Studies

Spirometry and the measurement of lung volume, pulmonary diffusion capacity, and blood gases should be carried out to exclude the possibility of intrinsic bronchopulmonary disease, which may be partly responsible for any sleep-disordered breathing in the presence of autonomic failure. To detect respiratory muscle weakness, it is important to measure the maximal static inspiratory and expiratory pressures. Factors that may be abnormal in patients with dysfunction of the metabolic respiratory control system include the chemical control of ventilation (72), and this can be assessed by determining the hypoxic and hypercapnic ventilatory responses. The mouth occlusion pressure ($P_{0.1}$) reflects central respiratory drive and inspiratory muscle strength independently of pulmonary mechanical factors (72).

Laryngeal EMG

It is important to obtain a laryngeal EMG (44) in patients with MSA and laryngeal stridor to detect possible laryngeal paresis.

Treatment of Sleep Apnea in Autonomic Failure

The purpose of treatment of sleep-related apnea and hypopnea in patients with autonomic failure is to improve the quality of sleep by preventing repeated arousals, sleep fragmentation, nocturnal episodes of hypoxemia associated with sleep apnea, and daytime hypersomnolence. Thus, treatment may improve the quality of life in patients with primary autonomic failure, but it may not necessarily alter the natural history of the underlying illness, such as MSA. The treatment may also prevent life-threatening cardiac arrhythmias and congestive cardiac failure. However, uncertainty regarding the pathogenesis of sleep apnea in the presence of autonomic failure makes the treatment of such patients problematic. Furthermore, the relentless progression of their illness despite treatment makes it difficult to justify the implementation of aggressive measures to treat sleep-disordered breathing. In my view, only palliative measures should be carried out in these cases. Such treatment may be divided into four categories: general, pharmacologic, mechanical, and surgical.

General Measures

The main purpose of general measures is to reduce or eliminate the risk factors that can precipitate sleep-related breathing disorders. The two most readily identifiable risk factors are alcohol and drugs, whose actions can interfere with breathing during sleep (24,80). Alcohol has been shown to depress the genioglossus and other upper-airway dilator muscles selectively, and also to depress arousal responses (52,56,90). The net effect is an increase in duration and frequency of apnea. These patients must therefore avoid alcohol consumption. Certain drugs, such as benzodiazepines, barbiturates, and narcotics, also have depressant effects on respiration and should be avoided (80).

Pharmacologic Agents

Protriptyline, a nonsedating tricyclic antidepressant, may reduce the duration and frequency of apnea when given in a dose of 5 mg to 20 mg at bedtime (24,80). This drug may be useful in mild cases of apnea associated with oxygen desaturation and may reduce daytime hypersomnolence. Its mechanism of action is not known exactly, but it may stem from a combination of factors (80): REM suppression when the most severe apnea arises, a specific alerting property, and a shift from apnea to hypopnea. Anticholinergic side effects and cardiac arrhythmias limit its use, particularly in patients with autonomic failure who show evidence of both parasympathetic and sympathetic dysfunction.

Medroxyprogesterone acetate may increase ventilatory drive and the hypercapnic ventilatory response but has not been found to be useful in most patients with sleep apnea (45,76,86,87).

Acetazolamide is of limited value in mild cases of central sleep apnea (82,95). It may reduce central apnea but lead to the development of obstructive apnea in such patients. Another danger associated with this drug, which is of particular concern in patients with autonomic failure, is that it may exacerbate orthostatic hypotension through its diuretic and natriuretic effects. The efficacy of this pharmacologic agent is difficult to assess in patients with autonomic failure, as it has not been used to treat a large number of them. The drug has not been helpful in treating patients with MSA because of the natural history of the illness, which is one of relentless progression despite treatment.

Nasal Continuous Positive Airway Pressure

Nasally administered continuous positive airway pressure represents an important therapeutic advance in the treatment of patients with obstructive sleep apnea syndrome (9,79,81,89). A dramatic reduction in the number and severity of episodes of obstructive and mixed apnea and increase in nocturnal oxygen saturation have been associated with improvement in the quality of sleep and amelioration of daytime symptoms in patients with the primary obstructive sleep apnea syndrome. However, its benefit in patients with autonomic failure, particularly those with MSA, has been less dramatic because of the natural history of the illness and the fact that central apnea is often an important component in MSA. Nevertheless, this treatment should be tried in patients with predominantly obstructive and mixed types of apnea to provide possible symptomatic improvement. The lowest pressure that effectively decreases the number and duration of episodes of apnea should be used. There are several types of home units available for treatment. The principal mechanism of action of this technique is that the continuous positive airway pressure functions as a pneumatic splint, thereby relieving upper-airway obstruction.

Surgical Treatment

A variety of surgical treatments have been used to treat patients with the primary sleep apnea syndrome, but all these measures, except tracheostomy (84), have been impractical in patients with autonomic failure whose illness has an unrelenting course.

Tracheostomy

Tracheostomy is the only form of treatment that has been used successfully in patients with MSA associated with severe laryngeal stridor. Tracheostomy remains the only form of treatment in patients with sudden respiratory arrest after resuscitation by intubation.

Electrophrenic Respiration

Electrophrenic respiration does not represent a viable option for treating sleep apnea in patients with autonomic failure. Diaphragm pacing or electrophrenic respiration has been used in some patients with central apnea (39), but this often precipitates obstructive apnea and therefore should be used only in conjunction with tracheostomy.

CONCLUSION

The treatment of sleep apnea in patients with autonomic failure remains highly unsatisfactory because the pathogenesis of sleep apnea in these conditions is uncertain and because a specific cause is lacking in the best-known form of autonomic failure (MSA), a disorder characterized by relentless progression despite treatment. Palliative measures may, however, temporarily improve a patient's quality of life and should therefore be used for sleep-related respiratory disturbances associated with any type of autonomic failure in accordance with the methods outlined in this chapter.

REFERENCES

1. Bannister R, et al. Defective autonomic control of blood vessels in idiopathic orthostatic hypotension. *Brain* 1984;90:725–746.
2. Bannister R, Oppenheimer DR. Degenerative disease of the nervous system associated with autonomic failure. *Brain* 1972;95:457–474.
3. Bannister R, et al. Laryngeal abductor paralysis in multiple system atrophy. *Brain* 1981;104:351–368.
4. Batini C, et al. Neural mechanisms underlying the enduring EEG and behavioral activation in the mid-pontine pretrigeminal cat. *Arch Ital Biol* 1959;97:13–25.
5. Batini C, et al. Effect of complete pontine transections on the sleep-wakefulness rhythm: the mid-pontine pretrigeminal preparation. *Arch Ital Biol* 1959;97:1–12.
6. Berger AF, et al. Regulation of respiration. *N Engl J Med* 1997;297:92–97; 138–143; 194–201.
7. Berthon-Jones M, Sullivan CE. Ventilatory and arousal response to hypoxia in sleeping humans. *Am Rev Respir Dis* 1982;125:632–639.
8. Berthon-Jones M, Sullivan CE. Ventilatory and arousal responses to hypercapnia in normal sleeping adults. *J Appl Physiol* 1984;57:59–67.
9. Block AJ, Hughs RL. Factors influencing upper airway closure. *Chest* 1984;86:114–122.
10. Bremer F. Cerveau "isolé" et physiologie du sommeil. *C R Soc Biol (Paris)* 1935;118:1235.
11. Bremer F. Cerebral hypnogenic centers. *Ann Neurol* 1977;2:1–6.
12. Briskin JG, et al. Shy-Drager syndrome and sleep apnea. In: Guilleminault C, Dement WC, eds. *Sleep Apnea Syndromes*. New York: Alan R Liss; 1978:316–322.
13. Brunt PW, McKusick V. Familial dysautonomia. *Medicine* 1970;49:343–374.
14. Bulow K. Respiration and wakefulness in man. *Acta Physiol Scand* 1963;59(Suppl 209):1–110.
15. Bulow K, Ingvar DH. Respiration and state of wakefulness in normals, studied by spirography, capnography and EEG. *Acta Physiol Scand* 1961;51:230–238.
15a. Carlson JT, et al. Augmented resting sympathetic activity in awake patients with obstructive sleep apnea. *Chest* 1993;103:1763–1768.
16. Carskadon MA, et al. Guidelines for the multiple sleep latency test (MSLT): a standard measure of sleepiness. *Sleep* 1986;9:519–524.
17. Castaigne P, et al. Syndrome de Shy et Drager avec troubles du rhythme respiratoire et de la vigilance. *Rev Neurol (Paris)* 1977;133:455–456.
18. Catterall JR, et al. Breathing, sleep and diabetic autonomic neuropathy. *Diabetes* 1984;33:1025–1027.
19. Cherniack N. Respiratory dysrhythmias during sleep. *N Engl J Med* 1981;305:325–330.
20. Cherniack NS, Longobardo GA. Abnormalities in respiratory rhythm. In: Fishman AF, Cherniack NS, Widdicombe JG, eds. *The Respiratory System*; vol II, part 2. Bethesda, MD: American Physiological Society; 1986:729–749 (*Handbook of Physiology*; section 3).
21. Chester CS, et al. Pathophysiological findings in a patient with Shy-Drager and alveolar hypoventilation syndromes. *Chest* 1988;94:212–214.
22. Chokroverty S. Phasic tongue movements in human rapid-eye-movement sleep. *Neurology* 1980;30:665–668.
23. Chokroverty S. Autonomic dysfunction in olivopontocerebellar atrophy. In: Duvoisin RC, Plaitakis A, eds. *The Olivopontocerebellar Atrophies*. New York: Raven Press; 1984:105–141.
24. Chokroverty S. Sleep and breathing in neurological disorders. In: Edelman, NH, Santiago TV, eds. *Breathing Disorders of Sleep*. New York: Churchill Livingstone; 1986:225–264.
25. Chokroverty S. The Shy-Drager syndrome. *Neurol Neurosurg Update* 1986;7:1–8.
26. Chokroverty S. Sleep apnoea and respiratory disturbances in multiple system atrophy with progressive autonomic failure (Shy-Drager syndrome). In: Bannister R, ed. *Autonomic Failure*. 2nd ed. London: Oxford University Press; 1988:432–450.
27. Chokroverty S. The spectrum of ventilatory disturbances in movement disorders. In: Chokroverty S, ed. *Movement Disorders*. Costa Mesa, CA: PMA Publishing; 1990:365–392.
28. Chokroverty S. Functional anatomy of the autonomic nervous system: autonomic dysfunction and disorders of the CNS. *American Academy of Neurology Course No 144*, Boston, 1991.
28a. Chokroverty S, et al. Autonomic dysfunction and sleep apnea in olivopontocerebellar degeneration. *Arch Neurol* 1984;41:926–931.
29. Chokroverty S, Sharp JT. Primary sleep apnoea syndrome. *J Neurol Neurosurg Psychiatry* 1981;44:970–982.
30. Chokroverty S, et al. Periodic respiration in erect posture in Shy-Drager syndrome. *J Neurol Neurosurg Psychiatry* 1978;41:980–986.
31. Chokroverty S, et al. The syndrome of primary orthostatic hypotension. *Brain* 1969;92:743–768.
31a. Consensus statement on the definition of orthostatic hypotension, pure autonomic failure, and multiple system atrophy. *Neurology* 1996;46:1470.
32. Douglas J, et al. Respiration during sleep in normal man. *Thorax* 1982;37:840–844.
33. Douglas NJ, et al. Hypoxic ventilatory response decreases during sleep in normal men. *Am Rev Respir Dis* 1982;125:286–289.
34. Douglas NJ, et al. Hypercapnic ventilatory response in sleeping adults. *Am Rev Respir Dis* 1982;126:758–762.
35. Duron B, Marlot D. Intercostal and diaphragmatic electrical activity during wakefulness and sleep in normal unrestrained adult cats. *Sleep* 1980;3:269–280.

35a. Eadie MJ. Olivopontocerebellar atrophy. In: Vinken PJ, Bruyn GW, eds. Amsterdam: Elsevier North-Holland; 1975:21:415–457 (*Handbook of Clinical Neurology*).
35b. Eisenberg E, et al. Plasma norepinephrine levels in patients with sleep apnea syndrome (Letter). *N Engl J Med* 1990;322:932–933.
36. Fink BR. Influence of cerebral activity in wakefulness on regulation of breathing. *J Appl Physiol* 1961;16:15–20.
36a. Fletcher EC, et al. Urinary catecholamines before and after tracheostomy in patients with obstructive sleep apnea and hypertension. *Sleep* 1987;10:35–44.
37. Frank Y, et al. Sleep apnea and hypoventilation syndrome associated with acquired nonprogressive dysautonomia: clinical and pathological studies in a child. *Ann Neurol* 1980;10:18–22.
38. Gadoth N, et al. Sleep structure and nocturnal disordered breathing in familial dysautonomia. *J Neurol Sci* 1983;60:117–125.
39. Glenn WL, et al. Diaphragm pacing in the management of central alveolar hypoventilation. In: Guilleminault C, Dement WC, eds. *Sleep Apnea Syndromes*. New York: Alan R Liss; 1978:333–344.
40. Goethe B, et al. Effect of quiet sleep on resting and CO_2- stimulated breathing in humans. *J Appl Physiol* 1981;57:59–67.
41. Guilleminault C. Sleep and breathing. In: Guilleminault C, ed. *Sleep and Waking Disorders: Indications and Techniques*. Menlo Park, CA: Addison-Wesley; 1982:155–182.
42. Guilleminault C, et al. Sleep apnoea syndrome: states of sleep and autonomic dysfunction. *J Neurol Neurosurg Psychiatry* 1977;40:718–725.
43. Guilleminault C, et al. The impact of autonomic nervous system dysfunction in breathing during sleep. *Sleep* 1981;4:263–278.
44. Guindi GM, et al. Laryngeal electromyography in multiple system atrophy with autonomic failure. *J Neurol Neurosurg Psychiatry* 1981;44:49–53.
44a. Hedner J, et al. Reduction in sympathetic activity after long-term CPAP treatment in sleep apnoea: cardiovascular implications. *Eur Respir J* 1995;8:222–229.
44b. Hedner J, et al. Is high and fluctuating muscle nerve sympathetic activity in the sleep apnea syndrome of pathogenetic importance for the development of hypertension? *J Hypertens* 1988;6(Suppl 4):S529–S531.
45. Hensley MJ, et al. Medroxyprogesterone treatment of obstructive sleep apnea. *Sleep* 1980;3:441–446.
46. Hess WR. Das Schlafsyndrom als Folge dieenzephaler Reizune. *Acta Physiol Pharmacol Helv* 1944;2:305.
47. Hobson JA, et al. Evolving concepts of sleep cycle generation: from brain centers to neuronal populations. *Behav Brain Sci* 1986;9:371–448.
48. Hobson JA, et al. Sleep cycle oscillation: reciprocal discharge by two brain stem neuronal groups. *Science* 1975;189:55–58.
49. Hudgel DW, et al. Mechanics of the respiratory system and breathing during sleep in normal humans. *J Appl Physiol* 1984;56:133–137.
50. Hugelin A, Cohen MI. The reticular activating system and respiratory regulation in cat. *Ann N Y Acad Sci* 1963;109:586–603.
51. Israel RH, Marino JM. Upper airway obstruction in the Shy-Drager syndrome. *Ann Neurol* 1977;2:83.
52. Issa FG, Sullivan CE. Upper airway closing pressures in snorers. *J Appl Physiol* 1984;57:528–535.
53. Jouvet M. Biogenic amines and the state of sleep. *Science* 1969;162:32–41.
54. Jouvet M. The role of monoamines and acetylcholine-containing neurons in the regulation of the sleep-waking cycle. *Ergeb Physiol* 1972;64:166–307.
55. Kenyon GS, et al. Stridor and obstructive sleep apnea in Shy-Drager syndrome treated by laryngofissure and cord lateralization. *Laryngoscope* 1984;94:1106–1108.
56. Krol RC, et al. Selective reduction of genioglossal muscle activity by alcohol in normal human subjects. *Am Rev Respir Dis* 1984;129:247–250.
57. Kryger MH. Monitoring respiratory and cardiac function. In: Kryger MH, Roth T, Dement WC, eds. *Principles and Practice of Sleep Medicine*. Philadelphia: WB Saunders; 1989:702–708.
58. Lehrman KL, et al. Sleep apnea syndrome in a patient with Shy-Drager syndrome. *Arch Intern Med* 1978;138:206–209.
59. Lockwood AH. Shy-Drager syndrome with abnormal respirations and antidiuretic hormone release. *Arch Neurol* 1976;33:292–295.
60. Lowey AD, Spyer KM. *Central Regulation of Autonomic Functions*. Oxford: Oxford University Press; 1990.
61. Martin JB, et al. Centrally mediated orthostatic hypotension. *Arch Neurol* 1968;19:163–173.
62. McNicholas WT, et al. Abnormal respiratory pattern generation during sleep in patients with autonomic dysfunction. *Am Rev Respir Dis* 1983;128:429–433.
63. Merrill EG. The lateral respiratory neurons of the medulla: their associations with nucleus ambiguus, nucleus retroambigualis, the spinal accessory nucleus and the spinal cord. *Brain Res* 1970;24:11.
63a. Micieli G, et al. Sleep-apnoea and autonomic dysfunction: a cardiopressor and pupillometric study. *Acta Neurol Scand* 1995;91:382–388.
64. Mitchell RA. Neural regulation of respiration. *Clin Chest Med* 1980;1:3–12.
65. Mondini S, Guilleminault C. Abnormal breathing patterns during sleep in diabetes. *Ann Neurol* 1985;17:391–395.
66. Moruzzi G. The sleep waking cycle. *Ergeb Physiol* 1972;64:1–165.
67. Munschauer FE, et al. Abnormal respiration and sudden death during sleep in multiple system atrophy with autonomic failure. *Neurology* 1990;40:677–679.
68. Newsom Davis J. Control of the muscles in breathing. In: Widdicombe JG, ed. *Respiratory Physiology*. London: Butterworth; 1974:221–246 (*MTP International Review of Science*; vol 2).
68a. Oppenheimer DR. Diseaess of the basal ganglia, cerebellum and motor neurons. In: Blackwood W, Corsellis JAN, eds. *Greenfield's Neuropathology*. 3rd ed. London: Edward Arnold; 1976:608–651.
69. Orem JM. Sleep. In: Rosenberg RN, ed. *The Clinical Neurosciences: Neurobiology*. New York: Churchill Livingstone; 1983:V589–V616.
69a. Parish JM, Shepard JW, Jr. Cardiovascular effects of sleep disorders. *Chest* 1990;97:1222–1226.
70. Phillipson EA. Control of breathing during sleep. *Am Rev Respir Dis* 1978;118:909–939.
71. Phillipson EA. Respiratory adaptions in sleep. *Annu Rev Physiol* 1978;40:133–156.
72. Phillipson EA, Bowes G. Control of breathing during sleep. In: Fishman AF, Cherniack NS, Widdicombe JG, eds. *The Respiratory System*; vol II, part 2. Bethesda, MD: American Physiological Society; 1986:649–689 (*Handbook of Physiology*; section 3).
73. Phillipson EA, et al. American Thoracic Society Consensus Conference on indications and standards for cardiopulmonary sleep studies. *Am Rev Respir Dis* 1989;139:559–568.
74. Plum F. Breathlessness in neurological disease: the effects of neurological disease on the act of breathing. In: Howell JBL, Campbell EJM, eds. *Breathlessness*. Oxford: Blackwell Scientific; 1966:203–222.
75. Pompeiano O. The neurophysiological mechanisms of the postural and motor events during desynchronized sleep. *Res Publ Assoc Res Nerv Ment Dis* 1967;45:351–423.
76. Rajagopal KR, et al. Effects of medroxyprogesterone acetate in obstructive sleep apnea. *Chest* 1986;90:815–821.
77. Rechtschaffen A, Kales A. *A Manual of Standardized Terminology, Techniques, and Scoring System for Sleep Stages of Human Subjects*. Los Angeles: University of California at Los Angeles Brain Information Service/Brain Research Institute; 1968.
78. Rees PJ, et al. Sleep apnoea in diabetic patients with autonomic neuropathy. *J R Soc Med* 1981;74:192–195.
79. Sanders MH. Nasal CPAP effect on patterns of sleep apnea. *Chest* 1984;86:839–844.
80. Sanders MH. The management of sleep-disordered breathing. In: Martin RJ, ed. *Cardiorespiratory Disorders during Sleep*. Mount Kisco, NY: Futura Publishing; 1990:141–187.
81. Sanders MH, et al. CPAP via nasal mask: a treatment for occlusive sleep apnea. *Chest* 1983;83:144–145.
82. Sharp JT, et al. Effect of metabolic acidosis upon sleep apnea. *Chest* 1985;87:619–624.
83. Shy GM, Drager GA. A neurological syndrome associated with orthostatic hypotension. *Arch Neurol* 1960;2:511–527.
84. Simmons FB, et al. Surgical management of airway obstructions during sleep. *Laryngoscope* 1977;87:326–338.
85. Skatrud JB, Dempsey JA. Airway resistance and respiratory muscle function in snorers during NREM sleep. *J Appl Physiol* 1985;59:328–335.

86. Skatrud JB, et al. Ventilatory response to medroxyprogesterone acetate in normal subjects: time course and mechanisms. *J Appl Physiol* 1978;44:939–944.
87. Strohl KP, et al. Progesterone administration and progressive sleep apneas. *JAMA* 1981;245:1230–1232.
88. Sullivan CE. Breathing in sleep. In: Orem J, Barnes CD, eds. *Physiology in Sleep*. New York: Academic Press; 1980:213–272.
89. Sullivan CE, et al. Reversal of obstructive sleep apnoea by continuous positive airway pressure applied through the nares. *Lancet* 1981;1:862–865.
89a. Svanborg E, et al. Autonomic nervous system function in patients with primary obstructive sleep-apnoea syndrome. *Clin Auton Res* 1991;1:125–130.
90. Taasan VC, et al. Alcohol increases sleep apnea and oxygen desaturation in asymptomatic men. *Am J Med* 1981;71:240–245.
90a. Veale D, et al. Autonomic stress tests in obstructive sleep apnea syndrome and snoring. *Sleep* 1992;15:505–513.
91. Von Economo C. Die Pathologie des Schlafes. In Bethe A, Bergmann G, Embden G, eds. *Handbuck der normalen und pathologischen Physiologie*. Berlin: Springer-Verlag; 1926:591–610.
91a. Waravdekar NV, et al. Influence of treatment on muscle sympathetic nerve activity in sleep apnea. *Am J Respir Crit Care Med* 1996;153:1333–1338.
91b. Watanabe T, et al. Enhanced muscle sympathetic nerve activity during sleep apnea in the elderly. *J Auton Nerv Syst* 1992;37:223–226.
92. White DP. Ventilation and the control of respiration during sleep: normal mechanisms, pathologic nocturnal hypoventilation, and central sleep apnea. In: Martin RJ, ed. *Cardiorespiratory Disorders During Sleep*. Mount Kisco, NY: Futura Publishing; 1990:53–108.
93. White DP, et al. Metabolic rate and breathing during sleep. *J Appl Physiol* 1985;59:384–391.
94. White DP, et al. Hypoxic ventilatory response during sleep in normal women. *Am Rev Respir Dis* 1982;126:530–533.
95. Whyte KF, et al. Role of protriptyline and acetazolamide in the sleep apnea/hypopnea syndrome. *Sleep* 1988;11:463–472.
96. Wiegand L, et al. Collapsibility of the human upper airway during normal sleep. *J Appl Physiol* 1989;66:1800–1808.
97. Williams A, et al. Vocal cord paralysis in the Shy-Drager syndrome. *J Neurol Neurosurg Psychiatry* 1979;42:151–153.
98. Williams RL, et al. *Electroencephalography (EEG) of Human Sleep: Clinical Applications*. New York: John Wiley; 1974.
99. Wooten V. Medical causes of insomnia. In: Kryger MH, Roth T, Dement WC, eds. *Principles and Practice of Sleep Medicine*. Philadelphia: WB Saunders; 1994:509–522.
100. Wyatt RJ, Gillin JC. Biochemistry and human sleep. In: Williams RL, Karacan I, eds. *Pharmacology of Sleep*. New York: John Wiley; 1976:239–274.

CHAPTER 48

Fainting: Approach to Management

Win-Kuang Shen and Bernard J. Gersh

1. Syncope is a common clinical syndrome that may occur at least once during a lifetime in up to one third of the general population.
2. Causes of syncope encompass a wide spectrum of physiologic and pathophysiologic conditions; these can be categorized generally as cardiovascular and noncardiovascular. The prognosis of a patient with syncope depends on the presence and severity of any associated or underlying organic disease.
3. After initial evaluation, including a complete history, a medical and neurologic examination, and a routine 12-lead electrocardiogram, a presumptive diagnosis can be established in approximately 50% of patients. In the remaining patients, the cause of syncope may require additional information.
4. The decision to proceed with noncardiac evaluation, such as electroencephalography (EEG), computed tomography (CT) of the head, cerebral angiogram, or psychiatric testing, can usually be reached after the initial evaluation.
5. Tilt-table testing in conjunction with isoproterenol infusion increases positive yield but degrades specificity in the diagnosis of vasovagal syncope.
6. For a patient with suspected cardiovascular syncope or unexplained syncope, the decision to proceed with more costly or invasive testing, such as electrophysiologic testing, depends on the patient's clinical presentation, severity of associated injury, presence or absence of underlying cardiac disease, and occupation (e.g., airline pilots and school bus drivers are considered to be at "high risk").
7. The goals of selecting a given test are as follows: (a) establish a diagnosis; (b) confirm a presumptive diagnosis by evaluating dynamic relationships between symptoms, cardiac rhythms, and hemodynamic changes; (c) assess prognosis; and (d) determine response to therapy.
8. Once the cause of syncope has been accurately identified, appropriate therapy is usually effective in preventing recurrent cardiogenic syncope. Treatment for vasodepressor syncope remains less than satisfactory.

INTRODUCTION

Syncope, a clinical manifestation of the temporary interruption of cerebral perfusion, is defined as a sudden and transient loss of consciousness with spontaneous recovery. The spectrum of physiologic and pathophysiologic conditions that may cause syncope ranges from common, benign faints to severe, life-threatening disturbances of cardiac rhythm. The prognosis for a patient with syncope depends on the presence and severity of any associated or underlying organic disease and the severity of any traumatic injuries that may be sustained following abrupt loss of consciousness. Because syncope is usually an episodic and infrequent event, establishing a cause-and-effect relationship can be difficult. The initial history, physical examination, and conventional noninvasive tests, such as electrocardiography (ECG) and Holter monitoring, may suggest a cardiovascular or a noncardiovascular cause of the index syncopal event; nevertheless, in a substantial number of patients, the cause of syncope remains unknown or is at best presumptive. Additional testing modalities, such as tilt-table testing, electrophysiologic testing, and provocative pharmacologic testing, hold promise for an improved diagnostic yield, but many issues concerning the optimal use and the sensitivity and specificity of these tests are yet to be established. Because of these uncertainties in correctly identifying the cause of syncope and the sporadic nature of the event, the outcome of therapy is also variable.

W.-K. Shen: Division of Cardiovascular Diseases and Internal Medicine, Mayo Clinic and Mayo Foundation, Rochester, Minnesota 55905.

B. J. Gersh: Division of Cardiology, Georgetown University Medical Center, Washington, D.C. 20007.

In this chapter, we provide an overview of the etiology, pathophysiology, diagnostic approach, and therapeutic strategies in the management of patients who have experienced syncope. Special attention is given to vagally mediated (neurally mediated) reflex syncope. Orthostatic hypotension, an important cause of syncope, is discussed in detail elsewhere in this book (Chapter 55) and is therefore not covered in this chapter.

ETIOLOGY AND PATHOPHYSIOLOGY

The evaluation of syncope requires a comprehensive consideration of many disease entities. The diagnostic classification of syncope has been correlated with eventual prognostic outcomes (51,66,128). Causes of syncope have been categorized as cardiovascular, noncardiovascular, and unexplained (Table 1). Cardiovascular syncope can be further subdivided into reflex, orthostatic, and cardiogenic syncope. Noncardiovascular causes of syncope include neurologic, metabolic, and psychologic disorders. Syncope is classified as unexplained or idiopathic when a firm diagnosis cannot be established.

Cardiovascular Syncope

Reflex Syncope

Knowledge of the regulatory mechanisms of homeostasis under physiologic conditions is essential to understanding the various mechanisms of reflex syncope. A detailed description of the neurohumoral control of the cardiovascular system can be found elsewhere in this volume (Chapters 4 and 5) and in many standard textbooks (83,106,142,273).

TABLE 1. *Major known causes of syncope*

Cardiovascular	Noncardiovascular
Reflex syncope	Neurologic
Vasovagal	Metabolic
Carotid sinus hypersensitivity	Psychiatric
Situational	
Micturition	
Deglutition	
Defecation	
Glossopharyngeal neuralgia	
Postprandial	
Tussive	
Valsalva	
Oculovagal	
Sneeze	
Instrumentation	
Diving	
After exercise	
Orthostatic hypotension (discussed elsewhere in this book)	
Cardiogenic syncope	
Structural heart disease	
Coronary artery disease	
Rhythm disturbances	

Vasovagal Syncope

The common faint is the prototype of vasovagal syncope. Vasodilation as a component of syncope was first suggested by John Hunter in 1773 (115) in reference to a patient undergoing phlebotomy. Vagally mediated cardioinhibition as a primary cause of syncope was noted in 1888 by Foster (84), who believed that profound bradycardia diminished cerebral blood flow to a level inadequate to maintain consciousness. Mechanisms of the syncopal reaction were probed in studies by Lewis (153), in which he observed that although the bradycardia associated with a faint was reversed by administration of atropine, hypotension and an altered level of consciousness persisted. The association of bradycardia and vasodilation led to his introduction of the term *vasovagal* to describe the circulatory alterations responsible for the syncopal reaction. A similar response has been observed in several animal species in threatening situations in which neither fight nor flight is possible—when the animal is "cornered." These animals exhibit bradycardia, loss of sympathetic vasoconstrictor tone, and motionlessness: they "play dead" (83).

The triggering mechanisms of the common faint have been thoroughly investigated in the past 40 years (3,20,22, 41,69,71,92,95,97,98,156,188,196,203,209,226,254,256,264, 269–271,277,300,303,305,306,313). The apparently paradoxic responses immediately preceding syncope can now be explained by the complex interactions that take place between the neurologic and cardiovascular systems. In general, situations that provoke fainting seem to be those likely to arouse anxiety, fear, emotional distress, and anticipation; these emotions are accompanied by hemodynamic changes associated with increased activity of the sympathetic nervous system. After an unspecified time, a decrease in heart rate (HR) typical of vagal stimulation and a sudden decrease in systemic resistance typical of sympathetic withdrawal supervene. The net result is a major impairment in the capacity to maintain adequate cerebral perfusion, with loss of consciousness as a result, particularly when the subject is in an erect position. The concept of a pre-existing vigorous cardiac contraction, particularly in the setting of decreased ventricular filling, as a predisposition to fainting has also been supported by indirect observation, as in patients with heart failure whose hearts cannot contract vigorously. However, not a single faint was observed in hundreds of patients with congestive heart failure during "threatening" procedures, including phlebotomy (256).

The first direct evidence of the neurophysiologic mechanism underlying syncope was recorded by Öberg and Thorén in 1972 (209). The induction of hypovolemia in an open-chest cat preparation was accompanied by a marked activation of ventricular receptor activity immediately preceding a reflex bradycardia. A marked initial tachycardia during blood withdrawal was an important antecedent condition to this ventricular fiber stimulation. Peripheral autonomic nervous system activity during vasovagal syncope was later documented by microelectrode recordings from peroneal nerve fascicles and reported in 1982 (306). Increased sympathetic activity was noted initially, but with the onset of syncope, sympathetic outflow suddenly ceased, providing direct evidence of an inhibition of vasoconstriction impulses. All these observations support the theory that before vasovagal syncope, there occurs a reflexogenic effort to maintain homeostasis by means of tachycardia and vasoconstriction. The progressive decrease of ventricular filling, increased HR, and powerful contractions can activate the ventricular mechanoreceptors proposed as the triggering mechanism of vasovagal syncope in humans.

Many sensory receptors can be found in various locations of the heart (163). The concept of depressor reflexes originating in the heart was introduced by von Bezold and Hirt (302) in 1867 and later revived by Jarisch and Richter (119) in 1939. The Bezold-Jarisch reflex originates in cardiac sensory receptors that respond to wall tension, chemical substances, or drugs. These sensory receptors are innervated by nonmyelinated (C-fiber) vagal afferent pathways (2,38,177,186,288,309). The left ventricle, particularly the inferoposterior wall, is the principal location for these sensory receptors. Stimulation of these inhibitory cardiac receptors increases parasympathetic activity and inhibits sympathetic activity, resulting in bradycardia, vasodilation, and hypotension (Bezold-Jarisch reflex) (177). It is believed that increased ventricular wall tension resulting from vigorous contraction and decreased ventricular filling in response to the "empty heart" activate these subendocardial mechanoreceptors and promote the inhibitory Bezold-Jarisch reflex, resulting in vasovagal syncope (Fig. 1). Stimulation of cardiac chemoreceptors—for example, during myocardial ischemia and infarction or reperfusion, especially in the inferoposterior region (213,291), or during coronary arteriography (37, 325)—may also activate this inhibitory reflex.

Although the left ventricle is believed to be the primary reflexogenic area that triggers vasovagal syncope, other mechanisms are implicated, including the input and interaction of afferent responses in the higher centers. During emotional stress, modulatory effects from higher centers, such as the forebrain and hypothalamus, could also play a role in patients with denervated ventricles (142,268).

Studies on cardiac transplant recipients suggest that a typical episode of vasodepressor syncope could occur in a presumably denervated heart (81,194,251). Figure 2 shows the response to tilt-table testing of a 50-year-old woman, who was seen with recurrent syncope following cardiac transplantation. During isoproterenol infusion in the upright position, a vasodepressor response without cardioinhibition was induced, and this was associated with a transient loss of consciousness until she was returned to the supine position. The lack of a cardioinhibitory response suggests that at least the efferent vagal reinnervation was not present. Although donor bradycardia was observed in three of the seven vasodepressor reactions induced in transplant recipients reported by Fitzpatrick et al. (81), this bradycardia may merely reflect sudden withdrawal of heightened sympathetic tone and does not necessarily reflect vagal reinnervation (194,251). These observations suggest that vasodepressor syncope could occur in patients with ventricular denervation. The afferent impulses might originate elsewhere, as in the remnant atria, venoatrial

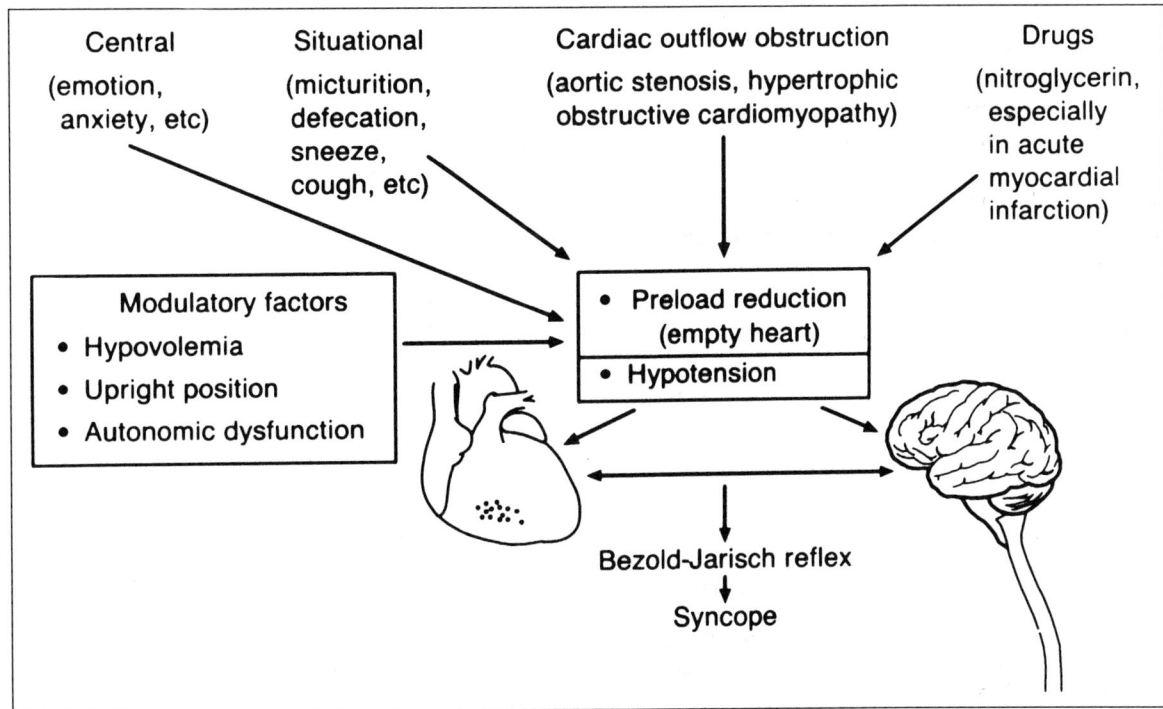

FIG. 1. Reflex syncope: "empty heart syndrome."

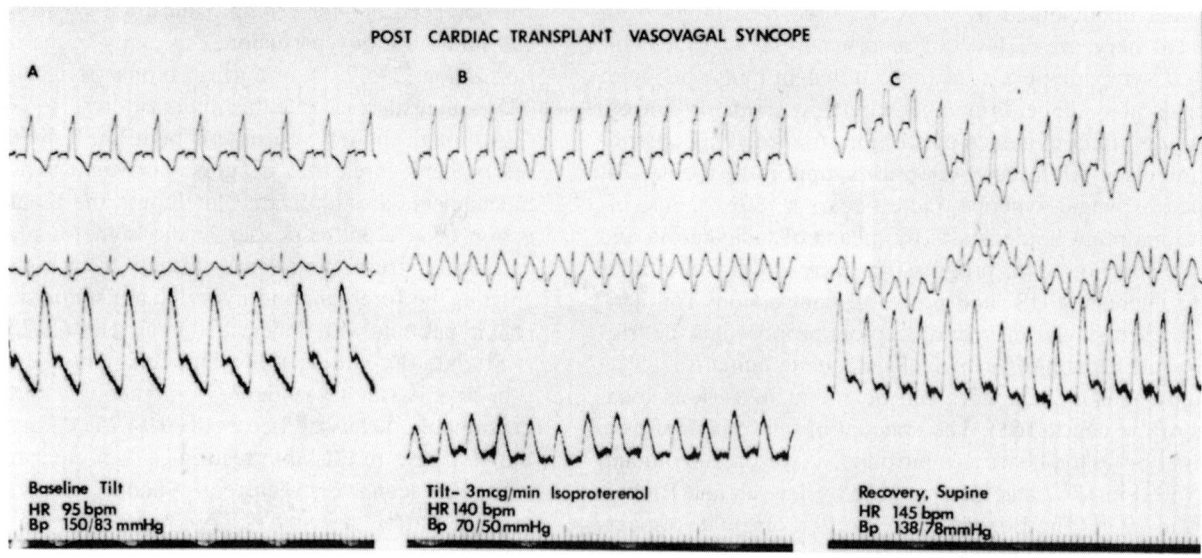

FIG. 2. A vasodepressor response induced during tilt-table testing with isoproterenol. The *top two tracings* are from surface electrocardiogram leads I and III. The *bottom tracing* is beat-to-beat arterial pressure. **A:** Parameters during baseline tilt. **B:** A vasodepressor response (without any bradycardia) induced during tilt combined with infusion of 3 μg of isoproterenol per minute. The patient experienced syncope before she was returned to the supine position. **C:** Recovery in the supine position. See text for discussion.

junction, pulmonary veins, arterial baroreceptors, and peripheral vasculature, because these structures are left intact in an orthotopic cardiac transplantation procedure. The sudden withdrawal of sympathetic tone was the probable result of stimulation by peripheral afferent impulses or central (forebrain or hypothalamus) modulation.

In addition to the multiple potential neurologic circuits involved in the vasodepressor syncope complex, several natural substances have been identified to modulate the triggering of a vasovagal response. In animal studies, serotonin (193) and cyclic adenosine monophosphate (AMP) (11) could induce a vasodepressor response when applied centrally. In clinical studies, serotonin reuptake blockers could prevent recurrent vasovagal syncope in selected patient populations (102,103,143). In the periphery, nitric oxide (241), endogenous opioids (197), and adenosine (264) are potential mediators in the triggering of the vasovagal response. We recently demonstrated that intravenous administration of adenosine could induce a typical vasovagal reaction in susceptible patients (264). The precise role of these neural chemical interactions awaits further investigation.

Carotid Sinus Hypersensitivity

The carotid sinus, containing both chemoreceptors and baroreceptors, plays an important role in the reflex regulation of HR, arterial blood pressure (BP), and peripheral vascular tone (4,168). Patients with carotid sinus hypersensitivity exhibit an exaggerated response to carotid sinus baroreceptor stimulation (73,198,200,282,287,307,312) that results in dizziness or syncope from transient diminished cerebral perfusion.

Responses to carotid sinus baroreceptor stimulation can be divided into three groups: (a) a predominantly cardioinhibitory response that produces marked but transient sinus bradycardia or atrioventricular (AV) block, or both; (b) a vasodepressor response that is manifested predominantly by pronounced hypotension in the absence of marked bradycardia; and (c) a mixed response in which both cardioinhibitory and vasodepressor factors contribute to hypotension (Fig. 3). The relative frequency of each type of response has been estimated to be 70%–75%, 5%–10%, and 20%–25% for cardioinhibitory, vasodepressor, and mixed-type responses, respectively (287,307); nonethe-

FIG. 3. Demonstration of carotid sinus hypersensitivity in patients with recurrent syncope. **Patient 1. A:** An 8.6-second pause and sinus bradycardia occurred during left carotid sinus massage (CSM) associated with syncope. **B:** During repeated CSM, temporary AV pacing at a cycle length of 800 milliseconds maintained a steady BP and prevented recurrent symptoms, suggesting that the cardioinhibitory component was predominant. **Patient 2. C:** Prolonged pause (4.8 seconds) during right CSM associated with near syncope. **D:** Vasodepressor response persisted during CSM with AV pacing at a cycle length of 700 milliseconds. BP remained low and the patient experienced near syncope despite pacing, suggesting a mixed response. *HBE*, His bundle electrogram; *HRA*, high right atrial electrogram; *RV*, right ventricular electrogram.

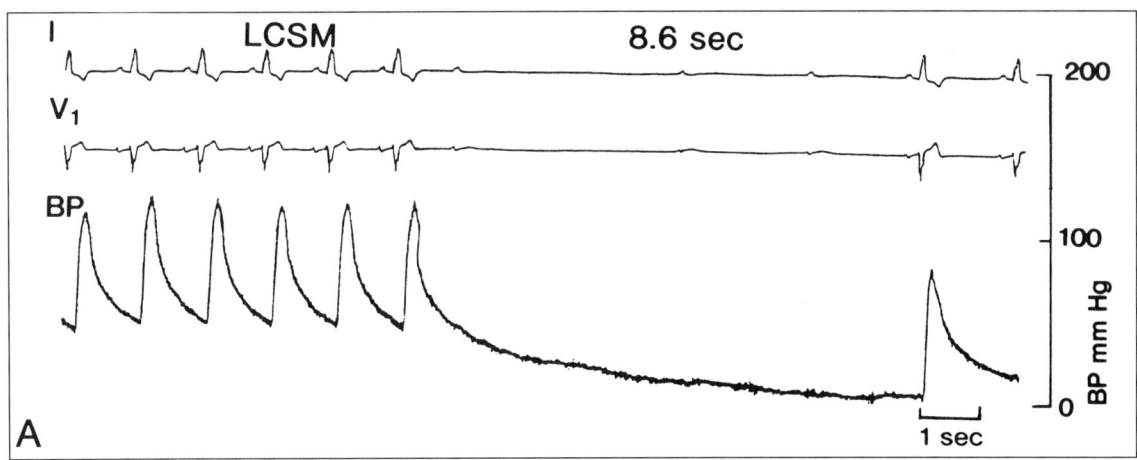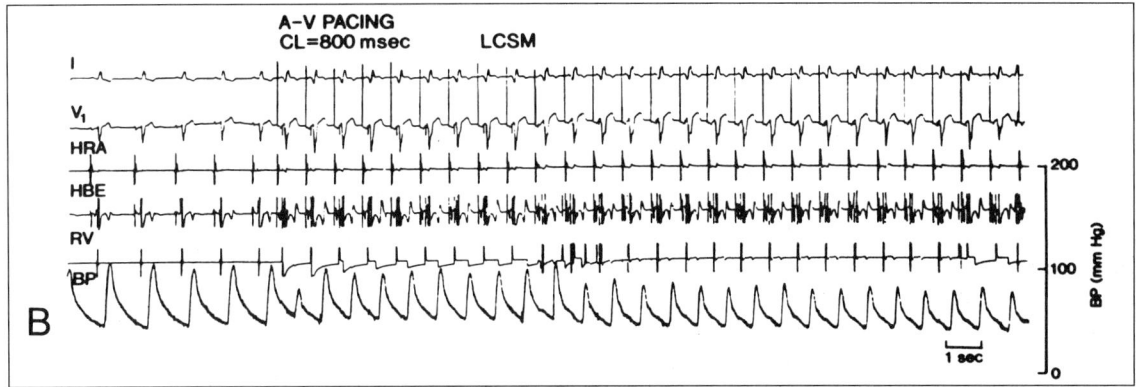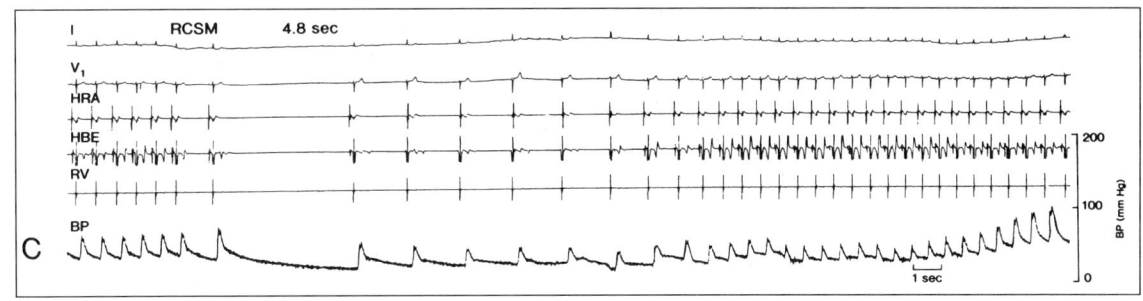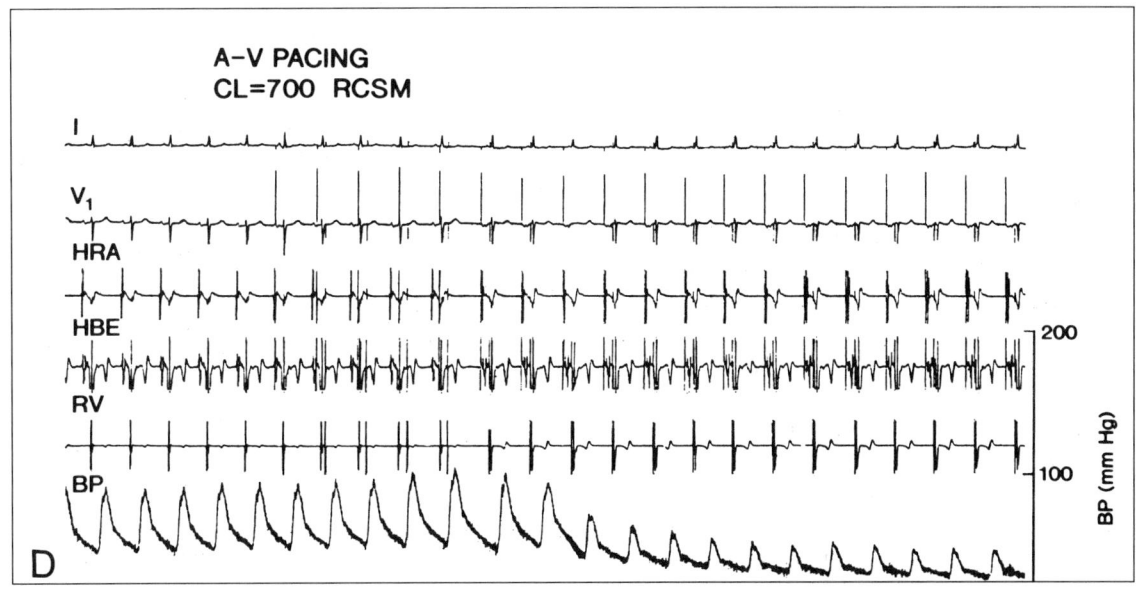

less, we and others have found that the reproducibility of these exaggerated cardiovascular responses may vary considerably in a given patient (114,283). The site of abnormality in the reflex arc of carotid sinus hypersensitivity has not been identified completely (200). A study (137) showed that arginine vasopressin release (which reflects afferent pathway activity) in patients with carotid sinus hypersensitivity was no different from that in controls, yet vagal activity (the efferent pathway activity) was considerably increased. These observations suggest that a central abnormality may exist in patients with carotid sinus hypersensitivity or, alternatively, that stimulation of the carotid sinus and vagus identifies a patient with heightened activity at the interface between the vagus and the heart.

Situational Syncope

Syncope is described as a consequence of many situations (some of which occur in normal daily life) that have in common a propensity to decrease preload, promote sympathetic withdrawal, and increase vagus nerve activity. The causes of situational syncope are listed in Table 1. The central and efferent pathways of the reflex arcs most likely resemble those of the Bezold-Jarisch reflex and the carotid sinus reflex, with various degrees of cardioinhibitory and vasodepressor effects. The afferent pathways can be multiple and differ, depending on the site of stimulation.

Micturition syncope is associated with rapid emptying of a distended bladder; this initiates the inhibitory reflex, which may be further accentuated by the upright standing position and Valsalva's maneuver during voiding (125, 253). Other causes of situational syncope, such as cough, defecation, ingestion of a meal, sneeze, Valsalva's maneuver, instrumentation, and diving, may also involve decreased cardiac filling during the precipitating event plus possible stimulation of local afferents (31,118,120,126, 129,151,152,159,160,227,318). Many of these situational syncopes are associated with a concomitant Valsalva's maneuver, during which transthoracic pressures and respiratory patterns change (6). Mechanoreceptors located in the pulmonary vasculature and parenchyma that are known to affect the cardiovascular system via the respiratory center in the brain stem may play a triggering role.

Glossopharyngeal syncope, which is triggered by pain in the posterior pharynx or external auditory canal, stems from activation of the dorsal motor nucleus of the vagus by afferent impulses originating in the glossopharyngeal nerve (141,151). Swallowing syncope is closely related to glossopharyngeal syncope (120). It is usually associated with an abnormality in the esophagus, such as diverticula, stricture, or tumor, although it also can occur in patients with a normal esophagus (152,318).

Syncope after exercise can occur in young and healthy patients. It has been attributed to an exaggerated vasovagal reflex that is precipitated by preceding sympathetic overactivity and decreased preload as a consequence of venous pooling immediately after exercise (68,82,116,211,216, 252,272).

Cardiogenic Syncope

Structural Heart Disease

The maintenance of a stable BP requires a fine balance between cardiac output and vascular resistance. A decrease in systemic vascular resistance is normally compensated for by the augmentation of cardiac output. In patients with significant structural heart disease (aortic stenosis, obstructive hypertrophic cardiomyopathy, ischemic heart disease, or dilated idiopathic cardiomyopathy with depressed cardiac function), cardiac output cannot increase in proportion to the decrease in vascular resistance, and there is a consequent profound decline in BP. Thus, exertional hypotension and syncope are characteristic features of virtually all forms of heart disease in which cardiac output is relatively fixed and fails to increase normally during exertion.

Exertional syncope is most characteristic of severe valvular aortic stenosis and other forms of obstruction to the left or right ventricular outflow (10,85,162,231). When obstruction of the left ventricular outflow tract is dynamic, hemodynamic instability is exacerbated by increased contractility, decreased chamber dimensions, and decreased afterload. Although exertional syncope in those patients who have severe structural heart disease can usually be explained by the hemodynamic derangement, it is extremely important to keep in mind that transient cardiac arrhythmias with spontaneous recovery (bradycardia or tachycardia) may also be the cause of syncope (145,183). Although an impairment in the increase of cardiac output, as in compensation for a decrease in systemic vascular resistance, is the major source of exertional hypotension and syncope in patients with outflow tract obstruction, a disproportionate reduction of systemic vascular resistance resulting from blunting of the carotid and aortic baroreceptor-mediated reflexes may also play a significant, if not dominant, role (85,177).

Patients with congenital heart disease characterized by right-to-left shunt or outflow tract obstruction, or both, as occurs in tetralogy of Fallot, may experience exertional hypotension or syncope brought about by similar underlying mechanisms. A significant obstruction in prosthetic valves can also cause episodic syncope. Systemic hypotension and syncope may be critical sequelae of massive pulmonary emboli or severe primary pulmonary hypertension. Both conditions produce significant right ventricular outflow tract obstruction and decreased left ventricular filling.

Coronary Artery Disease

Syncope in patients with coronary artery disease is the result of many factors. Arrhythmias (tachyarrhythmias or bradyarrhythmias) are probably the most common cause of syncope in patients with coronary artery disease. In patients with depressed left ventricular function and a prior myocardial infarction, ventricular tachycardia with spontaneous termination should always be considered. Involvement of the conduction system (sinus node, AV node, or His-Purkinje system) may occur during an acute episode of ischemia or as a sequela of severe long-standing disease.

Exertional syncope in a patient with coronary artery disease should alert the clinician to either the presence of severe exercise-induced ischemia or a limited cardiac reserve, with an inability to increase cardiac output during exercise in those patients with severe left ventricular dysfunction. Reflexogenic or vasovagal syncope may occur during acute ischemia or after reperfusion, with accompanying activation of the mechanoreceptors in the inferoposterior left ventricle. Nitroglycerin, which causes further preload reduction, may precipitate syncope in these "presensitized" individuals.

Rhythm Disturbances

Arrhythmia-mediated syncope may result from bradycardia or tachycardia. The syncope occurs because the cardiac output and cerebral perfusion are markedly diminished. The rate of bradycardia or tachycardia is one of the factors that determines the severity of the cerebral symptoms, but there is no absolute relationship between the HR and the occurrence of syncope (109). Whether syncope develops may depend on the complex interaction of many variables, including overall status of cardiac function, presence of obstructive cerebrovascular disease, intactness of autonomic regulation, body position, and status of intravascular volume at the time of the rhythm disturbance.

The conduction system of the heart is specialized, in that it possesses the inherent ability to initiate and conduct impulses to ensure a regular and orderly activation of atrial and ventricular myocardium. The origin of *bradycardia* can be localized to the sinoatrial (SA) node or to the AV conduction system, including the AV node and the His-Purkinje fibers. Pathologic changes associated with SA node dysfunction or AV conduction abnormalities have many common causes. As a result, patients with overt clinical SA node dysfunction frequently also have AV conduction disturbances (205,234). Ischemic heart disease and idiopathic fibrosis are the causes of most bradyarrhythmias. In addition to the structural abnormalities of the conduction system, metabolic abnormalities, such as electrolyte disturbances, acidosis, drugs, and autonomic dysfunction, can also provoke hemodynamically significant bradyarrhythmias (5,50,176,228,280,292).

Abnormal SA node function can be manifested as follows: persistent, inappropriate sinus bradycardia or chronotropic incompetence with exercise or stress; SA block; sinus arrest; inappropriately long pauses after a premature atrial contraction; chronic atrial fibrillation or flutter with a slow ventricular rate resulting from additional AV nodal disease; replacement of sinus rhythm by a subsidiary atrial or functional pacemaker; prolonged suppression of sinus rhythm after cardioversion; and bradycardia-tachycardia syndrome, in which bradycardia alternates with episodes of supraventricular tachycardia (18,26,50,64,75, 90,176,201,205,228,234,237,257,266,280,299). Frank syncope caused by SA node dysfunction usually results from a sudden, prolonged sinus pause caused by sinus arrest or sinus exit block. Sinus bradycardia at a rate of 40 to 60 beats/min seldom causes syncope, although this may contribute to a decrease in BP and cardiac output and the development of a more subtle and less easily recognized syncope.

Dysfunction of the AV conduction system has been traditionally classified electrocardiographically as first-, second-, and third-degree AV block (189). The development of the intracardiac His bundle catheter recording technique in the 1960s brought about major increases in our understanding of the pathophysiologic characteristics of AV conduction disturbances. By means of invasive electrophysiologic studies, AV block can be further categorized as occurring above, at, or below the His bundle recording site (suprahisian, intrahisian, and infrahisian blocks, respectively). The evaluation of AV conduction has been based on the premise that differentiating AV nodal from infranodal conduction delays provides useful prognostic information (59,181,249,250). When the block occurs distal to the AV node (intrahisian), the escape rhythm is generally slow and unreliable, and loss of consciousness (Stokes-Adams attacks) is frequent. In the setting of vagal hypertonia, however, the site of AV block is at the level of the AV node, which is richly innervated by the vagus. High-grade AV block, frequently associated with a sinus bradycardia, characterizes the cardioinhibitory component of vasovagal syncope.

Tachyarrhythmias, both supraventricular and, more commonly, ventricular, are important and potentially serious causes of syncope. Supraventricular *tachycardia,* as a rule, does not cause syncope, but it does occur, particularly in patients with very rapid rates and underlying cardiac dysfunction (49,94,110,170,182,232,233,284). In patients with Wolff-Parkinson-White syndrome, syncope may occur during atrial fibrillation when the ventricular response rate is particularly rapid, for example, 300 beats per min during anterograde conduction down the accessory pathway. Sudden death is an uncommon but nonetheless well-documented complication that results from the degeneration of rapid atrial fibrillation into ventricular fibrillation (139,232,323).

Ventricular arrhythmias are a relatively common and probably lethal cause of syncope (19,21,30,46,76,91, 150,179,214,286,301). Depending on the morphology and duration of the electrophysiologic signal, ventricular tachyarrhythmias can be classified as monomorphic or polymorphic ventricular tachycardia, torsades de pointes, or ventricular fibrillation, which can be either sustained (≥ 30 seconds)—with or without hemodynamic collapse—or nonsustained.

Most patients with sustained ventricular tachycardia have underlying left ventricular dysfunction, usually as a result of coronary artery disease. Torsades de pointes occur in an important subset of patients, in whom polymorphic ventricular tachycardia and sudden death occur in the setting of a prolonged QT interval. The causes for prolongation of the QT interval include congenital syndromes, such as the Romano-Ward and the Jervell and Lange-Nielsen (associated with deafness) syndromes, and acquired reversible conditions, such as ischemia, drug effects (117,150,179,294,316), and electrolyte imbalance (hypokalemia, hypomagnesemia) (150). Patients vary widely in their hemodynamic tolerance of ventricular arrhythmia and the propensity to faint as a result. The major determinants of tolerance are the rate of the tachycardia and the severity of the underlying cardiac dysfunction, but altered cardiovascular reflexes during tachyarrhythmias may exaggerate the hypotensive response. Based on studies using Holter monitoring, it appears that the most common mechanism of sudden death is degeneration of ventricular tachycardia into ventricular fibrillation.

Noncardiac Syncope

Neurologic Syncope

Neurologic causes of isolated syncope are uncommon (25,310). Brain stem ischemia from basilar artery insufficiency or transient ischemic attacks involving the posterior circulation may result in transient loss of consciousness in association with symptoms of brain stem dysfunction, such as diplopia, vertigo, ataxia, dysarthria, paresthesias, and weakness. Basilar migraine may similarly result in syncope. Compression of the vertebral arteries, such as by a cervical rib, cervical spondylosis, or osteoarthritis, and the subclavian steal syndrome during arm exercise are other uncommon causes of syncope related to cerebrovascular abnormalities. Transient ischemic attacks resulting from carotid artery disease almost never cause syncope (25). Seizure disorders, including classic grand mal, partial complex, or akinetic temporal lobe seizures, need to be differentiated from true syncope.

Metabolic Causes

Metabolic causes of syncope include hypocapnia, hypoxia, and hypoglycemia (242). Hyperventilation resulting from anxiety is the most frequent cause of hypocapnia, in which cerebral perfusion is decreased by vasoconstriction of the cerebral vasculature. Although lightheadedness and presyncope frequently occur during hyperventilation, complete loss of consciousness is infrequent. The mechanism of syncope in hypoxemia and hypoglycemia is an impairment of energy supplies to the brain, which, if profound and persistent, precipitates coma.

Psychogenic Syncope

Syncope may occur in patients with psychiatric disorders, such as anxiety, hysteria, panic, or major depression (132,155). Hyperventilation-mediated hypocapnia suffices to explain the syncope that can occur during an anxiety attack. Suprabulbar-mediated regulation of autonomic tone in patients with major depression or panic disorders also explains syncope. However, the episodic display of a dramatic loss of consciousness in a hysterical patient is more often found during hemodynamic monitoring to be associated with a normal BP or pulse rate.

INCIDENCE

The relative frequency of the various causes of syncope depends on the age and clinical characteristics of the patient population (Table 2) (51,66,121,128,178,265). The most common cause of syncope in patients evaluated in an emergency department or an outpatient clinic (51,66,121,128,178) is vasovagal or vasodepressor syncope; the incidence of this ranges from 8%–37%. Among other causes of syncope, it has been estimated that cardiogenic syncope occurs in 4%–26%, orthostatic hypotension in 4%–10%, neurologic disorders (excluding seizures) in 3%–9%, and metabolic or hysterical syncope in 1%–5% of this group of patients.

Cardiogenic causes are much more common in patients admitted to a medical intensive care unit for syncope; a vasovagal reaction is highly unusual in these patients (265). All studies have shown that in a large proportion of patients (13%–47%), a cause cannot be established even after a standardized evaluation, and the reasons for this diagnostic difficulty are multiple (123,124). The inability to identify a cause for syncope in such a high percentage of patients remains a source of frustration. Because of the episodic and infrequent nature of syncope, it is unlikely for an episode to recur during the period of evaluation, and this is a major reason why it is difficult to reach a diagnosis in most patients. Moreover, many patients evaluated after the syncopal event may not recall the details surrounding the episode, and if witnesses were not present, the cause of syncope may not be apparent. Furthermore, conventional noninvasive diagnostic tests, such as ECG and Holter monitoring, which are able to detect cardiac abnormalities only at one point in time, may be inadequate. Additional diagnostic tests, including tilt-table testing in conjunction with

TABLE 2. *Relative frequency of the causes of syncope*

Study (ref.)	No.	Patient population	Mean age, y	F/M	Recurrent, No. (%)	Vasovagal	Other reflex syncope	Orthostatic	Cardiac	Metabolic	Neuro	Psy	UC
Eagle et al. (66)	176	ER[a]	54	90/86	74(42)	64(36)	3(2)	11(6)	15(9)	7(4)	5(3)	2(1)	69(39)
Day et al. (51)	198	ER	44	111/87	73(37)	57(29)	2(1)	7(4)	17(9)	13(7)	5(4)[b]	14(7)	25(13)
Kapoor (121)	433	All (ER, Outpt, Adm)	56	261/172	212(49)	35(8)	37(9)	43(10)	110(26)	9(2)	17(4)	3(1)	179(41)
Martin et al. (178)	170	ER	41	...	...	63(37)	4(2)	13(8)	7(4)	3(2)	15(9)	1(1)	64(38)
Silverstein et al. (265)	108	ICU	67	53/55	...	1(1)	1(1)	4(4)	42(39)	4(4)	5(5)	...	51(47)

F, female; M, male; Adm, hospital admission; ER, emergency room; ICU, intensive care unit; Neuro, neurologic; Outpt, outpatient; Psy, psychiatric; UC, unknown cause.

[a]Excluding patients with obvious seizures.
[b]Excluding 58 patients with seizures.

provocative pharmacologic challenge, prolonged ambulatory cardiac rhythm evaluation with loop ECG and BP recordings, and invasive electrophysiologic testing, are extremely useful and enhance the yield of the diagnostic evaluation.

NATURAL HISTORY AND PROGNOSIS

When the presumed diagnosis is benign (e.g., vasodepressor or hyperventilation syncope in a young patient with a low risk for serious cardiovascular disease in whom an isolated syncopal event has not been associated with any traumatic injuries), few if any tests are needed, and the patient can be reassured that the event was not serious. In contrast, when a cardiac cause is suspected, a definitive diagnosis must be vigorously pursued with the objective of identifying a specific therapeutic approach. No cause can be established after the initial evaluation is completed in up to 50% of patients seen with syncope. The prognosis depends on the nature and severity of the underlying disease. To achieve the most favorable cost-benefit ratio for treatment, a detailed understanding of the natural history and prognosis of patients with syncope is important.

Syncope caused by cardiac disorders is associated with high mortality (51,65,66,128,178,265). In a large prospective study, Kapoor (121) reported a 5-year mortality of 51% in patients with a cardiac cause of syncope, compared with 30% in patients with noncardiac causes of syncope and 24% in patients with an unknown cause of syncope. At 5 years, the sudden death rate in patients with cardiogenic syncope (33%) was also significantly higher than that in patients with either noncardiogenic syncope (5%) or unexplained syncope (9%) (Fig. 4). Although noncardiac syncope is usually benign and self-limited, considerable morbidity can arise from the trauma sustained during abrupt loss of consciousness, particularly in elderly patients (129,157,158,173,178,202,265,317).

Patients with unexplained syncope create a dilemma. On the one hand, syncope may be a manifestation of a very poor prognosis among those with underlying heart disease. On the other hand, patients with a more benign cause of syncope may still be at considerable risk because of trauma or occupational hazards. Moreover, because of the intermittent and transient nature of syncope, a definitive diagnosis usually requires an expensive and invasive procedure. It is helpful, therefore, to stratify the patients into low- and high-risk groups as a guide to the need for therapy and the extent of the diagnostic evaluation (Table 3).

The prognosis for patients with an isolated syncopal event but no stigmata of concurrent neurologic, coronary, or other cardiovascular disease is excellent. In the Framingham study, when characteristic-matched groups with and without isolated syncope were compared during a 26-year follow-up, there was no significant increase in the risk for total mortality, sudden death, myocardial infarction, or stroke (246). A similar low-risk group, comprising patients who were generally healthy and had a negative cardiac evaluation, was identified in the Pittsburgh study (219).

Although nonlethal recurrent syncope is a troublesome clinical problem, most retrospective studies have shown that if the cause of the recurrent episodes cannot be identified, a life-threatening cause is unlikely (130,146,149), which suggests that arrhythmias are not the primary cause of syncope. In contrast, a prospective study from Pittsburgh documented recurrence in a third of the patients during a 5-year period (121). The recurrence rate did not differ among patients with cardiac, noncardiac, or unexplained syncope; in only 5% of patients with an initial diagnosis of syncope of unknown origin did further evaluation at the

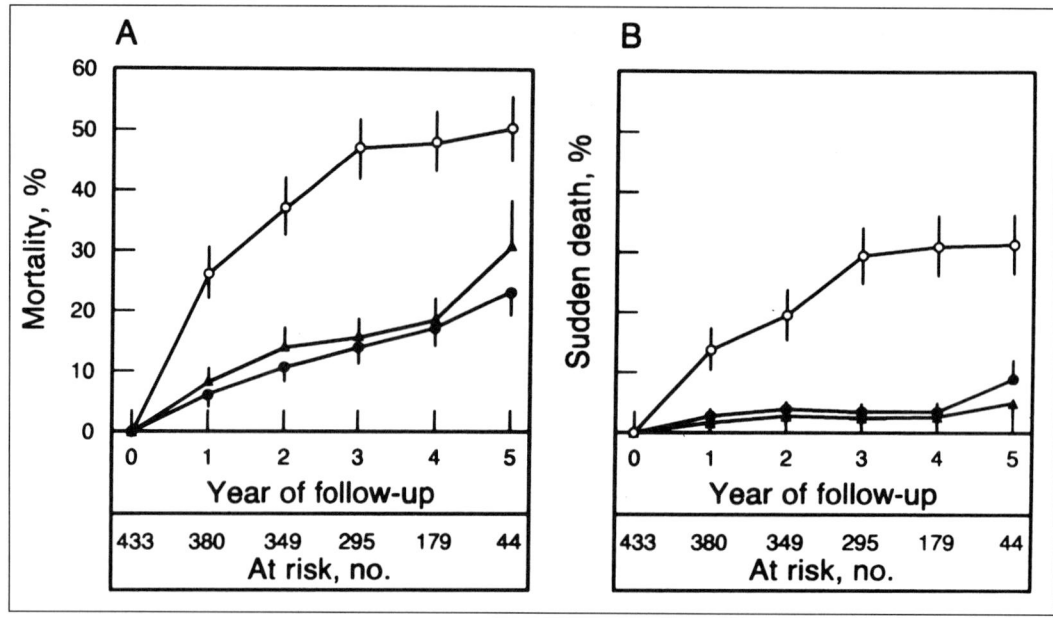

FIG. 4. Five-year actuarial mortality (**A**) and sudden death (**B**) rates from a prospective study in patients with syncope. Total mortality and sudden death in patients with a cardiac cause of syncope (▲) were both significantly higher than those in patients with a noncardiac cause (○) or patients with syncope of unknown cause (●). The patients were accrued from the emergency department, hospital admissions, and outpatient clinics. The mean ages were 61, 52, and 56 years for patients with cardiac, noncardiac, and unknown causes of syncope, respectively. (From Kapoor, ref. 121, with permission of Williams & Wilkins.)

time of recurrence establish a diagnosis, and recurrence did not predict either mortality or sudden death.

The presence of structural heart disease, a history of congestive heart failure, and left ventricular dysfunction are strong predictors of an arrhythmogenic cause of syncope, particularly of ventricular tachycardia (7,23,47,52,61–63, 104,112,146,190,191,230,285). In patients undergoing electrophysiologic testing for syncope of unknown cause, fewer than 5% with abnormal findings are free of underlying heart disease (146). A higher prevalence of arrhythmic syncope has been found in older patients as a group. The abrupt onset of symptoms with little or no warning or a history of palpitations, physical exertion, or emotional upset preceding syncope suggests a cardiogenic cause. The lack of palpitations does not exclude tachycardia as a cause.

A history of injuries resulting from syncope has been correlated with abnormal findings on electrophysiologic testing, suggesting an arrhythmogenic cause (108,146). However, older patients are more likely to sustain injury than are younger patients (45,175), as are patients who are standing or driving at the onset of syncope, compared with sitting (157).

TABLE 3. *Risk stratification in patients with unexplained syncope*

High-risk factors	Low-risk factors	Controversial
Coronary artery disease, prior myocardial infarction	Isolated syncope without underlying cardiovascular diseases	Recurrence[a]
Structural heart disease		
Left ventricular dysfunction	Younger age	
Congestive heart failure	Symptoms consistent with a vasovagal cause	
Older age	Normal electrocardiogram	
Abrupt onset		
Serious injuries		
Abnormal electrocardiogram (presence of Q wave, bundle-branch block, or atrial fibrillation)		
Abnormal signal-averaged electrocardiogram		

[a]See text for discussion.

EVALUATION OF PATIENTS WITH SYNCOPE

History and Physical Examination

The most important and fruitful elements of the evaluation are a detailed clinical history and a careful physical examination. Among patients in whom a diagnosis is eventually established, the diagnostic yield from the history and physical examination is high, ranging from 40%–75% in patients during the initial evaluation alone (51,65,66, 127,128,178,265).

Vasovagal syncope is a dramatic reaction occurring as a response to an emotionally disturbing event, but the sudden loss of consciousness without any period of warning is common. Information regarding the environmental circumstances at the time of syncope may be helpful. Because vasodepressor syncope may be precipitated by the sight of blood, loss of blood, sudden stressful or painful experiences, surgical manipulation, or trauma, a history of prior childhood syncope may provide a clue to vasovagal syncope in the adult. Premonitory signs and symptoms, if present, include pallor, weakness, lightheadedness, yawning, nausea, diaphoresis, hyperventilation, blurred vision, and impaired hearing immediately before the syncopal event. If the patient sits or lies down promptly, frank syncope may be aborted. When consciousness returns, the patient may have a persisting sensation of weakness, but syncope is not usually followed by a state of confusion.

Wearing a tight shirt collar or rotation or extension of the neck can induce syncope in patients with carotid sinus hypersensitivity. However, in a significant proportion of patients with carotid hypersensitivity syndrome, no mechanical trigger for the spontaneous episodes of syncope can be identified. Carotid sinus hypersensitivity usually occurs in the elderly and is more frequent in men than in women (282,283,307). Atherosclerosis, hypertension, diabetes mellitus, and local structures involving the carotid body (e.g., scars, lymph nodes, tumors) can predispose the patient to a hyperactive carotid sinus.

A history of syncope occurring shortly after rising from a lying or sitting position suggests that the cause may be orthostatic hypotension. Causes of secondary orthostatic hypotension should be sought. A complete drug history should be obtained to determine whether the patient is taking drugs that could cause hypotension. For situational syncope, establishing a relationship to meals, cough, swallowing, micturition, defecation, and invasive procedures confirms the diagnosis.

Arrhythmia-mediated syncope is usually sudden and may or may not be preceded by cardiac signs and symptoms, such as chest tightness, dyspnea, diaphoresis, apprehension, or palpitations. Syncope associated with abrupt termination of paroxysmal palpitations suggests a tachycardia-bradycardia or sick sinus syndrome. A history of coronary artery disease, congestive heart failure, and palpitations in a patient with syncope would significantly increase the possibility of ventricular tachyarrhythmias.

The relationship between exertion and syncope may point toward an obstructive cardiac lesion, ischemic heart disease, or catecholamine-mediated arrhythmias. Obtaining a detailed history of current medications is mandatory. If drugs are being taken that have negative chronotropic or dromotropic properties, this should alert the physician to the potential for bradycardia-related syncope, particularly in the elderly. Temporal relationships between taking class I antiarrhythmic agents and syncope suggest the possibility of drug-induced ventricular tachyarrhythmia. Chest pain or pressure may precede syncope. Significant ischemia, outflow tract obstruction, and pulmonary hypertension as well as hysteria and hyperventilation need to be included in the differential diagnosis. The frequency of previous events may give a clue to the possible diagnosis. Multiple episodes of syncope without any resultant injuries and a history of bizarre symptoms suggest hysterical syncope. A detailed family history should be obtained in patients suspected of having arrhythmia-mediated syncope. A positive family history for syncope or sudden cardiac death may point to the diagnosis of hypertrophic obstructive cardiomyopathy or congenital long-QT syndrome.

Seizures and cerebral ischemia can usually be differentiated from cardiovascular syncope. Clues suggesting seizures include the recollection of an aura preceding the sudden loss of consciousness. Seizures can occur with the patient in any position and even during sleep. A history of sporadic jerking movements does not differentiate seizures from syncope, because these may occur either with primary seizures or with cerebral hypoperfusion secondary to a prolonged arrhythmia. Urinary incontinence may also occur in either situation but is more commonly associated with seizures, as is tongue biting. A prolonged postictal state of mental confusion and drowsiness suggests seizures. Attacks of cerebral ischemia resulting from arteriosclerotic lesions are usually associated with other transient ischemic attacks characterized by neurologic symptoms, depending on the location of the lesions. There are often visual disturbances, hemiparesis, hemianesthesia, slurred speech, and impaired consciousness.

The physical examination in every patient should include an assessment of orthostatic vital signs. BP and HR should be measured in the supine, sitting, and standing positions. A postural decrease in BP of ≥20 mm Hg without an accompanying increase in HR should raise suspicion that the patient may have autonomic insufficiency, and further questions and diagnostic tests are appropriate to investigate this possibility.

A complete neurologic examination is required as part of the evaluation for syncope. Measurement of BP in both arms and listening for bruits in the carotid, subclavian, and temporal areas may identify patients with vascular disorders, such as cerebrovascular disease, Takayasu's disease, or subclavian steal syndrome. If subclavian steal syndrome is suspected, an attempt should be made to reproduce symptoms by having the patient perform arm exercises. Cardiac examination should focus specifically on identifying signs of overall cardiac function, aortic stenosis, hypertrophic cardiomyopathy, mitral valve prolapse, atrial myxoma, and pulmonary hypertension.

Carotid sinus massage should be a mandatory part of the evaluation of any patient with syncope. It is imperative, however, to exclude carotid bruits or peripheral vascular disease before performing massage. If these exist, the examination should be deferred, because the patient may be at a higher risk for cerebral complication during or after carotid sinus massage, although no data are available for the actual incidence of this complication. It is helpful to have atropine readily available for intravenous administration, although this measure is only rarely required. A pause of 3 sec or longer, a decrease in systolic BP of 50 mmHg without symptoms, or a decrease of 30 mmHg with symptoms is considered abnormal.

The diagnosis of carotid sinus hypersensitivity is, by and large, one of exclusion, but in the absence of any other identifiable cause, reproduction of the patient's symptoms during carotid sinus massage can provide evidence implicating carotid sinus hypersensitivity as the cause of syncope.

Diagnostic Testing

Electrocardiography

An abnormal result of 12-lead ECG was found in up to 50% of patients with syncope in one study (146). Most of the ECG abnormalities are nonspecific and are very rarely diagnostic. Nonetheless, certain ECG findings may point to a cause of syncope, such as Q waves, indicating prior myocardial infarction and possible ventricular tachyarrhythmias; prolongation of the QT interval, correlating with torsades de pointes; a short PR interval and ventricular pre-excitation, indicating the Wolff-Parkinson-White syndrome; bifascicular or trifascicular block, suggesting significant conduction system disease as a cause of bradycardia; and presence of left ventricular hypertrophy and intraventricular conduction disturbances, suggesting an underlying structural cardiac disease.

In contrast, a normal result of 12-lead ECG in a patient with syncope makes it unlikely that a cardiac cause will be identified (104,146). In one series, among patients whose initial ECG finding was normal, only approximately 10% had a significant abnormality revealed by an invasive electrophysiologic test. Only 6%–12% of patients with an initial normal ECG result had abnormalities considered to be definitive or potentially diagnostic on electrophysiologic testing. A 12-lead ECG should be performed in all patients.

Ambulatory Electrocardiographic Monitoring

When the cause of syncope is thought to be arrhythmogenic, continuous ambulatory (Holter) cardiac monitoring for a 24-hour period is strongly advised. Although the yield from ambulatory monitoring may be increased by prolonging the duration of monitoring, the likelihood that syncope or near syncope will recur during the period of monitoring remains extremely low (24,43,91,93,111,131,164,229,296). In one study, only 31 of 1512 Holter monitor recordings (2%) performed to evaluate syncope demonstrated findings considered to be diagnostic (91) (Fig. 5). When less strin-

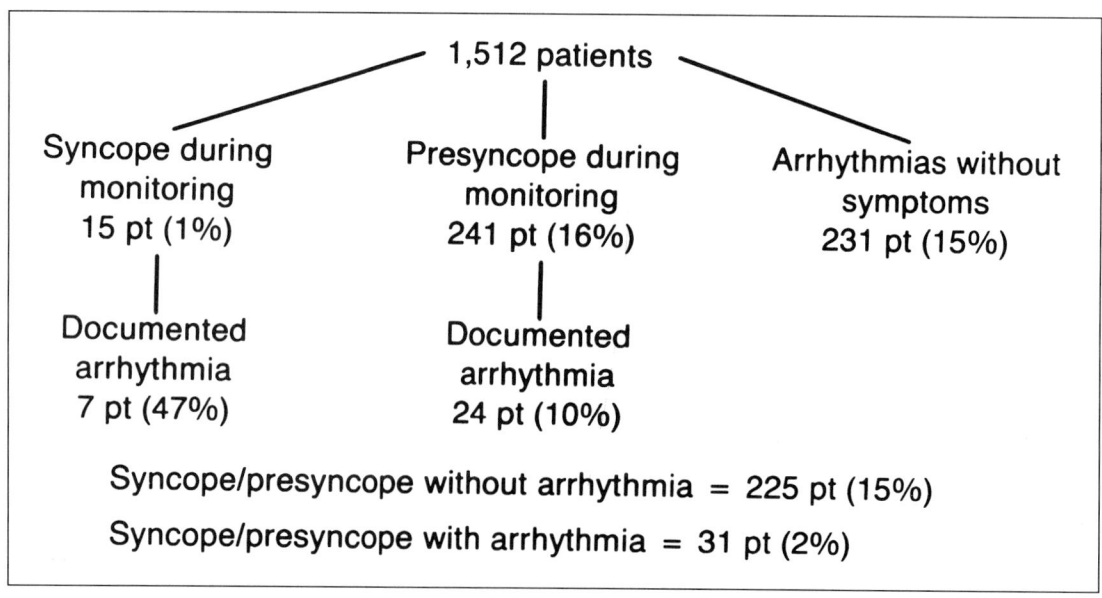

FIG. 5. Diagnostic efficacy of 24-hour Holter monitoring for syncope. *pt*, patients. (From Gibson and Heitzman, ref. 91.)

gent criteria were used for a positive correlation, a higher frequency of arrhythmia-related symptoms, including presyncope, lightheadedness, and dizziness, was reported (24, 93,196). Symptoms are often poorly correlated with ECG findings; however, typical symptoms with negative results from monitoring can be helpful (43,324). In some instances, the ECG abnormalities documented are not sufficiently severe to account for the symptoms (324). Symptoms may be noted without an arrhythmia being observed, or vice versa. However, unless syncope (or at least near syncope) occurs in association with an arrhythmia, it should not be assumed that the arrhythmia is the cause of syncope (9,324).

Patient-activated transtelephonic event recorders, with or without digital or solid-state memory loops, represent a promising new approach that can enhance the diagnostic yield of ambulatory monitoring (32,48,154,263). Cardiac rhythm disturbances during typical symptoms were reported in up to 35% of patients with previously undiagnosed syncope (154). The advantage of loop recorders is that they can be activated after the syncopal event, at which time they retrieve information about the cardiac rhythm during the preceding 4 minutes. These devices are small, nonobstructive, and inexpensive, and they can be worn for months at a time. Implantable monitoring devices are under development.

Signal-Averaged Electrocardiography

Signal-averaged ECG is a noninvasive, computerized method of detecting high-frequency, low-amplitude potentials at the end of QRS complexes (17,27,55,239,267) (Fig. 6). The ventricular late potential detected by a signal-averaged ECG represents an area of delayed depolarization from regions of slow conduction at the border zone of damaged myocardial tissue. These regions of delayed conduction constitute part of the nearby circuits, which are in turn the electrophysiologic substrate for ventricular arrhythmias (34,36,70,89,147,204,297,298,319,320). An abnormal signal-averaged ECG does not indicate the cause of syncope but can provide evidence that a substrate for ventricular arrhythmias exists.

A negative signal-averaged ECG does not exclude the possibility of cardiac disease or cardiogenic syncope, but it does correlate strongly with the ability to induce ventricu-

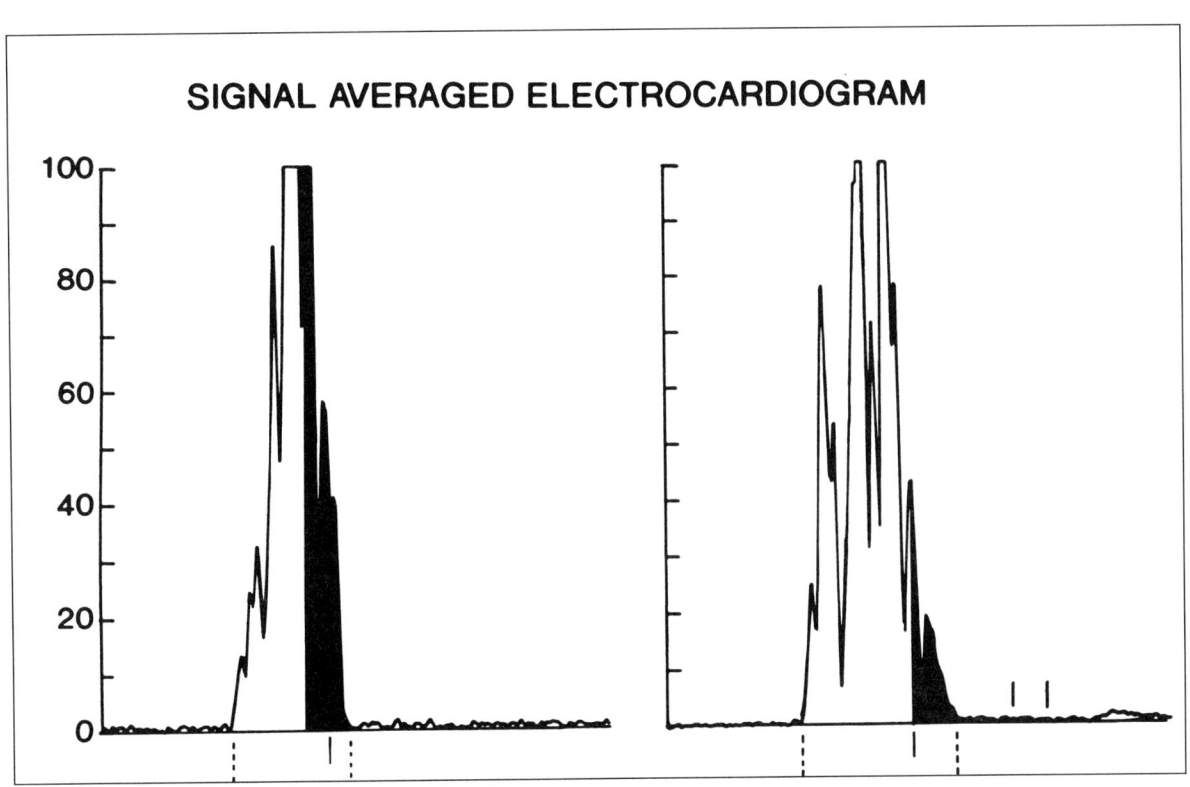

FIG. 6. Signal-averaged electrocardiograms (SA-ECGs) with (A) and without (B) late potentials. Late potentials are high-frequency, low-amplitude potentials at the terminal portion of QRS complexes. Both SA-ECGs were filtered with a 40-Hz bidirectional filter. Different criteria have been used for defining late potentials. Currently, late potentials are defined as "positive" when at least two of the following three criteria have been met: (a) QRS duration, >114 milliseconds; (b) root mean square (RMS) voltage of the terminal, 40 milliseconds of QRS <20 μV; and (c) duration of low-amplitude signal (LAS) defined as signals <40 μV, >38 milliseconds. (See Vatterott et al., ref. 298, for detailed explanation of QRSD, RMS, and LAS.)

lar tachycardia at the time of electrophysiologic study. The sensitivity of this technique for predicting inducible ventricular tachycardia during electrophysiologic studies in patients with unexplained syncope is variable and ranges from 30%–85%, depending on the characteristics of the patient population, the definition of inducibility (sustained versus nonsustained, monomorphic versus polymorphic ventricular tachycardia), and the stimulation protocols (89,147,298,319,320). Conversely, the specificity or negative predictive value of signal-averaged ECG has been uniformly high, ranging from 80%–100%, although the negative predictive value of signal-averaged ECG in patients with severely depressed left ventricular function remains to be determined.

In patients with bundle-branch block or marked intraventricular conduction delay on the surface ECG, standard techniques of signal-averaged ECG yield far less reliable and useful information, and it remains to be seen whether newer approaches incorporating spectral temporal mapping will enhance its role in this setting (34,70). From a practical standpoint, signal-averaged ECG has become more of a research tool in the assessment of ventricular arrhythmias and syncope.

Treadmill Exercise Text

A treadmill exercise test may be useful in selected patients with syncope, although the common purpose of the procedure has been to detect coronary artery disease in asymptomatic patients and assess prognosis among patients with known coronary artery disease. In a patient who has had syncope during or after exercise in association with chest pain, unless significant aortic stenosis or hypertrophic obstructive cardiomyopathy is present, a treadmill exercise test can be safely performed to evaluate ischemic signs and symptoms, and the results can be used to assess further the need for cardiac catheterization and coronary angiography (244). Exercise-induced rhythm disturbances, bradycardia, or tachycardia may identify a specific connotation not revealed by Holter or electrophysiologic testing (1,45,113,274,301,311,321). An inappropriately slow sinus rate during exercise may suggest chronotropic incompetence and underlying sinus node dysfunction (1).

Other abnormalities during exercise testing that may be diagnostic include AV block at slow HR, indicating distal conduction disease (321), and exercise-induced supraventricular or ventricular arrhythmias. The latter may reflect the complex interactions between a static arrhythmogenic substrate, such as a fixed myocardial scar (after infarction), and a dynamic process that can modulate arrhythmias, such as fluctuation of autonomic tone or even exercise-induced ischemia (45,274,311). It is mandatory that cardiac rhythm and BP be carefully monitored during stress testing in a patient with exertional syncope.

Other Cardiac Tests

Echocardiography, cardiac catheterization, and coronary angiography should be considered when structural or coronary artery disease is the suspected cause of syncope. Any decision to pursue an invasive diagnostic approach is based on the findings obtained from the initial clinical history and physical examination.

Tilt-table and Pharmacologic Provocative Test

Tilt-table testing represents an exciting addition to the diagnostic evaluation of patients with unexplained syncope, particularly if caused by vasodepression. The use of upright tilt testing is rapidly expanding as a provocative maneuver in patients with unexplained syncope (8,38,77,80,99,110,122,136,165,167,185,186,224,225,259–261,275,278,309).

This test is performed using a specially designed tilt table with a footboard. The patient is tilted to an upright position of 60° to 80° after having been supine for 10 to 60 min; a supplemental intravenous infusion of isoproterenol is given if baseline passive tilt fails to provoke a positive response. It is believed that upright tilt from a supine position precipitates vasovagal syncope in a predisposed patient. As discussed earlier in this chapter, the proper hemodynamic adjustment to venous pooling associated with gravitational stress results in stabilization of BP by an increase in HR and contractility, as well as peripheral vasoconstriction. In predisposed patients, this stimulus presumably activates the Bezold-Jarisch reflex, which results in an abrupt withdrawal of varying degrees of peripheral sympathetic tone or a sudden surge of vagal discharge, or both, predominantly causing hypotension (vasodepressor) or bradycardia (cardioinhibitory), respectively, or both.

Although a strict definition of positivity remains controversial, a positive response is defined by the reproduction of symptoms (syncope or near syncope) in association with either hypotension or bradycardia, or both (Fig. 7). If symptoms develop without accompanying bradycardia or hypotension, a cardiovascular or vasovagal cause can probably be excluded. A diagnosis of vasovagal or vasodepressor syncope cannot be made with certainty if symptoms are not reproduced, even though moderate hypotension or a relative bradycardia, or both, may be provoked by tilt-table testing.

The sensitivity and specificity of tilt-table testing in detecting vagally mediated syncope are difficult to determine, because the true incidence of vasovagal syncope is unknown in most patient groups and the diagnosis is usually based on a history of a typical prodrome and the exclusion of other conditions. In one study, the tilt-table test produced positive results in 67% of patients (10 of 15) with unexplained syncope, suggesting vagally mediated syn-

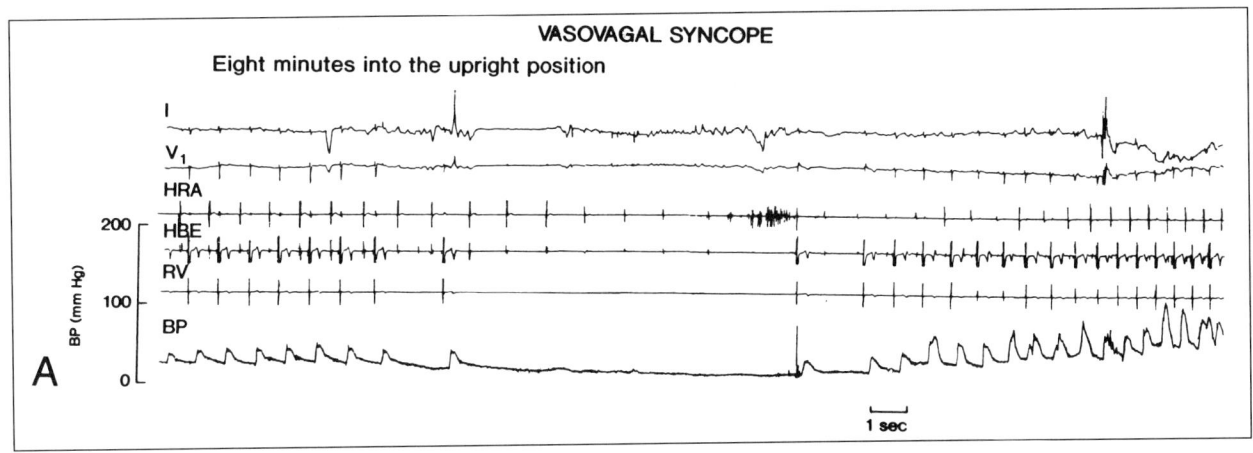
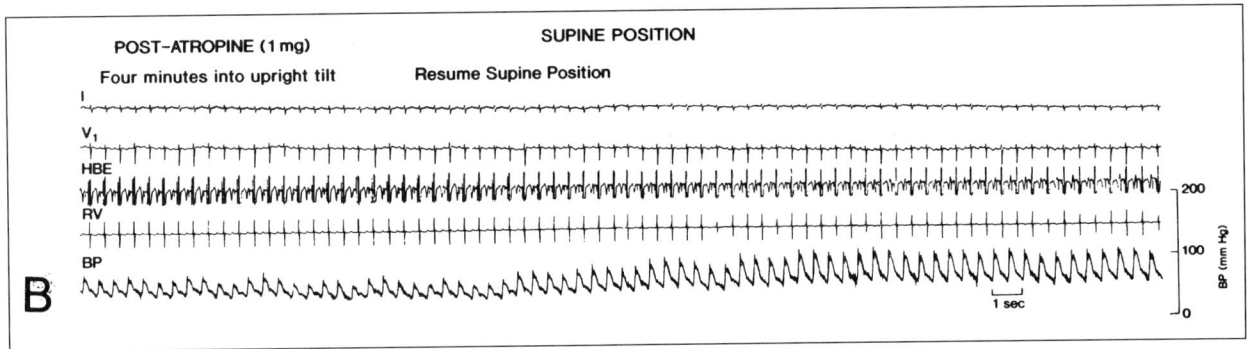
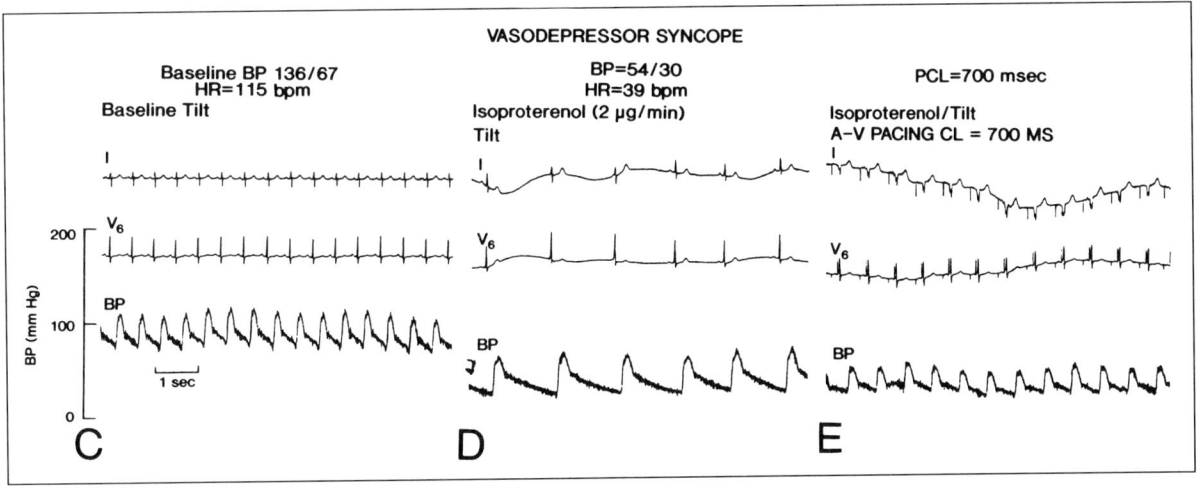

FIG. 7. Demonstration of vasovagal reaction in patients with recurrent syncope. **Patient 1. A:** Bradycardia/asystole and significant hypotension associated with syncope occurred at 8 minutes in the tilted upright position. The patient spontaneously recovered immediately after being returned to the supine position. **B:** After 1 mg of atropine was administered, syncope was again reproduced with the patient in the upright position, which was associated with hypotension but no significant bradycardia (see text for discussion). **Patient 2. C:** Results of tilt-table test at baseline were normal. The HR was 115 beats per minute, and BP remained stable at 136/67 mm Hg in the upright position. **D:** During isoproterenol infusion (2 μg/min) in the upright position, the patient became nauseated, and this was followed by bradycardia (30 to 60 beats per minute), hypotension (54/30 mm Hg), and presyncope. **E:** AV sequential pacing at three different cycle lengths (800, 700, and 600 milliseconds) did not relieve the hypotension or the patient's symptoms. *I*, surface lead I; *HBE*, His bundle electrogram; *HRA*, high right atrial electrogram; *RV*, right ventricular electrogram; *MS*, milliseconds.

cope, compared with 10% (1 of 10) in the control population (136). In another large study, 74% of patients (53 of 71) with unexplained syncope had positive test results, compared with 7% (2 of 27) in the asymptomatic age-matched control group (77). The findings from several other small series that compared patients who had vasovagal syncope with healthy controls further suggest that the specificity of the tilt-table test for vasodepressor syncope is high (around 90%) (8,38,309).

The addition of isoproterenol infusion to standard tilt-table testing was advocated as a means of increasing the sensitivity of the test (8,38,309). The rationale was based on earlier studies of the hemodynamic profile of vasovagal reactions, which documented that HR and BP frequently increase immediately *before* the onset of symptoms, indicating a period of increased sympathetic activity (69,92,97). Moreover, measurements of circulating catecholamine concentrations immediately before syncope further implicated catecholamine excess as a probable trigger of the neurally mediated vasovagal response.

Results of several series attest to the increased sensitivity of isoproterenol infusions in combination with tilt-table testing. Almquist et al. (8) reported that upright tilt testing alone induced significant vasovagal symptoms in only 4 of 15 patients with unexplained syncope who had negative electrophysiologic findings (27%). Among the remaining 11 patients, 9 had syncope during tilt with isoproterenol infusion. Similarly, Waxman et al. (309) were able to reproduce symptoms in 67% of their patients with vasodepressor syncope when they combined isoproterenol infusion with tilt-table testing. The same authors also reported that muscarinic receptor blockade with atropine prevented the vagally mediated bradycardia but, of more importance, did not prevent either hypotension or symptoms of fainting. However, β-adrenergic receptor blockade inhibited all aspects of the isoproterenol-induced faint. Grubb et al. (99) reported a 24% yield during baseline tilt and an additional 36% yield during isoproterenol infusion. The total positive yield was 60%.

These observations support the notion that vagally induced bradycardia is but one arm of a neurally mediated reflex loop and that muscarinic receptor blockade has minimal impact on the peripheral vascular tone. However, β-adrenergic blocking agents may act in several ways: (a) by decreasing the intensity of the catecholamine-mediated stimulus to the afferent arc of the reflex; (b) by decreasing ventricular contractility with its attendant stimulation of myocardial mechanoreceptors; and (c) by possibly modifying centrally mediated neurogenic responses.

The tilt test combined with isoproterenol infusion appears to represent a valuable clinical technique for evaluating patients with unexplained syncope. Many important issues related to tilt-table testing remain to be resolved. Although most of the tilt-table tests have been performed at angles between 60° and 80°, the optimal angle and duration of tilting have not been determined. Isoproterenol as well as other provocative agents, including adenosine (264), nitroglycerin (225), and edrophonium (165), may enhance the positive yield of tilt-table testing. This is likely accomplished at the expense of specificity. Several studies have observed that isoproterenol-induced vasovagal response during tilt-table testing can be significantly less specific, especially in the younger patient population (122,208,260). Furthermore, reproducibility of tilt-table testing (35,39,101,262), and therefore its utility in guiding the evaluation of therapy, remain to be defined. Currently, we perform the tilt/isoproterenol test in conjunction with electrophysiologic testing once an arrhythmogenic cause has been excluded. The intracardiac electrodes can be used for pacing, either to prevent prolonged bradycardia and thereby minimize potential complications, or to assess the response to atrial, ventricular, or dual-chamber pacing during induced syncope. The effectiveness and safety of the tilt/isoproterenol test without continuous intracardiac monitoring and the availability of temporary pacing are not well defined, but it is likely that tilt-table testing with or without isoproterenol will be utilized increasingly as a single procedure without the use of prior invasive electrophysiologic testing in selected patients.

Electrophysiologic Testing

Although in many patients syncope is nonarrhythmogenic in origin and the prognosis is favorable, there is a substantial subset of patients in whom life-threatening bradyarrhythmias and tachyarrhythmias are a potential mechanism and in whom invasive electrophysiologic testing is the diagnostic procedure of choice.

There are several reasons to perform an electrophysiologic test in patients with syncope: (a) to establish the diagnosis; (b) to evaluate dynamic relationships among symptoms, dysrhythmias, and hemodynamic changes; (c) to assess the response to different pacing modalities in bradyarrhythmias; and (d) to determine the response to therapy in the case of tachyarrhythmias. Depending on the patient population studied and endpoints for diagnosis, the yield of electrophysiologic testing has been reported to range from 18%–75% (7,12,47,52,56,61,63,104,112,146,285) (Table 4). An arrhythmogenic cause of unexplained syncope disclosed by electrophysiologic studies in patients without underlying heart disease is generally less common, ranging from 10%–20% (7,104,190,191). In patients with underlying heart disease, particularly in association with left ventricular dysfunction as a consequence of coronary artery disease or prior myocardial infarction (or both), the yield from an electrophysiologic study is likely higher (12,24, 52,56,60,62,63,88,104,112,123,146,190,212,315). A stepwise approach for selecting patients to undergo electrophysiologic study is outlined in Fig. 8.

Physicians need to address the following questions before subjecting a patient to invasive electrophysiologic

TABLE 4. *Role of electrophysiologic testing in patients with unexplained syncope*

			Diagnostic yield						Follow-up outcome				
											Recurrent syncope		Mortality (sudden death)	
Study (ref.)	No.	HD, No.	Brady	VT	SVT	Vasovagal CSH	Total (%)	HD+/HD−	No.	Duration, y	Total	EP+/EP−	Total	EP+/EP−
DiMarco et al. (62)	25	15	4	9	1	3	17(68)	11(73)/6(60)	25	18	7	18/50	—	—/—
Gulamhusein et al. (104)	34	0	3	0	3	0	6(18)	—/6(18)	34	15	14	16/46	—	—/—
Hess et al. (112)	32	17	6	12	—	—	18(56)	12(71)/6(40)	32	21.3	6	11/29	2	2/—
Akhtar et al. (7)	30	18	5	11	0	—	16(53)	15(83)/1(8)	30	16	13	12/79	—	—/—
Morady et al. (191)	53	38	2	28	—	—	30(57)	27(71)/3(20)	53	27.5	18	27/43	1	0/1
Teichman et al. (285)	150	75	88	36	18	20	112(75)	64(85)/48(64)	137	31	31	15/47	3	—
Doherty et al. (63)	119	62	14	31	23	15	78(66)	—/—	85	27	15	19/14	3	—
Denes and Ezri (52)	50	35	28	4	6	12	37(74)	—/—	50	23	4	13/4	2	—
Krol et al. (146)	104	66	8	21	2	—	31(30)	30(46)/1(3)	—	—	—	—	—	—
Crozier et al. (47)	94	42	22	2	0	3	26(28)	16(38)/10(20)	92	52	34	30/41	3	—
Denes et al. (56)	89	61	74	13	13	15	64(71)	—/—	82	47	9	11/18	18	15/3
Bass et al. (12)	70	—	3	31	3	—	37(53)	—/—	70	30	20	32/24	26	23/3

Brady, bradycardia; CSH, carotid sinus hypersensitivity; EP, electrophysiologic testing; HD, heart disease; SVT, supraventricular tachycardia; VT, ventricular tachycardia; —, not done.

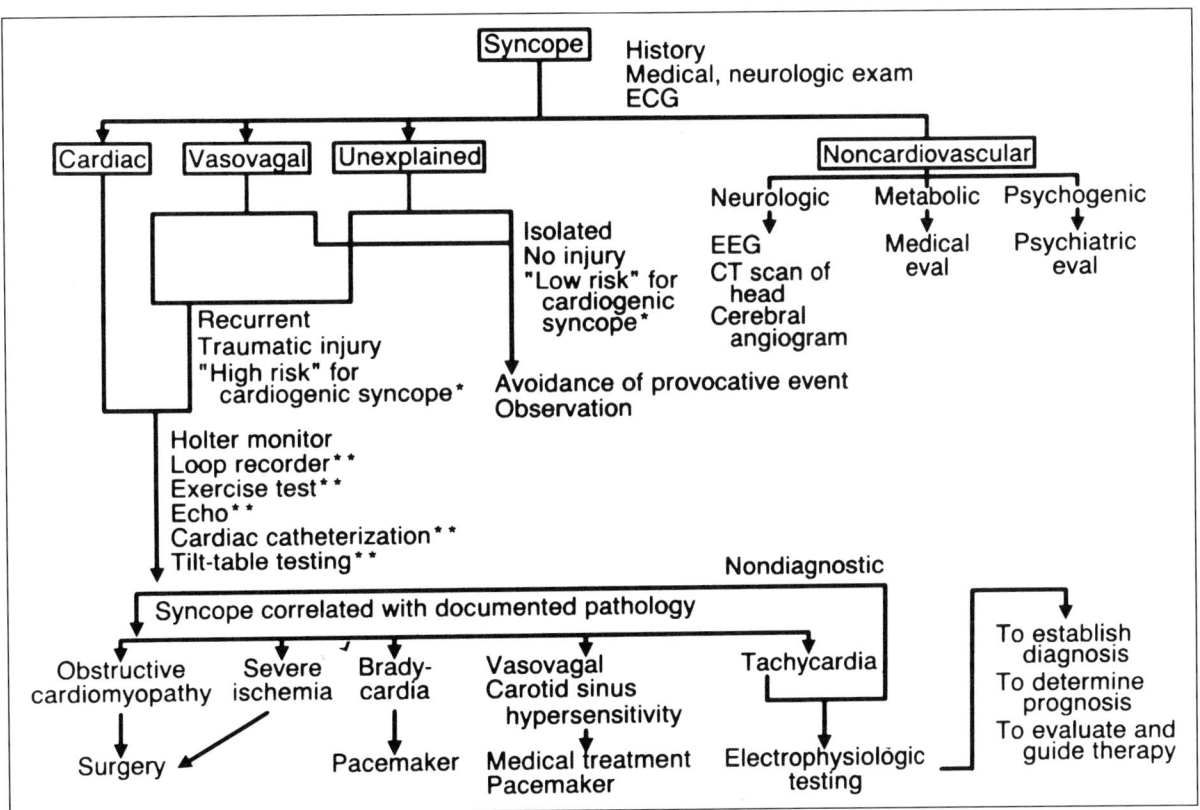

FIG. 8. Stepwise approach in the evaluation of syncope and the decision to obtain an electrophysiologic test. (*) High- and low-risk factors associated with cardiogenic syncope are summarized in Table 3 and discussed in the text. (**) The selection of various tests should be individualized. The significance of these test results is also discussed in detail in the text. *CT*, computed tomography; *ECG*, electrocardiogram; *Echo*, echocardiogram; *EEG*, electroencephalogram; *eval*, evaluation.

study: (a) Is the information obtained from the history and noninvasive tests adequate to explain the patient's clinical presentation? (b) Could the results of an invasive electrophysiologic study offer additional prognostic information? (c) Can the results of the electrophysiologic study affect and direct therapy? A complete electrophysiologic study should include assessment of (a) sinus node function; (2) AV node and His-Purkinje system conduction; (c) inducibility of supraventricular arrhythmias, including atrial fibrillation or flutter, or ventricular tachycardia by programmed stimulation; and (d) carotid sinus hypersensitivity. It should also evaluate therapeutic modalities, such as drugs, antitachycardia pacing, and different pacing modalities for bradycardia.

Evaluation of Sinus Node Function

The prevalence of sinus node dysfunction increases with advanced age. It is a relatively frequent cause of presyncope and syncope (134,322). ECG abnormalities that suggest sinus node dysfunction, as discussed earlier, can usually be demonstrated on a 12-lead ECG or during continuous ambulatory monitoring. Only when the symptoms of near syncope or syncope can be clearly correlated with a significant bradycardia—that is, prolonged sinus pause (>3 seconds) caused by sinus exit block, sinus arrest, or persistent severe sinus bradycardia (<40 beats per minute)—can permanent pacemaker implantation be recommended without additional electrophysiologic studies being performed (235, 236,257). Because most instances of sinus node disease are diagnosed by a noninvasive technique, it is not surprising that only 5%–10% of patients undergoing electrophysiologic study for unexplained syncope ultimately are shown to have sinus node abnormalities as the presumed cause of syncope (7,12,56,61–63,112,146,190,191,289). Not infrequently, especially in elderly patients with syncope, signs of sinus node dysfunction may be documented during ambulatory monitoring without associated symptoms, and therefore it cannot be assumed that syncope is caused by the sick sinus syndrome.

Although the electrophysiologic study may confirm an abnormality in sinus node function or other evidence of conduction disease or arrhythmias, it is equally valuable for its ability to exclude electrophysiologic mechanisms as the cause of syncope. The test result is most definitive when symptoms can be correlated with the electrophysiologic findings, but in patients with syncope and evidence of sinus node dysfunction in whom other causes can be excluded, electrophysiologic testing may provide the best (albeit circumstantial) evidence for sinus node dysfunction as the cause of syncope.

Sinus node dysfunction is evaluated during electrophysiologic study by determining the sinus node recovery time (SNRT), sinoatrial conduction time (SACT), and sinus node refractoriness. SNRT measures sinus node automaticity (169). It evolved from experiments that documented a suppression of node automaticity after a period of atrial pacing (Fig. 9). The rapid atrial pacing technique is implemented by pacing the high right atrium for a fixed period (30 seconds) at rates ranging from 100 to 200 beats/min, allowing for 60-second rest periods between pacing. The rapid atrial depolarizations should conduct in retrograde fashion into the sinus node and repeatedly depolarize it, thereby suppressing its automaticity. The interval between the last paced response and the first spontaneous high atrial response is the SNRT. One corrects for the variability in spontaneous cycle length (SCL) by subtracting SCL from the SNRT to derive a corrected SNRT (CSNRT). A range of normal values for CSNRT has been proposed (375 to 533 millisec). We currently accept 525 millisec as the upper limit of normal. Techniques for evaluating sinus node conduction (206,279) and refractoriness (138) are not discussed here.

Sinus node dysfunction may result from disturbances in one or more of these underlying mechanisms. The sensitivity and specificity of SNRT and SACT vary, depending on the different criteria used in defining abnormal values and the different patient populations in various studies (15). The SACT is less sensitive than the SNRT. Fewer than 50% of patients with clinical findings of SA node dysfunction have a prolonged SACT. The overall sensitivity and specificity of the measurements, either alone or in combination, are

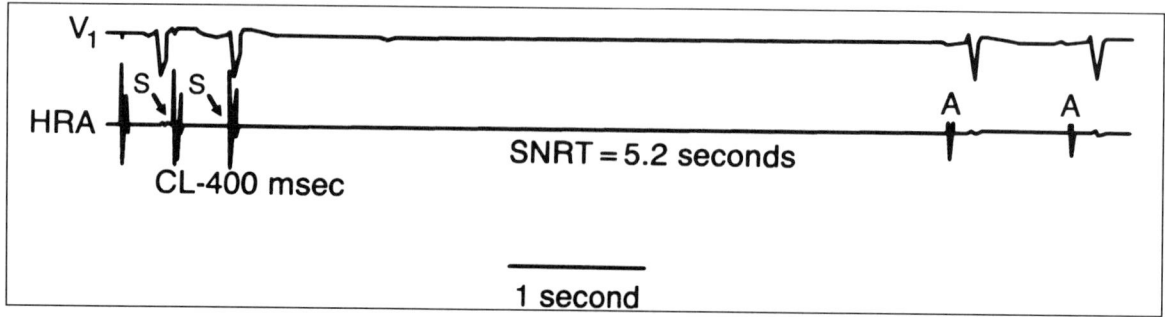

FIG. 9. Prolonged sinus node recovery time (SNRT) in a patient with two episodes of syncope. Results of noninvasive testing were nondiagnostic. The only abnormal finding during electrophysiologic testing was a markedly prolonged SNRT (5.2 seconds) that was associated with near syncope. *A*, atrial deflection; *HRA*, high right atrial electrogram; *S*, pacing stimulus; *CL*, cycle lengths.

low (88). Measurement of SA node refractoriness has not become a standard part of the SA node evaluation; however, it may be a more sensitive index of node dysfunction than are the SNRT and SACT determinations (138).

Dysfunction of the Atrioventricular Conduction System

As in sinus node dysfunction, treatment of syncope can be initiated without electrophysiologic studies if symptoms can be documented in concordance with a high-grade AV block using noninvasive techniques. Episodes of high-grade AV block (Adams-Stokes attacks) are often intermittent and unpredictable, and it may not be possible to establish a diagnosis despite repeated ambulatory recordings. Electrophysiologic study can be helpful in identifying patients with unexplained syncope without documented AV block in whom intermittent high-grade AV block is suspected (52,146). In one study of 190 patients with syncope of unknown cause, after prolonged cardiac monitoring, only five patients (2.6%) were found to have AV conduction system diseases that were considered severe enough to account for the event (43). In addition, electrophysiologic testing is useful in patients with unexplained syncope who also have documented asymptomatic AV block, because it can determine the site of the conduction disturbance. Differentiating supranodal from infranodal conduction delays provides important prognostic information.

The evaluation of AV node conduction during electrophysiologic study includes determining the baseline AV node-to-His bundle conduction time (AH interval), the His bundle-to-ventricle conduction time (HV interval), and the duration of His bundle deflection (Fig. 10). These intervals are obtained from a His bundle electrogram, which is recorded from a multipolar electrode catheter with the tip positioned near the His bundle. Although measurements may vary somewhat for different laboratories, normal intervals generally have been well established (Fig. 10).

The most useful information is provided by the HV interval, which is determined by the His bundle electrogram. An HV interval of more than 55 millisec is considered abnormal (Fig. 11). The prognostic value of measuring the HV interval in patients with chronic bifascicular block, with or without symptoms, generated a considerable degree of controversy in the 1970s (59,181,250). It was believed by some investigators that prolongation of the HV interval indicated more diffuse and significant disease in the conduction system and would identify patients at high risk for complete heart block, for whom permanent pacing was indicated.

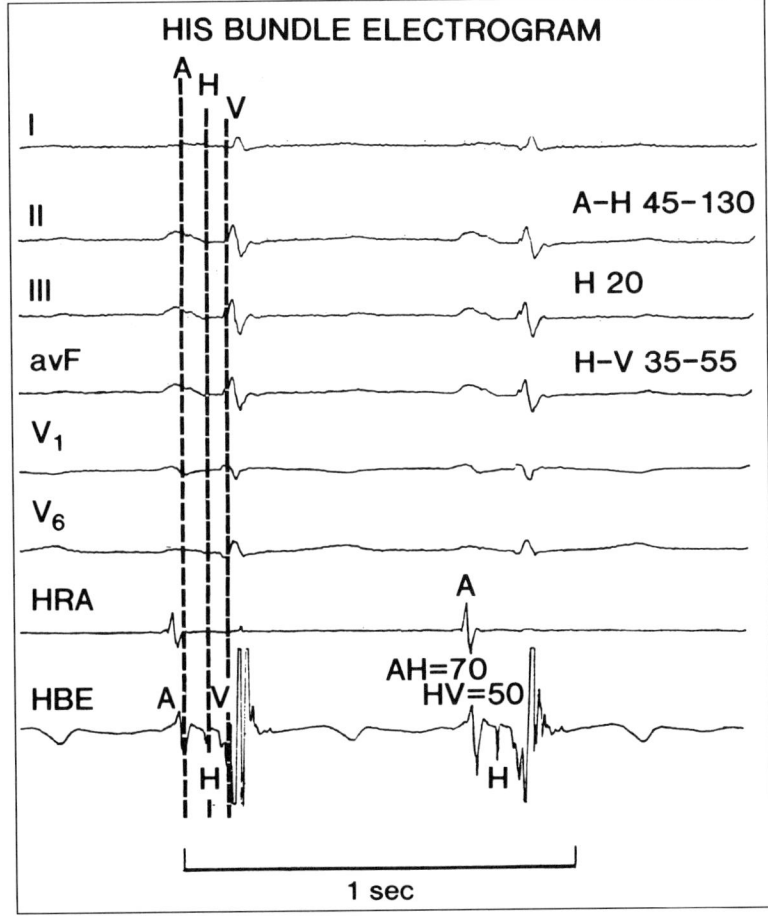

FIG. 10. Intracardiac His bundle electrogram. *Top six tracings* are from surface electrogram leads I, II, III, aVF, V_1, and V_6. AH and HV intervals are shown. Normal values for AH and HV intervals and duration of H deflection are shown *on the right*. All numbers are in milliseconds. *HRA*, high right atrial electrogram; *HBE*, His bundle electrogram (records low right atrial and ventricular activity sequentially). *A*, *H*, and *V* denote atrial, His bundle, and ventricular deflections, respectively.

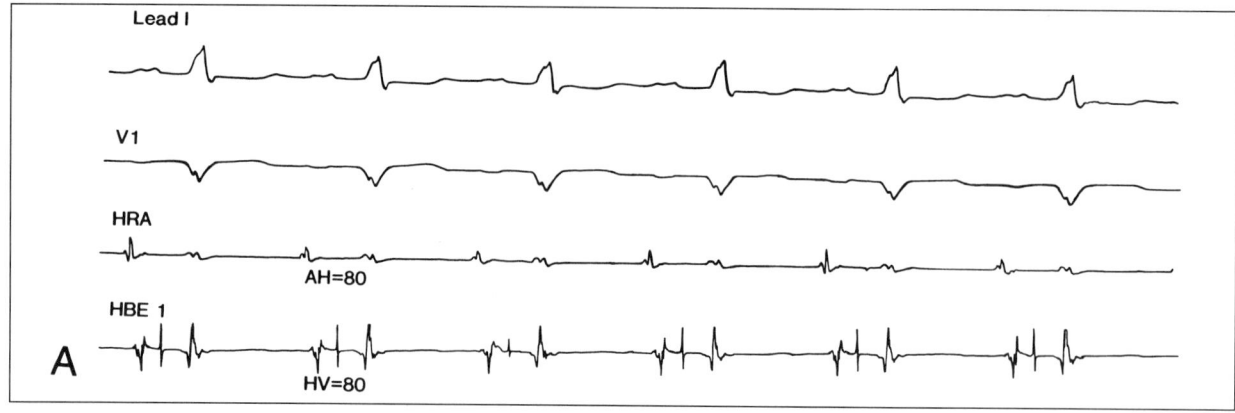
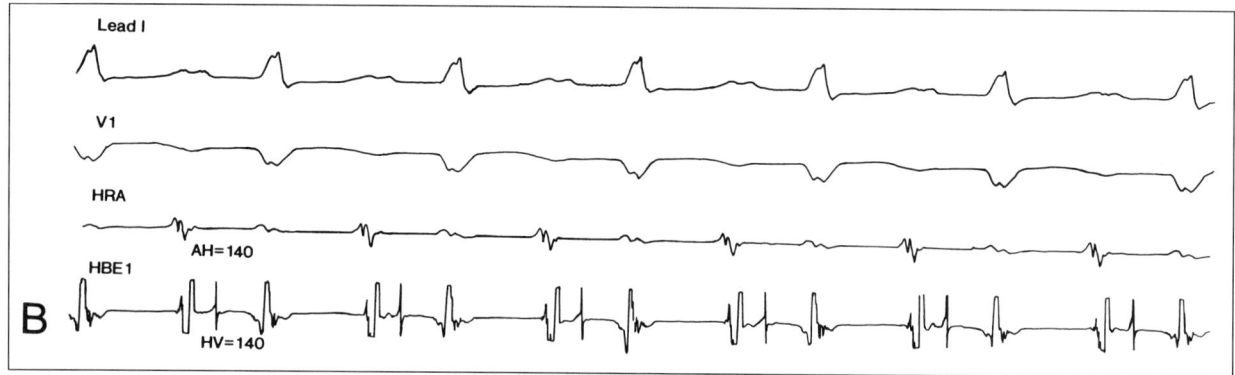
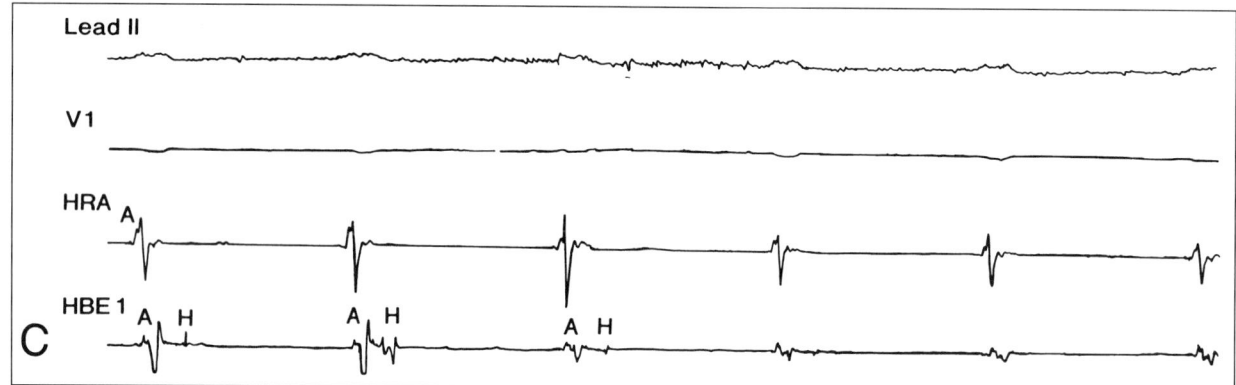

FIG. 11. Significant infranodal conduction system disease. **Patient 1.** A 12-lead electrocardiogram showed a left bundle-branch block. A 24-hour ambulatory monitoring interval was nondiagnostic. **A:** During electrophysiologic testing, baseline HV interval was significantly prolonged (80 milliseconds). No other abnormalities were detected during atrial and ventricular programmed stimulation. **B:** After procainamide injection (50 mg/min, maximal dose of 15 mg/kg), HV interval increased further (140 milliseconds). **C:** This was followed by spontaneous infrahisian block without any ventricular escape rhythm, which was associated with complete loss of consciousness. Temporary pacing was required for approximately 5 to 10 minutes before AV conduction was re-established (see text for discussion).

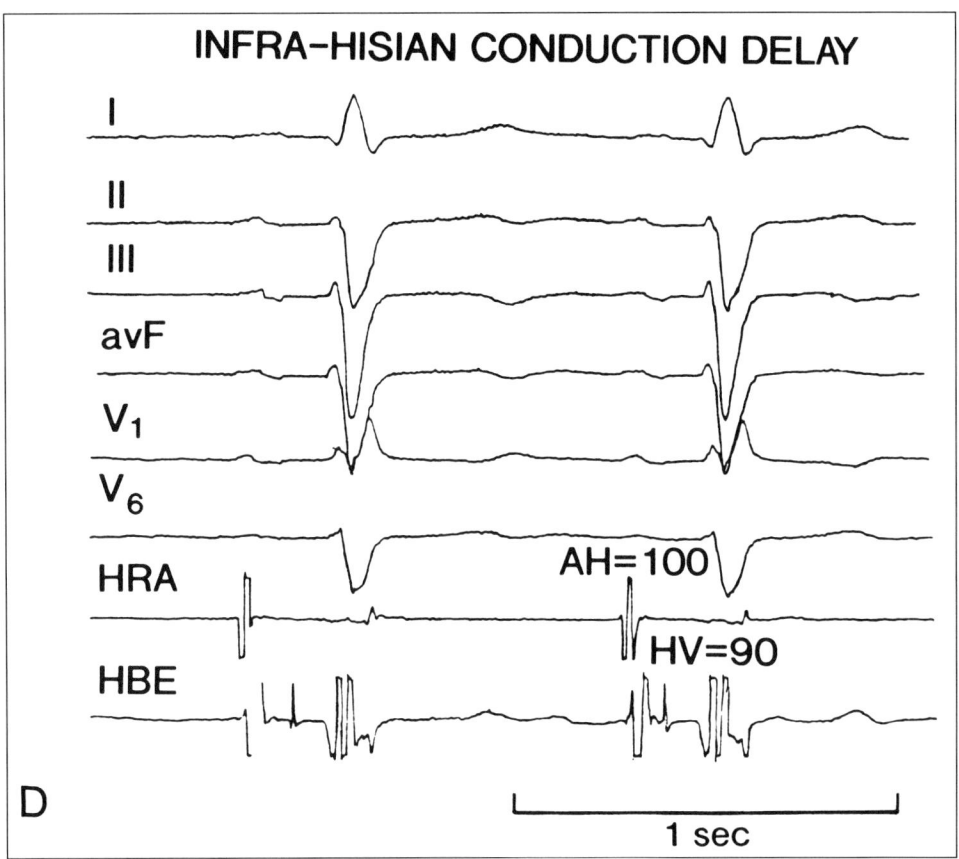
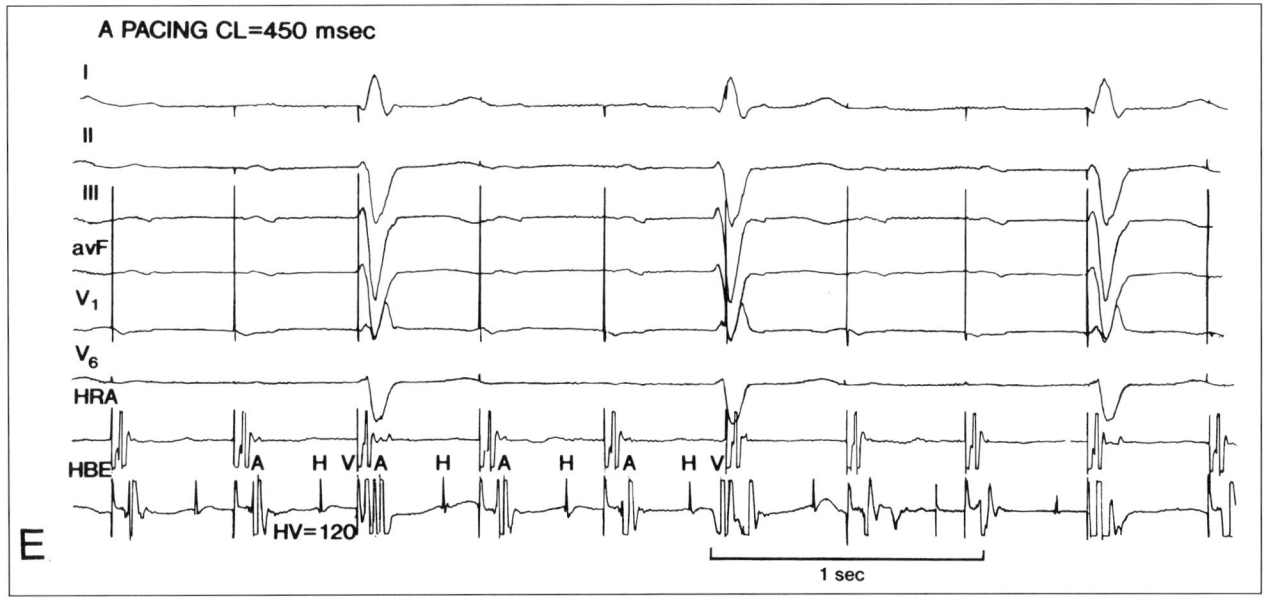

Patient 2. D: Baseline HV interval was significantly prolonged (90 milliseconds). **E:** Infrahisian 3:1 AV block occurred during atrial decremental pacing (cycle length of 450 milliseconds), suggesting significant conduction system disease. *I*, *V$_1$*, surface electrocardiogram; *AH*, atrioventricular node-to-His bundle conduction time; *HRA*, high right atrial electrogram; *HBE*, His bundle electrogram; *HV*, His bundle-to-ventricle conduction time; *A PACING CL*, atrial decremental pacing cycle length. (All numbers are in milliseconds.)

Late follow-up reports from three large studies of patients with chronic bifascicular block have, for the most part, resolved these controversies (59,181,250). These studies have shown the following: (a) Prolongation of the HV interval is positively correlated with the severity of underlying heart disease, and the HV interval is probably not an independent predictor of cardiovascular mortality; (b) the high mortality is associated with the severity of the underlying heart disease; (c) the majority of cardiovascular deaths most likely reflect the severity of the underlying cardiac dysfunction and are the consequence of ventricular arrhythmias in most patients; and (d) although the rate of development of complete heart block is low, it depends on the degree of HV interval prolongation, and in the majority of patients with marked HV prolongation (>100 millisec) at rest, progression to complete AV block occurs at a rate of 8% per year. Permanent pacing may be of prophylactic benefit in these patients.

Atrial programmed extrastimulation and decremental pacing are additional maneuvers that may expose latent conduction system disease (58) (Fig. 11D,E). The site of the block (above, below, or within the His bundle), rather than the pacing rate at which the block occurs, appears to have more prognostic significance. Intrahisian or infrahisian blocks are associated with a much worse prognosis than are blocks at a more proximal site in the conduction system. Pharmacologic maneuvers may also be used to expose latent conduction system disease (133) (Fig. 11C). A vagolytic agent such as atropine should be used if distal conduction system disease is suspected; however, proximal block develops at long atrial cycles, which may also prevent the detection of distal block (258). Antiarrhythmia agents (e.g., procainamide, ajmaline) may also be used to "stress" the distal conduction system because of their sodium channel-blocking properties (40,180,210,212,248, 290,293). Procainamide, because it can produce peripheral vasodilation, may also possess reflex vagolytic properties.

The yield from electrophysiologic testing is particularly high in patients with bundle-branch block. At one time, it was assumed that syncope in the presence of bundle-branch block, bifascicular block, or trifascicular block was the result of conduction disease. Furthermore, permanent pacemaker implantation was shown to be strongly indicated and highly effective in alleviating symptoms and improving prognosis among such patients (44,74,114). Nonetheless, it has also been documented that many such patients have inducible ventricular tachycardia as the likely cause of syncope, and the conduction disturbance in these patients is simply a manifestation of the severity of the underlying cardiac disease. In this subgroup of patients, therapy should be directed against the responsible ventricular tachyarrhythmia, although permanent pacemaker implantation may also be required if the antiarrhythmia drugs further depress conduction to a potentially lethal level. Although invasive electrophysiologic testing is extremely useful in patients with presumed conduction disease, negative test findings do not exclude the possibility of intermittent, high-grade AV block or sinus node dysfunction (88,116).

Supraventricular Tachycardia

Supraventricular tachycardia manifested as syncope alone, without a history of palpitations, is not common (94). Electrophysiologic studies may be helpful as a diagnostic tool in a few patients who experience sporadic episodes of syncope secondary to supraventricular tachycardia and in whom ambulatory monitoring is unrevealing. Overall, supraventricular tachycardia is established as a cause of unexplained syncope in from none to 15% of patients (56,146). Electrophysiologic studies may also be useful in assessing the hemodynamic response during induced supraventricular tachycardia in patients with presumed supraventricular tachycardia-mediated syncope when such a cause-and-effect relationship cannot be confirmed by noninvasive means.

Although supraventricular tachycardia is a relatively uncommon cause of syncope, electrophysiologic testing is invaluable in those subjects in whom a supraventricular arrhythmia is the presumed cause. A detailed electrophysiologic study, including programmed stimulation of both the atria and the ventricles, is required to reveal the presence of an accessory pathway (221,304), dual AV nodal pathways (53), enhanced AV node conduction (14), or various other forms of supraventricular arrhythmias, including atrial fibrillation or atrial flutter. Common forms of supraventricular tachycardia, such as AV re-entry tachycardia or AV nodal re-entry tachycardia involving a macroscopic re-entry mechanism, are usually inducible during electrophysiologic study. If supraventricular tachycardia is not inducible during a baseline study in a patient suspected of having it (by a history of rapid palpitations or documentation of short runs of supraventricular tachycardia during ambulatory monitoring), repeated programmed stimulation should be performed in conjunction with isoproterenol infusion.

In patients with Wolff-Parkinson-White syndrome, a detailed evaluation of the conduction properties of the accessory pathway must be included in the electrophysiologic study. The capacity of the accessory pathway to sustain rapid antegrade conduction during atrial fibrillation and various other indirect measures of rapid pathway conduction have been shown to be associated with sudden death (140,255). The development of surgical and catheter ablation techniques aimed at interrupting conduction down the accessory pathway has extended the application of electrophysiologic testing, and a precise determination of the location of the accessory pathway has now become a major objective of the study.

Supraventricular tachycardia is unlikely to be the cause of syncope unless associated symptoms, such as hypotension and near syncope, are present. The patient should be tilted to the upright position during induced tachycardia if symptoms do not develop in the supine position (Fig. 12). Studies have shown that tilt-table testing during an arrhythmia episode is able to reproduce symptoms and confirm the diagnosis in a small but significant subgroup (approximately 20%) of patients (110,172). Supraventricular tachy-

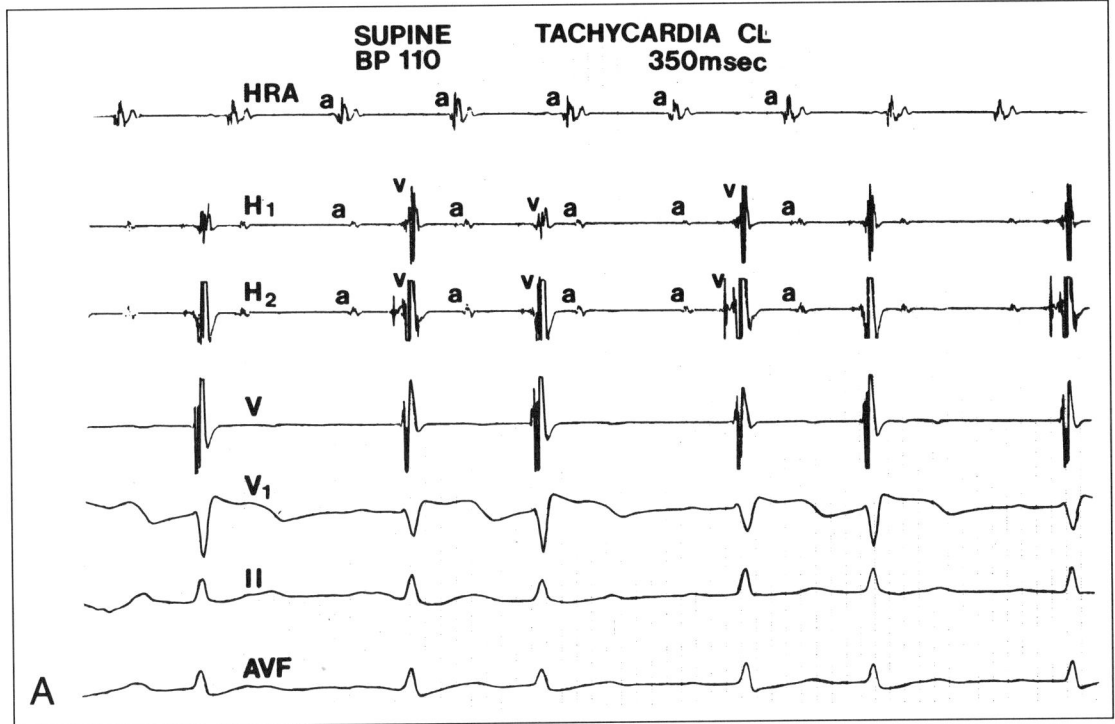
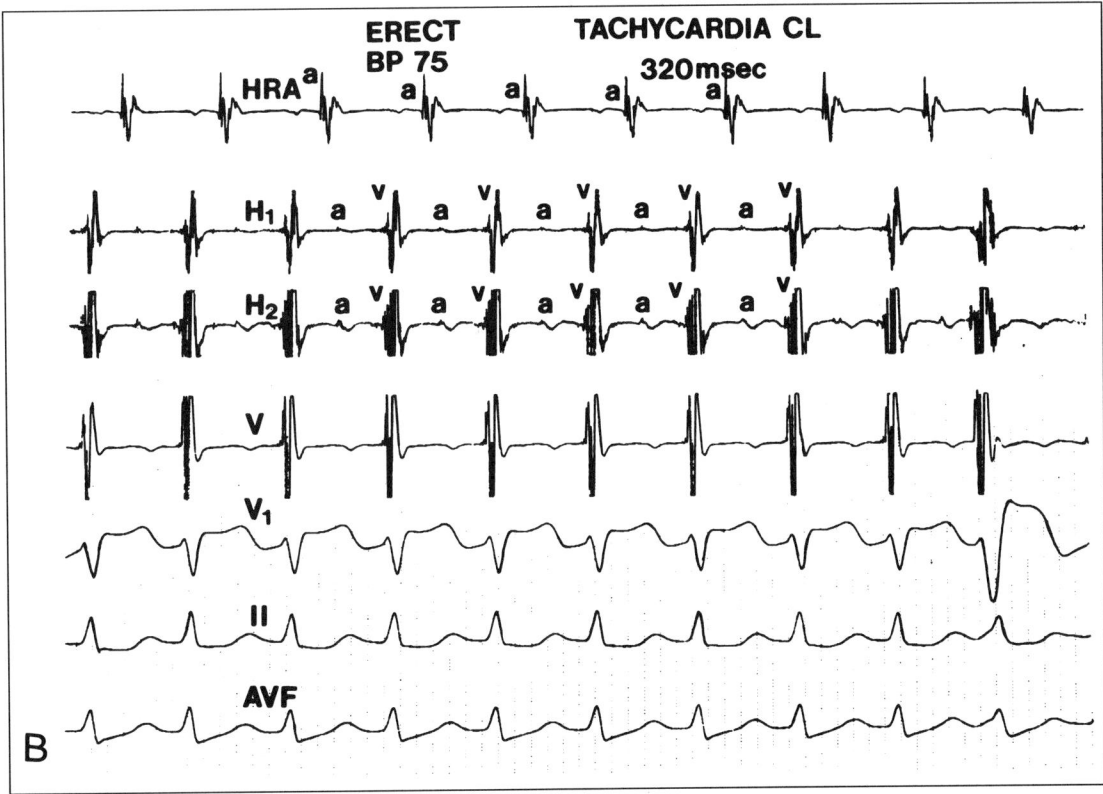

FIG. 12. Supraventricular tachycardia associated with near syncope. The patient had experienced recurrent palpitations associated with lightheadedness. An atrial tachycardia was inducible during electrophysiologic testing. A: In the supine position, the atrial cycle length was 350 milliseconds with 3:2 Wenckebach AV block; the patient was hemodynamically stable (systolic BP of 110 mm Hg). B: Immediately after upright tilt, atrial cycle length accelerated to 320 milliseconds with 1:1 AV conduction. Systolic BP decreased to 75 mm Hg and was associated with lightheadedness and near syncope. HRA, H_1, H_2, and V are intracardiac electrograms corresponding to high right atrial, His bundle 1 and 2, and ventricular recordings, respectively. V_1, II, and aVF denote surface electrocardiographic leads.

cardia may be an incidental finding unrelated to syncope during electrophysiologic studies, especially when symptoms of syncope or presyncope are not observed (53,54).

Ventricular Tachycardia

The most common abnormality or arrhythmia detected by electrophysiologic study in patients with unexplained syncope is ventricular tachycardia (7,62,190,191). Sustained monomorphic ventricular tachycardia, rarely a false-positive finding, can be induced in 2%–20% of patients with unexplained syncope (33,56,161,171,192,295). Sustained monomorphic ventricular tachycardia, if inducible, is the probable cause of unexplained syncope (Fig. 13). The optimal stimulation protocol for induction of ventricular tachycardia in patients with unexplained syncope has not yet been determined (308). More aggressive stimulation protocols are bound to increase the sensitivity of electrophysiologic studies in detecting ventricular arrhythmias; however, the increased sensitivity will be at the expense of specificity (314).

MANAGEMENT

The most appropriate treatment for syncope is usually quite obvious once the cause has been determined. However, in some situations the diagnosis is presumptive, as when electrophysiologic abnormalities cannot be correlated with symptoms. In this setting therapeutic decisions are difficult. The specific treatment of noncardiovascular causes of syncope and orthostatic hypotension are not discussed here.

Vasovagal Syncope/Carotid Sinus Hypersensitivity

In all types of vagally mediated syncope, an important consideration before treatment is recommended is whether syncope is primarily the result of a cardioinhibitory or a vasodepressor response. Both components of the abnormal reflexes are active in most patients, although one component is usually dominant. Unfortunately, this may vary at any given time, which compounds the therapeutic decision, as treatment must be targeted against either the cardioinhibitory response (bradycardia) or the vasodepressor response (hypotension), or both.

In patients with a predominantly cardioinhibitory response, implantation of a pacemaker should be considered if vagally mediated syncope is recurrent or has caused traumatic injuries (16,28,72,78,148,166,199,203,215,218,243,245,276). Despite the hemodynamic advantages of dual-chamber AV pacing over single-chamber ventricular demand pacing, neither pacemaker modality can prevent hypotension in patients in whom the vasodepressor component of the response is dominant. Nonetheless, dual-chamber pacing may blunt the hypotensive response, which may be sufficient to prevent syncope even though symptoms may not be entirely abolished. Unfortunately, the treatment

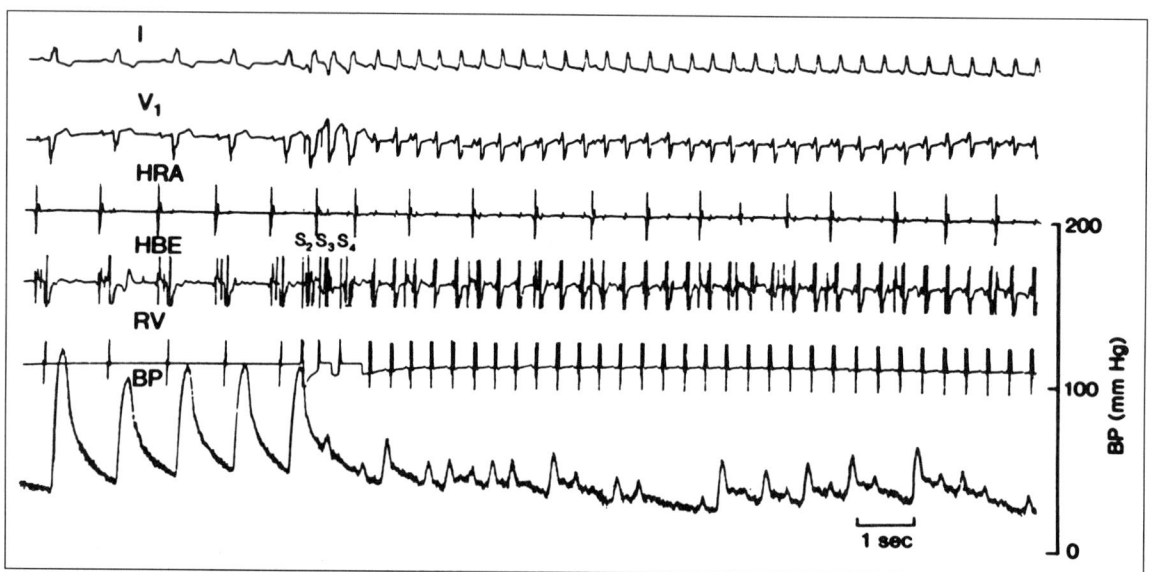

FIG. 13. Monomorphic ventricular tachycardia (VT) induced by triple extrastimuli (S_2, S_3, S_4) during sinus rhythm in a patient with coronary artery disease and a prior history of myocardial infarction and two episodes of syncope. The induced VT had a cycle length of 360 milliseconds. The systolic BP was 55 mm Hg during VT and the patient experienced near syncope. The induced VT was terminated by overdrive pacing (cycle length of 280 milliseconds). The patient was successfully treated with quinidine, and the VT was not inducible during repeated electrophysiologic testing. Syncope did not recur during a follow-up period of 18 months. *HBE*, His bundle electrogram; *HRA*, high right atrial electrogram; *RV*, right ventricular electrogram.

for primarily vasodepressor syncope remains unsatisfactory, and the theoretical advantages of many drugs require documentation in prospective studies. Effects of newer pacemakers with sudden rate drop response algorithms (rate hysteresis) in the treatment of vasovagal syncope remain to be determined.

Pharmacologic therapy with agents having anticholinergic effects (e.g., disopyramide, propantheline) and with β-adrenergic blockers may be effective in some patients (29,67,79,184,195,217). Although the exact mechanisms of these drugs in the prevention of vasodepressor response are not known, it has been postulated that their negative inotropic effect may inhibit the triggered stimulus (vigorous ventricular contractions) to the afferent limb of the Bezold-Jarisch reflex arc. Other therapies, such as the wearing of tight stockings (decreased venous pooling) or the administration of fludrocortisone (increased intravascular volume) (100,238), α-adrenergic agonists such as ephedrine (vasoconstrictor) (281), theophylline (adenosine blocker) (207), or fluoxetine or sertraline (serotonin reuptake blockers) (102,103), may also be effective in selected patient populations. We believe that the variable responses to pharmacologic and pacing therapy reflect the heterogeneous nature of the vasovagal syndrome complex. Improved clinical responses can be achieved when mechanisms underlying the vasovagal reaction can be individually defined and therapy can be designed with target specificity.

Syncope Caused by Arrhythmias

Pharmacologic treatment has little place in the treatment of bradycardia. Atropine or isoproterenol is indicated only in emergencies and temporary situations before cardiac pacing can be introduced. The mainstay of treatment for sinus node dysfunction or high-grade AV block is pacemaker implantation. Permanent pacing is clearly indicated when syncope or near syncope is correlated with bradycardia, regardless of the site of block (87). The critical HV interval above which a pacemaker should be implanted remains controversial. Among patients with syncope and bifascicular block, those with an HV interval of 70 millisec or longer or an infrahisian block may benefit from pacemaker treatment. Those with an HV interval of 100 millisec or longer show a high incidence of progression to heart block, which merits pacemaker treatment.

Treatment of ventricular tachycardia as the cause of syncope should be guided by the results of electropharmacologic testing (96,174,187,222). Empiric drug therapy for patients with malignant ventricular tachycardia has no proven benefit. When pharmacologic therapy guided by electrophysiologic testing fails to eliminate ventricular tachycardia, an implantable cardioverter defibrillator is highly effective in aborting ventricular arrhythmias by overdrive pacing or cardioversion (13,86,220,223,240). Supraventricular tachycardia, especially of the AV node reentry type or the AV re-entry type with concealed conduction in the accessory pathway, can usually be treated successfully with antiarrhythmia agents given orally. Pharmacologic therapy guided by electrophysiologic testing is usually not necessary. For patients with syncope, patients at higher risk of sudden death, or young patients who do not wish to be committed to long-term drug therapy, radiofrequency ablation of the arrhythmogenic target is highly effective and potentially provides a "cure" for the supraventricular tachycardia and tachycardia-associated syncope (42,57,105,107,135,144,247).

CONCLUSION

Syncope is a common clinical disorder with a wide variety of causes. The history, physical examination, and initial noninvasive tests are key components of patient evaluation. A presumptive diagnosis can be achieved in approximately 50% of patients after the initial evaluation. A high percentage of patients have vagally mediated syncope, and the prognosis is usually excellent. Tilt-table evaluation done in conjunction with isoproterenol infusion may improve the diagnostic capability in patients with vasovagal syncope. In patients with unexplained syncope, cardiac syncope is the most feared cause because of the attendant high morbidity and mortality. Invasive electrophysiologic studies should be performed in those who show a high pretest probability of arrhythmic causes of syncope (patients with organic heart disease) or those in whom serious injury has occurred. Results from any diagnostic studies should be interpreted in light of the following considerations: (a) Specificity and sensitivity of the study may vary depending on the patient population and the study protocol used to elicit the abnormality; (b) false-negative results can occur; and (c) abnormal findings may not necessarily relate to the actual cause of the syncope, and multiple abnormalities may coexist. Once the cause of syncope has been identified, appropriate treatment of the cardiac arrhythmia will be effective in preventing arrhythmia-mediated syncope. Treatment for vasodepressor syncope remains less than satisfactory.

REFERENCES

1. Abbott JA, et al. Graded exercise testing in patients with sinus node dysfunction. *Am J Med* 1977;62:330–338.
2. Abboud FM. Ventricular syncope: is the heart a sensory organ? (Editorial). *N Engl J Med* 1989;320:390–392.
3. Abboud FM. Neurocardiogenic syncope (Editorial). *N Engl J Med* 1993;328:1117–1120.
4. Abel FL, McCutcheon EP. *Cardiovascular Function: Principles and Applications*. Boston: Little, Brown; 1979:319–320.
5. Agruss NS, et al. Significance of chronic sinus bradycardia in elderly people. *Circulation* 1972;46:924–930.
6. Aicardi J, et al. Syncopal attacks compulsively self-induced by Valsalva's maneuver associated with typical absence seizures: a case report. *Arch Neurol* 1988;45:923–925.
7. Akhtar M, et al. Role of cardiac electrophysiologic studies in patients with unexplained recurrent syncope. *PACE Pacing Clin Electrophysiol* 1983;6:192–201.

8. Almquist A, et al. Provocation of bradycardia and hypotension by isoproterenol and upright posture in patients with unexplained syncope. *N Engl J Med* 1989;320:346–351.
9. Antman EM, et al. Transtelephonic electrocardiographic transmission for management of cardiac arrhythmias. *Am J Cardiol* 1986;58:1021–1024.
10. Atwood JE, et al. Exercise testing in patients with aortic stenosis. *Chest* 1988;93:1083–1087.
11. Baccaro R, et al. Cardiovascular effects of micro injection of cyclic AMP into the tractus solitarius of rats. *Med Sci Res* 1987;15:1123–1124.
12. Bass EB, et al. Long-term prognosis of patients undergoing electrophysiologic studies for syncope of unknown origin. *Am J Cardiol* 1988;62:1186–1191.
13. Beauregard LA, et al. Perceived and actual risks of driving in patients with arrhythmia control devices. *Arch Intern Med* 1995;155:609–613.
14. Benditt DG, et al. Enhanced atrioventricular nodal conduction in man: electrophysiologic effects of pharmacologic autonomic blockade. *Circulation* 1984;69:1088–1095.
15. Benditt DG, et al. Sinus node dysfunction: pathophysiology, clinical features, evaluation, and treatment. In: Zipes DP, Jalife J, eds. *Cardiac Electrophysiology from Cell to Bedside*. Philadelphia: WB Saunders; 1990:708–734.
16. Benditt DG, et al. Cardiac pacing for prevention of recurrent vasovagal syncope. *Ann Intern Med* 1995;122:204–209.
17. Berbari EJ, et al. Recording from the body surface of arrhythmogenic ventricular activity during the S-T segment. *Am J Cardiol* 1978;41:697–702.
18. Bigger JT Jr, Reiffel JA. Sick sinus syndrome. *Annu Rev Med* 1979;30:91–118.
19. Bigger JT Jr, Sahar DI. Clinical types of proarrhythmic response to antiarrhythmic drugs. *Am J Cardiol* 1987;59:2E–9E.
20. Blair DA, et al. Excitation of cholinergic vasodilator nerves to human skeletal muscles during emotional stress. *J Physiol (Lond)* 1959;148:633–647.
21. Blomström-Lundqvist C, et al. A long-term follow-up of 15 patients with arrhythmogenic right ventricular dysplasia. *Br Heart J* 1987;58:477–488.
22. Bloomfield DM, et al. Vagal modulation of RR intervals during head-up tilt and the infusion of isoproterenol. *Am J Cardiol* 1995;75:1145–1150.
23. Borbola J, et al. Correlation between the signal-averaged electrocardiogram and electrophysiologic study findings in patients with coronary artery disease and sustained ventricular tachycardia. *Am Heart J* 1988;115:816–824.
24. Boudoulas H, et al. Comparison between electrophysiologic studies and ambulatory monitoring in patients with syncope. *J Electrocardiol* 1983;16:91–95.
25. Bousser MG, et al. Pertes de connaissance brèvesu cours des accidents ischémiques cérébraux: étude de 557 accidents. *Ann Med Interne (Paris)* 1981;132:300–305.
26. Breithardt G, et al. Sinus node recovery time and calculated sinoatrial conduction time in normal subjects and patients with sinus node dysfunction. *Circulation* 1977;56:43–50.
27. Breithardt G, et al. Non-invasive detection of late potentials in man—a new marker for ventricular tachycardia. *Eur Heart J* 1981;2:1–11.
28. Brignole M, et al. Pacing for carotid sinus syndrome and sick sinus syndrome. *PACE Pacing Clin Electrophysiol* 1990;13:2071–2075.
29. Brignole M, et al. A controlled trial of acute and long-term medical therapy in tilt-induced neurally mediated syncope. *Am J Cardiol* 1992;70:339–342.
30. Brooks R, Burgess JH. Idiopathic ventricular tachycardia: a review. *Medicine (Baltimore)* 1988;67:271–294.
31. Brophy CM, et al. Defecation syncope secondary to functional inferior vena caval obstruction during a Valsalva maneuver. *Ann Vasc Surg* 1993;7:374–377.
32. Brown AP, et al. Detection of arrhythmias: use of a patient-activated ambulatory electrocardiogram device with a solid-state memory loop. *Br Heart J* 1987;58:251–253.
33. Brugada P, et al. Results of a ventricular stimulation protocol using a maximum of 4 premature stimuli in patients without documented or suspected ventricular arrhythmias. *Am J Cardiol* 1983;52:1214–1218.
34. Buckingham TA, et al. Effect of conduction defects on the signal-averaged electrocardiographic determination of late potentials. *Am J Cardiol* 1988;61:1265–1271.
35. Buitleir M de, et al. Immediate reproducibility of the tilt-table test in adults with unexplained syncope. *Am J Cardiol* 1993;71:304–307.
36. Cameron J, et al. The signal-averaged vectorcardiogram in syncope: a noninvasive predictor of induction of ventricular tachycardia at electrophysiologic study. *Circulation* 1985;72(Suppl 3):III-434(abst).
37. Carson RP, Lazzara R. Hemodynamic responses initiated by coronary stretch receptors with special reference to coronary artery arteriography. *Am J Cardiol* 1970;25:571–578.
38. Chen MY, et al. Cardiac electrophysiologic and hemodynamic correlates of neurally mediated syncope. *Am J Cardiol* 1989;63:66–72.
39. Chen XC, et al. Reproducibility of head-up tilt-table testing for eliciting susceptibility to neurally mediated syncope in patients without structural heart disease. *Am J Cardiol* 1992;69:755–760.
40. Chiale PA, et al. Usefulness of the ajmaline test in patients with latent bundle branch block. *Am J Cardiol* 1982;49:21–26.
41. Chosy JJ, Graham DT. Catecholamines in vasovagal fainting. *J Psychosom Res* 1965;9:189–194.
42. Chun HM, Sung RJ. Supraventricular tachyarrhythmias. Pharmacologic versus nonpharmacologic approaches. *Med Clin North Am* 1995;79(Sept):1121–1134.
43. Clark PI, et al. Arrhythmias detected by ambulatory monitoring: lack of correlation with symptoms of dizziness and syncope. *Chest* 1980;77:722–725.
44. Click RL, et al. Role of invasive electrophysiologic testing in patients with symptomatic bundle branch block. *Am J Cardiol* 1987;59:817–823.
45. Coehlo A, et al. Tachyarrhythmias in young athletes. *J Am Coll Cardiol* 1986;7:237–243.
46. Cregler LL, Mark H. Cardiovascular dangers of cocaine abuse. *Am J Cardiol* 1986;57:1185–1186.
47. Crozier IG, et al. Cardiac electrophysiological assessment and the natural history of unexplained syncope. *N Z Med J* 1988;101:106–108.
48. Cumbee SR, et al. Cardiac loop ECG recording. A new noninvasive diagnostic test in recurrent syncope. *South Med J* 1990;83:39–43.
49. Curry PVL, et al. The relationship between posture, blood pressure and electrophysiological properties in patients with paroxysmal supraventricular tachycardia. *Arch Mal Coeur Vaiss* 1978;71:293–299.
50. Davis JC, et al. Sinus node dysfunction caused by methyldopa and digoxin. *JAMA* 1981;245:1241–1243.
51. Day SC, et al. Evaluation and outcome of emergency room patients with transient loss of consciousness. *Am J Med* 1982;73:15–23.
52. Denes P, Ezri MD. The role of electrophysiologic studies in the management of patients with unexplained syncope. *PACE Pacing Clin Electrophysiol* 1985;8:424–435.
53. Denes P, et al. Demonstration of dual A-V nodal pathways in patients with paroxysmal supraventricular tachycardia. *Circulation* 1973;48:549–555.
54. Denes P, et al. Dual atrioventricular nodal pathways: a common electrophysiological response. *Br Heart J* 1975;37:1069–1076.
55. Denes P, et al. Quantitative analysis of the high-frequency components of the terminal portion of the body surface QRS in normal subjects and in patients with ventricular tachycardia. *Circulation* 1983;67:1129–1138.
56. Denes P, et al. Clinical predictors of electrophysiologic findings in patients with syncope of unknown origin. *Arch Intern Med* 1988;148:1922–1928.
57. Deshpande S, et al. Catheter ablation in supraventricular tachycardia. *Annu Rev Med* 1995;46:413–430.
58. Dhingra RC, et al. Significance of block distal to the His bundle induced by atrial pacing in patients with chronic bifascicular block. *Circulation* 1979;60:1455–1464.
59. Dhingra RC, et al. Significance of the HV interval in 517 patients with chronic bifascicular block. *Circulation* 1981;64:1265–1271.
60. DiMarco JP. Electrophysiologic studies in patients with unexplained syncope. *Circulation* 1987;75(Suppl 3):III-140–III-145.
61. DiMarco JP, et al. Approach to the patient with recurrent syncope of unknown cause. *Mod Concepts Cardiovasc Dis* 1983;52:11–16.
62. DiMarco JP, et al. Intracardiac electrophysiologic techniques in recurrent syncope of unknown cause. *Ann Intern Med* 1981;95:542–548.

63. Doherty JU, et al. Electrophysiologic evaluation and follow-up characteristics of patients with recurrent unexplained syncope and presyncope. *Am J Cardiol* 1985;55:703–708.
64. Dreifus LS, et al. Bradyarrhythmias: clinical significance and management. *J Am Coll Cardiol* 1983;1:327–338.
65. Eagle KA, Black HR. The impact of diagnostic tests in evaluating patients with syncope. *Yale J Biol Med* 1983;56:1–8.
66. Eagle KA, et al. Evaluation of prognostic classifications for patients with syncope. *Am J Med* 1985;79:455–460.
67. Editorial. Vasovagal syncope? *Lancet* 1986;1:594–595.
68. Eichna LW, et al. Cardiac asystole in a normal young man following physical effort. *Am Heart J* 1947;33:254–262.
69. Engel GL. Psychologic stress, vasodepressor (vasovagal) syncope, and sudden death. *Ann Intern Med* 1978;89:403–412.
70. Engel TR, et al. Signal-averaged electrocardiograms in patients with atrial fibrillation or flutter. *Am Heart J* 1988; 115:592–597.
71. Epstein SE, Stampfer M, Beiser GD. Role of the capacitance and resistance vessels in vasovagal syncope. *Circulation* 1968;37:524–533.
72. Estes NAM III, et al. Pacemakers and exercise: current status, future developments and practical implications of physiological pacemakers. *Sports Med* 1989;8:1–8.
73. Evans E. The carotid sinus: its clinical importance. *JAMA* 1952;149:46–50.
74. Ezri M, et al. Electrophysiologic evaluation of syncope in patients with bifascicular block. *Am Heart J* 1983;106:693–697.
75. Ferrer MI. The sick sinus syndrome in atrial disease. *JAMA* 1968;206:645–646.
76. Fields CD, et al. "Quinidine syncope" without lengthening of Q-Tc interval in the presence of left bundle branch block. *Chest* 1988;94:111–114.
77. Fitzpatrick A, Sutton R. Tilting towards a diagnosis in recurrent unexplained syncope. *Lancet* 1989;1:658–660.
78. Fitzpatrick A, et al. Dual chamber pacing aborts vasovagal syncope induced by head-up 60 degrees tilt. *PACE Pacing Clin Electrophysiol* 1991;14:13–19.
79. Fitzpatrick AP, et al. A randomized trial of medical therapy in malignant vasovagal syndrome or neurally-mediated bradycardia/hypotension syndrome. *Eur J Cardiac Pacing Electrophysiol* 1991;2:99–102.
80. Fitzpatrick AP, et al. Methodology of head-up tilt testing in patients with unexplained syncope. *J Am Coll Cardiol* 1991;17:125–130.
81. Fitzpatrick AP, et al. Vasovagal reactions may occur after orthotopic heart transplantation. *J Am Coll Cardiol* 1993;21:1132–1137.
82. Fleg JL, Asante AVK. Asystole following treadmill exercise in a man without organic heart disease. *Arch Intern Med* 1983;143:1821–1822.
83. Folkow B, Neil E. *Circulation*. New York: Oxford University Press; 1971.
84. Foster M. *Textbook of Physiology*. London: Macmillan; 1888:297, 345.
85. Frenneaux MP, et al. Abnormal blood pressure response during exercise in hypertrophic cardiomyopathy. *Circulation* 1990;82:1995–2002.
86. Friedman PA, Stanton MS. The pacer-cardioverter-defibrillator: function and clinical experience. *J Cardiovasc Electrophysiol* 1995;6:48–68.
87. Frye RL, et al. Guidelines for permanent cardiac pacemaker implantation, May 1984: a report of the Joint American College of Cardiology/American Heart Association Task Force on Assessment of Cardiovascular Procedures (Subcommittee on Pacemaker Implantation). *Circulation* 1984;70:A331–A339.
88. Fujimura O, et al. The diagnostic sensitivity of electrophysiologic testing in patients with syncope caused by transient bradycardia. *N Engl J Med* 1989;321:1703–1707.
89. Gang ES, et al. Detection of late potentials on the surface electrocardiogram in unexplained syncope. *Am J Cardiol* 1986;58:1014–1020.
90. Gann D, et al. Electrophysiologic evaluation of elderly patients with sinus bradycardia: a long-term follow-up study. *Ann Intern Med* 1979;90:24–29.
91. Gibson TC, Heitzman MR. Diagnostic efficacy of 24-hour electrocardiographic monitoring for syncope. *Am J Cardiol* 1984;53:1013–1017.
92. Glick G, Yu PN. Hemodynamic changes during spontaneous vasovagal reactions. *Am J Med* 1963;34:42–51.
93. Goldberg AD, et al. Ambulatory electrocardiographic records in patients with transient cerebral attacks or palpitation. *Br Med J* 1975;4:569–571.
94. Goldreyer BN, et al. The hemodynamic effects of induced supraventricular tachycardia in man. *Circulation* 1976;54:783–789.
95. Goldstein DS, et al. Circulatory control mechanisms in vasodepressor syncope. *Am Heart J* 1982;104:1071–1075.
96. Gottlieb C, Josephson ME. The preference of programmed stimulation-guided therapy for sustained ventricular arrhythmias. In: Brugada P, Wellens HJJ, eds. *Cardiac Arrhythmias; Where to Go From Here?* Mount Kisco, NY: Futura Publishing; 1987:421–434.
97. Graham DT, et al. Vasovagal fainting: a diphasic response. *Psychosom Med* 1961;23:493–507.
98. Grubb BP, et al. Cerebral vasoconstriction during head-upright tilt-induced vasovagal syncope. A paradoxic and unexpected response. *Circulation* 1991;84:1157–1164.
99. Grubb BP, et al. Utility of upright tilt-table testing in the evaluation and management of syncope of unknown origin. *Am J Med* 1991;90:6–10.
100. Grubb BP, et al. The use of head-upright tilt table testing in the evaluation and management of syncope in children and adolescents. *PACE Pacing Clin Electrophysiol* 1992;15:742–748.
101. Grubb BP, et al. Reproducibility of head-upright tilt-table test results in patients with syncope. *PACE Pacing Clin Electrophysiol* 1992;15:1477–1481.
102. Grubb BP, et al. Usefulness of fluoxetine hydrochloride for prevention of resistant upright tilt-induced syncope. *PACE Pacing Clin Electrophysiol* 1993;16:458–464.
103. Grubb BP, et al. Use of sertraline hydrochloride in the treatment of refractory neurocardiogenic syncope in children and adolescents. *J Am Coll Cardiol* 1994;24:490–494.
104. Gulamhusein S, et al. Value and limitations of clinical electrophysiologic study in assessment of patients with unexplained syncope. *Am J Med* 1982;73:700–705.
105. Gursoy S, Schluter M, Kuck KH. Radiofrequency current catheter ablation for control of supraventricular arrhythmias. *J Cardiovasc Electrophysiol* 1993;4:194–205.
106. Guyton AC. *Textbook of Medical Physiology*. 8th ed. Philadelphia: WB Saunders; 1991.
107. Haissaguerre M, Saoudi N. Role of catheter ablation for supraventricular tachyarrhythmias, with emphasis on atrial flutter and atrial tachycardia. *Curr Opin Cardiol* 1994;9:40–52.
108. Haissaguerre M, et al. Étude électrophysiologique des syncopes prévision du résultat. *Presse Med* 1989;18:212–220.
109. Hamer AWF, et al. Factors that predict syncope during ventricular tachycardia in patients. *Am Heart J* 1984;107:997–1005.
110. Hammill SC, et al. Electrophysiologic testing in the upright position: improved evaluation of patients with rhythm disturbances using a tilt table. *J Am Coll Cardiol* 1984;4:65–71.
111. Hertzeanu H, et al. Holter monitoring in dizziness and syncope. *Acta Cardiol* 1979;34:375–383.
112. Hess DS, et al. Electrophysiologic testing in the evaluation of patients with syncope of undetermined origin. *Am J Cardiol* 1982;50:1309–1315.
113. Holden W, et al. Characterisation of heart rate response to exercise in the sick sinus syndrome. *Br Heart J* 1978;40:923–930.
114. Huang SKS, et al. Carotid sinus hypersensitivity in patients with unexplained syncope: clinical, electrophysiologic, and long-term follow-up observations. *Am Heart J* 1988;116:989–996.
115. Hunter J. *Works of John Hunter*. London: JF Palmer; 1837 (vol 3).
116. Huycke EC, et al. Postexertional cardiac asystole in a young man without organic heart disease. *Ann Intern Med* 1987;106:844–845.
117. Jackman WM, et al. The long QT syndromes: a critical review, new clinical observations, and a unifying hypothesis. *Prog Cardiovasc Dis* 1988;31:115–172.
118. Jansen RW, Lipsitz LA. Postprandial hypotension: epidemiology, pathophysiology, and clinical management. *Ann Intern Med* 1995;122:286–295.
119. Jarisch A, Richter H. Die afferenten Bahnen des Veratrineffektes in den Herznerven. *Arch Exp Pathol Pharmakol* 1939;193:355–371.
120. Kadish AH, et al. Swallowing syncope: observations in the absence of conduction system or esophageal disease. *Am J Med* 1986;81:1098–1100.
121. Kapoor WN. Evaluation and outcome of patients with syncope. *Medicine (Baltimore)* 1990;69:160–175.

122. Kapoor WN, Brant N. Evaluation of syncope by upright tilt testing with isoproterenol. A nonspecific test. *Ann Intern Med* 1992;116: 358–363.
123. Kapoor WN, et al. Diagnosis and natural history of syncope and the role of invasive electrophysiologic testing. *Am J Cardiol* 1989;63: 730–734.
124. Kapoor W, et al. Issues in evaluating patients with syncope (Editorial). *Ann Intern Med* 1984;100:755–757.
125. Kapoor WN, et al. Micturition syncope: a reappraisal. *JAMA* 1985; 253:796–798.
126. Kapoor WN, et al. Defecation syncope: a symptom with multiple etiologies. *Arch Intern Med* 1986;146:2377–2379.
127. Kapoor WN, et al. Syncope of unknown origin: the need for a more cost-effective approach to its diagnostic evaluation. *JAMA* 1982; 247:2687–2691.
128. Kapoor WN, et al. A prospective evaluation and follow-up of patients with syncope. *N Engl J Med* 1983;309:197–204.
129. Kapoor W, et al. Syncope in the elderly. *Am J Med* 1986;80: 419–428.
130. Kapoor WN, et al. Diagnostic and prognostic implications of recurrences in patients with syncope. *Am J Med* 1987;83:700–708.
131. Kapoor WN, et al. Prolonged electrocardiographic monitoring in patients with syncope. *Am J Med* 1987;82:20–28.
132. Kapoor W, et al. Psychiatric illnesses in patients with syncope. *Clin Res* 1989;37:A316(abst).
133. Kaul U, et al. Evaluation of patients with bundle branch block and "unexplained" syncope: a study based on comprehensive electrophysiologic testing and ajmaline stress. *PACE Pacing Clin Electrophysiol* 1988;11:289–297.
134. Kay R, et al. Primary sick sinus syndrome as an indication for chronic pacemaker therapy in young adults: incidence, clinical features, and long-term evaluation. *Am Heart J* 1982;103:338–342.
135. Kay GN, et al. Role of radiofrequency ablation in the management of supraventricular arrhythmias: experience in 760 consecutive patients. *J Cardiovasc Electrophysiol* 1993;4:371–389.
136. Kenny RA, et al. Head-up tilt: a useful test for investigating unexplained syncope. *Lancet* 1986;1:1352–1355.
137. Kenny RA, et al. Enhanced vagal activity and normal arginine vasopressin response in carotid sinus syndrome: implications for a central abnormality in carotid sinus hypersensitivity. *Cardiovasc Res* 1987;21:545–550.
138. Kerr CR, Strauss HC. The measurement of sinus node refractoriness in man. *Circulation* 1983;68:1231–1237.
139. Klein GJ, et al. Ventricular fibrillation in the Wolff-Parkinson-White syndrome. *N Engl J Med* 1979;301:1080–1085.
140. Klein GJ, et al. Asymptomatic Wolff-Parkinson-White: should we intervene? *Circulation* 1989;80:1902–1905.
141. Kong Y, et al. Glossopharyngeal neuralgia associated with bradycardia, syncope, and seizures. *Circulation* 1964;30:109–113.
142. Korner PI. Integrative neural cardiovascular control. *Physiol Rev* 1971;51:312–367.
143. Kosinski D, et al. The use of serotonin reuptake inhibitors in the treatment of neurally mediated cardiovascular disorders. *J Serotonin Res* 1994;1:85–90.
144. Kou WH, Morady F. Radiofrequency catheter ablation in the treatment of cardiac arrhythmias. *Adv Intern Med* 1995;40:533–571.
145. Kowey PR, et al. Sustained arrhythmias in hypertrophic obstructive cardiomyopathy. *N Engl J Med* 1984;310:1566–1569.
146. Krol RB, et al. Electrophysiologic testing in patients with unexplained syncope: clinical and noninvasive predictors of outcome. *J Am Coll Cardiol* 1987;10:358–363.
147. Kuchar DL, et al. Late potentials detected after myocardial infarction: natural history and prognostic significance. *Circulation* 1986; 74:1280–1289.
148. Kus T, et al. Vasovagal syncope: management with atrioventricular sequential pacing and beta-blockade. *Can J Cardiol* 1989;5:375–378.
149. Kushner JA, et al. Natural history of patients with unexplained syncope and a nondiagnostic electrophysiologic study. *J Am Coll Cardiol* 1989;14:391–396.
150. Laakso M, et al. Diseases and drugs causing prolongation of the QT interval. *Am J Cardiol* 1987;59:862–865.
151. Lagerlund TD, et al. An electroencephalographic study of glossopharyngeal neuralgia with syncope. *Arch Neurol* 1988;45:472–475.
152. Levin B, Posner JB. Swallow syncope: report of a case and review of the literature. *Neurology* 1972;22:1086–1093.
153. Lewis T. A lecture on vasovagal syncope and the carotid sinus mechanism: with comments on Gowers's and Nothnagel's syndrome. *Br Med J* 1932;1:873–876.
154. Linzer M, et al. Recurrent syncope of unknown origin diagnosed by ambulatory continuous loop ECG recording. *Am Heart J* 1988; 116:1632–1634.
155. Linzer M, et al. Psychiatric syncope: a new look at an old disease. *Psychosomatics* 1990;31:181–188.
156. Lippman N, Stein KM, Lerman BB. Failure to decrease parasympathetic tone during upright tilt predicts a positive tilt-table test. *Am J Cardiol* 1995;75:591–595.
157. Lipsitz LA. Syncope in the elderly. *Ann Intern Med* 1983; 99:92–105.
158. Lipsitz LA. Syncope in the elderly patient. *Hosp Pract (Off Ed)* 1986 Oct 30;21:33–44.
159. Lipsitz LA, et al. Postprandial reduction in blood pressure in the elderly. *N Engl J Med* 1983;309:81–83.
160. Lipsitz LA, et al. Cardiovascular and norepinephrine responses after meal consumption in elderly (older than 75 years) persons with postprandial hypotension and syncope. *Am J Cardiol* 1986;58: 810–815.
161. Livelli FD Jr, et al. Response to programmed ventricular stimulation: sensitivity, specificity and relation to heart disease. *Am J Cardiol* 1982;50:452–458.
162. Lombard JT, Selzer A. Valvular aortic stenosis: a clinical and hemodynamic profile of patients. *Ann Intern Med* 1987;106:292–298.
163. Longhurst JC. Cardiac receptors: their function in health and disease. *Prog Cardiovasc Dis* 1984;27:201–222.
164. Lopes MG, et al. Comparison of 24 versus 12 hours of ambulatory ECG monitoring. *Chest* 1975;67:269–273.
165. Lurie KG, et al. Evaluation of edrophonium as a provocative agent for vasovagal syncope during head-up tilt-table testing. *Am J Cardiol* 1993;72:1286–1290.
166. Madigan NP, et al. Carotid sinus hypersensitivity: beneficial effects of dual-chamber pacing. *Am J Cardiol* 1984;53:1034–1040.
167. Maloney JD, et al. Malignant vasovagal syncope: prolonged asystole provoked by head-up tilt. *Cleve Clin J Med* 1988;55:542–548.
168. Mancia G, et al. Control of blood pressure by carotid sinus baroreceptors in human beings. *Am J Cardiol* 1979;44:895–902.
169. Mandel W, et al. Evaluation of sino-atrial node function in man by overdrive suppression. *Circulation* 1971;44:59–66.
170. Mann DE, Reiter MJ. Effects of upright posture on atrioventricular nodal re-entry and dual atrioventricular nodal pathways. *Am J Cardiol* 1988;62:408–412.
171. Mann DE, et al. Induction of clinical ventricular tachycardia using programmed stimulation: value of third and fourth extrastimuli. *Am J Cardiol* 1983;52:501–506.
172. Mann DE, et al. Effects of upright posture on antegrade and retrograde atrioventricular conduction in patients with coronary artery disease, mitral valve prolapse or no structural heart disease. *Am J Cardiol* 1987;60:625–629.
173. Manolis AS. Syncope in the elderly. *Compr Ther* 1989;15:31–42.
174. Manolis AS, et al. Prognostic value of early electrophysiologic studies for ventricular tachycardia recurrence in patients with coronary artery disease treated with amiodarone. *Am J Cardiol* 1989;63: 1052–1057.
175. Marcus FI, et al. Arrhythmias. *J Am Coll Cardiol* 1987;10(Suppl A): 66–73.
176. Margolis JR, et al. Digitalis and the sick sinus syndrome: clinical and electrophysiologic documentation of a severe toxic effect on sinus node function. *Circulation* 1975;52:162–169.
177. Mark AL. The Bezold-Jarisch reflex revisited: clinical implications of inhibitory reflexes originating in the heart. *J Am Coll Cardiol* 1983;1:90–102.
178. Martin GJ, et al. Prospective evaluation of syncope. *Ann Emerg Med* 1984;13:499–504.
179. Martinez R. Torsades de pointes: atypical rhythm, atypical treatment. *Ann Emerg Med* 1987;16:878–884.
180. Masterson M, et al. Value of procainamide administration during a nondiagnostic cardiac electrophysiologic study in patients with recurrent undiagnosed syncope. *PACE Pacing Clin Electrophysiol* 1988;11:837(abst).

181. McAnulty JH, et al. Natural history of "high-risk" bundle-branch block: final report of a prospective study. *N Engl J Med* 1982; 307:137–143.
182. McIntosh HD, Morris JJ Jr. The hemodynamic consequences of arrhythmias. *Prog Cardiovasc Dis* 1965;8:330–363.
183. McKenna W, et al. Syncope in hypertrophic cardiomyopathy. *Br Heart J* 1982;47:177–179.
184. McLaran CJ, et al. Increased vagal tone as an isolated finding in patients undergoing electrophysiological testing for recurrent syncope: response to long-term anticholinergic agents. *Br Heart J* 1986;55: 53–57.
185. McMichael J, Sharpey-Schafer EP. Cardiac output in man by a direct Fick method: effects of posture, venous pressure change, atropine, and adrenaline. *Br Heart J* 1944;6:33–40.
186. Milstein S, et al. Upright body tilt for evaluation of patients with recurrent, unexplained syncope. *PACE Pacing Clin Electrophysiol* 1989;12:117–124.
187. Mitchell LB, et al. A randomized clinical trial of the noninvasive and invasive approaches to drug therapy of ventricular tachycardia. *N Engl J Med* 1987;317:1681–1687.
188. Mizumaki K, et al. Left ventricular dimensions and autonomic balance during head-up tilt differ between patients with isoproterenol-dependent and isoproterenol-independent neurally mediated syncope. *J Am Coll Cardiol* 1995;26:164–173.
189. Morady F, et al. Bradyarrhythmias and bundle branch block. In: Scheinman MM, ed. *Cardiac Emergencies.* Philadelphia: WB Saunders; 1984:135–151.
190. Morady F, Scheinman MM. The role and limitations of electrophysiologic testing in patients with unexplained syncope. *Int J Cardiol* 1983;4:229–234.
191. Morady F, et al. Long-term follow-up of patients with recurrent unexplained syncope evaluated by electrophysiologic testing. *J Am Coll Cardiol* 1983;2:1053–1059.
192. Morady F, et al. Programmed ventricular stimulation in patients without spontaneous ventricular tachycardia. *Am Heart J* 1984;107: 875–882.
193. Morgan DA, et al. Serotonergic mechanisms mediate renal sympathoinhibition during severe hemorrhage in rats. *Am J Physiol* 1988; 255:H496–H502.
194. Morgan-Hughes NJ, et al. Vasodepressor reactions after orthotopic cardiac transplantation: relationship to reinnervation status. *Clin Auton Res* 1994;4:125–129.
195. Morillo CA, et al. A placebo-controlled trial of intravenous and oral disopyramide for prevention of neurally mediated syncope induced by head-up tilt. *J Am Coll Cardiol* 1993;22:1843–1848.
196. Morillo CA, et al. Time and frequency domain analyses of heart rate variability during orthostatic stress in patients with neurally mediated syncope. *Am J Cardiol* 1994;74:1258–1262.
197. Morita H, et al. Opiate receptor-mediated decrease in renal nerve activity during hypotensive hemorrhage in conscious rabbits. *Circ Res* 1988;63:165–172.
198. Morley CA, Sutton R. Carotid sinus syncope (Editorial Review). *Int J Cardiol* 1984;6:287–293.
199. Morley CA, et al. Carotid sinus syncope treated by pacing: analysis of persistent symptoms and role of atrioventricular sequential pacing. *Br Heart J* 1982;47:411–418.
200. Morley CA, et al. Is there a difference between sick sinus syndrome and carotid sinus syndrome? *Br Heart J* 1983;49:620–621.
201. Moss AJ, Davis RJ. Brady-tachy syndrome. *Prog Cardiovasc Dis* 1974;16:439–454.
202. Murdoch BD. Loss of consciousness in healthy South African men: incidence, causes and relationship to EEG abnormality. *S Afr Med J* 1980;57:771–774.
203. Naccarelli GV. Evaluation of the patient with syncope. *Med Clin North Am* 1984;68:1211–1230.
204. Nalos PC, et al. The signal-averaged electrocardiogram as a screening test for inducibility of sustained ventricular tachycardia in high-risk patients: a prospective study. *J Am Coll Cardiol* 1987;9: 539–548.
205. Narula OS. Atrioventricular conduction defects in patients with sinus bradycardia: analysis by His bundle recordings. *Circulation* 1971;44:1096–1110.
206. Narula OS, et al. A new method for measurement of sinoatrial conduction time. *Circulation* 1978;58:706–714.
207. Nelson SD, et al. The autonomic and hemodynamic effects of oral theophylline in patients with vasodepressor syncope. *Arch Intern Med* 1991;151:2425–2429.
208. Newman D, et al. Head-up tilt testing with and without isoproterenol infusion in healthy subjects of different ages. *PACE Pacing Clin Electrophysiol* 1993;16:715–721.
209. Öberg B, Thorén P. Increased activity in left ventricular receptors during hemorrhage or occlusion of caval veins in the cat—a possible cause of the vasovagal reaction. *Acta Physiol Scand* 1972;85:164–173.
210. Ogunkelu JB, et al. Electrophysiologic effects of procainamide in subtherapeutic to therapeutic doses on human atrioventricular conduction system. *Am J Cardiol* 1976;37:724–731.
211. Osswald S, et al. Asystole after exercise in healthy persons. *Ann Intern Med* 1994;120:1008–1011.
212. OteroCagide M, et al. Syncope of undetermined etiology: value of procainamide administration during a nondiagnostic cardiac electrophysiologic study. *J Electrophysiol* 1988;2:437–447.
213. Pantridge JF. Autonomic disturbance at the onset of acute myocardial infarction. In: Schwartz PJ, et al, eds. *Neural Mechanisms in Cardiac Arrhythmias.* New York: Raven Press; 1978:7–17.
214. Patt MV, et al. Spontaneous reversion of ventricular fibrillation. *Am Heart J* 1988;115:919–923.
215. Pavlovic SU, et al. The etiology of syncope in pacemaker patients. *PACE Pacing Clin Electrophysiol* 1991;14:2086–2091.
216. Pedersen WR, et al. Post-exercise asystolic arrest in a young man without organic heart disease: utility of head-up tilt testing in guiding therapy. *Am Heart J* 1989;118:410–413.
217. Perry JC, Garson A, Jr. The child with recurrent syncope: autonomic function testing and beta-adrenergic hypersensitivity. *J Am Coll Cardiol* 1991;17:1168–1171.
218. Petersen ME, et al. Permanent pacing for cardioinhibitory malignant vasovagal syndrome. *Br Heart J* 1994;71:274–281.
219. Peterson J, Karpf M, Kapoor W. Long-term follow-up of patients with isolated syncope. *Clin Res* 1988;36:716A(abst).
220. Pinski SL, Trohman RG. Implantable cardioverter-defibrillators: implications for the nonelectrophysiologist. *Ann Intern Med* 1995;122:770–777.
221. Prystowsky EN. Diagnosis and management of the pre-excitation syndrome. *Curr Probl Cardiol* 1988;13:225–310.
222. Prystowsky EN. Electrophysiologic-electropharmacologic testing in patients with ventricular arrhythmias. *PACE Pacing Clin Electrophysiol* 1988;11:225–251.
223. Raitt MH, Bardy GH. Advances in implantable cardioverter-defibrillator therapy. *Curr Opin Cardiol* 1994;9:23–29.
224. Raviele A, et al. Usefulness of head-up tilt test in evaluating patients with syncope of unknown origin and negative electrophysiologic study. *Am J Cardiol* 1990;65:1322–1327.
225. Raviele A, et al. Value of head-up tilt testing potentiated with sublingual nitroglycerin to assess the origin of unexplained syncope. *Am J Cardiol* 1995;76:267–272.
226. Rea RF, Thames MD. Neural control mechanisms and vasovagal syncope. *J Cardiovasc Electrophysiol* 1993;4:587–595.
227. Reddy K, et al. Painless glossopharyngeal "neuralgia" with syncope: a case report and literature review. *Neurosurgery* 1987;21:916–919.
228. Reiffel JA. Drugs to avoid in patients with sinus node dysfunction. *Drug Ther* 1982;6:99–106.
229. Reiffel JA, et al. Ability of Holter electrocardiographic recording and atrial stimulation to detect sinus node dysfunction in symptomatic and asymptomatic patients with sinus bradycardia. *Am J Cardiol* 1977;40:189–194.
230. Reiffel JA, et al. Electrophysiologic testing in patients with recurrent syncope: are results predicted by prior ambulatory monitoring? *Am Heart J* 1985;110:1146–1153.
231. Richards AM, et al. Syncope in aortic valvular stenosis. *Lancet* 1984;2:1113–1116.
232. Rinne C, et al. Relation between clinical presentation and induced arrhythmias in the Wolff-Parkinson-White syndrome. *Am J Cardiol* 1987;60:576–579.
233. Robinson BF, et al. Control of heart rate by the autonomic nervous system: studies in man on the interrelation between baroreceptor mechanisms and exercise. *Circ Res* 1966;19:400–411.
234. Rosen KM, et al. Cardiac conduction in patients with symptomatic sinus node disease. *Circulation* 1971;43:836–844.

235. Rosenqvist M, et al. Long-term pacing in sinus node disease: effects of stimulation mode on cardiovascular morbidity and mortality. *Am Heart J* 1988;116:16–22.
236. Rosenqvist M, Obel IWP. Atrial pacing and the risk for AV block: is there a time for change in attitude? *PACE Pacing Clin Electrophysiol* 1989;12:97–101.
237. Rosenqvist M, et al. Clinical and electrophysiologic course of sinus node disease: five-year follow-up study. *Am Heart J* 1985;109:513–522.
238. Ross BA, et al. Orthostatic versus electrophysiologic testing in unexplained syncope in children and adolescence. *J Cardiovasc Electrophysiol* 1992;3:418–422.
239. Rozanski JJ, et al. Body surface detection of delayed depolarizations in patients with recurrent ventricular tachycardia and left ventricular aneurysm. *Circulation* 1981;63:1172–1178.
240. Saksena S, et al. Clinical investigation of antiarrhythmic devices. A statement for healthcare professionals from a joint task force of the North American Society of Pacing and Electrophysiology, the American College of Cardiology, the American Heart Association, and the Working Groups on Arrhythmias and Cardiac Pacing of the European Society of Cardiology. *Eur Heart J* 1995;16:446–459.
241. Sakuma I, et al. NG-methyl-L-arginine, an inhibitor of L-arginine-derived nitric oxide synthesis, stimulates renal sympathetic nerve activity in vivo. A role for nitric oxide in the central regulation of sympathetic tone? *Circ Res* 1992;70:607–611.
242. Salins PC, et al. Hypoglycemia as a possible factor in the induction of vasovagal syncope. *Oral Surg Oral Med Oral Pathol* 1992;74:544–549.
243. Samoil D, et al. Comparison of single and dual chamber pacing techniques in prevention of upright tilt-induced vasovagal syncope. *Eur J Cardiac Pacing Electrophysiol* 1993;3:36–41.
244. Sanmarco ME, et al. Abnormal blood pressure response and marked ischemic ST-segment depression as predictors of severe coronary heart disease. *Circulation* 1980;61:572–578.
245. Sapire DW, et al. Vasovagal syncope in children requiring pacemaker implantation. *Am Heart J* 1983;106:1406–1411.
246. Savage DD, et al. Epidemiologic features of isolated syncope: the Framingham study. *Stroke* 1985;16:626–629.
247. Scheinman M. Supraventricular tachyarrhythmias: drug therapy versus catheter ablation. *Clin Cardiol* 1994;17(9 Suppl 2):II11–II15.
248. Scheinman MM, et al. Electrophysiologic effects of procainamide in patients with intraventricular conduction delay. *Circulation* 1974;49:522–529.
249. Scheinman MM, et al. Prognostic value of infranodal conduction time in patients with chronic bundle branch block. *Circulation* 1977;56:240–244.
250. Scheinman MM, et al. Value of the H-Q interval in patients with bundle branch block and the role of prophylactic permanent pacing. *Am J Cardiol* 1982;50:1316–1322.
251. Scherrer U, et al. Vasovagal syncope after infusion of a vasodilator in a heart-transplant recipient. *N Engl J Med* 1990;322:602–604.
252. Schlesinger Z. Life-threatening "vagal reaction" to physical fitness test (Letter to the Editor). *JAMA* 1973;226:1119.
253. Schoenberg BS, Kuglitsch JF, Karnes WE. Micturition syncope—not a single entity. *JAMA* 1974;229:1631–1633.
254. Shalev Y, et al. Echocardiographic demonstration of decreased left ventricular dimensions and vigorous myocardial contraction during syncope induced by head-up tilt. *J Am Coll Cardiol* 1991;18:746–751.
255. Sharma AD, et al. Sensitivity and specificity of invasive and noninvasive testing for risk of sudden death in Wolff-Parkinson-White syndrome. *J Am Coll Cardiol* 1987;10:373–381.
256. Sharpey-Schafer EP, et al. Mechanism of acute hypotension from fear or nausea. *Br Med J* 1958;2:878–880.
257. Shaw DB, et al. Survival in sinoatrial disorder (sick-sinus syndrome). *Br Med J* 1980;280:139–141.
258. Shaw DB, et al. Survival in second degree atrioventricular block. *Br Heart J* 1985;53:587–593.
259. Sheldon R. Evaluation of a single-stage isoproterenol-tilt table test in patients with syncope. *J Am Coll Cardiol* 1993;22:114–118.
260. Sheldon R. Effects of aging on responses to isoproterenol tilt-table testing in patients with syncope. *Am J Cardiol* 1994;74:459–463.
261. Sheldon R, Killam S. Methodology of isoproterenol-tilt table testing in patients with syncope. *J Am Coll Cardiol* 1992;19:773–779.
262. Sheldon R, et al. Reproducibility of isoproterenol tilt-table tests in patients with syncope. *Am J Cardiol* 1992;69:1300–1305.
263. Shen W-K, et al. Transtelephonic monitoring: documentation of transient cardiac rhythm disturbances. *Mayo Clin Proc* 1987;62:109–112.
264. Shen W-K, et al. Adenosine: potential modulator for vasovagal syncope. *J Am Coll Cardiol* (in press).
265. Silverstein MD, et al. Patients with syncope admitted to medical intensive care units. *JAMA* 1982;248:1185–1189.
266. Simon AB, Zloto AE. Symptomatic sinus node disease: natural history after permanent ventricular pacing. *PACE Pacing Clin Electrophysiol* 1979;2:305–314.
267. Simson MB. Use of signals in the terminal QRS complex to identify patients with ventricular tachycardia after myocardial infarction. *Circulation* 1981;64:235–242.
268. Smith OA. Reflex and central mechanisms involved in the control of the heart and circulation. *Annu Rev Physiol* 1974;36:93–123.
269. Sneddon JF, et al. Assessment of autonomic function in patients with neurally mediated syncope: augmented cardiopulmonary baroreceptor responses to graded orthostatic stress. *J Am Coll Cardiol* 1993;21:1193–1198.
270. Sneddon JF, et al. Do patients with neurally mediated syncope have augmented vagal tone? *Am J Cardiol* 1993;72:1314–1315.
271. Sneddon JF, et al. Impaired immediate vasoconstrictor responses in patients with recurrent neurally mediated syncope. *Am J Cardiol* 1993;71:72–76.
272. Sneddon JF, et al. Exercise-induced vasodepressor syncope. *Br Heart J* 1994;71:554–557.
273. Sobel RE, Roberts R. Hypotension and syncope. In: Braunwald E, ed. *Heart Disease: A Textbook of Cardiovascular Medicine*. 3rd ed. Philadelphia: WB Saunders; 1988:884–895.
274. Sokoloff NM, et al. Plasma norepinephrine in exercise-induced ventricular tachycardia. *J Am Coll Cardiol* 1986;8:11–17.
275. Sra JS, et al. Unexplained syncope evaluated by electrophysiologic studies and head-up tilt testing. *Ann Intern Med* 1991;114:1013–1019.
276. Sra JS, et al. Comparison of cardiac pacing with drug therapy in the treatment of neurocardiogenic (vasovagal) syncope with bradycardia or asystole. *N Engl J Med* 1993;328:1085–1090.
277. Sra JS, et al. Circulatory and catecholamine changes during head-up tilt testing in neurocardiogenic (vasovagal) syncope. *Am J Cardiol* 1994;73:33–37.
278. Strasberg B, et al. The head-up tilt-table test in patients with syncope of unknown origin. *Am Heart J* 1989;118:923–927.
279. Strauss HC, et al. Premature atrial stimulation as a key to the understanding of sinoatrial conduction in man: presentation of data and critical review of the literature. *Circulation* 1973;47:86–93.
280. Strauss HC, et al. Electrophysiologic effects of propranolol on sinus node function in patients with sinus node dysfunction. *Circulation* 1976;54:452–459.
281. Strieper MJ, Campbell RM. Efficacy of alpha-adrenergic agonist therapy for prevention of pediatric neurocardiogenic syncope. *J Am Coll Cardiol* 1993;22:594–597.
282. Sugrue DD, et al. Carotid sinus hypersensitivity and syncope. *Mayo Clin Proc* 1984;59:637–640.
283. Sugrue DD, et al. Symptomatic "isolated" carotid sinus hypersensitivity: natural history and results of treatment with anticholinergic drugs or pacemaker. *J Am Coll Cardiol* 1986;7:158–162.
284. Swiryn S, et al. Assessment of left ventricular function by radionuclide angiography during induced supraventricular tachycardia. *Am J Cardiol* 1981;47:555–561.
285. Teichman SL, et al. The value of electrophysiologic studies in syncope of undetermined origin: report of 150 cases. *Am Heart J* 1985;110:469–479.
286. Thiene G, et al. Right ventricular cardiomyopathy and sudden death in young people. *N Engl J Med* 1988;318:129–133.
287. Thomas JE. Hyperactive carotid sinus reflex and carotid sinus syncope. *Mayo Clin Proc* 1969;44:127–139.
288. Thoren P. Role of cardiac vagal C-fibers in cardiovascular control. *Rev Physiol Biochem Pharmacol* 1979;86:1–94.
289. Tonkin AM, Heddle WF. Electrophysiological testing of sinus node function. *PACE Pacing Clin Electrophysiol* 1984;7:735–748.
290. Tonkin AM, et al. Intermittent atrioventricular block: procainamide administration as a provocative test. *Aust N Z J Med* 1978;8:594–602.

291. Toubes DB, Brody MJ. Inhibition of reflex vasoconstriction after experimental coronary embolization in the dog. *Circ Res* 1970;26:211–224.
292. Tresch DD, Fleg JL. Unexplained sinus bradycardia: clinical significance and long-term prognosis in apparently healthy persons older than 40 years. *Am J Cardiol* 1986;58:1009–1013.
293. Twidale N, et al. Procainamide administration during electrophysiology study—utility as a provocative test for intermittent atrioventricular block. *PACE Pacing Clin Electrophysiol* 1988;11:1388–1397.
294. Tzivoni D, et al. Torsades de pointes versus polymorphous ventricular tachycardia. *Am J Cardiol* 1983;52:639–640.
295. Vandepol CJ, et al. Incidence and clinical significance of induced ventricular tachycardia. *Am J Cardiol* 1980;45:725–731.
296. Van Durme JP. Tachyarrhythmias and transient cerebral ischemic attacks (annotation). *Am Heart J* 1975;89:538–540.
297. Vatterott PJ, et al. Improving the predictive ability of the signal-averaged electrocardiogram with a linear logistic model incorporating clinical variables. *Circulation* 1990;81:797–804.
298. Vatterott PJ, et al. Signal-averaged electrocardiography: a new noninvasive test to identify patients at risk for ventricular arrhythmias. *Mayo Clin Proc* 1988;63:931–942.
299. Vera Z, Mason DT. Detection of sinus node dysfunction: considerations of clinical application of testing methods. *Am Heart J* 1981;102:308–312.
300. Vingerhoets AJJM. Biochemical changes in two subjects succumbing to syncope. *Psychosom Med* 1984;46:95–103.
301. Vlay SC. Catecholamine-sensitive ventricular tachycardia. *Am Heart J* 1987;114:455–461.
302. von Bezold A, Hirt L. Uber die physiologischen Wirkungen des essigsauren veratrins. Untersuchungen aus dem physiologischen laboratorium. *Wurzburg* 1867;1:75–156.
303. Wahbha MMAE, et al. Cardiovascular reflex responses in patients with unexplained syncope. *Clin Sci* 1989;77:547–553.
304. Waldo AL, et al. Appropriate electrophysiologic study and treatment of patients with the Wolff-Parkinson-White syndrome. *J Am Coll Cardiol* 1988;11:1124–1129.
305. Wallbridge DR, et al. Increase in plasma beta endorphins precedes vasodepressor syncope. *Br Heart J* 1994;71:597–599.
306. Wallin BG, Sundlöff G. Sympathetic outflow to muscles during the vasovagal syncope. *J Auton Nerv Syst* 1982;6:287–291.
307. Walter PF, Crawley IS, Dorney ER. Carotid sinus hypersensitivity and syncope. *Am J Cardiol* 1978;42:396–403.
308. Ward DE. Can the technicalities of electrophysiological testing for ventricular tachycardia be simplified? (Editorial). *Br Heart J* 1987;58:437–440.
309. Waxman MB, et al. Isoproterenol induction of vasodepressor-type reaction in vasodepressor-prone persons. *Am J Cardiol* 1989;63:58–65.
310. Wayne HH. Syncope. Physiological considerations and an analysis of the clinical characteristics in 510 patients. *Am J Med* 1961;30:418–438.
311. Weiner DA, et al. Ventricular arrhythmias during exercise testing: mechanism, response to coronary bypass surgery and prognostic significance. *Am J Cardiol* 1984;53:1553–1557.
312. Weiss S, Baker JP. The carotid sinus reflex in health and disease: its role in the causation of fainting and convulsions. *Medicine (Baltimore)* 1933;12:297–354.
313. Weissler AM, et al. Vasodepressor syncope. Factors influencing cardiac output. *Circulation* 1957;15:875–882.
314. Wellens HJJ, et al. Programmed electrical stimulation of the heart in patients with life-threatening ventricular arrhythmias: what is the significance of induced arrhythmias and what is the correct stimulation protocol? *Circulation* 1985;72:1–7.
315. Westveer DC, et al. The role of electrophysiologic studies in the evaluation of recurrent, unexplained syncope. *Cardiovasc Rev Rep* 1984;5:770–780.
316. Wharton JM, et al. Torsade de pointes during administration of pentamidine isethionate. *Am J Med* 1987;83:571–576.
317. Whiteside-Yim C. Syncope in the elderly: a clinical approach. *Geriatrics* 1987;42:37–41.
318. Wik B, Hillestad L. Deglutition syncope. *Br Med J* 1975;3:747.
319. Winters SL, Stewart D, Gomes JA. Signal averaging of the surface QRS complex predicts inducibility of ventricular tachycardia in patients with syncope of unknown origin: a prospective study. *J Am Coll Cardiol* 1987;10:775–781.
320. Winters SL, et al. Role of signal averaging of the surface QRS complex in selecting patients with nonsustained ventricular tachycardia and high-grade ventricular arrhythmias for programmed ventricular stimulation. *J Am Coll Cardiol* 1988;12:1481–1487.
321. Woelfel AK, et al. Exercise-induced distal atrioventricular block. *J Am Coll Cardiol* 1983;2:578–581.
322. World Survey on Cardiac Pacing. *PACE Pacing Clin Electrophysiol* 1983;6:A157.
323. Yee R, Klein GJ. Syncope in the Wolff-Parkinson-White syndrome: incidence and electrophysiologic correlates. *PACE Pacing Clin Electrophysiol* 1984;7:381–388.
324. Zeldis SM, et al. Cardiovascular complaints: correlation with cardiac arrhythmias on 24-hour electrocardiographic monitoring. *Chest* 1980;78:456–462.
325. Zelis R, et al. Reflex vasodilation induced by coronary angiography in human subjects. *Circulation* 1976;53:490–493.

CHAPTER 49

Postural Tachycardia Syndrome

Phillip A. Low, Ronald Schondorf, Vera Novak, Paola Sandroni,
Tonette L. Opfer-Gehrking, and Peter Novak

1. POTS is defined as the development of orthostatic symptoms associated with a heart rate increment ≥30 to an orthostatic heart rate ≥120 beats/min without orthostatic hypotension. A known autonomic neuropathy is exclusionary.
2. Females predominate over males by 5:1. The mean age of onset is about 30 years, and most patients are between the ages of 20 and 40 years.
3. Symptoms of orthostatic intolerance comprise those due to brain hypoxia and those due to sympathetic overaction.
4. Other symptoms are poor exercise tolerance and episodic worsening of orthostatic intolerance. Some patients have paroxysmal nonorthostatic symptoms.
5. About one half of patients have a postviral mild autonomic neuropathy. Laboratory tests demonstrate orthostatic tachycardia and distal impairment of sudomotor and vasomotor function.
6. Pathophysiologic mechanisms (not mutually exclusive) include increased capacitance, hypovolemia, venous pooling, β-receptor supersensitivity, and presumed impairment of brain stem regulation.
7. Orthostatic intolerance can be a feature of a number of other conditions, including chronic fatigue syndrome (CFS) and mitral valve prolapse (MVP). CFS is characterized by overwhelming symptoms of physical and mental fatigue and poor exercise tolerance. Additional subjective symptoms include headaches, poor sleep, cognitive symptoms, and pseudoinfectious (sore throat, lymphadenopathy) symptoms. Orthostatic intolerance is not a core feature.
8. All patients with POTS require a high-salt diet, copious fluids, and postural training. Many require β-receptor antagonists in small doses.

DEFINITION AND PERSPECTIVE

Orthostatic intolerance is defined as the development of symptoms during standing that are relieved by recumbency. Patients with orthostatic intolerance often present with complaints of exercise intolerance, dizziness, diminished concentration, tremulousness, nausea, and recurrent syncope and may be incorrectly labeled as having panic disorder or chronic anxiety (55). Simple activities such as eating, showering, or low-intensity exercise may profoundly exacerbate these symptoms and may significantly impair even the most rudimentary activities of daily living. Somewhat paradoxically, the magnitude of these symptoms is often significantly greater than that observed in patients with clinically detectable autonomic failure. Despite these symptoms, clinical examination alone is often unrevealing because florid autonomic failure is not present; therefore, these disorders are sometimes considered "benign."

Postural tachycardia syndrome (POTS) is defined as the development of orthostatic symptoms associated with a heart rate increment of 30 beats/min (bpm) or greater (Table 1). We chose these practical and reasonable criteria rather than requiring an increment that relates to our nor-

P. A. Low, V. Novak, P. Novak, P. Sandroni, T. L. Opfer-Gehrking: Department of Neurology, Mayo Clinic, Rochester, Minnesota, 55905.

R. Schondorf: Department of Neurology, McGill Universuty, Montreal, Quebec H3T 1E2.

V. Novak and P. Novak: Autonomic Disorders Center, Mayo Clinic, Rochester, Minnesota 55905.

TABLE 1. *Criteria for Postural Tachycardia Syndrome*

Heart rate increment ≥30 bpm within 5 minutes of standing or tilt-up
Heart rate ≥120 bpm within 5 minutes of standing or tilt-up
Orthostatic symptoms consistently develop
Absence of a known cause of autonomic neuropathy
Absence of orthostatic hypotension

bpm, beats per minute.

mative data by age and gender. Considering the age range of most patients with POTS (15 to 50 years), an increment of 30 bpm exceeds the 99th percentile for female control subjects from 10 to 83 years but is more stringent in terms of the absolute orthostatic heart rate. Some patients might have a heart rate increment of 30 bpm with a standing heart rate below 120 bpm, criteria that we would previously have accepted (56,77). These patients are best considered to have mild orthostatic intolerance. Mild orthostatic intolerance can occur in a heterogeneous group of patients. These include otherwise normal subjects under conditions of mild hypovolemia, patients experiencing deconditioning with prolonged bed rest, patients with reduced orthostatic tolerance sometimes associated with mitral valve prolapse (MVP), and patients at certain phases of the menstrual cycle.

Neurogenic orthostatic hypotension can be due to autonomic neuropathies, such as diabetes and amyloidosis (see Chapter 36), and to non-neuropathic disorders, such as MSA (multiple system atrophy, Shy-Drager syndrome) and PAF (pure autonomic failure, idiopathic orthostatic hypotension; see Chapter 42). Neurogenic orthostatic hypotension is relatively uncommon. POTS, in contrast, is much more common, but is unassociated with orthostatic hypotension. Improved recognition of lesser degrees of orthostatic intolerance came with the observation that the most common and earliest manifestation of orthostatic intolerance is an excessive tachycardia (83). These subjects have disorders that are sometimes termed "benign" disorders of reduced orthostatic tolerance. The unifying feature is the development of orthostatic symptoms without consistent orthostatic hypotension. Investigators and clinicians have been impressed with different aspects of the conditions and have approached orthostatic intolerance from different perspectives. Terms such as effort syndrome, neurasthenia, idiopathic hypovolemia (27), sympathotonic orthostatic hypotension, emphasizing sympathetic overactivity (37), and MVP syndrome (12) exemplify the concentration on particular components of the patient's disease. Postural tachycardia with or without syncope can be present in several of the disorders. Most patients with MVP do not have florid dysautonomia (22), and the "dysautonomic" patients with MVP are indistinguishable from those with similar complaints and normal echocardiographic examinations (87); therefore, the implication that MVP is somehow mechanistically involved, when POTS is present, is questionable. Similarly, most patients who have vasovagal syncope do not have POTS. About half the patients with POTS have an autonomic neuropathy (77, 78). Some patients with chronic fatigue syndrome (CFS) have orthostatic intolerance with tilt-induced syncope, and a subset will respond to treatment directed at syncope (3); however, most patients with CFS do not have POTS.

We have focused on orthostatic tachycardia because an excessive heart rate increment appears to be the earliest and most consistent of the easily measured indices of orthostatic intolerance (85). Most of the other terms focus on manifestations that are not consistently present. Most patients with orthostatic intolerance do not have florid autonomic failure and do not have orthostatic hypotension. The term idiopathic hypovolemia is unsatisfactory because most patients do not have reduced plasma volumes or red cell mass. As discussed earlier, most patients with MVP do not have dysautonomia. The emphasis on postural tachycardia does, however, have a disadvantage in that it ignores nonorthostatic symptoms such as paroxysmal episodes of autonomic dysfunction, including sinus tachycardia, blood pressure (BP) fluctuations, vasomotor (especially acral) symptoms, and fatigue.

A classification of disorders of orthostatic intolerance not associated with florid orthostatic hypotension is shown in Table 2. Mild orthostatic intolerance was described earlier. We prefer this term to mild POTS because it is unsatisfactory to have a syndrome that is variably present. Several conditions (syncope, CFS, MVP) are sometimes but not invariably associated with orthostatic intolerance. The classification recognizes this variable association. Neurocardiogenic syncope is discussed in detail in Chapter 48. The two conditions are not mutually exclusive. We believe it is preferable to designate the condition as POTS with syncope when a patient consistently has orthostatic tachycardia and also has the propensity for syncope. Most patients with syncope do not have excessive tachycardia. Similarly, orthostatic intolerance and CFS are not synonymous. This will be discussed further, as will orthostatic intolerance associated with prolonged bed rest.

TABLE 2. *Classification of orthostatic intolerance*

Mild orthostatic intolerance
POTS (postural tachycardia syndrome)
Secondary POTS
Neurocardiogenic (vasovagal) syncope
Orthostatic intolerance associated with CFS (chronic fatigue syndrome)
Orthostatic intolerance associated with mitral valve prolapse
Orthostatic intolerance associated with reduced gravity
Constitutional orthostatic intolerance

TABLE 3. *Orthostatic symptoms as frequency percentage in patients with Postural Tachycardia Syndrome and Orthostatic Hypotension*

	Postural Tachycardia Syndrome (N = 15)	Orthostatic Hypotension (N = 11)
Dizziness	100%	100%
Blurred vision	80%	82%
Tiredness	80%	91%
Nausea	66%	18%
Palpitations	60%	9%
Tremulousness	47%	18%
Breathing difficulties	40%	0%
Sweating	27%	9%
Anxiety	20%	18%
Gastrointestinal symptoms	20%	36%
Vasomotor symptoms	13%	0%
DSFN	7%	44%

DSFN, Distal small fiber neuropathy.

POSTURAL ORTHOSTATIC TACHYCARDIA SYNDROME

Clinical Features

The age of presentation of POTS is most commonly between 15 and 50 years (77,78). Most patients we have evaluated have had the symptoms for about 1 year. The orthostatic symptoms consist of lightheadedness, visual blurring or tunneling, palpitations, tremulousness, and weakness (especially of the legs). Less common symptoms are hyperventilation, anxiety, chest wall pain, nausea, acral coldness or pain, and headaches. The symptoms these patients experience differ from those of patients with orthostatic hypotension in that there are significant symptoms of sympathetic activation (Table 3). There may be an over-representation of migraine and sleep disorders (55). There is a clear preponderance of women (56,71,74,77,78), although some earlier studies were at variance (27,37). The age and sex distribution of 88 patients with the diagnosis of POTS is shown in Table 4. We have found a consistent female-to-male ratio of 5 : 1.

About half of patients have an antecedent presumed viral illness (56,77,78). Another feature of POTS is the cyclical nature of the symptoms. Some females will have marked deterioration of their symptoms at certain stages of their menstrual cycle associated with significant weight and fluid changes. Typically, these patients have large fluctuations in their weight, sometimes up to 5 pounds. Others have cycles of several days of intense orthostatic intolerance followed by a similar period when their symptoms are less severe. Some patients have episodic symptoms at rest associated with changes in BP and heart rate (HR) that are unrelated to arrhythmias. The HR alterations are typically a sinus tachycardia, although a bradycardia can occur. Fatigue can be a problem during these episodes. Some describe periods when they have trouble retaining fluid, in spite of heavy intake. Studies of fluid balance and antidiuretic hormone levels are not well documented. Orthostatic intolerance with low BP requiring repeat visits to the emergency room for intravenous saline infusions is uncommon but by no means rare.

The relationship to anxiety and panic is uncertain. The patient with typical anxiety/panic disorder is easy to differentiate from the patient with POTS, and the orthostatic anxiety symptoms are easy to differentiate from an anxiety disorder in most patients. However, the relationship can be more complicated. Many of the symptoms of anxiety are mediated by the autonomic nervous system. Orthostatic stress can evoke anxiety/panic symptoms in predisposed subjects. Patients with panic disorders and POTS patients share certain clinical features. These include an intense fear or discomfort at the onset of symptoms, shortness of breath with hyperventilation, dizziness or faintness, palpitations, trembling, numbness or tingling sensations, flushes or chills, chest pain, and generalized weakness. In a minority of patients there seems to be a coexistence of the two disorders. There may be an overlap in proposed central mechanisms for both POTS and panic disorders. The noradrenergic system is involved in both disorders (93). Other central neurotransmitters that potentially affect the production of panic disorders include gamma-aminobutyric acid (GABA) (39), serotonin (96), and adenosine (5). Their role in POTS needs evaluation. Finally, both conditions share common treatments, including phenobarbital, benzodiazepines, β-blockers (91), and clonidine (92).

TABLE 4. *Postural Tachycardia Syndrome by age and gender*

Number of patients: 88
Age: 31.5 ± (SD) 7.0 years
Gender: F = 75; M = 13

SD, standard deviation.

TABLE 5. *Pathophysiologic types of Postural Tachycardia Syndrome (POTS)*

Mild orthostatic intolerance
Idiopathic POTS
Neurogenic POTS (associated with idiopathic autonomic neuropathy)
Secondary POTS
POTS associated with mitral valve prolapse
Hypertensive POTS

Clinical examination reveals an excessive heart rate increment. Pulse pressure may be excessively reduced. One clinical correlate is the difficulty in palpating a radial pulse with continued standing, or with the performance of a Valsalva maneuver (Flack sign). Another clinical sign is the development of acral coldness. With continued standing there may be venous prominence resulting in blueness and even swelling of the feet (85).

Etiology

Postural Orthostatic tachycardia syndrome appears to be heterogeneous in both etiology and pathophysiology. Some suggested etiopathologic mechanisms and a tentative classification of POTS are shown in Table 5. Mild orthostatic intolerance is listed here again. POTS that is clearly associated with an idiopathic autonomic neuropathy (typically postviral, peripheral denervation with absent late phase II of the Valsalva maneuver and peripheral anhidrosis; failure of systemic peripheral resistance to increment on tilt-up) is recognized. The term secondary POTS is used for patients who have a known autonomic disorder with peripheral denervation and relative cardiac autonomic preservation. These might be autonomic neuropathies (such as diabetic, amyloid, or idiopathic) or, less commonly, a stage in the evolution of pure autonomic failure or multiple system atrophy. Clearly, the preferable diagnosis is the primary diagnosis. POTS associated with MVP is also of less certain value. We have retained it for certain practical clinical reasons. The relationship could still be important. It is also helpful to be cognizant of an associated condition that might need antibiotic coverage during dental and related procedures. The term hypertensive POTS is used for the patient who has supine normotension and an increase in diastolic BP of at least 20 mmHg. Suggested mechanisms of POTS are listed in Table 6 and described below.

PERIPHERAL DENERVATION, POOR VASOMOTOR TONE, AND VENOUS POOLING

Vasomotor, especially venomotor, tone could be impaired as part of a length-dependent autonomic neuropathy (77,78), although a separate end-organ defect (of venomotor tone) cannot be excluded. The presence of peripheral denervation with intact cardiac autonomic innervation is well documented (56,77,78; also see below). Related to this mechanism is the excessive venous pooling seen in some patients. Streeten (85) made careful clinical observations that these patients develop a bluish discoloration of the lower extremities on continued standing, and he also noted that their orthostatic intolerance can be overcome by pressure garments at a pressure that reduces venous capacitance. Excessive venous pooling was documented by the use of isotope labeling, which demonstrated that these patients had excessive sequestration of the isotope to their calves with standing; the abnormality was corrected after venous compression (83,85). Our own studies, showing an excessive fall in end-diastolic volume and stroke volume on tilt-up, also suggest venous pooling (56). Venous pooling would cause a reduction in preload, excessive baroreceptor unloading in the upright position, and a resultant increase in sympathetic outflow. Indeed, mild hypovolemia after hemorrhage in young healthy subjects is typically associated with a surge of sympathetic outflow, mild tachycardia, lower BP, and large, slow oscillations in BP and HR (90).

β-RECEPTOR SUPERSENSITIVITY

β-Receptor supersensitivity is often inferred from the clinical symptoms of tremulousness, anxiety, tachycardia, and palpitations with continued standing (78). Whether this supersensitivity is a primary or secondary denervation supersensitivity is unclear. During the Valsalva maneuver, these patients have an excessive phase IV BP overshoot, which is normalized by intravenous propranolol (Figs. 1 and 2) (76,77). We have preliminary results on the HR response to isoproterenol infusion with the patient supine. In five patients with POTS infused with a dose of 0.01 mg/kg/min of isoproterenol, the tachycardic response (an index of β-receptor supersensitivity) regressed with the heart rate increment during tilt-up ($Y = 3.29X - 24.19$; $R = 0.88$; significance of slope, $P < 0.05$). (Y = heart rate response to tilt-up and X is the increment to isoproterenol.) This relationship suggests that the tachycardic response to tilt represents β-receptor supersensitivity or reduced vagal braking, although a compensatory heart rate response to exaggerated β-adrenergic–mediated vasodilatation is also

TABLE 6. *Some suggested mechanisms of Postural Tachycardia Syndrome*

Length-dependent autonomic neuropathy
Excessive venous pooling
β-receptor supersentivity
α-receptor hyper- or hyposensitivity
Altered sympathetic–parasympathetic balance
Brain stem dysregulation

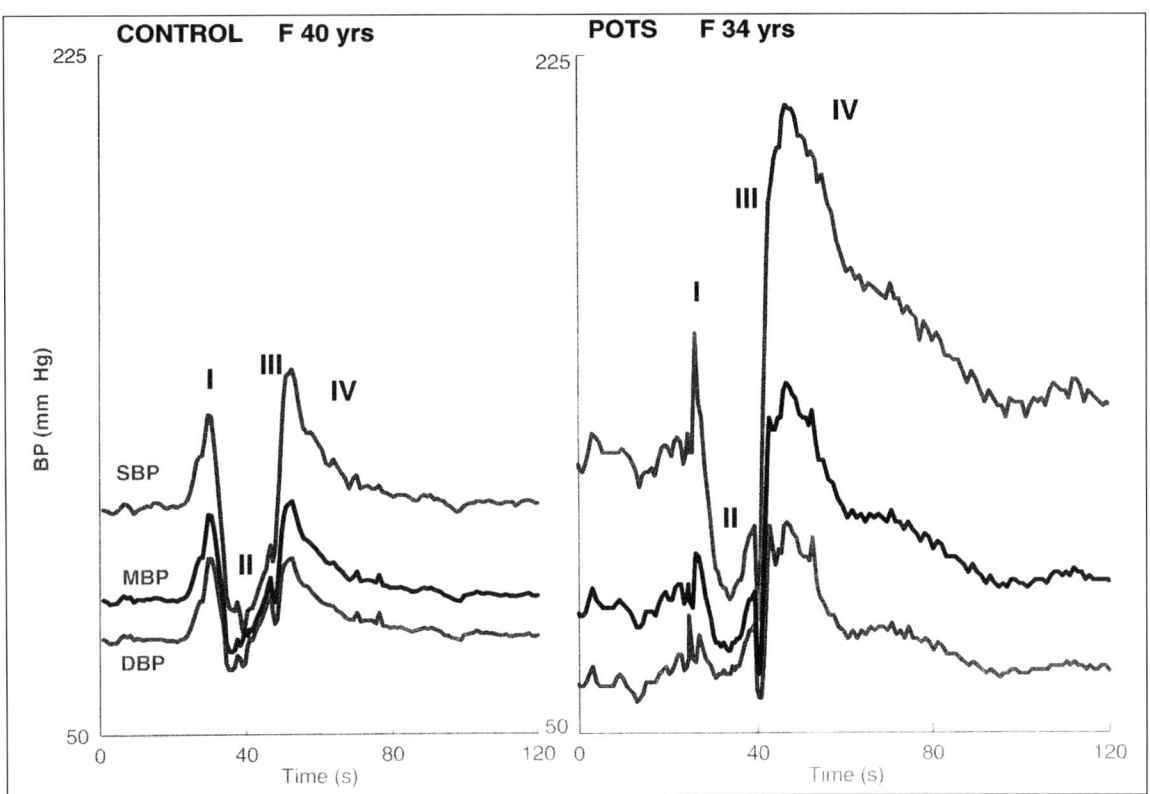

FIG. 1. Normal Valsalva maneuver and Valsalva maneuver from a patient with POTS. The patient with POTS has an excessive phase IV.

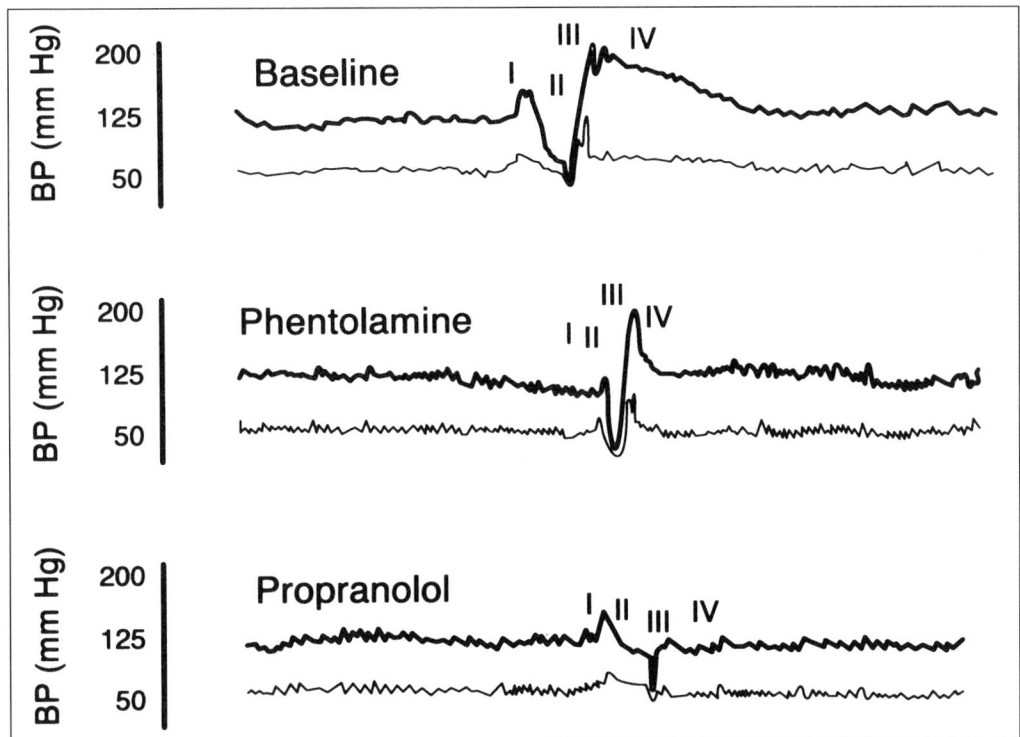

FIG. 2. Continuous BP recordings in a patient with hypertensive POTS. A large fluctuation in BP is seen.

possible. The BP response to intravenous norepinephrine is usually normal (21,82), although a reduced response has been described in four patients (71).

HYPOVOLEMIA

Hypovolemia has been reported in some patients (27, 43,74). Although most of our patients have normal plasma volumes, this etiologic feature is important to recognize because it is treatable. On a cautionary note, given the propensity for venous pooling and transudation of plasma volume to the interstitial space, plasma volume should be measured only after the patient has been recumbent for a minimum of 45 min.

SYMPATHETIC–PARASYMPATHETIC IMBALANCE

The question of altered sympathetic–parasympathetic balance has been systematically addressed (see Chapter 26). Patients with POTS have increased sympathetic tone. The sympathetic overactivity is likely secondary to peripheral denervation, venous pooling, or end-organ dysfunction. These alterations result in increased capacitance and a hyperadrenergic state. In some patients the additional contributions of brain stem dysregulation or receptor upregulation (β-receptor) may aggravate the symptoms. It is possible that the sympathotonic state not only causes some of the symptoms in POTS but also perpetuates the condition by constricting plasma volume.

BRAIN STEM MECHANISMS

Streeten and colleagues (84) described the entity of orthostatic hypertension and advanced reasons why this was secondary to peripheral venous pooling. They described a subset of patients with orthostatic intolerance associated with an excessive rise in BP. This subset consisted of 181 patients out of 1800 referred hypertensive patients. These patients had recumbent diastolic BP below 90 mm Hg and standing diastolic BP above 90 mm Hg. In 12 patients studied in greater detail, the orthostatic fall in cardiac output was double that in 8 normotensive subjects. An inflated pressure suit over the pelvis and lower limbs prevented the excessive fall in cardiac output and significantly reduced ($P < 0.02$) the excessive rise in standing diastolic BP in orthostatic hypertensive patients. Gravitational pooling of blood in the legs was significantly greater ($P < 0.01$) than in controls, and the magnitudes of orthostatic pooling and orthostatic increases in diastolic BP were closely correlated (r = +0.85). Plasma norepinephrine concentrations were similar in recumbency and after sustained handgrip exercise but were significantly greater ($P < 0.01$) in the patients than in the normotensive subjects after 5 to 60 min of standing. These authors suggested that orthostatic hypertension is common and that its mechanism involves excessive orthostatic blood pooling, which results in decreased venous return, decreased cardiac output, increased sympathetic stimulation (presumably through low-pressure cardiopulmonary receptors), and excessive arteriolar, but not venular, constriction.

We have seen four patients with marked orthostatic hypertension, markedly labile blood pressures, and trouble-

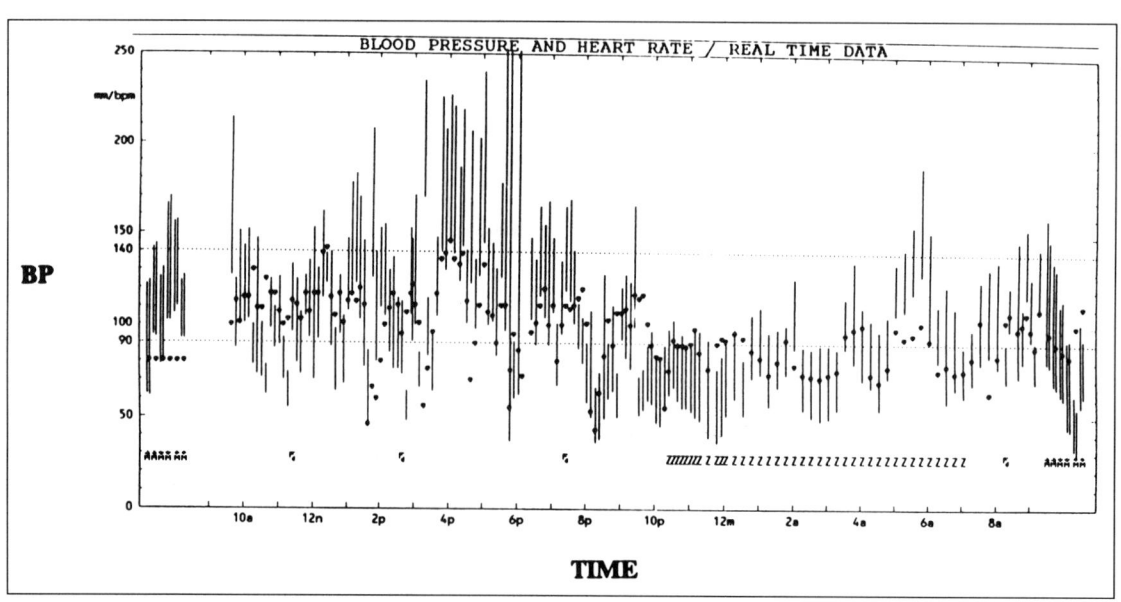

FIG. 3. Representative pharmacologic dissection of the Valsalva maneuver in POTS. Note absent late phase II and excessive phase IV (*top*). Phentolamine (10 mg intravenously) affects the duration but not the amplitude of phase IV. Propranolol (10 mg intravenously) completely blocks phase IV.

some orthostatic symptoms, including headaches (Fig. 3). These disorders superficially resemble the syndrome of baroreflex failure (73) but differ in that the baroreflexes are operative. Although Streeten and associates (84) emphasized peripheral denervation, we are more impressed with the dysregulation. A normal individual subjected to increased baroreceptor activation responds appropriately. These patients respond excessively; they have large BP fluctuations (see Fig. 3), and the surges in BP are associated with other symptoms of sympathetic excess (nausea, acral skin vasoconstriction, sweating, tachycardia), which suggests the problem of central (presumably brain stem) dysregulation. They may respond to clonidine, but the response can be inadequate. One patient responded for 5 months after microvascular decompression at the region of the left upper medulla. We have tentatively assigned a brain stem localization of the dysautonomia.

EVALUATION

Autonomic Studies

One half to two thirds of patients have a restricted autonomic neuropathy, typically a length-dependent type (56, 77,78). The term length-dependent neuropathy refers to one in which the ends of the longer fibers are affected before the shorter ones. The original belief (11) was that the defect was in the cell body, and that the distal ends of the longest and largest fibers, because they have the largest metabolic demands and are the most compromised (because of their distance), were the most affected. The term length-dependent neuropathy was subsequently modified (63). It still applies to the greater involvement of the distal processes (not necessarily the ends) of the longest fibers, and the processes can be either axonal or neuronal. As applied to the autonomic nervous system, the postganglionic sympathetic adrenergic fibers to the limbs and splanchnic–mesenteric bed have the longest fibers. Next are the vagal fibers to the heart, which have a long preganglionic path. The cardiac adrenergic fibers, in contrast, are relatively short fibers.

Cardiovagal Tests

The HR response to deep breathing is usually normal and is often large (43,56,78). The Valsalva ratio is normal and often excessively large, with a prominent and sustained undershoot during phase IV. Heart rate variability to deep breathing is normal and is often very large. A few patients with POTS have impaired cardiovagal function on standard tests of cardiovagal function (Table 7). There is an overall loss of heart period variability in the respiratory frequency, with both the resting and tilt-up positions (see Chapter 26), and an increased score in the cardiovagal subset of the composite autonomic scoring scale (CASS) (56). Khurana (43) reported mild abnormalities in cardiovagal function in a minority of patients. Intravenous atropine-induced tachycardia was subnormal in two out of eight patients. The site of the lesion was postganglionic because the quantitative sudomotor axon reflex test (QSART) was often absent and because dilute pilocarpine-induced miosis, which detects denervation supersensitivity as an indicator of postganglionic denervation, was found in three of six patients.

Adrenergic Tests

The BP_{BB} responses to the Valsalva maneuver are abnormal in about two thirds of patients (56,78). The pulse pressure falls by more than 50% and may be obliterated. Early phase II of the Valsalva maneuver is exaggerated, and late phase II may be reduced or absent (see Fig. 2). Phase IV is normal but usually is excessively large (see Figs. 1 and 2). The cardiovascular responses to tilt-up are abnormal. The heart rate response varies from 120 to 170 bpm on tilt-up; these values are typically attained by 2 min. The HR response may oscillate excessively; in patients with significant peripheral denervation, the variability may be reduced. The BP responses occur in several patterns. Patients with prominent venous pooling may have an excessive reduction in pulse pressure. Some have a prominent hypertensive response with increases in diastolic BP of up to 50 mmHg, with large fluctuations. Some patients have relatively normal BP responses but have tachycardia and symptoms. The pattern of responses with peripheral sudo-

TABLE 7. *Severity of autonomic deficits by systems*

Parameter	Control	Orthostatic hypotension (OH)	Postural tachycardia syndrome (POTS)
$CASS_{Vag}$	0.0 ± 0.0	2.0 ± 0.2[b]	0.2 ± 0.2δ
$CASS_{Adr}$	0.1 ± 0.1	3.4 ± 0.3[b]	1.2 ± 0.3[b]; δ
$CASS_{Sud}$	0.0 ± 0.0	2.4 ± 0.2[b]	0.9 ± 0.3[a]; δ
CASS	0.1 ± 0.1	7.7 ± 0.5[b]	2.3 ± 0.6[b]; δ

vs CON, [a]$P < 0.05$
[b]$P < 0.001$
POTS vs OH, δ, $P < 0.001$
$CASS_{Vag}$, ; $CASS_{Adr}$, ; $CASS_{Sud}$, ; CASS, ; CON,

motor deficits (absent late phase II of the Valsalva maneuver with intact phase IV) and normal forced respiratory sinus arrhythmia is consistent with a length-dependent autonomic neuropathy.

Plasma norepinephrine is normal when patients are supine and is normal and often increased when patients are erect (77,78,83), likely secondary to increased baroreceptor unloading. Concomitant with the orthostatic surge in norepinephrine, slow adrenergic vasomotor rhythms in blood pressure are preserved (see Chapter 26), and with the reduction in parasympathetic function, marked sympathovagal imbalance is present, with sympathetic overbalance, manifested as a dramatic increase in the sympathovagal index (NONRF_SBP/RFR_RRI; $P < 0.001$).

There is a contradiction between peripheral autonomic failure (including adrenergic failure) and apparent systemic adrenergic overactivity (as indicated by an excessive norepinephrine response to tilt-up, increased total peripheral resistance [76], and increased sympathovagal balance on power spectral analysis). In fact, this contradiction is more apparent than real. Peripheral denervation hypovolemia or venous pooling results in increased vascular capacitance and a reduction in preload, resulting in a fall in pulse pressure, unloading baroreflexes, and an increased sympathetic efferent drive. This exaggerated norepinephrine response is in fact the expected response to partial denervation. There are a number of manifestations of peripheral adrenergic denervation. There is denervation supersensitivity, which is manifested as intense vasoconstriction of the hands and feet in response to normal or increased levels of plasma norepinephrine. The orthostatic accentuation of these symptoms, associated with a normal (or more often excessive) increase in norepinephrine (78), suggests that central sympathetic drive is not impaired and that some receptors (e.g., skin vessels) respond normally or excessively (?denervation supersensitivity). Selective muscle beds clearly do not, as indicated by the total loss of late phase II of the Valsalva maneuver (78), a component that is driven primarily by sympathetic efferents to muscle (75) and the transient orthostatic hypotension. α-Adrenoreceptor density of microvessels in POTS has not been reported. Kafka and co-workers (40) evaluated α-adrenergic receptor function in platelets and found that patients with POTS had normal receptor number and cAMP production.

The response to intravenous norepinephrine has been normal (21,82) or reduced (71). Suggestions of altered contractile responses of foot veins to infused norepinephrine in POTS and neurogenic orthostatic hypotension (82) were not confirmed in a subsequent study by the same laboratory (60), and no group differences in platelet α_2-adrenergic receptor densities and dissociation constants were found.

Sudomotor Tests

One half to two thirds of patients with POTS have sudomotor impairment. The actual percentages vary depending on the particular center and case selection. Presumed postviral cases have a larger percentage than nonpostviral cases. These patients have an impairment of QSART volumes in the lower extremity distally, typically involving the foot and distal leg sites. The sudomotor score is typically about 1 (out of a maximum of 3; see Table 7). The description in our earlier reports included more neuropathic cases (78). With the wider recognition of POTS, cases now appear to have less severe neuropathic deficits. All of these cases have a neuropathic distribution of anhidrosis on QSART and the thermoregulatory sweat test. In the latter, sweat impairment involves the lower extremities to varying degrees; the feet are typically anhidrotic and the remainder of the legs are somewhat involved. The distribution of anhidrosis can be patchy or more widespread. Khurana (43) reported a segmental or patchy anhidrosis in six out of eight patients. Skin potential abnormalities with a loss of skin potentials in the lower extremity have also been described (36).

Blood Volume Measurements

As noted earlier, plasma volume is generally normal in POTS, although some patients with intravascular plasma volume depletion have been described (27,43). Two modifications of the plasma volume measurement have been suggested. The first is the recording of venous pooling by scintillographic determinations of calf isotope counts with the patient supine and then tilted up (83). Another recent suggestion is to evaluate the time course of change of plasma volume (26). Once baseline plasma volume is determined with the use of Evans blue or radiolabeled albumin, changes in plasma volume are measured by noting changes in hematocrit during head-up tilt. An excessive rate of decline would suggest extravasation into subcutaneous tissue. El-Sayed and Hainsworth (24) reported a modification of the standard Evans blue indicator method that increased the sensitivity of the method to detect small changes in plasma volume. They also recorded the 24-hr urine sodium excretion in patients with neurocardiogenic syncope and noted that patients with a urinary sodium excretion <170 mmol/24 hrs were more likely to have reduced plasma volume and responded better to salt loading.

Cardiologic Studies

The early studies on POTS had much information on cardiac function and heart rhythms. Twenty-four-hour Holter monitor recordings have been unrewarding and have usually been normal, except for sinus tachycardia. Echocardiographic studies have demonstrated normal ejection fractions and normal valvular function, except for MVP. Cardiac electrophysiologic studies have been unrewarding for patients with normal electrocardiograms (ECGs). Continuous BP monitoring has been useful in a subset of patients with large oscillations in BP. It is our im-

TABLE 8. *The grading of orthostatic intolerance*

Grade 0:
  Normal orthostatic tolerance
Grade I:
  Orthostatic symptoms are infrequent or occur only under conditions of increased orthostatic stress
  Subject is able to stand >15 minutes on most occasions
  Subject typically has unrestricted activities of daily living
Grade II:
  Orthostatic symptoms are frequent, developing at least once a week. Orthostatic symptoms commonly develop with orthostatic stress
  Subject is able to stand >5 minutes on most occasions
  Some limitation in activities of daily living is typical
Grade III:
  Orthostatic symptoms develop on most occasions and are regularly unmasked by orthostatic stresses
  Subject is able to stand >1 minute on most occasions
  There is marked limitation in activities of daily living
Grade IV:
  Orthostatic symptoms are consistently present
  Subject is able to stand <1 minute on most occasions
  Patient is seriously incapacitated, being bed- or wheelchair-bound because of orthostatic intolerance. Syncope/presyncope is common if patient attempts to stand

Symptoms may vary with time and state of hydration and circumstsances.
Orthostatic stresses include prolonged standing, a meal, exertion, and heat stress.

pression that subtle changes in P wave and T wave morphology can occur in some of these patients in response to tilt-up.

Grading of Orthostatic Intolerance

To minimize some of the subjectivity inherent in grading degrees of orthostatic intolerance, we have developed a grading system of orthostatic intolerance using the three-pronged criteria of: rapidity of development, severity of orthostatic symptoms, ability of the subject to withstand orthostatic stresses, and degree of interference with activities of daily living. We document the following: (1) the standing time (in min) to the onset of sustained orthostatic symptoms of sufficient severity to affect activities of daily living, (2) the resistance to orthostatic stresses such as prolonged standing, a meal, exertion, and heat stress, (3) the ability of the subject to perform activities of daily living in the home and at work. Four grades of orthostatic intolerance are defined (Table 8).

Differential Diagnosis

Postural tachycardia syndrome is differentiated mainly from neurogenic orthostatic hypotension, other causes of orthostatic intolerance, and anxiety–panic attacks. The differentiation from neurogenic orthostatic hypotension is straightforward and is summarized in Table 9. The symptoms of orthostatic hypotension are similar, but symptoms of sympathetic overactivity such as tremulousness, anxiety, nausea, sweating, and acral vasoconstriction are seen in POTS and not in neurogenic orthostatic hypotension. In the latter, orthostatic hypotension and evidence of generalized autonomic failure (cardiovagal, adrenergic, sudomotor) are found (see Table 7).

Differentiation from other causes of orthostatic intolerance is more difficult. Mild orthostatic intolerance secondary to recent illness with prolonged bed rest, dehydration, hypovolemia, or medication effect is usually straightforward. A related condition is constitutional orthostatic intolerance. Patients with this condition have always had some degree of orthostatic intolerance. They may have had syncopal episodes in their youth in response to prolonged standing or syncope in response to pain or the sight of blood. They may have had transient lightheadedness on standing up suddenly. These subjects are more prone to develop orthostatic intolerance after a period of bed rest or after a viral illness. The condition may be familial. Three

TABLE 9. *Comparison between generalized autonomic neuropathy patients and patients with postural orthostatic tachycardia syndrome*

Parameter	Neurogenic Orthostatic Hypotension	Postural Orthostatic Tachycardia Syndrome
Orthostatic dizziness	Variably present	Present
Orthostatic tremulousness	Absent	Common
Orthostatic palpitations	Absent	Common
Orthostatic hypotension	Consistent	Usually absent
Orthostatic tachycardia	Reduced	Exaggerated
Supine norepinephrine	Usually reduced	Normal or increased
Standing norepeniphrine	Reduced	Increased or normal
HR response to deep breathing	Reduced	Normal
Valsalva ratio	Reduced	Normal or increased
BP_{BB} to VM:		
Early phase II	Markedly increased	Increased
Late phase II	Absent	Normal or reduced
Phase IV	Absent	Increased

HR, Heart Rate; BP_{BB}, Beat-to-Beat blood pressure; VM, Valsalva Maneuver.

conditions (prolonged bed rest, CFS, and MVP) deserve special attention and will be described later. POTS can be differentiated from CFS by the predominance of *orthostatic* symptoms. CFS affects the sexes less unevenly, is dominated by nonorthostatic symptoms, and has many quasi-infectious symptoms. Some patients with CFS do have orthostatic intolerance, including tachycardia. Both groups have marked worsening of symptoms after syncope or presyncope. One possible suggestion is that the nonorthostatic symptoms are a continuation of postsyncopal symptoms. We recommend that when the features of fatigue predominate, the condition should be designated as POTS associated with CFS. Similarly, orthostatic intolerance should not be considered an integral part of MVP. When orthostatic intolerance is a feature of MVP, the condition should be recognized as orthostatic intolerance or POTS associated with MVP. The effects of microgravity and prolonged bed rest are detailed in Chapter 33. CFS and MVP are described in greater detail below.

CHRONIC FATIGUE SYNDROME

Chronic fatigue syndrome is defined by the Centers for Disease Control and Prevention (CDC) as fatigue of at least 6 months' duration that seriously interferes with the patient's life—without evidence of various organic or psychiatric illnesses that can produce chronic fatigue. The criteria include myalgias, postexertional malaise, headaches, and a group of infectious-type symptoms (chronic fever and chills, sore throat, lymphadenopathy). These criteria appear to distinguish CFS patients from healthy control subjects and from the comparison groups with multiple sclerosis and depression (45). In addition to chronic fluctuating fatigue, these patients have somatic, cognitive, depressive, and sleep dysfunction. These patients are often separated into postviral and nonpostviral fatigue syndrome groups. Attempts have also been made to quantitate the severity of fatigue (67). The condition affects both sexes, and demographic, clinical, and psychosocial factors do not distinguish male from female CFS patients (8). The diurnal fluctuations have also been evaluated. The pattern is similar to that of normal subjects, but the energy levels are lower (97). The history of CFS has recently been reviewed (44).

Investigations

Disorders of sleep are not uncommon, but there is no specific pattern of involvement (59,62). Abnormalities such as alpha rhythm disturbance (7.5–11 Hz) in the electroencephalogram (EEG) (61,95) are nonspecific and reflect a lack of refreshing sleep. The circadian thermic pattern has been studied in CFS and has been reported to be altered (10).

Cardiologic abnormalities, typically subtle, have been reported. These include abnormal left ventricular myocardial dynamics and orthostatic T-wave changes (49).

Gibson and colleagues (29) evaluated exercise performance and fatigability in patients with CFS. These patients showed normal muscle physiology before and after exercise. Raised perceived exertion scores during exercise suggested that central factors were limiting exercise capacity in these patients. Essentially similar conclusions were reached by Kent-Braun and associates (42). Gait kinematics confirm an impairment of gait, a finding of uncertain specificity (2).

Single-fiber EMG studies reportedly showed increased jitter or altered fiber density in CFS (13).

Although cognitive complaints are common, and complaints of memory impairment dominate, Grafman and co-workers (32) studied 20 CFS patients using a clinical and experimental battery composed of memory and cognitive tests and found generally negative results. They concluded that memory impairment in CFS patients is typically mild and involves primarily memory processes that participate in conceptualizing information. Similar conclusions were reached by DeLuca and colleagues (20), who found normal cognitive function, although information processing speed was reduced.

The possibility of a continued postviral mechanism, such as Lyme disease (30) or Epstein-Barr virus (95), has been considered, but studies have been either negative or equivocal.

Brain perfusion has been studied with the use of ^{99m}Tc-hexamethylpropyleneamine oxime (^{99m}Tc-HMPAO) single photon emission computed tomography (SPECT). Impaired perfusion is relatively common, but no specific pattern has emerged. Impairment of both cortical (38) and brain stem (18) hypoperfusion has been reported.

Ultrastructural mitochondrial abnormalities have been reported in CFS patients, but these observations were not confirmed in a quantitative study by Plioplys and Plioplys (69). Barnes and associates (1) studied skeletal muscle bioenergetics and control of intracellular pH in 46 patients with CFS by phosphorus magnetic resonance spectroscopy. The results have been compared with results from healthy controls and from a group of patients with mitochondrial cytopathies affecting skeletal muscle. No consistent abnormalities of glycolysis, mitochondrial metabolism, or pH regulation were identified in the group when taken as a whole, although in 12 of the 46 patients the relationship between pH and phosphocreatine use during exercise fell outside the normal range. These findings do not support any specific metabolic underlying abnormality in this syndrome.

Edwards and co-workers (23) reviewed muscle biopsy specimens from 108 patients with CFS and found no consistent correlation between symptoms and changes in fiber type or fiber size, degenerative or regenerative features, glycogen depletion, or mitochondrial abnormalities. Physiologic contractile properties were also examined before and for up to 48 hrs after a symptom-limited incremental cycle ergometer exercise test in 12 CFS patients and 12 normal volunteers. The authors concluded that voluntary and stimulated force characteristics were normal at rest and during recovery. Exercise duration was similar in the two groups, although CFS patients had higher perceived exertion scores in relation to heart rate during exercise, indicating a reduced effort sensation threshold. They were confident that CFS was not a myopathy. Psychological/psychiatric factors appear to be of greater importance in this condition.

Because these symptoms are exacerbated by physical exertion, the effect of exercise on serum cytokine and cerebral blood flow abnormalities has been studied (50,68). One study (68) reported that serum transforming growth factor beta (TGF-β) levels were elevated in the CFS group compared with the control group, although exercise did not cause a significant alteration (50,68).

Sisto and colleagues (80) reported that vagal tone was reduced during paced breathing in patients with CFS. Twelve women between the ages of 32 and 59 years with the diagnosis of CFS were compared with healthy age-matched women. Paced breathing at 8, 12, and 18 breaths/min were performed in the sitting and standing postures. Heart rate variability was used to evaluate vagal function. With this method, overall vagal power was significantly lower ($P < 0.034$) in the CFS group versus the healthy controls.

Evoked potential studies have been normal (70). A role for serotonin has been suggested, however neuroendocrine assessment of serotonin function in CFS was normal (98).

Bou-Holaigah and colleagues (3) reported a study of 23 patients with CFS (5 men and 18 women; mean age, 34 years) who were compared with 14 healthy controls (4 men and 10 women; mean age, 36 years). Each subject completed a symptom questionnaire and underwent a tilt-table test, which was then followed by infusion of isoproterenol. Patients were offered therapy with fludrocortisone, β-adrenergic blocking agents, and disopyramide, alone or in combination, directed at neurally mediated hypotension. An abnormal response to upright tilt was observed in 22 of 23 patients with CFS versus 4 of 14 controls ($P < 0.001$). Seventy percent of CFS patients, but no controls, had an abnormal response to tilt-up without isoproterenol ($P < 0.001$). Nine patients reported complete or nearly complete resolution of CFS symptoms after therapy directed at neurally mediated hypotension. The authors concluded that CFS is associated with neurally mediated hypotension and that its symptoms may be improved in a subset of patients by therapy directed at this abnormal cardiovascular reflex.

Strayer and associates (81) reported a randomized, multicenter, placebo-controlled, double-blind study of 92 patients with CFS in which the response to an antiviral and immunomodulatory drug, poly(I).poly(C12U), was determined. Measures of clinical response included Karnofsky performance score, a cognition scale derived from a self-administered instrument assessing symptomatology (SCL-90-R), an activities of daily living scale, and exercise treadmill performance. After 24 weeks, patients receiving poly(I).poly(C12U) had higher scores for both global performance and perceived cognition than did patients receiving placebo. In particular, patients given poly(I).poly(C12U) had increased Karnofsky performance scores ($P < 0.03$), exhibited a greater ability to do work during exercise treadmill testing ($P = 0.01$), displayed an enhanced capacity to perform the activities of daily living ($P < 0.04$), had a reduced cognitive deficit ($P = 0.05$), and required less use of other medications ($P < 0.05$).

Outcome

Limited information is available on the outcome of CFS. Maffulli and co-workers (58) concluded from a longitudinal study in eight varsity endurance runners with postviral fatigue syndrome that both aerobic and anaerobic exercise variables are seriously affected by postviral fatigue syndrome, and these subjects were not fully recovered by 1 year. Bonner and colleagues reported a follow-up study of 46 patients with CFS and offered treatment 4 years previously. Twenty-nine patients were interviewed, 3 patients refused an interview, and information on the remaining 14 was obtained from their general practitioners. All of the instruments used during the interview had been used in the initial study. The long-term prognosis for patients with CFS who initially responded to treatment was good. Spontaneous recovery in those who declined treatment or did not benefit from treatment was poor. Patients who continued to have CFS 4 years later had more somatic complaints, were more fatigued, and were more likely to have had a previous psychiatric history when they were initially assessed.

MITRAL VALVE PROLAPSE

Mitral valve prolapse is the most common human abnormality of heart valves, affecting roughly 4% of the population (22). The term MVP syndrome is loosely applied to patients who have a number of somatic and autonomic symptoms. The autonomic symptoms described in the literature are those of POTS in patients with MVP. Patients with MVP are reported to be sympathotonic. They have high urinary epinephrine and norepinephrine excretion, high plasma catecholamine concentrations (19), an abnormal catecholamine response to volume expansion, and a hyperresponse to adrenergic stimulation (4,28,87). Resting heart rate is increased and pulse pressure is excessively reduced on standing (28).

These patients may also have β-receptor supersensitivity. Davies and associates (19) studied nine women with MVP and symptoms and signs of β-adrenergic hypersensitivity and seven normal volunteer women. The heart rate and plasma norepinephrine increment was greater in these patients than in normal subjects. The dose of isoproterenol required to increase heart rate 25 bpm or to decrease mean arterial pressure 20 mm Hg was significantly less in the patients with MVP than in the volunteers.

Patients with MVP differed from control subjects by their widely oscillating HR during the upright posture and their exaggerated and prolonged bradycardia during the recovery phase of the Valsalva maneuver and after their return to recumbency in the postural test (12). This bradycardia persisted for 30 to 90 sec after BP returned to control values. Patients also showed a greater respiratory variation of the R-R interval (12). Coghlan and co-workers (12) postulate an abnormal central modulation of baroreflexes as the best explanation for the dysautonomic responses of symptomatic patients with prolapsed mitral valves.

Symptoms suggesting altered autonomic regulation of cardiovascular function have been noted in some patients with MVP and in patients with other disorders. Taylor and colleagues (87) evaluated cardiovascular responses in 118 patients with dysautonomia (78 of whom had MVP and 40 of whom did not) to determine if unique patterns of these responses distinguished patients in one symptomatic subgroup from patients in another. The responses of patients to standing, Valsalva maneuver, facial immersion in ice water, and administration of isoproterenol, phenylephrine, and tyramine were compared with those of 12 asymptomatic patients with MVP and 23 normal volunteers. Constitutional, cardiovascular, and neuropsychiatric symptoms occurred with similar frequency in the two symptomatic patient groups. The most common pattern of abnormal responses in symptomatic patients with or without MVP consisted of (1) an increased heart rate and elevated plasma norepinephrine levels while supine and then while standing quietly for 5 minutes, (2) an exaggerated increase in heart rate during phase II of the Valsalva maneuver, (3) a diminished bradycardic response during phase IV of the Valsalva maneuver, and (4) an exaggerated heart rate response to the administration of isoproterenol. The increased heart rate during Valsalva, but not the exaggerated sensitivity to isoproterenol, was correlated with the magnitude of the chronotropic response to standing only in symptomatic patients with MVP. Exaggerated hypertensive overshoot during phase IV of the Valsalva maneuver was observed in only a few symptomatic patients. No consistent pattern of these abnormalities, however, was noted in any of the patient subgroups. Hemodynamic responses in asymptomatic MVP patients were generally indistinguishable from those observed in normal subjects. The authors concluded that abnormal responses can occur in any patient with dysautonomia regardless of the presence or absence of MVP and that the pattern of these abnormal responses is not characteristic of MVP. Therefore, it is important to characterize the pattern of altered autonomic regulation of cardiovascular function in each patient when making therapeutic decisions about these patients.

The MVP syndrome is associated with a variety of atrial and ventricular arrhythmias. Some patients have bradyarrhythmias, which may be the cause of lightheadedness and syncope. Gonzalez (31) detailed the clinical and electrophysiologic characteristics of seven patients with symptomatic MVP and atrioventricular (AV) node dysfunction. The electrophysiology study demonstrated either a prolonged AH interval or abnormal response to atrial pacing in six of seven patients. A significant proportion of these patients had abnormalities of sinus node function and distal His–Purkinje conduction in addition to AV node dysfunction.

Management of the MVP syndrome is varied, and its efficacy appears to be dependent on the symptoms in the particular patient. Some symptoms are related to the arrhythmias. Some patients respond to the maintenance of adequate fluid intake and a generous salt intake, and postural training. Additional approaches are based on the observations of β-supersensitivity and α-adrenergic overactivity. Certain patients with MVP syndrome and high adrenergic tone may benefit from β-blockade (4).

Using the hypothesis that there is α-adrenergic overactivity, Gaffney and associates (28) measured hemodynamic and neuroendocrine responses to long-term oral clonidine therapy in eight women, aged 36 ± 1.8 years. None had responded favorably to β-blockers. Heart rate, blood pressure, oxygen consumption, cardiac output, and plasma norepinephrine levels were measured in both supine and standing positions, before and after 1 to 4 weeks of clonidine (0.3 to 0.4 mg daily). Clonidine reduced standing plasma norepinephrine levels, total peripheral resistance, and diastolic blood pressure; a smaller decrease in cardiac output on standing was noted. Plasma volumes increased 12%. Mild reductions in plasma catecholamines and total peripheral resistance are associated with fewer, not more, orthostatic symptoms in this group of patients. Another approach involved an attempt to desensitize β-receptors. Symptomatic patients with MVP were desensitized by a 4-hr isoproterenol infusion, whereas the sensitivity in normal control subjects did not change.

PROGNOSIS OF POSTURAL ORTHOSTATIC TACHYCARDIA SYNDROME

Limited information is available on prognosis. Our own experience has not yet been analyzed in sufficient detail. The variability in severity and the number of confounding variables are factors that render prognostication difficult. About one in four patients makes a good practical recovery, defined as the relative absence of orthostatic intolerance and the ability to perform activities of daily living with no or only minimal restriction. Khurana (43) reported a small experience with six patients. A follow-up of these patients 8 to 17 years after the autonomic evaluation showed spontaneous and complete improvement in two out of six, partial improvement in one out of six, and persistence of symptoms in three out of six patients.

MANAGEMENT OF POSTURAL ORTHOSTATIC TACHYCARDIA SYNDROME

Step 1: On the basis of a detailed history, an examination, and a general medical evaluation including ECG, it should be possible to decide if further evaluation is warranted. The patient with POTS (standing heart rate >120 bpm, consistent orthostatic symptoms, significant impairment in ability to perform activities of daily living—i.e., grade 3 or 4 by symptoms) should be further evaluated and treated. Many of the patients with mild orthostatic intolerance have a recognizable mechanism for orthostatic intolerance and may not need detailed evaluation. Such a patient might be an individual with constitutional orthostatic intolerance, deconditioning (patients confined to bed for more than a few days; debilitating illness), or hypovolemia.

Step 2: Once a decision is made to evaluate the patient, the study should include a cardiologic and autonomic laboratory evaluation. The cardiologic evaluation usually consists of a cardiologic interview and examination, an ECG, a chest x-ray, 24-hour Holter monitoring, and a decision as to whether cardiac electrophysiologic studies should be undertaken. Electrophysiologic testing is most useful in patients with heart disease that manifests as:

Abnormal ventricular function (reduced ejection fraction)
Abnormal ECG (conduction defect, ischemia, arrhythmia, multifocal ventricular ectopic beats)
Cardiac arrhythmia on Holter monitor (41)

It is likely that the value of electrophysiologic studies will follow the same guidelines used in patients with syncope. These studies are least useful in patients without heart disease, with an ejection fraction >40%, and with a normal ECG and normal Holter monitoring (79).

Step 3: The neurologic evaluation comprises a neurologic history, an examination (52), and tests (51,53,54), all looking for evidence of an autonomic neuropathy. The autonomic laboratory evaluation follows and consists of a modified autonomic reflex screen and thermoregulatory sweat test. The laboratory evaluation has two specific aims. The first aim is to establish if an autonomic neuropathy is present. The next aim is to seek, during an 80° tilt test of up to 20 min evidence of orthostatic intolerance (Chapter 15). Oscillations in BP are an index of sympathetic compensation, and a loss is indicative of adrenergic failure. Nevertheless, one of the manifestations of orthostatic intolerance is excessive oscillations, presumably indicating sympathovagal imbalance. The subsequent loss of these oscillations indicates pending presyncope. Finally, if the patient becomes presyncopal, the dramatic HR and BP fall should be documented. There is typically a gradual decline in BP for about 2 min before frank presyncope. Anxiety and tremulousness are also noted. We measure plasma volume and red cell mass, although these are usually normal. A 24-hr urinary sodium should be performed. Normal subjects should excrete >150 mmol/24 hrs. It may be helpful to measure venous pooling in the calf (85). This could be done after injection of the isotope for plasma volume estimations. One modification of the Streeten approach is to undertake repeated measurements of plasma volume with continued standing. There is some suggestion that patients with POTS will have a progressive fall in plasma volume, presumably reflecting a slow transudation of fluid into subcutaneous tissue.

Step 4: In selected subjects, additional studies are warranted. These include the isoproterenol infusion test for evidence of sympathetic β-adrenergic supersensitivity and the phenylephrine infusion test for α-adrenergic supersensitivity and establishment of the baroreflex gain. The HR response to tilt regresses with the response to isoproterenol infusion and therefore appears to be an indicator of β-receptor sensitivity. This can be used by clinicians who do not wish to undertake invasive testing. Supine and standing plasma norepinephrine values can be estimated as an index of adrenergic response, but they may be less sensitive than BP_{BB} recordings to the Valsalva maneuver.

Step 5: The cardiologic and autonomic evaluations are synthesized, and treatment is planned. POTS is best considered a syndrome of orthostatic intolerance rather than a disease sui generis. It is reasonable to document the presence and severity of POTS and to seek evidence of associated autonomic neuropathy, MVP, deconditioning, or a history of vasovagal syndrome. The severity of POTS, the plasma volume, the degree of vagotonia (degree and duration of reflex bradycardia with Valsalva maneuver and tilt-back, Valsalva ratio, and heart rate range), β-adrenergic supersensitivity (heart rate increment, anxiety, tremor, and reduction of muscle peripheral resistance), and central integration (blood pressure and heart rate oscillations) are determined. The patient is segregated to mechanistic categories, and treatment is individualized.

a. The deconditioned hypovolemic patient will do well sleeping with the head of the bed elevated and with plasma volume expanded with generous salt intake and fludrocortisone. The salt intake should be between 150 and 250 mEq of sodium (10–20 g of salt). Some patients are intensely sensitive to salt intake and can fine-tune their plasma volume and BP control with salt intake alone. Foods with a high salt content include fast foods like hamburgers, hot dogs, chicken pieces, fries, and fish fries. Canned soups, chili, ham, bacon, sausage, additives like soy sauce, and commercially processed canned products also have a high sodium content. The patient should have at least one glass or cup of fluids with their meals and at least two at other times each day to obtain 2 to 2.5 L/day. Fludrocortisone, with doses up to 1 mg in young subjects, can be used initially, with the dose adjusted downward to a maintenance dose of 0.1 to 0.4 mg/day. These patients should sleep with the head of the bed elevated 4 to 6 inches, a maneuver that can be highly beneficial for the patient's symptoms.

b. The patient with venous pooling needs a different approach to treatment. Body stockings may help as a temporary measure, but they are inconvenient and unphysiologic for long-term use. The best approach needs to be defined. Several approaches appear to work in some patients. Midodrine is efficacious in some patients, sometimes dramatically. In others, supplemental octreotide can be used for periods of orthostatic decompensation. Physical countermaneuvers (6,94) appear to be especially efficacious in venous poolers. Some patients seem to benefit with a 3-month program of graduated training. Resistance training may be more beneficial than endurance training but remains to be better documented. Although progressive heavy-strength training combined with explosive types of exercise clearly leads to considerable increases in maximal strength, in explosive force production, and in muscular.hypertrophy (35), the effects on orthostatic intolerance need to be better documented.

c. The patient with peripheral adrenergic failure, manifested as a loss of late phase II of the Valsalva maneuver or frank orthostatic hypotension, is best treated with fludrocortisone and an α-agonist. Midodrine appears to work best in terms of absorption, predictable duration of action, and lack of central nervous system side effects. An alternative agent is ephedrine, but this is poorly tolerated in POTS because it causes tachycardia and has central side effects. Phenylpropanolamine at a dose of 12.5 mg to 25 mg bid to tid can be used. An alternative agent is methylphenidate (e.g., Ritalin) at a dose of 5 mg to 10 mg bid or tid. The patient with florid POTS is likely β-receptor supersensitive. These patients respond to, but are sometimes exquisitely sensitive to, β-antagonists. At conventional doses, fatigue is a major problem. We use propranolol (e.g., Inderal), which may be more efficacious than the β-selective nonlipophilic agents at a dose of 10 mg per day, increasing over 2 to 3 weeks to 30 mg to 60 mg per day. The aim is to maintain the heart rate increment at about 50% of the pretreatment level. For patients with bronchospasm, a β-selective lipophilic agent such as metoprolol (e.g., Lopressor) can be used at a beginning dose of 25 mg daily and increased to a typical dose of 50 mg bid. For patients who have central side effects such as lethargy or depression, a nonlipophilic agent is preferred. Nadolol at a beginning dose of 10 mg every day, increasing as necessary to 40 mg, is a useful nonselective agent. β-Selective agents such as atenolol (e.g., Tenormin), betaxolol (e.g., Kerlone), and acebutolol (e.g., Sectral) can be used. Their beginning doses are 25 mg, 10 mg, and 200 mg, respectively.

d. A particularly difficult subset of patients have unstable hypertensive responses to tilt. Some of these patients have BP responses up to 250/150 on standing. Some of these patients with autonomic instability respond to oral phenobarbital, beginning with 60 mg at night and 15 mg every morning. An alternative treatment is clonidine or another $α_2$-agonist. Clonidine is administered at a dose of 0.1 mg bid and is increased to the maximally tolerated dose. Reports of a response to microvascular decompression of the brain stem have been reported, but its role is as yet undefined.

e. Some patients are seen during the acute postviral phase of the illness. Treatment with prednisone, plasma exchange, or intravenous gamma globulin may be considered, especially if there is additional evidence of an acute autonomic neuropathy. We recently adopted an aggressive laboratory-based approach to evaluate the mechanisms that are operative and to select the optimal approach to treatment. Patients are systematically evaluated with tilt studies before and after the administration of test agents. Cardiovascular indices are acquired with the use of BOMED and Finapres with the patient supine and then tilted for up to 20 min. The study is then repeated after administration of the test agent. The end points are symptomatic relief and improvement in cardiovascular parameters.

Step 1: Intravenous infusion of 1 L of isotonic saline over 30 to 60 min.
Step 2: Midodrine 10 mg po.
Step 3: Propranolol 40 mg po.
Step 4: Phenobarbital 120 mg po.
Step 5: Clonidine 0.2 mg po.

A minimum interval of 1 day is allowed to elapse before the next procedure. Intravenous saline is chosen as the first agent to rule out the effects of hypovolemia, although patients with increased capacitance due to venous pooling or poor vasomotor tone may also respond. Midodrine does not cross the blood–brain barrier, and the elimination of orthostatic tachycardia with midodrine suggests a primary peripheral adrenergic defect. Midodrine's actions are primarily on the resistance bed, but because it has some venoconstrictor effects (89), an effect on the capacitance bed cannot be excluded. If midodrine is ineffective or only partially beneficial, octreotide, which reduces splanchnic capacitance, is used, and normalization provides indirect evidence of a venomotor defect.

A correction of orthostatic tachycardia in response to propranolol is a pharmacologic effect of the drug and does not demonstrate the presence of β-receptor supersensitivity. In preliminary studies, patients who have β-receptor supersensitivity lose their orthostatic intolerance and tachycardia after the administration of propranolol, whereas those with compensatory cardioacceleration, because of peripheral adrenergic failure, lose their tachycardia but become more orthostatic and may develop orthostatic hypotension after the administration of propranolol. Patients whose orthostatic intolerance is normalized tend to have their supine and orthostatic power spectrum returned to normal after propranolol administration. Phenobarbital at the doses mentioned is centrally acting. Its actions in brain are complex, and its precise site or mode of action in improving POTS is unknown. The drug tends to suppress polysynaptic responses and has potent effects on the brain stem (57,72). Clonidine at the dose mentioned has primarily a central mode of action, diminishing central sympathetic outflow.

The global score for the improvement in orthostatic tolerance is graded as follows: 1 = mild; 2 = moderate; 3 = excellent degree of improvement. We have graded nine patients. The mean improvements in orthostatic tolerance in descending order were: midodrine 1.7 ± 1.2; saline 1.2 ± 0.8; Inderal 0.3 ± 1.7; phenobarbital −0.1 ± 1.1; and clonidine −0.8 ± 1.6. There is considerable individual variation.

CONCLUSION

The present approach is imperfect and will be supplanted by better approaches with new insights into POTS. Several approaches hold promise for elucidating pathophysiology and improving treatment. The first is the relation of cardiovascular parameters to indices of brain perfusion (e.g., transcranial Doppler) and oxygenation (EEG). Preliminary reports of a paradoxical vasoconstrictor rather than vasodilator response to tilt-up in patients with orthostatic intolerance are of interest (33,34,46). Coupled with transcranial Doppler studies is the quantitative evaluation of the EEG using power spectral analysis to relate changes in vasoregulation to brain oxygenation. Although very limited information is available on brain stem rhythms, the importance of especially the brain stem reticular formation has been appreciated by a number of authors (9,47,48). The medial brain stem reticular formation belongs to a common brain stem system for the integration of somatosensory and autonomic functions. All neurons are located in the medial two thirds of the reticular formation of the lower brain stem. These neurons are modulated by inputs from baroreceptors. They are subject to respiratory modulation, and their activity can be correlated with rhythms of the electrocorticogram. These neurons are also responsible for generating rhythmic discharges (48). The background EEG activity is modulated by certain slow rhythms, which may be of brain stem origin (64–66). These authors have characterized the periodic slower components as having average frequencies of 0.024 and 0.06 Hz. They hypothesize that this modulation reflects periodic discharges from the brain stem, because these frequencies are similar to the 20-second (0.05 Hz) and 1-minute (0.016 Hz) rhythms that have been recorded from brain stem cardiovascular and respiratory centers for BP regulation and respiratory movement in the cat and rabbit.

One mechanism that is potentially amenable to treatment is venous pooling (16) that results from known changes in the bulk, structure, and function of striated muscles that support the encased veins and propel venous return (7,17). Venous pooling is especially troublesome in POTS (56,85). Resistance training may be beneficial in reversing several of these abnormalities. Resistance exercise has been reported to result in an increase in plasma volume (16), and it results in an increase in simulated orthostatic tolerance. Resistance training has been reported to increase baroreflex gain (86). By increasing the size and strength of supporting muscles (14,15) in the legs and abdominal wall, resistance training is potentially efficacious in reducing orthostatic intolerance in POTS, perhaps by increasing the efficiency and capacity of this muscle pump (25, 88).

REFERENCES

1. Barnes PR et al. Skeletal muscle bioenergetics in the chronic fatigue syndrome. *J Neurol Neurosurg Psychiatry* 1993;56:679–683.
2. Boda WL et al. Gait abnormalities in chronic fatigue syndrome. J. Neurol. Sci. 131:156-161, 1995.
3. Bou-Holaigah I et al. The relationship between neurally mediated hypotension and the chronic fatigue syndrome (see comments). *JAMA* 1995;274:961–967.
4. Boudoulas H, Wooley CF. Mitral valve prolapse syndrome. Evidence of hyperadrenergic state (review). *Postgrad Med* 1988;152–162.
5. Boulenger JP et al. Increased sensitivity to caffeine in patients with panic disorders. Preliminary evidence. *Arch Gen Psychiatry* 1984; 41:1067–1071.
6. Bouvette CM et al. Role of physical countermaneuvers in the management of orthostatic hypotension: efficacy and biofeedback augmentation. *Mayo Clin Proc* 1996;71:847–853.
7. Buchanan P, Convertino VA. A study of the effects of prolonged simulated microgravity on the musculature of the lower extremities in man: an introduction. *Aviat Space Environ Med* 1989;60:649–652.
8. Buchwald D et al. Gender differences in patients with chronic fatigue syndrome. *J Gen Intern Med* 1994;9:397–401.
9. Calaresu FR, Yardley CP. Medullary basal sympathetic tone (review). *Annu Rev Physiol* 1988;50:511–524.
10. Camus F et al. Unexplained fever and chronic fatigue: abnormal circadian temperature pattern. *Eur J Med* 1992;1:30–36.
11. Cavanagh JB. Peripheral nerve changes in orthocresyl phosphate poisoning in the cat. *J Pathol Bacteriol* 1964;87:365–383.
12. Coghlan HC et al. Dysautonomia in mitral valve prolapse. *Am J Med* 1979;67:236–244.
13. Connolly S et al. Chronic fatigue: electromyographic and neuropathological evaluation. *J Neurol* 1993;240:435–438.
14. Convertino V, Hoffler GW. Cardiovascular physiology. Effects of microgravity. *J Fla Med Assoc* 1992;79:517–524.
15. Convertino VA. Neuromuscular aspects in development of exercise countermeasures. *Physiologist* 1991;34:S125–S128.
16. Convertino VA. Endurance exercise training: conditions of enhanced hemodynamic responses and tolerance to LBNP. *Med Sci Sports Exerc* 1993;25:705–712.
17. Convertino VA et al. Changes in volume, muscle compartment, and compliance of the lower extremities in man following 30 days of exposure to simulated microgravity. *Aviat Space Environ Med* 1989; 60:653–658.
18. Costa DC, et al. Brainstem perfusion is impaired in chronic fatigue syndrome. *Q J Med* 1995;88:767–773.
19. Davies AO et al. Mitral valve prolapse with symptoms of beta-adrenergic hypersensitivity. Beta 2-adrenergic receptor supercoupling with desensitization on isoproterenol exposure. *Am J Med* 1987;82:193–201.
20. DeLuca J et al. Neuropsychological impairments in chronic fatigue syndrome, multiple sclerosis, and depression. *J Neurol Neurosurg Psychiatry* 1995;58:38–43.
21. Demanet JC. Usefulness of noradrenaline and tyramine infusion tests in the diagnosis of orthostatic hypotension. *Cardiology* 1976;61 (suppl 1):213–224.

22. Devereux RB, et al. Mitral valve prolapse: causes, clinical manifestations, and management. *Ann Intern Med* 1989;111:305–317.
23. Edwards RH et al. Muscle histopathology and physiology in chronic fatigue syndrome. *Ciba Found Symp* 1993;173:102–117; discussion 117–123.
24. El-Sayed H, Hainsworth R. Salt supplementation increases plasma volume and orthostatic tolerance in patients with unexplained syncope. *Heart* 1996;75:134–140.
25. Epperson WL, et al. The influence of differential physical conditioning regimens on simulated aerial combat maneuvering tolerance. *Aviat Space Environ Med* 1982;53:1091–1097.
26. Ertl AC, et al. Postural effects on plasma volume in patients with orthostatic intolerance (abstr). *Clin Auton Res* 1995;5: 330A.
27. Fouad FM et al. Idiopathic hypovolemia. *Ann Intern Med* 1986; 104:298–303.
28. Gaffney FA et al. Abnormal cardiovascular regulation in the mitral valve prolapse syndrome. *Am J Cardiol* 1983;52:316–320.
29. Gibson H et al. Exercise performance and fatigability in patients with chronic fatigue syndrome (see comments). *J Neurol Neurosurg Psychiatry* 1993;56:993–998.
30. Goldenberg DL. Fibromyalgia, chronic fatigue syndrome, and myofascial pain syndrome (review). *Curr Opin Rheumatol* 1994;6:223–233.
31. Gonzalez ER. Pandora's box of autonomic ills found in some heart patients (news). *JAMA* 1981;245:107–108.
32. Grafman J et al. Analysis of neuropsychological functioning in patients with chronic fatigue syndrome. *J Neurol Neurosurg Psychiatry* 1993;56:684–689.
33. Grubb BP et al. Cerebral vasoconstriction during head-upright tilt-induced vasovagal syncope. A paradoxic and unexpected response. *Circulation* 1991;84:1157–1164.
34. Grubb BP et al. Head-upright tilt-table testing: a useful tool in the evaluation and management of recurrent vertigo of unknown origin associated with near-syncope or syncope. *Otolaryngol Head Neck Surg* 1992;107:570–576.
35. Hakkinen K, Hakkinen A. Neuromuscular adaptations during intensive strength training in middle-aged and elderly males and females. *Electromyogr Clin Neurophysiol* 1995;35:137–147.
36. Hoeldtke RD, Davis KM. The orthostatic tachycardia syndrome: evaluation of autonomic function and treatment with octreotide and ergot alkaloids. *J Clin Endocrinol Metab* 1991;73:132–139.
37. Hoeldtke RD et al. Sympathotonic orthostatic hypotension: a report of four cases. *Neurology* 1989;39:34–40.
38. Ichise M et al. Assessment of regional cerebral perfusion by 99Tcm-HMPAO SPECT in chronic fatigue syndrome. *Nucl Med Commun* 1992;13:767–772.
39. Insel TR et al. A benzodiazepine receptor-mediated model of anxiety. Studies in nonhuman primates and clinical implications. *Arch Gen Psychiatry* 1984;41:741–750.
40. Kafka MS et al. Alpha-adrenergic receptors in orthostatic hypotension syndromes. *Neurology* 1984;34:1121–1125.
41. Kapoor WN, et al. Diagnosis and natural history of syncope and the role of invasive electrophysiologic testing. *Am J Cardiol* 1989;63: 730–734.
42. Kent-Braun JA et al. Central basis of muscle fatigue in chronic fatigue syndrome (see comments). *Neurology* 1993;43:125–131.
43. Khurana RK. Orthostatic intolerance and orthostatic tachycardia: a heterogeneous disorder. *Clin Auton Res* 1995;5:12–18.
44. Kim E. A brief history of chronic fatigue syndrome. *JAMA* 1994; 272:1070–1071.
45. Komaroff AL et al. An examination of the working case definition of chronic fatigue syndrome. *Am J Med* 1996;100:56–64.
46. Krajewski A et al. Transcranial Doppler assessment of the cerebral circulation during postprandial hypotension in the elderly. *J Am Geriatr Soc* 1993;41:19–24.
47. Langhorst P, et al. Common brainstem system (CBS): a multifunctional "centre." In: Rother M, Zwiener U (eds). *Quantitative EEG Analysis—Clinical Utility and New Methods.* Jena: Universitatverlag Jena. 1993;228–239.
48. Langhorst P et al. Convergence of visceral and somatic afferents on single neurones in the reticular formation of the lower brain stem in dogs. *J Auton Nerv Syst* 1996;57:149–157.
49. Lerner AM, et al. Repetitively negative changing T waves at 24-h electrocardiographic monitors in patients with the chronic fatigue syndrome. Left ventricular dysfunction in a cohort. *Chest* 1993;104:1417–1421.
50. Lloyd A et al. Cytokine production and fatigue in patients with chronic fatigue syndrome and healthy control subjects in response to exercise. *Clin Infect Dis* 1994;18(suppl 1):S142–S146.
51. Low P et al. Measurement of endoneurial fluid pressure with polyethylene matrix capsules. *Brain Res* 1977;122:373–377.
52. Low PA. Clinical evaluation of autonomic function. In: Low PA (ed). *Clinical Autonomic Disorders: Evaluation and Management.* Boston: Little, Brown & Company. 1993;157–167.
53. Low PA. Autonomic nervous system function. *J Clin Neurophysiol* 1993;10:14–27.
54. Low PA. Laboratory evaluation of autonomic failure. In: Low PA (ed). *Clinical Autonomic Disorders: Evaluation and Management.* Boston: Little, Brown & Company. 1993;169–195.
55. Low PA et al. Postural tachycardia syndrome (POTS). *Neurology* 1995; 45(suppl 5):S19–S25.
56. Low PA et al. Comparison of the postural tachycardia syndrome (POTS) with orthostatic hypotension due to autonomic failure. *J Auton Nerv Syst* 1994;50:181–188.
57. Macdonald RL, McLean MJ. Cellular bases of barbiturate and phenytoin anticonvulsant drug action. *Epilepsia* 1982;23(suppl 1):S7–S18.
58. Maffulli N, et al. Post-viral fatigue syndrome. A longitudinal assessment in varsity athletes. *J Lab Clin Med* 1993;115: 549–558.
59. Manu P et al. Alpha-delta sleep in patients with a chief complaint of chronic fatigue (see comments). *South Med J* 1994;87:465–470.
60. Miller JW, Streeten DH. Vascular responsiveness to norepinephrine in sympathicotonic orthostatic intolerance. *J Lab Clin Med* 1990; 115:549–558.
61. Moldofsky H. Fibromyalgia, sleep disorder and chronic fatigue syndrome (review). *Ciba Found Symp* 1993;173:262–271;discussion 272–279.
62. Morriss R et al. Abnormalities of sleep in patients with the chronic fatigue syndrome. *Br Med J* 1993;306:1161–1164.
63. Mozes M, et al. Saphenous nerve entrapment simulating vascular disorder. *Surgery* 1975;77:299–303.
64. Novak P, Lepicovska V. Slow modulation of EEG. *Neuroreport* 1992; 3:189–192.
65. Novak P, et al. Periodic amplitude modulation of EEG. *Neurosci Lett* 1992;136:213–215.
66. Novak P, Novak V. Time/frequency mapping of the heart rate, blood pressure and respiratory signals. *Med Biol Eng Comput* 1993;31: 103–110.
67. Packer TL, et al. Fatigue secondary to chronic illness: postpolio syndrome, chronic fatigue syndrome, and multiple sclerosis. *Arch Phys Med Rehabil* 1994;75:1122–1126.
68. Peterson PK et al. Effects of mild exercise on cytokines and cerebral blood flow in chronic fatigue syndrome patients. *Clin Diagn Lab Immunol* 1994;1:222–226.
69. Plioplys AV, Plioplys S. Electron-microscopic investigation of muscle mitochondria in chronic fatigue syndrome. *Neuropsychobiology* 1995;32:175–181.
70. Polich J, et al. P300 assessment of chronic fatigue syndrome. *J Clin Neurophysiol* 1995;12:186–191.
71. Polinsky RJ et al. Pharmacologic distinction of different orthostatic hypotension syndromes. *Neurology* 1981; 31: 1–7.
72. Richter JA, Holtman JR Jr. Barbiturates: their in vivo effects and potential biochemical mechanisms. *Prog Neurobiol* 1982;18:275–319.
73. Robertson D et al. The diagnosis and treatment of baroreflex failure (see comments). *N Engl J Med* 1993;329:1449–1455.
74. Rosen SG, Cryer PE. Postural tachycardia syndrome. Reversal of sympathetic hyperresponsiveness and clinical improvement during sodium loading. *Am J Med* 1982;72:847–850.
75. Sandroni P, Benarroch EE, Low PA. Pharmacological dissection of components of the Valsalva maneuver in adrenergic failure. *J Appl Physiol* 1991;71:1563–1567.
76. Sandroni P et al. Early cardiovascular predictors of syncope (abstr). *Neurology* 1995;45:A396.
77. Schondorf R, Low PA. Idiopathic postural tachycardia syndrome. In: Low PA (ed). *Clinical Autonomic Disorders: Evaluation and Management.* Boston: Little, Brown & Company. 1993;641–652.
78. Schondorf R, Low PA. Idiopathic postural orthostatic tachycardia syndrome: an attenuated form of acute pandysautonomia? *Neurology* 1993; 43:132–137.

79. Shen W-K, Gersh BJ. Syncope: mechanisms, approach, and management. In: Low PA (ed). *Clinical Autonomic Disorders: Evaluation and Management.* Boston: Little, Brown & Company. 1993;605–640.
80. Sisto SA et al. Vagal tone is reduced during paced breathing in patients with the chronic fatigue syndrome. *Clin Auton Res* 1995;5:139–143.
81. Strayer DR et al. A controlled clinical trial with a specifically configured RNA drug, poly(I).poly(C12U), in chronic fatigue syndrome. *Clin Infect Dis* 1994; 18(suppl 1):S88–S95.
82. Streeten DH. Pathogenesis of hyperadrenergic orthostatic hypotension. Evidence of disordered venous innervation exclusively in the lower limbs. *J Clin Invest* 1990; 86:1582–1588.
83. Streeten DH et al. Abnormal orthostatic changes in blood pressure and heart rate in subjects with intact sympathetic nervous function: evidence for excessive venous pooling. *J Lab Clin Med* 1988;111:326–335.
84. Streeten DH et al. Orthostatic hypertension. Pathogenetic studies. *Hypertension* 1985;7:196–203.
85. Streeten DHP. *Orthostatic Disorders of the Circulation: Mechanisms, Manifestations and Treatment.* New York: Plenum Press. 1987.
86. Tatro DL, Dudley GA, Convertino VA. Carotid-cardiac baroreflex response and LBNP tolerance following resistance training. *Med Sci Sports Exerc* 1992;24:789–796.
87. Taylor AA et al. Spectrum of dysautonomia in mitral valvular prolapse. *Am J Med* 1989;86:267–274.
88. Tesch PA, et al. Effects of strength training on G tolerance. *Aviat Space Environ Med* 1983;54:691–695.
89. Thulesius O, et al. Vasoconstrictor effect of midodrine, ST 1059, noradrenaline, etilefrine and dihydroergotamine on isolated human veins. *Eur J Clin Pharmacol* 1979;16:423–424.
90. Triedman JK, et al. Mild hypovolemic stress alters autonomic modulation of heart rate. *Hypertension* 1993;21:236–247.
91. Tyrer P. Current status of beta-blocking drugs in the treatment of anxiety disorders. *Drugs* 1988;36:773–783.
92. Uhde TW et al. Behavioral and physiologic effects of short-term and long-term administration of clonidine in panic disorder. *Arch Gen Psychiatry* 1989;46:170–177.
93. Uhde TW, Tancer M. Chemical models of panic: a review and critique. In: Tyrer P (ed). *Psychopharmacology of Anxiety.* New York: Oxford University Press. 1988;110–131.
94. van Lieshout JJ, et al. Physical manoeuvres for combating orthostatic dizziness in autonomic failure. *Lancet* 1992; 339:897–898.
95. Whelton CL, et al. Sleep, Epstein-Barr virus infection, musculoskeletal pain, and depressive symptoms in chronic fatigue syndrome. *J Rheumatol* 1992;19:939–943.
96. Wise CD, et al. Benzodiazepines: anxiety-reducing activity by reduction of serotonin turnover in the brain. *Science* 1972; 177:180–183.
97. Wood C, et al. Fluctuations in perceived energy and mood among patients with chronic fatigue syndrome (see comments). *J R Soc Med* 1992;85:195–198.
98. Yatham LN et al. Neuroendocrine assessment of serotonin (5-HT) function in chronic fatigue syndrome. *Can J Psychiatry* 1995;40:93–96.

CHAPTER 50

Distal Small-Fiber Neuropathy

Michael J. Giuliani, John D. Stewart, and Phillip A. Low

1. Small-fiber neuropathy (SFN) results from pathologic processes causing preferential damage to small-diameter peripheral nerves.
2. Dysesthesias are common; clinical signs are minimal and frequently limited to reduced sensation of pinprick and temperature in the distal regions of the legs.
3. SFN and painful sensory neuropathy are not synonymous.
4. The most commonly diagnosed specific cause of SFN is diabetes mellitus.
5. Results of electromyographic (EMG) studies are normal; tests that specifically evaluate small nerve fibers are more valuable.
6. The causes of SFN are relatively few.
7. Symptomatic and specific treatment is available for SFN.

INTRODUCTION

As early as 1860, Brown-Séquard (16) stated, "We think . . . that the (peripheral) nerve fibers employed for the transmission of . . . sensitive impressions are as distinct from the others as they all are from the nerve fibers employed in the transmission of the orders of the will to muscles. . . . The kinds of sensitive impressions which have different conductors are those giving the sensations of touch, tickling, pain, heat and cold." This clear realization of the correlation between the morphology and function of peripheral nerve fibers was followed by the concept that peripheral neuropathies can selectively involve certain populations of nerve fibers. In a brilliant article published 25 years later, Pavy (79) observed that whereas some diabetic patients have an ataxic, "pseudotabetic" neuropathy, others have burning "neuritic" pain in the feet without ataxia. In the former situation, predominant involvement of the large-diameter, myelinated peripheral nerve fibers with the loss of proprioception gives rise to ataxia; the latter condition results from predominant involvement of small-diameter nerve fibers.

Some may question the need for a separate category for SFN, as this category may be incorporated within the realm of sensory neuropathy. A separate distinction is justified for two reasons: The differential diagnosis for an SFN is more restricted than that for sensory neuropathy, which limits diagnostic options and testing. The second theoretical justification is that the size of the involved fiber may determine the choice of experimental treatments for various neuropathies. For example, nerve growth factor (NGF) has preferential trophic effects on small fibers. NGF and other trophic factors with similar properties may be logical choices for therapeutic intervention in SFNs.

Certain misconceptions are widely held with respect to SFNs. The most common misconception is that the presence of pain indicates the presence of an SFN. Large-fiber neuropathies can be painful, and conversely, some SFNs do not have pain as a major feature. Another major misconception is that SFN represents an early phase of a sensory neuropathy. Part of this misconception is that an SFN will evolve into a more typical pattern of large- and small-fiber dysfunction. There are well-documented cases of patients followed for many years in whom progression to involvement of large sensory fibers did not occur (91). Another misconception is that the presence of any evidence of large-fiber dysfunction, either clinically or histopathologically, excludes the diagnosis of SFN. Frequently, with careful investigation, some minimal evidence of large-fiber dysfunction will be found, either clinically or, even more often, histopathologically. If most of the evidence falls

M. J. Giuliani: Department of Neurology, University of Pittsburgh-Presbyterian University Hospital, Pittsburgh, Pennsylvania 15213.
J. D. Stewart: Department of Neurology and Neurosurgery, McGill University, Montreal, Quebec H3A 2B4, CANADA.
P. A. Low: Department of Neurology, Mayo Clinic, Rochester, Minnesota 55905.

TABLE 1. Morphology and function of peripheral nerve fibers

Morphology	Function
Large-diameter myelinated fibers	Skeletal muscle efferents (α motoneurons)
	Tendon reflex afferents
	Vibration and proprioception afferents
	Some skin touch afferents
Small-diameter myelinated fibers	Preganglionic sympathetic efferents
	γ Efferents to intrafusal spindle muscle fibers
	Cold sensory afferents
Small-diameter unmyelinated fibers	Warm sensory afferents
	Pain afferents
	Some skin touch afferents
	Autonomic efferents
	Sympathetic postganglionic
	Parasympathetic pre- and postganglionic
	Autonomic afferents

From Light and Perl, ref. 60; Mackenzie et al., ref. 67; and Valbo et al., ref. 100.

within the domain of small-fiber dysfunction, the classification into a category of SFN is warranted.

Small-fiber dysfunction can be defined as a generalized peripheral neuropathy in which the small-diameter myelinated and unmyelinated nerve fibers are affected, either exclusively or to a much greater degree than the large-diameter myelinated fibers (7,95). Although this definition is adequate for a conceptual image of SFN, it is not specific enough to apply in the clinical and research settings. A good working definition was established by Stewart et al. (91). It encompasses features of dysesthesia along with abnormalities on neurologic examination limited principally to small-fiber dysfunction. Exclusion criteria include proprioceptive loss in the toes, vibration loss at or above the ankles, any distal wasting or weakness, generalized areflexia, or abnormal findings on EMG. Although this definition is quite specific and applicable, both clinically and for research, these delineations are empiric. A challenge to investigators and clinicians is to determine how much large-fiber dysfunction can be allowed within the category of SFN while retaining the important implications of this category for diagnosis and treatment.

By correlating the morphology of peripheral nerve fibers with their functions (Table 1), it can be seen that in SFN the sensations of pain and temperature are mainly depressed. In addition, patients often have dysesthesias, consisting of sensations of tingling, prickling, and burning (40). As in many other peripheral neuropathies, the longest nerve fibers are involved first, so the earliest symptoms and signs arise in the feet. Because autonomic functions are also mediated mainly by unmyelinated fibers, sweating and sometimes vasomotor abnormalities may occur in the feet as well. Other autonomic functions, such as blood pressure, heart rate, gastrointestinal and genitourinary function, and glandular secretions, are sometimes affected.

In the past 40 years, it has become apparent that the neuropathy associated with some types of familial amyloidosis also has a predilection for small-diameter fibers. These two disorders, diabetic and amyloid neuropathy, are therefore the "clinical prototypes" of SFN. Other causes are limited; recognition that a neuropathy is mainly small-fiber in type is a first step in the search for the cause (Table 2).

TABLE 2. Causes of small-fiber neuropathy

Common causes
  Diabetes mellitus
  Primary systemic amyloidosis
  Idiopathic
  Hereditary
    HSAN types I, IV, and V
    Burning foot dominantly inherited sensory neuropathy
    Tangier disease (hereditary high-density-lipoprotein deficiency)
    Fabry's disease (α-galactosidase A deficiency)
Rare causes
  Nutritional neuropathies
  AIDS
  Alcohol
  Toxins and drugs
  Monoclonal gammopathy/antisulfatide antibodies
  Hyperlipidemia
  Cancer
  Primary biliary cirrhosis

HSAN, hereditary sensory and autonomic neuropathy.

CAUSES OF SMALL-FIBER NEUROPATHY

Diabetic Small-Fiber Neuropathy

Diabetes mellitus may be the most common single diagnosed cause of SFN. It has been estimated that SFN comprises about 10% of the different varieties of diabetic peripheral neuropathies (15). Diabetic distal symmetric polyneuropathy ranges from chiefly small-fiber to mainly large-fiber involvement, but most patients have varying combinations of both (Chapter 37). Many of these patients may have positive symptoms regardless of the fiber type involved, although those denoting pure larger-fiber neuropathy are infrequent. Therefore, it is difficult to judge specifically whether the neuropathy is exclusively small-fiber in type. Furthermore, evidence of small-fiber dysfunction can be detected by testing diabetic patients with no neuropathic symptoms, showing that small-fiber damage can be asymptomatic (38,56,88,105).

SFN has general medical implications in diabetes regarding mortality. Autonomic neuropathy in diabetes is an important risk factor for sudden death (9b,28b,28c,35a,74). The presence of autonomic cardiovascular abnormalities has been correlated with the development of diabetic foot ulcers. The extent of neuropathy correlates positively with the risk for development of foot ulcers. Most patients with diabetic foot ulcers have both large- and small-fiber neuropathy (1). However, the loss of nociceptive function is particularly important (39a,76).

Diabetic SFN can be divided clinically into three subtypes: pure SFN, pseudosyringomyelic SFN, and acute painful neuropathy.

Pure Small-Fiber Neuropathy

Pure SFN is the most common type of diabetic SFN. The presenting symptoms and signs are those just described. Reduced or absent ankle reflexes and mild vibration impairment in the big toes are usual findings. Sural nerve sensory action potentials are also often abnormal, reflecting mild associated large-fiber dysfunction. Biopsy specimens of nerves from patients with pure diabetic SFN have shown a moderate loss of large myelinated fibers and a severe depletion of unmyelinated fibers (15a). Most patients with pure SFN do not have generalized autonomic dysfunction except for erectile impotence, which is common in male patients. This may well be an early symptom of SFN involving the sympathetic and parasympathetic nerve fibers that control erection and ejaculation (30,90).

Adequate longitudinal studies have not been performed in these patients, but it is generally thought that small peripheral nerve fibers are damaged earlier than are the large ones (37,56,105), and that diabetic SFN evolves into a mixed large- and small-fiber sensorimotor neuropathy. However, there are case reports of objective improvement when the diabetes is rigorously controlled (36).

Pseudosyringomyelic Small-Fiber Neuropathy

Said et al. (83) have described a group of diabetic patients with type I disease who had profound suppression of pain and temperature sensations in the hands and often the feet, with sparing of other sensations. This dissociation of sensations, characteristically seen in syringomyelia, is the basis for the name of this type of diabetic SFN. Autonomic symptoms and signs were frequent in this group of patients, as was the case in one subgroup of the patients described by Brown et al. (15a). Painless burns and gangrene of the toes stemming from arterial disease, plantar ulcers, and neurogenic arthropathy were also present. All patients had mild but definite clinical and electrophysiologic evidence of large-fiber dysfunction. Nerve biopsy specimens showed a severe loss of unmyelinated and small myelinated fibers and a mild to moderate depletion of large myelinated fibers.

Acute Painful Neuropathy

Acute painful neuropathy occurs in patients with diabetes of short duration. It is characterized by the acute onset of burning neuropathic pain, mainly in the distal regions of the legs (2). Associated symptoms include severe weight loss, erectile impotence, insomnia, and depression. Neurologic examination generally shows reduced sensation of light touch, pinprick, and temperature in the toes, feet, or legs, hypersensitivity to touch but no sensory loss, or normal sensory findings. Testing of heart rate reveals abnormalities in about half the patients. Nerve conduction studies also show mild abnormalities. Evidence of active degeneration of both myelinated and unmyelinated nerve fibers is seen in nerve biopsy specimens. With good control of the diabetes, these patients usually gain weight and the neuropathic symptoms and signs abate remarkably.

Amyloidosis

The amyloidoses are multisystem diseases caused by deposition of the complex protein amyloid in various tissues throughout the body (see also Chapter 36). The three major types are primary systemic amyloidosis, heredofamilial amyloidosis, and secondary amyloidosis. Primary systemic amyloidosis is probably always the result of a plasma cell dyscrasia. Twenty percent of such patients have multiple myelomas, whereas most of the others have a nonmyeloma monoclonal protein in either the serum or urine, or both (50). The heredofamilial amyloidoses are divided into five types based on clinical and genetic differences (19). Secondary amyloidosis is seen in the context of chronic inflammatory illnesses, some tumors, and familial Mediterranean fever. SFN is seen in patients with primary systemic amyloidosis and heredofamilial amyloidosis types I, II, and III.

Primary Systemic Amyloidosis

The clinical presentation of primary systemic amyloidosis depends on the organs involved. About 15% of patients have peripheral neuropathy (50). The clinical features of this group have been reviewed by Kelly et al. (45). In their series, 13 of 31 patients were initially seen with evidence of predominant peripheral neuropathy, and the other 18 had symptoms and signs involving the peripheral nervous system as well as other organ systems. Patients in whom peripheral neuropathy is the sole presenting manifestation of amyloidosis have a better prognosis (22c). The neuropathic symptoms are typically the same as those described earlier in this chapter, and symptoms of carpal tunnel syndrome are frequently present. Most patients also have symptoms of generalized autonomic dysfunction.

The clinical signs of neuropathy usually include prominent impairment of pinprick and temperature sensation, with lesser involvement of vibration sensation and proprioception. Kelly et al. (45) found that sensations of pinprick and temperature were predominantly affected in 52% of their patients, vibration and position loss were the most marked signs in 16%, and all senses were equally affected in 32%. In addition, patients frequently displayed some distal weakness and ankle areflexia. Signs of autonomic involvement, such as poorly reactive pupils and orthostatic hypotension, were common.

Electrophysiologic studies often reveal evidence of the involvement of the large myelinated motor and sensory fibers. Tests of sweating show impairment in the extremities. Nerve biopsy specimens have shown a marked loss of both myelinated and unmyelinated nerve fibers (96).

In summary, at the time of presentation, the neuropathy of primary systemic amyloidosis is usually characterized by prominent features of small-fiber dysfunction, but often some coexisting large-fiber damage as well. Autonomic involvement, both of the distal limbs and other organs, is usually clearly evident. It is possible that very early on the peripheral neuropathy is exclusively small-fiber in type, but as the disease progresses, all fiber types become involved to produce a severe sensorimotor peripheral neuropathy (45,96).

Familial Amyloidosis Types I, II, and III

The onset of the neuropathy in familial amyloidosis types I, II, and III occurs earlier than in primary systemic amyloidosis, and the progression is slower. The clinical features of the peripheral neuropathy and dysautonomia are similar to those of primary systemic amyloidosis. With time, a severe sensorimotor type of neuropathy develops (19,24). Nerve biopsy specimens show a moderate loss of myelinated nerve fibers with a profound depletion of unmyelinated fibers (24). Familial amyloid polyneuropathy can be identified by several techniques that measure variant transthyretin from sera. Several proteins have been associated with inherited amyloid polyneuropathy, including transthyretin, gelsolin, and apolipoprotein A-I. Genetic screening resulting in the identification of point mutation is also possible (70b,81b).

Alcoholic Neuropathy

The neuropathy of alcoholics can be categorized into purely sensory and sensorimotor types (9,101). Of 37 patients in their study, Behse and Buchthal (9) found that half had mainly sensory signs. All modalities were affected, and the ankle reflexes were absent, indicating large- and small-fiber involvement. EMG studies showed subclinical motor involvement. In Victor's series of 189 cases (101), 26% had sensory neuropathy, and about 25% of these had involvement of mainly small fibers. Paresthesias, including "burning feet," are a common symptom in patients with alcoholic neuropathy, regardless of the clinical pattern of the neuropathy (9,101). Histologic studies of nerve biopsy specimens from patients with alcoholic neuropathy show changes of axonal degeneration that involve both myelinated and unmyelinated fibers (9,99,103). It is therefore common for the small nerve fibers to be affected in patients with alcoholic neuropathy, but most patients with alcoholic neuropathy have evidence of large-fiber involvement. However, in one series with sophisticated screening, 20% of the patients had only small-fiber dysfunction. Investigators have concluded that thermal testing significantly contributes to the diagnosis of alcoholic neuropathy, frequently because of the involvement of small fibers (39b,39c).

Nutritional Neuropathies

In times of famine and war, large numbers of people are afflicted by neuropathies, a topic that was well reviewed by Victor (101). Symptoms begin with dysesthesias in the feet, which often become exceedingly painful—hence the term *burning foot*. Neurologic signs vary from those of SFN to severe sensorimotor neuropathy. Variably associated signs consist of nutritional amblyopia and dermatitis. The likely cause is a deficiency of a variety of B vitamins and other nutrients.

In one study, beriberi neuropathy was diagnosed in 32 individuals imprisoned in Japanese war camps during World War II. These prisoners were studied and evaluated both clinically and electrophysiologically. Most of them had evidence of large-fiber neuropathy. Only one patient in this series had neuropathy on clinical examination with no evidence of peripheral neuropathy on EMG and nerve conduction studies. The authors postulated that the patient's symptoms were related to small-fiber dysfunction. No tests to confirm small-fiber dysfunction were performed. In conclusion, nutritional neuropathy may cause pure SFN, but there is much more likely to be concomitant large-fiber involvement (39d).

Hereditary Neuropathies

With the exception of hereditary sensory and autonomic neuropathy (HSAN) type I, the hereditary neuropathies are all rare (23).

Hereditary Sensory and Autonomic Neuropathy Type I

HSAN type I is probably dominantly inherited. The clinical manifestations vary from one patient to another, but onset is usually in the second decade with symptoms in the feet, and progress is insidious. Dysesthesias and neuropathic pains may be manifested early, as well as reduced pain and thermal sensation. Because of the dysesthesias, ulcers and other damage to the feet develop. In the early stages, sensations of pinprick and temperature as well as sweating are reduced in the feet. Other sensations are involved in more severely affected patients, and there is some distal muscle wasting and weakness. Nerve biopsy specimens show a marked loss of unmyelinated nerve fibers, a moderate loss of small myelinated fibers, and a minimal loss of large myelinated fibers. Patients in later stages of the disease show a substantial depletion of large myelinated fibers.

Familial Dysautonomia

Familial dysautonomia, also known as *Riley-Day syndrome* and *HSAN type III*, is a rare disorder. One of its many features is a lack of pain sensation that can lead to damage from burns, trauma, and infection. However, the many additional symptoms and signs resulting from widespread abnormalities in the autonomic nervous system outweigh the features of SFN.

Congenital Sensory Neuropathy with Anhidrosis

Children affected by congenital sensory neuropathy with anhidrosis (HSAN type IV) usually have widespread loss of pain and temperature sensation that may lead to mutilation, ulceration, and bone fractures. Associated features include motor and mild mental retardation. Nerve specimens obtained at biopsy show a mild reduction in the number of small myelinated fibers and a marked loss of unmyelinated fibers.

Hereditary Sensory and Autonomic Neuropathy Type V

HSAN type V represents a less well-defined group of disorders, but the essential features are selective loss of pain perception and sweating in a peripheral distribution, with disease onset in childhood.

Other, Unclassified Hereditary Sensory and Autonomic Neuropathies

Some forms of HSAN are quite rare. Descriptions of these neuropathies are usually case reports or small series. In one report, HSAN has been described in which loss of pain was the only evident symptom (63a). HSANs are not exclusively seen in young patients and rarely onset occurs later in older patients (67a).

Burning Foot Dominantly Inherited Sensory Neuropathy

The inherited sensory neuropathy with the dominant symptom of burning foot has not yet been included in Dyck's classification of HSANs (28). These patients have chronic burning dysesthesias in the feet. The few who have been examined carefully, with one exception, showed no clinical evidence of a neuropathy, but a nerve biopsy specimen showed minor abnormalities in one patient.

Hereditary Neuropathies with Specific Metabolic Defects

Tangier Disease

Tangier disease is also known as *hereditary high-density-lipoprotein deficiency*. Neurologic involvement is common. There are several prototypes of neuropathy: a relapsing and asymmetric neuropathy, a syringomyelia-like syndrome, and a slowly progressive symmetric neuropathy. Acute presentations are rare (29a). The generalized neuropathy may initially be manifested as extensive loss of pain and temperature sensations, but other sensory modalities are not involved. The pattern of distribution is highly unusual in that the distal parts of the limbs are usually spared. Coexisting signs of this disorder are facial and intrinsic hand muscle weakness (39).

Fabry's Disease

The main symptom of Fabry's disease, which results from a deficiency of α-galactosidase A, is burning pain in the extremities, which is often severe. Patients have characteristic skin lesions, angiokeratoma corporis diffusum. Neurologic examination findings are usually normal, but nerve biopsy tissue shows a loss of small myelinated and unmyelinated fibers (14). Abnormalities in cutaneous thermal sensation are common, with elevations of cold sensitivity thresholds preceding and surpassing the elevations of heat sensation thresholds (70a).

Acquired Immunodeficiency Syndrome

Peripheral neuropathies of different types occur in the various stages of infection with human immunodeficiency virus (20,78). Patients with both distal sensorimotor and painful sensory peripheral neuropathy always first have dysesthesias and pain in the feet (8,20,33,52,69,80). Clinical examination reveals abnormalities of distal muscles and of all sensations in patients with distal sensorimotor neuropathy, and abnormalities of all sensations in those with painful sensory peripheral neuropathy, in addition to absence of ankle reflexes. Nerve biopsy specimens show involvement of large and small fibers. However, a few patients with AIDS may actually have SFN.

Toxic Neuropathies

The degree of motor, sensory, and autonomic involvement varies with the toxic agent or drug and the degree of exposure. In many cases, a patient with a toxic neuropathy first has sensory symptoms that include dysesthesias, but by the time the patient is evaluated, the neuropathy involves both motor and sensory large- and small-diameter fibers. It is possible that these sensorimotor neuropathies go through a phase of SFN. Neuropathies associated with exposure to arsenic, thallium, disulfiram, gold, isoniazid, perhexiline, and cisplatinum all fall into this category (53, 54,104).

The most conspicuous toxic cause of SFN is prolonged treatment with metronidazole. Nerve biopsy specimens from such patients have shown involvement of both myelinated and unmyelinated fibers (13). Neurologic assessment of patients with Crohn's disease who take metronidazole on a long-term basis demonstrates quantitative abnormalities on sensory testing. These consist of elevated thresholds of perception for discriminating warmth from cold; at the same time, results of vibration testing remain normal. Whether these findings represent an effect of metronidazole or of Crohn's disease could not be ascertained (88a).

Pyridoxine toxicity typically affects large-fiber sensory axons. However, when pyridoxine was administered to healthy volunteers, the earliest abnormality in subjects given low doses was an elevation of the thermal threshold in the toes. These quantitative abnormalities on sensory testing preceded nerve conduction abnormalities in low-dose subjects (10a). High doses of pyridoxine also caused large-fiber dysfunction and therefore did not show the same tendency to involve small fibers. This observation may predict the development of SFN with appropriate doses and duration of pyridoxine therapy.

Propafenone hydrochloride is a new antiarrhythmic agent. In one case report, the development of SFN has been attributed to this compound. Results of thermoregulatory sweat test and autonomic tests were abnormal, confirming the clinical diagnosis of SFN. Pathologic examination of the sural nerve revealed widespread loss of the unmyelinated fibers (33a). As a result of this observation, the short list of toxic agents known to cause SFN has been expanded.

Monoclonal Gammopathy/Antisulfatide Antibodies

Monoclonal gammopathy is usually thought to cause large-fiber demyelinating neuropathy. However, neuropathies associated with monoclonal antibodies are heterogeneous. Most of these neuropathies significantly involve large fibers. Small-fiber function has been investigated in these patients and found to be abnormal (8a). Whether monoclonal gammopathy without amyloid production leads to the development of SFN and whether this association is causal are important questions for further investigation.

The presennce of antisulfatide antibodies represents an important subgroup of monoclonal gammopathies. Antisulfatide antibodies are not specific for any neurologic condition. However, they have been reported to occur in predominantly sensory axonal neuropathies. Whether these antibodies are important in the pathogenesis of any form of neuropathy remains unproven. The association of antisulfatide antibodies with SFN has been reported (79a,100a). Whether this observation represents a specific syndrome with treatment implications must be clarified.

Neuropathy Associated with Hyperlipidemia

In a recent report, six patients with markedly increased triglyceride levels had clinical features of SFN. However, there was frequent evidence of large-fiber dysfunction in this group. One patient showed symptomatic improvement after the serum triglycerides were lowered. Confirmation of the existence of a specific syndrome based on the findings in this report, and particularly its response to treatment, will necessitate further investigation with a larger patient population (68c).

Lyme Disease

A single patient infected with *Borrelia burgdorferi* in whom a large-fiber neuropathy developed has been reported by Hughes et al. (39e). Eight months after treatment, the patient was found to have only a residuum of small-fiber dysfunction. The evidence is vague regarding whether small-fiber dysfunction is ever a presenting feature of Lyme disease.

Cancer

Several types of neuropathy commonly develop as a neuromuscular complication of malignancy. Large-fiber involvement is most prevalent. Small-fiber dysfunction has been investigated in cancer patients. Quantitative sensory testing demonstrated a very high proportion of patients with elevated thermal thresholds (61b), with 50% demonstrating such abnormalities. The majority of patients with small-fiber dysfunction did not have concomitant large-fiber dysfunction. Therefore, with careful screening, SFN appears to be relatively common with malignancy. The etiology of small-fiber damage is unknown (61b). The relevance of the frequent finding of subclinical small-fiber involvement to the occasional patient with symptomatic SFN needs to be determined.

Primary Biliary Cirrhosis

SFN can develop in patients with primary biliary cirrhosis, which is associated with prominent dysesthesias that are usually painful. By the time the neuropathy appears, the signs of liver failure are evident (98). Neuropathy is common in these patients, manifested in possibly up to 40% of cases. The presence of SFN in primary biliary cirrhosis may have important implications. As in diabetes, prolongation of the QT interval in chronic liver disease is an indicator of the severity of autonomic neuropathy and appears to be an important risk factor for death (38a). A plausible treatment is available for the neuropathy associated with primary biliary cirrhosis; plasmapheresis has been used successfully to treat this neuropathy (19a,92a).

Vasculitis

Vasculitis usually presents as multiple mononeuropathies or a distal sensory motor axonopathy with significant large fiber involvement. Recently, a small case series was reported where small fiber neuropathy was attributed to vasculitis. *(Arthritis & Rheumatism* 1997;40:1173–77.)

Idiopathic Small-Fiber Neuropathy

In previous reports of SFN, diabetes, postviral infection, alcohol abuse, nutritional defects, and heredity were considered as etiologic factors. In most cases, however, the cause was not determined (41,91). The diagnosis, management, and treatment of idiopathic distal SFN is one of the most vexing problems facing clinicians. Routinely, the treatment of SFN depends on its pathogenesis. Tight control of diabetes is pivotal in the prevention of diabetic neuropathy (22b). SFN of other causes, such as amyloidosis, toxins, and alcohol, is also best approached through its primary pathogenesis. With idiopathic SFN, this approach is not possible. Such patients are frequently referred to a neurologist because of their significant morbidity. They also pose a diagnostic dilemma because idiopathic SFN is a diagnosis of exclusion. These patients have significant complaints without many of the classic signs of peripheral neuropathy. Therefore, their problems are misunderstood as being as functional, or they are thought to be embellishing a minor physical ailment. Information about prognosis, treatment, and the evolution of this disorder is of great importance.

Retrospective Review of Idiopathic Small-Fiber Neuropathy

Methods

Although information is available regarding distal SFN, it is not known whether this knowledge is applicable to idiopathic distal SFN. To determine the prognosis, clinical features, and evolution of idiopathic distal SFN, a retrospective review was conducted of all patients referred to the autonomic laboratory at the Mayo Clinic between 1986 and 1995. More than 300 patients were referred for the evaluation of neuropathy or SFN during this period. All cases considered for inclusion had an onset of distal symmetric symptoms in the feet with a lack of large-fiber sensory loss or weakness. Reflexes had to be preserved, except at the ankle. No evidence of large-fiber neuropathy could be revealed by nerve conduction studies. Patients with prominent bladder dysfunction, gastrointestinal disorders, or orthostatic hypotension were excluded to eliminate cases of pandysautonomia. Patients with other neurologic conditions that could obscure the analysis of clinical symptoms and prognosis were also excluded. These conditions included radiculopathy, lumbar canal stenosis, Guillain-Barré syndrome, peripheral vascular disease, porphyria, myelopathy, spinal cord arteriovenous malformation, multiple sclerosis, and syrinx. Sixty-one patients were excluded for signs of large-fiber neuropathy on examination. Seventy patients were excluded because nerve conduction studies indicated large-fiber involvement. Large-fiber neuropathy as evidenced by EMG or clinical examination was the cause of exclusion in the largest group. Twenty patients were excluded because of diabetes. Thirty-nine patients were identified as appropriate candidates for further analysis. The remaining patients were excluded for any of the following: lack of distal onset, concomitant conditions, or a known cause of neuropathy.

Of the 39 patients included in this review, 23 were women and 16 were men. Their mean age was age 58 years. The age range was 25 to 82 years, with a standard deviation of 13.7. The patients' subjective characterization of the clinical symptoms resulted in many descriptors. In this series, 15 descriptors were elicited from the patients. However, six descriptors were most commonly reported (Table 3).

Presentation/Onset/Course

Of the 39 patients, 27 had constant discomfort. Eight patients originally had intermittent discomfort that progressed to become constant, and only four described intermittent sensory phenomena. A number of patients described a certain physical modality that gave them significant relief. However, the physical modality that provided relief was not constant in this group of patients. Thir-

TABLE 3. *Clinical symptoms of idiopathic small-fiber neuropathy in 39 patients*

Descriptor	Patients affected, No.
Type of burning	30
Tingling	15
Numbness	12
Aching	8
Prickling	6
Cold	5

teen of the 39 patients obtained significant relief by either lowering or raising the temperature of the extremity, or massaging the extremity. Seven of the 13 patients found cold to be the modality that gave the most relief. Five obtained significant relief with heat, and one with massage. The gradual onset of symptoms in the majority of patients was also stereotypic. Four patients described an acute onset, whereas two had relapsing symptoms.

The average duration of symptoms was 4 years, and the time to diagnosis was 3.4 years. All patients had significant morbidity. Seven of the 39 patients had decreased functional scales and problems with the activities of daily living.

In summary, positive symptoms usually predominate. However, rare patients are first seen with only negative symptoms. Often, pain is the major presenting manifestation of large-fiber neuropathy. Painful sensory neuropathy and SFN are not equivalent. A history of symptomatic relief obtained by physical modalities should be specifically sought, and this may be helpful in both the management and diagnosis of this disorder. Frequently, a long time elapses before the diagnosis is made, with no evidence of a progression to large-fiber neuropathy. Morbidity in this group of patients is significant, with some occasional minor disability.

Results of Examination

Mild impairment of vibratory sensation was permitted in the toes and feet, and 13 of the 39 patients had mild deficits. Proprioception abnormalities were limited, by design, to the toes and had to be only partial. Only 2 of the 39 patients had any deficit of proprioception. The most common deficit was a reduced sensation of pinprick, and 23 of the 39 patients had clinical deficits involving pinprick. Most abnormalities were limited to the level of the toes or feet. Four patients had involvement in both the hands and feet. Five patients had deficits that extended more proximally. It should be noted that these examination features were biased by the fact that they were utilized as part of the exclusion criteria. The reflex examination was also part of the exclusion criteria and was therefore also biased. Two patients had slightly reduced knee reflexes. Of particular interest, only two patients had absent ankle jerks. Eight had slightly reduced ankle reflexes.

Conclusion

Several features of SFN are forthcoming from this analysis. Loss of pinprick sensation is not universal, and allodynia can be present without the ability to document loss of pinprick sensation at the bedside. Although subtle features of large-fiber neuropathy can be present, a significant disparity exists between large- and small-fiber findings. The term *small-fiber neuropathy* is a clinical designation that denotes a marked significant preferential involvement of the small fibers.

Treatment

Treatment of SFN is problematic, reflected by the various medications prescribed. Side effects were frequent and often resulted in dose limitations or noncompliance. Medications utilized included narcotics, tricyclics, steroids, capsaicin, anticonvulsant agents (valproic acid, carbamazepine, phenytoin, clonazepam), antiarrhythmic agents (lidocaine hydrochloride, mexiletine hydrochloride), antipsychotics (fluphenazine), and skeletal muscle relaxants (baclofen). Only 20 patients had adequate documentation of treatment response. Nine of 20 patients responded, but only partially. No patient had complete relief of symptoms. Tricyclic agents were the most frequently reported efficacious therapy.

Testing

All patients were referred to the autonomic laboratory to confirm the diagnosis of SFN. Sudomotor testing was one of the most useful tests to confirm the diagnosis. Sudomotor testing in this series involved either the quantitative sudomotor axon reflex test (QSART) or thermoregulatory testing (see Chapters 15 and 19).

Eighty percent of the patients (31 of 39) had an abnormality on QSART, which represented the single most sensitive test for the confirmation of SFN. Fewer thermoregulatory sweat tests were performed. Results were abnormal for 75% of the patients (15 or 20). Occasionally, a greater deficit on thermoregulatory sweat testing was detected than would otherwise be predicted by the clinical examination. With both tests combined to yield a single composite score, 37 of the 39 patients had an abnormality (61c). When both tests were combined, the sensitivity for detection of SFN approached a level appropriate for an adequate screening examination.

Cardiovagal testing consisted of determination of the Valsalva ratio and heart rate changes related to deep breathing. For the purposes of analysis, these two measures were combined into the cardiovascular heart rate index, which assigns point values for abnormalities obtained with either test. Results were abnormal in approximately 66% of the patients (23 of 36). Three of the 39 had atrial fibrillation and were therefore omitted from the analysis. This value is somewhat higher than previously reported (91). Cardiovagal abnormalities may be more prevalent than formerly recognized, or this may represent a referral bias.

The Valsalva ratio and the presence of orthostatic hypertension were evaluated to identify adrenergic abnormalities. These measures were not particularly useful for the evaluation of idiopathic SFN. Of the 39 patients, this type of testing revealed an abnormality in only four.

Quantitative sensory testing was not performed in all patients in this group, limiting conclusions regarding sensitivity and specificity. Cold thermal testing was performed in 15 patients and vibratory testing in 14. Five abnormalities were noted with each of the testing modalities. Only two patients had abnormal results with both modalities. Eight patients had an abnormality on one of the two tests. Quantitative sensory testing was therefore just as likely to show large-fiber dysfunction as small-fiber dysfunction. Neither cold testing nor vibratory testing was sufficiently sensitive in this group of patients to allow utilization as a screening test.

An unexpected observation was that 15 of the 39 patients in this series had evidence of an increased risk for autoimmune disease. These risks included the presence of monoclonal antibodies, a positive result on antinuclear antibody test, and a history of autoimmune thyroid disease, leukocytoclastic vasculitis, idiopathic thrombocytopenic purpura, recent mycoplasma infection, or Bell's palsy. This observation provides indirect evidence that SFN may result from an autoimmune process. There have been recent reports of beneficial results of immune-modulating therapy in a subgroup of patients with SFN (35b). Whether idiopathic SFN warrants an empiric trial of immune modulation warrants further consideration.

EVOLUTION OF SMALL-FIBER NEUROPATHY

SFN may evolve in one of four ways. In the first pattern, the large fibers become involved and give rise to a pansensory or sensorimotor neuropathy. Many SFNs fall into this category: diabetes, amyloidosis, alcohol-related and nutritional neuropathies, and HSAN type I.

In the second pattern, diffuse involvement of the autonomic nervous system gives rise to widespread autonomic dysfunction. (Both the first and second patterns can occur together, as is seen in some patients with diabetes and primary amyloidosis.)

In the third pattern, the neuropathy is restricted to the distal small fibers. This was the case in 28 of 40 patients with chronic idiopathic SFN and in the five patients suspected of having burning foot familial neuropathy in the one series of patients with SFN discussed previously in this chapter (91). Fabry's disease also follows this course.

In the fourth pattern, the neuropathy can resolve, particularly if a toxic cause is identified and eliminated. Some patients with alcohol-related (101) and diabetic neuropathy show improvement with treatment (2,36).

PATHOGENESIS OF SYMPTOMS AND SIGNS

The cause of lessened cutaneous sensitivity and autonomic hypofunction is a failure of transmission of impulses along diseased or degenerated small peripheral nerve fibers. The cause of the positive symptoms is less clear. Numerous clinical observations and some studies that correlated clinical findings with those from biopsies of nerve specimens have linked the dysesthesias to small rather than large nerve fibers (6,15,25,83,86). The general concept is that damaged small fibers, probably the nociceptive ones, produce excessive nerve action potentials that arrive in abnormal numbers and patterns in the central nervous system areas, where such signals are decoded. They are perceived as aberrant sensations, such as dysesthesias and neuropathic pain.

Three sites have been implicated as possible generators of these abnormal impulses: (a) damaged small-fiber axons; (b) regenerating sprouts that arise from damaged axons; and (c) dorsal root ganglion cells that become activated following damage to their peripheral axons. Most studies showing excessive neuronal discharges have been done in animals with neuromas (the mass of regenerating nerve axon sprouts that develops following nerve transection), with congenital disorders of myelination, or with diabetic neuropathy. Mainly large myelinated nerve fibers, not unmyelinated fibers, have been studied. (For more details, see ref. 89.) Extrapolations from these experimental laboratory findings to patients with SFN are somewhat tenuous.

DIAGNOSTIC TESTS

The investigations to be considered in a patient with probable SFN can be categorized as follows: (a) tests of peripheral nerve function, both somatic and autonomic; (b) tests for autonomic dysfunction involving other organs (Chapters 15 and 19); and (c) investigations aimed at establishing a cause.

Investigation of Peripheral Nerves

Standard nerve conduction studies and needle EMG recordings of muscles are valuable to rule out subclinical large-fiber involvement. Normal results of an EMG study in the presence of clinical signs of neuropathy provide preliminary evidence of SFN.

A variety of techniques can be used to assess small-diameter peripheral nerve fibers.

Histologic Evaluation

Electron microscopy is required to perform histologic evaluation, and quantification, particularly of the unmyelinated fibers, is difficult and time-consuming (75,97). A nerve biopsy specimen, except in the case of amyloidosis, seldom helps to identify the specific cause of SFN. This topic is also discussed in Chapter 28.

Skin Biopsy

Small-caliber C fibers and Aδ nerve fibers innervate the skin. Punch biopsies of the skin allow further histologic examination of these nerve fibers. After fixation of the skin tissue, the sections are stained with monoclonal antibody to neuron-specific ubiquitin hydrolase. The nerve fibers are then counted within the sections of tissue and the numbers compared with control values. This technique represents a method for quantification of small cutaneous sensory fibers. The method may allow for histopathologic evaluation of the response of cutaneous nerve fibers to treatment with NGFs or other compounds (68b).

In Vitro *Evaluation of Compound Action Potentials*

Freshly excised sural nerve is used for the measurement of compound action potentials of the small fibers (51). Disadvantages of this technique include the need for a nerve biopsy and special equipment, and the ultimate poor sensitivity of the test.

Microneurography

Microneurography involves recording from very fine needles inserted into peripheral nerves (Chapter 18). It can be used to study function in small-fiber sensory afferents and sympathetic efferents. Impairment in both has been shown in patients with a variety of neuropathies, including very mild diabetic sensory neuropathy (29,65,66). However, this technique lends itself better to the study of the normal physiology of peripheral nerves than to the detection of abnormalities. It is also invasive and time-consuming, so it is unlikely to become a standard diagnostic test (102).

Current Perception Threshold

Measurement of current perception thresholds is another technique used to evaluate the presence of peripheral neuropathy. Three frequencies are used: 5, 250, and 2000 Hz. The system enables rapid screening and is quite mobile. It is unclear if the three frequencies employed test fiber-size populations entirely independently (44b,68a).

Somatosensory Evoked Potential

Carbon dioxide laser pulses stimulate afferent fibers in the outermost layers of the skin, the C and Aδ fibers. The technique produces cortical evoked potentials from these specific receptors instead of from the large 1A afferent fibers responsible for the classic somatosensory evoked potential. This unique method was developed to study the functional integration of small-fiber tracks and their central projections (14b).

Sympathetic Penile Skin Response

Several physiologic techniques have been identified to study the relationship of the somatic nervous system to erectile dysfunction. A new technique allows for the assessment of the nerve fibers most important for erection, that is, the small myelinated and unmyelinated fibers. It involves recording the sympathetic skin response directly from penile tissue. Long latencies reportedly reflect neuropathy of these regional autonomic fibers. A drawback of this procedure is that only 80% of normal controls have recordable potentials (22a).

Skin Flare Responses

Pain-mediating (nociceptive) unmyelinated fibers can be assessed by the intradermal injection of histamine, which elicits a flare response mediated through an axon reflex (44). This is one of the few tests of small-fiber function that can be done without specialized equipment. A normal response is a reddening of the skin involving an area greater than 1 cm in diameter. However, the flare can be variable in size and shape, difficult to see on dark skin, and hard to quantitate. Flare responses are reduced in patients with diabetic neuropathy (5). One way of improving the test is to use a laser-Doppler skin blood flow device to measure the increased cutaneous blood flow that gives rise to the flare. Additionally, it has been found that iontophoresis of the test agent is superior to injection. Le Quesne et al. (56,76,77) developed the technique of iontophoresis of acetylcholine (which works equally as well as histamine) through a small plastic skin capsule; the flare and vasodilation response are recorded with a laser-Doppler probe. Abnormalities have been found in diabetic patients with Charcot's joints using this technique. When applied in patients representing a wider spectrum of severity of diabetic and other neuropathies, however, the test appears to have two major faults (10): First, normal individuals and patients with mild to moderate neuropathy may have normal or increased adrenergic activity that causes vasoconstriction, thus counteracting the flare response. Second, sensitivity of the test appears to be low.

Sweat Testing

A variety of methods can be used to detect a peripheral reduction in sweating. The thermoregulatory sweat test (Chapter 19) was found to reveal abnormalities in 72% of patients (18 of 25) with SFN (91). Testing of sympathetic skin response (Chapter 17) in diabetic patients with sensorimotor neuropathy but not specifically SFN showed abnormalities in 60%–83% (68,73,85,87). However, when the sensitivity of this test was examined in isolated SFN, the yield was low. When EMG results were normal and SFN was suspected clinically, only 10% of the patients demonstrated an abnormality (28a). Acetylcholine or pilocarpine can be introduced by injection or iontophoresis into the skin, and sweat production can then be recorded by direct observation, moisture sensitive paper, Silastic imprint (46) (Chapter 15), or the quantitation of water vapor following evaporation of sweat (QSART) (62) (Chapter 15).

The pilocarpine-Silastic imprint method has been reported to show abnormalities in the feet of 53% of unselected diabetic patients with type I disease (72). A modification, using Silastic imprint recording but measuring the axon-mediated indirect response to acetylcholine, has improved the sensitivity of the test (47,62,92). A fairly reliable reading of the imprint can be done with a low-power microscope, but more accurate quantification requires specialized scanning techniques. Quantitative sweat evaporimetry testing was shown to reveal defective sweating patterns in 80% of patients (32 of 40) with SFN (91). QSART evaluation has the added advantages of excellent reproducibility and lack of dependence on patient cooperation (62).

Of these various sweat tests, the easiest to perform in the setting of the EMG laboratory is the sympathetic skin response test. This is a simple but insensitive test that requires no specialized equipment. It consists of the intradermal injection of acetylcholine or pilocarpine; sweating is observed through a magnifying glass or by using paper impregnated with a moisture-sensitive compound that is applied to the skin (44). A relatively simple thermoregulatory sweat test can be done by applying a moisture-sensitive compound to parts of the patient's body, warming the patient by either heating the room or placing the patient under a makeshift cradle mounted with heating lamps, and observing sweating as indicated by color changes in the compound. However, to do this with accuracy, a purpose-built heat cradle or chamber with close monitoring of temperature and humidity is required. Drawbacks of this procedure are that it is messy and time-consuming. The equipment used for iontophoresis and the Silastic sweat imprint methods is relatively simple, but the precise quantification requires specialized scanning techniques. The QSART is undoubtedly the most accurate method of testing sweat production from a small area of skin, but specialized and expensive equipment is necessary.

Temperature Threshold Testing

Temperature threshold testing involves the use of a thermode in which the temperature is raised and lowered. There are several approaches to testing these thresholds. The "Marstock" technique employs the principle of limits: subjects press a button when they sense the warmth or coolness of the thermode, and the temperature of the thermode then reverses. This is repeated about 10 times, until the warm and cool thresholds are consistent (32). This technique relies entirely on patient cooperation and is liable to patient bias. Another approach is the "forced choice" method of psychophysical analysis, in which patient bias is probably reduced (4,27,28,31,42). Commercial thermal threshold testers using one or the other of these approaches are available.

One thermal threshold machine heats and cools the thermode to the extent that hot and cold pain thresholds can be determined. These devices are thought to test unmyelinated nociceptor nerve fibers (32,60,61). In a study of unselected patients with type I diabetes, these hot and cold pain thresholds were found to be abnormal considerably less frequently than the thermal thresholds (71).

Abnormalities of thermal thresholds have been found in several studies conducted in patients with asymptomatic and symptomatic diabetes (1,11,30,37,38,57,58,71,88,105). In one study of 25 patients with SFN, many of whom had diabetes, abnormal warm or cool thermal thresholds, or both, were found in all subjects (41).

The difficulty with all quantitative sensory testing is the significant variability for both vibration testing and thermal testing (81a,44a). The variability is greater for thermal threshold testing than for vibratory threshold testing. In patients with neuropathy, variability is increased in comparison with normal subjects. With respect to thermal testing, cold threshold testing is more reproducibile than warm threshold testing (14a). Interobserver and intraobserver reliability are important issues in studies of treatment efficacy. The true sensitivity of thermal testing in distal SFN is a subject of much controversy, with wide variations of sensitivity (40%–100%) reported (41,86a).

Pain Threshold Testing

Besides measurement of thermal pain, other methods have been used to evaluate pain thresholds in patients with neuropathies, but no entirely satisfactory technique has evolved. In one study of diabetic patients who had neuropathies of varying severity, the pain threshold, as measured by a pinch stimulus, was abnormal in about half (55). A new technique to measure heat-pain thresholds has good reproducibility and may augment the evaluation of pain associated with SFN. Studies to confirm its utility in SFN will be necessary (27a).

Skin Blood Flow

Skin blood flow can be measured either by plethysmography (34,35) or by laser-Doppler techniques (63,81) (Chapter 15). Various stimuli, such as a deep inspiratory gasp, cough, startle, application of cold to the skin, body tilting, and lowering one leg, normally provoke vasoconstriction and reduced skin blood flow. Most studies have been done in patients with diabetic sensorimotor neuropathy, not SFN, and abnormalities have been found (35,49, 63,81,84). Archer et al. (3) studied eight diabetic patients with the acute painful form of SFN (described earlier in this chapter). All had abnormally elevated temperatures and skin blood flow in the big toes.

Choice of Test

Testing small-fiber function is important for diagnosing SFN, following the course of the neuropathy, and assessing response to treatment. When deciding which tests to perform and what equipment to purchase, the following information should be borne in mind:

1. Most tests evaluate only a single type of small fiber. However, it is quite possible that in a patient with SFN, other small fibers, such as somatic unmyelinated nociceptive afferents, may also be affected. Testing only one type of fiber may therefore yield misleading results, and is analogous to doing nerve conduction studies (testing large fibers) in a patient with SFN.
2. As stated by Le Quesne et al. (56), "The capacity of a test to detect abnormality is influenced both by the nature and design of these tests as well as the range of biological variability in control subjects." There is a wide variation in these factors in the tests described herein. To continue with the quotation from Le Quesne et al. (56), "Because of this lack of comparability of the different tests, the results of a variety of tests of different small-fiber populations cannot be taken as an indication of damage to different types of nerve fibers."
3. Practical issues are important: availability, reliability, ease of use, cost, comfort to the patient, and time required to perform the test are all factors to be considered when buying or building testing equipment.

It is difficult to recommend with confidence any of the simple bedside tests. The intradermal histamine flare response has potential. The discomfort of the injection can largely be overcome by using iontophoresis, and a machine for doing this is simple and inexpensive to make. However, the value of the test and choice of indices need to be evaluated more critically before the test can be recommended. For the electromyographer, the sympathetic skin response is a test that can be done without any extra equipment.

In regard to tests that require specialized equipment, the thermal threshold testing devices may be the easiest to set up. Thresholds for warming have been reported to be abnormal in large numbers of asymptomatic and neuropathic diabetic patients and, more importantly, in a very high number of patients with SFN (41). Most machines test for cold perception, which represents another group of fibers, and this increases the diagnostic yield. Other devices also allow for testing of hot and cold pain, which assesses a third population of fibers. The value of the test will be better known when such devices have been used in multiple centers for a longer period of time. In fully equipped autonomic laboratories, the sudomotor fibers are the best small-fiber group to evaluate. QSART is the most accurate technique for accomplishing this, particularly when recordings are made simultaneously from four sites (Chapter 15). The thermoregulatory sweat test is also a sensitive assessment for small-viber dysfunction.

Investigating the Cause of Small-Fiber Neuropathy

The patient's history has to be probed to determine the existence of other family members with diabetes, neuropathy, or both. As Dyck has emphasized, the search for such relatives often requires a careful examination and investigation of persons who may have few or no neuropathic symptoms (23). In cases of suspected SFN, the shortcomings of the physical examination have to be offset by the use of tests of small-fiber function, as outlined previously in this chapter.

A personal history of diabetes, excessive alcohol intake, inadequate diet, medication use, symptoms of generalized autonomic dysfunction, and symptoms suggesting other medical problems are all relevant. Symptoms of generalized dysautonomia strongly imply amyloidosis. Generalized autonomic failure rarely develops in diabetes, but when it does, affected patients usually have a severe sensorimotor peripheral neuropathy, not SFN.

Blood should be sent for routine hematologic and biochemical analyses, plus thorough testing for diabetes if the patient is not known to have the disease. If amyloidosis is suspected, then investigations for multiple myeloma and benign gammopathy should be done. These include serum and urine immunoelectrophoresis for monoclonal proteins, bone scan or skeletal survey, and bone marrow biopsy. A biopsy specimen of abdominal fat pad, rectal mucosa, or sural nerve provides a definitive diagnosis. Apart from confirming this diagnosis, there is usually no other reason to do a nerve biopsy in patients with SFN, particularly as improved noninvasive methods for testing small-fiber function are becoming increasingly available.

TREATMENT

Treatment of SFN can be categorized as primary therapy of the underlying disorder, symptomatic therapy, and therapy with experimental agents that may reverse nerve damage and promote repair of small fibers. Approaches to primary therapies include tight control of diabetes, abstinence from alcohol, measures to correct nutritional deficiencies, and removal of toxins.

In addition to primary therapy, many patients require symptomatic treatment for neuropathic pain. Simple but often effective measures are cooling the feet with towels soaked in cold water or immersing the feet in a tub of cool water. Gentle massaging with skin creams is also helpful, as may be transcutaneous nerve stimulation. A cradle to keep bedclothes off the feet at night is essential for the patient with exquisitely painful and sensitive feet. The regular application of capsaicin-containing cream has been reported to benefit some patients with painful diabetic neuropathy (59,94). Capsaicin is of limited or questionable benefit in SFN. In one study, it was found to have no benefit over placebo (63b). Another topical agent that may be used for this indication is EMLA (eutectic mixture of lidocaine anesthetics, which contains 2.5% lidocaine and 2.5% prilocaine). This agent awaits approval and further investigation for use in neuropathic pain (33b).

There are very few well-designed studies to determine the effectiveness of drugs in patients with neuropathic pain (64). It seldom responds adequately to mild analgesics, such as acetaminophen and acetylsalicylic acid, but these may be effective when combined with codeine. Such a combination, taken at bedtime and then again during the night if necessary, often provides some relief, and it can be taken during the day as well. Carbamazepine has been shown to be effective in some patients with diabetic neuropathy (82). It is important to build up the dose gradually during 1 or 2 weeks, so that the maintenance dose can be decided from the patient's response and blood levels of the drug. Using a higher dose at night is often effective in controlling nocturnal pain; minor toxic side effects go unnoticed during sleep. Carbamazepine activates the hepatic enzymes involved in its catabolism, so that blood levels fall and pain returns after several weeks; a slight increase in the dose is then required. An alternative agent is phenytoin, and its dose also has to be individualized (93). It is important to be aware of the saturation kinetics of phenytoin, in that small increments in doses can cause marked elevations in blood levels and toxicity. The tricyclic antidepressants also have analgesic properties and can be effective in relieving neuropathic pain. It is advisable to start with a low dose and increase it gradually, balancing symptom relief against the anticholinergic and other side effects. Some authors have advocated the concomitant use of either phenothiazines or a butyrophenone drug, such as haloperidol, for enhanced analgesic effect (21,48,70). Clonazepam, a benzodiazepine, has also been used with success to treat a variety of neuropathic pains, and it is sometimes given in combination with carbamazepine (93). Clonidine has been shown to be useful in cases of painful diabetic neuropathy. The greatest effect of clonidine is on sharp and shooting pain (17). It has recently been reported that mexiletine, a drug used in the treatment of cardiac arrhythmias, is effective in reducing neuropathic pain (22). Some investigators believe that intravenous lidocaine can be used as a diagnostic test to indicate whether a patients's neuropathic pain will respond to a sodium channel blocker, such as mexiletine or carbamazepine (94a). Other compounds that have been investigated in the treatment of neuropathic pain include adenosine and ketamine (68d). Adenosine has certain modulatory effects on nociceptive reflexes. It is thought to have a central site of action, and in a small series has been shown to alleviate neuropathic pain (9a). Venlafaxine, nefazodone, gabapentin, and lamotrigine all may be efficacious in the management of neuropathic pain based on their pharmacologic actions (33b). Further investigations are necessary to explore their potential in this area.

Experimental agents under clinical investigation in the United States and Europe involve the use of neurotrophic factors. These factors promote growth and development and repair of specific populations of nerve fibers. Several neurotrophic factors are the focus of clinical trials of the treatment of diabetic neuropathy: NT-3, IGF-1, BDNF, and NGF. Some of these trophic agents, such as NGF, have a particular affinity for small fibers (1a,61a).

In conclusion, drugs are often more effective in combination than when given singly. In particular, it is useful to combine the classic analgesics, such as acetaminophen and codeine, with carbamazepine, phenytoin, or a tricyclic antidepressant. When none of these measures effectively relieve severe pain, narcotics should be used.

REFERENCES

1. Ali Z, et al. The extent of small-fibre sensory neuropathy in diabetics with plantar foot ulceration. *J Neurol Neurosurg Psychiatry* 1989;63:94–98.
1a. Apfel SC, et al. Nerve growth factor administration protects against experimental diabetic sensory neuropathy. *Brain Res* 1994;634:7–12.
2. Archer AG, et al. The natural history of acute painful neuropathy in diabetes mellitus. *J Neurol Neurosurg Psychiatry* 1983;46:491–499.
3. Archer AG, et al. Blood flow patterns in painful diabetic neuropathy. *Diabetologia* 1984;27:563–567.
4. Arezzo JC, et al. Thermal sensitivity tester. Device for quantitative assessment of thermal sense in diabetic neuropathy. *Diabetes* 1986;35:590–592.
5. Aronin N, et al. Diminished flare response in neuropathic diabetic patients. *Diabetes* 1987;36:1139–1143.
6. Asbury AK, Fields HL. Pain due to peripheral nerve damage: an hypothesis. *Neurology* 1984;34:1587–1590.
7. Asbury AK, Gilliatt RW. The clinical approach to neuropathy. In: Asbury AK, Gilliatt RW, eds. *Peripheral Nerve Disorders: A Practical Approach*. London: Butterworth; 1984:1–20.
8. Bailey RO, et al. Sensory motor neuropathy associated with AIDS. *Neurology* 1988;38:886–891.
8a. Barbieri S, et al. Small-fiber involvement in neuropathy associated with IgG, IgA and IGM monoclonal gammopathy. *Electromyogr Clin Neurophysiol* 1995;35:39–44.
9. Behse F, Buchthal F. Alcoholic neuropathy: clinical, electrophysiological, and biopsy findings. *Ann Neurol* 1977;2:95–110.
9a. Belfrage M, et al. Systematic adenosine infusion alleviates spontaneous and stimulus-evoked pain in patients with peripheral neuropathic pain. *Anesth Analg* 1995;81:713–717.

9b. Bellavere F, et al. Prolonged QT period in diabetic autonomic neuropathy: a possible role in sudden death? *Br Heart J* 1988;59:379–383.
10. Benarroch EE, Low PA. The acetylcholine-induced flare response in evaluation of small-fiber dysfunction. *Ann Neurol* 1991;29:590–595.
10a. Berger AR, et al. Dose response, coasting and differential fiber vulnerability in human toxic neuropathy: a prospective study of pyridoxine neurotoxicity. *Neurology* 1992;42:1367–1370.
11. Bertelsmann FW, et al. Thermal discrimination thresholds in normal subjects and in patients with diabetic neuropathy. *J Neurol Neurosurg Psychiatry* 1985;48:686–690.
12. Bourque PR, Windebank AJ. Thoracic myelopathy presenting as peripheral neuropathy. *Can J Neurol Sci* 1989;16:264.
13. Bradley WG, et al. Metronidazole neuropathy. *Br Med J* 1977;2:610–611.
14. Brady RO. Fabry disease. In: Dyck PJ, et al, eds. *Peripheral Neuropathy*. 2nd ed. Philadelphia: WB Saunders; 1984:1717–1727.
14a. Bravenboer B, et al. Thermal threshold testing for the assessment of small-fiber dysfunction: normal values and reproducibility. *Diabet Med* 1992;9:546–549.
14b. Bromm B, et al. Laser-evoked brain potentials in patients with dissociated loss of pain and temperature sensibility. *Electroencephalogr Clin Neurophysiol* 1991;80:284–291.
15. Brown MJ, Asbury AK. Diabetic neuropathy. *Ann Neurol* 1984;15:2–12.
15a. Brown MJ, et al. Painful diabetic neuropathy. A morphometric study. *Arch Neurol* 1976;33:164–171.
16. Brown-Séquard CE. *Lectures on the Physiology and Pathology of the Central Nervous System*. Philadelphia: Collins; 1860.
17. Byas-Smith MG, et al. Transdermal clonidine compared to placebo in painful diabetic neuropathy using a two-stage "enriched enrollment" design. *Pain* 1995;60:267–274.
18. Charron L, et al. Sensory neuropathy associated with primary biliary cirrhosis. *Arch Neurol* 1980;37:84–87.
19. Cohen AS, Rubinow A. Amyloid neuropathy. In: Dyck PJ, et al, eds. *Peripheral Neuropathy*. 2nd ed. Philadelphia: WB Saunders; 1984:1866–1898.
19a. Cohen LB, et al. Role of plasmapheresis in primary biliary cirrhosis. *Gut* 1985;26:291–294.
20. Cornblath DR, McArthur JC. Predominantly sensory neuropathy in patients with AIDS and AIDS-related complex. *Neurology* 1988;38:794–796.
21. Davis JL, et al. Peripheral diabetic neuropathy treated with amitriptyline and fluphenazine. *JAMA* 1977;238:2291–2292.
22. Dejgaard A, et al. Mexiletine for treatment of chronic painful diabetic neuropathy. *Lancet* 1988;29:9–11.
22a. Derouet H, et al. Penile sympathetic skin response in erectile dysfunction. *Eur Urol* 1995;28:314–319.
22b. Diabetes Control and Complications Trial (DCCT) Research Group. Effect of intensive diabetes treatment on nerve conduction in the diabetes control and complications trial. *Ann Neurol* 1995;38:869–880.
22c. Duston MA, et al. Peripheral neuropathy as an early marker of AL amyloidosis. *Arch Intern Med* 1989; 149:358–360.
23. Dyck PJ. Neuronal atrophy and degeneration predominantly affecting peripheral sensory and autonomic neurons. In: Dyck PJ, et al, eds. *Peripheral Neuropathy*. 2nd ed. Philadelphia: WB Saunders; 1984:1557–1599.
24. Dyck PJ, Lambert EH. Dissociated sensation in amyloidosis. *Arch Neurol* 1969;20:490–507.
25. Dyck PJ, et al. Pain in peripheral neuropathy related to rate and kind of fiber degeneration. *Neurology* 1976;26: 466–471.
26. Dyck PJ, et al. "Burning feet" as the only manifestation of dominantly inherited sensory neuropathy. *Mayo Clin Proc* 1983;58:426–429.
27. Dyck PJ, et al. Detection thresholds of cutaneous sensation in humans. In: Dyck PJ, et al, eds. *Peripheral Neuropathy*. 2nd ed. Philadelphia: WB Saunders; 1984:1103–1138.
27a. Dyck PJ, et al. A standard test of heat-pain responses using case IV. *J Neurol Sci* 1996;136:54–63.
28. Dyck PJ, et al. Comparison of algorithms of testing for use in automated evaluation of sensation. *Neurology* 1990;40:1607–1613.
28a. Evans BA, et al. The peripheral autonomic surface potential in suspected small-fiber peripheral neuropathy. *Muscle Nerve* 1988;11:982.
28b. Ewing DJ, et al. Autonomic neuropathy, at interval lengthening and unexpected deaths in most diabetic patients. *Diabetologia* 1991;34:182–185.
28c. Ewing DJ, et al. The natural history of diabetic autonomic neuropathy. *Q J Med* 1980;193:95–108.
29. Fagius J. Microneurographic findings in diabetic polyneuropathy with special reference to sympathetic nerve activity. *Diabetologia* 1982;23:415–420.
29a. Fazio R, et al. Acute presentation of Tangier polyneuropathy: a clinical and morphological study. *Acta Neuropathol* 1993;86:90–94.
30. Fowler CJ, et al. The value of testing for unmyelinated fibre, sensory neuropathy in diabetic impotence. *Br J Urol* 1988;61:63–67.
31. Fowler CJ, et al. A portable system for measuring cutaneous thresholds for warming and cooling. *J Neurol Neurosurg Psychiatry* 1987;50:1211–1215.
32. Fruhstorfer H, et al. Method for quantitative estimation of thermal thresholds in patients. *J Neurol Neurosurg Psychiatry* 1976;39:1071–1075.
33. Fuller GN, et al. Association of painful peripheral neuropathy in AIDS with cytomegalovirus infection. *Lancet* 1989; 2:937–941.
33a. Galasso PJ, et al. Propafenone-induced peripheral neuropathy. *Mayo Clin Proc* 1995;70:469–472.
33b. Galer BS. Neuropathic pain of peripheral origin: advances in pharmacologic treatment. *Neurology* 1995;45(12 Suppl 9):S17–S25; discussion, S35–S36..
34. Gilliatt RW. Vaso-constriction in the fingers after deep inspiration. *J Physiol (Lond)* 1948;107:76–88.
35. Goadby HK, Downman CBB. Peripheral vascular and sweat-gland reflexes in diabetic neuropathy. *Clin Sci Mol Med* 1973;45:281–289.
35a. Gonin JM, et al. Corrected Q-T interval prolongation as diagnostic tool for assessment of cardiac autonomic neuropathy in diabetes mellitus. *Diabetes Care* 1990;1368–1371.
35b. Gorson KC, et al. Idiopathic small-fiber neuropathy. *Neurology* 1994;44(Suppl 2):A181.
36. Greene DA, et al. Comparison of clinical course and sequential electrophysiological tests in diabetics with symptomatic polyneuropathy and its implications for clinical trials. *Diabetes* 1981;30:139–147.
37. Guy RJC, et al. Evaluation of thermal and vibration sensation in diabetic neuropathy. *Diabetologia* 1985;28:131–137.
38. Heimans JJ, et al. Large and small nerve fiber function in painful diabetic neuropathy. *J Neurol Sci* 1986;74:1–9.
38a. Hendrickse MT, Triger DR. Autonomic and peripheral neuropathy in primary biliary cirrhosis. *J Hepatol* 1993;19:401–407.
39. Herbert PN. Abetalipoproteinemia, hypobetalipoproteinemia, and Tangier disease. In: Dyck PJ, et al, eds. *Peripheral Neuropathy*. 2nd ed. Philadelphia: WB Saunders; 1984:1728–1744.
39a. Hilz MJ, et al. Early diagnosis of diabetic small-fiber neuropathy by disturbed cold perception. *J Diab Comp* 1992;1:35–43.
39b. Hilz MJ, et al. Is heat hypoalgesia a useful parameter in quantitative thermal testing of alcoholic polyneuropathy? *Muscle Nerve* 1994;17;1456–1460.
39c. Hilz MJ, et al. Thermal threshold determination in alcoholic polyneuropathy: an improvement of diagnosis. *Acta Neurol Scand* 1995;91:389–393.
39d. Hong CZ. Electrodiagnostic findings of persisting polyneuropathies due to previous nutritional deficiency in former prisoners of war. *Electromyogr Clin Neurophysiol* 1986;26:351–363.
39e. Hughes PJ, et al. Small-fiber dysfunction in a *Borrelia burgdorferi* infection. *Muscle Nerve* 1993;16:221–222.
40. IASP Subcommittee on Taxonomy. Pain terms: a list with definitions and notes on usage. *Pain* 1979;6:249–252.
41. Jamal GA, et al. The neurophysiologic investigation of small-fiber neuropathies. *Muscle Nerve* 1987;10:537–545.
42. Jamal GA, et al. An improved automated method for the measurement of thermal threshold. 2. Patients with peripheral neuropathy. *J Neurol Neurosurg Psychiatry* 1985;48:361–366.
43. Jaspan JB, et al. Hypoglycemic peripheral neuropathy in association with insulinoma: implication of glucopenia rather than hyperinsulinism. *Medicine* 1972;61:33–44.
44. Johnson RH, Spalding JMK. *Disorders of the Autonomic Nervous System*. Philadelphia: FA Davis; 1974:124–125.
44a. Kahn R. Quantitative sensory testing. *Diabetes Care* 1992;15 (Suppl 3):1092–1094.

44b. Katims JJ, et al. Constant current sine wave transcutaneous nerve stimulation for the evaluation of peripheral neuropathy. *Arch Phys Med Rehabil* 1987;68:210–213.
45. Kelly JJ, et al. The natural history of peripheral neuropathy in primary systemic amyloidosis. *Ann Neurol* 1979;6:1–7.
46. Kennedy WR, et al. Quantitation of the sweating deficiency in diabetes mellitus. *Ann Neurol* 1984;15:482–488.
47. Kihara M, et al. Comparison of directly stimulated with axon reflex-mediated sudomotor responses in human subjects. *Ann Neurol* 1989; 26:169.
48. Kocher R. The use of psychotropic drugs in the treatment of chronic, severe pains. *Eur Neurol* 1976;14:458–464.
49. Koltringer P, et al. A new measuring design for autonomic dysfunction of skin in neuropathies: hyperthermal laser-Doppler flowmetry. *Acta Neurol Scand* 1989;80:589–592.
50. Kyle RA, Greipp PR. Amyloidosis (AL). Clinical and laboratory features in 229 cases. *Mayo Clin Proc* 1983;58:665–683.
51. Lambert EH, Dyck PJ. Compound action potentials of sural nerve in vitro in peripheral neuropathy. In: Dyck PJ, et al, eds. *Peripheral Neuropathy*. 2nd ed. Philadelphia: WB Saunders; 1984:1030–1044.
52. Lange DJ, et al. The neuromuscular manifestations of human immunodeficiency virus infections. *Arch Neurol* 1988;45:1084–1088.
53. Le Quesne PM. Toxic neuropathies. In: Asbury AK, Gilliatt RW, eds. *Peripheral Nerve Disorders: A Practical Approach*. London: Butterworth; 1984:1–20.
54. Le Quesne PM. Neuropathy due to drugs. In: Dyck PJ, et al, eds. *Peripheral Neuropathy*. 2nd ed. Philadelphia: WB Saunders; 1984: 2162–2179.
55. Le Quesne PM, Fowler CJ. A study of pain threshold in diabetics with neuropathic foot lesions. *J Neurol Neurosurg Psychiatry* 1896;49F:1191–1194.
56. Le Quesne PM, et al. Peripheral neuropathy profile in various groups of diabetics. *J Neurol Neurosurg Psychiatry* 1990;53:558–563.
57. Levy DM, et al. Small- and large-fiber involvement in early diabetic neuropathy: a study with the medial plantar response and sensory thresholds. *Diabetes Care* 1987;10: 441–447.
58. Levy D, et al. Comparison of two methods for measuring thermal thresholds in diabetic neuropathy. *J Neurol Neurosurg Psychiatry* 1989;52:1072–1077.
59. Levy D-M, et al. Topical capsaicin in the treatment of painful diabetic neuropathy. *N Engl J Med* 1991;324: 776.
60. Light AR, Perl ER. Peripheral sensory systems. In: Dyck PJ, et al, eds. *Peripheral Neuropathy*. 2nd ed. Philadelphia: WB Saunders; 1984:210–230.
61. Lindholm U. Quantitative testing of sensibility including pain. In: Stalberg E, Young R, eds. *Neurology 11, Clinical Neurophysiology*. London: Butterworth; 1981:168–190.
61a. Lindsey RM. Neurotrophic growth factors and neurodegenerative diseases: therapeutics potential of the neurotrophins and ciliary neurotrophic factor. *Neurobiol Aging* 1994;15:249–251.
61b. Lipton RB, et al. Large and small fiber type sensory dysfunction in patients with cancer. *J Neurol Neurosurg Psychiatry* 1991;54:706–709.
61c. Low PA. Composite autonomic scoring scale for laboratory qualifications of general autonomic failure. *Mayo Clin Proc* 1993;68: 748–752.
62. Low PA, et al. Quantitative sudomotor axon reflex test in normal and neuropathic subjects. *Ann Neurol* 1983;14:573–580.
63. Low PA, et al. Evaluation of skin vasomotor reflexes by using laser Doppler velocimetry. *Mayo Clin Proc* 1983;58:583–592.
63a. Low PA, et al. Congenital sensory neuropathy with selective loss of small myelinated fibers. Ann Neurol 1978; 3:179–182.
63b. Low PA, et al. Double-blind, placebo-controlled study of the application of capsaicin cream in chronic distal painful polyneuropathy. *Pain* 1995; 62:163–168.
64. Maciewicz R, et al. Drug therapy of neuropathic pain. *Clin J Pain* 1985;1:39–49.
65. Mackel R. Properties of cutaneous afferents in diabetic neuropathy. *Brain* 1989;112:1359–1376.
66. Mackenzie RA, et al. A micro-electrode study of peripheral neuropathy in man. *J Neurol Sci* 1977;34:157–174.
67. Mackenzie RA, et al. Fibre function and perception during cutaneous nerve block. *J Neurol Neurosurg Psychiatry* 1975;38:865–873.
67a. Marbini A, et al. Hereditary sensory and autonomic neuropathy with ataxia and late onset. *Clin Neurol Neurosurg* 1994;96:191–196.
68. Maselli RA, et al. Comparison of sympathetic skin response with quantitative sudomotor axon reflex test in diabetic neuropathy. *Muscle Nerve* 1989;12:420–423.
68a. Masson EA, et al. Current perception thresholds: a new, quick, and reproducible method for the assessment of peripheral neuropathy in diabetes mellitus. *Diabetologia* 1989;32:724–728.
68b. McCarthy BG, et al. Cutaneous innervation in sensory neuropathies: evaluation by skin biopsy. *Neurology* 1995;45:1848–1855.
68c. McManis PG, et al. Neuropathy associated with hyperlipidemia. *Neurology* 1994;44:2185–2186.
68d. Mercadante S, et al. Long-term ketamine subcutaneous continuous infusion in neuropathic cancer pain. *J Pain Symptom Manage* 1995; 10:564–568.
69. Miller RG, et al. The spectrum of peripheral neuropathy associated with ARC and AIDS. *Muscle Nerve* 1988;11:857–863.
70. Monks R, Merskey H. Psychotropic drugs. In: Wall PD, Melzack R, eds. *Testbook of Pain*. Edinburgh: Churchill Livingstone; 1984:526–537.
70a. Morgan SH, et al. The neurological complications of Anderson-Fabry disease (alpha-galactosidase A deficiency)—investigation of symptomatic and presymptomatic patients. *Q J Med* 1990;75: 491–507.
70b. Murakami T, et al. Genetic abnormalities and pathogenesis of familial amyloidotic polyneuropathy. *Pathol Int* 1995;45: 1–9.
71. Navarro X, Kennedy WR. Evaluation of thermal and pain sensitivity in type I diabetic patients. *J Neurol Neuroaurg Psychiatry* 1991; 54:65–67.
72. Navarro X, et al. Small nerve fiber dysfunction in diabetic neuropathy, *Muscle Nerve* 1989;12:498–507.
73. Niakan E, Harati YI. Sympathetic skin response in diabetic peripheral neuropathy. *Muscle Nerve* 1988;11:261–264.
74. O'Brien IA, et al. The influence of autonomic neuropathy on mortality in insulin-dependent diabetes. *Q J Med* 1991;290:495–502.
75. Ochoa J. Recognition of unmyelinated fiber disease: morphologic criteria. *Muscle Nerve* 1978;1:375–387.
76. Parkhouse N, Le Quesne PM. Impaired neurogenic vascular response in patients with diabetes and neuropathic foot lesions. *N Engl J Med* 1988;318:1306–1309.
77. Parkhouse N, Le Quesne PM. Quantitative objective assessment of peripheral nociceptive C fibre function. *J Neurol Neurosurg Psychiatry* 1988;51:28–34.
78. Parry GJ. Peripheral neuropathies associated with human immunodeficiency virus infection. *Ann Neurol* 1988;23:S49–S53.
79. Pavy FW. Introductory address to the discussion on the clinical aspect of glycosuria. *Lancet* 1885;2:1085–1087.
79a. Quattrini A, et al. Antisulfatide antibodies in neurological disease: binding to rat dorsal root ganglia neurons. *J Neurol Sci* 1992;112: 152–159.
80. Rance NE, et al. Gracile tract degeneration in patients with sensory neuropathy and AIDS. *Neurology* 1988;38:265–271.
81. Rayman G, et al. Blood flow in the skin of the foot related to posture in diabetes mellitus. *Br Med J* 1986;292:87–90.
81a. Redmond J, et al. Variability of quantitative sensory testing: implications for clinical practice. *Henry Ford Hosp Med J* 1990;38:62–67.
81b. Reilly M, Staunton H. Peripheral nerve amyloidosis. *Brain Pathol* 1996;6:163–177.
82. Rull JA, et al. Symptomatic treatment of peripheral diabetic neuropathy with carbamazepine (Tegretol): double cross-over study. *Diabetologia* 1969;5:215–220.
83. Said G, et al. Progressive centripetal degeneration of axons in small-fiber diabetic polyneuropathy. *Brain* 1983;106:791–807.
84. Sefton M, et al. The venoarteriolar reflex in diabetic and other neuropathies. *Neurology* 1989;39:1490–1492.
85. Shahani BT, et al. RR interval variation and the sympathetic skin response in the assessment of autonomic function in peripheral neuropathy. *Arch Neurol* 1990;47:659–664.
86. Sivak M, Ochoa J. Positive manifestations of nerve fiber dysfunction: clinical, electrophysiologic, and pathologic correlates. In: Brown WF, Bolton CF, eds. *Clinical Electromyography*. Boston: Butterworth; 1987:3–30.

86a. Smith SJ, et al. Cutaneous thermal thresholds in patients with painful burning feet. *J Neurol Neurosurg Psychiatry* 1991;54:877–881.
87. Soliven B, et al. Sympathetic skin response in diabetic neuropathy. *Muscle Nerve* 1987;10:711–716.
88. Sosenko JM, et al. Specific assessments of warm and cool sensitivities in adult diabetic patients. *Diabetes Care* 1988;11:481–483.
88a. Stahlberg D, et al. Neurophysiologic studies of patients with Crohn's disease on long-term treatment with metronidazole. *Scand J Gastroenterol* 1991;26:219–224.
89. Stewart JD. *Focal Peripheral Neuropathies*. New York: Elsevier; 1987:30–37.
90. Stewart JD, Lal S. Autonomic and somatic neurologic dysfunction in impotent type 11 diabetic men. *Can J Neurol Sci* 1990;17:222.
91. Stewart JD, et al. Distal small-fiber neuropathy: results of tests of sweating and autonomic cardiovascular reflexes. *Muscle Nerve* 1992;15:661–665.
92. Stewart JD, et al. Modified quantitative sweat axon reflex testing (QSART) in diabetic neuropathy. *Can J Neurol Sci* 1991;18:262–263.
92a. Surrenti C, et al. Effects of plasma exchange (PE) in primary biliary cirrhosis (PBC). A pilot study. *Hepatogastroenterology* 1990;37:128–130.
93. Swerdlow M, Cundill JG. Anticonvulsant drugs used in the treatment of lancinating pain: a comparison. *Anaesthesia* 1981;36:1129–1132.
94. Tandan R, et al. Topical capsaicin in painful diabetic polyneuropathy. *Neurology* 1990;40:(Suppl 1):380.
94a. Tanelian DL, Brose WG. Neuropathic pain can be relieved by drugs that are use-dependent sodium channel blockers: lidocaine, carbamazepine, and mexiletine. *Anesthesiology* 1991;74:949–951.
95. Thomas PK. Clinical features and differential diagnosis. In: Dyck PJ, et al, eds. *Peripheral Neuropathy*. 2nd ed. Philadelphia: WB Saunders; 1984:1169–1190.
96. Thomas PK, King RHM. Peripheral nerve changes in amyloid neuropathy. *Brain* 1974;97:395–406.
97. Thomas PK, Ochoa J. Microscopic anatomy of peripheral nerve fibers. In: Dyck PJ, et al, eds. *Peripheral Neuropathy*. 2nd ed. Philadelphia: WB Saunders; 1984:39–96.
98. Thomas PK, Walker JG. Xanthomatous neuropathy in primary biliary cirrhosis. *Brain* 1965;88:1079–1092.
99. Tredici G, Minazzi M. Alcoholic neuropathy. An electron-microscopic study. *J Neurol Sci* 1975;25:333–346.
100. Valbo AB, et al. Somatosensory, proprioceptive, and sympathetic activity in human peripheral nerves. *Physiol Rev* 1979;59:919–965.
100a. van den Berg LH, et al. Anti-sulphatide antibodies in peripheral neuropathy. *J Neurol Neurosurg Psychiatry* 1993;56:1164–1168.
101. Victor M. Polyneuropathy due to nutritional deficiency and alcoholism. In: Dyck PJ, et al, eds. *Peripheral Neuropathy*. 2nd ed. Philadelphia: WB Saunders; 1984:1899–1940.
102. Wallin BG. New aspects of sympathetic function in man. In: Stalberg E, Young R, eds. *Neurology 11, Clinical Neurophysiology*. London: Butterworth, 1981:145–167.
103. Walsh JC, McLeod JG. Alcoholic neuropathy. An electrophysiological and histological study. *J Neurol Sci* 1970;10:457–469.
104. Windebank AJ, et al. In: Dyck PJ, et al, eds. Metal neuropathy. *Peripheral Neuropathy*. 2nd ed. Philadelphia: WB Saunders; 1984:2133–2161.
105. Ziegler D, et al. Evaluation of thermal, pain, and vibration sensation thresholds in newly diagnosed type I diabetic patients. *J Neurol Neurosurg Psychiatry* 1988;51:1420–1424.

CHAPTER 51

Mechanisms of Normal and Abnormal Facial Flushing and Sweating

Peter D. Drummond and James W. Lance

1. Facial flushing can result from the release of tonic sympathetic vasoconstriction, active sympathetic vasodilatation, parasympathetic vasodilatation mediated by the facial and glossopharyngeal nerves, and the release of vasoactive neuropeptides from the trigeminal nerve.
2. The part played by each of these mechanisms differs in various parts of the face and depends on the nature of stimulation.
3. Sympathetic fibers responsible for cutaneous vasomotor activity and sweating in the face emerge from the spinal cord in the second and third thoracic segments. They accompany branches of the carotid artery to the periphery and are distributed to the skin with branches of the trigeminal nerve or facial blood vessels.
4. Sympathetic fibers that supply the skin in the supraorbital region travel with the internal carotid artery, whereas those for the remainder of the face accompany branches of the external carotid artery.
5. Sweat glands in the forehead may receive dual innervation from cervical sympathetic fibers and fibers emerging from the brain stem with the facial nerve.
6. Irritative gustatory stimulation induces parasympathetic vasodilatation in the forehead, releases sympathetic vasoconstrictor tone in the forehead, and increases sympathetic sudomotor activity. Pain in the first division of the trigeminal nerve also induces parasympathetic vasodilatation in the forehead.
7. Sympathetic denervation, denervation supersensitivity, and inappropriate reinnervation account for the various forms of pathologic gustatory sweating and flushing, harlequin syndrome, and Ross's syndrome.
8. The ocular Horner's syndrome in cluster headache and some cases of migraine may be caused by the greater superficial petrosal nerve releasing vasoactive peptides from the carotid ganglion, producing edema of the wall of the internal carotid artery, and thus compromising sympathetic fibers in the periarterial plexus.

SYMPATHETIC PATHWAY TO THE FACE

The cervical sympathetic pathway descends from the hypothalamus through the posterolateral part of the medulla and pons to the posterior angle of the anterior horn in the spinal cord (93). Occasionally, facial sweating and flushing is normal in patients with ocular signs of a central sympathetic lesion (33,93), indicating that vasomotor, oculomotor, and sudomotor fibers may take slightly different routes in the brain stem. Pathways may also vary slightly in the spinal cord. For example, Johnson and colleagues (64) reported that the toes were warmer on the operated side by 2 to 5°C in three patients after an incision was made in the anterolateral part of the spinal cord, but sweating in the lower part of the body was not affected.

Preganglionic sympathetic fibers leave the intermediolateral column of the spinal cord with the ventral thoracic roots and synapse with cells in the superior cervical ganglion. Most fibers destined for the pupil and eyelid leave the spinal cord in the first thoracic root, whereas fibers to sweat glands and blood vessels exit in the second and third thoracic roots (Fig. 1).(48) Thus, a sympathectomy below the first thoracic root usually reduces thermoregulatory sweating in the face and hands without producing undesirable effects on the eyes. Conversely, damage to the first thoracic root will produce a small pupil and drooping eyelid (the oc-

---

P. D. Drummond: Department of Psychology, Murdoch University Western Australia.

J. W. Lance: Institute of Neurological Sciences, Prince of Wales Hospital, Sydney, New South Wales, Australia.

The work described in this paper received support from the National Health and Medical Research Council of Australia, the Australian Brain Foundation, the J.A. Perini Family Trust, Warren and Cheryl Anderson, and Murdoch University.

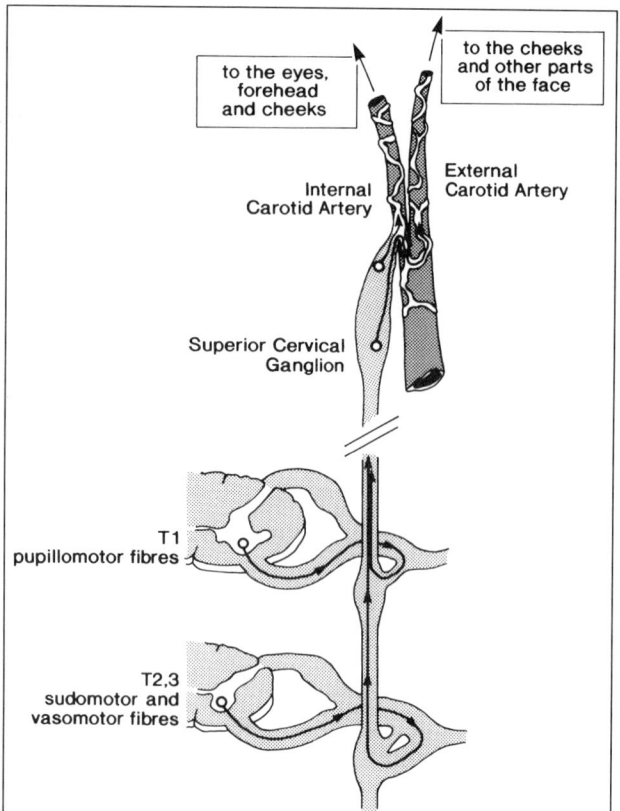

FIG. 1. Origin of pre- and postganglionic fibers in the cervical sympathetic pathway. The preganglionic supply of the eyelids and eyes leaves the spinal cord in the first thoracic root, whereas preganglionic sudomotor and vasomotor fibers leave below T1. Postganglionic fibers supplying the eyes, forehead, and cheeks project from the caudal part of the superior cervical ganglion into the internal carotid nerve, whereas postganglionic fibers supplying the cheeks and other parts of the face project from the rostral part of the ganglion into the external carotid nerve. (Reprinted with permission from Drummond PD. Sweating and vascular responses in the face: normal regulation and dysfunction in migraine, cluster headache and harlequin syndrome. *Clin Autonom Res* 1994;4:273–285.)

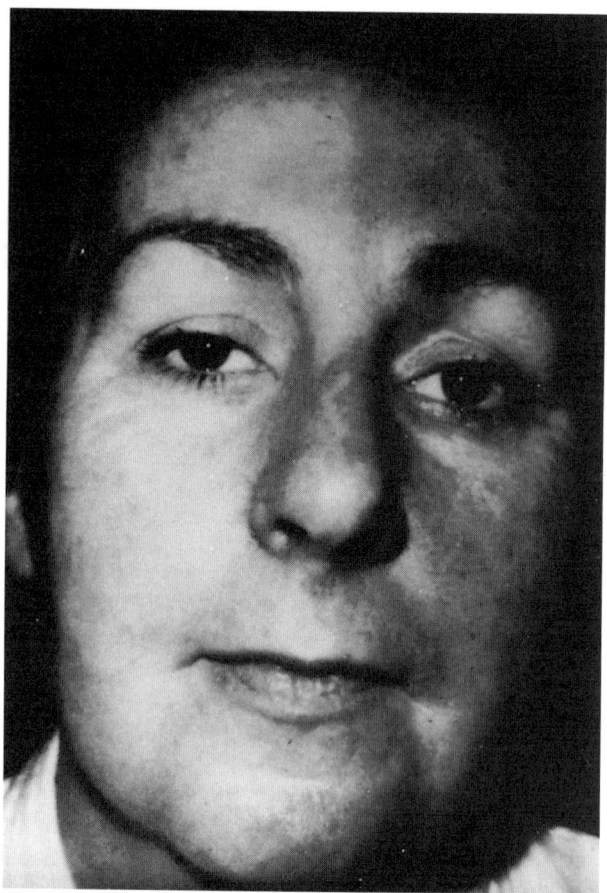

FIG. 2. Unilateral flushing observed after body heating on the side opposite Horner's syndrome. (Reprinted with permission from Drummond PD, Lance JW. Facial sweating and flushing mediated by the sympathetic nervous system. *Brain* 1987;110:793–803.)

ular signs of Horner's syndrome) without affecting facial sweating or flushing (32,91). A few sympathetic fibers may leave the spinal cord with the cervical roots and form intermediate sympathetic microganglia (90). These fibers could account for residual sweating in the central mask area of the face after cervical sympathectomy (90,130).

Neurons that innervate the eyes and lower part of the forehead project from the rostral part of the superior cervical ganglion into the internal carotid nerve (37,86) and course along the internal carotid artery through the carotid canal to the cavernous sinus. Here, they join the sixth cranial nerve for a short distance before following the first division of the trigeminal nerve to the skin (84,101). Fibers destined for other parts of the face project into the external carotid nerve from the caudal part of the superior cervical ganglion (see Fig. 1); these fibers are distributed to the skin by branches of the second and third divisions of the trigeminal nerve. Fibers to the cheeks travel by either route in the rat (37) and possibly also in humans (33). Thus, after damage to sympathetic fibers surrounding the internal carotid artery, thermoregulatory facial sweating and flushing is normal except in the lower part of the forehead, the side of the nose, and occasionally the cheek (32,33,91). A more proximal lesion will interrupt sweating and flushing hemifacially (Fig. 2).

SYMPATHETIC CONTROL OF FACIAL SWEATING AND FLUSHING

The effect of damage to cervical sympathetic pathways on facial sweating and flushing was described with great clarity by Wier Mitchell in 1872 (89). A patient of Dr. William Ogle was thought to have "probable destruction of the right cervical sympathetic chain by abscesses. In this case the eyeball was retracted, the right side of the face redder and hotter than the left in repose, but after violent fever or exercise colder. The left side of the face alone sweated...."

Since then, studies have confirmed that cutaneous blood flow through the ears, nose, and lips is regulated primarily by changes in sympathetic vasoconstrictor tone, whereas active sympathetic vasodilatation predominates in other parts of the face (27). Various nasal (54,100) and ocular structures (50,81), the gums (63), and the lacrimal and salivary glands (50) are innervated by sympathetic vasoconstrictor fibers. Blair and associates (4) observed release vasodilatation after cutaneous nerves supplying the ear were blocked with a local anesthetic agent. In other parts of the face, blocking cutaneous nerves caused only a minor release of vasoconstrictor tone but prevented vasodilatation and sweating during body heating (4,38). Evidence that active cutaneous vasodilatation is mediated by the sympathetic nervous system was obtained in an investigation of patients with a lesion in the sympathetic pathway to the face (32,33). Sweating and flushing during body heating were impaired on the denervated side of the forehead in most patients, and also in the cheek in some instances (see Fig. 2). Exceptions included a man with a brachial plexus injury affecting outflow through the first thoracic root and another with a glioma extending down to the first thoracic segment, confirming that sudomotor and vasomotor fibers usually leave the spinal cord below this level.

Active sympathetic vasodilatation during heat stress was studied after pharmacologic blockade of the stellate ganglion in 10 patients (27). Release of sympathetic vasoconstrictor tone after stellate ganglion blockade caused an increase in orbital and cheek temperature in all patients and an increase in temperature of the forehead, lips, and chin in some cases. Blood flow increased 40% on the blocked side of the forehead, consistent with the release of minor sympathetic vasoconstrictor tone. Patients were then heated until facial sweating was visible. Blood flow increased over 200% on the intact side of the forehead but did not change contralaterally, indicating that sympathetic blockade had interrupted active sympathetic vasodilatation. The neurotransmitter for active sympathetic vasodilatation has not been identified, but the process probably involves an endothelium-derived relaxing factor such as nitric oxide (120). Postganglionic sudomotor fibers contain potent vasodilator neuropeptides, including vasoactive intestinal peptide (VIP) and calcitonin gene-related peptide (CGRP) (72). These peptides may enhance cholinergic sweating (72) and increase cutaneous blood flow when released from sudomotor nerves.

Blushing is sometimes impaired on the sympathectomized side of the face (55,83). In our studies, sweating and increases in blood flow were diminished on the sympathetically denervated side of the forehead when patients with a pre- or postganglionic lesion sang childish songs (32). Emotional vasodilatation was symmetrical in patients with a central sympathetic lesion, suggesting that there is more than one central pathway for emotional blushing. A high density of β-adrenergic receptors in facial blood vessels might influence blushing (65,88), because stimulation of β-adrenoreceptors induces vasodilatation. We recently identified β-adrenoreceptors in forehead vessels (22); blocking these receptors with propranolol inhibited a minor component of emotional vasodilatation, indicating that stimulation of β-adrenoreceptors by circulating catecholamines may contribute to blushing (unpublished observations). However, most of the response is likely to be mediated neurally by active sympathetic vasodilatation.

Nordin (97) measured sympathetic activity in the supraorbital nerve directly with tungsten microelectrodes. His studies confirmed that increases in sympathetic activity during body heating, mental stress, and arousal stimuli preceded increases in forehead sweating and cutaneous blood flow. Forehead blood flow decreased during body cooling, but this was not accompanied by an increase in the rate of sympathetic discharge in the supraorbital nerve. Sympathetic vasoconstrictor nerves may take another route to the forehead, perhaps along blood vessels or branches of the facial nerve (87). In contrast to recordings from the supraorbital nerve, sympathetic activity was never encountered in infraorbital nerve recordings (98), indicating that sympathetic fibers to the cheek are not distributed with this nerve.

SYMPATHETIC DENERVATION SUPERSENSITIVITY

After sympathetic nerves have been injured, blood vessels and sweat glands often develop supersensitivity to autonomic neurotransmitters. Sudomotor fibers release acetylcholine as their peripheral neurotransmitter, whereas sympathetic pupillary and vasoconstrictor fibers release noradrenaline. Sweating after a subcutaneous injection of pilocarpine 0.1 mg/kg body weight (which stimulates cholinergic receptors) was investigated in five patients with central Horner's syndrome and in three patients with Horner's syndrome after a brachial plexus injury (105). In contrast to the response to body heating, sweating in response to pilocarpine was symmetrical or greater on the denervated side in patients with central Horner's syndrome. These patients also showed a supersensitive pupillary response to dilute phenylephrine eye drops. Because phenylephrine stimulates postsynaptic adrenergic receptors, this finding suggests that denervation supersensitivity develops even in patients with a central sympathetic lesion. The sweating response to pilocarpine was less clear-cut in patients with brachial plexus injuries involving the first thoracic root, possibly because most sudomotor fibers leave the spinal cord through T2 and T3.

Sweat gland and pupillary responsiveness was investigated in two patients with probable dysfunction in postganglionic cervical sympathetic pathways (104). Sweating during body heating was reduced on the symptomatic side of the forehead close to the midline but was normal in other areas. Sweating in response to a subcutaneous injection of pilocarpine was greater in the affected supraorbital region in one case, consistent with denervation supersensitivity of sweat glands. Pupillary dilatation to 1% phenylephrine eye drops was greater on the symptomatic side in both patients.

Taken together, these observations document that denervation supersensitivity can develop in sweat glands and blood vessels after central or peripheral sympathetic nerve injury. Thus, denervation supersensitivity may contribute to autonomic disturbances in patients with a long-standing lesion in the cervical sympathetic pathway.

PARASYMPATHETIC VASODILATATION

A major function of parasympathetic reflexes in the face is to dilute and wash away sources of irritation in the eyes, nose, and mouth. Vasodilator reflexes increase blood flow to the lacrimal, nasal, and salivary glands to enhance secretion; blood flow also increases in the surrounding tissues and skin, presumably as part of a protective reflex.

Parasympathetic vasodilator neurons in the superior salivatory nucleus project through the nervus intermedius of the facial nerve to the sphenopalatine and otic ganglia (71,77,92,116,122). Postganglionic fibers are distributed to intracranial vessels, the lacrimal glands and skin of the forehead, the nasal vasculature, and orofacial tissues (17, 20,60,61,109,118,129). A second parasympathetic vasodilator pathway traversing the glossopharyngeal nerve and otic ganglion supplies intracranial vessels, the parotid gland, the lower lip, the gums, and the tongue (61,62,66, 103,110). A separate vasodilator center for the glossopharyngeal nerve has not been identified; however, Gonzalez and co-workers (49) reported that stimulating discrete sites in the facial and trigeminal nuclei increased the temperature of the supraorbital ridge and the upper or lower lips, suggesting that more than one vasodilator center exists in the brain stem.

The parasympathetic vasodilator response to ocular irritation with soapy water was studied in the forehead and cheeks of 15 normal subjects and 15 patients with a facial nerve lesion produced during removal of an acoustic neuroma (17). In normal subjects, blood flow increased ipsilaterally in the forehead for several minutes after stimulation; the persistence of vasodilatation is consistent with the release of VIP, a long-acting vasodilator (47). Vasodilatation was limited mainly to the forehead, with an occasional increase in cheek blood flow. A facial nerve lesion prevented the vasodilator response to ocular irritation (17) and also the vasodilator response to pinching the nasal septum with forceps (20). In normal subjects, pinching the nasal ala induced lacrimation and an increase in blood flow on the ipsilateral side of the forehead; substantial co-variation between these two responses suggests that they are end products of the same reflex (20).

Pinching the upper lip occasionally induced lacrimation and vasodilatation in the forehead but did not influence cheek blood flow, indicating that stimulation of the maxillary division of the trigeminal nerve does not evoke a separate parasympathetic vasodilator response in the cheek (20). Similarly, stimulation of the vidian nerve in dogs increased blood flow through nasal tissues but not through cutaneous branches of the maxillary artery (117). Thus, increases in cheek blood flow during trigeminal nerve stimulation are probably mediated by local axon reflexes (see later).

Orofacial stimulation triggers parasympathetic vasodilator reflexes by way of the otic ganglion (60,67). In human subjects, painful electrical or thermal stimulation of the upper lip increases blood flow in the pulp of the ipsilateral upper central incisor; conversely, painful stimulation of the tooth increases blood flow in the ipsilateral upper lip (69). These reflexes probably have a protective function in the mouth. The effect of sympathetic vasoconstrictor tone on parasympathetic vasodilator reflexes in the cat lip was investigated by Karita and Izumi (68). Simultaneous stimulation of sympathetic and parasympathetic nerves induced opposing responses; vasoconstriction predominated when vasoconstrictor tone was low, whereas vasodilatation predominated when vasoconstrictor tone was high. One of the roles of parasympathetic vasodilator reflexes might be to protect orofacial tissues from frost damage in extreme cold (117).

The facial nerve reflex might influence sweating in the forehead. In normal subjects, ocular irritation with soapy water induced an ipsilateral increase in electrodermal activity (which reflects subclinical sweating) (17). The response was not mediated by sympathetic sudomotor fibers because stellate ganglion blockade enhanced electrodermal activity to the soapy eye drop (18). Attenuation of the response in patients with a facial nerve lesion suggests that forehead sweat glands receive input from the superior cervical ganglion and the facial nerve (17). The facial nerve does not supply conventional sudomotor fibers because sweating increases in response to pain, not thermal stress, after sympathetic blockade (18). The putative neurotransmitter for parasympathetic vasodilatation, VIP (47), potentiates sweat secretion (131). Perhaps release of substances such as VIP from parasympathetic terminals augments forehead sweating as a by-product of the trigeminal–facial nerve reflex. This process seems to be disinhibited by sympathetic blockade (18).

THE ROLE OF VASODILATOR PEPTIDES IN FACIAL FLUSHING

A small component of the vasodilator response to trigeminal nerve stimulation persists after section of the trigeminal root in cats; this component of the response is probably caused by antidromic activation of trigeminal fibers releasing vasodilator peptides (77). Thermocoagulation of the trigeminal ganglion in human patients causes flushing in the distribution of the division or divisions affected (28). Goadsby and colleagues (45) found that levels of CGRP and substance P increased in external jugular venous blood only in those patients who flushed after this procedure. Parallel studies in the cat showed that the same peptides were released after electrical stimulation of the trigeminal nerve. De Marinis and associates (11) noted that the facial flushing response to intravenous injection of histamine was diminished on the side of a previous trigeminal ganglion thermocoagulation, suggesting that release of vasodilator peptides from trigeminal nerve terminals normally played a part in this reaction, and that these peptides were depleted postoperatively. In the rat, stimulation of the trigeminal ganglion evoked an increase in cheek blood flow that was markedly inhibited by a CGRP receptor antagonist, $CGRP_{8-37}$ (36). As noted earlier, trigeminal–parasympathetic reflexes have not been identified in the cheek; thus, release of CGRP from trigeminal nerve terminals probably increases cheek blood flow during painful stimulation.

Such observations may have relevance to the extracranial vasodilatation that sometimes accompanies vascular headache. Zagami and co-workers (133) reported that blood levels of CGRP and VIP rose in the external jugular vein of cats after stimulation of the superior sagittal sinus, a potent cause of headache in human subjects. In patients with migraine, the external jugular levels of CGRP (but not substance P or VIP) were found to be increased on the side affected by headache (46). During attacks of cluster headache, levels of CGRP and VIP were raised in the external jugular vein, indicating antidromic activation of trigeminal nerves (CGRP) and activation of trigeminal–parasympathetic reflexes (VIP) (44). Serum concentrations of CGRP also increase during menopausal flushes (7). It is therefore probable that vasodilator peptides are of importance in mediating normal and pathologic flushing.

PHYSIOLOGIC GUSTATORY FLUSHING AND SWEATING

Almost everyone has experienced facial sweating and flushing after eating chilies or spicy curries. Lee (82) found that physiologic gustatory sweating induced by eating chilies was bilateral and symmetric. The size of the re-

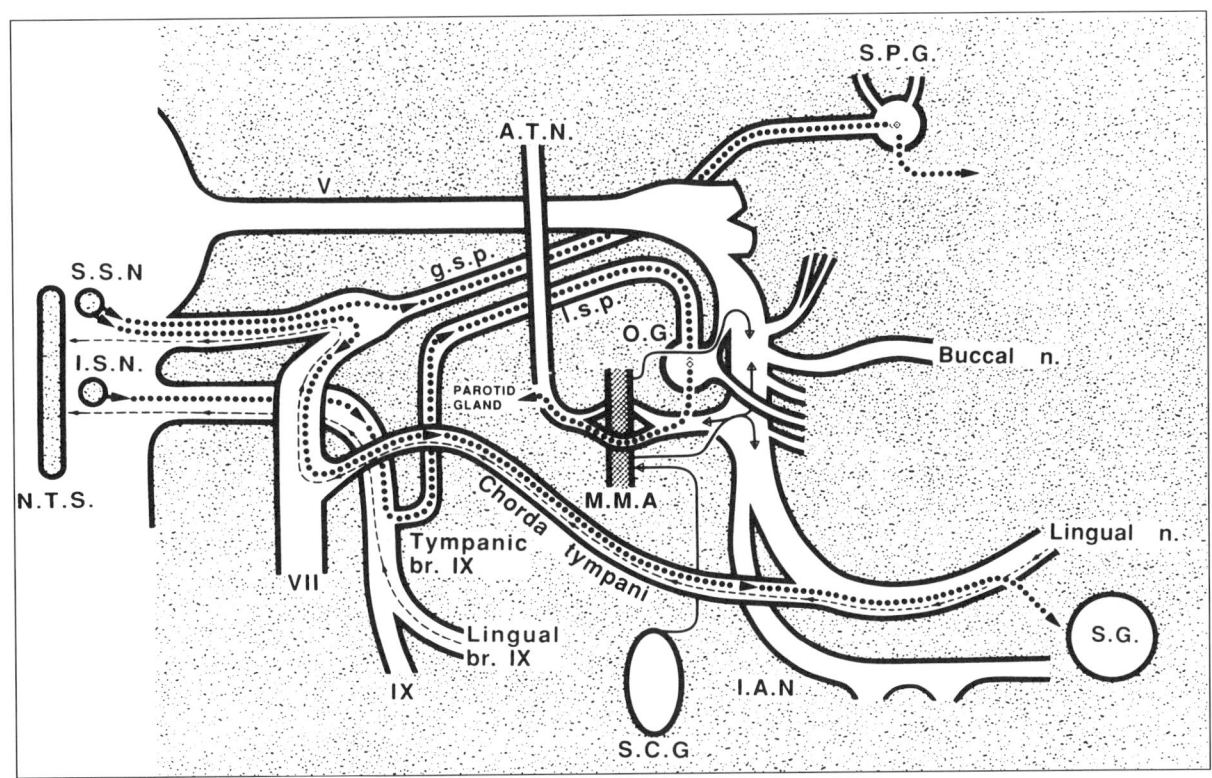

FIG. 3. Autonomic pathways relevant to gustatory flushing and sweating. Afferent fibers (*interrupted lines*) from the anterior two thirds of the tongue follow the lingual nerve and chorda tympani, whereas those from the posterior one third travel in the lingual branch of the glossopharyngeal nerve (*IX*) to the nucleus tractus solitarius (*N.T.S.*). Efferent parasympathetic fibers (*dotted lines*) innervate the parotid gland from the inferior salivatory nucleus (*I.S.N.*) by way of the tympanic branch of the glossopharyngeal nerve, lesser superficial petrosal (*l.s.p.*) nerve, otic ganglion (*O.G.*), and auriculotemporal nerve (*A.T.N.*). Efferents from the superior salivatory nucleus (*S.S.N.*) (*dotted lines*) travel with the facial nerve (*VII*) to the greater superficial petrosal (*g.s.p.*) nerve and sphenopalatine ganglion (*S.P.G.*), to be distributed to the lacrimal gland and extracranial circulation. Other fibers from the S.S.N. travel by way of the chorda tympani and lingual nerve to the submandibular ganglion (*S.G.*) to innervate the sublingual and submandibular glands. Sympathetic fibers (*continuous lines*) from the superior cervical ganglion (*S.C.G.*) are distributed from the plexus around the middle meningeal artery (*M.M.A.*) to branches of the submandibular nerve after passing through the otic ganglion without synapsing. *I.A.N.*, inferior alveolar nerve. (Reprinted with permission from Drummond PD, Boyce GM, Lance JW. Postherpetic gustatory flushing and sweating. *Ann Neurol* 1987;21:559–563.)

sponse varied with the intensity of burning sensation in the mouth, suggesting that pain fibers formed part of the afferent mechanism. Cooling the body reduced or completely inhibited gustatory sweating, whereas warming the body had the opposite effect. Thus, gustatory stimulation apparently caused sweat secretion in glands already activated to a subthreshold level of thermal sweating.

The facilitation of gustatory sweating by thermal stimuli suggests that the reaction is mediated by the sympathetic nervous system. This was confirmed in 13 patients undergoing diagnostic blockade of the stellate ganglion (21); sympathetic blockade clearly prevented increases in electrodermal activity on the ipsilateral side of the forehead when patients tasted Tabasco sauce. In addition, increases in blood flow were greater on the blocked side of the forehead than contralaterally, indicating that release of sympathetic vasoconstrictor tone augmented vasodilatation.

Eating chilies makes the eyes and mouth water and the nose run. These secretory responses are normally mediated by trigeminal–parasympathetic reflexes in the facial and glossopharyngeal nerves (Fig. 3). To determine whether parasympathetic vasodilatation contributes to gustatory flushing, forehead blood flow was monitored in patients with a facial nerve lesion while they ate chilies (21). The facial nerve lesion inhibited vasodilatation on the denervated side of the forehead, indicating that parasympathetic fibers in the facial nerve contribute to this response. Thus, central connections between the maxillary or mandibular divisions of the trigeminal nerve (which relay nociceptive sensations from the mouth) and vasodilator and lacrimal centers in the superior salivatory nucleus appear to mediate gustatory flushing and lacrimation.

PATHOLOGIC GUSTATORY FLUSHING AND SWEATING

Three main types of pathologic gustatory sweating have been described. The first, termed idiopathic hemifacial hyperhidrosis, is provoked by heat, emotion, and eating (5,90,102,111,119). This condition can be associated with hypertrophy of sweat glands (9) and is interrupted by blocking the stellate ganglion (90,119). Tankel (119) reported that sweating was provoked on the affected side of the face in one patient by subcutaneous injection of 0.5 mg histamine. Conversely, gustatory sweating was inhibited by antihistamines. No explanation of the role of histamine was put forward, but the development of adaptive supersensitivity in this condition seems possible because responses to cholinergic agents were exaggerated.

Two other types of gustatory sweating and flushing develop after damage to pre- or postganglionic neurons in the cervical sympathetic pathway. Gustatory sweating develops in up to 70% of patients after bilateral cervicothoracic sympathectomies (57,74) and can be associated with tingling or pilomotion in the scalp and gooseflesh and vasoconstriction in the arms or trunk (5,74). Sweat glands are supersensitive in affected areas (55), but this cannot be solely responsible for the condition because sweating and flushing are reduced on the affected side during body heating. Furthermore, gustatory responses are inhibited by cervical sympathetic blockade (2,55). The most reasonable explanation for this condition is that denervated neurons in the superior cervical ganglion are reinnervated by preganglionic sympathetic fibers originally destined for orofacial tissues.

Gustatory sweating may also develop after local damage to autonomic fibers traveling with peripheral branches of the trigeminal nerve. The auriculotemporal (8,40,41,43) and submental syndromes (125,132) appear to be caused by reinnervation of sympathectomized sweat glands and blood vessels by parasympathetic vasodilator fibers traveling originally to salivary glands. Thus, gustatory responses can be prevented by blocking parasympathetic pathways for salivation but are unaffected by stellate ganglion blockade (41,43,125,132). The syndrome most often develops after parotid or submandibular injury or surgery but was observed in one patient after an attack of herpes zoster in the distribution of the third division of the trigeminal nerve (25). In rare cases, gustatory responses are accompanied by aching or burning pain, or by brief paroxysms of shooting pain (10). Pain could be due to cross talk between sensory and autonomic fibers, or to partial deafferentation or sensitization of sensory nerves. Applying anticholinergic agents to the affected skin is the simplest way to treat the abnormal sweating (56,75), but local injections of botulinum toxin may also be an effective long-term treatment (12).

ROSS'S SYNDROME

The tonic pupil in Holmes-Adie syndrome is commonly associated with loss of tendon jerks, and more rarely with autonomic disturbances such as loss of sweating (Ross's syndrome). The tonic pupil responds to changes in light intensity only after prolonged exposure, and it constricts slowly during near focus. Because the tonic pupil displays supersensitivity to cholinergic agents, the mechanism of the disturbance is thought to be denervation of iris muscles, followed by misdirected reinnervation by parasympathetic fibers originally destined for the ciliary muscle (85). Signs of degeneration in the ciliary and dorsal root ganglia were detected during an autopsy examination of a patient with Holmes-Adie syndrome (124).

We investigated pupillary responses in a 51-year-old woman with tonic pupils, areflexia, and hemifacial loss of sweating and flushing (26). Pupillary dilatation to cocaine and tyramine eye drops was less on the nonflushing side, indicating that outflow was disrupted in postganglionic fibers of the ocular sympathetic pathway. Unlike previous cases (123), there was no evidence of any other neurologic disease. Sweating and flushing during body heating were diminished on the forehead, cheek, and chin, indicating that the sympathetic lesion was proximal to the bifurcation of the common carotid artery, possibly in the superior cervical ganglion. The pathologic process responsible for Holmes-Adie syndrome can thus affect sympathetic as well as parasympathetic outflow and the stretch reflex arc.

HARLEQUIN SYNDROME

Harlequin syndrome was originally described in five patients who complained of the sudden onset of sweating and flushing on one side of the face (80). In one patient, the pupil was slightly smaller on the nonflushing side, and the eyelid sometimes drooped, indicating a partial Horner's syndrome. However, the pupils were symmetric or larger on the nonflushing side in the other four patients. In each of these patients, gustatory sweating was observed on the side that did not sweat during body heating, thus resembling findings in patients with surgical resection of the second and third thoracic segments of the sympathetic chain (32,33). In one case of harlequin syndrome, latency of contraction of the intercostal muscles to electrical stimulation of the motor cortex and spinal cord was delayed on the nonflushing side, indicating that motor fibers in the third thoracic root had been compromised. Thus, loss of thermoregulatory sweating and flushing was probably due to a lesion in this region.

The nature of autonomic deficit in harlequin syndrome was investigated in more detail in two patients from the original series and in two new patients (34). No abnormality was detected on magnetic resonance imaging scans of the upper spinal cord in any of the four patients. However, in two patients, the pupil was larger on the nonflushing side by 0.8 mm and 0.9 mm, respectively, in dim light, well outside the range of simple anisocoria (up to 0.4 mm) (76). Byrne and Clough (6) described signs of increased sympathetic activity in the eye that occurred after damage to the sympathetic plexus around the carotid artery in one patient. This was termed the Pourfour Du Petit syndrome (121), in recognition of a French physician who described signs of sympathetic hyperactivity in the face after sword injuries to the neck. The pupillary signs in harlequin syndrome may be caused by irritation of the sympathetic chain in the neck (121), or they may be due to supersensitivity after partial sympathetic denervation of the iris. In favor of the latter hypothesis, pupillary dilatation to dilute phenylephrine eye drops was greater on the nonflushing side in three patients (34).

The parasympathetic innervation of the pupils may also be compromised in harlequin syndrome. In three of our patients, one or both pupils constricted excessively to dilute pilocarpine eye drops, consistent with ocular parasympathetic deficit (34). Thus, both harlequin syndrome and Ross's syndrome are associated with a patchy sympathetic and parasympathetic neuropathy, although the parasympathetic deficit is more developed in Ross's syndrome. Most evidence implicates fallout of postganglionic autonomic fibers in both syndromes; perhaps a viral infection or autoimmune process targets susceptible neurons in autonomic ganglia. The sympathetic disturbances are mimicked by a lesion of preganglionic fibers emerging from the spinal cord through the second and third thoracic roots (32,33,96).

THE RED EAR SYNDROME

The complaint of a painful, burning red ear has recently been described (78). It is usually unilateral, and pain may radiate to the occiput or to a strip behind and below the mandible that is innervated by the second and third cervical segments of the spinal cord, respectively, or occasionally to the ipsilateral forehead. It is often brought on by exercise, heat, touch, chewing, or neck movement. It is commonly associated with an irritative lesion of the third cervical root, but an association with atypical glossopharyngeal neuralgia and temporomandibular joint dysfunction is described. Some patients have no demonstrable underlying lesion.

The mechanism is uncertain but could involve the antidromic discharge of impulses along the third cervical root, causing pain and vasodilatation in the ear by the release of vasodilator peptides in those patients with a disorder of the upper cervical spine. The relationship of temporomandibular joint dysfunction to redness and burning pain experienced in the ipsilateral ear might depend on a local axon reflex that could also explain idiopathic cases in which the symptoms are provoked by heat or touch. Ochoa (99) identified this phenomenon as "cross modality receptor threshold modulation" because temperature changes alter the threshold for pain induced by mechanical stimulation. He termed this the "ABC syndrome" (angry backfiring C-nociceptor syndrome), of which the red ear syndrome may be an example.

MIGRAINE AND CLUSTER HEADACHE

Cluster headache is associated with an array of autonomic disturbances. Attacks are accompanied by ipsilateral signs of parasympathetic overactivity (lacrimation and nasal discharge), sympathetic overactivity (forehead sweating), and ocular sympathetic paralysis (miosis and ptosis) (73,112). Skin temperature and capillary pulsation increase on the painful side (24,30), more so in areas of sympathetic deficit (14). Furthermore, ocular and thermoregulatory signs of sympathetic deficit persist during the headache-free interval in some cluster headache patients (79,107), and supersensitivity to adrenergic and cholinergic agents develops in symptomatic areas of the face (106,107).

Persistent subclinical sympathetic deficit sometimes develops on the usual side of unilateral migraine headache in patients with frequent or severe episodes (15,16). Increases in blood flow at the site of unilateral migraine (29,31,59) are most apparent in patients with ocular signs of sympathetic deficit (15).

The most probable site of involvement of ocular sympathetic fibers in migraine and cluster headache is the periarterial plexus of the internal carotid siphon. A lesion at this site would compromise ocular sympathetic fibers and the sudo- and vasomotor innervation of the forehead; occasional loss of thermoregulatory flushing in the symptomatic cheek of cluster headache patients (32,33) is consistent with injury to vasomotor fibers that sometimes follow the internal carotid artery before branching off to the cheek (37). Kunkle and Anderson (73) and Nieman and Hurwitz (95) postulated that dilatation, engorgement, or edema of the vessel wall could compress the sympathetic plexus in the carotid canal. Ekbom and Greitz (35) reported the angiographic appearance of localized narrowing of the lumen of the internal carotid artery, just beyond the entry to the skull, at the height of an attack of cluster headache. This was attributed to edema or spasm of the vessel wall and persisted after pain ceased. Similar angiographic findings have been reported for patients with ophthalmoplegic migraine (3). Magnetic resonance imaging angiography of two patients during an attack of cluster headache did not identify swelling of the internal carotid artery (115,128); however, neither patient had ocular signs of Horner's syndrome during their attack. Hannerz and Jogestrand (51) recently reported that moderate unilateral pain developed in 2 of 11 patients studied during a bout of cluster headaches when they were tilted head down for up to 30 minutes; this maneuver increased the diameter of the common carotid artery, as measured by pulsed Doppler ultrasound in the neck. Slight unilateral pain developed in 4 other patients but not in controls or in patients studied outside a bout. In 4 of 8 patients studied during a bout, signs of ocular sympathetic deficit developed during head-down tilting independently of pain. These findings suggest that an intracranial vascular disturbance mediates Horner's syndrome and contributes to the pain of cluster headache. Speculation that sympathetic deficit in cluster headache is of central origin is not consistent with symmetric sudomotor and vasomotor startle reflexes in the hands of cluster headache patients with persistent Horner's syndrome (23).

Hardebo and colleagues (53) studied a group of 100 to 150 nerve cells containing vasodilator peptides situated where the greater superficial petrosal nerve makes contact with the internal carotid artery (Fig. 4). Fibers from this carotid ganglion project to the proximal part of the middle cerebral artery. The greater superficial petrosal nerve continues on as the vidian nerve to the sphenopalatine ganglion, from which second-order neurons are distributed to the lacrimal gland, submandibular and sublingual salivary glands, and the vascular supply of the nasal mucosa, conjunctiva, and cheek. Some fibers loop back from the sphenopalatine ganglion to the internal carotid artery (129) (Fig. 5) and presumably play a part in intracranial vasodilatation.

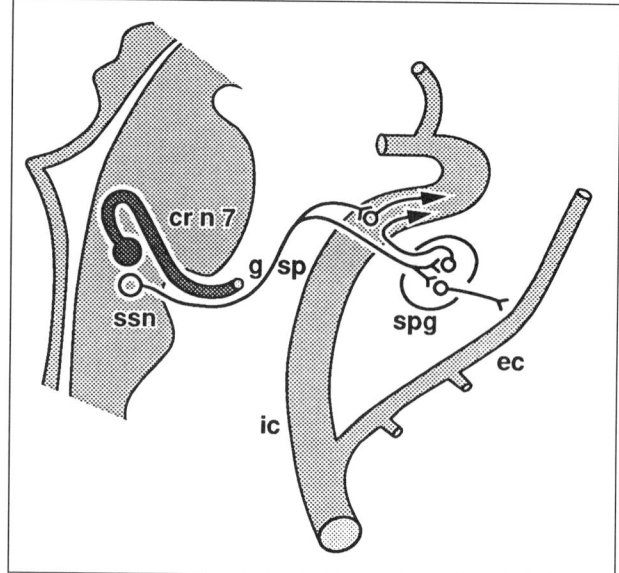

FIG. 4. Parasympathetic fibers from the superior salivatory nucleus (SSN) emerge with the facial nerve (cr n 7) and continue as the greater superficial petrosal (gsp) nerve to the sphenopalatine ganglion (spg). Some fibers from the spg loop back to the internal carotid (ic) artery, whereas others proceed peripherally to the external carotid (ec) circulation.

There is no doubt that the greater superficial petrosal nerve mediates the lacrimation that is so characteristic of cluster headache (and is occasionally seen in migraine), because this symptom is abolished by section of that nerve (42). It is quite possible that antidromic activation of the trigeminal nerve, and parasympathetic discharge along the greater superficial petrosal nerve to the carotid ganglion cells studied by Hardebo and associates (53), could induce edema of the carotid wall by the release of substance P, CGRP, and VIP, thus causing pain felt behind the eye and a partial Horner's syndrome. What has been described as a primary inflammatory vasculitis in the cavernous sinus region in patients with cluster headache (52) may develop in response to antidromic release of neuropeptides from trigeminal terminals during attacks of cluster headache. Deactivation of intranasal trigeminal fibers with repeated applications of capsaicin appears to interrupt the cluster headache cycle (39).

The paradox of an ocular sympathetic paresis and an increase in forehead sweating on the affected side during attacks of cluster headache (106,107,112) remains to be explained. Sweating is normally mediated by an increase in sympathetic outflow, but it can also be provoked by aberrant parasympathetic outflow, as, for example, in postganglionic gustatory sweating. Van Weerden and co-workers

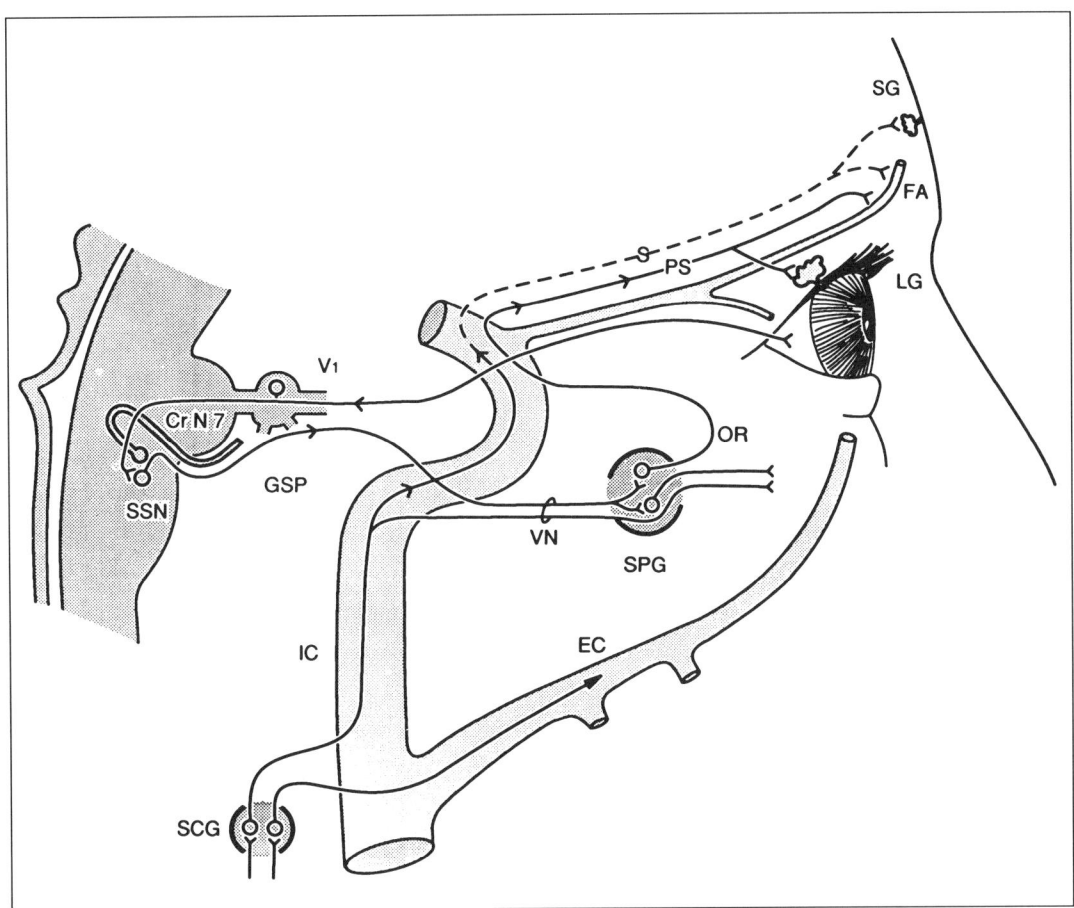

FIG. 5. Postulated explanation for forehead sweating associated with the ocular Horner's syndrome of cluster headache and other postganglionic sympathetic lesions. Sympathetic fibers (S) arising from the superior cervical ganglion (SCG) are injured in the wall of the internal carotid artery (IC), causing their peripheral distribution to the frontal arteries (FA) and sweat glands (SG) to degenerate. Parasympathetic fibers, originating in the superior salivatory nucleus (SSN), traverse the facial nerve (CrN7) and the greater superficial petrosal nerve (GSP) to join the vidian nerve (VN) and synapse in the sphenopalatine ganglion (SPG); postganglionic fibers then loop back as orbital rami (OR) to the cavernous sinus and internal carotid artery, where they form a retro-orbital plexus with sympathetic and trigeminal fibers before advancing to supply the lacrimal glands (LG) and cutaneous circulation of the forehead. Discharge of afferent fibers in the first division of the trigeminal nerve (V1) in response to conjunctival irritation and during attacks of cluster headache reflexly activates parasympathetic outflow to the lacrimal glands and forehead circulation. The *interrupted line* represents the route taken by parasympathetic fibers that occupy the denervated sympathetic pathway and cause frontal sweating and flushing in response to trigeminal discharge. (Reprinted with permission from Drummond PD, Lance JW. Pathological sweating and flushing accompanying the trigeminal lacrimal reflex in patients with cluster headache and in patients with a confirmed site of cervical sympathetic deficit: evidence for parasympathetic cross-innervation. *Brain* 1992; 115: 1429–1445.)

(126) reported that, contrary to the usual findings in Horner's syndrome, sweating was extensive in the right frontal region of a patient who had right-sided Horner's syndrome and a history of continuous mild pain over the right eye and temple for 3 years. Sweating was much more profuse in the right frontal region after Schirmer's strips were inserted under the eyelids. Van Weerden and colleagues (126) postulated that sweating was caused by parasympathetic lacrimal fibers that had sprouted into vacant sympathetic sudomotor pathways. We investigated this possibility in cluster headache patients and in patients with a lesion in the cervical sympathetic pathway from some other cause (32). Ocular irritation with soapy water induced a substantial increase in electrodermal activity on the symptomatic side of the forehead in patients with a postganglionic lesion, including those with cluster headache. In contrast, electrodermal responses generally were small and symmetric in patients with a preganglionic or

central sympathetic lesion. Thus, discharge of parasympathetic fibers that occupy denervated sympathetic pathways to forehead sweat glands could initiate sweating during attacks of cluster headache (see Fig. 5). Denervation supersensitivity of sweat glands in cluster headache (106,107) could amplify sweating during attacks.

Mechanisms similar to those just described may be responsible for the array of autonomic disturbances in variants of cluster headache, such as chronic paroxysmal hemicrania (13,58), the cluster-tic syndrome (1), hemicrania continua (94), and short-lasting, unilateral, neuralgiform headaches associated with conjunctival injection and tearing (SUNCT) (113). In these syndromes, increases in periocular blood flow, lacrimation, and rhinorrhea are probably mediated by trigeminal–parasympathetic reflexes. Fully developed ocular sympathetic deficit is rare in SUNCT and chronic paroxysmal hemicrania, although weak signs such as minor miosis or ptosis may be present during attacks. The symptomatic side of the forehead usually sweats during the SUNCT syndrome (70) and occasionally sweats during attacks of chronic paroxysmal hemicrania (114); unlike cluster headache, however, the symptomatic side of the forehead sweats normally during thermal stress, indicating that sympathetic sudomotor innervation is grossly intact. Irritation of the cervical sympathetic tract may provoke local sweating during SUNCT and chronic paroxysmal hemicrania, as in the Pourfour du Petit syndrome (108); however, sweating is not associated with other signs of cervical sympathetic discharge. Sweating possibly develops in response to VIP, released from parasympathetic vasodilator fibers that innervate the forehead microcirculation during trigeminal–parasympathetic discharge (17,18).

Local pain, tension headache, or migraine occasionally develops after injury to the head or neck. Vijayan and Dreyfus (127) described five cases of post-traumatic migraine that started weeks or months after injury to the soft tissues of the neck in the region of the carotid artery. During episodes of headache, facial sweating and pupillary dilatation were observed on the symptomatic side. No clear-cut disturbance in sweating could be detected between attacks, possibly because the method used (the starch–iodine test) was not sensitive enough to detect minor abnormalities. However, in each case the symptomatic pupil showed evidence of partial sympathetic denervation and adaptive supersensitivity. Because these post-traumatic headaches responded to β-adrenergic blockade, Vijayan and Dreyfus (127) suggested that episodes of headache were due to intermittent bursts of sympathetic overactivity.

In summary, several mechanisms may interact to influence autonomic disturbances during episodes of headache. Vascular disturbances probably arise from activation of trigeminal–parasympathetic reflexes and antidromic release of vasoactive peptides from trigeminal terminals. Injury to sympathetic fibers may lead to parasympathetic or sensory cross-innervation and may increase the sensitivity of sympathetically denervated effector tissues (including blood vessels) to neurotransmitters and circulating substances. A vicious circle of autonomic disturbance and pain may then develop.

REFERENCES

1. Alberca R, Ochoa JJ. Cluster tic syndrome. *Neurology* 1994;44: 996–999.
2. Ashby WB. Gustatory sweating and pilomotor changes. *Br J Surg* 1960;47:406–410.
3. Bickerstaff ER. Complicated migraine. In: Rose FC (ed). *Progress in Migraine Research, Vol. 2*. Bath: Pitman Press. 1984;83–101.
4. Blair DA, et al. Cutaneous vasomotor nerves to the head and trunk. *J Appl Physiol* 1961;16:119–122.
5. Bloor K. Gustatory sweating and other responses after cervico-thoracic sympathectomy. *Brain* 1969;92:137–146.
6. Byrne P, Clough C. A case of Poufour Du Petit syndrome following parotidectomy. *J Neurol Neurosurg Psychiatry* 1990;53:1014.
7. Chen JT, et al. Menopausal flushes and calcitonin gene-related peptide. *Lancet* 1993;342(8862):49.
8. Coldwater KB. Surgical treatment of the auriculotemporal syndrome. *Arch Surg* 1948;69:54–57.
9. Cunliffe WJ, et al. Localized unilateral hyperhidrosis—a clinical and laboratory study. *Br J Dermatol* 1972;86:374–378.
10. De Benedittis G. Auriculotemporal syndrome (Frey's syndrome) presenting as tic douloureux: report of two cases. *J Neurosurg* 1990;72:955–958.
11. De Marinis M, et al. Trigeminal control of cranio-facial vasomotor response: I. Histamine test in patients with unilateral gasserian ganglion lesions. *Cephalalgia* 1984;4:243–251.
12. Drobik C, Laskawi R. Frey's syndrome: treatment with botulinum toxin. *Acta Otolaryngol* 1995;115:459–461.
13. Drummond PD. Thermographic and pupillary asymmetry in chronic paroxysmal hemicrania. A case study. *Cephalalgia* 1985;5:133–136.
14. Drummond PD. Autonomic disturbances in cluster headache. *Brain* 1988;111:1199–1209.
15. Drummond PD. Disturbances in ocular sympathetic function and facial blood flow in unilateral migraine headache. *J Neurol Neurosurg Psychiatry* 1990;53:121–125.
16. Drummond PD. Effect of body heating and mental arithmetic on facial sweating and blood flow in unilateral migraine headache. *Psychophysiology* 1991;28:172–176.
17. Drummond PD. The mechanism of facial sweating and cutaneous vascular responses to painful stimulation of the eye. *Brain* 1992;115:1417–1428.
18. Drummond PD. The effect of sympathetic blockade on facial sweating and cutaneous vascular responses to painful stimulation of the eye. *Brain* 1993;116:233–241.
19. Drummond PD. Sweating and vascular responses in the face: normal regulation and dysfunction in migraine, cluster headache and harlequin syndrome. *Clin Autonom Res* 1994;4:273–285.
20. Drummond PD. Lacrimation and cutaneous vasodilatation in the face induced by painful stimulation of the nasal ala and upper lip. *J Autonom Nerv Syst* 1995;51:109–116.
21. Drummond PD. Mechanisms of physiological gustatory sweating and flushing in the face. *J Autonom Nerv Syst* 1995;52:117–124.
22. Drummond PD. Adrenergic receptors in the forehead microcirculation. *Clin Autonom Res* (In press, 1996)
23. Drummond PD. The site of sympathetic deficit in cluster headache. *Headache* (In press, 1996)
24. Drummond PD, Anthony M. Extracranial vascular responses to sublingual nitroglycerin and oxygen inhalation in cluster headache patients. *Headache* 1985;25:70–74.
25. Drummond PD, et al. Postherpetic gustatory flushing and sweating. *Ann Neurol* 1987;21:559–563.
26. Drummond PD, Edis RH. Loss of facial sweating and flushing in Holmes-Adie syndrome. *Neurology* 1990;40:847–849.
27. Drummond PD, Finch PM. Reflex control of facial flushing during body heating in man. *Brain* 1989;112:1351–1358.

28. Drummond PD, et al. Facial flushing after thermocoagulation of the gasserian ganglion. *J Neurol Neurosurg Psychiatry* 1983;46:611–616.
29. Drummond PD, Lance JW. Extracranial vascular changes and the source of pain in migraine headache. *Ann Neurol* 1983;13:32–37.
30. Drummond PD, Lance JW. Thermographic changes in cluster headache. *Neurology* 1984;34:1292–1298.
31. Drummond PD, Lance JW. Facial temperature in migraine, tension-vascular and tension headache. *Cephalalgia* 1984;4:149–158.
32. Drummond PD, Lance JW. Facial sweating and flushing mediated by the sympathetic nervous system. *Brain* 1987;110:793–803.
33. Drummond PD, Lance JW. Pathological sweating and flushing accompanying the trigeminal lacrimal reflex in patients with cluster headache and in patients with a confirmed site of cervical sympathetic deficit: evidence for parasympathetic cross-innervation. *Brain* 1992;115:1429–1445.
34. Drummond PD, Lance JW. Site of autonomic deficit in harlequin syndrome: local autonomic failure affecting the arm and face. *Ann Neurol* 1993;34:814–819.
35. Ekbom K, Greitz T. Carotid angiography in cluster headache. *Acta Radiol Diag* 1970;10:177–186.
36. Escott KJ, et al. Trigeminal ganglion stimulation increases facial skin blood flow in the rat: a major role for calcitonin gene-related peptide. *Brain Res* 1995;669:93–99.
37. Flett DL, Bell C. Topography of functional subpopulations of neurons in the superior cervical ganglion of the rat. *J Anat* 1991;177:55–66.
38. Fox RH, et al. Cutaneous vasomotor control in the human head, neck and upper chest. *J Physiol* 1962;161:298–312.
39. Fusco BM, et al. Preventative effect of repeated nasal applications of capsaicin in cluster headache. *Pain* 1994;59:321–325.
40. Gardner WJ. Cross talk—the paradoxical transmission of a nerve impulse. *Arch Neurol* 1966;14:149–156.
41. Gardner WJ, McCubbin JW. Auriculotemporal syndrome: gustatory sweating due to misdirection of regenerated nerve fibers. *JAMA* 1966;160:272–277.
42. Gardner WJ, et al. Resection of the greater superficial petrosal nerve in the treatment of unilateral headache. *J Neurosurg* 1947;4:105–114.
43. Glaister DH, et al. The mechanism of post-parotidectomy gustatory sweating (the auriculotemporal syndrome). *Br Med J* 1958;2:942–946.
44. Goadsby PJ, Edvinsson L. Human *in vivo* evidence for trigeminovascular activation in cluster headache: neuropeptide changes and effects of acute attacks therapies. *Brain* 1994;117:427–434.
45. Goadsby PJ, et al. Release of vasoactive peptides in the extracerebral circulation of humans and the cat during activation of the trigeminovascular system. *Ann Neurol* 1988;23:193–196.
46. Goadsby PJ, et al. Vasoactive peptide release in the extracranial circulation of humans during migraine headache. *Ann Neurol* 1990;28:183–187.
47. Goadsby PJ, Macdonald GJ. Extracranial vasodilatation mediated by vasoactive intestinal polypeptide (VIP). *Brain Res* 1985;329:285–288.
48. Goetz RH. The surgical physiology of the sympathetic nervous system with special reference to cardiovascular disorders. *Int Abstr Surg* 1948;87:417–439.
49. Gonzalez G, et al. Vasodilator system for the face. *J Neurosurg* 1975;42:696–703.
50. Granstam E, Nilsson SFE. Non-adrenergic sympathetic vasoconstriction in the eye and some other facial tissues in the rabbit. *Eur J Pharmacol* 1990;175:175–186.
51. Hannerz J, Jogestrand T. Effects of increasing the intracranial blood volume in cluster headache patients and controls. *Cephalalgia* 1995;15:499–503.
52. Hardebo JE. How cluster headache is explained as an intracavernous inflammatory process lesioning sympathetic fibers. *Headache* 1994;34:125–131.
53. Hardebo JE, et al. Morphological and functional substrates for neurogenic inflammation in the human internal carotid artery. Implication for cluster headache. *Cephalalgia* 1989;9(suppl 10):17–18.
54. Hashimoto M, et al. Sympathetic control of blood flow to AVAs and capillaries in nasal and facial tissues supplied by the internal maxillary artery in dogs. *Pflugers Arch* 1987;410:589–595.
55. Haxton HA. Gustatory sweating. *Brain* 1948;71:16–25.
56. Hays LL. The Frey syndrome: a review and double blind evaluation of the topical use of a new anticholinergic agent. *Laryngoscope* 1978;88:1796–1824.
57. Herbst F, et al. Endoscopic thoracic sympathectomy for primary hyperhidrosis of the upper limbs: a critical analysis and long-term results of 480 operations. *Ann Surg* 1994;220:86–90.
58. Horven I, Sjaastad O. Cluster headache syndrome and migraine. Ophthalmological support for a two-entity theory. *Acta Ophthalmol* 1977;55:35–51.
59. Iversen HK, et al. Arterial responses during migraine headache. *Lancet* 1990;336:837–839.
60. Izumi H, Karita K. Vasodilator responses following intracranial stimulation of the trigeminal, facial and glossopharyngeal nerves in the cat gingiva. *Brain Res* 1991;560:71–75.
61. Izumi H, Karita K. Somatosensory stimulation causes autonomic vasodilatation in cat lip. *J Physiol* 1992;450:191–202.
62. Izumi H, Karita K. The parasympathetic vasodilator fibers in the trigeminal portion of the distal lingual nerve in the cat tongue. *Am J Physiol* 1994;266:R1517–R1522.
63. Izumi H, et al. The nervous control of gingival blood flow in cats. *Microvasc Res* 1990;39:94–104.
64. Johnson DA, et al. Autonomic pathways in the spinal cord. *J Neurosurg* 1952;9:599–605.
65. Johnstone M. Facial vasomotor behaviour. *Br J Anaesth* 1974;46:765–769.
66. Kaji A, et al. Parasympathetic innervation of cutaneous blood vessels examined by retrograde tracing in the rat lower lip. *J Autonom Nerv Syst* 1991;32:153–158.
67. Karita K, Izumi H. Somatosensory afferents in the parasympathetic vasodilator reflex in cat lip. *J Autonom Nerv Syst* 1992;39:229–234.
68. Karita K, Izumi H. Effect of baseline vascular tone on vasomotor responses in cat lip. *J Physiol* 1995;482:679–685.
69. Kemppainen P, et al. Blood flow increase in the orofacial area of humans induced by painful stimulation. *Brain Res Bull* 1994;33:655–662.
70. Kruszewski P, et al. SUNCT syndrome: forehead sweating pattern. *Cephalalgia* 1993;13:108–113.
71. Kuchiiwa S, et al. Origins of parasympathetic postganglionic vasodilator fibers supplying the lips and gingivae; an WGA-HRP study in the cat. *Neurosci Lett* 1992;142:237–240.
72. Kumazawa K, et al. Modulatory effects of calcitonin gene-related peptide and substance P on human cholinergic sweat secretion. *Clin Autonom Res* 1994;4:319–322.
73. Kunkle EC, Anderson WB. Significance of minor eye signs in headache of migraine type. *Arch Ophthalmol* 1961;65:504–508.
74. Kurchin A, et al. Gustatory phenomena after upper dorsal sympathectomy. *Arch Neurol* 1977;34:619–623.
75. Laccourreye O, et al. Treatment of Frey's syndrome with topical 2% diphemanil methylsulphate (Prantal): a double-blind evaluation of 15 patients. *Laryngoscope* 1990;100:651–653.
76. Lam BL, et al. The prevalence of simple anisocoria. *Am J Ophthalmol* 1987;104:69–73.
77. Lambert GA, et al. Decreased carotid arterial resistance in cats in response to trigeminal stimulation. *J Neurosurg* 1984;61:307–315.
78. Lance JW. The red ear syndrome. *Neurology* (In press, 1996)
79. Lance JW, Drummond PD. Horner's syndrome in cluster headache. In: Rose FC (ed). *Advances in Headache Research.* London: John Libbey. 1987;169–174.
80. Lance JW, et al. Harlequin syndrome: the sudden onset of unilateral flushing and sweating. *J Neurol Neurosurg Psychiatry* 1988;51:635–642.
81. Lanigan LP, et al. The effect of cervical sympathectomy on retinal vessel responses to systemic autonomic stimulation. *Eye* 1990;4:181–189.
82. Lee TS. Physiological gustatory sweating in a warm climate. *J Physiol* 1954;124:528–542.
83. Lewis T, Landis EM. Some physiological effects of sympathetic ganglionectomy in the human being and its effect in a case of Raynaud's malady. *Heart* 1930;15:151–176.
84. List CF, Peet MM. Sweat secretion in man. IV. Sweat secretion of the face and its disturbances. *Arch Neurol Psychiatry* 1938;40:443–470.
85. Loewenfeld IE, Thompson HS. The tonic pupil: a re-evaluation. *Am J Ophthalmol* 1967;63:46–87.

86. Luebke JI, Wright LL. Characterization of superior cervical ganglion neurons that project to the submandibular glands, the eyes, and the pineal gland in rats. *Brain Res* 1992;589:1–14.
87. Matthews B, Robinson PP. The course of postganglionic sympathetic fibres distributed with the facial nerve in the cat. *Brain Res* 1986;382:55–60.
88. Mellander S, et al. Neural beta-adrenergic dilatation of the facial vein in man: possible mechanism in emotional blushing. *Acta Physiol Scand* 1982;114:393–399.
89. Mitchell SW. *Injuries of Nerves and Their Consequences*. Philadelphia: JB Lippincott. 1972.
90. Monro PAG. *Sympathectomy*. London: Oxford University Press. 1959;157–186.
91. Morris JGL, et al. Facial sweating in Horner's syndrome. *Brain* 1984;107:751–758.
92. Nakai M, et al. Parasympathetic cerebrovasodilator centre of the facial nerve. *Circ Res* 1993;72:470–475.
93. Nathan PW, Smith MC. The location of descending fibres to sympathetic neurons supplying the eye and sudomotor neurons supplying the head and neck. *J Neurol Neurosurg Psychiatry* 1986;49:187–194.
94. Newman LC, et al. Hemicrania continua: ten new cases and a review of the literature. *Neurology* 1994;44:2111–2114.
95. Nieman EA, Hurwitz LJ. Ocular sympathetic palsy in periodic migrainous neuralgia. *J Neurol Neurosurg Psychiatry* 1961;24:369–373.
96. Noda S. Harlequin syndrome due to superior mediastinal neurinoma. *J Neurol Neurosurg Psychiatry* 1991;54:744.
97. Nordin M. Sympathetic discharges in the human supraorbital nerve and their relation to sudo- and vasomotor responses. *J Physiol* 1990;423:241–255.
98. Nordin M, Thomander L. Intrafascicular multi-unit recordings from the human infra-orbital nerve. *Acta Physiol Scand* 1989;135:139–148.
99. Ochoa JL. The human sensory unit and pain: new concepts, syndromes and tests. *Muscle Nerve* 1993;16:1009–1016.
100. Olsson P, Bende M. Sympathetic neurogenic control of blood flow in human nasal mucosa. *Acta Otolaryngol (Stockh)* 1986;102:482–487.
101. Parkinson D, et al. Sympathetic connections to the fifth and sixth cranial nerves. *Anat Rec* 1978;191:221–226.
102. Pearce JMS. Abnormal facial sweating. *Br J Clin Pract* 1964;18:409–412.
103. Ruskell GL. Distribution of otic postganglionic and recurrent mandibular nerve fibres to the cavernous sinus plexus in monkeys. *J Anat* 1993;182:187–195.
104. Salvesen R, et al. Horner's syndrome: sweat gland and pupillary responsiveness in two cases with a probable 3rd neurone dysfunction. *Cephalalgia* 1989;9:63–70.
105. Salvesen R, et al. Sweat gland and pupillary responsiveness in Horner's syndrome. *Cephalalgia* 1987;7:135–146.
106. Salvesen R, et al. Cluster headache: combined assessment with pupillometry and evaporimetry. *Cephalalgia* 1988;8:211–218.
107. Saunte C, et al. Cluster headache: on the mechanism behind attack-related sweating. *Cephalalgia* 1983;3:175–185.
108. Saunte C, et al. Chronic paroxysmal hemicrania. IX. On the mechanism of attack-related sweating. *Cephalalgia* 1983;3:191–199.
109. Segade LAG, Quintanilla JS. Distribution of postganglionic parasympathetic fibers originating in the pterygopalatine ganglion in the maxillary and ophthalmic nerve branches of the trigeminal nerve; HRP & WGA-HRP study in the guinea pig. *Brain Res* 1990;522:327–332.
110. Segade LAG, Saurez-Quintanilla D. Otic ganglion parasympathetic neurons innervate the pulp of the mandibular incisor of the guinea pig. *Neurosci Lett* 1988;90:33–38.
111. Shafar J. The syndromes of the third neurone of the cervical sympathetic system. *Am J Med* 1966;40:97–109.
112. Sjaastad O, et al. Cluster headache. The sweating pattern during spontaneous attacks. *Cephalalgia* 1981;1:233–244.
113. Sjaastad O, et al. SUNCT syndrome: VII. Ocular and related variables. *Headache* 1992;32:489–495.
114. Sjaastad O, et al. Chronic paroxysmal hemicrania. VIII. The sweating pattern. *Cephalalgia* 1983;3:45–52.
115. Somerville B. MRI angiography of a patient before and during alcohol-induced cluster headache. *Headache* 1994;34:463–466.
116. Spencer SE, et al. CNS projections to the pterygopalatine parasympathetic preganglionic neurons in the rat: a retrograde transneuronal viral cell body labeling study. *Brain Res* 1990;534:149–169.
117. Sugahara M, Pleschka K. Nutrient and shunt flow responses to vidian nerve stimulation in nasal and facial tissues of the dog. *Eur Arch Otorhinolaryngol* 1992;249:79–84.
118. Suzuki N, Hardebo JE. Anatomical basis for a parasympathetic and sensory innervation of the intracranial segment of the internal carotid artery in man. *J Neurol Sci* 1991;104:19–31.
119. Tankel HI. A case of gustatory sweating. *J Neurol Neurosurg Psychiatry* 1951;14:129–133.
120. Taylor WF, Bishop VS. A role for nitric oxide in active thermoregulatory vasodilation. *Am J Physiol* 1993;264:H1355–H1359.
121. Teeple E, et al. Poufour Du Petit syndrome—hypersympathetic dysfunctional state following a direct non-penetrating injury to the cervical sympathetic chain and brachial plexus. *Anesthesiology* 1981;55:591–592.
122. Ten Tusscher MPM, et al. Pre- and post-ganglionic nerve fibres of the pterygopalatine ganglion and their allocation to the eyeball of rats. *Brain Res* 1990;517:315–323.
123. Trend PStJ, et al. A tonic pupil with Horner's syndrome. *J Neurol Neurosurg Psychiatry* 1986;49:841.
124. Ulrich J. Morphological basis of Adie's syndrome. *Eur Neurol* 1980;19:390–395.
125. Uprus V, et al. Localized abnormal flushing and sweating on eating. *Brain* 1934;57:443–453.
126. van Weerden TW, et al. Lacrimal sweating in a patient with Raeder's syndrome. *Clin Neurol Neurosurg* 1979;81:119–121.
127. Vijayan N, Dreyfus PM. Posttraumatic dysautonomic cephalalgia: clinical observations and treatment. *Arch Neurol* 1975;32:649–652.
128. Waldenlind E, et al. MR-angiography during spontaneous attacks of cluster headache: a case report. *Headache* 1993;33:291–295.
129. Walters BB, et al. Cerebrovascular projections from the sphenopalatine and otic ganglia to the middle cerebral artery of the cat. *Stroke* 1986;17:488–494.
130. Wilson WC. Observations relating to the innervation of the sweat glands of the face. *Clin Sci* 1936;2:273–286.
131. Yamashita Y, et al. Local effect of vasoactive intestinal polypeptide on human sweat-gland function. *Jpn J Physiol* 1987;37:929–936.
132. Young AG. Unilateral sweating of the submental region after eating (chorda tympani syndrome). *Br Med J* 1956;2:976–979.
133. Zagami AS, et al. Stimulation of the superior sagittal sinus in the cat causes release of vasoactive peptides. *Neuropeptides* 1990;16:69–75.

CHAPTER 52

Autonomic Failure and AIDS

Roy Freeman

1. Human immunodeficiency virus (HIV) infection is associated with a variety of symptoms of autonomic dysfunction that involve the cardiovascular, gastrointestinal, and urogenital systems.
2. Tests that evaluate autonomic function frequently reveal abnormal findings in this patient population.
3. Autonomic dysfunction is most severe in the late stages of illness, although some seropositive patients and patients with AIDS-related complex have signs and symptoms of dysautonomia.
4. The cause, natural history, and neuroanatomic features of autonomic dysfunction accompanying HIV infection are not established.

INTRODUCTION

Human immunodeficiency virus (HIV-1), the causative agent of the acquired immunodeficiency syndrome (AIDS), is a retrovirus from the subfamily lentiviruses. HIV-1 infects mononuclear phagocytes and CD4 + T lymphocytes. Intracellular replication of the virus produces cytopathic effects and subsequently evolves into the immune deficiency syndrome (5,33). The HIV-1–infected mononuclear phagocytes also disseminate systemically. These cells may migrate into the central nervous system and infect neuronal cells (38,47). HIV can thus produce a spectrum of neurologic diseases involving every level of the neuraxis, both directly or secondary to opportunistic infections and neoplasms (10,48,55). Neurologic disease may manifest at any stage of infection from seroconversion to established AIDS. In retrospective reports, 10% of patients with AIDS are cited to have neurologic symptoms at presentation, 40% develop neurologic symptoms during the course of the illness, and 75% to 95% have evidence of central or peripheral nervous system pathology at autopsy (10,48,55). Although the symptoms of autonomic dysfunction are common, particularly in well-established cases of AIDS, the prevalence of dysautonomia accompanying HIV infection is unknown.

R. Freeman: Department of Neurology, Deaconess Hospital, The Department of Neurology, Beth Israel Hospital, Harvard Medical School, Boston, Massachusetts 02115.

AUTONOMIC SYNDROMES

Lin-Greenberger and Taneja-Uppal (49) first drew attention to the association between HIV infection and autonomic dysfunction. They described a patient with AIDS who had orthostatic hypotension, impotence, and anhidrosis. Several additional case reports expanded upon their description. Symptoms of dysautonomia in this group of patients have included orthostatic hypotension, syncope and presyncope, proximal body hyperhidrosis, diminished sweating, diarrhea, bladder dysfunction, and impotence (20,22,30,49,59,70).

Cohen and colleagues (16) reported five HIV-infected patients with orthostatic hypotension. Four patients had AIDS and one had AIDS-related complex (ARC). Concurrent infection, severe vomiting, and diarrhea were not present. The patients did not have a significant tachycardia with postural change. A variety of neurologic signs were noted, including cognitive abnormalities, extrapyramidal dysfunction, reduced coordination, and peripheral neuropathy. Autonomic evaluation of these patients revealed abnormal heart rate variation with deep breathing (in four patients) and an abnormal quantitative sudomotor axonal reflex test (in three patients). All patients improved on therapy with fludrocortisone. Four patients remained asymptomatic once fludrocortisone was discontinued, suggesting a transient cause of orthostatic hypotension, at least in these patients.

Orthostatic symptoms typically respond to standard therapies, such as fludrocortisone, sympathomimetic agents, and other pressors, although the patients in the above series responded to fludrocortisone alone. Because autonomic dysfunction is often accompanied by a painful peripheral neuropathy and other symptoms of motor dysfunction, supportive stockings are poorly tolerated. Orthostatic hypotension frequently occurs when a tricyclic antidepressant is introduced as therapy for a painful neuropathy or depression. Nortriptyline and desipramine are tricyclic agents with a relatively low incidence of postural hypotension, and their use may minimize this problem (69). If orthostatic symptoms persist, the addition of fludrocortisone or a pressor agent is usually sufficient to control all symptoms.

Hypotension may also be a manifestation of adrenal insufficiency, which has been reported in a number of patients with HIV infection (42,56). In these patients, hypotension may be associated with weakness, weight loss, mucocutaneous pigmentation, and hyponatremia. Characteristically, these patients have low plasma cortisol levels with a blunted plasma cortisol response to adrenocorticotropic hormone (ACTH) stimulation (42,56), although some patients are reported to have high plasma cortisol values. These high cortisol values have been interpreted as a stress response to illness (65), ectopic production of adrenal cortex stimulating factors by lymphocytes or monocytes (90), or peripheral resistance to glucocorticoids (63).

Hemodynamic lability has also been reported in HIV-infected patients. Luginbuhl and associates (52) drew attention to the presence of episodic hypotension in 20% and episodic hypertension in 19% of their cohort of HIV-infected children. Eleven percent of the patients had episodes of both hypotension and hypertension. Other reports have also documented episodic hypotension, particularly in association with medication administration (37,40,51). Heart rate and rhythm abnormalities including a resting tachycardia (64%), sinus bradycardia (11%), marked sinus arrhythmia (17%), ventricular tachycardia, and torsades de pointes were also observed (52). Ventricular tachycardia and torsades de pointes have often been associated with the administration of medications (12,21,28,79,88).

Patients with HIV infection often report bowel, bladder, and erectile dysfunction (1). Diarrhea is a particularly troublesome symptom for HIV-infected patients. Griffin and co-workers (35) suggested that autonomic denervation of the jejunum might be responsible for nonpathogen diarrhea in some patients. They documented structural abnormalities of the axons and Schwann cells of the autonomic nerves of the jejunal mucosa using transmission electron microscopy. Batman and colleagues (6) used the neuron-specific polyclonal antibody PGP 9.5 to quantify the depletion of autonomic axons in the villi and lamina propria of the jejunum. These histologic abnormalities were present at all stages of HIV infection, and they were also present in asymptomatic patients. Abnormalities of the rectal autonomic nerves have also been documented on rectal biopsy

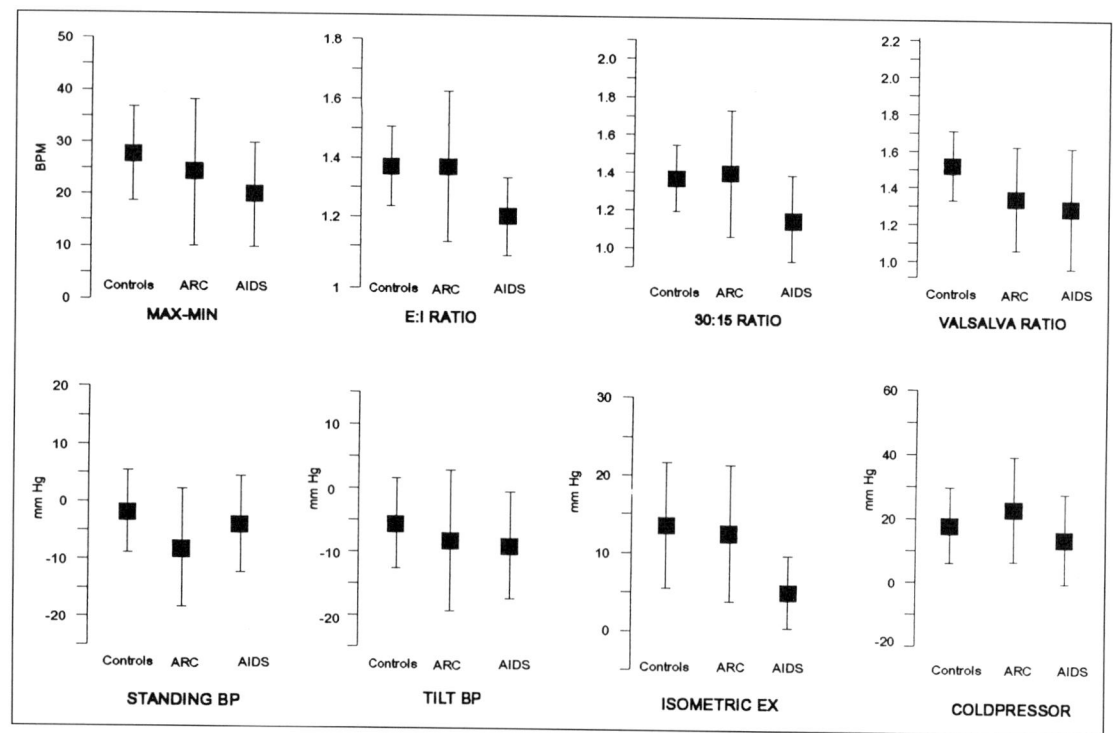

FIG. 1. Results of tests of autonomic function. AIDS, acquired immunodeficiency syndrome; ARC, AIDS-related complex; MAX-MIN, maximum–minimum heart rate difference on deep respiration; E : I, expiratory/inspiratory ratio; BP, blood pressure; EX, exercise.

(9). Increased gut parasympathetic nervous system activity may be an alternate mechanism for nonpathogen diarrhea (17). Incontinence of bowel and bladder is characteristically a late symptom of AIDS. The incontinence is typically associated with a severe neuropathy, myelopathy, or polyradiculopathy and may be exacerbated by an accompanying dementia.

TESTS OF AUTONOMIC FUNCTION

Autonomic testing of seropositive and AIDS patients has been the subject of several reports and case studies (15, 16,22,30,49,59,83,84). In a controlled study, we used multiple tests of the autonomic nervous system and demonstrated significant differences in autonomic function between controls and HIV-infected patients. A steady decline in autonomic function was noted across diagnostic groups (controls, ARC, AIDS), with the most severe autonomic dysfunction found in the patients with AIDS. The abnormalities in autonomic function correlated with signs of HIV-associated nervous system disease. The three patients with the most severe autonomic dysfunction all had evidence of dementia, myelopathy, and distal sensory neuropathy (31).

The autonomic abnormalities were most prominent in tests of heart rate variation. These tests, which principally assess vagus nerve function, included the expiratory/inspiratory ratio (E : I ratio), the standard deviation of heart rate (SD HR), the HR means square successive difference (MSSD), and the maximum–minimum HR difference on deep respiration (MAX-MIN) (Fig. 1; Table 1). There was a significant difference between the resting heart rate in patients with AIDS and that in control subjects. A resting tachycardia is also commonly observed in diabetic patients with a vagal neuropathy and most likely represents unopposed cardiac sympathetic activity (89). A similar mechanism may exist in HIV-infected patients. No patient had clinical or laboratory evidence of dehydration or cardiac failure, either of which might result in an increased resting heart rate. There was also a low correlation between the resting heart rate and the fall in blood pressure with orthostatic change, which would not occur if hemodynamic factors were solely responsible for the resting tachycardia. We could not, however, exclude the possibility that myocardial dysfunction or myocarditis due to HIV infection might be partially responsible for this resting tachycardia (2,14,50). Comparison of the heart rate response to postural change (30 : 15 ratio) and the Valsalva ratio between controls and AIDS patients also revealed a trend toward declining autonomic function in the AIDS patients (see Fig. 1 and Table 1).

Of the tests for assessing sympathetic nervous system function, the blood pressure response to isometric exercise and the fall in mean arterial pressure on tilt-table testing revealed a statistically significant difference in findings among the study groups. In addition, one patient with AIDS was taking fludrocortisone for the treatment of symptomatic orthostatic hypotension, and three patients with ARC exhibited pathologic falls (>20 mm Hg) in systolic BP in response to standing or passive tilting. None of the controls showed comparable declines in BP. Intergroup comparisons showed that these differences were largely a result of significantly more abnormal test results in the AIDS subgroup. A trend toward declining autonomic function was noted in AIDS patients compared with controls, in the systolic BP fall on standing, the systolic BP fall on passive tilting, and the BP response to a cold stimulus (see Fig. 1 and Table 1).

All subjects were assigned an overall measure of autonomic function, called the mean autonomic deviation score. This statistically based summary measure used the control sample to establish normal variability. For each

TABLE 1. Results of tests of autonomic function[a]

Test	Controls	ARC	AIDS
E:I ratio	1.37 ± 0.14[b,c]	1.37 ± 0.27	1.20 ± 0.13
MAX-MIN	27.3 ± 9.12	24.47 ± 15.03	21.17 ± 10.19
SD HR	3.79 ± 1.33[c]	3.41 ± 1.62	2.60 ± 1.70
MSSD	3385 ± 3181.5[b,c]	2725.6 ± 3527[d]	413.1 ± 652.3
30/15 ratio	1.31 ± 0.23	1.39 ± 0.36	1.25 ± 0.24
Valsalva ratio	1.48 ± 0.25	1.33 ± 0.30	1.38 ± 0.35
ST MAP	4.59 ± 9.51	1.63 ± 3.78	5.20 ± 9.77
Tilt MAP	5.36 ± 6.57[b,c]	−1.63 ± 6.80	0.39 ± 6.89
Isometric exercise	13.57 ± 8.35[b,c]	−12.43 ± 9.47[d]	5.17 ± 4.79
Cold pressor	17.90 ± 12.02	23.00 ± 17.94	13.71 ± 14.48

[a]Mean ± SD; [b]$P < 0.05$ (ANOVA); [c]$P < 0.017$ (Bonferroni corrected t-test—controls to AIDS); [d]$P < 0.017$ (Bonferroni corrected t-test—AIDS to ARC).

ARC, AIDS-related complex; AIDS, acquired immunodeficiency syndrome; E:I, expiratory to inspiratory; MAX-MIN, maximum-minimum heart rate difference on deep respiration; SD HR, standard deviation of the heart rate; MSSD, heart rate mean square successive difference; ST MAP, systolic mean arterial pressure; tilt MAP, mean arterial pressure on tilt-table testing; BP, blood pressure; ANOVA, analysis of variance.

test, an individual deviation score (sample Z score) was determined by measuring the distance of the observed result from the control mean, rendered in units of standard deviation. The mean autonomic deviation score was then computed from the sample Z scores of two tests of sympathetic function (the systolic blood pressure responses to tilt-table testing and isometric exercise) and two tests of parasympathetic function (the E : I ratio and the Valsalva ratio) (Fig. 2).

The mean autonomic deviation scores were -0.005, -0.321, and -0.823 in the control, ARC, and AIDS subgroups, respectively. There was a significant difference in the scores across the diagnostic groups ($P = 0.001$). Analysis of intergroup comparisons revealed that this difference largely stemmed from abnormalities in the AIDS patients, whose mean autonomic deviation score differed significantly from that of controls ($P < 0.005$). Of the 10 most abnormal scores, 8 were in AIDS patients and 2 were in ARC patients; there were none in the controls (see Fig. 2).

These test results have been replicated in a number of studies of similar design (70,83,85,87). The HIV-positive subjects studied have included homosexual males and drug users. Homosexuals and drug users who were not HIV positive served as controls in some studies (70,85). Autonomic test abnormalities were demonstrated in 5.6% to 33.3% of HIV-negative intravenous-drug abusers (70,85).

Villa and associates (86) demonstrated that the corrected QT interval (QT_c) was significantly prolonged in a cohort of HIV-positive subjects with autonomic neuropathy. The QT_c was ≥440 millisec in 24 out of 37 (64.8%) patients with autonomic neuropathy but only 5 of 20 (25%) HIV-positive patients without autonomic neuropathy. There were no clinical signs of cardiac disease in any of these patients, although echocardiographic studies were not performed. Others have observed a prolonged QT interval associated with pentamidine administration (78). These observations may underlie the predisposition of HIV-infected patients to cardiac arrhythmias such as ventricular tachycardia and torsades de pointes (often in association with medication administration) and the observed incidence of unexpected cardiorespiratory arrest (12,22,28,52,79,88).

The pupil cycle time provides a noncardiac measure of parasympathetic nervous system function. Maclean and Dhillon (53) reported significant differences in the pupil cycle time between HIV-positive patients and controls. The average pupil cycle time in the HIV-positive group was 1370 millisec compared with 840 millisec in the controls. About half of the AIDS patients developed irregular jerky pupillary movements or hippus, which could not be quantified, after about 10 pupil cycles. Although patients with cytomegalovirus (CMV) and HIV retinopathy were excluded from the study, the authors acknowledged that subclinical optic neuropathy may have influenced their test results. In an earlier uncontrolled report, Scott and associates (71) noted normal pupil cycle times in 15 of 16 HIV-positive subjects in the early stages of infection.

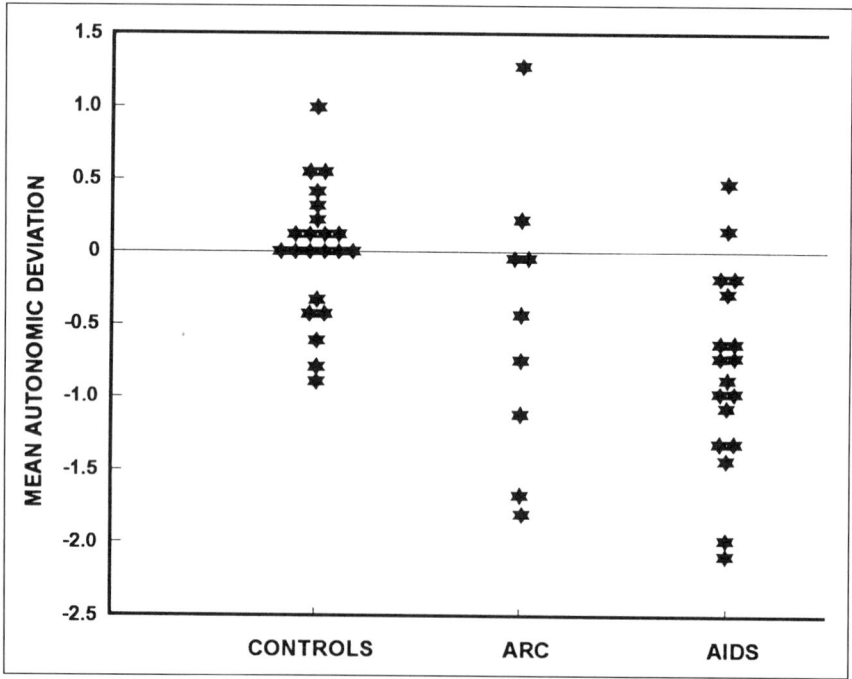

FIG. 2. Mean autonomic deviation scores. *AIDS*, acquired immunodeficiency syndrome; *ARC*, AIDS-related complex.

NATURAL HISTORY

Although autonomic dysfunction appears to occur more often and with greater severity in AIDS patients, several reports suggest that seropositive patients and patients in the early stages of infection exhibit evidence of dysautonomia (43,59,70,83–85). This is not surprising, because both peripheral and central neurologic syndromes may be the presenting or sole manifestation of HIV infection (62,75). The appearance of autonomic dysfunction in the early stage of infection, before the occurrence of opportunistic infections and tumors, implicates HIV or a virus–host interaction in the causation of the dysautonomia. Autonomic dysfunction, however, appears to constitute a continuum from the early to later stages of HIV infection (31,34,70, 85). Toxins, medications, vitamin deficiency, and malnutrition may therefore play a role in the manifestations of this syndrome in the later stages of illness.

We noted that the patients with ARC were a heterogeneous group, and several results exhibited a bimodal distribution with a large variance (see Fig. 1) (31). On the one hand, some tests of parasympathetic nervous system function (the E:I ratio, the SD HR, and the MSSD) showed a significant difference between the various stages of disease (from controls to ARC to AIDS), and there was a trend toward declining autonomic function from the controls to ARC patients to the AIDS patients in the MAX-MIN heart rate change to deep respiration. On the other hand, several patients in the ARC group showed exaggerated normal responses to autonomic testing (see Fig. 1). These findings in patients with ARC are consistent with the demonstration by others that tachycardia, marked heart rate variability, and cardiac arrest are associated with mildly symptomatic HIV infection (52). Bannister (3) has drawn attention to the transient appearance of hyperactive autonomic function occurring for a limited period over weeks to months in patients with autonomic nervous system degeneration. This phenomenon has been attributed to denervation supersensitivity. The exaggerated normal response observed in several ARC patients may well reflect this phenomenon.

In a small longitudinal study of autonomic function in patents with HIV infection, 12 patients in the early stages of infection (seropositive or persistent generalized lymphadenopathy) underwent repeated autonomic testing over the course of 9 to 18 months (71). During this time, no patient had a significant deterioration in autonomic function. This may reflect either the early stage of HIV infection of the patients in this report or the short duration of the follow-up period, or both. In contrast, in a longitudinal study of more advanced HIV infection, progression of autonomic test abnormalities occurred in 9 of 17 patients retested after an average of 11.2 months (85). In this time period, only two of the patients changed their CDC stage.

There is no prospective study of the effect of treatment on autonomic function. There is at present only anecdotal evidence that treatment with zidovudine results in improved autonomic function (18,71).

The relationship between autonomic dysfunction and the CD4+ cell count is unresolved. Welby and co-workers (87) noted an association between CD4+ cell counts <100 cells/mm^3 and the presence of autonomic dysfunction. Scott and colleagues (71) did not find this association in their prospective study, although the mean CD4+ cell count in their cohort of patients in the early stages of infection was considerably higher—512 cells/mm^3 when first evaluated and 314 cells/mm^3 at follow-up.

THE NEUROPATHOLOGIC BASIS OF AUTONOMIC DYSFUNCTION

The underlying neuroanatomic cause of the dysautonomia accompanying HIV infection is not established. HIV-1 can involve the central and peripheral nervous system at multiple sites, producing a variety of neurologic syndromes. Furthermore, there are several characteristic neuropathologic processes associated with AIDS, each having multiple potential sites of involvement. Therefore, in a given patient there is probably more than one cause of the dysautonomia. In our study, abnormalities revealed by autonomic testing correlated with the presence of neurologic signs (31). There was, however, no correlation between a specific neurologic sign and autonomic abnormalities. The three patients with the most severe autonomic dysfunction all had evidence of dementia, myelopathy, and distal sensory neuropathy. The following anatomic regions and neurologic syndromes are those most likely to be responsible for the autonomic dysfunction in HIV-infected patients (Table 2).

The Central Nervous System

The Cerebrum

The AIDS dementia complex is characterized by psychomotor slowing, poor attention, apathy, memory loss, and, less often, mania and psychosis. Motor abnormalities that accompany the dementia include pyramidal and extrapyramidal tract dysfunction, tremor, ataxia, incoordination, and frontal release signs (60). The coexistence of these motor system disorders with autonomic dysfunction may result in this disorder being confused with multiple system atrophy, but this is rare (57). The anatomic territories involved in this process include the subcortical cerebral regions, such as the basal ganglia, subcortical white matter, thalamus, and other deep brain nuclei (61). Dysfunction of these structures could constitute a central neuroanatomic basis for the dysautonomia. The central nervous system may also be affected by opportunistic infections and neoplasms. The clinical manifestations of these disor-

TABLE 2. *HIV and the nervous system*

Cerebrum
  AIDS dementia complex
  Opportunistic infections
    Viruses
      Cytomegalovirus
      Papovavirus
      Herpes simplex virus I and II
      Adenovirus
      Herpes varicella zoster
    Protozoa
      Toxoplasma gondii
    Fungi and yeasts
      Cryptococcus neoformans
      Candida albicans
      Aspergillus
      Coccidioidomycosis
      Histoplasmosis
    Bacteria
      Mycobacterium tuberculosis hominis
      Mycobacterium avium–intracellulare
      Nocardia
  Opportunistic neoplasms
    Primary central nervous system lymphoma
    Metastatic lymphoma
    Metastatic Kaposi's sarcoma
Spinal cord and cauda equina
  Vacuolar myelopathy
  Cytomegalovirus myelitis
  Varicella zoster virus myelitis
  Herpes simplex I and II myelitis
  Neurosyphilis
  Toxoplasma gondii
Peripheral nerve
  Distal sensorimotor neuropathy
  Acute inflammatory demyelinating polyneuropathy (AIDP)
  Chronic inflammatory demyelinating polyneuropathy (CIDP)
  Mononeuritis multiplex

ders will thus depend on the specific sites of involvement. Although these disorders have no predilection for central autonomic structures, the autonomic nervous system may, nevertheless, be involved with these diseases.

Hypothalamus

Purba and associates (68), using immunocytochemical methods to analyze vasopressin and oxytocin neurons in the paraventricular nucleus of the hypothalamus, noted that the number of oxytocin-expressing neurons was 40% lower in the AIDS patients than in the controls. There was no difference between the two groups in the number of vasopressin-expressing neurons in the paraventricular nucleus. On the basis of animal studies, which have shown that central vasopressin and oxytocin play a role in the expression of autonomic functions such as eating, cardiovascular regulation, nociception, and thermoregulation, the authors hypothesized that the selective changes in the oxytocin neurons of the paraventricular nucleus may be the basis for part of the neuroendocrine, autonomic dysfunction, and vegetative symptoms in AIDS.

Spinal Cord and Cauda Equina

HIV-1–associated myelopathy (vacuolar myelopathy) presents as a spastic paraparesis of the lower extremities, although the ankles are often less severely affected than the knees because of a concurrent peripheral neuropathy. Pathologic examination reveals vacuolation of the myelin sheath caused by the enlargement of the periaxonal spaces and splitting of the myelin lamella due to intramyelinic edema. This process involves predominantly the posterior and lateral columns of the middle and lower thoracic spinal cord. Intravacuolar macrophages that may contain HIV-1 are present in the involved areas (23,67,80).

Symptoms of bladder and bowel dysfunction, including urinary retention and loss of sphincter control that results in urinary and fecal incontinence, also occur as a feature of a polyradiculomyelopathy in AIDS patients. The bladder and bowel symptoms are accompanied by progressive, flaccid, areflexic lower extremity weakness and paralysis, with pain, paresthesias, and numbness of the legs and perineum. Most cases are due to infection by CMV, which can be cultured from the cerebrospinal fluid. The characteristic cerebrospinal fluid formula consists of a mixed pleocytosis with prominent polymorphonuclear leukocytes, hypoglycorrhachia, and elevated protein. CMV inclusions are noted at neuropathologic examination of the lumbosacral nerve roots and lower spinal cord (27,55). Therapy with intravenous ganciclovir or foscarnet, or both, may result in improvement of this disorder (13,58,76).

A similar clinical picture can occur with other opportunistic infections of the lumbosacral nerve roots and spinal cord, such as *Toxoplasma gondii* (39,64), herpes simplex virus type 2 (91) and neurosyphilis (8,45), and leptomeningeal spread of systemic lymphoma (41).

Peripheral Nervous System

The peripheral nervous system is involved in up to 80% of patients with AIDS, with a 95% involvement noted postmortem (24). The most common syndrome is the distal sensorimotor polyneuropathy. Symptoms of this neuropathy include numbness, burning, paresthesias, contact hypersensitivity, and walking difficulties. Although it may present at any stage of HIV infection (46), the distal sensory polyneuropathy is relatively uncommon early in the course of HIV disease and becomes more prevalent in immunologically compromised HIV infected persons (4). The pathologic changes include loss of myelinated and unmyelinated fibers, wallerian degeneration, and a mononuclear inflammatory infiltrate (24,32,46,54).

The prominence of neuropathic pain accompanying this neuropathy is similar to that seen in patients with diabetic neuropathy—a disorder in which pain and autonomic dysfunction may be associated with loss of small myelinated and unmyelinated fibers (81). Griffin and colleagues (36) described extensive loss of unmyelinated fibers in two patients who died shortly after the onset of neuropathic pain. Findings from such morphometric studies suggest that the distal sensorimotor neuropathy of AIDS may be a potential cause of autonomic dysfunction.

Because patients with either ARC or AIDS who have an acute inflammatory demyelinating polyneuropathy are clinically indistinguishable from non–HIV-infected patients, the well-described autonomic symptoms associated with the acute inflammatory demyelinating polyneuropathy are also likely to exist in HIV-infected patients (82). Chronic inflammatory demyelinating polyradiculoneuropathy and mononeuritis multiplex, two other neuropathic accompaniments of HIV infection, are not likely to cause autonomic dysfunction (66).

Pathologic examination of the sympathetic and sensory ganglia has revealed a mild ganglionitis consisting of macrophages, T lymphocytes, and an increase in the amount of major histocompatibility complex class II antigen expression. In addition, HIV-1 p24 core protein antigen and HIV-1 gp41 envelope protein antigen were found within macrophages in the ganglia of HIV-infected subjects. These findings were present in HIV-positive cases but were more prominent in cases with clinical AIDS (29).

MEDICATIONS AND TOXINS

Several medications commonly used to treat AIDS-related complications have recognized neurologic side effects, and new therapies may have unknown neurotoxic effects (73). Thus, treatment with these agents may produce the symptoms of autonomic dysfunction or may be responsible for some of the abnormalities in autonomic testing. Vincristine, a component of the drug regimen prescribed for Kaposi's sarcoma, is associated with orthostatic hypotension. In a prospective study, however, only 1 of 26 patients treated with vincristine suffered from orthostatic hypotension (11,25). Pentamidine (37,72), zidovudine (51), and trimethoprim-sulfamethoxazole (40) have also been associated with orthostatic hypotension. The antiretroviral nucleoside analogues 2'3'-dideoxyinosine (ddI or +didanosine) (19,44), 2'3'-dideoxycytidine (ddC or zalcitabine) (7,26), and 2'3'-dihydro 3'-deoxythymidine (d4T or stavudine) (74,77) all have peripheral nervous system neurotoxic effects, although dysautonomia has not been associated with the use of these agents. Dapsone and isoniazid are other recognized neurotoxic agents that are used to treat opportunistic infections in HIV-positive patients. We did not show a significant correlation between the use of any therapeutic agent and autonomic dysfunction; however, the relatively small number of subjects may have limited the predictive ability of our study (31).

CONCLUSION

Autonomic dysfunction is a common and disabling complication of AIDS. This manifestation of HIV infection has been the subject of several controlled studies and case reports. Characteristic features include syncope and presyncope, blood pressure and heart rate lability, cardiac arrhythmias, impotence, bowel dysfunction, bladder dysfunction, incontinence, and anhidrosis. HIV-infected patients are sensitive to the autonomic side effects of antidepressant and antihypertensive agents. To date, there has been no large prospective study of autonomic failure in patients with AIDS. Our knowledge of the prevalence of this disorder, its association with other neurologic and nonneurologic complications of AIDS, and its relationship to therapeutic interventions using potentially neurotoxic agents is still limited. The impact of this disorder on the natural history of HIV infection is unknown. These questions continue to represent areas for fruitful study.

REFERENCES

1. Ali ST, et al. HIV-1 associated neuropathies in males; impotence and penile electrodiagnosis. *Acta Neurol Belg* 1994; 94:194–199.
2. Anderson DW, et al. Prevalent myocarditis at necropsy in the acquired immunodeficiency syndrome. *J Am Coll Cardiol* 1988;11: 792–799.
3. Bannister R. Clinical features of autonomic failure. In: Bannister R (ed). *Autonomic Failure.* Oxford: Oxford University Press. 1988; 267–281.
4. Barohn RJ, et al. Peripheral nervous system involvement in a large cohort of human immunodeficiency virus–infected individuals (published erratum appears in *Arch Neurol* 1993; 50(4): 388). *Arch Neurol* 1993;50:167–171.
5. Barre-Sinoussi F, et al. Isolation of T-lymphotropic retrovirus from a patient at risk of acquired immunodeficiency syndrome (AIDS). *Science* 1983;220:868–871.
6. Batman PA, et al. Autonomic denervation in jejunal mucosa of homosexual men infected with HIV. *Aids* 1991;5:1247–1252.
7. Berger AR, et al. 2',3'-dideoxycytidine (ddC) toxic neuropathy: a study of 52 patients. *Neurology* 1993;43: 358–362.
8. Berger JR. Spinal cord syphilis associated with human immunodeficiency virus infection: a treatable myelopathy. *Am J Med* 1992;92: 101–103.
9. Blanshard C, et al. Electron microscopy of rectal biopsies in HIV-positive individuals. *J Pathol* 1993;169:79–87.
10. Bredesen DE, et al. The neurology of human immunodeficiency virus infection. *Q J Med* 1988;68:665–677.
11. Carmichael SM, et al. Orthostatic hypotension during vincristine therapy. *Arch Intern Med* 1970;126: 290–293.
12. Cohen AJ, et al. Ventricular tachycardia in two patients with AIDS receiving ganciclovir (DHPG). *Aids* 1990;4: 807–809.
13. Cohen BA, et al. Neurologic prognosis of cytomegalovirus polyradiculomyelopathy in AIDS (review) (see comments). *Neurology* 1993;43(Pt 1):493–499.
14. Cohen IS, et al. Congestive cardiomyopathy in association with the acquired immunodeficiency syndrome. *N Engl J Med* 1986;315:628–630.
15. Cohen JA, Laudenslager M. Autonomic nervous system involvement in patients with human immunodeficiency virus infection. *Neurology* 1989;39:1111–1112.
16. Cohen JA, et al. Orthostatic hypotension in human immunodeficiency virus infection may be the result of generalized autonomic nervous system dysfunction. *J Acquir Immune Defic Syndr* 1991 4:31–33.
17. Coker RJ, et al. Increased gut parasympathetic activity and chronic diarrhoea in a patient with the acquired immunodeficiency syndrome. *Clin Auton Res* 1992;2:295–298.

18. Confalonieri F, Villa A. Human immunodeficiency virus–associated autonomic neuropathy, drug addiction, and zidovudine treatment (letter; comment). *Arch Intern Med* 1993;153:400–401.
19. Cooley TP, et al. Once-daily administration of 2′3′-dideoxyinosine (ddI) in patients with the acquired immunodeficiency syndrome or AIDS-related complex. Results of a phase I trial. *N Engl J Med* 1990;322:1340–1345.
20. Cornblath DR, et al. Inflammatory demyelinating peripheral neuropathies associated with human-cell lymphotropic virus type III infection. *Ann Neurol* 1987;21:32–40.
21. Cortese LM, et al. Prolonged recurrence of pentamidine-induced torsades de pointes (review). *Ann Pharmacother* 1992;26:1365–1369.
22. Craddock C et al. Cardiorespiratory arrest and autonomic neuropathy in AIDS. *Lancet* 1987;2:16–18.
23. Dal Pan GJ, et al. Clinicopathologic correlations of HIV-1–associated vacuolar myelopathy: an autopsy-based case-control study. *Neurology* 1994;44:2159–2164.
24. de la Monte SM, et al. Peripheral neuropathy in the acquired immunodeficiency syndrome. *Ann Neurol* 1988;23: 485–492.
25. DiBella NJ. Vincristine-induced orthostatic hypotension: a prospective clinical study. *Cancer Treat Rep* 1980;62:2–3,359–360.
26. Dubinsky RM et al. Reversible axonal neuropathy from the treatment of AIDS and related disorders with 2'3'-dideoxycytidine (ddC). *Muscle Nerve* 1989;12:856–860.
27. Eidelberg D, et al. Progressive polyradiculopathy in acquired immune deficiency syndrome. *Neurology* 1986;36:912–916.
28. Eisenhauer MD, et al. Incidence of cardiac arrhythmias during intravenous pentamidine therapy in HIV-infected patients. *Chest* 1994; 105:389–395.
29. Esiri MM, et al. Sensory and sympathetic ganglia in HIV-1 infection: immunocytochemical demonstration of HIV-1 viral antigens, increased MHC class II antigen expression and mild reactive inflammation. *J Neurol Sci* 1993;114:178–187.
30. Evenhouse M, et al. Hypotension infection with the human immunodeficiency virus (letter). *Ann Intern Med* 1987;107: 598–599.
31. Freeman R, et al. Autonomic function and human immunodeficiency virus infection. *Neurology* 1990;40:575–580.
32. Fuller GN, Jacobs JM. Axonal atrophy in the painful peripheral neuropathy in AIDS. *Acta Neuropathol (Berl)* 1990;81:198–203.
33. Gallo RC, et al. Frequent detection and isolation of cytopathic retroviruses (HTLV-III) from patients with AIDS and at risk for AIDS. *Science* 1984;224:500–503.
34. Gastaut JL, et al. Study of sensory involvement and dysautonomia in HIV infected patients. A prospective study of 55 cases (French). *Neurophysiol Clin* 1992;22:417–430.
35. Griffin GE, et al. Damage to jejunal intrinsic autonomic nerves in HIV infection. *Aids* 1988;2:379–382.
36. Griffin JW, et al. Predominantly sensory neuropathy in AIDS: distal axonal degeneration and unmyelinated fiber loss. *Neurology* 1991; 41(suppl 1):374.
37. Helmich CG, Green JK. Pentamidine-associated hypotension and route of administration. *Ann Intern Med* 1985;103:480.
38. Ho DD, et al. Isolation of HTLV-III from cerebrospinal fluid and neural tissues of patients with neurological syndromes related to the acquired immunodeficiency syndrome. *N Engl J Med* 1985;313: 1493–1479.
39. Kayser C, et al. Toxoplasmosis of the conus medullaris in a patient with hemophilia A–associated AIDS. Case report. *J Neurosurg* 1990; 73:951–953.
40. Kelly JW, et al. A severe, unusual reaction to trimethoprim-sulfamethoxazole in patients infected with human immunodeficiency virus (review) (see comments). *Clin Infect Dis* 1992;14:1034–1039.
41. Klein P, et al. Primary CNS lymphoma: lymphomatous meningitis presenting as a cauda equina lesion in an AIDS patient. *Can J Neurol Sci* 1990;17:329–331.
42. Klein RS, et al. Adrenocortical function in the acquired immunodeficiency syndrome (letter). *Ann Intern Med* 1983;99:566.
43. Kumar M, et al. Norepinephrine response in early HIV infection. *J Acquir Immune Defic Syndr* 1991;4: 782–786.
44. Lambert JS, et al. 2'3'-dideoxyinosine (ddI) in patients with the acquired immunodeficiency syndrome or AIDS-related complex. A phase I trial. *N Engl J Med* 1990;322:1333–1340.
45. Lanska MJ, et al. Syphilitic polyradiculopathy in an HIV-positive man. *Neurology* 1988;38:1297–1301.
46. Leger JM, et al. The spectrum of polyneuropathies in patients infected with HIV. *J Neurol Neurosurg Psychiatry* 1989;52:1369–1374.
47. Levy JA, et al. Isolation of AIDS associated retroviruses from the cerebrospinal fluid and brains of patients with neurological symptoms. *Lancet* 1985;2:586–588.
48. Levy RM, et al. Neurological manifestations of the acquired immunodeficiency syndrome (AIDS): experience at UCSF and review of the literature. *J Neurosurg* 1985;62: 475–795.
49. Lin-Greenberger A, Taneja-Uppal N. Dysautonomia and infection with the human immunodeficiency virus (letter). *Ann Intern Med* 1987;106:167.
50. Lipshultz SE, et al. Cardiovascular manifestations of human immunodeficiency virus infection in infants and children. *Am J Cardiol* 1989; 63:1489–1497.
51. Loke RH, et al. Postural hypotension related to zidovudine in a patient infected with HIV. *Br Med J* 1990;300: 163–164.
52. Luginbuhl LM, et al. Cardiac morbidity and related mortality in children with HIV infection. *JAMA* 1993; 269:2869–2875.
53. Maclean H, Dhillon B. Pupil cycle time and human immunodeficiency virus (HIV) infection. *Eye* 1993;7:785–786.
54. Mah V, et al. Abnormalities of peripheral nerve in patients with human immunodeficiency virus infection. *Ann Neurol* 1988;24:713–717.
55. McArthur JC. Neurologic manifestations of AIDS. *Medicine* 1987; 66:407–437.
56. Membreno L, et al. Adrenocortical function in acquired immunodeficiency syndrome. *J Clin Endocrinol Metab* 1987; 65:482–487.
57. Miller RF, Semple SJ. Autonomic neuropathy in AIDS. *Lancet* 1987; 2:343–344.
58. Miller RG, et al. Ganciclovir in the treatment of progressive AIDS related polyradiculopathy. *Neurology* 1990;40:569–574.
59. Mulhall B, Jennens I. Testing for neurological involvement in HIV infection (letter). *Lancet* 1987;II:1531.
60. Navia BA, et al. The AIDS dementia complex. I. Clinical features. *Ann Neurol* 1986;19:517–524.
61. Navia BA, et al. The AIDS dementia complex. II. Neuropathology. *Ann Neurol* 1986;19:525–532.
62. Navia BA, Price RW. The acquired immunodeficiency syndrome dementia complex as the presenting or sole manifestation of human immunodeficiency virus infection. *Arch Neurol* 1987;44:65–69.
63. Norbiato G, et al. Cortisol resistance in acquired immunodeficiency syndrome. *J Clin Endocrinol Metab* 1992; 74:608–613.
64. Overhage JM, et al. Conus medullaris syndrome resulting from *Toxoplasma gondii* infection in a patient with the acquired immunodeficiency syndrome. *Am J Med* 1990;89:814–815.
65. Parker LN, et al. Evidence for adrenocortical adaptation to severe illness. *J Clin Endocrinol Metab* 1985;60:947–952.
66. Parry GJ. Peripheral neuropathies associated with human immunodeficiency virus infection. *Ann Neurol* 1988; 23(suppl P):S49–S53.
67. Petito CK, et al. Vacuolar myelopathy pathologically resembling subacute combined degeneration in patients with the acquired immunodeficiency syndrome. *N Engl J Med* 1985;312:874–879.
68. Purba JS, et al. Decreased number of oxytocin neurons in the paraventricular nucleus of the human hypothalamus in AIDS. *Brain* 1993;116:795–809.
69. Roose SP, et al. Comparisons of imipramine and nortriptyline induced orthostatic hypotension: a meaningful difference. *J Clin Pathol* 1981; 1:316–319.
70. Rüttimann S, et al. High frequency of human immunodeficiency virus–associated autonomic neuropathy and more severe involvement in advanced stages of human immunodeficiency virus disease (see comments). *Arch Intern Med* 1991;151: 2441–2443.
71. Scott G, et al. Sequential autonomic function tests in HIV infection. *Aids* 1990;4:1279–1281.
72. Siddiqui MA, Ford PA. Acute severe autonomic insufficiency during pentamidine therapy (letter). *South Med J* 1995;88:1087–1088.
73. Simpson DM, Tagliati M. Nucleoside analogue-associated peripheral neuropathy in human immunodeficiency virus infection (review). *J Acquir Immune Defic Syndr Hum Retrovirol* 1995;9:153–161.
74. Skowron G. Biologic effects and safety of stavudine: overview of phase I and II clinical trials (review). *J Infect Dis* 1995;171(suppl 2): S113–S117.
75. Smith T, et al. Symptomatic polyneuropathy in human immunodeficiency virus antibody seropositive men with and without immune de-

76. So YT, Olney RK. Acute lumbosacral polyradiculopathy in acquired immunodeficiency syndrome: experience in 23 patients. *Ann Neurol* 1994;35:53–58.
77. Sommadossi JP. Comparison of metabolism and in vitro antiviral activity of stavudine versus other 2',3'-dideoxynucleoside analogues (review). *J Infect Dis* 1995;171(suppl 2):S88–S92.
78. Stein KM, et al. Incidence of QT interval prolongation during pentamidine therapy of *Pneumocystis carinii* pneumonia. *Am J Cardiol* 1991;68:1091–1094.
79. Stein KM, et al. Ventricular tachycardia and torsades de pointes complicating pentamidine therapy of *Pneumocystis carinii* pneumonia in the acquired immunodeficiency syndrome. *Am J Cardiol* 1990;66:888–889.
80. Tan SV, et al. AIDS-associated vacuolar myelopathy. A morphometric study. *Brain* 1995;118:1247–1261.
81. Thomas PK, Tomlinson DR. Diabetic and hypoglycemic neuropathy. In: Dyck PJ, Thomas EH, Lambert RB et al (eds). *Peripheral Neuropathy*. Philadelphia: WB Saunders. 1993;1219–1250.
82. Tuck RR, McLeod JG. Autonomic dysfunction in the Landry-Guillain-Barré syndrome. *Clin Exp Neurol* 1978;15:197–203.
83. Villa A, et al. HIV related functional involvement of autonomic nervous system. *Acta Neurol* 1990;12:14–18.
84. Villa A, et al. Autonomic neuropathy and HIV infection (letter). *Lancet* 1987;1:915.
85. Villa A, et al. Autonomic nervous system dysfunction associated with HIV infection in intravenous heroin users. *Aids* 1992;6:85–89.
86. Villa A, et al. Autonomic neuropathy and prolongation of QT interval in human immunodeficiency virus infection. *Clin Auton Res* 1995;5:48–52.
87. Welby SB, et al. Autonomic neuropathy is common in human immunodeficiency virus infection. *J Infect* 1991; 23:123–128.
88. Wharton JM, et al. Torsades de pointes during administration of pentamidine isethionate. *Am J Med* 1987; 83:571–576.
89. Wheeler T, Watkins PJ. Cardiac denervation in diabetes. *Br Med J* 1973;4:584–586.
90. Whitcomb RW, et al. Monocytes stimulate cortisol production by cultured human adrenocortical cells. *J Clin Endocrinol Metab* 1988; 66:33–38.
91. Wiley CA, et al. Acute ascending necrotizing myelopathy caused by herpes simplex virus type 2. *Neurology* 1987;37:1791–1794.

The preceding text begins with: "ficiency: a comparative electrophysiological study. *J Neurol Neurosurg Psychiatry* 1990;53:1056–1059."

CHAPTER 53

Postprandial Hypotension

Robert D. Hoeldtke

1. Ingestion of food may cause severe hypotension in patients with autonomic neuropathy. Less severe forms of postprandial hypotension are common in the very elderly.
2. Patients with severe postprandial hypotension typically describe dizziness or blurred vision, or experience syncope after eating.
3. Postprandial hypotension is probably mediated by a vasodilating factor in the gut, most likely a peptide or prostaglandin, that is released in response to ingestion of food.
4. Eating stimulates the sympathetic nervous system in normal subjects. In patients with autonomic neuropathy, especially those with multiple-system atrophy (MSA), ingestion of food fails to activate the adrenergic nervous system normally. An inadequate sympathetic response to the vasodilating effects of ingestion of food is the most likely cause of postprandial hypotension.
5. Caffeine and the somatostatin analogue octreotide have vasoconstrictor effects on the splanchnic circulation and can be used to treat patients with postprandial hypotension.
6. Although octreotide suppresses the secretion of insulin, a potential vasodilator in patients with autonomic neuropathy, this is not the mechanism of the hemodynamic effects of octreotide in patients with autonomic neuropathy.

INTRODUCTION

Although it has been recognized since 1925 that the act of standing may cause hypotension in patients with autonomic dysfunction (5), it has only recently been discovered that ingestion of food also can lower blood pressure (BP) in patients with autonomic neuropathy (58). In extreme cases, profound hypotension and syncope may occur after eating, even while patients are supine. Less severe postprandial hypotension occurs commonly in the very elderly (42). It has also been described in patients with parkinsonism (61) and paraplegia (6), and in patients with renal failure who are undergoing hemodialysis (62).

DEFINITION

Guidelines for testing patients for postprandial hypotension have not been developed, and diagnostic criteria for this disorder are unavailable. Patients have been evaluated in a supine position (58) or sitting in a chair (44). The supine posture is theoretically advantageous because it ensures that hemodynamic changes that develop after eating are the result of ingestion of food and not of the orthostatic stress of prolonged sitting (58). Lipsitz et al. (40,44) have studied this question and shown that before ingestion of food, most patients with postprandial hypotension can maintain a stable sitting BP for 90 min. Therefore, they have recommended measuring the hemodynamic response to ingestion of food while patients are sitting, which is the usual posture for eating. Although we endorse this recommendation, it should be recognized that patients with severe autonomic neuropathy may not be able to tolerate sitting for long enough to permit evaluation of the impact of ingestion of food. Such patients should therefore be tested while semirecumbent, with the head of the bed raised to at least 30°.

The nutritional challenge also needs to be standardized. Mathias et al. (49) have shown that a mixed meal provokes a more pronounced hypotensive response than does ingestion of any single nutritional component. When nutritional components were tested individually, ingestion of carbohydrates lowered BP more than did ingestion of fat or protein. Thus, it is best to test the hemodynamic response to food consumption after the patient has had a mixed meal with a

R. Hoeldtke: Department of Medicine/Endocrinology, West Virginia University, Robert C. Byrd Health Sciences Center North, Morgantown, West Virginia 26506.

high carbohydrate content. A liquid meal is preferable, as many elderly patients require inordinate amounts of time to eat a solid meal. For these reasons, we recommended that the high-carbohydrate liquid meal developed by Lipsitz et al. (a 425-kcal meal consisting of 75% carbohydrate, 23% protein, 2% fat, and no caffeine) be adopted generally for both clinical and research testing of postprandial hypotension. The test meal should be served at room temperature and ingested during a period of 10 min in the morning after an overnight fast, as postprandial hypotension is most apt to occur during the first 2 hours after breakfast (54).

Identifying an abnormal response is difficult, particularly in the very elderly, for whom a postprandial decline in BP may be the rule rather than the exception (42). Patients with essential hypertension show a greater reduction in BP after eating than do their normotensive counterparts (29,40). In patients with hypertension, the postprandial decline in BP is generally asymptomatic and may actually be beneficial. The small minority of patients who experience symptoms of cerebral hypoperfusion after eating exhibit large changes in BP. Patients with documented postprandial syncope show an average reduction in mean BP of 26 mm Hg 60 min after eating (44). Similarly, in patients with autonomic neuropathy, we have observed that symptomatic hypotension is unlikely unless there has been a postprandial decline in the mean BP of at least 20 mm Hg. This degree of hypotension, even if asymptomatic, places patients at increased risk for falls and subsequent injury (43). On the basis of this reasoning, we suggest that until more rigorous guidelines become available, postprandial hypotension should be defined as a decrease in the mean BP of at least 20 mm Hg during the first 2 hrs after breakfast.

PATHOPHYSIOLOGY

The cardiovascular events responsible for the decline in BP in patients with postprandial hypotension are poorly understood. Because some patients with postprandial hypotension also have orthostatic hypotension, it is possible that the pathophysiologic characteristics of the two disorders are similar. In patients with orthostatic hypotension, failure of reflex vasoconstriction causes pooling of blood in the legs during standing. This naturally led to the speculation that excessive splanchnic pooling of blood following ingestion of food was the cause of postprandial hypotension. There is currently no evidence to support this (31). If splanchnic pooling of blood was a critical feature of postprandial hypotension, then it might be expected to compromise cardiac filling and decrease cardiac output, which would lower BP (58). We tested this hypothesis in a patient with severe postprandial hypotension (19). After performing cardiac catheterization in this patient, we measured the cardiac filling pressures, cardiac output, and systemic vascular resistance before and after an oral glucose challenge. We observed that ingestion of food lowered the BP by de-

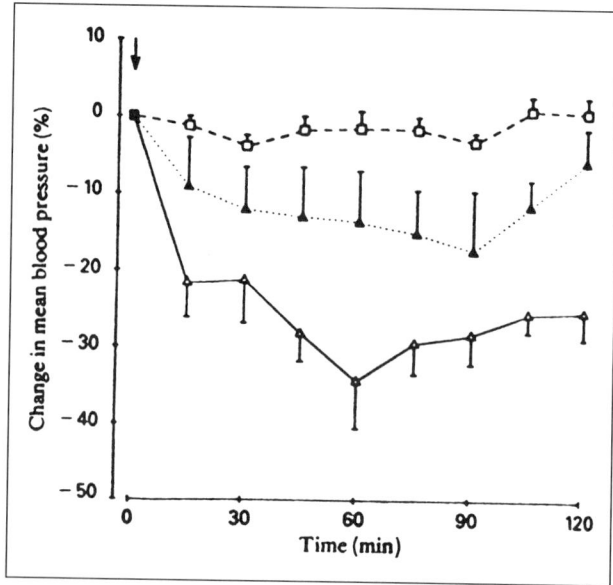

FIG. 1. Percentage change in mean blood pressure in 8 normal subjects after glucose administration *(open squares)* and in 6 patients with autonomic failure after glucose *(open triangles)* or xylose *(closed triangles)* administration. The differences between the fall in blood pressure after glucose and xylose administration in the patients, calculated as the area under the curve, were highly significant ($p < 0.001$). The arrow indicates ingestion of glucose or xylose. Results are mean SEM. (From Mathias, et al. [41]. Reproduced with permission.)

creasing systemic vascular resistance, whereas cardiac filling and cardiac output were unaffected. Noninvasive studies of cardiac function in similar patients have likewise shown that postprandial hypotension is not associated with changes in cardiac output (56).

The hormonal signal that triggers vasodilation during the postprandial period may be a pancreatic or gastrointestinal peptide. In the first known published case report of postprandial hypotension, Seyer-Hansen (61) noted an inverse relationship between the serum insulin level and BP, and suggested that insulin mediated the postprandial decline in BP. Thus, the ingestion of carbohydrates such as glucose, which are potent insulin secretogogues, causes postprandial hypotension; conversely, the ingestion of xylose (52) (Fig. 1) or fructose (27), which are both weak insulin secretogogues, does not provoke hypotension. The vasodilator effects of insulin are well documented in dogs (39) and normal human subjects (8), and there is evidence that insulin may inhibit baroreflex sensitivity, particularly in the elderly (1). The hypotensive effect of both insulin and glucose, administered intravenously, has been confirmed in patients with autonomic neuropathy (51). These data therefore indicate that insulin may mediate, or at least play a contributory role in, the development of postprandial hypotension in patients with autonomic neuropathy. Other evidence, however, contradicts this explanation, particularly in regard to the milder variant of postprandial hypotension that occurs in very elderly patients who do not have overt autonomic neuropathy. Postprandial serum insulin concentrations in very elderly patients do not correlate with the hemodynamic response to eating (44). Moreover, studies of the hemodynamic response to intravenously administered insulin in elderly patients have revealed that the physiologic concentrations of insulin never become high enough to lower BP in this group of patients (41). Similarly, Jansen and Hoefnagels (25) observed that the intravenous administration of glucose elicited a prompt insulin response (mean serum level of insulin, 51.1 ± 10 mU/L in 15 min) in a group of elderly patients with hypertension, yet there was no lowering of BP. By contrast, orally administered glucose precipitated a decrease of 17 ± 3 mm Hg in BP (Fig. 2). This finding suggests that a gastrointestinal factor, possibly a gastrointestinal peptide, is the hormonal signal responsible for lowering BP during the postprandial period. Accordingly, somatostatin, a known inhibitor of gastrointestinal hormone secretion (21), and octreotide, a somatostatin analogue, have been found to prevent the postprandial decline in BP in patients with autonomic neuropathy (22), as well as in those with age-related postprandial hypotension (29). Because somatostatin inhibits the secretion of insulin, other pancreatic peptides, gastrointestinal hormones, and other peptides, its effect on postprandial BP can potentially be interpreted many ways.

The plasma concentrations of some peptides (neurotensin, enteroglucagon, and pancreatic polypeptide) are higher after a meal in patients with autonomic neuropathy than in normal subjects. The plasma concentrations of other peptides (vasoactive intestinal peptide, cholecystokinin, and somatostatin) are similar in control subjects and patients with autonomic neuropathy, before as well as after eating (21,29,50). Of the peptides secreted excessively in patients with autonomic neuropathy, only neurotensin has known vasodilating effects. It is inhibited by octreotide and could be the hormonal signal that triggers postprandial hypotension (50,56). Ingestion of xylose, however, also causes a marked elevation in the plasma level of neurotensin in patients with autonomic neuropathy, but it fails to lower BP (49). Moreover, we have encountered a patient with profound postprandial hypotension in whom neurotensin was undetectable in the plasma (21).

The reversal of postprandial hypotension with somatostatin and octreotide does not necessarily mean that postprandial hypotension is mediated by a peptide hormone. There are a number of alternative explanations for the somatostatin effect. For example, a direct effect of somatostatin on venous tone has been described (63). Exogenous somatostatin and octreotide both decrease splanchnic blood flow (65,66). It is possible that endogenous somatostatin is a locally active splanchnic vasoconstrictor, a deficiency of which is manifested clinically as postprandial hypotension. Moreover, other drugs, such as indomethacin, also prevent postprandial hypotension (22,58). A specific

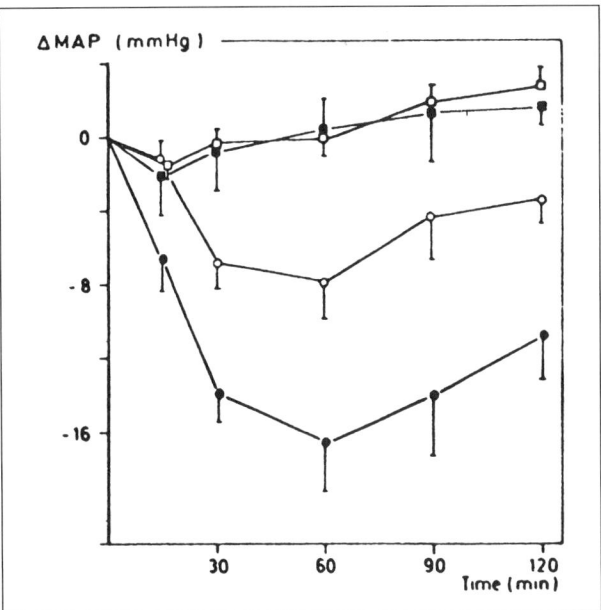

FIG. 2. Change in mean arterial pressure (ΔMAP) in mm Hg, after oral glucose loading in hypertensive (closed circles) and normotensive (open circles) elderly subjects and after intravenous glucose loading in hypertensive (closed squares) and normotensive (open squares) elderly subjects. Data represent mean SE. (From Jansen and Hoefnagels[18]. Reproduced with permission.)

prostaglandin with vasodilating properties has not been implicated, however, and attempts to identify abnormalities in prostaglandin production or metabolism in patients with autonomic neuropathy have thus far been unsuccessful (15).

Identifying the hormonal or neurohumoral signal that lowers BP in patients with postprandial hypotension would not fully explain this disorder. It is still necessary to elucidate its association with autonomic neuropathy and its predilection for the very elderly. These relationships are of fundamental importance, and understanding them will further our appreciation of the impact of eating on autonomic nervous system function and the regulation of vascular tone.

A number of effects of ingestion of food on autonomic function have been described. The impact of eating on baroreceptor function is of particular importance, because elderly patients with decreased baroreceptor sensitivity are particularly prone to a postprandial decline in BP (29,40). Appenzeller and Gross (1) were the first to study this question. They observed that ingestion of glucose led to a decreased baroreceptor response to Valsalva's maneuver in patients with neuropathy or cerebrovascular disease, and postulated that insulin mediated this effect. This mechanism, which provides a possible explanation for postprandial hypotension in the elderly, has recently been reassessed (42). Jansen and Hoefnagels (26) determined baroreceptor sensitivity by measuring the hemodynamic response to graded doses of phenylephrine and nitroglycerin in a group of elderly hypertensive patients before and after a glucose challenge. Although the glucose lowered BP significantly in these patients, it had no effect on baroreceptor sensitivity.

Eating has other effects on autonomic function. In rats, ingestion of food accelerates turnover of norepinephrine (36). This response is possibly mediated by insulin, as intravenous insulin has been shown to increase the plasma level of norepinephrine, at least in dogs (39). It is unclear, however, whether insulin stimulates the sympathetic nervous system directly (36) or whether sympathetic activation represents a compensatory response to insulin-mediated vasodilation (8,39). In some studies of this phenomenon, insulin has been observed to interfere with the action of norepinephrine (37,67) or to enhance its uptake into adrenergic nerve terminals (4).

Observations from clinical studies have confirmed that ingestion of food triggers sympathetic activity, as reflected by plasma concentrations of norepinephrine (68). The intravenous administration of insulin has also been shown to increase the plasma norepinephrine level, at least in some clinical studies (60). However, there are also indications that the adrenergic response to eating is unrelated to insulin secretion. The ingestion of glucose increases the plasma norepinephrine concentration even when the circulating insulin level is fixed and the blood glucose concentration is controlled with a euglycemic clamp (64). These results indicate that the sympathetic activation that occurs after eating represents a compensatory response to splanchnic vasodilation during the postprandial period. Microneurographic recordings from sympathetic neurons in the sural nerve have confirmed that the ingestion of a mixed meal or a solution of pure glucose increases sympathetic activity (3,13); the intravenous administration of glucose and concomitant hyperinsulinemia do not (3). The findings from these studies, taken together, establish that ingestion of food activates the adrenergic nervous system. The mechanism that mediates this effect is probably independent of insulin secretion.

The evidence that eating stimulates sympathetic activity in humans has led to the concept that an inadequate sympa-

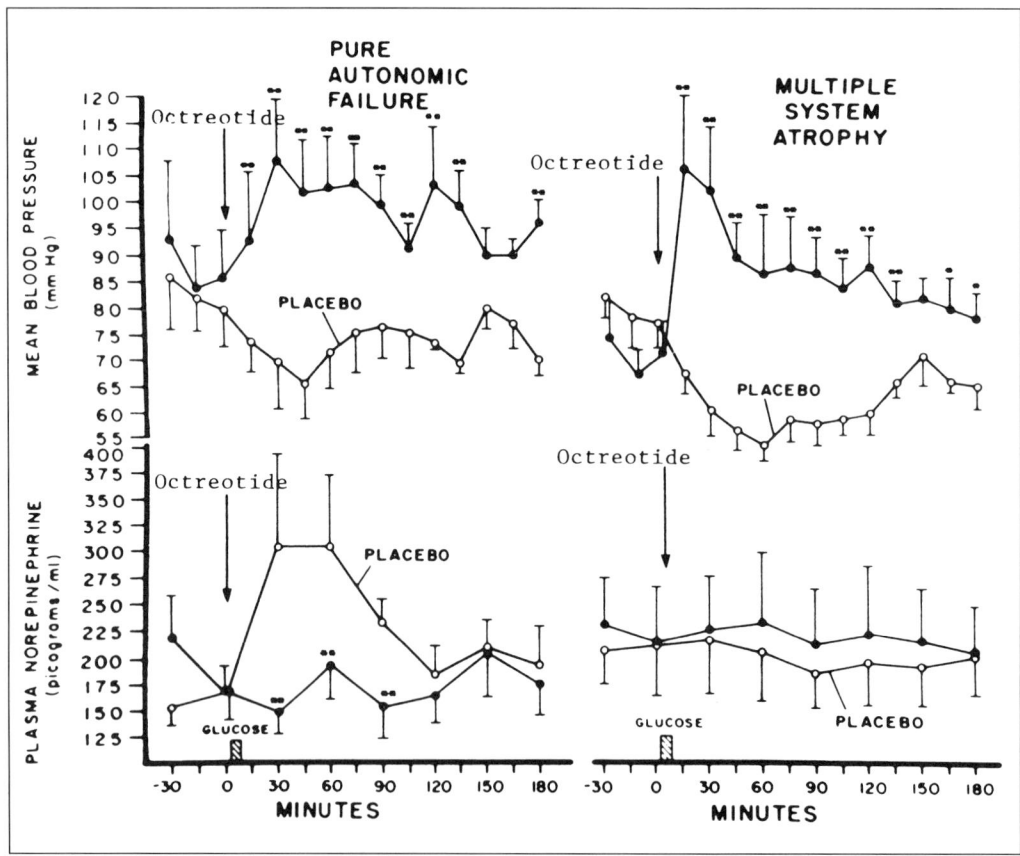

FIG. 3. Effect of octreotide on the plasma norepinephrine response to glucose ingestion. Patients with pure autonomic failure (N = 5) and multiple-system atrophy (N = 6) were given either octreotide subcutaneously (0.8 μg/kg) *(closed circles)* or a placebo *(open* circles) immediately before ingesting glucose. The *hatched area* indicates when patients were ingesting glucose. Data represent mean (no symbol) SE. Drug treatment (*) is different from placebo: $p < 0.05$, **$p < 0.01$. (From Hoeldtke, et al.[16]. Reproduced with permission.)

thetic response to ingestion of food may cause postprandial hypotension (23,44). This is an attractive hypothesis, because degeneration and loss of preganglionic splanchnic sympathetic neurons have been documented in both patients with autonomic failure and those with MSA (46). This concept has been corroborated by direct evidence gathered in patients with overt autonomic neuropathy and severe postprandial hypotension. In the study of Mathias et al. (50), ingestion of food did not elevate the plasma norepinephrine level of patients with autonomic neuropathy, even though eating increased norepinephrine levels by 40% in control subjects. We have made similar observations, but noted a difference between patients with pure autonomic failure (PAF), who generally show evidence of an appropriate adrenergic response to ingestion of food, and those with MSA, who do not (23) (Fig. 3). Hakusui et al. (17) have confirmed by microneurography that patients with MSA lack the normal increment in sympathetic activity following glucose ingestion.

The evidence for postprandial sympathetic dysfunction has been less convincing in those studies that focused on very elderly patients, most of whom did not have clinically apparent autonomic neuropathy. Lipsitz et al. (44) found that patients with postprandial hypotension had an initially normal but subsequently blunted plasma norepinephrine response to eating, and interpreted their data to indicate that the sympathetic response to the hypotensive effect of ingestion of food was inadequate in these patients. The plasma norepinephrine concentrations of patients with postprandial hypotension were only slightly lower than those of controls (approximately 25%), and the changes were evident at only one time point (90 minutes after eating). Robinson et al. (59) and later Jansen et al. (27) found that elderly patients with postprandial hypotension show a normal increment in plasma norepinephrine level following a glucose challenge. When the BP is decreasing, however, or in the setting of hypotension, even a "normal" plasma norepinephrine concentration may be inappropriately low and indicate an inadequate sympathetic response (9). Moreover, the norepinephrine concentration in venous blood, which derives largely from the sympathetic nerves in the forearm (16), may not reflect sympathetic activity (or the lack thereof) in the splanchnic neurons that modulate vascular tone during the digestion and absorption of nutrients.

CLINICAL PRESENTATION

Patients with postprandial hypotension typically experience dizziness or syncope after eating. Although hypotension occurs predictably after breakfast, the hemodynamic response to lunch and supper is variable. Blurred vision, the predominant symptom of the index patient (61), affects approximately one third of patients. In many patients, however, the symptoms of hypotension are nonspecific, consisting of weakness and malaise, and low BP is not diagnosed. This is especially true in patients with diabetic autonomic neuropathy, whose symptoms of postprandial hypotension are easy to confuse with those of hypoglycemia. Although postprandial hypotension is relatively uncommon in diabetic autonomic neuropathy, most patients with PAF or MSA have a significant (>20 mm Hg) decline in BP after eating, and this is symptomatic in approximately one third. In patients without overt autonomic neuropathy, who are generally elderly and hypertensive before ingestion of food, the BP decreases postprandially but stays in the normal range, and most such patients remain asymptomatic.

A minority of patients with postprandial hypotension (≤10%) have chest pain when their BP is low. It has been reported that postprandial hypotension can precipitate transient ischemic attacks (32). Although there has been speculation that ingestion of food may precipitate myocardial infarction or cerebrovascular accidents in the elderly (1), we are unaware of evidence to support this. Despite the increased recognition of postprandial hypotension as an entity, it remains underdiagnosed (30). It may account for as many as one half of all syncopal episodes that occur in nursing homes, but typically it is recognized only after an expensive battery of nondiagnostic neurologic and cardiovascular tests has been performed (30,31). Undiagnosed or improperly treated postprandial hypotension places patients at risk for syncope, falls, and serious injuries.

MANAGEMENT

Patients with postprandial hypotension should be warned about the danger associated with low BP, particularly the possibility of syncope or falling. The first therapeutic goal is to maintain intravascular volume. We generally start our patients with fludrocortisone (0.1 mg/d to 0.3 mg/d). Many symptomatic patients require additional therapy. Caffeine should be tried initially, because of its ready availability and excellent safety record. Although caffeine is only a weak pressor agent in healthy subjects, it can augment the mean BP by approximately 10 mm Hg in patients with autonomic neuropathy and prevents the BP from decreasing after ingestion of food (54). This latter effect most likely stems from a splanchnic vasoconstrictor action of the drug (43). Although tolerance to the pressor effect of caffeine develops rapidly in normal subjects, this may not be the case for patients with autonomic neuropathy, provided they abstain from caffeine ingestion for 24 hours before each treatment. Onrot et al. (54) conducted a short-term trial of caffeine treatment (250 mg administered as a pill 30 minutes before breakfast) and documented that the therapeutic effect was sustained for at least 7 days.

The pressor effect of caffeine in patients with autonomic neuropathy has been attributed to blockade of vasodilatory adenosine receptors, although the drug may have a direct vasoconstrictor effect (54,55). Caffeine also exhibits a pressor effect in patients with age-related postprandial hypotension, but it does not effectively prevent BP from declining during the postprandial period in these patients (38). Two recent studies have indicated caffeine therapy is ineffective in patients with symptomatic postprandial hypotension (2,45).

Indomethacin has also been shown to prevent postprandial hypotension in patients with autonomic neuropathy (58), and we have confirmed that some patients display a reproducible pressor response to this agent (22). One practical limitation to both caffeine and indomethacin stems from the fact that many patients with symptomatic postprandial hypotension also have orthostatic hypotension and need to be treated for both conditions. Even though caffeine and indomethacin may stabilize supine or sitting BP during the postprandial period, they are generally not sufficiently potent to normalize BP when patients assume an upright posture (20,34). Midodrine, an orally active α-adrenergic agonist, is being used increasingly to treat orthostatic hypotension (14). Although its pressor effect is attenuated by the hypotensive effect of ingestion of food (18), it nevertheless prevents symptomatic hypotension during the postprandial period in some patients.

Octreotide, a somatostatin analogue, can be used to treat patients who do not respond satisfactorily to the oral medications mentioned above. Octreotide needs to be given subcutaneously; because its plasma half-life is only 100 minutes, two or more daily injections may be necessary (22). It is primarily indicated for patients with severe autonomic neuropathy who have recurrent episodes of postprandial syncope. Octreotide, however, also prevents the milder form of postprandial hypotension typically present in the very elderly (29), although the hemodynamic responses to the drug are slightly different for the two groups of patients. In patients with autonomic neuropathy, octreotide has a prompt pressor effect, generally evident in 5 minutes, which is demonstrable even when patients are fasting (23). By contrast, in elderly patients with postprandial hypotension who do not have autonomic neuropathy, octreotide has no pressor effect but nevertheless prevents the BP from decreasing after ingestion of food (29).

Automatic BP monitoring should be performed whenever possible during the initiation of octreotide therapy, particularly in patients with severe autonomic neuropathy, who are at risk for having an excessive pressor response to the drug. An initial dose of 0.2 µg/kg is safe in the vast majority of patients, although we encountered one individual with diabetic autonomic neuropathy whose systolic BP increased by 80 mm Hg within 5 min after the administration of a very small dose of octreotide (0.1 µg/kg). When hypertensive responses occur, they can be reversed by having the patients stand, which normalizes the BP within a few minutes. The optimal morning dose of octreotide for patients with postprandial hypotension varies between 0.1 and 0.8 µg/kg. Larger doses (up to 2.0 µg/kg) may be required when patients wish to walk after eating (20). Smaller doses of octreotide (0.2 to 0.6 µg/kg) may be given with lunch or

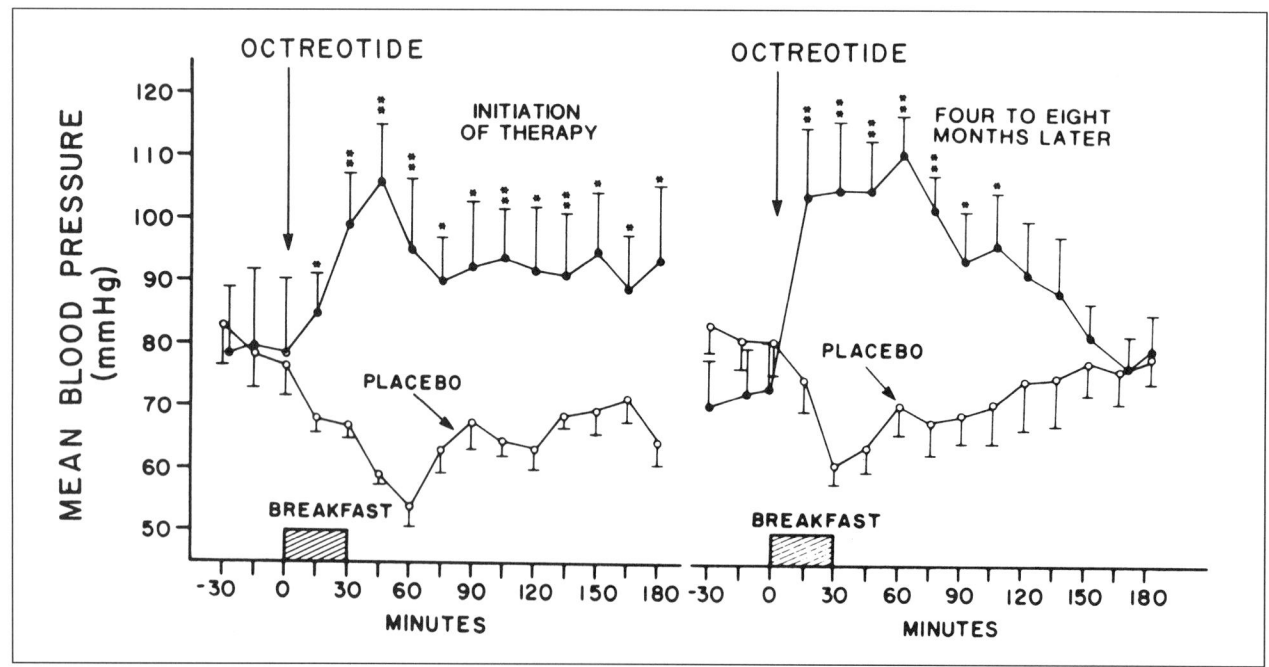

FIG. 4. Long-term therapy of postprandial hypotension with octreotide. The patients received an injection of octreotide (0.4 µg/kg) *(closed circles)* or a placebo *(open circles)* at the beginning of breakfast *(hatched area)*, both at the initiation of therapy and following four to eight months of therapy. Data represent mean SE. Drug treatment (*) is different from placebo: $p < 0.05$, **$p < 0$.

supper. Many patients with autonomic neuropathy have a satisfactory response to only one injection per day, as BP tends to increase spontaneously during the afternoon and evening because of the distinct circadian variations in vascular tone associated with this disorder (47,54). In patients with erratic BP, it may be useful to administer octreotide with an ambulatory infusion pump. This decreases the need for multiple injections and makes it possible to treat unexpectedly low BPs with either higher infusion rates or supplemental bolus doses (20).

We have assessed the efficacy of long-term octreotide therapy in seven patients with severe autonomic neuropathy; four had PAF, two had MSA, and one had diabetic autonomic neuropathy. The efficacy of treatment was evaluated initially by comparing the hemodynamic response to octreotide (0.4 µg/kg injected subcutaneously at the beginning of a 550-kcal caffeine-free breakfast) with that to administration of placebo (Fig. 4, left panel). These treatments were administered in a random sequence on separate days. Following completion of this protocol, patients underwent 4 to 8 months of octreotide treatment (generally given only once per day in a total daily dose of 0.4 to 2.0 µg/kg). Thereafter, the effect of octreotide on the postprandial BP was reassessed after a 24-hr drug-free period using the same protocol followed at the initiation of therapy. We observed that the therapeutic effect of octreotide persisted during long-term therapy and made it possible for bedridden patients to walk or use a wheelchair. When long-term therapy was interrupted with placebo administration, hypotension once again became evident after breakfast (Fig. 4, right panel). The pressor effect of octreotide at the end of 4 to 8 months of therapy resembled that observed at the initiation of treatment. Interestingly, however, postprandial hypotension was not as severe after long-term therapy as before, and two patients were switched from octreotide to caffeine at the end of the study. Neither patient had shown a satisfactory response to caffeine before the octreotide trial.

Although there was no evidence of tolerance to the pressor effect of octreotide in this group of patients, we have observed others who required increasing doses of octreotide to maintain its therapeutic effect. This problem is most likely to occur when patients take either multiple daily injections of octreotide or large doses (>2.0 µg/kg/d). Such individuals should be advised to take just one injection of octreotide per day, before or immediately after breakfast.

Mechanism of Effect of Octreotide in Postprandial Hypotension

The mechanism of the therapeutic effect of octreotide is poorly understood. We have postulated that a specific peptide hormone lowers the postprandial BP (21), and that the hypotension is analogous to that associated with carcinoid crisis, which can also be reversed with octreotide (35). As discussed previously, the vasodilating factor that causes lowered vascular resistance after ingestion of food has not yet been identified.

Although there is evidence implicating insulin as the hormonal signal that triggers postprandial hypotension (51), the hemodynamic effects of octreotide are not attributable to the suppression of insulin secretion. We tested this hypothesis by administering both insulin and octreotide simultaneously in two patients. The insulin dose was estimated so that the circulating insulin concentrations following octreotide treatment approximated those resulting from endogenous insulin secretion. We observed that octreotide effectively prevented postprandial hypotension despite the coadministration of insulin (22). The coadministration of insulin has similarly been shown not to alter the effect of octreotide in patients with age-related postprandial hypotension (28). Finally, we have documented that octreotide prevents postprandial hypotension in patients with autonomic neuropathy secondary to long-standing insulin-dependent diabetes mellitus (Fig. 5). Because endogenous insulin secretion was absent in these patients, the effect of octreotide could not have resulted from an effect on insulin.

Dudl et al. (11) have suggested that the pressor effect of octreotide is secondary to increased norepinephrine secretion. Somatostatin exists in sympathetic neurons (7), and *in vitro* evidence indicates it may activate tyrosine hydroxy-

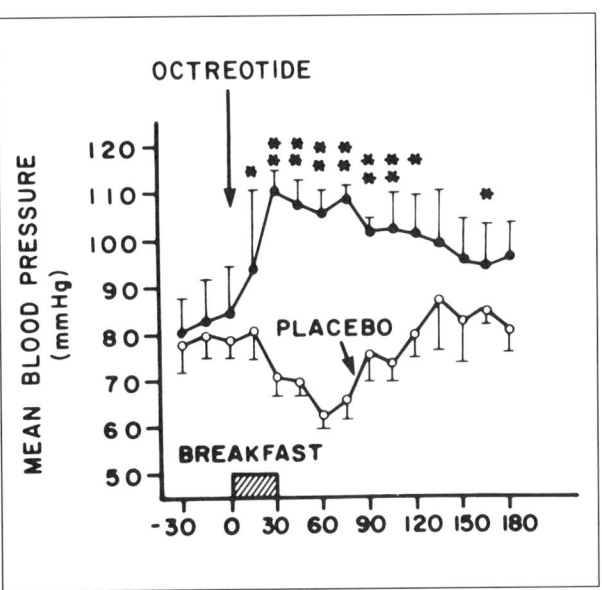

FIG. 5. Treatment of postprandial hypotension with octreotide in patients with diabetic autonomic neuropathy. Patients with postprandial hypotension secondary to diabetic autonomic neuropathy (N = 5) were given octreotide (0.4 µg/kg) *(closed* circles) or a placebo *(open circles) simultaneously with insulin immediately before breakfast *(hatched area)*. Data represent mean (no symbol) SE. Drug treatment (*) is different from placebo: $p < 0.05$; **$p < 0.001$.

lase (33). The findings from clinical studies, however, have not supported this hypothesis. Octreotide administration has no effect on the plasma norepinephrine concentrations in patients with MSA (23). It may even suppress adrenergic activity in patients with PAF, particularly during the postprandial period (Fig. 3). Thus, the pressor effect of octreotide appears to be independent of adrenergic control mechanisms, and in this regard it is distinct from most vasoconstrictor drugs that have been advocated for the treatment of hypotension in patients with autonomic neuropathy.

The mechanism that underlies prevention of postprandial hypotension by octreotide may be distinct from the mechanism responsible for its systemic pressor effect, which can be demonstrated even in fasting patients. Insofar as postprandial hypotension is most likely triggered by eating-related relaxation of splanchnic vascular tone, the splanchnic vasoconstrictor effect of octreotide is of particular interest. Both somatostatin (66) and octreotide (65) cause a decrease in splanchnic blood flow, as extrapolated from clearance of indocyanine green in healthy subjects. We have confirmed that clearance of indocyanine green decreases after administration of octreotide in patients with autonomic neuropathy, and estimated that octreotide causes at least a twofold increase in splanchnic vascular resistance during the postprandial period (24). We have observed other hemodynamic effects of the drug in patients with autonomic neuropathy. Octreotide administration produced an increase in forearm vascular resistance in fasting as well as fed patients. Moreover, octreotide treatment led to increased cardiac output, an effect that we have interpreted to indicate that octreotide may accentuate venous tone (63) and enhance cardiac filling (24). This may be an important action of octreotide, as decreased cardiac filling is one of the major causes of hypotension in patients with autonomic neuropathy.

Adverse Effects of Octreotide

Despite the multiple effects of octreotide on gastrointestinal and endocrine function, this agent is well tolerated by some patients during long-term administration. Loose bowel movements are common during the initial weeks of therapy; the stool fat content may be increased, but not to a clinically significant extent. If diarrhea persists into the third week of therapy, oral administration of exocrine pancreatic enzymes may be helpful. It has been reported that 88% of patients with acromegaly have nausea, cramps, or diarrhea with the initiation of octreotide, but after 6 months only 10% of patients still have these side effects (12). Gastrointestinal side effects nevertheless necessitate the use of a very low dose of octreotide (0.1 µg/kg) in some patients with autonomic neuropathy. Nausea and diarrhea cause at least 25% of patients to discontinue therapy. Gastrointestinal side effects are much more common in patients with diabetic autonomic neuropathy than in those with PAF or MSA, and long-term therapy is rarely successful in diabetic patients. Hyperglycemia develops in approximately 40% of nondiabetic patients. This can be managed by having patients inject the octreotide 10 to 20 minutes after the beginning of breakfast; sufficient insulin will have been secreted by that time to maintain plasma glucose concentrations below 200 mg/dL postprandially (23). As with any pressor drug, supine hypertension is a potential problem in patients with autonomic neuropathy. This can best be avoided by instructing patients not to lie down for the first 4 to 6 hours after octreotide administration.

Cholelithiasis may develop during long-term octreotide therapy. This has been well documented in patients with acromegaly (8), although they generally take larger doses of octreotide (150 to 500 µg/d) than are required by patients with autonomic neuropathy. We have administered octreotide on a long-term basis to 23 patients. The duration of therapy has varied between 4 months and 8 years. Acute cholecystitis developed in two patients during this time interval. Withdrawal of octreotide therapy for 24 to 96 hrs causes a rebound hypermobility of the gallbladder, which may facilitate clearing of sludge and prevent cholelithiasis (57). Periodic drug-free days, as perhaps 1 day each week, therefore seems prudent in patients on long-term therapy (57). Imaging studies of the gallbladder should be performed annually and new gallstones treated with ursodeoxycholic acid (53).

REFERENCES

1. Appenzeller O, Gross JE. Glucose and baroreceptor function. *Arch Neurol* 1970;23:137–146.
2. Armstrong E, et al. Effects of oral caffeine on postprandial and postural hypotension in chronic autonomic failure. *J Auton Nerv Syst* 1990;31:174–175.
3. Berne C, et al. Sympathetic response to oral carbohydrate administration: evidence from microelectrode nerve recordings. *J Clin Invest* 1989;84:1403–1409.
4. Bhagat B, et al. Insulin-induced enhancement of uptake of noradrenaline in atrial strips. *Br J Pharmacol* 1981;74:325–332.
5. Bradbrury S, Eggleston C. Postural hypotension: a report of three cases. *Am Heart J* 1925;1:73–86.
6. Catz A, et al. Symptomatic postprandial hypotension in high paraplegia. Case report. *Paraplegia* 1992;30:582–586.
7. Costa M, Furness JB. Somatostatin is present in a subpopulation of noradrenergic nerve fibers supplying the intestine. *Neuroscience* 1984;13:911–919.
8. Creager MA, et al. Beta-adrenergic-mediated vasodilator response to insulin in the human forearm. *J Pharmacol Exp Ther* 1985; 235: 709–714.
9. Creager MA, et al. Vasopressin response to hypotension in normal subjects. *Clin Res* 1987;35:271A(abst).
10. Daughaday WH. Octreotide is effective in acromegaly but often results in cholelithiasis. *Ann Intern Med* 1990;112–159.
11. Dudl RJ, et al. Treatment of diabetic diarrhea and orthostatic hypotension with somatostatin analogue SMS-201-995. *Am J Med* 1987;83:584–588.
12. Ezzat S, et al. Octreotide treatment of acromegaly: a randomized, multicenter study. *Ann Intern Med* 1992;117:711–718.

13. Fagius J, Berne C. Increase in muscle nerve sympathetic activity in humans after food intake. *Clin Sci* 1994;86:159–167.
14. Fouad-Tarazi FM, et al. Alpha sympathomimetic treatment of autonomic insufficiency with orthostatic hypotension. *Am J Med* 1995;99:604–610.
15. Goldberg MR, et al. Prostacyclin biosynthesis and platelet function in autonomic dysfunction. *Neurology* 1985;35:120–123.
16. Hilsted J, et al. Whole body clearance of norepinephrine: the significance of arterial sampling and surgical stress. *J Clin Invest* 1983;71:500–505.
17. Hakusui S, et al. Postprandial hypotension: microneurographic analysis and treatment with vasopressin. *Neurology* 1991;41:712–715.
18. Hirayama M, et al. Treatment of postprandial hypotension with selective α_1 and β_1 adrenergic agonists. *J Auton Nerv Syst* 1993;45:149–154.
19. Hoeldtke RD, Carabello B. Hemodynamic changes during food ingestion in a patient with postprandial hypotension. *J Am Geriatr Soc* 1987;35:354–356.
20. Hoeldtke RD, Israel B. Treatment of orthostatic hypotension with octreotide. *J Clin Endocrinol Metab* 1989;68:1051–1059.
21. Hoeldtke RD, et al. Prevention of postprandial hypotension with somatostatin. *Ann Intern Med* 1985;103:889–890.
22. Hoeldtke RD, et al. Treatment of autonomic neuropathy with a somatostatin analogue SMS-201-995. *Lancet* 1986;2: 602–605.
23. Hoeldtke RD, et al. Effect of the somatostatin analogue SMS-201-995 on the adrenergic response to glucose ingestion in patients with postprandial hypotension. *Am J Med* 1989;86:673–677.
24. Hoeldtke RD, et al. Hemodynamic effects of octreotide in patients with autonomic neuropathy. *Circulation* 1991;84:168–176.
25. Jansen RWMM, Hoefnagels WHL. Influence of oral and intravenous glucose loading on blood pressure in normotensive and hypertensive elderly subjects. *J Hypertens* 1987;5(Suppl 5):S501–S503.
26. Jansen RWMM, Hoefnagels WHL. The influence of oral glucose loading on baroreflex function in the elderly. *J Am Geriatr Soc* 1989;37:1017–1022.
27. Jansen RWMM, et al. Blood pressure reduction after oral glucose loading and its relation to age, blood pressure and insulin. *Am J Cardiol* 1987;60:1087–1091.
28. Jansen RWMM, et al. Influence of octreotide (SMS-201-995) and insulin administration on the course of blood pressure after an oral glucose load in hypertensive elderly subjects. *J Am Geriatr Soc* 1989;37:1135–1139.
29. Jansen RWMM, et al. Somatostatin analog octreotide (SMS-201-995) prevents the decrease in blood pressure after oral glucose loading in the elderly. *J Clin Endocrinol Metab* 1989;68:752–756.
30. Jansen RW, et al. Postprandial hypotension in elderly patients wtih unexplained syncope. *Arch Intern Med* 1995;155:945–952.
31. Jansen RW, Lipsitz LA. Postprandial hypotension: epidemiology, pathophysiology and clinical management. *Ann Intern Med* 1995;122:286–295.
32. Kamata T, et al. Cerebral ischemic attack caused by postprandial hypotension. *Stroke* 1994;25:511–513.
33. Kessler JA, et al. Substance P and somatostatin regulate sympathetic noradrenergic function. *Science* 1983;221:1059–1061.
34. Kochaar SM, Itzkovitz HD. Treatment of orthostatic hypotension (Shy-Drager syndrome) with indomethacin. *Lancet* 1978;1:1011–1014.
35. Kvols LK, et al. Treatment of the malignant carcinoid syndrome: evaluation of a long-acting somatostatin analogue. *N Engl J Med* 1986;315:663–666.
36. Landsberg L. Diet, obesity and hypertension: an hypothesis involving insulin, the sympathetic nervous system and adaptive thermogenesis. *Q J Med* 1986;236:1081–1090.
37. Lee JC, Downing SE. Effects of insulin on cardiac muscle contraction and responsiveness to norepinephrine. *Am J Physiol* 1976;230:1360–1365.
38. Lenders JWM, et al. The effects of caffeine on the postprandial fall of blood pressure in the elderly. *Age Ageing* 1988;17:236–240.
39. Liang C, et al. Insulin infusion in conscious dogs: effects on systemic and coronary hemodynamics, regional blood flows, and plasma catecholamines. *J Clin Invest* 1982;69:1321–1336.
40. Lipsitz LA, Fullerton KJ. Postprandial blood pressure reduction in healthy elderly. *J Am Geriatr Soc* 1986;34:267–270.
41. Lipsitz LA, et al. Does insulin play a role in postprandial blood pressure reduction in the elderly? *Clin Res* 1987; 35:509A(abst).
42. Lipsitz LA, et al. Postprandial reduction in blood pressure in the elderly. *N Engl J Med* 1983;309:818–883.
43. Lipsitz LA, et al. Syncope in institutionalized elderly: the impact of multiple pathological conditions and situational stress. *J Chronic Dis* 1986;39:619–630.
44. Lipsitz LA, et al. Cardiovascular and norepinephrine responses after meal consumption in elderly (older than 75 years) persons with postprandial hypotension and syncope. *Am J Cardiol* 1986;58:810–815.
45. Lipsitz LA, et al. Haemodynamic and neurohumoral effects of caffeine in elderly patients with symptomatic postprandial hypotension: a double-blind randomized, placebo-controlled study. *Clin Sci* 1994;87:259–267.
46. Low PA, Thomas JE, Dyck PJ. Splanchnic autonomic outflow in Shy-Drager syndrome and idiopathic orthostatic hypotension. *Ann Neurol* 1978;4:511–514.
47. Mann S, et al. Circadian variation in blood pressure in autonomic failure. *Circulation* 1983;68:477–483.
48. Mathias CJ, et al. Desmopressin reduces nocturnal polyuria, overnight weight loss and improves morning postural hypotension in autonomic failure. *Br Med J* 1986;293:353–354.
49. Mathias CJ, et al. Postcibal hypotension in autonomic disorders. In: Bannister R, ed. *Autonomic Failure: A Textbook of Clinical Disorders of the Autonomic Nervous System*. 2nd ed. New York: Oxford University Press; 1988:367–380.
50. Mathias CJ, et al. Cardiovascular biochemical and hormonal changes during food-induced hypotension in chronic autonomic failure. *J Neurol Sci* 1989;94:225–269.
51. Mathias CJ, et al. Hypotensive and sedative effects of insulin in autonomic failure. *Br Med J* 1987;295:161–163.
52. Mathias CJ, et al. Differential blood pressure and hormonal effects after glucose and xylose ingestion in chronic autonomic failure. *Clin Sci* 1989;77:85–92.
53. Montini M, et al. Cholelithiasis and acromegaly: therapeutic strategies. *Clin Endocrinol* 1994;40:401–406.
54. Onrot J, et al. Hemodynamic and humoral effects of caffeine in autonomic failure: therapeutic implications for postprandial hypotension. *N Engl J Med* 1985;313:549–554.
55. Onrot J, et al. Reduction of liver plasma flow by caffeine and theophylline. *Clin Pharmacol Ther* 1986;40:506–510.
56. Raimbach SJ, et al. Prevention of glucose-induced hypotension by the somatostatin analogue octreotide (SMS-201-995) in chronic autonomic failure: haemodynamic and hormonal changes. *Clin Sci* 1989;77:623–628.
57. Rhodes M, et al. Gallbladder function in acromegalic patients taking long-term octreotide: evidence of rebound hypermotility on cessation of treatment. *Scand J Gastroenterol* 1992;27:115–118.
58. Robertson E, et al. Postprandial alterations in cardiovascular hemodynamics in autonomic dysfunction states. *Am J Cardiol* 1981;48:1048–1052.
59. Robinson BJ, et al. Autonomic responses to glucose ingestion in elderly subjects with orthostatic hypotension. *Age Ageing* 1985;14:168–173.
60. Rowe JW, et al. Effects of insulin and glucose infusions on sympathetic nervous system activity in normal man. *Diabetes* 1981;30:219–225.
61. Seyer-Hansen K. Postprandial hypotension. *Br Med J* 1977;12:1262.
62. Sherman RA, Torres F, Cody RP. Postprandial blood pressure changes during hemodialysis. *Am J Kidney Dis* 1988;12:37–39.
63. Sicuteri F, et al. Venospastic activity of somatostatin in vivo in man: naloxone-reversible tachyphylaxis. *Int J Clin Pharmacol Res* 1984;4:253–257.
64. Tonino RP, et al. Splanchnic factors enhance the norepinephrine response to oral glucose in aged man. *Exp Gerontol* 1986;21:413–422.
65. Wahren J, Eriksson LS. The influence of a long-acting somatostatin analogue on splanchnic hemodynamics and metabolism in healthy subjects and patients with liver cirrhosis. *Scand J Gastroenterol* 1986;21(Suppl 119):103–108.

66. Wahren J, et al. Influence of somatostatin on splanchnic glucose metabolism in postabsorptive and 60-hour fasted humans. *J Clin Invest* 1977;59:299–307.
67. Yagi S, et al. Effects of insulin on vasoconstrictive responses to norepinephrine and angiotensin II in rabbit femoral artery and vein. *Diabetes* 1988;37:1064–1067.
68. Young JB, et al. Enhanced plasma norepinephrine response to upright posture and oral glucose administration in elderly human subjects. *Metabolism* 1980;29:532–539.

CHAPTER 54

Hyperthermia and Hypothermia

Timothy J. Ingall

1. Hyperthermia and hypothermia both occur commonly; when severe, they are life-threatening medical emergencies.
2. Impaired thermoregulation in the elderly contributes significantly to the increased occurrence of disturbances of body temperature in older age groups. Chronic diseases and medication use also contribute to the development of alterations in body temperature in the elderly.
3. There are many medications that can affect thermoregulation and lead to alterations in body temperature, especially in the elderly and those exposed to environmental extremes. The neuroleptic malignant syndrome and malignant hyperthermia are the two most specific disturbances of body temperature due to medications.
4. There are many diseases of the nervous system, especially those affecting the hypothalamus, that are associated with disturbances of body temperature. Patients with high thoracic or cervical cord lesions are also prone to develop altered body temperatures.

INTRODUCTION

Significant abnormalities of body temperature can result from a diverse number of causes. Abnormal body temperatures may be due to exposure to environmental extremes, diseases affecting thermoregulatory systems, or, not infrequently, a combination of both. Severe abnormalities, either hyperthermia or hypothermia, can result in life-threatening medical emergencies.

HYPERTHERMIA

As described in the chapters on thermoregulation, the temperature regulation systems of the human body function to maintain a body temperature close to 37°C (98.6°F). Body temperature may be elevated in normal circumstances, such as during the normal response to exercise in the heat in individuals not acclimated to the heat. This response also includes increases in heart rate (HR) and plasma volume and a decrease in stroke volume (199). There are many pathologic causes of increased body temperature (Table 1), the most common of which is fever resulting from an infection. Whatever the underlying cause of hyperthermia, the human body can tolerate increases in core body temperature up to about 40.5°C (104.9°F); above that temperature, the body tissues, and the brain in particular, are at risk of thermal damage (31).

HEAT STRESS DISORDERS

Thermoregulatory dysfunction during exposure to environmental heat leads to a number of important disorders, including heat syncope, heat edema, heat cramp, heat exhaustion, and heatstroke (131).

Excluding infants, there are two groups in the population that are at risk of developing heat stress disorders (65). The largest group is the elderly population, especially those from the lower socioeconomic groups, those with chronic diseases (such as diabetes mellitus, obesity, malnutrition, congestive heart failure, chronic alcohol abuse, and dementia), and those using medications that interfere with thermoregulation (Table 2). The elderly have less efficient thermoregulation, including reduced perception of environmental temperature changes, reduced vasodilation when exposed to heat, and reduced sweating (Table 3) (41,42,70).

The elderly poor living in urban areas are particularly prone to develop hyperthermia during heat waves (8,119, 203). A number of factors contribute to this increased risk.

T. J. Ingall: Department of Neurology, Mayo Clinic Scottsdale, Scottsdale, Arizona 85259.

TABLE 1. *Causes of hyperthermia*

Heat stress disorders after exposure to environmental heat	Drugs (see Table 2)
Heat syncope	Drug fever
Heat edema	Endocrine disorders
Heat cramp	Hyperthyroidism
Heat exhaustion	Adrenocortical insufficiency
Heatstroke	Growth hormone deficiency
Malignant hyperthermia	Adrenocortical carcinoma
Neuroleptic malignant syndrome	Pheochromocytoma
Fever	Diagetes insipidus
Central nervous system disorders	Insulinoma
Spinal cord lesions (cervical or high thoracic)	Familial Mediterranean fever
Hypothalamic lesions	Familial Hibernian fever
Head injuries	Hodgkin's disease
Seizures	Hyperimmunoglobulinemia D and periodic fever syndrome
Alcohol withdrawal	
Acute hydrocephalus	
Agenesis of the corpus callosum	

Urban areas generate a greater radiant heat load and often have less wind, resulting in a smaller differential between day and night temperatures compared with rural areas. Thus, urban dwellers are exposed to a greater thermal load (37). Also, many urban persons live in poorly ventilated apartments, which leads to prolonged exposure to high temperatures. Economic factors may contribute to the increased vulnerability of the elderly poor to hyperthermia. There is evidence that even though older people may be aware of their inability to judge the thermal environment, some consciously threaten their own health by decreasing the use of air conditioners and fans to save money on electric bills (156). Alcoholism is a problem in the elderly population and is a major risk factor predisposing to heat stress disorders (124). Apart from the malnutrition and general debilitation associated with chronic alcohol abuse, acute exposure causes vasodilation (117), which, when combined with high environmental temperature, could lead to an increase in body heat that could result in hyperthermia (131).

The second group at risk of developing heat stress disorders consists of essentially healthy young individuals who undertake prolonged exercise in a hot environment. Heat stress disorders have been reported in marathon runners (85,104,251), football players and other sportsmen (11, 178), armed forces personnel (17,28), and workers undertaking strenuous activity in the heat (211,222). Heat stress disorders have also been well documented in Moslems attending the Mekkah Pilgrimage (4,252). The presence of heat intolerance in younger persons predisposes to the development of heat stress disorders. Epstein (65) has reviewed the mechanisms underlying heat intolerance in the young active population and has defined three broad

TABLE 2. *Drugs associated with impaired thermoregulation*

Hyperthermia	Hypothermia
Alcohol	Alcohol
Benztropine mesylate	Vasodilators
Atropine	Bromocriptine
Phenothiazines	Phenothiazines
Butyrophenones	Neuroleptic drugs
Antihistamines	Barbiturates
Beta-blockers	Diazepam
Diuretics	Imipramine
Methyldopa	Reserpine
MAO inhibitors	Paracetamol
Tricyclic antidepressants	
Vasoconstrictors	
Amphetamines	
Cocaine	
LSD	
Opiates	
Cannabinoids	

MAO, monoamine oxidase

TABLE 3. *Factors associated with old age and impaired thermoregulation*

Hyperthermia
Reduced perception of environmental temperature changes
Reduced vasodilation
Reduced sweating
Drugs interfering with thermoregulation (see Table 2)
Underlying systemic diseases
Hypothermia
Reduced perception of environmental temperature changes
Reduced vasoconstriction
Lower metabolic rates
Decreased heat production when exposed to the cold
Excessive heat loss when exposed to the cold
Decreased subcutaneous fat insulation
Decreased muscle mass for shivering
Drugs interfering with thermoregulation (see Table 2)
Underlying systemic diseases

groups of predisposing factors: congenital, functional, and acquired. Congenital causes include ectodermal dysplasia and a rare condition called "chronic idiopathic anhidrosis" (152), both of which cause altered sweat production. Functional factors related to heat intolerance include low physical fitness, lack of acclimatization, low work efficiency, and reduced skin area to body mass ratio. Acquired heat intolerance consists of sweat gland dysfunction, including miliaria (prickly heat) and sweat gland damage following total body radiation. Other causes of acquired sweat gland dysfunction include barbiturate poisoning (141) and scleroderma (29). Other acquired causes of heat intolerance include dehydration, infectious diseases, and possibly previous heatstroke.

Heat Syncope

Syncope, or orthostatic symptoms, can occur in patients suffering from heat stress. These symptoms have been attributed to thermogenic vasodilatation, postural pooling of blood, diminished venous return to the heart, reduction of cardiac output, and global reduction in cerebral perfusion (131).

Heat Edema

Mild dependent edema has been described in unacclimatized persons exposed to a hot climate. It occurs typically in women and resolves with acclimatization. Possible underlying causes include salt supplementation, oliguria secondary to heat-induced vasodilatation, and increased aldosterone production (131).

Heat Cramps

Skeletal muscle cramps can occur in muscles subjected to intensive work and fatigue. It has been postulated that they are caused by hyponatremia and possibly hypochloremia (131).

Heat Exhaustion

Heat exhaustion is the most common heat stress disorder (131). Heat exhaustion is usually due to a combination of dehydration and salt depletion. The core body temperature is elevated, and the patient is clinically dehydrated and oliguric. Symptoms include thirst, weakness, and fatigue. Skeletal muscle cramps may occur. Affected persons are often agitated and frequently hyperventilate, with resulting paresthesias and tetany. Delirium and incoordination may develop. Untreated, heat exhaustion may progress to heatstroke.

Heatstroke

The term classical heatstroke is reserved for cases of heatstroke that develop in persons who undertake normal activities while exposed to prolonged periods of high environmental temperatures (129). Exertional heatstroke is the type of heatstroke that occurs in association with physical exertion in young active persons (207).

Heatstroke is considered present if three criteria are met (38): (1) there is severe hyperthermia with core body temperature above 41°C (105.8°F), (2) there are disturbances of the central nervous system, and (3) the skin is hot and dry and is pink or ashen, depending on the circulatory state. Although the diagnosis of heatstroke is easy to establish when all three criteria are present, the diagnosis may be missed if there has been a delay in the measurement of core temperature and the temperature has fallen (214). Similarly, the diagnosis may not be considered if the patient is seen early after the onset of exertional heatstroke when profuse sweating may still be present, because dry skin is a late development of heatstroke (214).

Although the hyperthermia itself is probably the major cause of tissue injury, the exact pathogenic mechanisms of heatstroke tissue damage are unknown. Metabolic acidosis, disseminated intravenous coagulation (DIC), circulatory failure, hypoxia, and myoglobinuria are associated disturbances contributing to the pathogenesis of organ damage (216). Circulating endotoxins may also contribute to the pathogenesis of heatstroke (61,84).

Heatstroke Complications

Central Nervous System

Coma is present in all cases of heatstroke. Early manifestations may include headache, drowsiness, confusion, agitation, and irrational behavior. Seizures occur in up to 60% of patients (207). Flaccidity, hemiplegia, cerebellar symptoms, and papilledema may also be present (216). Pinpoint pupils are present in over 50% of patients (252). Survivors of heatstroke may have residual neurologic deficits, including cerebellar ataxia, dysarthria, dysmetria, and peripheral neuropathy (145,170). All fatal cases of heatstroke have evidence of central nervous system damage (164). Autopsy reveals diffuse petechial hemorrhages, edema, and diffuse neuronal degeneration most obvious in the Purkinje fibers in the cerebellum.

Skeletal Muscle

Creatine kinase (CK) levels are elevated in virtually all cases of heatstroke. However, rhabdomyolysis is uncommon in classic heatstroke, although it is present in virtually every case of exertion-induced heatstroke with CK levels in the range of 100,000 to 2,500,000 IU/L (131).

Kidneys

Acute renal failure is seen in about 25% of exertion-induced heatstroke cases (207) but is seen in less than 5% of classic heatstroke cases (128). Multiple factors contribute to the development of renal failure, including decreased renal blood flow, direct thermal injury to renal tissue, intravascular clotting due to DIC, and myoglobinuria (187, 193,202).

Liver

Laboratory testing often reveals elevations in aspartate aminotransferase and alanine aminotransferase (122), although these increases may not occur until 24 to 48 hrs after the onset of heatstroke (216). The prothrombin level is often low, reaching its nadir on day 2 or 3 of the illness (214). Cholestasis associated with centrilobular perisinusoidal edema and patchy necrosis has been described (121).

Cardiovascular System

A number of cardiovascular changes are seen, including low cardiac output, low diastolic pressure, and high pulse pressure (216). Cardiac failure may occur (253). Electrocardiographic (ECG) changes, including inverted or flattened T waves and transient conduction disturbances, have been described (46). The myocardium may be damaged, with characteristic changes of subendocardial hemorrhage occurring beneath the left side of the ventricular septum (120).

Pulmonary System

Hyperventilation is common and may lead to respiratory alkalosis and tetany (207). Pulmonary edema has been observed before any treatment has been instituted and has been postulated to be caused by either acute left ventricular failure or a disturbance of pulmonary vascular permeability (131). In the presence of DIC, the development of adult respiratory distress syndrome has been observed (63). Postmortem studies have identified pulmonary infarctions in many cases (164).

Gastrointestinal System

Diarrhea and vomiting occur frequently (207), although in severe cases massive hematemesis and melena may occur (216). Serum amylase activity is usually elevated, and pancreatitis has been observed (131).

Hemostasis

Coagulation disorders are common, with DIC occurring almost universally in severe cases (35). Clinical manifestations include melena, bloody diarrhea, purpura, conjunctival hemorrhage, hematuria, and hemoptysis (164). The coagulopathy of heatstroke is probably related to multiple factors, including impaired production of clotting factors in the liver (15,214), direct thermal activation of clotting factors (213), thrombocytopenia (250), and fibrinolysis (213). It has recently been postulated that the coagulopathy of heatstroke may be triggered by direct heat activation of platelets (76).

Laboratory Findings in Heatstroke

Abnormalities of liver function tests, hemostasis, serum amylase, and CK levels were described earlier. In addition to these abnormalities, hypoglycemia may occur (46), and many electrolyte abnormalities have been observed. Hypocalcemia may develop and occurs initially when there has been extensive damage to skeletal muscle (131). Hypercalcemia may develop as a late complication in patients with rhabdomyolysis (143). Hypophosphatemia is seen early in the course of heatstroke (130). Hypokalemia develops early in the course of the illness (46), whereas hyperkalemia may develop later (214). Serum sodium levels are related to the state of hydration and are usually slightly elevated or normal (207). Acid–base balance is almost always abnormal. Nearly all cases of classic heatstroke have a respiratory alkalosis (23). In severe cases, lactic acidosis may develop (94). In exertional heatstroke, a primary respiratory alkalosis is seen early and is followed by the development of a metabolic acidosis (207). A leukocytosis of 20,000 to 30,000 per milliliter or higher is often seen (98).

Treatment of Heatstroke

Heatstroke is a medical emergency that requires the prompt institution of measures to reduce the body temperature. Immediate measures include removing the patient from the hot environment, removing constricting clothing, dousing the patient with water, applying ice packs, and fanning the patient to increase heat dissipation.

Once the patient has reached a medical facility, the mainstay of treatment is immersion in an ice water bath combined with vigorous skin massage (47,131). Core body temperature should be measured by a rectal thermistor probe. Additional measures include continuous cardiac monitoring, the administration of intravenous fluids, and the drawing of blood (venous and arterial) to determine serum electrolytes and blood gases. Other management may include tracheal intubation, insertion of a central line to estimate central venous pressure, placement of a nasogastric tube, and insertion of a urinary catheter. The management of heatstroke may be complicated by the development of DIC, renal failure, pulmonary edema, rhabdomyolysis, hypoglycemia, hyperglycemia, or electrolyte abnormalities. Apart from reducing the body temperature, these complications are managed by standard medical treatment. As the core body temperature falls, seizures may occur. Intravenous Valium in repeated doses of 5 mg to 10 mg should be administered until the convulsions are controlled (207). If shivering develops, either chlorpromazine (131) or diazepam (207) can be used. Medications that have been proposed, but not substantiated, as temperature-reducing agents include phenothiazines (183) and dantrolene (34, 154). One study of dantrolene (22), however, showed no beneficial effect from its use in heatstroke. Heparin has been reported to be effective in the treatment of heatstroke complicated by DIC (45), but other authors argue against its use (215). Exchange transfusion in combination with heparin has also been used successfully in the treatment of DIC associated with heatstroke (224).

Although ice water immersion is the standard recommended treatment, there is a conflict of opinion in the literature as to the most effective method of reducing body temperature in heatstroke victims (123). Ice water immersion has been criticized because it may be associated with shivering, fecal incontinence, aspiration of vomitus, and convulsions (131). Moreover, it has been theorized that the ice water may induce cutaneous vasoconstriction and impair cooling efficiency (162). Alternative methods of cooling include hand immersion in cool water (234), wetting the body with water and then rubbing the body surface with plastic bags containing ice (131), immersion in tap water (207), iced peritoneal lavage (105), warm air spray (243), and the use of a helicopter rotary blade downdraft (192). Costrini (47) has recommended that ice water immersion remain the treatment of choice at this time. Many of these alternative methods have been developed by tests on healthy subjects and have not been validated in the treatment of patients with heatstroke. None has been compared directly with ice water immersion.

With early recognition and appropriate management, the mortality rate from heat stroke can be kept as low as 5% to 10% (131,207), although in the past mortality rates as high as 52% have been reported (17). Duration of hyperthermia, body temperature above 41°C (105.8°F), prolonged coma, oliguric renal failure, hyperkalemia, and high levels of serum transaminases have been recognized as predictors of a poor outcome (214,252). Those who survive heatstroke usually recovery completely without any residual problems (214,252).

MALIGNANT HYPERTHERMIA

Malignant hyperthermia (MH) is a rare hereditary disease that presents during anesthesia and is characterized clinically by the rapid development of hyperthermia, acidosis, and muscle rigidity (71). MH can develop immediately after induction, several hours after initiation, or shortly after cessation of general anesthesia (52). It is now known that MH can be triggered by all potent inhalational general anesthetics and by succinylcholine (95).

During anesthesia, unexplained ventricular arrhythmia, tachycardia, sweating, patchy cyanosis of the skin, falling blood pressure, and increased respiratory rate are indicative of a developing MH crisis. MH is associated with the development of hypercarbia, metabolic acidosis, hypoxia, hyperglycemia, hyperphosphatemia, hypercalcemia, hypermagnesemia, and hyperkalemia. Large increases in CK levels and myoglobinuria are observed (26,194). DIC may develop and is often severe (64).

The exact nature of the genetic defect underlying MH has not been determined. However, there is good evidence that the regulation of intracellular free calcium ion concentration is defective (151). Current evidence indicates that the calcium channel of the sarcoplasmic reticulum of MH muscle is abnormally sensitive to calcium and halothane (95).

With earlier diagnosis and the use of dantrolene, the mortality rate has dropped from 70% to 10% in recent series (93). Dantrolene sodium is a lipid-soluble hydantoin derivative that relaxes skeletal muscle by acting directly on the muscle, probably by inhibiting calcium release from the sarcoplasmic reticulum (241). Apart from starting dantrolene therapy, the other components of the management of MH include: cessation of the anesthetic agent, hyperventilation with 100% oxygen, and the institution of appropriate cooling measures while monitoring core temperature (134). The patient should be on a cardiac monitor, and the following parameters should be monitored closely: hydration, electrolytes, acid–base balance, and coagulation status (134).

NEUROLEPTIC MALIGNANT SYNDROME

Neuroleptic malignant syndrome (NMS) is a rare but potentially lethal complication of neuroleptic medication characterized by hyperthermia, muscular rigidity, autonomic dysfunction, and impaired consciousness (19). The exact cause of the disease is unknown, but 1% of patients taking neuroleptic agents may be affected (33). Any of the neuroleptic drugs can cause NMS, including phenothiazines, butyrophenones, thioxanthenes, and miscellaneous antipsychotic agents such as loxapine (88). NMS has also been described in patients receiving neuroleptic drugs in combination with lithium, and there may be an increased risk for developing NMS receiving this combination of medications (40). NMS has occurred in patients receiving non-neuroleptic drugs, including metoclopramide (74,99), tetrabenazine (30), alpha-methyl tyrosine (30), and desipramine (10). Sudden withdrawal from treatment with dopamine agonists such as levodopa, amantadine, or bromocriptine can give rise to NMS (69,90,205,236). NMS can occur at any time during treatment with neuroleptic medication (19,33). The onset may be hours or months after the institution of therapy or after an increase in dose, but it is seen most often within 2 weeks of such changes. The symptoms of NMS usually progress rapidly over 1 to 3 days. Hyperthermia is a major feature, as is a movement disorder (19). In one series of 52 patients (138), all developed fever and a movement disorder; 70% to 80% of them had impaired consciousness and evidence of autonomic dysfunction, such as tachycardia (80%), sweating (60%), or labile blood pressure (54%). These signs of autonomic dysfunction may indeed be the first signs of NMS. Parkinsonism is the most common movement disorder with major signs of rigidity and resting tremor (19). Other movement disorders such as dystonia or chorea are found in about one third of patients, whereas catatonia is less common (19). Mental status varies from confusion to coma, and a wide range of associated neurologic signs appears in half the patients, with disorders of speech and swallowing being the most common (33). Once symptoms and signs develop, they intensify rapidly within 24 to 72 hrs. The disorder may last from 8 hrs to 30 days, but the average duration is over 2 weeks. Although most NMS patients make a complete recovery, there is a high mortality rate of approximately 20% (33). Serious complications that are associated with NMS include acute renal failure due to either dehydration or myoglobinuria, or both, pulmonary embolism, and acute myocardial infarction with pulmonary edema (62). Persisting neurologic sequelae have been seen in about 10% of all NMS patients, with parkinsonism, dyskinesia, dementia, and ataxia being described (40,62). In six patients who were rechallenged with neuroleptic medication, four developed features of NMS again (138).

There are no diagnostic tests for NMS, but a number of abnormalities are found frequently, including elevated creatine kinase levels and a white cell count of up to 30,000 per mL. Other findings include abnormal liver function tests, acidosis, hypoxia, hypercarbia, and elevated plasma and urinary catecholamine levels. Examination of cerebral spinal fluid is unremarkable, computed tomography scans of the brain show no abnormalities, and changes on the electroencephalogram (EEG) have been nonspecific, with generalized slowing in some cases (138).

Neuroleptic malignant syndrome is managed by first withdrawing the offending drug. Supportive treatment to control hyperthermia and dehydration and to treat complications appropriately is then instituted. A number of specific pharmacotherapies have been tried, including anticholinergics (19), levodopa (137), bromocriptine (177), and amantadine (168). Their use is based on theoretic considerations rather than empirical evidence of their efficacy. As discussed later, disturbed dopaminergic function is thought to be involved in the etiology of NMS, and dopamine agonists have been used for that reason. Anticholinergics have been advocated to overcome the increased central cholinergic activity that often accompanies altered dopaminergic activity (19). Dantrolene sodium is reported to be effective in some patients by controlling muscle contraction (20). Rosenberg and Green (198) have reviewed the literature on the treatment of NMS and have concluded that in addition to traditional supportive care, specific therapy with either bromocriptine or dantrolene is warranted.

Although the cause of NMS is not known, there is good evidence that it is related to disturbed dopaminergic function. NMS could result from a number of different alterations in dopaminergic function. First, it has been suggested that NMS could result from dopamine receptor blockade (19,100). Neuroleptic agents produce a competitive blockade of postsynaptic dopamine receptors, leading initially to increased dopamine turnover (166). Decreased dopamine turnover occurs with long-term use and is associated with hypersensitivity of the receptors to both dopamine agonists and antagonists (166). An increase in neuroleptic drug dose, or the substitution or addition of a more potent neuroleptic agent, could therefore produce a profound dopaminergic blockade that cannot be compensated for by increased turnover. Second, it has been postulated that a decrease in the number of dopamine receptors in the striatum may be the cause of NMS associated with withdrawal of dopaminergic therapy for Parkinson's disease (69). Lastly, NMS may be related in some cases to a central imbalance between norepinephrine and dopamine (10).

FEVER

Hyperthermia is the term used to describe any unspecified or unidentified elevation in body temperature above the normal resting range of body temperature (225). Fever has been given the specific connotation of an increase in body temperature (usually produced by the action of pyrogens) in which the thermoregulatory responses are functional but are acting to sustain an elevated body temperature (225).

Fever associated with infections is the most common cause of an abnormally raised body temperature. The concept of fever as a regulated body temperature was first raised in the late 1800s by Liebermeister (127) and has been substantiated by others in the 20th century (44,208). Thus, during the development of a fever when the body temperature is below the new, higher set-point, the thermoregulatory system regards the body as being relatively hypothermic. At this point, the individual feels cold, and a number of both heat-producing and heat-conserving changes occur in the body to raise the body temperature to the new set-point.

Fever results from exposure to exogenous pyrogens such as bacteria, viruses, or their products. However, there is little evidence that the fever is due to the direct action of exogenous pyrogens on the anterior hypothalamus. Current evidence favors an indirect effect of such pyrogens on the hypothalamus that is mediated by endogenous pyrogens produced by phagocytic leukocytes (127,157). In turn, it is believed that the endogenous pyrogens cause the brain to produce prostaglandin E_2, which has a direct pyrogenic effect on the anterior hypothalamus (18,39,126,226).

Endogenous pyrogen is produced by many different types of cells, including macrophages, Kupffer cells, astrocytes and glial cells, keratinocytes, and others (126). Within the last few years it has become apparent that endogenous pyrogen, leukocyte endogenous mediator, lymphocyte-activating factor, and mononuclear cell factor are the same or closely related proteins now known as interleukin-1 (126,157). Interleukin-1 probably represents a family of polypeptides with a wide range of biologic activities (other than producing fever), such as hypoferremia, synthesis of acute phase proteins, activation of T and B lymphocytes, and enhancement of natural killer cell activity (56,126). Interleukin-1 is, however, not the only endogenous pyrogen, and there is evidence that interleukin-6, tumor necrosis factor, interferon, and other cytokines all participate in the febrile response (127).

Once interleukin-1 reaches the brain by way of the cerebral circulation, it acts at or near the preoptic anterior hypothalamus to produce changes in the thermoregulatory pathways that result in fever (226). Stitt (226) has postulated that interleukin-1 stimulates mesenchymal cells in the organum vasculosum of the lamina terminalis (OVLT), causing the release of prostaglandin E_2 (PGE_2). It is thought that PGE_2 then activates other neurons in the OVLT or the surrounding preoptic area (201). These neurons are presumed to have axonal processes contacting other cell groups in the hypothalamus and brain stem that coordinate the autonomic, endocrine, and behavioral components of the febrile response (201).

Although fever plays an important role in host defense and the immune response (58), it is important that the body temperature not be allowed to rise too high. It is possible that several endogenous cryogens are involved in helping to regulate body temperature (49,173). Putative endogenous cryogens include arginine vasopressin, α-melanocyte-stimulating hormone, uromodulin, febrile inhibitor, and tumor necrosis factor (127). The antipyretic action of aspirin and other drugs, such as the nonsteroidal anti-inflammatory drugs, is thought to be mediated primarily through inhibition of the production of PGE (226). However, there are now data that indicate that antipyretic drugs may have multiple actions, including stimulating the release of endogenous cryogens such as arginine vasopressin or α-melanocyte-stimulating hormone (3,75).

DISORDERS OF THE CENTRAL NERVOUS SYSTEM

Patients with lesions of the spinal cord at the cervical or high thoracic cord level are at risk for hyperthermia, especially if the ambient temperature is high (191). These patients have sustained damage to the intermediolateral column that interferes with the efferent pathways of the thermoregulatory reflexes. Johnson and Spalding (110) have shown that vasodilatation in the hand does not occur in response to a rise in central temperature in a patient with cervical cord transection. Lesions in the region of the hypothalamus may result in hyperthermia (14,16,242,254). Tumors (14,51,254), stroke (242,254), and encephalitis (14,242) involving the hypothalamus have been associated with the occurrence of hyperthermia. Periodic fever has been reported in a patient with agenesis of the corpus callosum (reverse Shapiro's syndrome) (102). It was postulated that the hyperthermia was caused by dopaminergic denervation of the hypothalamic thermoregulatory center resulting in supersensitivity of its dopaminergic receptors (102). Hyperthermia has been described after both head injuries and operations involving the pituitary fossa, the region of the third ventricle, and the posterior fossa (66). Both seizures (239) and alcohol withdrawal (107,249) have been documented as causing hyperthermia not related to infection. Hyperthermia has been documented in patients with acute hydrocephalus (231). This could be due to a number of mechanisms, including the release of neuropeptides, disturbed central dopamine transmission, or compression of the hypothalamus (231).

IMPAIRED THERMOREGULATION DUE TO DRUGS

There are many drugs that can impair thermoregulation and lead to hyperthermia. Hyperthermia could result from a number of different drug effects, including increased heat production from hyperactivity, increased metabolic rate, or impaired heat dissipation (183). Impaired thermoregulation has been documented in patients taking benztropine mesylate, atropine and other anticholinergic drugs, phenothiazines, butyrophenones, antihistamines, β-blockers, diuretics, laxatives, methyldopa, monoamine oxidase inhibitors, tricyclic antidepressants, and vasoconstrictors (see Table 2) (36,83,146,148,238).

Abuse of drugs, including amphetamines, cocaine, LSD, opiates, and cannabinoids, has been associated with an increased risk of developing hyperthermia (32,149). In particular, there have been many reported cases since the late 1980s of hyperthermia associated with the illegal use of amphetamines. Hyperthermia has been reported with the use of both 3,4-methylenedioxymethamphetamine (MDMA, "Ecstasy") and 3,4-methylenedioxyethamphetamine (MDEA, "Eve") (182,233). It has been postulated that MDMA and MDEA induce hyperthermia by causing the central nervous system release of 5-hydroxytryptamine and dopamine (182,233).

Drug fever has been described in relation to the administration of many drugs and in most cases is thought to be due to an immune-mediated response to the drugs (157).

OTHER CAUSES OF HYPERTHERMIA

Hyperthermia can also be seen in a wide range of endocrine disturbances, including hyperthyroidism, growth hormone deficiency, adrenocortical insufficiency, diabetes insipidus, pheochromocytoma, and insulinoma (116,180, 184,217,235). In adrenocortical carcinoma, periodic fever may develop; this has been related to elevated levels of unconjugated etiocholanolamine (21).

Other noninfectious causes of hyperthermia include familial Mediterranean fever (97), familial Hibernian fever (245), Hodgkin's disease (82), and hyperimmunoglobulinemia D and periodic fever syndrome (57). Familial Mediterranean fever is characterized by recurrent fever, abnormal pain, and leukocytosis; it is believed to be an autosomal recessive inherited disease (97,220). Familial Hibernian fever is characterized by attacks of fever, localized myalgia, and painful erythema (245). Attacks may also include abdominal pain, pleurisy, leukocytosis, and an elevated erythrocyte sedimentation rate. It differs from familial Mediterranean fever in its prompt response to steroids and its autosomal dominant inheritance pattern. The pathogenesis of both familial Mediterranean fever and familial Hibernian fever is unknown.

The exact cause of the fever seen in Hodgkin's disease is unclear (195). It has been postulated that activated macrophages produce interleukin-1 (82), which then acts on the anterior hypothalamus to elevate the set-point for temperature regulation (55). Patients with hyperimmunoglobulinemia D and periodic fever syndrome present with a long history of recurrent attacks of fever, which are frequently preceded by chills and accompanied by headache, cervical lymphadenopathy, and occasionally abdominal pain and diarrhea (57). An uncontrolled type III hypersensitivity reaction related to IgD–containing complexes is thought to play an etiologic role in the syndrome (57).

HYPOTHERMIA

Hypothermia is a condition that occurs when the core body temperature falls below 35°C (95°F) (196). Hypothermia occurs most commonly after accidental exposure to low environmental temperatures, but it can also be associated with other causes, such as disorders of the central nervous system, alcohol or other drug use, and endocrine and metabolic disorders (Table 4). Hypothermia is conventionally divided into three levels: mild hypothermia (32°C to 35°C; 89.6°F to 95°F), moderate hypothermia

TABLE 4. *Causes of hypothermia*

Accidental hypothermia after exposure to low environmental temperatures
Disorders of the central nervous system
  Spinal cord lesions (cervical or high thoracic)
  Hypothalamic lesions
  Wernicke's encephalopathy
  Multiple sclerosis
  Parkinson's disease
  Mesodiencephalic lesions
  Agenesis of the corpus callosum
  Diencephalic epilepsy
  Episodic spontaneous hypothermia with hyperhidrosis
Alcohol
Drugs (see Table 2)
Endocrine and metabolic disorders
  Hyperglycemia
  Hypoglycemia
  Hypothyroidism
  Pituitary dysfunction
  Adrenocortical insufficiency
Hodgkin's disease
Systemic lupus erythematosus
Reye's syndrome
Electrical shock

(28°C to 32°C; 82.4°F to 89.6°F), and severe hypothermia (<28°C; 82.4°F) (176). There is disagreement in the literature regarding the temperature below which severe hypothermia is considered to occur. Although the author mentioned above used 28°C (82.4°F), other authors have used 32°C (89.6°F) (53), 30°C (86°F) (150), and 26°C (78.8°F) (210) as the temperature below which severe hypothermia develops. This disagreement, however, has little clinical consequence because all authors agree that low core body temperatures are associated with significant clinical problems.

Pathophysiology of Hypothermia

The pathophysiologic changes that occur in hypothermia are related to the severity of the hypothermia as well as the premorbid health of the patient and associated predisposing factors. With mild hypothermia, there is extensive shivering and a decrease in the level of consciousness (59). The respiratory rate shows an initial increase (59). There is also an initial tachycardia with vasoconstriction and a rise in blood pressure associated with an increased cardiac output (59,230). There are no specific ECG changes with mild hypothermia (150). Exposure to cold increases urine output even before the body temperature falls (142). Peripheral vasoconstriction, by shunting blood centrally, is at least partly responsible for the early increase in urine output. With a fall in body temperature there is a further increase in urine output, which is thought to be due to an osmotic diuresis accompanied by increased urinary electrolyte excretion (13,141). Dehydration and an increased hematocrit may also be present (1,196).

With moderate hypothermia there is a further decrease in the level of consciousness, with unconsciousness developing when the brain temperature is between 30°C and 32°C (86°F to 89.6°F) (43). Shivering decreases gradually, and there is subsequent stiffness of joints and muscles (150). Triphasic waves may be seen on the EEG (197). Cardiac output, systemic blood pressure, heart rate, and respiratory rate all decrease (175,196). Reduced myocardial contractility has been reported (155). ECG changes include bradycardia, lengthened PR and QT intervals, broadened QRS complexes, T-wave inversion, the appearance of J waves (Osborn waves), nodal rhythm, second-degree atrioventricular (AV) block, and atrial fibrillation or flutter (108, 185,221). Decreased renal perfusion results in a fall in glomerular filtration rate (118). Hypothermia causes decreased conduction in peripheral nerves (114), and peripheral neuropathy has been reported (2). Pancreatitis with significant amylase elevations may occur (59). Cerebral infarction attributed directly to hypothermia has been described in one patient (204).

With severe hypothermia, most of the changes seen in moderate hypothermia occur in an exaggerated form (150). Clinically, the skin is ice cold; muscles and joints are stiff; respirations, pulse, and blood pressure are difficult to detect; heart sounds are inaudible; and pupillary light reflexes and deep tendon reflexes are absent (109). Deep coma develops, and the EEG shows high-amplitude, bilateral sharp and slow wave complexes, and a burst suppression pattern may occur (186). Profound bradycardia is seen with rates falling as low as four beats per minute (182). Arrhythmias are common and include atrial fibrillation, high-grade AV block, multifocal ventricular extrasystoles followed by ventricular fibrillation, and, at extremely low temperatures (<15°C [68°F]), asystole (12,221). The respiratory rate may fall as low as one to two gasps per minute (150). Acute renal failure may develop (200).

Metabolic, Biochemical, and Hematologic Changes in Hypothermia

For every 10°C (18°F) fall in temperature, the metabolic rate is reduced by 50% (171). Coagulation defects, including prolonged prothrombin and partial thromboplastin times, are seen in neonates and may occur in adults, particularly the elderly (25). DIC is seen uncommonly in adults (163). Serum creatine kinase, lactate dehydrogenase, aspartate aminotransferase, alanine aminotransferase, and amylase may be moderately increased (59,158–160,165), although the level of the enzyme elevation does not correlate with the severity of the hypothermia (158,160). Hyperglycemia is common and is thought to be due, in part, to a decrease in insulin secretion (48). Free fatty acids, ketones, and cortisol levels are increased (91,227). Thyroid function tests (thyroid-stimulating hormone, T3, T4), growth hormone levels, and thyroid-releasing hormone and adrenocorticotropic hormone stimulation tests have been shown to be normal (248).

Serum sodium, calcium, and magnesium concentrations remain stable (59,118,150). There are conflicting reports regarding changes in serum potassium in association with hypothermia. Some authors have stated that no change in serum potassium occurs (59,150), whereas Britt and colleagues (27) have stated that the potassium level may rise during hypothermia and then fall after rewarming. In experimental work with dogs, a fall in serum potassium in association with hypothermia has been observed (118). Hepatic function is depressed, resulting in a decreased ability to metabolize drugs (27). A moderate leukopenia and thrombocytopenia is commonly seen (210). A moderate metabolic acidosis caused by reduced tissue perfusion with an associated accumulation of lactate is seen with moderate to severe hypothermia (150,165,196).

Pathologic Findings

Hypothermic injury does not produce any specific pathologic changes (219). Fatty infiltration as well as hemorrhagic and thrombotic lesions have been found in heart, liver, brain, lung, spleen, bowel, adrenal glands, and kidneys (27,59,219). Pancreatitis has been described (59), and bronchopneumonia is a common complication (196).

Management of Hypothermia

The treatment of hypothermia involves the initial resuscitation of the patient and then rewarming. Initial measures include removing the patient from the cold environment, removing any wet clothing, and wrapping the patient in a blanket. Patients who are in ventricular fibrillation or asystole should have cardiopulmonary resuscitation started. Once the patient is in the emergency room, an intravenous line and a Foley catheter should be inserted and a cardiac monitor attached to monitor cardiac rhythm. Core body temperature should be measured with a rectal thermistor probe. Hematology and chemistry groups, coagulation studies, arterial blood gases, and blood cultures should be drawn. Continuous monitoring of vital signs and serial measurement of electrolytes and arterial blood gases should be undertaken during rewarming. Thiamine should be administered, especially if chronic alcohol abuse is suspected.

Rewarming should be started only after cardiopulmonary resuscitation is under way. There are a number of rewarming techniques available to treat the hypothermic patient. A full discussion of the advantages, disadvantages, and contraindications of each of these techniques is beyond the scope of this review; the reader is directed to a number of recent articles for comprehensive reviews of each topic (27,50,53,77,81,113,140,150,176). Patients with mild hypothermia may be rewarmed by passive techniques, such as blanket insulation and placement in a warm environment. Patients with moderate hypothermia can be treated by active external rewarming, such as the use of warm blankets, mattresses, water bottles, forced-air rewarming, or immersion of all or part of the body in warm water. Gautam and associates (77) have described the use of a purpose-built rewarming chamber in the treatment of accidental hypothermia in the elderly. Severe cases of hypothermia and some cases of moderate hypothermia require internal rewarming. Internal or core rewarming involves techniques that allow the core temperature to be elevated without peripheral vascular collapse occurring. These techniques include warmed intravenous solutions, warmed peritoneal lavage, gastric–colonic lavage with a balloon filled with warm water, mediastinal lavage after thoracotomy, diathermy, breathing warm air, and extracorporeal blood rewarming. Hemodialysis (10l) and continuous arteriovenous rewarming (80) have also been used effectively in some patients.

Active external rewarming may be associated with a phenomenon known as "after-drop," in which the core temperature falls after the start of rewarming. Both shunting of cold acidotic blood from the periphery and conduction of heat from the cold central core to the rewarmed periphery contribute to this phenomenon (150). It was thought previously that after-drop carried a risk of precipitating hypovolemic shock or ventricular fibrillation, but it is now believed that after-drop does not induce any clinically significant problems (26,150). There are a number of well-recognized complications that occur during rewarming, including hypokalemia, lung edema, infections, and the late onset of AV block (26,150). Patients must be monitored closely for these complications, even after rewarming has been completed and treated appropriately.

The mortality rates in accidental hypothermia range from 30% to 80% (196). Mortality increases with age (176). Associated underlying diseases are thought to be more important in determining mortality than is the magnitude of the hypothermia (106).

CAUSES OF HYPOTHERMIA

Accidental Hypothermia

Accidental hypothermia occurs with exposure to low environmental temperatures. Often, there is an associated contributing factor such as an endocrine–metabolic disorder, infection, malnutrition, drug or alcohol exposure, or neurologic disease (59,196). Accidental hypothermia can occur in otherwise healthy individuals exposed to a cold environment, including outdoor workers (218) and outdoor enthusiasts (147). Hypothermia is a common problem in patients with severe injuries, even in temperate climates (153).

The elderly are particularly susceptible to accidental hypothermia (59,78,133,196,247). Apart from being more likely to have predisposing conditions, as detailed earlier (59,196), the elderly have impaired thermoregulatory mechanisms, including reduced vasoconstriction in response to cold (41,42,240), lower metabolic rates (240), and decreased heat production and excessive heat loss when exposed to the cold (see Table 3) (161). The elderly also have decreased levels of subcutaneous fat insulation, decreased muscle mass for shivering, and decreased awareness of environmental temperature changes (41,196). Disturbed glucose metabolism in the elderly, both hyperglycemia (179) and hypoglycemia (174), is associated with an increased risk for hypothermia.

Disorders of the Central Nervous System

Impaired temperature regulation occurs as a complication of tetraplegia (see section under Hyperthermia also) (111), and hypothermia can develop, occurring particularly soon after spinal cord transection (191).

Lesions localized to the region of the hypothalamus are well documented as being related to abnormal temperature regulation, causing either hypothermia or hyperthermia (see earlier). Hypothermia in association with hypothalamic lesions, including tumors, sarcoidosis, and strokes, has been well documented (14,24,51,72,112). Hypothermia can occur in patients with Wernicke's encephalopathy (89,190). This is thought to result from damage to the hypothalamus (92), and particularly the posterior hypothalamus (190). Hypothermia has also been documented in patients with multiple sclerosis (139,229). Sullivan and co-workers (229) postulated that hypothermia could be due to a plaque of demyelination affecting the hypothalamus, but neuropathologic examination of a case reported by Lammens and colleagues (139) showed no hypothalamic abnormality, raising the possibility that involvement in other areas of the brain or spinal cord could lead to hypothermia. Accidental hypothermia has been documented in patients with Parkinson's disease (86). Appenzeller and Goss (7) have documented abnormalities of thermoregulation in Parkinson's disease patients that are consistent with dysfunction of the hypothalamus; this could underlie a tendency of Parkinson's disease patients to develop hypothermia. Poikilothermic patients with hypothermia have been described (5,103) who have no obvious underlying neurologic lesion but have been postulated to have hypothalamic dysfunction, in one case suspected to be vascular in nature (5).

Other neurologic diseases may be associated with hypothermia. Hypothermia has been described in a patient with a mesodiencephalic hematoma (79). Recurrent hypothermia occurs in patients with Shapiro's syndrome (agenesis of the corpus callosum) (206) and in patients with diencephalic epilepsy (73). Arroyo and colleagues (9) described patients with an intact corpus callosum who had episodic hyperhidrosis, hypothermia, and bradycardia; the authors postulated that these were caused by dysfunction of central serotonergic pathways. This syndrome has also been called episodic spontaneous hypothermia with hyperhidrosis (212) and spontaneous periodic hypothermia (125). Hypothermia thought to be due to a lesion in the anterior hypothalamus may occur in patients with subarachnoid hemorrhage (223).

Drugs and Alcohol

Many drugs are believed to cause hypothermia and to contribute to the development of accidental hypothermia. Alcohol in particular is often associated with accidental hypothermia (132,196,244). Alcohol is known to have a hypothermic effect in man (117) that is related to decreased stores of glycogen for heat production, heat loss due to vasodilation, obtundation, and an increased risk of immobilizing trauma (117,135,196). In addition to these effects of alcohol, patients with Wernicke's encephalopathy are at risk for developing hypothermia (see earlier).

Drugs can cause hypothermia by either acting on the brain and disrupting central thermoregulation or increasing heat loss by causing peripheral vasodilation (196,246). Hypothermia has been documented with vasodilatory drugs (246), bromocriptine (189), phenothiazines (196), neuroleptic drugs (54,96,172), barbiturates (68), diazepam (67), imipramine (169), and reserpine (167) (see Table 2). Hypothermia has also been described in cancer patients receiving intraventricular morphine (228). Hypothermia may occur as an unusual side effect of paracetamol (237).

Metabolic and Other Causes of Hypothermia

As described previously, hypothermia can occur with both hypoglycemia and hyperglycemia (87,174,179). Hypothermia occurs in myxedema coma (6) as a result of decreased calorigenesis (60), and it may occur without exposure to low environmental temperatures (59). Hypothermia can also occur with pituitary dysfunction (209) and adrenal insufficiency (188).

Hypothermia thought to be due to central thermoregulatory dysfunction has been described in patients with Hodgkin's disease (115) and systemic lupus erythematosus (136). Hypothermia of uncertain etiology has been described in patients with Reye's syndrome (232). Severe electric shock may cause hypothermia and has been treated successfully with lithium (144).

REFERENCES

1. Adolph EF, Molnar GW. Exchanges of heat and tolerances to cold in men exposed to outdoor weather. *Am J Physiol* 1946;146: 07–537.
2. Afifi AK, et al. Hypothermia-induced reversible polyneuropathy: electrophysiologic evidence of axonopathy. *Pediatr Neurol* 1988; 4:49–53.
3. Alexander SJ, et al. Sodium salicylate: alternate mechanism of central antipyretic action in the rat. *Pflugers Arch* 1989;413:451–455.
4. Al-Harthi SS, et al. Metabolite and hormonal profiles in heat stroke patients at Mecca Pilgrimage. *J Intern Med* 1990;228:343–346.
5. Allen J, et al. Poikilothermia in a 68-year-old female. A risk factor for accidental hypothermia, or hyperthermia. *Q J Med* 1989;70: 103–112.
6. Angel JH, Sash L. Hypothermic coma in myxoedema. *Br Med J* 1960;1:1855–1859.
7. Appenzeller O, Goss JE. Autonomic deficits in Parkinson's syndrome. *Arch Neurol* 1971;24:50–57.
8. Applegate WB, et al. Analysis of the 1980 heat wave in Memphis. *J Am Geriatr Soc* 1981;29:337–342.
9. Arroyo HA, et al. A syndrome of hyperhidrosis, hypothermia, and bradycardia possibly due to central monoaminergic dysfunction. *Neurology* 1990;40:556–557.
10. Baca L, Martinelli L. Neuroleptic malignant syndrome: a unique association with a tricyclic antidepressant. *Neurology* 1990;40: 1797–1798.
11. Barcenas C, et al. Obesity, football, dog days and siriasis: a deadly combination. *Am Heart J* 1976;92:237–244.
12. Bashour TT, et al. Atrioventricular block in accidental hypothermia—a case report. *Angiology* 1989;40:63–66.
13. Bass DE. Electrolyte excretion during cold diuresis. *Fed Proc* 1954;13:8.
14. Bauer HG. Endocrine and other clinical manifestations of hypothalamic disease. A survey of 60 cases, with autopsies. *J Clin Endocrinol Metab* 1954;14:13–31.
15. Beard MEJ, Hickton CM. Haemostasis in heat stroke. *Br J Haematol* 1982;52:269–274.
16. Beaton LE, et al. Neurogenic hyperthermia and its treatment with soluble pentobarbital in the monkey. *Arch Neurol Psychiatry* 1943; 49:518–536.
17. Beller GA, Boyd AE III. Heat stroke: a report of 13 consecutive cases without mortality despite severe hyperpyrexia and neurologic dysfunction. *Mil Med* 1975;140:464–467.
18. Bernheim HA. Is prostaglandin E_2 involved in the pathogenesis of fever? Effects of interleukin-1 on the release of prostaglandins. *Yale J Biol Med* 1986;59:151–158.
19. Birkhimer LJ, DeVane CL. The neuroleptic malignant syndrome: presentation and treatment. *Drug Intell Clin Pharm* 1984;18: 462–465.
20. Bismuth C, et al. Dantrolene—a new therapeutic approach to the neuroleptic malignant syndrome. *Acta Neurol Scand* 1984;70(suppl 100):193–198.
21. Bondy PK, et al. Etiocholanolone fever. *Medicine* 1965;44:249–262.
22. Bouchama A, et al. Ineffectiveness of dantrolene sodium in the treatment of heatstroke. *Crit Care Med* 1991; 19:176–180.
23. Boyd AE, Beller GA. Heat exhaustion and respiratory alkalosis. *Ann Intern Med* 1975;83:835.
24. Branch EF, et al. Hypothermia in a case of hypothalamic infarction and sarcoidosis. *Arch Neurol* 1971;25:245–255.
25. Breen EG, et al. Impaired coagulation in accidental hypothermia of the elderly. *Age Ageing* 1988; 17:343–346.
26. Britt BA. Etiology and pathophysiology of malignant hyperthermia. *Fed Proc* 1979;38:44–48.
27. Britt LD, et al. New horizons in management of hypothermia and frostbite injury. *Surg Clin North Am* 1991; 71:345–370.
28. Brown JR. Heat illness and army recruits. *Lancet* 1986;1:496.
29. Buchwald I, Davis PJ. Scleroderma with fatal heat stroke. *JAMA* 1967;201:270–271.
30. Burke RE, et al. Neuroleptic malignant syndrome caused by dopamine-depleting drugs in a patient with Huntington disease. *Neurology* 1981;31:1022–1026.
31. Cabanac M. Face fanning: a possible way to prevent or cure brain hyperthermia. In: Khogali M, Hales JR (eds). *Heat Stroke and Temperature Regulation.* New York: Academic Press. 1983;213–221.

32. Campbell BG. Cocaine abuse with hyperthermia, seizures and fatal complications. *Med J Aust* 1988;149:387–388.
33. Caroff SN. The neuroleptic malignant syndrome. *J Clin Psychiatry* 1980;41:79–83.
34. Channa AB, et al. Is dantrolene effective in heat stroke patients? *Crit Care Med* 1990;18:290–292.
35. Chao TC, et al. Acute heat stroke deaths. *Pathology* 1981;13:145–156.
36. Chapman J, Bean WB. Iatrogenic heatstroke. *JAMA* 1956;161:1375–1377.
37. Clarke JF. Some effects of the urban structure on heat mortality. *Environ Res* 1972;5:93–104.
38. Clowes GHA, O'Donnell TF. Heat stroke. *N Engl J Med* 1974;291:564–567.
39. Coceani F, et al. Further evidence implicating prostaglandin E_2 in the genesis of pyrogen fever. *Am J Physiol* 1988; 254:R463–R469.
40. Cohen WJ, Cohen NH. Lithium carbonate, haloperidol, and irreversible brain damage. *JAMA* 1974;230:1283–1287.
41. Collins KJ, et al. Accidental hypothermia and impaired temperature homeostasis in the elderly. *Br Med J* 1977;1:353–356.
42. Collins KJ, Exton-Smith AN. Thermal homeostasis in old age. *J Am Geriatr Soc* 1983;31:519–524.
43. Conn AW. Near-drowning and hypothermia. *Can Med Assoc J* 1979;120:397–399.
44. Cooper KE, et al. Temperature regulation during fever in man. *Clin Sci* 1964;27:345–356.
45. Cornell CJ, et al. Heparin therapy for heat stroke. *Ann Intern Med* 1974;81:702–703.
46. Costrini AM, et al. Cardiovascular and metabolic manifestations of heat stroke and severe heat exhaustion. *Am J Med* 1979;66:296–302.
47. Costrini A. Emergency treatment of exertional heatstroke and comparison of whole body cooling techniques. *Med Sci Sports Exerc* 1990;22:15–18.
48. Curry DL, Curry KP. Hypothermia and insulin secretion. *Endocrinology* 1970;87:750–755.
49. D'Alecy LG, Kluger MJ. Avian febrile response. *J Physiol* 1975;253:223–232.
50. Danzl DF, Pozos RS. Accidental hypothermia. *N Engl J Med* 1994;331:1756–1760.
51. Davison C, Demuth EL. Disturbances in sleep mechanism: a clinicopathologic study. III. Lesions at the diencephalic level (hypothalamus). *Arch Neurol Psychiatry* 1946;55: 11–125.
52. Denborough MA. The pathopharmacology of malignant hyperpyrexia. *Pharmacol Ther* 1980;9:357–365.
53. Dexter WW. Hypothermia. Safe and efficient methods of rewarming the patient. *Postgrad Med* 1990;88:55–58,61–64.
54. Dilsaver SC. Effects of neuroleptics on body temperature. *J Clin Psychiatry* 1988;49:78–79.
55. Dinarello CA. Interleukin-1 and the pathogenesis of the acute-phase response. *N Engl J Med* 1984;311:1413–1418.
56. Dinarello CA, et al. Effects of human interleukin-1 on natural killer cell activity: is fever a host defense mechanism for tumor killing? *Yale J Biol Med* 1986;59:97–106.
57. Drenth JP, et al. Hyperimmunoglobulinemia D and periodic fever syndrome. *Medicine* 1994;73:133–144.
58. Duff GW. Is fever beneficial to the host: a clinical perspective. *Yale J Biol Med* 1986;59:125–130.
59. Duguid H, et al. Accidental hypothermia. *Lancet* 1961;2:1213–1219.
60. Edelman IS. Thyroid thermogenesis. *N Engl J Med* 1974;290:1303–1308.
61. Editorial. Endotoxins in heatstroke. *Lancet* 1989;2:1137–1138.
62. Eiser AR, et al. Acute myoglobinuric renal failure. A consequence of the neuroleptic malignant syndrome. *Arch Intern Med* 1982;142:601–603.
63. El-Kassimi FA, et al. Adult respiratory distress syndrome and disseminated intravascular coagulation complicating heat stroke. *Chest* 1986;90:571–574.
64. Ellis FR, Heffron JJA. Clinical and biochemical aspects of malignant hyperpyrexia. *Recent Adv Anesth Analg* 1985;15:173–207.
65. Epstein Y. Heat intolerance: predisposing factor or residual injury? *Med Sci Sports Exerc* 1990;22:29–35.
66. Erickson TC. Neurogenic hyperthermia (a clinical syndrome and its treatment). *Brain* 1939;62:172–192.
67. Fell RH, Dendy PR. Severe hypothermia and respiratory arrest in diazepam and glutethimide intoxication. *Anaesthesia* 1968;23:636–640.
68. Fell RH, et al. Severe hypothermia as a result of barbiturate overdose complicated by cardiac arrest. *Lancet* 1968;1:392–394.
69. Figa-Talamanca L, et al. Hyperthermia after discontinuance of levodopa and bromocriptine therapy: impaired dopamine receptors a possible cause. *Neurology* 1985;35:258–261.
70. Foster KG, et al. Sweat responses in the aged. *Age Ageing* 1976;5:91–101.
71. Foster PS. Malignant hyperpyrexia. *Int J Biochem* 1990;22:1217–1222.
72. Fox RH, et al. Hypothermia in a young man with an anterior hypothalamic lesion. *Lancet* 1970;2:185–188.
73. Fox RH, et al. Spontaneous periodic hypothermia: diencephalic epilepsy. *Br Med J* 1973;2:693–695.
74. Friedman LS, Weinrauch LA. Metoclopramide-induced neuroleptic malignant syndrome. *Arch Intern Med* 1987;147:1495–1497.
75. Fyda DM, et al. The effectiveness of arginine vasopressin and sodium salicylate as antipyretics in the Brattleboro rat. *Brain Res* 1990;512:243–247.
76. Gader AMA, et al. Direct activation of platelets by heat is the possible trigger of the coagulopathy of heat stroke. *Br J Haematol* 1990;74:86–92.
77. Gautam PC, et al. Hypothermia in the elderly: management in a purpose-built chamber. *Gerontology* 1988;34:145–150.
78. Gautam P, et al. Hypothermia in the elderly: sociomedical characteristics and outcome of 86 patients. *Public Health* 1989;103:15–22.
79. Gaymard G, et al. Hypothermia in a mesodiencephalic haematoma. *J Neurol Neurosurg Psychiatry* 1990;53: 1014–1015.
80. Gentilello LM, et al. Continuous arteriovenous rewarming: rapid reversal of hypothermia in critically ill patients. *J Trauma* 1992; 32:316–327.
81. Gentilello LM. Advances in the management of hypothermia. *Surg Clin North Am* 1995;75:243–256.
82. Gobbi PG, et al. Night sweats in Hodgkin's disease. A manifestation of preceding minor febrile pulses. *Cancer* 1990;65:2074–2077.
83. Gottschalk PG, Thomas JE. Heat stroke. *Mayo Clin Proc* 1966;41:470–482.
84. Graber CD, et al. Fatal heat stroke. Circulating endotoxin and gram-negative sepsis as complications. *JAMA* 1971;216:1195–1196.
85. Green LH, et al. Fatal myocardial infarction in marathon racing. *Ann Intern Med* 1976;84:704–706.
86. Gubbay SS, Barwick DD. Two cases of accidental hypothermia in Parkinson's disease with unusual E.E.G. findings. *J Neurol Neurosurg Psychiatry* 1966;29:459–466.
87. Guerin JM, et al. Hypothermia in diabetic ketoacidosis. *Diabetes Care* 1987;10:801–802.
88. Guze BH, Baxter LR Jr. Neuroleptic malignant syndrome. *N Engl J Med* 1985;313:163–166.
89. Haak HR, van Hilten JJ, Roos RAC, Meinders AE. Functional hypothalamic derangement in a case of Wernicke's encephalopathy. *Neth J Med* 1990;36:291–296.
90. Hamburg P, et al. Relapse of neuroleptic malignant syndrome with early discontinuation of amantadine therapy. *Compr Psychiatry* 1986;27:272–275.
91. Hanhela R, et al. Plasma catecholamines, corticosterone, glucose and fatty acids concentrations and mean arterial pressure and body temperature in haemorrhagic hypovolaemia, hypothermia and a combination of these in the rabbit. *Acta Physiol Scand* 1990;139:441–449.
92. Harper C. Wernicke's encephalopathy: a more common disease than realised. *J Neurol Neurosurg Psychiatry* 1979;42:226–231.
93. Harrison GG. Dantrolene—dynamics and kinetics. *Br J Anaesth* 1988;60:279–286.
94. Hart GR, et al. Epidemic classical heat stroke: clinical characteristics and course of 28 patients. *Medicine* 1982;61:189–197.
95. Heffron JJA, McCarthy TV. Current views of the molecular basis of the malignant hyperthermia syndrome. *Acta Anaesth Belg* 1990;41:73–78.
96. Heh CW, et al. Neuroleptic-induced hypothermia associated with amelioration of psychosis in schizophrenia. *Neuropsychopharmacology* 1988;1:149–156.
97. Heller H, et al. Familial Mediterranean fever. *Arch Intern Med* 1958;102:50–71.

98. Henderson A, et al. Heat illness. A report of 45 cases from Hong Kong. *J R Army Med Corps* 1986;132:76–84.
99. Henderson A, Longdon P. Fulminant metoclopramide induced neuroleptic malignant syndrome rapidly responsive to intravenous dantrolene. *Aust N Z J Med* 1991;21:742–743.
100. Henderson VW, Wooten GF. Neuroleptic malignant syndrome: a pathogenetic role for dopamine receptor blockade? *Neurology* 1981; 31:132–137.
101. Hernandez E, et al. Hemodialysis for treatment of accidental hypothermia. *Nephron* 1993;63:214–216.
102. Hirayama K, et al. Reverse Shapiro's syndrome. A case of agenesis of corpus callosum associated with periodic hyperthermia. *Arch Neurol* 1994;51:494–496.
103. Hockaday TDR, et al. Temperature regulation in chronic hypothermia. *Lancet* 1962;2:428–432.
104. Holman ND, Schneider AJ. Multi-organ damage in exertional heat stroke. *Neth J Med* 1989;35:38–43.
105. Horowitz BZ. The golden hour in heat stroke: use of iced peritoneal lavage. *Am J Emerg Med* 1989;7:616–619.
106. Hudson LD, Conn RD. Accidental hypothermia. Associated diagnoses and prognosis in a common problem. *JAMA* 1974;227:37–40.
107. Isbell H, et al. An experimental study of the etiology of "rum fits" and delirium tremens. *Q J Stud Alcohol* 1955; 16:1–33.
108. Jacob AI, et al. A-V block in accidental hypothermia. *J Electrocardiol* 1978;11:399–402.
109. Jessen K, Hagelsten JO. Peritoneal dialysis in the treatment of profound accidental hypothermia. *Aviat Space Environ Med* 1978; 49:426–429.
110. Johnson RH, Spalding JMK. The effect of surface and central temperature on hand blood flow in subjects with complete transection of the cervical cord. *J Physiol* 1964;171:14P–15P.
111. Johnson RH. Temperature regulation in paraplegia. *Paraplegia* 1970;9:137–145.
112. Johnson RH, et al. Do thermoregulatory reflexes pass through the hypothalamus? Studies of chronic hypothermia due to hypothalamic lesion. *Aust N Z J Med* 1990;20:154–159.
113. Jolly BT, Ghezzi KT. Accidental hypothermia. *Emerg Med Clin North Am* 1992;10:311–327.
114. Joyner RW. Temperature effects on neuronal elements. *Fed Proc* 1981;40:2814–2818.
115. Jung M, et al. Hypothermia in Hodgkin's disease after exploratory laparotomy. *Klin Wochenschr* 1988;66:552–555.
116. Juul A, et al. Growth hormone deficiency and hyperthermia during exercise: a controlled study of sixteen GH-deficient patients. *J Clin Endocrinol Metab* 1995;80:3335–3340.
117. Kalant H, Le AD. Effects of ethanol on thermoregulation. *Pharmacol Ther* 1984;23:313–364.
118. Kanter GS. Renal clearance of sodium and potassium in hypothermia. *Can J Biochem Physiol* 1962;40:113–122.
119. Kenney WL, Hodgson JL. Heat tolerance, thermoregulation and ageing. *Sports Med* 1987;4:446–456.
120. Kew MC, et al. The heart in heatstroke. *Am Heart J* 1969; 77: 324–335.
121. Kew M, et al. Liver damage in heatstroke. *Am J Med* 1970; 49:192–202.
122. Kew M, et al. The diagnostic and prognostic significance of the serum enzyme changes in heatstroke. *Trans R Soc Trop Med Hyg* 1971;65:325–330.
123. Khogali M, et al. Management of heatstroke. *Lancet* 1982;2:1225.
124. Kilbourne EM, et al. Risk factors for heatstroke. A case-control study. *JAMA* 1982;247:3332–3336.
125. Kloos RT. Spontaneous periodic hypothermia. *Medicine* 1995; 74:268–280.
126. Kluger MJ. Is fever beneficial? *Yale J Biol Med* 1986;59:89–95.
127. Kluger MJ. Fever: role of pyrogens and cryogens. *Physiol Rev* 1991;71:93–127.
128. Knochel JP, et al. The renal, cardiovascular, hematologic and serum electrolyte abnormalities of heat stroke. *Am J Med* 1961;30:299–309.
129. Knochel JP. Environmental heat illness. An eclectic review. *Arch Intern Med* 1974;133:841–864.
130. Knochel JP, Caskey JH. The mechanism of hypophosphatemia in acute heat stroke. *JAMA* 1977;238:425–426.
131. Knochel JP. Heat stroke and related heat stress disorders. *Dis Mon* 1989;35:301–378.
132. Kortelainen M-L. Drugs and alcohol in hypothermia and hyperthermia related deaths: a retrospective study. *J Forensic Sci* 1987;32:1704–1712.
133. Kramer MR, et al. Mortality in elderly patients with thermoregulatory failure. *Arch Intern Med* 1989;149:1521–1523.
134. Krivosic-Horber R. Treatment of the acute episode. *Acta Anaesth Belg* 1990;41:83–86.
135. Kugelberg J, et al. Treatment of accidental hypothermia. *Scand J Thorac Cardiovasc Surg* 1967;1:142–146.
136. Kugler SL, et al. Hypothermia and systemic lupus erythematosus. *J Rheumatol* 1990;17:680–681.
137. Kurlan R, Shoulson I. Levodopa therapy for persistent neuroleptic-induced movement disorders. *Neurology* 1983;33(suppl 2):162.
138. Kurlan R, et al. Neuroleptic malignant syndrome. *Clin Neuropharmacol* 1984;7:109–120.
139. Lammens M, et al. Hypothermia in three patients with multiple sclerosis. *Clin Neurol Neurosurg* 1989;91:117–121.
140. Larach MG. Accidental hypothermia. *Lancet* 1995;345:493–497.
141. Leavall UW. Sweat gland necrosis in barbiturate poisoning. *Arch Dermatol* 1969;100:218–221.
142. Lennquist S, et al. Fluid balance and physical work capacity in humans exposed to cold. *Arch Environ Health* 1974;29:241–249.
143. Leonard A, Nelms RJ. Hypercalcemia in diuretic phase of acute renal failure. *Ann Intern Med* 1970;73:137–138.
144. Lieb J, et al. Lithium treatment of hypothermia caused by electric shock. *Med Hypotheses* 1980;6:769–772.
145. Lin J-J, et al. Permanent neurologic deficits in heat stroke. *Chin Med J (Engl)* 1991;47:133–138.
146. Litman RE. Heatstroke in parkinsonism. *Arch Intern Med* 1952; 89:562–567.
147. Lloyd EL, et al. Accidental hypothermia: an apparatus for central rewarming as a first aid measure. *Scot Med J* 1972;17:83–91.
148. Lomax P. Drug-induced changes in the thermoregulatory system. In: Khogali M, Hales JRS (eds). New York: Academic Press. 1983; 197–211.
149. Lomax P. Drug-abuse and heat stroke. In: Lomax, Schonbaum (eds). *Thermoregulation: Research and Clinical Applications.* Basel: Karger. 1989;42–45.
150. Lonning PE, et al. Accidental hypothermia. Review of the literature. 1986;30:601–613.
151. Lopez JR, et al. Intracellular ionized calcium concentration in muscles from humans with malignant hyperthermia. *Muscle Nerve* 1985;8:355–358.
152. Low PA, et al. Chronic idiopathic anhidrosis. *Ann Neurol* 1985; 18:344–348.
153. Luna GK, et al. Incidence and effect of hypothermia in seriously injured patients. *J Trauma* 1987;27: 1014–1018.
154. Lydiatt JS, Hill GE. Treatment of heat stroke with dantrolene. *JAMA* 1981;246:41–42.
155. Maaravi Y, Weiss AT. The effect of prolonged hypothermia on cardiac function in a young patient with accidental hypothermia. *Chest* 1990;98:1019–1020.
156. Macey SM, Schneider DF. Deaths from excessive heat and excessive cold among the elderly. *Gerontologist* 1993;33:497–500.
157. Mackowiak PA. Southwestern Internal Medicine Conference: Drug fever: mechanisms, maxims and misconceptions. *Am J Med Sci* 1987;294:275–286.
158. Maclean D, et al. Serum-enzymes in relation to electrocardiographic changes in accidental hypothermia. *Lancet* 1968; 2: 1266–1270.
159. Maclean D, et al. Acute pancreatitis and diabetic ketoacidosis in accidental hypothermia and hypothermic myxoedema. *Br Med J* 1973; 4:757–761.
160. Maclean D, et al. Serum enzyme activities in accidental hypothermia and hypothermic myxoedema. *Clin Chim Acta* 1974;52:197–201.
161. MacMillan AL, et al. Temperature regulation in survivors of accidental hypothermia of the elderly. *Lancet* 1967;2:165–169.
162. Magazanik A, et al. Tap water, an efficient method for cooling heatstroke victims—a model in dogs. *Aviat Space Environ Med* 1980; 51:864–867.
163. Mahajan SL, et al. Disseminated intravascular coagulation during rewarming following hypothermia. *JAMA* 1981; 245:2517–2518.
164. Malamud N, et al. Heat stroke. A clinico-pathologic study of 125 fatal cases. *Military Surgeon* 1946;99:397–449.

165. Marcus P, Edwards R. Serum enzyme levels during experimental hypothermia in man. *Q J Exp Physiol* 1978;63:371–381.
166. Marsden CD, Jenner P. The pathophysiology of extrapyramidal side-effects of neuroleptic drugs. *Psychol Med* 1980;10:55–72.
167. Mathews JA. Accidental hypothermia. *Postgrad Med J* 1967;43:662–667.
168. McCarron MM, et al. A case of neuroleptic malignant syndrome successfully treated with amantadine. *J Clin Psychiatry* 1982;43:381–382.
169. McGrath MD, Paley RG. Hypothermia induced in a myxoedematous patient by imipramine hydrochloride. *Br Med J* 1960;2:1364.
170. Mehta AC, Baker RN. Persistent neurological deficits in heat stroke. *Neurology* 1970;20:336–340.
171. Meriwether WD, Goodman RM. Severe accidental hypothermia with survival after rapid rewarming. Case report, pathophysiology and review of the literature. *Am J Med* 1972;53:505–510.
172. Millan MJ, et al. Evidence that dopamine D_3 receptors participate in clozapine-induced hypothermia. *Eur J Pharmacol* 1995;280:225–229.
173. Morimoto A, et al. Suppression of antipyretic response in rabbits by intraventricular protein synthesis inhibitor, anisomycin. *Pflugers Arch* 1987;408:414–416.
174. Morley JE, et al. Diabetes mellitus in elderly patients. Is it different? *Am J Med* 1987;83:533–544.
175. Morris DL, et al. Hemodynamic characteristics of patients with hypothermia due to occult infection and other causes. *Ann Intern Med* 1985;102:153–157.
176. Moss J. Accidental severe hypothermia. *Surg Gynecol Obstet* 1986;162:501–513.
177. Mueller PS, et al. Neuroleptic malignant syndrome. Successful treatment with bromocriptine. *JAMA* 1983;249:386–388.
178. Murphy RJ. Heat illness in the athlete. *Am J Sports Med* 1984;12:258–261.
179. Neil HAW, et al. Risk of hypothermia in elderly patients with diabetes. *Br Med J* 1986;293:416–418.
180. Newell K, et al. Pheochromocytoma crisis. *Am J Hypertens* 1988;1:189S–191S.
181. Niazi SA, Lewis FJ. Profound hypothermia in man. Report of a case. *Ann Surg* 1958;147:264–266.
182. O'Connor B. Hazards associated with the recreational drug ecstasy. *Br J Hosp Med* 1994;52:507–514.
183. Olson KR, Benowitz NL. Environmental and drug-induced hyperthermia. Pathophysiology, recognition, and management. *Emerg Med Clin North Am* 1984;2:459–474.
184. Ongphiphadhanakul B, Rajatanavin R. Diabetes insipidus: another cause of hormonal hyperthermia. *J Med Assoc Thai* 1992;75:127–132.
185. Osborn JJ. Experimental hypothermia: respiratory and blood pH changes in relation to cardiac function. *Am J Physiol* 1953;175:389–398.
186. Pagni CA, Courjon J. Electroencephalographic modifications induced by moderate and deep hypothermia in man. *Acta Neurochir Suppl (Wien)* 1964;13:35–49.
187. Pattison ME, et al. Exertional heat stroke and acute renal failure in a young woman. *Am J Kidney Dis* 1988;11:184–187.
188. Petersdorf RG. Hypothermia and hyperthermia. In: Wilson JD, Braunwald E, Isselbacher KJ et al (eds). *Harrison's Principles of Internal Medicine.* New York: McGraw-Hill. 1991;2194–2200.
189. Pfeiffer RF. Bromocriptine-induced hypothermia. *Neurology* 1990;40:383.
190. Philip G, Smith JF. Hypothermia and Wernicke's encephalopathy. *Lancet* 1973;2:122–124.
191. Pledger HG. Disorders of temperature regulation in acute traumatic tetraplegia. *J Bone Joint Surg* 1962;44B:110–113.
192. Poulton TJ, Walker RA. Helicopter cooling of heatstroke victims. *Aviat Space Environ Med* 1987;58:358–361.
193. Raju SF, et al. The pathogenesis of acute renal failure in heat stroke. *South Med J* 1973;66:330–333.
194. Ranklev-Twetman E. Malignant hyperthermia: the clinical syndrome. *Acta Anaesth Belg* 1990;41:79–82.
195. Ree HJ, Pezzullo JC. Inflammation and/or necrosis of tumors cannot account for fever in most febrile patients with Hodgkin's disease. *Cancer* 1987;60:1787–1789.
196. Reuler JB. Hypothermia: pathophysiology, clinical settings, and management. *Ann Intern Med* 1978;89:519–527.
197. Reutens DC, et al. Triphasic waves in accidental hypothermia. *Electroencephalogr Clin Neurophysiol* 1990;76:370–372.
198. Rosenberg MR, Green M. Neuroleptic malignant syndrome. *Arch Intern Med* 1989;149:1927–1931.
199. Rowell LB. Human cardiovascular adjustments to exercise and thermal stress. *Physiol Rev* 1974;54:75–159.
200. Sandhu JS, et al. Acute renal failure in severe hypothermia. *Ren Fail* 1992;14:591–594.
201. Saper JS, Breder CD. The neurologic basis of fever. *N Engl J Med* 1994;330:1880–1886.
202. Schrier RW, et al. Renal, metabolic, and circulatory responses to heat and exercise. *Ann Intern Med* 1970;73:213–223.
203. Schuman SH. Patterns of urban heat-wave deaths and implications for prevention: data from New York and St. Louis during July, 1966. *Environ Res* 1972;5:59–75.
204. Semsarian C. Cold exposure, frostbite and acute cerebral infarction. *Aust N Z J Med* 1994;24:217.
205. Shalev A, Munitz H. The neuroleptic malignant syndrome: agent and host interaction. *Acta Psychiatr Scand* 1986;73:337–347.
206. Shapiro WR, et al. Spontaneous recurrent hypothermia accompanying agenesis of the corpus callosum. *Brain* 1969;92:423–436.
207. Shapiro Y, Seidman DS. Field and clinical observations of exertional heat stroke patients. *Med Sci Sports Exerc* 1990;22:6–14.
208. Sharp FR, Hammel HT. Effects of fever on salivation response in the resting and exercising dog. *Am J Physiol* 1972;223:77–82.
209. Sheehan HL, Summers VK. Treatment of hypopituitary coma. *Br Med J* 1952;1:1214–1215.
210. Shenaq SA, et al. Effect of profound hypothermia on leukocytes and platelets. *Ann Clin Lab Sci* 1986;16:130–133.
211. Sherman R, et al. Occupational death due to heat stroke: report of two cases. *Can Med Assoc J* 1989;140:1057–1058.
212. Sheth RD, et al. Episodic spontaneous hypothermia with hyperhidrosis: implications and pathogenesis. *Pediatr Neurol* 1994;10:58–60.
213. Shibolet S, Israel Defense Army, Fisher S et al. Fibrinolysis and hemorrhages in fatal heatstroke. *N Engl J Med* 1962;266:169–173.
214. Shibolet S, et al. Heatstroke: its clinical picture and mechanism in 36 cases. *Q J Med* 1967;36:525–547.
215. Shibolet S, Farfel Z. Heparin therapy for heatstroke. *Ann Intern Med* 1975;82:857–858.
216. Shibolet S, Lancaster MC, Danon Y. Heat stroke: a review. *Aviat Space Environ Med* 1976;47:280–301.
217. Simon HB, Daniels GH. Hormonal hyperthermia. Endocrinologic causes of fever. *Am J Med* 1979;66:257–263.
218. Sinks T. Hazards of working in cold weather include frostbite, hypothermia. Treatment for frostbite may be complex, including procedures to prevent infection. *Occup Health Saf* 1988;57:20–25.
219. Smith LW. Pathologic changes observed in human tissues subjected to subcritical temperatures. *Arch Pathol* 1940;30:424–438.
220. Sohar E, et al. Genetics of familial Mediterranean fever (FMF). A disorder with recessive inheritance in non-Ashkenazi Jews and Armenians. *Arch Intern Med* 1961;107:529–538.
221. Solomon A, et al. The electrocardiographic features of hypothermia. *J Emerg Med* 1989;7:169–173.
222. Spain WH, et al. Knowledge of causes, controls aids prevention of heat stress. *Occup Health Saf* 1985;54:27–33.
223. Spiro SG, Jenkins JS. Adipsia and hypothermia after subarachnoid haemorrhage. *Br Med J* 1971;3:411–412.
224. Srichaikul T, et al. Clinical manifestations and therapy of heat stroke: consumptive coagulopathy successfully treated by exchange transfusion and heparin. *Southeast Asian J Trop Med Public Health* 1989;20:479–491.
225. Stitt JT. Fever versus hyperthermia. *Fed Proc* 1979;38:39–43.
226. Stitt JT. Prostaglandin E as the neural mediator of the febrile response. *Yale J Biol Med* 1986;59:137–149.
227. Stoner HB, et al. Metabolic aspects of hypothermia in the elderly. *Clin Sci* 1980;59:19–27.
228. Su CF, Liu MY, Lin MT. Intraventricular morphine produces pain relief, hypothermia, hyperglycaemia and increased prolactin and growth hormone levels in patients with cancer pain. *J Neurol* 1987;235:105–108.

229. Sullivan F, et al. Chronic hypothermia in multiple sclerosis. *J Neurol Neurosurg Psychiatry* 1987;50:813–815.
230. Talbott JH. The physiologic and therapeutic effects of hypothermia. *N Engl J Med* 1941;224:281–288.
231. Talman WT, et al. A hyperthermic syndrome in two subjects with acute hydrocephalus. *Arch Neurol* 1988;45:1037–1040.
232. Taly AB, et al. Hypothermia: an unusual manifestation of Reye's syndrome. *Indian J Med Sci* 1990; 44:237–238,243.
233. Tehan B, et al. Hyperthermia associated with 3,4-methylenedioxyethamphetamine ("Eve"). *Anaesthesia* 1993; 48:507–510.
234. Tipton MJ, et al. Hand immersion as a method of cooling and rewarming: a short review. *J R Nav Med Serv* 1993;79:125–131.
235. Tornblom N. Hyperinsulinism with fatal postoperative hyperthermia. *Acta Med Scand* 1961;170:757–761.
236. Toru M, et al. Neuroleptic malignant syndrome-like state following a withdrawal of antiparkinsonian drugs. *J Nerv Ment Dis* 1981;169:324–327.
237. Van Tittelboom T, Govaerts-Lepicard M. Hypothermia: an unusual side effect of paracetamol. *Vet Hum Toxicol* 1989;31:57–59.
238. Vassallo SU, Delaney KA. Pharmacologic effects of thermoregulation: mechanisms of drug-related heatstroke. *Clin Toxicol* 1989;27:199–224.
239. Wachtel TJ, et al. Natural history of fever following seizure. *Arch Intern Med* 1987;147:1153–1155.
240. Wagner JA, et al. Age and temperature regulation of humans in neutral and cold environments. *J Appl Physiol* 1974;37:562–565.
241. Ward A, et al. Dantrolene. A review of its pharmacodynamic and pharmacokinetic properties and therapeutic use in malignant hyperthermia, the neuroleptic malignant syndrome and an update of its use in muscle spasticity. *Drugs* 1986;32:130–168.
242. Wechsler IS. Hypothalamic syndromes. *Br Med J* 1956;2:375–378.
243. Weiner JS, Khogali M. A physiological body-cooling unit for treatment of heat stroke. *Lancet* 1980;1:507–509.
244. Weyman AE, et al. Accidental hypothermia in an alcoholic population. *Am J Med* 1974;56:13–21.
245. Williamson LM, et al. Familial Hibernian fever. *Q J Med* 1982;204:469–480.
246. Wollersheim H, et al. Decreased rectal body temperature induced by different vasodilatory drugs. *Neth J Med* 1989; 34:189–193.
247. Wongsurawat N, et al. Thermoregulatory failure in the elderly. St. Louis University Geriatric Grand Rounds. *J Am Geriatr Soc* 1990;38:899–906.
248. Woolf PD, et al. Accidental hypothermia: endocrine function during recovery. *J Clin Endocrinol* 1972;34: 460–466.
249. Wrenn KD, Larson S. The febrile alcoholic in the emergency department. *Am J Emerg Med* 1991;9:57–60.
250. Wright DO, et al. Purpuric manifestations of heatstroke. Studies of prothrombin and platelets in 12 cases. *Arch Intern Med* 1946;77:27–36.
251. Wyndham CH. Heat stroke and hyperthermia in marathon runners. *Ann N Y Acad Sci* 1977;301:128–138.
252. Yaqub BA, et al. Heat stroke at the Mekkah Pilgrimage: clinical characteristics and course of 30 patients. *Q J Med* 1986;59.
253. Zahger D, et al. Evidence of prolonged myocardial dysfunction in heat stroke. *Chest* 1989;95:1089–1091.
254. Zimmerman HM. Temperature disturbances and the hypothalamus. *Res Publ Assoc Res Nerv Ment Dis* 1940;20:824–840.

CHAPTER 55

Management of Orthostatic Hypotension

Robert D. Fealey and David Robertson

1. A working knowledge of the mechanisms of postural blood pressure (BP) regulation helps in the planning of treatment strategies.
2. Varying criteria exist for the diagnosis of orthostatic hypotension (OH). The most recent consensus is a fall in BP of at least 20 mmHg systolic or 10 mmHg diastolic within 3 min of standing or of head-up tilt of at least 60°. Treatment is initiated for symptomatic OH.
3. Robertson has used the practical "standing time" criteria to characterize the severity of OH and as a parameter to monitor response to treatment.
4. Reversible causes of OH (volume depletion, medications, chronic anemia) must be identified and corrected; reversible causes often coexist with neurogenic mechanisms and must be appreciated for ideal management.
5. Rare syndromes for which there are highly specific and successful treatments (e.g., the dopamine β-hydroxylase deficiency syndrome treated with dihydroxyphenylserine) must be identified. Symptomatic improvement is achievable in most patients with neurogenic OH, even if the underlying disorder is not reversible.
6. Nonpharmacologic measures for treating patients with OH include elevating the head of the bed, increasing dietary salt and water intake, eating smaller and more frequent meals, using countermaneuvers (squatting, standing with legs crossed) and reconditioning exercises, and wearing elastic leotards or abdominal wraps.
7. Pharmacologic agents include nonsteroidal anti-inflammatory drugs, volume expanders, caffeine, sympathomimetics (including midodrine), erythropoietin (epoetin alfa), and ergotamine derivatives. In special situations, the antihypertensive drugs propranolol and clonidine can be helpful, as can the somatostatin analogue octreotide and the gastrointestinal prokinetic drugs metoclopramide and cisapride.
8. Patients with severe OH due to autonomic failure generally require simultaneous use of pharmacologic and nonpharmacologic therapy. A typical regimen consists of wearing elastic leotards or an abdominal binder, consuming 2 L of fluid and 175 mEq to 250 mEq of sodium daily, elevating the head of the bed, regularly using physical countermaneuvers, and taking fludrocortisone (0.1 mg bid) and phenylpropanolamine hydrochloride (50 mg tid).
9. Care is focused on producing symptomatic improvement (e.g., increasing the standing time from 1 to 3 min and not completely eliminating the OH). Supine hypertension is a common problem that occasionally requires treatment but seldom leads to disastrous consequences, such as central nervous system hemorrhage.

INTRODUCTION

Patients with autonomic disorders most often present with symptoms of orthostatic hypotension (OH). Commonly, the OH is secondary to a known disorder of the central or peripheral nervous system (e.g., cervical myelopathy due to trauma or demyelinating disease, or an autonomic neuropathy caused by a systemic disease such as diabetes mellitus) (32). Treatment of OH, therefore, may necessarily involve therapy of the associated illness, and the clinician must be aware of some conditions that can cause OH (Table 1). (Case Study 2 in the Appendix is an unusual and dramatic example of OH due to a removable posterior fossa tumor).

It is also helpful to keep in mind the physiologic mechanisms regulating postural blood pressure (BP), because many of the treatment modalities replace or augment these reflexes when they are affected by disease. These are ex-

R. D. Fealey: Department of Neurology, Mayo Clinic, Rochester, Minnesota 55905.
D. Robertson: Department of Neurology, Vanderbilt University School of Medicine, Nashville, Tennessee 37232.

TABLE 1. *Classification of disorders causing orthostatic hypotension*

Generalized primary autonomic failure
    Pure autonomic failure or idiopathic orthostatic hypotension (Bradbury-Eggleston syndrome)
    Pure autonomic failure with multiple-system atrophy or Shy-Drager syndrome
    Acute pandysautonomia (panautonomic neuropathy)
    Familial dysautonomia (Riley-Day syndrome)
Partial primary autonomic failure
    Dopamine β-hydroxylase deficiency
    Postural orthostatic tachycardia syndrome (length-dependent autonomic neuropathy)
    Monoamine oxidase deficiency
    Pure vasomotor failure
Disorders of idiopathic orthostatic intolerance
    Postural orthostatic tachycardia syndrome
    Mitral valve prolapse
    Due to prolonged bed rest or space flight
    Due to asthenic habitus
Disorders of the central nervous system
    Tumors (hypothalamic, parasellar, posterior fossa)
    Multiple cerebral infarcts
    Wernicke's encephalopathy
    Tabes dorsalis
    Traumatic and inflammatory myelopathies
    Parkinson's disease
    Hereditary system degenerations
    Syringomyelia
    Dysautonomia of advanced age
    Multiple sclerosis
Systemic diseases with autonomic neuropathy
    Botulism
    Diabetic neuropathy
    Primary systemic amyloidosis
    Guillain-Barré syndrome
    Porphyria
    Lambert-Eaton myasthenic syndrome
    Paraneoplastic autonomic neuropathy
    Uremic neuropathy
    Connective tissue disease
    Tangier and Fabry's diseases
    Vincristine and heavy metal neuropathies
    Leprosy
    B_{12} deficiency
    Chronic Chagas' disease
    Propafenone neuropathy (16)
Endorcine–metabolic disorders
    Primary and secondary adrenocortical insufficiency
    Pheochromocytoma
    Marked potassium depletion
    Severe hypoaldosteronism
Iatrogenic causes
    Antihypertensive drugs (α-methyldopa, guanethidine, prazosin, β blockers)
    Psychotropic drugs (phenothiazines, butyrophenones)
    Antiparkinsonian drugs (Sinemet, Parlodel)
    Vasodilator drugs (nitrates)
    Certain illicit drugs (marijuana)
    Thoracolumbar sympathectomy
Disorders with diminished cardiac output
    Reduced intravascular volume
    Acute and chronic blood loss
    Fluid loss due to vomiting, diarrhea, diuretics
    Gastrectomy with the dumping syndrome
    Salt-losing nephropathy
    Altered capillary permeability
    Impaired venous return
    Severe varicose veins
    Venous obstruction (late pregnancy)
    Reflex and pharmacologic vasodilatation
    Muscle wasting and prolonged recumbency
    Intrinsic cardiac disease
    Myocardial infarct
    Arrhythmias
    Restrictive pericardial/myocardial diseases
Miscellaneous causes
    Hyperbradykinnism
    Chronic renal hemodialysis
    Anorexia nervosa
    Reduced aortic compliance
    Mastocytosis
    Baroreflex failure

tensively reviewed in Chapters 5 and 6 and are briefly summarized below.

Under normal circumstances, assumption of the upright position in humans results in the following:

1. Reflex arteriolar constriction and increased total peripheral resistance mediated by baroreceptors and efferent sympathetic pathways within the brain stem, spinal cord, and pre- and postganglionic adrenergic fibers. Release of the neurotransmitter norepinephrine at smooth muscle synapses.
2. Reflex venous constriction and augmentation of respiration mediated by the sympathetic and parasympathetic nerves. Adrenomedullary release of epinephrine to resist further pooling of blood and to facilitate venous return.
3. Reflex acceleration of the heart rate due primarily to withdrawal of vagal parasympathetic tone.
4. An increase in muscle tone and tissue pressure in the legs and abdominal muscles.
5. An immediate increase in plasma catecholamine levels and delayed activation of the renin-angiotensin-aldosterone system, both due mainly to activation of sympathetic visceral efferents.
6. The release of vasopressin from the neurohypophysis, mediated by atrial stretch receptor reflexes.

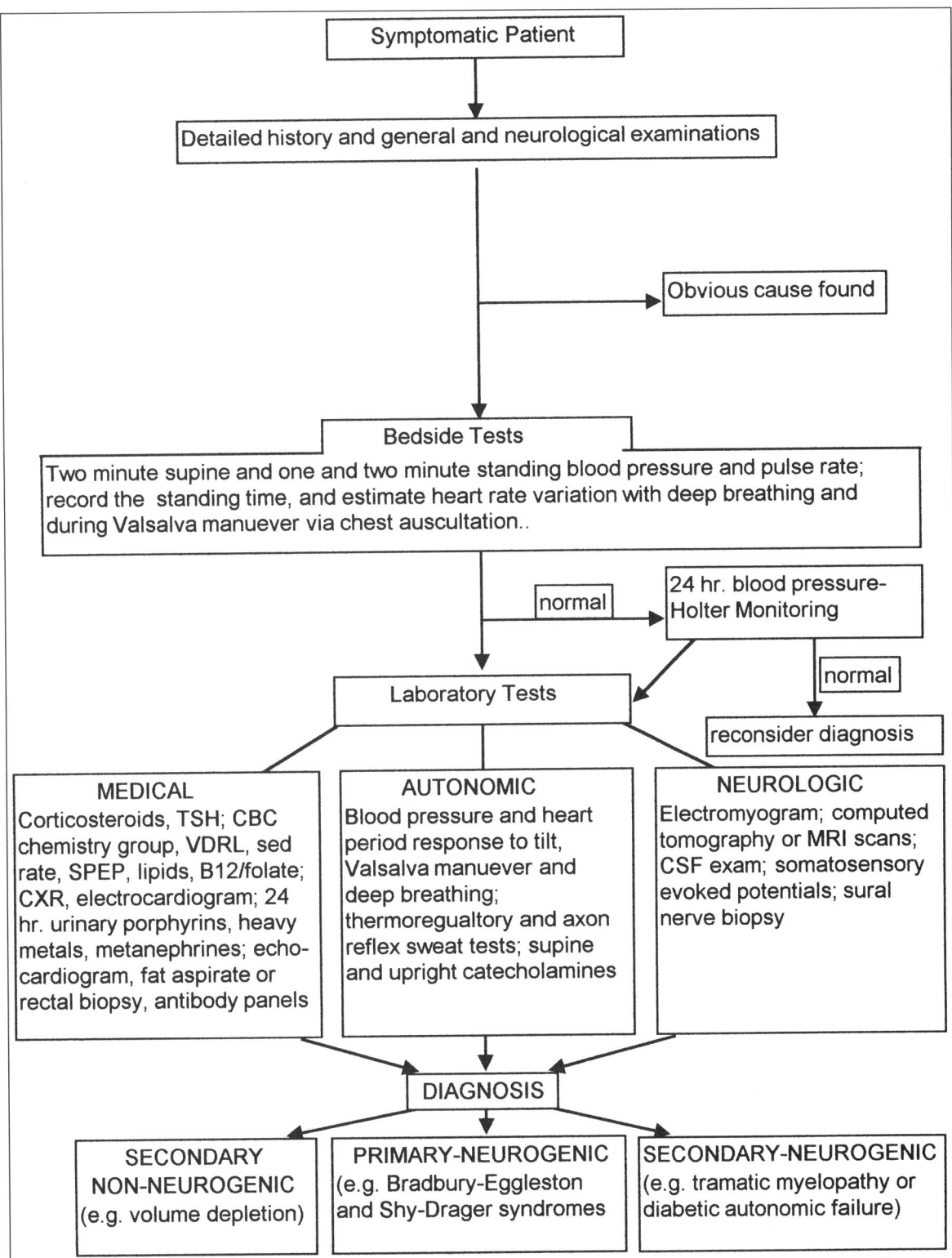

FIG. 1. Steps in diagnosis of a patient with orthostatic hypotension. (TSH = thyroid-stimulating hormone; CBC = complete blood count; VDRL = Venereal Disease Research Laboratory test for syphilis; SPEP = serum protein electrophoresis; CXR = chest x-ray study; MRI = magnetic resonance imaging; CSF = cerebrospinal fluid.) Note: Bradbury-Eggleston and Shy Drager syndromes should be pure autonomic failure and multiple system atrophy.

DIAGNOSIS OF ORTHOSTATIC HYPOTENSION

Not everyone with a postural BP drop deserves treatment, nor does everyone with posturally induced symptoms have OH. Therefore, guidelines have been developed pertaining to BP criteria for the diagnosis of OH. When one changes from a supine to a standing position, there is usually a drop in systolic BP of up to 5 to 19 mmHg. This is accompanied by either no change in diastolic pressure or a slight rise in diastolic pressure. These BP changes are usually accompanied by an acceleration of the heart rate of 5 to 25 beats/min (bpm). Varying criteria exist for the diagnosis of (OH) (3,37,42); the most recent consensus is a fall in BP of at least 20 mmHg systolic or 10 mmHg diastolic within 3 min of either standing or head-up tilt of at least 60°. Treatment is initiated for symptomatic OH (2). Alternatively, an operational definition for significant OH is any BP drop on standing that causes symptoms (34).

The OH should be reproducible with an accepted technique for determining postural BP. One technique includes a 2-min supine reading and pulse rate followed by a 2-min standing BP and pulse rate by way of standard cuff sphygmomanometry. The criteria for a significant BP drop with standing have already been mentioned. However, the degree of postural BP drop may vary substantially during the day, at times existing only postprandially, in the morning upon arising, or after standing still following vigorous exercise (27,35).

It is helpful to monitor the standing time, defined as the amount of time a patient can stand still before symptoms force him or her to sit. A standing time of <30 seconds is associated with severe OH and an inability to perform activities of daily living. A standing time of >1 min is usually associated with independent living (34). Either a 2-min supine/2-min standing BP or the standing time, or both, can be used to monitor patient response to treatment.

Although the treatment of OH may be similar regardless of the cause, the most effective treatment usually depends on the identification of a specific cause. Therefore, the diagnostic evaluation is the first step in treatment. A scheme depicting this process is illustrated in Fig. 1 and is described next. Often a detailed history and general medical and neurologic exam will point to the obvious cause. More commonly, bedside and laboratory studies need to be done.

The medical laboratory studies listed in Table 1 are familiar to most physicians. Neurologic tests include some that should be done only if recommended by a consulting neurologist. The specific tests of autonomic function constitute a battery of procedures that are described in Chapter 15. They are useful for confirming whether OH is due to autonomic failure and, if so, whether the site of the lesion is preganglionic or postganglionic. This factor is sometimes used to select the proper pressor agent for treating the OH. Assessing the integrity of autonomic neuronal pathways is therefore another important early step in the management of OH.

As shown in Table 1, disorders resulting in OH can be divided into primary and secondary causes. Secondary causes can be neurogenic or non-neurogenic (i.e., a normally functioning autonomic nervous system unable to compensate for another dysfunction, such as severe volume depletion). Primary causes consist of some form of autonomic neuronal failure.

Knowledge of the natural history of the diseases mentioned in Table 1, a thorough medical and neurologic examination, and specific laboratory tests to confirm or exclude secondary causes are also crucial in reaching the correct diagnosis and administering treatment. The clinical features of these disorders can be found elsewhere in this textbook.

Patients with symptomatic OH may complain of lightheadedness, cognitive impairment, faintness, blurred vision or even loss of vision, and a sense of profound weakness and unsteadiness after standing or walking. This constellation of symptoms collectively referred to as "orthostatism" is often worse in the morning and is aggravated by prolonged recumbency, heat and humidity, a heavy meal, and exercise. In severe cases, syncope results and the patient is unconscious for a short time, usually awakening once recumbent. Accompanying symptoms such as cold perspiration, pallor, and nausea are prominent in non-neurogenic causes of OH, whereas lack of sweating, impotence, and bladder dysfunction are common when there is autonomic neuronal failure.

SPECIFIC DISORDERS

Therapy is directed primarily toward the OH in pure autonomic failure and toward the OH and extrapyramidal symptoms in multiple system atrophy. Disorders that cause secondary OH syndrome can be placed into six categories, as indicated in Table 1. Many of the primary disorders of the central and peripheral nervous system have no specific treatment, so therapy is also directed toward alleviating the symptoms of the OH. This will be described later in this chapter. Several disorders, such as posterior fossa brain tumors, have treatment available, and these conditions must be recognized, because the primary treatment usually improves or relieves the autonomic failure and obviates the need for additional treatment. Treatment of the BP fluctuations that occur acutely with the Guillain-Barré syndrome differs from that adopted for other primary and secondary disorders and is discussed in Chapters 56 and 57.

The rare condition of dopamine β-hydroxylase (DBH) deficiency is a primary autonomic disorder for which there is a unique and most effective treatment. In DBH deficiency, adult patients have usually survived a complicated perinatal period and are seen because of severe OH, ejaculatory failure, nocturia, ptosis, hyperextensible joints, and nasal congestion, but they exhibit normal sweating patterns and no somatic neurologic deficit. Their serum norepinephrine to dopamine ratio is <0.1 (normal is about 10), and dopamine instead of norepinephrine is released from otherwise intact adrenergic nerve terminals. The administration of dihydroxyphenylserine (L-DOPS) causes the endogenous replacement of dopamine by norepinephrine and a remarkable improvement in BP regulation (6,8,26,36).

Many of the systemic diseases with autonomic failure are characterized by a sensorimotor neuropathy in addition to autonomic involvement. Some of the systemic conditions and neuropathies are reversible and require specific treatment. Examples include renal transplant for uremic neuropathy and B_{12} replacement for the treatment of the dysautonomia of pernicious anemia (see Chapter 31).

The OH due to adrenocortical insufficiency and severe hypoaldosteronism is related to reduced intravascular volume and sodium depletion and thus responds to rehydration and replacement therapy.

One should always ascertain if antihypertensive or psychotropic drugs are being used, because many agents in both categories can cause OH. Of the antihypertensive drugs, guanethidine, prazosin hydrochloride, methyldopa, and clonidine are frequently causative, particularly when combined with diuretics, which cause sodium and volume depletion. Reduced intravascular volume due to blood or fluid loss generally causes systolic OH with prominent tachycardia, pallor, and sweating. This is treated by finding the source of blood or fluid loss while replacing intravascular volume.

Mastocytosis is an uncommon disorder characterized by attacks of mast cell activation. This is often triggered by heat, exercise, narcotics, or emotional stimuli. Symptoms include flushing, pruritus, paresthesia, palpitations, dyspnea, dizziness, diarrhea, headaches, and occasionally syncope due to hypotension (31). Diagnosis is established by the finding of marked elevations of urinary methylhistamine and prostaglandin D_2 levels. The determinations of serum tryptase and spot urinary histamine level 2 hrs after a spell may also be diagnostic. Treatment is unique and consists of administering H_1- and H_2-receptor antagonists, sometimes in combination with aspirin. Severe attacks must be managed in the hospital and may require initial treatment with intravenous epinephrine.

THERAPEUTIC MEASURES

As has already been mentioned, reversible causes of OH must be identified and eliminated. Blood loss and other causes of volume depletion, drug-induced hypotension, and adrenal insufficiency are all examples of reversible causes. If the cause of OH is not reversible, symptomatic treatment measures are used. Most patients in this latter group will have neurogenic OH due to one of the primary or secondary neurologic disorders noted in Table 1.

Nonpharmacologic Measures

Diet

Neurogenic OH is much more critical when patients are sodium depleted and/or dehydrated. To avoid this, patients should have a daily dietary intake of at least 175 mEq of sodium and (in an adult) 2.0 to 2.5 L of fluid. Foods with a high salt content include canned soups, chili, ham, bacon, sausage, additives like soy sauce, fast food, and commercially processed canned products. Patients on high doses of Florinef, which causes hypokalemia, should eat high-potassium foods such as fruits and vegetables, No-salt, poultry, fish, beef, and pork. Water can be given in amounts of 400 mL with meals and 200 to 300 mL in between major meals and with a snack at bedtime. Because patients are often constipated and may develop syncope with straining, a high-fiber diet is recommended. Postprandial aggravation of OH can be offset by eating smaller, more frequent meals with a reduced carbohydrate content (34). In patients with supine hypertension, a bedtime snack can help reduce BP for several hours. Vasodilators such as alcohol should be avoided.

Head-Up Tilt and Other Positions

Sleeping with the head of the bed elevated (25) 6 to 12 inches (15 to 30 cm) or sleeping in the sitting position (3) moderates the sudden pooling of blood on arising in the morning and can reduce dangerous supine hypertension. The head-up position may stimulate endogenous renin, angiotensin, and aldosterone production and increase blood volume in patients who can still release renin (4,5). Patients should sit for several minutes on the edge of the bed before standing up and should postpone activities such as shaving until they have been up for a while, or they should accomplish the activity while sitting. Crossing the legs while standing and raising the feet on a stool while eating may be helpful. When presyncopal symptoms occur, quickly squatting may prevent loss of consciousness and falling. A handy mechanical aid used in severely affected patients who are still ambulatory is a "darby chair," (see pg. 776) which is a cane when folded and a chair when unfolded. When presyncopal symptoms arise, patients can sit for a brief period until asymptomatic and then resume walking.

Elastic Supports

For years, we have used a custom-fitted commercially available elasticized garment extending from the metatarsals to the costal margin, which allows a gradient of counterpressure to be applied with maximal pressure at the ankles and slight counterpressure at the top. This garment can be made with an open crotch to facilitate urination and should be donned while the patient is still recumbent (39).

TABLE 2. *Rx. of orthostatic hypotension (mechanical, dietary methods)*

Treatment	Details of treatment	Side effects/complications
Head-up tilt of bed	45 degree head-up tilt of hospital bed; front legs up on 6–12" blocks; a recliner can also be used.	Hypotension; sliding down in bed (may) need foot board); may be ineffective unless patient sits.
Elastic body garment: Jobst: (800-537-1063) Barton-Carey: (800-421-0444) Sigvaris: (800-322-7744) Camp: (800-492-1088) Medi: (800-633-6334) Abdominal binder: Professional Products' Easy-wraps	Jobst or Barton-Carey custom fit leotard; Medi, Sigvaris or Camp "off the shelf" leotard; 30–40 mm Hg ankle counterpressure; put on using rubber gloves with finger grips and sliding in foot; donn while still recumbant in am; remove and hand wash (Ivory liquid soap) h.s.; if incontinent use open crotch; avoid zippers; don't powder skin or wear "nylons" underneath; get two pair, wear on alternate days. On hot days use lighterweight Medi stocking or just an abdominal binder.	Hard to get on; last about 6 mo. @ $150 to $250/pair; may be intolerable in hot climates; may reduce action of leg 'muscle pump and prevent the helpful water jacket effect of perivascular edema.
Physical maneuvers (Clinical Autonomic Research, 1993;3;57-66)	Patients are taught to quickly squat, flex forward, stand cross-legged and step up with one leg at the first sign of hypotension.	May be hard to perform in patients with Multiple System Atrophy and compromised balance.
Exercise	Mild exercise, i.e. walking may facilitate venous return; avoid overheating and straining.	If too vigorous may further lower blood pressure.
Dietary	175-250 mEq Na+ (salt tablets may be needed); 24 hr urinary Na+ and K+ loss replaced; 2–2.5 L of fluid intake per day. Smaller more frequent meals with low carbohydrate content for post-prandial hypotension; avoid alcohol (a vasodilator).	Peripheral edema and supine hypertension may develop.

Several companies manufacture these, and we continue to use them even though they are somewhat difficult to put on and their constant counterpressure reduces the muscular pump action for venous return and may prevent the formation of edema (thought by some to provide a helpful extravascular water jacket of counterpressure). Zippers should be added only if the garment is impossible to get on otherwise. Some patients have more success with thigh-high supports plus an abdominal binder. Professional Products makes one such binder, known as Easy Wrap (see Table 2 for more information).

Exercise and Postural Countermaneuvers

A mild degree of exercise is desirable, but vigorous exercise often lowers the standing BP and aggravates the orthostatism. Swimming, aerobic exercise while in water, stationary bike riding, and, in milder cases, walking are potentially beneficial activities. Prolonged recumbency should be avoided. Isotonic exercise is preferable to isometric. Postural countermaneuvers such as squatting, standing with the legs crossed, placing one leg up on a step, and forward flexion with abdominal and pelvic muscle tightening have been shown to significantly raise BP and fend off impending syncope (45). Patients can be taught these techniques in just 10 min, and they can be used with or without the elastic support.

Pharmacologic Measures (Table 3)

Independently introduced by Hickler and Liddle (34) some 40 years ago, fludrocortisone acetate (Florinef) has been the drug of choice in the treatment of OH. Fludrocortisone may sensitize blood vessels to the effect of endogenous catecholamines at low doses, increasing the fluid content of blood vessel walls. It increases vascular resistance to stretching and may decrease the volume of blood pooled. Evidence suggests that fludrocortisone may even increase the number of α-adrenoreceptors that can interact with the remaining endogenous norepinephrine. At higher doses, fludrocortisone can expand the blood volume, improve cardiac output, and reduce postural hypotension; however, such dosages pose the threat of fluid overload and congestive heart failure (12), severe supine hypertension, and hypokalemia. For patients with severe symptoms and normal cardiac function, we use a dose of 0.5 to 1.0 mg bid for 2 to 3 days, subsequently reducing the dose to a maintenance level of 0.2 mg daily to twice daily. In less se-

TABLE 3. Rx. of orthostatic hypotension (pharmacologic methods)

Treatment	Details of treatment	Side effects/complication
Florinef (a-fluorocortisone); fludrocortisone	Start 0.05 mg p.o. b.i.d.; increase to 0.1–0.3 mg p.o. b.i.d. @ 7am, 2pm. A 3–6 lb. weight gain is desirable.	Hypokalemia, peripheral edema, steroid effects, congestive heart failure.
Sodium Chloride (salt tablets)	50 mEq or 1200 mg p.o. t.i.d.	Peripheral edema; congestive heart failure.
Ephedrine sulfate	Start 12.5 to 25 mg p.o. t.i.d.; increase to 50–75 mg t.i.d. prn.	Nervousness, tachycardia, supine hypertension, tachyphalaxis.
Phenylpropanolamine (Propagest)	25 mg tablets; same dose as above for ephedrine.	Nervousness, tachycardia, supine hypertension, tachyphalaxis.
Yohimbine (Yohimex)	Presynaptic α-adrenergic blocker, given as 5.4 mg p.o. t.i.d.; used early in course of autonomic failure, impotence Rx.	Anxiety, tremor, palpitations, diarrhea and supine hypertenstion.
Midodrine (ProAmatine)	5 mg tablet size; 1–2 tablets q-3hr to q-4hr, up to 40 mg a day.	Approved by FDA for OH Rx. 9/96; now available; supine hypertension, scalp pruritis, tachyphalaxis; weight loss, increased urinary Na+ loss.
Dihydroergotamine (DHE-45)	5.0 mg tablets; 2.5–10 mg p.o. b.i.d. to q.i.d.; parenteral use (0.5–1 mg) provides more predictable pressor effect.	Poor oral absorption; supine hypertension; ergotism; an investigational drug for this indication.
Ergotamine tartrate	1 mg tablets, 2 mg suppository or sublingual; 1–2 mg b.i.d. to t.i.d.; inhalation Rx (Medihaler) under investigation.	Same as above for dihydroergotamine.
Clonidine (Catapress)	0.1–0.3 mg tablets given as 0.2–0.8 mg b.i.d. to t.i.d. Used for severe efferent sympathetic failure with dysautonomic diarrhea.	Drowsiness, dry mouth, constipation hypertension, hypotension.
Propranolol (Inderal)	10–40 mg p.o. q.i.d. Used selectively in POTS, hyperbradykinism and beta-adrenergic vasodilation syndromes.	Hypotension, depression, congestive heart failure, bradycardia.
Pindolol (Viskin)	2.5–5.0 mg b.i.d. to t.i.d. Used in same situations as Propranolol.	Same as Propranolol.
Indomethacin (Indocin)	25–75 mg t.i.d. with meals; useful itself or combined with florinef for post-prandial hypotension.	Nausea, vomiting, gastric irritation, constipation, rash.
Ibuprofen (Motrin)	200–600 mg p.o. q.i.d. taken 30 min before each meal and hs.	Nausea, vomiting, gastric irritation, constipation, rash.
Caffeine	250 mg (2 cups) each morning. Used in ameliorating post-prandial hypotension.	Tachyphalaxis
Octreotide (Sandostatin)	25 mcg. sub q b.i.d. initially; up to 100–200 m.c. t.i.d. may be required. May be very useful in diabetic autonomic neuropathy with OH and diarrhea; very effective in prevention of postprandial hypotension.	Nausea, abdominal pain, muscle cramps injection site pain, fat malabsorption, hypertension.
Dihydroxyphenylserine (DOPS)	Only L-DOPS isomer biologically active 250–500 mg p.o. twice daily; mainly for Dopamine B-Hydroxylase syndrome.	Use is primarily for a rare disorder DBH deficiency.
Erythropoietin (epoetin alfa)	Rx. of anemia of autonomic failure; dose: 25–50 units/kg body wt. sub q 3x a week Fe supplementation often needed.	Expensive, parenteral medication; can cause supine hypertension.

vere cases, we begin with 0.1 mg once or twice daily, increasing as necessary up to 0.3 mg once or twice a day. In patients susceptible to fluid overload or recumbent hypertension, therapy can be initiated with a smaller dose, such as 0.05 mg once or twice daily, with careful observation of the clinical response. Standing time, body weight, supine BP, chest auscultation, and plasma potassium and magnesium should be monitored. One must try to avoid persistent supine BP above 200/110. Well-treated patients often have supine pressures in the range of 140 to 180/90 to 100.

A novel therapy that selectively increases intravascular volume has been published by several authors (8,20,29,33). Recombinant erythropoietin (epoetin alfa) has been used to successfully treat the mild anemia that is often seen in patients with autonomic failure. Both the hematocrit and the BP rise when this drug is given as 25 to 50 U/kg body weight subcutaneously three times a week. Maintenance doses given once weekly may be effective. Iron supplements are often needed when beginning the dosage. This drug's high cost, its availability only in parenteral form, and the fact that it exacerbates supine hypertension may limit its use to the hospital setting for patients with severe disease.

The earliest sympathomimetic drugs used included ephedrine, phenylephrine (13), and vasopressin. The latter was given by intramuscular injection or nasal inhalation of its lysine-S-vasopressin derivative. The combination of hydroxyamphetamine hydrobromide (Paredrine) and the monoamine oxidase (MAO) inhibitor tranylcypromine sulfate (Parnate) was introduced by Seller (38). Other sympathomimetics used with tranylcypromine included methylphenidate (Ritalin) and levodopa. Others advocated the use of cheese (containing the indirect-acting tyramine) plus an MAO inhibitor. Because of the erratic BP response and inherent danger of severe supine hypertension, we have avoided using most of these drugs in recently diagnosed patients. Ephedrine, 25 to 50 mg tid, may still be useful in mild cases. Nervousness, tachycardia, supine hypertension, and tachyphylaxis occur as side effects. A new agent, midodrine (see later), proved superior to ephedrine in a double-blind crossover study recently reported by Fouad-Tarazi and colleagues (15).

Biaggioni and associates (7) have demonstrated significant pressor effects using phenylpropanolamine (available without prescription), starting with doses of 12.5 mg tid. Doses two- to threefold higher may be necessary. Side effects are similar to those of ephedrine.

The investigational sympathomimetic drug midodrine, a direct-acting α-agonist, has the desirable characteristic of complete oral absorption but a half-life of only about 2 to 3 hrs (38,46). This drug causes vasoconstriction in arterioles and venous capacitance vessels without cardiac or central nervous system stimulation. Initial experience with midodrine has been encouraging, although not all patients respond. Recently reported multicenter trials (15,17,21,30) have confirmed its utility in neurogenic OH, and expedited FDA approval occurred September 6, 1996. The drug is widely available. Supine hypertension, piloerection, and scalp itching have been observed as side effects. Midodrine is started at a dose of 2.5 mg. Doses are given 4 hrs apart, 30–45 min. before meals, with a dose given just before meals. This regimen is usually ineffective, although some patients may respond to as little as 2.5 mg bid. We generally do not exceed 40 mg/day, often the first daily dose is the largest (i.e. 7.5–10.0 mg). The drug is safe and usually well tolerated. Worsening supine hypertension, weight loss, and urinary sodium loss may be predictors of a poor response to midodrine.

Dihydroergotamine (DHE 45) and ergotamine itself exhibit direct action on peripheral α-receptors and theoretically are useful. However, poor oral absorption makes the dose unpredictable from patient to patient. With DHE 45 it is best to start off with a low dose of 2.5 mg bid, increasing gradually to a maximum dose of 10 mg given bid to qid. Some patients may require a higher dose if oral absorption is very poor. Supine hypertension and signs of ergotamine excess may occur at the higher dosages. Biaggioni (9) has described the administration of ergotamine by inhalation, in which bioavailability was good and responses were dramatic. These drugs are not generally approved for the treatment of OH.

Clonidine, an α_2-agonist, is useful when OH is due to an efferent sympathetic lesion because its peripheral action on α_2-receptors (predominating in venous capacitance vessels) causes increases in BP. Patients who have non-neurogenic OH or OH due to an afferent lesion will likely become hypotensive with clonidine, so care is required when using this drug. Clonidine is usually given as 0.1 to 0.2 mg orally in the morning with a gradual increase in the dose to 0.2 to 0.8 mg bid. Drowsiness, dry mouth, constipation, supine hypertension, and hypotension may occur. Clonidine is of particular use when sympathetic failure causes both OH and diarrhea. Case Study 3 in the Appendix exemplifies this therapeutic situation.

Beta-blockers have been used recently in the treatment of orthostatic intolerance syndromes, especially florid postural tachycardia syndrome (24). They also have some role in the treatment of OH, particularly when the BP disturbance is due to hyperbradykininism (41) or the so-called hyperadrenergic state. The latter has been reported in diabetes and has been associated with mitral valve prolapse. It is occasionally seen in individuals who are otherwise normal. β-blockers may also be useful to treat severe supine hypertension. β-blocker use in peripheral autonomic neuropathies or efferent sympathetic lesions, such as occur in the primary OH syndromes, is more controversial. Pindolol and xamoterol, β-blockers with some intrinsic sympathomimetic activity, may be a better choice than propranolol, which has more undesirable myocardial depressant effects. Propranolol can be tried with a dose of 10 mg qid with a gradual increase, if tolerated, up to 40 mg qid. Pindolol is given at a dose of 2.5 to 5 mg bid to tid, and xamoterol is given at a dose of 200 mg bid. In addition to hypotension, these drugs may cause depression and congestive heart failure.

Tranylcypromine (Parnate) is an MAO inhibitor that has been used in combination with Ritalin, tyramine, and other sympathomimetics to raise the BP in OH. Most authors use this therapy as a last resort because the combination of the two drugs may lead to severe hypertensive crises and because tyramine is not readily available in a preparation for oral administration. Eating foods rich in tyramine content is too unreliable with respect to the dose of drug delivered to advocate it strongly in treatment. The use of prostaglandin inhibitors (indomethacin 25 to 50 mg tid with meals or ibuprofen 400 to 600 mg bid to qid with meals) has some support in the literature, particularly in the treatment of postprandial exacerbation of OH. This interesting phenomenon is illustrated by Case Study 1 in the Appendix. Uncommonly, gastrointestinal ulceration or interstitial nephritis occurs with these drugs. Their effectiveness in

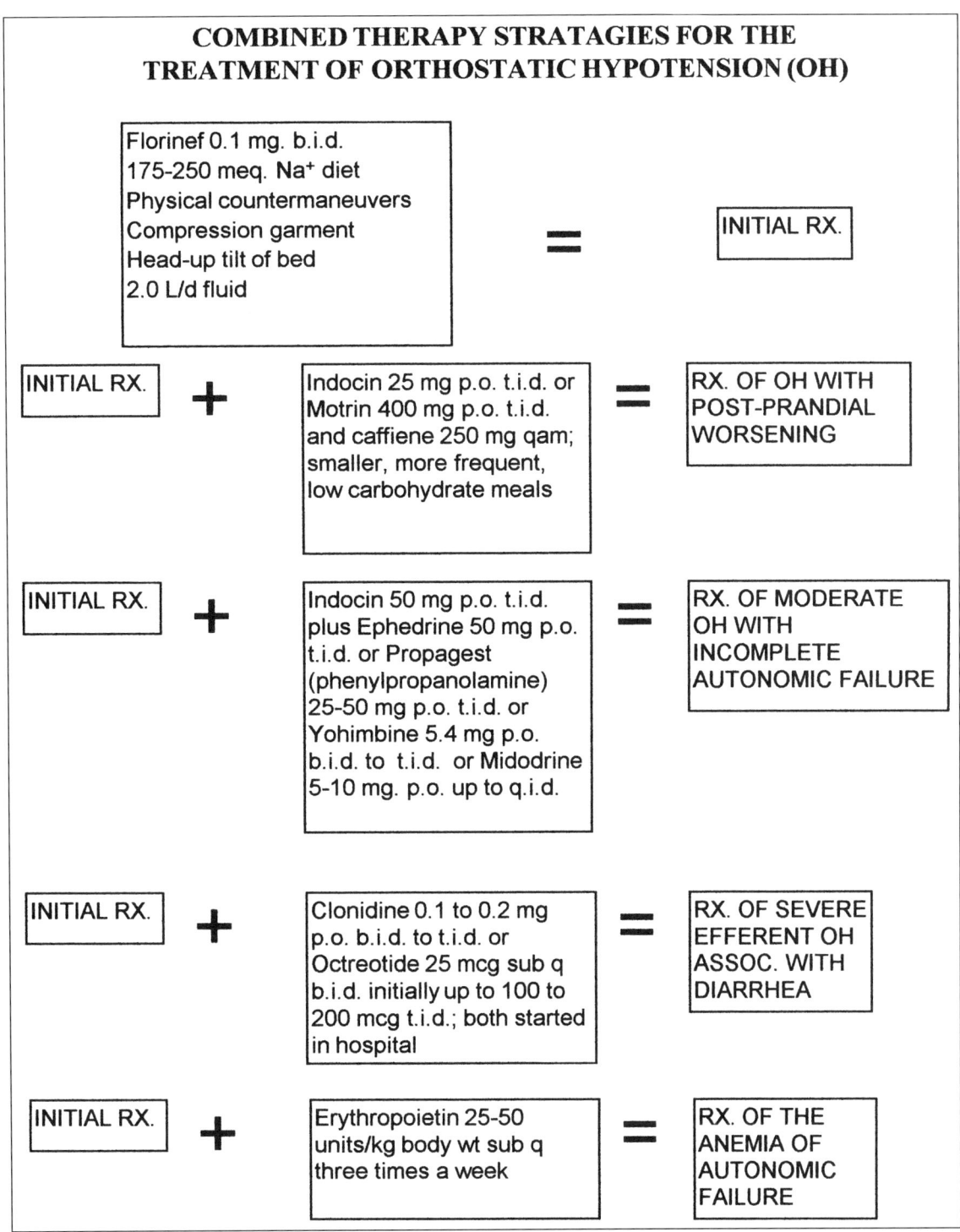

FIG. 2. Combined-therapy strategies for the treatment of orthostatic hypotension (OH). (RX = treatment; S = seconds; sub q = subcutaneously.

preventing postprandial hypotension can be monitored in the hospital setting with supine BPs obtained at 10-min intervals just before meals and up to 2 hours postprandially. Two cups of coffee each morning, or 250 mg of caffeine, has been reported to be helpful with postprandial hypotension. The caffeine is given no more than once a day to prevent tachyphylaxis (28).

Metoclopramide (Reglan) is useful in the treatment of OH in the uncommon and specific situation in which patients are found to have excessive supine and upright serum dopamine levels (14,23). Another use of the drug is for patients with dysautonomia of the upper gastrointestinal tract characterized by hypomotility, nausea, and anorexia. The dose is 5 to 10 mg given just before meals tid to qid. Because dyskinesias and an extrapyramidal syndrome may occur as side effects of the drug, it should be used quite cautiously in patients with OH due to multiple system atrophy; cisapride 10 to 20 mg qid should be considered instead. Before using the prokinetic drugs, the upper gastrointestinal tract should be visualized to rule out obstruction. Ideally, a gastroduodenal motility study should be performed, with documentation of antral hypomotility and abnormalities of interdigestive and postprandial motor activity. Case Study 3 exemplifies the use of Reglan.

The extrapyramidal symptoms of multiple system atrophy (MSA) (43) can be treated with levodopa, the combination of carbidopa and levodopa (Sinemet), or low doses of the dopamine agonists pergolide or bromocriptine. The response to these drugs is often poor (44), and at the highest doses exacerbation of OH often occurs. The role of stereotactic pallidotomy is not established in MSA. Anecdotal experience in two patients with severe rigidity that improved after the procedure and the occasional response reported in the neurosurgical literature may justify its consideration in young patients with MSA.

Our approach in the treatment of symptomatic and moderate to severe OH due to a neurogenic cause is to first try the head-up position of the bed, a liberal dietary salt (≥175 mEq), and 2.0 L/day fluid intake, along with the elasticized abdominal binder or leotard and fludrocortisone (Florinef) 0.2 mg every morning. If the patient has not had a history of gastrointestinal ulceration or bleeding and still has significant postural hypotension, particularly postprandial, ibuprofen or indomethacin is added for a 1-week trial. If control is still inadequate, indomethacin is stopped and we then add one of the sympathomimetic drugs, often starting with ephedrine or phenylpropanolamine hydrochloride (Propagest), 25 to 50 mg, given 45 minutes before meals or scheduled upright activities. Midodrine (now approved and available for use) is begun as 5 mg po tid about 1 hour before meals; the first two doses are then often titrated upward to 10 mg and 7.5 mg, respectively. Yohimbine 5.4 mg tid is used primarily in the early stages of the degenerative disorders (9).

If the patient is still symptomatic from OH, an attempt is made to further expand the blood volume by adding more dietary salt, increasing Florinef, and initiating erythropoietin injections for a 3- or 4-week period.

If the patient has fluid loss due to dysautonomic diarrhea and severe postganglionic sympathetic failure, we cautiously try clonidine and octreotide, beginning usually in the hospital setting where BP can be monitored. These combination treatment schemes are summarized in Fig. 2.

Treatment of Supine Hypertension

Not infrequently, severe dysautonomia with profound standing hypotension is complicated by a worrisome degree of supine hypertension. The hypertension typically produces sustained BPs in the range of 200/120. It rarely produces catastrophic cerebral hemorrhage or myocardial strain with left ventricular hypertrophy. It is necessary to treat this supine hypertension in some patients, particularly those who have lost their baroreceptor buffering capacity secondary to their disease and need to be on large doses of pressor medications and Florinef. One approach involves the use of short-acting antihypertensive drugs at bedtime, such as Apresoline 25 mg or Procardia 10 mg. The former, with its sodium-retaining properties, may be particularly useful in patients with excessive nocturnal sodium loss during recumbency (1). Patients who have lost their ambulatory status as a result of a somatic neurologic deficit are best managed by reducing or stopping pressor drugs, as long as an adequate supine and sitting BP is maintained. Patients with supine hypertension can develop left ventricular hypertrophy; an echocardiogram performed yearly can monitor this potential complication.

It is worth re-emphasizing that patients with neurogenic OH often have a concomitant, non-neurogenic contribution (i.e., volume depletion from vomiting or poor fluid intake) to their postural BP disturbance. Treatment of volume depletion with intravenous saline infusion and increased dietary salt and water intake will often lead to a marked improvement in BP management. Sepsis from a pulmonary or urologic infection is occasionally a cause of rapid deterioration in BP control; this must be identified and treated promptly to avoid a fatal outcome.

Most of the treatment measures discussed here provide symptomatic improvement rather than a reversal of the underlying disorder causing the OH (40). Much work needs to be done to elucidate the underlying mechanisms of neuronal loss, including the susceptibility and identification of additional neurotransmitter/receptor systems that are abnormal and potentially amenable to specific replacement therapy. Nevertheless, it is essential to pursue treatment because there is often a marked improvement in the quality of life of both the patient and caregiver with even a modest improvement in standing BP and standing time.

Appendix

CASE STUDY 1. MULTIPLE SYSTEM ATROPHY WITH POSTPRANDIAL HYPOTENSION

History

In 1964, this 62-year-old woman with multiple system atrophy underwent a left thalamotomy for an action tremor in the right upper extremity, with subsequent improvement. During the 1960s and 1970s, a parkinsonian syndrome gradually developed with bradykinesia, loss of associated movements, hypokinetic speech, micrographia, and so on. During 1978 and 1979, she began to be plagued by syncopal episodes that were almost exclusively associated with hypotension in the immediate postprandial state (onset 15 to 20 min after the start of the meal, lasting 15 to 20 min). At these times, her sitting systolic BPs were below 60 mmHg, and standing postural faints were also occurring. Decreased sweating and urinary urgency, incontinence, frequency of urination, and supine hypertension were noted. Treatment with fludrocortisone (Florinef), salt tablets, carbidopa/levodopa (Sinemet), and bromocriptine mesylate (Parlodel) somewhat helped her mobility but did not affect her syncope.

The neurologic examination revealed marked OH with a supine BP of 220/110 mmHg, falling to 110/80 mmHg at 2 min of quiet standing, and falling further to 90/60 mmHg after moderate exercise. Corresponding pulse rates were 75 bpm supine and 98 bpm after exercise. There were moderate to marked extrapyramidal features, some hyperreflexia, a positive Babinski sign, upper motor neuron type weakness (particularly on the left side), and some decreased coordination of the hands and feet. Sensation was largely normal except for difficulty with traced figure recognition in the left hand. Her mentation was intact except for some impairment of retentive memory.

In the hospital, the patient underwent frequent BP monitoring. Her levels decreased from about 200/110 to 90/50 mmHg. All measurements were taken in the supine position, beginning 15 min after meal ingestion and lasting for approximately 2 hrs. These decreases were most apparent with breakfast and lunch and less so in the evening. Standing BPs were almost unobtainable during the postprandial period of hypotension but otherwise ranged from 70/40 to 120/80 mmHg (average, 90/70 mmHg) between meals. Indomethacin treatment was begun, and the dosage was rapidly increased from 25 to 75 mg tid taken with meals. Parlodel therapy was discontinued, and the patient was placed on an anticholinergic, ethopropazine hydrochloride (Parsidol), 50 mg bid. The patient was fitted for a Jobst leotard.

On this regimen, her nonpostprandial BPs ranged from 160/100 to 220/130 mmHg supine and 100/60 to 140/100 mmHg standing. Typical post-treatment postprandial supine BP reductions were 170/110 down to 110/60 mmHg and 200/100 down to 120/80 mmHg. Her other medications included Sinemet (carbidopa/levodopa, 25/100 mg, 1 tablet qid) and Florinef (0.1 mg in the morning and 0.05 mg at noon). The patient was on a sodium diet of 175 mEq/day. Subjectively, the patient felt mildly improved, particularly postprandially.

Laboratory Studies

A chest x-ray study showed a mild cardiomegaly. Plasma norepinephrine levels were 237 pg/ml supine and 333 pg/ml after standing for 10 minutes. A thermoregulatory sweat test showed absent sweating over most of her body surface. The quantitative sudomotor axon reflex test yielded normal results in the forearm and a normal volume but relatively reduced response in the foot.

Follow-Up

The patient continued to respond to antihypotensive treatment for an additional year; she then became progressively bedridden and died of her illness 4 years later.

CASE STUDY 2. ORTHOSTATIC HYPOTENSION DUE TO A POSTERIOR FOSSA TUMOR

This patient was admitted to our hospital on May 5, 1975, after an 8-month history of orthostatic dizziness and episodic syncope associated with progressive gait ataxia.

History

In October 1974, the patient's gait had become shuffling and he had difficulty climbing stairs. He then suffered orthostatic lightheadedness that abated when he lay down. From November 1974 to February 1975, the orthostatic lightheadedness became more frequent and was accompanied by a staggering gait. By March 1975, he suffered almost constant orthostatic dizziness, marked gait ataxia, decreased sweating, slurred speech, headaches, and nausea. Neurologic examination revealed truncal ataxia, a progressive fall in BP while standing in place (decreasing from 160/96 mmHg supine to 80/58 mmHg at 10 minutes upright), and no change in his pulse rate of 88 bpm. His strength and deep tendon reflexes were normal. There was slight left-sided limb ataxia and mild distal sensory loss in the lower extremities.

Laboratory Studies

Initial laboratory evaluation included a tilt-table study, which reproduced the BP findings already mentioned, as well as a thermoregulatory sweat test that showed absent sweating over the entire body. Three days after admission, the patient became confused and somnolent and developed hiccups. An MRI (magnetic resonance imaging) scan showed a 4 × 4 cm mass in the left posterior fossa with dilatation of the lateral and third ventricles.

Treatment

On May 12, 1975, a large posterior fossa meningioma was removed through suboccipital craniectomy. On May 23, 1975, the patient was discharged from the hospital in an improved condition. In November 1975, the patient's balance was near normal, postural hypotension was absent, and the thermoregulatory sweat test showed normal total body sweating. In May 1977, the patient continued to do well with no signs of autonomic dysfunction.

CASE STUDY 3. IDIOPATHIC AUTONOMIC NEUROPATHY: MANAGEMENT OF SEVERE OH AND NEUROGENIC DIARRHEA

This patient was a 69-year-old woman who was admitted to our hospital on July 27, 1987, in a markedly debilitated state due to intractable diarrhea and marked OH with syncope when in the sitting position.

History

The patient had been well until April 1987, when she suffered an upper respiratory illness. She experienced some improvement after antibiotic therapy; however, crampy abdominal pain, loose stools, nausea, anorexia, fecal incontinence, and generalized malaise developed, and this prompted an extensive gastrointestinal evaluation that revealed essentially normal findings. There was no evidence of malabsorption or inflammatory or infectious bowel disease. Profound postural hypotension was noted, and treatment consisted of elastic stockings, Florinef, hydration, and steroids. Antidiarrheal drugs were not effective. Syncope in the sitting position, continued diarrhea, and mild congestive heart failure developed, and the patient was transferred to our hospital.

Initial examination showed an undernourished and debilitated woman who was incontinent of stool and unable to sit up for more than 20 seconds because of profound hypotension. There was mild, diffuse weakness with no atrophy. Her deep tendon reflexes were normal to slightly brisk. There was a decrease in pinprick and vibratory sensations in the feet, a mild essential tremor of the hands, and some masking of the face. Supine BP was 90/60 mmHg, and her pulse was 100 bpm; BP could not be obtained at 20 seconds of sitting. General examination revealed no specific abnormalities, and findings from the cardiac examination were considered to be within normal limits. Bowel sounds were somewhat hyperactive.

Hospital Course

The patient was hydrated and begun on parenteral nutrition. A battery of autonomic tests showed a primarily sympathetic autonomic failure. Radiographic studies of the intestine were normal and a small-bowel biopsy specimen was histologically normal, but interdigestive and postprandial upper gastrointestinal motility were markedly abnormal. General medical tests yielded essentially normal findings, except for mild anemia, hyponatremia, and hypokalemia. A feeding gastrojejunal tube was placed in August 1987; however, nausea, intestinal cramping, and diarrhea developed during tube feedings. Therefore, the patient was given loperamide hydrochloride (Imodium) tid to qid. This was unhelpful, so clonidine was started. Her diarrhea was controlled with 0.1 to 0.3 mg of clonidine tid. Metoclopramide (Reglan, 10 mg po qid) relieved the patient's nausea and did not worsen the diarrhea. Conventional treatment with Florinef, a prostaglandin inhibitor, hyperalimentation, and rehydration failed to prevent syncope while sitting, so treatment with the investigational drug midodrine was begun. The patient's sitting blood pressure became audible and was consistently above 90/50 mmHg. She was able to sit in a chair for several hours and to stand briefly. She was discharged from the hospital on September 24, 1987.

In October 1987 the patient was free of diarrhea and suffered mild constipation. She could walk for short distances and could sit for 1 hour at a time but could not stand in place. Her blood pressure was 150 to 160/90 mmHg supine, 130/70 mmHg sitting for 1 minute, and 55 mmHg systolic after standing for 1 minute, when she would also experience lightheadedness. Her mild muscle weakness was somewhat improved, and deep tendon reflexes were normal. There were minimal extrapyramidal features and an essential tremor. Treatment with Florinef (0.2 mg bid), clonidine (0.3 mg tid), potassium chloride (20 mEq bid), midodrine (7.5 mg qid), and Reglan (10 mg po qid) was continued. Gastrojejunal tube feedings were well tolerated, and the patient continued to gain weight. She was advised to wear an elastic support body stocking and to keep the head of her bed at home elevated to about a 30° to 45° angle. She was also instructed to drink fluids and to use salt on whatever she could take by mouth.

REFERENCES

1. Bachman DM, Youmans WB. Effects of posture on renal excretion of sodium and chloride in orthostatic hypotension. *Circulation* 1953;7: 413–421.
2. Bannister R, Schatz I. (co-chairs). Consensus statement on the definition of orthostatic hypotension, pure autonomic failure and multiple system atrophy. *Clin Auton Res* 1996;6:125–126.
3. Bannister R. Treatment of progressive autonomic failure. In: Bannister R (ed). *Autonomic Failure: A Textbook of Clinical Disorders of the Autonomic Nervous System*. New York, London: Oxford University Press. 1983;323.
4. Bannister R, et al. An assessment of various methods of treatment in idiopathic orthostatic hypotension. *Q J Med* 1969;38: 377–395.
5. Bannister R, et al. Cardiovascular reflexes and biochemical responses in progressive autonomic failure. *Brain* 1977;100: 327–344.
6. Biaggioni I, et al. Dopamine-beta-hydroxylase deficiency and dopamine. *N Engl J Med* 1987;314:1415–1416.
7. Biaggioni I et al. The potent pressor effect of phenylpropanolamine in patients with autonomic impairment. *JAMA* 1987;258:236–239.
8. Biaggioni I, et al. The anemia of primary autonomic failure and its reversal with recombinant erythropoietin. *Ann Intern Med* 1994;121: 181–186.

9. Biaggioni I, et al. Manipulation of norepinephrine metabolism with yohimbine in the treatment of autonomic failure (review). *J Clin Pharmacol* 1994;34(5):418–423.
10. Camilleri M et al. Gastrointestinal motility disturbances in patients with orthostatic hypotension. *Gastroenterology* 1985;88:1852–1859.
11. Chobanian AV et al. Use of propranolol in the treatment of idiopathic orthostatic hypotension. *Trans Assoc Am Physicians* 1977;90:324–334.
12. Chobanian AV et al. Mineralocorticoid-induced hypertension in patients with orthostatic hypotension. *N Engl J Med* 1979;301:68.
13. Davies B, et al. Pressor amines and monoamine oxidase inhibitors for treatment of postural hypotension in autonomic failure: limitations and hazards. *Lancet* 1978;1:172–175.
14. de Caestecker JS et al. Evaluation of oral cisapride and metoclopramide in diabetic autonomic neuropathy: an eight week double-blind crossover study. *Aliment Pharmacol Ther* 1989;3:69–81.
15. Fouad-Tarazi FM, et al. Alpha sympathomimetic treatment of autonomic insufficiency with orthostatic hypotension. *Am J Med* 1995; 99(6):604–610.
16. Galaso PJ, et al. Propafenone-induced peripheral neuropathy. *Mayo Clin Proc* 1995;70(5):469–472.
17. Gilden JL. Midodrine in neurogenic orthostatic hypotension. A new treatment. *Int Angiol* 1993;12(2):125–131.
18. Hickler RB et al. Successful treatment of orthostatic hypotension with 9-alpha-fluorohydrocortisone. *N Engl J Med* 1959;261:788.
19. Hirayama M, et al. Treatment of postprandial hypotension with selective alpha 1 and beta 1 adrenergic agonists *J Auton Nerv Syst* 1993; 45(2):149–154.
20. Hoeldtke RD, Streeten DH. Treatment of orthostatic hypotension with erythropoietin. *N Engl J Med* 1993;329(9):611–615.
21. Jankovic J, et al. Neurogenic orthostatic hypotension: a double-blind, placebo controlled study with midodrine. *Am J Med* 1993; 95(1):38–48.
22. Kochar MS, et al. Treatment of orthostatic hypotension with indomethacin. *Am Heart J* 1979;98:271–280.
23. Lopes de Faria et al. Peripheral dopaminergic blockade for the treatment of diabetic orthostatic hypotension. *Clin Pharmacol Ther* 1988; 44:670–674.
24. Low PA, et al. Comparison of the postural tachycardia syndrome (POTS) with orthostatic hypotension due to autonomic failure. *J Auton Nerv Syst* 1994;50(2):181–188.
25. MacLean AR, Allen EV. Orthostatic hypotension and orthostatic tachycardia: treatment with the "head-up" bed. *JAMA* 1940;115:2162.
26. Man in't Veld AJ et al. Congenital dopamine-beta-hydroxylase deficiency. A novel orthostatic syndrome. *Lancet* 1976;1:183–187.
27. Mathias CJ et al. Cardiovascular biochemical and hormonal changes during food-induced hypotension in chronic autonomic failure. *J Neurol Sci* 1989;94:255–269.
28. Onrot J et al. Hemodynamic and humoral effects of caffeine in human autonomic failure. *N Engl J Med* 1985;313:549–554.
29. Perara R, et al. Effect of recombinant erythropoietin on anemia and orthostatic hypotension in primary autonomic failure. *Clin Auton Res* 1995;5(4):211–213.
30. Puchmayer V, et al. Midodrine, a new therapeutic agent: recent experience. *Int Angiol* 1993;12(2):113–118.
31. Roberts LJ, Oates JA. Mastocytosis. In: Wilson JD, Foster DW (eds). *Williams Textbook of Endocrinology.* Philadelphia: WB Saunders. 1985;1363–1379.
32. Robertson D, et al. Classification of autonomic disorders. *Int Angiol* 1993;12(2):93–102.
33. Robertson D, Davis TL. Recent advances in the treatment of orthostatic hypotension. *Neurology* 1995;45(suppl 5):526–532.
34. Robertson D. Orthostatic hypotension in clinical pharmacology. In: Melmon KL et al (eds). *Melmon and Morrelli's Clinical Pharmacology, 3rd ed.* New York: Pergamon Press. 1991.
35. Robertson D, et al. Postprandial alterations in cardiovascular hemodynamics in autonomic dysfunctional states. *Am J Cardiol* 1981; 48:1048–1052.
36. Robertson D et al. Isolated failure of autonomic noradrenergic neurotransmission: evidence for impaired beta-hydroxylation of dopamine. *N Engl J Med* 1986;314:1494–1497.
37. Schatz J. Orthostatic hypotension: II. Clinical diagnosis and treatment. *Arch Intern Med* 1984;144:1037.
38. Schirger A et al. Midodrine: a new agent in the management of idiopathic orthostatic hypotension and Shy-Drager syndrome. *Mayo Clin Proc* 1981;56:429–433.
39. Sheps SG. Use of an elastic garment in the treatment of orthostatic hypotension. *Cardiology* 1976;61(suppl 1):271–279.
40. Stumpf JL, Mitrzyk B. *Am J Hosp Pharm* 1994;51(5):648–660; quiz 697–698.
41. Streeten DHP et al. Hyperbradykininism: a new orthostatic syndrome. *Lancet* 1972;2:1048–1053.
42. Tarazi RC, Fouad FM. Circulatory dynamics in progressive autonomic failure. In: Bannister R (ed). *Autonomic Failure: A Textbook of Clinical Disorders of the Autonomic Nervous System.* New York, Oxford: Oxford University Press. 1983;97.
43. Thomas JE, Schirger A. Idiopathic orthostatic hypotension: a study of its natural history in 57 neurologically affected patients. *Arch Neurol* 1970;22:289–293.
44. Thomas JE et al. Orthostatic hypotension. *Mayo Clin Proc* 1981;56: 117–125.
45. Wieling W, van Lieshout JJ. Investigation and treatment of autonomic circulatory failure (review). *Curr Opin Neurol Neurosurg* 1993;6(4): 537–543.
46. Zacharia PK et al. Pharmacodynamics of midodrine, an antihypotensive agent. *Clin Pharmacol Ther* 1986;39(5):586–591.

CHAPTER 56

Syndromes of Autonomic Overactivity

Jan Fagius

1. Temporary overactivity of the autonomic nervous system, with a risk of circulatory arrest and sudden death, may arise in a number of acute diseases of the nervous system, such as the Guillain-Barré syndrome, porphyric neuropathy, and tetanus.
2. Sympathetic hyperactivity, with accompanying spells of tachycardia and hypertension, may predominate or alternate with episodes of bradycardia, hypotension, and asystole, probably stemming from vagal hyperactivity.
3. One proven underlying mechanism is acute baroreceptor deafferentation, but parts of the pathophysiology remain obscure.
4. Detailed monitoring of heart rate (HR) and blood pressure (BP) is compulsory in the assessment of these patients, who usually need to be cared for in an intensive care unit.
5. Pharmacologic blocking of the effects of sympathetic and parasympathetic activity may be helpful, as may the use of a temporary pacemaker, to avoid sudden cardiac death.

INTRODUCTION

When autonomic dysfunction occurs, irrespective of its origin, the main outcome tends to be reduced function, with defective maintenance of postural blood pressure as a major cardiovascular consequence. One important and impressive exception to this rule is the massive sympathoadrenergic discharge that accompanies an acute increase in intracranial pressure (which is further dealt with in Chapter 57). However, there are other clinical situations in which cardiovascular symptoms and signs suggest unimpeded activity in the sympathetic and parasympathetic nervous systems. Such a disorder may be an uncommon feature of a few relatively rare diseases. Nevertheless, it is very important to detect and manage the disorder because it carries a high risk for cardiovascular collapse and may have a fatal outcome. The diseases listed in Table 1 may give rise to clinical cardiovascular states that are known or suspected to stem from autonomic overactivity.

All of the diseases listed in Table 1 are serious ones that compel the patient to seek medical attention because of the pronounced acute disability; many patients are managed in an intensive care unit, irrespective of the occurrence of a severe autonomic disturbance. On the other hand, in Guillain-Barré syndrome (GBS) there may be a striking lack of correlation between the severity of the disease and the sudden development of pronounced hypertension and tachycardia, with their accompanying risk of sudden death. The clinician must be aware of this risk and must monitor the patient appropriately.

CLINICAL PICTURE

Acute Inflammatory Polyneuropathy— the Guillain-Barré Syndrome

Guillain-Barré syndrome (GBS) is an acute, immunologically mediated disease characterized by flaccid paralysis that develops over the course of days or a couple of weeks. The paralysis may progress to total tetraparesis with respiratory failure and involvement of cranial nerves (2). As described in Chapter 36 and detailed in a 1994 review by Zochodne (77), overt involvement of autonomic function is relatively common in GBS, and, with the help of autonomic tests, some degree of dysfunction can be detected in most cases. Usually the autonomic involvement

---

J. Fagius: Department of Neurology, University Hospital S-751 85 Uppsala, Sweden.

The author's quoted research is supported by The Swedish Medical Research Council, grant no. 10839.

TABLE 1. *Diseases giving rise to clinical states consistent with autonomic overactivity*

CNS damage
   Subarachnoid hemorrhage, intracerebral hemorrhage, closed head injury
   Acute upper spinal cord compression/injury
   Chronic upper spinal cord injury: autonomic dysreflexia
Acute inflammatory polyneuropathy (Guillain-Barré syndrome, GBS)
Porphyric neuropathy
Diphtheria (?)
Thallium intoxication
Tetanus
Neuroleptic malignant syndrome
Malignant hyperthermia
Poliomyelitis (?)
Delirium tremens

Question mark indicates that autonomic overactivity is not established.
The acute CNS disorders are described in Chapter 59. The spinal cord disorders are described in Chapter 36.

means reduced function, but in some instances this autonomic dysfunction can include signs of overactivity.

Cardiovascular instability, with spells of pronounced hypertension and simultaneous marked resting tachycardia, was described by Lampen (41) in 1949 as a feature of acute polyneuritis. In the survey by Haymaker and Kernohan (34), 11 of 50 deaths were associated with acute hypertension and tachycardia. In a subsequent study of 35 cases by Marshall (49), fluctuating hypertension was noted as a prominent feature of the disease in some cases. Eiben and Gersony (17) reported that hypertension occurred during the course of the illness in 29 of 48 cases, including both children and adults. In a review by Goulon and colleagues (28) of 172 GBS cases, 28 patients were reported to display particularly severe autonomic symptoms, including symptoms suggestive of autonomic overactivity. Andersson and Sidén (1), in a survey of 60 consecutive patients with GBS, reported 4 deaths attributable to cardiac or thromboembolic events, and they described an additional 5 patients who displayed nonfatal cardiac tachy- or bradyarrhythmia.

The multifaceted, clinically overt cardiovascular expressions of GBS, including those in which parts of the autonomic nervous system are seemingly overactive, were described in detail in a number of papers published during the 1970s (6,14,28,45). Elevation of BP and HR may appear within a few days of the onset of the disease. Blood pressure may become extremely high, with readings possibly exceeding 300/150 mmHg, and the simultaneous resting HR may reach 150 beats/min (bpm) or more in adults. Hypertension may persist for days or, in some instances, weeks. Rapidly fluctuating blood pressure and heart rate (Fig. 1) are also often noted, with spells of hypertension alternating with recumbent hypotension and a postural blood pressure that decreases with head-up tilt. As illustrated in Figure 1, this situation carries a definite risk of circulatory collapse and sudden death (6,45). Some patients exhibit profuse paroxysmal generalized perspiration of 10 to 15 min duration, with signs of peripheral cutaneous vasoconstriction. These may occur with or without pronounced hypertension and tachycardia. In a few instances, such attacks have immediately preceded sudden death (6,45).

The hyperadrenergic cardiovascular state should carry a risk for ventricular fibrillation, but it is not clear from the literature whether the most common cause of circulatory failure after marked tachycardia and hypertension is ventricular fibrillation or sudden cardiac arrest. Conversely, spells of bradycardia can arise that may or may not be followed by asystole, and such events may be fatal. Bradycardia episodes can be precipitated by sudden changes in the patient's body position during nursing or by tracheal suction (6,28), and these can persist for up to half an hour. Prophylactic atropine treatment does not reliably prevent subsequent attacks (28).

Profuse paroxysmal sweating can also occur without being directly related to sudden death, as already described (6,14,28,45). Hypersalivation and bronchial hypersecretion are noted occasionally (28). Goulon and associates (28) emphasized that the combination of symptoms may be very complex. This is illustrated by a patient who exhibited arterial hypertension, tachycardia (but with cardiac arrest upon ocular bulb compression), profuse sweating and salivation, urinary retention, and paralytic ileus (28).

The duration of the cardiovascular instability varies considerably from a few days to several weeks, but more than 3 weeks appears to be uncommon. Lichtenfeld (45) reported a mean duration of 7 days with a range of 2 to 21 days.

There is no consistent correlation between the severity of peripheral paresis in GBS and the risk of acute hyperten-

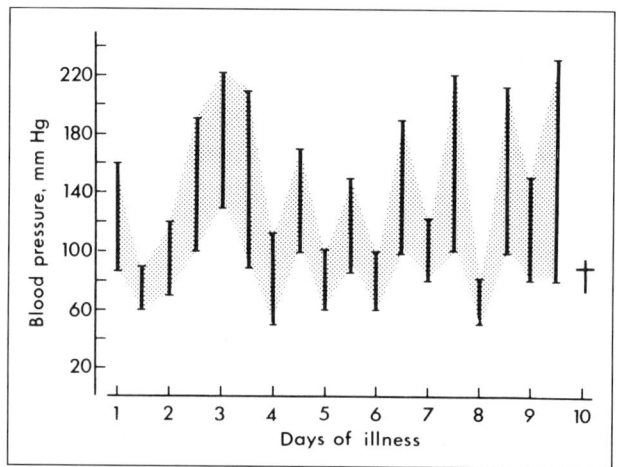

FIG. 1. Blood pressure recordings from a 34-year-old woman with acute Guillain-Barré syndrome. She was normotensive before onset of the acute disease. Progression of peripheral paresis ceased on day 6 and she died suddenly on day 10. (Redrawn with permission from Lichtenfeld P. Autonomic dysfunction in the Guillain-Barré syndrome. *Am J Med* 1971; 50: 772–780.)

sion and cardiac dysrhythmias, with the latter possibly occurring in an otherwise minimally disabled patient (45). Statistically, severely ill patients are at higher risk, and patients requiring artificial respiration are the most prone to suffer from autonomic overactivity (11,14). Even in these patients, the autonomic symptoms usually precede respiratory failure (6).

Disordered autonomic function, resulting in the cardiovascular symptoms described, probably is the most common cause of death in patients with GBS, at a time when modern intensive care techniques can manage even longstanding respiratory failure. In Lichtenfeld's series (45) of 28 patients, 6 died, 4 of them from circulatory arrest (45). Bredin (6) reported 5 deaths among 24 cases, 2 of which were undoubtedly attributable to autonomic dysfunction; none were due to respiratory failure.

Porphyric Neuropathy

The acute hepatic porphyrias (acute intermittent porphyria, variegate porphyria, and hereditary coproporphyria) produce episodes of acute, widespread polyneuropathy that may be indistinguishable from GBS but that are usually characterized by involvement of proximal nerves, including cranial nerves (62). Acute hypertension with concomitant tachycardia is characteristic of this uncommon disease (3,40,41,63). Tachycardia is reported to be a consistent finding in porphyric neuropathy (63), and hypertension has been observed in more than 50% of patients with acute intermittent porphyria (3). Blood pressures of 180/135 mmHg and heart rates approaching 140 bpm during supine rest have also been reported. In 1954, Kezdi (40) had already labeled this hypertension *neurogenic*. The severity of the autonomic disorder seems to follow the degree of peripheral polyneuropathy more closely than that reported for GBS, but detailed reports on this relationship are scanty.

Diphtheria and Thallium Intoxication

There are occasional anecdotal reports of acute hypertension and tachycardia that accompany diphtheritic polyneuropathy, which is now a very rare disease (41). This is mentioned here because diphtheria involves predominantly cranial nerves and thus may share a common pathophysiologic mechanism with GBS and the porphyrias (this will be discussed later). The same is true for the polyneuropathy induced by thallium intoxication, which may include cranial nerve palsies and hypertension with tachycardia, the latter two symptoms being of moderate degree (5,41, 52,53).

Tetanus

Extreme and fluctuating hypertension and tachycardia (in the absence of secondary infection and pyrexia), with a high systemic vascular resistance, are well-known characteristics of severe tetanus (12,16,39,46,47,75). Profuse sweating and marked peripheral cutaneous vasoconstriction, with icy cold extremities, are other features indicative of sympathetic overactivity (39,46,75). Cardiac arrest has occurred when a patient was turned during nursing (39), and it has also occurred during tracheal suction. In the latter case, the patient had been treated with a low dose of the nonselective β-blocking agent propranolol to control tachycardia (16).

Increased salivation and bronchial secretion are also common (75). Thus, there may be symptoms that suggest both sympathetic and parasympathetic overactivity, as described for GBS. Long-standing and sometimes refractory hypotension, without signs of shock, may also develop (9).

The autonomic disorder constitutes a major threat to the patient's life in severe tetanus (75).

Neuroleptic Malignant Syndrome and Malignant Hyperthermia

Neuroleptic malignant syndrome is a rare, occasionally fatal disorder due to an adverse reaction to antipsychotic therapy with major tranquilizers (especially butyrophenones, but any neuroleptic may induce the state). Hyperpyrexia and muscular rigidity are the main features. Abrupt discontinuation of antiparkinsonian drugs may also evoke the reaction, which is generally considered to be due to central dopamine blockade or depletion (15,33).

Clinical signs suggesting autonomic overactivity are common in the neuroleptic malignant syndrome and may precede the onset of hyperthermia, thereby possibly acting as warning signals. These symptoms include skin pallor, sweating, moderately increased and labile blood pressure, and tachycardia. If untreated, the condition carries a mortality risk of 20% to 30%. The major causes of death are reported to be respiratory failure and cardiovascular collapse (33).

Neuroleptic malignant syndrome has some features in common with malignant hyperthermia, a genetic disorder with subclinical myopathy that gives rise to acute, vigorous muscular rigidity and extreme hyperpyrexia on exposure to certain muscle relaxants and inhalation anesthetics (13). The fulminant syndrome also comprises hypertension, tachycardia, and cardiac arrhythmias, including ventricular tachycardia and fibrillation (13).

Poliomyelitis

Relatively mild hypertension, usually lasting for a few days but sometimes persisting for months, was noted during the acute stage of poliomyelitis in almost half of a prospectively studied group of patients (51). Hypertension was most pronounced and of longest duration in patients who needed artificial respiration; the average blood pressure in this subgroup was 164/104 mmHg, and the maximum blood pressure cited in this report was 235/110 mmHg. A close relationship between respiratory insufficiency and episodes of hypertension has also been reported (73).

Transient hypertension was reported to be a frequent feature of bulbar poliomyelitis in children (51 out of 70 cases), with a lower incidence of elevated blood pressure in cases of spinal poliomyelitis and an even lower, but still not negligible (14 of 36 patients), incidence in nonparalytic poliomyelitis (30). Tachycardia coinciding with increased SGP has not been reported in the context of poliomyelitis.

No reports on the cardiovascular manifestations of poliomyelitis have appeared since the 1950s. This must be ascribed to the successful vaccination programs undertaken in the industrialized parts of the world, which have effectively made poliomyelitis a rare disease.

Autonomic Dysreflexia in Chronic Upper Spinal Cord Lesion

Autonomic dysreflexia, first recognized in the 1910s (35), is a clinical problem encountered in patients with a complete or nearly complete spinal cord lesion above T5 (31,50). When such a patient is exposed to manipulation of the urinary bladder or the bowel or to noxious stimulation below the lesion, a reaction may occur, consisting of spells of hypertension (sometimes to extreme levels, with a risk of intracranial hemorrhage), headache, bradycardia, skin vasodilation above the lesion, diaphoresis above the lesion, and piloerection. (See Chapters 32 and 35.)

Alcohol Withdrawal and Delirium Tremens

Some of the well-known symptoms that occur in alcoholics upon withdrawal after prolonged alcohol abuse are consistent with sympathetic hyperactivity. These are most markedly manifested during delirium tremens and include tachycardia, moderately increased blood pressure, sweating, and dilated pupils (36,65,68). Death may result from cardiovascular collapse. Increased urinary excretion of catecholamines and high arterial levels of norepinephrine have also been observed (7,19,26,66). A correlation has been noted between norepinephrine levels and the severity of symptoms, and a return to normal values after recovery from alcohol withdrawal and delirium tremens has been reported (7,26).

Congestive Heart Failure, Renal Failure, and Cyclosporine Treatment

To complete the list of syndromes known to be associated with sympathetic hyperactivity, it should be mentioned that well-known features of heart failure include high peripheral vascular resistance and high plasma levels of norepinephrine. These changes are paralleled by a very high output of muscle nerve sympathetic activity, as revealed by microneurography (44). In addition, patients with chronic renal failure on hemodialysis who had not undergone nephrectomy exhibited a 2.5 times higher outflow of baroreflex-governed sympathetic nerve discharge to muscle vessels at rest than did healthy control subjects and patients with renal failure after nephrectomy (8). Furthermore, chronic hypertension complicating immunosuppressive cyclosporine treatment has been shown to be associated with increased sympathetic vasoconstrictor outflow to resistance vessels (64). These phenomena are beyond the scope of this chapter.

PATHOPHYSIOLOGY

Hypertension and Tachycardia

Acute hypertension accompanied by tachycardia suggests sympathetic overactivity, as do attacks of diaphoresis and cutaneous vasoconstriction. Detailed hemodynamic data are scarce, but tachycardia with high cardiac output and simultaneous increased systemic vascular resistance has been reported in the context of GBS (14) and tetanus (12,46). This combination implies a high level of sympathetic outflow to the heart and resistance vessels.

High urinary excretion and elevated plasma levels of catecholamines are common, although not invariable, findings in GBS patients with this clinical presentation (10,11, 14,28,54,55,69,76), as well as in cases of porphyric neuropathy (3,5), thallium intoxication (5,52), and tetanus (12, 38,39,47). Repeated measurements have demonstrated normalization of catecholamine levels with clinical improvement of the patient.

In the neuroleptic malignant syndrome, elevation of urinary catecholamines has been observed as an inconsistent feature (31). More recently, increased cerebrospinal fluid levels of norepinephrine and its metabolites were reported (57). High levels of arterial catecholamines signify fulminant malignant hyperthermia (29).

Thus, indices of increased sympathetic activity are observed for a number of the mentioned diseases. In *GBS*, microelectrode recordings of muscle nerve sympathetic activity (i.e., baroreflex-governed vasoconstrictor signals to resistance vessels in striated muscle) (70) (see Chapter 18) have provided direct evidence of increased sympathetic activity (22). Recordings were performed in three GBS patients with acute hypertension and resting tachycardia who uniformly displayed very high levels of sympathetic outflow in the acute stage of the disease (Fig. 2). The sympathetic nerve activity exhibited normal pulse synchrony, indicating preserved arterial baroreceptor influence on outflow. When the patients recovered from the disease, the level of sympathetic outflow was markedly reduced (see

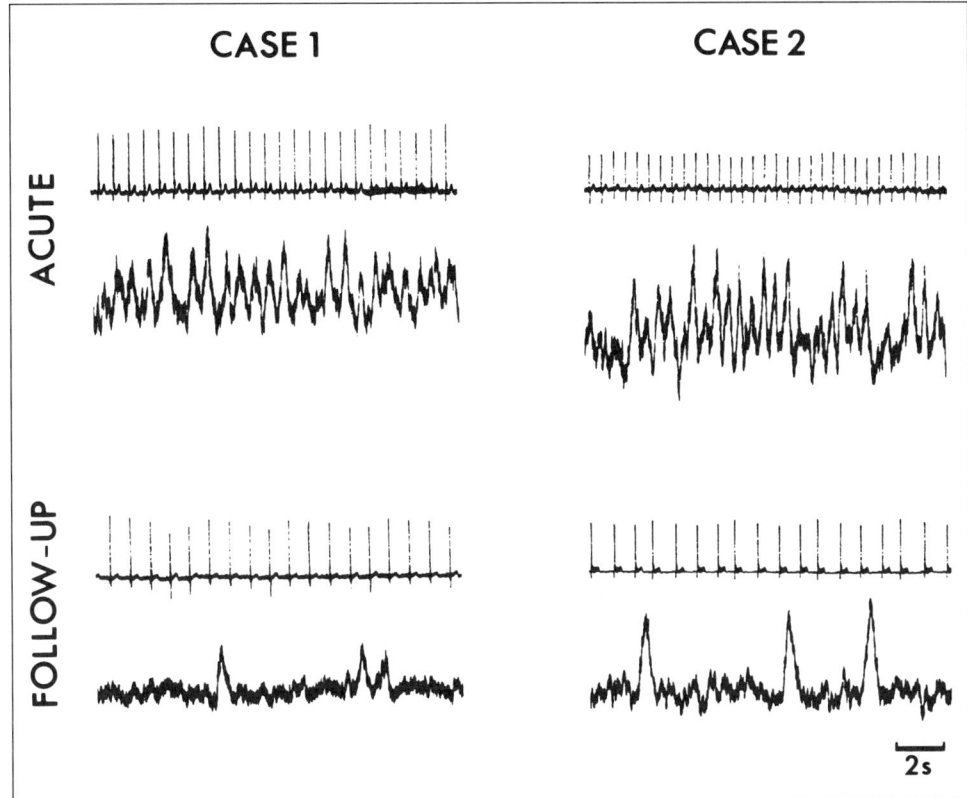

FIG. 2. Electrocardiogram (*upper traces*) and muscle nerve sympathetic activity (mean voltage neurogram; microneurographic recording from the peroneal nerve; *lower traces*) in the acute phase and at follow-up after recovery in two patients with acute Guillain-Barré syndrome. Both exhibited acute hypertension and resting tachycardia during the acute stage of the disease. Note the enhanced outflow of sympathetic activity with preservation of cardiac rhythmicity in the acute phase. The same time scale was used in all panels. (Reprinted with permission from Fagius J, Wallin BG. Microneurographic evidence of excessive sympathetic outflow in the Guillain-Barré syndrome. *Brain* 1983;106:589–600.)

Fig. 2). This lower outflow was reproducible at a second follow-up recording, indicating that the activity had reverted to normal, because outflow of this type of sympathetic activity is normally stable from one recording to another (Fig. 3). Thus, the elevation of blood pressure in the acute stage of GBS represents true neurogenic hypertension.

Guillain-Barré syndrome predominantly affects the peripheral nerves. The consequences of this are a failure of impulse transmission and a loss of function (2). Because the baroreflex regulation of blood pressure mediated by sympathetic nerve activity is an inhibitory reflex, sympathetic hyperactivity can be assumed if the afferent nerves from the baroreceptors are blocked by the pathologic process. The involvement of such short nerves is consistent with the patchy nature of the disease.

Such an underlying mechanism was suggested as early as 1949 by Lampen (41), who, in a series of papers, reported *Entzügelungshochdruck* (unbridled hypertension) to be an uncommon feature of different types of acute polyneuropathy and demonstrated that the symptoms could be experimentally imitated after local anesthesia of the baroreceptor afferents (41–43). Strong evidence for the same pathophysiologic mechanism underlying acute hypertension and tachycardia in porphyria was provided by Kezdi (40), who demonstrated that further increases in blood pressure were not induced by procaine block of the baroreceptor afferents in a *porphyric* patient. This indicated that the nerves were already blocked by the disease process itself (Fig. 4). The fact that an interruption of the afferent arc of the baroreflex might underlie tachycardia and hypertension was also suggested by the neuropathologic findings in three fatal cases of porphyria (27). These results also emphasized the patchy nature of peripheral nerve involvement in porphyria, which, in this respect, is similar to GBS.

Many years later, the technique used to block afferent signals in the vagus and glossopharyngeal nerves, which causes cardiovascular symptoms that imitate those of GBS, was combined with microneurographic recordings of sympathetic nerve signals (23). This confirmed the presence of sympathetic hyperactivity, identical to that found in GBS (Fig. 5). With complete experimental block, the ordinary cardiac rhythm of muscle nerve sympathetic activity was

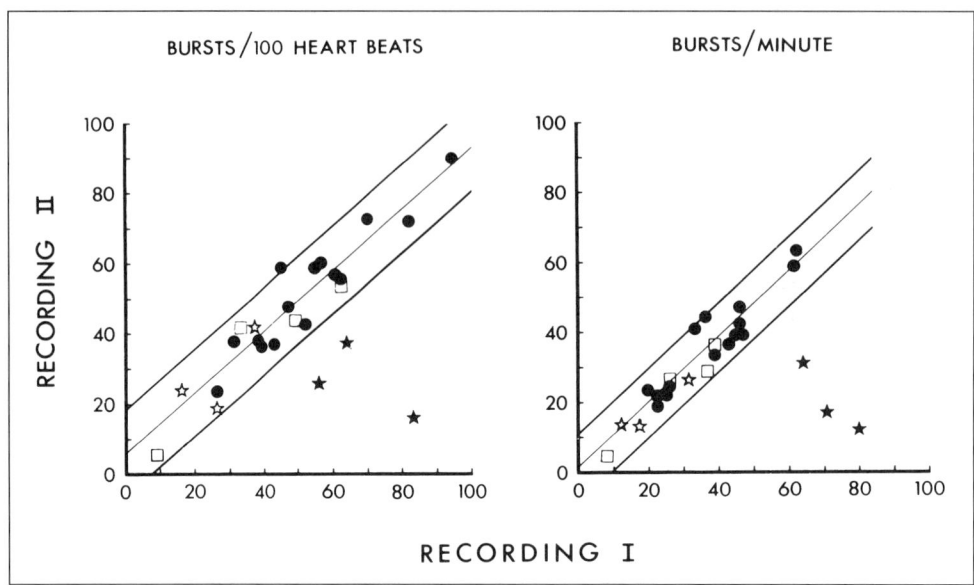

FIG. 3. Quantity of muscle nerve sympathetic activity, counted as bursts/100 heart beats (*left*) and bursts/min (*right*), in patients with acute Guillain-Barré syndrome and healthy controls. The results from two consecutive microneurographic recordings were plotted against each other. Regression lines (± 2 SD; r = 0.94 in both graphs) represent the correlation between the first and second recordings in the healthy subjects. Note the clear aberration of the three Guillain-Barré patients, with hypertension and tachycardia recorded during their acute illness. *Closed stars*, Guillain-Barré patients with acute tachycardia and hypertension, acute and first follow-up recordings made after recovery from the disease; *open stars*, the same patients, with both recordings made after recovery; *open squares*, Guillain-Barré patients without clinical signs of autonomic involvement, recordings made in the acute stage and after recovery; *closed circles*, healthy subjects. (Reprinted with permission from Fagius J, Wallin BG. Microneurographic evidence of excessive sympathetic outflow in the Guillain-Barré syndrome. *Brain* 1983;106:589–600.)

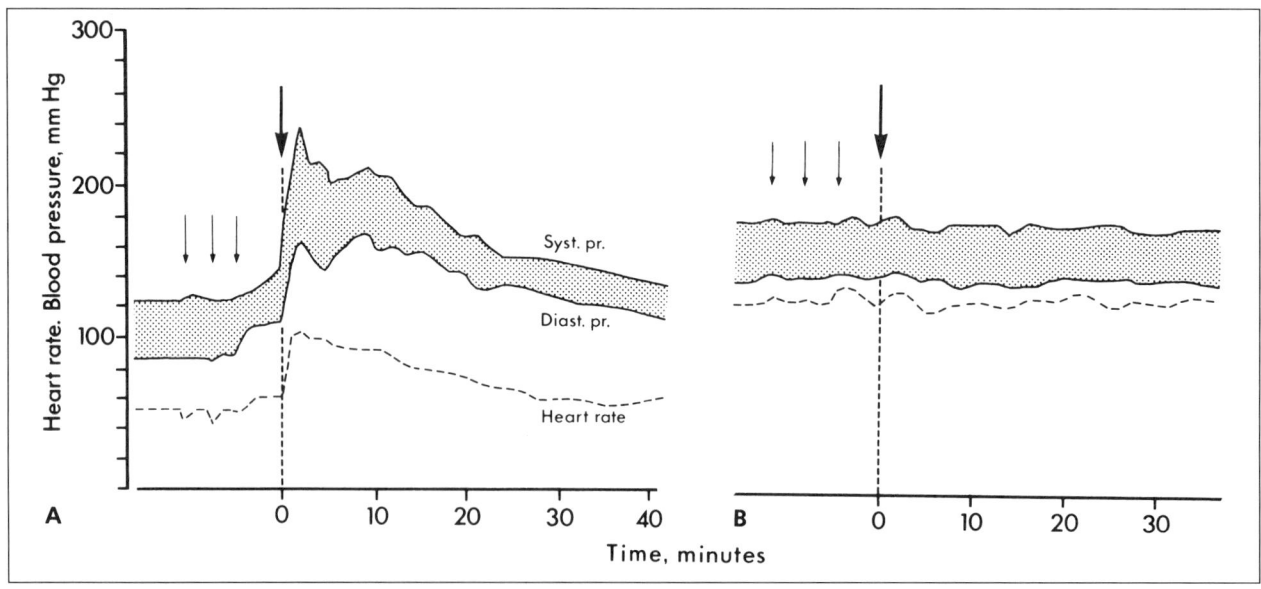

FIG. 4. Course of blood pressure and heart rate after carotid sinus pressure (*small arrows*) and procaine block of the baroreceptor afferent nerves (*thick arrow and dashed line at time 0*) in a healthy subject (**A**) and a 24-year-old woman (**B**) with acute porphyric neuropathy who had high blood pressure and resting tachycardia. Note the missing cardiovascular response in the patient after block, indicating spontaneous baroreceptor deafferentation. (Redrawn from Kezdi P. Neurogenic hypertension in man in porphyria. Transient hypertension and tachycardia caused by disruption of the carotid sinus; review of buffer nerve mechanism. *Arch Intern Med* 1954;94:122–130.)

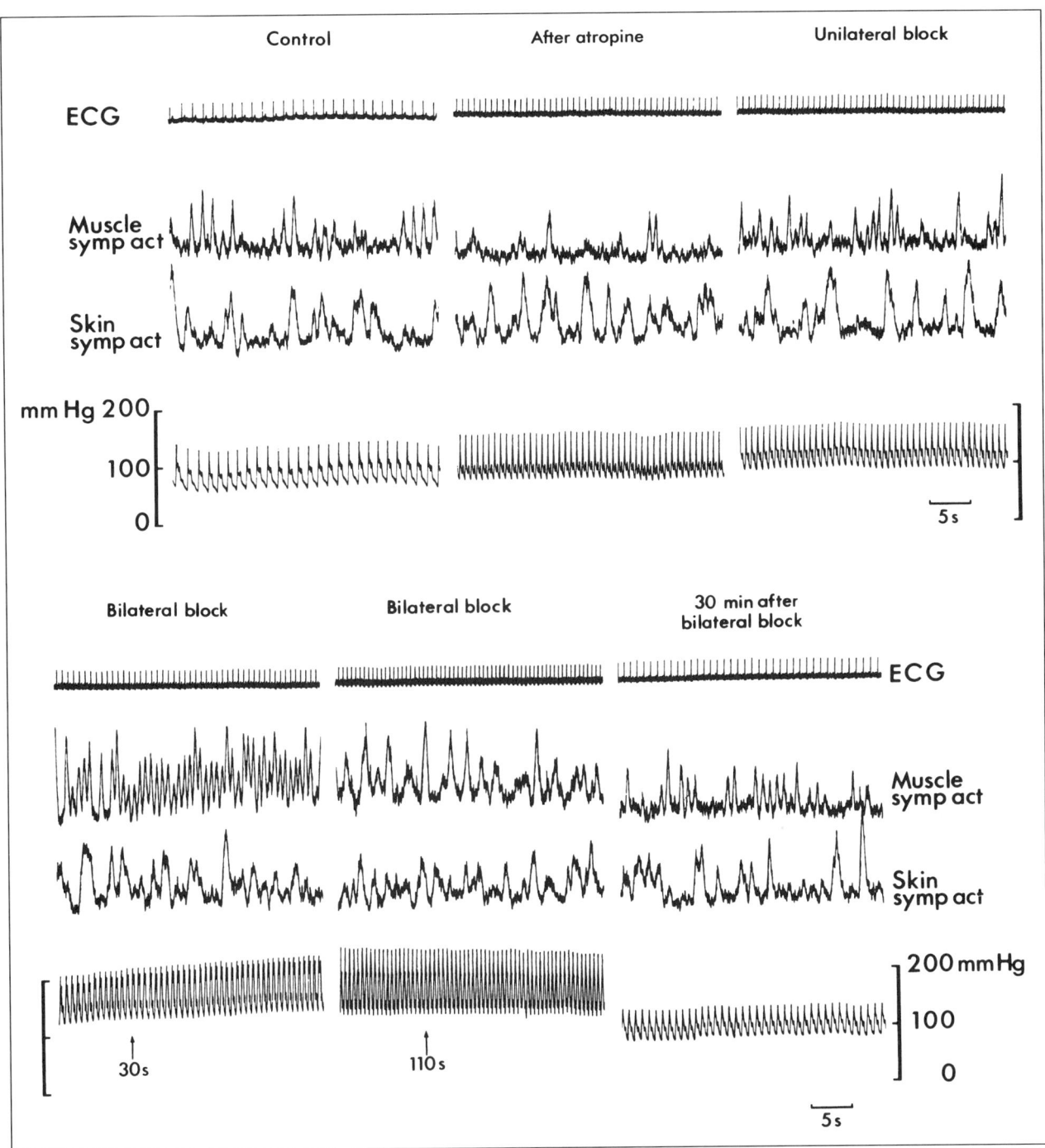

FIG. 5. Microneurographic recordings of muscle nerve sympathetic activity (baroreceptor governed and involved in blood pressure homeostasis) and skin nerve sympathetic activity (not involved in blood pressure regulation) before, during, and after experimental block of baroreceptor afferent nerves in a healthy subject. Traces from top: electrocardiogram (ECG), mean voltage neurograms of muscle and skin nerve sympathetic activity, and intra-arterially recorded blood pressure. Time notations in panels 4 and 5 indicate the interval after bilateral injection of lidocaine was completed. The same time scale was used in all panels.

Note the strong increase in muscle nerve sympathetic activity, with a simultaneous increase in heart rate and blood pressure, after block. Cardiac rhythmicity of muscle nerve sympathetic activity was initially preserved after block (panel 4), presumably stemming from some delay before the block was complete. This yielded an outflow resembling that observed in Guillain-Barré patients (see Fig. 2). Skin nerve sympathetic outflow was not affected by the procedure. (Reprinted with permission from Fagius J, Wallin BG, Sundlöf G et al. Sympathetic outflow in man after anaesthesia of the glossopharyngeal and vagus nerves. *Brain* 1985;108:423–438.)

totally lost, which is not the case in GBS patients (see Fig. 2) (22). Thus, it seems likely that there is only a partial block of baroreceptor inflow in these patients, such that the cardiac rhythm of the sympathetic activity is maintained (see Fig. 5, fourth panel). It has been suggested that the enhanced sympathetic activity observed in GBS (see Fig. 2) might be attributed to a decrease in afferent inflow from volume (low-pressure) receptors, in conjunction with preserved arterial baroreceptor regulation (22). Such partial baroreceptor denervation is also consistent with reports that carotid sinus pressure may induce some slowing of the heart rate in patients with GBS (10,45,55).

A common feature of GBS and the acute neuropathy seen with *porphyria, diphtheria,* and *thallium intoxication* is that short and proximal, including cranial nerve, are often involved in the disease process. Thus, it is conceivable that a lesion of baroreceptor afferents could constitute a common pathophysiologic mechanism underlying the sympathetic hyperactivity seen in these diseases.

Another possible mechanism is a brain stem lesion that could affect the baroreflex arc or give rise to direct central excitatory phenomena. The lack of other signs of central nervous system involvement in most cases of GBS makes this mechanism less likely, however. Moreover, the observation that ocular pressure usually induces a reduced heart rate in GBS patients with tachycardia, and can even induce spells of bradycardia (28), shows that other receptors that influence the baroreflex arc can exert their ordinary effect on the central vasomotor system (and even exert an amplified effect, which could be due to a lack of baroreceptor buffering).

Hypoxia and hypercapnia provoked by respiratory insufficiency might induce an increase in blood pressure due to sympathetic activation, but the increase in BP should be accompanied by bradycardia. Many observers have stated that respiration and blood oxygenation were normal in reported cases of hypertension in GBS (6,45,49,55) and tetanus (39,47), thus ruling out the possibility that hypoxia is the cause of sympathetic activation.

Direct involvement of the cardiac conduction system, due to myocarditis, has been proposed as a factor that contributes to the cardiac arrhythmia in GBS. Haymaker and Kernohan (34), in their review of 50 fatal cases of GBS, observed sparse and small foci of myocarditis, unrelated to cardiovascular symptoms. Signs of myocarditis were sought but not found at autopsy in a number of fatal cases associated with autonomic hyperactivity (6). Direct involvement of the heart as a main contributor to cardiac dysrhythmia in GBS seems unlikely.

In the context of *diphtheria*, direct myocardial involvement is common (48). The possibility that the mechanism just described for GBS might be operative in diphtheria neuropathy is hypothetical, because adequate experimental and clinical substantiation is lacking.

A vagus nerve lesion, leading to efferent vagal denervation of the heart, would certainly contribute to the development of tachycardia, but the unstable clinical state, including attacks of bradycardia, strongly suggests that vagal efferent activity is present (and sometimes even increased, as will be discussed).

In *tetanus*, another mechanism may be at work. Baroreceptor sensitivity was recently shown to be normal (normal heart period response to phenylephrine-induced rise in blood pressure) in a case of tetanus with signs of sympathetic hyperactivity (47). The authors concluded that the intact baroreflex was overruled by some mechanism that gave rise to primary sympathetic overactivity. This conclusion agrees with the suggestion that autonomic overactivity in tetanus is due to a direct central tetanospasmin action, resulting in disinhibition of autonomic efferent neurons. This resembles the widespread disinhibition of motor neurons that results in the muscle spasms typical of the disease (75).

Neuroleptic malignant syndrome and *malignant hyperthermia* are considered to have distinctly different pathophysiology despite common clinical features (13,15,33). The former is due to central dopamine blockade; the muscular stiffness is of central origin, and the sympathetic overactivity can be understood as a primary central feature as well. The disease process of malignant hyperthermia is almost certainly confined to skeletal muscle (13), and the hyperadrenergic state is best understood as a secondary consequence of the extreme disturbance of muscle metabolism.

The mechanism underlying the hypertension seen in cases of *poliomyelitis* is unknown. Direct involvement of autonomic motoneurons or interneurons in bulbar poliomyelitis has been suggested (51), but bulbar involvement is not a prerequisite for hypertension, which may occur even in nonparalytic poliomyelitis (30). The absence of an increased HR during the hypertensive periods indicates a pathophysiology different from those discussed. Some investigators have suggested that underestimated hypoxia may be a possible basis for the short-lived hypertension in poliomyelitis (73). The long-standing increase in blood pressure observed after the acute phase of poliomyelitis in patients with persistent muscle atrophies remains unexplained (59).

Bradycardia could be due to parasympathetic hyperactivity (45). Theoretically, efferent vagal "paresthesia," or spells of aberrant impulse generation, could occur in nerve fibers with altered conduction properties. Another possibility is the occurrence of episodes of abnormal impulse production in the sinus nerves. These could evoke a sudden arrest of the blood pressure defense, similar to what is known to occur in glossopharyngeal neuralgia with fainting (72). In such cases, a total and sudden inhibition of sympathetic vasoconstrictor outflow is evoked along with simultaneous vagal slowing of the heart. A related mechanism in GBS would account for both the bradycardia and the pronounced hypotensive episodes appearing even in the recumbent position. This is a more likely explanation than

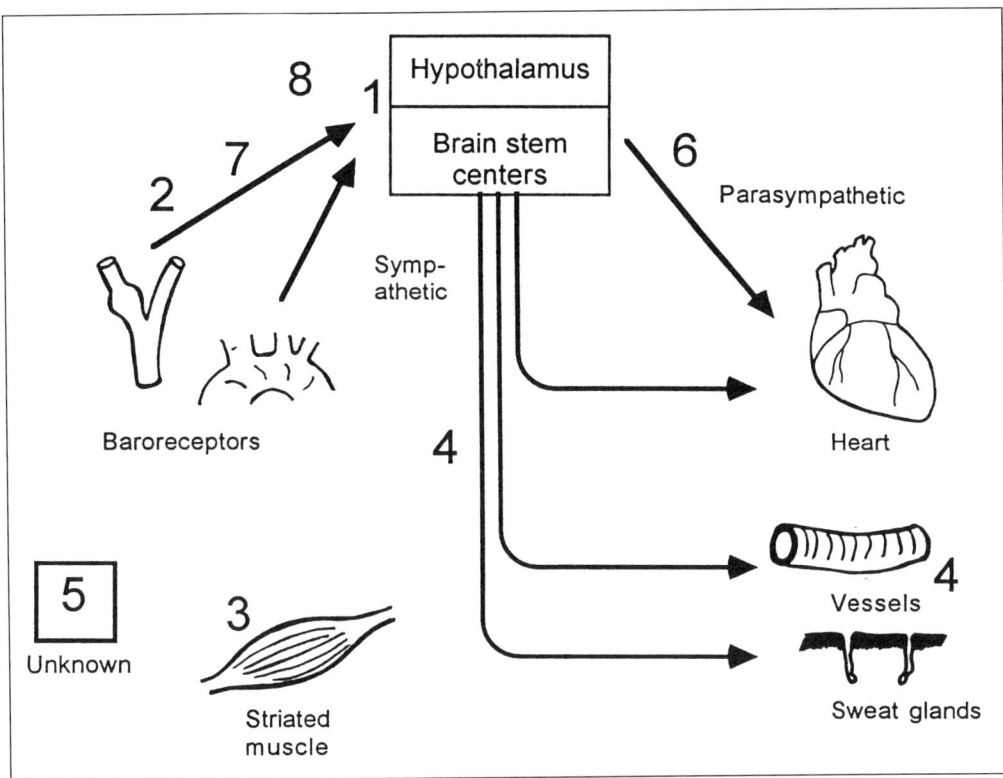

FIG. 6. Autonomic overactivity; known or postulated pathophysiologic mechanisms.

Hypertension and tachycardia—sympathetic hyperactivity
1. Primary cerebral activation
    Activation due to acute increase in intracranial pressure
        Intracranial hemorrhage, cerebral contusion (**see Chapters 32 and 57**)
    Activation due to neurotransmitter perturbation
        Neuroleptic malignant syndrome
    Activation following action of tetanospasmin
        Tetanus
    Activation, unknown mechanism
        Alcohol withdrawal syndrome
2. Baroreceptor deafferentation
    GBS, porphyria (thallium intoxication? diphtheria?)
3. Muscle activation with secondary sympathetic hyperactivity
    Malignant hyperthermia
4. Spinal cord activation plus effector organ hypersensitivity (?)
    Autonomic dysreflexia in upper spinal cord lesion
5. Unknown
    Poliomyelitis

Bradycardia—parasympathetic hyperactivity
6. Vagal "paresthesia"?
    GBS
7. Aberrant sinus nerve impulse generation evoking strong vagal activation?
    GBS

Perspiration, cutaneous vasoconstriction
1. Primary cerebral activation
    Activation due to acute increase in intracranial pressure
        Intracranial hemorrhage, cerebral contusion (**see Chapters 32 and 57**)
    Activation following action of tetanospasmin
        Tetanus
8. Generalized activation related to baroreceptor deafferentation (cf. vasovagal syncope)?
    GBS

paresthesia arising in the efferent part of the vagus. The fact that asystole may occur as the result of body turning (with redistribution of blood volume) or tracheal suction is also consistent with an abnormally strong activation of baroreceptor afferents.

To summarize, the labile cardiovascular state sometimes encountered in GBS might be due to alternating blockade and overactivity (the latter due to local aberrant impulse generation) in afferent nerves from the baroreceptors.

Perspiration and Cutaneous Circulation

The spells of sweating experienced in GBS are not well understood. Abnormal, paresthesia-like signal production in peripheral postganglionic fibers is not expected to occur simultaneously throughout the entire body. A primary central disinhibition or excitation cannot be ruled out, but, as stated earlier, other signs of central nervous system involvement are usually not present in GBS patients who exhibit this clinical feature. A more likely mechanism, although not precisely understood, is that the marked diaphoresis might be related to the sweating that occurs in vasovagal syncope, which is part of the peculiar, undifferentiated sympathetic mass activation that immediately precedes vasovagal fainting. This includes sweating, cutaneous vasoconstriction, and mydriasis. In this context, the finding that sudomotor (but not vasoconstrictor!) sympathetic nerve activity to the skin in healthy humans displays a nonovert but detectable cardiac rhythmicity (indicating a possible relationship to baroreceptors) may be relevant (4).

In tetanus, attacks of sweating and cutaneous vasoconstriction are understandable as direct central disinhibition phenomena, provided the mechanism referred to earlier exists (60).

The pathophysiology of *autonomic dysreflexia* is complex, comprising both sympathetic and parasympathetic functions. A massive, uninhibited sympathetic discharge of spinal origin was previously suggested to be operative (32). The attacks are associated with an acute increase in plasma norepinephrine levels, although not to high levels (compared with intact subjects). This increase ranges from very low levels at rest to low levels during the attack (50). Microneurographic recordings of sympathetic outflow below the lesion in such patients (67,71) have demonstrated an absence of spontaneous sympathetic outflow at rest (explaining the marked postural hypotension but not the dysreflexia). A massive discharge was never observed, but noxious stimuli below the lesion or increasing bladder pressure induced single, strong sympathetic bursts simultaneously in skin and muscle nerve fascicles, which is a change comparable to the normal situation (70). These few bursts were accompanied by strong skin vasoconstriction and a rise in BP, indicating an effector organ hypersensitivity (67,71). The bradycardia can be regarded as an attempt of the intact vagus nerve to buffer the high blood pressure after inflow from the likewise intact baroreceptor afferents.

The mechanism responsible for the sympathetic hyperactivity seen in the alcohol withdrawal syndromes is not clear. There is no reason, however, to suspect a defective baroreflex afferent function, as discussed earlier. Instead, a primary central effect is plausible, possibly as part of the cerebral hyperexcitability and the simultaneous increase in cerebral blood flow that have been observed in alcohol withdrawal (36). It has been hypothesized that the physical signs of withdrawal, including the symptoms of sympathetic hyperactivity, are directly related to recent drinking, whereas the psychotic symptoms and seizures are related to a long history of alcohol abuse (36).

Acute ethanol administration has been shown to increase plasma norepinephrine levels by reducing its circulatory clearance, without signs of increased neuronal release (18). However, this observation is probably not related to the pathophysiologic mechanism of alcohol withdrawal.

The pathophysiologic mechanisms, demonstrated or postulated, for the disorders discussed in this chapter are summarized in Figure 6.

ASSESSMENT

The cornerstone in the evaluation of patients with disorders that may be complicated by autonomic hyperactivity is simple heart rate and blood pressure monitoring. In GBS and porphyric neuropathy, for which mildly and moderately affected patients are treated in an ordinary ward, heart rate and blood pressure must be recorded repeatedly at brief intervals. Continuous electrocardiographic monitoring should be instituted if signs of cardiovascular instability appear, and the patient should be transferred to the intensive care unit. Patients with tetanus are probably without exception initially treated in an intensive care unit, where extensive monitoring of vital functions can be routinely applied. Constant surveillance of the patient's clinical state, with special emphasis on sweating spells and changes in cutaneous circulation, is essential.

Repeated application of a simple autonomic test such as the R-R interval variation (61,74) (see Chapter 24) has been suggested for identifying those patients with GBS most at risk of developing dangerous heart arrhythmia (58). However, abnormal results from such testing are much more frequent in GBS than are signs of autonomic overactivity. Moreover, the abnormal functioning of the autonomic nervous system may develop abruptly. Serial measurement of plasma norepinephrine levels might disclose sympathetic overactivity, but this is a relatively slow diagnostic procedure that cannot, in any instance, replace the direct monitoring of HR and BP. Intra-arterial measurement of BP is probably indicated only exceptionally, but the noninvasive technique for continuous recording of finger arterial BP that is now available (Finapres) (37) will certainly be of value.

Diagnostic blockade of the baroreceptor afferent pathways in cases of acute hypertension (to test whether it is possible to further increase blood pressure) (40) has enhanced our understanding of the underlying pathophysiologic mechanisms (see earlier), but this is a potentially hazardous procedure that must not be undertaken in light of current knowledge of the risk of fatal circulatory failure in these patients.

In summary, close monitoring of heart rate and blood pressure and the patient's overall clinical state is imperative and generally sufficient in the assessment of disorders that carry a risk for the development of autonomic overactivity.

MANAGEMENT

Patients who have developed a cardiovascular state consistent with autonomic overactivity should be treated in an intensive care unit, where resources for the immediate management of circulatory arrest and access to a temporary pacemaker exist. As stated earlier, many of these patients are so severely ill, with a risk of respiratory insufficiency, that they are primarily under intensive medical care.

Because tracheal suction and sudden changes in body posture during nursing carry a documented risk for provoking asystole in these patients, such procedures should be performed with great care and under intensified cardiac monitoring. Anesthetic procedures have also been implicated as a cause of asystole (60). The administration of suxamethonium (for muscle relaxation in conjunction with anesthesia, as in tracheostomy) has been reported to elicit immediate ventricular fibrillation or tachycardia in patients with severe, long-standing, and progressive polyneuropathy, presumably of the chronic inflammatory type. This has not been noted in patients with acute GBS (25).

The aim of management is to prevent circulatory arrest and the development of complications from severe hypertension. Pharmacologic treatment of sympathetic and parasympathetic overactivity as well as pacemaker assistance has been suggested. The cardiac effects of sympathetic hyperactivity can be reduced by β-adrenergic blocking treatment, and neurogenic hypertension can be managed by α-adrenergic blockade. The nonselective β-adrenergic blocker propranolol has been recommended and tried by many authors. The combined α- and β-adrenergic blocking agent labetalol has been successfully used in a case of severe tetanus (12). Conversely, adrenergic blockade may increase the risk of bradycardia and asystole (16,47), which is not unexpected in view of the spontaneous fluctuations between signs of sympathetic and parasympathetic overactivity in GBS and tetanus. The central sympathetic inhibitor clonidine was not effective according to one case report (54).

The use of atropine has been suggested for managing and preventing bradycardia (1,6,45), but is not fully reliable in preventing further attacks (28). Moreover, the administration of atropine alone may aggravate the episodes of tachycardia.

Temporary, on-demand (ventricular rate–inhibited) pacemakers have been recommended and used in a number of patients with bradyarrhythmias and asystolic episodes (1,16,20,24,56). An overall impression gleaned from the literature is that pharmacologic treatment of the cardiovascular complications, alone, is unreliable; consequently, ready recourse to a pacemaker may be justified. Theoretically, an appropriate treatment for intense, acute tachycardia and hypertension should be the use of labetalol (i.e., combined α- and β-adrenergic blockade) and the addition of atropine, if bradycardia occurs, along with ready use of a pacemaker, if necessary.

In the neuroleptic malignant syndrome, immediate withdrawal of the neuroleptic is essential. Sodium dantrolene (to relieve muscle contractions) and bromocriptine (to activate dopamine receptors) constitute the current drug treatment (15,33). With these measures, even the autonomic overactivity is usually managed, but the addition of a β-adrenergic blocking agent is recommended in some instances. Dantrolene is also the specific treatment for malignant hyperthermia, but the reader is referred to textbooks in intensive care for the management of this hyperacute disorder (13).

The management of autonomic dysreflexia in tetraplegia is described in Chapters 32 and 35.

The treatment of alcohol withdrawal syndromes relies on sedation (preferably with high doses of diazepam), fluid and electrolyte control (and administration of thiamine), and close surveillance for respiratory and cardiovascular depression (68). There is no general agreement that adrenergic blocking drugs are beneficial in the management of alcohol withdrawal syndromes and delirium tremens (65), but many centers use propranolol for the treatment of severe tachycardia (and tremor), according to general principles applied in intensive medical care (21).

REFERENCES

1. Andersson T, Sidén Å. A clinical study of the Guillain-Barré syndrome. *Acta Neurol Scand* 1982;66:316–327.
2. Arnason BGW, Soliven B. Acute inflammatory demyelinating polyradiculoneuropathy. In: Dyck PJ, Thomas PK, Griffin JW et al (eds). *Peripheral Neuropathy, 3rd ed.* Philadelphia: WB Saunders. 1993; 1437–1497.
3. Beattie AD, et al. Acute intermittent porphyria: response of tachycardia and hypertension to propranolol. *Br Med J* 1973;3:257–260.
4. Bini G, et al. Cardiac rhythmicity of skin nerve sympathetic activity recorded from peripheral nerves in man. *J Autonom Nerv Syst* 1981; 4:17–24.
5. Bock KD, et al. Zur Pathogenese von Hypertonie und Tachykardie bei der akuten Thalliumvergiftung und bei akuter intermittierender Porphyrie. *Dtsch Med Wochenschr* 1968;93: 2119–2124.
6. Bredin CP. Guillain-Barré syndrome: the unsolved cardiovascular problems. *Ir J Med Sci* 1977;146:273–279.

7. Carlsson C, Häggendal J. Arterial noradrenaline levels after ethanol withdrawal. *Lancet* 1967;II:889.
8. Converse RL Jr, et al. Sympathetic overactivity in patients with chronic renal failure. *N Engl J Med* 1992;327: 1912–1918.
9. Corbett JL, et al. Hypotension in tetanus. *Br Med J* 1973;2:423–428.
10. Davidson DLW, Jellinek EH. Hypertension and papilloedema in the Guillain-Barré syndrome. *J Neurol Neurosurg Psychiatry* 1977;40:144–148.
11. Davies AG, Dingle HR. Observations on cardiovascular and neuroendocrine disturbance in the Guillain-Barré syndrome. *J Neurol Neurosurg Psychiatry* 1972;35:176–179.
12. Domenighetti GM, et al. Hyperadrenergic syndrome in severe tetanus: extreme rise in catecholamines responsive to labetalol. *Br Med J* 1984;288:1483–1484.
13. Donahue PL, Gronert GA. Malignant hyperthermia. In: Grande CM et al (eds). *Textbook of Trauma, Anesthesia, and Critical Care.* St. Louis: CV Mosby.1993;1140–1159.
14. Durocher A, et al. Autonomic dysfunction in the Guillain-Barré syndrome. Hemodynamic and neurobiochemical studies. *Intensive Care Med* 1980;6:3–6.
15. Editorial. Neuroleptic malignant syndrome. *Lancet* 1984; I:545–546.
16. Edmondson RS, Flowers MW. Intensive care in tetanus: management, complications, and mortality in 100 cases. *Br Med J* 1979;1:1401–1404.
17. Eiben RM, Gersony WM. Recognition, prognosis and treatment of the Guillain-Barré syndrome (acute idiopathic polyneuritis). *Med Clin North Am* 1963;47:1371–1380.
18. Eisenhofer G, et al. Effects of ethanol on plasma catecholamines and norepinephrine clearance. *Clin Pharmacol Ther* 1983;34:143–147.
19. Eisenhofer G, et al. Plasma catecholamine responses to change in posture in alcoholics during withdrawal and after continued abstinence from alcohol. *Clin Sci* 1985;68:71–78.
20. Emmons PR, et al. Cardiac monitoring and demand pacemaker in Guillain-Barré syndrome. *Arch Neurol* 1975;32: 59–61.
21. Erstad BL, Cotugno CL. Management of alcohol withdrawal. *Am J Health Syst Pharm* 1995;52:697–709.
22. Fagius J, Wallin BG. Microneurographic evidence of excessive sympathetic outflow in the Guillain-Barré syndrome. *Brain* 1983;106:589–600.
23. Fagius J, et al. Sympathetic outflow in man after anaesthesia of the glossopharyngeal and vagus nerves. *Brain* 1985;108:423–438.
24. Favre H, et al. Use of demand pacemaker in a case of Guillain-Barré syndrome. *Lancet* 1970;I:1062–1063.
25. Fergusson RJ, et al. Suxamethonium is dangerous in polyneuropathy. *Br Med J* 1981;282:298–299.
26. Giacobini E, et al. Urinary norepinephrine and epinephrine excretion in delirium tremens. *Arch Gen Psychiatry* 1960;3:289–296.
27. Gibson JB, Goldberg A. The neuropathology of acute porphyria. *J Pathol Bacteriol* 1956;71:495–509.
28. Goulon M, et al. La dysautonomie des polyradiculonévrites aiguës primitives. *Rev Neurol (Paris)* 1975;131: 96–119.
29. Gronert GA, et al. Dantrolene in porcine malignant hyperthermia. *Anesthesiology* 1976;44:488–495.
30. Grulee CG Jr, Panos TC. Epidemic poliomyelitis in children: clinical study with special reference to symptoms and management of bulbar polioencephalitis. *Am J Dis Child* 1948;75:24–39.
31. Gurrera RJ, Romero JA. Sympathoadrenomedullary activity in the neuroleptic malignant syndrome. *Biol Psychiatry* 1992;32:334–343.
32. Guttman L, Whitteridge D. Effects of bladder distention on autonomic mechanisms after spinal cord injuries. *Brain* 1947;70:361–404.
33. Guzé BH, Baxter LR. Neuroleptic malignant syndrome. *N Engl J Med* 1985;313:163–166.
34. Haymaker W, Kernohan JW. The Landry-Guillain-Barré syndrome. A clinicopathologic report of fifty fatal cases and a critique of the literature. *Medicine* 1949;28:59–141.
35. Head H, Riddoch G. The autonomic bladder, excessive sweating and some other reflex conditions, in gross injuries of the spinal cord. *Brain* 1917;40:188–263.
36. Hemmingsen R, Kramp P. Delirium tremens and related clinical states. Psychopathology, cerebral pathophysiology and psychochemistry: A two-component hypothesis concerning etiology and pathogenesis. *Acta Psychiatr Scand* 1988;78(suppl 345):94–107.
37. Imholz BPM, et al. Continuous finger arterial pressure: utility in the cardiovascular laboratory. *Clin Autonom Res* 1991;1:43–53.
38. Keilty SR, et al. Catecholamine levels in severe tetanus. *Lancet* 1968; II:195.
39. Kerr JH, et al. Involvement of the sympathetic nervous system in tetanus. *Lancet* 1968;II:235–241.
40. Kezdi P. Neurogenic hypertension in man in porphyria. Transient hypertension and tachycardia caused by disruption of the carotid sinus; review of buffer nerve mechanism. *Arch Intern Med* 1954;94:122–130.
41. Lampen H. Über Entzügelungshochdruck bei Polyneuritis. *Dtsch Med Wochenschr* 1949;74:536–540.
42. Lampen H, et al. Entzügelungshochdruck am Menschen. *Klin Wochenschr* 1949;27:272–278.
43. Lampen H, et al. Experimenteller Entzügelungshochdruck bei arterieller Hypertonie. *Z Kreislaufforsch* 1949;38:577–592.
44. Leimbach WN, et al. Direct evidence from intraneural recordings for increased central sympathetic outflow in patients with heart failure. *Circulation* 1986;73:913–919.
45. Lichtenfeld P. Autonomic dysfunction in the Guillain-Barré syndrome. *Am J Med* 1971;50:772–780.
46. van Lieshout JJ, et al. Hyperadrenergic syndrome with hypertension, hypotension and myocardial necrosis in tetanus. *Neth J Med* 1988; 33:33–36.
47. van Lieshout JJ, et al. Cardiovascular instability and baroreflex activity in a patient with tetanus. *Clin Autonom Res* 1991;1:5–8.
48. Lupton MD, Klawans HL. Neurological complications of diphtheria. In: Vinken PJ, Bruyn GW (eds). *Handbook of Clinical Neurology, Vol. 33. Infections of the Nervous System, Part I.* Amsterdam: North-Holland Publishing Company. 1978;479–489.
49. Marshall J. The Landry-Guillain-Barré syndrome. *Brain* 1963;86:55–66.
50. Mathias CJ, Frankel HL. Cardiovascular control in spinal man. *Annu Rev Physiol* 1988;50:577–592.
51. McDowell FH, Plum F. Arterial hypertension associated with acute anterior poliomyelitis. *N Engl J Med* 1951;245:241–246.
52. Merguet P, et al. Untersuchungen zur Pathogenese von Hypertonie und Sinustachykardie bei der Thalliumvergiftung des Menschen. *Arch Klin Med* 1969;216:1–20.
53. Mertens HG. Die vegetativen Syndrome der Thalliumvergiftung. *Klin Wochenschr* 1952;30:843–849.
54. Minami N, et al. The mechanism responsible for hypertension in a patient with Guillain-Barré syndrome. *Clin Exp Hypertens* 1995;17: 607–617.
55. Mitchell PL, Meilman E. The mechanism of hypertension in the Guillain-Barré syndrome. *Am J Med* 1967;42:986–995.
56. Narayan D, et al. Bradycardia and asystole requiring permanent pacemaker in Guillain-Barré syndrome. *Am Heart J* 1984;108:426–428.
57. Nisijima K, Ishiguro T. Cerebrospinal fluid levels of monoamine metabolites and gamma-aminobutyric acid in neuroleptic malignant syndrome. *J Psychiatr Res* 1995;29:233–244.
58. Oakley CM. The heart in the Guillain-Barré syndrome. *Br Med J* 1984;288:94.
59. Ostfeld AM. Sustained hypertension after poliomyelitis. *Arch Intern Med* 1961;107:551–557.
60. Perel A, et al. Anaesthesia in the Guillain-Barré syndrome. *Anaesthesia* 1977;32:257–260.
61. Persson A, Solders G. R-R variations in the Guillain-Barré syndrome: a test of autonomic dysfunction. *Acta Neurol Scand* 1983;67:294–300.
62. Ridley A. Porphyric neuropathy. In: Dyck PJ, Thomas PK, Lambert EH, Bunge R (eds). *Peripheral Neuropathy, 2nd ed.* Philadelphia: WB Saunders. 1984;1704–1716.
63. Ridley A, et al. Tachycardia and the neuropathy of porphyria. *Lancet* 1968;II:708–710.
64. Scherrer U, et al. Cyclosporine-induced sympathetic activation and hypertension after heart transplantation. *N Engl J Med* 1990;323: 693–699.
65. Schuckit MA. *Drug and Alcohol Abuse. A Clinical Guide to Diagnosis and Treatment, 3rd ed.* New York: Plenum Medical Book Company. 1989.
66. Smith AJ, et al. Plasma noradrenaline, platelet alpha-2-adrenoceptors, and functional scores during ethanol withdrawal. *Alcohol Clin Exp Res* 1990;14:497–502.
67. Stjernberg L, et al. Sympathetic activity in man after spinal cord injury. Outflow to muscle below the lesion. *Brain* 1986;109:695–715.

68. Taylor RW, Bush HS. Substance abuse and withdrawal: alcohol, cocaine, and opioids. In: Cavetta JM, Taylor RW, Kirby RR (eds). *Critical Care*. Philadelphia: JB Lippincott. 1988.
69. Ventura HO, et al. Norepinephrine-induced hypertension in the Guillain-Barré syndrome. *J Hypertens* 1986;4:265–267.
70. Wallin BG, Fagius J. Peripheral sympathetic neural activity in conscious humans. *Annu Rev Physiol* 1988;50:565–576.
71. Wallin BG, Stjernberg L. Sympathetic activity in man after spinal cord injury. Outflow to skin below the lesion. *Brain* 1984;107:183–198.
72. Wallin BG, et al. Syncope induced by glossopharyngeal neuralgia: sympathetic outflow to muscle. *Neurology* 1984;34:522–524.
73. Weinstein L, Shelokov A. Cardiovascular manifestations in acute poliomyelitis. *N Engl J Med* 1951;244: 281–285.
74. Wieling W, et al. Reflex control of heart rate in normal subjects in relation to age: a data base for cardiac vagal neuropathy. *Diabetologia* 1982;22:163–166.
75. Wright DK, et al. Autonomic nervous system dysfunction in severe tetanus: current perspectives. *Crit Care Med* 1989;17:371–375.
76. Yao H, et al. Neurogenic hypertension in the Guillain-Barré syndrome. *Jpn Heart J* 1985;26:593–596.
77. Zochodne DW. Autonomic involvement in Guillain-Barré syndrome: a review. *Muscle Nerve* 1994;17:1145–1155.

CHAPTER 57

Management of the Autonomic Storm

Allan H. Ropper

---

1. Hypersympathetic states resulting from cerebral lesions may be mediated by any one of four different mechanisms: (a) sympathoadrenal discharge, (b) the Cushing response, (c) "diencephalic seizures," or (c) epileptic discharges.
2. Subarachnoid hemorrhage is a frequent cause of arrhythmias, hypertension, and electrocardiographic alterations.
3. Mild or moderate hypertension that appears after an ischemic stroke should not be treated, although treatment may be needed if the mean arterial pressure persistently exceeds 120 mmHg.
4. The best index of blood pressure (BP) is the mean arterial pressure.
5. The choice of antihypertensive medication in extreme dysautonomia is best based on the underlying neurologic condition.
6. Treatment for an overdose of street drugs is generally supportive.
7. Profound fluctuations of BP in patients with Guillain-Barré syndrome are uncommon, and treatment should not be too aggressive.
8. Patients with severe dysautonomia often require admission to intensive care units because of the severity of their primary illness and because of the extreme alterations in BP that accompany the illness.

INTRODUCTION

Most of the acute and dramatic disturbances of autonomic function seen in clinical practice result from catastrophic diseases of the central nervous system, such as cerebral hemorrhage or head injury. Others stem from diseases of the peripheral nervous system, such as Guillain-Barré syndrome, or from spinal cord transection. This chapter reviews the causes and treatment of extreme autonomic dysfunction and focuses on the secondary hypersympathetic state, or "autonomic storm," which has mainly cardiovascular manifestations. Despite its clinical impact, autonomic storm is often overshadowed by the underlying cerebral, spinal, or peripheral nerve disease. A general distinguishing feature between central and peripheral autonomic storm is the tendency for central types to begin soon after onset of the acute brain or spinal cord disease, then fluctuate and persist for several hours or days; peripheral dysautonomia is more often paroxysmal and recurs over longer periods.

MECHANISMS OF SYMPATHETIC STORM RESULTING FROM CEREBRAL LESIONS

The hypersympathetic state that accompanies acute and massive damage to the central nervous system may be mediated by any one of four different mechanisms: (a) an acute sympathoadrenal discharge; (b) the Cushing response, which results from secondary distortion of the medulla; (c) "diencephalic seizures," which may accompany the acute decorticate state after head injury (but was first described in third ventricular tumor); or (c) true electrocerebral seizures, which result from spontaneous or induced (electroconvulsive) epilepsy.

Sympathoadrenal Discharge

When encountered in neurologic practice, acute hypertension is most commonly the result of a sympathoadrenal discharge precipitated by an acute intracranial event (71). Excessive sympathetic activity also plays a role in producing the electrocardiographic (ECG) changes and neurogenic pulmonary edema seen in patients after an acute cerebral injury. The findings from several series of head-

---

A. H. Ropper: Department of Neurology, St. Elizabeth's Medical Center, Boston, Massachusetts, 02135.

injured patients suggest that the hypertension, tachycardia, and increased cardiac output, with either normal or decreased peripheral vascular resistance, are the result of a hyperadrenergic state brought about by a combined sympathetic neural discharge and excessive adrenal activity (20, 21,66,115,133). Severe neural injury is associated with the most intense adrenergic discharge and the highest plasma and urinary concentrations of catecholamines. Raised intracranial pressure or medullary tissue shifts, discussed later in this chapter, are not necessary for this type of intense adrenergic overactivity to occur (110).

Cushing Response

The Cushing response, reflex, or, as Cushing called it, "reaction" (27,28) consists of the triad of hypertension, bradycardia, and slow irregular breathing. Direct pressure applied to a restricted area of the paramedian caudal medulla produces the response in animals (65), pontomesencephalic section exaggerates it, and similar pressure-sensitive areas in the upper spinal cord are responsible for the hypertension elicited by increased intraspinal pressure (97). In clinical circumstances, acute distortion of the lower brain stem is the unifying clinical feature of the Cushing response (125), but supratentorial masses, typically cerebral hematomas, are the most common cause of secondary compression of the brain stem. It is not known whether transmission of pressure indirectly through the fourth ventricle can also elicit a Cushing response. A Cushing response may also be seen in patients with masses of the posterior fossa, such as edematous cerebellar infarction (81), tumors (17,43), or a basilar arterial aneurysm (93). Many patients with subacutely evolving masses of the posterior fossa, such as cerebellar infarction, exhibit hypertension before the bradycardia, and this briefly resembles the sympathoadrenal discharge of acute injury.

Diencephalic Seizures

Diencephalic seizure is an ambiguous term that has been used to describe episodes of acute hypertension, tachycardia, intense diaphoresis, and pupillary dilatation. These phenomena are associated with centrally placed cerebral tumors and were called *diencephalic autonomic seizures* by Penfield (98,99). However, the term has been applied to describe an identical phenomenon that is associated with spontaneous or induced epileptic discharges, and also with the extreme decorticate state that may appear after head trauma. Penfield proposed that these paroxysms were caused by epilepsy, although his first patient had a tumor at the foramen of Monro (85), so that the cause of the spells was uncertain. Numerous similar cases have been reported under different names, most with lesions near the third ventricle (3,5,13,18,47,87,119), but none has exhibited convincing evidence of an epileptic discharge. Additional features in some cases have included a rise in temperature just before an episode, cyclic respirations, lacrimation, or shivering. During episodes that last up to several minutes, the systolic blood pressure may exceed 200 mm Hg, the pulse rate is approximately 150 beats/min, and the respiratory rate may approach 40 breaths/min. The bed is often soaked in sweat, and large beads of perspiration form on the patient's forehead.

Most instances of this syndrome encountered in clinical practice are the result of closed head injury, usually associated with a decorticate state and widespread axonal injury of the white matter. The syndrome appears days or longer after the injury. Acute hydrocephalus, the likely explanation for one of Penfield's original cases, in which paroxysms ceased with ventricular shunting (18), may provoke similar episodes, typically after subarachnoid hemorrhage. The release of the hypothalamus from inhibitory cortical control is the mechanism that has been been proposed to account for these episodes, rather than direct hypothalamic damage or the synchronized electrical discharge of sympathetic neurons in the hypothalamus. Anticonvulsant medications have no consistent effect on the paroxysms and the electroencephalogram generally fails to show epileptic activity. Morphine may curtail individual episodes, but bromocriptine has been reported to have a more sustained beneficial effect (13).

The autonomic effects of epilepsy and electrographic seizures have been studied extensively, but the findings have been inconsistent. Generalized convulsions cause a hypersympathetic state coupled with hypertension (73,90); however, the effect of electrical discharges on limbic and hypothalamic structures is unclear. Blood pressure is commonly increased for up to 30 min in the immediate postictal period, and persistent or severe hypertension suggests that a seizure has been triggered by an acute cerebral hemorrhage. Antihypertensive treatment is rarely needed to control the hypertension of typical epilepsy. Patients with temporal lobe epilepsy that causes paroxysmal hypertension and tachycardia have been described (89). Experimentally induced seizures without clinically apparent convulsions have generally not led to increased central or peripheral sympathetic activity (40,109), but electrical spread to the hypothalamus may be necessary for these autonomic effects.

The autonomic nervous system also plays a poorly understood role in the genesis of arrhythmias, sudden death, and pulmonary edema that arise with seizures (30,34,116). The sympathetic effector limb has been implicated in all these infrequent but serious complications.

Electroconvulsive Therapy

One of the most interesting models for the study of the autonomic effects of seizures is electroconvulsive therapy (ECT). Cardiovascular complications are the leading cause of death in patients treated with ECT, and severe hypertension (39,72,83) or pulmonary edema are rare consequences (12). From these observations has emerged the concept of "diencephalic seizures," discussed above, which can be elicited experimentally by stimulating the hypothalamus (49), abolished by β-adrenergic blockade (64), and incompletely suppressed by adrenalectomy (22). Clinical studies have shown abrupt increases in sympathetic activity and circulating catecholamine levels in patients undergoing ECT, similar to observations in head trauma (39,51,91, 100,131).

Attention has also been directed toward the ECG abnormalities evoked by ECT; these include frequent T-wave changes and an initial parasympathetic discharge that can cause asystole. Because of these observations, it has become customary for the attending anesthesiologist at an ECT session to induce combined vagal and β-adrenergic blockade, or adrenergic blockade alone, in the patient undergoing the procedure.

Subarachnoid Hemorrhage as a Special Cause of Sympathetic Storm

Subarachnoid hemorrhage and head trauma are associated with acute autonomic phenomena, but the complexity and varied pathologic presentation of head trauma make subarachnoid hemorrhage a better model for understanding the clinical aspect of the hypersympathetic state. Some of the manifestations of sympathoadrenal discharge after subarachnoid hemorrhage, particularly hypertension and ECG changes, can influence outcome and pose problems in diagnosis (45). Experimental adrenalectomy or cervical cord section prevents most of the systemic changes from occurring, suggesting that direct neural and indirect endocrine overactivity are responsible. The irritating effects of subarachnoid blood on the hypothalamus (53), posterior hypothalamic infarction (25,37), or transmitted pressure to medullary vasopressor centers are possible stimuli to the adrenergic discharge.

Arterial blood pressures up to 210/110 mmHg (mean, 140 mmHg) are common after large hemorrhages, particularly if there is acute hydrocephalus, and hypertension may increase the risk for repeated hemorrhage (6,126). The latter notion has not been proved systematically but is supported by anecdotal experience. Overtreatment of the hypertension, however, has been linked to stroke caused by delayed vasospasm. Without hydrocephalus, hypertension usually subsides spontaneously over several days.

ECG changes that simulate cardiac ischemia are found in approximately 50% of patients after subarachnoid hemorrhage (11) and in a smaller but still important proportion of patients with intracerebral hemorrhage. Similar changes occur in conjunction with other catastrophic central lesions, including head trauma (60), tumors (59), and meningitis (46,54,59,88). For further details, readers are referred to published reviews, particularly the ones by Marion et al. (86) and Oppenheimer et al. (95), and to original descriptions of these phenomena (14,15,26,70,79). Abnormalities that have been reported in patients with subarachnoid hemorrhage, in approximate order of frequency, are as follows: depression or, less often, elevation of the ST segment; broad inverted or biphasic T waves; QT prolongation; upright peaked T waves; U waves; peaked P waves; Q waves; short PR interval; and an S wave in V_1. The repolarization changes are particularly likely to be mistaken for myocardial ischemia (56,61,82), whereas deep symmetric T-wave inversion, peaked T waves, and peaked P waves are most characteristic of subarachnoid or intracerebral hemorrhage.

Morphologic ECG changes can be produced by stimulating electrically various cortical and subcortical areas, but most observations suggest that the repolarization and other ECG changes are caused by a surge of norepinephrine released locally from sympathetic nerve terminals adjacent to the myocardium, and by elevated levels of circulating catecholamines. The ECG changes, although reversible, are often accompanied by moderate elevations in the MB fraction of creatine phosphokinase (1,55,94). This rise in the creatine phosphokinase level, some of the ECG changes, and muscle fiber damage may be partially prevented by adrenergic blockade. The role of subendocardial ischemia in the cause of morphologic ECG changes and in the genesis of arrhythmias is still controversial, but most evidence suggests that focal areas of subendocardial damage are extremely common, although often overlooked in pathologic studies (52,59,75,118).

Various arrhythmias also may reappear after subarachnoid hemorrhage; the most frequent, although innocuous, are sinus bradycardia (11) and supraventricular tachyarrhythmias related to the hyperadrenergic state in the first days after hemorrhage (33). Ventricular tachycardia occurs in a very few instances (63). Although the mechanisms for these arrhythmias are thought to be neurogenic, microscopic areas of damaged cardiac muscle damage could also constitute foci of electrical instability that precipitate arrhythmias. A prolonged QT interval is apparently a predictor of the serious arrhythmias that underlie some cases of sudden death observed in patients with subarachnoid hemorrhage (41,42,95,130), although apnea and disorders of respiratory rhythm have been reported to be more common than cardiac arrhythmias (63).

Because catecholamine blockade has been found to reduce experimentally induced subendocardial damage and ventricular arrhythmias in subarachnoid hemorrhage, labetalol or propranolol are recommended as antihypertensive agents, especially in patients with tachycardia. Clonidine has been used as an alternative agent. When a patient cannot take oral medications, or if the mean BP is above 140 mm Hg, sodium nitroprusside may be used to lower the mean pressure to approximately 100 to 110 mm Hg (see later discussion and Table 1). However, excessive treatment may produce ischemia distal to regions of cerebral

TABLE 1. *Antihypertensive drugs for use in acute conditions in neurologic practice*

Drug	Dose range	Method	Duration	ICP potential increase
Sodium nitroprusside	1–10 μg/kg/min	Continuous IV	2–5 min	+
Nitroglycerin	5–100 μg/min	Continuous IV	3–5 min	++
Labetalol	20–80 mg	Bolus every 20 min IV	30 min–4 h	0
	0.5–2 mg/min	Continuous IV		
Esmolol	50–200 μg/min over 4 min	IV	2–5 min	0
Pentobarbital	50–150 mg	Slow bolus IV	30 min–2 h	—
Nicardipine	5–15 mg/h	Continuous IV	1–4 h	0/+
Nifedipine	10–20 mg	Orally every 10–15 min	2–4 h	++
Clonidine	0.05–0.15 mg	Orally every 1 h	4–8 h	0
α-Methyldopa	250–500 mg	Orally or IV bolus	2–6 h	0

ICP, intracranial pressure; IV, intravenous; +, mild; ++, moderate; —, reduces ICP; 0, none.

vasospasm. Nitroglycerin has become popular in the management of hypertensive patients with subarachnoid hemorrhage because of its putative beneficial effect on vasospasm, but its value as an antihypertensive agent is inconsistent in these circumstances. In many patients, particularly those with milder hemorrhages who remain conscious, narcotic treatment for pain lowers BP.

Treatment of Extreme Hypertension Resulting from Acute Cerebral Lesions

Hypertension Associated with an Intracranial Mass

The management of hypertension during the first hours after an acute intracranial catastrophe is complex, because exaggerated cerebral blood flow in areas of brain damage may enhance regional edema (77,113,114) and because most antihypertensive medications are cerebral vasodilators that raise the intracranial pressure (7,105,106) (Table 1). The goal of treatment is to prevent edema in regions surrounding acute lesions and avoid ischemia in other areas (Fig. 1). An alternative view, proposed by Rosner and colleagues (110,111), holds that hyperperfusion is infrequent or clinically unimportant and that the net cerebral perfusion pressure should be maintained, even if this requires the use of pressor agents. This view is supported by observations that episodes of raised intracranial pressure (plateau waves) may be induced by a slight degree of hypotension, which leads to cerebral vasodilation, and that raised intracranial pressure may be either stabilized by preventing hypotension or terminated by raising the BP iatrogenically. If this concept proves true, then hypertension, particularly if it is episodic and occurs with raised intracranial pressure, may not require treatment.

Factors that must be considered in the decision to treat hypertension include the mean level of BP, presence of cardiac disease, likelihood of rebleeding from a parenchymal or subarachnoid hemorrhage, size and location of the mass and edema as shown by radiologic studies, and associated risk for clinical deterioration from progressive edema. Only an estimate of the ideal BP can be rendered in individual circumstances, but it is generally agreed that even minimal hypotension should be avoided. A reasonable approach in acute situations is to reduce the mean BP only to approximately 20% above normal, or 20% above premorbid levels. This reduction should be achieved slowly to avoid hypotension that would produce ischemia in areas of raised intracranial pressure or induce plateau waves (110), particularly as the acute sympathoadrenal discharge associated with stroke, hemorrhage, and trauma usually abates spontaneously over several days.

The intracranial pressure usually falls passively when the mean arterial pressure is reduced by medications. The *cerebral perfusion pressure*, which is the difference between the mean arterial and intracranial pressures, remains unchanged in these circumstances unless the antihypertensive agent used is a cerebral vasodilator that increases the intracranial blood volume. The ideal antihypertensive medication in patients with intracranial masses should therefore lower the intracranial pressure more than it reduces BP, fostering a net increase in the perfusion pressure. Lowering the intracranial pressure may also suppress the sympathoadrenal or Cushing response that initially led to the hypertension. Short-acting barbiturates, such as thiopental or pentobarbital, are the only medications that consistently produce this beneficial combination of effects on intracranial pressure and BP (57), but they are practical to use only in comatose, intubated patients, and they must be administered slowly to prevent hypotension (Table 1). Other potent antihypertensive drugs that do not adversely affect intracranial pressure include adrenergic blockers such as propranolol (45) and labetalol (132), both of which are particularly effective in patients with tachycardia, and possibly, angiotensin-converting enzyme inhibitors. Additional agents that may be employed are clonidine (67) and the now outdated ganglionic blockers, such as trimethaphan, which are nonetheless safe in patients with raised

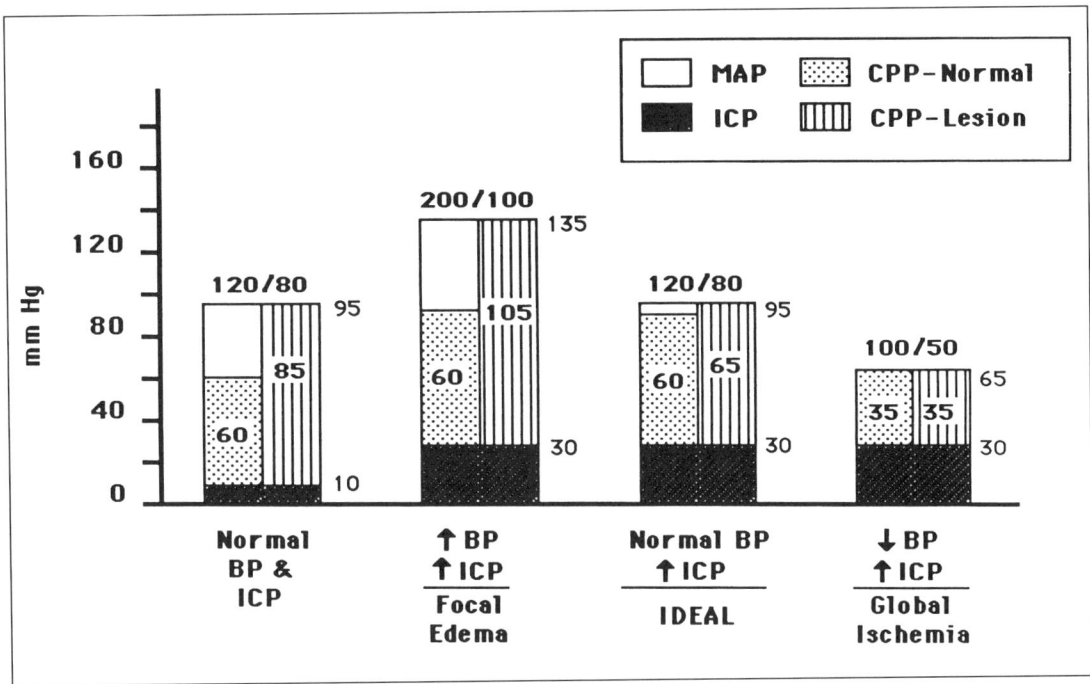

FIG. 1. BP in different regions of the brain under different BP conditions. MAP, mean arterial pressure; ICP, intracranial pressure; CPP, cerebral perfusion pressure. (From Ropper and Rockoff, ref. 106, with permission.)

intracranial pressure. Loop diuretics, such as furosemide, may produce parallel reductions in BP and intracranial pressure in some circumstances but are frequently ineffective after repeated use.

Sodium nitroprusside, the most potent agent, is used when the mean arterial pressure exceeds 140 mm Hg in awake or comatose patients because it is easily titrated, allowing for rapid withdrawal if BP begins to fluctuate. It has cerebral vasodilating effects (24) but does not usually raise intracranial pressure. Nonetheless, monitoring of intracranial pressure is advisable if there is a risk for progressive mass effect. Risks associated with continuous use of sodium nitroprusside for days include cyanide toxicity with hepatic failure, and thiocyanate toxicity with renal failure (Table 1). An alternative is continuous infusion of a short-acting adrenergic blocking agent, such as labetalol. This has become the mainstay of treatment of severe hypotension in the setting of the intensive care unit. Nitroglycerin, an erratic antihypertensive agent to which patients develop tolerance, may also cause decompensation of intracranial dynamics (23). Other antihypertensive drugs that have been associated with neurologic deterioration in patients with intracranial masses include diazoxide and hydralazine (96) and some calcium channel blockers, such as nifedipine, with the possible exception of nicardipine (9,67,92,124). These agents are recommended in special circumstances, such as control of hypertension in cases of stable subarachnoid hemorrhage, in which an increase in the cerebral blood volume and intracranial pressure might not be detrimental (Table 1). Each medication is best suited to particular clinical situations (16) (Table 1).

Hypertension After an Ischemic Stroke

Patients with acute stroke or transient ischemic attacks (TIAs) often have hypertension, usually as a pre-existing chronic condition rather than a centrally mediated result of the infarction. In one series, patients with pre-existing hypertension had higher BPs on the day of the stroke than did control subjects (129). However, a contrasting report on five patients with TIAs suggested that BP was normal or minimally elevated at the time of the acute episode (117).

The risks for precipitating complete occlusion of a stenotic vessel as a result of lowering BP are well known (10,79), but the ill-advised practice of rapidly treating mild or moderate hypertension after ischemic stroke still occurs. Hypertension abates slowly in most patients during several days after a stroke, even without treatment, and this drop in BP is most conspicuous in patients with pre-existing hypertension (129). Treatment of hypertension is therefore not recommended unless the mean pressure exceeds approximately 120 mmHg. Oral medications such as nifedipine (which may cause reflex tachycardia), propranolol, labetalol, or clonidine may be used after stroke (Table 1) if there is no imminent risk for basilar or carotid arterial occlusion. The patient's usual antihypertensive medications should be reintroduced slowly.

Neuroleptic Malignant Syndrome and Lethal Catatonia

Autonomic instability accompanies some cases of neuroleptic malignant syndrome and lethal catatonia, which is a similar but much rarer condition in psychotic patients who have not received phenothiazines. The core syndrome of muscle stiffness and rigidity in conjunction with hyperthermia has been treated with dantrolene, administered intravenously, but may also be amenable to treatment with amantadine, dopaminergic agonists such as bromocriptine or levodopa, or lorazepam. Hypertension and tachycardia may be early signs of the syndrome (2), or they may occur as an abortive form in some patients (19). The addition of β-adrenergic-blocking drugs to the primary treatments has been successful according to anecdotal accounts.

SYMPATHETIC STORM CAUSED BY SPINAL CORD LESIONS

Acute compression of the upper cervical spinal cord may rarely produce a Cushing response, isolated hypertension, cardiac arrhythmias, including cardiac arrest (44,103), or neurogenic pulmonary edema (80). All these disorders presumably stem from acute sympathetic overactivity elicited by pressure on the upper cord, and not from the more common segmental reflexive hypertension seen in the subacute and chronic stages after cord transection.

Transection of the cord above the midthoracic segments is associated with autonomic dysreflexia, including severe hypertension, in approximately half of patients (58,84). Episodes usually begin in the first few months after injury, typically as the orthostatic hypotension resolves. Paroxysms of hypertension with systolic pressures above 200 mm Hg that last several min to hrs may be precipitated by any of a number of noxious stimuli, especially bladder or bowel distention or manipulation of the viscera (4,112). Episodes are often accompanied by intense diaphoresis and piloerection. Acute headache is common and heralds a hypertensive crisis in patients with high-spinal transection.

If a precipitating factor can be identified and eliminated, BP can usually be lowered within 2 to 10 min. Many drugs have been used, with varying success, to abort the acute hypertensive state. Propantheline or oxybutynin, both anticholinergic agents, may reverse episodes, and ganglionic blockers have been popular but are rarely necessary. α-Adrenergic blockers have not proved consistently beneficial.

DYSAUTONOMIA IN NEUROMUSCULAR DISEASES

Guillain-Barré Syndrome

Acute inflammatory polyneuropathy is frequently associated with cardiovascular dysautonomia, but only a few patients have such profound fluctuations in BP that they require special attention and monitoring. Half the patients with Guillain-Barré syndrome have sinus tachycardia, sustained or paroxysmal hypertension, "vagal spells" with flushing, bronchorrhea and hypotension, or major cardiac arrhythmias (127). The most profound abnormalities occur in patients with severe weakness and respiratory failure. Only four of our approximately 250 patients with Guillain-Barré syndrome, described elsewhere (108), had severe cardiovascular dysautonomia that required special monitoring for this reason alone. All were almost fully ventilated and virtually quadriplegic.

Episodes of acute and severe hypotension seen in Guillain-Barré syndrome appear to be caused by a vasodepressor response with an accompanying drop in the systemic vascular resistance, but the pulse rate (usually 70 to 90 beats/min) is unchanged or only slightly slowed (29,107) (Fig. 2). The hypotension may last from 1 to 20 min and at times is resistant to administration of fluids and pressor agents. Nevertheless, the only treatment is crystalloid infusion and administration of an alpha agonist, such as phenylephrine. Maintaining elevated cardiac filling pressures with the guidance of a Swan-Ganz catheter reverses some episodes. Vagotonic stimuli, such as suctioning, bladder manipulation, or pain, often incite hypotensive episodes, but these episodes may also occur spontaneously. When the vasodepressor effect alternates with extreme hypertension, overtreatment with antihypertensives sometimes compounds the problem. The mechanism of dysautonomic vasodepressor episodes in Guillain-Barré syndrome is unknown.

Severe paroxysmal hypertension is a more dangerous and dramatic problem that can either coexist with hypotension or occur independently. A few exceptional cases have been reported in conjunction with papilledema and retinal hemorrhages (62,120), and possibly as a cause of subarachnoid hemorrhage (32). Hypertension may be a consequence of loss of the baroreflex buffering capacity caused by an afferent neuropathy (31). Elevated circulating levels of catecholamines and atrial natriuretic factor have been noted during both hypertensive and hypotensive episodes in patients with Guillain-Barré syndrome (32,107). Pressor agents often have erratic effects on the hypotension of Guillain-Barré syndrome and other peripheral nerve diseases. Loss of baroreflex buffering is a more likely explanation than is denervation hypersensitivity for the excessive response to pressors and rebound hypertension.

Treatment of extreme hypertension should not be too aggressive in patients with Guillain-Barré syndrome unless there is cardiovascular decompensation or myocardial ischemia. Most episodes are brief and asymptomatic and are often followed by hypotension. If the mean arterial pressure exceeds approximately 120 mmHg, sodium nitroprusside may be administered, but the BP should be closely monitored and the infusion stopped as soon as this level is reached. We have had limited experience with rapidly acting beta blockers, such as esmolol, but paroxysmal hypertension has not been precluded by the administration of longer-acting agents. Sustained severe hypertension is infrequent, but it does occur and may be more amenable to conventional antihypertensive drugs, including calcium channel blockers. When hypertension has been associated with increased renin levels, propranolol has been effective when hydralazine or diuretics have not (78).

Tetanus

Generalized tetanus produces increased muscle tone and generalized spasms, often beginning with the classic symptom of trismus, or "lockjaw." An accompanying hypersympathetic state resembles the syndromes seen with head injury; features include labile or sustained hypertension, tachycardia, profuse diaphoresis, and fever, associated with increased circulating catecholamine levels. Hypotension and bradycardia may be later findings. Tetanus toxin probably has a direct effect on the autonomic nervous system, because adrenergic overactivity persists when muscle activity is eliminated with curare (74).

In addition to administration of antitoxin and therapies directed at easing the muscle spasms (diazepam, barbiturates, neuromuscular blockade, and baclofen have all been used alone or in combination), combined α- and β-adrenergic blockers, such as labetalol, have been effective (35, 101); however, a few instances of sudden hypotension and death have been associated with their use. The hypertension has been reported to be lowered by morphine (104, 123), magnesium sulfate (128), clonidine (123), neuromuscular blockade, and intrathecally or epidurally administered anesthetic agents (122,134), even when adrenergic or ganglionic blockade was unsuccessful.

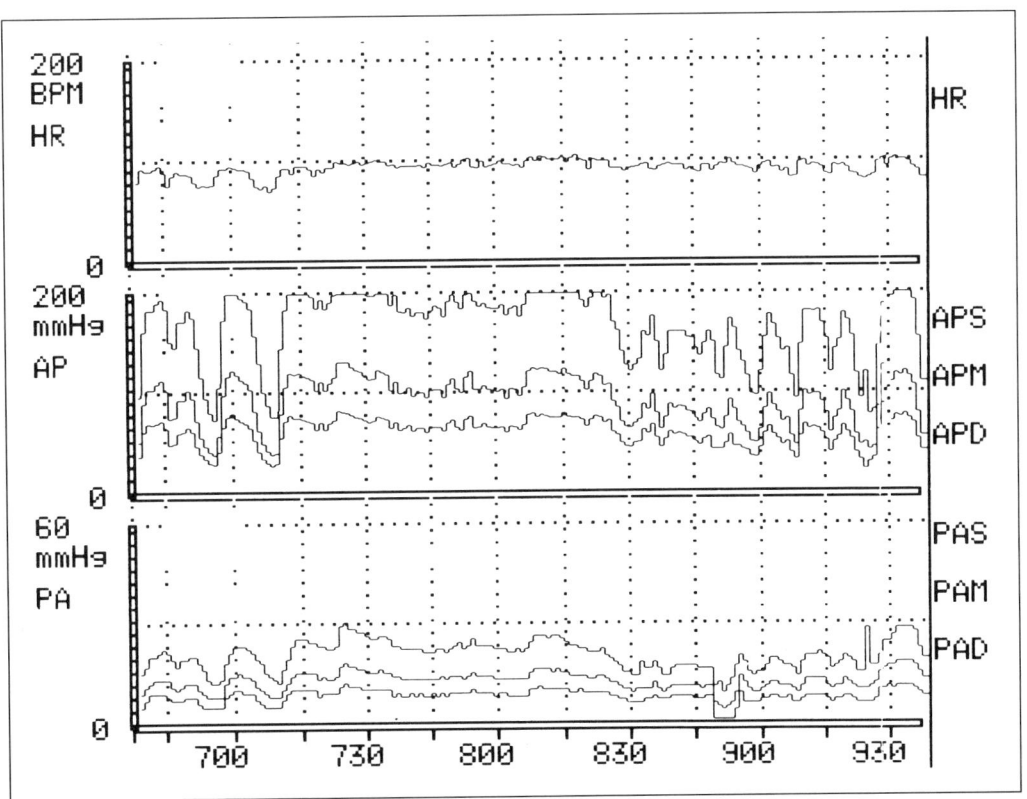

FIG. 2. BP fluctuations in a patient with dysautonomia of Guillain-Barré syndrome. There is no change or slight slowing of the pulse rate (*top panel*; *BPM*) with each episode of hypotension (*middle panel*; *AP*), suggesting a vasopressor response. Extremes of hypertension may exceed 200 mmHg systolic pressure. *Bottom panel* shows pulmonary arterial (*PA*) pressuring. *HR*, heart rate; *S*, systole; *D*, diastole; *M*, mean.

Porphyria

Attacks of acute porphyria may be accompanied by dysautonomia, including hypertension and tachycardia. The mechanism responsible is unclear, but both sympathetic and parasympathetic defects have been observed (50,76). The occurrence of labile hypertension and postural hypotension in some attacks suggests that baroreceptor afferents are disordered, as probably occurs in Guillain-Barré syndrome. Treatment with large intravenous doses of propranolol is usually successful in reducing hypertension and tachycardia (8,38,121), and it has been suggested that other neurologic deficits abate as well. Guanethidine and reserpine are among the other "safe" antihypertensive drugs for use in patients with porphyria.

Botulism

An anticholinergic state is characteristic in patients with botulism; blurred vision and dry mouth are usually present (69). These symptoms rarely represent an emergency, but there may be associated hypertension and sympathetic hyperactivity. Control of BP and heart rate are impaired early in some cases, possibly because of loss of the parasympathetic baroreflex buffering capacity (135). The autonomic component of the illness may recover more slowly than the neuromuscular blockade.

Drug Overdose

Severe hypertension, sometimes accompanied by a seizure, is an important component of the overdose syndrome associated with several illicitly used sympathomimetic drugs. The presence of hypertension may help in the prompt recognition of drug ingestion, but, as discussed earlier, coma or seizures in the presence of hypertension should first be attributed to a cerebral hemorrhage, particularly if accompanied by the bradycardia of a Cushing response.

Phenylpropanolamine, an amphetamine-like sympathomimetic, is used in over-the-counter diet aids and nasal congestion preparations; it is called "street speed," "magnums," or "pink hearts." It is often combined with caffeine, is rapidly absorbed from the gastrointestinal tract, and has a variable half-life of 3 to 6 hrs. Enzyme-multiplied immunoassay techniques (EMIT) for toxic screening may misidentify the drug as amphetamine. The toxicity syndrome consists of confusion, occasional psychosis, headache, blurred vision, and hypertension (68) simulating hypertensive encephalopathy. Numerous cases of small intracranial hemorrhages have been reported. Treatment is supportive, because the toxicity is brief, but extreme hypertension is treated with phentolamine or nitroprusside.

Overdose of cocaine, including "crack," may cause hypertension that is usually not as severe as with phenylpropanolamine. It is overshadowed by features of central nervous system stimulation, including pupillary dilatation, tachycardia, and psychosis. Supraventricular or ventricular tachycardias are common, and seizures or intracranial hemorrhage have been reported. Treatment of the hypertension is pre-empted by the need to control the arrhythmias, but several agents, such as beta blockers, may accomplish both. The reported paroxysmal hypertension that followed propranolol treatment of a cocaine overdose (102) may have been caused by unopposed α-adrenergic activity.

An overdose of a tricyclic antidepressant precipitates an anticholinergic state that is accompanied by peripheral, central, and cardiac dysautonomia. Besides the well-known signs of flushing, tachycardia, fever, mydriasis, and absent sweating, there may be an acute toxic psychosis, myoclonus, movement disorders, seizures, and coma. The main morbidity is associated with arrhythmias and quinidine-like effects (increased QT interval, prolonged QRS interval, and heart block). Hypotension occurs with extreme overdoses (serum concentrations above 1000 ng/mL), but some patients with intermediate syndromes also have hypertension. The earlier enthusiasm for treatment with physostigmine has waned because of adverse effects, including seizures and bradycardia. It is now used cautiously as a diagnostic test. Rare severe hypertension is treated with nitroprusside, and hypotension is treated with any of several pressor agents. The arrhythmias are often resistant to treatment with the usual medications (48).

INTENSIVE CARE AND SECONDARY EFFECTS OF SEVERE AUTONOMIC DYSFUNCTION

Patients with severe dysautonomia usually require admission to an intensive care unit because of the severity of their primary illness; a few who otherwise have relatively mild intracranial or peripheral nervous system disease are admitted solely because of BP fluctuations. The most compelling reason for admission is the risk for secondary damage to systemic organs caused by extremes of BP. The cardiovascular management of hypotension or hypertension, bradycardia or tachycardia, and arrhythmias is generally the same regardless of the underlying disease.

Unlike the situation in most other areas of medicine, the hypertension associated with dysautonomia is more common and more treacherous than hypotension; most of the diseases discussed in this chapter do not produce life-threatening hypotension until they are so advanced that death is imminent. Severe hypertension, with a mean arterial pressure above 140 mmHg, precipitates a complex set of changes in all organs that may lead to myocardial damage, and it exaggerates the mass effect and increased intracranial pressure that initially generated the hypertension. Signs of hypertensive encephalopathy, a theoretical risk and rare secondary phenomenon in dysautonomia, may be obscured by the clinical signs of an intracranial mass.

The cardiac risks of severe hypertension are related to age, coexistent valvular disease, and, most importantly, coronary artery disease. Acute hypertension may precipitate congestive heart failure, brought about by the increased afterload. One hypothesized mechanism for the *neurogenic pulmonary edema* arising from brain lesions incorporates the effects of hypertension and acute left ventricular overload on the pulmonary circulation. A few poorly documented cases of neurogenic pulmonary edema have been reported in conjunction with severe paroxysmal hypertension caused by the peripheral dysautonomia of Guillain-Barré syndrome.

Mean arterial blood pressure falling below 80 mmHg can cause coronary, renal, or bowel hypoperfusion, especially in the presence of pre-existing atherosclerotic occlusive disease. Hypotension that is severe enough to cause organ failure, manifested as coma, angina, ECG changes denoting ischemia, or decreased urinary volume, justifies surveillance in an intensive care unit and treatment with fluids and pressor agents. Depending on how rapidly the BP is declining, patients generally become unresponsive when the mean arterial pressure falls below 45 mmHg. Global or watershed infarction of the brain from paroxysmal hypotension is rare without additional reduction of flow from carotid arterial stenosis. For example, I have encountered three patients with Guillain-Barré syndrome, each of whom had no lasting neurologic deficit after more than 20 episodes of paroxysmal hypotension that caused transient unresponsiveness.

Patients at risk for cardiovascular complications, particularly if hypertension or severe hypotension is likely to precipitate angina, myocardial ischemia, or heart failure, should be observed in an intensive care unit with continuous ECG and BP monitoring.

TECHNIQUES OF MEASURING BLOOD PRESSURE IN ACUTE DYSAUTONOMIA

Measurements of systolic and diastolic BP may differ depending on the techniques used, but mean arterial pressure readings remain relatively consistent and usually serve as the best guide to the appropriate acute therapy. In hypersympathetic states, when pressure is monitored through an arterial cannula, an apparent overshoot may be detected as a result of increased cardiac output and peripheral vasoconstriction, which generate higher systolic and lower diastolic pressures than are measured with occlusion (cuff) methods. The occlusion systolic pressures in these circumstances may be lower by 15 mmHg to 20 mmHg than intraluminally recorded arterial pressures. Both pressures are "real," but they represent different mechanical properties of the arterial system. Distortions may also be introduced by resonance originating from low-compliance catheter-transducer systems. A typical radial arterial cannula configuration with 4 feet (1.2 meters) of low-compliance tubing has a resonant frequency of approximately 20 Hz to 30 Hz, which is normally higher than the components of the arterial pressure wave. However, in patients in the hypersympathetic states discussed in this chapter, the rapid arterial pressure upstrokes produce pressure waveform frequencies that approach the system's resonant frequency, rarely causing "ringing" with spuriously raised systolic pressures.

Cannulation of the radial or other peripheral arteries is currently the most commonly used technique for the continuous monitoring of BP fluctuations, or for monitoring of BP when pressor agents or intravenously administered antihypertensive drugs are necessary. Self-cycled oscillometric cuff devices, however, suffice for monitoring in many neurologic patients. The more recently introduced continuous noninvasive fiberoptic plethysmographic techniques (36) are often useful for neurologic applications, but in patients in hypersympathetic vasoconstricted states, the pressures registered are 10 mmHg or more lower than those shown by oscillometric devices. Noninvasive techniques do not allow access for blood sampling, and until recently they have not allowed monitoring of arterial blood gas levels, but they do track BP accurately and continuously (fiberoptic) or nearly continuously (oscillometric). Trend monitoring, which is an important adjunct to any method of BP and pulse rate recording in an intensive care unit, can assess the frequency of acute BP changes, effects of therapy, and the relationship between BP, clinical signs, and other physiologic measurements, such as intracranial or pulmonary arterial pressures.

REFERENCES

1. Acheson J, et al. Serum creatine kinase levels in cerebral vascular disease. *Lancet* 1965;1:1306–1307.
2. Adityanjee PD. Neurologic malignant syndrome and early autonomic dysfunction (Letter). *Acta Psychiatr Scand* 1987;75:447–448.
3. Andy OJ, Jurko M. Diencephalic seizures. Case report. *Appl Neurophysiol* 1983;46:62–67.
4. Arieff AJ, et al. Acute hypertension induced by urinary bladder distension. *Arch Neurol* 1962;6:248–256.
5. Aring CD, Engle GL. Hypothalamic attacks with thalamic lesion. II. Anatomic considerations. *Arch Neurol Psychiatry* 1945;54:44–50.
6. Artiola A, et al. Long-term prognosis in surgically treated intracranial aneurysms. *J Neurosurg* 1981;54:26–34.
7. Barry DI. Cerebrovascular aspects of antihypertensive treatment. *Am J Cardiol* 1989;63:14C–18C.
8. Beattie AD, et al. Acute intermittent porphyria: response of tachycardia and hypertension to propranolol. *Br Med J* 1973;3:257–260.
9. Bedford RF, et al. Adverse impact of a calcium entry-blocker (verapamil) on intracranial pressure in patients with brain tumors. *J Neurosurg* 1983;59:800–802.
10. Britton M, et al. Hazards of therapy for excessive hypertension in acute stroke. *Acta Med Scand* 1980;207:253.
11. Broumers PJAM, et al. Serial electrocardiographic recordings in aneurysmal subarachnoid hemorrhage. *Stroke* 1989;20:1162–1167.
12. Buisseret P. Acute pulmonary edema following *grand mal* epilepsy and as a complication of electric shock therapy. *Br J Dis* 1982;76:198.

13. Bullard DE. Diencephalic seizures: responsiveness to bromocriptine and morphine. *Ann Neurol* 1987;21:609–611.
14. Burch GE, et al. A new electrocardiographic pattern observed in cerebrovascular accidents. *Circulation* 1954;9: 719–723.
15. Byer E, et al. Electrocardiogram with large upright T waves and long Q-T intervals. *Am Heart J* 1947;33:796–799.
16. Calhoun DA, Oparil S. Treatment of hypertensive crisis. *N Engl J Med* 1990;323:1177–1183.
17. Cameron SJ, Doig A. Cerebellar tumors presenting with clinical features of pheochromocytoma. *Lancet* 1970;1:492–494.
18. Carmel PW. Vegetative dysfunctions of the hypothalamus. *Acta Neurochir* 1985;75:113–121.
19. Clark T, et al. On the early recognition of neuroleptic malignant syndrome. *Int J Psychiatry Med* 1985/1986;15:299–310.
20. Clifton GL, et al. Circulating catecholamines and sympathetic activity after head injury. *Neurosurgery* 1981;8: 10–14.
21. Clifton GL, et al. Cardiovascular responses to severe head injury. *J Neurosurg* 1983;59:447–454.
22. Colville KL, et al. Mechanism involved in the cardiovascular response to transcranial stimulation. *Arch Neurol Psychiatry* 1958;80: 374–379.
23. Cottrell JE, et al. Intracranial pressure during nitroglycerine-induced hypotension. *J Neurosurg* 1980;53:309–311.
24. Cottrell JE, et al. Intracranial pressure elevations induced by sodium nitroprusside in patients with intracranial mass lesions. *J Neurosurg* 1978;48:329–331.
25. Crompton MR. Hypothalami lesions following the rupture of cerebral berry aneurysms. *Brain* 1963;86:301–314.
26. Cropp GJ, Manning GW. Electrocardiographic changes simulating myocardial ischemia and infarction associated with spontaneous intracranial hemorrhage. *Circulation* 1960;22:25–38.
27. Cushing H. Some experimental and clinical observations concerning states of increased intracranial tension. *Am J Med Sci* 1902; 124:375–400.
28. Cushing H. The blood pressure reaction of acute cerebral compression, illustrated by cases of intracranial hemorrhage. *Am J Med Sci* 1903;125:1017–1044.
29. Dalos NP, et al. Cardiovascular autonomic dysfunction in Guillain-Barré syndrome: therapeutic implications of Swan-Ganz monitoring. *Arch Neurol* 1988;45:115–117.
30. Darnell J, Jay SJ. Recurrent postictal pulmonary edema. A case report and review of the literature. *Epilepsia* 1982;23:71–83.
31. Davidson DL, Jellinek EH. Hypertension and papilledema in the Guillain-Barré syndrome. *J Neurol Neurosurg Psychiatry* 1977;40: 144–148.
32. Davies AG, Dingle H. Observations on cardiovascular and neuroendocrine disturbance in Guillain-Barré syndrome. *J Neurol Neurosurg Psychiatry* 1972;35:176–179.
33. Dispaquale G, et al. Holter detection of cardiac arrhythmias in intracranial subarachnoid hemorrhage. *Am J Cardiol* 1987;59:596–600.
34. Doba N, et al. Changes in regional blood flow and cardiodynamics associated with electrically and chemically induced epilepsy in cat. *Brain Res* 1975;90:115–132.
35. Domenighetti GM, et al. Hyperadrenergic syndrome in severe tetanus: extreme rise in catecholamines responsive to labetalol. *Br Med J* 1984;288:1483–1484.
36. Dorlas JC, et al. Effects of peripheral vasoconstriction on the blood pressure in the finger, measured continuously by a new non-invasive method (the Finapres). *Anesthesiology* 1985;62:342–345.
37. Doshi R, Nei-Dwyer G. A clinicopathological study of patients following a subarachnoid hemorrhage. *J Neurosurg* 1980;52:295–301.
38. Douer D, et al. Treatment of acute intermittent porphyria with large doses of propranolol. *JAMA* 1978;240:766–768.
39. Drop LJ, et al. Arterial hypertension and multiple cerebral aneurysms in a patient treated with electroconvulsive therapy. *J Clin Psychiatry* 1988;49:280–282.
40. Eshel Y, et al. Effect of electroconvulsive treatment on serum beta-hydroxylase activity in man. *Experientia* 1978;34:212–213.
41. Estanol BV, Marin OSM. Cardiac arrhythmias and sudden death in subarachnoid hemorrhage. *Stroke* 1975;6:382–385.
42. Estanol BV, et al. Cardiac arrhythmias in experimental subarachnoid hemorrhage. *Stroke* 1977;8:440–447.
43. Evans CH, et al. Astrocytoma mimicking the features of pheochromocytoma. *N Engl J Med* 1972;286:1397–1399.
44. Evans DE, et al. Cardiac arrhythmias accompanying acute compression of the spinal cord. *J Neurosurg* 1980;52: 52–59.
45. Feibel JH, et al. Catecholamine-associated refractory hypertension following acute intracranial hemorrhage: control with propranolol. *Ann Neurol* 1980;9:340–343.
46. Fentz V, Gormsen J. Electrocardiographic patterns in patients with cerebrovascular accidents. *Circulation* 1962;25:22–28.
47. Fox RH, et al. Spontaneous periodic hypothermia: diencephalic epilepsy. *Br Med J* 1973;2:693–695.
48. Frommer DA, et al. Tricyclic antidepressant overdose. A review. *JAMA* 1987;257:521–526.
49. Fuster JM, Weinberg SJ. Bioelectric changes of the heart cycle induced by stimulation of diencephalic regions. *Exp Neurol* 1960; 2:26–39.
50. Goto J, et al. Autonomic dysfunctions in acute intermittent porphyria. *Rinsho Shinkeigaku* 1989;29:774–777.
51. Gravenstein JS, et al. Catecholamine and cardiovascular response to electro-convulsion therapy in man. *Br J Anaesth* 1965;37:833–839.
52. Greenhoot JH, Reichenbach DD. Cardiac injury and subarachnoid hemorrhage: a clinical pathological and physiological correlation. *J Neurosurg* 1969;30:521–531.
53. Hallpike JF, et al. Glucose tolerance and plasma insulin levels in subarachnoid hemorrhage. *Brain* 1971;94:151–164.
54. Hansson L, Larsson O. The incidence of ECG abnormalities in acute cerebrovascular accidents. *Acta Med Scand* 1974;195:45–47.
55. Hammer WJ, et al. Observations on the electrocardiographic changes associated with subarachnoid hemorrhage with special reference to their genesis. *Am J Med Sci* 1975; 59:427–433.
56. Harrison MT, Gibb BH. Electrocardiographic changes associated with myocardial damage in patients with acute cerebrovascular accidents. *Stroke* 1977;8:448–455.
57. Hayashi M, et al. Treatment of systemic hypertension and intracranial hypertension in cases of brain hemorrhage. *Stroke* 1988;19: 314–321.
58. Head H, Riccoch G. The autonomic bladder, excessive sweating and some other reflex conditions in gross injuries of the spinal cord. *Brain* 1917;40:188–263.
59. Heinrich D, Muller W. Focal myocardial necrosis in cases of increased intracranial pressure. *Eur Neurol* 1974;12:369–376.
60. Hersch C. Electrocardiographic changes in head injuries. *Circulation* 1961;23:853–869.
61. Hersch C. Electrocardiographic changes in subarachnoid hemorrhage, meningitis, and intracranial space-occupying lesions. *Br Heart J* 1964;26:785–793.
62. Hewer RL, et al. Acute polyneuritis requiring artificial respiration. *Q J Med* 1966;37:479–491.
63. Hijdra A, et al. Respiratory arrest in subarachnoid hemorrhage. *Neurology* 1984;34:1501–1503.
64. Hockman CH, et al. ECG changes resulting from cerebral stimulation. II. A spectrum of ventricular arrhythmias of sympathetic origin. *Am Heart J* 1966;71:695–700.
65. Hoff JT, Reis DJ. Localization of regions mediating the Cushing response in CNS of cat. *Arch Neurol* 1970;23:228–240.
66. Hortnagl H. The activity of the sympathetic nervous system following severe head injury. *Intensive Care Med* 1980;6:169–177.
67. Houston MC. The comparative effects of clonidine hydrochloride and nifedipine in the treatment of hypertensive crisis. *Am Heart J* 1983;115:152–159.
68. Howrie DL, Watson JH. Phenylpropanolamine-induced hypertensive seizures. *J Pediatr* 1983;102:143–145.
69. Jenzer G, et al. Autonomic dysfunction in botulism B: a clinical report. *Neurology* 1975;25:150–153.
70. Johnson RH, et al. *Neurocardiology.* London: Saunders; 1984.
71. Jones JV. Differentiation and investigation of primary versus secondary hypertension. *Am J Cardiol* 1989;63:10C–13C.
72. Jones RM, Knight PR. Cardiovascular and hormonal responses to electroconvulsive therapy. *Anesthesia* 1981;36:795–799.
73. Kennedy PGE, Moxham J. Transient severe hypertension following alcohol withdrawal seizures. *Postgrad Med J* 1980;56:252–253.
74. Kerr JH. Involvement of the sympathetic nervous system in tetanus. *Lancet* 1968;2:236–241.
75. Koskelo P, et al. Subendocardial hemorrhage and ECG changes in intracranial bleeding. *Br Med J* 1964;1:1479–1480.
76. Laiwah AC, et al. Autonomic neuropathy in acute intermittent porphyria. *J Neurol Neurosurg Psychiatry* 1985;48:1025–1030.

77. Langfitt JW, et al. The pathophysiology of brain swelling produced by mechanical trauma and hypertension. *Scand J Clin Lab Invest* 1968;22(Suppl 102):144.
78. Laufer J, et al. Raised plasma renin activity in the hypertension of Guillain-Barré syndrome. *Br Med J* 1981;282:1272–1273.
79. Lavin P. Management of hypertension in patients with acute stroke. *Arch Intern Med* 1980;146:66–68.
80. Lee DS, Korbrine A. Neurogenic pulmonary edema associated with ruptured spinal cord arteriovenous malformation. *Neurosurgery* 1983;12:691–693.
81. Lehrich JR, et al. Cerebellar infarction with brainstem compression. *Arch Neurol* 1970;22:490–498.
82. Levine H. Non-specificity of the electrocardiogram associated with coronary artery disease. *Am J Med* 1953;15:344–354.
83. Lewis WH, et al. Cardiovascular disturbances and their management in modified electrotherapy for psychiatric illness. *N Engl J Med* 1955;252:1016–1020.
84. Lindan R, et al. Incidence and clinical features of autonomic dysreflexia in patients with spinal cord injury. *Paraplegia* 1980;18:285–292.
85. Magnus O, et al. Cerebral mechanisms and neurogenic hypertension in man, with special reference to baroreceptor control. In: DeJong W, Provost AP, Shapiro AP, eds. *Hypertension and Brain Mechanisms*. Amsterdam; Elsevier; 1977:199–218 (*Progress in Brain Research*; vol 47).
86. Marion DW, et al. Subarachnoid hemorrhage and the heart. *Neurosurgery* 1986;18:101–106.
87. McLean AJ. Autonomic epilepsy. Report of a case with observations at necropsy. *Arch Neurol Psychiatry* 1934;32:1891–1897.
88. Menon IS. Electrocardiographic changes simulating myocardial infarction in cerebrovascular accident. *Lancet* 1964;2:433–434.
89. Metz SA, et al. Autonomic epilepsy: clonidine blockade of paroxysmal catecholamine release and flushing. *Ann Intern Med* 1978;88:189–193.
90. Mosier JM, et al. Cerebroautonomic and myographic changes accompanying induced seizures. *Neurology* 1957;7:204–210.
91. Mulgoakar GD, et al. Noninvasive assessment of electroconvulsive-induced changes in cardiac function. *J Clin Psychiatry* 1985;46:479–482.
92. Nishikawa T, et al. The effects of nicardipine on cerebrospinal fluid pressure in humans. *Anesth Analg* 1986;65:508–510.
93. Nogues M, et al. Unusual manifestations of basilar artery ectasia. *Eur Neurol* 1988;28:345–348.
94. Norris JW, et al. Serum cardiac enzymes in stroke. *Stroke* 1979;10:548–553.
95. Oppenheimer SM, et al. Cerebrogenic cardiac arrhythmias. Cerebral electrographic influences and their role in sudden death. *Arch Neurol* 1990;47:513–519.
96. Overgard J, Skinhoj E. A paradoxical cerebral hemodynamic effect of hydralazine. *Stroke* 1975;6:402–404.
97. Pasztor A, Pasztor E. Spinal vasomotor reflex and Cushing response. *Acta Neurochir* 1980;52:85–97.
98. Penfield W. Diencephalic autonomic epilepsy. *Arch Neurol Psychiatry* 1929;22:358–374.
99. Penfield H. *Epilepsy and the Functional Anatomy of the Human Brain*. Boston: Little, Brown; 1954.
100. Perrin GM. Cardiovascular aspects of electric shock therapy. *Acta Psychiatr Neurol Scand* 1961;36:1–45.
101. Prys-Roberts C, et al. Treatment of sympathetic overactivity in tetanus. *Lancet* 1969;1:542–546.
102. Ramoska E, Sachetti AD. Propranolol-induced hypertension in treatment of cocaine intoxication. *Ann Emerg Med* 1985;14:1112–1113.
103. Rayner PR. Cardiac arrhythmias during high spinal surgery. *Br Med J* 1983;287:182.
104. Rie MA, Wilson RS. Morphine therapy controls autonomic hyperactivity in tetanus. *Ann Intern Med* 1978;88:653–654.
105. Robertson CS, et al. Treatment of hypertension associated with head injury. *J Neurosurg* 1983;59:455–460.
106. Ropper AH, Rockoff MA. Treatment of intracranial hypertension. In: Ropper AH, ed. *Neurological and Neurosurgical Intensive Care*. New York: Raven Press; 1993.
107. Ropper AH, Wijdicks EFM. Blood pressure fluctuations in the dysautonomia of Guillain-Barré syndrome. *Arch Neurol* 1990;47:706–708.
108. Ropper AH, et al. *Guillain-Barré Syndrome*. Philadelphia: FA Davis; 1991.
109. Rosenbaum KJ, et al. Sympathetic nervous system response to lidocaine-induced seizures in cats. *Acta Anaesthesiol Scand* 1978;22:548–555.
110. Rosner NJ, et al. Mechanical brain injury: the sympathoadrenal response. *J Neurosurg* 1984;61:76–86.
111. Rosner NJ, Daughton S. Cerebral perfusion pressure management in head injury. *J Trauma* 1990;30:933–940.
112. Scher AT. Autonomic hyperreflexia: a serious complication of radiological procedures in patients with cervical or upper thoracic spinal cord lesions. *S Afr Med J* 1978;53:208–210.
113. Schrader H, et al. Influence of blood pressure on tolerance to an intracranial expanding mass. *Acta Neurol Scand* 1985;71:114–126.
114. Schutta EH, et al. Brain swelling produced by injury and aggravated by hypertension. *Brain* 1968;91:281–294.
115. Simard JM, Bellefleur M. Systemic arterial hypertension in head trauma. *Am J Cardiol* 1989;63:32–35.
116. Simon RP. Neurogenic pulmonary edema. *Semin Neurol* 1984;4:490–496.
117. Skinhoj E, et al. Regional cerebral blood flow and its autoregulation in patients with transient focal cerebral ischemic attacks. *Neurology* 1970;20:485–493.
118. Smith RP, Tomlinson BE. Subendocardial hemorrhages associated with intracranial lesions. *Br J Pathol Bacteriol* 1954;68:327–374.
119. Solomon GE. Diencephalic autonomic epilepsy caused by a neoplasm. *J Pediatr* 1973;83:277–280.
120. Spalding JMK, Smith AC. *Clinical Practice of Physiology of Artificial Respiration*. Oxford: Blackwell Scientific; 1963.
121. Srugo I, et al. Acute intermittent porphyria—an unusual case of "surgical" abdomen. Response to propranolol. *Eur J Pediatr* 1987;146:305–308.
122. Sugimoto H, et al. The use of continuous spinal anesthesia in severe tetanus with autonomic disturbance. *J Trauma* 1989;29:1423–1429.
123. Sutton DN, et al. Management of autonomic dysfunction in severe tetanus: the use of magnesium sulfate and clonidine. *Intensive Care Med* 1980;16:75–80.
124. Tateishi A, et al. Effects of nifedipine on intracranial pressure in neurosurgical patients with hypertension. *J Neurosurg* 1988;69:213–215.
125. Thompson RK, Malina S. Dynamic axial brain-stem distortion as a mechanism explaining the cardio-respiratory change in increased intracranial pressure. *J Neurosurg* 1959;16:664–675.
126. Torner JC, et al. Preoperative prognostic factors for rebleeding and survival in aneurysm patients receiving antifibrinolytic treatment: report of the Cooperative Aneurysm Study. *Neurosurgery* 1981;9:506–513.
127. Truax BT. Autonomic disturbances in the Guillain-Barré syndrome. *Semin Neurol* 1984;4:462–468.
128. Udwadia FE, et al. Tetanus and its complications: intensive care and management in 150 Indian patients. *Epidemiol Infect* 1987;99:675–684.
129. Wallace JD, Levy LL. Blood pressure after stroke. *JAMA* 1981;246:2177–2180.
130. Weintraub BM, McHenry LC. Cardiac abnormalities in subarachnoid hemorrhage: a resume. *Stroke* 1974;5:384–392.
131. Welch CA, Drop LJ. Cardiovascular effects of ECT. *Convulsive Ther* 1989;5:35–43.
132. Wilson DJ, et al. Intravenous labetalol in the treatment of severe hypertension. *Am J Med* 1983;75(Suppl 4):95–102.
133. Wortsman J, et al. Hyperadrenergic state after trauma to the neuraxis. *JAMA* 1980;243:1459–1460.
134. Wright DK, et al. Autonomic nervous system dysfunction in severe tetanus: current perspectives. *Crit Care Med* 1989;17:371–375.
135. Vita G, et al. Cardiovascular reflex testing and single-fiber electromyography in botulism. *Arch Neurol* 1987;44:202–206.

CHAPTER 58

Management of Male Sexual Dysfunction

John D. Stewart

1. The focus of this chapter is the treatment of organic erectile dysfunction.
2. Oral or buccal medications for erectile dysfunction include yohimbine, trazodone, and apomorphine.
3. Proerectile medications topically applied to the penis include nitroglycerin paste and minoxidil.
4. Substances injected into the corpora cavernosa are more effective than oral, buccal, or topical medications. Papaverine, phentolamine, prostaglandin E_1 (PGE_1), or combinations of these are effective in erectile impotence stemming from several causes.
5. Penile implants have also been used successfully in restoring erectile function. An alternative method for some patients is a vacuum device.
6. In some patients with arterial insufficiency, arterial revascularization of the penis can be effective. In patients with excessive venous leakage, venous occlusion can also restore erectile function.
7. Erectile dysfunction caused by hyperprolactinemia is treated with bromocriptine and pituitary surgery. Androgens are used for patients with hypogonadism.
8. Retrograde ejaculation is often best left untreated, but desipramine is sometimes helpful. Sperm release for the purpose of artificial insemination in men with anejaculation can be accomplished by using vibratory stimuli, subcutaneous physostigmine, or electrostimulation techniques.

INTRODUCTION

The physiology of sexual function is described in Chapter 11, and the evaluation of male patients with erectile failure is discussed in Chapters 21 and 22. This chapter deals with the management of male sexual dysfunction in the context of organic dysfunction, principally erectile impotence resulting from impairment of the autonomic nervous system.

CAUSES

In devising a rational management strategy for a male patient with sexual dysfunction, the first step is to classify his dysfunction according to type: diminished libido, erectile impairment, or ejaculatory disorder (Chapter 21, Table 1). Impairment of erection is the most common. A further, critical subdivision is made according to whether the dysfunction has a psychogenic or an organic cause. However, these are not mutually exclusive, in that organic impairment of erection often produces secondary psychologic problems, notably anxiety, which in turn aggravate the original problem of organic erectile dysfunction.

MANAGEMENT OF ORGANIC ERECTILE IMPOTENCE

Once the presence and cause of organic erectile dysfunction have been established, five preliminary steps should be taken before embarking on treatment:

1. Consideration should be given to whether specific treatment is required. Some couples, after being reassured that the man's impaired sexual performance does not have a psychologic or psychiatric cause, or is not related to extraconjugal sexual activities, are prepared to abstain from coitus or derive sexual pleasure from activities other than coitus.
2. It is important to treat secondary psychologic problems, principally anxiety. Confirming an organic cause goes a long way in doing this, but consulting with a psychologist, psychiatrist, or trained sex therapist may be additionally helpful.

J. D. Stewart: Department of Neurology and Neurosurgery, McGill University, Montreal, Quebec H3A 2B4, CANADA.

TABLE 1. *Treatment of organic erectile dysfunction*

General measures
  Decide if treatment is necessary
  Treat **secondary** psychological problems
  Remove aggravating factors (alcohol, medications)
  Address general medical problems
  Consider age
Specific measures
  Pharmacologic
    Oral medications
    Intracavernosal injections
  Mechanical
    Penile implants
    Vacuum devices
  Vascular
    Arterial revascularization
    Venous occlusion
  Hormonal
    Treat hyperprolactinemia
    Treat hypogonadism

TABLE 2. *Choice of treatment in organic male erectile dysfunction*

Medications
  Stop medications
Neurogenic
  Oral yohimbine, trazodone
  Intracavernosal injections of papaverine, phentolamine, prostaglandin E_1; mixtures of these
  Penile prostheses
Arterial insufficiency
  Revascularization
  Intracavernosal injections
  Penile prostheses
Venous leakage
  Venous occlusion
  Penile prostheses
Endocrine
  Bromocriptine
  Pituitary surgery
  Androgens

3. Factors that might aggravate erectile dysfunction should be eliminated. Alcohol and certain medications (see Chapter 21) are the principle culprits.
4. A variety of general medical factors may contribute to impaired sexual performance and should be addressed if possible. These include poor sleep, chronic pain, depression, malnutrition, hypothyroidism, and any other cause of general poor health.
5. It is well recognized that libido and frequency of erections decrease with age (42). Some patients' complaints of reduced sexual activity are merely a reflection of this normal age-related physiologic change and do not require treatment.

Specific treatments for dealing with organic erectile dysfunction are summarized in Tables 1 and 2.

Oral Pharmacologic Agents

Very few oral medications are available for the treatment of erectile dysfunction in men (33). Yohimbine, which is chemically related to reserpine, has long been reputed to be an aphrodisiac. It acts peripherally as an α-adrenergic antagonist, thus blocking sympathetic/adrenergic antierectile mechanisms. Yohimbine also readily enters the central nervous system, where it blocks α_2-adrenergic receptors, but whether this contributes to its role in improving erections is unclear.

A randomized, controlled study with partial crossover of yohimbine versus placebo in men with organic impotence from a variety of causes showed an overall improvement in 43% of the patients (complete response in 20%; partial response in 23%) (31). The authors concluded that a satisfactory "response rate . . . is at best marginal"; however, the drug may be more effective in higher doses than those used in that study. It is possible that this drug is more effective in certain subgroups of organically impotent men, but this has not yet been determined (47). In patients with primarily psychogenic impotence, yohimbine has been shown to be clearly better than placebo (40).

Used in larger amounts than the standard daily doses, yohimbine has been anecdotally reported as being effective as an "on demand" proerectile agent. The effectiveness of yohimbine may be enhanced by combining it with trazodone (see below), according to the results of a double-blind placebo-controlled study of men with *psychogenic* impotence (30). It is clear that further studies with yohimbine are required.

Because of its ease of administration and relative lack of major side effects, it is appropriate to use yohimbine as an initial therapy; it is also appropriate for patients who find more invasive methods unacceptable. The dose is 30 mg/d (31,33).

Trazodone is an antidepressant and anxiolytic drug that has complex pharmacologic actions, including antiserotoninergic effects. As a result of reports of increased libido and of priapism in both men and women taking this drug for depression, studies of its utility as a proerectile agent have been performed (1,9,15,18,37,41). Trazodone does seem capable of improving erectile ability in some patients, but controlled studies in patients rigorously categorized as to cause of erectile dysfunction are required before this drug can gain acceptance. It is widely believed that trazodone and yohimbine taken together have a synergistic effect, although supporting data are limited (30,33). Because of this belief, some physicians now use this combination as a first-line oral treatment for sexual dysfunction (15,33). As with yohimbine, it has yet to be clearly identified as to which types of sexual dysfunction are best treated with trazodone.

Apomorphine is a dopamine agonist that has long been known to produce erections when given subcutaneously. A buccal tablet that has been developed for "on demand" use shows promise, although side-effects can be troublesome (19).

Topical Agents

Nitroglycerin is a smooth muscle relaxant that has been used for years to treat angina pectoris. An early study suggested that nitroglycerin paste applied to the penis can produce erections (32). A more recent controlled trial has shown that this treatment produces better erections than placebo in 85% of patients (13,34). Unfortunately, the effects are not usually adequate to permit penetration. There are also concerns about side effects, such as headache, in both patient and partner, "with disastrous consequences for sexual performance," because the paste is readily absorbed (33). Minoxidil is a vasodilator used for the treatment of baldness. Although one report has shown it to be better than nitroglycerin as a topical agent, other studies have not found the drug to be effective (5,7,39).

Intracavernosal Injections

Intracavernosal injections can be effective treatment for patients with erectile dysfunction of vasculogenic, neurologic, psychogenic, and mixed causes. The principal drugs used are papaverine, phentolamine, and PGE_1. All three have a direct relaxing action on vascular and nonvascular smooth muscle; phentolamine may also work by inhibition of antierectile α-adrenergic receptors (4,12,50). Phentolamine when used alone produces erections that are too brief, so is often combined with papaverine (4). For several years, papaverine was the drug of choice (4,23), but it is being superseded by PGE_1. The latter is more effective than papaverine alone and has about the same efficacy as papaverine plus phentolamine (12); PGE_1 has fewer side effects than papaverine (22). The Alprostadil Study Group has reported that in 577 men using PGE_1 injections at home, 69% were still using the treatment at 6 months, and satisfactory sexual activity occurred after 87% of the injections (22).

Combinations of phentolamine, papaverine, and PGE_1 may produce even better results than a single agent or dual combination (27). Trials are currently under way to evaluate the efficacy of intraurethral administration of PGE_1 (36). Combining intracavernosal injections with the use of a vacuum device (see below) is a useful approach in men who have inadequate responses to the injections (8).

The dose of the intracavernous medication is established with test doses adjusted to the patient's response. Paraplegics may respond to very low doses (11). Then the patient or his partner is taught how to inject the drug. Patient and partner satisfaction is relatively high (12,22,54). Penile pain is the main side effect, occurring in up to 50% of men in a large PGE_1 study, although it occurred after only 11% of injections; however, 6% of men discontinued use of injections for this reason (22). Prolonged erections occur in 5% of men using PGE_1 and 11% of those using papaverine (22,57). Priapism is the most worrying complication; it occurs less frequently with PGE_1 (1%) and with the combination of all three medications than with papaverine alone or combined with phentolamine (12,22). Priapism can be reversed by aspiration of the corpora cavernosa and irrigation with an α-adrenergic agonist solution, such as ephedrine, epinephrine, or phenylephrine (23). The most serious long-term complication is scarring within the corpora cavernosa, which may eventually lead to ineffectiveness of injections and difficulty in later implantation of a penile prosthesis (6,57). The frequency of scarring with PGE_1 injections is 2% (22). Scarring can largely be prevented by restricting injections to 10 or fewer per month and rotating the injection sites. Further details of techniques for intracavernosal injections have been published elsewhere (17,23,54).

Penile Prostheses

These consist of paired, tubular devices that are inserted into the corpora cavernosa (28,38) (Chapter 11, Fig. 1). Two types are available: a semirigid/malleable and an inflatable device. The former is made of material that can withstand being bent many thousands of times. The penis is permanently rigid and may be bent upward or downward, whichever is most comfortable; for coitus, it can be bent into an intermediate position. These prostheses are reliable and durable, and breakage is uncommon with the modern versions.

Inflatable penile prostheses constitute a totally implanted system; a reservoir of fluid contained in a sac in the scrotum is used to pump fluid into the paired cavernosal implants. The fluid is released back through a valve mechanism into the reservoir after coitus. These hydraulic devices are associated with a higher incidence of mechanical failure than are the simpler rigid prostheses, but design refinements have lessened complications, and the devices can function satisfactorily for many years.

Penile prostheses are indicated in the treatment of erectile dysfunction that is neurogenic or vascular in origin. A high degree of satisfaction has been reported by both patients and their partners with the use of these implants (3,14,38). Further details have been published elsewhere (21,29,38).

Vacuum Devices

These devices use a vacuum to induce filling of the corpora cavernosa with blood; simultaneously, bands are applied to the base of the penis to impede venous return and so prolong erection (53,55). Major drawbacks are that they are cumbersome, require experience to use well, and may not produce adequate rigidity. Failure to remove the elastic band after coitus can dangerously prolong vascular engorgement. User satisfaction in several series is reported as high (2,10,48,53). These devices are useful in the treatment of patients with either neurogenic or venous leakage impotence, and they represent "an attractive alternative to either sexual abstinence or invasive therapy" (55).

Arterial Revascularization

When investigations demonstrate arterial blockage or stenosis between the common iliac artery and the dorsal artery of the penis, surgical revascularization should be considered (35,46,51). A variety of procedures exist; these have recently been comprehensively reviewed (45). Sometimes venous leakage is also present, and this must be treated as well (see below). The success rates of revascularization procedures are impossible to assess because of the varied selection criteria and poor diagnostic methods and follow-up (46). The best results are in young men who have had pelvic trauma (45). Arterial revascularization is unsuccessful in patients who also have severe diabetes mellitus, probably because of the autonomic neuropathy associated with diabetes. Vascular surgery is contraindicated in patients with other causes of neurogenic erectile dysfunction.

Treatment of Venous Leakage

Venous leakage occurs when blood shunts too rapidly out of the corpora cavernosa during erection. This can be demonstrated by a poor response to intracavernosal vasoactive drugs and by cavernosography (Chapter 21). Surgical treatment consists of ligating the veins draining the penis. Some patients have coexisting arterial insufficiency, which requires arterial revascularization. Results in terms of restoring potency have been variable (20). A newer approach is occlusion of penile draining veins by using sclerosing agents and coils (43,44).

Hormonal Treatment

The use of testosterone is indicated in patients with hypogonadism. Further details of this treatment have been published elsewhere (26). Improvement in libido rather than the other phases of the sexual cycle is the expected result. When hyperprolactinemia is diagnosed, temporary improvement can be obtained with bromocriptine, but the definitive treatment is to remove the prolactin-secreting pituitary adenoma.

Sex Therapy Techniques

Details are beyond the scope of this chapter; for further details see references 24, 25, and 49.

MANAGEMENT OF EJACULATORY DISORDERS

Disturbances of ejaculation include premature ejaculation, retarded ejaculation, retrograde ejaculation, and anejaculation (Chapter 21) (16,56).

Premature ejaculation is common, but it is not a neurologic disorder and is best treated by a sex therapist. Retrograde ejaculation is the propulsion of semen from the proximal urethra back into the bladder. Because retrograde ejaculation is usually accompanied by the sensation of orgasm, it is a problem only for those men who wish to procreate. If the problem is of recent onset or is partial, improvement may be brought about by the use of desipramine, a tricyclic antidepressant with both sympathomimetic and anticholinergic effects. Insemination using freshly voided postcoital urine is sometimes successful.

Patients with retarded ejaculation have the ability to ejaculate and achieve orgasm during masturbation but not during sexual activity. This rare disorder is psychogenic in origin and is treated by sex therapy.

Anejaculation, with or without failure of orgasm, can be associated with a variety of medications and with neurologic disorders, such as spinal cord injury. Treatment consists of stopping any medications causing the problem, if possible. Men with spinal cord injuries who wish to procreate pose an important challenge. Many years of research in veterinary medicine have led to the development of electrostimulation techniques for obtaining semen release for artificial insemination (56). These methods have now been adapted for use in human males and have led to successful pregnancies (56). Semen release may also be achieved with vibratory stimuli and subcutaneous injection of physostigmine (52).

REFERENCES

1. Abber JC, et al. Priapism induced by chlorpromazine and trazodone: mechanism of action. *J Urol* 1987;137:1039–1042.
2. Baltaci S, et al. Treating erectile dysfunction with a vacuum tumescence device: a retrospective analysis of acceptance and satisfaction. *Br J Urol* 1995;76:757–760.
3. Beutler L, et al. Women's satisfaction with partners' penile implant. *Urology* 1984;24:552–558.
4. Brindley, GS. Cavernosal alpha-blockade: a new technique for investigating and treating erectile impotence. *Br J Psychiatry* 1983;143:332–337.
5. Cavallini G. Minoxidil versus nitroglycerin: a prospective, double-blind controlled trial in transcutaneous erection facilitation for organic impotence. *J Urol* 1991;146:50–54.
6. Chan JCK, et al. Five- to seven-year follow-up of patients in a pharmacologic erection program: satisfaction and complications. *J Urol* 1992;147(2)Suppl:309A(abstract).
7. Chancellor MB, et al. Prospective comparison of topical minoxidil to vacuum constriction device and intracorporeal papaverine injection in treatment of erectile dysfunction due to spinal cord injury. *Urology* 1994;43:365–369.
8. Chen J, et al. Combining intracavernous injection and external vacuum as treatment for erectile dysfunction (see Comments). *J Urol* 1995;153:1476–1477.
9. Chiang PH, et al. The role of trazodone in the treatment of erectile dysfunction. *Kao Hsiung I Hsueh Ko Hsueh Tsa Chih* 1994;10:287–294.

10. Cookson MS, Nadig PW. Long-term results with vacuum constriction device. *J Urol* 1993;149:290–294.
11. Earle CM, et al. The role of intracavernosal vasoactive agents to overcome impotence due to spinal cord injury. *Paraplegia* 1992;30:273–276.
12. Fallon B. Intracavernous injection therapy for male erectile dysfunction. *Urol Clin North Am* 1995;22:833–845 (Melman A, ed. *Impotence*).
13. Heaton JPW, et al. Topical glyceryl trinitrate causes measurable penile dilatation in impotent men. *J Urol* 1990;143:729–731.
14. Kaufman JJ, et al. Physical and psychological results of penile prostheses: statistical survey. *J Urol* 1981;126:173–175.
15. Kurt U, et al. The efficacy of anti-serotoninergic agents in the treatment of erectile dysfunction. *J Urol* 1994;152:407–409.
16. Lakin M. The evaluation and nonsurgical management of impotence. *Semin Nephrol* 1994;14:544–550.
17. Lakin MM. Therapeutic pharmacologic erections. In: Montague DK, ed. *Disorders of Male Sexual Function*. Chicago: Year Book; 1988:223–229.
18. Lance R, et al. Oral trazodone as empirical therapy for erectile dysfunction: a retrospective review. *Urology* 1995;46:117–120.
19. Leonard M, et al. Hyperprolactinemia and impotence: why, when and how to investigate. *J Urol* 1989;142:992–995.
20. Lewis RW. Diagnosis and management of corporal veno-occlusive dysfunction. *Semin Urol* 1990;8:113–123.
21. Lewis RW. Long-term results of penile prosthetic implants. *Urol Clin North Am* 1995;22:847–856 (Melman A, ed. *Impotence*).
22. Lipshultz LI. Injection therapy for erectile dysfunction. *N Engl J Med* 1996;334:913–914.
23. Lue TF, Tanagho EA. Physiology of erection and pharmacological management of impotence. *J Urol* 1987;137:829–836.
24. Martin LM. Male sexual dysfunction: psychological assessment. In: Montague DK, ed. *Disorders of Male Sexual Function*. Chicago: Year Book; 1988:105–117.
25. Masters WH, Johnson VE. *Human Sexual Responses*. Boston: Little, Brown; 1966.
26. McClure RD. Endocrine evaluation and therapy. In: Tanagho EA, Lue TF, McClure RD, eds. *Contemporary Management of Impotence and Infertility*. Baltimore: Williams & Wilkins; 1988:84–94.
27. McMahon CG. A comparison of the response to the intracavernosal injection of a combination of papaverine and phentolamine, prostaglandin PGE_1 and a combination of all three agents in the management of impotence. *Int J Impot Res* 1991;3:113.
28. Montague DK. Penile prostheses. In: Montague DK, ed. *Disorders of Male Sexual Function*. Chicago: Year Book; 1988:154–191.
29. Montague DK, ed. *Disorders of Male Sexual Function*. Chicago: Year Book; 1988.
30. Montorsi F, et al. Effect of yohimbine-trazodone in psychogenic impotence: a randomized, double-blind, placebo-controlled study. *Urology* 1994;44:732–736.
31. Morales A, et al. Is yohimbine effective in the treatment of organic impotence? Results of a controlled trial. *J Urol* 1987;137:1168–1172.
32. Morales A, et al. Oral and transcutaneous pharmacologic agents in the treatment of impotence. *Urol Clin North Am* 1988; 15:87–93.
33. Morales A, et al. Oral and topical treatment of erectile dysfunction: present and future. *Urol Clin North Am* 1995;22:879–886 (Melman A, ed. *Impotence*).
34. Owen JA. Nitroglycerin in the treatment of impotence. *J Urol* 1989;141:546.
35. Padma-Nathan H, Goldstein IC. Arterial reconstruction. In: Tanagho EA, Lue TF, McClure RD, eds. *Contemporary Management of Impotence and Infertility*. Baltimore: Williams & Wilkins; 1988:163–174.
36. Padma-Nathan H, et al. Hemodynamic effect of intraurethral alprostadil: the medicated urethral system for erection (MUSE). *Int J Impot Res* 1994;6:A42.
37. Pescatori E, et al. Priapism of the clitoris: a case report following trazodone use. *J Urol* 1993;149:1558–1559.
38. Petrou SP, Barrett DM. The use of penile prostheses in erectile dysfunction. *Semin Urol* 1990;8:138–152.
39. Radomski SB, et al. Topical minoxidil in the treatment of male erectile dysfunction. *J Urol* 1994;151:1225–1226.
40. Reid K, et al. Double-blind trial of yohimbine in the treatment of psychogenic impotence. *Lancet* 1987;2:42–43.
41. Saenz de Tejada I, et al. Pathophysiology of prolonged penile erection associated with trazodone use. *J Urol* 1991;165:60–63.
42. Schiavi RC, Rehman J. Sexuality and aging. *Urol Clin North Am* 1995;22:711–726 (Melman A, ed. *Impotence*).
43. Schild HH, et al. Effectiveness of platinum wire microcoils for venous occlusion: a study on patients treated for venogenic impotence. *Cardiovasc Intervent Radiol* 1994;17:170–172.
44. Schild HH, et al. Percutaneous penile venoablation for treatment of impotence. *Cardiovasc Intervent Radiol* 1993;16:280–286.
45. Sharaby JS, et al. Penile revascularization. *Urol Clin North Am* 1995;22:821–832 (Melman A, ed. *Impotence*).
46. Sharlip ID. The role of vascular surgery in arteriogenic and combined arteriogenic and venogenic impotence. *Semin Urol* 1990;8:129–137.
47. Susset JG, et al. Effect of yohombine hydrochloride on erectile impotence: a double-blind study. *J Urol* 1989;141:1360–1363.
48. Tay KP, Lim PH. A prospective trial with vacuum-assisted erection devices. *Ann Acad Med Singapore* 1995;24:705–707.
49. Tiefer L, Schuetz-Mueller D. Psychological issues in diagnosis and treatment of erectile disorders. *Urol Clin North Am* 1995;22:767–773.
50. Virag R. Intracavernous injection of papaverine for erectile failure. *Lancet* 1982;2:938.
51. Virag R, et al. Vasculogenic impotence: a review of 92 cases with 54 surgical operations. *Vasc Surg* 1981;15:9.
52. Wheeler JS, et al. Anejaculation treated by vibratory stimulation. *Fertil Steril* 1988;50:377.
53. Wiles PG. Successful non-invasive management of erectile impotence in diabetic men. *Br Med J* 1988;296:161–162.
54. Williams G, et al. Impotence: treatment by autoinjection of vasoactive drugs. *Br Med J* 1987;295:595–596.
55. Witherington R. External penile appliances for management of impotence. *Semin Urol* 1990;8:124–128.
56. Witt MA, Grantmyre JE. Ejaculatory failure. *World J Urol* 1993;11:89–95.
57. Zentgraf M, et al. How safe is the treatment of impotence with intracavernous autoinjection? *Eur Urol* 1989;16:165–171.

CHAPTER 59

Acral Sympathetic Dysfunction and Hyperhidrosis

R. Khurana

1. The principal acral sympathetic functions are sudomotor, vasomotor, and pilomotor.
2. Localized hyperhidrosis may occur in patients with lesions of the brain, spinal cord, peripheral nerves, or sweat glands. Thoracic hyperhidrosis may indicate an underlying malignancy.
3. Generalized hyperhidrosis is usually primary and benign. Infrequently, it may be secondary to infections, malignancy, neuroendocrinopathies, or neurologic disease.
4. Treatment options for patients with disabling primary hyperhidrosis include the topical application of aluminum chloride, tap water iontophoresis, biofeedback, anticholinergic drugs, sympathectomy, and local surgical excision of sweat glands.
5. Vasomotor dysfunction is manifested either as a vasospasm or as vasomotor paralysis. Raynaud's phenomenon, acrocyanosis, and livedo reticularis are examples of vasospasm.
6. Raynaud's phenomenon may be primary or secondary in origin. The common causes of secondary Raynaud's phenomenon include drugs, recurrent trauma, and connective tissue disorders.
7. Raynaud's phenomenon is treated with simple physical measures, biofeedback, and pharmacotherapy. Plasmapheresis, sympathectomy, and spinal cord stimulation can be used in refractory cases.

INTRODUCTION

The principal acral sympathetic functions are sweating, vasoconstriction, and piloerection. Under normal physiologic conditions, these sympathetic functions maintain the core body temperature. Cutaneous blood flow regulates the convective transfer of heat, and sweat production by the eccrine sweat glands controls evaporative heat loss (38). The physiologic importance of pilomotor function in humans is not clearly understood. Sympathetic dysfunction can be characterized by both overactivity and underactivity. In disorders characterized by overactivity, treatment has consisted of selective lesions made in the peripheral autonomic pathways. Loss or reduction of activity is an important clinical sign that helps identify the level of the lesion along the sympathetic pathways (45,55).

Sympathetic nerves to the extremities originate from the spinal autonomic outflow. Preganglionic fibers to the upper extremities exit in the thoracic ventral spinal roots of T2-9, but may extend from the spinal roots of C8-T10 (62). Preganglionic fibers to the lower extremities emerge along the lower two or three thoracic and upper two lumbar ventral spinal roots (63). Postganglionic neurons of the sympathetic system are found in the prevertebral and paravertebral ganglia. These are catecholamine-containing neurons except for the sweat glands, which are cholinergic. Gibbins (25) demonstrated chemical subtypes of catecholaminergic neurons in the superior cervical ganglion of guinea pigs. The pilomotor neurons showed immunoreactivity to prodynorphin-derived peptides, and vasomotor neurons displayed immunoreactivity to neuropeptide Y. Postgangli-

R. Khurana: Department of Neurology, University of Maryland School of Medicine, Baltimore, Maryland 21201; and Department of Neurology, The Johns Hopkins University School of Medicine, Baltimore, Maryland 21287-0875.

onic fibers are distributed peripherally to the effector organs via gray rami and the cervical, intercostal, and lumbosacral nerves. Because sympathetic fibers accompany the somatic nerves, the distribution of sympathetic functions corresponds to the somatic sensory innervation (8). The conduction velocities of postganglionic sympathetic nerves in humans are 0.7 to 1 m/sec for cutaneous vasoconstrictor axons and 1.2 to 1.4 m/sec for sudomotor axons (39). Postganglionic sympathetic nerve fibers supply autonomic effector organs in the skin, muscles, and bones of the extremities. In the skin, they innervate sweat glands, erector pili muscles, blood vessels, the cutaneous receptors, and lipocytes (38). This chapter deals with dysfunction of the sudomotor, pilomotor, and vasomotor systems.

SUDOMOTOR SYSTEM

Human skin contains two functional types of eccrine sweat glands. Those on the general body surface serve thermoregulatory functions and respond to afferent thermal stimuli. Those on the palms, soles, and other areas, such as the forehead, respond to emotional, mental, and sensory stimuli (17). Sweat disorders are characterized by either excessive sweating (hyperhidrosis) or by reduced or absent sweating (hypohidrosis or anhidrosis). Hypohidrosis and anhidrosis are reviewed in other chapters.

Hyperhidrosis

Hyperhidrosis is defined as sweating that is increased above the normal level for a given stimulus (17). Hyperhidrosis may be either physiologic or pathologic in origin. Physiologic hyperhidrosis is well known in physically trained subjects. It is usually generalized and may be related to exercise or weather conditions. Recurrent heating of the body on one side, as may occur in stokers, can occasionally produce unilateral hyperhidrosis. Pathologic hyperhidrosis is a less frequent disorder, and it may be localized or generalized (41).

Localized Hyperhidrosis

Localized hyperhidrosis may be caused by lesions of the central or peripheral autonomic neural pathways. An inhibitory pathway has been proposed to explain hyperhidrosis of central origin. This pathway originates from the opercular cerebral cortex and traverses the hypothalamus, brain stem, and cervical spinal cord to terminate at the preganglionic sudomotor neurons of the contralateral thoracic spinal cord. Involvement of this inhibitory pathway at the level of the hemispheres, hypothalamus, pons, and medulla has been reported to cause contralateral hyperhidrosis. Hyperhidrosis caused by an infarct in the territory of the middle cerebral artery may be confined to the face, but it generally affects the neck and arm as well; this is usually self-limiting (47,49). A contralateral hyperhidrosis of the face, arm, and leg has been described in patients with medullary infarction and in patients with Arnold-Chiari malformation. In patients with Arnold-Chiari malformation, it has been attributed to compression of the inhibitory pathway by the herniated cerebellar tonsils (79). Bilateral facial hyperhidrosis has been reported in a patient with bilateral infarctions of the pons and cerebellum. Bassetti and Staikov (5) described a patient with an infarct in the territory of the proximal posterior cerebral artery who displayed ipsilateral Horner's syndrome and contralateral hemi-hyperhidrosis (hemiplegia vegetativa alterna), probably caused by involvement of ipsilateral excitatory and crossed inhibitory pathways. Hyperhidrosis has been well documented in patients with traumatic lesions of the spinal cord (45). It may be a presenting feature of posttraumatic syringomyelia (78) and usually appears in dermatomes where sensation is later altered by the syrinx. An area of hyperhidrosis surrounds the anhidrotic region produced by lesions involving the sympathetic ganglia or rami (3,78). Partial injury to the median and sciatic nerves is associated with hyperhidrosis; however, any nerve may be affected (41). Hatzis et al. (32) described a patient with paroxysmal hyperhidrosis of unknown cause that affected the ulnar aspect of the forearm and hand and awakened the patient from his sleep. Gitter and Sato (26) reported spontaneous localized hyperhidrosis in patients with pretibial myxedema. This was provoked either by a relatively high ambient temperature or by mild physical activity and was confined to the pretibial region. Tissue obtained from biopsy of the eccrine sweat glands demonstrated glandular hypertrophy. This was attributed to stimulation of the peripheral sympathetic nerves by the mucinous perineural infiltrate. Chan et al. (12) observed episodic hyperhidrosis on the dorsal aspect of hands. Exercise, direct heat, and the intradermal injection of cholinergic drugs precipitated the profuse sweating. Examination of the skin by light microscopy and electron microscopy revealed hyperplasia of the sweat glands and ducts, and an increased concentration of hyaluronic acid in the stroma.

Hyperhidrosis may rarely be unilateral and limited to other skin sites, namely the face or the thorax. Unilateral facial hyperhidrosis may be confined to the forehead alone or to one entire side of the face. It may be paroxysmal or persistent. It has been reported in association with central lesions, postganglionic sympathetic dysfunction, and hyperplasia and hypertrophy of the sweat glands (18,46,47, 48). Thoracic hyperhidrosis may involve a single dermatome or multiple segments. In addition, it may affect the face and arm. Although it has been reported in patients with osteoma of a vertebra or a cervical rib, several cases have been described in association with intrathoracic malignancy (57,64,82).

Generalized Hyperhidrosis

Generalized hyperhidrosis may be secondary or primary in origin.

Secondary Hyperhidrosis

Secondary hyperhidrosis has been observed in patients with infections, malignancy, neuroendocrine disorders, neurologic diseases, and other miscellaneous conditions.

The night sweats that occur in patients with brucellosis or tuberculosis probably serve to lower the body temperature. Night sweats and pruritus occur in patients with malignancy and may respond either to cimetidine, an H_2-receptor antagonist, or to plasmapheresis (3,41,65,72). Paroxysms of sweating are a characteristic feature of pheochromocytoma and thyrotoxicosis. In patients with pheochromocytoma, excess circulating catecholamine levels presumably stimulate thermoregulatory structures to trigger cholinergic sudomotor activity, as shown by the fact that sweating can be blocked by the local administration of hyoscine (3). In patients with thyrotoxicosis, inappropriate heat production resulting from increased body metabolism and increased sensitivity of the autonomic nerve fibers to circulating epinephrine may be the causative factors. Treatment with β-adrenergic blockade can alleviate this hyperhidrosis.

Hyperhidrosis also affects patients with acromegaly or carcinoid syndrome. Patients with diencephalic epilepsy have paroxysms of hyperhidrosis. Profuse sweating in patients with basilar occlusion and consequential pontine ischemia is a common finding, and is attributed to disinhibition of sudomotor structures. Severe anxiety, hypotension, hypoglycemia, and cholinergic agents can also precipitate profuse sweating (3,28,65).

Primary Hyperhidrosis

Primary or essential hyperhidrosis is defined as excessive sweating that affects either certain areas or the entire body without an obvious cause (3). The axillary, palmar, and plantar regions are commonly affected. Occasionally, sweating may affect the general body surface without increased sweating in the palmar region (44). Of all patients with axillary hyperhidrosis, only 25% have palmoplantar hyperhidrosis as well (69). Similarly, patients with palmoplantar hyperhidrosis usually do not have axillary hyperhidrosis. This condition predominantly affects adolescents and young adults and may be aggravated at the time of puberty.

Sweat glands on the palms and soles are activated predominantly by emotional stimuli, whereas axillary glands respond to thermal stimuli as well. This condition can be regarded as a quantitative exaggeration of the normal sweat response to emotional stimuli. The sweating is absent during sleep or sedation (65). The sweating can be profuse, and those affected may produce as much as 26 mL of sweat per hour from each axilla, necessitating frequent changes of clothes. Sweat may even drip from the fingers. When these subjects write, the paper becomes wet from the sweat and the ink runs, making this simple task impossible. The feet can become macerated with development of fungal infections. This condition can be socially and occupationally disabling and can ultimately turn the patient into a recluse.

No definite cause of this type of hyperhidrosis is known, hence the term *primary* or *essential hyperhidrosis*. It has been considered an autonomically mediated anxiety phenomenon. Lerer et al. (51) performed personality evaluations in 23 afflicted patients using the Shanan Sentence Completion test, the Stein Self-Description Questionnaire, the Taylor Manifest Anxiety Scale, and the Rorschach test. They observed a lower overall ability to cope, an avoidance pattern of defense, a tendency toward impulsiveness, and poorly integrated emotional responses in these subjects, but the levels of manifest anxiety were not significantly elevated. A family history of hyperhidrosis can be found in one-fourth to one-half the patients. In addition, hyperhidrosis is an associated feature of several other hereditary disorders, including nail-patella syndrome, Charcot-Marie-Tooth disease, and familial dysautonomia. This suggests that primary hyperhidrosis may have an autosomal dominant transmission with incomplete penetrance (37).

Studies intended to elucidate the pathophysiology of hyperhidrosis are few. In theory, hyperhidrosis that is limited to certain regions can result from an abnormality affecting either specific sectors of the sympathetic pathways or the end-organ. No abnormalities were demonstrated in the sweat constituents or in the morphology of the eccrine sweat glands (3). Rechardt et al. (66) evaluated tissue specimens obtained at surgery from the axillae of 10 patients and two normal controls. The innervation was primarily cholinergic and did not differ qualitatively or quantitatively from that seen in the normal controls. Palmer (61) demonstrated that anesthetizing the ulnar nerve abolished hyperhidrosis in that distribution in response to emotional and thermal stimuli. These findings indicate that a sweat gland abnormality is unlikely in patients with primary hyperhidrosis, and indirectly incriminate the sympathetic pathways. However, the question is whether the abnormality is postganglionic, preganglionic, or central in origin. The therapeutic success of preganglionic sympathectomy argues against the possibility of postganglionic dysfunction. Shih and Wang (74) studied autonomic functions in hyperhidrotic subjects. They observed less bradycardia in these subjects in response to Valsalva's maneuver and facial immersion, and these findings indicate reduced vagal activity. Also, cutaneous vasoconstriction in response to external cooling was increased in their subjects. These autonomic abnormalities abated following T2-3 sympathetic ganglionectomy, suggesting overactivity of the sympathetic fibers passing through the T2-3 ganglia (75). The involvement of all four extremities, symmetric distribution, response to psychic stimuli, and absence during sleep or sedation all favor an abnormality with a central origin (61). Additional evidence supporting a cortical origin includes hyperventilation-induced bursts of sharp waves on the electroencephalogram and hyperperfusion of the frontal areas, as demonstrated by an increased accumulation of the marker N-isopropyl-p-iodoamphetamine I^{123} on single-photon emission computed tomograms (69). In brief, the clinical and experimental evidence to date is inconclusive, but it points toward a functional derangement at the level of the premotor cortex (61,69).

Treatment of Hyperhidrosis

Hyperhidrosis caused by general medical disorders requires specific treatment of the precipitating factors. For mild to moderate primary hyperhidrosis, reassurance and hygiene in combination with cosmetic care may be sufficient. For plantar hyperhidrosis, appropriate nonocclusive footwear should be worn to avoid the complications of maceration and infection. For patients with disabling primary hyperhidrosis, treatment is directed at the emotional stimuli, the gland innervation, or the eccrine sweat gland itself. The use of sedatives and anxiolytics may provide only transient and partial benefit. Relaxation training combined with galvanic skin response biofeedback may reduce the magnitude of the sweat response (81). Surgical sympathectomy and computed tomography-guided percutaneous phenol block have been employed to interrupt innervation at the level of the T2-3 sympathetic ganglia (1,85). Systemic pharmacotherapy (anticholinergic drugs and diltiazem), topical agents (aluminum chloride, tap water iontophoresis, and tanning agents), and local surgical excision are used to disrupt excessive sweat gland activity (37,85). Commonly used modalities for the treatment of hyperhidrosis are discussed in the following paragraphs.

Aluminum Chloride

The topical application of 20% aluminum chloride hexahydrate (Drysol) is the first choice of treatment for patients with axillary hyperhidrosis. In 1916, Stillians first introduced aluminum salts as antiperspirants. They can reduce sweating by about 50% (73). This compound acts initially by mechanically blocking the eccrine sweat gland pore. Over a longer term, it produces vacuolization and atrophy of the secretory cells and dilatation of eccrine acini (34, 85). Its cationic properties may also have antibacterial and antifungal effects. It is a simple and relatively safe remedy when guidelines for its use are followed properly. It should be applied at night over dry skin. Because sweat glands are less active during sleep, it prevents the formation of hydrochloric acid, which irritates the skin and damages clothing. Application at night also ensures penetration into the sweat ducts for a period of several hours. To reduce irritation, the antiperspirant should be washed off in the morning and, if needed, a hydrocortisone cream applied (69,85).

Iontophoresis

Iontophoresis is the process of increasing the penetration of electrically charged drugs into surface tissue by the application of an electrical current. Tap water iontophoresis is an effective, safe, and inexpensive treatment for patients with palmar and plantar hyperhidrosis, for which aluminum chloride may not be effective because of the presence of thick local epidermis (17). Its mechanism of action is believed to be the transient mechanical obstruction of the sweat ducts at the level of the stratum corneum, as stripping of the stratum corneum by the repeated application and removal of adhesive tape restores the sweating response. Light microscopy and transmission electron microscopy have not revealed any resulting tissue abnormalities stemming from the treatment (33,85). Sato et al. (70) demonstrated that anodal current has more of an inhibitory effect than cathodal current, that distilled water is superior to saline solution, and that the inhibitory effect is a function of the amperage used. The reduction of active sweat pores was noted to be proportional to the amperage used, with 1 mA/cm^2 being the most effective current. Tap water iontophoresis using direct current may produce burning, skin irritation, erythema, and vesicles. This can be avoided if alternating current is combined with direct current for the iontophoresis (67). Proper use of the apparatus ensures safety and effectiveness. In a double-blind controlled clinical study, Dahl and Glent-Madsen (19) observed an 81% reduction in sweating in patients treated with this method.

Excision of Axillary Sweat Glands

Patients whose hyperhidrosis is refractory to medical therapy can benefit from the surgical excision of a sufficient number of eccrine sweat glands. There are approximately 25,000 eccrine sweat glands in each axillary vault (73). A qualitative assessment of the area of hyperhidrosis should precede surgical excision. Several surgical approaches are available, depending on the severity of the problem (53,85).

Sympathectomy

As essential hyperhidrosis is usually self-limiting by the fourth or fifth decade, sympathectomy should be reserved for those whose condition is extremely severe. Sympathectomy is the traditional surgical method for treating palmar hyperhidrosis; it involves resecting the T2-4 sympathetic ganglia. Although pupillary fibers usually exit from the T1 ganglion, the variability of this level can be assessed during the surgical procedure by stimulating the sympathetic trunk (40). Various surgical approaches have been advocated, all with good to excellent results. They include anterior and posterior approaches, stereotactic percutaneous thermocoagulation, and endoscopic transthoracic electrocautery (11,13,27,65,68,74,85). Results of studies comparing the morbidity, mortality, and long-term efficacy of the various procedures are not available. Horner's syndrome, pneumothorax, and nasal congestion are some of the early complications. Recurrence of hyperhidrosis, compensatory hyperhidrosis, gustatory hyperhidrosis, and hyperkeratosis with fissure of the anhidrotic region may also be sequelae (41,65).

Botulinum Toxin

Botulinum toxin type A denervates the sudomotor junction by binding to presynaptic cholinergic terminals. This eliminates local sweating for a period of several months. Drobik and Laskawi (21) used multiple intracutaneous injections to eliminate gustatory sweating. Cheshire (14) has demonstrated that this toxin can be delivered transcutaneously by iontophoresis, which may turn out to be a promising modality of treatment for localized hyperhidrosis.

PILOMOTOR SYSTEM

Pilomotor reflexes in animals help in temperature regulation. Human hairs function primarily as somatic sensory structures. Piloerection as an autonomic function in humans is rudimentary, taking the form of goose bumps in response to cold, deep pressure, sharp noises, and emotional stimuli (38). Pilomotor reflexes are most easily elicited from the neck and chest. Experimentally, stimulation of human skin induced by a strong faradic current or an intradermal injection of 0.1 mL of 1% acetylcholine produces goose bumps that involve an area extending 5 cm to 10 cm around the site of the stimulus. This axon reflex can be blocked by the intradermal injection of 1% procaine hydrochloride or by surgical division of the cutaneous nerve. Conversely, the local response to the application of ice or heavy stroking persists after cutaneous denervation. In 1927, Lewis and Marvin (52) reported on an experiment in which they divided a cutaneous nerve and tested the denervated region for local response to application of ice. Goose bumps persisted 32, 54, and 55 days after the surgical division. In clinical practice, the absence of axon reflex indicates degeneration of the sympathetic nerve supply to that area of skin. Bárány and Cooper (4) studied diabetic patients and reported loss of pilomotor reflexes in the region of their anhidrosis. Interruption of a peripheral nerve produced by an injury or disease can likewise abolish piloerection in the anesthetic region.

VASOMOTOR SYSTEM

Central sympathetic pathways from the hypothalamus, medulla oblongata, and spinal cord regulate acral blood flow via the intermediolateral cell column, sympathetic nerves, neurovascular synapses, and adrenergic receptors. Human digital vasculature contains α_1- and α_2-adrenergic receptors, of which the α_2-adrenergic receptors are more important during sympathetic vasoconstriction. Serotonin receptors have been demonstrated, but their role in vasoconstriction is not certain. Vasodilation may result from the withdrawal of sympathetic activity, but peptidergic and cholinergic mechanisms, as well as local axon reflexes, have also been postulated. Vasomotor dysfunction implies vasospasm or vasomotor paralysis of the acral vessels. Vasospasm may be episodic or persistent (15,16). Episodic vasospasm is discussed in the section on Raynaud's phenomenon. Acrocyanosis and livedo reticularis represent examples of possibly persistent vasospasm.

VASOSPASTIC DISORDERS

Raynaud's Phenomenon

Raynaud's phenomenon, originally described by Maurice Raynaud, is characterized by episodic, bilateral, and symmetric changes in acral skin color provoked by cold or emotional stimuli. This color change may be triphasic, beginning with pallor, progressing to cyanosis, and terminating in rubor on rewarming. Allen and Brown proposed the following criteria for identifying Raynaud's phenomenon: bilaterality, precipitation by cold or emotion, normal pulsations in the palpable arteries, absence of trophic changes, duration of 2 years or more, and negative findings on etiologic screening. The term *Raynaud's disease* is traditionally used to refer to the condition of patients without a known underlying disorder, and *Raynaud's phenomenon* denotes the presence of an associated disease (15).

Raynaud's disease is prevalent in 3%–4% of the population, and is mostly seen in 11- to 40-year-old female patients who are otherwise healthy (42). It primarily affects the fingers and sometimes the fingers and toes, but rarely the toes alone. Trophic digital effects, consisting of ulceration and scarring, are infrequent. The long-term prognosis in such patients is good, with disappearance or improvement in 46%, no change in 38%, and worsening in 16%. Light microscopy examination of the digital vessels has revealed no abnormality in patients with mild cases, but intimal hyperplasia, inflammatory destruction of the capillary bed in the superficial dermis, and segmental inflammation and edema in the walls of small blood vessels have been reported in severe cases. Electron microscopy has shown endothelial swelling, an increased number of intracytoplasmic filaments, and a thickened and multilayered basement membrane (15).

Color changes and digital ischemia are presumably caused by the episodic closure of the main digital arteries. The pathophysiologic features of this phenomenon remain to be elucidated. It is not clear if the pathophysiology of Raynaud's disease is the same as that of Raynaud's phenomenon. Raynaud ascribed it to "enormous exaggeration of the excitomotor energy of the gray parts of the spinal cord which control the vasomotor innervation" (84). Lewis suggested the existence of a "local fault" in the blood vessels (15). Raynaud's hypothesis is supported by the induction of attacks in response to emotional stimuli, cessation of attacks in the toes produced by sympathectomy, a severe vasoconstriction response to postural changes, and normal digital capillary flow with α-adrenergic-receptor blockade. Greenstein et al. (29) postulated central thermoregulatory dysfunction, studying the effects of central body cooling (13°C) and central body rewarming (35°C) on the core body temperature and the digital blood flow in patients. Core body temperature in the patients was lower than that in the normal subjects, and it dropped more in the patients following the cold challenge. The patients had significantly lower digital blood flow at all stages of the test; their digital rewarming response following central cooling was considerably prolonged when compared with that of controls (29). Data from several studies, however, militate against this hypothesis. Fagius and Blumberg (23) made direct microneurographic recordings of cutaneous sympathetic nerve activity from the median nerve in one hand of various patients and controls during different afferent stimuli: immersion of the contralateral hand in ice water, sudden shouts, air puffs to the face, electrical stimuli to the skin above the clavicle, and suprapubic pressure. The increase in the sympathetic outflow in the ipsilateral hand was similar in both patients and controls. No consistently demonstrable increase in the plasma and urinary catecholamine levels or an increase in the sensitivity of digital vessels to norepinephrine infusion has been found (15). Furthermore, BP responses to standing up, to 5 min of isometric handgrip, and to immersion of the hand in ice water did not demonstrate impairment of sympathetic cardiovascular reflexes (30).

Lewis proposed his "local fault" theory based on his observations that local cooling produced ischemic attacks in sympathetically denervated fingers and that vasospasm in the little finger was unaffected by anesthetization of the ulnar nerve (15). As Lewis performed the study on patients with advanced disease and gangrene (59), additional studies on a selected group of patients are needed to substantiate this hypothesis. Two different observations are of interest. Fagius and Blumberg (23) plotted the increase in sympathetic nerve activity against a reduction in pulse amplitude, and this correlated well in control subjects but not in patients. Halperin et al. (31) observed digital vasodilation and increased blood flow in patients with Raynaud's disease, compared with diminished blood flow and increased vascular resistance in normal subjects, during mental stress. This response was unaffected by the intraarterial administration of propranolol or atropine, or by digital nerve block. These observations suggest an abnormal interaction between the sympathetic nerves and adrenergic receptors (22).

Recent studies have shown that the mechanism of cutaneous vascular tone, which was thought to be under adrenergic control, is far more complex. It depends on perivascular autonomic and somatic nerves, neuropeptides, hemorrheologic factors, and endothelium. Noradrenaline and adenosine-5-triphosphate act as cotransmitters for vasoconstrictor nerves, whereas neuropeptide Y has a neuromodulatory role. Vasoactive intestinal polypeptide, stored with acetylcholine, and prostaglandins contribute to vasodilation. Calcitonin gene-related peptide (CGRP) and substance P coexist in sensorimotor nerves (afferent nerves have efferent functions during axon reflex). Neuropeptides interact with the vessel wall to produce spasm or relaxation. CGRP-containing nerve fibers are lost and the axon reflex vasodilator mechanism is reduced in patients with Raynaud's phenomenon. In regard to hemorrheologic factors, an increase in spontaneous, adenosine diphosphate- and collagen-induced whole-blood platelet aggregation has been described in patients with Raynaud's phenomenon (20,42,43).

An increase in the plasma levels of endothelin-1, a vasoconstrictor peptide, has been shown in patients with Raynaud's phenomenon, but there is no correlation between endothelin levels and severity of Raynaud's phenomenon. In addition to vasoconstriction, endothelin may also play a role in the axon reflex flare. CGRP activates nitric oxide synthase in endothelium via adenylate cyclase to produce vasodilation. Normal serum reduces the ionophore-stimulated release of prostaglandins. The serum from patients exerts a greater inhibitory effect, suggesting that a circulating inhibitor of prostaglandin release might contribute to vasoconstriction. Singh et al. (76) studied digital arterial diameter and cutaneous temperature in response to a sequential series of infusions with acetylcholine, L-arginine, prostacyclin, and glyceryl trinitrate. They demonstrated attenuation of dilation in response to acetylcholine (endothelium-dependent) and good vasodilation in response to glyceryl trinitrate (a donor of nitric oxide), indicating a dysfunction of endothelium-dependent vasodilation. Following 40 min of whole-body cooling, Leppert et al. (50) observed an increase in the venous levels of cyclic guanosine monophosphate in control subjects, which remained elevated after 20 min. This response was absent in patients with Raynaud's phenomenon, suggesting a local fault in the L-arginine-nitric oxide-cGMP pathway. In conclusion, the mechanisms that promote vasospasm and reduce vasodilation are still not clear. The recent data show an increase of vasoconstrictor peptide endothelin and inadequate vasodilation as a consequence of impaired endothelium-dependent vasodilation, reduction of the axon reflex vasodilator mechanism, and deficiency of CGRP vasodilator neuropeptide (20,50,76).

Diagnosis of Raynaud's disease depends on a careful history, as vasospastic phenomena cannot be reproduced consistently in the clinical or laboratory setting. In addition to fulfilling the criteria formulated by Allen and Brown, patients with Raynaud's disease can be identified by a normal sedimentation rate, negative findings on antinuclear antibody test, normal total immunoglobulins and electrophoresis, normal findings on nail fold capillaroscopy, and normal esophageal motility on esophageal scintigraphy. Men at any age, women past the age of 40, and patients with severe disease should be evaluated further to exclude various causes of Raynaud's phenomenon.

Raynaud's phenomenon secondary to drug therapy, connective tissue disorders, occupational trauma, thoracic outlet syndrome, and carpal tunnel syndrome has been described. Drug-induced Raynaud's phenomenon is a preventable problem. β-Adrenergic blockers are the most common offenders. The following pathophysiologic mechanism has been postulated for these agents: Their central cardiovascular depressant effects elicit increased reflex sympathetic vasoconstriction and increased sensitivity to α-adrenergic-receptor stimulation as a result of peripheral β-adrenergic blockade. Approximately 5% of patients taking beta blockers need to stop the treatment because of vasospastic phenomena. Ergot intoxication, usually resulting from dosages exceeding 10 mg/week, can cause Raynaud's phenomenon through stimulation of α-adrenergic receptors. Experimentally and clinically, this agent has been found to damage the endothelium, leading to stasis and thrombosis. Methysergide, vinblastine, bleomycin, nitroglycerin, amphetamines, bromocriptine, and cyclosporine can also precipitate Raynaud's phenomenon. Connective tissue disorders, such as scleroderma, polymyositis, dermatomyositis, rheumatoid arthritis, Sjögren's syndrome, and psoriasis, are associated with Raynaud's phenomenon. Raynaud's phenomenon occurs frequently in association with scleroderma; esophageal motility is also abnormal in these patients, and examination of the nail beds using wide-field microscopy reveals sparse, dilated, and convoluted capillaries and avascular areas (15,36,54).

Traumatic vasospastic disease is most frequently associated with the use of such machinery as pneumatic drill hammers, chain saws, riveting machines, road drills, and sewing machines. This disorder has also been reported in typists, pianists, and telephone operators. Raynaud's phenomenon develops in 30%–84% of operators of such machinery after 6.4 to 8 years, or after a total approximate exposure time of 6000 to 7000 hrs. Vibration at 125 Hz is more potent in producing vasospasm than are other frequencies (15,35). The hand exposed to the tool is more severely affected, but symptoms can appear in the absence of exposure to vibration immediately before they develop (59). It is believed that the pacinian corpuscles are most sensitive in the 125-Hz range and that excessive afferent activity in these receptors triggers reflex efferent sympathetic discharges. Okada et al. (58) demonstrated increased plasma guanosine 3',5'-monophosphate responses to the cold pressor test in these patients; the responses were abolished by administration of phentolamine or atropine, suggesting enhanced responses of α-adrenergic or cholinergic receptors, or both. Use of better tools and limited exposure are necessary to reduce the prevalence and severity of this disorder.

Raynaud's phenomenon may precede other somatic manifestations of carpal tunnel syndrome by 6 to 12 months; it may also be limited to fingers innervated by the median nerve and precipitated by wrist movement or Phalen's maneuver (71). No clinical correlation has been documented between the severity of the median nerve lesion and the occurrence of Raynaud's phenomenon. Median nerve decompression may not alleviate Raynaud's phenomenon (56). The thoracic outlet syndrome is presumed to cause Raynaud's phenomenon through irritation of sympathetic nerves in the neurovascular bundle or embolization of the digital arteries. Raynaud's phenomenon in patients with thromboembolism should last longer than a few minutes and should predominantly involve the radial artery distribution in conjunction with absent digital pulses (15).

Raynaud's phenomenon should be suspected in patients with the following characteristics: later age at onset, male sex, asymmetric attacks, painful attacks, evidence of tissue necrosis, occupational trauma, symptoms of connective tissue disease, use of drugs such as propranolol or ergotamine, and positional symptoms. Appropriate diagnostic studies should be conducted in such patients.

Because Raynaud's disease and phenomenon carry a relatively good prognosis, conservative treatment is preferred. Simple physical measures should be implemented first. These include wearing loose and warm clothing, using mittens, preventing dryness with proper skin care, stopping smoking, and limiting exposure to vibrating tools. Autogenic training and biofeedback can help reduce the frequency of attacks. These patients can learn to raise their finger temperature as readily as normal individuals and maintain it, even in cold environments (60).

Pharmacologic therapy should be reserved for patients whose activities of daily living continue to be affected after the adoption of simple physical measures or for patients who show trophic changes. No drug selectively dilates digital vessels. Several drugs, including sympatholytic agents, calcium channel blockers, serotonin antagonists, antiplatelet agents, and angiotensin-converting enzyme (ACE) inhibitors, have been tried, but there are no comparative studies that show which drug is better. Nifedipine and diltiazem are useful. Of the sympatholytic agents, reserpine, guanethidine, and prazosin appear to be more effective. Ketanserin, a selective 5-HT$_2$-receptor antagonist, blocks both the vasoconstricting and platelet-aggregating effects of serotonin. This drug is useful but unavailable in the United States (15). Captopril, an ACE inhibitor, permits the accumulation of bradykinin, and patients, especially those with scleroderma and hypertension, may benefit from its use.

Newer therapies include CGRP, prostacyclin and its analogue, and glyceryl trinitrate. Because patients have deficiency of CGRP in digital cutaneous perivascular nerves but exhibit vasodilation in response to CGRP, it should be a useful treatment. A daily 3-hour intravenous administration of CGRP at 0.6 µg/min for 5 days increased digital blood flow and healed ulcers. Prostaglandins dilate arterioles and inhibit platelet aggregation. Administration of prostacyclin or its stable synthetic analogue, iloprost, reduced the frequency and severity of attacks, but oral administration was of questionable benefit. Glyceryl trinitrate patches, 0.2 mg/h, placed on the chest wall for 12 hours a day, reduced the frequency and severity of attacks but lacked objective efficacy (6,7,10,80).

Plasmapheresis has been employed in refractory cases. Lumbar sympathectomy in the treatment of Raynaud's phenomenon of the toes has been reported to be quite effective. Sympathectomy in patients whose upper limbs are affected by Raynaud's disease produces immediate benefits, but relapse is common (15). Recently, spinal cord stimulation has been shown to reduce the frequency, severity, and duration of attacks, presumably through spinal or supraspinal inhibition of the sympathetic nervous system (24).

Acrocyanosis

In patients with acrocyanosis, cyanosis is persistent and symmetric, and may extend to the wrists and ankles. The cyanosis results from arteriolar constriction and is aggravated by exposure to cold. It can be relieved in the fifth digit by anesthetizing the ulnar nerve. Acrocyanosis is usually a benign disorder and carries only cosmetic consequences (15).

Livedo Reticularis

Livedo reticularis affects the extremities and sometimes the trunk; it appears as a mottled discoloration that assumes a lacelike pattern. It is attributed to vasospasm, obstruction of small perpendicular arterioles, or stasis of blood in superficial veins. It may be a benign disorder or associated with vasculitis, connective tissue disorders, hyperviscosity syndrome, thrombocythemia, and drugs. Immunoglobulins M and G, fibrin, and complement deposits have been demonstrated in the vessel walls of patients with livedo reticularis and ulceration. It is seen in patients who take amantadine. Laboratory evaluation and appropriate treatment are recommended, especially when the condition is associated with ulceration (15).

Vasomotor Paralysis

Vasomotor paralysis can occur in patients with lesions of the sympathetic pathways at the level of the spinal cord, preganglionic nerves, sympathetic ganglia, or postganglionic nerves. Surgical sympathectomy at the preganglionic or ganglionic level has been used to treat many circulatory disorders (84). At present, it is performed in selected patients with Raynaud's phenomenon, hyperhidrosis, and reflex sympathetic dystrophy. Trauma and tumor infiltration of the peripheral sympathetic structures are commonly associated with vasomotor paralysis. Involvement of peripheral vasomotor fibers has been observed in patients with carpal tunnel syndrome, ulnar nerve lesions, and peripheral neuropathies (2,40,77). Interruption of the cervical sympathetic pathways in patients with Pancoast's tumor is a well-known problem; it produces vasomotor paralysis along with sudomotor abnormalities and Horner's syndrome. A similar involvement of the sympathetic pathways in the lower extremities has also been described. Vasomotor paralysis that evokes a warm and flushed lower extremity is a useful diagnostic sign in patients with malignant retroperitoneal disease (9,83).

REFERENCES

1. Adler OB, et al. Palmar hyperhidrosis: CT-guided chemical percutaneous thoracic sympathectomy. *Fortschr Geb Rontgenstr Nuklearmed Erganzungsbd* 1990;153:400–403.
2. Aminoff MJ. Involvement of peripheral vasomotor fibers in carpal tunnel syndrome. *J Neurol Neurosurg Psychiatry* 1979;42:649–655.
3. Appenzeller O. *Clinical Autonomic Failure*. New York: Elsevier; 1986:23–98.
4. Bárány FR, Cooper EH. Pilomotor and sudomotor innervation in diabetes. *Clin Sci* 1956;15:533–540.
5. Bassetti C, Staikov IN. Hemiplegia vegetativa alterna (ipsilateral Horner's syndrome and contralateral hemihyperhidrosis) following proximal posterior cerebral artery occlusion. *Stroke* 1995;26:702–704.
6. Belch JJF, et al. Oral iloprost as a treatment for Raynaud's syndrome: a double-blind multicentre placebo-controlled study. *Ann Rheum Dis* 1995;54:197–200.
7. Bolster MB, et al. The evaluation and treatment of Raynaud's phenomenon. *Cleve Clin J Med* 1995;62:51–61.
8. Brodal A. *Neurological Anatomy*. 3rd ed. Oxford: Oxford University Press; 1981:698–787.
9. Brown RC, et al. Unilateral lumbar sympathectomy due to retroperitoneal tumors. *Br Med J* 1978;1:410.
10. Bunker CB, et al. Calcitonin gene-related peptide in treatment of severe peripheral vascular insufficiency in Raynaud's phenomenon. *Lancet* 1993;342:80–82.
11. Byrne J, et al. Endoscopic transthoracic electrocautery of the sympathetic chain for palmar and axillary hyperhidrosis. *Br J Surg* 1990; 77:1046–1049.
12. Chan P, et al. Episodic hyperhidrosis on the dorsum of hands. *J Am Acad Dermatol* 1985;12:937–942.
13. Chuang K-S, et al. New stereotactic technique for percutaneous thermocoagulation upper thoracic ganglionectomy in cases of palmar hyperhidrosis. *Neurosurgery* 1988;22:600–604.

14. Cheshire WP. Anhidrotic effect of botulinum toxin delivered by iontophoresis. *Clin Auton Res* 1995;5:339.
15. Coffman JD. *Raynaud's Phenomenon*. Oxford: Oxford University Press; 1989.
16. Coffman JD, Davies WT. Vasospastic disease: a review. *Prog Cardiovasc Dis* 1975;18:123–146.
17. Collins KJ. Autonomic control of sweat glands and disorders of sweating. In: Bannister R, ed. *Autonomic Failure*. 2nd ed. Oxford: Oxford University Press; 1988:748–765.
18. Cunliffe WJ, et al. Localized unilateral hyperhidrosis—a clinical and laboratory study. *Br J Dermatol* 1972; 86:374–378.
19. Dahl JC, Glent-Madsen L. Treatment of hyperhidrosis manuum by tap water iontophoresis. *Acta Derm Venereol (Stockh)* 1989;69: 346–348.
20. Dowd P. Raynaud's phenomenon. *Lancet* 1995;346:283–290.
21. Drobik C, Laskawi R. Frey's syndrome: treatment with botulinum toxin. *Acta Otolaryngol (Stockh)* 1995;115:459–461.
22. Engelhardt M. The effect of sympathetic blockade and cooling in Raynaud's phenomenon. *Clin Physiol* 1990;10:131–136.
23. Fagius J, Blumberg H. Sympathetic outflow to the hand in patients with Raynaud's phenomenon. *Cardiovasc Res* 1985;19:249–253.
24. Francaviglia N, et al. Spinal cord stimulation for the treatment of progressive systemic sclerosis and Raynaud's syndrome. *Br J Neurosurg* 1994;8:567–571.
25. Gibbins IL. Dynorphin-containing pilomotor neurons in the superior cervical ganglion of guinea pigs. *Neurosci Lett* 1989;51:45–50.
26. Gitter DG, Sato K. Localized hyperhidrosis in pretibial myxedema. *J Am Acad Dermatol* 1990;23:250–254.
27. Gjerris F, Olesen HP. Palmar hyperhidrosis. *Acta Neurol Scand* 1975;51:167–172.
28. Good JL, et al. Endplate degeneration in organophosphate poisoning. *Neurology* 1990;40 (Suppl 1):431.
29. Greenstein D, et al. Impaired thermoregulation in Raynaud's phenomenon. *Angiology* 1995;46: 603–611.
30. Gutrecht JA. Sympathetic cardiovascular reflexes in primary Raynaud's phenomenon. *Clin Auton Res* 1994;4:219.
31. Halperin JL, et al. Digital vasodilatation during mental stress in patients with Raynaud's disease. *Cardiovasc Res* 1983;17:671.
32. Hatzis J, et al. Local hyperhidrosis. *Dermatologica* 1980;161:45–50.
33. Hill CA, et al. Mechanism of action of iontophoresis in the treatment of palmar hyperhidrosis. *Cutis* 1981;28:69–70.
34. Holzle E, Braun-Falco O. Structural changes in axillary eccrine glands following long-term treatment with aluminum chloride hexahydrate solution. *Br J Dermatol* 1984;110:399–403.
35. Hyvarinen J, et al. Vibration frequencies and amplitudes in the aetiology of traumatic spastic disease. *Lancet* 1973;1: 791–794.
36. Isenberg DA, Black C. Raynaud's phenomenon, scleroderma, and overlap syndromes. *Br Med J* 1995;310:795–798.
37. James WD, et al. Emotional eccrine sweating—a heritable disorder. *Arch Dermatol* 1987;123:925–929.
38. Jänig W. Functions of the sympathetic innervation of the skin. In: Loewy AD, Speyer KM, eds. *Central Regulation of Autonomic Functions*. Oxford: Oxford University Press; 1990:334–348.
39. Jänig W, et al. Discharge patterns of sympathetic neurons supplying skeletal muscle and skin in man and cat. *J Auton Nerv Syst* 1983; 7:239–256.
40. Johnson RH, Spalding JMK. *Disorders of the Autonomic Nervous System*. Oxford: Blackwell Scientific; 1974:114–128.
41. Johnson RH, Spalding JMK. *Disorders of the Autonomic Nervous System*. Oxford: Blackwell Scientific; 1974:179–198.
42. Kahaleh MB. Raynaud's phenomenon and vascular disease in scleroderma. *Curr Opin Rheumatol* 1994;6:621–627.
43. Kahaleh B, Matucci-Cerinic M. Raynaud's phenomenon and scleroderma. *Arthritis Rheum* 1995;38:1–4.
44. Kenney MJ, et al. Characterization and quantification of sweating in a systemic hyperhidrotic patient. *Clin Exp Dermatol* 1986;2:543–552.
45. Khurana RK. Orthostatic hypotension-induced autonomic dysreflexia. *Neurology* 1987;37:1221–1224.
46. Khurana RK. Posttraumatic headache with ptosis, miosis, and chronic forehead hyperhidrosis. *Headache* 1990;30:64–68.
47. Kim-Beum-Saeng, et al. Contralateral hyperhidrosis after cerebral infarction—clinicoanatomic correlations in five cases. *Stroke* 1995;26: 896–899.
48. Kuritzky A, et al. Clonidine treatment in paroxysmal localized hyperhidrosis. *Arch Neurol* 1984;41: 1210–1211.
49. Labar DR, et al. Unilateral hyperhidrosis after cerebral infarction. *Neurology* 1988;38:1679–1682.
50. Leppert J, et al. Cold exposure increases cyclic guanosine monophosphate in healthy women but not in women with Raynaud's phenomenon. *J Intern Med* 1995;237:493–498.
51. Lerer B, et al. Personality features in essential hyperhidrosis. *Int J Psychiatry Med* 1980/81;10:59–67.
52. Lewis T, Marvin HM. Observations upon a pilomotor reaction in response to faradism. *J Physiol* 1927;64:87–106.
53. Lillis PJ, Coleman WP. Liposuction for treatment of axillary hyperhidrosis. *Dermatol Clin* 1990;8:479–482.
54. Limburg AJ, et al. Esophageal hypomotility in primary and secondary Raynaud's phenomenon: comparison of esophageal scintigraphy with manometry. *J Nucl Med* 1995;36:451–455.
55. List CF, Peet MM. Sweat secretion in man. II. Anatomic distribution of disturbances in sweating associated with lesions of the sympathetic nervous system. *Arch Neurol Psychiatry* 1938;40:27–43.
56. Loebe M, Heidrich H. The carpal tunnel syndrome—a disease underlying Raynaud's phenomenon? *Angiology* 1988;39:891–901.
57. McEvoy M, et al. Unilateral hyperhidrosis—an unusual presentation of bronchial carcinoma. *Ir J Med Sci* 1982;151:51–52.
58. Okada F, et al. Plasma guanosine 3'-5' monophosphate responses to the cold pressor test in patients with vibration disease. *Arch Environ Health* 1983;38:144–147.
59. Olsen N. Vibration-induced white finger. *Dan Med Bull* 1989;36: 47–64.
60. Orne MT. The efficacy of biofeedback therapy. *Annu Rev Med* 1979; 30:489–503.
61. Palmer AJ. Hyperhidrosis. *Arch Neurol Psychiatry* 1947;58:582–592.
62. Pick J. *The Autonomic Nervous System*. Philadelphia: JB Lippincott; 1970:341–349.
63. Pick J. *The Autonomic Nervous System*. Philadelphia: JB Lippincott; 1970:351–358.
64. Pleet DL, et al. Paroxysmal unilateral hyperhidrosis and malignant mesothelioma. *Arch Neurol* 1983;40:256.
65. Quinton PM. Sweating and its disorders. *Annu Rev Med* 1983;34: 429–452.
66. Rechardt L, et al. Innervation of human axillary sweat glands. *Scand J Plast Reconstr Surg* 1976;10:107–112.
67. Reinauer S, et al. Iontophoresis with alternating current and direct current offset (AC/DC iontophoresis): a new approach for the treatment of hyperhidrosis. *Br J Dermatol* 1993;129: 166–169.
68. Riolo J, et al. Surgical management of palmar hyperhidrosis. *South Med J* 1990;83:1138–1143.
69. Sato K, et al. Biology of sweat glands and their disorders. II. Disorders of sweat gland function. *J Am Acad Dermatol* 1989;20:713–726.
70. Sato K, et al. Generation and transit pathway of H^+ is critical for inhibition of palmar sweating by iontophoresis in water. *J Appl Physiol* 1993;75:2258–2264.
71. Serra G, et al. Raynaud's phenomenon and entrapment neuropathies. *Ann Neurol* 1985;18:519.
72. Shaw D, Trotter JM. Plasma exchange to control sweats and pruritis in malignant disease. *Br Med J* 1980;2:1459.
73. Shelley WB, Hurley HJ Jr. Studies on topical antiperspirant control of axillary hyperhidrosis. *Acta Derm Venereol (Stockh)* 1975;55:241–260.
74. Shih C-J, Wang YC. Thoracic sympathectomy for palmar hyperhidrosis. Report of 457 cases. *Surg Neurol* 1978;10:291–296.
75. Shih C-J, et al. Autonomic dysfunction in palmar hyperhidrosis. *J Auton Nerv Syst* 1983;8:33–43.
76. Singh S, et al. Response of digital arteries to endothelium dependent and independent vasodilators in patients with Raynaud's phenomenon. *Eur J Clin Invest* 1995; 25:182–185.
77. Smith GP, et al. Biochemical studies of pyridoxal and pyridoxal phosphate status and therapeutic trial of pyridoxine in patients with carpal tunnel syndrome. *Ann Neurol* 1986;15:104–107.
78. Stanworth PA. The significance of hyperhidrosis in patients with post-traumatic syringomyelia. *Paraplegia* 1982;20:282–287.
79. Stovner LJ, Sjaastad O. Segmental hyperhidrosis in two siblings with Chiari type I malformation. *Eur Neurol* 1995;35:149–155.

80. Teh LS, et al. Sustained-release transdermal glyceryl trinitrate patches as a treatment for primary and secondary Raynaud's phenomenon. *Br J Rheumatol* 1995;34:636–641.
81. Tsuhima WT, et al. Behavioral treatment of palmar hyperhidrosis. *Hawaii Med J* 1987;46:238;259–260.
82. Walsh JC, et al. Localized sympathetic overactivity: an uncommon complication of lung cancer. *J Neurol Neurosurg Psychiatry* 1976;39:93–95.
83. Watson CPN and Evans RJ. The hot foot sign in malignant retroperitoneal disease. *Neurology* 1980;30:358.
84. White JC. *The Autonomic Nervous System. Anatomy, Physiology, and Surgical Treatment*. New York: Macmillan; 1935:150–196.
85. White JW. Treatment of primary hyperhidrosis. *Mayo Clin Proc* 1986;61:951–956.

Subject Index

Note: a t following a page number denotes a table; an f denotes a figure; an n denotes a footnote.

A

A1 cell group, 54
A1-A3 and A5 neuron groups, 19
ABC (angry backfiring C nociceptor) syndrome, 11, 481, 721
Abdominal contraction, circulatory responses, 75, 76f
"Abdominal epilepsy," 423
Abdominal pressure, and circulatory response to standing up, 79
Acceleration index, 304
Accommodation, 260, 266
   see also Ciliary muscle
   autonomic disturbances affecting, 452–453
Acetylcholine, 29
   and assessing cholinergic function, 591–592
   as neurotransmitter, 586
   and vascular endothelium, 70
Acetylcholine iontophoresis, *see* Quantitative sudomotor axon reflex test; Neurogenic flare response; Flare response
Acetylcholinesterase, 29, 591
Acetylcholinesterase antibodies, use for sympathectomy, 413–414, 414f
Acidosis, and chemosensitive afferents, 69–70
Acquired immunodeficiency syndrome, *see* AIDS
Acquired neuromyotonia (Isaacs' syndrome), 519
Acquired nonprogressive dysautonomia syndrome, 642
Acral sympathetic dysfunction, 809–818
Acral sympathetic functions, 809
Acrocyanosis, 816
Acute autonomic neuropathies, *see under* Autonomic neuropathies; Panautonomic neuropathies
Acute inflammatory polyneuropathy, *see* Guillain–Barré syndrome
Adams-Stokes attacks, 655
   electrophysiologic studies, 667
Adhesion molecules, 149, 517
Adie's tonic pupil (Adie's syndrome; Holmes-Adie syndrome), 442t, 444, 474, 720
Adjuvant-induced arthritis, 152
Adrenal gland
   and immune system, 155
   and diabetes, 510, 511–512, 511f, 512f, 516
Adrenergic agonists, use in urinary bladder dysfunction, 626
α-Adrenergic agonists
   use in orthostatic hypotension, 569
   use in syncope, 673
   use in postural orthostatic tachycardia syndrome, 694
β-Adrenergic agonists, effects on immune system, 150–151
α-Adrenergic blockade, and autonomic function tests, 395
Adrenergic blocking agents
   effects on pupil, 448

use in urinary bladder dysfunction, 626
β-Adrenergic blocking agents
   and Raynaud's phenomenon, 815
   use in multiple system atrophy, 569
   use in orthostatic hypotension, 769t, 770
   use in postural orthostatic tachycardia syndrome, 694
   use in syncope, 673
Adrenergic failure
   focal, methods of study, 397
   vs. hypovolemia, 397
   problems in evaluation, 397–398
Adrenergic nervous system
   and exposure to low gravity, 436–437, 436f, 438f
   overactivity, from intracranial causes, 791–792
   in penile erection and detumescence, 133
   pitfalls in evaluation, 397–398
   and postprandial hypotension, 740–741, 743–744
   recommended tests, 291
   and sweating, 103, 104
Adrenergic neurons
   experimental injury, from 6-hydroxydopamine, 412
   postganglionic, guanethidine-induced destruction, 413
Adrenergic receptors
   and exposure to low gravity, 435–437
   on immune cells, 150, 153–154
   and postural orthostatic tachycardia syndrome, 684
β-Adrenergic sensitivity, in diabetes, 496
Adrenergic/sensory neuropeptide-deficient neuropathy, 474–475
Adrenocorticotropic hormone (ACTH)
   in multiple system atrophy and pure autonomic failure
     response to arecoline, 591–592, 593, 594f
     response to hypoglycemia, 589t, 593
   stimulation during stress, 22
Adrenomyeloneuropathy, 479
"After-drop," 756
Aging, 161–176
   see also Elderly
   and cardiovascular oscillations, 325–331, 331, 332f, 332f
   effects on baroreflexes, 166–167
   effects on blood pressure response to tilt-up, 196t
   effects on central autonomic functions, 167
   effects on exercise capacity, 167
   effects on forced sinus arrhythmia, 163, 164
   effects on ganglionic transmission, 167
   effects on heart rate
     effects on heart rate responses, 394
     to deep breathing, 193, 193t, 194f, 288, 301
     to tilt-up, 196t
   effects on resting heart rate, 162, 162f
   and heart rate variability, 331
   effects on norepinephrine levels, 167, 170, 171f

effects on orthostatic 30:15 ratio, 164, 166, 166f
   effects on pupil, 171–173, 172f, 265
   effects on skin vasomotor reflexes, 171, 172t
   effects on sudomotor neuraxis, 168–169
   effects on sweat glands, 93, 168, 169t
     effects on QSART, 193t
     effects on thermoregulatory sweat test, 248, 254
   effects on sympathetic function, 169–173
     effects on sympathetic cardiac function, 167
     effects on sympathetic skin response, 225
   effects on total power spectral density, 166
   effects on Valsalva ratio, 164, 165f, 194, 194t, 195f, 288, 303
   effects on venoarteriolar reflex, 171
   and heat stroke, 168
   heterogeneity of effects, 162
   and orthostatic hypotension, 167–168, 167t
   and spectral power, 337
AIDS, *see also* Human immunodeficiency virus INFECTION
   associated myelopathy, sweat test, 255f
   associated peripheral neuropathies, 703–704
   autonomic dysfunction
     clinical features, 733
     natural history, 731
   autonomic failure, 727–735
   autonomic function tests, 728f, 729–731, 729t
   dementia, 731–732
   distal sensorimotor polyneuropathy, 732–733
AIDS-related complex
   autonomic dysfunction, 731
   autonomic function tests, 728f, 729–731, 729t, 731
Airways, vagal innervation, 42
Alcohol ingestion
   and baroreflexes, 497f
   and erectile dysfunction, 270, 283
   and hypothermia, 757
   and multiple system atrophy, 565
   and pure autonomic failure, 565
   and sympathetic nerve activity, 238
Alcohol withdrawal
   autonomic overactivity, 780, 786
   management, 787
Alcoholic neuropathy, 480, 702
   histopathologic findings, 379
   pupillary findings, 453
Allodynia, 10, 211
Aluminum chloride, use in hyperhidrosis, 812
Alzheimer's disease
   cerebrospinal fluid antibodies, 568
   dysautonomia, 341, 341f
   electroencephalogram, 339, 341, 341f
   pupillary response to anticholinergics, 453
American Academy of Neurology Therapeutics and Technology Committee, grading of autonomic function testing, 291

Amplitude modulation, 353, 353f
  in electroencephalography (AM-EEG), 336, 339,
      352–358, 355t
    see also Electroencephalogram, -graphy
  during tilt-up, 356f, 357
Amplitude modulation rhythms, 354f
Amygdala, 17, 22
  and aversive stimuli, 21–22
  in stress response, 21, 21f
Amyloid neuropathy, 475–477, 701–702
  see also Distal small fiber neuropathy; Small fiber
      neuropathy
  amyloid deposition patterns, 375
  biochemistry and classification, 475
  gastrointestinal dysmotility, 608
    distinguishing neuropathic from myopathic, 608
  histopathologic findings, 375
  myeloma-associated, 476
  sural nerve compound action potential, 372f
  thermoregulatory sweat test, 253
  tissue biopsy, 10
Amyloid precursor proteins, 375
Amyotrophic lateral sclerosis (ALS), 426, 480
  gastrointestinal dysmotility, 605–606
  urinary bladder dysfunction, 622
  vs. multiple system atrophy: sacral motor neurons,
      566
  vs. Shy-Drager syndrome: sphincter
      electromyography, 563
Anal sphincter
  extrinsic neural control, 137t
  and urinary sphincter innervation, 122
  pudendal innervation, 121
Analysis of variability, in constituent frequencies,
    312–317
Anejaculation, 271, 806
Anemia, and exposure to low gravity, 432, 438f
Anesthesia
  and sympathetic nerve activity, 241
  complications
    in diabetes, 494–495
    in generalized autonomic failure, 570–571
    malignant hyperthermia, 751
  and pupillary dilatation, 265
Angiotensin, see Renin-angiotensin system
Angry backfiring C nociceptor (ABC) syndrome, 11,
    481, 721
Anhidrosis, 99–100
  causes, 248t
  chronic idiopathic, 473
    sweat test, 250, 250f, 251
  distal, sweat pattern, 248
  focal, sweat pattern, 249
  global, sweat pattern, 249
  in heat stroke, 99, 103
  iatrogenic, 248t
  mixed thermoregulatory sweat pattern, 249
  "normal," 248
  poral occlusion vs. lack of sweat secretion, 100
  from radiation damage, 254, 254f
  regional, sweat pattern, 249
  Ross' syndrome, 251
  segmental, sweat pattern, 248–249
  thermoregulatory sweat test, 248–249, 254
  in Tangier disease, 377, 377f
  with excessive localized sweating, 99
Anisocoria
  essential (simple, benign central), 266
  vs. Horner's syndrome, 444–445, 446, 450
  evaluation, 443f, 449–450
Anorexia, 155, 251
Anterior pituitary hormones, 593–594
Antibodies, 148
  see also Autoantibodies
  anti-adrenal, and diabetes, 511–512, 511f, 512f, 516

anti-glutamic acid dexarboxylase, in diabetes, 517
anti-islet cell, antigenic targets, 516–517
antineuronal, 509–510
  antigenic targets, 516–517
  antineuronal nuclear antibody (anti-Hu), 550
  and diabetes, 510, 517
  in nondiabetic polyglandular diseases, 518–519
antisulfatide, 704
anti-sympathetic ganglia
  and diabetes, 512, 513f
  and Parkinson's disease, 517
  and postural blood pressure changes, 514–515,
      515f
anti-vagus nerve, and diabetes, 512, 514f, 516, 517
in cerebrospinal fluid, in neurodegenerative
    disorders, 568
Antibody-mediated immunity, and diabetes, 511–514
Anticholinergic agents
  and autonomic function tests, 399
    and thermoregulatory sweat test, 254
  effects on eye, 447
    pupillary response in Alzheimer's disease, 453
  use in urinary bladder dysfunction, 626
Antidepressants, tricyclic
  overdosage, 798
  use in sleep apnea, 644
  use in small fiber neuropathy, 711
  use in urinary bladder dysfunction, 626
Antidiuretic hormone (ADH), see Vasopressin
Antigen-binding domains, 148
Antigen-presenting cells, 148
Antigen recognition by lymphocytes, 148
Antihypertensive agents
  for acute conditions, 794t
  for acute intracranial conditions, 794–795
  and intracranial pressure, 794
  and orthostatic hypotension, 767
Antineuronal nuclear antibody (anti-Hu), 550
Antionconeural immune response, 548
Antipyretic agents, 753
Aortic arch, baroreceptor efferents, 21f
Aortic baroreceptors, 64, 65–66, 79, 433, 434, 435,
    438f
Apnea, see also Sleep apnea
  central, 638, 639f
  during normal sleep, 638
  mixed, 638–639, 639f
  and sympathetic vasomotor outflow, 352
  upper-airway obstructive, 638, 639f
Apnea index, 638
Apnea-hypopnea index, 639
Apneic facial immersion, see Facial immersion test
Apneustic breathing, 639f, 640
Apneustic center, 636
Apocrine sweat glands, 91
Apocrinelike (trichial, hair-associated) sweat glands,
    98, 98f
Apoeccrine sweat glands, 100
Apoptosis, and aging, 162
Area under the curve, 312f
Arecoline, in autonomic failure syndromes
  ACTH response, 591–592, 593, 594f
  epinephrine response, 589, 592
Arginine vasopressin (AVP), see Vasopressin
Argyll Robertson pupils, 441–442, 442t, 444
Arnold-Chiari malformation, 425, 810
Arrector pili (arrectores pilorum) muscles, 110, 111f,
    113f, 114
Arrhythmias, see Cardiac arrhythmias
Arterial baroreceptors, 20
  and upright posture, 64–66, 74
Arterial baroreflexes
  and blood pressure, 64–66
  and exercise, 68–69, 69f
  set-point resetting, 65, 65f, 68

Arterial reflexes, interaction with cardiopulmonary
    reflexes, 66
Arterioles of skin, innervation, 111f, 112
Arteriovenous anastomoses, in thermoregulation, 89,
    90
Artificial insemination, after spinal cord injury, 460,
    806
Astronauts, see also Gravity, prolonged reduction
  motion sickness, 437
  and study of autonomic dysfunction, 429
Atopic diathesis, and sweating disorders, 100
Atrial decremental pacing, 669f, 670
Atrial natriuretic peptide (factor), 238, 592
Atrial programmed extrastimulation, 670
Atrichial (eccrine) sweat glands, see Sweat glands,
    eccrine
Atrioventricular (AV) conduction disturbances, and
    syncope, 655
  electrophysiologic studies, 667–670, 667f,
      668f–669f
  therapeutic management, 673
Atropine
  effect on blood pressure response to Valsalva
      maneuver, 190f
  effects on eye, 447
  effects on heart rate variability, 297–298, 298f
  mechanism of action, 447
Auerbach's (myenteric) plexus, 136, 138f, 139, 139f,
    140
Augmentation cystoplasty, 627f, 628
Auricular branch of vagus nerve, 40
Auriculotemporal syndrome, 92, 720
Auto Wigner distribution, 357
Autoantibodies, see also Antibodies
  antineuronal, 509–510
  and diabetes, 510, 511–514
    antigenic targets, 516–517
    and diabetics' relatives, 513–514
  in Lambert-Eaton myasthenic syndrome, 549
Autoimmune disorders
  experimental acetylcholinesterase autoimmunity,
      413–414, 414f
  experimental autoimmune myasthenia gravis
      (EAMG), 152
  and idiopathic small fiber neuropathy, 707
  polyglandular autoimmune syndrome type II, 510,
      517
Autoimmune mechanisms, 517
  in diabetic neuropathy, 509–524
Autoimmune responses, 148
Autonomic autoantibodies, and diabetes, 511–514
  antigenic targets, 516–517
  autonomic brake index, 516
  and diabetics' relatives, 513–514
  and pathophysiology, 514–516
  and postural catecholamine responses, 515f
  in type II diabetes, 514
Autonomic "brake," in gastrointestinal motility, 598
Autonomic brake index, 304, 516
Autonomic clinical neurophysiologist, training and
    experience, 294
Autonomic disorders
  see also Dysautonomias; other Autonomic entries,
      below, and specific disorder or site
  autonomic system review, 5–6
  central disorders, 421–428
  classification, 3–5, 4t
  clinical evaluation, see Clinical evaluation
  compensatory mechanisms, 7
  emergencies, 6
  episodic, 11, 12
  finding the cause, 12
  laboratory evaluation, see Autonomic function tests;
      Laboratory evaluation
  laboratory monitoring, 180, 291

choice of tests, 392–393
recognizing benign vs. life-threatening, 180
recognizing distribution, 5–6
recognizing treatable disorders, 6
site of lesion, pitfalls in deducing, 393
time frequency analysis, 333f, 334–336
Autonomic dysreflexia (hyperreflexia), 426, 458–459
  in spinal cord injury, 623, 780, 796
  stimuli, 458, 458t
  symptoms, 458–459, 458t
  thermoregulatory sweat test, 252
Autonomic evaluation in the frequency domain, 336–338
Autonomic failure, *see also* Pure autonomic failure; Dysautonomias; Multiple system atrophy
  and acute panautonomic neuropathy, 465
  and AIDS, 727–735
  erebral autoregulation, 362
  combined sympathetic-parasympathetic
    in acute panautonomic neuropathy, 465
    with clinically important autonomic dysfunction, 475–478
    with clinically unimportant autonomic dysfunction, 478–481
  distinguishing central vs. peripheral, 586–587, 589, 594
  electroencephalographic monitoring, 362–366
  episodic, 12
  functional, in diabetes, 496
  gastrointestinal peptides, 593
  generalized
    anesthesia problems, 570–571
    asymptomatic hypoglycemia, 559
    causes, 11–12
    laboratory studies, 180
    symptom pattern, 11
  hypoglycemia-associated, 496
  indications for laboratory tests, 180–181
  and lateral horn cell loss, 578
  neurochemical and pharmacologic abnormalities, 585–595
    responses to hypoglycemia, 589t
  and postprandial hypotension, 557f, 559, 559f
  primary syndromes, sweat test, 250–251
  primary vs. secondary, 638
  and sleep apnea, 638–645
  suspected, approach to management, 11–12
  treatment, 568–571
  and Valsalva maneuver, 189, 190t
  vasopressin responses, 594
  with sensory neuronopathy, 477–478
Autonomic function tests, *see also* Laboratory evaluation; Screening tests; *and specific test names*
  American Academy of Neurology test grades, 291
  clinical uses
    AIDS, 729–731
    clinical trials, 294
    gastrointestinal dysmotility, 609–611, 610t
    erectile dysfunction, 281–282
      indications, 284
    HIV infection, 728f, 729–731, 729t
    Lambert-Eaton myasthenic syndrome, 546, 547t, 548
    multiple system atrophy, 561–562
    Parkinson's disease, 579–581
    pure autonomic failure, 561–562
  concordance among tests, 393, 399
  criteria for good tests, 288–289, 399–400
  evaluating new tests, 288, 399
  factors affecting, 399
  indications for retesting, 294
  interpretation, 293–294
    interpretation problems, 392, 393
  justification, 287–288

less well validated tests, 291
normal values, 610t
patient preparation, 292, 294
pitfalls, 391–401
  "black-boxing," 392–393
  in blood pressure photoplethysmography, 398, 398f, 399f
  complexity of underlying reflexes, 392
  deducing lesion site, 393
  in evaluating adrenergic function, 397–398
  in frequency analysis, 396
  heart rate recording problems, 394–396
  importance of blood volume, 396
  inaccurate observations, 393–394
  oversimplifying assumptions, 391–392
  in skin potential recordings, 397
  standardization problems, 392
  true stimulus vs. test stimulus, 391, 392f
  in validation of tests, 399–400
rating of tests, 290t, 291t
recommendations of San Antonio Conference on Diabetic Neuropathy, 290–291
routine tests, 181–198, 182t
selecting individual tests, 289–290
  how many to use, 289
sensitivity vs. specificity, 288
standardization, 287–295, 392
stimuli used, 345
system review, 5–6
test batteries, 289, 292, 298, 385
  for clinical trials, 294
testing conditions, 181
tests with demonstrated sensitivity, 288
tests with low sensitivity, 288
validated tests, 291
Autonomic hyperactivity, *see* Autonomic overactivity
Autonomic hyperreflexia, *see* Autonomic dysreflexia
Autonomic laboratory, *see* Laboratory
Autonomic nervous system
  central components, *see* Central *entries*
  changes during sleep, 637–638
  in circulatory control, 61–71, 62f, 73–81
  clinical examination, 9–11
  information from frequency analysis, 320
  medications affecting, 4t
  and neuropeptides, 592–594
  regeneration after injury, 444
  spinal and peripheral components, 25–45
  system review, 5–6
Autonomic neuropathies, 463–486
  see also Neuropathies; Panautonomic neuropathies; *and specific disorders*
  acute, 12, 464–472
    classification, 464t
    medication-induced, 470–471
    restricted forms, 465
    somatic involvement, 465
  acute toxic, 472
  classification, 4t, 464t
  diagnosis, 180
  differential diagnosis, 564t
  effects of tilt-up, 365, 366
  experimental, 403–417
    acrylamide-induced, 406–410, 472
    cardiovascular system, 407–409, 408f
    esophagus, 409f, 410
    gastrointestinal system, 409f, 410
    histopathology, 407, 407f, 408f
    physiologic studies, 407–410
    renal sympathetic activity, 409
    respiratory system, 409–410
  diabetic, 403–406
  induced by sympathetic chain antigens with adjuvant, 414–415
  idiopathic (IAN), 465

case study, 774
thermoregulatory sweat test, 250
vs. pure autonomic failure, 564, 564t
neuropathology, 369–381
as paraneoplastic disorder, 552
pathologic findings, 374–379
in postural orthostatic tachycardia syndrome, 336
sleep apnea, 642
spectral analysis applications, 320
sural nerve biopsy, 372–374
urinary bladder dysfunction, 624
Autonomic overactivity (hyperactivity), *see also* Sympathetic disorders, overactivity
  from acute hydrocephalus, 424
  adrenergic, from intracranial causes, 791–792
  autonomic storm, 12, 791–801
  blood pressure measurements, 799
  disorders causing, 778t
  in Guillain-Barré syndrome, 777–779, 796–797
  paroxysmal, *see* Diencephalic seizures
  pathophysiology, 780–786, 785f
  from seizures, 792–793
  syndromes, 777–789
    management, 787
    monitoring, 786–787
Autonomic plexuses, 36
Autonomic reflex screen, 181, 182t, 292–293, 385
  and composite autonomic scoring scale (CASS), 191
  Finapres technique, 292
  personnel requirements, 384
Autonomic reflexes
  neural pathways, 199t
  problems in quantitating, 397–398
  testing, *see also* Autonomic reflex screen; Autonomic function tests
    interpretation problems, 392, 393
    testing conditions, 181
    true stimulus vs. test stimulus, 391, 392f
Autonomic storm, 12, 791–801
Autonomic symptom profile, 9
Autonomic system review, 5–6
Autoregressive modeling, 324f
  dynamic, 345
  in electroencephalography, 353–357, 354f
Autoregressive spectral estimation, 314–315, 316f
Autoregulatory failure, 360
Avitaminosis B^{12} neuropathy, 480
Axon flare response, *see* Neurogenic flare response
Axon reflex sweat response, *see* Quantitative sudomotor axon reflex test
Axonal (dying-back) neuropathy, 227, 228, 406

B

B cells, 148
  see also Lymphocytes
  antigen recognition, 148
  clonal expansion, 148
  effects of sympathetic ablation, 151
  proliferation, 149
    and β-adrenergic agonists, 150–151
  T-cell independent and T-cell dependent responses, 148
Bainbridge reflex, 299
Baroreceptor reflex, *see* Baroreflex *entries*
Baroreceptors, *see also* Baroreflexes
  afferent block, 781, 783f, 784
  aortic baroreceptors, 21f, 64, 65–66, 79, 433, 434, 435, 438f
    methods of study, 433
    and upright posture, 65
  arterial, 20
  and upright posture, 64–66, 74
  cardiopulmonary, 79, 434, 435
  of carotid sinus, 21f, 64–66, 79, 433
    and exercise, 68

Baroreceptors, of carotid sinus (contd.)
  innervation, 39, 40
  and syncope, 652–654
  effects of eating, 739
  set-point, 65
Baroreflex arc
  afferent and efferent pathways, 75f
  neural prosthesis, 570
Baroreflex failure, from medullary lesions, 424
Baroreflex sensitivity
  and heart rate variability, spectral analysis, 320
  quantitating, 201–202
Baroreflex stimulus, and reflex bradycardia, 394
Baroreflexes
  in alcoholism, 497f
  arterial
    and blood pressure, 64–66
    and exercise, 68–69, 69f
    set-point resetting, 65, 65f, 68
  and blood pressure variability, 318–319
  carotid sinus to sinoatrial node, 202
  central circuits, 20, 21f
  in diabetic neuropathy, 496–497, 497f
  effects of aging, 166–167
  effects of exposure to low gravity, 433–435, 434f, 435f, 438f
  and orthostatic hypotension, 55
Basal ganglia, and urinary bladder function, 119
bcl-2 proto-oncogene, 162
Beat-to-beat analysis, in transcranial Doppler monitoring, 351
Beat-to-beat blood pressure measurements
  Finapres technique, 188–189
    factors affecting, 188
  photoplethysmographic recording problems, 398
  and responses to upright posture, 190–191, 304
  and responses to Valsalva maneuver, 189–190, 302, 303
Beat-to-beat variability, see Heart rate variability
Bed rest, and orthostatic intolerance, see also Gravity, prolonged reduction
  prophylaxis before reambulation, 437, 438
Behavioral (voluntary) breathing system, 637
Benign central (simple, essential) anisocoria, vs. Horner's syndrome, 446, 450
Beta-adrenergic, see β–Adrenergic, in A's
Bethanechol, use in urinary bladder dysfunction, 625–626
Bethanechol test, in diabetes, 500
Bezold-Jarisch reflex, 651
Bier block, use in pain syndromes, 216
Biliary cirrhosis, and small fiber neuropathy, 705
Biofeedback therapy
  for gastrointestinal dysmotility, 611
  for urinary bladder dysfunction, 624–625
Birth injuries, and Horner's syndrome, 445
Bladder, see Urinary bladder
Blood flow velocity, see also Cerebral blood flow velocity
  in postural orthostatic tachycardia syndrome, 363f
  in static vs. rhythmic exercise, 67
  spectral analysis, 350, 350f
  transcranial Doppler waveform, 350f
Blood flow volume, in orthostatic hypotension and cerebral perfusion, 365
Blood pressure, see also Hypertension; Hypotension; Orthostatic hypotension; Postural normotension
  central factors, 53–55
  changes during sleep, 637
  clinical examination, 9–10
  diurnal variation, 61, 63f
    and multiple system atrophy, 557
  effects of aging, 331, 332f
  effects of exposure to low gravity, 438–439, 438f
  fractal dimension, 337
  monitoring techniques, 799
  and muscle sympathetic activity, 235, 238
  and nucleus tractus solitarii lesions, 53, 54f
  photoplethysmographic recordings, 188–189
  regulatory mechanisms, 61, 62f, 73–81, 429
    and caudate nuclei, 583
    neurotransmitters and neuropeptides, 592, 592t
  respiratory effects, 310, 317
  response to exercise
    in multiple system atrophy, 557
    in pure autonomic failure, 557
    static vs. rhythmic exercise, 67
  response to food, see Postprandial hypotension
  response to intravenous tyramine, 202
  response to mental stress, 203
  response to postural changes, and anti-sympathetic ganglia autoantibodies, 514–515, 515f
  response to pressor drugs, in pure autonomic failure vs. multiple system atrophy, 588
  response to prolonged tilt-up, 201
  response to standing, 61–62, 79–80, 396f
    after exposure to low gravity, 430
    homeostatic mechanisms, 62–66, 64f, 303
  response to tilt-up, 190–191, 191f, 292–293, 329f, 330, 330f, 334
    effects of pacemaker, 331, 331f
    normative data, 194, 196t
  response to Valsalva maneuver, 189–190, 190f, 292, 360, 360f
    in orthostatic hypotension, 361f, 362
    in postural orthostatic tachycardia syndrome, 363f
  and skin sympathetic activity, 237
  slow oscillations at non-respiratory frequencies (non-RF rhythms), 325, 353
    factors affecting, 328–331
    generating factors, 328–331
    structures involved, 353
  and spinal cord transection, 55
  after spinal cord trauma, 456
  supine, and orthostatic hypotension in elderly, 168
Blood pressure variability, 309–312, 310f, 311f
  causative mechanism, 318
  as cause of heart rate variability, 318, 320
  frequency analysis
    clinical applicability, 319–321
    physiologic interpretation, 317–319
  spectral analysis, 315–317, 316f
Blood volume, see also Circulation; Hypovolemia
  and autonomic function tests, 395–396, 399
  and body temperature, 87
  effects of exposure to low gravity, 431–432
  methods of measuring, 397
  orthostatic displacement, 73, 74f
  response to standing, 61–62, 63, 64f, 74, 75, 77, 81
    and autonomic function tests, 395–396
Blushing, 716–717
  see also Facial flushing
Body temperature, see Temperature, of body; Thermoregulation
Botulinum toxin, use in hyperhidrosis, 813
Botulism, 470, 798
Bowel, see Gastrointestinal; Intestinal
Brachial plexus, 36
  and Horner's syndrome, 445
Bradbury-Eggleston syndrome, 432
Bradycardia, mechanisms, 784, 785f
Bradycardia latency, 302
Bradytachyarrhythmias, 642
Brain, autonomic disorders, classification, 4t
Brain-dead patient, spectral analysis, 342–343, 343f
Brain injury, spectral analysis, 342–343
Brain tumors
  gastrointestinal dysmotility, 606, 606f
  urinary bladder dysfunction, 621
Brainstem
  and cardiovascular and respiratory oscillations, 353
  cardiovascular centers, 67–68
  central autonomic network, 633–636, 634f, 635f
  and Cushing response, 792
  and dysautonomia, 5
  evoked potentials, 563
  and gut motility, 136
  and postural orthostatic tachycardia syndrome, 686–687, 695
  and thermal afferents, 84
Brainstem-dead patient, 342–343, 343f
Brainstem disorders, 424–425
  classification, 4t
  and sweating, 90
Brake, autonomic, in gastrointestinal motility, 598
Brake index, autonomic, 304, 516
Breathing disorders, see Respiratory entries
Bulbar palsy, progressive, 605–606
Bulbocavernosus (bulbospongiosus) muscle
  in female, 130, 132
  in male, 129–130
Bulbocavernosus (BC) reflex, 278–279
  clinical utility, 279
Bulbocavernosus reflex latency, 620–621
"Burning feet" syndrome, sweat test, 254, 255f
Burning foot dominantly inherited sensory neuropathy, 703

C

C fibers, and nociception, see Neurogenic flare response; ABC syndrome
C1-C3 neuron groups, 19
Cajal's (deep muscular) plexus, 138f, 140
Cajal's interstitial cells, 140
Calcitonin gene-related peptide, 30f, 32, 112
Calcium channel blockers
  use in pain syndromes, 218
  use in urinary bladder dysfunction, 626
Calcium channels, 549
  in Lambert-Eaton myasthenic syndrome, 548–550
Cancer, see also Tumors and Paraneoplastic autonomic disorders
  of lung, 546, 606f, 608
Cancer-associated neuropathies, 704–705
Capillaries, of skin, innervation, 112, 113f
Carbon dioxide balance, and sweating, 87, 88f, 93
Cardiac, see also Heart; Myocardium; and Cardiovascular entries
Cardiac arrhythmias (dysrhythmias)
  in AIDS, 728, 730
  forced (respiratory) sinus arrhythmia, see Respiratory sinus arrhythmia
  from autonomic function tests, 204
  from exposure to low gravity, 432–433
  from intracranial causes, therapy, 48
  from seizure, 422
  from stroke, 422
  neurogenic, 47–50
    changing central mechanisms, 48
    electrocardiographic changes, 49, 50
    intracranial causes, 48
    pathophysiologic basis, 48–49, 49–50
    and peripheral nerve disease, 49
    and stellate ganglion, 49
  after subarachnoid hemorrhage, 793
  and syncope, 655–656
    electrophysiologic studies, 664–672
    therapeutic management, 673
Cardiac disorders, use of spectral analysis, 332
Cardiac enzymes, and ECG changes, 51
Cardiac monitoring, in syncope, 660–661, 660f
Cardiac nerves, 42
  and arrhythmias, 48–49
  and ECG changes, 53
Cardiac output

and baroreflexes, 69, 69f
and impedance cardiography, 202
response to standing, 79
in thermoregulation, 90
Cardiac plexus, 34, 36
Cardiodynamic parameters in impedance cardiography, 202
Cardiogenic syncope, 654–656
electrophysiologic studies, 664–672
Cardiopulmonary afferents, and baroreflex arc, 75f
Cardiopulmonary baroreceptors, 79, 434, 435
Cardiopulmonary plexuses, 42
Cardiopulmonary receptors, 62–63, 66, 74
in prolonged orthostatic stress, 81
response to standing, 79, 80f
Cardiopulmonary reflexes, 62
and exposure to low gravity, 434–435, 435f, 438f
interaction with arterial reflexes, 66
Cardiorespiratory central network, 20
Cardiovagal function
and 30:15 ratio, 395
and Valsalva ratio, 394
Cardiovagal function tests
comparison, 188
heart rate tests, 162–167
potential tests, 201
recommended tests, 290t, 292
sensitivity of new vs. established tests, 336–337
Cardiovagal neuropathy, with alcoholism, 453
Cardiovascular control system
neurotransmitters and neuropeptides, 592, 592t
spectral analysis, clinical applications, 320
unpredictability, 319
Cardiovascular disturbances
in diabetes, 337, 339
neurogenic, 47–55
from central lesions, 47–53
from natural events, 50
Cardiovascular dysautonomia
in Guillain–Barré syndrome, 778–779, 796–797, 797f
measuring blood pressure, 799
Cardiovascular heart rate tests
in diabetes, 488t, 493–494
and anesthesia complications, 494–495
recommended tests, 291
Cardiovascular oscillations (rhythms), 325, 353
see also Heart rate variability
in development and aging, 325–331, 332f
in disease, 332–345
factors affecting, 325
structures involved, 353
in young adults, 325f, 326f, 327–328, 327–328, 327f, 328f
Cardiovascular reflexes
in diabetes, 493–494
in Parkinson's disease, 580
in progressive supranuclear palsy, 583
Cardiovascular syncope, 650–654
Cardiovascular system, see also components, e.g., Heart; Circulation; Hemodynamics
autonomic control, vestibular effects, 437
central and cardiac control, 47–55
brainstem centers, 67–68
changes during sleep, 637
response to exercise, 66–70, 68f
response to head-up tilt, 77, 79, 334
contour map, 330f
time–frequency analysis, 330, 330
time series, 329f
response to standing, 61–62, 64f, 74–77, 78f, 79–80
as test of autonomic function, 188
effects of prolonged standing, 80–81
after exposure to low gravity, 430
homeostatic mechanisms, 73

vs. passive head-up tilt, 77
response to stress, central circuits, 21f
response to venous pooling, 63, 64f, 74, 75, 77
responses, in syncope, 334
time–frequency analysis, 334f
time–frequency analysis, 323–348
technical guidelines, 343–347
Carotid baroreceptors, 64–66, 79, 433
effects of standing, 65
and exercise, 68
Carotid body (carotid glomus), 39, 39f
Carotid-cardiac baroreflex function
effects of exposure to low gravity, 433–434, 434f, 438f
and vestibular stimulation, 437–438
Carotid sinus, 39, 40
baroreceptor efferents, 21f
Carotid sinus hypersensitivity (carotid hypersensitivity syndrome), 652–654, 652f–653f
predisposing factors, 659
therapeutic management, 672–673
Carotid sinus massage, 660
Carotid sinus nerve, 39, 39f
Carotid sinus to sinoatrial node baroreflex, assessment, 202
Carpal tunnel syndrome, and Raynaud's phenomenon, 815
Catatonia, lethal, 796
Catecholamines
of central autonomic network, 19
in dopamine bhydroxylase deficiency, 562f
and ECG changes, 51, 53
effect on pupil, 265
effects on sweat glands, 103
and exposure to low gravity, 435
kinetics, 587–588, 587f
and diagnosis of diabetic neuropathy, 492
in multiple system atrophy, 562f
myocardial toxicity, 53
and neurogenic arrhythmias, 49
plasma level testing, 10, 198
postural response, 81
in diabetes, and autonomic antibodies, 515–516, 515f
in pure autonomic failure, 562f
Catheterization, for urinary bladder dysfunction, 625
Cauda equina lesions
and sexual dysfunction, 278
bulbocavernosus reflex, 278–279
and urinary bladder dysfunction, 623
Caudate nuclei, and blood pressure, 583
Causalgia (complex regional pain syndrome type II)
characteristics, 211t
definition, 537–538
Cavernosography, 272
Cavernosometry, 272
CD surface markers, on T cells, 147, 148
CD2-fas transgene, and aging, 162
Celiac ganglion, 35f
Celiac plexus, 36
Central autonomic disorders, 421–428
cardiovascular time–frequency studies, 339, 341–343
central dysautonomia, and sympathetic nerve activity, 239
thermoregulatory sweat test, 251–254
Central autonomic network, 17–23, 633–636, 634f, 635f
afferent pathways, 18–19
components, 17–18, 18f
effectors, 19
electroencephalographic rhythms, 339
and emotions, 21–22
functional aspects, 20–22
neurochemistry, 19
paraventricular nucleus as controller, 22
and stress, 21–22

Central command, 67–68
Central nervous system
and AIDS autonomic dysfunction, 731–732
and blood pressure, 53–55
and cardiovascular disturbances, 47–55
and cytokines, 155
dopamine turnover, 590–591
dopaminergic pathways, 590
and electrodermal activity, 224–225, 226
and gastrointestinal motility, 136, 137t
and hyperthermia, 753
and hypothermia, 756–757
neurotransmitter function studies, 588–589
in sexual function, 131–132
supraspinal autonomic pathways, 425
supraspinal control of gut motility, 136
supraspinal modulation of perception, 144f, 145
supraspinal (psychogenic) erection, 132
and sympathetic skin response, 226–227, 229
thermoregulatory mechanisms, see under Thermoregulation
in urinary bladder innervation, 118, 122, 122f
Central sudomotor drive, 92
nonthermal modifiers, 92–93
Central venous pressure, set-point, 432, 438f
Cerebellum
autonomic disorders, 4t
and urinary bladder function, 119
hemorrhage, 343f
Cerebral blood flow, see also Cerebral perfusion
in diabetes, 365
in multiple system atrophy, 556–557
regulation, 359
Cerebral blood flow velocity, see also Blood flow velocity
Doppler approach, 350
effects of tilt-up, 362
in autonomic failure, 362, 366
effects of Valsalva maneuver, 360, 360f
in orthostatic hypotension, 361f, 362
in postural orthostatic tachycardia syndrome, 362
in multiple system atrophy, 365–366, 365f
Cerebral cortex
autonomic components, 17
autonomic disorders, 4t
and dysautonomia, 5
in urethral innervation, 119
in urinary bladder innervation, 118–119
Cerebral perfusion, see also Cerebral blood flow
autoregulation, 359–360
in autonomic failure, 362
and effects of Valsalva maneuver, 361f, 362
in multiple system atrophy, 365–366, 365f
in postural orthostatic tachycardia syndrome, 362
in orthostatic hypotension, and blood flow volume, 365
transcranial Doppler monitoring, 360
Cerebral perfusion pressure, and antihypertensive therapy, 794
Cerebral vasoconstriction, in syncope, 366–367
Cerebrospinal fluid antibodies, 568
Cerebrovascular disorders, see also Stroke; Hemorrhage, intracerebral and ECG changes, 51
Cervical spondylosis, urinary bladder dysfunction, 623, 623f
Cervical sympathetic ganglia, 34–36
Cervical sympathetic pathways, 715–716, 716f
Cervicothoracic (stellate) ganglion, 35–36
and arrhythmias, 49
and ECG changes, 53
Chagas' disease, 474
Chaos analysis, 319
Chaos theory
and analysis of cardiovascular variability, 311
and cardiovascular rhythms, 331

Charcot-Marie-Tooth disease, 478–479
  eye involvement, 453
  hypertrophic, 479
Charcot's joints, 10
Cheyne-Stokes breathing, 639f, 640–641
Cheyne-Stokes variant breathing, 639f, 640–641
Cholecystokinins (CCKs), 31–32
Cholinergic agents
  use in diabetic neuropathy, 608
  use in syncope, 673
  use in urinary bladder dysfunction, 625–626
Cholinergic blockade, effects on heart rate variability, 298, 298f
Cholinergic dysfunction
  in multiple system atrophy, 558, 562
  in pure autonomic failure, 558
Cholinergic function tests, 591
  cholinergic sweat rate, 104
  in multiple system atrophy, 562
Cholinergic nerves, in penile erection and detumescence, 133
Cholinergic neuropathies, 473–474
  acute, 468
    vs. acute panautonomic neuropathy, 466
  pure, symptom pattern, 11
Cholinergic stimulation of sweating, 103, 104
  and Na-K-Cl cotransporter model, 104–105, 105f
Cholinergic vasodilation, and central command, 68
Chorda tympani syndrome, 92
Chronic fatigue syndrome (CFS), 690–691
Chronic inflammatory demyelinating polyradiculoneuropathy (CIDP), 473, 479
  in diabetes, 489
  with tonic pupil, 474
Chronic pain syndromes, see also Complex regional pain syndromes
  sympathetic nerve activity, 241
  with autonomic features, 209–220
    diagnostic considerations, 211–214
    terminology, 210
    treatment modalities, 214–218
Chronic sensory and autonomic neuropathy of unknown cause, 608, 609f
Ciliary body, 260
  disorders, 441–454
  innervation, 260–261
Ciliary ganglion, 37f, 38, 260–261
Ciliary muscle, 260, 261, 262f
  effects of anticholinergics, 447
  and nerve regeneration, 444
Ciliospinal reflex, 265
Circadian rhythms, 594
  and autonomic function, 20–21
  of blood pressure, 61, 63f, 310, 310f
  of heart rate, 310, 310f, 493
Circulation
  autonomic regulation, 61–71, 62f
  neurohumoral reflex adjustments, 77–81
  response to standing, 73, 74f
Circumventricular organs, 19
Cisplatin, neuropathy from, 470–471, 478
Clinical autonomic laboratory, see Laboratory
Clinical autonomic neurophysiologist, 294
Clinical evaluation of autonomic disorders, 3
  aims, 5–7
  autonomic examination, 9–11
  autonomic symptom profile, 9
  bedside or office vs. laboratory studies, 7
  diagnostic checklist, 14–15
  distribution of dysfunction, 5–6
  effects of dysfunction, 7
  for gastroparesis, 9
  genitourinary symptoms, 9
  guiding principles, 7–11
  history-taking, 7–9
  indications for laboratory studies, 12
  level of involvement, 11
  need for more studies, 6–7
  pupillomotor symptoms, 9
  sexual dysfunction, 9
  specialized organ system tests, 11
  sudomotor symptoms, 9
  in suspected autonomic failure, 11–12
  syndrome patterns, 6, 7, 11–12
  treatable disorders, 6
  vasomotor changes, 8–9
  when symptoms occur, 7
Clinical trials, 290, 290t, 294
Clitoris, 130, 133
Cluster headache, 721–724
  variants, 724
Cluster-tic syndrome, 724
Cocaine
  effects on eye, 446, 448
  overdosage, 798
Cocaine test, in Horner's syndrome, 446
Cocktail-party posture, 76f
Coefficient of variation, in time domain heart rate tests, 300
Cognition (mentation), see also Mental stress
  in multiple system atrophy, 556, 558
Coherence, in spectral analysis, 316–317, 316f
Cold, see also Temperature, ambient; Shivering
  vascular responses, 89
Cold face test, 164, 204, 304–305
  see also Facial immersion test
Cold pressor test, 236, 395
Cold-sensitive neurons, 84, 85, 86f
Collagen vascular disease neuropathy, 253
Combined adrenergic/sensory neuropeptide-deficient neuropathy, 474–475
Combined sympathetic and parasympathetic failure, see under Autonomic failure
Complement activation, in diabetes, 514
Complement-fixing (CF) autoantibodies, in diabetes, 510, 511, 512
  antigenic targets, 516–517
Complement-dependent sympathectomy, 413–414
Complete ophthalmoplegia, 443
Complex regional pain syndromes (CRPS), 209–220
  see also Pain, sympathetically maintained; Reflex sympathetic dystrophy
  autonomic features, 211–212
  clinical presentations, 211–212
  diagnostic algorithm, 540t
  diagnostic considerations, 211–214
  identifying sympathetic-based pains, 214
  Kozin's criteria, 214, 214t
  laboratory studies, 212–214
  pain characteristics, 211
  radiographic findings, 213
  taxonomy, 210–211, 211t
  treatment modalities, 214–218
  type II (causalgia)
    characteristics, 211t
    definition, 537–538
  types I and II, 211–212
Composite autonomic scoring scale (CASS), 191, 192t, 491–492, 492t
  in multiple system atrophy, 561f, 562
  in Parkinson's disease, 561f, 562
Condom catheters, 625
Conduction system disease, see Atrioventricular conduction disturbances
Congestive heart failure, see Heart failure
Connective tissue diseases, 479
Constant current generators, 387
  commercial sources, 389
Constipation, 602–604, 608
Constitutional orthostatic intolerance, 689
Continuous positive airway pressure therapy, 642, 644
Contour maps, of time–frequency distributions, 330f
Conus medullaris, and urinary bladder, 120, 623
Coronary artery disease, and syncope, 654–655
Coronary cardiac nerves, 42
Corpus cavernosum (corpora cavernosa), 129, 130f
  electromyography, 283–284, 283f
Corpus spongiosum, 129, 130f
Cortex, see Cerebral cortex
Cortical evoked potentials, see Evoked potentials
Corticotropin-releasing factor (CRF), 155
Cotransmitter, 29
Coughing, physiologic effects, 201, 304
Covariance method, modified, see Method of forward–backward least squares
Craniosacral parasympathetic pathways, (craniosacral outflow), 37, 37f, 601f
Crocodile tears (gustolacrimal reflex), 451
Crohn's disease, and small fiber neuropathy, 704
Cross modality receptor threshold modulation, 721
Cross-spectral analysis, 315–317, 316f
Cross-time–frequency distributions, 345
Cryogens, 753
Cushing response (Cushing reflex), 53–54, 792
Cutaneous, see also Skin entries
Cutaneous nerves
  abnormalities, 114–115
  how to quantify, 114
  methods of study, 109–110
Cutaneous thermal threshold testing, in erectile dysfunction, 282
Cycloplegia, from medications, 447
Cystic fibrosis, 97–98
Cystometry, 118, 615–617, 616f, 617f
Cytokines, 148, 149
  and central nervous system, 155
  effects on sympathetic nervous system, 154–156
  and nonneuronal supporting cells, 155–156
Cytomegalovirus, and AIDS incontinence, 732
Cytotoxic T cells, 148

D

Data acquisition, in spectral analysis, 344
Data stationarity (signal stationarity)
  and autonomic function studies, 345
  and electroencephalographic monitoring, 357
Deep muscular plexus of Cajal, 138f, 140
Defecation, 602, 603f
  neural dysfunction, 602
  in spinal cord injuries, 607
  testing methods, 605
Defense reaction, 21
Degenerative autonomic disorders, see also Neurodegenerative disorders
  and gastrointestinal dysmotility, 606–607
  time–frequency studies, 341
Degenerative central dysautonomia, and sympathetic nerve activity, 239
Dehydration, see also Blood volume; Hypovolemia
  and sweating, 87, 88f, 92, 399
Delayed-type hypersensitivity (DTH), 149
Delirium tremens, 780
Delta functions (spikes), in spectral analysis, 313f
Dementia, urinary bladder dysfunction, 621
Demyelinating neuropathies, 227, 228, 473
Denervation hypersensitivity (supersensitivity), 497
  and diabetic neuropathy, 288, 497
  evaluation, 202
  in progressive multiple sclerosis, 154
  sympathetic, 717–718
  and vasoactive agents, 288
"Derby chair," use in orthostatic hypotension, 767
Dermal nerves, 110
Dermal papillae, 110, 111f
Dermatoepidermal basement membrane, 110, 111f

Dermatomes, and thermoregulation, 90
Des-glymidodrine, 569
Detrusor muscle
    anatomy, 124
    areflexia, 617
        bethanechol therapy, 625–626
        cystometrogram, 616f
    collagen architecture, 124
    contraction
        anatomy, 124
        coordination, 124
        cystometrogram, 616f
    hyperreflexia, 118, 122, 617
        anticholinergic therapy, 626
        cystometrogram, 616f
        surgical denervation, 626, 628
    hypocontractility, 617
    innervation, 122–124
        afferent axons, 120
        motor axons, 120, 122
        nuclei, 120, 123f
            distribution, 121
    laboratory studies, 615
    neurotransmitters, 124
    reflex micturition pathways, 122, 122f
    thoracolumbar spinal innervation, 121–122
    true pressure, 615, 617f
Detrusor reflex, 119, 616f
Detrusor-sphincter dyssynergia
    diagnostic tests, 619
    sphincterotomy, 628
Diabetes
    animal models, 517
    autonomic function tests, 288
    cardiovascular accidents, 337, 339
    cerebral blood flow changes, 365
    constipation, 602
    esophageal disorders, 499
    fractal dimension of heart rate and blood pressure, 337
    functional autonomic failure, 496
    general anesthesia complications, 494–495
    glucagon response, 495
    heart rate response to squatting, 304
    heart rate variability analyses, 300–301
    MIBG-SPECT study results, 200
    ocular autonomic findings, 453
    skin vasomotor reflex tests, 200
    spectral power, 337
    thermoregulatory sweat test, 255f
        sweat distribution patterns, 247f, 248–249
    transfer function analysis of respiratory sinus arrhythmia, 337
    type I (insulin-dependent, IDDM)
        activated T cells, 511
        anti-adrenal medullary antibodies, 511–512, 511f, 512f
        anti-glutamic acid dexarboxylase antibodies, 517
        anti-sympathetic ganglia antibodies, 512, 513f
            and postural blood pressure changes, 514–515, 515f
        anti-vagus nerve antibodies, 512, 514f
        antibody-mediated immunity, 511–514
        autonomic antibodies
            antibody correlations, 512
            and postural catecholamine responses, 515–516, 515f
            in relatives, 513–514
        complement-fixing (CF) autoantibodies, 510, 511, 512
            neuronal and islet antigenic targets, 516–517
        parasympathetic function and anti-vagus nerve antibodies, 516
        sympathetic ganglia autoantibodies, 512, 513f
        vagus nerve autoantibodies, 512, 514f
    vs. non-insulin-dependent (NIDDM, type II), 488–489, 489t
    type II (non-insulin-dependent, NIDDM), autonomic antibodies, 514
    with oculomotor palsies, lesion site, 260
    with orthostatic hypotension, 494
        effects of tilt-up, 365, 365f, 366
        mechanism, 494
        time–frequency analysis, 337, 338f
Diabetes Control and Complications Trial (DCCT), 502
Diabetic autonomic neuropathy, 487–507
    see also Diabetic neuropathy; Distal small fiber neuropathy; Small fiber neuropathy
    β-adrenergic sensitivity, 496
    biochemical and neurophysiologic markers, 492–493
    complement activation and immune complexes, 514
    course and prognosis, 501–502
    diagnostic symptom patterns, 6
    epinephrine kinetics, 496
    epinephrine response, 495
    experimental, 403–406
        cardiovascular system, 405
        gastrointestinal tract, 406
        histopathology, 403–405, 404f, 405f, 406f
        physiologic studies, 405–406
        symptoms, 403
        urinary bladder function, 405–406
    gastrointestinal dysmotility, 608
        treatment, 608
    glucagon response, 495
    glucose counterregulation, 496
    hormonal and metabolic aspects, 495–496
    immune mechanisms, 509–524
    immunosuppressive therapy, 517
    involvement by system, 492–501
    and iritis, 517–518
    and measurement of heart rate variability, 320
    natural history, 501–502
    and neurogenic arrhythmias, 49
    pancreatic polypeptide test, 495
    pathogenesis, 502
    pathology, 510–511
    postprandial hypotension, use of octreotide, 743, 743f
        adverse effects, 744
    power spectral analysis, 493–494
    prevalence, 488–489, 488t
    San Antonio Conference test recommendations, 290–291
    sleep apnea, 642
    spectral analysis applications, 320
    symptoms and signs, 6, 501
    thermoregulatory sweat test, 252–253
    urinary bladder dysfunction, 624
Diabetic cystopathy, 500
Diabetic diarrhea, 499–500
Diabetic lumbosacral radiculoplexopathies, 490
Diabetic neurogenic bladder, 500
Diabetic neuropathy, see also Diabetic autonomic neuropathy; Distal small fiber neuropathy; Small fiber neuropathy
    asymmetric, 489
    baroreflexes, 496–497, 497f
    and bulbocavernosus reflex, 279
    cardiovascular, and anesthesia complications, 494–495
    classification, 489, 489t
    clinical features, 491t
    denervation supersensitivity, 288, 497
    effects of autonomic dysregulation, 336
    electrocardiographic findings, 501–502
    false assumptions, 393
    ganglioside therapy, 517
    gastric, 499
    gastrointestinal, 498–500
        manometry, 600f
        treatment, 503
    histopathologic findings, 375–377
    insulin-induced, 489, 490
    intestinal, 499–500
    and male sexual dysfunction, 270, 500–501
        associated factors, 281
        autonomic function tests, 281–282
        treatment, 503
    painful types, 489t
        acute, 489t, 490–491
        chronic, 489t, 491–492
    peripheral reflexes, 497–498, 498f
    prevention, 502
    proximal, 489, 491–492
    pupillary function studies, 498
    skin biopsy, 114–115
    skin blood flow testing, 398
    spectral power, 337
    sudomotor function tests, 496
    sympathetic skin response, 228
    thermoregulatory sweat test, 252–253, 252f
    treatment, 502–503, 502t
    vasomotor function tests, 496–498
Diabetic painful radiculopathies, 480
Diabetic pseudotabes, 489
Dialysis, and sweating, 92
Diarrhea
    in diabetes, 499–500, 608
    in HIV infection, 728–729
Diencephalic seizures (episodic autonomic paroxysms, diencephalic epilepsy), 423–434, 792, 793
    and thermoregulation, 102
Diencephalic syndrome, 5
Diencephalon, disorders, 423–424
Diet
    high-salt (high-sodium) foods, 693
    in treating orthostatic hypotension, 767, 768t
Dihydroxyphenylalinine, see Dopa
Dihydroxyphenylglycol, 587
    as marker of sympathetic neuropathy, 492
Dimension of a signal, 319
Diphtheritic neuropathy, 479, 779
Distal painful neuropathy, chronic, 491
Distal sensorimotor polyneuropathy, 732–733
Distal sensory and sensorimotor neuropathy, 489, 491
Distal small fiber neuropathy, 472–473, 699–714
    see also Small fiber neuropathy; Neuropathies; Diabetic neuropathy; Amyloid neuropathy
    autonomic examination, 472, 473f
    in diabetes, 489, 490, 491
    laboratory diagnosis, 180
Distal sympathetic failure, 11
Distal sympathetic neuropathies, 11, 472–473
Distal sympathetic overactivity, 11
Diuresis, during exposure to low gravity, 432
Diuretics, in elderly
    and orthostatic hypotension, 168
    and thermoregulatory changes, 169
Diurnal rhythms, see Circadian rhythms
Dive reflex response, Diving reflex, see Facial immersion test; Cold face test
Dogiel neurons, 139f, 140
Dopa (dihydroxyphenylalinine), 587
    in diabetic autonomic neuropathy, 492
    in Riley-Day syndrome, 530, 532f
Dopamine, 590–591
    see also Catecholamines
    in diabetic autonomic neuropathy, 492
    effects on eye, 448
    in neuroleptic malignant syndrome, 752
    as neurotransmitter, 586
Dopamine agonists, use in multiple system atrophy, 569
Dopamine bhydroxylase, sural nerve content, 373t
Dopamine bhydroxylase deficiency, 590, 766–767
    and catecholamines, 10, 562f
    and pure adrenergic neuropathy, 474

Dopaminergic central pathways, 590
Dopaminergic therapy, in striatonigral degeneration, 581
Doppler shift, 350
Doppler studies, see Transcranial Doppler
Dorsal nerve of penis, evoked potentials, 118, 620, 622f
Drug fever, 754
Drugs, see Medications; Street drugs
Dry eye, 451, 452
Dying-back (axonal) neuropathy, 227, 228, 406
Dynamic autoregressive modeling, 345
Dynamic (rhythmic) exercise, 66–67, 67f, 68f
Dysarthria, in multiple system atrophy, 558
Dysautonomias, see also Pandysautonomias
   acquired nonprogressive, 642
   in Alzheimer's disease, 341, 341f
   familial, see Riley-Day syndrome
   in Guillain–Barré syndrome, 379
   intermediolateral column neurons, 379t
   morphometric studies, 378–379
   τ-motoneurons, 378, 378f
   neurogenic (axon) flare, 528f
   in paraneoplastic neurologic syndromes, 545–546
   paroxysmal (intermittent), 12, 481
   in porphyria, 379
   selective, gastrointestinal dysmotility, 606–607
   and sleep apnea, 641–642
   and sympathetic skin response, 227
   tongue, 537f
"Dysautonomic crisis," in Riley-Day syndrome, 534
Dysphagia, 598, 598t, 599f, 605–606
Dystrophy, see Reflex sympathetic dystrophy

E

Ear, vagal innervation, 40
Eating, see also Postprandial hypotension; Diet; Gustatory
   effects on autonomic function, 739–740
Eccrine sweat glands, see under Sweat glands
Eccrine sweating, see Sweating, thermoregulatory
Edge-light pupil cycle time test, 450
Edinger–Westphal nucleus, 260, 261f, 262f
Edrophonium
   catecholamine response, 610f
   norepinephrine response, 202
Effector failure, heart rate variability patterns, 339
E:I (E/I) ratio, see Expiration:inspiration ratio
Ejaculation, 132
   anejaculation, 271, 806
   disorders, 271
     causes, 270t
     classification, 271, 806
     in diabetes, 501
     management, 806
   premature, 271, 806
     sympathetic skin responses, 283
   retarded, 806
   retrograde, 271, 806
   after spinal cord injury, 460
Elastic supports, use in orthostatic hypotension, 767–768, 768t
Elderly, see also Aging
   accidental hypothermia, 756
   heat stress disorders, 747–748
   impaired thermoregulation, 747, 748t
   post-glucose baroreceptor sensitivity, 739–740
   postprandial hypotension, 737–746
     role of sympathetic dysfunction, 741
     testing difficulties, 738
     use of octreotide, 742
   postprandial insulin levels, 739
   sweat response, 248
   thermoregulatory sweat test, 169, 246, 254
Electrical pacemakers, see under Pacemakers
Electrical stimulation
   in fecal incontinence, 605
   in gastrointestinal dysmotility, 611
Electrocardiogram, -graphy
   in diabetic neuropathy, 501–502
   in diagnosing syncope, 660–662
     signal-averaged, 661–662, 661f
   monitor used, 388
     commercial sources, 389
   neurogenic changes, 50–53
     arrhythmias, 49, 50
     and cardiac enzymes, 51
     common abnormalities, 50, 51f, 52f
     common causes, 51
     and hypothalamus, 52
     pathophysiologic mechanisms, 51–53
     from peripheral sympathetic nervous system, 52–53
     resembling ischemic heart disease, 50
     and ventrolateral medulla, 52
   after subarachnoid hemorrhage, 793
   use in spectral analysis, 312, 313f
Electroconvulsive therapy, autonomic effects, 792–793
Electrodermal activity (EDA), see also Sympathetic skin responses; Skin potentials
   central modulation, 223–227
   clinical utility, 227–229
   definition, 221
   diphasic potential, 222
     morphologic modifications, 222
   and emotive vs. thermoregulatory sudomotor activity, 223
   endosomatic vs. exosomatic, 221
   evoked, 225–226
   generator, 221–223
   recording skin sites, 223
   spontaneous, 222f, 223–225
   synchronized spontaneous, 223
   tightly synchronized spontaneous, 223f, 224f
Electrodermal skin response, hand vs. penis vs. foot, 283f
Electrodiagnostic tests, of urinary tract, 620–621
Electroencephalogram, -graphy
   alpha, beta, and theta band powers, 353, 354f, 355t
   amplitude modulation (AM-EEG), 336, 339, 352–358, 355t
     during tilt-up, 356f, 357, 362–367, 364f
   central autonomic rhythms, 339
     in Alzheimer's disease, 341, 341f
     and neurodegenerative disorders, 339, 341
   clinical applictions, 351–352
     in autonomic failure, 362–366
     in orthostatic syncope, 367, 367f
     in postural orthostatic tachycardia syndrome, 362, 363f
     in presyncope, 356f, 357
     in syncope, 357
     in vasodepressor syncope, 366f, 367
   modulating rhythms, 354f, 355, 355f, 355t
   and neuronal synchronization, 358, 359f
   technical aspects, 353–359
   time–frequency analysis, 357
Electrophrenic respiration, 645
Electrophysiologic studies
   in complex regional pain syndromes, 213
   in Lambert-Eaton myasthenic syndrome, 546
   in syncope, 664–672
     AV conduction, 667–670
     choice of patients, 664–666, 665f
     His bundle electrogram, 667, 667f
     sinus node dysfunction, 666–667, 666f
     supraventricular tachycardia, 670–672, 671f
     test components, 666
     ventricular tachycardia, 672, 672f
Emotional stimuli
   central autonomic responses, 21–22
   effect on pupil, 265
   and sympathetic vs. parasympathetic nervous system, 37–38
Emotional stress, and sweating, 91, 92
Emotive sudomotor activity, and electrodermal activity, 223
   see also Mental sweating
"Empty heart" syndrome, 651f
End-organ failure, heart rate variability patterns, 339
β-Endorphin, in autonomic failure syndromes, 589t, 593
Endothelial factors, in sexual function, 133
Endothelium, vascular, 70
Enkephalins, 30f, 33
Enteric brain, 136f
Enteric (intrinsic) nervous system, 136, 136f, 139–142, 597–598
   anatomy, 139
   integrative circuits, 140f, 141
   interaction with extrinsic system, 140f, 142
   overall functions, 140–141
   specific functions, 141–142
Enteric neuronopathy, 551–552
Enteric plexuses, 136, 138f, 139–140, 139f
Entropy, and signal complexity, 331
Envelope, spectral, in transcranial Doppler monitoring, 351
Envelope of spindles, in amplitude modulation, 353, 353f
Envelope slow modulation, in electroencephalography, 354f
Environmental signals, central afferent pathways, 19
Environmental temperature, see Temperature, ambient
Ephapse, 239
Epidermal nerves, 110, 111f, 371–372
   in diabetic neuropathy, 114–115
   types, 112
Epidermis, 110, 111f, 112
   in diabetes, 114
   and electrodermal activity, 222–223
Epididymis, 130
Epilepsy, see Seizures; Pseudoseizures; Diencephalic seizures
Epinephrine, 589–590
   see also Catecholamines
   in diabetic autonomic neuropathy, 495, 496
   metabolic functions, 495
   response to arecoline, 589, 592
   response to edrophonium, 610f
   supine plasma levels: effects of aging, 170, 171f
Epitopes, 148
Epitrichial (apocrine) sweat glands, 91
Equidistant data sampling, in spectral analysis, 344
Equidistant interpolation, 344
Erectile dysfunction, 269–275
   approach to diagnosis, 273–274
   arterial revascularization, 806
   arteriographic studies, 272
   autonomic function tests, 281–282
   causes, 270, 270t
   clinical evaluation, 9, 271
   in diabetes, 270, 500–501
     associated factors, 281
     bulbocavernosus reflex, 279
     treatment, 503
   electromyography, 281, 283–284, 283f
   erotic stimulation testing, 273
   intracavernosal (intracorporeal) vasoactive injections, 272, 278, 805
   laboratory tests, 271–273, 272t
   management, 803–806, 804t
     preliminary steps, 803–804
     oral medications, 804
     topical medications, 805
     use of penile prostheses, 805
     use of testosterone, 806

use of vacuum devices, 805–806
in multiple sclerosis, 280f, 281
need for neurophysiologic studies, 284
pudendal cortical evoked potentials, 280–281
clinical utility, 281
and small fiber neuropathy, 708
in spinal cord disorders, 281
sympathetic skin responses, 282–283, 282f
venous leakage, treatment, 806
Erection, 130f, 132
clinical evaluation, 9
counterpart in female, 133
neural and neurotransmitter control, 132–133
nocturnal, 272, 273
proerectile neuropharmacologic mechanisms, 133
reflexogenic (spinal) vs. psychogenic (supraspinal), 132
tumescence vs. rigidity, 273
Ergoreceptors, 69–70
Erythromelalgia, 472, 481
Erythropoiesis, and exposure to low gravity, 432, 438f
Erythropoietin (epoetin alfa), use in orthostatic hypotension, 769–770, 769t
Esophagus
in diabetes, 499
extrinsic neural control, 137t
vagal innervation, 42
Essential hypertension, 55, 153
see also Hypertension
Essential (primary) hyperhidrosis, 811–812
Essential (simple, benign central) anisocoria, vs. Horner's syndrome, 444–445, 446, 450
Evoked electrodermal activity (EDA), see Electrodermal activity; Sympathetic skin responses; Skin potentials
Evoked potentials
brain stem, 563
dorsal nerve of penis, 118, 620, 622f
pelvic nerve, 118, 620
pudendal, 118, 279f, 280–281, 280f, 620, 622f, 623, 623f
clinical utility, 281
tibial, 279f, 280f, 281
urethroanal, 620, 621f
uses
in cervical spondylosis, 623, 623f
in genitourinary studies, 118, 620, 621f, 622f, 623f
in multiple sclerosis, 280f, 281
in multiple system atrophy, 563
in Parkinson's disease, 563
in pure autonomic failure, 563
in small fiber neuropathy, 708
Exercise
and β-adrenergic receptors on lymphocytes, 153
and arterial baroreflexes, 68–69, 69f
and baroreflex resetting, 65, 68
and body temperature, 86
and chemosensitive afferents, 69–70
and heat stress disorders, 748–749
hemodynamic effects, 78f, 79, 80f
and muscle sympathetic activity, 235–236
physiologic responses, 66–70, 66f, 68f
in diabetic autonomic neuropathy, 494
static (isometric) vs. rhythmic (dynamic), 66–67, 67f
and sweating, 92
syncope from, 654
Exercise capacity, effects of aging, 167
Exercise testing, in diagnosing syncope, 662
Exertional syncope, in heart disease, 654, 655
Experimental acetylcholinesterase autoimmunity, 413–414, 414f
Experimental allergic encephalomyelitis (EAE), 152
Experimental allergic neuritis (EAN), 410–412
effects of β–adrenergic agonist, 152

histopathology, 410, 410f, 411f, 412f
Experimental autoimmune myasthenia gravis (EAMG), 152
Experimental autonomic neuropathy, see under Autonomic neuropathies
Experimental diabetes, 517
see also Diabetic autonomic neuropathy, experimental
Expiration:inspiration (E:I) ratio, 187, 187t, 300
factors affecting, 301
interpretation problems, 394
Extended amygdala, 17, 22
External environment, central afferents, 19
External ophthalmoplegia, 443
External urinary sphincter, 122, 123, 123f, 124
Extrapyramidal disorders, with autonomic dysfunction, 577–584
Extremities
sympathetic innervation, 809
sympathetic dysfunction, 809–818
Extrinsic nervous system of gut, 136–138, 136f, 137t
disorders causing gastrointestinal dysmotility, 605–609
identification, 609–611
and gastrointestinal motility, 598
interaction with intrinsic system, 140f, 142
Eyes, see also specific components and disorders
accommodation, 260, 266
autonomic disturbances affecting, 452–453
anatomy, 259–264
changes, in seizures, 423
clinical examination, 10
dry eye, 451, 452
eliciting symptoms, 9
near response, 266
parasympathetic innervation, 38, 260–263
sympathetic innervation, 263–264, 264f

F

Fabry's disease, 479, 703
Face
parasympathetic fibers, 38
sweat glands, innervation, 90
sympathetic pathway, 715–716, 716f
Facial flushing, 715–726
gustatory, 719–720
autonomic pathways, 719f
pathologic, 720
role of vasodilator peptides, 718–719
sympathetic control, 716–717
Facial hyperhidrosis, 810
Facial immersion test, 164, 201, 304–305
in Parkinson's disease, 580–581
Fainting, 649–679
see also Syncope
common faint, 652
Familial amyloid polyneuropathy (FAP), 375, 476–477
Familial amyloidosis, 608, 702
Familial dysautonomia, see Riley-Day syndrome
Familial Hibernian fever, 754
Familial insomnia, fatal (FFI), 5, 424
Familial Mediterranean fever, 754
Familial olivopontocerebellar atrophy, 559
Fas CD95, and aging, 162
Fast Fourier transform, 313–314
see also Fourier transform; Periodogram
in electroencephalographic monitoring, 353–357
in transcranial Doppler monitoring, 351
Fastigial nucleus, and urinary bladder function, 119
Fatal familial insomnia (FFI), 5, 424
Fatigue
chronic fatigue syndrome (CFS), 690–691
effect on pupil, 265
Fecal incontinence, 604–605, 608
Feeding behavior, and body temperature, 86

Feeding center, 87
Feet, see also Soles
thermoregulation, 89
Females, see also Gender
anhidrosis, in elderly, 248, 254
bulbospongiosus (bulbocavernosus) muscle, 132
erection counterpart, 133
ischiocavernosus muscle, 132
orgasm, 133
postural orthostatic tachycardia syndrome, 683, 683t
pudendal cortical evoked response, 620
sexual dysfunction, 278
in diabetes, 501
sexual organs, 130, 133
sexual response cycle, 133
spinal cord injuries, 460
sweating capacity, 93
urethral pressure profile, 619, 619f
urinary stress incontinence, 614, 626
Fetal distress
detecting by heart rate variability, 297
indicators, 325
Fetus, respiratory and vasomotor rhythms, 325
Fever, 85, 86f, 752–753
noninfections forms, 754
and prostaglandin E, 87
and sympathetic nervous system, 155
Fibromyalgia, 241
Filtering, in spectral analysis, 344–345
Finapres technique, 188–189
see also Photoplethysmographic blood pressure recordings
commercial sources, 389, 390
computer setup, 385, 386
effects of tilt-up, 399f
effects of vasoconstriction, 398, 398f, 399f
use in autonomic reflex screen, 292
Fingers, thermoregulation, 89, 90
Flack sign, 684
Flare response, see Neurogenic flare response
Fludrocortisone (Florinef)
use in autonomic failure, 570
use in orthostatic hypotension, 768–769, 769t
risks, 503
Fluorescence microscopy, 371f
Flushing, see Facial flushing
Food, see Postprandial hypotension; Eating; Diet; Gustatory
Forced (respiratory) sinus arrhythmia, see Respiratory sinus arrhythmia
Forward–backward least squares method, 345, 347
Fourier analysis, 312, 344
Fourier power spectrum, 324
Fourier spectrum
comparison with modified Wigner distribution, 345, 346f
methods of computing, 312–317
Fourier transform, see also Fast Fourier transform; Periodogram
in electroencephalographic monitoring, 354f, 355f
of heart rate variability, 314f
distorting factors, 314, 315f
shortcomings, 345
smoothed vs. unsmoothed, 314f
zero padding, 314
Fractal dimension (FD), 337
Fractals, 319
Frequency analysis, see also Spectral analysis; Time–frequency analysis
for cardiovagal function testing, 336–337
effects of aging, 166
in electroencephalographic monitoring, 353–357, 354f, 355f
of heart rate and blood pressure variability
clinical applicability, 319–321

Frequency analysis, of heart rate and blood pressure variability *(contd.)*
    physiologic interpretation, 317–319
    problems, 396
Frequency domain
    autonomic evaluation in the frequency domain, 336–338
    methods of interpretation, 344
    in transcranial Doppler monitoring, 351
Frequency smoothing, 345
Frey's syndrome, 92
Friedreich's ataxia, 479
Functional autonomic failure, in diabetes, 496
Functional gastrointestinal disorders
    and autonomic dysfunction, 608, 609f
    identifying neurologic cause, 609–611

G

Gain, in cardiovascular homeostasis, 73
Galanin, 30f, 32
Gallbladder, vagal innervation, 42
Galvanic skin response, 98
Ganglia, 34
    cervical sympathetic, 34–36
    in control of gastrointestinal motility, 137t, 138–139
    effects of aging, 167, 170
    glossopharyngeal, 38
    lumbar sympathetic, 36
    parasympathetic, 28, 37f, 38, 40
    of paravertebral sympathetic chain, 27, 28f
    paravertebral vs. prevertebral vs. intermediate, 34
    pelvic sympathetic, 36
    sympathetic, 34–36, 35f
    thoracic paravertebral, 36
    of vagus nerve, 40
Ganglion defects, in Riley-Day syndrome, 528, 529, 529f
Ganglionitis, in paraneoplastic neuropathy, 608
Gangliosides, in diabetes
    as autoantibody targets, 516
    as therapy, 517
Gastric pacing, 611
Gastric stasis, *see* Gastroparesis
Gastrin, 589t, 593
Gastrointestinal diabetic neuropathy, 498–500
    gastric, 499
    intestinal, 499–500
    treatment, 503
Gastrointestinal dysmotility, 597–612
    and bioavailability of medications, 605
    biofeedback therapy, 611
    diagnostic evaluation, 609–611
    functional, and autonomic dysfunction, 608, 609f
    intestinal pseudo-obstruction, 551–552, 599–600, 602
    of lower tract, evaluation, 602–604, 603f
    manometry, 600f
    neurologic causes, 605–609
    in neurologic disorders, 598–605, 601f, 602t
    of upper tract, evaluation, 600f
Gastrointestinal motility, control mechanisms, 135–145, 597–598
    centers involved, 136
    extrinsic neural control, 136–138, 136f, 137t
        interaction with intrinsic system, 140f, 142
    inhibitory reflexes, 139
    intrinsic neural control, *see* Enteric nervous system
    levels of neural control, 138t
    sphincteric vs. nonsphincteric muscle, 141
    supraspinal control, 136
Gastrointestinal peptides, 592–593, 738–739
Gastrointestinal syndromes, and visceral afferents, 145
Gastrointestinal tract
    bacterial overgrowth, 602
    homeostatic pathways, 142
    intrinsic vs. extrinsic nerves, 136
    layers, 135
    pacemakers, 140, 141
    sensory information, 142–145
    smooth muscle, electrical properties, 597
    vagal innervation, 42
Gastroparesis, 598–599
    causes, 599, 599t
    clinical features, 9, 598–599
    in diabetes, 499, 608
    scintigraphic study, 606f
    treatment, 599
Gender
    and cardiovascular rhythms, 331
    and heart rate response to tilt-up, 196t
    and orthostatic hypotension in elderly, 167, 167t
    and QSART, 193t
    and sweat glands, 93, 169t
    and Valsalva ratio, 164, 165f, 194, 194t, 195f
    and venoarteriolar reflex, 171
Generalized autonomic failure, *see under* Autonomic failure
Genitourinary tract, *see also* Sexual organs; Urinary bladder
    electrodiagnostic studies, 620–621
Gestation, *see* Pregnancy; Fetus
Global Fourier transform, *see* Fourier transform
Global periodogram, Global spectrum, *see* Periodogram
Glomerulonephritis, 153
Glossopharyngeal ganglia, 38
Glossopharyngeal nerve, 38–40, 39f
    branches, 39–40, 39f
    parasympathetic fibers, 38–40, 39f
Glossopharyngeal syncope, 239, 654
Glucagon, 495, 593
    in diabetes, 495
    in multiple system atrophy, 589t, 593
Glucose
    and baroreceptor sensitivity, 739–740
    counterregulation, 495–496
    and postprandial hypotension, 738–739, 738f, 739–740, 739f
    and sympathetic nerve activity, 237–238
Glutamic acid decarboxylase antibodies, in diabetes, 517
Glycoproteins, of skin, 110
Glycosylation, of myelin proteins, 510
Gonadotropins, 132
Goose bumps, 813
Gravity, *see also* Venous pooling; Venous return; Standing up; Upright posture; Head-up tilt
    and cardiovascular hemodynamics, 74–77
    effects on circulation, 73, 74f
    prolonged reduction, autonomic effects, 429–440
    overview, 438–439, 438f
Greater splanchnic nerve, 36, 377
Growth and development, cardiovascular oscillations, 325–331, 332f
Growth hormone, 495, 565, 589t, 593
Guanethidine-induced sympathectomy, 412–413
Guillain-Barré syndrome, 468–469
    see also Landry-Guillain-Barré syndrome
    autonomic function tests, 469
    cardiovascular dysautonomia, 778–779, 796–797, 797f
    clinical features, 777–779
    experimental, 152, 410–412
    gastrointestinal dysmotility, 607
    histopathologic findings, 379
    management, 787
    monitoring, 786–787
    and neurogenic arrhythmias, 49
    sweat test, 252
    sweating, pathophysiologic mechanisms, 785f, 786
    sympathetic nerve activity, 238
    sympathetic overactivity, 780–781, 781f, 782f, 784–786
    vs. acute panautonomic neuropathy, 466
Gustatory fibers, 265
Gustatory lacrimation, 720
Gustatory sweating, 91–92, 719–720, 719f, 813
Gustolacrimal reflex (crocodile tears), 451

H

Hair, *see* Pilomotor system
Hair-associated (apocrinelike, trichial) sweat glands, 98, 98f
Hair follicles, 110, 111f
    innervation, 112, 113f, 114
Handgrip, sustained, 198
    interpretation problems, 395
    potential risks, 204
Handgrip contraction, 235
Hands, *see also* Palms
    thermoregulation, 89, 90
Harlequin syndrome, 721
Head-down tilt, and gravity studies, 429
Head injury
    autonomic effects, 791–792, 793–794
    gastrointestinal dysmotility, 605
    sympathetic effects, 342
Head-up tilt
    in autonomic failure, 362, 366, 580
    blood pressure response, 190–191, 292–293
        normative data, 194, 196t
    cardiovascular effects, 77
    cardiovascular responses, 334
        contour map, 330f
        initial response, 77, 79
        time–frequency analysis, 329f
    and cerebral blood flow velocity, 362, 366
    in diabetic orthostatic hypotension, 365, 365f, 366
    electroencephalographic monitoring, 356f, 357
    in Finapres study, 399f
    heart rate response, 191, 292–293, 304
        effects of pacemaker, 331, 331f
        normative data, 194, 196t
        time–frequency analysis, 328f, 330
    hemodynamic changes, 78f
    in multiple system atrophy, 365f, 366, 580
    orthostatic intolerance grade, 191, 191t
    in Parkinson's disease, 579, 580
    potential risks, 204
    prolonged
        blood pressure response, 201
        circulatory adjustments, 80–81
        heart rate response, 201
        potential risks, 204
    vs. standing up, circulatory responses, 77
    in syncope, 662–664, 663f
    testing requirements, 384
    tilt table, 388
        commercial sources, 390
    transcranial Doppler and electroencephalogram, 362–367, 364f
    in treating orthostatic hypotension, 767, 768t
Headache
    migraine and cluster headache, 721–724
    short-lasting, unilateral, neuralgiform, with conjunctival injection and tearing (SUNCT), 724
    and vasodilator peptides, 719
Heart, *see also* Cardiac *entries*; Cardiovascular *entries*
    excitability, sympathetic-parasympathetic influences, 48
    monitoring, in syncope, 660–661, 660f
    myocardial infarction, and heart rate variability, 298
    myocardial injury, 50–53
        from catecholamines, 53

study by MIBG-SPECT, 199–200
sympathetic function, effects of aging, 167
vagal innervation, 42
Heart disease, and syncope, 654–656
Heart failure
autonomic overactivity, 780
heart rate variability patterns, 339
peripheral sympathoexcitation, 339
Poincare plots, 339
and sympathetic nerve activity, 240f, 241
time–frequency changes, 339, 340f
Heart period
cross-spectral analysis, 315–317, 316f
variation, 299, 299f
vs. heart rate, 394
Heart period range, 394
Heart rate, see also RR interval
clinical examination, 9–10
diurnal variations, 310, 310f, 493
during sleep, 637
and exposure to low gravity, 430, 430f, 432–433, 436, 436f, 438f
fractal dimension, 337
intrinsic, 163
laboratory studies
effects of aging, 162–167
equipment used, commercial sources, 389–390
procedure details, 292
in postural orthostatic tachycardia syndrome, 681–682, 682t
recordings, 186–188
problems, 394
techniques, 186
respiratory effects, 310, 317
resting variation, 201
slow oscillations at non-respiratory frequencies (non-RF rhythms), 325, 353
factors affecting, 328–331
generating factors, 328–331
structures involved, 353
and vasomotor rhythms, 330–331
and vestibular stimulation, 437–438
vs. heart period, 394
Heart rate range, 293, 394
factors affecting, 394–395
Heart rate responses
averaged vs. nonaveraged, 394
factors affecting, 394–395
to coughing, 164, 201, 304
to deep breathing, 186–187, 299–301
see also Heart rate variability; Respiratory sinus arrhythmia
determinants, 299
effects of age, 301
effects of aging, 163–164, 163t, 164f, 193, 193t, 194f, 288
evaluation, 187, 187t, 293, 293t
factors affecting, 186, 187t, 301, 394–395
interpretation problems, 392
normative data, 193–194, 193t
problems, 394–395
procedure, 186–187, 292
test conditions, 300
to drinking fluids, 201
to exercise
and arterial baroreflexes, 69, 69f
effects of aging, 167
to facial cold stimulus, 164
to facial immersion, 201, 304–305
to head-up tilt, 191, 191f, 292–293, 304
contour map, 330f
effects of pacemaker, 331, 331f
normative data, 194, 196t
time–frequency analysis, 328, 329f, 330
with prolonged tilt, 201
to intravenous tyramine, 202
to lying down, 304
to mental stress, 203
to squatting, 201, 304
to standing, 79–80, 164, 188, 303–304, 396f
bimodal nature, 303
and exposure to low gravity, 433, 437
factors affecting, 303–304
to Valsalva maneuver, 301–303, 302f
effects of aging, 165t
and Valsalva ratio, 302–303
Heart rate variability, 309–312, 310f, 311f
and blood pressure variability, 318, 320
in children vs. adults, 327
circadian distribution, 337
development of tests, 297–299
effects of aging, 162–163, 162f, 331
effects of propranolol and atropine, 297–298, 298f
factors affecting, 301
Fourier transform, 314f
distorting factors, 314, 315f
frequency analysis
clinical applicability, 319–321
physiologic interpretation, 317–319
low-frequency changes, 313
and myocardial infarction, 298
in end-organ failure, 339
spectral analysis, 312–315
clinical applications, 320
signal test, 312
vs. simple statistical methods, 319–320
stimuli used in testing, 298
testing in AIDS, 728f, 729, 729t
time domain tests, 297–307
list of tests, 298f
Heat acclimatization, in elderly, 169
Heat exchange, between body and environment, 87
Heat loss, evaporative, 90
Heat-related illnesses (heat stress disorders), 98–99, 747–751
heat cramps, 749
heat edema, 749
heat exhaustion, 749
heat intolerance
in active young, 748–749
causes, 749
and decreased sweating, 99
heat syncope, 749
heatstroke, 98–99, 103, 749–751
and aging, 168
classical, 749
complications, 749–750
diagnosis, 749
exertional, 749
laboratory findings, 750
treatment, 750–751
populations at risk, 747–749
Hemicrania, 724
Hemifacial hyperhidrosis, 720
Hemihidrosis, 92
Hemiplegia vegetativa alterna, 423, 810
Hemodialysis, and sweating, 92
Hemodynamics
effects of exercise, 78f, 79, 80f
effects of head-up tilt, 78f
effects of upright posture, 78f, 80f
influence of gravity, 74–77
effects of Valsalva maneuver, 301, 302f, 360–362, 360f
factors affecting, 302, 303
in orthostatic hypotension, 361f, 362
Hemorrhage, see also Stroke
cerebellar, 343f
electrocardiographic changes, 51, 52f
intracerebral, 51
subarachnoid, 48
Hereditary high-density-lipoprotein deficiency, see Tangier disease
Hereditary neuropathies, 478–479, 703
hereditary motor and sensory neuropathy (HMSN), 520
see also Charcot-Marie-Tooth disease
hereditary sensory and autonomic neuropathies (HSANs), 525, 703
type III, see Riley-Day syndrome
type IV (congenital sensory neuropathy with anhidrosis), 703
hereditary sensory neuropathy, 479
Hering-Breuer reflex, 299, 409
Herniation, intracranial, 54
Heterochromia iridis, in Horner's syndrome, 445
Hidromeiosis, 93
Hines-Bannick syndrome, 102
Hippus (pupillary unrest), 266
His bundle electrogram, 667, 667f
see also HV interval
Histamine test, see also Neurogenic flare response
in Riley-Day syndrome, 526, 528f
Histogram of the RR intervals, 300
History-taking, 7–9
HIV, see Human immunodeficiency virus
Hodgkin's disease, thermoregulatory disorders, 754, 757
Holmes-Adie syndrome, see Adie's tonic pupil
Holter (cardiac) monitoring, in syncope, 660–661, 660f
Holter recordings, of heart rate variability, time–frequency analysis, 320
Horner's syndrome, 444–447, 445t
acquired, 445–447
catecholamine effects on pupil, 265
central, 445
in childhood, 446
and cluster headache, 722, 723f
congenital, 445
finding lesion site, 446
ocular signs, 715–716, 716f
pharmacologic tests, 446–447
postganglionic, 445–446
preganglionic, 445–446
in stroke, 423
sweat test, 255f
and sympathetic block, 213
vs. essential (simple, benign central) anisocoria, 444–445, 446, 450
HR$_{DB}$, see Heart rate responses, to deep breathing
5-HT, see Serotonin
Human immunodeficiency virus (HIV-1), 727
HIV-1–associated myelopathy, 732
Human immunodeficiency virus (HIV) infection, see also AIDS
autonomic dysfunction
and CD4- cell count, 731
clinical features, 733
incidence, 727
from medications, 733
natural history, 731
neuropathologic basis, 731–733, 732t
autonomic function tests, 728f, 729–731, 729t
autonomic syndromes, 727–729
distal sensorimotor polyneuropathy, 732–733
skin biopsy findings, 372
Humoral signals, central afferents, 19
Humoral system, and upright posture, 63, 81
Hunting reaction, 89
Huntington's disease, 583
HV interval (His bundle-to-ventricle conduction time), and syncope, 667–670, 667f, 668f–669f, 673
Hydrocephalus, 55, 424
6-Hydroxydopamine (6OHDA), for sympathectomy, 151, 412

5-Hydroxyindoleacetic acid (5-HIAA), 591
Hyperalgesia, 10
Hyperhidrosis, 99–100, 810–813
  see also Sweating
  in autonomic hyperreflexia, 252
  causes, 248t
  and central inhibitory pathway, 810
  episodic, 12
  episodic with hypothermia, 423
  generalized, 811–812
  gustatory, 813
  in hereditary disorders, 811
  idiopathic hemifacial, 720
  localized, 99–100, 810
  palmar and plantar, 91, 811
    use of iontophoresis, 812
    use of sympathectomy, 813
  pathophysiology, 811
  primary (essential), 253f, 254, 811–812
  secondary, 811
  treatment, 812–813
Hyperimmunoglobulinemia D, 754
Hyperlipidemia-associated neuropathies, 704
Hyperpathia, 211
Hypertension, see also Blood pressure
  acute neurogenic
    from brainstem disorders, 424–425
    from cerebral lesions, treatment, 794–796, 794t
  and apnea, 352
  and baroreflex resetting, 65, 65f
  dysautonomic, clinical consequences, 798–799
  essential, 55, 153
  in Guillain–Barré syndrome, 469, 796–797
  and increased intracranial pressure, 54
  intracranial, 424
  and ischemic stroke, 795–796
  and medulla, 54
  in multiple system atrophy, 557
  neurogenic, 53–55
  neurotransmitter mechanisms, 55
  and normal pressure hydrocephalus, 55
  and nucleus tractus solitarii lesions, 53
  paroxysmal, from brainstem tumors, 425
  in poliomyelitis, 779–780
    pathophysiology, 784
  and posterior fossa lesions, 54
  in pure autonomic failure, 557
  from seizures, 792–793
  after spinal cord injury, 796
  from subarachnoid hemorrhage, 793–794
    management, 793–794
  supine, 557, 744
  and sympathetic nerve activity, 239, 241
  from sympathoadrenal discharge, 791–792
  with tachycardia, 780–786, 781f, 782f, 785f
Hypertensive postural orthostatic tachycardia syndrome (POTS), 684
Hyperthermia, 98–99, 747–761
  body cooling methods, 751
  causes, 747, 748t, 754
  in elderly, 747–748, 748t
  malignant, 751, 779, 784
  medications and drugs causing, 748t, 753–754
  in quadriplegics, 459
  vs. fever, 752
Hyperventilation
  effect on electroencephalogram, 357–358, 358f
  and orthostatic intolerance, 352
  and syncope, 656
Hypnosis, and analgesia, 145
Hypocapnia (hypocarbia), circulatory effects, 75, 395, 395f
Hypogastric plexus, 36
Hypoglycemia
  in autonomic failure, 496, 559

insulin-induced, 589, 589t
  in adrenergic insufficiency, 590f
  hormonal and peptide responses, in autonomic failure syndromes, 589, 589t, 593
  normal response, 589, 590f
  pancreatic polypeptide response, 495
    adrenal medullary response, 565
  somatostatin response, 495
Hypohidrosis, 99–100, 100f
  with excessive localized sweating, 99, 100
Hypopnea, sleep-related, 639
Hypotension, see also Blood pressure; Orthostatic hypotension; Postprandial hypotension
  in Alzheimer's disease, 341
  and central lesions, 55
  in Guillain–Barré syndrome, 796–797
  in HIV infection, 727, 728
  and intracranial pressure, 794
  neurogenic, 53, 55
  paroxysmal, 799
  after spinal cord trauma, 456
  supine, treatment, 772
  after Valsalva maneuver, 189, 189f
Hypothalamic-pituitary-adrenal axis, 593
  cholinergic function studies, 591
  and cytokines, 155
  and stress, 22
Hypothalamus
  and AIDS autonomic dysfunction, 732
  autonomic components, 17–18
  autonomic disorders, 5, 423–424
    classification, 4t
    sweat test, 251, 251f
  and electrocardiographic changes, 52
  and feeding behavior, 86, 87
  and hypertension, 54–55
  and hyperthermia, 753
  and hypothermia, 423, 756
  and immune system, 155
  and modulation of sensory pathways, 144, 144f, 145
  and pain, 144
  paraventricular (parvicellular) nucleus, 22
  in pupillary function, 264f, 265
  in sexual function, 131, 132
  in stress response, 21, 21f
  in thermoregulation, 84, 85–86, 90, 102
Hypothermia, 747–761
  accidental, 756
  causes, 754, 754t, 756–757
  in elderly, 748t
  episodic spontaneous, with hyperhidrosis, 757
  of hypothalamic origin, 423, 756
  levels, 754
  management, 755–756
  medications causing, 748t, 757
  metabolic causes, 757
  mild
    physiologic changes, 754, 755
    temperature range, 754
  moderate
    physiologic changes, 755
    temperature range, 754
  pathophysiology, 754–755
  rewarming techniques, 755–756
  severe
    physiologic changes, 755
    temperature range, 754
  after spinal cord injury, 459
Hypoventilation, from medullary lesions, 425
Hypovolemia, see also Blood volume
  from exposure to low gravity, 431–432, 431f, 438f
  and peripheral vascular resistance, 434–435, 435f
  idiopathic, 682
  therapeutic measures, 693–694
  vs. adrenergic failure, 397

I
Ictus emeticus, 423
Ileal conduit, for treating urinary bladder dysfunction, 628, 629f
Ileocecal sphincter, extrinsic neural control, 137t
Immune complexes, in diabetic neuropathy, 514
Immune system, 147–149
  autonomic regulation, 147–159
  in diabetic neuropathy, 509–524
  effects of adrenergic agonists and antagonists, 150–151
  effects of glycosylation and vascular disease, 510
  effects of sympathetic ablation, 151–153
  inductive and effectory phases, 148
  in Lambert-Eaton myasthenic syndrome, 548–550
  in multiple sclerosis, 426
  and neurotransmitters, 150, 156
  in paraneoplastic gastrointestinal neuropathy, 608
  and parasympathetic nervous system, 154
  and sympathetic nervous system, 149–156
    in human disease, 153–156
Immunocytes, see Lymphocytes
Immunoglobulins, 148
  antigen-binding domains, 148
Immunosuppressive therapy
  in diabetic autonomic neuropathy, 517
  in Lambert-Eaton myasthenic syndrome, 550
Immunosympathectomy, 413
Impedance cardiography, 202
Impotence, see Erectile dysfunction; Sexual dysfunction
Inclusion bodies, in multiple system atrophy, 567–568, 567f
Incontinence
  fecal 604–605, 608
  urinary
    in dementia, 621
    from stress, 614, 626
Indwelling catheters, 625
Infants, see Neonates
Infections
  associated neuropathies, 479
  and cytokine–sympathetic effects, 156
  gastrointestinal dysmotility, 607
Inferior vagal (nodose) ganglion, 40
Inflammatory neuropathy, 519
Inflammatory polyneuropathy, 519–520
Infrahisian block, 655
Infrared thermometry, 196, 197f
Innocent bystanders, in immune response, 149
Insensible water loss, 90
Insomnia, fatal familial (FFI), 5, 424
Inspiratory gasps, 640
Inspiratory-expiratory ratio, see Expiration:inspiration ratio
Instantaneous coherence, 357
Insular cortex, 19
Insulin
  and baroreceptor sensitivity, 739–740
  and nerve growth factor, 517
  and postprandial hypotension, 738–739, 739–740, 743
  and sympathetic nerve activity, 237–238
Insulin-induced hypoglycemia, 589, 589t, 590f, 593
Insulin neuropathy (neuritis), 489, 490
Interdigestive migrating motor complex, 600f
Interleukins, 148
  interleukin-1, and fever, 753
  nterleukin-1B(IL-1B), 155, 156
Intermediate ganglia, 34
Intermediolateral cell columns, 25–27, 26f, 28–29
  in amyloid neuropathy, 375, 375f
  in diabetic neuropathy, 376f, 377
  in dysautonomia, 379t
  in Tangier disease, 375f

neuropeptides and neurotransmitters, 29
Intermediomedial cell columns, 25–27, 26f, 28–29
  neuropeptides and neurotransmitters, 29
Interspindle sequences of thalamus, 358
Interstitial cells of Cajal, 140
Intestinal motility, *see* Gastrointestinal motility
Intestinal neuropathy, in diabetes, 499–500
Intestinal pseudo-obstruction, 551–552, 599–600, 602
Intracardiac His bundle electrogram, 667, 667f
Intracavernosal (intracorporeal) therapy
  pharmacotherapy, 272, 278, 805
  vasoactive injections, 272, 278, 805
Intracranial herniation, 54
Intracranial hypertension, 424
Intracranial pressure
  and antihypertensive therapy, 794
  and hypertension, 54
Intradural anesthetic blocks, and sympathetic activity, 241
Intraepidermal eccrine sweat duct unit, 106
Intrahisian block, 655
Intraneural recordings, 233–234
Intraocular pressure, in Horner's syndrome, 445
Intravascular pressure, response to standing, 74
Intravesical pressure, 615, 616f
Intrinsic heart rate, 163
Intrinsic nervous system, *see* Enteric nervous system
Ion transport, during sweating, 104–106, 105f, 107f
Iontophoresis
  of acetylcholine, *see* Quantitative sudomotor axon reflex test; Neurogenic flare response
  of pilocarpine, *see* Sweat imprint test
  potential risks, 204
  use in hyperhidrosis, 812
Iris, *see also* Pupil
  anatomy, 259–260
  effects of aging, 172
  effects of anticholinergics, 447
  innervation, 260
  isolated paralysis, 443
  and nerve regeneration, 443–444, 444
  pigmentation
    in Horner's syndrome, 445
    and medications, 448
    and sympathetic nervous system, 445
  in syphilis, 442
Iris dilator muscle, 264f
  cortical and subcortical regulation, 265–266
  sympathetic innervation, 263
Iris sphincter, innervation, 260–261, 262f
Iritis, in diabetes, 517–518
Irritable bowel syndrome, and autonomic dysfunction, 608, 609f
Isaacs' syndrome (acquired neuromyotonia), 519
Ischiocavernosus muscle
  in female, 130, 132
  in male, 129–130
Islet cell autoantibodies, antigenic targets, 516
Isometric (static) exercise, 66–67, 67f, 70
Isoproterenol infusion test, 202, 663f, 664

J
Jugular (superior vagal) ganglion, 40

K
Keratoconjunctivitis sicca, 452
Kidney failure
  autonomic overactivity, 780
  and sweating, 92

L
Laboratory, 383–390
  air flow, 384
  computer configurations, 385–386
  computer software, 385, 386
  commercial sources, 389
  data acquisition and analysis, 385–386
  equipment, 385, 386, 386–388, 386f
    commercial sources, 389–390
  modules, 384
  office requirements, 384
  personnel, 384
  room temperature, 384, 387
  space requirements, 384
  technician training, 384
Laboratory evaluation of autonomic function, 179–208
  see also Autonomic function tests *and specific tests*
  aims, 181
  approach, 204
  blood pressure photoplethysmography, 188–189
  blood pressure response tests, 189–190, 190–191
  cardiovagal function tests, 188, 201
  categories of tests, 181
  in complex regional pain syndromes, 209–220
  composite autonomic scoring scale (CASS), 191, 192t
  frequency analysis, 332
  heart rate recordings, 186–188
  indications, 12, 180–181
  less common tests, 199–203
  less useful tests, 203–204
  MIBG-SPECT study, 199–200
  neural pathways, 199t
  normative data, 191–194
  orthostatic stress tests, 200
  pitfalls, 391–401
  plasma catecholamines, 198
  potential risks, 204
  recent advances, 179–180
  responses to standing, 188
  routine tests, 181–198, 182t
  skin vasomotor reflex tests, 200
  sudomotor function tests, 185–186, 185t, 186t
  in suspected autonomic failure, 11–12
  sustained handgrip, 198
  for sympathetically maintained pain, 196–198
  synthesis with clinical data, 198
  testing conditions, 181
  Valsalva ratio, 187–188
  vs. bedside or office evaluation, 7
Lacrimal apparatus, 260
  evaluation, 259–268
Lacrimal disorders, 451–454
Lacrimal glands, 260
  parasympathetic innervation, 261–263, 262f
  sympathetic innervation, 263, 263f, 264f
Lacrimal reflex, sensory afferents, 263f
Lacrimal sac, 260
Lacrimation, 267
  see also Tear production
  autonomic disturbances affecting, 452–453
  gustatory, 451, 720
Lacunae (sinusoids) of penis, 129, 130f
Lambert-Eaton myasthenic syndrome (LEMS), 519, 546–550, 547t
  autoantibodies, 549
  autonomic function tests, 546, 547t, 548
  autonomic manifestations, 546
  clinical features, 546, 547t
  electrophysiologic abnormalities, 546
  immunosuppressive drug regimens, 550
  pathogenesis, 548–550
  pupillary findings, 453
  treatment, 548, 550
  voltage-sensitive calcium channels, 548–550
Landry-Guillain–Barré syndrome, *see also* Guillain–Barré syndrome
  Fisher variant, pupillary findings, 452–453
Langerhans' cells, 112
Large-fiber-type neuropathy, 489

Laryngeal disorders, 640, 645
Larynx, vagal innervation, 40, 42
Latency, in cardiovascular homeostasis, 73
Least squares, forward–backward method, 345, 347
Leg-crossing, circulatory effects, 75, 76f
Legs, and circulatory response to standing up, 75, 79
Length-dependent autonomic neuropathy, 336, 684, 687
Lens, *see* Accommodation
Leprosy, 253, 253f, 255f, 479
Lewis' reaction, 89
Lewy body disease, 578
Libido, 132
  diminished, causes, 269–270, 270t
Lie detector tests, 98
Light-near dissociation
  in Argyll Robertson pupils, 442
  evaluation, 450
Light-near dissociation syndrome, 442, 442t
Light reflex, *see* Pupillary light reflex; Light-near dissociation
Limbic system
  autonomic disorders, 4t
  rostral, 21
  and seizures, 5
  and urinary bladder function, 119
Livedo reticularis, 816
Liver disease, associated neuropathy, 480
"Long QT syndrome," 49, 502
Longitudinal muscle plexus, 140
Low-frequency oscillations, *see* Slow oscillations; Vasomotor rhythms; Nonrespiratory oscillations
Lumbar sympathetic ganglia, 36
Lumbosacral radiculoplexopathies, in diabetes, 490
Lung cancer, 546, 606f, 608
Lungs, vagal innervation, 42
Lyme disease, 704
Lymphocytes, *see also* B cells; T cells
  β-adrenergic receptors, 150
    in human diseases, 153–154
  muscarinic receptors, 154
Lymphoid organs, sympathetic innervation, 149
  postnatal development, 150

M
Möbius' syndrome, 451
Macrophages, 149
  effects of sympathetic ablation, 152
Madelung's disease (multiple symmetric lipomatosis), 480–481
Magnetic resonance imaging, in multiple system atrophy, 560–561, 560f
Magnetoelectric stimulation
  in fecal incontinence, 605
  in gastrointestinal dysmotility, 611
Major histocompatibility complex (MHC), 148, 149, 519–520
Male erectile dysfunction (MED), *see* Erectile dysfunction
Malignant hyperthermia, 751, 779, 784
Manometry, in gastrointestinal dysmotility, 600f
Mastocytosis, 767
Mayer waves, 310
Mayo Autonomic Reflex Laboratory
  computer configuration, 385
  routine test battery, 292
Mayo Clinic Neurophysiology Technology Program, 294
McArdle's disease, 69
Mean autonomic deviation score, 729–730
  in AIDS, 730, 730f
Mean circular resultant, 293, 301
  technique, 301
Mean square successive difference (MSSD), 300
Mean successive difference (MSD), 300
Mean vasoconstrictor response, 497

832 / SUBJECT INDEX

Medications, *see also* specific categories, e.g., Adrenergic agonists; Anticholinergic agents
  affecting autonomic function tests, 399
  affecting autonomic regulation, 4t
  affecting pupils, 447–449
    systemic agents, 448–449
  affecting sweat glands, 103–104
  affecting tear secretion, 452
  affecting urinary bladder function, 614
  bioavailability, and gastrointestinal dysmotility, 605
  causing acute autonomic neuropathies, 470–471
  causing anhidrosis, 248t
  causing autonomic neuropathies, 464t
  causing diminished libido, 270
  causing ejaculation disorders, 271
  causing erectile dysfunction, 270–271
  causing erythromelalgia, 481
  causing gastroparesis, 599
  causing impaired thermoregulation, 748t, 753–754, 757
  causing intestinal pseudo-obstruction, 602
  causing neuroleptic malignant syndrome, 424, 751–752
  causing orthostatic hypotension, 6, 767
  causing Raynaud's phenomenon, 815
  causing serotonin syndrome, 424
  causing small fiber neuropathy, 704
  causing syncope, 659
  neurotransmitter modulators, 217
  overdoses, autonomic consequences, 798
  prokinetic agents, 599, 611
  for treating AIDS, neurologic side effects, 733
  for treating complex regional pain syndromes, 216, 217–218
  for treating hyperhidrosis, 812
  for treating hypotension, 568–570, 768–772, 769t, 771t
  for treating intestinal pseudo-obstruction, 602
  for treating male sexual dysfunction, 804–805, 804t, 806
  for treating neuropathic pain, 711
  for treating Raynaud's phenomenon, 815–816
  for treating syncope, 673
  for treating urinary bladder dysfunction, 625–626
Medulla
  A1 cell group, 54
  autonomic components, 18, 18f
  and blood pressure, 54, 55
  and Cushing response, 54
  lesions, 424–425
  role in sympathetic control, 20
  rostral ventrolateral, 20, 22, 54, 55
  tumors, and gastrointestinal dysmotility, 606
  ventrolateral, 20, 52, 54
  ventromedial, 20
Medullary (autonomic) respiratory neurons, 636, 636f
Medullary reflexes, 20
Meissner's (submucosal, submucous) plexus, 136, 138f, 139–140
Melatonin
  and circadian rhythms, 594
  and distinguishing central vs. peripheral lesions, 594
Mental stress
  and electrodermal activity, 224, 224f
  and muscle sympathetic activity, 236
  pressor response, 203
  and skin sympathetic activity, 237
  and sweating, 91, 92
Mental sweating, 91, 92
  see also Emotive sudomotor activity
Merkel's cells, 112
Mesenteric ganglia, 35f
Metabolic neuropathies, 479–480
Metaiodobenzylguanidine (MIBG) uptake test, 199–200
Method of forward–backward least squares, 345, 347

3-Methoxy-4-hydroxyphenylglycol (MHPG)
  cerebrospinal fluid levels, 588–589, 589f
  in autonomic failure syndromes, 565–566, 589
MIBG-SPECT study, 199–200
Microneurography, 233–243
  see also Sympathetic nerve activity
  in baroreceptor afferent block, 781, 783f, 784
  in diabetes, 493
  as diagnostic tool, 238
  methods, 233–234
  quantitative vs. qualitative abnormalities, 238
  in small fiber neuropathy, 708
  uses, 233–234
Micturition, *see also* Urinary bladder function
  reflex pathways, 122
    real-time evaluation, 619, 620f
  voiding diary, 614
Micturition cycle, 615
Micturition syncope, 654
Midbrain, autonomic components, 18
Middle cervical ganglion, 34–35
Midodrine (ProAmatine), use in hypotension, 569, 742, 769t, 770
Migraine, 721–724
Migrating motor complex, interdigestive, 600f
Minnesota Multiphasic Personality Inventory (MMPI), in male sexual dysfunction studies, 273
Miosis, 447, 447t, 449
Mitochondria, of sweat gland, 101, 101f, 102f
Mitochondrial DNA, and aging, 161–162
Mitral valve prolapse (MVP), 682, 691–692
Mitral valve prolapse (MVP) syndrome, 691
Mixed apnea, 638, 639f
Mixed connective tissue diseases, 479
Mixed (somatic) blocks, use in pain syndromes, 216–217
Modified covariance method, *see* Method of forward–backward least squares
Modified Wigner distribution, 345
  comparison with Fourier spectrum, 345, 346f
  formula, 357
  in transcranial Doppler monitoring, 351
  use with electroencephalographic data, 357
Monoamine oxidase (MAO) inhibitors, use in orthostatic hypotension, 770
Monoclonal gammopathy-associated neuropathies, 473, 704
Mononucleosis, infectious, 607
Motion sickness, in astronauts, 437
τ-Motoneurons, 19
  in dysautonomia, 378, 378f
Moving periodogram, *see* Periodogram
Mucosa (mucous membranes)
  clinical examination, 10
  gastrointestinal, 135
Mucosal plexus, 138f, 140
Muller's muscle, 445
Multiple myeloma, and amyloid neuropathy, 476
Multiple sclerosis
  affecting nucleus tractus solitarius, 425
  affecting spinal cord, 426
  and breathing disorders, 352
  effects of terbutaline, 154
  erectile dysfunction, evoked potentials, 280f, 281
  gastrointestinal dysmotility, 607
  hypothermia, 756
  immune and sympathetic nervous systems, 153–154
  parasympathetic nervous system, 154
  sympathetic skin response, 229
  thermoregulatory sweat test, 251–252
  urinary tract dysfunction, 622
    artificial sphincter, 628
Multiple sleep latency test, 643
Multiple symmetric lipomatosis, 480–481
Multiple system atrophy (MSA), 555–575

  see also Striatonigral degeneration; Shy-Drager syndrome
  afferent and central pathways, pharmacologic tests, 565–566
  arecoline tests
    ACTH response, 591–592, 593, 594f
    epinephrine response, 589, 592
  atrial natriuretic peptide, 592
  autonomic function tests, 561–562
  blood pressure response to pressor drugs, 588
  and breathing disorders, 352
  catecholamine kinetics, 587f
  catecholamine plasma levels, 562f
  as central autonomic failure, 589, 594
  and cerebral autoregulation, 362
    effects of tilt-up, 365–366, 365f
  cerebrospinal fluid findings
    acetylcholinesterase levels, 591
    antibodies, 568
    5-hydroxyindoleacetic acid (5-HIAA) levels, 591
  cholinergic dysfunction, 558, 562
  cholinergic function studies, 591–592
  clinical features, 556–558, 571t
  cognition (mentation), 556, 558
  Consensus Panel definition, 555–556
  course and prognosis, 571
  diagnosis, 556, 563–564
  differential diagnosis, 564, 564t
  distinguishing from Parkinson's disease, 342, 556, 564, 567
    brain stem evoked potentials, 563
    composite autonomic scoring scale (CASS), 561f, 562
    magnetic resonance imaging, 560
    positron emission tomography, 561
    sphincter electromyography, 563
    urologic evaluation, 563
    voice changes, 558
  dopamine metabolism, 590–591
  erectile dysfunction, 270
    sphincter electromyography, 281
  extrapyramidal symptoms, 772–773
  ganglionic changes, 566–567
  glial cytoplasmic inclusions, 567–568, 567f
  histopathologic findings, 378, 378t
  laryngeal findings, 640
    tracheostomy, 645
  magnetic resonance imaging, 560–561, 560f
  nerve cells affected, 566
  neuropathologic findings, 566–568
  neuropharmacologic abnormalities, 585–595
  nocturnal diuresis, 592
  nomenclature problems, 578
  nonspecific, 556
  norepinephrine metabolism, 587, 589
  norepinephrine plasma levels, 562–563, 562f, 563t, 586
  norepinephrine response to acetylcholine, 591
  ocular signs, 452
  original description, 555
  orthostatic hypotension, 556–558
  peripheral neuropathy, 559
  positron emission tomography, 561
  postprandial hypotension, 741, 772–773
    use of octreotide, 743
      adverse effects, 744
  prognosis, 564
  pyramidal lesion, 559
  respiratory irregularities, 563
  responses to hypoglycemia, 589, 589t, 593
  sleep abnormalities, 563
  sleep-related respiratory disorders, 638–639, 639–641, 639f, 640f
  somatic deficits, 638
  spinal cord neuropathology, 566

sweat test, 249f, 250, 342f
time–frequency studies, 341, 342f
treatment, 568–571
  medications, 568–570
types, 556, 558–559
urologic disorders, 558, 563
vasopressin responses, 594
vs. olivopontocerebellar atrophy, 581
Muscarinic agonists, and immune response, 154
Muscle, see also Smooth muscle; Sympathetic nerve activity, of muscle; and specific muscles
  acidosis, and chemosensitive afferents, 69–70
  and venous return on standing, 74, 75
Muscle chemoreflex, 70
Muscle relaxants, use in urinary bladder dysfunction, 626
Muscularis mucosae, 135
Muscularis propria (externa), 135
Mutations, in mitochondrial DNA, and aging, 161–162
Myasthenia gravis
  experimental autoimmune (EAMG), use of sympathetic ablation, 152
  and polyglandular autoimmune syndrome type II, 517
  pupillary findings, 453
Mydriasis, pharmacologic causes, 447, 448–449
Myelin proteins, glycosylation, 510
Myelinated fibers, see under Nerve fibers
Myelopathy, in HIV infection, 732
Myenteric (Auerbach's) plexus, 136, 138f, 139, 139f, 140
Myocardial infarction, and heart rate variability, 298
Myocardium
  adrenergic function, study by MIBG-SPECT, 200
  injury, 50–53
    from catecholamines, 53
Myotonic dystrophy, pupillary findings, 453

N

(Na, K)-ATPase–dependent Na$^+$ pump, and sweat gland, 104, 105f, 106
Na-K-Cl cotransporter model of sweating, 104–105, 105f
Natural killer (NK) cells, 153
  effects of sympathectomy, 153
Near response, 266
  see also Light-near dissociation
  in Argyll Robertson pupils, 442
Near syncope, and supraventricular tachycardia, 670, 671f
Neonates
  sweating capacity, 93
  thermoregulation, 89
Nerve biopsy, see also Sural nerve biopsy
  clinical uses, 374
  complications, 373–374
  indications, 373–374
  procedure, 374
  research uses, 374
Nerve blocks, use in pain syndromes, 216–217
Nerve fibers
  action potentials, 372f, 373
  intraepidermal, in HIV-positive patients, 372
  morphology and function, 699, 700, 700t
  myelinated, 700t
    composition and type, 370t
    in diabetic neuropathy, 376f, 377
    norepinephrine content, 373, 373t
    single-teased-fiber studies, 374
  in skin, 371–372
  sympathetic adrenergic, 370, 370t
  unmyelinated, 700t
    composition and type, 369, 370t
    degeneration and regeneration, 369–370, 371f
    distribution in skin, 371–372
    findings on sural nerve biopsy, 373, 374f
    morphology, 370f, 371f
Nerve growth factor (NGF), 413
  deprivation, 475
  and insulin, 517
  in Riley-Day syndrome, 530
Neuritis (neuropathy), insulin-induced, in diabetes, 489, 490
Neurochemistry, see also Neurotransmitters; Neuropeptides; and specific substances
  of central autonomic network, 19
  changes in autonomic failure syndromes, 585–595
  of medulla, 20
Neurodegenerative disorders, see also Degenerative entries
  cerebrospinal fluid antibodies, 568
  electroencephalographic rhythms, 339, 341
Neuroendocrine tests, 202–203
Neurogenic bladder, 459–460, 500, 503
Neurogenic flare response, 203, 528f, 708
  in diabetic neuropathy, 498
  equipment used, 388
  limitations, 288, 396–397
  mechanism, 397
Neurokinins, of spinal cord, 30–31
Neuroleptic malignant syndrome, 424, 751–752, 779, 780, 796
  management, 787
  pathophysiology, 784
Neurologic disorders
  affecting gastrointestinal motility, 598–605, 601f, 602t, 605–609
    identification, 609–611
  affecting urinary bladder, 613–614, 623–624
  spectral analysis, 332
Neuromodulators, 29
  in thermoregulation, 87
Neuromyotonia, acquired (Isaacs' syndrome), 519
Neuronal autoantibodies, 509–510
  antigenic targets, 516
  and diabetes, 510, 517
  in nondiabetic polyglandular diseases, 518–519
Neuronal Charcot-Marie-Tooth disease, 479
Neuronal paucity, in Riley-Day syndrome, 528–529, 529f
Neuron staining properties, effects of aging, 169
Neuropathies, see also Autonomic neuropathies; Panautonomic neuropathies; Peripheral neuropathies; Polyneuropathy; and specific neuropathies
  in alcoholics, 480, 702
    histopathologic findings, 379
    pupillary findings, 453
  autonomic overactivity, 779–780
  pathophysiology, 784
  axonal (dying-back)
    experimental, 406
    and sympathetic skin response, 227, 228
  chronic sensory and autonomic, of unknown cause, 608, 609f
  combined adrenergic/sensory neuropeptide-deficient, 474–475
  congenital sensory, with anhidrosis, 703
  distal sympathetic, symptom patterns, 11
  enzymes in sural nerve biopsy, 373t
  gastrointestinal dysmotility, 602t
  hereditary, 703
  in hyperlipidemia, 704
  inflammatory, 519
  laboratory monitoring
    choice of tests, 392–393
    during therapy, 180–181
  large-fiber-type, 489
  mixed somatic and autonomic, ocular findings, 453
  nutritional, 480, 702
  pure adrenergic, 11
  pure cholinergic, 11
  skin blood flow testing, 398
  and sympathetic skin response, 227–229
  toxic, 6, 472, 704
Neuropeptide Y, 30f, 32
  as marker of sympathetic adrenergic neuropathy, 492
Neuropeptides, 29–33
  see also Neurotransmitters; Vasoactive peptides; and specific peptides
  anatomic sites
    central autonomic network, 19
    medulla, 20
    paraventricular nucleus, 22
    paraventriculospinal tract, 22
    spinal cord, 29, 30f
    sweat glands, 100, 103
  and autonomic nervous system, 592–594
  in cardiovascular control, 592, 592t
  clinical studies, 585–586
  and cluster headache, 722
  and cutaneous vascular tone, 814
  and facial flushing, 718–719
  and facial sweating, 717, 718
  and postprandial hypotension, 738–739
  in thermoregulation, 87
Neurophysiology training, 294
Neurosyphilis, Argyll Robertson pupils, 441–442
Neurotransmitters, 586–592
  see also Neuropeptides
  anatomic sites
    central autonomic network, 19
    detrusor muscle, 124
    gastrointestinal enteric plexuses, 140
    intermediolateral and -medial cell columns, 29
  in cardiovascular control, 592, 592t
  clinical studies, 585–586
  and denervation supersensitivity, 717–718
  effects of aging, 167
  and gastrointestinal motility, 597, 598
  and hypertension, 55
  and immune system, 150, 156
  modulators, use in pain syndromes, 217
  and muscle sympathetic activity, 236
  neuromodulator vs. cotransmitter, 29
  in penile erection and detumescence, 132–133
  in peristaltic reflex, 141f, 142
  in sexual function, 132
  in supraspinal modulation of pain, 145
  and sweat glands, 100, 103
  in thermoregulation, 87
Neurovestibular system, and exposure to low gravity, 437–438
Newborn, see Neonates
Night sweats, 811
Nigrostriatal system, 590
Nitric oxide, 33–34
  autonomic-induced release, 70
  and central autonomic network, 19
  and central command, 68
  in penile erection and detumescence, 133
Nitric oxide synthase, 33–34
Nociceptive pathways, see also Pain
  visceral, 142–144
  visceral afferents, 143f
Nociceptive stimuli
  effects on sympathetic nerve activity, 236, 241
  physiologic responses, 209
Nocturnal penile tumescence studies, 272–273
Nodose (inferior vagal) ganglion, 40
Nondiabetic polyglandular diseases, 518–519
Nonneuronal supporting cells
  and cytokines, 155–156
  and neurotransmitters, 156
Non-REM (slow-wave, synchronized) sleep, 637
  respiratory changes, 637–638

Nonrespiratory oscillations, see also Slow oscillations
  in blood pressure, 334
    in mild orthostatic tachycardia, 334
    periodogram (global spectrum), 326f
  in RR interval (RRI), 328f, 334
    time–frequency maps, 326f
  in young adults, 326f, 328, 328f
Nonshivering thermogenesis (NST), 89
Nonspecific multiple system atrophy, 556
Norepinephrine (noradrenaline), 586–589
  see also Catecholamines
  assessing neuronal uptake, 587–588, 587f
  central metabolism, 588–589, 589f
    in autonomic failure syndromes, 589
  and central vs. peripheral autonomic failure, 586–587
  effects on eye, 446
  and exposure to low gravity, 435, 437
  hormonal functions, 495
  levels in neural tissue, 373, 373t
  levels in spleen, 149–150
    and cytokines, 155
    effects of 6-hydroxydopamine, 151
  plasma levels
    in automatic hyperreflexia, 459
    and diagnosis of diabetic autonomic neuropathy, 492
    effects of aging, 167, 170, 171f
    effects of standing, 586
    as index of adrenergic function, 198
    as marker of sympathetic neuropathy, 492
    in multiple system atrophy, 562–563, 562f, 563t, 586
    normal, 586
    and postprandial hypotension, 740–741, 740f, 743–744
    in pure autonomic failure, 562–563, 562f, 563t, 586, 588
    response to acetylcholine, 591
  testing, 10
  use in laboratory evaluation, 198
  response to edrophonium, 202, 610f
  and vascular pooling, 586
Norepinephrine spillover, 167, 170, 198
  and muscle sympathetic activity, 236, 240f, 241
Normal pressure hydrocephalus, and hypertension, 55
Normal-to-normal (NN) RR intervals, 300
Normative data, for laboratory tests, 191–194
Normetanephrine, 586–587
Nuclei, see also specific nuclei
  of central autonomic network, 18, 18f
  in control of gastrointestinal motility, 137t
  for eye innervation, 260, 260f, 261f, 262f
  for urinary bladder innervation, 119, 120–121, 122
  of vagus nerve, 40
Nucleus locus coeruleus, and detrusor reflex contraction, 119–120
Nucleus of solitary tract (of tractus solitarius, solitarii)(NTS), 633–636, 634f, 635f
  afferent pathways, 19
  afferents and efferents, 636
  and baroreceptor reflexes, 20, 21f
  and medullary reflexes, 20
  lesions, and blood pressure, 53, 54f
Nutritional neuropathies, 480, 702

O

Obstructive (primary) sleep apnea syndrome (OSAS), 642–643
  continuous positive airway pressure therapy, 642, 644
  surgical therapy, 644–645
Octreotide
  adverse effects, 744
  and hypotension, 559, 559f
  in postprandial hypotension

effects, 739, 742
mechanism of effects, 743–744
therapeutic use, 168, 742–743, 742f
use in autonomic failure syndromes, 570
Ocular motor nuclei, 260, 260f
Oculomotor nerve
  aberrant regeneration, 442t, 443–444
  in Horner's syndrome, 446
  parasympathetic fibers, 38
Oculosympathetic spasm (sympathetic irritation), 447, 447t
Oligodendroglial cytoplasmic inclusions, in multiple system atrophy, 567–568, 567f
Olivopontocerebellar atrophy (OPCA), 558–559, 581–582
  autonomic deficits, 641
  familial, 559
  familial vs. sporadic, 581, 582
  and multiple system atrophy, 581, 582
  nomeclature problems, 578
  site of lesion, 582
  sleep apnea, 641
  sporadic
    clinical features, 581
    Consensus Panel definition, 556
  vs. Shy-Drager syndrome, 641
Onuf's nucleus, 121, 131, 281
Operating point, see Set-point
Ophthalmoplegia, 442t, 443
Opiate receptors, 33
Opioids, endogenous, in thermoregulation, 87
Organ failure, selective, 12
Orgasm
  in female, 133
  in male, 132
Original variance, see Total variance
Orthostasis, see Upright posture; Head-up tilt; Standing up
Orthostatic disorders, classification, 4t
Orthostatic hypertension, 686–687
Orthostatic hypotension, see also Orthostatic intolerance; Orthostatic stress
  in AIDS, from medications, 733
  and autonomic dysreflexia, 426
  and autonomic failure, 397
  and baroreflex, 55
  from brainstem disorders, 425
  case studies, 773–774
  causes
    disorders causing, 764t
    medications causing, 767
    primary vs. secondary, 764t
  and central lesions, 55
  and cerebral autoregulation, 359–360, 361f, 362
  cerebral perfusion and blood flow volume, 365
  clinical examination, 10
  compensatory mechanisms, 7
  in diabetes, 494
    anti-sympathetic ganglia autoantibodies, 514–515, 515f
    effects of tilt-up, 365, 365f, 366
    false assumptions, 393
    mechanism, 494
    postural catecholamine responses, 515–516, 515f
    time–frequency analysis, 337, 338f
    treatment, 503
  diagnostic algorithm, 765f
  diagnostic criteria, 766
  diagnostic evaluation, 6
    tests needed, 10–11
  effects of Valsalva maneuver, 361f, 362
  in elderly, 167–168, 167t
  and head movements, 437–438
  head-up tilt effects on electroencephalographic data, 364f

history-taking, 7–8
in HIV infection, 727, 728
idiopathic, and gastrointestinal dysmotility, 607
management, 763–775
in multiple system atrophy, 556–558, 560
operational definition, 766
postprandial, 168
and preganglionic neuron attrition, 375
in pure autonomic failure, 560
in Riley-Day syndrome, 526t
and spinal cord injury, 456
and splanchnic outflow, 374
symptoms, 766
  time of occurrence, 7
therapeutic measures, 767–772
  nonpharmacologic, 570, 767–768, 768t
    mechanical corrective maneuvers, 75, 76f
    sympathetic neural prosthesis, 570
  pharmacologic, 568–570, 768–772, 769t
    pharmacologic combinations, 771t, 772
    use of midodrine, 569
in HIV infection, 727, 728
in specific disorders, 766–767
in postural orthostatic tachycardia syndrome, 694
vs. postural orthostatic tachycardia syndrome, 7, 683, 683t, 687t, 689, 689t
Orthostatic intolerance (instability, incompetence)
  aggravating factors, 8, 8t
  causes, 334
  classification, 682t
  constitutional, 689
  definition and perspective, 681–682
  evaluation, 180
  from exposure to low gravity, 430
    and adrenergic sensitivity, 437
    and baroreflex changes, 434
    mechanisms, 429–440, 438f
  grading, 7, 8t, 689, 689t
  and hyperventilation, 352
  standing time, 8, 8t
  symptoms, 8, 8t, 334
  time frequency analysis, 333f, 334–336
  transcranial Doppler monitoring, 349–368
    clinical applications, 359–362
  vs. postural orthostatic tachycardia syndrome, 689
Orthostatic intolerance grade to tilt-up, 191, 191t
Orthostatic stress
  cardiovascular responses, 61–66, 303
  circulatory responses, 77–81, 77f
  prolonged, circulatory adjustments, 80–81
Orthostatic stress tests, 200, 303–304
  see also specific tests
Orthostatic tachycardia, see Postural orthostatic tachycardia syndrome (POTS); Heart rate responses
Orthostatic 30:15 ratio, 188, 303
  effects of aging, 164, 166, 166f
  and erectile dysfunction, 282
  limitations, 289, 395
"Orthostatism," 766
Otic ganglion, 37f, 39f, 40, 265
Oxidative stress, and aging, 161–162
Oxytocin, 30f, 32–33

P

Paced-breathing tests, 320
Pacemakers
  electrical, use in syncope, 672, 673
  of gut, 140, 141
Pacinian corpuscles, in detrusor muscle, 124
Pain
  and afferent fiber types, 143f, 144
  in diabetic neuropathy, 490
  effects on sympathetic nerve activity, 236, 241
  in extremity, consequences, 542

"first" vs. "second," 144
in neuropathies, treatment, 710–711
nociceptive pathways, 142–144, 143f
physiologic responses, 209
referred, 142, 144
in reflex sympathetic dystrophy, treatment, 541–542
and small fiber neuropathy, 699
supraspinal modulation, 145
sympathetic involvement, mechanisms, 210t, 538
sympathetically independent (SIP), 538, 542
sympathetically maintained (SMP), 11, 538, 541–542
  laboratory evaluation, 181, 196–198
    patient preparation, 196
  threshold testing, 709
  visceral, 142–144
Pain syndromes, chronic, *see also* Complex regional pain syndromes
  sympathetic nerve activity, 241
  with autonomic features, 209–220
    diagnostic considerations, 211–214
    terminology, 210
    treatment modalities, 214–218
  false assumptions, 393
  QSART recordings, 393f
Pallidotomy, use in multiple system atrophy, 772
Palms, *see also* Hands
  sweat glands, 98
  sweating, 91
    expulsion rhythm, 92
Palsy
  progressive bulbar, 605–606
  progressive supranuclear, 582–583, 605
Panautonomic neuropathies, *see also* Autonomic neuropathies
  acute, 465, 465–468
    autonomic function tests, 466, 467t
    clinical features, 465
    course and prognosis, 466, 468
    differential diagnosis, 466
    etiology, 466
    forme fruste, 468
    investigations, 465–466
    neurologic examination, 465
    site of lesion, 465
    sural nerve biopsy, 466, 466f
    sural nerve potentials, 467f
    treatment, 468
  chronic vs. acute, 476
  histopathologic findings, 377
  pupillary findings, 452
  sweat test, 250
Pancoast (apical lung) tumor, 252, 252f, 816
Pancreas, vagal innervation, 42
Pancreatic polypeptide, 593
  in diabetes, 492–493, 495
  in hypoglycemia, 495
  in autonomic failure syndromes, 589t, 593
  measurement, 202–203
Pandysautonomia, *see also* Panautonomic neuropathies; Autonomic neuropathies
  chronic, 476
  gastrointestinal dysmotility, 606–607
  and pancreatic polypeptide, 593
  sweat test, 250
Panic disorders, and postural orthostatic tachycardia syndrome, 683
Panting, for heat dissipation, 90
Papillary dermis, 110, 111f, 112
Paradoxic sleep, *see* REM sleep
Paralimbic circuit, 4t
  and seizures, 5
Paraneoplastic autonomic disorders, 545–554
  see also Cancer-associated neuropathies *and specific syndromes*

gastrointestinal dysmotility, 608
immunologic findings, 377
neurologic syndromes, 545–546
sweat test, 253
Parasympathetic disorders
  biochemical and neurophysiologic markers, 492–493
  pupillary, 441–444, 442t, 447, 447t
  sympathetic-parasympathetic combined failure, *see under* Autonomic failure
Parasympathetic function tests, 289, 290, 291, 611t
  in diabetes, spectral power vs. conventional tests, 337
  in Lambert-Eaton myasthenic syndrome, 547t
Parasympathetic ganglia, 28, 37f
Parasympathetic nerves
  efferent neurons, pre- and postganglionic, 37f
  facial fibers, 38
  glossopharyngeal fibers, 38–40, 39f
  innervation to eye, 260–263
  ocular motor nuclei, 260, 260f
  oculomotor fibers, 38
  preganglionic neurons, 19, 37f, 425
  in sexual function, 131
Parasympathetic nervous system, 37–42, 37f
  and anti-vagus nerve antibodies, in type I diabetes, 516
  in cardiac control, 299
  and exposure to low gravity, 430–431, 438f
  and facial vasodilatation, 718
  in gastrointestinal motility, 601f, 137t, 598
  in heart rate variability, 318
  and immune response, 154
  and myocardial damage, 53
  origin, 27–28
  and pancreatic polypeptide, 593
  and progressive multiple sclerosis, 154
  in Riley-Day syndrome, 528–529
  sympathetic-parasympathetic vagal network, 40
  and vestibular stimulation, 437
  vs. sympathetic nervous system, 29f, 37–38
Parasympatholytic agents, *see* Anticholinergic agents
Paraventricular (parvicellular) nucleus (PVN) of hypothalamus, 22
Paraventriculospinal tract, 22
Paravertebral ganglia, 34
  of sympathetic chain, 27, 27f
  thoracic, 36
Parinaud's syndrome, 450
Parkinson's disease, 579–581
  autonomic function tests, 579–581
  blood pressure, 579
  cardiovascular reflexes, 580
  central vs. peripheral dysautonomia, 580–581
  cerebrospinal fluid antibodies, 568
  gastrointestinal dysmotility, 605
    and medications, 605
  hypothermia, 756
  and neuroleptic malignant syndrome, 424
  neuropathologic findings, 566
  and polyneuroendocrine autoimmunity, 517
  urinary bladder dysfunction, 621
  vs. multiple system atrophy, *see* Multiple system atrophy, distinguishing from Parkinson's disease
  vs. striatonigral degeneration, 558
Parkinsonism
  autonomic dysfunction, 577–578
  gastrointestinal dysmotility, 605
  and medications, 605
Parkinsonism-plus, 556, 581
Parotid gland, and sweating, 92
Paroxysmal autonomic hyperactivity, *see* Diencephalic seizures
Paroxysmal hemicrania, 724
Paroxysmal (intermittent) dysautonomia, 12, 481
Parvicellular, *see* Paraventricular
Passive head-up tilt, *see* Head-up tilt

Pelvic detrusor nerves, afferent pathways, 119, 122
Pelvic nerve, cortical evoked response, 118, 620
Pelvic nuclei, of conus medullaris, in urinary bladder innervation, 120
Pelvic plexuses, 36
  in sexual function, 131
  and urinary bladder innervation, 123
Pelvic sympathetic trunk, 36
Pelvic urethral nerve, *see also* Pelvic nerve; Pelvic detrusor nerves
  evoked-potential studies, 118
Penile brachial index, 272
Penile emission, 132
Penile erection, *see* Erection
Penile prostheses, 805
  vacuum devices, 805–806
Penis
  see also Erection; Erectile dysfunction
  anatomy, 124, 129, 130f
  detumescence
    neural and neurotransmitter control, 132–133
    physiology, 132
  dorsal nerve, evoked-potential studies, 118, 620, 622f
  rigidity studies, 273
  skin response, in small fiber neuropathy, 708
  smooth muscle electromyography, 283, 283f
  tumescence studies, 272–273
    postage stamp test, 9
    tumescence vs. rigidity, 273
  vascular studies, 272
Peptides, *see* Neuropeptides; Vasoactive peptides
Perforin, 148
Periaqueductal gray matter, 18, 22
  in stress response, 21, 21f
Peridural anesthetic blocks, and sympathetic nerve activity, 241
Perineum, muscles of sexual function, 129–130
Periodic fever syndrome, 754
Periodogram (global spectrum), 324f
  comparison with Wigner distribution, 345
  filtering window, 345
  of RR interval, 326f
  shortcomings, 345
Peripheral adrenergic impairment, in postural orthostatic tachycardia syndrome (POTS), 336, 688
Peripheral autonomic neuropathies, *see also* Peripheral neuropathies; Autonomic neuropathies
  chronic, 464t, 472–481
  classification, 4t, 464t
Peripheral autonomic surface potential (PASP), 221
  see also Sympathetic skin response
Peripheral cholinergic agonists, in diabetic neuropathy, 608
Peripheral nerve blocks, use in pain syndromes, 216–217
Peripheral nerves, *see also* Nerve fibers
  composition, 369–370, 370t
Peripheral nervous system
  and AIDS autonomic dysfunction, 732–733
  and ECG changes, 52–53
  responses to tissue damage, 538
  sympathetic outflow, effects of pulmonary vagal afferents, 63–64
Peripheral neuropathies, *see also* Autonomic neuropathies; Neuropathies; Polyneuropathy; *and specific type*
  in amyloidosis, 701–702
  autonomic, 4t, 464t, 472–481
  autonomic evaluation in the frequency domain, 336–338
    technical factors affecting, 337
  and bulbocavernosus reflex, 279
  evaluation of autonomic involvement, 181
  gastrointestinal dysmotility, 607–609

Peripheral neuropathies *(contd.)*
   justification for autonomic testing, 287–288
   and male sexual dysfunction, 270
   in multiple system atrophy, 559
   and neurogenic arrhythmias, 49
   skin vasomotor reflex tests, 200
   sympathetic nerve activity, 238
   and sympathetic skin response, 227–229
Peripheral reflexes, in diabetic neuropathy, 497–498, 498f
Peripheral vascular resistance
   and exposure to low gravity, 434–435, 435f, 436f, 438f
   response to standing, 79, 303
Peripheral vasoconstriction, effects on blood pressure photoplethysmography, 398
Peristaltic reflex, 141–142, 141f
Periurethral striated muscle, 124
Persistent sweat activity (PSA), 185
Perspiration, *see* Sweating
Pharmacologic abnormalities, in autonomic failure syndromes, 585–595
Pharmacologic agents, *see* Medications *and specific types*
Pharmacologic tests
   of central pathways, 565–566
   in Horner's syndrome, 446–447
   in multiple system atrophy, 565
   in pure autonomic failure, 565
   responses to hypoglycemia, 589, 589t, 593
      normal response, 589, 590f
Pharyngeal branch of vagus nerve, 40
Phase, in spectral analysis, 316–317, 316f
Phase angle, in spectral analysis, 316
Phasic sleep stage, 637
Phenytoin, use in small fiber neuropathy, 711
Pheochromocytoma
   hypertension, vs. Guillain-Barré syndrome, 469
   sweating, 811
Photoplethysmographic blood pressure recordings, 188–189
   see also Finapres
   problems, 398
Pilocarpine iontophoresis, *see* Sweat imprint test
Pilomotor reflexes, testing, 813
Pilomotor seizures, 423
Pilomotor system, 813
Pink disease (mercury poisoning), 472
Pituitary gland
   and immune system, 155
   in sexual function, 132
Pituitary hormones, 593–594
   see also Hypothalamic-pituitary-adrenal axis
Placebo effects, 541
Plantar, *see* Soles; Feet
Plasma volume, *see* Blood volume
Plethysmography, *see* Photoplethysmographic blood pressure recordings; Finapres
Plexuses, *see also specific plexuses*
   autonomic, 36
   gastrointestinal, 136, 138f, 139–140, 140f
   in sexual function, 131, 131f
   in urinary bladder control, 123
Pneumotaxic center, 636
POEMS syndrome, 519
Poincare plots, 339
Poisons, autonomic disorders from, 6, 472, 704
Poliomyelitis
   dysphagia, 606
   hypertension, 779–780
      pathophysiology, 784
   medullary effects, 425
Polyglandular autoimmune syndrome type II, 510, 517
   and diabetes, 510, 511
Polyglandular diseases, nondiabetic, 518–519
Polymodal C nociceptor, *see* Neurogenic flare response; ABC syndrome

Polyneuroendocrine autoimmunity, and Parkinson's disease, 517
Polyneuropathy, *see also* Peripheral neuropathies
   acute inflammatory, *see* Guillain–Barré syndrome
   chronic inflammatory, 519–520
   distal sensorimotor, in HIV infection, 732–733
   sympathetic nerve activity, 238
Polyradiculoneuropathy, 252f
Polysomnography, 640f, 643
Pontine nuclei, and urinary bladder innervation, 119–120, 122
Pontine tegmentum, in urinary bladder innervation, 120
Poral occlusion, 100
Porphyria, 470
   dysautonomia, 798
   gastrointestinal dysmotility, 609
   histopathologic findings, 379
Porphyric neuropathy, 779
Positron emission tomography (PET), 561
Postage stamp test, 9
Posterior fossa, and blood pressure, 54
Postganglionic disorders
   autonomic function test results, 611t
   postganglionic vs. preganglionic failure, norepinephrine test, 198
   sympathetic lesion, and QSART results, 185, 185t
Postganglionic neurons
   age-related attrition, 170
   parasympathetic, 37f
   sympathetic, 35f, 809–810
      conduction velocity, 810
      edrophonium testing, 610f
      thermoregulatory fibers, 90
Postpolio syndrome, dysphagia, 606
Postprandial hypotension, 737–746
   in autonomic failure, 557f, 559, 559f, 560
   clinical presentation, 741
   guidelines for testing, 737–738
   management, 741–744
      use of octreotide, 742–743
   in Parkinson's disease vs. multiple system atrophy vs. pure autonomic failure, 580
   pathophysiology, 738–741
      and octreotide therapy, 743–744
      role of gastrointestinal peptides, 738–739
      role of glucose, 738–739, 738f, 739–740, 739f
      role of insulin, 738–739, 739–740, 743
      role of sympathetic dysfunction, 740–741, 743–744
   prophylaxis, 771
   with multiple system atrophy, 772–773
Postprandial orthostatic hypotension, 168
Postural hypotension, *see* Orthostatic hypotension
Postural normotension, 73–81, 397
   control system, 73–74, 74t
   neurohumoral reflex adjustments, 77–81
Postural orthostatic tachycardia syndrome (POTS), 681–697
   blood pressure and heart rate examination, 9–10
   and blood volume, 395–396
   cerebral autoregulation, 362
   clinical features, 683–684
   criteria, 681–682, 682t
   definition and perspective, 681–682
   differential diagnosis, 689–690
   effects of Valsalva maneuver, 362, 363f, 684, 685f, 687, 688
   etiology, 684
   evaluation, 687–690
   future research, 695
   hypertensive, 684
   management, 693–695
   mild, 333f, 334
   orthostatic response, 333f, 334, 336
   pathophysiologic mechanisms, 684–687

   peripheral adrenergic impairment, 336, 688
   postviral, management, 694
   prognosis, 692–693
   role of brain stem, 686–687, 695
   secondary, 684
   severe, 333f, 336
   sudomotor impairment, 688
   symptoms, 7, 8, 336
   time–frequency maps, 333f
   types, 684t
   vs. orthostatic hypotension, 683, 683t, 687t, 689, 689t
Postviral fatigue syndrome, 690–691
Pourfour Du Petit syndrome, 721, 724
Power spectral (power-spectrum) analysis, *see* Spectral analysis
Power spectrum
   effects of respiration, 396
   in syncope, 356f, 357
   of systolic blood pressure variability, 312f
Preganglionic autonomic neurons, 19, 425
   age-related attrition, 169–170, 170f, 375
   medullary modulation, 20
   parasympathetic, 19, 37f, 425
   selective destruction
      induced by acetylcholinesterase antibodies, 413
      and QSART results, 184–185, 185t
   sympathetic, 19, 27, 27f, 33f, 35f, 809
   in thermoregulation, 90
Preganglionic vs. postganglionic failure, norepinephrine test, 198
Pregnancy, *see also* Birth; Fetus
   after spinal cord injury, 460
   autonomic dysreflexia, 426
Premature ejaculation, 271, 806
   sympathetic skin responses, 283
Prenalterol, use in autonomic failure, 568
Preoptic area, and thermoregulation, 84, 85, 90, 102
Presyncope, electroencephalography, 356f, 357
Prevertebral ganglia, 34
   sympathetic, and gastrointestinal motility, 138–139
ProAmatine, *see* Midodrine
Progesterone, and body temperature, 85
Programmed circuits, in control of gastrointestinal motility, 598
Prolonged QT syndrome, *see* Long QT syndrome
Propafenone, and small fiber neuropathy, 704
Propranolol
   effect on blood pressure response to Valsalva maneuver, 190f
   effects on heart rate variability, 298, 298f
Prostaglandin inhibitors, use in orthostatic hypotension, 770–771
Prostaglandins
   effects on eye, 448
   E, and fever, 87
   E_1, use in male sexual dysfunction, 805
Prostatectomy, for urinary bladder dysfunction, 628
Protein glycosylation, 510
Protriptyline, use in sleep apnea, 644
Proximal diabetic neuropathy, 489, 491–492
Pseudomembranous colitis, 602
Pseudoseizures, and neurogenic arrhythmias, 50
Pseudosyringomyelic small fiber neuropathy, 701
Psychiatric disorders, and syncope, 656
Psychogenic (supraspinal) erection, 132
Psychogenic (emotion-induced) sweating, 91, 92
Psychogenic tearing, 267
Pterygopalatine (sphenopalatine) ganglion, 37f, 38, 262, 264
Ptosis, 445
Pudendal cortical evoked potentials, 118, 279f, 280–281, 280f, 620, 622f
   clinical utility, 281
   in cervical spondylosis, 623, 623f

Pudendal motor neurons, 121, 123, 123f
Pudendal nerves, 131
  somatic, in sexual function, 131
  urethral, afferent pathways, 119
Pudendal nuclei, 121, 123f
  in reflex micturition pathways, 122
  in urinary bladder innervation, 120
Pulmonary carcinoid, 608
Pulmonary edema, neurogenic, 799
Pulmonary plexuses, 36, 42
Pulmonary stretch receptors, 63–64
Pulmonary vagal afferents, 63–64
Pulsatility index, in transcranial Doppler monitoring, 351
Pupil, 259–260
  see also Iris, Anisocoria; Light-near dissociation
  aberrant nerve regeneration, 442t, 443–444
  Adie's, 442t, 444, 474
  in Alzheimer's disease, 453
  Argyll Robertson, 441–442, 442t, 444
  autonomic disturbances affecting, 452–453
  clinical examination, 10
  constrictors, 448
  in diabetic neuropathy, 498
  diagnostic tests, 449–451
    in diabetic neuropathy, 498
  diameter, measuring technique, 498
  direct and consensual light reflexes, 266
  disorders, 441–454
  effects of aging, 171–173, 172f
  effects of anticholinergics/parasympatholytics, 447
  effects of parasympathomimetics, 448
  effects of sympatholytics, 448
  effects of sympathomimetics, 448
  evaluation, 9, 259–268
  factors affecting, 265–266, 447–449
  in Horner's syndrome, 444–445
  loss of constriction (ophthalmoplegia), 442t, 443
  medications affecting, 447–449
    systemic medications, 448–449
  parasympathetic deficiencies, 441–444, 442f
  redilation speed, as test in diabetic neuropathy, 498
  physiology, 265–266
  spastic paralysis, 442
  supranuclear regulation, 265–266
  sympathetic and parasympathetic balance, 265
  sympathetic deficiencies, 444–447
  tonic, 442t, 444, 474, 720
Pupil cycle time, 450
  in AIDS, 730
  in diabetic autonomic neuropathy, 498
Pupillary dilator muscle, innervation, 264, 264f
Pupillary dilators, 447–448
Pupillary light reflex, 266, 267f
  see also Light-near dissociation
  in Argyll Robertson pupils, 442
  assessment, 449–450, 449f
  clinical utility, 266
  quantitation, 450
Pupillary unrest (hippus), 266
Pupillography, 449f, 451
Pupillometric tests, 498
Pupillomotor symptoms, evaluation, 9
Pure adrenergic failure, 474
Pure adrenergic neuropathy, 11, 474
Pure autonomic failure (PAF), 555–575
  see also Autonomic failure
  arecoline tests
    ACTH response, 591–592, 593, 594f
    epinephrine response, 589, 592
  atrial natriuretic peptide, 592
  autonomic function tests, 561–562
  blood pressure, response to pressor drugs, 588
  brain stem evoked potentials, 563
  catecholamines, plasma levels, 562f
  and cerebral autoregulation, 362
  cholinergic function studies, 591–592
  clinical features, 560, 571t
  course and prognosis, 571
  cerebrospinal fluid findings
    acetylcholinesterase levels, 591
    homovanillic acid levels, 591
    5-hydroxyindoleacetic acid (5-HIAA) levels, 591
  differential diagnosis, 564–565, 564t
  erectile dysfunction, 270
  ganglionic changes, 566–567
  lesion site, pharmacologic evidence, 588, 588t, 594
  neurochemical and pharmacologic abnormalities, 585–595
  neuropathologic findings, 566–568
  nocturnal diuresis, 592
  norepinephrine
    metabolism, 587, 589
    neuronal uptake, 587, 587f
    plasma levels, 562–563, 562f, 563t, 586, 588
  original description, 555
  as peripheral autonomic failure, 589, 591
  pharmacologic tests, 565
    of afferent and central pathways, 565–566
    responses to hypoglycemia, 589, 589t, 593
  positron emission tomography, 561
  postprandial hypotension, 741
    use of octreotide, 743
      adverse effects, 744
  spectral analysis findings, 565
  spinal cord neuropathology, 566
  thermoregulatory sweat test, 249f, 250
  tilt-up effects on cerebral blood flow, 362, 366
  treatment, 568–571
    medications, 568–570
  urologic disorders, 558, 563
Pure cholinergic neuropathies, 11, 473–474
Pure small fiber neuropathy, 701
Pyramidal lesions, in multiple system atrophy, 559
Pyridoxine neuropathy, 478, 704
Pyrogens, 85, 753

Q

Quantitative sudomotor axon reflex test (QSART), 182–186, 186f
  in complex regional pain syndromes, 212–213, 213f
  effects of age and gender, 169t, 193t
  equipment needed, 387–388, 387f
    commercial sources, 389
  false assumptions, 393
  interpretation, 184–185
  and lesion site, 184–185, 185t
  normative data, 193, 193t
  principle, 182f
  recording sites, 183–184, 183f
  response patterns, 184, 184f
  in sympathetically maintained pain, 197
  technique details, 292
QSART index, for reflex sympathetic dystrophy, 197t
QT lengthening, in diabetes, 502
Quadriplegia, nonrespiratory oscillations, 343

R

Radiculoplexopathies, in diabetes, 490
Rapid eye movement sleep, see REM sleep
Raynaud's disease, 813–816
  clinical features, 813
  diagnosis, 815
  management, 815–816
  pathophysiology, 813–814
  vs. Raynaud's phenomenon, 813
Raynaud's phenomenon, 813–816
  causes, 815
  clinical features, 813
  criteria, 813
  management, 815–816
  pathophysiology, 814
Rectoanal inhibitory reflex, 602
Red ear syndrome, 721
Referred pain, visceral, 142, 144
Reflex bradycardia, 391–392, 394
Reflex heating, 398
Reflex sympathetic dystrophy (RSD), 537–542
  see also Complex regional pain syndromes
  autonomic symptoms, 539
  clinical characteristics, 211t, 212t, 538–539, 538t, 540t
  clinical probability scoring system, 198t
  definition, 211t, 212t, 537
  diagnostic criteria, 214t, 538, 538t, 539–541, 540t
  diagnostic tests, 182t, 212t, 385
  false assumptions, 393
  grading scale, 197t
  Kozin's criteria, 214t
  laboratory evaluation, 197t, 198
  physical rehabilitation, 542
  prevention, 542
  and sympathetic skin response, 229
  treatment, 541–542
Reflex sympathetic dystrophy (RSD) screen, 182t, 385
  see also Sympathetic dysfunction screen
Reflex syncope, 650–654, 651f
  types, 650t
Reflex tears, 267
Reflex vasoconstriction, in head-up tilt, 79
Reflex vasodilation, in standing up, 79
Reflexes, see Autonomic reflexes and specific reflexes
Reflexogenic (spinal) erection, 132
Regional intravenous blockade, use in pain syndromes, 216
Regional pain syndromes, see Complex regional pain syndromes
Rehydration, and sweating, 92
REM (rapid eye movement, paradoxic) sleep, 637
  respiratory changes, 638
Renal failure
  autonomic overactivity, 780
  and sweating, 92
Renal (least splanchnic) nerve, 36
Renal sympathetic activity, and exposure to low gravity, 432
Renin-angiotensin system, 592
  in autonomic failure, 592
  response to upright posture, 63, 81
Research studies, see also Experimental entries
  clinical trials, 290, 290t, 294
  computer configurations, 385
  nerve biopsy, 374
  tests used, 181
Respiration
  central cardiorespiratory network, 20
  changes during sleep, 637–638
  control systems, 636–637
  effects on power spectra, 396
  electrophrenic, 645
  monitoring, clinical applications, 352
  normal time series, 325f
  periodogram (global spectrum), 326f
  spectral analysis, technical aspects, 344
  time–frequency maps, 326f
  and upright posture, 64, 75
Respiratory control abnormalities, in Riley-Day syndrome, 533
Respiratory disturbance index, 639
Respiratory frequency, 325f, 326f
  tracking changes, technical aspects, 345–347
  in young adults, 327–328
Respiratory function studies, in sleep-disordered breathing, 643–644

Respiratory irregularities, dysrhythmias
  sleep-related, 352
    see also Sleep apnea
  in multiple system atrophy, 563, 638–639, 639–641, 639f, 640f
  respiratory function studies, 643–644
  respiratory monitoring, 352
Respiratory-mediated heart rate variability, *see* Heart rate responses, to deep breathing
Respiratory neurons, autonomic (medullary), 636
Respiratory oscillations
  and electroencephalogram, 357
  in heart rate and blood pressure, 325, 353
    frequencies, 325, 326f, 327
  in RR interval (RRI), 325
    see also Respiratory sinus arrhythmia
    changes during development, 325, 327
    effects of aging, 332f
    effects of tilt-up, 334
    technical aspects, 345
    in young adults, 326f, 327–328, 327f, 328f, 328f
Respiratory power, in children vs. adults, 327
Respiratory pump, and venous return, 75
Respiratory rate, and heart rate range, 394–395
Respiratory (forced) sinus arrhythmia, 299–301
  see also Heart rate variability; Heart rate responses, to deep breathing; Respiratory oscillations, in RR interval
  definition, 299
  effects of aging, 163, 164
  factors affecting, 301, 396
  transfer function analysis, in diabetes, 337
Respiratory variations
  in blood pressure and heart rate, 310, 317
  in heart period, 299, 299f
Resting heart rate, effects of aging, 162, 162f
Resting skin temperature, measurement, 196–197
Resting sweat activity (RSA), 185
Resting sweat index, in reflex sympathetic dystrophy, 197t
Resting sweat output (RSO)
  in complex regional pain syndromes, 212–213, 213f
  measurement, 196
  normative data, 193, 193t
Retarded ejaculation, 806
Reticular activating (arousal) system, 636
Reticular formation
  and respiration, 20
  and urinary bladder innervation, 120
Reticulospinal tracts
  and respiration, 636
  and urinary bladder innervation, 120
Retrograde ejaculation, 132, 271, 501, 806
Reverse Shapiro's syndrome, 753
Rexed lamination of spinal cord, 26f, 27n
Rheumatoid arthritis, 479
  and lymphocyte β–adrenergic receptors, 154
  animal model, sympathetic ablation, 152
Rhythmic (dynamic) exercise, 66–67, 67f, 68f
Rhythms, *see also* Circadian rhythms; Cardiovascular oscillations; Slow oscillations; Vasomotor rhythms; Nonrespiratory oscillations; Respiratory oscillations
  in blood pressure and heart rate, 309–312, 310f, 311f
  in fetus, 325
  electroencephalographic, 339, 354f, 355, 355f, 355t
  in sweat expulsion, 92
Rigiscan method, 273
Riley-Day syndrome (familial dysautonomia), 478, 525–535
  autonomic dysfunction, 526t, 532–534
  cardiovascular manifestations, 526t, 527, 533
  catechol levels, 530, 531f
  central defects, 528, 529, 529f, 530
  clinical manifestations, 526–527, 526t, 530–534
  diagnostic criteria, 526–527
  DOPA:DHPG ratios, 530, 532f
  "dysautonomic crisis," 534
  dysautonomic manifestations, 641
  emotional reactivity, 534
  ganglion defects, 528, 529, 529f
  gastrointestinal manifestations, 526t, 532
  genetics, 526
  histopathologic findings, 378–379
  management, 530–534
  nerve growth factor, 530
  neurochemical and pharmacologic abnormalities, 530, 531f, 532f
  neuropathology, 528–530, 529f
  ocular manifestations, 452, 526t, 533–534
  peripheral defects, 528, 530
  prognosis, 534
  renal problems, 526t, 533
  respiratory manifestations, 526t, 532–533, 641
  sensory manifestations, 526t, 530
  sleep apnea, 641
  small fiber neuropathy, 703
  spinal cord defects, 529–530, 529f
  substance P axons, 529
  sural nerve findings, 529, 529f
Rochester Diabetic Neuropathy Study, 501
Ross syndrome, 100f, 251, 473, 474, 720–721
RR counts, 300
RR interval (RRI), *see also* Heart rate *entries and under* Respiratory oscillations
  and amplitude modulation of electroencephalogram, 357
  data acquisition, technical aspects, 344
  in diabetic neuropathy, 501
  and exposure to low gravity, 430, 430f
  methods of evaluating, 344
  normal time series, 325f
  periodogram (global spectrum), 326f
  in postural orthostatic tachycardia syndrome (POTS), 333f
  response to head-up tilt, 334
    time–frequency analysis, 330, 330f
  spontaneous fluctuations, 311f
  in syncope, 334f
  time–frequency maps, 326f
  use in spectral analysis, 313f
  use in time domain measurements, 300
  in young adults, 326f, 327–328, 327f, 328f
Rubor, episodic, 11

S

Sacral anterior root stimulation, for constipation, 604
Sacral parasympathetic nerves, in sexual function, 131
Sacral reflex pathways, electrodiagnostic studies, 620–621
Salivary glands
  innervation, 263f, 265
  parasympathetic, 262f
  and sweating, 92
Salivary reflex, sensory afferents, 263f
Salivation test, procedure, 196
San Antonio Conference on Diabetic Neuropathy, 290–291
Satiety center, 86
Schirmer's test, 452
Schwann cells, 110, 519–520
Sciatic nerve, fluorescence microscopy, 371f
Screening tests
  autonomic reflex screen, 181, 182t, 292–293, 385
    and composite autonomic scoring scale (CASS), 191
    personnel requirements, 384
    use of Finapres technique, 292
  reflex sympathetic dystrophy (RSD) screen, 182t, 385
  sympathetic dysfunction screen, 181
  test batteries, 289, 292, 298, 385
    for clinical trials, 294
SDANN, SDNN, *see* Standard deviation *entries*
Sebaceous glands, 110, 111f
Secretion, *see* Stimulus–secretion coupling
Secretory coil, of sweat glands, 98f, 100, 101, 101f
  and Na-K-Cl cotransporter model of sweating, 104–105
Seizures, 422–423
  see also Pseudoseizures; Diencephalic seizures
  autonomic manifestations, 422–423; 792
  cardiovascular manifestations, 422–423
  cerebral autonomic sites, 5
  distinguishing from syncope, 659
  electroencephalographic monitoring, 352
  and neurogenic arrhythmias, 49
  respiratory manifestations, 423
  thermoregulatory responses, 423
Self-catheterization, 625
Semicircular canals, and parasympathetic nerve output, 437
Semihidrosis, 92
Seminal vesicles, 130
Sensory and autonomic neuropathies, *see also* Riley-Day syndrome
  chronic, of unknown cause, 608, 609f
Sensory neuronopathy, 477–478
Sensory neurons, of enteric nervous system, 140
Sensory neuropathies, vs. small fiber neuropathy, 699
Sensory pathways, descending modulation, 144f
Serotonin (5-HT), 591
  as neurotransmitter, 586
Serotonin syndrome, 5, 424
Set-point (operating point)
  of baroreceptors, 65
  for body temperature, 85, 86f, 102, 102f
    and changes in homeostasis, 103
    in fever, 752–753
    and sleep, 92
Sex, *see* Gender
Sexual dysfunction, *see also* Erectile dysfunction
  clinical evaluation, 9
  in diabetic neuropathy, 500–501
    treatment, 503
  in female, 278, 501
  in male, 269–275
    approach to diagnosis, 273–274
    categories, 269
    causes, 269–271, 270t
    electrophysiologic evaluation, 277–285
      indications, 284
    evaluation, 271–273
    management, 803–807
    neurologic causes, 278
    organic causes, 269
    psychogenic vs. organic, 269, 271, 278
      erotic stimulation testing, 273
      psychological testing, 273
    psychogenic vs. spinal cord disease, 281
    in temporal lobe disease, 278
Sexual function
  autonomic regulation, 129–134
  central nervous system components, 131–132
  hormonal control, 132
Sexual organs
  in female, 130, 133
  in male, 129–130
  innervation, 130–131, 131f
  neurotransmitters, 132–133
Sexual response cycle, 129
  in females, 133
  in males, 132–133
Shapiro's syndrome, 5, 102, 423, 756
  symptom pattern, 12

Shapiro's syndrome in reverse, 753
Shivering, 86, 87–89
   after spinal cord injury, 459
Short-term Fourier transform, 345
Shy-Drager syndrome, see also Multiple system atrophy; Striatonigral degeneration
   Consensus Panel definition, 556
   and gastrointestinal dysmotility, 607
   glial cytoplasmic inclusions, 567
   nomenclature problems, 578
   original description, 578
   prognosis, 564
   and sympathetic nerve activity, 239
   vs. amyotrophic lateral sclerosis, 563
   vs. olivopontocerebellar atrophy (OPCA), 641
Signal-averaged electrocardiography, in diagnosing syncope, 661–662, 661f
Signal complexity, and approximate entropy, 331
Signal stationarity, see Data stationarity
Signals, in Fourier analysis, 312
Silastic (sweat) imprint test, 185, 186t, 709
Simple (essential, benign central) anisocoria, vs. Horner's syndrome, 444–445, 446, 450
Single-photon-emission computed tomography (SPECT), 199–200
Single-potential analysis of cavernosus electrical activity (SPACE), 283
Single-teased-fiber studies, 374
Sinoatrial (SA) node dysfunction, and syncope, 655
Sinus arrhythmia, forced (respiratory), see Respiratory sinus arrhythmia
Sinus node dysfunction, and syncope
   electrophysiologic studies, 666
   therapeutic management, 673
Sinusoids (lacunae) of penis, 129, 130f
Sjögren's syndrome, 474, 477–478
   evaluation, 10
   immune findings, 478
   patterns of neuropathy, 477–478
   sural nerve biopsy, 478
   thermoregulatory sweat test, 253
   vasculitis, 478
Skeletal muscle, see Muscle
Skin, see also Cutaneous; Dermal; Epidermal; Electrodermal; Sympathetic nerve activity, of skin; Sympathetic skin responses
   blood flow
      abnormalities, in experimental autonomic neuropathy, 415
      measurements, 200, 709
         in complex regional pain syndromes, 212
         methods of testing, 397
         equipment used, 388
         problems in testing, 397
         in neuropathies, 398
      and skin sympathetic activity, 237
      and vasomotor asymmetry, 196
   clinical examination, 10
   dermatoepidermal basement membrane, 110, 111f
   dystrophic changes, 10
   electrical resistance, 237, 237f
   epidermis, 110, 111f
   galvanic (sympathetic, conductance) response, 98
   glycoproteins, 110
   innervation, 109–115
      general features, 110–114
      types of nerves, 109
   papillary dermis, 110, 111f, 112
   sympathetic neuroeffector transfer, 237
   temperature
      asymmetry, 196, 197t
      in complex regional pain syndromes, 212
      in Horner's syndrome, 445
      recording, 387, 388
      regulation, 89–90

      in thermoregulation, 93, 102–103, 102f
   and thermal afferents, 85
   thermal threshold testing, 282
   vascular innervation, 111f, 112, 113f
   vascular tone, mechanism, 814
   vasomotor abnormalities, in experimental neuropathy, 415
   visualization of structures, 110, 111f
Skin biopsy
   clinical utility, 114
   normal findings, 371–372
   in sensory neuropathies, 372
   in small fiber neuropathy, 708
Skin potentials, 221–231
   see also Electrodermal activity
   recordings, 186t, 397
Skin vasomotor (vasoconstrictor) reflexes
   and blood pressure photoplethysmography, 398, 398f
   in diabetic neuropathy, 497–498
   effects of aging, 171, 172t
   factors affecting, 397–398
   methods of study, 200
   test limitations, 288
Sleep, 637
   autonomic changes, 637–638
   control of breathing, 636–637
   and cytokines, 155
   proposed physiology, 637
   pupillary changes, 265
   respiratory changes, 638
   stages, 637
   and sweating, 92
Sleep apnea, 633–647
   see also Sleep-related breathing disorders
   in acquired dysautonomia, 641–642
   in autonomic failure, 638–645
      diagnosis, 643–644
      laboratory assessment, 643–644
      treatment, 644–645
         goals, 644
   in autonomic neuropathies, 642
   central, 638, 639f
   dire consequences, 643
   during normal sleep, 638
   from medullary lesions, 425
   mixed, 638–639, 639f
   in multiple system atrophy, 638–641
   obstructive (primary) sleep apnea syndrome (OSAS), 642–643
      continuous positive airway pressure therapy, 644
      surgical therapy, 644–645
   in olivopontocerebellar atrophy, 641
   in Riley-Day syndrome, 641
   spectral analysis, 320–321
   and sympathetic nerve activity, 239, 241
   symptoms, 352
   types, 638
   upper-airway obstructive, 638, 639f
Sleep latency, 643
Sleep-related abnormalities, in multiple system atrophy, 563
Sleep-related breathing disorders (sleep-disordered breathing)
   see also Sleep apnea
   clinical manifestations, 643
   and hypertension, 352
   hypopnea, 639
   laboratory assessment, 643–644
   in multiple system atrophy, 563, 638–639, 639–641, 639f, 640f
   related conditions, 352
   respiratory monitoring, 352
Sleep-wake cycle
   see also Circadian rhythm
   and autonomic function, 20–21

Sleepiness, in daytime, 643
Slow amplitude modulation, 336, 339, 353, 353f, 354f, 355f
   centers involved, 359f
   during tilt-up, 356f
   orthostatic effects, 336
Slow oscillations (non-RFs; non-RF rhythms), see also Vasomotor rhythms; Nonrespiratory oscillations
   in heart rate and blood pressure, 325, 353
   effects of aging, 331, 332f
   effects of pacemaker, 330–331, 331f
   factors affecting, 328–331
   generating factors, 328–331
   structures involved, 353
Slow-wave sleep, see Non-REM sleep
Small-cell lung cancer
   and gastrointestinal dysmotility, 606f, 608
   and Lambert-Eaton myasthenic syndrome, 546
Small fiber neuropathy, 699–714
   see also Amyloid neuropathy; Distal small fiber neuropathy
   in amyloidosis, 701–702
   in cancer, 704–705
   causes, 490, 700–705, 700t
   choice of tests, 710
   clinical course, 707
   in diabetes, 490–491, 700–701
      subtypes, 701
   diagnostic approach, 710
   diagnostic tests, 707–710
   and erectile dysfunction, laboratory testing, 282
   idiopathic, 705–707
      and autoimmune disease, 707
      autonomic testing, 706–707
      symptoms, 705–706, 706t
      treatment, 706
   misconceptions, 699
   pathogenesis, 707
   peripheral nerve tests, 707–710
   skin biopsy, 708
   and sympathetic skin response, 227
   thermoregulatory sweat test, 254, 255f
   toxic causes, 704
   treatment, 710–711
   vs. sensory neuropathy, 699
   working definition, 700
Small intensely fluorescent (SIF) cells, 34
Smoking, and male sexual dysfunction, 271
Smooth muscle, see also Muscle
   gastrointestinal, 135, 141–142
      electrical properties, 141, 597
Smooth muscle electromyography, of penis, 283, 283f
Smoothing, in spectral analysis, 344, 345
Sodium chloride, reabsorption by sweat gland duct, 106, 107f
Sodium intake, high-salt (high-sodium) foods, 693
Sodium pump, and sweat gland activity, 104, 105f, 106
Soles, see also Feet
   sweat glands, 98
   sweating, 91
      expulsion rhythm, 92
Somatic (mixed) blocks, use in pain syndromes, 216–217
Somatostatin, 30f, 31, 495
   and postprandial orthostatic hypotension, 168, 739
Spaceflight, see also Gravity, prolonged reduction
   motion sickness, 437
   and study of autonomic dysfunction, 429
Spastic miosis, 442–443, 442t
Spectral analysis, see also Frequency analysis; Time–frequency analysis
   artifacts, 344
   of cardiovascular parameters, technical guidelines, 343–347
   clinical uses, 293, 320, 332–345

Spectral analysis *(contd.)*
   coherence, 316–317, 316f
   delta functions (spikes), 313f
   in diabetic autonomic neuropathy, 493–494
   minimum guidelines for adequate studies, 344–345
   notation used, 317f
   phase, 316–317, 316f
   technical aspects, 309–317, 344–345, 345–347
   techniques, 312–317
      for blood pressure variability, 315–317
      for heart rate variability, 312–315
      for spectrum estimation, 312–315
   of two signals, 315–317, 316f
   zero padding, 314
Spectral envelope, in transcranial Doppler monitoring, 351
Spectral power, 337
Spectrum, *see also* Fourier spectrum
   definition, 312
Spectrum estimation
   autoregressive method, 314–315, 316f
   fast Fourier transform, 313–314
Sphenopalatine (pterygopalatine) ganglion, 37f, 38, 262, 264
Sphincter electromyography, 281, 563, 619
Sphincteric muscle, in gut, 141
Sphincterotomy, urinary, 628
Spikes (delta functions), in spectral analysis, 313f
Spinal cord
   afferent pathways, 19
   autonomic components, 25–29, 26f
      descending fibers, 25
         distribution, 27
      intermediolateral and intermediomedial cell columns, 25–27, 26f, 28–29
      neurotransmitters, 29
   lateral horn cells, and autonomic failure, 578
   nerve fiber tracts, 26f
   neurokinins, 30–31
   neuropeptides, 29, 30f
   pathways in urinary bladder control, 120
   Rexed lamination (laminar architecture), 26f, 27n
   sympathetic neurons, age-related attrition, 169–170, 170f
   tachykinins, 30–31
   and thermal afferents, 84–85
   thoracolumbar, innervation of detrusor and urethra, 121–122
Spinal cord disorders, 4t, 5, 425–427
   in AIDS, 732
   changes in Riley-Day syndrome, 529–530, 529f
   and erectile dysfunction, 281
   lesions
      autonomic dysreflexia, 780
      causing sexual dysfunction, 270, 278
      gastrointestinal dysmotility, 604, 605, 607
      and hyperthermia, 753
      and hypothermia, 756
      spectral analysis, 342–343
      thermoregulatory sweat test, 251, 251f, 252
   neuropathology
      and autonomic failure, 578
      in multiple system atrophy, 566
      in pure autonomic failure, 566
   nontraumatic injury, major causes, 456
   transection
      and hypotension, 55
      and sympathetic nerve activity, 239
   traumatic injury, 425–426, 455–461
      blood pressure consequences, 456
      cardiovascular consequences, 456
      and cerebral blood flow autoregulation, 456
      disruption of autonomic pathways, 456
      effects of postural change, 456
      ejaculation, 460, 806

evaluation principles, 456
in females, 460
and hyperhidrosis, 810
immediate consequences, 456
major causes, 455
mortality rates, 456
penile engorgement, 456, 460
sites, 455
sympathetic consequences, 456
sympathetic storm, 796
thermoregulatory consequences, 459
urogenital consequences, 459–460, 622–623, 806
and urinary tract dysfunction
   artificial sphincter, 628
   sphincterotomy, 628
   from trauma, 459–460, 622–623
   from tumors, 623
Spinal (reflexogenic) erection, 132
Spinal shock, 456
   urinary bladder dysfunction, 622
Spinobulbospinal pathway, in micturition, 120, 122
Spinoreticular tract, visceral afferents, 144
Spinothalamic tract, visceral afferents, 144
   and pain, 143f, 144
Spinovascular disease, 623
Splanchnic blood flow, and postprandial hypotension, 738, 744
Splanchnic capacitance vessels, and circulatory homeostasis, 63
Splanchnic-mesenteric bed, evaluation, 203, 494
Splanchnic nerves, 36, 377
Splanchnic outflow
   morphometric studies, 374–375
   neuron and axon counts, 378t
Splanchnic resistance vessels, effects of head-up tilt, 79
Spleen
   norepinephrine levels, 149–150
      and cytokines, 155
      effects of 6-hydroxycatecholamine dopamine, 151
   and sympathetic nervous system, 149
   T-cell and B-cell numbers, effects of sympathectomy, 153
Sports physiology, and thermoregulation, 97
Standard deviation of average RR intervals (SDANN), 300
Standard deviation of normal-to-normal RR intervals (SDNN), 300
Standard deviation of the mean RR interval, 300
Standard deviation of the RR intervals, 300
Standard deviation of the successive differences (SDSD), 300
Standing time, 766
   in orthostatic intolerance, 8, 8t
Standing up, *see also* Upright posture; Postural normotension; Orthostatic stress; Orthostatic 30:15 ratio; Head-up tilt
   cardiovascular effects, 74, 188, 396f
   and autonomic function tests, 395–396
   after exposure to low gravity, 430
   effects on blood volume, 61–62, 64f, 73, 74f, 75, 77
   and exposure to low gravity, 432
   initial circulatory response, 79–80, 80f
   physiologic effects, 64f, 75, 77, 303, 764
   vs. passive head-up tilt, circulatory responses, 77, 77f
Static (isometric) exercise, 66–67, 67f
   and ergoreceptors, 70
Stellate ganglion, *see* Cervicothoracic ganglion
Stereotactic pallidotomy, in multiple system atrophy, 772
Steroids, use in pain syndromes, 217
Stiff-man syndrome, 426–427, 517
Stimulus–secretion coupling, 104
   in eccrine sweat secretion, 104
Stokes-Adams attacks, 655

electrophysiologic studies, 667
Stomach
   delayed emptying, 598–599
      scintigraphic study, 606f
   extrinsic neural control, 137t
   vagal innervation, 42
Street drugs
   causing dysautonomia, 6
   and male sexual dysfunction, 271
   overdose, autonomic consequences, 798
Stress, *see also* Orthostatic stress; Mental stress
   central autonomic responses, 21–22
   effects on heart, 50
   effects on immune function, 153
   effects on muscle sympathetic activity, 236
Stress response, 21–22
   central circuits, 21f
Stress urinary incontinence, 614, 626
Striatonigral degeneration, 558, 581
   see also Multiple system atrophy; Shy-Drager syndrome
   Consensus Panel definition, 556
   nomeclature problems, 578
   two kinds, 578–579
   vs. Parkinson's disease, 558
Stroke, *see also* Hemorrhage, intracerebral
   in brainstem region, 425
   in frontal cortex, 422
   hypertension, 795–796
   swallowing problems, 605
   urinary bladder dysfunction, 621
Subacute combined degeneration, 480
Subacute proximal diabetic motor neuropathy, 492
Subacute sensory neuronopathy, 550–551
Subarachnoid hemorrhage
   and cardiac arrhythmias, 48
   complications from sympathoexcitation, 424
   and ECG changes, 51, 52f
   sympathetic storm, 793–794
Subepidermal plexus, 110, 111f
   in diabetes, 114
Submandibular ganglion, 37f, 38
Submental syndrome, 720
Submucosa, gastrointestinal, 135
Submucosal (Meissner's, submucous) plexus, 136, 138f, 139–140
Substance K (neurokinin A), 30–31
Substance P, 29–31, 30f
   and immune system, 150, 156
   in Riley-Day syndrome, 529
Substance P immunoreactive nerves, 112
Sudden death
   and cardiac arrhythmias, 49, 50, 655, 656
   in Guillain–Barré syndrome, 778, 778f
   and seizures, 423
   and stress, 50
   in stroke, 423
   and syncope, 655, 656, 657, 658f
Sudden infant death syndrome, 49
Sudomotor drive, 92–93
Sudomotor dysfunction, and sympathetic skin response, 228, 229
Sudomotor function, *see also* Sweat entries
   and aging, 168–169
   clinical examination, 10
   eliciting symptoms, 9
Sudomotor function tests, *see also specific tests*
   comparison, 185–186, 185t, 186t, 709
   in complex regional pain syndromes, 212
   concordance among tests, 393, 399
   in diabetic neuropathy, 496
   factors affecting, 399
   recommended tests, 291
   in small fiber neuropathy, 708–709
   sweat capsules, sweat cells (equipment), 387, 387f

multicompartmental, 182–183
commercial sources, 389
Sudomotor nerves, 111f, 112
Sudomotor pathway, 90
Sudomotor system, 810–813
Sudorometry
   equipment, 182, 183f, 387, 387f
      commercial sources, 389
   personnel requirements, 384
Summation, 211
Superior cervical ganglion, 34, 39f, 263–264
Superior mesenteric flow, measurement, 203
Superior vagal (jugular) ganglion, 40
Supine blood pressure, and orthostatic hypotension in elderly, 168
Supine hypertension
   in multiple system atrophy, 557
   from octreotide, 744
   in pure autonomic failure, 557
Supine hypotension, treatment, 772
Suppressor T cells, 148
Suprahisian block, 655
Supranuclear palsy, 605
Supraspinal, *see* Central nervous system
Sural nerve
   compound action potential, 372f, 373
   dopamine–bhydroxylase content, 373, 373t
   in Riley-Day syndrome, 529, 529f
Sural nerve biopsy
   in autonomic neuropathies, 372–374, 377
   complications, 373–374
   in diabetic neuropathy, 376, 376f
   enzyme content, 373t
   indications, 373–374
   unmyelinated fiber findings, 373, 374f
Surgical procedures, and sympathetic activity, 241
Surgical sympathectomy, use in pain syndromes, 217
Swallowing, extrinsic neural control, 137t
Swallowing syncope, 654
Sweat capsules, sweat cells (equipment), 387, 387f
   multicompartmental, 182–183
   commercial sources, 389
Sweat center, 102–103
Sweat gland dysfunction, 97–108
   see also Hyperhidrosis; Hypohidrosis; Anhidrosis
   atrophy, 100, 100f
   and heat intolerance, 749
Sweat glands, 111f
   see also Sudomotor *entries*
   acrosyringium, 106
   adaptation, 93
   in apes, 98, 98f
   apocrine (epitrichial) vs. eccrine (atrichial), 91
   apocrinelike (trichial, hair-associated), 98f
   apoeccrine, 100
   basal cell, 101f, 102
   clear cell, 101, 101f, 102f
      and Na-K-Cl cotransporter, 104–105, 105f
      and cyclic AMP, 103, 104
      and cyclic GMP, 104
   dark cell, 101, 101f
   in diabetes, 114
   distribution and density, 91
   duct, 98f, 100, 101f, 102, 106, 112, 113f
      and ion transport, 106
   eccrine, 91, 97–99, 98f
      anatomy, 100–102, 101f
      pharmacologic responsiveness, 103–104
      stimulus–secretion coupling, 104
      and thermoregulation, 98–99
   effects of aging, 168, 169t, 248
   and thermoregulatory sweat test, 254
   and electrodermal activity, 222–223
   excision, 812–813
   innervation, 91, 112

on face, 90
location, 110, 111f
luminal cell, 101f, 102
myoepithelial cell, 101–102, 102f
nerve fibers, 372
normal and abnormal function, 97–108
of palms and soles, 98
periglandular nerves, 103
periglandular neurotransmitters, 100, 103
regulators, 100
regulatory peptides, 100, 103
secretory coil, 98f, 100, 101, 101f
   and Na-K–Cl cotransporter model of sweating, 104–105
secretory tubule, 110, 111f, 112
size, 100–101
   relation to sweat rate, 100
Sweat (Silastic) imprint test, 185, 185t, 186t
Sweat-inhibitory efferents, 90
Sweat loss, *see* Anhidrosis
Sweat rate, 88f, 92, 101
   factors affecting, 92–93
   and local temperature, 103, 103f
   relation to gland size, 100
   and temperature set-point, 102, 102f
   as test of sweat gland activity, 104
Sweat response
   in elderly, 248
      and thermoregulatory sweat test, 169, 246, 254
   normal distribution patterns, 247f, 248, 249
   pathways, 245, 246f
Sweat retention syndrome, 100
Sweat-spot test, 185–186, 185t
Sweat tests, *see* Sudomotor function tests *and specific tests*
Sweating, *see also* Hyperhidrosis; Hypohidrosis; Anhidrosis; *and* Sudomotor *entries*
   adrenergic stimulation, 103, 104
   autonomic regulation, 83–93
   axillary, 91, 811
   and brainstem lesions, 90
   central and peripheral control, 102–103
   cholinergic stimulation, 103, 104
      and Na-K-Cl cotransporter model, 104–105, 105f
   clinical examination, 10
   cold sweat, physiologic basis, 237
   and core temperature, 102–103
   and cyclic AMP, 103, 104
   and cyclic GMP, 104
   and dehydration, 87, 92
   effects of gender and age, 93
   effects of posture, 92
   effects of pressure, 92
   emotive, and electrodermal activity, 223
   and evaporation, 90
   expulsion rhythm, 92
   facial, 715–726
      and cluster headache, 722–724, 723f
      sympathetic control, 716–717
   factors affecting, 88f, 92–93, 399
   in Guillain–Barré syndrome, 785f, 786
   gustatory, 91–92, 719–720, 813
      autonomic pathways, 719f
   and membrane transport, 104–105
   mental, 91
   Na-K-Cl cotransporter model, 104–105, 105f
   palmar and plantar, 91
   recruitment patterns, 92
   stress-induced, 91, 92
   in stroke, 423
   thermoregulatory (thermal, eccrine), 91, 92, 97
      and electrodermal activity, 223
      in multiple sclerosis, 426
      pathways, 245, 246f
      and sports physiology, 97

testing for, 99–100, 99f
and vasoactive peptides, 93
and vasodilation, 89
volume, *see* Sweat rate
Sympathectomy
   experimental, 412–414
      complement-dependent, 413–414
      guanethidine-induced, 412–413
      6-hydroxydopamine-induced, 412
      induced by acetylcholinesterase antibodies, 413–414, 414f
      induced by nerve growth factor antibodies, 413
   Telford's operation, 36
   use in hyperhidrosis, 812–813
Sympathetic blockade
   effects on heart rate variability, 297–298, 298f
   by peri- and intradural anesthesia, 241
   use in pain syndromes, 215–216
Sympathetic disorders, *see also* Reflex sympathetic dystrophy; Pain, sympathetically maintained
   acral, 809–818
   autonomic function test results, 611t
   combined sympathetic-parasympathetic failure, *see under* Autonomic failure
   denervation supersensitivity, 717–718
   distal sympathetic failure, 11
   distinguishing central vs. peripheral lesions, 586–587
   by melatonin secretion, 594
   Horner's syndrome, 444–447
   neuropathies, *see also specific neuropathies*
      biochemical and neurophysiologic markers, 492
      distal sympathetic, 11, 472–473
      symptom patterns, 11
   overactivity, *see also* Autonomic overactivity
      distal, 11
      in Guillain–Barré syndrome, 780–781, 781f, 782f, 784–786
      measuring blood pressure, 799
      pathophysiology, 780–786
      in sleep apnea, 352
      in tetanus, 784
      and cardiac excitability, 48
      and exposure to low gravity, 430–431
      and pupillary function, 265
   sympathetic irritation (oculosympathetic spasm), 447, 447t
   sympathetic storm
      from cerebral lesions, mechanisms, 791–796
      from spinal cord lesions, 796
      from subarachnoid hemorrhage, 793–794
      from sympathoadrenal discharge, 791–792
Sympathetic dysfunction screen, 181, 385
Sympathetic function tests
   in AIDS, 728f, 729, 729t
   problems, 395
   screening tests, 181, 385
   suitable tests, 290, 291
   in Lambert-Eaton myasthenic syndrome, 547t
Sympathetic ganglia, 27, 27f, 28f, 34–36, 35f
   autoantibodies
      and diabetes, 512, 513f
      and Parkinson's disease, 517
      and postural blood pressure changes, 514–515, 515f
   cervical, 34–36
   prevertebral, and gastrointestinal motility, 138–139
Sympathetic ganglionectomy
   induced by nerve growth factor antibodies, 413
   and thermoregulatory sweat test, 254, 255f
Sympathetic nerve activity, 234–237
   see also Microneurography
   during anesthesia, 241
   bursting patterns, 234, 235, 236
   in central autonomic network, and electroencephalographic rhythms, 339

Sympathetic nerve activity (contd.)
  in central dysautonomia, 239
  after closed head injury, 342
  effect of Valsalva maneuver, 234f
  and exposure to low gravity, 430–431, 438f
  hormonal influences, 237–238
  and low-frequency oscillations, 328–331
  of muscle, 235–236
    and blood pressure, 235, 238
    burst incidence, 235
    cardiac and respiratory rhythmicity, 235
    conduction velocity, 235
    in Guillain-Barré syndrome, 238
    and neurotransmitter release, 236
    reflex regulation, 235–236
  in pain, 236, 241
  in pathologic conditions, 238–241
  in polyneuropathies, 238
  recording methods, 233–234
  of skin, 236–237
    cardiac rhythmicity, 237
    conduction velocity, 236
    effects of ambient and body temperatures, 236
    effects of sleep, 236
    reflex regulation, 236–237
    vasomotor and sudomotor components, 236
  in sleep apnea, 239, 241
  in spinal cord transection, 239
  in syncope, 239
Sympathetic neurons
  adrenergic, 370, 370t
  innervation of eye, 263–264, 264f
  innervation of face, 715–716, 716f
  innervation of lymphoid organs, 149–150
  origin, 27
  postganglionic, 35f, 809–810
    conduction velocity, 810
    edrophonium testing, 610f
  preganglionic, 19, 27, 27f, 33f, 35f, 809
    age-related attrition, 169–170, 170f, 375
    medullary modulation, 20
    selective destruction
      induced by acetylcholinesterase antibodies, 413
      and QSART results, 184–185, 185t
  in thermoregulation, 90
Sympathetic nervous system
  ablation, effects on immune system, 151–153
  acral functions, 809
  and ECG changes, 52–53
  effects of aging, 169–173
  effects of cytokines, 154–156
  effects of eating, 740–741
  and fever, 155
  in heart failure, 240f, 241
  and heart rate variability, 318
  in hypertension, 239, 241
  and gastrointestinal motility, 137t, 598, 601f
  interactions with immune system, 149–156
    in human disease, 153–156
  and iris pigmentation, 445
  and myocardial damage, 53
  neural prosthesis, 570
  in pain, mechanisms, 210t, 538
  in postprandial hypotension, 740–741, 743–744
  in Riley-Day syndrome, 528
  in sexual function, 131
  sympathetic-parasympathetic vagal network, 40
  and T-cell and epithelial adhesion molecules, 149
  and urinary bladder function, 122
  vs. parasympathetic nervous system, 29f, 37–38
Sympathetic outflow
  during exercise, and ergoreceptors, 69–70
  functional organization, 234–235
  peripheral, effects of pulmonary vagal afferents, 63–64

vasomotor
  activators, and blood pressure variability, 318
  and apnea, 352
Sympathetic ratio, 304
Sympathetic skin responses (SSR), 98, 221–231, 225f
  see also Electrodermal activity
  and central nervous system disease, 229
  central organization, 226–227
  clinical utility, 227–229
  comparison with thermoregulatory sweat test, 225f, 228
  criteria of abnormality, 227
  electrophysiologic properties, 225–226
  in erectile dysfunction, 282–283, 282f
  as index of sympathetic sudomotor dysfunction, 228
  penile, in small fiber neuropathy, 708
  and peripheral neuropathies, 227–229
Sympathetic skin response test, 709
Sympathetic tone, 234
Sympathetically independent pain (SIP), 538, 542
Sympathetically maintained pain (SMP), 11, 538, 541–542
  see also Reflex sympathetic dystrophy
  laboratory evaluation, 181, 196–198
  patient preparation, 196
Sympathoadrenal discharge, 791–792
  after subarachnoid hemorrhage, 793–794
Sympathoexcitation, indicators, 339
Sympathoexcitatory cold pressor test, 236
  interpretation problems, 395
Sympatholytic agents, 448
Sympathomimetic agents, 448
  effects on eye, 448
  for treating orthostatic hypotension, 769t, 770
  for treating urinary bladder dysfunction, 626
Sympathovagal balance
  conventional tests vs. spectral analysis, 336–337
  spectral analysis, 320
Sympathovagal index, 688
Synaptotagmin, and calcium channels, 549
Synchronization, and electroencephalogram, 358, 359f
Synchronized sleep, see Non-REM sleep
Syncope, 62, 649–679
  cardiac receptors, 651
  cardiogenic, 654–656
    arrhythmia-induced, 655–656
    electrophysiologic studies, 664–672
    therapeutic management, 673
  cardiovascular, 650–654
  cardiovascular responses, 334
    time–frequency analysis, 334f
  cerebrovascular changes, 366–367
  course and prognosis, 657–658, 658f, 658t
  diagnostic algorithm, 665f
  diagnostic evaluation, 180, 659–672
    electrocardiography, 660–662
      signal-averaged, 661–662, 661f
    electrophysiologic studies, 664–672
      AV conduction, 667–670
      choice of patients, 664–666, 665f
      His bundle electrogram, 667, 667f
      sinus node dysfunction, 666–667, 666f
      supraventricular tachycardia, 670–672, 671f
      test components, 666
      ventricular tachycardia, 672, 672f
    exercise testing, 662
    history, 659
    physical examination, 659–660
    tilt-table testing, 662–664, 663f
  distinguishing from seizures, 659
    electroencephalographic monitoring, 352
  during seizures, 422
  electroencephalographic changes, 367, 367f
  electroencephalography, 335f, 336, 356f, 357
  episodic syndromes, 12

etiology, 650–656, 650t
  cardiogenic, 654–656
  cardiovascular, 650–654
  metabolic causes, 656
  neurologic causes, 656
  noncardiovascular causes, 656
  psychogenic causes, 656
  relative frequencies, 656–657, 657t
exercise-induced, 654
exertional, in heart disease, 654, 655
heat-induced, 749
impending, 334f, 336
near syncope, 670, 671f
pathophysiology, 650–656
postprandial, 741
premonitory signs, 191
presyncope, electroencephalography, 356f, 357
reflex, 650–654, 651f
  types, 650t
in response to tilt-up, 191
  and isoproterenol infusion test, 202, 663f, 664
situational, 654
causes, 650t
and sudden death, 655, 656, 657, 658f
suggested pathophysiology, 336
and sympathetic nerve activity, 238–239
therapeutic management, 672–673
unexplained
  course and prognosis, 657–658
  diagnostic difficulties, 656
  likely causes, 658
  risk stratification, 658t
and upright posture, 64, 75, 77
vasodepressor, 651–652, 652f
  autonomic mechanism, 366
  electroencephalography, 366f, 367
  hypoperfusion, 360
  neurophysiologic mechanisms, 662, 664
  therapeutic management, 673
  tilt-up reaction, 662–664, 663f
  vs. bradycardiac syncope, 662
vasomotor rhythms, 334
vasovagal, 650–652
  neurophysiologic mechanisms, 650–652, 651f, 654
  premonitory signs, 659
  and respiration, 64, 75
  and sympathetic nerve activity, 238–239
  therapeutic management, 672–673
  tilt-up reaction, 662–664, 663f
  triggers, 650
Syndrome of episodic hyperhidrosis with hypothermia, 423
Syndromes, see also specific syndromes
  pattern recognition, 6, 7, 11–12
Syntaxin, and calcium channels, 549
Syphilis, Argyll Robertson pupils, 441–442
Syringobulbia, 425
Syringomyelia, 426
System failure, selective, 12
Systemic lupus erythematosus, 153, 479
Systemic sclerosis, manometry, 600f
Systemic sympatholytic procedures, use in pain syndromes, 216
Systolic pressure, see Blood pressure

T

T cells, see also Lymphocytes
  activated, 149
  in diabetes, 511
  antigen recognition, 148
  CD4:CD8 ratio in spleen, effects of sympathectomy, 153
  CD4-positive, 148
    and sympathetic nervous system, 152
  CD8-positive, 148

clonal expansion, 148
cytotoxic type, 148
effects of sympathetic ablation, 151–152
proliferation, 149
and β-adrenergic agonists, 150–151
receptors for antigens, 148
suppressor type, 148
surface marker proteins, 147, 148
T helper type 2 (Th2) cells, 148
Th1 cells, 149
Tachycardia
with hypertension, 781f, 782f, 785f
supraventricular
and near syncope, 670, 671f
and syncope, 655, 670–672
therapeutic management, 673
Tachycardia latency, 302
Tachycardia ratio, 302
Tachykinins, see also Substance P
of spinal cord, 30–31
Taeniae coli, 135
Tangier disease
associated neuropathies, 703
histopathologic findings, 377
intermediolateral column neurons, 375f
Taste, sensory afferents, 264–265
Taste receptors, and lacrimation, 451
Tear osmolarity test, 452
Tear production, tear secretion, see also Lacrimation
central abnormalities, 451
decreased, 451, 452
effects of medications, 452
peripheral abnormalities, 451
quantitation, 452
Tears, crocodile, (gustolacrimal reflex), 451
Telencephalon, disorders, 422–423
Telethermography
in complex regional pain syndromes, 212
equipment, 388
laboratory requirements, 384
for measuring resting skin temperature, 196–197, 197f
vs. thermometry, 198
Telford's sympathectomy operation, 36
Temperature, see also Heat; Cold; Shivering; and Thermal entries
ambient
in autonomic laboratory, 384, 387
and electrodermal activity, 223, 224f
and number of sweat glands, 91
and thermoregulation, 86, 89, 90, 102–103, 103f
of body, see also Thermoregulation; Thermal entries; Sweating; Hypothermia; Hyperthermia
"after-drop," 756
autonomic regulation, 83–93
central blood temperature, 246
clinical examination, 9–10
core temperature, 102–103
and exercise, 86
factors affecting, 86–87
and feeding behavior, 86, 87
heat exchange with environment, 87
maximal tolerated, 747
and menstrual cycle, 85, 93
methods of lowering, 751
methods of rewarming, 755–756
of skin
in Horner's syndrome, 445
recording, 387, 388
regulation, 89–90
in thermoregulation, 93, 102–103, 102f
Temperature (thermal) threshold testing, 709
Temporal lobe disorders, and sexual dysfunction, 278
Testes, 130

Tests, see Laboratory evaluation; Autonomic function tests; Screening tests
Tetanus, 425, 426, 779
management, 787, 797
sympathetic overactivity, pathophysiologic mechanisms, 784
Tetraplegia
blood pressure, 425, 456
from lesions above T5, 425–426
Th1, Th2 cells, see under T cells
Thalamic nuclei
and urinary bladder innervation, 119
visceral afferents, 144
and pain, 143f, 144
Thalamic spindles, 358
Thallium-induced neuropathy, 472, 779
Thermal afferents, 84–85, 85f
central integration, 85–87
Thermal sensitivity testing, in erectile dysfunction, 282
Thermal (thermoregulatory) sweating, see under Sweating
Thermal threshold testing, 709
Thermogenesis
by shivering, 87–89
after spinal cord injury, 459
nonshivering mechanisms (NST), 89
Thermography, see Telethermography
Thermometry, 196, 197f
vs. telethermography, 198
Thermoreceptors, 84–85, 85f
Thermoregulation, see also Sweating
and aging, 168–169
and autonomic function, 20–21
central and peripheral control, 102–103
central mechanisms, 85–87
hypothalamic–higher brain connections, 86
nonthermal factors, 86
regulatory factors, 86–87
and eccrine sweat glands, 98–99
effector mechanisms, 87–90
efferent autonomic pathways, 90
and fluid balance, 87
in neonates, 89
neurotransmitters and neuropeptides, 87
nonthermal modifiers, 92–93
peripheral modifiers, 93
and preoptic hypothalamic area, 102
in seizures, 423
set-point for body temperature, 85, 86f, 102, 102f
and changes in homeostasis, 103
and fever, 752–753
and sleep, 92
after spinal cord injury, 459
and sports physiology, 97
thermal afferents, 84–85
thermoreceptors, 84–85, 85f
vasomotor response, 89–90
Thermoregulatory disorders, and hypothalamus, 423
Thermoregulatory sweat test (TST), 99–100, 99f, 186t, 245–257
clinical uses, 249–250
comparison with sympathetic skin response, 225f, 228
in dermatologic disorders, 254
in elderly, 169, 246, 254
end point, 246
in functional gastrointestinal disorders, 609f
indications, 293
interpretation problems, 254–255
in multiple system atrophy, 342f
normal data, 246, 247f
patient preparation, 254
in peripheral disorders, 252
potential risks, 204
reporting results, 249
in secondary autonomic disorders, 251–254

sweat distribution patterns, 247f, 248–249
normal, 247f, 249
in specific autonomic disorders, 250–254
technique, 246–248
testing conditions, 246
unwanted effects, 247, 254, 256
and cord lesions, 251, 252
use with QSART, 184–185, 185t
Thermoregulatory sweating, see under Sweating
Thermoregulatory system, 84f
Thermosensitive neurons, 84, 85, 86f
30:15 ratio, 188, 303
effects of aging, 164, 166, 166f
and erectile dysfunction, 282
limitations, 289, 395
Thoracic bioimpedance, 202
Thoracic hyperhidrosis, 810
Thoracic outlet syndrome, 815
Thoracic paravertebral ganglia, 36
Thoracolumbar outflow, 27
Thoracolumbar sympathetic nerves, in sexual function, 131
Threatening stimuli, responses, 209
Three-phase bone scan, 214
Thymus, and sympathetic nervous system, 149
Thyroid function, and sympathetic nerve activity, 238
Thyrotoxicosis, and sweating, 811
Thyrotropin-releasing hormone (TRH), 30f, 31
and sweating, 88f
in thermoregulation, 87
Tibial evoked potentials, 279f, 280f, 281
Tightly synchronized spontaneous electrodermal activity, 223, 223f, 224f
Tilt-up, see Head-up tilt
Time and frequency smoothing, 345
Time constant, in cardiovascular homeostasis, 73
Time domain
methods of interpretation, 344
in transcranial Doppler monitoring, 351
Time domain measures of heart rate, mathematical measurements, 300–301
Time domain measures of heart rate variability, 297–307
list of tests, 298t
Time–frequency analysis, see also Spectral analysis; Frequency analysis; Wigner distribution
of cardiovascular function, 323–348
technical guidelines, 343–347
of electroencephalographic data, 357
new techniques, 345
sympathoexcitation indicators, 339
technical aspects, 345–357
in transcranial Doppler monitoring, 351
what it does, 324
Time–frequency distributions, see also Time-frequency maps
concept, 345–357
contour map, 330f
Time–frequency maps, 324, 324f
changes, in end-organ failure, 339, 340f
of respiration, 326f
of RR interval, 326f
Time of day, and dysautonomic symptoms, 7
Time-related analysis, 201
Time series, 324f
of electroencephalographic band powers, 354f
of respiration and RR intervals, 325f
Tissue damage
peripheral responses, 538
and sympathetic involvement in pain, 538
Toes, thermoregulation, 89
Tongue, in dysautonomia, 537f
Tonic pupil, 442t, 444, 474
in Holmes-Adie syndrome, 720
with chronic inflammatory demyelinating polyradiculoneuropathy, 474

Tonic sleep stage, 637
Torsades de pointes, 656
Total area under the curve, 312f
Total peripheral resistance, response to standing, 79
Total power spectral density, effects of aging, 166
Total variance, 312f
Tourney's phenomenon, 266
Toxic neuropathies, 6, 472, 704
Trabeculae of penis, 129
Training
  for autonomic clinical neurophysiologists, 294
  for autonomic laboratory technicians, 384
Transcapillary fluid shift, on standing up, 74
Transcranial Doppler (TCD) monitoring
  beat-to-beat analysis, 351
  blood flow velocity waveform, 350f
  clinical applications, 349
  effects of tilt-up, 362–367
  effects of Valsalva maneuver, 360–362, 360f
  in failed cerebral autoregulation, 362
  frequency domain, 351
  in impaired cerebral perfusion, 360
  insonation approaches, 350–351, 351f
  limitations, 360
  momentum statistics, 351
  in orthostatic intolerance, 349–368
    clinical applications, 359–362
  spectral envelope, 351
  technical aspects, 349–351
  time domain, 351
  time–frequency analysis, 351
  "ultrasound windows," 350
Transfer dysphagia, 598, 598t
  diagnostic evaluation, 599f
Transfer function analysis of respiratory sinus arrhythmia, 337
Transient ischemic attacks, 425, 795–796
Transmitters, see Neurotransmitters; Neuropeptides
Transthyretin, 375, 476
Traumatic vasospastic disease, 815
Trichial (apocrinelike, hair-associated) sweat glands, in apes, 98, 98f
Tricyclic antidepressants, see Antidepressants
Trigeminal nerve, in Horner's syndrome, 446
Trigeminal pathways, and diving reflex, 304–305
Trigone, anatomy, 124
Trinitroglycerin stress test, 200
TST%, 249
  in diabetic neuropathy, 252–253
Tumor necrosis factor α (TNF-α), and hypothalamus, 155
Tumors, see also Cancer and Paraneoplastic autonomic disorders
  of brain
    gastrointestinal dysmotility, 606, 606f
    urinary bladder dysfunction, 621
  of brainstem region, 425
  Pancoast (of apical lung), 252, 252f, 816
  of spinal cord, and urinary tract dysfunction, 623
  of temporal lobe, and seizures, 423
Tunica albuginea, 129, 130f
Tympanic plexus, 264, 265
Tyramine, blood pressure and heart rate response, 202

U

Ultrasound, see Transcranial Doppler
Uninhibited bladder, in stroke, 423
Unmyelinated fibers, see under Nerve fibers
Upper-airway obstructive apnea, 638, 639f
Upright posture, see also Standing up; Head-up tilt; Postural normotension; and Orthostatic entries
  circulatory effects, 61–62, 64f, 73, 74f
  and circulatory homeostasis, 61–66, 73–81
  early stabilization phase, 80
  effects on humoral system, 63, 81

hemodynamic changes, 78f, 80f
initial circulatory adjustment, 78f
loss of consciousness, electroencephalographic changes, 367, 367f
prolonged, circulatory adjustments, 80–81
and respiration, 64, 75
venous return, mechanical aids, 75
Urban elderly, hyperthermia, 747–748
Uremia, 479–480
Urethra
  anatomy, 124
  innervation
    cerebral, methods of study, 119
    of external sphincter, and reticular formation, 120
    sensory and motor, 124–125
    thoracolumbar spinal, 121–122
Urethral function tests, 615, 617–619, 618f, 619f
Urethral pressure profile, 618–619, 619f
Urethral surgery, 628
Urethroanal evoked response, 620, 621f
Urinary bladder
  anatomy, 124–125
  autonomic regulation, 117–127
  bivalved, 627f
  compliance, 615
  filling
    responses to filling, 121–122
    electroencephalographic responses, 118
  filling and emptying, normal physiology, 615
  innervation
    afferents to pontine nuclei, 120
    central, 122, 122f
    cerebral cortical, 118–119
    by pontine nuclei, 119–120
    cat vs. human, 118
    pelvic nerve cortical evoked response, 118, 620
    peripheral, 122–125
    principal nuclei, 120–121
    sensory afferents, 122
    spinobulbospinal pathway, 120
    and thalamic nuclei, 119
  role of sympathetic nervous system, 122
Urinary bladder dysfunction, 613–631
  in diabetes, 500
  diagnosis, 613–621, 624
    general physical examination, 614
    history, 614
    laboratory studies, 614–621, 614t
    neurologic examination, 614
  evaluating symptoms, 9
  neurogenic bladder, 459–460
    in diabetes, 500
    treatment, 503
  neurologic disorders causing, 613–614, 623–624
  outlet obstruction
    adrenergic antagonist therapy, 626
    pathognomonic sign, 617
  after spinal cord injury, 459–460
  therapy, 624–628
    alternative measures, 624, 624t
    artificial sphincter, 628
    augmentation cystoplasty, 627f, 628
    behavior modification, 624–625
    in diabetes, 503
    medications, 625–626
    self-catheterization, 625
    surgical measures, 626–628, 627f, 629f
    urine collection devices, 625
  uninhibited bladder, in stroke, 423
Urinary bladder function, see also Micturition
  animal vs. human, 117
  and basal ganglia, 119
  cerebellar control, 119
  and limbic system, 119
  methods of study, 118

reflex pathways, 122, 122f
voiding diary, 614
Urinary detrusor, see Detrusor
Urinary flow rate
  measurement, 617–618, 618f
  obstruction vs. detrusor contractility, 618
Urinary incontinence
  in dementia, 621
  from stress, 614, 626
Urinary sphincter
  artificial device, 628
  external, 124
  innervation, 122, 123, 123f
Urine collection devices, 625
Uroflowmetry, 617–618, 618f
Urogenital system, after spinal cord injury, 459–460
Urologic problems
  in diabetes, 500
  in multiple system atrophy, 558, 563
  in pure autonomic failure, 558, 563
Ussing's leak-pump model, 106, 107f

V

Vacuolar myelopathy, in HIV infection, 732
Vagal ratio, 304
Vagina, 130, 133
Vagovagal reflexes, and high cervical spinal lesions, 425
Vagus nerve, 40–42, 41f
  see also Cardiovagal entries
  and baroreflex arc, 75f
  branches, 40t, 41f
  connections with other cranial nerves, 40
  in diabetes, 377, 608
  ganglia, 40
  gastrointestinal afferents, 138, 142, 143
  in gastrointestinal motility, 137t, 140f, 141, 142, 598
    diagnostic evaluation, 609
  and myocardial damage, 53
  and neurogenic arrhythmias, 49
  nuclei, 40
  relation to glossopharyngeal nerve, 39f
  and Valsalva ratio, 391, 394
Vagus nerve autoantibodies, and diabetes, 512, 514f, 517
  and parasympathetic function, 516
Valsalva maneuver
  in activities of daily living, 189
  and autonomic failure, 189, 190t
  blood pressure response, 189–190, 189f, 190f, 292
  effects on cerebral blood flow velocity, 360
  effects on skin and muscle sympathetic activity, 234f, 235
  equipment used, 388
  heart rate response, 301–303, 302f
    effects of aging, 165t
  hemodynamic responses, 301, 302f, 360–362, 360f
    factors affecting, 302, 303
  in orthostatic hypotension, 361f, 362
  and peripheral adrenergic dysfunction, 336
  phases, 189–190, 189f, 190f, 190t, 301–302, 302f, 360–361
  see also Valsalva ratio
  in postural orthostatic tachycardia syndrome, 362, 363f, 684, 685f, 687, 688
  potential risks, 204
  and syncope, 654
  and transcranial Doppler monitoring, 360–362, 360f
Valsalva ratio, 187–188, 293, 302–303
  definition, 302
  effects of aging, 164, 165f, 194, 194t, 195f, 288, 303
  effects of gender, 194, 194t, 195f
  factors affecting, 187t
  and heart rate response to Valsalva maneuver, 302–303
  interpretation, 187–188

problems in interpreting, 391, 394, 395
normative data, 194, 194t
procedure, 187
Variance, total, 312f
Variegate porphyria, 470
Vas deferens, 130
Vascular endothelium, interaction with autonomic nerves, 70
Vascular headache, and vasodilator peptides, 719
Vascular tone, cutaneous, mechanism, 814
Vasoactive agents
and denervation supersensitivity, 288
and vascular endothelium, 70
Vasoactive intestinal polypeptide (VIP), 30f, 31
and immune system, 150
Vasoactive intracavernosal (intracorporeal) injections, 272, 278, 805
Vasoactive peptides, *see also* Neuropeptides; Vasoactive intestinal polypeptide
and facial flushing, 718–719
and Raynaud's phenomenon, 814–815
and sweating, 93, 717, 718
Vasoconstriction, *see also* Skin vasomotor reflexes
effects on Finapres, 398, 398f, 399f
in initial responses to head-up tilt, 79
mechanisms, 814–815
from standing up, 62–63
in thermoregulation, 89, 90
Vasoconstrictive reserves, and exposure to low gravity, 434–435, 438f
Vasoconstrictor pathway, 90
Vasodepressor syncope, *see under* Syncope
Vasodilation
cholinergic, and central command, 68
in initial responses to standing up, 79
parasympathetic, facial, 718
in Raynaud's phenomenon, 814–815
in thermoregulation, 89
Vasodilator B^1-adrenergic response, and exposure to low gravity, 436f
Vasomotor asymmetry, and skin blood flow, 196
Vasomotor changes
history-taking, 8–9
in reflex sympathetic dystrophy, 539
Vasomotor control, in Horner's syndrome, 445
Vasomotor function tests
in diabetic neuropathy, 496–498
equipment used, 388
Vasomotor index, for reflex sympathetic dystrophy, 197t
Vasomotor paralysis, 816
Vasomotor pathway, 90
Vasomotor reflexes, in skin, effects of aging, 171, 172t

Vasomotor response, in thermoregulation, 89–90
Vasomotor rhythms, *see also* Slow oscillations
effects of aging, 331
and heart rate, 330–331
in neurally mediated syncope, 334
patterns in end-organ failure, 339
Vasomotor system, 813
Vasopressin (antidiuretic hormone [ADH], arginine vasopressin [AVP]), 593–594
and hypothalamic lesions, 5
in multiple system atrophy, 556, 565
and orthostatic hypotension in elderly, 168
in pure autonomic failure, 565
and response to stress, 22
response to upright posture, 81
use in treating autonomic failure, 570
Vasopressor pathway, 90
Vasospasm
episodic vs. persistent, 813
mechanisms, 814–815
Vasospastic disorders, 813–816
traumatic causes, 815
Vasovagal syncope, *see under* Syncope
Veins, heat exchange with arteries, 89
Venoarteriolar axon reflexes, 62, 77
Venoarteriolar reflex
in diabetic neuropathy, 497–498, 498f
effects of aging, 171
effects on blood pressure photoplethysmography, 398
equipment used, 388
false assumptions, 393
measurement, 203
Venoconstriction, *see* Vasoconstriction
Venous compliance, and exposure to low gravity, 438f
Venous hydrostatic indifference point (HIP), 74
Venous pooling
approach to treatment, 694, 695
cardiovascular responses, 63, 64f, 74, 75, 77
and exposure to low gravity, 431
mechanical corrective maneuvers, 75, 76f
and orthostatic hypertension, 686–687
and postural orthostatic tachycardia syndrome, 684, 695
Venous return, during upright posture, 73, 74f
and exposure to low gravity, 431
mechanical aids, 75
Ventricular arrhythmias, and syncope, 655–656
Ventricular outflow tract obstruction, syncope from, 654–656
Ventricular tachycardia, and syncope
electrophysiologic studies, 672, 672f
therapeutic management, 673

Venules of skin, innervation, 112
Vertebral plexus, 35
Vestibular-autonomic interactions, 437–438
Vestibular (Bartholin's) glands, 130
Vestibular disturbances, from exposure to low gravity, 437–438, 438f
Vestibule of vagina, 130, 133
Videourodynamics, 615, 619–620, 620f
Vigilance reaction, 21
Viral illnesses
gastrointestinal dysmotility, 607
and cytokine–sympathetic effects, 156
Viscera, and thermoregulation, 85
Visceral afferents, 18–19
functions, 142–145
pathways, 142, 144
relevance to gastrointestinal syndromes, 144
Visceral referred pain, 142, 144
Visceral stimuli, perception, 142–144
Vitamin B^{12} deficiency, 480
Vocal cords, in multiple system atrophy, 558
Voiding, *see* Micturition; Urinary bladder function
Voltage-sensitive calcium channels (VSCCs), in Lambert-Eaton myasthenic syndrome, 548–550
Voluntary (behavioral) breathing system, 637
Vomiting, in seizures, 423

W

Wakefulness, control of breathing, 636–637
Wallenberg's syndrome, 90, 425
Warm-sensitive neurons, 84, 85, 86f
Wavelet transform, 345
Wernicke-Korsakoff syndrome, central lesions, 5
Wernicke's encephalopathy, 423, 480
and hypothermia, 756, 757
Wheal and flare reaction, *see* Neurogenic flare response
Wigner distribution (Wigner map), *see also* Time–frequency analysis
comparison with periodogram, 345
modified, 345
comparison with Fourier spectrum, 345, 346f
formula, 357
in transcranial Doppler monitoring, 351
use with electroencephalographic data, 357, 358f
Wigner-Ville distribution, 345
Wolff-Parkinson-White syndrome, and syncope, 655
electrophysiologic studies, 670
Women, *see* Females

Z

Zero padding, in spectrum analysis, 314